D1295320

ARTHRITIS
and Allied Conditions

The Contributing Editors

K. Frank Austen, M.D.
John Baum, M.D.
Theodore B. Bayles, M.D.
Morris A. Bowie, M.D.
John J. Calabro, M.D.
Evan Calkins, M.D.
C. William Castor, M.D.
Charles L. Christian, M.D.
Glenn M. Clark, M.D.
Alan S. Cohen, M.D.
George E. Ehrlich, M.D.
Richard H. Ferguson, M.D.
Adrian E. Flatt, M.D.
George J. Friou, M.D.
Ernest Gardner, M.D.
John A. Goldman, M.D.
A. McGehee Harvey, M.D.
Louis A. Healey, M.D.
Evelyn V. Hess, M.D.
Donald F. Hill, M.D.
S. Richardson Hill, Jr., M.D.
Howard L. Holley, M.D.
David S. Howell, M.D.
Ruth Jackson, M.D.
Ralph A. Jessar, M.D.
David B. Levine, M.D.
L. Maxwell Lockie, M.D.
Edward W. Lowman, M.D.
William Martel, M.D.
Victor A. McKusick, M.D.
Clifton K. Meador, M.D.
William M. Mikkelsen, M.D.
Roland W. Moskowitz, M.D.
Metro A. Ogryzlo, M.D.
Carl M. Pearson, M.D.
Robert S. Pinals, M.D.
Gerald P. Rodnan, M.D.
John L. Sbarbaro, M.D.
Frank R. Schmid, M. D.
H. Ralph Schumacher, M.D.
John T. Sharp, M.D.
John W. Sigler, M.D.
Hugh A. Smythe, M.D.
Leon Sokoloff, M.D.
Otto Steinbrocker, M.D.
Norman Talal, M.D.
Angelo Taranta, M.D.
John H. Vaughan, M.D.
Philip D. Wilson, Jr., M.D.
James B. Wyngaarden, M.D.
Morris Ziff, M.D.
Nathan J. Zvaifler, M.D.

ARTHRITIS

and Allied Conditions

A TEXTBOOK OF RHEUMATOLOGY

Editor-in-Chief

JOSEPH LEE HOLLANDER, M.D.

Associate Editor

DANIEL J. McCARTY, JR., M.D.

Section Editors

Edward W. Boland, M.D.	Theodore A. Potter, M.D.
John L. Decker, M.D.	Charles A. Ragan, Jr., M.D.
Ephraim P. Engleman, M.D.	William D. Robinson, M.D.
Richard H. Freyberg, M.D.	Lawrence E. Shulman, M.D.
Currier McEwen, M.D.	Charley J. Smyth, M.D.

Eighth Edition
902 Illustrations on 606 Figures

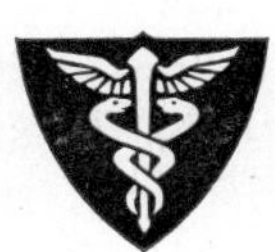

LEA & FEBIGER *Philadelphia*

First Edition, 1940
Second Edition, 1941
Third Edition, 1944
Fourth Edition, 1949
Fifth Edition, 1953
Sixth Edition, 1960
Seventh Edition, 1966
Eighth Edition, 1972
Reprinted, March, 1974
Reprinted, January, 1976

Published in Great Britain by Henry Kimpton Publishers, London

Library of Congress Catalog Card Number: 72-79349

PRINTED IN THE UNITED STATES OF AMERICA

ISBN 0-8121-0392-0

Foreword

THE opportunity offered to me by Joseph Lee Hollander to write a foreword for the eighth edition of *Arthritis and Allied Conditions* came as a great pleasure because I deem it a privilege to add a word of comment to such an excellent book. It has had an impressive history since it first appeared thirty-two years ago. The subject of this book, arthritis and allied conditions, comprises a collection of disorders which has commanded a large part of my professional life. These disorders continue to pose a challenge which has generated interest in the fields of clinical care, investigation and research. Studying the several editions of this book gives an insight into the history of the rheumatic diseases of the period. Each successive edition has shown an increase in the number of subjects covered and the number of writers, each an authority, who have written on their subjects.

When Dr. Bernard I. Comroe published the first edition in 1940, the book was immediately recognized as an outstanding treatise on arthritis and rheumatic diseases. He published two more successful revisions before his untimely death in 1945. It was a monumental task for one man.

After Dr. Comroe's death, Dr. Hollander assumed the responsibility of editorship. He organized a group of distinguished collaborators who completely reorganized and largely rewrote the book for the fourth edition in 1949. Interest in this field is still growing, more and more attention is devoted to its problems, more money is spent on research, investigation and patient care, and a broader comprehension of the problem has been attained as is proven by the fact that the number of chapters, the number of subject headings and the number of authors continue to increase in successive editions. The subjects have been chosen with judgment, the writers have been selected with discrimination, their contributions have been made compatible and have been properly coordinated into a unified presentation by careful editing. Dr. Hollander thus has been able to control the size of the book and keep it within bounds. The book has achieved a preeminent place in medicine, a place which it promises to hold. What Dr. Comroe started Dr. Hollander has continued with great success.

This book has been written by the leading authorities on the subject who are living today. Many of the giants in the field have left their marks on previous editions, although they themselves have passed away. Their presence and their words will be missed, but their messages have been continued by younger men who are filling their places.

Inasmuch as the first edition of this book was published in 1940, *Arthritis and Allied Conditions* in its various stages has been available during the professional life of every doctor living today who has an interest in these problems; and probably everyone interested in these problems has profited from studying it. The book has been kept up-to-date; it has covered the subject; it has been adequate to such an extent that few competitors have survived. The editors, the authors and the publishers are to be congratulated on their success.

ROBERT M. STECHER, M.D.

Shortly after the above Foreword had been set in type, the Editors were saddened to learn that Robert M. Stecher, M.D., had died on March 13, 1972. A fine friend and able colleague has been lost. The Editors felt his last message as it appears above would be most fitting to introduce this volume as he had introduced the Seventh Edition with a previous version.

"Bob" Stecher has done much for Rheumatology throughout the many years of his career. He was one of the great pioneers of American Rheumatology. He was the first to introduce genetics into the field in his classic research on Heberden's nodes. It was his foresight and instigation which led to the establishment of the first American journal of Rheumatology *Arthritis and Rheumatism*. He was an organizing member of the American Rheumatism Association and served as President 1947–48. His enthusiasm and leadership increased the membership and stature of the Ligue Internationale contre le Rhumatisme, and he served as its President from 1953 to 1957. He was beloved and revered by rheumatologists all over the World.

Perhaps the best way to express our loss is to paraphrase his own words above by saying: "His presence and his words will be missed, but his message will be continued by younger men who will try to fill his place."

The Editors

In Memoriam

Deceased Contributors to Previous Editions

BERNARD I. COMROE, M.D.
RALPH H. BOOTS, M.D.
JOSEPH J. BUNIM, M.D.
RUSSELL L. CECIL, M.D.
WALLACE GRAHAM, M.D.
W. PAUL HOLBROOK, M.D.
JOHN G. KUHNS, M.D.

Preface

MORE than thirty-two years have passed since Bernard I. Comroe, M.D., wrote and published the first edition of this textbook in 1940. The increasing popularity of *Arthritis and Allied Conditions* throughout the years has confirmed the wisdom of his effort to organize and present the current knowledge of Rheumatology. This subspecialty of Medicine was in its infancy when this book was first written. Empiricism was the basis for most of its contents. Although Dr. Comroe wrote the book alone, he acknowledged to the present editor that much of it was based on the *Rheumatism Reviews*. This series of comprehensive, authoritative and critical reviews of the American and English literature was organized and written by Philip S. Hench, M.D., with the active collaboration of Walter Bauer, M.D., and others. The first Review, covering the literature of rheumatism and arthritis for 1932 and 1933, appeared in the *Annals of Internal Medicine* in 1935. Subsequent Reviews have since appeared there until 1964. They have been invaluable in the preparation of subsequent editions of this textbook as well.

Dr. Comroe's untimely death in 1945 after the appearance of the third edition of this book might have meant the termination of this effort, except that Dr. O. H. Perry Pepper convinced the present editor it should be carried on. The awesome assignment was accepted with many misgivings, but the carrying forward of this project of a departed friend has yielded a lasting satisfaction.

Interest and research in the field of Rheumatology have expanded almost explosively since 1948 when the nucleus of the present group of collaborators first took over the task of preparing the fourth edition. Even at this time the present editor found that the only way to achieve an authoritative and up-to-date text was to have the sections rewritten simultaneously by a *group* of rheumatologists. The widespread acceptance of *Arthritis and Allied Conditions* all over the world has been convincing evidence that this step was justified. Not only does this convey great honor upon the collaborators, but also it puts upon them a much increased responsibility for keeping the volume authoritative and up-to-date. The steadily increasing complexity of Rheumatology has necessitated the invitation of more contributors to report on newer fields and on changes in older fields of Rheumatology. Each contributing editor is intimately associated with his subject and reviews not only what has appeared in the literature, but has added recent developments from reports at medical meetings, from conversations and correspondence with others in the same line of research, and from his own as yet unpublished experience and research those points which he feels will stand the critical test of time. This would appear the only way the textbook can keep pace with the rapid developments in a field as expanding as Rheumatology.

In planning this eighth edition the effort has been to obtain an outstanding competent contributor on each subject, not necessarily chosen for the neutrality of his point of view. A review of the list of contributors on the following pages will reveal their responsibilities and attainments which should attest the background and experience necessary for formulation of authoritative opinions. The editor takes full responsibility for the choice of contributors. The number of the contributors who are deans, chairmen of departments of medicine, and professors of medicine in their respective medical schools would appear to reflect the increasing importance of Rheumatology as a subspecialty of Internal Medicine. Many of the leaders in the field of Rheumatology, of the American Rheumatism Association, of The Arthritis Foundation, and of the National Institute of Arthritis and Metabolic Diseases, as well as editors of the *Rheumatism Reviews*, the *Bulletin on Rheumatic Diseases* and *Arthritis and Rheumatism* are contributing editors to this volume.

Review of the literature has been aided not only by the continued use of the *Rheumatism Reviews*, as mentioned earlier, but also by the *Bulletin on Rheumatic Diseases*, the American Rheumatism Association journal: *Arthritis and Rheumatism*, the British journal: *Annals of the Rheumatic Diseases*, the *Index of Rheumatology*, *Arthritis and Rheumatic Diseases Abstracts*, and *Excerpta Medica-Arthritis and Rheumatism* in which much of the newer material has been presented or reviewed. When the small trickles of new information in widely scattered journals are compiled and placed in perspective as in this volume, the combined impact often provides a new concept of the diseases studied.

Entirely new chapters, 12 in number, have been added because of new developments in the field. These are: The Acute Inflammatory Response, Pathogenetic Mechanisms in Rheumatoid Arthritis, Extra-articular Manifestations of Rheumatoid Disease, Cytotoxic Drug Therapy in Rheumatic Diseases, Synovectomy in Rheumatoid Arthritis, Intermittent and Periodic Arthritic Syndromes, Enteropathic Arthritis, Sjögren's Syndrome and Connective Tissue Diseases with Other Immunologic Disorders, Relapsing Polychondritis, Polymyalgia Rheumatica, Principles of Diagnosis and Treatment of Infectious Arthritis, and Heritable and Developmental Disorders of Connective Tissue and Bone.

Entirely rewritten chapters, 18 in number, are: Organization of an Arthritis Center, Radiology in the Rheumatic Diseases, Endocrinology of the Rheumatic Diseases, Salicylate Therapy for Rheumatoid Arthritis, Corticosteroid and Corticotropin Therapy of Rheumatoid Arthritis, Ankylosing Spondylitis, Polymyositis and Dermatomyositis, Progressive Systemic Sclerosis (Scleroderma) and Calcinosis, Symptoms and Laboratory Findings in Osteoarthritis, Treatment of Osteoarthritis, Hemochromatosis, Ochronosis and Wilson's Disease, Gonococcal Arthritis, Reiter's Syndrome, Tuberculous Arthritis, Unusual Features and Special Types of Infectious Arthritis, Sarcoidosis, Arthritis with Hematologic Disorders, Storage Diseases and Dysproteinemias and Traumatic Arthritis.

Thirty-one more of the 82 chapters have been extensively revised and partly rewritten, and *every* chapter has been carefully reviewed to be certain newer facts and concepts are included. *More than 200 new illustrations* have been added or substituted, and many new tables and summaries have been inserted because of the tremendous growth and complexity of Rheumatology. This eighth edition of *Arthritis* is virtually a new book.

Because of the tremendous segment of medical knowledge bearing on Rheumatology, the editor again is indebted to 10 Section Editors, each with particular knowledge and experience, who have checked the accuracy, completeness, compatibility and coherence of the material in each section. Not only multiple authors but multiple editors have been necessitated by the growth of this field.

A list of former collaborators who have died appears on page vi. They have been sorely missed, but younger men and women have filled the gap. Other former contributors, who have resigned because of health or other pressures, are: Nathan R. Abrams, M.D., Eörs Bajusz, Ph.D., Victor G. Balboni, M.D., Roger L. Black, M.D., Denys K. Ford, M.D., Rosaline R. Joseph, M.D., Ronald W. Lamont-Havers, M.D., John Lansbury, M.D., Bernard M. Norcross, M.D., and Hans Selye, M.D. Their contributions to previous editions were great, and the editor is grateful to them for their help.

While this volume presents a comprehensive view of Rheumatology, it is not written only for the rheumatologist, but also as a source of information for researchers, internists, orthopedic surgeons, and particularly graduate students of medicine. The editors have kept in mind the fact that many physicians use this volume as a reference and have, therefore, continued the extensive bibliographies and "box summaries" for those with too limited time for reading an entire chapter. In those subjects discussed too briefly for the needs of a particular reader, adequate source references are given for obtaining further details.

In this age of increasing permissiveness it is consistent that the Editors have allowed more latitude to the contributors than formerly. Limitation of assignments of space have been relaxed somewhat for those whose contributions were longer than assigned but seemed to deserve the extra space. In chapters dealing with a *group* of topics, e.g. Chapters 30, 45, 47 and 61, bibliographies have been divided to list references separately for each subject. Titles of papers referred to are still not listed in order to conserve space. Certain redundancies in subject matter have been permitted so that the reader does not constantly have to cope with references to other chapters while reading. Roentgenograms are often referred to as *x rays* in this volume, but *x-ray* treatment, etc., remains hyphenated. Some contributors have preferred the original spelling of *anulus* rather than the usual *annulus*. The Editor, who has mellowed with age, also tires more readily.

The collaborators have worked many hours in the preparation of this edition, hours stolen from leisure with families and recompensed by little more than personal satisfaction. Although most of the 224 new illustrations presented in this edition come from the contributors' own files, some are borrowed from friends to whom the editors make grateful acknowledgment. The editors are grateful to the authors and publishers of many recent articles and monographs for permission to reproduce material. The publishers of this volume have been most cooperative and helpful.

The present editor, after organizing and assembling 5 editions of this textbook, has decided to pass on the responsibility to a younger man for subsequent editions. *Dr. Daniel J. McCarty, Jr.*, who has distinguished himself in Rheumatology in many ways since he first trained in this field with the present editor 12 years ago, has been persuaded to accept editorship of *Arthritis and Allied Conditions*. He has been of tremendous help in the planning and execution of this edition as Associate Editor. His extensive experience as former editor of *Arthritis and Rheumatism* has fitted him admirably for the job ahead.

J.L.H.

Philadelphia, Pennsylvania

Contributors

K. FRANK AUSTEN, M.D., F.A.C.P., Boston, Massachusetts.
Professor of Medicine, Harvard Medical School. Physician-in-Chief, Robert B. Brigham Hospital. Physician, Peter Bent Brigham Hospital.

JOHN BAUM, B.A., M.D., Rochester, New York.
Associate Professor of Medicine, Pediatrics, and Preventive Medicine and Public Health, University of Rochester School of Medicine and Dentistry. Senior Associate Physician, Strong Memorial Hospital. Director of Arthritis and Clinical Immunology Unit, Monroe Community Hospital.

THEODORE B. BAYLES, B.S., M.D., F.A.C.P., Boston, Massachusetts.
Associate Clinical Professor of Medicine, Harvard Medical School. Lecturer in Medicine, Boston University School of Medicine. Visiting Physician and Director of Training Program, Robert B. Brigham Hospital. Senior Associate in Medicine, Peter Bent Brigham Hospital.

EDWARD W. BOLAND, B.S., M.D., M.S. (Med.), F.A.C.P., Los Angeles, Calif.
Clinical Professor of Medicine, University of Southern California School of Medicine. Director, Department of Medicine, St. Vincent's Hospital. Past-President, American Rheumatism Association (1954–55).

MORRIS A. BOWIE, A.B., M.D., Swarthmore, Pennsylvania.
Assistant Professor of Clinical Medicine, Assistant Professor of Physical Medicine and Rehabilitation, School of Medicine, University of Pennsylvania. Consulting Physician, Arthritis Service, Bryn Mawr Hospital.

JOHN J. CALABRO, B.S., M.D., F.A.C.P., Worcester, Massachusetts.
Clinical Professor of Medicine, University of Massachusetts Medical School. Director of Rheumatology, Saint Vincent Hospital. Clinical Professor of Medicine and Pediatrics, Tufts University School of Medicine; Associate Visiting Physician, Tufts Medical Service, Boston City Hospital; Consultant in Pediatrics, New England Medical Center (Boston Floating Hospital), Boston, Massachusetts. Consultant in Rheumatology, Jersey City Medical Center.

EVAN CALKINS, M.D., F.A.C.P., Buffalo, New York.
Professor and Chairman, Department of Medicine, State University of New York at Buffalo. Director of Medicine, Edward J. Meyer Memorial Hospital. Attending Physician, Buffalo General Hospital. Past-President, American Rheumatism Association (1967–68).

C. WILLIAM CASTOR, Jr., M.D., F.A.C.P., Ann Arbor, Michigan.
Professor of Internal Medicine and Member, Rackham Arthritis Research Unit, University of Michigan Medical School.

CHARLES L. CHRISTIAN, M.D., New York, New York.
Professor of Medicine, Cornell University College of Medicine. Physician-in-Chief, The Hospital for Special Surgery. Editor, Seventeenth to Nineteenth *Rheumatism Reviews*. Editor, Arthritis and Rheumatism (1971–76).

GLENN M. CLARK, M.S., M.D., F.A.C.P., Memphis, Tennessee.
Assistant Dean in Charge of Hospital Affairs, University of Tennessee. Chief of Staff, City of Memphis Hospitals. Professor of Medicine, University of Tennessee. Consultant in Internal Medicine, U.S. Navy. Active Staff, City of Memphis Hospitals and Baptist Memorial Hospital. Consulting Staff, Methodist Hospital and St. Joseph Hospital, Memphis, Tennessee.

ALAN S. COHEN, M.D., Boston, Massachusetts.
Professor of Medicine, Boston University School of Medicine; Head, Arthritis and Connective Tissue Disease Section, University Hospital, Boston University Medical Center.

JOHN L. DECKER, B.A., M.D., F.A.C.P., Bethesda, Maryland.
Chief, Arthritis and Rheumatism Branch, National Institute of Arthritis and Metabolic Diseases, National Institutes of Health. Consultant, Walter Reed Army Medical Center, Washington, D.C., and National Naval Medical Center, Bethesda, Maryland. President, American Rheumatism Association (1972–73).

GEORGE E. EHRLICH, A.B., M.B., M.D., F.A.C.P., Philadelphia, Pennsylvania.
Professor of Medicine and Associate Professor of Rehabilitation, Temple University School of Medicine. Chief of Section of Rheumatology and Director of the Arthritis Center, Albert Einstein Medical Center and Moss Rehabilitation Hospital. Editor, *Arthritis and Rheumatic Diseases Abstracts* (1969–71).

EPHRAIM P. ENGLEMAN, M.D., F.A.C.P., San Francisco, California.
Clinical Professor of Medicine, University of California School of Medicine. Head, Rheumatic Disease Group, University of California Medical Center. Secretary-General, La Ligue Internationale contre le Rhumatisme. Consultant in Medicine and Rheumatic Diseases for Western States Area, Veterans Administration and for Letterman Hospital, United States Army. Past-President, American Rheumatism Association (1962–1963).

RICHARD H. FERGUSON, M.D., F.A.C.P., Rochester, Minnesota.
Assistant Professor of Medicine, Mayo Graduate School, University of Minnesota. Consultant in Internal Medicine and Head of a Section of Rheumatology, Mayo Clinic.

ADRIAN E. FLATT, M.A., M.D., F.R.C.S., F.A.C.S., Iowa City, Iowa.
Professor of Orthopedic Surgery, Director of Hand Surgery, University of Iowa Medical School. Hunterian Professor of the Royal College of Surgeons of England. Civilian National Consultant in Hand Surgery to U.S. Air Force at Wilford Hall Hospital, San Antonio, Texas.

RICHARD H. FREYBERG, A.B., M.S., M.D., F.A.C.P., New York, New York.
Emeritus Clinical Professor of Medicine, Cornell University Medical College. Emeritus Director, Department of Rheumatic Diseases, Hospital for Special Surgery, New York. Past-President, American Rheumatism Association (1948–49).

GEORGE J. FRIOU, B.S., M.D., F.A.C.P., Los Angeles, California.
Professor of Medicine, University of Southern California School of Medicine. Director of the Rheumatic Disease and Immunology Section, Department of Medicine, Los Angeles County–University of Southern California Medical Center.

ERNEST GARDNER, M.D., Detroit, Michigan.
Professor of Anatomy, Wayne State University College of Medicine.

JOHN A. GOLDMAN, M.D., Major, M.C., U.S. Army, Fort Gordon, Georgia.
Chief of Division of Immunology and Rheumatology and Officer-in-Charge of Immunology and Rheumatology Clinic, U.S. Army Hospital Specialized Treatment Center, Fort Gordon. Clinical Instructor in Medicine, Medical College of Georgia, Augusta, Georgia.

A. McGEHEE HARVEY, M.D., F.A.C.P., Baltimore, Maryland.
Professor and Director of the Department of Medicine, The Johns Hopkins University School of Medicine. Physician-in-Chief, The Johns Hopkins Hospital.

LOUIS A. HEALEY, M.D., F.A.C.P., Seattle, Washington.
Clinical Associate Professor of Medicine, University of Washington School of Medicine. Associate, The Mason Clinic, Seattle.

EVELYN V. HESS, M.D., F.A.C.P., Cincinnati, Ohio.
McDonald Professor of Medicine and Director, Division of Immunology, Department of Internal Medicine, University of Cincinnati Medical Center.

DONALD F. HILL, B.S., M.S., M.D., F.A.C.P., Tucson, Arizona.
President, Southwestern Clinic and Research Institute, Inc. Senior member Holbrook-Hill Medical Group. Consultant, Governing Staff Tucson Medical Center. Consultant, Honorary Staff, Saint Mary's Hospital and Saint Joseph's Hospital. Past-President American Rheumatism Association (1966–67).

S. RICHARDSON HILL, JR., B.A., M.D., F.A.C.P., Birmingham, Alabama.
Vice-President for Health Affairs and Professor of Medicine, The University of Alabama in Birmingham.

JOSEPH L. HOLLANDER, A.B., M.D., M.A.C.P., Philadelphia, Pennsylvania.
Professor of Medicine, School of Medicine, University of Pennsylvania. Chief of Arthritis Section, Department of Medicine, Hospital of the University of Pennsylvania (1946–72). Consultant in Medicine (Rheumatology) at Pennsylvania Hospital, Children's Hospital, Veterans Administration Hospital and U.S. Naval Hospital. Past-President, American Rheumatism Association (1961–62).

HOWARD L. HOLLEY, B.S., M.D., F.A.C.P., Birmingham, Alabama.
Waters Professor of Medicine in Rheumatology, University of Alabama School of Medicine.

DAVID S. HOWELL, M.D., F.A.C.P., Miami, Florida.
Professor of Medicine and Director of Arthritis Training Program, University of Miami School of Medicine. Attending Physician, Jackson Memorial Hospital and Coral Gables Veterans Administration Hospital.

RUTH JACKSON, B.A., M.D., F.A.C.S., F.I.C.S., Dallas, Texas.
Assistant Professor of Orthopedic Surgery, Southwestern Medical School of the University of Texas, Attending Orthopedic Surgeon, Baylor Medical Center. Consulting Orthopedic Surgeon, Parkland Memorial Hospital.

RALPH A. JESSAR, B.A., M.D., Philadelphia, Pennsylvania.
Assistant Professor of Clinical Medicine, School of Medicine, University of Pennsylvania; Chief of Arthritis Section, Department of Medicine, Graduate Hospital, University of Pennsylvania.

DAVID B. LEVINE, M.D., F.A.C.S., New York, New York.
Clinical Associate Professor of Surgery (Orthopaedics), Cornell University Medical College, Associate Attending Orthopaedic Surgeon, Hospital for Special Surgery. Assistant Attending Orthopaedic Surgeon, New York Hospital.

L. MAXWELL LOCKIE, M.D., F.A.C.P., Buffalo, New York.
Clinical Professor of Medicine, State University of New York at Buffalo. Consulting Physician in Medicine, Buffalo General Hospital. Past-President, American Rheumatism Association (1957–58).

EDWARD W. LOWMAN, M.D., F.A.C.P., New York, New York.
Professor of Rehabilitation Medicine, New York University School of Medicine. Clinical Director, Institute of Rehabilitation Medicine, New York University Medical Center.

WILLIAM MARTEL, B.S., M.D., Ann Arbor, Michigan.
Professor of Radiology, University of Michigan School of Medicine. Director of Diagnostic Radiology, University Hospital. Consultant Radiologist, Wayne County General Hospital and Veterans Administration Hospital.

DANIEL J. McCARTY, Jr., B.S., M.D., F.A.C.P., Chicago, Illinois.
Professor of Medicine, School of Medicine, University of Chicago. Head, Section of Arthritis and Metabolism, Department of Medicine, University of Chicago Hospitals. Editor, *Arthritis and Rheumatism* (1965–70).

CURRIER McEWEN, B.S., M.D., D.Sc. (Hon.), M.A.C.P., South Harpswell, Maine.
Professor Emeritus of Medicine, New York University School of Medicine. Consulting Physician, Bellevue and University Hospitals, New York. Consulting Physician to Regional Memorial Hospital, Brunswick, Maine Medical Center, Portland, Central Maine General Hospital, Lewiston, and Veterans Administration Hospital, Togus, Maine. Past-President, American Rheumatism Association (1952–53).

VICTOR A. McKUSICK, M.D., F.A.C.P., Baltimore, Maryland.
Professor of Medicine and Director, Division of Medical Genetics, Department of Medicine, Johns Hopkins University School of Medicine. Physician, The Johns Hopkins Hospital.

CLIFTON K. MEADOR, B.A., M.D., F.A.C.P., Birmingham, Alabama.
Dean and Professor of Medicine, University of Alabama School of Medicine.

WILLIAM M. MIKKELSEN, M. D., F.A.C.P., Ann Arbor, Michigan.
Professor of Internal Medicine and Associate Physician, Rackham Arthritis Research Unit, University of Michigan Medical School. Consultant, Veterans Administration Hospital and Wayne County General Hospital.

ROLAND W. MOSKOWITZ, M.D., M.S. (Med.), F.A.C.P., Cleveland, Ohio.
Associate Professor of Medicine, Case Western Reserve University School of Medicine. Associate Physician, University Hospitals, Cleveland. Consultant in Arthritis, Cleveland Veterans Administration Hospital.

METRO A. OGRYZLO, M.D., F.R.C.P.(C.), Toronto, Ontario, Canada.
Professor of Medicine, Faculty of Medicine, University of Toronto. Director, University of Toronto Rheumatic Disease Unit, Wellesley Hospital. Past-President, Canadian Rheumatism Association (1961–63).

CARL M. PEARSON, A.B., M.D., F.A.C.P., Los Angeles, California.
Professor of Medicine and Director of Division of Rheumatology, School of Medicine, University of California, Los Angeles. Consultant in Medicine, Wadsworth Hospital, Veterans Administration Center, Los Angeles, California.

ROBERT S. PINALS, B.A., M.D., F.A.C.P., Syracuse, New York.
Associate Professor of Medicine and Rehabilitation Medicine and Director of Rheumatic Disease Section, State University of New York, Upstate Medical Center.

THEODORE A. POTTER, M.D., F.A.C.S., Boston, Massachusetts.
Clinical Professor of Orthopedic Surgery, Tufts University School of Medicine. Visiting Surgeon, New England Medical Center, Boston City Hospital and New England Baptist Hospital.

CHARLES A. RAGAN, Jr., A.B., M.D., M.A.C.P , New York, New York.
Lambert Professor of Medicine and Chairman, Department of Medicine, Columbia University College of Physicians and Surgeons. Director of Medical Service, Presbyterian Hospital. Past-President, American Rheumatism Association (1953–54).

WILLIAM D. ROBINSON, A.B., M.D., F.A.C.P., Ann Arbor, Michigan.
Professor and Chairman, Department of Internal Medicine, and Consultant to Rackham Arthritis Research Unit, University of Michigan Medical School. Editor, Tenth and Eleventh *Rheumatism Reviews*. Past-President, American Rheumatism Association (1956–57).

GERALD P. RODNAN, M.D., F.A.C.P., Pittsburgh, Pennsylvania.
Professor of Medicine and Chief of Section on Rheumatic Diseases, University of Pittsburgh School of Medicine. Attending Physician, Presbyterian-University and Veterans Administration Hospitals. Editor, *Bulletin of the Rheumatic Diseases* since 1966.

JOHN L. SBARBARO, B.S., M.D., F.A.C.S., Philadelphia, Pennsylvania.
Assistant Professor of Orthopaedic Surgery, School of Medicine, University of Pennsylvania. Attending Orthopaedic Surgeon, Hospital of the University of Pennsylvania. Consultant in Orthopaedic Surgery, Veterans Administration Hospital, Philadelphia General Hospital and Children's Seashore House.

FRANK R. SCHMID, M.D., F.A.C.P., Chicago, Illinois.
Professor of Medicine, Northwestern University Medical School. Chief of Section on Arthritis-Connective Tissue Diseases, Department of Medicine, and Director of Arthritis Clinical Center, Northwestern University Medical Center. Attending Physician, Passavant Memorial Hospital and Veterans Administration Research Hospital. Consulting Physician, Rehabilitation Institute of Chicago, Children's Memorial Hospital and Chicago Wesley Memorial Hospital.

H. RALPH SCHUMACHER, Jr., M.D., Philadelphia, Pennsylvania.
Associate Professor of Medicine, University of Pennsylvania School of Medicine. Director of Research, Arthritis Section, Department of Medicine, Hospital of the University of Pennsylvania. Chief, Arthritis Section, Philadelphia Veterans Administration Hospital.

JOHN T. SHARP, M.D., F.A.C.P., Houston, Texas.
Professor of Medicine and Chief of Rheumatic Disease Section, Department of Medicine, Baylor College of Medicine, Texas Medical Center.

LAWRENCE E. SHULMAN, M.D., Ph.D., F.A.C.P., Baltimore, Maryland.
Associate Professor of Medicine, The Johns Hopkins University School of Medicine. Director, Connective Tissue Division, Department of Medicine, The Johns Hopkins University School of Medicine. Physician, The Johns Hopkins Hospital. Physician, Arthritis and Connective Tissue Clinics, The Johns Hopkins Hospital. Physician, The Good Samaritan Hospital.

JOHN W. SIGLER, A.B., M.D., F.A.C.P., Detroit, Michigan.
Chief, Division of Rheumatology, Department of Medicine, Henry Ford Hospital.

CHARLEY J. SMYTH, M.B., M.S., M.D., M.A.C.P., Denver, Colorado.
Professor of Medicine, University of Colorado School of Medicine. Head, Division of Rheumatic Diseases, Colorado General and Denver General Hospitals. Editor, Twelfth to Sixteenth *Rheumatism Reviews*. Past-President, American Rheumatism Association (1959–60).

HUGH A. SMYTHE, M.D., F.R.C.P.(C), Toronto, Ontario, Canada.
Assistant Professor, Faculty of Medicine, University of Toronto. Consultant, Rheumatic Disease Units at Wellesley Hospital and Sunnybrook Hospital. Chairman, Medical and Scientific Committee, Canadian Arthritis and Rheumatism Society.

LEON SOKOLOFF, M.D., Bethesda, Maryland.
Chief, Section on Rheumatic Diseases, Laboratory of Experimental Pathology, National Institute of Arthritis and Metabolic Diseases, National Institutes of Health.

OTTO STEINBROCKER, M.D., New York, New York.
Consulting Physician (Rheumatology), Hospital for Joint Diseases and Lenox Hill Hospital. Past-President, American Rheumatism Association (1950–51).

NORMAN TALAL, M.D., San Francisco, California.
Associate Professor of Medicine and Microbiology, University of California Medical Center. Chief, Division of Clinical Immunology, Veterans Administration Hospital, San Francisco.

ANGELO TARANTA, M.D., New York, New York.
Associate Professor of Medicine, New York University School of Medicine. Associate Attending in Medicine, University Hospital and Bellevue Hospital.

JOHN H. VAUGHAN, A.B., M.D., F.A.C.P., La Jolla, California.
Adjunct Professor of Medicine, University of California, San Diego. Chairman of the Clinical Divisions, Scripps Clinic and Research Foundation, La Jolla. Past-President, American Rheumatism Association (1970–71).

PHILIP D. WILSON, JR., M.D., F.A.C.S., New York, New York.
Clinical Professor of Surgery (Orthopaedics), Cornell University Medical College. Attending Orthopaedic Surgeon, New York Hospital and Hospital for Special Surgery.

JAMES B. WYNGAARDEN, M.D., F.A.C.P., Durham, North Carolina.
Frederic M. Hanes Professor and Chairman, Department of Medicine, Duke University School of Medicine. Chief of Medical Services, Duke University Medical Center.

MORRIS ZIFF, B.S., Ph.D., M.D., F.A.C.P., Dallas, Texas.
Professor of Internal Medicine, University of Texas Southwestern Medical School. Chief of Section on Rheumatic Diseases, Department of Internal Medicine. Director, Arthritis Clinical Center, Parkland Memorial Hospital. Attending Physician, Parkland Memorial Hospital and Dallas Veterans Administration Hospital. Past-President, American Rheumatism Association (1965–66).

NATHAN J. ZVAIFLER, M.D., F.A.C.P., San Diego, California.
Professor of Medicine, University of California, San Diego, School of Medicine. Physician, University Hospital.

Contents

CHAPTER PAGE

Part I

The Study of the Rheumatic Diseases

EDITOR: CHARLES A. RAGAN, M.D.

Part II

Factors Influencing the Onset or Course of the Rheumatic Diseases

EDITOR: WILLIAM D. ROBINSON, M.D.

CHAPTER PAGE

Part X

Arthritis Caused by or Occurring with Specific Infections

EDITOR: EPHRAIM P. ENGLEMAN, M.D.

Part XI

Miscellaneous Conditions Complicating or Producing Arthritis

EDITOR: JOHN L. DECKER, M.D.

Part XII

Regional Disorders of Joints and Related Structures

EDITOR: THEODORE A. POTTER, M.D.

PART I

The Study of the Rheumatic Diseases

Editor: Charles Ragan, M.D.

Chapter 1

Introduction to Arthritis and the Rheumatic Diseases

By JOSEPH LEE HOLLANDER, M.D.

THE term "rheumatism" is derived from the Greek word *rheumatismos*, which designated mucus (catarrh) as an evil humor which was thought to flow from the brain to the joints and other portions of the body, producing pain.[11] Since many studies[14,16,17] have shown that an alteration of an important constituent of the joint mucin (the mucopolysaccharide: hyaluronic acid) actually occurs in at least some of the "rheumatic diseases," the term, at long last, may be somewhat appropriate. The *Rheumatic Diseases* are those conditions in which pain and stiffness of some portion of the musculoskeletal system are prominent. *These include diseases of connective tissue.*

Arthritis is the general term used when the joints themselves are the major seat of the rheumatic disease. *Fibrositis* denotes inflammation of connective tissue in any location, particularly around joints, and in or near muscles and tendons. *Rheumatology* is the study of the rheumatic diseases, including arthritis, rheumatic fever, fibrositis, neuralgia, myositis, bursitis, gout, and other conditions producing somatic pain, stiffness and soreness.

Arthritis is one of the oldest known, yet most neglected, diseases. The earliest known example of multiple arthritis in a fossil vertebrate is in a skeleton of a platycarpus (a large swimming reptile), which lived about 100,000,000 years ago. This now resides in the Museum of Natural History in the University of Kansas.[12] Chronic arthritis of the spine was present in the Ape Man of 2,000,000 years ago as well as in our ancestors, the Java and Lansing men of 500,000 years ago, and Egyptian mummies dating to 8000 B.C.[13] The Romans built extensive baths throughout their empire because of this disease.

Baillou (1538–1616) was the first to use the term rheumatism to designate a form of acute arthritis (as distinguished from gout); he also was the first to regard rheumatism as a clinical entity. (Further historical data are presented in appropriate sections.)

CLASSIFICATION OF ARTHRITIS

There are many different forms of joint disease, some caused by known etiologic agents, others from unknown etiologic factors. Some types are characterized by certain pathological and clinical features which makes their differentiation relatively easy. In other forms of joint disease the clinical pattern varies considerably, and identification may depend on detailed study. There are also numerous terms for certain types which are confusing. A few types of arthritis even remain unproved as distinct clinical entities.

It is impossible to divide arthritis into acute and chronic forms, as almost any acute arthritis can pass into a subacute or chronic stage, and many cases of chronic arthritis began acutely or are subject to acute exacerbations.

Most cases of arthritis fall into one of

Nomenclature and Classification of Arthritis and Rheumatism
(Tentatively Accepted by American Rheumatism Association)[1]

I. Polyarthritis of unknown etiology

A. Rheumatoid arthritis
B. Juvenile rheumatoid arthritis (Still's disease)
C. Ankylosing spondylitis
D. Psoriatic arthritis
E. Reiter's syndrome
F. Others

II. "Connective tissue" disorders

A. Systemic lupus erythematosus
B. Polyarteritis nodosa
C. Scleroderma (progressive systemic sclerosis)
D. Polymyositis and dermatomyositis
E. Others

III. Rheumatic fever

IV. Degenerative joint disease (osteoarthritis, osteoarthrosis)

A. Primary
B. Secondary

V. Non-articular rheumatism

A. Fibrositis
B. Intervertebral disc and low back syndromes
C. Myositis and myalgia
D. Tendinitis and peritendinitis (bursitis)
E. Tenosynovitis
F. Fasciitis
G. Carpal tunnel syndrome
H. Others
(See also shoulder-hand syndrome, VIII E)

VI. Diseases with which arthritis is frequently associated

A. Sarcoidosis
B. Relapsing polychondritis
C. Henoch-Schönlein syndrome
D. Ulcerative colitis
E. Regional ileitis
F. Whipple's disease
G. Sjögren's syndrome
H. Familial Mediterranean fever
I. Others
(See also psoriatic arthritis, I D)

VII. Associated with known infectious agents

A. Bacterial
  1. Brucella
  2. Gonococcus
  3. Mycobacterium tuberculosis
  4. Pneumococcus
  5. Salmonella
  6. Staphylococcus
  7. Streptobacillus moniliformis (Haverhill fever)
  8. Treponema pallidum (syphilis)
  9. Treponema pertenue (yaws)
  10. Others
B. Rickettsial
C. Viral
D. Fungal
E. Parasitic
(See also rheumatic fever, III)

VIII. Traumatic and/or neurogenic disorders

A. Traumatic arthritis (viz., the result of direct trauma)
B. Lues (tertiary syphilis)
C. Diabetes
D. Syringomyelia
E. Shoulder-hand syndrome
F. Mechanical derangements of joints
G. Others
(See also degenerative joint disease, IV; carpal tunnel syndrome, VG)

IX. Associated with known biochemical or endocrine abnormalities

A. Gout
B. Ochronosis
C. Hemophilia
D. Hemoglobinopathies (e.g., sickle cell disease)
E. Agammaglobulinemia
F. Gaucher's disease
G. Hyperparathyroidism
H. Acromegaly
I. Hypothyroidism
J. Scurvy (hypovitaminosis C)
K. Xanthoma tuberosum
L. Others
(See also multiple myeloma, XG;
Hurler's syndrome, XII C).

Nomenclature and Classification of Arthritis and Rheumatism (*Continued*)
(Tentatively Accepted by American Rheumatism Association)[1]

X. Tumor and tumor-like conditions

A. Synovioma
B. Pigmented villonodular synovitis
C. Giant cell tumor of tendon sheath
D. Primary juxta-articular bone tumors
E. Metastatic
F. Leukemia
G. Multiple myeloma
H. Benign tumors of articular tissue
I. Others

XI. Allergy and drug reactions

A. Arthritis due to specific allergens (e.g., serum sickness)
B. Arthritis due to drugs (e.g., hydralazine syndrome)
C. Others

XII. Inherited and congenital disorders

A. Marfan's syndrome
B. Ehlers-Danlos syndrome
C. Hurler's syndrome
D. Congenital hip dysplasia
E. Morquio's disease
F. Others

XIII. Miscellaneous disorders

A. Amyloidosis
B. Aseptic necrosis of bone
C. Behcet's syndrome
D. Chondrocalcinosis (pseudo-gout)
E. Erythema multiforme (Stevens-Johnson syndrome)
F. Erythema nodosum
G. Hypertrophic osteoarthropathy
H. Juvenile osteochondritis
I. Osteochondritis dissecans
J. Reticulohistiocytosis of joints (lipoid dermato-arthritis)
K. Tietze's disease
L. Others

five major groups:[8] (1) the frankly infectious cases caused by a specific microorganism; (2) cases that are possibly infectious but of unproved etiology; (3) cases representing degenerative forms of joint disease, which in Europe are termed arthroses; (4) cases in which the arthritis results from direct trauma to the joint; (5) cases of metabolic arthritis (e.g., gout).

Many classifications of diseases of joints and related structures have been suggested. All have certain disadvantages. For the sake of simplification, clarity, and unification of terminology the classification tentatively approved by the American Rheumatism Association in 1963 is recommended for general use.[1] The International League Against Rheumatism, at the 9th Congress in Toronto in 1957, tentatively adopted another grouping of arthritis and rheumatic disorders which is summarized also on page 6.

Until the etiology of all types of arthritis is known, no grouping can be accurate. The present classifications are based on clinical patterns, pathological change in the tissues, and etiology when known. The arrangement of this book itself (see Table of Contents) is another attempt at classification.

A comprehensive *Thesaurus of Rheumatology*, which should standardize the terms used in this field, has recently been compiled and published.[15] This epic work is indispensable for reference, particularly for identification of rare entities, and for the many conditions previously described under multiple names, such as ankylosing spondylitis, so that unanimity of terminology can be achieved.

Nomenclature and Classification of Arthritides and Other Rheumatic Disorders
(Tentatively Adopted by International League Against Rheumatism, 1957)

I. *Diseases and Disorders of Connective Tissue Accepted as Rheumatic*
  A. Articular
    1. Inflammatory
      Idiopathic
      (a) Rheumatic fever
      (b) Rheumatoid arthritis
      (c) Atypical forms
        Arthritis with psoriasis—psoriatic arthropathy
        Juvenile rheumatoid arthritis (Still-Chauffard disease)
        Rheumatoid arthritis with hypersplenism (Felty's syndrome)
        Polyarthritis with keratoconjunctivitis sicca (Sjögren's syndrome)
      (d) Special forms
        Ankylosing spondylitis (rheumatoid spondylitis)
        Intermittent hydrarthrosis
        Palindromic rheumatism
      Infectional—Arthritis due to specific infection
    2. Degenerative
      (a) Osteoarthritis, degenerative joint disease (osteoarthrosis)
      (b) Osteochondrosis
      (c) Intervertebral disc syndromes
  B. Nonarticular
    1. Bursitis
    2. Fasciitis
    3. Fibrositis
    4. Myositis, myalgia
    5. Neuritis, neuropathy, neuralgia
    6. Periarthritis
    7. Tendinitis, peritendinitis
    8. Tenosynovitis, tendovaginitis
    9. Disorders of fatty tissue (Panniculitis)

II. *Diseases and Disorders with Rheumatic Features*
    1. Inflammatory, idiopathic (Diffuse Collagen Diseases)
      (a) Dermatomyositis
      (b) Polyarteritis nodosa, diffuse arteritis
      (c) Systemic lupus erythematosus
      (d) Scleroderma
    2. Hypersensitivity states with musculoarticular reactions to serum, drugs, etc.
    3. Traumatic
      (a) Postural syndromes
      (b) Traumatic arthropathy
    4. Associated with:
      (a) Cutaneous or mucosal features
        Erythema multiforme
        Erythema nodosum
        Purpura (various types), Purpura rheumatica
        Polyarthritis with urethritis and conjunctivitis (Reiter's syndrome)
      (b) Metabolic disturbances
        Alcaptonuria
        Gout
      (c) Endocrine disturbances
        Acromegaly
        Hyperparathyroidism
        Myxedema, etc.
        Menopause
        Osteoporosis: Menopausal, senile, and others
      (d) Blood diseases: Hemophilia, Leukemia, etc.
      (e) Pulmonary diseases: Hypertrophic pulmonary osteoarthropathy, Sarcoidosis, etc.
      (f) Nervous system disease: Neuroarthropathy, Reflex dystrophy
      (g) Psychiatric states and psychologic syndromes
      (h) Neoplastic diseases of articular or periarticular tissues
      (i) Osteochondrodystrophies

THE PREVALENCE AND PROBLEM OF RHEUMATIC DISEASE

Numerous population studies have been made to determine prevalence of rheumatic diseases, but difficulties are many. Large-scale surveys are inaccurate because they depend on answers to set questions, permitting guesswork by the people surveyed. Smaller population samplings, with strict diagnostic criteria and medical examination, are far more accurate but represent such a local segment that doubt is thrown on the projection of the figures to cover the general population.

In spite of the handicaps, the realization that rheumatic diseases form a tremendous segment of chronic disability all over the world has become more widespread in recent years. The epidemiology of rheumatic diseases has become a major project for research and will be discussed in a separate chapter in this volume (see Chapter 12).

A fairly recent population sampling survey in the United States was conducted from 1957 to 1959 by the U.S. Department of Health, Education and Welfare as part of a National Health Survey.[6] The data from this were based on answers to questions put by lay interviewers to adults, and eliminated any who were confined to hospitals, nursing homes, etc. From this survey a total of 10,845,000 persons were estimated to have arthritis or rheumatism in the United States, an incidence of about 6.4 per cent of those in the country over fifteen years of age. Whereas nearly 30 per cent of those over seventy-five years were reported to have rheumatism or arthritis, only 0.2 per cent of those from fifteen to twenty-five years of age had such complaints. Forty-two per cent of those having rheumatic disease were not under medical care at the time of interview, and an additional 19 per cent had never received medical care for their rheumatism.

With a total of nearly 11 million persons in the United States suffering from some form of rheumatism or arthritis, it is most important to determine the extent of disability in order to estimate the true socioeconomic impact on the country. From the National Health Survey figures[7] it appears that 26 per cent of those having rheumatic disease were definitely limited in their activities, and 10 per cent were grossly disabled. This means that more than a million persons are rendered unemployable by arthritis and rheumatism.

About 27 million work days are lost annually because of arthritis. About 1 in every 5 chronically house-bound invalids had arthritis. Arthritis and rheumatism were the second greatest cause of chronic limitation of major activity with a relative incidence of 16 per cent. Heart disease, with an incidence of 17 per cent, was the only disease group exceeding arthritis.

Although arthritis cripples a tremendous number of persons each year, it kills relatively few. *There is no other group of diseases which causes so much suffering by so many for so long.* Because of the tendency to cripple without killing, arthritis and rheumatism belong at the head of the list of chronic diseases from the standpoint of social and economic importance.

Industry has recognized the importance of the problem of rheumatic diseases. Both the necessity for job changes and the time lost from work have received attention. At the Second Conference on Rheumatic Diseases in Industry,[5] which was sponsored by the Arthritis and Rheumatism Foundation and other groups concerned with industrial medicine in 1961, the questions of compensability, disability, employability, placement of handicapped arthritics, incidence of rheumatic disease in industry, and many other specific problems, such as low back pain, were extensively discussed. Those physicians practicing industrial medicine are concerned directly, and the Proceedings of this Second Conference would be of great use to them.[5]

In an extensive survey of musculoskeletal complaints in industry, Brown and Lingg[2] chose to study the employees of the Consolidated Edison Company of New York for one year. By random sampling of 25 per cent of all daily medical records for the period, they found that 15 per cent of all employees requested medical care because of rheumatic complaints during the year. Of the 805 sample records studied, a third had definite and diagnosable rheumatic disease, ranging from bursitis, disc disease, and fibrositis to osteoarthritis, gout, and rheumatoid arthritis. A total of 15,040 days were lost from work that year in that company alone from rheumatic diseases, and 20,800 medical visits were needed for treatment. This constituted about 10 per cent of the total employee days lost from work from all illnesses that year, or more than $300,000 lost to that company alone in one year from rheumatic diseases.[2] By projecting such data to all of industry, one can see the enormity of the problem.

The National Health Survey[6,7] showed that during the period of study (1957–1959) there were 30,000 persons unable to work because of arthritis for a minimum of six months, and therefore became eligible for Social Security benefits. Of these, 78 per cent were over fifty years of age, and 20 per cent were women. Osteoarthritis was present in 56 per cent and rheumatoid arthritis in 27 per cent.

RELATIVE INCIDENCE OF THE RHEUMATIC DISEASES

In civilian populations many attempts have been made to determine the relative frequency of the various types of arthritis and related conditions. The difficulties are great.[3,4] Actually the majority of all persons who live beyond middle life have some rheumatic complaints—mostly due to degenerative joint disease.[4] The complaints usually are not severe enough, nor the duration of painful periods long enough to force many of these individuals to seek medical attention, but degenerative joint disease (osteoarthritis) is the most common form of rheumatic disease observed in several large arthritis clinics[10] (see also Chapter 12).

Statistics for the relative incidence of osteoarthritis and rheumatoid arthritis among non-institutionalized adults in the United States were obtained from a careful study of 6,672 persons, selected nationwide as a highly stratified multistage probability sample.[4a] These persons ranged in age from 18 to 79 years, and were all examined between 1960 and 1962 as a part of the United States Health Examination Survey. In addition to a detailed rheumatologic history, a complete physical examination, test for rheumatoid factor and x-ray examination of hands and feet were performed on each. Osteoarthritis was diagnosed in 37 per cent of these persons, with incidence of 4 per cent among the younger up to 85 per cent among the oldest group. About 23 per cent of those with osteoarthritis had a moderate to severe form of the disease. The incidence of rheumatoid arthritis was 3.2 per cent, with 30 per cent of these satisfying ARA criteria for classic or definite forms of the disease. Incidence was about equal between whites and blacks, but was higher in women than men and increasingly common at older ages.

Another common form of rheumatic disease is fibrositis. Nearly everyone at some time has experienced a stiff neck, a siege of lumbago, a stiff shoulder, or simply "morning stiffness" in many of the muscles. Only those with severe or persistent complaints of this type seek medical attention, so that hospital, clinic, or even medical statistics obtained from all physicians would not reflect the true incidence of such a disorder.

The most common of the more severe forms of rheumatic disease are *rheumatoid arthritis* and *rheumatic fever*. The latter was the chief cause of death from disease in children aged five through nineteen,[8] and produced more chronic heart disease than all other causes combined. Rheumatoid arthritis, though it most commonly attacks later (twenty to fifty years of age at onset), and seldom causes death directly, is still the greatest cause of crippling deformity from disease. These patients form a great proportion of the population attending arthritis clinics because of the long duration and severity of the process. Although patients with rheumatoid arthritis actually number only 27 per cent of the total patients registered in the Arthritis Clinic of the Hospital of the University of Pennsylvania,[10] 82 per cent of the revisits to the clinic are by this group.

It is with *rheumatoid arthritis*, the great crippler, that physicians should be concerned most. Here is the greatest problem of the rheumatic diseases, from the standpoint of severity and prolonged disability. It is no wonder that patients at the mention of "arthritis" think of rheumatoid arthritis, and begin to look forward with dread to crippling deformities and a wheel-chair existence. It is because of the dread that "arthritis" conjures up in the minds of most, that physicians should know how to diagnose correctly the forms of rheumatic disease. *Reassurance, to a patient who has a milder form of arthritis than the rheumatoid type, may be the best treatment the physician can give.* For this reason also, the term degenerative joint disease is preferable to osteoarthritis when explaining the condition to a patient.

THE RHEUMATIC DISEASES AS A MILITARY PROBLEM

Among the 4,000,000 soldiers in the American Army of the First World War there were reported 33,613 instances of rheumatoid arthritis and degenerative joint disease, 24,770 cases of acute articular rheumatism (rheumatic fever), 12,093 instances of fibrositis (muscular rheumatism), 7895 cases of gonorrheal arthritis, 2671 cases of tenosynovitis, 188 instances of tuberculous arthritis, and only 82 cases of gouty arthritis.

In the British Expeditionary Forces (1940), 26 per cent of all medical patients admitted to several General Hospitals had rheumatic disorders, the most common of which was fibrositis (70 per cent), with 15 per cent of those affected having rheumatic fever and 9 per cent having rheumatoid arthritis; only 6 per cent had degenerative joint disease—usually traumatic.

Military factors which may be expected to cause an increase in the incidence of rheumatoid arthritis include emotional disturbances, exposure to dampness, prolonged chilling, exposure to respiratory infections, etc.

To care for the large numbers of soldiers in the Army expected to acquire rheumatic fever or other rheumatic diseases in World War II, five army hospitals were designated, staffed and equipped for proper treatment. Three were for treatment of rheumatic fever, and two for various types of arthritis and allied conditions.

Complete figures on the incidence of rheumatic fever in World War II were not made available, but from 1942 to 1944 inclusive nearly 15,000 cases had been reported in the United States Army.[9]

Over 14,000 cases of arthritis and related diseases were treated at the Army Rheumatism Centers at Army and Navy General Hospital, Hot Springs, Arkansas, and Ashburn General Hospital, McKinney, Texas.[10]

The relative incidence of the rheumatic diseases among soldiers was not as anticipated, in some instances because the advent of sulfonamides and penicillin had reduced septic arthritis (particularly gonococcal) to a very low rate of occurrence, and because better understanding of the difference between fibrositis and psychogenic rheumatism (psychoneurosis with musculoskeletal reference of symptoms) was emphasized in the training of medical officers in the Rheumatism Centers.[9]

The methods of group treatment in teaching large numbers of arthritis pa-

Principal Diagnosis in over 5200 Patients Admitted to the Army Rheumatic Disease Center at Ashburn General Hospital[10]

Diagnosis	Cases	%
Rheumatoid Arthritis	1840 cases	35%
Involving peripheral joints alone	988 cases	
Involving both spinal and peripheral joints	256 cases	
Involving spine and/or sacroiliac joints only	499 cases	
Involving spine and hips or shoulders only	97 cases	
Degenerative Joint Disease (osteoarthritis) (Some had multiple involvement)	1449 cases	28%
Involving spine	955 cases	
Involving knees	404 cases	
Involving feet	325 cases	
Involving hips	83 cases	
Involving fingers	43 cases	
Involving other joints (shoulders, elbows, etc.)	42 cases	
Psychogenic Rheumatism (psychoneurosis with musculo-skeletal reference of symptoms)	893 cases	17%
Fibrositis (including bursitis, lumbago, etc.)	151 cases	3%
Specific Infectious Arthritis	115 cases	2%
Gonococcal arthritis (proved)	41 cases	
Reiter's Syndrome	57 cases	
Tuberculous Arthritis	4 cases	
Septic Arthritis (Staph. or Strept.)	8 cases	
Miscellaneous infectious types	5 cases	
Orthopedic Conditions	644 cases	12%
Spinal Deformities and Backstrain	362 cases	
Footstrain or Deformity	119 cases	
Ruptured Intervertebral Disc	89 cases	
Internal Derangement of Joint	51 cases	
Miscellaneous Deformities, tumors, etc.	23 cases	
Rheumatic Fever*	36 cases	0.7%
Gout	21 cases	0.4%
Miscellaneous and Undiagnosed	72 cases	1.4%

* Soldiers with rheumatic fever were usually sent to other hospitals, so the relative incidence was very low.

tients how to " live with the disease" and how to "help themselves" used at the Army Arthritis Centers have established a pattern for civilian clinics. The Reconditioning Programs emphasized proper physical therapy, exercise, and mental reorientation for all the soldiers with rheumatic disease. This emphasis on convalescent care and training also has been carried over into civilian medical practice to the great benefit of arthritic patients.

THE CAMPAIGN AGAINST ARTHRITIS AND RHEUMATISM

Rheumatology has recently become one of the most active fields in Medicine. Original research has geometrically increased with the expansion and addition of many laboratories devoted to this broad subject. There has been a tremendous influx of new personnel into Rheumatology, stimulated by the many recent discoveries in this relatively virgin field of Medicine, and made possible by increasing financial support from governmental and voluntary health agencies. Whereas in 1945 there were only about 12 centers in the United States for the study of rheumatic diseases, there are now more than 100. The "Renaissance of Rheumatology" began shortly after World War II, when many young physicians who had been trained in the Army Arthritis Centers returned to practice. It was given tremendous impetus by the founding of the Arthritis and Rheumatism Foundation in 1948, the discovery of the effects of cortisone in 1949, the Seventh International Congress on Rheumatic Diseases at New York in 1949, and the founding of the National Institute of Arthritis and Metabolic Diseases in 1953. This same growth trend in Rheumatology has been obvious in most countries throughout the world.

World and National Organizations

La Ligue Internationale contre le Rheumatisme, the worldwide organization in Rheumatology, noted tremendous increase in membership, both in numbers of physicians (nearly 5000), and numbers of national and regional organizations affiliated. Nearly a thousand physicians attended and participated in the Tenth International Congress on Rheumatic Diseases in Rome in 1961, presenting hundreds of scientific papers. Large attendance and participation were also recorded at the Eleventh Congress in Mar del Plata, Argentina, in December 1965, and at the Twelfth International Congress on Rheumatic Diseases in Prague, Czechoslovakia, in October 1969. The Thirteenth Congress will be held in Kyoto, Japan, in October 1973.

The World Health Organization (WHO) has had an Expert Committee on Rheumatic Diseases since 1953. This Committee has contact with the International League Against Rheumatism and seeks to establish uniformity of terminology, classification, to set up studies of prevalence of rheumatic diseases, research and education in this field as well as prevention and control. Liaison between the League and the WHO has improved through the years, but, as yet, there has not been much emphasis on rheumatic diseases by the World Health Organization.

The International League Against Rheumatism is composed of three regional Leagues. The European League is the oldest of these, consisting of 24 national rheumatism societies to which have been added those of Turkey, Israel and Egypt as neighboring groups. The European League has a congress every four years, the latest of which was held in Brighton, England in June 1971.

The Pan-American League Against Rheumatism embraces fourteen national rheumatism societies of North and South America. This League has also been active with congresses every four years, the last held at Punte del Este, Uruguay, in December 1970, with the next one planned for Toronto, Canada, in June 1974.

The Southeast Asia and Pacific Area League Against Rheumatism, established in 1963 from the national societies of Australia, New Zealand, India, Japan and the Philippines, has conducted two congresses. The first was in Bombay, India, in 1968 and the second in Aukland, New Zealand, in February 1972. Other regions are also showing increasing interest in rheumatic diseases; for example a second South African Congress on Rheumatism and Arthritis was held in Cape Town in March 1970.

The American Rheumatism Association is the largest single national society in Rheumatology with more than 2000 active members. Two meetings are held each year, at which more than a hundred original scientific papers are read to the more than 500 members who attend each meeting. Large and active memberships in such societies as the Japan Rheumatism Association, the Australian Rheumatism Association, the Society of Rheumatology of Chile, of Mexico, of Argentina, of Brazil, of New Zealand, and many others have joined with the older societies of Great Britain, France, Italy, Holland, Germany, Belgium, U.S.S.R., the Scandinavian countries and Canada in the effort to learn more of the crippling ailments. More societies are being formed each year, and existing ones are enlarging. All are important in the dissemination of knowledge in this field. All are actively providing more and better training for physicians, and most are seeking and obtaining government cooperation in coping with the social and economic problems imposed by rheumatic diseases. Many also sponsor research programs.

Government and Voluntary Agencies

The Arthritis and Rheumatism Council in Great Britain, The Canadian Arthritis and Rheumatism Society, the Australian Rheumatism Council, and other agencies throughout the World have been active in raising money and sponsoring research and education programs in Rheumatology. In the United States the National Institute of Arthritis and Metabolic Diseases, a unit of the National Institutes of Health of the United States Department of Health, Education and Welfare, is the largest single agency devoted to study and control of the rheumatic disease problem. In 18 years this agency has established tremendous intramural research programs at the Clinical Center, and sponsored hundreds of extramural research projects all over the country. The appropriation for the budget of this Institute has been increased, but the many millions made available are still far short of the need.

The Arthritis and Rheumatism Foundation, a voluntary health agency, was formed in 1948 and raises and allocates about four million dollars yearly for arthritis training, research, care and public education. The National Foundation entered the field of Rheumatology in 1959, but the programs it sponsored were given over to the Arthritis Foundation in 1964 in order to create a single, powerful agency in the field of Arthritis. The American Rheumatism Association also joined with the Arthritis Foundation in 1965 to direct the medical portion of the programs.

Publications in Rheumatology

An increasing number of medical journals devoted exclusively to the subject of rheumatic disease is further evidence of the growth and activity in Rheumatology. An increasing number of rheumatologic articles in other journals also attests the amount of research going on in this field.

There are journals of Rheumatology in many languages. The main ones in English are the *Annals of the Rheumatic Diseases*, published in Great Britain; *Arthritis and Rheumatism*, published by the American Rheumatism Association; the *Acta Rheumatologica Scandinavica*; and the *Bulletin on Rheumatic Diseases*, published by the Arthritis Foundation.

In addition, the American Rheumatism Association compiles almost yearly the *Rheumatism Reviews*, originated by Hench *et al.* in 1935. Heretofore published in the *Annals of Internal Medicine* including the Sixteenth Review in 1964,[17] subsequent reviews appeared in *Arthritis and Rheumatism.*[3a,b,c] Periodically the ARA also compiles and publishes the *Primer on Rheumatic Diseases* in the *Journal of the American Medical Association.*[4] The Association also began in 1965 to publish the *Index of Rheumatology*, a semimonthly bibliographic listing of world literature in Rheumatology in cooperation with the National Library of Medicine. This brings almost the complete world literature within reach of all who seek it, and within a few months of publication.

The year 1964 also saw a new development in Rheumatology when the N.I.A.M.D. and the Excerpta Medica Foundation began publication of a monthly abstract journal of world literature in Rheumatology, entitled *Arthritis and Rheumatic Diseases Abstracts.* In 1965 another abstract journal, *Arthritis and*

Rheumatism (Excerpta Medica), with an international board of editors also began publication, using the same abstracting facilities. These additions to the regular scientific journals facilitate the task of retrieving research findings in this active field of endeavor.

Rheumatology as a Specialty

The tremendous interest in and growth of Rheumatology have stimulated much thought and discussion concerning the place of this field of research and clinical effort in Medicine. Rheumatologists have been Internists, Orthopedic Surgeons, Physiatrists or Pediatricians, but there have been also some physicians interested in this field who are Radiologists, Pathologists or from other clinical disciplines of Medicine. The general feeling has been that Rheumatology should not be split off into a separate specialty, such as Dermatology, Psychiatry or Ophthalmology, but should be regarded as a *subspecialty* of Internal Medicine, Orthopedic Surgery, Physical Medicine and Rehabilitation, Pediatrics, etc. Even this designation has been objected to on the ground that it further splinters each specialty.[18] Committees to study the question have been appointed by the American Rheumatism Association, the Canadian Rheumatism Association, and the Heberden Society (Great Britain). In the United States the American Board of Internal Medicine has already recognized Rheumatology as a subspecialty of Internal Medicine by appointing, from candidates suggested for this task by the American Rheumatism Association, a panel to formulate examinations in Rheumatology. Thus, the ARA will have a voice in determining the training requirements and subjects in which a candidate should be proficient in this field without having to set up a separate examining board. Other subspecialties of Internal Medicine have already followed suit.

Progress in training in Rheumatology, and problems in teaching this subject were thoroughly reviewed during the Third National Conference on Education in the Rheumatic Diseases.[18]

Opportunities in Rheumatology

The foregoing discussion should illustrate the tremendous advances and possibilities. This field of Medicine is still underpopulated by physicians and the number of sufferers needing better care is very large. Although many and substantial advances in knowledge in Rheumatology will become evident to those who read this book, there is still a dearth of knowledge about rheumatic diseases and a great need for careful, thorough study. The opportunities for "pathfinding research" are endless and open to any interested physician, even though the complexities of the many intricate disciplines may limit his ability to carry new findings forward into all the ramifications needed to substantiate their full meaning. This latter type is "surveying research," the careful mapping out of new findings in complete detail, which needs the efforts of research workers trained in specific disciplines. Both types of research are needed for further development of Rheumatology.

The American Rheumatism Association, with the Arthritis Foundation, compiles a listing of such opportunities for training and for academic and research positions. This is available on request from The Arthritis Foundation, 1212 Avenue of the Americas, New York, N.Y., 10036. Many physicians, both in the U.S. and abroad, have found opportunities for study and work from this pamphlet. The ranks are filling out, and the campaign against arthritis and rheumatism steadily increases in power.

BIBLIOGRAPHY

1. Blumberg, B. S., Bunim, J. J., Calkins, E., Pirani, C. L. and Zvaifler, N. J.: Bull. Rheum. Dis., *14*, 340, 1964.
2. Brown, R. and Lingg, C.: Arth. & Rheum., *4*, 283, 1961.

3. Cobb, S., Merchant, W. R. and Warren, J. E.: J. Chron. Dis., *2*, 50, 1955.

3a. Christian, C. L. *et al.*: (Seventeenth Rheumatism Review), Arth. & Rheum., *9*, 93–266, 1966.

3b. ————: (Eighteenth Rheumatism Review), Arth. & Rheum., *11*, 525–732, 1968.

3c. ————: (Nineteenth Rheumatism Review), Arth. & Rheum., *13*, 455–711, 1970.

4. Decker, J. L., Bollet, A. J., Duff, I. F., Shulman, L. E. and Stollerman, G. H.: (Primer on Rheumatic Diseases), J.A.M.A., *190*, 127; 425; 509; 741, 1964.

4a. Engel, A., and Burch, T. A.: Arth. & Rheum., *10*, 61, 1967.

5. Goldstein, D. H., Klein, I., Roemmich, W. *et al.*: (Second Conference on Rheumatic Diseases in Industry), Arch. Environ. Health, *5*, 487–527, 1962.

6. Health Statistics, Series B, No. 20, U.S. Dept. of Health, Education and Welfare, 1960. (Arthritis and Rheumatism.)

7. Health Statistics, Series B, No. 36, U.S. Dept. of Health, Education and Welfare, 1962. (Chronic Conditions Causing Limitation of Activities.)

8. Hench, P. S. *et al.*: (Ninth Rheumatism Review), Ann. Int. Med., *28*, 66, 1948.

9. Hench, P. S. and Boland, E. W.: Ann. Int. Med., *26*, 808, 1946.

10. Hollander, J. L.: Unpublished data.

11. Hormell, R. S.: New Engl. J. Med., *223*, 754, 1940.

12. Murphy, G. E.: Bull. Hist. Med., 14, 123, 1940.

13. Osgood, R. B.: Am. J. Med. Sci., *200*, 429, 1940.

14. Ragan, C. A. and Meyer, K.: Ann. Rheum. Dis., *7*, 35, 1948.

15. Ruhl, M. J. and Sokoloff, L.: (A Thesaurus of Rheumatology), Arth. & Rheum., *8*, 97, 1965.

16. Smyth, C. J. *et al.*: (Fifteenth Rheumatism Review), Ann. Int. Med., *59*, Suppl. 4, (Nov.), 1963.

17. ————: (Sixteenth Rheumatism Review), Ann. Int. Med., *61*, Suppl. 6, (Nov.), 1964.

18. Stollerman, G. H.: Proceedings of the Third National Conference on Education in the Rheumatic Diseases. Arth. & Rheum., *11*, 209–376, (Suppl.), 1968.

Chapter 2

Examination of the Arthritic Patient

By L. Maxwell Lockie, M.D.

An accurate diagnosis is essential in the care of the patient with joint disease. A complete study is necessary even though the diagnosis may seem obvious or the joint involvement trivial. In fact, thorough investigation is of the greatest importance in patients who have only one joint involved and the etiology is obscure. As the physician always looks for a cause of "fever," he should also seek the cause of "arthritis" as neither of these terms is a diagnosis. Inasmuch as there are so many underlying physical conditions which produce manifestations of "arthritis," the examining physician should exercise patience and tact, as well as take enough time for a thorough initial study.

The work-up consists of a detailed history, complete physical examination, certain laboratory data and x-rays as necessary. Only by proper assessment of all factors can the examining physician arrive at an accurate total diagnosis and use sound judgment as to the treatment indicated. After completion of these studies, the results of the physical examination as well as interpretation of laboratory and x-ray data are discussed with the patient. The program of management is then explained in detail, preferably with a responsible member of the family at the conference. A written outline frequently is given, in order that the patient understands clearly the projected plan of therapy. In this frank discussion, the general course of the disease is anticipated as far as possible, and the patient is made to realize that his cooperation is absolutely necessary. In fact, without the enthusiastic willingness of the patient to enter into the program, the examination and the treatment following will result in little gain.

THE HISTORY IN JOINT DISEASE

The following suggestions will aid in obtaining a complete history referable to joint disease.

I. General Information—For Record

1. Name, address, age, sex, color, occupation, marital status, source of referral, and medical insurance status.

2. If medical legal problems are involved, detailed data must be obtained in order to file a complete report.

II. Specific Information Relative to the Articular Structures

1. Inquire with careful detail concerning the involved joint structures including:

a. Prodromes or preceding illnesses.
b. Date of onset of symptoms.
c. Description of the pattern of the onset including the rapidity of progression of symptoms, severity of pain, amount and location of swelling, symmetry of joints involved, extent of limitation of motion, persistence of complaints and the degree of disability.
d. General pattern of joint involvement since onset.

2. Inquire into precipitating or aggravating circumstances.

3. Record amount, location, and duration of morning stiffness; also occurrence and degree of fever, anorexia, or loss of weight (see Chapter 26).

4. Ask about previous disability of a similar or allied nature.

5. Discuss past treatment, including the names of drugs or modalities, concerning effectiveness, dosage, duration of administration, why discontinued, evidence of sensitivity or reaction.

6. Date and interpretation of previous x-ray studies.

III. Items of a General Nature

1. The family history may suggest gouty arthritis, ankylosing spondylitis, rheumatoid arthritis, Heberden's nodes, etc.

2. The marital status and living conditions at home, including the ages of children (if any) aid in evaluation of responsibilities when outlining a program of treatment for those with rheumatoid arthritis or ankylosing spondylitis. For instructions in ambulation, it is helpful to know the type of home in which the patient lives, whether it is an apartment, ranch style or a house with sleeping rooms on another floor.

3. Personal habits, including diet, exact amount of liquor and cigarettes used, and the number of hours rest and sleep should be recorded.

4. Allergies to drugs must be known in detail in order to avoid them in the future. Many patients are unable to tolerate one or more such as: salicylates, gold, adrenal cortical steroids, butazolidin, codeine or indomethacin.

5. Inquire concerning past injuries and surgical procedures.

GENERAL PHYSICAL EXAMINATION

The physician needs no instruction on the procedure for the general physical examination of a patient. However, there are some physical signs of special importance in arthritic patients.[1]

1. The general appearance, including a description of gait and posture.

2. Skin lesions suggestive of psoriasis, lupus erythematosus, erythema nodosum, scleroderma, or purpura.

3. The cold, moist extremities as in rheumatoid arthritis, or marked heat, as in gouty or specific infectious arthritic joints.

4. Subcutaneous swellings, such as nodules in the elbow area in rheumatoid arthritis, or subcutaneous tophi of gout in margin of ear, in finger pads or elsewhere.

5. Cardiac abnormalities, such as aortic lesions in ankylosing spondylitis and syphilis, etc.

6. Lymphadenopathy, splenomegaly and hepatomegaly as in juvenile rheumatoid arthritis, or Felty's types of rheumatoid arthritis, or in lupus erythematosus.

7. Moon face, striae, acne, purpuric spots on arms or legs, supraclavicular fat deposits, or other evidence of previous steroid therapy.

PHYSICAL SIGNS OF JOINT DISEASE

As one proceeds to examine the joints individually, it is advisable to recall that the synovial membranes and the peri-articular structures are primarily involved in rheumatoid diseases, infectious arthritis and gout, while the cartilage and bone are mainly affected in osteoarthritis and in some rarer varieties.

The important physical signs of joint diseases are:

1. Abnormalities of *color*, *consistency*, *temperature*, or amount of *sweating* of the *overlying skin*. Skin lesions or ulcers near the joints occur in some types.

2. *Joint swelling* or enlargement, which may be one or more of four types:

A. *Peri-articular edema*, a *diffuse* edema of subcutaneous tissue about a joint, extending beyond the reflections of the synovium, or *localized* in adjacent bursae or tendon sheaths.

B. *Synovial or capsular thickening*, recognized as a doughy enlargement confined to the areas where the joint capsule and synovial reflections are near the surface.

C. *Effusion*, or hydrops, which is identified by the demonstration of fluctuation in the joint sac, or by bulging limited to the reflections of the synovium. (In the knee, effusion is readily demonstrable by ballottement of the "floating patella" against the femur.) Bursal effusion, as in "housemaid's knee," is extra-articular.

D. *Bony enlargement.—Osteophytes* of sufficient size to be palpable are commonly found at the articular margins in degenerative joint disease (osteoarthritis). Spur formation at the articular margins of the terminal phalangeal joints of the fingers accounts for much of the enlargement of Heberden's nodes. Gross distortion of the bone ends may be noted in acromegaly, or locally in osteogenic sarcoma or other bone tumors arising near a joint.

3. *Tenderness* may be *localized* (as at a point of injury), or *diffuse*, about the entire joint. The *degree of tenderness* is important.

4. *Crepitation on motion.*—"Grating" or "grinding" on motion is common in degenerative joint disease. Presence of this finding usually indicates a roughening of the opposing cartilages, which may be from age changes, chondromalacia, injuries, abnormal strains, previous inflammatory changes, osteochondritis, or other conditions which have caused irregularities in the surface of the articular cartilage. This must be differentiated as:

A. *Fine "rubbing" crepitation* felt over rheumatoid arthritic joints from presence of granulation tissue (pannus), or from bone ends denuded of cartilage by pannus.

B. *Coarse crepitation* or "crackling" so commonly felt in the knees from age changes or "wearing" of the subpatellar surface. (This is the type usually noted in degenerative joint disease.)

C. *Joint cracking* or *snapping*. This may connote nothing more than slipping of tendons or ligaments over a bony prominence when the joint is flexed. Many people can "crack" their fingers, yet have no demonstrable joint disease. (Generally, the coarser the crepitation, the less significant.)

5. *Deformity*, from gross joint destruction or injury, producing actual *dislocation* or *subluxation* of the articulating bones, with demonstrable malalignment.

6. *Limited motion.*—Limitation may be due to trauma, joint effusion, spasm, contracture of periarticular structures, fibrous or bony ankylosis.

7. *Muscle changes.—Weakness*, hyperactive stretch reflex (*spasm*), *atrophy*, and *shortening* are usually more prominent in the flexor muscles of a diseased joint, and produce marked deformity or limitation of motion.

8. *Nodules.—Rheumatoid nodules* are frequently found adjacent to finger, elbow or knee joints, as are the *tophi* of gout. Small *loose bodies* or "joint mice" can occasionally be felt in the knee—these can be moved under the finger, and frequently disappear when palpated. Nodules or tophi near joints are usually subcutaneous, or fixed to the joint capsule, and are not usually freely movable. *Ganglia*, or synovial cysts, are often found at the wrist, and occasionally behind the knee (Baker's cysts).

TECHNIQUE OF JOINT EXAMINATION

The technique for examination of joints is presented in some detail on the following pages, arranged by specific joint or group of joints to be studied. Normal ranges of joint motion are presented graphically in Figures 2–1 and 2–2. For those desiring more detail on joint anatomy and abnormal physical signs of joint disease, an excellent monograph is available, is copiously and well illustrated, and is highly recommended especially for those undertaking Rheumatology as a specialty.[1] Greater detail on ranges of joint motion in determination of disabilities may also be obtained from a special manual.[2]

The Fingers and Hands.—Identification of anatomical landmarks, for concise and complete record:

a. Distal interphalangeal joint (DIP).

b. Proximal interphalangeal joint (PIP).

c. Metacarpal phalangeal joint (MCP).

d. Number of finger (Thumb 1—little finger 5).

1. *Observe* for: swelling, skin lesions,

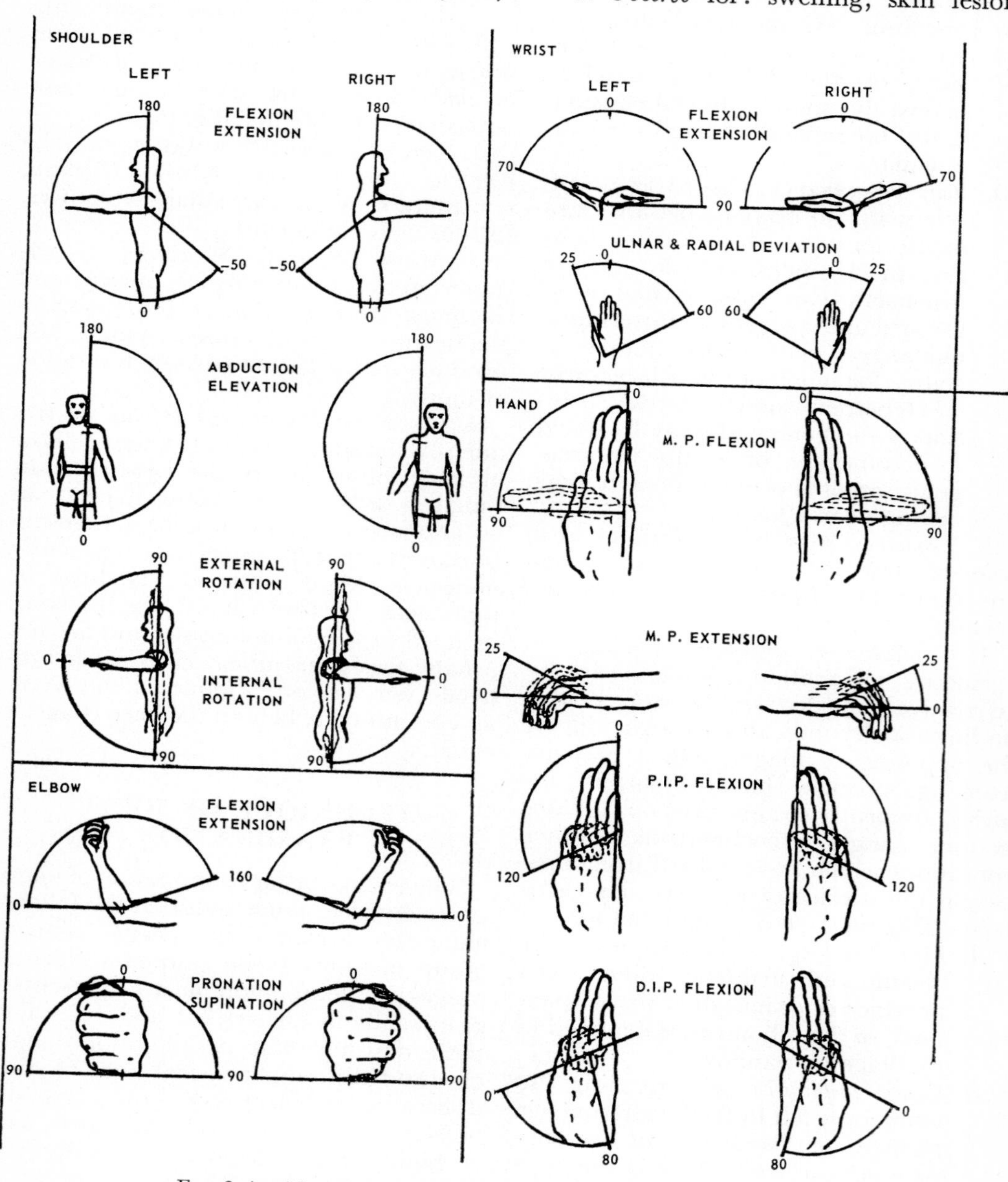

FIG. 2–1.—Normal range of motion diagrams (upper extremity). (From chart used at Children's Hospital of Buffalo.)

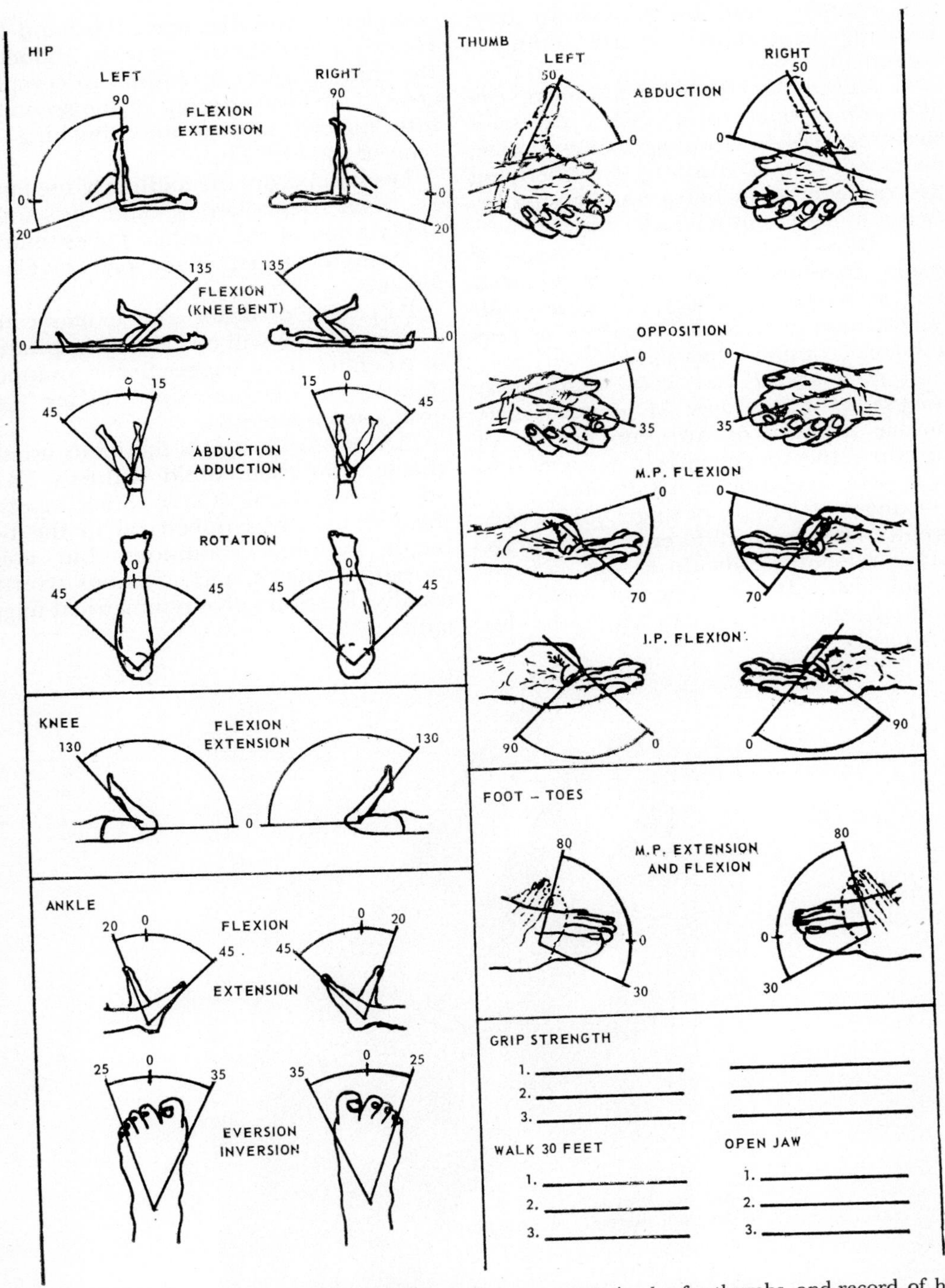

Fig. 2–2.—Normal range of motion diagrams (lower extremity), also for thumbs, and record of hand grip strength, walking time and temporomandibular function. (From chart used at Children's Hospital of Buffalo.)

nail changes, skin or muscle atrophy, sweating, deformities, or shortened fingers (brachydactylia).

2. *Palpate for: degree of tenderness, type of swelling,* heat or coldness, excessive sweating, *nodules* (noting location, size, consistency, and fixation to underlying tissues), edema, or hardness of tissues between joints (as in scleroderma).

3. *Move joints to determine: range of motion,* existence of *contractures, subluxations, pain on motion, instability, fibrous ankylosis* (slight motion possible, usually), or *bony ankylosis* (complete fixation).

4. *Have patient move joints to determine: strength of grip, range of active motion,* muscle *weakness* or atrophy, or loss of certain active movements (*e. g.*, extension of fingers, deviation of MCP joints).

Ranges of motion of finger joints vary greatly between different individuals. Measurement is difficult, except by functional tests. If the range of motion is normal, the patient can close the fist completely and can open the hand flat. He can spread the fingers wide, abducting the thumb, and can adduct to complete contact or even overlap of the second to fifth fingers, with thumb touching the base of the fifth finger.

Deviation from the midline of the hand, as ulnar deviation, should be noted. Description of the method for estimation of strength of grip is set forth in Chapter 26.

Palpation of flexor and extensor tendons in motion will reveal any crepitation or catching, as in trigger finger, snapping thumb, or DeQuervain's disease (stenosing tenosynovitis).

Figure 2–3 illustrates the joints usually affected by rheumatoid arthritis (RA) and osteoarthritis (OS). Such involvement is usually symmetrical in the two hands in these conditions, but gout, psoriatic arthritis, and infectious arthritis usually do not involve symmetrical finger joints.

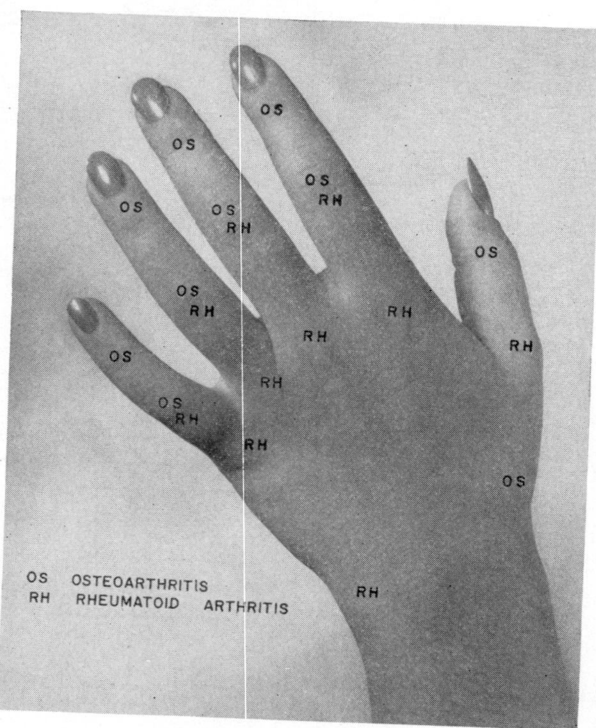

Fig. 2–3.—Joints usually affected by rheumatoid arthritis and osteoarthritis.

Distal interphalangeal joint involvement (DIP) is common in osteoarthritis, psoriatic arthritis, and occasionally gout. Proximal interphalangeal (PIP) involvement usually means rheumatoid arthritis if there is effusion or soft, tender swelling of the joint, but firm non-tender enlargement of these joints characterizes the so-called "Bouchard's nodes" of osteoarthritis. These are the counterpart of the Heberden's nodes of the DIP finger joints. Metacarpal phalangeal joints (MCP) are rarely involved *except* in rheumatoid arthritis.

Examination of the Wrists.—The wrist is a compound joint—a *group* of joints. *Inspection* quickly reveals the presence or absence of swelling or deformity. Predominance of flexor muscle strength in severe arthritis of the wrist usually produces deformity in palmar flexion and ulnar deviation in rheumatoid arthritis. *Palpation* reveals the type of swelling, degree of tenderness, and particularly localized swellings, such as ganglia (synovial cysts). Comparison with the opposite wrist, if not also involved, or estimation by comparison with the examiner's own movements may be satisfactory enough for ordinary clinical record, but, for later reference, measurements made with a goniometer (an instrument for measuring angles) are much more accurate in noting actual degrees of motion. *Weakness* and *atrophy* of *forearm muscles* should be noted. Measurements of circumference of the forearm at a given distance below the elbow give a valuable record of degree of atrophy. Infectious arthritis, such as the gonococcal and tuberculous forms, may involve *one* wrist, but rheumatoid arthritis often will involve *both.* Localized pain and tenderness at the radial styloid indicates stenosing tenosynovitis (DeQuervain's disease). This latter condition may be further diagnosed by the "Finklestein test," in which the thumb of the patient is held in his clenched fist and the examiner forces the wrist into ulnar deviation. This motion produces acute pain if DeQuervain's disease is present.

Pain and swelling in the ulnar styloid area are highly suggestive of the presence of rheumatoid arthritis. They may occur early and appear as a harbinger of widespread rheumatoid arthritis later.

Examination of the Elbow

The elbow joint has two distinct functions. The humero-ulnar joint is a hinge joint permitting *flexion* and *extension.* The humero-radial joint permits rotation of the head of the radius, making possible *supination* and *pronation* of the forearm. Mild to moderate degrees of *swelling* and *tenderness* are most noticeable on the extensor surface, just medial and lateral to the olecranon. *Nodules* should be looked for *in the olecranon bursa* and *along the ulna* distal to the olecranon. *Effusion* into the *olecranon bursa* is frequently found after *trauma* and in *gout.* The first nodules in a patient with rheumatoid arthritis are nearly always found near the elbow. Limitation of motion at the elbow is usually noted first as decreased extension and supination. Ankylosis of the elbow joint is fairly common in severe rheumatoid arthritis. *Active motion* of the elbow reveals any weakness of the biceps, triceps, or brachialis muscles. Atrophy in rheumatoid arthritis may be severe, and muscle tenderness is sometimes marked. The *carrying angle*, or angle the ulna makes with the humerus anteriorly, should be compared on the two sides.

Examination of the Shoulder

The shoulder joint proper, or *scapulohumeral joint* is a ball and socket joint permitting motion in all directions, including rotation. Shoulder movement as we know it is more complex than simple scapulohumeral motion, however. Motion is assisted by *sliding* of the *scapula* over the posterior chest wall, with some movement of the *acromioclavicular* and *sternoclavicular* joints. *Inspection* of the shoulder reveals abnormalities in position and muscular development. In arthritis of the shoulder, visible *atrophy* of the deltoid, scapular or pectoral muscles may be observed. *Palpation* will often confirm the presence of moderate degrees of *muscle atrophy*, and *tenderness*, usually localized, may be elicited. *Swelling* is *rarely palpable* over the true shoulder joint. Swelling and tenderness, however, are readily noted over the sternoclavicular joints and acromioclavicular joints when present. *Motion* will quickly reveal limitations in range in *abduction* (raising to the side), *anterior elevation* (or flexion forward), *posterior elevation* (extension backward), *external rotation* (flex elbow, rotate arm laterally), *internal rotation* (place arm across back—"reach for the hip pocket"). *Pain on motion*, and particularly *location* and *position* of arm when pain is noted, or visible *muscle spasm* or involuntary contraction produced by sudden pain, should be noted. *Crepitation* is commonly noted on shoulder motion. This may be felt over the scapulohumeral joint, over the sternoclavicular joint, or over the angle of the scapula (fibrous crepitation). *Abduction*, and *internal* and *external rotation* are usually all painful and limited with inflammation of the true shoulder (scapulohumeral joint), or closely adjacent structures (as in periarthritis, subdeltoid bursitis, or supraspinatus tendinitis). (For further details, see Chapter 80 on The Painful Shoulder.)

Examination of the Temporomandibular Joints

Involvement of the articulation of the jaw is rather uncommon in rheumatoid arthritis. Attention has been focused on the problems related to this area and an excellent textbook has appeared concerned solely with the temporomandibular joint.[4] One main point made in this book is that a tight masseter muscle is frequently found associated with the painful joint and that local anesthesia to the area of the muscle may provide satisfactory relief. The incidence of organic disease in patients with symptoms referable to this joint is small. Particularly, a plea is made to dentists and physicians to hesitate before undertaking major dental work *to correct malocclusion* as this is frequently the seat of the trouble.

Examination of the Cervical Spine

Abnormal attitudes are easily detected by observation. *Torticollis* may be congenital or may result from spasm (guarding contraction) of neck muscles, pulling the neck to one side. In abnormalities of the lower spine, the cervical curve, normally lordotic, may become exaggerated or may be lost. *Scoliosis* and *kyphosis* of the neck may result from disorders of the spine. *Palpation* will reveal local areas of *tenderness*, and perhaps *crepitation* on rotation when osteoarthritic changes are present. *Spasm* may be palpable, particularly over the trapezius muscle, or the scalenus anticus. *Arthritic changes in the cervical spine* frequently account for *pain in the shoulder and arm* (brachial neuralgia). *Motion* of the cervical spine should be observed in forward *flexion*, backward *extension*, *rotation* to left and right, and *deviation* to left and right. (A convenient examining routine is to direct the patient to move "chin to chest, chin to left and right shoulder, ear to left and right shoulder, and head back".) Measurements of degrees of motion are difficult, but painful motions should be noted, and estimations may be made of per cent of normal motion possible (see also Chapter 37).

Examination of the Spine

The details of this somewhat complicated examination are given in the chapters on Spondylitis and on Backache. A few general pointers will be given here.

1. With the patient standing, note *posture*—viewed laterally. In the dorsal (thoracic) spine, increased forward curve, or *kyphosis*, or decreased curve, or flattening may be noted. In the lumbar area, increased forward curvature, or *lordosis*, may be noted, or *flattening*, with the pelvis rotated forward and upward.

2. With the patient standing, and viewing from behind, note presence of

scoliosis, or deviation from a straight line. *Tilting of the pelvis*, from short leg or flexion deformity of a knee or hip, will produce a lateral curvature of the spine to compensate for the imbalance. The paravertebral muscles (erector spinae) on the shortened side will appear more prominent. *Sharp angulation* may be noted from structural abnormality of the vertebrae. Measure *leg length* from anterior superior iliac spine to internal malleolus.

3. *Motion* of the spine should be tested by having patient bend (*flexion*) with knees straight, noting the *curve* of the back in flexion (see chapter on Spondylitis), and whether sections of the back are held rigid. Tenderness along the spine may be palpated for in this position. *Hyperextension* of the spine is usually the first function limited by disease.

Lateral deviation (bending to left and right) is principally a motion of the *lumbar vertebrae* when the patient *stands*. When *sitting*, the *dorsal*, or thoracic, vertebral joints are called into play. (Have patient sit on table, shoulders hunched forward, and elbows bent. Direct patient to touch point of elbow to table beside him without raising opposite buttock from table.) *Rotation* of the spine should be tested both sitting and lying supine. In sitting, the patient is directed to turn to left and right (pelvis fixed), and limited motion or spasm thus elicited is noted. In lying supine the patient is directed to keep shoulders flat on table, while pelvis is rotated to left and right (flex right hip and knee to rotate pelvis to left, and vice versa). *Limited motion*, *muscle atrophy*, or *spasm* are all important signs.

4. With patient supine, test *straight leg raising* (flexion of hip with knee extended) (Lasegue's test).

5. *Measure chest expansion.*—This is a composite motion of the costovertebral joints. (For other important tests for spinal disorders, see Chapter 82.)

Examination of the Hips

With the patient lying supine the legs normally lie flat with slight rotation of the pelvis producing some lumbar lordosis. If the hips are slightly flexed, the lordosis flattens out. *Patrick's sign* for hip function is the "heel to knee test." The hip and knee are flexed so that the heel lies beside the opposite knee, then the hip is externally rotated as if to place the lateral surface of the bent knee on the table. This movement combines *flexion*, *abduction*, and *external rotation*. *Pain*, *limitation*, and *spasm* of the *adductor muscles* indicate a hip disorder. In hip disease, hyperextension is nearly always the first movement limited or lost completely. Ankylosis of the hip occurs in various degrees of flexion, usually with adduction and perhaps internal rotation. *Spasm* or *atrophy* of the gluteal muscles is common with hip disease.

Examination of the Knee

With the patient standing, observe for *knock-knee* (genu valgum), or *bow-leg* (genu varum), and for *contracture*. With the patient lying supine, look for *atrophy* of the quadriceps muscles, and observe contour of the knees. *Swelling* is usually easily detected by loss of visible bony landmarks, and lateral bulging of the capsule above and below the patella. *Palpation* reveals the nature of swelling, which may be localized over the patella in prepatellar bursitis, below the patella in hypertrophy of the infrapatellar fat pad, or above the patella (under the quadriceps in the suprapatellar pouch) in villous degeneration of the synovium. In synovial cysts at the knee, the usual site of the swelling is into the popliteal space. *Palpable spurs* or *lipping* of the articular margins are common in degenerative joint disease. In rheumatoid involvement *synovial thickening* and *effusion* are commonly found in both of the knees. The presence of *effusion* may be demonstrated by feeling *fluctuation*, or by *ballotting* the patella against the femur (*floating patella*). In lesser degrees of effusion, the suprapatellar pouch should be compressed with one hand to press fluid into the knee joint proper, then the patella is tapped against the femur to reproduce this sign.

Another useful method for detection of minor degrees of knee effusion is as follows: With the leg fully extended and relaxed, all fluid is milked from the medial portion of the knee joint by stroking. The lateral aspect of the knee is then stroked, and *a bulge* will immediately appear medial to the patella if even small amounts of effusion are present. *Thickening* of the synovium is recognized by doughy enlargement confined to the bursae of the knee joint, or by loss of ability to palpate the bony landmarks—femoral condylar outline, or margin of tibia beside the patella. *Tenderness* should be investigated for severity and location. This may be confined to the region of one inflamed *bursa*, may be at the point of *attachment* of the *medial* or *lateral collateral ligaments* to the tibia, about the patellar ligament, or at the tibial tuberosity. (In degenerative changes of the knee secondary to knock-knee and flat feet, the usual point of tenderness is at the attachment of the internal collateral ligament of the tibia. In meniscus injury the point of tenderness is just below the medial femoral condyle.)

Testing for *instability* is important (ligamentous tears—chronic sprains). To check the *external collateral ligament* one of the examiner's hands is placed on the inside of the patient's knee, to make countertraction to the other hand of the examiner, which pulls the extended lower leg toward the midline. For testing the *internal collateral ligament*, one hand is braced against the lateral surface of the knee, while the other pulls the lower leg away from the midline. *Cruciate ligament relaxation* is demonstrable by grasping the leg just below the knee (flexed to 90°), and pulling forward and pushing back ("rocking" the knee). The unstable knee joint permits increased lateral mobility and abnormal slipping of the tibia on the femur. Both knees should be compared.

Crepitation on motion is common in the knee. Coarse crepitation is felt in knees following trauma, with degenerative changes, and with subpatellar chondromalacia. Finer rubbing crepitus is felt in the rheumatoid arthritic knee. *Muscle spasm* is usually most marked in the hamstring muscles, *atrophy* is first noticed in the quadriceps. *Contractures* and *ankylosis* usually occur in a position of partial flexion. (See also Chapter 77.)

Examination of the Ankle

At this location *periarticular swelling* (edema) from causes other than joint disease is common. Painless, pitting edema of the lower legs and about the ankle is often from old phlebitis, or varicosities if unilateral, or from nutritional, cardiac, or renal deficiency if bilateral. *Swelling* from arthritis of the ankle joint is *tender*, or, in low-grade chronic swelling, is usually limited to the reflections of the synovium of the ankle (particularly below the malleoli). *Effusion* may be demonstrable as fluctuation below the malleoli. *Crepitation* may be noted on motion. *Motion* of the *ankle proper* is possible as *dorsiflexion* and *plantar flexion*. Motion of the *sub-astragalar joint* is possible as *inversion* and *eversion* (lateral deviation) of the foot. *Pronation* of the foot on standing may be the result of weakened and stretched ligaments about the sub-astragalar joint.

Examination of the Foot

This is described fully in the chapter on Painful Feet. A few points will be set forth here.

1. With the patient standing, note shape of the foot. *Pronation*, with flattened long arch, is common (*pes planus*). *Splay foot*—spreading and flattening of the metatarsal arch—is also common. Note presence of *hallux valgus* (bunion deformity of great toe), *hammer toes* (hyperextension contracture), corns or calluses.

2. *Color* of skin should be noted, and *arterial* (dorsalis pedis and posterior tibial) *pulsations* palpated.

3. *Swelling* and *tenderness* should be investigated for severity and location (*e. g.*, over the heel in inflammation of tendo achilles, under heel at attachment of plantar fascia, under heads of meta-

tarsals, over dorsum of foot, or in toe joints). The metatarsophalangeal (MTP) joints are commonly involved in rheumatoid arthritis, and are also tender in weak feet and other conditions. *Skin lesions* about the feet and toes should be noted—the presence of dermatophytosis, keratosis, psoriatic nail changes, and ulcers may give diagnostic hints. *Excessive sweating* usually accompanies the swelling of the feet from active rheumatoid arthritis.

4. *Movements* of the feet, particularly for joint mobility can be checked first with the patient standing. *Raising* on the metatarsal heads or "standing on the toes" should be attempted, standing on the heels, and grasping, or flexion of the toes, will often quickly reveal limitations. *Manipulation* of the tarsometatarsal, and metatarsophalangeal joints will elicit tenderness if tenosynovitis or arthritis is present. (See also Chapter 78 on Painful Feet.)

In most patients with joint complaints, the history and a quick survey will reveal which joints are involved, so that attention can be focused at these points. If the examiner quickly observes and palpates the joints while he and the patient carry them through normal range of motion, he can spot which joints are abnormal, and examine them in detail after checking all the others.

IBM CARDS FOR RECORDS

During a thorough examination of the patient a great amount of data is recorded. It is necessary on subsequent visits, for determination of changes in the arthritis, to refer to this record (see Chapter 26). A convenient chart-finding system has been devised by the author and found through experience to be helpful. Separate code sheets are available for ankylosing spondylitis, rheumatoid arthritis and gout.[3] The data, in turn, are taken from the code sheets and put on an appropriate IBM punch card, which includes the patient's code number and name. Tabulation of data is simple, by putting the IBM punch cards in a sorting machine. In this way, in those patients with unusual findings, diagnoses or other data, the chart can be easily located. In the future, it is anticipated that many clinics will use this method. From such combined efforts, a large amount of statistical data will be available for teaching and research purposes.*

* We regret that space does not permit reproduction of the code sheets and punch cards here. —Ed.

BIBLIOGRAPHY

1. Beetham, W. P., Polley, H. F., Slocumb, C. H. and Weaver, W. F.: *Physical Examination of Joints*, Philadelphia, W. B. Saunders Company, 1965.
2. Committee on Medical Rating of Physical Impairment: A Guide to the Evaluation of Permanent Impairment of the Extremities and Back. J.A.M.A., Special Edition, Feb. 15, 1958.
3. Lockie, L. M.: President's Address—American Rheumatism Association, Mass Tabulation of Data on Arthritic Patients; June 1958 (San Francisco).
4. Schwartz, L.: *Disorders of the Temporomandibular Joint*, Philadelphia, W. B. Saunders Company, 1959.

Chapter 3

Organization of An Arthritis Center

By Metro A. Ogryzlo, M.D.

The recent trend in the United Kingdom and other countries of Europe has been toward the development of centers specifically designed to deal with the problems of arthritis. Such centers usually include facilities for outpatient care, research laboratories and facilities for inpatient treatment as well. Usually located in relation to centers of higher learning, they foster a close collaboration between various clinical and basic science disciplines, providing total patient care, rehabilitation, education and research. This trend is now apparent in Canada and there are indications that it is beginning to take hold in the United States. Perhaps the biggest obstacle to its acceptance in a society which favors a voluntary health system is the enormous cost of hospitalization.

The concept of developing special centers for the rheumatic diseases is not a new one; rheumatic patients still flock to the various spas of Europe as they have for centuries. However, until the early part of this century, there was no attempt to develop special centers in the modern sense. The earliest development along this line was the founding of the Landesbad Hospital in Aachen, Germany, in 1912, as a special hospital for rheumatic diseases. The modern concept of the rheumatic disease center probably had its origin in the United Kingdom in 1928, in the report of J. Allison Glover.[4] The arthritis center, he stated, should be part of an existing, fully equipped general hospital preferably affiliated with a School of Medicine, thus enabling it to fulfill the purpose of research and education as well as treatment. From 1935 to 1938 a British Committee on Chronic Rheumatic Diseases appointed by the Royal College of Physicians published a series of reports on the rheumatic diseases. In the fourth volume was a report entitled, "Can the Voluntary Hospital Solve the Problem of Rheumatic Disease?"[1] Recognizing the importance of economic considerations, the authors believed they could not, as the title implied.

While this sort of planning was going on in Britain, a voluntary women's organization financed a rheumatic disease hospital in Oslo, Norway, in 1938. It is an interesting commentary on the time to note that the gift of this hospital was initially rejected by the local university. Similarly in the United States, the Robert Breck Brigham Hospital was established in Boston, as an institution devoted solely to the rheumatic diseases. The concept of Rheumatic Disease Centers or Rheumatic Disease Units has also received high priority in Canada during recent years.[7] Since 1960, ten such units have been established in major teaching hospitals across Canada, actively supported by the Canadian Arthritis and Rheumatism Society.

THE ARTHRITIS CENTER

A rheumatic disease unit may be defined as a segregated group of beds reserved for the rheumatic diseases in a well-equipped general hospital affiliated with a School of Medicine. These should be supplemented by an active outpatient clinic and, if possible, with research facilities. Several aspects of this arrangement are of particular importance to the arthritic:

1. The segregation of patients enables a more efficient delivery of health care for a group of diseases that differ materially from illnesses affecting systems other than the musculoskeletal.

2. The unit concept ensures that patients with rheumatic diseases are not in competition for beds with patients with acute illnesses.

3. The general hospital setting provides the necessary facilities and disciplines for a thorough investigation of these diseases and the efficient treatment of complications.

4. The university affiliation provides for participation in a variety of research endeavors, designed to improve the understanding and management of rheumatic diseases.

5. Coupled with an outpatient arthritis clinic, it provides for continuity of treatment and greater efficiency of follow-up, in collaboration with the patient's own physician.

Such a unit has a special role in the delivery of medical care. Most important is that it provides a team approach to the management of these diseases. It permits close collaboration between rheumatologist, orthopedist, physiatrist, psychiatrist, medical social worker and other paramedical personnel. The development of new techniques and approaches to treatment are facilitated, and follow-up and assessment of the results of treatment are made easier. Improved recording and documentation procedures permit a more accurate definition of the natural history and prognosis of these diseases. Greater opportunity is provided for the education of the patient into the nature of the illness, its potential complications and the preventive measures that may be taken. The ready access to a large group of patients with specific types of rheumatic disease assures the laboratory and the clinical investigator a rich source of patient material. Finally, it provides an excellent opportunity for leadership in professional training and education. The objectives of such a unit should be:

1. to set the highest standards of medical care for patients requiring treatment.

2. to provide opportunity for observation and a clearer definition of the natural history of the rheumatic diseases.

3. to provide the facilities and resources for original clinical investigation and basic research.

4. to enhance undergraduate and graduate instruction in medicine, physical and occupational therapy, public health and social work.

The development of a rheumatic disease center requires the collaboration of government, universities, local hospital boards, voluntary agencies and the medical profession. The community environment is of considerable importance, especially the attitude towards the rheumatic diseases within the institution and in the community itself. In some areas resistance to the development of such centers may be anticipated, due to prejudices within the profession against the provision of special facilities for a select few. But the specialized unit concept is now accepted in other special fields, e.g., coronary care unit, respiratory disease unit and renal dialysis units.

INPATIENT FACILITIES

The rheumatic diseases, in common with other diseases that tend to run a chronic course, confront the physician with problems in management that differ markedly from the more definitive treatment directed toward acute illnesses. This is particularly true of rheumatoid arthritis and related disorders, which result in structural damage to joints, lifelong disability and serious socioeconomic difficulties. The treatment of these patients requires special skills relating to medical care, nursing, counselling and rehabilitation, not usually available in the setting of a general medical service. In fact, the traditional organization of medical services hinders the team approach to treatment. It accentuates difficulties in communication between the medical, surgical, nursing, physiotherapy and social service members of the therapeutic team, particularly when these members are often pre-occupied with the problems of the patients with life-threatening diseases. The random distribution of arthritis patients throughout the medical wards of hospitals tends to complicate rather than facilitate the administration of a coordinated rheumatic disease program.

It is abundantly clear that a radical revision in our concept of treatment for the rheumatic diseases is required. Experience has shown that the needs of these patients can best be met in a segregated setting within the broader framework of general medicine, making possible the provision of the special skills that are needed, and to provide these more economically, both in terms of professional time expended as well as of cost. Many of the less complicated cases should continue to be treated within the setting of standard general medical services. The need for designated beds for the treatment of arthritis within a community is approxiately 5 beds per 100,000 population.

Such a unit should be considered for the major teaching institutions and for some of the larger, non-teaching hospitals. The inpatient facilities may consist of:

1. 10 to 40 segregated beds, located within a single location, in close relation to other medical services of the hospital. Any combination of one, two or four-bed rooms will suffice. While larger wards may be equally satisfactory, modern hospital construction tends to favor a greater degree of privacy. The use of standard four-bed rooms, along with semi-private and private accommodation within the same unit, has certain advantages. It ensures that private patients receive the same high standards of investigation and treatment as standard ward patients and also provides for a richer source of teaching material in institutions where private cases are used for teaching purposes.

2. the segregated unit might differ from the general medical wards in certain respects. Bathrooms should be larger to accommodate a wheelchair, toilets may be installed at a higher level or designed to permit use with a wheelchair, and showers instead of bath tubs.

3. a treatment room in the unit for group physiotherapy and occupational therapy classes such as activities of daily living.

4. a room for the physical and occupational therapists, as a base from which to operate within the unit and where equipment may be stored.

5. an intercom system with speakers at the bedside to facilitate group exercises in bed, especially where the patients are located in individual rooms. In this way a therapist or a taped program calls out the exercises and instructions, and other therapists move from patient to patient to provide individual supervision.

6. a room for one or two social workers attached specifically to the unit.

7. a number of examining or treatment rooms as well as offices for resident house staff and fellows in training.

8. a seminar room with facilities for teaching.

The resident staff rotating through the unit can thus obtain a more complete and intensive experience in the rheumatic diseases than was previously possible. They become better oriented to the problems and tend to develop an interdisciplinary approach to the management of these diseases. The patients obtain a more thorough diagnostic investigation, including a social history and an assessment by a physiotherapist. This system facilitates early, accurate diagnosis and prompt application of proper therapy. Patients improve more rapidly when they follow a scheduled daily routine and learn a good deal from their association with other patients with similar diseases. The patient becomes a part of the team.

OUTPATIENT FACILITIES

A well organized outpatient clinic specifically designed for consultation, examination, investigation and treatment of ambulatory patients, and for patient recall and long term follow-up, is a necessary adjunct to any rheumatic disease center. In hospitals without a segregated inpatient service, it is the focal point around which most patient care, clinical investigation and teaching will be centered. A detailed guide to clinic organization is to be found in the *Manual for Arthritis Clinics*, issued by the Arthritis Foundation.[5]

Certain basic requirements must be met for efficient operation:

1. a number of private consultation or examining rooms.
2. specialized laboratory and x-ray facilities providing for a thorough investigation of problems relating to rheumatic diseases.
3. adequate facilities for physical medicine, occupational therapy and rehabilitation.
4. access to consultation with other special outpatient clinics as well as general medicine.
5. an appointment system similar to that used in private practice.
6. a unit record system, which may be incorporated into the inpatient hospital record.
7. social services for patients requiring this form of assistance.
8. provision, where possible, of transportation for indigent or more severely disabled patients.

In a rheumatic disease center the outpatient clinic complements and enhances the work of the inpatient service by providing continuity of treatment. Many of the administrative difficulties previously encountered in managing an outpatient rheumatic disease program are automatically eliminated.[3]

RESEARCH FACILITIES

It is well recognized that the standards and quality of treatment as well as the effectiveness of a training program, are enhanced when these are closely integrated with an active research program.[6] This does not imply that extensive research laboratory facilities with sophisticated basic equipment, computers and highly trained personnel are necessarily required, although these can provide obvious advantages. An individual with an enquiring mind and a willingness to pursue a problem to a stated objective is sufficient to start a research program. Even a modest outpatient clinic, combined with well kept records, can contribute valuable information on the natural history of disease, evaluation, diagnostic and treatment methods and on health care delivery. While the success of any research program depends on many factors, the foremost is the scientific curiosity and imagination of the investigators.

STAFF OF THE UNIT

In North America, rheumatology has traditionally functioned as a division within internal medicine. For this reason, the overall management of rheumatic diseases has been considered the responsibility of the internist.

There is a growing feeling that the increasing complexity and broad scope of rheumatology now demands that it be formally recognized as a specialty. Advances in this special field require that those who devote themselves to rheumatology be exposed to intensive training and experience designed to develop a high degree of skill, leaving less time for undertaking additional responsibilities within the broader field of general medicine.[2] At the moment there is no adequate mechanism or standard by which it may be determined whether a physician is proficient in rheumatology (*see also* Chapter 1, p. 13). The care of patients in this area of medicine varies greatly in different parts of the world. These deficiencies make it apparent that there is a need for a better definition of minimum training requirements and qualifications.

Since it is presumed that the comprehensive rheumatic disease centers will plan to include training programs, it follows that the staff members must be of high caliber, particularly if the center is to be accredited for training by the higher examining bodies.

Medical Staff

The *chief* of the arthritis unit should be a physician of stature. The special interests of the chief will determine the particular direction along which the center will develop, both from the clinical as well as the research point of view. He must be an intimate part of the medical staff of the institution, the medical school with which it is affiliated and the national rheumatism association, to provide leadership in relation to patient care, teaching at all levels and clinical investigation. He must be familiar with community services as they relate to treatment and rehabilitation, as well as work closely with local chapters in the field of arthritis and with other voluntary health agencies.

The staff of the unit or center may include one or more *associate rheumatologists*. In general, they should hold qualifications similar to the chief and have similar objectives. Wherever possible, all members should also participate actively in the research program of the unit. There should be a close working arrangement with general *internal medicine* and other specialties, including *orthopedics*, in order to provide free access for consultation and management of various complications. There must be a close working arrangement with the department of *physical medicine and rehabilitation*. It is desirable therefore, that a *physiatrist* be attached to the unit. It is also necessary to have the services of a *psychiatrist*, preferably one with an interest in arthritis. The rheumatic disease unit ideally should have a *resident house physician*, committed to a career in rheumatology. Together with *assistant residents* who may rotate through the unit, he should be responsible for the day to day care of patients, under the supervision of the medical staff. *Fellows in training* can also take part in the activities of the unit, and have much to contribute through their participation in clinical investigation and research projects. Finally the facilities of the unit must be available for teaching, in respect to *clinical clerks* and *undergraduate students*, to ensure that they receive an adequate exposure to the rheumatic diseases.

Paramedical Staff

An adequate staff of *physiotherapists* and *occupational therapists* is the most urgent requirement. Since they are fundamental to the rehabilitation of these patients, an arthritis unit requires a higher ratio of therapists, approximately one for every six to eight patients, compared to the ratio of one for every thirty to fifty patients usually found in general hospitals. There is much to be gained from having the physiotherapists and occupational therapists perform as much of their function as possible on the wards of the unit, reserving the facilities of their department for more cumbersome procedures. A *rehabilitation officer*, experienced in industry, is an additional asset. The *medical social worker* is an important member of the team, preferably stationed in close proximity to the patient area. Depending on the size of the unit, the work load of the social worker can be expected to be heavier than in other departments of the hospital, with the possible exception of psychiatry. The *unit nurse* is an important member of the team. In many instances they may also serve the role of patient recall for follow-up as well as case work. While not essential, the services of a *podiatrist* and *clinical psychologist* can also be helpful. A *unit secretary* is essential to the efficient operation of the unit. *Volunteer workers*, such as members of women's auxiliaries, can relieve the staff of many routine tasks.

In conclusion, the progressive medical center will develop a comprehensive arthritis unit. It can be predicted with confidence that the centers that succeed in this venture will set the standards of excellence in patient care, and will become the leaders in clinical research and in education in the rheumatic diseases.

BIBLIOGRAPHY

1. Davidson, L. S. T. and Duthie, J. J. R.: in *Reports on Chronic Rheumatic Diseases*, London, H. K. Lewis & Co., Volume 4, 1938, p. 1.
2. Duthie, J. J. R.: Scottish Med. J., *15*, 165, 1970.
3. Engleman, E. P., Sellinger, E. and Mettier, S. R.: Arth. & Rheum., *6*, 78, 1963.
4. Glover, J. A.: *Reports on Public Health and Medical Subjects*, *#52*, London, Ministry of Health, 1928.
5. Manual for Arthritis Clinics—prepared by a Subcommittee of the A.R.A.: New York, The Arthritis Foundation 1964.
6. Means, J. H.: *Ward 4, The Mallinckrodt Research Ward of the Massachusetts General Hospital*, Cambridge, Harvard University Press, 1958.
7. Ogryzlo, M. A., Gordon, D. A. and Smythe, H. A.: Arth. & Rheum., *10*, 479, 1967.

Chapter 4

The Structure and Function of Joints

By Ernest Gardner, M.D.

In anatomical usage, a joint has been described as "the connexion subsisting in the skeleton between any of its rigid component parts, whether bones or cartilages."[11] Joints may be classified on the basis of their most characteristic structural features into three main types: fibrous, cartilaginous, and synovial. The present account deals mainly with synovial joints.

FIBROUS JOINTS

The bones of a fibrous joint (sometimes called a *synarthrosis*) are united by fibrous tissue. There are two types of fibrous joints, *sutures* and *syndesmoses*. The joint between a tooth and the bone of its socket is termed a *gomphosis* and is sometimes classed as a third type of fibrous joint. Little if any movement occurs at fibrous joints.

CARTILAGINOUS JOINTS

The bones of a cartilaginous joint are united either by hyaline cartilage or by fibrocartilage.

Hyaline Cartilage Joints

In this type of joint, which is sometimes called a *synchondrosis*, and sometimes a primary cartilaginous joint, the bones are temporarily united by hyaline cartilage. This cartilage is a persistent part of the embryonic cartilaginous skeleton, and it serves as a growth zone for one or both of the bones that it joins. Most hyaline cartilage joints are obliterated; that is, the cartilage is replaced by bone when growth ceases. Examples of hyaline cartilage joints include epiphysial plates, and the spheno-occipital and neurocentral synchondroses.

Fibrocartilaginous Joints

In this type of joint, which is sometimes called a secondary cartilaginous joint and sometimes an *amphiarthrosis*, and to which the term *symphysis* has also been applied, the skeletal elements are united by fibrocartilage during the later phases of their existence, and the fibrocartilage is usually separated from the bones by thin plates of hyaline cartilage. Fibrocartilaginous joints include the pubic symphysis and the intervertebral discs between the bodies of the vertebrae.

Intervertebral discs.—In a young adult man a disc consists of the *anulus fibrosus*, the *nucleus pulposus*, and two *hyaline cartilage* plates.[2] The anulus fibrosus consists of a series of lamellae of collagenous bundles, which are arranged spirally. The bundles in adjacent lamellae lie at right angles with respect to each other. Above and below, the fibers of the anulus are anchored to the ring epiphysis and to the margins of the hyaline plates. The outermost fibers of the anulus blend with the longitudinal ligaments of the vertebral column; fibrocartilage is present in the innermost lamellae. The nucleus pulposus, which occupies the center of the disc, is white, glistening, and semigelatinous. It contains fine bundles of collagenous fibers, connective tissue cells, cartilage cells, and much amorphous, intercellular material. The nucleus is highly plastic, and it is held in shape by the cartilage plates and by the anulus fibrosus. The hyaline cartilage plates are thin and cover the upper and lower aspects of the vertebral bodies. In growing bone, they form the 2 zones from which the vertebral body grows in height.

The intervertebral discs have few, if any, blood vessels or nerve fibers. Vasomotor and sensory (mostly pain) fibers supply the longitudinal ligaments of the vertebral column[65] and a few of these fibers may enter the peripheral part of the anulus.

At birth, the nucleus pulposus is mucoid. It contains notochordal cells and fine strands of fibrous tissue and fibrocartilage. The fibrous elements, which are probably derived from the anulus, proliferate and replace the notochordal tissue. The process of replacement continues throughout life. With advancing age, the entire disc tends to become fibrocartilaginous, and the structural differences between the anulus and the nucleus are often lost.[64,74]

The intervertebral discs have a high water content, which is maximal at birth and decreases with advancing age. Diurnal changes in water content probably account for the diurnal variation in stature (1 to 2 cm.); the stature decreases during the day. The decrease in water content with age, together with other factors, results in a permanent thinning of the discs and a permanent decrease in stature. With advancing age also, the fibers become coarse and hyalinized. The disc is also subject to pathological changes, which consist of degenerative changes in the anulus and nucleus pulposus, changes that in some respects seem to be exaggerations of those that normally occur with advancing age.

Each component of the intervertebral disc subserves several functions. The nucleus pulposus is a shock-absorbing mechanism; it equalizes stresses, it is important in fluid exchange, and it serves as the axis of movement between adjacent vertebrae. The anulus fibrosus binds the vertebral bodies together and provides stability; it permits motion between vertebral bodies (because of the spiral arrangement of its fibers); it acts as a check ligament; it retains the nucleus pulposus, and it is a shock-absorbing mechanism. The hyaline cartilage plates, in addition to serving as growth zones for the bodies of vertebrae, permit the diffusion of fluid between the discs and capillaries in the vertebrae. (For further details on spinal anatomy, see Chapters 74 and 77.)

The pubic symphysis is a fibrocartilaginous joint characterized by a thick mass of fibrocartilage, the interpubic disc. A sagittal cleft is often present in this disc after childhood, but it has no synovial lining. In many mammals, probably including human beings also, a relaxation of the ligaments and a loosening of the interpubic disc may occur during pregnancy. These changes result from the influence of the hormone relaxin and, by allowing for the enlargement of the pelvis, facilitate the passage of the fetus.

SYNOVIAL JOINTS

The term *synovia* was introduced in the 16th century by Paracelsus for various body fluids. The use of the term synovia is now confined to the fluid present in certain joints, which are consequently termed synovial. Similar fluid is present in bursae and synovial tendon sheaths.

Synovial joints, which are often termed *diarthrodial* joints, possess a cavity and are specialized to permit more or less free movement. They have the following chief characteristics, which have been dealt with in detail in monographs and reviews.[7,25,27,28,35,36]

The articular surfaces of the bones are covered with cartilage, which is usually hyaline in type. The bones are united by a *joint capsule* and by ligaments. The inner surface of the capsule is lined by a vascular connective tissue, the *synovial membrane*, sometimes called synovial tissue, which produces the synovial fluid that fills the joint cavity and lubricates the joint. The remainder of the capsule consists of a *fibrous layer* (the term joint capsule is often used to refer specifically to the fibrous layer). The joint cavity is sometimes partially or completely subdivided by fibrous or fibrocartilaginous *discs* or *menisci*. These are not covered by synovial membrane except to a certain extent at their periphery. However, intra-articular ligaments or tendons are usually lined by synovial membrane.

As mentioned above, synovial joints are specialized to permit more or less free movement. The effects of friction are minimized by the lubrication mechanisms of these joints. Effective lubrication depends upon many factors, including the nature and geometry of the articulating surfaces and of synovial membrane, the physical and chemical properties of the lubricating fluid (synovial fluid), the load on a joint, and the rate and degree of movement.

Synovial joints, by virtue of proprioceptive nerve endings in their capsules and ligaments, are key components of the kinesthetic sense.

Types of Synovial Joints.—Synovial joints may be classified as *simple* or *compound*, according to the number of articulating surfaces. A finger joint (one pair of surfaces) is a simple joint, the elbow a compound one.

Synovial joints may also be classified according to whether they have but one axis of movement (and, therefore, movement in but one plane), two axes (two degrees of freedom), or three axes (three degrees of freedom; all movements permitted).

More commonly, however, synovial joints are classified according to the shapes of the articular surfaces of the constituent bones. These shapes determine the types of movements and are partly responsible for determining the range of movement. The most common types are *plane*, *hinge*, and *condylar*. Less common are *ball-and-socket*, *ellipsoidal*, *pivot*, and *saddle* joints. These classifications indicate as simply as possible the shapes of the articular surfaces and the movements that can occur at the joints. They do not, however, take into account the complexity of joint mechanics and the fact that articular movements must be appreciated in terms of spherical as well as plane geometry.

The articular surfaces of a plane joint are usually slightly curved; they permit gliding or slipping in any direction, or the twisting of one bone in relation to the other. The term hinge joint is self-explanatory. In a condylar joint, the articular area of each bone consists of two distinct surfaces, each called a condyle. A condylar joint resembles a hinge joint in movement, but nevertheless permits several kinds of movements (for example, the knee joint). In a ball-and-socket joint, there are three degrees of freedom, and, therefore, all movements and combinations of movements are permitted. An ellipsoidal joint resembles a ball-and-socket joint, but the articulating surfaces are much longer in one direction than in the direction at right angles so that the circumference of the joint margin forms an ellipse (for example, the radiocarpal joint). In a pivot joint, the single axis is vertical, and one bone pivots within a bony or an osseoligamentous ring. A saddle joint is shaped like a saddle and has two axes of movement.

Movements and Lubrication Mechanisms.—The movements that can occur or can be produced at joints may be classified as active, passive, and accessory.

There are three types of active movements. These are (1) gliding or slipping movements, (2) angular movements about a horizontal axis (flexion and extension) or about an anteroposterior axis (abduction and adduction), and (3) rotary movements about a longitudinal axis (medial and lateral rotation). Whether one, several, or all of the movements occur at a particular joint depends upon the shape and ligamentous arrangement of that joint. The range of movement at joints is limited by muscles, by ligaments and capsule, and by the shapes of the bones. Not so important is the opposition of soft parts, such as the meeting of the front of the arm and forearm during full flexion at the elbow.

Passive movements are produced by the examiner, when the subject is relaxed. For example, the examiner holds the subject's wrist so as to immobilize it. He can then flex, extend, adduct, and abduct the subject's hand at the wrist, movements that the subject can normally carry out actively. By careful manipulation, the examiner can also produce a slight degree of gliding and rotation at the wrist, movements that the subject cannot actively carry out himself. The gliding and rotation are examples of accessory movements, defined as movements for which the muscular arrangements are not suitable, but which can be brought about by manipulation.

The lubricating mechanisms of synovial joints are such that the effects of friction on articular cartilage are minimized. These mechanisms are extremely effective, so much so that the coefficient of friction during movement is less than that of ice sliding on ice. As mentioned above, a variety of factors are involved; the result is that they permit a replaceable fluid to protect a nearly irreplaceable bearing.

Joint lubrication has usually been considered to be an example of hydrodynamic lubrication (also termed fluid-film or "floating" lubrication). This type of lubrication requires incongruous bearing surfaces, a viscous lubricating fluid, and a relative speed of movement. Incongruity is present in synovial joints where the male component has a greater degree of curvature than the female; no two joint surfaces fit perfectly. Consequently, wedge-shaped spaces are said to exist. Synovial fluid circulates through the joint during movement. As this incompressible fluid flows through the narrower part of the wedge, its rate of circulation increases and its pressure rises. The intra-articular pressure becomes sufficient to keep the moving surfaces apart. Synovial fluid is non-Newtonian, that is, with increasing shear rates its viscosity decreases. This has been thought to facilitate circulation (aided by menisci, fat pads, and synovial folds). Conversely, the increased viscosity at lower speeds has been thought to reduce friction.

However, hydrodynamic mechanisms do not explain many features of lubrication. It is not suited to reciprocating motions (which characterize animal joints), especially with heavy loads, and it has been shown that under certain conditions the viscosity of the lubricant is unimportant compared with the nature of the sliding surfaces. Consequently, boundary lubrication has been proposed as a mechanism.[14,15,58] Here, the moving surfaces are separated by a layer of lubricant which is adherent to, or incorporated into, the surfaces. The layer is but a few molecules thick. Under such conditions, the coefficient of friction is independent of the velocity of movement. Boundary lubrication would seem to be well adapted for slowly moving, heavily loaded joints with reciprocating movements.

To the mechanisms cited above must be added further complexities, with particular consideration being given to microstructural and ultrastructural features of articular cartilage and synovial membrane. An important mechanism is "weeping" lubrication.[51,57] This term arises from the fact that synovial fluid, which is absorbed by articular cartilage, oozes from cartilage under pressure. It may be considered to be a special kind of hydrostatic lubrication, a condition in which fluid is pumped in under pressure to keep moving surfaces apart. The continuous film of fluid provided by weeping lubrication is considered to supplement both hydrodynamic lubrication and, under special conditions, boundary lubrication also.[6,53,54] Moreover, elastic deformation of the cartilage is yet another important factor.[19,20,54] In all of these mechanisms, the protein component of the hyaluronate protein of synovial fluid seems to be the chief lubricating factor in that fluid.[55,56] Finally, the microstructure of articular surfaces has to be taken

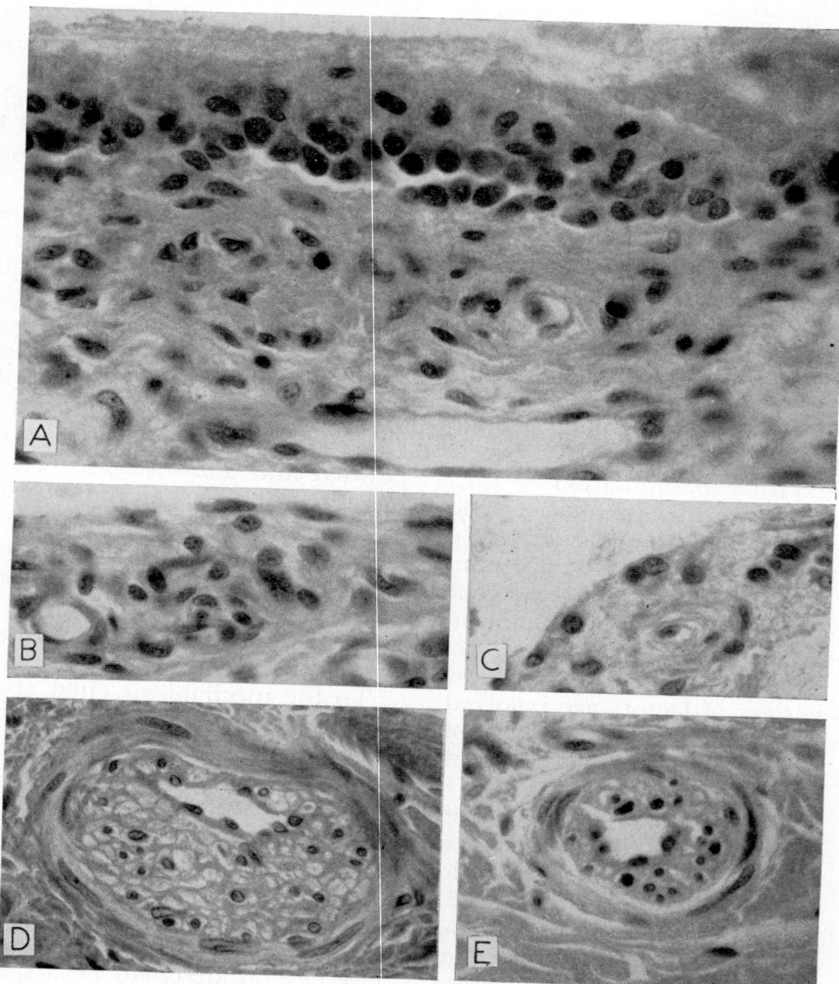

FIG. 4–1.—General features of human synovial membrane and joint capsule, as shown by light microscopy. Tissues are from an adult knee joint obtained following amputation for crushing injury of the leg; Bouin's fixative was injected into the knee joint. Section in A stained with hematoxylin and eosin; remaining sections with a modified Papanicolaou's stain. All sections 7 microns thick; magnification × 300. *A*, synovial membrane with cellular surface and precipitated synovial fluid. Cytoplasmic outlines of many cells can be distinguished. Note capillaries and venule in subsurface tissue. This section is from tissue lining the capsule at the side of the joint. *B* and *C*, sections from the same region as *A*, but showing fewer cells, arranged irregularly. *D* and *E*, arteriovenous anastomoses in the joint capsule, with a thick layer of longitudinal smooth muscle and a thin outer circular layer. From Gardner, Figures 1 and 2, Instructional Course Lectures, *9*, 162, 1952, J. W. Edwards, Publisher, Inc., with permission of the American Academy of Orthopaedic Surgeons.

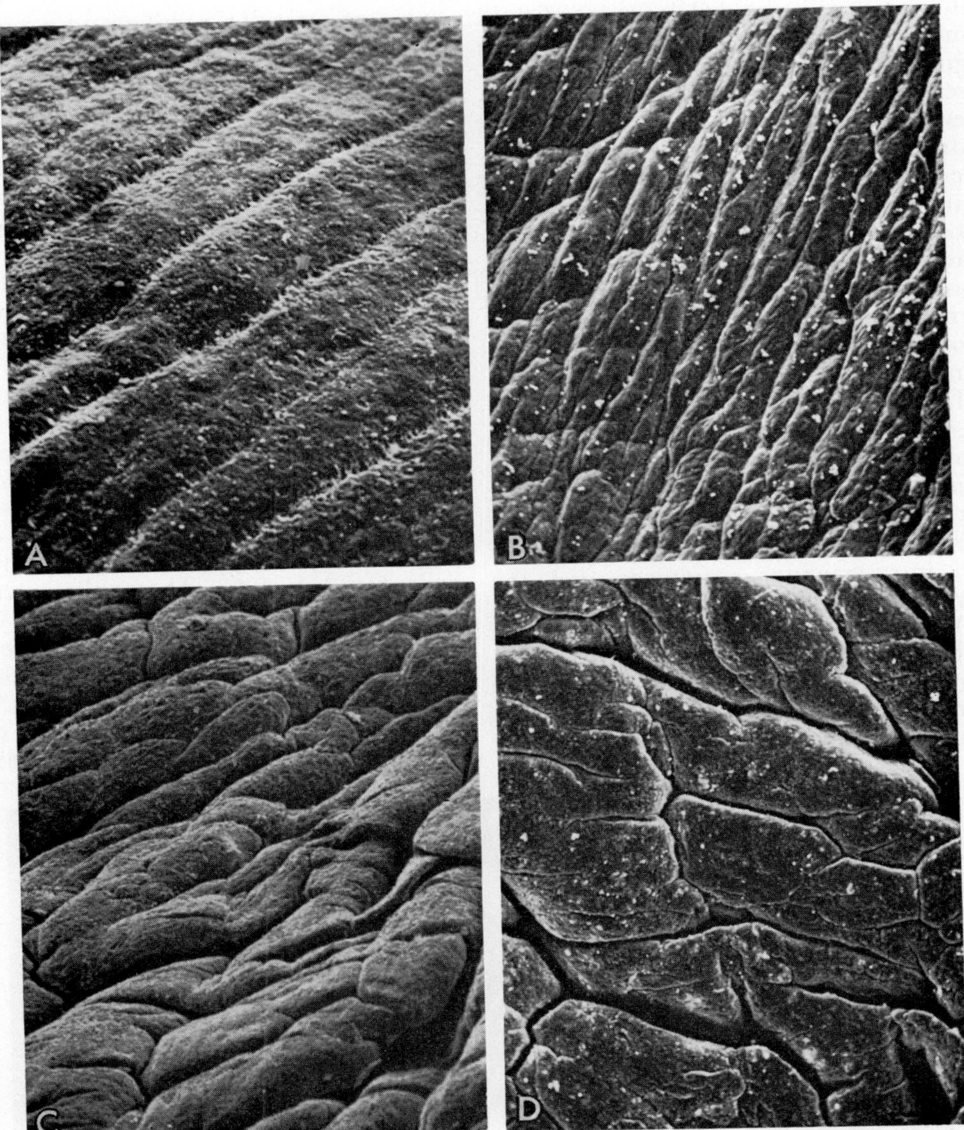

FIG. 4–2.—The surface topography of near-normal synovial membrane as viewed at low magnification with the scanning electron microscope. These specimens and those of Figures 4–3 and 4–4 were obtained after surgical procedures, such as above-the-knee amputation or meniscus repair, in which the joint showed no demonstrable significant pathological changes. *A*, the surface shows nearly parallel, shallow undulations. × 54. *B*, as in *A*, the surface shows many approximately parallel shallow folds. × 54. *C*, (× 41) and *D*, (× 54) both show somewhat larger but still roughly parallel, shallow folds. All four views suggest an arrangement designed to permit flexible adjustment and expansion, perhaps also related to lubrication mechanisms. These findings, as well as those illustrated in Figures 4–3 and 4–4, are by Dr. Jeanne M. Riddle, Department of Pathology, Wayne State University. Her work was supported by the Michigan Chapter of the Arthritis Foundation, and was carried out in the Bargman Laboratory for Cell and Molecular Research. The normal features of Figures 4–2 to 4–4 show significant changes in rheumatoid arthritis.

into account in the development of fluid films. Normal cartilage surfaces are significantly rougher than normal engineering bearings. Its minute surface elevations make possible the formation of entrapped pools of synovial fluid. In these pools, pressure causes the escape of water and other low molecular weight substances into the cartilage matrix,[56] leaving behind complex gels. These gel pools in turn contribute to a mechanism termed "boosted" lubrication,[72,73] which is of obvious importance in load-bearing joints such as the hip and knee.

It is clear, therefore, that lubrication in synovial joints includes special mechanisms related to load and special features of movement and depending upon boundary conditions, microstructural and ultrastructural features of joint surfaces and intra-articular structures, and the physicochemical nature of the lubricant.

Any moving mechanical system wears with time, and human joints are no exception. Some use-destruction (wear and tear) is inevitable during normal activity. The most common result is the wearing away of articular cartilage to a varying degree, sometimes to the extent of exposing, eroding, and polishing (eburnating) underlying bone.[5,59] Use-destruction may be hastened or exaggerated by many factors, of which the most important are trauma, disease, and structural and biochemical changes in articular cartilage.

Synovial Membrane and Synovial Fluid.—Synovial membrane, also called synovial tissue, is a vascular connective tissue which lines the inner surface of the capsule, but does not cover articular cartilage. It consists of formed elements such as cells and fibers, together with intercellular matrix or ground substance. Synovial membrane is characterized by its surface cells and by the capillary network immediately subjacent to the surface cells (Fig. 4–1, *A–C*). These cells resemble other connective tissue cells, at least with ordinary histological stains. However, even with light microscopy they exhibit certain distinguishing characteristics.[13,50] Forming a surface layer one to three cells deep, they resemble fibroblasts, but differ

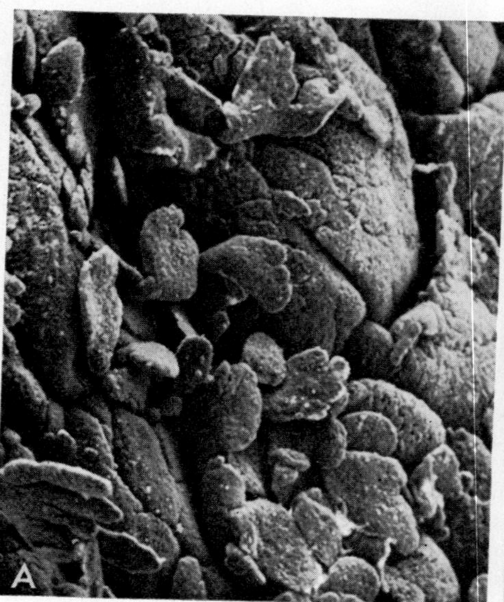

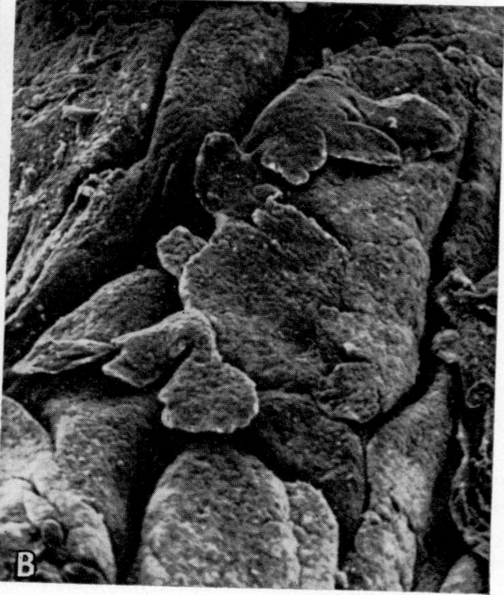

Fig. 4–3.—The surface morphology of synovial villi as viewed by scanning electron microscopy. Villi are found chiefly near the articular margins at the attachments of the capsule and synovial membrane. *A*, thin but stubby or finger-like villous projections. × 54. *B*, villous projections, characteristically short and flat, as in *A*. × 54. Courtesy of Dr. Jeanne M. Riddle (see Fig. 4–2).

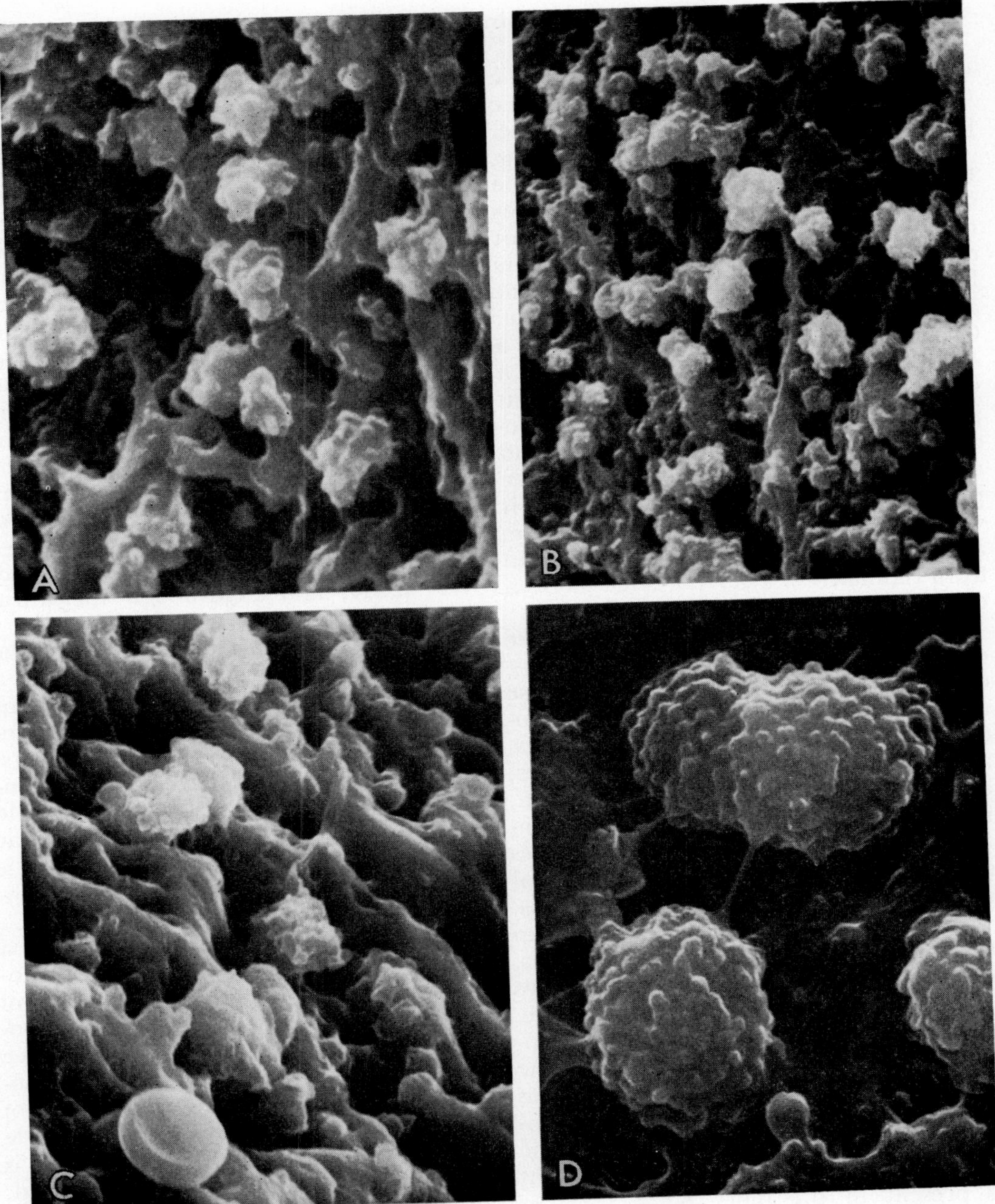

Fig. 4–4.—The surface of near-normal synovial membrane, as viewed by the scanning electron microscope at higher magnifications than in Figures 4–2 and 4–3. *A*, individual synoviocytes are clearly visualized. They are relatively uniform in size, exhibit an activated surface with knobby and fold-like processes, are evenly distributed, and are separated by wide expanses of matrix. × 2860. *B*, from another part of the same joint; similar findings. × 2860. *C*, similar findings from the synovial membrane of another joint. In addition, a red blood cell is visible at the lower left. Its characteristic shape and smooth surface are in striking contrast to the ruffled, activated surface of the adjacent synoviocytes. × 2290. *D*, the surface details of individual synoviocytes at higher magnification, and exhibiting a previously undiscovered association, namely, that some synoviocytes are connected by narrow, cytoplasmic spans which extend across the surrounding matrix. Courtesy of Dr. Jeanne M. Riddle (see Fig. 4–2) × 5720.

in their detailed structure and metabolic activities. They have long cytoplasmic processes which overlap and intertwine. They do not form a continuous lining, that is, some intercellular matrix may be directly adjacent to the joint cavity. This matrix is generally free of collagen, but does contain fine fibrils. Collagen fibers lie more deeply, and become prominent adjacent to and within the fibrous capsule. Grossly, the synovial membrane forms a relatively smooth surface from which a variable number of villi, folds, and fat pads project into the joint cavity, especially near the capsular attachment around the joint. The tissue deep to the surface may be fibrous, fatty, or areolar, and it varies in thickness. Synovial membrane, after surgical removal, may form again from remnants of synovial tissue or from cells in the underlying capsule.

Important microstructural details are revealed by scanning electron microscopy[67,76] (Figs. 4–2 to 4–4). These three-dimensional features, including undulations, folds, villi, surface openings, and special characteristics of synoviocytes, are of obvious importance in diffusion, mechanical properties, and lubrication mechanisms. Moreover, these features show significant changes in pathological conditions such as rheumatoid arthritis.

Ultrastructural studies[3,33,36,49] confirm the fact that the surface or lining cells, termed *synoviocytes*, form a discontinuous layer which lacks a basement membrane. The cell processes, which may interdigitate, project toward the surface. The amorphous intercellular matrix contains hyaluronic acid. It generally lacks collagen fibers but contains thin, non-periodic branching fibrils or filaments (collagen is present in the more basal parts of synovial tissue). Two distinct kinds of synoviocytes may be recognized (some authors discount the importance of this finding[46]). Type A cells are characterized by the presence of abundant processes, by a prominent Golgi apparatus, many smooth-walled vacuoles, mitochondria, intracellular fibrils (branched and aperiodic), and micropinocytic vesicles and by a relatively scanty endoplasmic reticulum. Type B cells have an abundant endoplasmic reticulum, but only occasional mitochondria, and scanty Golgi apparatus, vacuoles, and vesicles. The functional implications of these structural features are not yet clear. Type A cells have been implicated in phagocytic activity. Moreover, intermediate cell types are common, suggesting that Types A and B are different functional phases of one type of cell. What is clear, however, from the morphological and from biochemical and other studies, is that the synoviocytes are distinct cells serving specific functions, and are not to be considered simply as surface aggregates of fibroblasts or macrophages. Figure 4–5 illustrates fundamental features of synovial tissue, and Figure 4–6 the ultrastructure of Type A and Type B cells.

As mentioned previously, one of the characteristics of synovial tissue is a capillary network adjacent to the joint cavity.[18] The tissue also contains lymphatic vessels and a few nerve fibers. The immediately subjacent tissue contains fibroblasts, mast cells, and variable amounts of collagenous fibers, areolar tissue, and fat. The capillary network is directly related to the formation of synovial fluid.

Synovial fluid can be considered as a fluid ground substance. All ground substances contain complex compounds of high molecular weight, including mucopolysaccharides, of which at least five different kinds are known. Most contain sulfate and are found in a variety of tissues, including cartilage. The single mucopolysaccharide of synovial fluid is a sulfate-free compound, hyaluronic acid. It imparts to synovial fluid its characteristic stickiness and viscosity, being much like egg white in consistency. All mucopolysaccharides are complex, asymmetric, long-chain compounds which form viscous sols or even gels. They are attacked by a variety of enzymes usually called hyaluronidases. It is thought that basic units, perhaps disaccharides, are formed elsewhere and are brought to connective

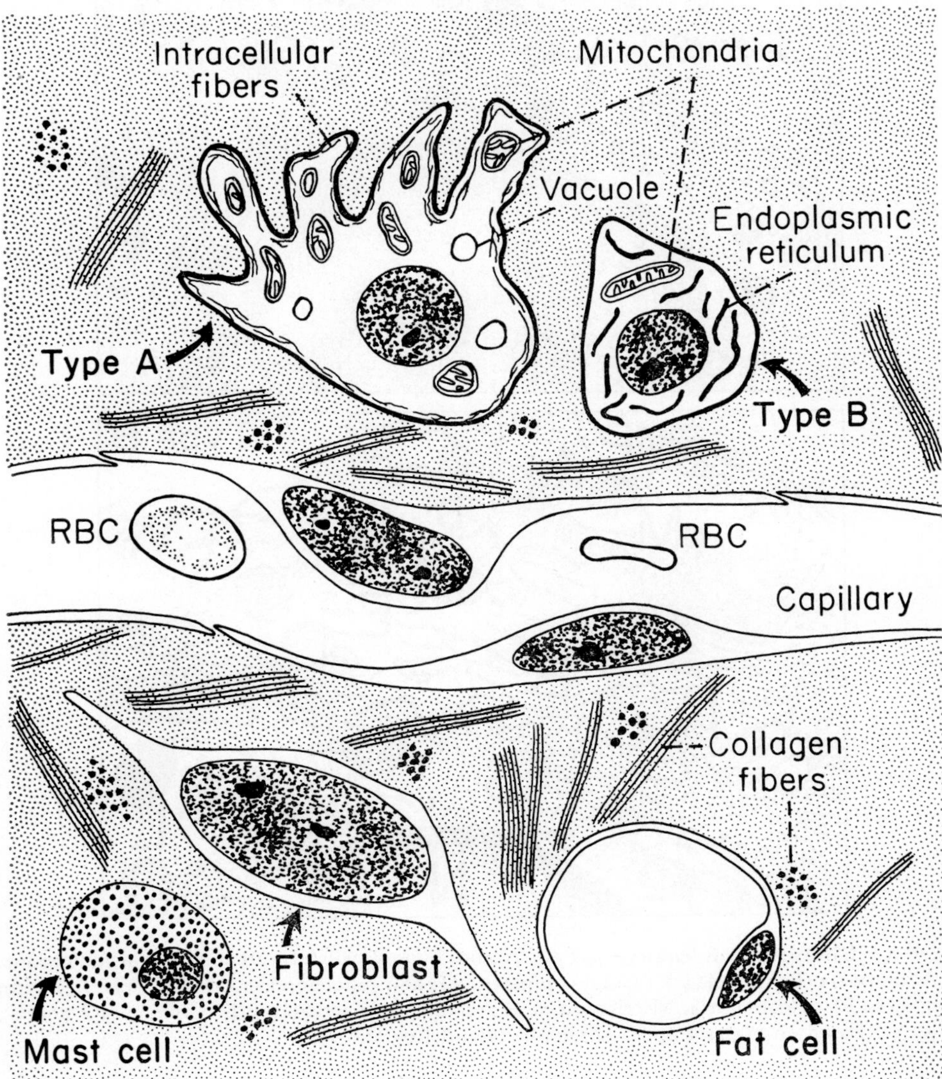

Fig. 4–5.—Schematic representation of some of the major features of synovial membrane and joint capsule. Type A and Type B cells are shown with a capillary separating them from the joint capsule. Few, if any, collagenous fibers are present in the surface part of synovial membrane. The intercellular ground substance is mostly amorphous. Based in part on Barland, Novikoff and Hamerman (1962); also on Ghadially and Roy (1969).

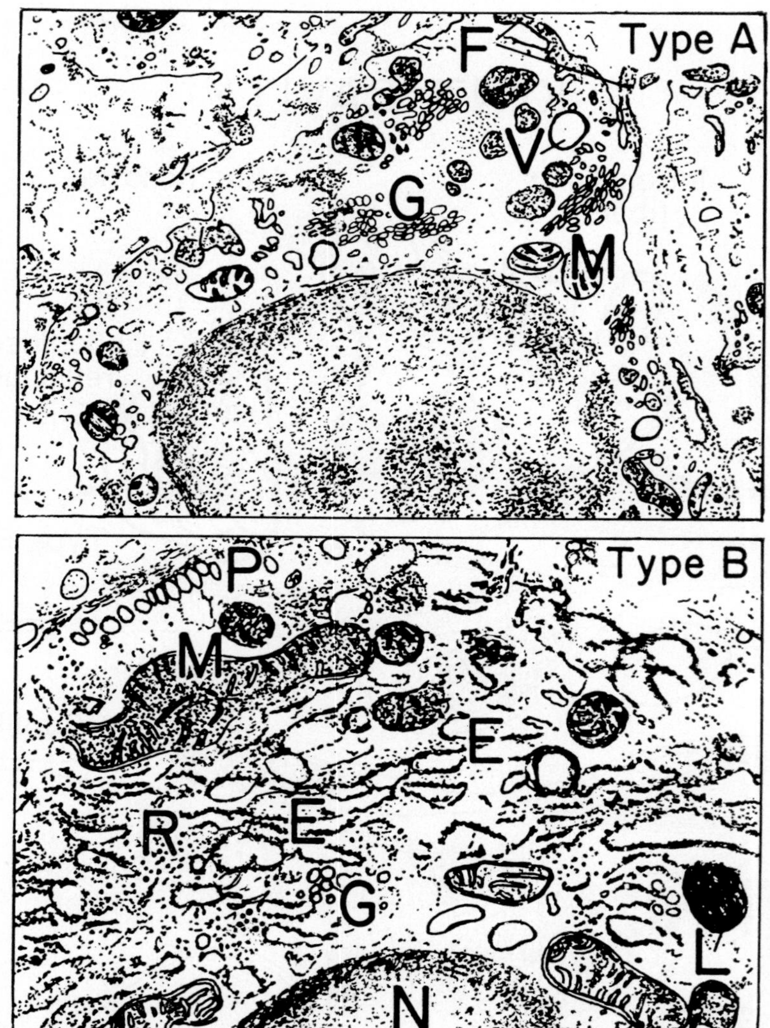

FIG. 4–6.—Ultrastructural features of Type A and Type B cells of human synovial membrane. In Type A, filopodia, F; vacuoles, V; Golgi complexes, G; and mitochondria, M. In Type B, micropinocytic vesicles, P; mitochondria, M; ribosomes, R; endoplasmic reticulum, E; Golgi complexes, G; and nucleus, N. Based on Plates 4 and 5 of Ghadially and Roy (1969).

tissue by the blood stream. Synoviocytes synthesize these units into hyaluronic acid, probably chiefly by polymerization, that is, by a linking together of the basic units.[7,25,36,71] That this is an active process, specifically involving synoviocytes, is indicated by tissue culture experiments and immunofluorescent and other studies.[9,12,37] It is not yet known, however, whether Type A cells alone, or Type B, or both, are responsible.

Synovial fluid is usually slightly alkaline, ranges from colorless to deep yellow, and is sticky and viscous. Its viscosity is due almost entirely to the presence of hyaluronic acid which, when precipitated with acetic acid, forms what is called mucin. The viscosity of solutions of hyaluronic acid increases exponentially with increasing concentration. Solutions of more than 1 per cent may form gels. The viscosity of synovial fluid decreases to that of water if the hyaluronic acid is removed by precipitation with acid, if it is hydrolyzed by enzymes, or if its polymerization is destroyed by enzymes or by physical processes. The viscosity also varies with temperature; the lower the temperature the more viscous the fluid. One of the factors that may contribute to joint stiffness with cold is an increase in synovial fluid viscosity.[40,41] Viscosity may also vary with species and according to type of joint. For example, fluid from large joints is usually less viscous than that from smaller joints.

It must be emphasized that hyaluronic acid is normally bound to protein to form what is termed hyaluronate-protein. The binding is also a specific function of synoviocytes.[9,36] Moreover, the protein moiety is an important lubrication factor (trypsin digestion destroys lubricating properties).[55,66] Hyaluronate-protein, in diffusing into the joint cavity, comprises a significant part of the intercellular matrix of synovial membrane. Together with cytoplasmic processes it constitutes a barrier to diffusion of other substances, especially proteins (some solutes are sterically excluded from the volume occupied by hyaluronate chains[63]).

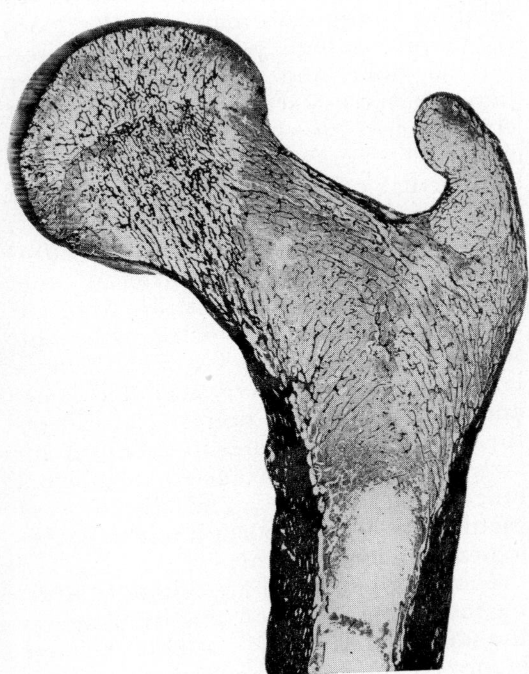

Fig. 4–7.—Frontal section of human femur to show its characteristic architecture and the extent of articular cartilage (see Figure 4–8).

The other constituents of synovial fluid are those that are normally present in blood plasma. In fact, synovial fluid, aside from its hyaluronate-protein content, can be considered as a dialysate of blood plasma. However, a number of proteins are present in synovial fluid in concentrations such that factors of molecular shape and charge seem important, as well as molecular weight.[8,62] Synovial fluid also normally contains a few cells, mostly mononuclear, derived from the lining tissue. Pathological processes that affect synovial membrane alter the cellular content of the fluid. Withdrawal of synovial fluid and determination of its cellular and chemical content and physical characteristics can be a valuable diagnostic aid.[24,68] (See also Chapter 6.)

The chief function of synovial fluid is related to joint lubrication, but it has other functions, including the nourishment of articular cartilage.

Articular Cartilage. — Cartilage is a tough, resilient connective tissue which is composed of cells and fibers embedded in a firm, gel-like matrix, which consists chiefly of chondroitin sulfate A and C. Adult cartilage lacks nerves, and it usually lacks blood vessels. Metabolic substances must, therefore, diffuse through the matrix to reach the cells.

The most plentiful type of cartilage is hyaline cartilage, so-named because, owing to the character of its matrix, it has a glassy, translucent appearance. The matrix and the collagenous fibers embedded in it have about the same index of refraction. The fibers are, therefore, not visible in ordinary microscopic preparations. Articular cartilage is usually hyaline; the part adjacent to bone is usually calcified (Figs. 4–7, 4–8). Articular cartilage, except for its calcified zone, is not visible in ordinary radiograms. Hence, the so-called "radiological joint space" is wider than the true joint space.

Cartilage is a resilient and elastic tissue. When it is compressed, it becomes thinner. When the pressure is released, the cartilage slowly regains its original thickness. There is also evidence that intermittent pressure causes cartilage to thicken by taking up fluid.[43] Thus, cartilage has the spongelike property of being able to absorb synovial fluid which diffuses through cartilage matrix. Moreover, this absorption may involve chiefly water and other low molecular weight substances. As discussed earlier, these physical and physicochemical properties of articular cartilage are important in lubrication mechanisms.

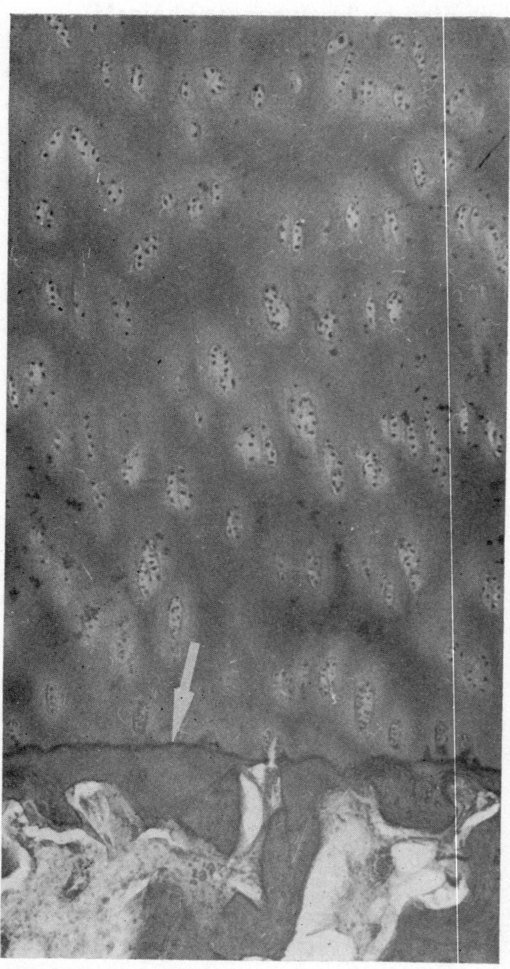

Fig. 4–8.—Microscopic section of articular cartilage and subchondral bone from the femoral head shown in Figure 4–7; the superficial part of the cartilage is not included. Note the thin layer of calcified cartilage (arrow) separating the cartilage above from subchondral bone below. Note also at the right the vascular marrow spaces approaching the cartilage through the subchondral bone. About 60 ×.

With regard to the physical and ultrastructural features of cartilage, its stiffness and strength depend upon the orientation of surface collagen, whose fibers resist tensile stresses. The surface of cartilage is comprised of undulating, tightly woven fiber bundles which in turn exhibit microundulations, the total pattern contributing to the normal surface roughness. In general terms, then, articular cartilage resembles a stiff sponge, capable of resisting tensile stresses, exhibiting elastic deformation under load, containing a high proportion of extracellular fluid, and exuding fluid under pressure, thereby serving as an important component of lubrication mechanisms.[17,36,48,51,61,67,75]

Articular cartilage probably derives its main nourishment from synovial fluid, but other possible sources include diffusion from capillaries in the arterial circle at the periphery of the joint, and diffusion from epiphysial vessels which loop through subchondral bone (Fig. 4–8).[22,42] Articular cartilage is a relatively acellular tissue, and its rate of respiration is low. Nevertheless, its nutrition and metabolism are factors of prime importance in the normal functioning of joints, and disorders of cartilage play an important role in pathological changes in joints.

Cartilage grows by apposition, that is, by the laying down of new cartilage on the surface of the old. The new cartilage is formed by chondrocytes derived from the deeper cells of the perichondrium. Cartilage also grows interstitially, that is, by the increase in size and number of existing cells and by the increase in amount of intercellular material. The cells of adult cartilage, especially hyaline cartilage, have usually lost the power of mitotic activity. Consequently, unless the cartilage possesses a perichondrium, repair or regeneration after injury is inadequate. This is especially true of articular cartilage, which lacks a perichondrium. However, there is evidence that, in normal use, some replacement of articular cartilage may occur.[23,70] Furthermore, a peripheral lesion of articular cartilage may be repaired by adjacent connective tissue, and a central lesion, if deep enough, may be filled in with fibrous tissue or fibrocartilage from connective tissue in the underlying bone marrow. Also, growth of cartilage is directly involved in the remodeling of adult joints that may result from mechanical or pathological stress.[44,60]

Joint Capsule and Ligaments.—In a few joints (middle ear) the capsule and ligaments are composed almost entirely of elastic fibers. In most joints the capsule is composed of bundles of collagenous fibers, which are arranged somewhat irregularly, in contrast to their more regular arrangement in tendons and many ligaments. These bundles, and the bundles in some ligaments, tend to spiral. Such an arrangement renders them sensitive to tension in most positions that the joint happens to occupy. Hence, the slightest movement alters the tension or torsion in the bundles, and this change stimulates proprioceptive nerve endings in the capsule and ligaments. Thus, in addition to their mechanical functions, most ligaments serve as sense organs in that nerve endings in them are important in reflex mechanisms and in the perception of movement and position.

Intra-articular Structures.—Menisci, intra-articular discs, fat pads, and synovial folds are structures that aid in spreading synovial fluid throughout the joint. Thus, they are of importance in joint lubrication. Intra-articular discs and menisci, which are composed mostly of fibrous tissue, but may contain some fibrocartilage, have other important functions. They are attached at their periphery to the joint capsule, and they are usually present in joints where flexion and extension are associated with gliding, a combination that requires a rounded male surface and a relatively flattened female surface.[4] The menisci and discs, the mobility of which is usually under ligamentous or muscular control, help to prevent instability and yet allow a considerable range of gliding.

Peri-articular Tissues.—The term peri-articular tissues is a general one, and refers to fascial investments around the joint. These investments blend with capsule and ligaments, with the musculotendinous expansions that pass over or blend with joint capsules, and with the looser connective tissue that invests the vessels and nerves approaching the joint. The peri-articular tissues contain many elastic fibers, blood vessels, and nerves. Increased fibrosis of the peri-articular tissues may limit movement almost as much as fibrosis within a joint.

Blood and Lymphatic Supply.—The blood vessels that supply a joint and adjacent bone arise more or less in common (Fig. 4–9). Most of those that supply bone (epiphysial and metaphysial vessels in the case of long bones) enter the bone at or near the line of capsular attachment and form a prominent arterial circle around the joint. The vessels that supply the joint ultimately break up into a rich capillary network, which is especially prominent in the cellular and areolar areas of synovial membrane. Lymphatic vessels accompany blood vessels and form plexuses in the synovial membrane and capsule.

The capillary network and lymphatic plexus in synovial membrane are adjacent to the joint cavity. Diffusion takes place readily between these vessels and the joint cavity.[1,21] Most substances in the blood stream, normal or pathological, easily enter the joint cavity. Conversely, many substances injected into the joint readily enter the blood. When true solu-

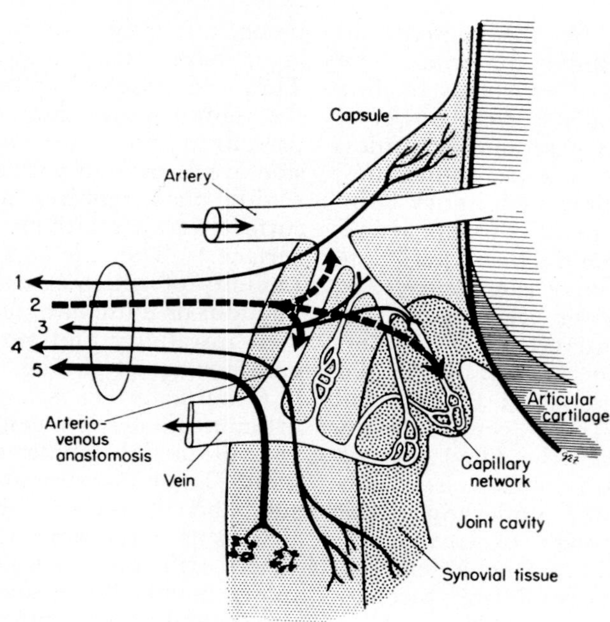

FIG. 4–9.—Schematic representation of blood and nerve supply of joints. The arterial supply to epiphysis, capsule, and synovial tissue is shown, as well as capillary networks, venous drainage, and an arteriovenous anastomosis. An articular nerve is shown enclosed by a circle. Such a nerve contains various fibers, indicated by numbers, with direction of conduction shown by arrows. (1) Afferent (pain) from the capsule. (2) Efferent (postganglionic sympathetic or vasomotor) to smooth muscle of blood vessels. (3) Afferent (pain) and others with unknown functions from adventitia of vessels. (4) Afferent (pain) from the capsule and synovial tissue. (5) Afferent (proprioceptive) from the capsule. These fibers form Ruffini endings and small lamellated corpuscles (not shown). (From Gardner, Figure 2, Instructional Course Lectures, *10*, 251, 1953, J. W. Edwards, Publisher, Inc., with permission of the American Academy of Orthopaedic Surgeons.)

tions are injected into a joint cavity, they enter the subsynovial tissue rapidly, and are removed by blood and lymphatic capillaries, mainly by the former. When colloidal solutions and fine suspensions are injected, they also enter subsynovial tissue, but these, including proteins, are removed mainly by lymphatics. Large molecules leave the joint cavity with difficulty, and for large colloidal particles and particulate matter there is no way of exit, except for a few particles that may reach regional lymph nodes after being phagocytized (phagocytosis seems to be a particular property of Type A lining cells). The rate of absorption of solutions is increased if the intra-articular pressure is increased, either by injection under high pressure or by movement.

There have been relatively few experimental studies of articular blood vessels and their control.[52] Some investigators have reported that temperature changes in the human knee joint may be the reverse of those in the skin after the application of hot or cold to the skin over the joint.[38,39] Others, however, have found a direct correspondence between joint temperature and skin temperature, but in smaller joints (fingers).[40] Arteriovenous anastomoses are present in joints[16,52] and their structure and arrangement (Fig. 4–1, *D–E*) indicate that they can shunt blood past capillary networks. It therefore seems likely that they play an important role in the regulation of blood flow through joints, and perhaps through adjacent bone, but this remains to be determined physiologically. Thus, important unsolved problems in joint physiology include the study of the normal pattern of blood flow, and the alterations in flow under various physiological, experimental, and pathological conditions.

Nerve Supply.—The importance of joint nerve supply lies in two main factors: (1) the marked subjective effects (pain) and reflex changes that may accompany joint disease, and (2) the role of joint nerves in posture, locomotion, and the kinesthetic sense. Articular nerves, which carry fibers derived from several spinal nerves, vary in number and in course. An articular nerve may supply more than one joint. Upon entering a joint, an articular nerve has a wide distribution to ligaments, capsule, and synovial membrane. Furthermore, each major articular nerve overlaps in distribution with one or more articular nerves. The proximal joints, such as the hip and shoulder, and the joints of the vertebral column, also receive fibers that arise in sympathetic trunks and course along blood vessels to the joints.

Articular nerves contain autonomic fibers and sensory fibers of varying size (Fig. 4–9). Although a considerable amount of experimental work has been done on the functions of these fibers, most of it has been carried out in animals such as the cat, and much remains to be done, especially in man and other primates.

The larger sensory fibers in articular nerves form proprioceptive endings (Ruffini endings and small lamellated corpuscles) in the capsule and ligaments.[25,26,29] These endings are very sensitive to position and movement. Their central connections (in the spinal cord and brain stem) are such that they are concerned in the reflex control of posture and locomotion, and in the perception of position and movement.[10,25,29,69]

Most of the smaller sensory fibers form pain endings (free nerve endings) in the capsule and ligaments, and in the adventitia of blood vessels. The most effective painful stimulus of the capsule and ligaments is twisting or stretching. Studies of human joints opened under local anesthesia indicate that the capsule and ligaments are highly sensitive, whereas synovial membrane is relatively insensitive (most of the fibers that enter synovial membrane supply blood vessels).[47] Whether arising from the capsule or from synovial membrane, joint pain is diffuse and poorly localized. When severe, it may be felt over much of the limb, especially distally. When severe and sudden in onset, there may be reflex reactions, including slowing of the pulse, fall in blood pressure, nausea, and vomiting. Joint pain commonly leads to reflex contractions of muscles, especially those that flex or adduct. These reflex contractions may take the form of spasm. Antagonistic muscles (extensor) may relax reflexly, to the extent that if the pain is long continued, the extensor muscles may atrophy. Joint pain is often referred, just as any deep or visceral pain may be. For example, in some hip disorders, pain may be felt in an uninvolved knee (both joints are supplied by the femoral and obturator nerves). Joint nerves may be sectioned to relieve pain in a joint. Owing to overlap, however, section of a single nerve will not completely denervate even part of a joint, and the section thus often fails to relieve pain. Furthermore, section of as many nerves to a joint as possible may not relieve pain completely or permanently. Regeneration may occur, and the possibility must also be considered that some pain fibers may course along blood vessels to sympathetic trunks, and then pass through the trunks to enter dorsal roots. Such fibers would not be affected by section of articular nerves.

It is ordinarily believed that changes in temperature, humidity, or pressure make joints more sensitive or painful, and there is undoubtedly some truth in these beliefs. It may well be that such changes reflexly alter blood flow, but, as mentioned above, little is known about the control of blood flow through joints, or about the possible effect of changes in blood flow upon joint sensitivity.

If the sensory fibers to a limb are lost

(by surgery, by disease of dorsal roots, or by peripheral nerve disease) the joints of that limb may undergo a progressive destruction, an affliction known as a neuropathic joint. It has been suggested that it is the specific loss of sensory or so-called trophic fibers to a joint that causes the destruction. However, section of just the nerves supplying a joint does not cause a neuropathic change. Neuropathic joints occur only when the denervation is extensive enough to eliminate reflexes and leave a joint unprotected and liable to mechanical damage. Neuropathic joints do not inevitably occur after denervation, but when they do, the rapidity of destruction sometimes seen is a phenomenon as yet unexplained.

The autonomic fibers in joint nerves are vasomotor fibers. They supply the blood vessels, but little is known of their pattern of activity. Some of the small sensory fibers in joint nerves are pain fibers that end in the adventitia of blood vessels, as mentioned above. A few small sensory fibers form more complex endings in the adventitia. The functions of these fibers are unknown; possibly they are concerned with reflex vascular mechanisms.

Development of Joints

Most studies of the development of joints have been concerned with the synovial joints of the limbs.[25,30,31,32,34] Shortly after limb buds appear in the human embryo, an axial condensation or blastema develops within them. The blastema then becomes chondrified in the regions of the future bones, the chondrification proceeding in a proximodistal sequence. The process of chondrification begins at about five postovulatory weeks.

The early development of the large joints of the limbs involves two chief phases: the formation of interzones and the appearance of cavities. The blastema that remains between the chondrifying skeletal elements forms homogeneous cellular areas termed interzones. Very often these interzones become three-layered as an intermediate, loose layer forms. The mesenchyme which surrounds the joint (synovial mesenchyme) becomes vascularized, and the capsule and most intra-articular structures (ligaments, menisci, synovial membrane) differentiate from it. By the end of the embryonic period (eight postovulatory weeks), the developing joints closely resemble adult joints in form and arrangement.

In the larger synovial joints, minute spaces appear in the interzone and synovial mesenchyme by the end of the embryonic period or early in the fetal period. These spaces coalesce and form a joint cavity. The onset of cavitation appears to be an enzymatic process; it is independent of joint movement. Early in fetal life, the synovial membrane forms a relatively smooth lining with a subjacent vascular network. Synovial fluid begins to be formed at this time.

It should be emphasized that the differentiation of bones and joints proceeds very rapidly from a generalized blastema to structures having a form and arrangement characteristic of the adult. There is no recapitulation in the sense that structures characteristic of adult lower forms appear as an intermediate phase. It must also be emphasized that differentiation is not only rapid, but occurs in a precise sequence.

The normal number and arrangement of skeletal elements are determined genetically before the appearance of limb buds. Congenital defects characterized by a true increase or decrease in the number of skeletal elements are produced by causes, whether genetic or environmental, which operate during or preceding differentiation, during what are termed critical periods.[45] The critical period for limb joints is during the 3 to 6 weeks after conception (5 to 8 menstrual weeks), from just before the limb buds appear until the bones and joints are well differentiated. Once the skeletal elements are present, neither true increase or decrease in elements is possible. However, certain congenital defects may begin later in prenatal development. Whatever their nature, they result from interference with the growth, development, and maturation of skeletal elements already formed.

Experimental and biochemical studies of limb development, both normal and abnormal, comprise an important and expanding field, one that is necessary for the proper interpretation of many skeletal and muscular abnormalities.

BIBLIOGRAPHY

1. Adkins, E. W. O. and Davies, D. V.: Quart. J. Exp. Physiol., *30*, 147, 1940.
2. Armstrong, J. R.: *Lumbar Disc Lesions*, Edinburgh, Livingstone, 2nd ed., 1958.
3. Barland, P., Novikoff, A. B. and Hamerman, D.: J. Cell Biol., *14*, 207, 1962.
4. Barnett, C. H.: J. Anat., *88*, 363, 1954.
5. ———: J. Bone & Joint Surg., *38B*, 567, 1956.
6. Barnett, C. H. and Cobbold, A. F.: J. Bone & Joint Surg., *44B*, 662, 1962.
7. Barnett, C. H., Davies, D. V. and MacConaill, M. A.: *Synovial Joints*, London, Clowes and Sons, 1961.
8. Binetti, J. P. and Schmidt, K.: Arth. & Rheum., *8*, 14, 1965.
9. Blau, S., Janis, R., Hamerman, D. and Sandson, J.: Science, *150*, 353, 1965.
10. Browne, K., Lee, J. and Ring, P. A.: J. Physiol., *126*, 448, 1954.
11. Bryce, T. H.: *Osteology and Arthrology*, Vol. 4, pt. 1 of Quain's *Elements of Anatomy*, London, Longmans, 11th ed., 1915.
12. Castor, C. W.: Proc. Soc. Exp. Biol. Med., *94*, 51, 1957.
13. ———: Arth. & Rheum., *3*, 140, 1960.
14. Charnley, J.: *The Lubrication of Animal Joints*, Institution of Mechanical Engineers, Proceedings of Symposium on Biomechanics, April 17, 1959, p. 12.
15. ———: Ann. Rheum. Dis., *19*, 10, 1960.
16. Clara, M.: *Die Arterio-Venösen Anastomosen*, Vienna, Springer, 2nd ed, 1956.
17. Davies, D. V., Barnett, C. H., Cochrane, W. and Palfrey, A. J.: Ann. Rheum. Dis., *21*, 11, 1962.
18. Davies, D. V. and Edwards, D. A. W.: Ann. Roy. Coll. Surg., *2*, 142, 1948.
19. Dintenfass, L.: J. Bone & Joint Surg., *45–A*, 1241, 1963.
20. ———: Fed. Proc., *25*, 1054, 1966.
21. Edlund, T.: Acta Physiol. Scand., Suppl., *62*, 1949.
22. Ekholm, R.: Acta Anat., Suppl. *15*, 1951.
23. Ekholm, R. and Norbäck, B.: Acta Orthop. Scand., *21*, 81, 1951.
24. Furey, J. G., Clark, W. S. and Brine, K. L.: J. Bone & Joint Surg., *41–A*, 167, 1959.
25. Gardner, E.: Physiol. Rev., *30*, 127, 1950.
26. ———: Bull. Hosp. Joint Dis., *21*, 153, 1960.
27. ———: J. Bone & Joint Surg., *45–A*, 856, 1963.
28. ———: J. Bone & Joint Surg., *45–A*, 1061, 1963.
29. ———: In *Myotatic, Kinesthetic and Vestibular Mechanisms*, Ciba Foundation Symposium, eds. A. V. S. de Reuds and J. Knight, London, J. and A. Churchill Limited, 1967.
30. ———: In *The Biochemistry and Physiology of Bone*, ed. G. H. Bourne, New York, Academic Press, 2nd ed., in press, 1972.
31. Gardner, E. and Gray, D. J.: Amer. J. Anat., *129*, 121, 1970.
32. Gardner, E. and O'Rahilly, R.: J. Anat., *102*, 289, 1968.
33. Ghadially, F. N. and Roy, S.: *Ultrastructure of Synovial Joints in Health and Disease*, London, Butterworth, 1969.
34. Gray, D. J. and Gardner, E.: Amer. J. Anat., *124*, 431, 1969.
35. Hamerman, D., Barland, P. and Janis, R.: In *The Biological Basis of Medicine*, ed. E. E. Bittar and N. Bittar, New York, Academic Press, 1969, Vol. 30, p. 269.
36. Hamerman, D., Rosenberg, L. C. and Schubert, M.: J. Bone & Joint Surg., *52–A*, 725, 1970.
37. Hedberg, H. and Moritz, V.: Proc. Soc. Exp. Biol. Med., *98*, 80, 1958.
38. Hollander, J. L. and Horvath, S. M.: Amer. J. Med. Sci., *288*, 543, 1949.
39. Horvath, S. M. and Hollander, J. L.: J. Clin. Invest., *28*, 469, 1949.
40. Hunter, J., Kerr, E. H. and Whillans, M. G.: Canad. J. Med. Sci., *30*, 367, 1952.
41. Hunter, J. and Whillans, M. G.: Canad. J. Med. Sci., *29*, 255, 1951.
42. Ingelmark, B. E.: Acta Orthop. Scand., *20*, 144, 1950.
43. Ingelmark, B. E. and Ekholm, R.: Upsala Läk Fören Förh., *53*, 51, 1948.
44. Johnson, L. C.: Lab. Invest., *8*, 1223, 1959.
45. Kalter, H. and Warkany, J.: Physiol. Rev., *39*, 69, 1959.
46. Kanie, R.: Nagoya Med. J., *11*, 77, 1965.
47. Kellgren, J. A. and Samuel, E. P.: J. Bone & Joint Surg., *32B*, 84, 1950.
48. Kempson, G. E., Freeman, M. A. R. and Swanson, S. A. V.: Nature, *220*, 1127, 1968.

49. Langer, E. and Huth, F.: Z. Zellforsch., *51*, 545, 1960.
50. Lever, J. D. and Ford, E. H. R.: Anat. Rec., *132*, 525, 1962.
51. Lewis, P. R. and McCutchen, C. W.: Nature, *184*, 1285, 1959.
52. Lindström, J.: Acta Rheum. Scand., Suppl., *7*, 1963.
53. Linn, F. C.: J. Bone & Joint Surg., *49–A*, 1079, 1967.
54. ————: J. Biomechanics, *1*, 193, 1968.
55. Linn, F. C. and Radin, E. L.: Arth. & Rheum., *11*, 674, 1968.
56. Maroudas, A.: Proc. Inst. Med. Eng., *181*, 122, 1967.
57. McCutchen, C. W.: New Scientist, *301*, 412, 1962.
58. ————: Fed. Proc., *25*, 1061, 1966.
59. Meyer, A. W.: Calif. West. Med., *47*, 375, 1937.
60. Moffett, Jr., B. C., Johnson, L. C., McCabe, J. B. and Askew, H. C.: Amer. J. Anat., *115*, 119, 1964.
61. Muir, H., Bullough, P. and Maroudas, A.: J. Bone & Joint Surg., *52B*, 554, 1970.
62. Neuhaus, O.: J. Mich. State Med. Soc., *61*, 458, 1962.
63. Ogston, A. G. and Phelps, C. F.: Biochem. J., *78*, 827, 1961.
64. Peacock, A.: J. Anat., *86*, 162, 1952.
65. Pedersen, H. E., Blunck, C. F. J. and Gardner, E.: J. Bone & Joint Surg., *38–A*, 377, 1956.
66. Radin, E. L., Swann, D. A. and Weisser, P. A.: Nature, *228*, 377, 1970.
67. Redler, I. and Zimny, M. L.: J. Bone & Joint Surg., *52–A*, 1395, 1970.
68. Ropes, M. W. and Bauer, W.: *Synovial Fluid Changes in Joint Disease.* Cambridge, Harvard University Press, 1953.
69. Rose, J. E. and Mountcastle, V. B.: In *Handbook of Physiology*, Vol. 1, Sect. 1, Ed., J. Field, H. W. Magoun and V. E. Hall. American Physiological Society, 1959.
70. Sääf, F. J.: Acta Orthop. Scand., Suppl., *7*, 1950.
71. Sundblad, L.: Acta Soc. Med. Ups., *58*, 113, 1953.
72. Walker, P. S., Dowson, D., Longfield, M. D. and Wright, V.: Ann. Rheum. Dis., *27*, 512, 1968.
73. Walker, P. S., Sikorski, J., Dowson, D., Longfield, M. D., Wright, V. and Buckley, T.: Ann. Rheum. Dis., *28*, 1, 1969.
74. Walmsley, R.: Edinburgh Med. J., *60*, 341, 1953.
75. Weiss, C., Rosenberg, L. and Helfet, A. J.: J. Bone & Joint Surg., *50–A*, 663, 1968.
76. Woodward, D. H., Gryfe, A. and Gardner, D. L.: Experientia, *25*, 1301, 1969.

Chapter 5

The Study of the Connective Tissue

By C. William Castor, M.D.

Connective tissue was once visualized as an inert fabric serving to support and bind together the parenchymal, vascular, and neural structures of the living organism. Spurred by interest in disease states characterized by pathologic alteration of the supporting tissues, numerous investigators have outlined a new concept which emphasizes the complex, dynamic nature of these tissues and their important roles in the physiology of multicellular organisms. The embryonic mesoderm generates mesenchymal cells which differentiate to form the several types of connective tissue. A partial list would include loose (areolar) and dense fibroelastic connective tissue, reticular, adipose, and elastic connective tissue as well as cartilage, bone, and synovial membrane.

In examining the concept of a "connective tissue" it is convenient to divide it into *cellular* and *intercellular* components, and to subdivide the latter category into *fibrillar* and *ground substance* materials. The proportion of these three constituents varies with anatomic location and functional requirements. Thus, tendon and fascia have a disproportionate fibrillar component, while Wharton's jelly of the umbilical cord is predominantly ground substance with infrequent cells and fibers. Cartilage and synovial membrane are connective tissues with a marked cellular content.

Mechanical support and protection are among the more important functions performed by the connective tissues. The osteoblast, a specialized connective tissue cell, provides a matrix of fibers and ground substance suitable for deposition of calcium salts. The bone thus formed protects viscera from mechanical injury, and its rigidity preserves intricate pressure relationships necessary for the life of the organism. In addition, the long bones serve as a lever system to which tendons and fascia transmit the mechanical energy derived from muscle contraction. The smooth transmission of mechanical energy, used to move the organism or its parts, is facilitated by lubrication from ground substance components located in the gliding planes of the tendon sheaths, bursae, and joints. Since connective tissue is everywhere interposed between the vascular system and epithelial structures, it must function as an organ of transport, conveying essential nutrients to the periphery and returning metabolic wastes. The role of connective tissue in selecting or modifying nutrients, or determining their rate of transport, is largely unexplored. Energy reserves in the form of neutral fat are stored in and released from adipose connective tissue in response to direct hormonal influence, but the role of other metabolically active constituents, such as the glycoproteins of the ground substance, is less obvious.

No summary of the general functions of connective tissue would be complete without noting its reparative potential. When injury disrupts the anatomic continuity of an organism, connective tissue rapidly bridges the defect. The cellular components effectively neutralize or destroy any noxious agents, remove debris, and produce a framework of fibers and ground substance which restores anatomic continuity and (usually) functional capacity to the injured part.

COMPOSITION OF THE CONNECTIVE TISSUE

Cellular Components

The *cellular elements* of connective tissue control the formation, maintenance, and breakdown of the extracellular components. Microscopic study discloses a heterogeneous mixture of cells whose proportions vary from one anatomic site to another. The origin and genetic relationships of these cell types are an unsettled matter.[66] Available evidence is largely derived from morphologic studies of inflammation, tissue culture, and extramedullary hematopoiesis. Primordial mesenchymal cells, believed to retain potentiality for differentiation into many specialized cell types, are found around the adventitia of vascular elements traversing the connective tissue. Such cells may differentiate in several directions to become macrophages (histiocytes), mast cells, plasma cells, lymphocytes, and probably fibroblasts. There is little doubt, however, that fibroblasts and macrophages are capable of mitotic division and do not depend on a "stem cell" for the perpetuation of their respective species. Whether small lymphocytes are fully differentiated cells or are essentially totipotential and capable of transformation into various hematopoietic and connective tissue cellular elements remains controversial. Tissue culture studies[119] in particular have led to the suggestion that tissue macrophages, or blood monocytes, and fibroblasts may be interconvertible. Morphologic studies attempt to document the transformation of one cell type to another by demonstrating suitable intermediate forms, a difficult task in view of the imperfect cytologic criteria now available. Where tissue culture techniques have been used, the possibility that the final cell type results from *selection* in a mixed cell population, rather than a cellular *transformation*, has not been adequately eliminated.

Morphologic criteria may be too crude for the accurate identification of many cell types in certain functional or pathologic states. The growing discipline of histochemistry should provide helpful supplementary information at the level of the tissue section. In addition, cultured cells of diverse origins, although of similar appearance, can be shown to be functionally and metabolically different.

Fibroblasts and their specialized variants, the *chondrocytes*, *osteocytes*, and *synoviocytes* are credited with the formation and maintenance of fibroelastic connective tissue, cartilage, bone, and synovial membrane, respectively. Under the light microscope the fibroblast appears as a stellate or spindle-shaped cell with a large pale nucleus and scanty, faintly stained cytoplasm. Histochemical methods show cytoplasmic particles in proliferating fibroblasts, interpreted to represent ribonucleic acid,[67] glycogen,[3] and acid phosphatase.[74] Oxidative enzymes demonstrable by histochemical methods in fibroblasts include: succinic dehydrogenase, lactic dehydrogenase, DPN diaphorase, malic dehydrogenase, and cytochrome c oxidase.[4] Tissue culture evidence[45] indicates that the fibroblast synthesizes the acid mucopolysaccharides of the ground substance. *In vitro* studies further indicate that alterations in the physiologic state of fibroblasts may be reflected by striking changes in the molecular weight of hyaluronic acid, one of the ground substance mucopolysaccharides formed by these cells.[21] In addition, the fibroblast produces collagen which is first clearly detected in aggregated form outside the cell periphery.[104]

Diffusely distributed *tissue macrophages* ingest foreign substances and remove tissue debris in their "scavenger" role. Tissue *mast cells* are also widely distributed throughout the connective tissue and, like the blood basophil, have large basophilic, metachromatic granules. These morphologically distinctive cells may often be present in significant numbers, as in the superficial aspect of the synovial membrane where they constitute approximately 3 per cent of the cellular population.[17] It is now reasonably well established that the mast cells contain heparin, histamine, and 5-hydroxytryptamine,[99,105] but their role in the physiology of connective tissue remains obscure. *Plasma cells*, *lymphocytes*, and *eosinophilic leukocytes* are sparsely and irregularly distributed among the connective tissues. The latter, at least, are probably derived from the circulating blood.

Fibrillar Components

The fibrillar elements of the connective tissue have been intensively studied and a growing body of information is available concerning them.[31,88,104] With the aid of staining techniques and visible light microscopy, one can distinguish collagen, reticulin, and elastic fibers. *Collagen* is present in impressive amounts in the body, composing approximately one-third of the body protein. Conventional histologic methods stain it with eosin and acid aniline dyes, such as aniline blue. Inspection shows wavy fibers arranged in bundles whose smallest units are non-branching fibers with a uniform diameter of 0.3 to 0.5 microns. Electron microscopy reveals that collagen fibers are composed of submicroscopic fibrils with a characteristic 640 Å band period. Tropocollagen particles, measuring 2000 to 3000 Å in length and 15 Å in width, are believed to aggregate outside the connective tissue cell to produce the banded fibril.

Collagen possesses many interesting physical properties, including the tendency to swell in dilute acid and to form solutions with heat-dependent viscosity. Warming a solution of collagen converts it to gelatin with an irreversible fall in viscosity. In mammalian tissues the thermal instability of collagen is manifested by shrinkage on heating to 64° C. Physical-chemical measurements, employing osmotic pressure, light scattering, viscosity, and flow birefringence, suggest that the molecular weight of the collagen macromolecule is approximately 300,000. From such studies and from x-ray diffraction came the suggestion that the molecule is composed of three polypeptide strands wound around each other in an extended helical pattern.

Detailed study of denatured collagen indicates that the triple helical array is usually composed of two similar (α_1) polypeptide strands and one dissimilar (α_2) unit. These three α chains, each with a molecular weight of about 100,000, have the spatial configurations of polyproline-II type helices which are then coiled together to form a super helix (tropocollagen). The highly ordered packing of the polypeptide chains in these tropocollagen molecules requires that every third amino acid residue be glycine. One can visualize the amino acid sequence in the α chains as a series of triplets of the form: glycine-X-Y, where X and Y are often proline or hydroxyproline. Chemical analyses of purified collagen preparations show that glycine (30 per cent), hydroxyproline (13 per cent), and proline (16 per cent) combined constitute more than half of the collagen macromolecule, while the proportion of aromatic and sulfur-containing amino acids is small. Most of the hydroxyproline, the "chemical fingerprint" of the collagen family, is 4-hydroxyproline although traces of 3-hydroxyproline have been found.[80] About 0.6 per cent of collagen is hexose in nature, with more galactose being found than glucose. Isolation of glucosylgalactosylhydroxylysine and galactosylhydroxylysine from hydrolysates of collagen indicates that the carbohydrate is covalently linked to collagen at hydroxylysine sites and that some of the bound hexose occurs as disaccharide side chains.[16,100]

While interchain hydrogen bonding has been considered primarily responsible for the stability of the collagen triple helix, there is now clear evidence for covalent cross-links between α chains within tropocollagen molecules (intramolecular) as well as between them (intermolecular). An *intramolecular* site has been located in α_1 and α_2 chains at the fifth amino acid residue from the N-terminal end of the chains, where aldehydes derived from lysine residues on adjacent chains are believed to undergo aldol condensation to form a cross-link.[12] *Intermolecular* cross-linking substances, lysinonorleucine and hydroxylysinonorleucine, have been isolated from calf skin collagen.[111,112] These cross-linking materials arise when α-aminoadipic semialdehyde (derived from lysine) spontaneously condenses with lysine or hydroxylysine in a neighboring polypeptide chain to form a Schiff base which is reduced to yield lysinonorleucine or hydroxylysinonorleucine.

Understanding of the detailed chemical structure of collagen has been aided by the cyanogen bromide technique for disruption of the collagen molecule. Cyanogen bromide cleaves polypeptide chains at methionyl residues, yielding eight peptide fragments from the α_1 chain and six fragments from the α_2 chain of collagen.[81,49,54] The order of the peptide fragments within the respective α chains is now established, and the amino acid composition of the fragments has been determined.

It is clear from recent work that the picture of a tropocollagen molecule composed of two α_1 chains and one α_2 chain is not universally correct. Codfish skin collagen, for example, consists of three distinct α chains (α_1, α_2, α_3), and chick cartilage exhibits collagen with three identical α_1 chains in addition to the conventional variety.[82,113] The newly described collagen from chick cartilage has an additional peculiarity in that it possesses 5.5 per cent hexose, far more than that associated with conventional collagen. The relationship of such subtle molecular differences to genetic defects and acquired pathology involving skeletal tissue awaits further study.

Early studies suggested that collagen was not a potent antigen, although it could be rendered more strongly antigenic by acetylation.[52] It is now clear that species-specific antibody can be developed in rabbits against bovine, guinea pig, and rat collagen.[61,72] Both precipitating and complement-fixing antibodies have been described.[61] Antibody to collagen appears to be directed primarily towards determinants in the α_2 chain, and studies with cyanogen bromide cleavage products indicate that the major determinant occurs in the N-terminal peptide fragment, a region that probably lacks helical structure.[72]

Reticulin fibers are virtually ubiquitous, being found around blood and lymph vessels, nerve and muscle fibers, in basement membranes, and the lymphoid organs. Microscopically the reticular fibers are of smaller diameter than collagen fibers and frequently branch. Like collagen they can be stained with acid aniline blue, but are distinguished by their affinity for silver stains (argyrophilia) and intense staining by the PAS procedures. Electron microscopic pictures of reticulin preparations show the same 640 Å banding seen in collagen, and supporting chemical evidence indicates that the protein component has a similar amino-acid pattern. Approximately 4 per cent of reticulin is carbohydrate, and chromatographic studies suggest that glucose, galactose, mannose, and, to a lesser extent fucose, are the sugars present.[40] Fatty acids, mostly myristic acid with a minor amount of palmitic acid, account for about 11 per cent of the dry weight of reticulin. The pattern of susceptibility of reticulin to enzymatic degradation resembles that of collagen. Studies employing fluorescent antibody techniques suggest that something in the reticulin complex behaves as a potent antigen.

Elastic fibers appear under the microscope as curling, branching, refractile fibers or as fenestrated sheets. Selective stains such as Gomori's aldehyde fuchsin, orcein, or Weigert's resorcin-fuchsin are useful for their demonstration. They are widely distributed, being found in the vascular tunics, in the dermis, and in fibrous structures such as ligamentum nuchae and ligamenta subflava. While elastic fibers do not have the tensile strength of collagen fibers, they have greater ability to return to their previous fiber length after removal of a distorting force, i.e., "elasticity." Electron microscopy discloses no evidence of periodic banding, and the x-ray diffraction pattern is unlike that which characterizes the collagen family. The protein portion of the elastic fiber has been separated into α and β fractions, differing in their molecular weights which are about 80,000 and 5,500 respectively. Amino-acid analyses of the two protein components are similar and reveal large amounts of glycine, alanine, valine, proline, leucine, and isoleucine, while little hydroxyproline is found.[76,78]

Elastin may be thought of as a three-dimensional mesh of polypeptide chains embedded in a cementing substance wherein the polypeptide strands are joined by covalent cross-links composed of unusual amino acid derivatives. These cross-linking substances include lysinonorleucine (as in collagen), desmosine, and isodesmosine.[58,115,38] Desmosine is visualized as a pyridinium ring with side chains at the 1,3,4, and 5 positions. Each side chain has a terminal carboxyl and α amino group which may enter into peptide linkage with the primary polypeptide strands. The cementing matrix is believed to contain sulfated and nonsulfated acid mucopolysaccharides, unsaturated fatty acid, and a yellow pigment responsible for the gross color of elastic tissue. Pancreatic elastase digests elastic fibers, apparently hydrolyzing both the cementing matrix and fibrillar material. The source of elastic fibers (an "elastoblast") has never been adequately identified, although both fibroblasts and muscle cells have been suggested as candidates for this synthetic function. In view of amino acid and cross-linking similarities, collagen has been proposed as a possible evolutionary precursor of elastin.[83] In this connection it is of interest that while collagen is found in the earliest animal forms, elastin appears to be confined to vertebrates.

Ground Substance Components

The amorphous ground substance is a gelatinous continuum in which the cellular and fibrillar components of the connective tissue are embedded. When viewed in routine histologic preparations, where many of the ground substance materials have been leeched out, one assigns the empty spaces between cells and fibers to the "ground substance." Special fixation followed by a variety of histochemical procedures produces dramatic coloration of the ground substance. Colloidal iron, alcian blue, and metachromatic dyes such as azure A and toluidine blue O are some of the materials used to achieve this effect. Although it is frequently stated that the stainable substances are acid mucopolysaccharides, there is little evidence to suggest that the staining methods are specific for this class of chemical substances.

The nature of the ground substance is incompletely understood. Limited information is available concerning its general chemical composition, let alone specialized variations with anatomical site or alterations related to aging or disease. It is recognized that this optically structureless gel is an aqueous solution of electrolytes, proteins, mucoproteins, acid mucopolysaccharides, and lipids.

The *protein content* of both human and rat connective tissue has been studied by multiple extractive procedures supplemented by amino-acid analyses and paper electrophoresis.[55] Approximately 30 per cent of the connective tissue protein proved to be saline soluble and amino-acid analyses of this extract showed significant amounts of tyrosine and relatively little hydroxyproline, proline, or glycine. Electrophoresis of this noncollagenous protein fraction of connective tissue yielded a pattern resembling human serum. The proportion of α_1 and α_2 globulins was higher than in serum, while albumin was somewhat decreased. The relative amounts of β and γ globulin were similar in connective tissue saline extract and serum. Though estimates

TABLE 5–1. COMPOSITION OF CARBOHYDRATE COMPONENT OF SOME MAMMALIAN MUCOPOLYSACCHARIDES

Glycosaminoglycan	*Hexosamine*	*Hexuronic Acid*	*Hexose*	*Sulfate*
Hyaluronic Acid	N-acetyl-D-glucosamine	D-glucuronic acid	—	—
Chondroitin-4-Sulfate, (CS-A)	N-acetyl-D-galactosamine	D-glucuronic acid	—	+
Dermatan-4-Sulfate, (CS-B)	N-acetyl-D-galactosamine	L-iduronic acid (D-glucuronic acid, 5–15%)	—	+
Chondroitin-6-Sulfate, (CS-C)	N-acetyl-D-galactosamine	D-glucuronic acid	—	+
Heparin	D-glucosamine	D-glucuronic acid (L-iduronic acid, trace)	—	+
Chondroitin	N-acetyl-D-galactosamine	D-glucuronic acid	—	?
Heparitin Sulfate	D-glucosamine (acetyl)*	D-glucuronic acid	—	+*
Keratosulfate	N-acetyl-D-glucosamine	—	D-galactose	+

* The acetyl and sulfate content of heparitin sulfate varies in different preparations. Expressed as a molar ratio in relation to hexosamine, acetyl varies from 0.4 to 1.0 and sulfate varies from 0.6 to 1.8.

suggest that 50 per cent or more of the plasma proteins are in an extravascular site, there is a possibility that part of the saline-soluble glycoproteins of the connective tissue, while electrophoretically similar to the plasma glycoproteins, may possess significant chemical or physical differences. There is now evidence that at least some of the acid-soluble glycoproteins of connective tissue are synthesized by the cellular components of this tissue.[7]

Acid mucopolysaccharides (*glycosaminoglycans*) have been the most intensively studied components of the ground substance. This class of substances is capable of binding water and cations, and is responsible for at least part of the viscosity of ground substance. Mucopolysaccharides consist of high molecular weight polymers of carbohydrate, frequently associated with protein, but separable from it by mild chemical methods. The carbohydrate, or polysaccharide portion, is frequently a large polymer of a basic disaccharide unit which usually contains a hexosamine and a hexuronic acid moiety linked via a glycosidic bond. Table 5–1 records the composition of the carbohydrate component of some important mucopolysaccharides found in mammalian organisms, including man. The detailed chemistry of "linkage" areas connecting protein and polysaccharide in these protein polysaccharide complexes (*proteoglycans*) is becoming clearer. (See Fig. 5–1.) Chondromucoprotein, a tyrosine-rich, hydroxyproline-free protein found in cartilage, exists in a complex with chondroitin sulfate.[77,102]

Present evidence indicates that the carbohydrate side chains are linked via glycosidic bonds to the hydroxyl groups of serine moieties in the protein chain.[1] Study of the carbohydrate chains near the sites of attachment to the protein core shows that xylose is the initial sugar, followed by two galactose molecules, glucuronic acid, and finally by the disaccharide-repeating units of chondroitin sulfate.[62] The viscosity exhibited by solutions of this macromolecule depends not only on the carbohydrate side chains, but also on the preservation of the intact protein core. When the protein component is disrupted *in vitro* by papain digestion, a fall in viscosity ensues.[73] Intra-

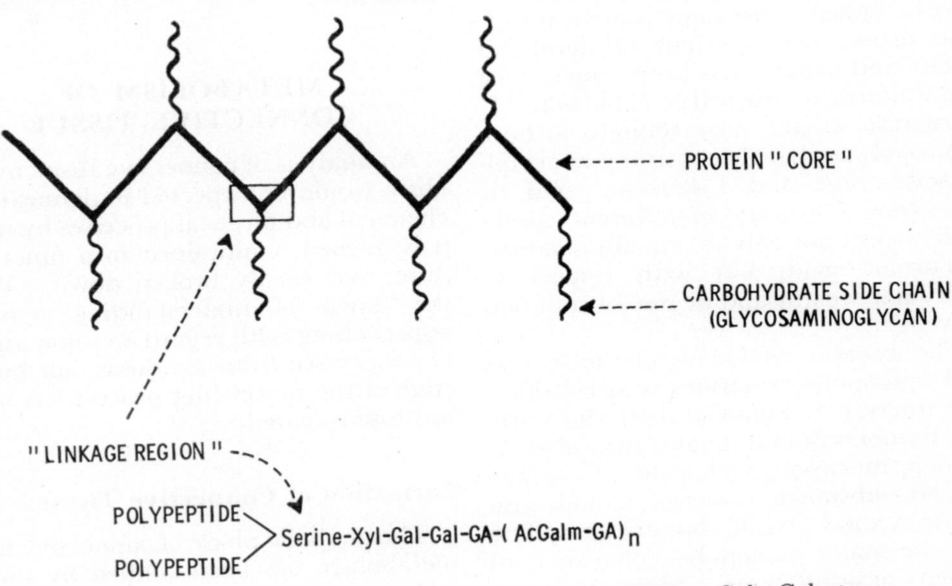

Fig. 5–1.—The linkage area of a proteoglycan. Xyl = Xylose, Gal = Galactose, GA = Glucuronic Acid, and AcGalm = Acetyl Galactosamine.

venous administration of papain to rabbits leads to loss of sulfated mucopolysaccharide from cartilage and to physical collapse of some cartilaginous structures.[68]

The schematic diagram of a typical proteoglycan macromolecule (Fig. 5–1) corresponds to electronmicrographs of protein-polysaccharide from nasal cartilage showing carbohydrate chains radiating in a perpendicular manner at regular intervals from a central protein filament.[93] While the "linkage" region illustrated (Fig. 5–1) appears correct for chondroitin-4-sulfate, dermatan sulfate, and heparin, the picture is less clear for other mucopolysaccharides. The variability in pentoses, hexoses, and apparent amino acid branch points suggests that some glycosaminoglycans may have different "linkage" structures in different tissues. For instance, the hyaluronate isolated from brain includes traces of arabinose, glucose, and galactose, while that from umbilical cord lacks arabinose.[117,91] There is also evidence that keratosulfate from human rib cartilage is bound to protein via N-acetylgalactosamine linked to serine and threonine.[14] Complicating matters yet further are data indicating that in some tissues keratosulfate and chondroitin-4-sulfate may be linked to the same protein core.[94] The uronic acid content of dermatan sulfate and heparin has been shown to be non-uniform as recorded in Table 5–1.[36,63] Dermatan sulfate, once thought to be a heteropolysaccharide consisting of acetylgalactosamine and L-iduronic acid, is now known to vary in different tissues with respect not only to amount of added glucuronic acid, but with respect to molecular weight and degree of sulfation as well.[37]

The *anatomic distribution* of the several acid mucopolysaccharides is of considerable interest.[70] Synovial fluid and vitreous humor contain hyaluronic acid as the sole mucopolysaccharide. Cartilage ground substance possesses chondroitin sulfate A and C, while chondroitin sulfate A is the major mucopolysaccharide constituent of adult bone. Mixtures of the chondroitin sulfates and hyaluronic acid occur in such diverse locations as umbilical cord, skin, tendon, heart valve, and aorta. Heparitin sulfate, a family of compounds with variable acetyl and sulfate content, has been isolated from aorta, lung, liver, and amyloid tissue.[69,27] In addition, this class of compounds is excreted in the urine in large amounts by some patients with Hurler's syndrome, a hereditary disease involving connective tissue. Heparin may be recovered from liver, lung, and aorta. Keratosulfate has been identified in cornea, nucleus pulposus, aging cartilage, and in small amounts in growing bone. Chondroitin has been identified only in the cornea.

Lipid is found in connective tissue formed in response to polyvinyl sponge implantation where as much as 20 to 30 per cent of the dry weight is reported to consist of fatty acids, phospholipids, and cholesterol.[15] Autoradiographic studies using glycerol-1,3-^{14}C indicate that substantial amounts of the lipidic materials formed by such granulomata are deposited in the ground substance.[8] The structural configurations, functions, and metabolism of ground substance lipids in normal and pathologic tissue are not understood.

METABOLISM OF CONNECTIVE TISSUE

An analysis of connective tissue metabolism would be expected to delineate the chemical and physical processes by which it is formed, maintained in a functional state, and finally broken down. While the dawn of understanding may be approaching with regard to some aspects of connective tissue synthesis, our knowledge of the succeeding processes is much less sophisticated.

Formation of Connective Tissue

The anabolic phase of connective tissue metabolism has been studied by several techniques which provoke a host inflammatory response, including first an exudative and then a proliferative or reparative phase. One profitable experimental model has been the healing wound where combined histochemical and analytical chemical techniques have illuminated the orderly sequence of connective tissue formation. After wounding, the connective tissue defect is flooded with plasma proteins and leukocytes from the circulatory system. As the reparative phase is initiated, the microscopist is impressed with the sudden numerical increase in cellular elements. During early wound repair, the active proliferation of connective tissue cells is accompanied by an impressive tinctorial alteration in the ground substance, characterized by prominent metachromatic staining which may reflect high local concentrations of acid mucopolysaccharides. Soon one can detect fine intercellular argyrophilic reticular fibers (more likely small collagen fibers than true reticulin). As the reparative phase continues, the fibers become more numerous and individually larger, while the cellular elements decrease in number and in their individual cytoplasmic mass, and the metachromatic hue of the ground substance subsides. Chemical analyses made along the time course of the connective tissue reparative process show the hexosamine content (from glycoproteins and acid mucopolysaccharides) to fall steadily after an early peak, while hydroxyproline, as a measure of collagen, rises steadily.[32] Similar results have been obtained from studies of newly formed connective tissue stimulated by implantation of polyvinyl sponges. Where uronic acid has been measured instead of hexosamine as an indicator of acid mucopolysaccharide content, the peak values and period of decline appear to occur later in the reparative process.[11]

Protein depletion of an animal prior to wounding is known to retard healing and reduce wound tensile strength. Analysis of wound-induced granulation tissue from protein-depleted animals revealed decreased amounts of hexosamine and hydroxyproline, suggesting that fibroblastic synthesis of ground substance and collagenous elements had been retarded. This retardation of connective tissue formation in the protein-depleted animal can apparently be reversed by supplementation with methionine.[116] Failure of collagen fiber formation after wounding can also be induced in guinea pigs by ascorbic acid deficiency, possibly by preventing the hydroxylation of proline.[41]

The biosynthesis of collagen may be considered as a sequence involving: 1) polypeptide synthesis, 2) hydroxylation of proline and lysine residues, 3) carbohydrate addition, 4) extracellular aggregation into fibrils, and 5) development of cross-links. Polypeptide synthesis takes place on polyribosome aggregates of the endoplasmic reticulum in connective tissue cells. In chick corium, collagen polypeptide synthesis has been shown to be associated with very large polyribosomal aggregates which sediment at rates of 350–1600 S. These large aggregates appeared to be stabilized by the newly formed polypeptides, since they were extensively disrupted by bacterial collagenase.[35] This newly formed "protocollagen" serves as a substrate for a post-ribosomal hydroxylation reaction which converts many proline and lysine residues to hydroxyproline and hydroxylysine, thus forming molecules which resemble α chains. The protocollagen hydroxylase which carries out this reaction requires oxygen, ascorbic acid, ferrous iron, and α ketoglutarate.[87] Extracellular aggregation of α chains into tropocollagen molecules may occur spontaneously as a consequence of steric characteristics of the α chains, although a role for ground substance mucopolysaccharides and glycoproteins in regulating this process has not been excluded. An important development in understanding the collagen cross-linking process was the demonstration of a soluble enzyme in chick bone which converts peptide-bound lysine to α amino-adipic semialdehyde.[84] As noted earlier, this reactive aldehyde forms cross-links via aldol condensation reactions and

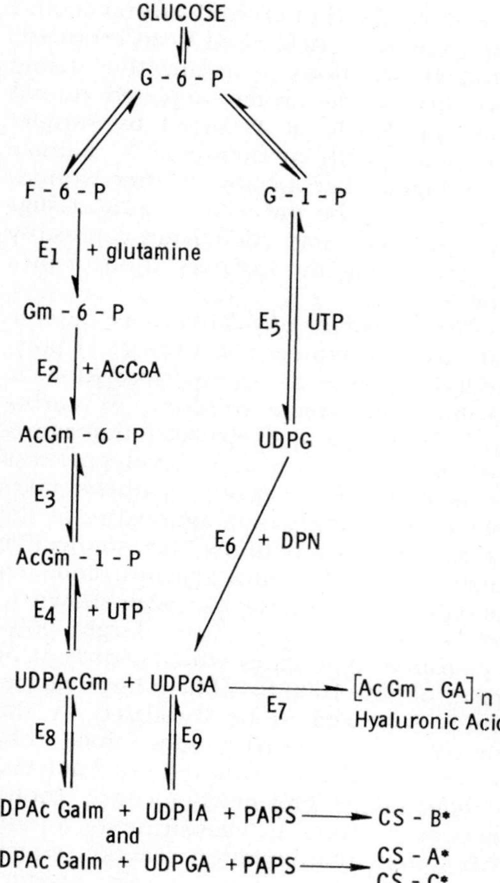

FIG. 5–2.—Hypothetical scheme for enzymatic synthesis of glycosaminoglycans from glucose. Abbreviations: G-6-P = glucose-6-PO_4; G-1-P = glucose-1-PO_4; Gm-6-P = glucosamine-6-PO_4; AcGm-6-P = N-acetylglucosamine-6-PO_4; AcGm-1-P = N-acetylglucosamine-1-PO_4; UTP = uridine triphosphate; AcCoA = acetyl coenzyme A; UDPG = uridine diphosphoglucose; UDPAcGm = uridine diphosphoacetylglucosamine; UDPGA = uridine diphosphoglucuronic acid; UPDAcGalm = uridine diphosphoacetylgalactosamine; UDPIA = uridine diphosphoiduronic acid; GA = glucuronic acid; DPN = diphosphopyridine nucleotide; PAPS = 3′-phosphoadenosine-5′-phosphosulfate; F-6-P = fructose-6-PO_4; "E" represents the enzyme responsible for each reaction. The majority of the enzymes noted were originally described in microbial systems. References describing the individual enzymes are as follows:

E_1 (60,6); E_2 (28); E_3 (89); E_4 (64); E_5 (53); E_6 (109); E_7 (65); E_8 (39,51); E_9 (50).

formation of Schiff bases with amino groups of lysine and hydroxylysine in adjacent chains.

The biosynthesis of ground substance acid mucopolysaccharides includes synthesis of the protein core, linkage region, and the repeating disaccharide units of the side chains. Formation of the "linkage" region (as in Fig. 5–1) may be initiated by an enzyme which transfers xylose from UDPXyl to the protein core.[90] Galactose residues are then added to "xylosyl-protein" by another transferase enzyme.[48] Recently, a glucuronosyltransferase has been described in chick brain which transfers glucuronic acid from UDPGA to the final galactose, thus completing formation of the linkage region.[13]

The biosynthetic pathways leading to *formation of the glycosaminoglycan chains* of repeating disaccharide units have been illuminated largely by research employing microbiological systems. Isotope studies carried out with a hyaluronic acid-producing group A streptococcus demonstrated conversion of glucose to both the glucosamine and glucuronic acid moieties without scission of the glucose carbon skeleton.[92] Figure 5–2 is a diagrammatic summary of some proven enzymatic reactions which represent possible routes for glycosaminoglycan biosynthesis.

Whether such pathways are operative, or important, in the formation of mucopolysaccharides in higher forms of life is not known. Such information is of obvious importance since it must precede the detection of possible pathologic alterations in disease states. As we have already seen, numerous studies of *in vivo* granuloma formation have outlined the general nature and sequence of many major events leading to the formation of

* CS-A, B, and C refer to the three varieties of chondroitin sulfate. The schematic summary equation ignores the uncertainties relevant to the mechanism of sulfation and formation of the protein-polysaccharide complex. It may be noted that UDPGA can be enzymatically converted to UDP-xylose, which is required to initiate the "linkage region."

a connective tissue. In an effort to further explore the fundamental nature of these "major events," investigators have exploited the *in vivo* granuloma, tissue slice, and cell culture techniques.

Studies of polyvinyl sponge granulomas induced in guinea pigs provide evidence for a pyrophosphorylase that converts glucose-1-PO_4 and UTP to UDPG. The same experimental system served to demonstrate the existence of a UDPG dehydrogenase which catalyzes the formation of uridine diphosphoglucuronic acid (UDPGA). These enzymes, which may play a role in mammalian mucopolysaccharide biosynthesis, have both been identified in human synovial tissue.[10]

When slices of rabbit subcutaneous tissue were incubated in a saline medium, hexosamine synthesis appeared to be glucose dependent.[9] Confirmatory evidence came from isotope experiments where human synovial slices were briefly incubated in a buffer with uniformly labeled glucose-C^{14} and showed incorporation of radioactivity into a substance tentatively identified as hyaluronic acid.[120] Cell culture experiments using connective tissue cells from many sources have also demonstrated *in vitro* synthesis of acid mucopolysaccharides.[45] Cultures of human synovial tissue synthesize hyaluronic acid from the components of a chemically defined medium.[19] In general, the data support the idea that connective tissue cells synthesize glycosaminoglycans locally from simple precursors.

The process by which sulfate is incorporated into glycosaminoglycans has intrigued many investigators. There is considerable evidence that sulfate is enzymatically transferred from 3′-phosphoadenosine-5′-phosphosulfate (PAPS) to the polymerized glycosaminoglycan.[110,103] A newly described enzyme of considerable interest is a sulfotransferase which catalyzes the sulfation of UDPAcGalm to form uridinediphosphate-N-acetylgalactosamine-4 sulfate.[114] Whether this material serves as an immediate precursor for the formation of sulfated glycosaminoglycans is not yet known.

Maintenance and Catabolism of Connective Tissue

The nature of the energy metabolism required to maintain a functional connective tissue, once formed, has been explored in a fragmentary manner. Oxygen consumption as measured in the Warburg apparatus appears to be meager in guinea pig skin and normal synovium of human and equine origin. However, careful measurements of oxygen and glucose uptake and lactate formation by normal synovium revealed appreciable aerobic and anaerobic glycolysis.[29] Malate, fumarate, and succinate markedly stimulated oxygen uptake of normal synovium, suggesting that the enzymes of the tricarboxylic acid cycle required for their oxidation are present, even though playing a minor role in the energy metabolism of the normal tissue.[75] This is of interest, since inflamed rheumatoid synovium appeared to develop a significant oxidative metabolism as well as a more robust rate of glycolysis than normal tissue.

Isotope techniques provide a convenient method for *measuring the turnover rates of constituents of connective tissue*. In the case of collagen, at least three fractions are recognized; a neutral salt or alkali-soluble fraction, a citric acid-soluble fraction, and an insoluble residue. Except in rapidly growing animals, neutral salt- or alkali-soluble material represents a small fraction of the total collagen mass. When labeled with glycine ^{14}C, this material, which presumably includes tropocollagen, exhibits a half-life of one or two days' duration, and probably represents the precursor of mature, insoluble collagen.[104] Thus neutral salt-soluble collagen, a relatively small component of the collagen mass, is more active in a metabolic sense than even the plasma proteins. On the other hand, the insoluble collagen is by far the largest fraction and has a prolonged half-life. Such data suggest that most of the fibrous collagen is relatively inert metabolically. Acid-soluble collagen behaves like the insoluble residue material in isotope experiments, but is probably less highly cross-linked than the insoluble material.

Collagenase has been demonstrated in association with living cells in regions of active collagen resorption, as in the tail fin of the tadpole during metamorphosis, the involuting uterus, in remodeling bone, rheumatoid synovial tissue, and human polymorphonuclear leukocytes.[42,44,95,34,59] This long-sought degradative enzyme cleaves native collagen into one-quarter length and three-quarter length molecules. Collagen degraded by this enzyme shows partial loss of its viscous property, a reduction in denaturation temperature, and loss of immunity to attack by less specific proteases. While the importance of this enzyme in physiologic remodeling processes has been stressed, it is also clear that it is a candidate for a major role in tissue destruction by pathologic processes. There is already evidence that collagenase-producing rheumatoid synovium has the capacity, *in vitro*, to invade and destroy connective tissue.[46] Rheumatoid synovial fluid is now known to harbor two kinds of collagenase. The "B" form resembles that produced in tissue culture and is inhibited by serum. The "A" form has twice the molecular weight (40–50,000), and will degrade collagen in solution or as fibers in the presence of serum.[47]

Mucopolysaccharides of rodent skin were labeled with ^{14}C-acetate, ^{35}S-sulfate, and ^{14}C-glucose, and the biologic half-life of different components was computed.[97,98] The biological half-life of hyaluronic acid was two to four days, while that of chondroitin sulfate extended from seven to ten days. A double-labeled experiment, using $^{35}SO_4$ and lysine-l-^{14}C, respectively, to label the carbohydrate and protein portions of chondromucoprotein, was interpreted as indicating that the complex was metabolized as a unit.[43] Definition of the relative significance of tissue polysaccharidases, glycosidases, and specific proteases may be expected to clarify the mechanism of degradation of mucopolysaccharide-protein complexes.

It is clear that collagen is a relatively static material with an active capacity for repair or replacement, and that the mucopolysaccharides of connective tissue are continuously in active flux. Information concerning quantitative changes in the nature and turnover rates of the various constituents in different physiologic and pathologic situations may be of fundamental importance. In this connection, study of the composition of polyvinyl sponge granulomas revealed that with *aging* the proportion of total protein represented by collagen increased as did the concentration of lipids.[55] In a related vein are the results from chemical analyses of human costal cartilage of varying ages.[71,108] Whereas the mucopolysaccharide of neonatal cartilage was chondroitin sulfate, the relative amount of keratosulfate increased with aging while the proportion of chondroitin sulfate fell. In human aortic tissue the relative amounts of hyaluronate and chondroitin sulfate C decreased with aging, while heparitin sulfate and chondroitin sulfate B increased.[57] Such data led to the suggestion that "differentiation" rather than degeneration might characterize the aging process in this connective tissue.[56]

REGULATION OF THE CONNECTIVE TISSUE

Regulation of the metabolic activities of connective tissue is an intricate process requiring a balanced interplay of many agents. Where hormonal alterations of connective tissue have been reported, the effect noted has been a quantitative alteration of some or all of the components of the connective tissue. Stimulation of mucopolysaccharide formation is said to follow administration of androgen, estrogen, thyrotropin, and somatotropin.[2,33] Somatotropin may also promote collagen formation, and aldosterone is said to stimulate granulation tissue around foreign bodies, while suppression of mucopolysaccharide synthesis has been attributed to thyroid hormone. These generalizations must be viewed with caution, particularly as to their applicability to human physiology. Some of the effects reported may be species specific, and frequently the method of quantitative assay of the connective tissue components has been nonspecific.

Adrenal glucocorticoids are the most adequately studied of the "suppressive" hormones. An excess of adrenal glucocorticoid will suppress both the oxidative and glycolytic metabolism of rheumatoid synovium *in vitro*,[30] interfere with *in vivo* formation of granulation tissue,[5] reduce the cellularity and dermal thickness of rat skin following local application,[22] reduce the hexosamine to collagen ratio in rat connective tissue,[106] and suppress the uptake of labeled sulfate into the sulfated mucopolysaccharides of rodents.[96] Data supporting a local action of hydrocortisone on connective tissue also come from cell culture experiments which show that near physiologic concentrations of this hormone induce multiple effects in human fibroblasts. These include accelerated mitosis, suppression of collagen deposition, and depression of the specific rate of hyaluronate formation.[19,20] Such effects have been maintained for up to four months *in vitro* without evidence of either accumulative action or escape from the hormone, and all measured evidence of hormone effect was promptly reversible on steroid omission from the cultures.[18]

Information concerning the role of vitamins in the regulation of connective tissue metabolism is limited. The importance of ascorbic acid at the local connective tissue level for collagen fiber formation has been noted. Vitamin A apparently has an effect on connective tissue since intoxication with this substance is associated with osteoclastic bone resorption, a lesion which can be aggravated by concurrent administration of adrenal glucocorticoids.[101] A role for trace metals is suggested by findings in copper-deficient chicks where aortic elastic tissue was quantitatively reduced and qualitatively altered with respect to solubility properties and lysine content.[107] The speculation that copper deficiency may induce a cross-link defect, perhaps involving the desmosines, is under study in several laboratories. Among the nonphysiologic substances known to alter the connective tissues, the active principal of the sweet pea (Lathyrus odoratus) is important as an investigative tool. The β-amino-proprionitrile-glutamine conjugate (BAPN) found in the sweet pea induces widespread defects in the supporting tissues of weanling rats, including proliferative and degenerative lesions of cartilage and bone.[85,86] A major action of BAPN in causing these connective tissue lesions may be its capacity to block the enzymatic formation of aldehydes required for cross-linking of collagen and elastin. Penicillamine not only inhibits cross-linking, but may actually cleave newly formed intermolecular cross-links.

Regulation of hyaluronate synthesis in human synovial tissue may be at least partially dependent on a "connective tissue activating peptide" (CTAP) which is widely distributed in mammalian cells, including leukocytes and connective tissue cells.[23,24] This interesting polypeptide markedly stimulates glycolysis in synovial cells *in vitro* and increases the rate of hyaluronic acid formation by 10 to 40 times the basal rate in unstimulated cultures. Of special interest is the fact that hyaluronate formed as a consequence of intense activation of synovial cells is of low molecular weight, as in most inflammatory synovial effusions. Increased amounts of CTAP in cultured rheumatoid synovial cells may offer a partial explanation for the many propagatable "abnormalities" that have been demonstrated in cultivated rheumatoid synovial cells.[25,26] The idea that CTAP mediates the transition from the exudative stage of inflammation to the proliferative (reparative) stage is now supported by evidence from *in vivo* granulomata showing an early peak of CTAP activity corresponding with maximal elaboration of hyaluronate into the ground substance.

The mechanism of the anti-inflammatory action of drugs such as phenylbutazone and salicylates remains an unsolved mystery. Clinical studies[79] indicate that the anti-inflammatory effect of salicylates is independent of the adrenal cortex. Emphasis has been placed recently on the capacity of these anti-inflammatory organic acids to uncouple oxidative phosphorylation, thereby presumably limiting the energy supply available to execute the operational sequences of the inflammatory process.[118]

More than anything else, the investigations to date have emphasized the complexity of the connective tissue and spotlighted approaches to understanding its structure and function. It is reasonable to hope that by utilizing improving methodology, continued exploration of the composition and metabolism of the connective tissues will provide us with sufficient understanding to permit identification of the defects in the rheumatic diseases.

BIBLIOGRAPHY

1. Anderson, B., Hoffman, P., and Meyer, K.: J. Biol. Chem., *240*, 156, 1965.
2. Asboe-Hansen, G.: Amer. J. Med., *26*, 470, 1959.
3. Bangle, R. J.: Amer. J. Path., *28*, 1027, 1952.
4. Baker, B. L. and Han, S. S.: *Transactions of the Conference on The Biology of Connective Tissue Cells*, New York, The Arth. and Rheum. Foundation Conference Series No. 7, 1962, pp. 1–25.
5. Baker, B. L. and Whitaker, W. L.: Endocrinol., *46*, 544, 1950.
6. Blumental, H. J., Horowitz, S. T., Hemmerline, A., and Roseman, S.: Bact. Proc., *137*, 82, 1955.
7. Bole, G. G.: The University of Michigan Med. Center J., Dec., 1968, p. 283.
8. Bole, G. G.: Arth. & Rheum., *9*, 295, 1966.
9. Bollet, A. J., Boas, N. F., and Bunim, J. J.: Science, *120*, 348, 1954.
10. Bollet, A. J., Goodwin, J. F., and Brown, A. K.: J. Clin. Invest., *38*, 451, 1959.
11. Bollet, A. J., Goodwin, J. F., Simpson, W. F., and Anderson, D. V.: Proc. Soc. Exp. Biol. and Med., *99*, 418, 1958.
12. Bornstein, P. and Piez, K. A.: Biochemistry, *5*, 3460, 1966.
13. Brandt, A. E., Distler, J., Jourdian, G. W.: Proc. Nat. Acad. Sci., *64*, 374, 1969.
14. Bray, B. A., Lieberman, R., and Meyer, K.: J. Biol. Chem., *242*, 3373, 1967.
15. Boucek, R. J. and Noble, N. L.: Arch. of Path., *59*, 553, 1955.
16. Butler, W. T. and Cunningham, L. W.: J. Biol. Chem., *241*, 3882, 1966.
17. Castor, C. W.: Arth. & Rheum., *3*, 140, 1960.
18. ———: J. Lab. Clin. Med., *65*, 490, 1965.
19. Castor, C. W. and Fries, F. F.: J. Lab. Clin. Med., *57*, 394, 1961.
20. Castor, C. W. and Muirden, K. D.: Lab. Invest., *13*, 560, 1964.
21. Castor, C. W. and Prince, R. K.: Biochim. Biophys. Acta, *83*, 165, 1964.
22. Castor, C. W. and Baker, B. L.: Endocrinol., *47*, 234, 1950.
23. Castor, C. W., Smith, S. F., Ritchie, J. C., and Dorstewitz, E. L.: Arth. & Rheum., *14*, 41, 1971.
24. Castor, C. W., Dorstewitz, E. L., Smith, S. F., and Ritchie, J. C.: Arth. & Rheum., *14*, 55, 1971.
25. Castor, C. W. and Dorstewitz, E. L.: J. Lab. Clin. Med., *68*, 300, 1966.
26. Castor, C. W., Dorstewitz, E. L., Rowe, K., and Ritchie, J. C.: J. Lab. Clin. Med., *77*, 65, 1971.
27. Cifonelli, J. A. and Dorfman, A.: J. Biol. Chem., *235*, 3283, 1960.
28. Davidson, E. A., Blumenthal, H. J., and Roseman, S.: J. Biol. Chem., *226*, 125, 1957.
29. Dingle, J. T. M. and Page Thomas, D. P.: Brit. J. Exp. Path., *37*, 318, 1956.
30. ———: Ann. Rheum. Dis., *16*, 464, 1957.
31. Doty, P. M.: *Transactions of Second National Conference on Research and Education in Rheumatic Diseases* (1956) Arth. and Rheum. Foundation, 1957, p. 21–32.
32. Dunphy, J. E. and Udupa, K. N.: New Eng. J. Med., *253*, 847, 1955.
33. Edwards, L. C. and Dunphy, J. E.: New Eng. J. Med., *259*, 275, 1958.
34. Evanson, J. M., Jeffrey, J. J., and Krane, S. M.: J. Clin. Invest., *47*, 2639, 1968.
35. Fernández-Madrid, F.: J. Cell Biol., *33*, 27, 1967.
36. Fransson, L. A. and Rodén, L.: J. Biol. Chem., *242*, 4170, 1967.
37. Fransson, L. A., Anseth, A., Antonopoulos, C. A., and Gardell, S.: Carbohydrate Research, *15*, 73, 1970.

38. Franzblau, C. and Lent, R. W.: Brookhaven Symposium in Biology, *21*, 358, 1968.
39. Glaser, L.: J. Biol. Chem., *234*, 2801, 1959.
40. Glegg, R. E., Eidinger, D., and Leblond, C. P.: Science, *118*, 614, 1953.
41. Gould, B. S. and Woessner, J. F.: J. Biol. Chem., *226*, 289, 1957.
42. Gross, J. and Lapiere, C. M.: Proc. Nat. Acad. Sci., *48*, 1014, 1962.
43. Gross, J. I., Mathews, M. B., and Dorfman, A.: J. Biol. Chem., *235*, 2889, 1960.
44. Gross, J. and Nagai, Y.: Proc. Nat. Acad. Sci., *54*, 1197, 1965.
45. Grossfeld, H., Meyer, K., Godman, G., and Linker, A.: J. of Biophys. and Biochem. Cytol., *3*, 3, 391, 1957.
46. Harris, E. D., Evanson, J. M., DiBona, D. R., and Krane, S. M.: Arth. & Rheum., *13*, 83, 1970.
47. Harris, E. D., DiBona, D. R., and Krane, S. M.: J. Clin. Invest., *48*, 2104, 1969.
48. Helting, T. and Rodén, L.: Biochem. Biophys. Res. Comm., *31*, 786, 1968.
49. Igarashi, S., Kang, A. H., and Gross, J.: Biochem. Biophys. Res. Comm., *38*, 697, 1970.
50. Jacobson, B. and Davidson, E. A.: J. Biol. Chem., *237*, 638, 1962.
51. ———: Biochim. Biophys. Acta, *73*, 145, 1963.
52. Jasin, H. E. and Glynn, L. E.: Arth. & Rheum., *7*, 740, 1964.
53. Kalkar, H. M.: Science, *125*, 105, 1957.
54. Kang, A. H., Igarashi, S., and Gross, J.: Biochemistry, *8*, 3200, 1969.
55. Kao, K. T., Boucek, R. J., and Noble, N. L.: J. of Gerontol., *12*, 153, 1957.
56. Kaplan, D. and Meyer, K.: *Report at the Second Pan American Congress on Rheumatic Diseases*, Washington, June, 1959.
57. ———: Proc. Soc. Exp. Biol. Med., *105*, 78, 1960.
58. Lansing, A. I., Rosenthal, T. B., Alex, M., and Dempsey, E. W.: Anat. Rec., *114*, 555, 1952.
59. Lazarus, G. S., Brown, R. S., Daniels, J. R., and Fullmer, H. M.: Science, *159*, 1483, 1968.
60. Leloir, L. F. and Cardini, C. E.: Biochim. Biophys. Acta, *12*, 15, 1953.
61. LeRoy, E. C.: Proc. Soc. Exp. Biol. Med., *128*, 341, 1968.
62. Lindahl, U. and Rodén, L.: Biochem. and Biophys. Res. Comm., *17*, 254, 1964.
63. Lindahl, U.: Biochim. Biophys. Acta, *130*, 368, 1966.
64. Maley, F. and Lardy, H. A.: Science, *124*, 1207, 1956.
65. Markovitz, A., Cifonelli, J. A., and Dorfman, A.: Biochim. Biophys. Acta, *28*, 453, 1958.
66. Maximow, A. A. and Bloom, W.: *A Textbook of Histology*, Ed. 7, Philadelphia, W. B. Saunders Co., 1957, p. 113.
67. McManus, J. F. A.: in *Connective Tissue in Health and Disease* ed. by Asboe-Hansen, G., Copenhagen, Munksgaard, 1954, p. 45.
68. McCluskey, R. T. and Thomas, L.: J. Exp. Med., *108*, 371, 1958.
69. Meyer, K.: *Small Blood Vessel Involvement in Diabetes Mellitus*, The American Institute of Biological Sciences, 1964.
70. Meyer, K., Davidson, E., Linker, A., and Hoffman, P.: Biochim. Biophys. Acta, *21*, 506, 1956.
71. Meyer, K., Hoffman, P., and Linker, A.: Science, *128*, 896, 1958.
72. Michaeli, D., Martin, G. R., Kettman, J., Benjamini, E., Leung, D. V. K., and Blatt, B. A.: Science, *166*, 1522, 1969.
73. Muir, H.: Biochem. Jour., *69*, 195, 1958.
74. Noback, C. R. and Paff, G. H.: Anat. Rec., *109*, 71, 1951.
75. Page Thomas, D. P. and Dingle, J. T.. Biochem. J., *68*, 231, 1958.
76. Partridge, S. M. and Davis, H. F.: Biochem. J., *61*, 21, 1955.
77. ———: Biochem. J., *68*, 298, 1958.
78. Partridge, S. M., Davis, H. F., and Adair, G. S.: Biochem. J., *61*, 11, 1955.
79. Peterson, R. E., Black, R. L., and Bunim, J. J.: Arth. & Rheum., *1*, 29, 1958.
80. Piez, K. A., Eigner, E. A., and Lewis, M. S.: Biochemistry, *2*, 58, 1963.
81. Piez, K. A., Bladen, H. A., Lane, J. M., Miller, E. J., Bornstein, P., Butler, W. T., and Kang, A. H.: Brookhaven Symp. in Biol., *21*, 345, 1968.
82. Piez, K. A.: Biochemistry, *4*, 2590, 1965.
83. Piez, K. A.: *Annual Review of Biochemistry*, ed. P. D. Boyer, Palo Alto, Calif.: Annual Review Inc., 1968, p. 547.
84. Pinnell, S. R. and Martin, G. R.: Proc. Nat. Acad. Sci., *61*, 708, 1968.
85. Ponseti, I. V. and Shepard, R. S.: J. Bone & Joint Surg., *36A*, 1031, 1954.
86. Ponseti, I. V., Wawzonek, S., Shepard, R. S., Evans, T. C., and Stearns, G.: Proc. Soc. Exp. Biol. & Med., *92*, 366, 1956.
87. Prockop, D. J. and Kivirikko, K. I.: Chapter 5, *Treatise on Collagen*, Vol. 2, Part A, Ed. B. S. Gould, New York, Academic Press, 1968, p. 220.

88. Randall, J. T.: *Nature and Structure of Collagen*, New York, Academic Press, Inc., 1953.
89. Reissig, J. L.: J. Biol. Chem., *219*, 753, 1956.
90. Robinson, H. C., Telser, A., and Dorfman, A.: Proc. Nat. Acad. Sci., *56*, 1859, 1966.
91. Rodén, L.: *Symposium, 7th International Congress of Biochemistry*, Abstracts I., 1967, p. 69.
92. Roseman, S., Moses, F. E., Ludowieg, J., and Dorfman, A.: J. Biol. Chem., *203*, 213, 1953.
93. Rosenberg, L., Hellman, W., and Kleinschmidt, A. K.: J. Biol. Chem., *245*, 4123, 1970.
94. Rosenblum, E. L. and Cifonelli, J. A.: Fed. Proc., *26*, 282, 1967.
95. Sakai, T. and Gross, J.: Biochemistry, *6*, 518, 1967.
96. Schiller, S. and Dorfman, A.: Endocrinol., *60*, 376, 1957.
97. Schiller, S., Mathews, M. B., Cifonelli, J. H., and Dorfman, A.: J. Biol. Chem., *218*, 139, 1956.
98. Schiller, S., Mathews, M. B., Goldfaber, L., Ludowieg, J., and Dorfman, A.: J. Biol. Chem., *212*, 531, 1955.
99. Schindler, R., Day, M., and Fischer, G. A.: Cancer Res., *19*, 47, 1959.
100. Segrest, J. P. and Cunningham, L. W.: J. Clin. Invest., *49*, 1497, 1970.
101. Selye, H.: Arth. & Rheum., *1*, 87, 1958.
102. Shatton, J. and Schubert, M.: J. Biol. Chem., *211*, 565, 1954.
103. Silbert, J. E.: J. Biol. Chem., *242*, 5133, 1967.
104. Slack, H. G. B.: Amer. J. Med., *26*, 113, 1959.
105. Smyth, C. J. and Gum, O. B.: Arth. & Rheum., *1*, 178, 1958.
106. Sobel, H., Gabay, S., and Johnson, C.: Proc. Soc. Exp. Biol. Med., *99*, 296, 1958.
107. Starcher, B., Hill, C. H., and Matrone, G.: J. Nutr., *82*, 318, 1964.
108. Stidworthy, G., Masters, Y. F., and Shetlar, M. R.: J. Gerontol., *13*, 10, 1958.
109. Strominger, J. L., Maxwell, E. S., Axelrod, J., and Kalkar, H. M.: J. Biol. Chem., *224*, 79, 1957.
110. Suzuki, S. and Strominger, J. L.: J. Biol. Chem., *235*, 257, 1960.
111. Tanzer, M. L. and Mechanic, G.: Biochem. and Biophys. Res. Comm., *39*, 183, 1970.
112. Tanzer, M. L., Mechanic, G., and Gallop, P. M.: Biochim. Biophys. Acta, *207*, 548, 1970.
113. Trelstad, R. L., Kang, A. H., Igarashi, S., and Gross, J.: Biochemistry, *9*, 4993, 1970.
114. Tsuji, M., Shimizu, S., Nakanishi, Y., and Suzuki, S.: J. Biol. Chem., *245*, 6039, 1970.
115. Thomas, J., Elsden, E. F., and Partridge, S. M.: Nature (London), *200*, 651, 1963.
116. Udupa, K. N., Woessner, J. F., and Dunphy, J. E.: Surg. Gyn. and Obst., *102*, 639, 1956.
117. Wardi, A. H., Allen, W. S., Turner, D. L., and Stary, Z.: Arch. Biochem. Biophys., *117*, 44, 1966.
118. Whitehouse, M. W.: In *International Symposium on Non-Steroidal Anti-Inflammatory Drugs*, Amsterdam, Excerpta Medica Foundation, 1965, p. 52.
119. Willmer, E. N.: *Tissue Culture*, Ed. 2, London, Methuen and Co., Ltd., 1954, p. 121.
120. Yielding, K. L., Tomkins, G. M., and Bunim, J. J.: Science, *125*, 1300, 1957.

Chapter 6

The Study of Synovial Fluid

By Ralph A. Jessar, M.D.

The knowledge of the presence of the viscid fluid within the joint cavity dates from the 16th century when it was first noted by Paracelsus.[84] This viscous, pale yellow, clear fluid lying within diarthrodial joints and resembling egg white, is known as synovia or synovial fluid. The synovial fluid, its components and its source, the surrounding synovial membrane, has been the subject of much fruitful study and the subject of several excellent reviews.[6,25,31,80,84]

Synovial fluid is formed as a dialysate of blood plasma. It is clear yellow and contains protein; hyaluronate, a secretory product of the synovial cells is added to this transudate.

SYNOVIAL FLUID CONSTITUENTS

Hyaluronate

The hyaluronate imparts to the synovial fluid its characteristic sticky and

Normal Synovial Fluid[84]

	Range	*Average*
Amount in Knee, cc.	0.13 — 3.5	1.1
Relative Viscosity at 25° C	5.7 —1160.	235
pH	7.2 — 7.4	7.4
Leukocyte Count, per cu. mm.	13 — 180	63
Differential—per cent		
Polymorphonuclears	0 — 25	6.5
Lymphocytes	0 — 78	24.6
Monocytes	0 — 71	47.9
Clasmatocytes	0 — 26	10.1
Unclassified phagocytes	0 — 21	4.9
Synovial Lining Cells	0 — 12	4.3
Total solids, gm. per 100 gm.	2.4 — 4.83	3.41
Total albumin and globulin, gm. per 100 cc.	1.07 — 2.13	1.72
Albumin, gm. per 100 cc.		1.02
Globulin, gm. per 100 cc.		.05
Mucin nitrogen, gm. per 100 cc.	0.068— 0.135	0.104
Mucin glucosamine, gm. per 100 cc.	0.012— 0.132	0.074
Fibrinogen	0	
Glucose	Approximately the same as in plasma	
Non-protein nitrogen	Approximately the same as in plasma	
Electrolytes	Approximately the same as plasma dialysate	
Uric Acid	Approximately the same as in plasma	

viscid qualities. The normal concentration of hyaluronate is about 3.5 mg. per gram of fluid[31,32] and this has been shown to decrease with advancing age.[31,32,46] In normal joints the amount of synovial fluid present is quite limited and no more than 3 ml. of fluid should be present in a knee joint. The hyaluronate exists *in vivo* covalently bound to protein. A complex isolated from synovial fluid found to contain hyaluronate and approximately 2 per cent protein was shown to have anomalous viscosity and the same intrinsic viscosity as the fluid from which it was obtained.[31,87]

Hyaluronate is composed of equimolar proportions of glycosamine and glucuronic acid and exists in normal synovial fluid in long linear chains consisting of 2500 units which randomly coil and kink on themselves so that the molecule in solution occupies a spherical pattern.[31] Molecular weight of hyaluronate of synovial fluid is estimated at 6.5 to 10.9 million[3] and is reduced in rheumatoid arthritis to 1.4 to 2.1 million.[2a] With this large size and the volume of the domain (calculated at 3000 to 4000 Å) occupied by them, the molecules of hyaluronate interlace and show high relative viscosities.[3,31,70]

In the presence of inflammatory disease, particularly rheumatoid arthritis, the viscosity falls paralleled by a decrease in the concentration of the hyaluronate in the synovial fluid,[11,17,33] and a decrease in the size of at least some of the hyaluronate molecules[31,77] either because of a defect in production by synovial cells or degradation by enzymes released into synovial fluid by leukocytes or synovial membrane cells.[42,100] Regardless of the techniques used for its measurement, the hyaluronate is found to be of low concentration (1.29 mg./gm. or less) in active rheumatoid arthritis;[11,18,33] but since the total amount of fluid increases in the synovial effusions the total hyaluronate production is increased.[77] Polymerization of the hyaluronate measured turbidometrically is known to be decreased in rheumatoid fluids and is believed to increase on treatment with salicylates or indomethacin.[42a]

Mucin Clot

The addition of acetic acid to normal synovial fluid leads to the formation of a white ropy clot[84] which contains all the synovial hyaluronate and is 60 to 70 per cent protein.[32] In normal fluid this protein is albumin.[73] A normal mucin clot is tight as opposed to the loose, easily fragmenting, friable clot or flocculent precipitate seen in synovial fluids obtained from the joints of patients with rheumatoid arthritis or other joint inflammation.[40,84] The treatment of normal synovial fluid with hyaluronidase prior to the performance of the mucin clot test leads to the formation of the inflammatory type of precipitate and suggests that the type of clot seen in rheumatoid arthritis may be the result of depolymerization of the hyaluronate.[84] However, dilution of hyaluronate may also lead to the formation of a flocculent precipitate; in the synovial fluid of rheumatoid arthritis the concentration of both albumin and hyaluronate is decreased.[31]

Proteins

In the normal synovial fluid, proteins are present in low concentration, usually approximating one-third that of serum proteins.[33,72] Partition of the protein by paper and moving zone electrophoresis establishes differences in distribution of the synovial fluid protein compared to serum. Synovial fluid protein is 60 to 75 per cent albumin and contains only 6 to 7 per cent alpha 2 globulin.[89] This unusual distribution of protein prevails so long as the synovial membrane is normal, even in the presence of systemic disease in which alpha 2 globulin and acute phase reactants are elevated. In inflammatory synovial fluids the pattern resembles and approaches that of the serum;[8,65,72,91,92] the total protein is increased as are the alpha 2 and other globulin components.[31] By immunoelectrophoresis, Schur and Sandson[94] were able to show that all factors present in serum appeared in inflammatory synovial fluid. This supports the thesis that size of molecules governs the passage of protein across the normal synovial membrane. Fibrinogen is present[94] and these inflammatory synovial fluids will clot. Normal fluids, however, will not clot because of the absence of fibrinogen, as well as other clotting factors normally found in serum.[14]

In rheumatoid arthritis 19S globulins may be increased in the synovial fluid as well as in the serum.[8] Various studies have demonstrated the presence of rheumatoid factor in synovial fluids of rheumatoid patients, some of whom had negative test results for the presence of rheumatoid factor in serum.[82] All immunoglobulin types are produced in rheumatoid synovium. IgG accounts for 79 per cent; less than 10 per cent of IgM is rheumatoid factor.[94c] As much as 100 mg. of IgG can be made daily in a rheumatoid knee.[94b] One observer was able to produce intra-articular dissociation of rheumatoid factor by the use of penicillamine.[45] Recently, hemolytic complement[71] has been shown to be reduced in the synovial fluids of rheumatoid arthritis.[37] This finding suggests the local utilization of complement in an antigen-antibody reaction in rheumatoid arthritis.[37,71] Complement (C′) levels in most other inflammatory fluids are elevated in proportion to the elevated joint fluid protein, i.e. they approximate one third to one half the C′ levels in serum obtained simultaneously. In Reiter's syndrome, for example, joint fluid C′ is usually very high, but only because the serum C′ is also greatly elevated.[37,70c,71,71a]

Other Components

Many chemical components of the synovial fluid have been investigated. It is possible to measure quantitatively: hyaluronate hexosamine[33,96] or hexuronic acid,[11,12] non-dialyzable hexose,[88] sialic acid,[74] glycoproteins,[18,66] total protein,[18] its distribution by electrophoresis[18,65] and ultracentrifugation[94] as well as nonelectrolytes including urea, bilirubin and urates. These varied tests, while helping to separate normal from abnormal joint fluids, give little aid in the practical differential diagnosis of the arthritides.[31]

Lipids in joint fluid have recently been studied by Chung *et al.*[15] and Bole.[10] They have been found in low concentration in normal synovial fluid but equal to 40 to 60 per cent of serum concentration in both osteoarthritic and rheumatoid disease. A direct relationship seems to exist between total protein and lipid constituents in synovial fluid, suggesting that the lipids come from the blood due to increased permeability. However, local production cannot be completely ruled out.

In septic arthritis markedly lowered glucose values related to the presence of organisms which utilize sugar may be of differential help. Rheumatoid fluids containing cell counts in excess of 20,000 tend to have lower glucose levels than that of the serum, and, as would be expected, with counts of over 40,000 per cubic millimeter, glucose levels may be less than 50 mg. per cent due to the glucolytic metabolism of white cells.[84]

The electrolytes in normal fluid are distributed as expected in accordance with the Donnan theory of equilibrium across a semipermeable membrane. Those substances present in the blood plasma, and permeable through capillary endothelium, will be found in synovial fluid in concentrations somewhat lower than those in the serum.

Synovial fluids of rheumatoid arthritics show increased copper, iron and aluminum, while their sera show a decreased concentration of iron, aluminum and chromium and an increase in rubidium and copper[68] confirming early reports that abnormal trace metal metabolism is present in rheumatoid arthritis. Its significance is unknown.

Deviations from normal findings seen in fluids from diseased joints may tend to be reversed toward normal by the local intra-articular instillation of hydrocortisone.[33,47,58] Despite this, rheumatoid synovium does not metabolize radioisotopic labeled cortisol to the same degree[21,22] or as rapidly[64,96b] as osteoarthritic joints.

Enzymes found in synovial fluid have included beta glucuronidase,[44] pepsin, trypsin,[97] amylase, lipase,[75] peroxidase[84] the transaminases, and alkaline and acid phosphatase.[86,95] These may be directly correlated with the increase in polymorphonuclear leukocytes seen with effusions of active synovitis.[95] The presence of these lysosomal hydrolytic enzymes may be accompanied by the degradation of hyaluronate and the digestion of cartilage matrix.[19] Synovial fluid lactic dehydrogenase, but not transaminase, was found by Cohen[16] to be elevated in patients with inflammatory joint disease. The isozyme LDH-5 was markedly elevated in rheumatoid, gouty and septic fluids.

Pyruvic kinase,[47b] lysozyme muramidase,[47b,75a] cathepsin[4] and catalase[1a] were noted to be elevated in inflammatory synovial fluids.

Collagenase has been found present in fresh synovial fluid of some patients with rheumatoid arthritis,[34] in young growing granulation tissue,[23,24,51] rheumatoid synovium and tissue cultured from non-inflamed and inflamed non-rheumatic sources.[35] Synovial cell cultures from rheumatoid patients may attack fragments of cartilage matrix *in vitro* and lyse collagen substrate.[23,29] The origin of collagenase remains unclear but has been suggested to be the synovial cells of mesenchymal origin.[35]

Kinins were found in inflammatory synovial fluids[63] and may be related to inflammatory reactions by virtue of their ability to produce vasodilatation, increased capillary permeability, warmth, contraction of smooth muscle and pain.[63]

Formation and Removal of Synovial Fluid

Knowledge about the formation and absorption of synovial fluids is scanty and fragmentary. Studies on the passage of heterologous proteins into the joints of laboratory animals were carried out as early as 1933 when Bauer *et al.*[7] noted the rapid appearance of egg albumin and horse serum albumin in the knee joints promptly after their intravenous administration. Furthermore, these studies showed that albumin was rapidly detectable in the lymph of the thoracic duct following the intra-articular injection of these substances, but globulins were removed with more difficulty from the joint and could not thus be demonstrated. Removal to local lymph nodes of colloids and fine particulate matter with particle sizes larger than those of serum globulin has demonstrated the problem to be other than one of mere size.[1] In normals, radio-active tagged albumin and globulin were absorbed from the joint space with little difference in rate. Both appeared in the peripheral blood within fifteen minutes of their intra-articular injection, but approximately one-third remained in the knee joints for as long as seventy-two hours.[83] When IgG was reduced and heat aggregated its removal from the joint was enhanced[94a] in both rheumatoid and osteoarthritic joints. Radiosodium and heavy water absorption from the knees was prompt, but sodium was absorbed more slowly in both healthy and rheumatoid knees. The rate of sodium absorption was slower in rheumatoids than in normals.[90] Intra-articular hydrocortisone slowed the absorption rate of heavy water in rheumatoids. The study of the dynamics of joint fluid exchange in terms of osmotic and colloidal pressure gradients shows a decrease in the total osmotic pressure of the synovial fluid compared to that of plasma in rheumatoid effusions.[53] The colloid osmotic pressure in joint effusion favors the flow of fluid out of joint space into the circulation.[70a,70b] This situation is reversed with local articular or general systemic improvement when the total osmotic pressure of both synovial fluid and plasma tend to increase and that of the synovial fluid may rise to equal or exceed that of the plasma. Exercise has been shown to increase the rate of removal of isotope-tagged red blood cells from the knee joint.[81] The rate of red blood cell clearance from the joint is not altered by intra-articular hyaluronidase or corticosteroid or repeated red blood cell injections. Recently a technique using ^{133}Xenon has shown an increase in clearance in rheumatoid joints compared with normals.[96b] Other studies with phenolsulfonphthalein (PSP) showed increased clearance rate from involved joints in rheumatoid arthritis, osteoarthritis and traumatic arthritis (meniscal injury).[64a]

The functions of synovial fluid, although yet ill-defined, are the subject of discussion and investigation. Lubrication has been thought to be one important function.[5,9,13] Other functions include nutrition of cells in under-

Synovial Fluid Examination

Gross Appearance	Clarity	Can print be read through it?
	Turbidity	The cloudier the fluid, the higher the leukocyte count, and the greater the evidence of inflammation.
	Color Range	Straw, yellow, xanthochromic. Creamy, milky, grayish, greenish. Blood tinged to sanguineous.
Viscosity	Drop Test	Drop by drop from a syringe. High-viscosity fluids form a string several inches long. Low-viscosity fluids drip like water.
	Stringing	A drop of fluid placed between thumb and forefinger will form a "string" several inches in length when the fingers are separated if the viscosity is high. Low-viscosity fluids will not string.
	Viscosimeter	Ostwald viscosimeter can be used to compare the viscosity of synovial fluid to water.
"Ropes Test"	Acetic Acid Clotting	Addition of synovial fluid (dropwise) to dilute acetic acid in beaker forms clot. Shake after 1 minute to determine friability.
Microscopic	Cell Count	WBC with saline dilution RBC Differential WBC of stained smear
	Formed Elements	Cartilage fibrils or fragments Crystals: Urate Pyrophosphate Cholesterol
	Special Cells	"Rheumatoid cells" "L.E." cells

TABLE 6-1.—SYNOVIANALYSIS IN ARTHRITIS

	Disease	*Color*	*Clarity*	*Viscosity*	*Mucin clot*	*Cell WBC/mm³ % Polys*	*Cartilage Debris*	*Crystals*	*"R.A." Cells**	***Bact.***
Group I non-inflammatory	Normal	Straw	Transparent	High	Good	<200 WBC; <25%	0	0	0	0
	Traumatic arthritis	Straw to bloody to xanthochromic	Transparent to turbid	High	Good	<2000 WBC; few to many RBC; <25%	0 or +	0	0	0
	Osteoarthritis	Yellow	Transparent	High	Good	1000 WBC; <25%	+	0	0	0
Group II inflammatory	Systemic lupus erythematosus	Straw	Sl. cloudy	High	Good	5000 WBC; 10%	0	0	0 †	0
	Rheumatic fever	Yellow	Sl. cloudy	Low	Good	10,000 WBC to 12,000; 50%	0	0	0 or +	0
	Pseudo-gout	Yellow	Sl. cloudy (if acute)	Low (if acute)	Good to poor	1000 to 5,000 WBC; 25 to 50%	+	Calcium Pyro-phosphate +	0	0
	Gout	Yellow to milky	Cloudy	Low	Poor	10,000 to 12,000 WBC; 60 to 70%	0	Urate +	0	0
	Rheumatoid arthritis	Yellow to greenish	Cloudy	Low	Poor	15,000 to 20,000 WBC; 75%	0	Occ. cholesterol	+	0
Group III septic	Tuberculous arthritis	Yellow	Cloudy	Low	Poor	25,000 WBC; 50 to 60%	0	0	0	+
	Septic arthritis	Grayish or bloody	Turbid Purulent	Low	Poor	80 to 200,000; 75%	0	0	0	+

* "R.A." cells—Rheumatoid cells are not morphologically specific, but these inclusion-bearing cells are most frequently seen in high concentration in rheumatoid arthritis.

† "L.E." cells may be demonstrated in Wright stained smears of sediment from centrifuged synovial fluid in S.L.E.

lying articular cartilage,[20,36] protection of articular cartilage from mechanical damage and joint stabilization. (*See also* Chapter 4.)

SYNOVIANALYSIS

The many changes in synovial fluid previously discussed have been known for many years since the publications of the work of Kling in 1938,[49] Ropes and Bauer in 1953[84] and many others. Unfortunately, these excellent works and their implications in the diagnosis of joint disease were largely ignored and neglected by clinicians until recently.[39] An orderly application of the multiple techniques available for examination of the synovial fluid is called synovianalysis.[40] It should be carried out on the fluid of any effused joint as a routine diagnostic procedure.

Technique of Joint Aspiration

The approaches to specific joint aspiration are discussed in detail elsewhere (Chapter 32). The collection of synovial fluid from any involved joint is not difficult and is now readily performed using a rigid aseptic technique.[40] The skin over the site of the joint to be aspirated is carefully and completely cleansed using pHisoHex and alcohol and then painted with tincture of iodine which is allowed to dry for two minutes. The site of aspiration is then anesthetized with ethyl chloride spray and aspiration of a large joint is carried out using sterile disposable or autoclaved 20 gauge needles and sterile syringes. Fluid can often be obtained from any swollen joint, but the knee is by far the most frequent site of aspiration and the most easily accessible joint. At the time of joint aspiration, all the fluid present within a joint may be removed; but it is possible to obtain valuable information from even a few drops of joint fluid. For example, it is occasionally possible to aspirate a drop of synovial fluid from an involved small joint of the hand and foot in which the microscopic observation of urate crystals may make an immediate and definite diagnosis of gouty arthritis possible.[57,61]

From a practical viewpoint, examination of synovial fluid is a useful aid in the differential diagnosis of arthritis and its follow-up. Synovianalysis is easily performed as an office procedure using a minimum of equipment. It is as useful and important in differential diagnosis of joint disease as is urinalysis in genitourinary tract disease.

Methods of Examination

Gross Appearance. — *Clarity.* — Observations on the clarity of the fluid under examination are important. Normal fluid is crystal clear and print can be read easily through a test tube containing it. In the presence of inflammation, this clarity is lost and it is replaced by turbidity which is related to, and a direct but rough measure of, the cell count and hence the degree of inflammation present.[40] As the white cell count rises, clarity is lost and turbidity increases. However, in synovial fluid of traumatic arthritis the presence primarily of red cells leads to a decrease in clarity despite the absence of frank inflammation. Fluid of degenerative joint disease closely resembles that of normal fluid in its clarity, although occasionally flecks of cartilage fragments may be seen suspended in it. Early rheumatoid arthritic fluid may be clear, but as the inflammation increases, clarity is lost; in severe active rheumatoid arthritis the fluid is extremely turbid and may be almost purulent in appearance. Gouty and purulent fluids are often quite turbid. Any fluid which is quite cloudy, or is unexpectedly grossly bloody, should be sent for bacterial culture, particularly if on prior examination it has been relatively clear and subsequently increased in turbidity.

Color.—Normal synovial fluid is colorless or straw colored. In degenerative joint disease the fluid is often yellow or amber; in rheumatoid arthritis it is usually yellow to greenish.[40,84] Gouty synovial fluid may be yellow to white. If it contains many urate crystals, it may be milky white in appearance and consistency. Septic fluid usually has a creamy or grayish appearance. Traumatic fluids are often sanguineous in the acute phase and may appear xanthrochromic later. Fluid from osteoarthritic, rheumatoid arthritic and septic arthritic patients may be bloody on occasion, secondary to superimposed trauma. The presence of blood streaks in the joint fluid is usually due to puncture of a small blood vessel in the course of arthrocentesis.

Viscosity.—For the purpose of investigation, viscosity of synovial fluid relative to water may be measured using the Ostwald viscosimeter; but in the office, viscosity may be easily estimated by allowing the fluid to drip slowly drop-by-drop from the aspirating syringe, and observing the length of the string made by each drop before it separates. With high viscosity fluids the string thus formed may be one to several inches in length before separating. Similarly, a drop of fluid may be placed between thumb and forefinger and the fingers separated. With high viscosity fluids the fingers may be spread more than an inch before the string breaks. Normal, osteoarthritic and traumatic joint fluids are usually noted to have high viscosity as are the fluids of patients with systemic lupus erythematosus.[71a] Decreased viscosity is noted with synovial fluids of rheumatoid arthritis, gout and septic arthritis. Viscosity is a function of the concentration and the quality of hyaluronate in synovial fluid.[77] A decrease in synovial fluid viscosity can occur if the mucin is diluted by the presence of edema fluid or rapid effusion after trauma.

Mucin Clot.—The dropwise addition of glacial acetic acid to a test tube containing synovial fluid leads to the formation of a mucin clot which varies in consistency and friability with the process involving the joint. Conversely, the Ropes test[84] may be performed by adding a few drops of synovial fluid to a small beaker containing 10 ml. of a 5 per cent solution of acetic acid and allowing the clot to form. This test performed by either technique gives a good indication of the character of the protein-polysaccharide complex of the synovial fluid. In general, this test seems to be dependent upon the degree of polymerization of the mucin complex, although the concentration of the mucin in the synovial fluid may play a role.[31] In the presence of high quality mucin as in normal, traumatic, osteoarthritic, rheumatic fever, and SLE joint fluids, a firm, hard, ropy, and non-friable clot is formed. Synovial fluids of rheumatoid arthritis, gout and septic arthritis form clots which are loose and friable or only a flocculent precipitate.

Microscopic Examination. — Microscopic examination of synovial fluid is

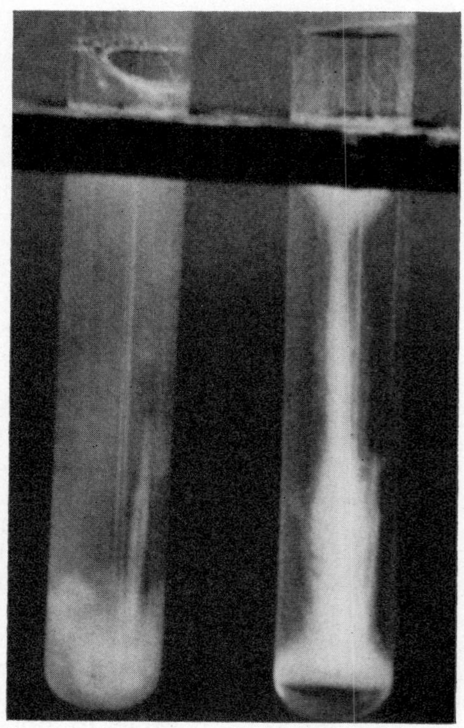

FIG. 6–1.—Dropwise addition of glacial acetic acid to synovial fluid leads to formation of a firm dense ropy clot in osteoarthritic fluid on the right in contrast to flocculent precipitate formed in rheumatoid fluid on the left.

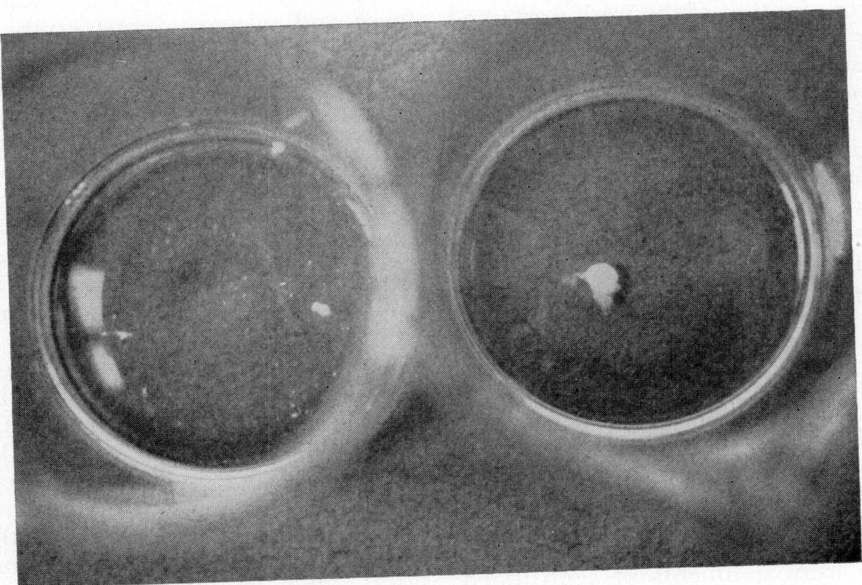

Fig. 6–2.—Addition of several drops of synovial fluid to diluted acetic acid leads to a firm clot in osteoarthritis (on the right) and a friable clot, easily fragmenting, in rheumatoid arthritis (on the left)

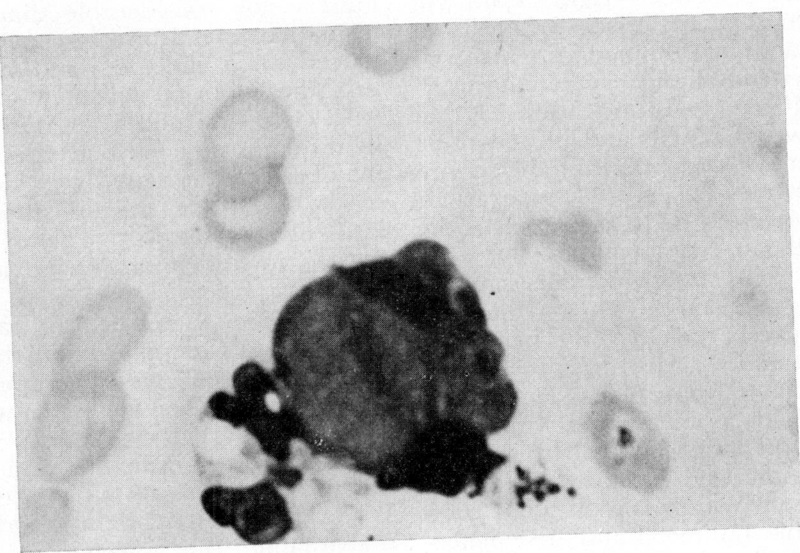

Fig. 6–3.—LE cells often can be demonstrated in sediment of centrifuged synovial fluid from lupus erythematosus patients using ordinary Wright's stain (×1200). Here two juxtaposed LE cells overlap. (Photomicrograph courtesy Dr. George Backer.)

divided into two parts; 1. cell count; 2. the examination of the fresh unstained fluid for formed elements. On occasion, examination of a stained preparation of cells from the sediment of centrifuged synovial fluid may give additional information.

Cell Counts.—The use of ordinary white cell counting solution with synovial fluid is impractical since its acidic properties lead to mucin clot formation. Therefore, physiologic saline solution is used as a diluent in white cell counts on freshly aspirated synovial fluids. In those fluids which are grossly bloody, a hypotonic solution of saline (0.3 per cent) hemolyzes the red cells but spares the leukocytes.[40] In all other respects the white cell count is carried out using the standard technique.

Differential leukocyte counts on smears prepared from sediments of centrifuged synovial fluid and stained with Wright's stain are useful in determining the predominant cell type seen in the various types of joint effusion. Such smears stained with ordinary Wright's stain will reveal many characteristic LE cells in the synovial fluids obtained from involved joints of systemic lupus erythematosus.[41b] Seven of 10 synovial fluids from LE patients showed LE cells and in one these were present when absent from the serum. The presence of LE cells in preparations made immediately upon aspiration of the fluid suggests *in vivo* formation.[41b,43]

Normal joint fluids contain no red blood cells and rarely show white cell counts in excess of 300 WBC per cubic millimeter and 25 per cent or less of these are polymorphonuclear leukocytes. Synovial fluids from persons with traumatic arthritis, osteochondritis dissecans, Charcot's joints and osteoarthritis rarely show leukocyte counts of more than 2000 cells per cubic millimeter and these generally have the same differential count as normal fluid. In fluids from rheumatoid arthritics, cell counts vary between 5,000 and 60,000 per cubic millimeter depending upon the severity of the inflammation; 65 per cent or more of these cells are polymorphonuclear leukocytes. Rheumatic fever and systemic lupus erythematosus fluids yield cell counts between 2,000 and 10,000 WBC per cubic centimeter of which 10 to 50 per cent are polymorphonuclear leukocytes. Acute gouty and pseudogouty joint fluid will show leukocyte counts similar to those for rheumatoid arthritis. In septic joint fluids the white cell counts may be in excess of 100,000 per cubic millimeter with 90 or more per cent polymorphonuclear leukocytes.[84]

Normal and osteoarthritic-type fluids (group I) and acute gouty and rheumatoid fluids (group II) are, of course, sterile while septic types (group III) have bacterial organisms present which may be demonstrated on smear or culture. Any group II or group III fluid goes through a group I phase as inflammation subsides; synovianalysis, like all laboratory procedures, must be interpreted in the context of the clinical picture.

Formed Elements.—Examination of a fresh, unstained, wet specimen of synovial fluid yields considerable diagnostic information. A drop of synovial fluid is placed on a slide, covered by a cover slip, the edges of which may be sealed with clear nail polish.[57] With ordinary light microscopy, various types of crystals may be seen and tentatively identified at 450 to 1200 times magnification. Polarized light microscopy helps to make crystal identification easier and more positive.

Urate Crystals.—The appearance of urate crystals in polarized light using a first order red plate compensator is definitive.[61] When viewed in wet preparation they are rod shaped.[61] Rarely, they are more needle-like and resemble the urate crystals obtained from tophi. When a polarized light microscope is unavailable, the insertion of polaroid discs into the ocular and condenser of a standard light microscope is satisfactory for polarized light viewing.[57] The urate crystals show strong *negative* birefringence with extinction on their long axis whether seen floating free in the fluid or lying within the white cells.[56] When seen, these crystals are pathognomonic of the diagnosis of gouty arthritis.[57] Any doubt as to the chemical composition of the urate crystal may be resolved by specific digestion of the crystals with uricase.[61]

The presence of urate crystals free or within leukocytes is an essential feature of gouty attacks. When electron microscopic study of ultrastructure is carried out, the crystals are noted to be free in the cytoplasm of the white cell and not membrane contained.[19a,79a]

Calcium Pyrophosphate Crystals. — The presence of non-urate crystals in joint fluids of a gout-like arthritis has been noted repeatedly. Crystals have been identified as calcium pyrophosphate.[50,59,62] By light microscopy the crystals appear as a rod-like or rhomboid forms with sharp corners. Using polarized light microscopy, they demonstrate weak *positive* birefringence or are non-refractile and are easily distinguished from urate; these appear in the syndrome of chondrocalcinosis or pseudo-gout (discussed in Chapter 60).

Cholesterol Crystals. — These crystals,

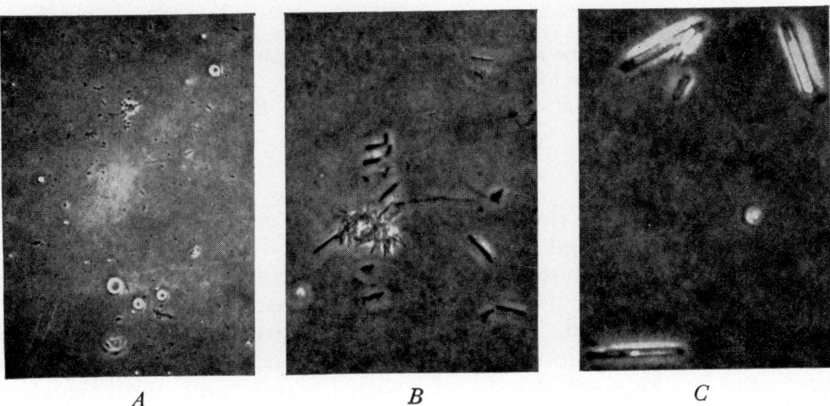

FIG. 6–4.—Crystals of sodium urate in the synovial fluid from the knee of a patient with acute gout. *A*, Tiny, dark crystals under low power (× 100). *B*, Crystals under middle power (× 450). *C*, Crystals magnified 1200 times, showing marked refractiveness. Note rounded ends of crystals in synovial fluid, whereas crystals of urate from tophi show more pointed ends. (Hollander.)

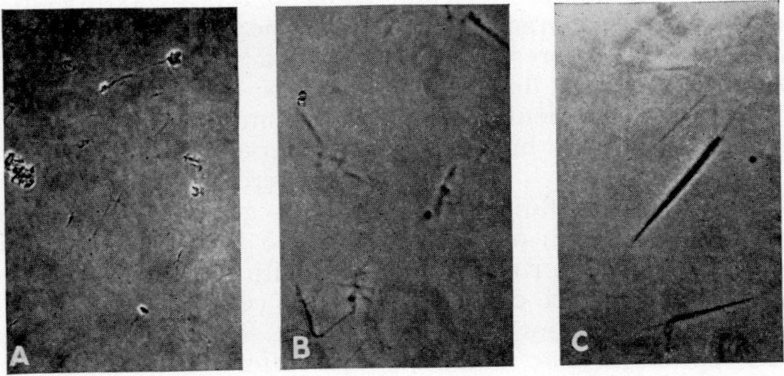

FIG. 6–5.—Fragments of cartilage fibrils from knee synovial fluid of patient with osteoarthritis. *A*, Under low power (× 100), these might easily be confused with urate crystals. *B*, Higher magnification (× 450) shows smaller caliber, branched or tapered ends, and much less refractiveness than urate crystals. *C*, High power (× 1200) shows marked difference from urate crystals, and typical fibrillar contour. (Hollander.)

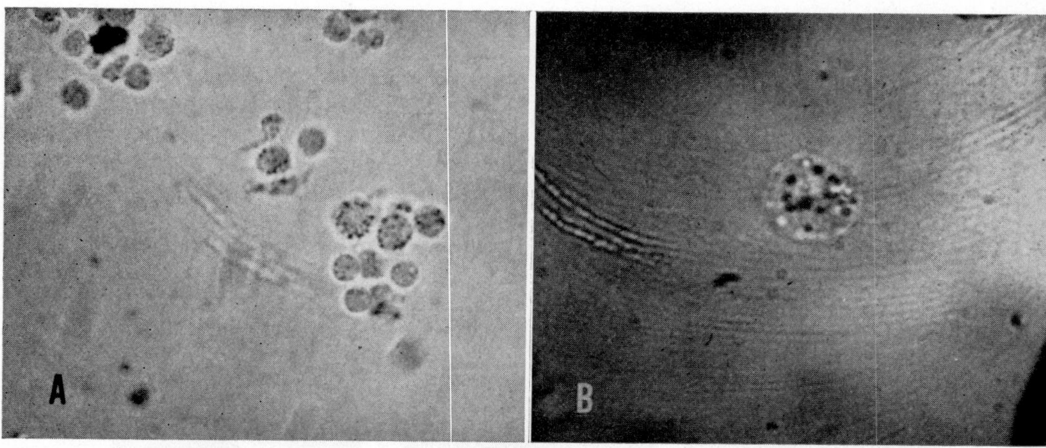

Fig. 6–6.—*A*, "R.A." cells may be seen in the fresh wet preparations of synovial fluid by ordinary light microscopy using unstained specimens or, as in this instance, using the Sternheimer-Malbin supravital stain which renders inclusion granules dark gray, × 430. *B*, Magnified × 1200. (Photomicrographs courtesy Dr. George Backer.)

which have a characteristic flat, plate-like appearance with notched corners, have been reported in rheumatoid joint fluids by several workers.[85,101] Their source, as yet undetermined, may be related to chronicity of effusion,[29] local hemorrhage[2] and/or local synthesis of lipid material by synovial tissue[67] or leukocytes.[12]

In joints into which intra-articular corticosteroid had been injected, steroid crystals have been described.[60] Studies of steroid crystal suspensions in synovial fluid have delineated the characteristics of these crystals.[47a] The presence of metallic fragments in synovial fluids and synovial biopsies from patients with metallic prostheses in knees has been reported.[48a]

Cartilage Debris.—Synovial fluids from osteoarthritic joints have been observed to contain many irregularly formed elements.[39] These desquamated cartilage fragments at high magnifications may be seen to contain typical lacunae, if from deeper layers. The number of such fragments is a rough index of the rate of cartilage destruction in the joint. After the matrix of such fragments has been dissolved by leukocytic enzymes, the reticular collagen fibrils remain (Fig. 6–5).

These collagen fibers have been identified in synovial fluid by phase contrast and electron microscopy and chemical analysis and have been shown to coexist with fibrin strands with which they may be confused on examination with ordinary light microscopy.[48] Total hydroxyproline levels were highest in osteoarthritic and traumatic fluids.

The "Rheumatoid Arthritis Cell."—In the course of repeated synovianalysis over the past nine years, Hollander *et al.*[41] have observed that leukocytes in the joint fluids of rheumatoid arthritics contain cytoplasmic inclusions which in unstained wet preparations viewed with ordinary light microscopy under high power appear as dark granules. The inclusions vary from 0.5 to 2 microns in size, and will stain with oil red O or supravitally with 0.2 per cent brilliant cresyl blue which can be counterstained with Wright's stain after centrifuging, smearing and drying. Supravital staining in wet preparations with a drop of Sternheimer-Malbin stain renders the inclusion granules dark gray with blue cytoplasm and purple nuclei. These cells were noted in

95 per cent of all rheumatoid fluids examined. From 3 to 97 per cent of the cells showed these cytoplasmic inclusions. Similar inclusion-bearing cells have sometimes been seen in inflammatory fluids other than rheumatoid arthritis.[11a,96a,98] However, only in the fluid from patients with rheumatoid arthritis and its variants has it been possible to demonstrate a rise in the synovial fluid rheumatoid factor titer when these cells have been fractured.[41] Subsequent studies of the rheumatoid cells by Rawson *et al.*,[78] and later confirmed by Vaughan *et al.*,[98] using fluorescent antibody techniques, have demonstrated that the intracytoplasmic inclusion bodies carry antigenic determinants for both 7S and 19S gamma globulin. Other materials found in synovial fluid leukocyte inclusions include complement,[11a,98] nucleoprotein,[11a] fibrin,[4] albumin, DNA bodies[55] and triglycerides.[38] The extension of these observations to show that autologous 7S gamma globulin may be specifically irritating in the rheumatoid arthritic joint[79] seems to support the hypothesis that the pathogenesis of rheumatoid joint inflammation is related to the deposition of complexes of rheumatoid factor and 7S gamma globulin within the joint leading to leukocytosis, phagocytosis and the release of lysosomal enzymes with further joint inflammation. The finding of these cells in individuals with rheumatoid arthritis or its variants in which the rheumatoid factor of the serum may be negative has added an additional tool for the diagnosis of rheumatoid disease.[41a]

BIBLIOGRAPHY

1. Adkins, E. W. D. and Davies, D. V.: Quart. J. Exper. Physiol., *30*, 147, 1940.
1*a*. Arai, M.: J. Exper. Med., *91*, 35, 1967.
2. Avres, W. N. and Haymaker, W.: J. Neuropath. Exper. Neurol., *19*, 280, 1960.
2*a*. Balazs, E. A., Watson, D. and Duff, I. F.: Arth. & Rheum., *10*, 357, 1967.
3. Balzacs, E.: Fed. Proc., *17*, 1086, 1958.
4. Barnhardt, M. I., Riddle, J. M. and Bluhm, G. B.: Ann. Rheum. Dis., *26*, 281, 1967.
5. Barnett, C. H., Davies, D. V. and MacCaill, M. A.: *Structure and Mechanics*, Springfield, Ill., Chas. C Thomas, 1961.
6. Bauer, W., Ropes, M. W. and Waine, H.: Physiol. Rev., *20*, 272, 1940.
7. Bauer, W., Short, C. L. and Bennett, G. A.: J. Exper. Med., *57*, 419, 1933.
8. Binette, J. P. and Schmid, K.: Arth. & Rheum., *8*, 14, 1965.
9. Blumberg, B. S., Ogston, A. G.: Ciba Symposium on *Chemistry and Biology of Mucopolysaccharides*, Boston, Little, Brown and Co., 1958.
10. Bole, G. G.: Arth. & Rheum., *5*, 589, 1962.
11. Bollet, A. J.: J. Lab. Clin. Med., *48*, 721, 1956.
11*a*. Brandt, K., Cathcart, E. S. and Cohen, A. S.: J. Lab. Clin. Med., *72*, 631, 1968.
12. Buchanan, A. A.: Biochem. J., *75*, 315, 1960.
13. Charnley, J.: Ann. Rheum. Dis., *19*, 10, 1960.
14. Cho, M. H. and Newhaus, O. W.: Thromb. Diath. haem., *5*, 108, 1960.
15. Chung, A. C., Shanahan, R., and Brown, E. M., Jr.: Arth. & Rheum., *5*, 176, 1962.
16. Cohen, A. S.: Arth. & Rheum., *7*, 490, 1964.
17. Decker, B., McGuckin, W. F., McKenzie, B. F.: Clin. Chem., *5*, 465, 1959.
18. Decker, B., McKenzie, B. F., McGuckin, W. F., and Slocumb, C. H.: Arth. & Rheum., *2*, 162, 1959.
19. Dingle, J. T.: Proc. Roy. Soc. Med., *55*, 109, 1962.
19a. Duncan, H., Bluhm, G. B., Riddle, J. M., *et al.*: Clin. Orthop., *59*, 277, 1968.
20. Ekholm, R.: Acta Anat., *24*, 329, 1955.
21. Elattar, T. M. A., Gustafson, G. M., and Wong, D. G.: Bioch. Biophys. Acta, *137*, 375, 1967.
22. Elattar, T. M. A., Murray, W. R., and Anderson, C. E.: Arth. & Rheum., *11*, 178, 1968.
23. Evanson, J. M., Jeffrey, J. J., and Krane, S. M.: Science, *158*, 499, 1967.
24. ———: J. Clin. Invest., *47*, 2639, 1968.
25. Gardner, E.: Physiol. Rev., *30*, 127, 1950.
26. Genecin, A.: Amer. J. Med., *26*, 496, 1959.
27. Ghadially, F. H. and Roy, S.: Ann. Rheum. Dis., *26*, 426, 1967.
28. ———: Nature, *213*, 1041, 1967.
29. Hamerman, D., Jones, R., and Smith, C.: J. Exper. Med., *126*, 1005, 1967.
30. Hamerman, D. and Sandson, J.: Arth. & Rheum., *4*, 420, 1961 (abstr.).

31. Hamerman, D. and Schubert, M.: Amer. J. Med., *33*, 555, 1962.
32. Hamerman, D. and Schuster, H.: J. Clin. Invest., *37*, 57, 1958.
33. ———: Arth. & Rheum., *1*, 523, 1958.
34. Harris, E. D., DiBona, D. R., and Krane, S. M.: J. Clin. Invest., *48*, 2104, 1969.
35. Harris, E. D., Evanson, J. M., DiBona, D. R., and Krane, S. M.: Arth. & Rheum., *13*, 83, 1970.
36. Harrison, M. H. M., Schajowicz, F. and Trueta, J.: J. Bone Joint Surg., *35B*, 598, 1953.
37. Hedberg, H.: Acta Rheum. Scand., *10*, 109, 1964.
38. Hersko, C., Michaeli, D., and Shaboletz, S., *et al.*: Israel J. Med. Sci., *3*, 838, 1967.
39. Hollander, J. L.: Arth. & Rheum., *3*, 364, 1960.
40. Hollander, J. L., Jessar, R. A., McCarty, D. J.: Bull. Rheum. Dis., *12*, 263, 1961.
41. Hollander, J. L., McCarty, D. J., Astorga, G. and Castro-Murillo, E.: Ann. Intern. Med., *62*, 271, 1965.
41*a*. Hollander, J. L., McCarty, D. J., and Rawson, A. J.: Bull. Rheumat. Dis., *16*, 382, 1965.
41*b*. Hollander, J. L., Reginato, A., Torralba, T. P.: Med. Clin. N. Am., *50*, 1281, 1966.
42. Holmes, W. F., Keefer, C. S. and Myers, W. K.: J. Clin. Invest., *14*, 124, 1935.
42*a*. Holt, P. J. L., How, M. J., Long, V. J. W., *et al.*: Ann. Rheum. Dis., *27*, 264, 1968.
43. Hunder, G. G. and Pierre, R. V.: Arth. & Rheum., *13*, 448, 1970.
44. Jacos, R. F. and Feldmann, A.: J. Clin. Invest., *34*, 263, 1955.
45. Jaffee, I. A.: J. Lab. and Clin. Med., *60*, 409, 1962.
46. Jeffrey, M. R.: Amer. J. Med. Sci., *239*, 154, 1960.
47. Jessar, R. A., Ganzell, M. A. and Ragan, C.: J. Clin. Invest., *32*, 480, 1953.
47*a*. Kahn, C. B., Hollander, J. L., and Schumacher, H. R.: J.A.M.A., *211*, 807, 1970.
47*b*. Kerby, G. P. and Taylor, S. M.: Proc. Soc. Exper. Biol. & Med., *126*, 865, 1967.
48. Kitridou, R., McCarty, D. J., Prockop, D. J. and Hummeler, K.: Arth. & Rheum., *12*, 580, 1969.
48*a*. Kitridou, R., Schumacher, H. R., Sbarbaro, J. and Hollander, J. L.: Arth. & Rheum., *12*, 520, 1969.
49. Kling, D. J.: *The Synovial Membrane and the Synovial Fluid*, Los Angeles, Medical Press, 1938.
50. Kohn, N., Hughes, R., McCarty, D. J. and Faires, J. S.: Ann. Intern. Med., *56*, 738, 1962.
50*a*. Lawrence, C. and Seife, B.: Ann. Intern. Med., *74*, 740, 1971.
51. Lazarus, G. S., Decker, J. L., Oliver, C. H., *et al.*: New Engl. J. Med., *279*, 914, 1968.
52. Linn, F. C.: J. Bone and Joint Surg., *49A*, 1079, 1967.
53. Lipson, R. L. and Baldes, E. J.: Arth. & Rheum., *8*, 29, 1965.
54. Luckenbill, L. M. and Cohen, A. S.: Arth. & Rheum., *10*, 517, 1967.
55. Malinin, T. I., Pekin, T. J. and Zvaifler, N.: Am. J. Clin. Path., *47*, 203, 1967.
56. McCarty, D. J., Jr.: Amer. J. Med. Sci., *243*, 288, 1962.
57. ———: Post. Grad. Med., *33*, 142, 1963.
58. McCarty, D. J., Jr. and Faires, J. S.: Current Therapy Res., *5*, 284, 1963.
59. McCarty, D. J., Jr., and Gatter, R. A.: Bull. Rheum. Dis., *14*, 331, 1964.
60. McCarty, D. J., Jr. and Hogan, J. M.: Arth. & Rheum., *7*, 359, 1964.
61. McCarty, D. J. and Hollander, J. L.: Ann. Intern. Med., *54*, 452, 1961.
62. McCarty, D. J., Kohn, N. and Faires, J.: Ann. Intern. Med., *56*, 711, 1962.
63. Melman, K. L., Webster, M. E., Goldfinger, S. E., *et al.*: Arth. & Rheum., *10*, 13, 1967.
64. Murphy, D. and West, H. F.: Arth. & Rheum., *11*, 696, 1968.
64*a*. Nakanura, R., Asai, H., Sonozaki, H., *et al.*: Ann. Rheum. Dis., *26*, 246, 1967.
65. Nettelbladt, E. and Sundblad, L.: Arth. & Rheum., *2*, 144, 1959.
66. ———: Arth. & Rheum., *4*, 161, 1961.
67. Newcombe, D. S. and Cohen, A. S.: Program Amer. Soc. for Clin. Invest. 55th Annual Meet. Atlantic City, 1963.
68. Niedermeier, W., Creitz, E. E., and Holley, H. L.: Arth. & Rheum., *5*, 439, 1962.
69. Nies, A. S. and Melman, K. L.: Bull. Rheum. Dis., *19*, 512, 1968.
70. Ogston, A. G. and Phelps, C. F.: Biochem. J., *78*, 827, 1961.
70*a*. Olson, M. E., Kubicek, W. G. and Sampson, G. R.: Arth. & Rheum., *10*, 180, 1967.
70*b*. Palmer, D. J. and Myers, D. F.: Arth. & Rheum., *11*, 745, 1968.
70*c*. Pekin, T. J., Malinin, T. I. and Zvaifler, N. J.: Ann. Intern. Med., *66*, 1628, 1967.
71. Pekin, T. J. and Zvaifler, N. J.: J. Clin. Invest., *43*, 1372, 1964.
71*a*. ———: Arth. & Rheum., *13*, 777, 1970.

71*b*. PELTIER, A. P., DELBARRE, F. and KRASSININE, G.: Ann. Rheum. Dis., *26*, 528, 1967.
72. PERLMANN, G. E., ROPES, M. W., KAUFMAN, D., and BAUER, W.: J. Clin. Invest., *33*, 319, 1954.
73. PIGMAN, W., GROWLING, E., PLATT, D. and HOLLEY, H. L.: Biochem. J., *71*, 201, 1959.
74. PIGMAN, W., HAWKINS, W. L., BLAIR, M. G., HOLLEY, H. L.: Arth. & Rheum., *1*, 151, 1958.
75. PODKAMINKSY, N. A.: Arch. Klin. Chir., *165*, 383, 1931.
75*a*. PRUZANSKI, W., SAITOS, S. and OGRYZLO, M.: Arth. & Rheum., *13*, 389, 1970.
76. RADIN, E. L.: Arth. & Rheum., *11*, 693, 1968.
77. RAGAN, C. and MEYER, K.: J. Clin. Invest., *28*, 56, 1949.
78. RAWSON, A. J., ABELSON, N. J., HOLLANDER, J. L.: Ann. Intern. Med., *62*, 281, 1965.
79. RESTIFO, R. A., LUSSIER, A. J., RAWSON, A. J., ROCKEY, J. H. and HOLLANDER, J. L.: Ann. Intern. Med., *62*, 285, 1965.
79*a*. RIDDLE, J. M., BLUHM, G. B. and BARNHART, M. I.: Ann. Rheum. Dis., *26*, 389, 1967.
80. RIZZO, T. D.: Bull. Hosp. Spec. Surg., *4*, 98, 1961.
81. RODNAN, G. P.: Arth. & Rheum., *3*, 195, 1960.
82. RODNAN, G. P., EISENBEIS, C. and CREIGHTON, A. S.: Arth. & Rheum., *5*, 316, 1962 (abstr.).
83. RODNAN, G. P. and MACLACHLAN, M. J.: Arth. & Rheum., *3*, 152, 1960.
84. ROPES, M. W. and BAUER, W.: *Synovial Fluid Changes in Joint Disease.* Cambridge, Massachusetts, Harvard University Press, 1953.
85. ROPES, M. W., MULLER, A. F. and BAUER, W.: Arth. & Rheum., *3*, 496, 1960.
86. SALOMONE, G. and QUARTINI, V.: Bull. Soc. Ital. Biol. Sper., *37*, 41, 1961.
87. SANDSON, J. and HAMERMAN, D.: J. Clin. Invest., *41*, 1817, 1962.
88. ————: J. Clin. Invest., *39*, 364, 1958.
89. ————: Proc. Soc. Exper. Biol. & Med., *98*, 364, 1958.
90. SCHOLER, J. F., LEE, P. R. and POLLEY, H. F.: Arth. & Rheum., *2*, 426, 1959.
91. SCHMID, K. and MACNAIR, M. B.: J. Clin. Invest., *35*, 814, 1956.
92. ————: J. Clin. Invest., *37*, 708, 1958.
93. SCHUMACHER, H. R.: Arth. & Rheum., *11*, 426, 1968.
94. SCHUR, P. H. and SANDSON, J.: Arth. & Rheum., *6*, 115, 1963.
94*a*. SLIWINSKI, A. J. and ZVAIFLER, N. J.: Arth. & Rheum., *12*, 504, 1969.
94*b*. ————: J. Lab. Clin. Med., *76*, 304, 1970.
94*c*. SMILEY, J. D., SACHS, S. C. and ZIFF, M.: J. Clin. Invest., *47*, 624, 1968.
95. SMITH, CAROL and HAMERMAN, D.: Arth & Rheum., *5*, 411, 1962.
96. SMITH, J. E., CROWLEY, G. T., GILES, R. B.: Arth. & Rheum., *3*, 409, 1960.
96*a*. SONES, D. A., MCDUFFIE, F. C. and HUNDER, G. G.: Arth. & Rheum., *11*, 500, 1968.
96*b*. ST.ONGE, R. A., DICK, W. C., BELL, G., *et al.*: Ann. Rheum. Dis., *27*, 163, 1968.
96*c*. TAKASUGI, K. and HOLLINGSWORTH, J. W.: Arth. & Rheum., *10*, 495, 1967.
97. VARTIO, T.: Ann. Med. Exper. & Biol. Fenniae, *38*, 94, 1960.
98. VAUGHAN, J. H., BARNETT, E. V. and SOBEL, M. V.: Arth. & Rheum., *11*, 125, 1968.
99. YIELDING, K. L. and TOMPKINS, G. M.: Science, *125*, 1300, 1957.
100. ZIFF, M., GRIBETZ, H. J. and LOSPALLUTO, J.: J. Clin. Invest., *39*, 405, 1960.
101. ZUCKNER, J., UDDIN, J., JAMAL, L., GANTNER, G. and DORNER, R.: Ann. Intern. Med., *60*, 436, 1964.

Chapter 7

Radiology of the Rheumatic Diseases

By William Martel, M.D.

The radiologic manifestations of the rheumatic diseases reflect the gross pathology of these conditions and are extremely important. A specific radiologic diagnosis is possible more often than is realized and is particularly valuable when clinical manifestations are nonspecific or atypical. Obviously, the skeletal system can react to disease in limited ways and it is therefore not surprising that different pathologic conditions may, to some extent, exhibit similar radiologic features. However, it is the *pattern* of skeletal lesions that is important and the radiologic diagnosis will often depend on a characteristic combination of findings, a predilection for particular anatomic sites and a characteristic evolution.

This chapter will concern itself with the radiologic manifestations of the more common rheumatic diseases with emphasis on some distinguishing features. It is beyond the scope of this section to dwell on atypical cases or discuss in detail a most important aspect of the radiology of any group of diseases, namely, the differential diagnosis. Many of these diseases are systemic and affect multiple organs but no attempt will be made to cover *all* of their radiologic manifestations; skeletal lesions will be stressed inasmuch as these are usually the most conspicuous in these diseases.

RHEUMATOID ARTHRITIS

Extremities.—Any synovial joint of the extremities may be affected but there is a predilection for the small joints of the hand, wrist and foot with the exception of the distal interphalangeal joints. The metacarpophalangeal and proximal interphalangeal joints are commonly involved (Fig. 7–1). The carpal joints become involved more or less as a group so that extensive destruction of some of these joints with complete sparing of others is unusual. It is axiomatic in this disease that joints which communicate with one another tend to be affected together.[89] Except for the pisi-triquetral joint, the joints between the carpal bones often share a common synovial cavity (the mid-carpal joint). The latter generally communicates with the intermetacarpal and carpometacarpal joints which in turn connect with each other (except for that of the thumb). The distal radio-ulnar and radiocarpal joints are also often involved simultaneously. Communication between adjacent joints is a frequent consequence of articular destruction.[55,102] The feet are affected about as often as the hands and when the radiologic findings in the latter are equivocal or non-specific, these joints should be examined. The earliest and most frequently affected joints are the metatarsophalangeal (Fig. 7–2), particularly the first and fifth. It is claimed that the first three joints are the most commonly involved.[158] As in the carpus, all of the tarsal joints are affected more or less uniformly. The calcaneus is often affected near the retrocalcaneal bursa (Fig. 7–3) and at the posterior attachment of the plantar aponeurosis.[12,90] Arthritis of the acromioclavicular and sternoclavicular joints is common but involvement of the sternomanubrial synchondrosis is rare.

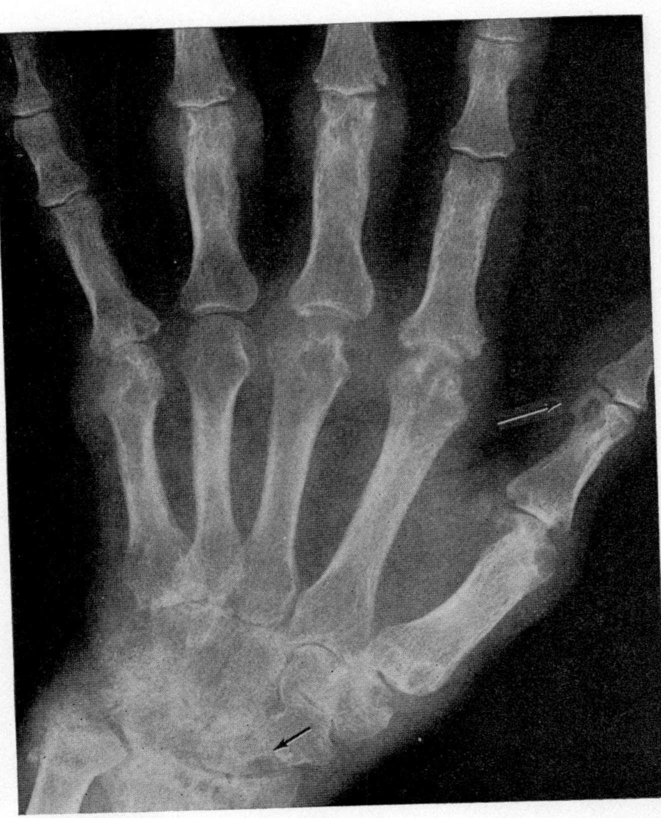

FIG. 7–1.—Characteristic distribution of arthritis in rheumatoid disease; the other hand and wrist were similarly affected. Note articular soft tissue swelling, uniform narrowing of interosseous spaces and typical distribution of marginal erosions, some of which are projected "*en face*" (arrow). Compare with Fig. 7–5. The navicular is rotated into the hollow of the distal radius and there is an erosion in its midportion (small arrow). The ulna is slightly displaced distally.

The arthritis may be asymmetrical at first but as the disease progresses, some degree of radiologic symmetry is usually evident. Occasionally, pronounced asymmetry persists even in long-standing cases and, rarely, the disease may remain monarticular for months. Persistent monarticular disease is probably more common in children[28,103] than in adults.

Soft tissue swelling[144] is due to joint effusion, hyperplastic synovitis, both of joints and tendon sheaths, and periarticular edema (Fig. 7–1). It is an early finding which is easily detected in the hands and feet but may also be visualized in large joints by virtue of displacement of normal periarticular fat. It is usually fusiform and characteristically involves all aspects of the affected joints. It may appear lobulated if there is much synovial hyperplasia, particularly when this involves tendon sheaths. Occasionally, discrete subcutaneous nodules develop but these are not usually juxta-articular in the hands and feet. Nodular periarticular swelling in rheumatoid arthritis often represents herniated synovial tissue rather than "rheumatoid nodules." Calcification in rheumatoid nodules used to be noted after continuous massive doses of vitamin D but is nowadays rare. The radiologic detection of subtle soft tissue swelling may be helpful in differential diagnosis.[12,144] For example, thickening of the subcutaneous tissue adjacent to the ulnar styloid or the retrocalcaneal soft tissue is characteristic.

Generalized soft tissue atrophy is typical in the later stages. Regional osteoporosis or bone atrophy is an early finding and tends to be juxta-articular but may be spotty. How much can be attributed to the restricted use or immobility of joints because of pain and how much to neuro-

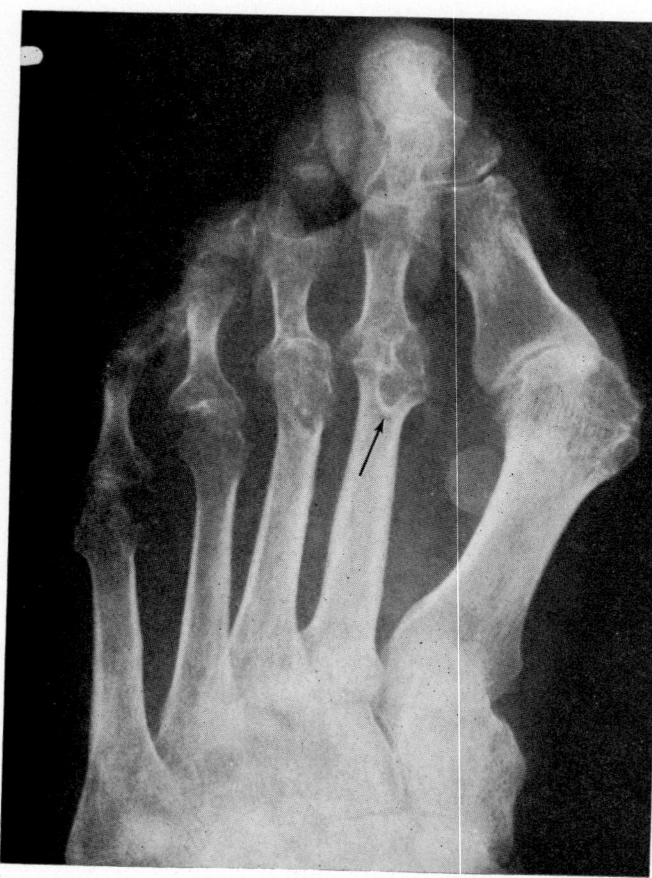

Fig. 7–2.—Advanced rheumatoid arthritis showing hallux valgus, metatarsophalangeal subluxations and erosions of the metatarsal heads. In the lateral projection the latter were plantar-depressed and the toes were slightly cocked-up. Minimal sclerosis at the margin of the erosion in the second metatarsal (arrow) indicates it has been present for some time. Note uniform narrowing of tarsal interosseous spaces. (Reproduced with permission of J.A.M.A.).

genic or hyperemic factors is not clear. Chronic hyperemia is probably an important factor in the early phase. However, as the disease progresses, the bones become more or less uniformly osteoporotic and while this may be influenced by long-term steroid therapy, it appears to be a reflection of a general inhibition of osteogenesis due to the disease itself.

An early and irreversible change in the articular cartilage is reflected in narrowing of the interosseous "joint space" (Figs. 7–1, 7–2 and 7–4). This narrowing is virtually always uniform since all of the articular cartilage of an involved joint is affected at the same time. Thus, in the knee joint one may expect more or less uniform narrowing of the interosseous spaces of the medial, lateral and retropatellar compartments (Fig. 7–4). On the other hand, in osteoarthritis of the knee, one almost never finds uniform narrowing of all three compartments but rather of only one or two and virtually never of both medial and lateral compartments in the same joint.[3] Interosseous space narrowing may occur without bone erosion particularly in certain joints such as the interphalangeal, carpal, tarsal and radiocarpal. However, erosion of the metacarpal and metatarsal heads is often an early finding[145] in metacarpophalangeal and metatarsophalangeal arthritis, and it is unusual to find the interosseous spaces of many of these joints to be narrowed without bone erosions. Occasionally, slight interosseous space widening occurs,

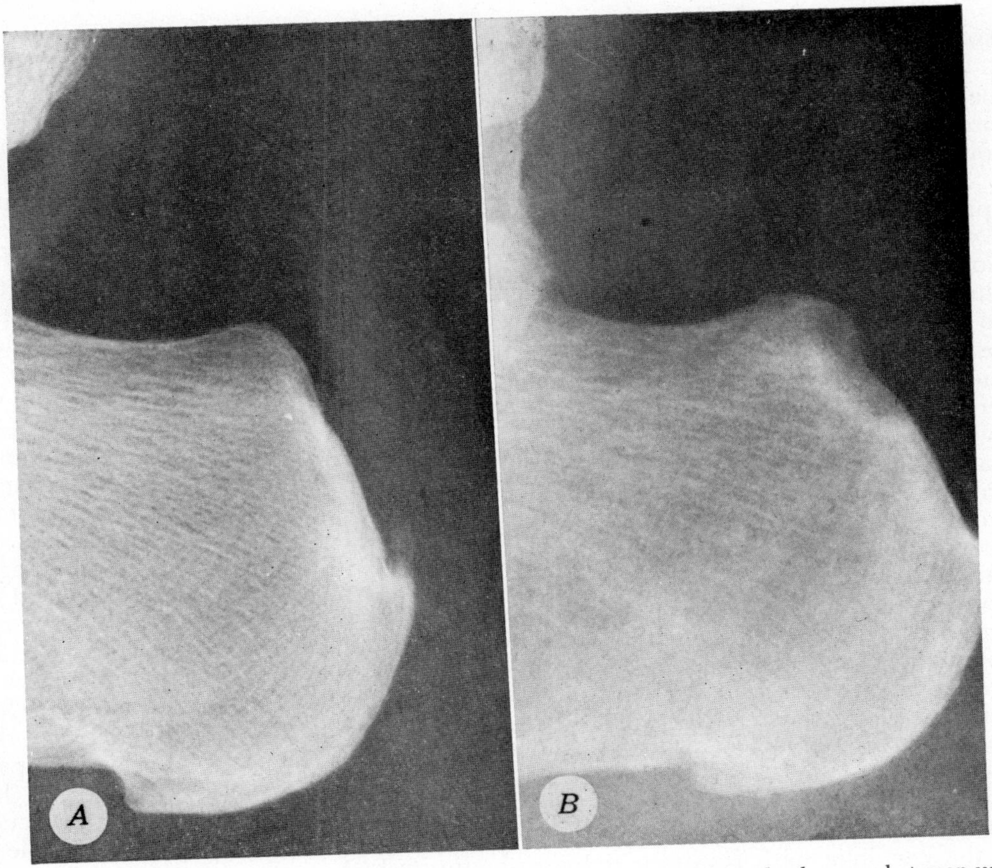

FIG. 7–3.—Rheumatoid arthritis. *A*. Normal appearance showing triangular lucency between upper calcaneus and Achilles tendon due to fatty bursa at this site. *B*. Same patient months after onset of heel pain. Note thickening of Achilles tendon, obliteration of retrocalcaneal lucency and adjacent calcaneal erosion.

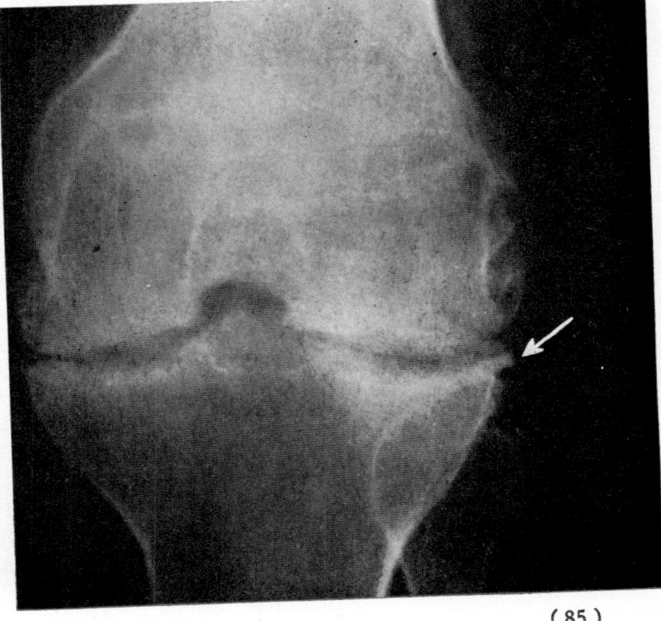

FIG. 7–4.—Rheumatoid arthritis. Uniform narrowing of interosseous spaces of *both* medial and lateral compartments. The retropatellar space was also narrowed. Note subchondral sclerosis and *minimal* marginal osteophyte (arrow).

particularly in the hands and feet, and probably reflects ligamentous laxity and joint effusion.

Narrowing of an interosseous joint space occurs in many arthropathies. *Uniform* narrowing is characteristic, though not pathognomonic, of rheumatoid arthritis. This is presumed to correspond to actual erosion of the joint surface with resultant thinning of the cartilage inasmuch as surface erosions are demonstrable in pathologic specimens. However, the characteristic evenness of this narrowing suggests that the earliest change may be a biochemical one with secondary dehydration or atrophy of the articular cartilage. It is probable that this is responsible for the radiologic appearance and that it precedes surface erosion. It has been suggested that in rheumatoid arthritis there occurs a degradation of the mucoprotein ground substance by enzymes liberated in the course of breakdown of cells present in the inflamed synovial membrane.[174] This could conceivably result in a significant diminution in the water-binding capacity of the cartilage with resultant dehydration corresponding to the narrowing seen radiologically. This may explain why such uniform narrowing may be seen in chronic inflammatory conditions other than rheumatoid arthritis.

Although subperiosteal bone apposition is common in children, it is only rarely seen in adults.[89] When it does occur in adults, it is invariably *subtle* and tends to be found at capsule and tendon attachments. In some cases it probably reflects tenosynovitis rather than joint disease. The relative lack of bone formation, despite advanced and often dramatic joint destruction, is a hallmark of the disease. This lack of reactive bone formation is so characteristic that the presence of exuberant bone apposition in adults should suggest another diagnosis.

Malalignment and subluxation are typical and occur in a characteristic manner.[146] Inflammation of the periarticular ligaments with resultant edema and laxity alters the relationship of tendons and the joints across which they act. Tenosynovitis is a conspicuous feature of the disease.[89] These factors change the action of certain muscle groups so that the normal muscular balance is no longer maintained and the restraints of the weakened articular ligaments are easily overcome.[142] Thus in the hand, the terminal interphalangeal joints may become hyperflexed and the proximal ones hyperextended, or vice versa. In the thumb, the terminal phalanx is often displaced dorsally and a flexion deformity of the metacarpophalangeal joint may be seen. The tendency toward ulnar deviation and volar subluxation of the metacarpophalangeal joints is well known. Less recognized but frequent is deviation of the radiocarpal joint such that the carpus is rotated and the navicular lies within the hollow of the distal radius. This deformity is characteristic but may also be seen in other conditions. The normal relationships of the carpal bones are altered.[5,102] The expected rotary motion of the navicular in radioulnar deflection, for example, is diminished or absent and the lunate is often malpositioned. Occasionally, there is volar dislocation of the radiocarpal joint. Diastasis of the distal radioulnar joint is commonly evident and the lateral view may show dorsal displacement of the distal ulna. The deformities in the foot are somewhat analogous to those in the hands. Progressive hallux valgus is the most frequent deformity (Fig. 7–2) and "fibular deviation" of the metatarsophalangeal joints is characteristic, except for the fifth joint which usually remains in a normal or varus position.[158] Subluxation is especially common in these joints and the metatarsal heads may become spread apart due to soft tissue swelling. Plantar depression of the metatarsal heads is common. Both the distal and proximal interphalangeal joints become flexed, giving either the "cocked-up" or "hammer-toe" deformities depending on whether there are concomitant hyperextension deformities of the metatarsophalangeal joints. The mid-foot characteristically shows planovalgus deformity. Flexion deformities of the knees and elbows and glenohumeral subluxation are common. The head of the humerus may be displaced craniad so that it impacts against the acromion process. This finding indicates rupture or extreme laxity of the rotator cuff.

The most conspicuous sites of bone erosion early in the disease correspond to those parts of the bone within the joint that are bare of articular cartilage.[102] These "marginal erosions" can be found near the attachments of the joint capsule, where the articular cartilage ends and the synovial reflection begins (Fig. 7–5). The anatomy of a particular joint appears to determine the distribution of these erosions. In the proximal interphalangeal joints of the fingers, for example, the erosion usually involves a larger area on the proximal side of the joint than on the distal side. This reflects the larger area of bone between the edge of the articular cartilage and the proximal attachment of the capsule. In the metacarpophalangeal joints the erosions tend to develop first and most extensively in the metacarpal head, particularly at the radial-volar aspect (Fig. 7–6). The fifth metacarpal may exhibit the earliest erosions on its lateral aspect. Erosions of the proximal phalanges generally develop late, compared to the metacarpals, with the exception of the index finger where an erosion often develops first at the base of the radial aspect. Metacarpophalangeal erosions often develop earliest in the index and middle fingers. They commonly occur in the proximal interphalangeal joint of the middle finger before other interphalangeal joints. A deep notch-like erosion often develops at the ulnar side of the volar aspect of the base of the thumb's distal phalanx. The ulnar styloid is quite commonly eroded and there is often a characteristic broad erosion of the radius at the distal radioulnar joint.[8] The triquetrum is characteristically eroded on the proximal ulnar surface. An erosion frequently develops at the mid-radial aspect of the carpal navicular and capitate, respectively. The latter should not be confused with a normal notch commonly present at this site. Metatarsophalangeal joint erosions tend to occur on the medial-plantar aspect of the metatarsal head. The lateral aspect of the fifth metatarsal may be selectively eroded. Calcaneal erosions occur at the posterosuperior aspect (Fig. 7–3), and, occasionally, at the posterior plantar surface where, subsequently, a well-marginated bony spur often develops.

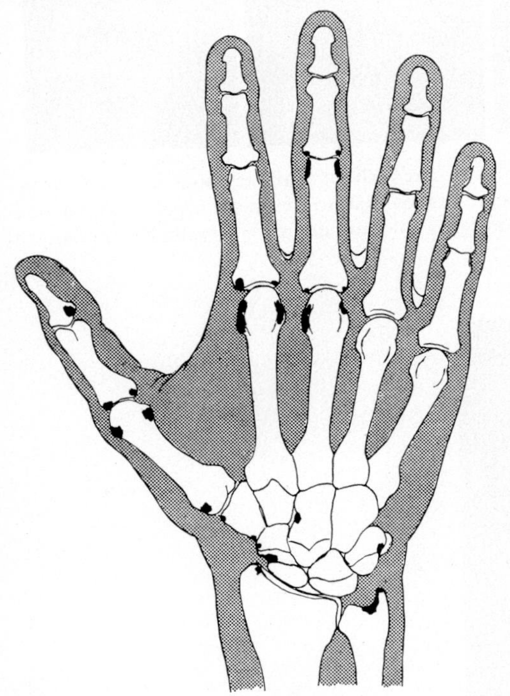

Fig. 7–5.—Diagram of sites of predilection for marginal erosions in rheumatoid arthritis. All of the proximal interphalangeal and metacarpophalangeal joints may exhibit these erosions but the latter are depicted in only three of these joints.

In other joints such as the ankles, knees, hips, elbows, and shoulders[34,78] (Fig. 7–7) erosions also develop near the capsular attachment; their distribution is analogous to the marginal erosions in the hands and feet. Inward protrusion of the acetabulum is common and may be severe (Fig. 7–8). This reflects acetabular remodeling coincident with pressure

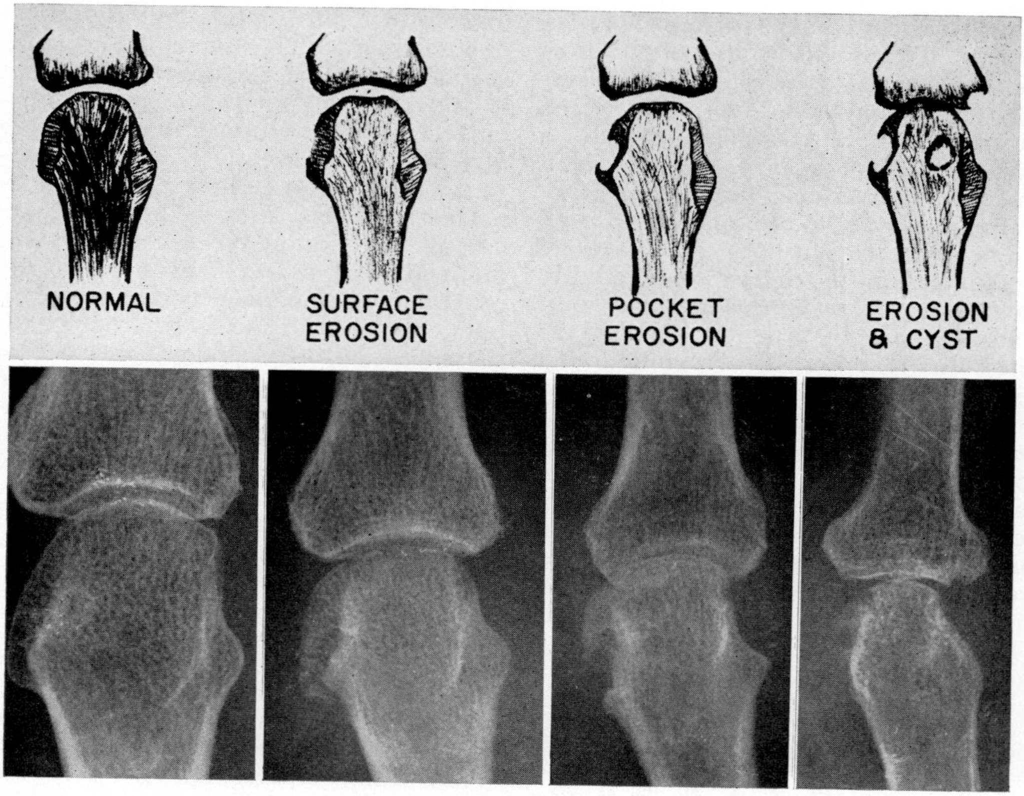

NORMAL
SURFACE EROSION
POCKET EROSION
EROSION & CYST

FIG. 7–6.—Roentgenograms and schematic drawings of progressive marginal erosions in a metacarpophalangeal joint in rheumatoid arthritis. The erosions are first evident in the metacarpal head, particularly at the radial-volar aspect, producing a hook-like configuration, and are often seen on the phalangeal side of the joint in the advanced stage.

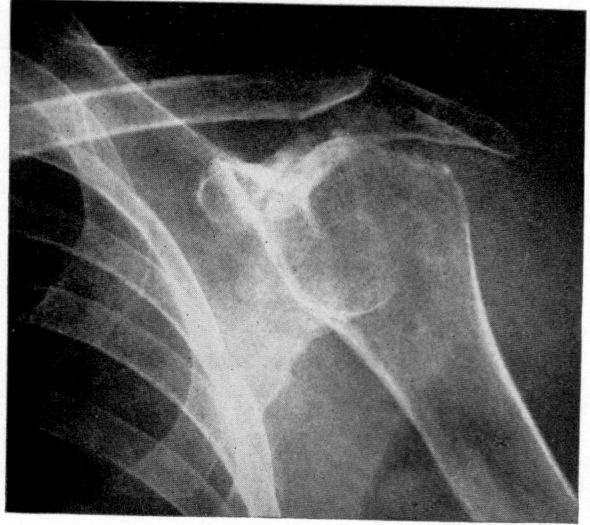

FIG. 7–7.—Advanced rheumatoid arthritis involving the glenohumeral and acromioclavicular joints. Note marginal erosions in the head of the humerus and "tapering" of distal clavicle.

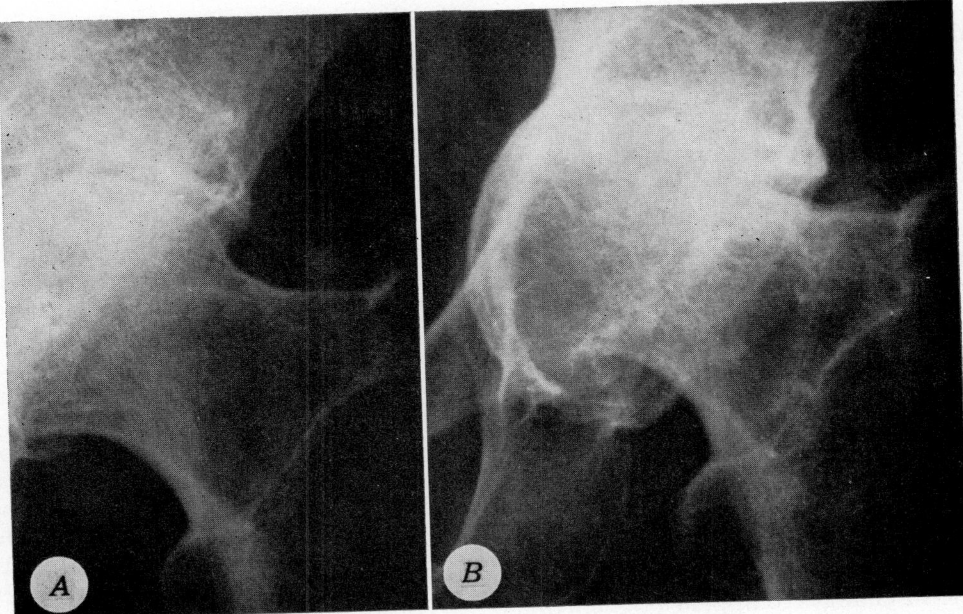

FIG. 7–8.—Progressive acetabular protrusion in rheumatoid arthritis. *A*. Early. *B*. Years later. There is some subchondral sclerosis but the narrowing of interosseous space is uniform and the absence of osteophytes is conspicuous.

resorption due to impaction by the femoral head. An erosion in the central part of the medial femoral condyle is occasionally observed. Acromioclavicular erosions characteristically begin at the outer end of the clavicle often producing a tapered appearance (Fig. 7–7). Occasionally, there is resorption of the posterior aspects of the ribs, particularly the upper ones. Erosions at extra-articular sites, such as the ischial margins may be associated with contiguous soft tissue masses.

Most marginal erosions can be projected either in profile or "en face" and may be sharply marginated. Some erosions are "pocketed" and, although adjacent to the subchondral bone, appear unconnected to the joint in all projections. On pathologic examination they can usually be seen to communicate with the joint. Some pocketed erosions are "cyst-like" in appearance[22,29,89] and quite large, and are particularly common in patients with massive synovial proliferation. When such cyst-like lesions are present in one joint, they generally occur in other joints as well. It is possible that these "pseudocysts" become filled with granulation tissue that undergoes liquefaction necrosis with secondary erosion of the bone. Their pathogenesis may be analogous to the lesions of villonodular synovitis, in this instance, superimposed on the basic rheumatoid process. A healing phase may take place and the pseudocysts may eventually develop thin, sclerotic margins which should not be confused with the subchondral cyst-like lesions of osteoarthritis. Although marginal erosions and pseudocysts may, to a minimal extent, be filled in by bone during a quiescent period, they virtually never disappear (Fig. 7–2). Erosions may be associated with an adjacent tenosynovitis, particularly in the hands and wrists; these appear as a subtle, superficial surface resorption of the cortex.[102] They develop, not only at tendon attachments, but apparently also at sites contiguous to chronically swollen tendon sheaths.

Tarsal, carpal and interphalangeal ankylosis is frequent but bony ankylosis of the metacarpophalangeal joints is rare. Interphalangeal ankylosis was noted in 5% of 100 consecutive clinic cases.[102] To the extent that any inflammatory arthropathy, particularly a chronic one such as rheumatoid arthritis, may irreversibly alter a joint so as to interfere with its subsequent mechanical function, secondary osteoarthritis may supervene. Hence, marginal osteophytes and subchondral sclerosis occur in long-standing rheumatoid arthritis but the osteophytes tend to be small and atypical in location compared to those seen in primary osteoarthritis. Furthermore, the distribution of joint involvement and the pattern of bone erosion provide a basis for radiologic differentiation. In most patients it takes at least three months for irreversible joint changes to appear (e.g. cartilage thinning or bone erosion). Occasionally, these may not be evident for six months or longer but it is unusual to see them within weeks after the onset of disease.

Spine.—The spondylitis of rheumatoid arthritis[30,86,87,88,96,137] is distinctive and differs significantly from ankylosing spondylitis with which it has often been confused. There is a predilection for the cervical segment and, other than osteoporosis, there are usually no obvious, specific radiologic changes in the dorsolumbar spine. Sacroiliac arthritis is relatively uncommon and is usually clinically inconspicuous. Reactive sclerosis, as is seen in ankylosing spondylitis, is typically absent and there is little bone formation. The spondylitis tends to occur in those who have had the disease for years and it is unusual for it to be evident at the onset of peripheral arthritis.

Cervical subluxation is common particularly at the atlanto-axial joints (Fig. 7–9). The frequency of atlanto-axial subluxation reflects the unique anatomic character of the occipito-atlanto-axial joints.[86] The atlanto-axial joints are primarily concerned with rotary motion and, consequently, the supporting ligaments must be lax with the exception of the transverse ligament.[166] The latter is primarily responsible for the integrity of the atlanto-odontoid joint and when it becomes lax, as it often does in rheumatoid disease,[93] the atlas will fall forward when the head is flexed. Inasmuch as this is largely a mechanical effect, atlanto-axial subluxation is almost always bilateral in this condition.[92] If roentgenograms are not routinely obtained with the neck in flexion, this instability will often go undetected. Flexion must be such that the center of gravity of the head lies anterior to the coronal plane of the lateral atlanto-axial joints. The upper limit of the atlanto-odontoid inter-

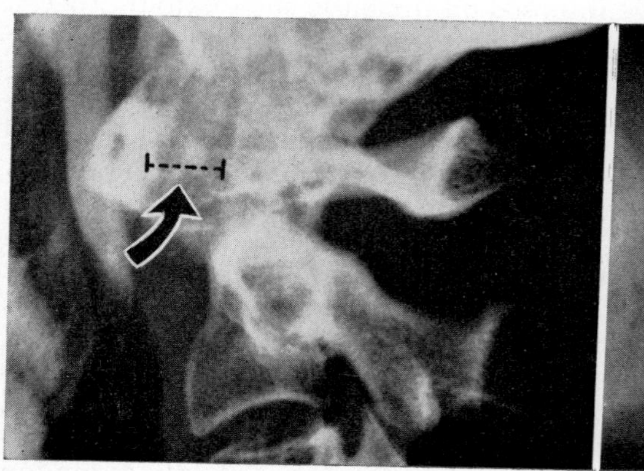
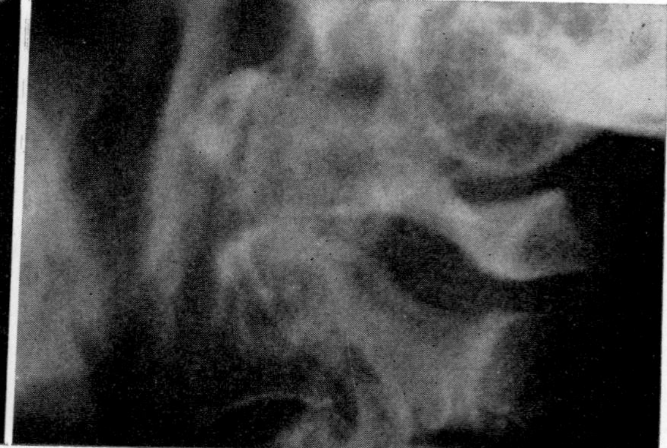

Fig. 7–9.—Bilateral subluxation of the atlanto-axial joints in rheumatoid arthritis. (Left) Flexion. (Right) Neutral. The atlanto-odontoid interval (arrow) is increased in flexion and exceeds 2.5 mm. This is common in this disease and is due to ligamentous laxity.

val in adults, measured at the inferior aspect of the atlanto-odontoid joint in the lateral projection, is 2.5 mm. This figure varies somewhat with age[60] but should be constant in flexion and extension.

Odontoid erosions, best seen on laminagrams, are common. They tend to develop earliest at the posteroinferior aspect, at the articulation with the transverse ligament.[86] A pathologic fracture of the odontoid process may develop secondary to deep erosion.[94] The tips of the spinous processes are also eroded, particularly at C-6, C-7 and T-1, and erosions commonly develop in the apophyseal joints. Early erosions in the latter may be difficult to detect on conventional views but they may progress to extensive destruction of the subchondral bone and laminae (Fig. 7–10). Occasionally, apophyseal joints ankylose at one or two levels,[88,95] but ankylosis of *all* the cervical apophyseal joints is unusual in adults. Cervical intervertebral disc narrowing is common, both in the upper and lower segments, and is not usually associated with hypertrophic spur formation. Disc narrowing often occurs at the levels of apophyseal ankylosis suggesting that the former is a consequence of the latter and a reflection of atrophy rather than inflammation. On the other hand, cervical vertebral endplate erosions are common and may be widespread and dramatic (Fig. 7–10). Such erosions often occur at those levels where apophyseal joint destruction is most marked. In the early stages they may have the appearance of Schmorl's nodes (intravertebral disc prolapses).[92] It is possible that they may in part be a consequence of increased cervical mobility secondary to the apophyseal joint destruction and ligamentous laxity. It is conceivable that cervical immobilization may retard the development of vertebral endplate destruction.[88]

Occasionally, the sacroiliac joints in rheumatoid arthritis exhibit minimal ero-

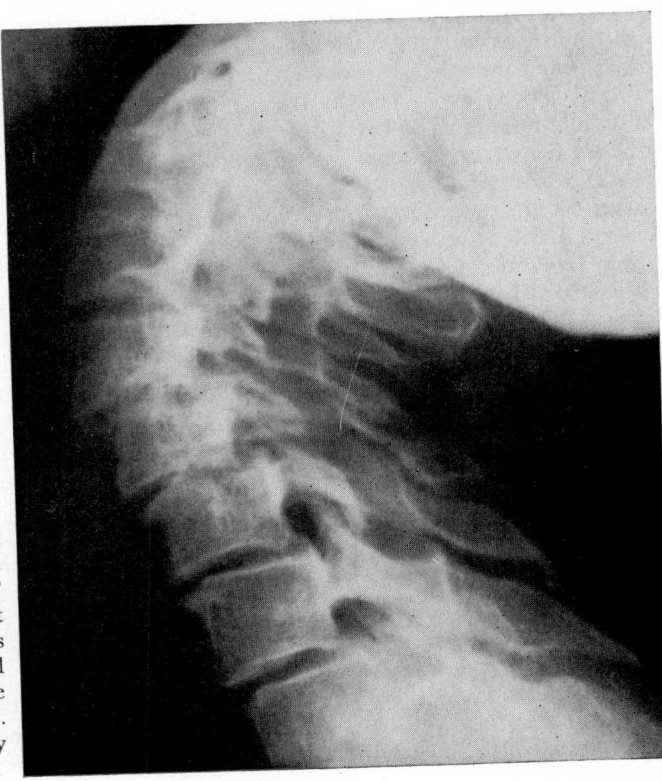

FIG. 7–10.—Advanced rheumatoid arthritis. Cervical spine, lateral view. There are multiple, "step-ladder" subluxations with reduction in height of the intervertebral discs and erosions of the vertebral endplates, apophyseal joints and posterior arches. Note tapering of lower spinous processes. The odontoid process (not clearly depicted) was almost totally destroyed

sions and interosseous space narrowing but reactive sclerosis, a feature of ankylosing spondylitis, is characteristically absent.[95] Sacroiliac joint involvement may be unilateral or asymmetric. Rarely, the cartilage spaces are completely obliterated making it difficult to differentiate from advanced ankylosing spondylitis. In such cases the remainder of the spine and peripheral joints form the basis for differentiation. Minimal irregularities in the subchondral bone may be due to focal cortical compression and should not be confused with sacroiliac arthritis. These compression deformities are associated with osteoporosis and are best shown with laminagraphy.

Idiopathic pleural effusion is common in rheumatoid arthritis and may be unilateral or bilateral. It tends to be minimal to moderate and transient although, occasionally, it persists for long periods without change. It may occur early in the disease and may even antedate the arthritis, although it is more usual in cases of well-established polyarthritis. Pericardial effusion may coexist. Discrete *pulmonary rheumatoid nodules* are occasionally present. These are generally multiple and tend to be subpleural, varying in size from several millimeters to a few centimeters. Only rarely are these lesions solitary. They may cavitate, occasionally leading to pneumothorax, or they may regress spontaneously. Chronic interstitial pneumonitis is not infrequent with or without these discrete nodules, and progressive fibrosis usually ensues. The radiologic and pathologic findings are nonspecific. In the acute stage the appearance is indistinguishable from a viral pneumonitis whereas in the later stages it may resemble a number of chronic fibrosing diseases, such as scleroderma and idiopathic pulmonary fibrosis. A "honeycomb" appearance due to bronchiolar ectasia is indicative of severe interstitial fibrosis. Occasionally, bullous emphysema and bronchiectasis develop. Patients with chronic interstitial pneumonitis and fibrosis often exhibit respiratory symptoms whereas those with only discrete pulmonary nodules are frequently asymptomatic.

There is little correlation between the clinical severity of the arthritis and the development of these pulmonary and pleural lesions.[106] Whereas rheumatoid patients exposed to dust-producing occupations seem prone to develop these lesions, there are many cases without such occupational exposures. Furthermore, these patients need not have particularly high titers of rheumatoid factor nor subcutaneous rheumatoid nodules.

JUVENILE RHEUMATOID ARTHRITIS

Most would agree that the pathologic process in rheumatoid arthritis in children is basically the same as in adults but the clinical picture is modified by severe constitutional and visceral reactions and growth disturbances. (*See also* Chapter 24.) Certain roentgenologic manifestations are also significantly different and merit special consideration.[51,103]

There is a predilection for the knees, ankles and wrists (Fig. 7–11) and it is not uncommon for the small joints of the hands and feet to be spared early in the disease. As the disease continues and the patients get older, the hands and feet are more likely to be affected. Monarticular arthritis is not uncommon, particularly in the knee (Fig. 7–12) and the disease may remain monarticular for many months before involving other joints. The roentgenographic abnormality may consist of soft tissue swelling and regional rarefaction for long periods without cartilage or bone destruction. This is particularly true of monarticular disease.[28] Nonspecific, band-like zones of metaphyseal rarefaction, not unlike those seen in childhood leukemia, may occasionally develop at the growth plate adjacent to involved joints. These probably represent zones of acute trabecular atrophy secondary to intense chronic hyperemia.[103]

Subperiosteal bone apposition is common, particularly in the phalanges,

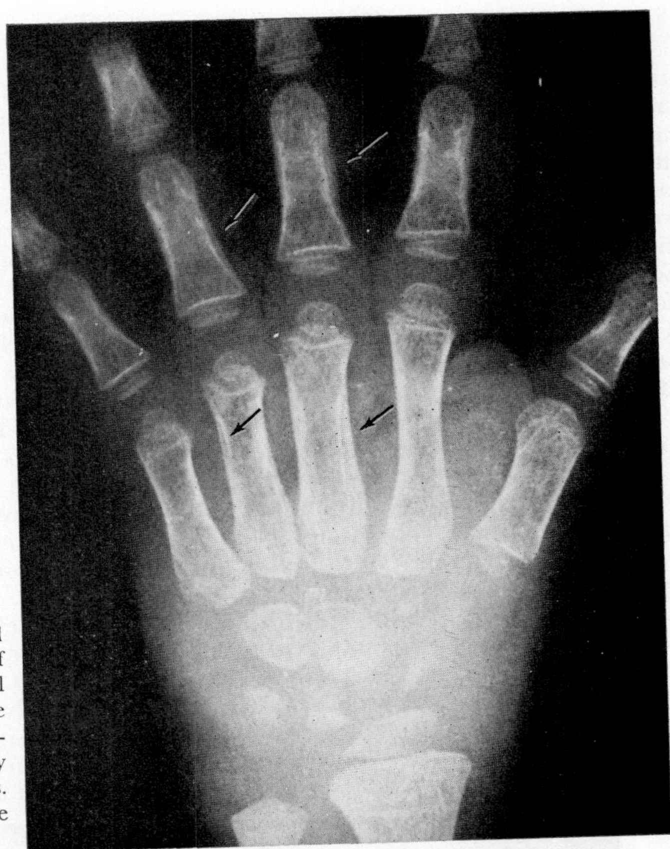

Fig. 7–11.—Juvenile rheumatoid arthritis. Note soft tissue swelling of wrist with accelerated epiphyseal maturation and subperiosteal bone apposition in phalanges and metacarpals (arrows) adjacent to minimally affected metacarpophalangeal joints. The opposite hand and wrist were similarly involved.

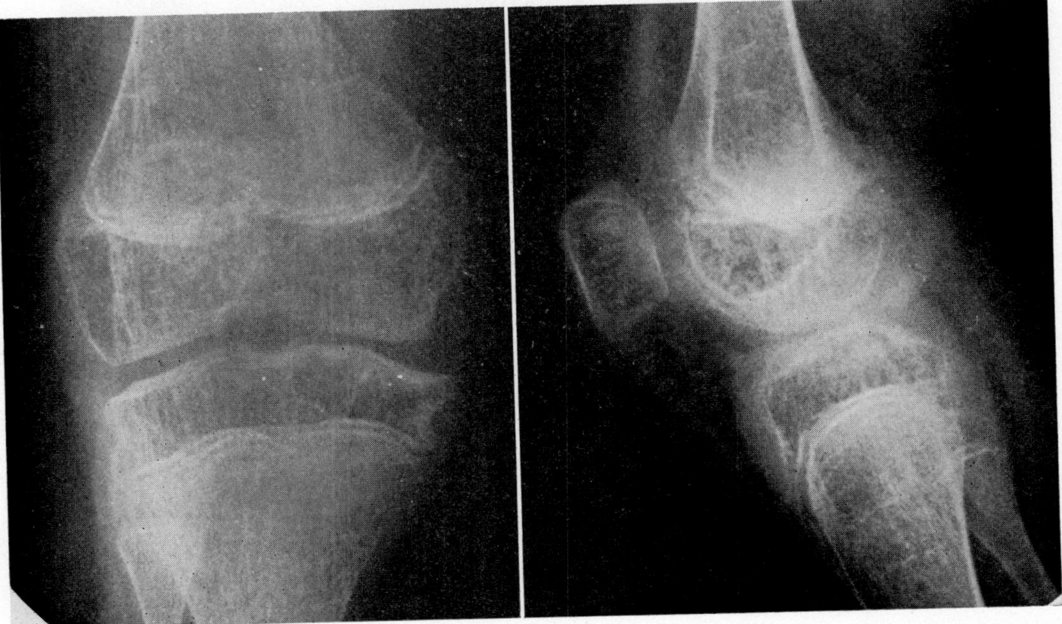

Fig. 7–12.—Juvenile rheumatoid arthritis with knee involvement of several years duration. Note enlargement of epiphyseal ossification centers with "squaring" of patella, bone atrophy and moderate, uniform narrowing of interosseous space.

metacarpals and metatarsals adjacent to affected joints[103,109,131] (Fig. 7–11). It is an early finding and although it may indicate inflammation of the joint capsule and adjacent periosteum, it may also represent a nonspecific effect of chronic hyperemia; this reflects the ease with which the periosteum is stimulated to form new bone in the immature skeleton. Occasionally, the cortex of an involved bone remains thickened but more often it becomes thin due to concomitant endosteal resorption. Generalized osteoporosis is characteristic.

Subluxations are not limited to small joints, as in adults, but often also involve large joints. Hip subluxation is not rare[65,103] and should not be confused with congenital dislocation. Bony ankylosis of involved joints may develop rapidly, and is frequent in the carpal joints. It should not be confused with congenital malformations. In rheumatoid disease many carpal bones usually fuse together, whereas in isolated congenital malformations it is usually two bones that fuse, most often the lunate and triquetrum and, less commonly, the capitate and hamate. Carpal fusions have also been described in various congenital malformation syndromes.[127]

As in adults, attenuation of the articular cartilage is seen as a uniform narrowing of the interosseous space. Cartilage destruction and bone erosion follow and may develop rapidly. In addition one often finds "cupping" of the ends of the bones, particularly in the hands and feet.[103] This is due to bone compression similar to that seen in adults but in children it may cause an inhibiting effect on the growth plate; this may be responsible for the characteristic brachydactyly. The inhibition of bone growth associated with the ancient Chinese custom of binding children's feet is analogous. Premature fusion of growth plates is usually *not* found in patients with generalized brachydactyly. Frank compression fractures may occur in the epiphyseal ossification centers of weight-bearing joints and in the spine, particularly the

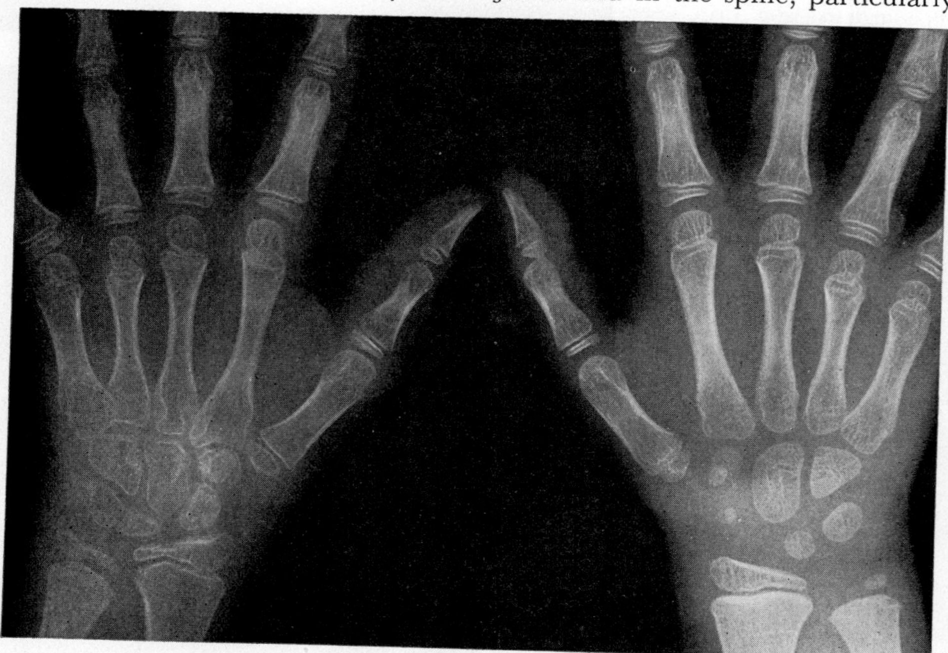

Fig. 7–13.—Long-standing juvenile rheumatoid arthritis with involvement of the left wrist. There is increased maturation of the bones on the affected side but they will probably be smaller than on the unaffected side in adult life. Note bone atrophy on the left.

dorsal region. Diaphyseal fractures[9] are a complication of advanced disease associated with severe bone atrophy. These fractures occur principally in association with prolonged steroid therapy but may develop in any patient who has osteoporosis.

Growth disturbances are often outstanding and not necessarily related to the severity of the arthritis[4,103] (Fig. 7–13). The epiphyseal ossification centers of affected joints often show an accelerated maturation[16] and certain ossification centers, particularly those about the knee, are often enlarged, presenting a characteristic "ballooned appearance" with relative constriction just above and below the articular surfaces (Fig. 7–12). It is as though that part of the epiphysis covered with articular cartilage participates less in this hypertrophy than the remainder, near the hyperemic joint capsule. The patella is often enlarged and may have a "squared" appearance as in hemophilic arthropathy. The ends of the long bones often present a striking contrast to the atrophic, slender diaphyses. Generalized inhibition of long bone growth may be so severe as to mimic a bone dysplasia. However, there may be an *overgrowth* in the length of a long bone adjacent to an involved joint such as the knee. In such cases one extremity may be longer than the contralateral one or there may be a disparity in growth rate of adjacent long bones causing bowing deformities. Monarticular disease involving the knee may be associated with pronounced atrophy of all bones of the ipsilateral extremity including the foot and innominate bone. Premature epiphyseal fusion may involve one or several bones but it is not a generalized effect. It is unrelated to joint destruction and is often symmetrical, sometimes affecting only a portion of the growth plate; the fourth metatarsal is frequently involved.

Young adults with a long history of rheumatoid arthritis in childhood may show remarkable, often bizarre, skeletal deformities. These reflect uncoordinated, stunted bone growth which in part is secondary to the mechanical effects on the joints themselves. Bones grow and model as a response to mechanical requirements and joint destruction with subluxation, inflammation of periarticular tissues, ligamentous laxity and alteration in muscle action all produce abnormal stresses which are bound to lead to modeling deformities.

Temporomandibular arthritis is common in adults and children. Micrognathia is characteristic of the disease in children, particularly when it starts early in life, and may be secondary to temporomandibular arthritis.[103] The length of the mandible and the height of its ramus are determined largely by its condylar growth center. Unlike the epiphyses of the long bones, growth of the condylar cartilage, in which bone arises, is derived by apposition from a layer of precartilaginous connective tissue which lies beneath the fibrous articular surface. Since the fibrous layer lines the joint cavity there is no cartilaginous barrier to protect the precartilaginous zone. This delicate construction suggests that there may be a particular susceptibility to injury especially in early life. Temporary cessations in condylar growth are not compensated and a significant period of arrest will be reflected in the final size of the mandible. However, the disparity between severe growth retardation and minimal temporomandibular arthritis suggests that micrognathia is *indirectly* related to such arthritis or that it is a consequence of some other factor, such as cervical spondylitis.

As in adults, the spondylitis in children primarily affects the cervical region and atlanto-axial subluxation is common (Fig. 7–9). The normal upper limit of the atlanto-odontoid interval may be as much as 4.5 mm. and there may be a 1 mm. difference between extension and flexion. There is a more pronounced tendency toward apophyseal joint ankylosis than in adults. This may involve the entire cervical spine, including the atlanto-axial joints; the latter may fuse in the subluxed position. Apophyseal ankylosis has caused confusion between this disease and ankylosing spondylitis. However, "squaring" of the vertebral bodies and syndesmophyte formation do not occur even when these patients are followed into adult life. Although the sacroiliac joints may be involved, it is quite uncommon and clinically insignificant. The vertebral bodies are characteristically small and the intervertebral discs are atrophic at those cervical levels where the apophyseal joints have fused. The discs and vertebral bodies assume more normal proportions where the apophyseal joints are not fused. Vertebral endplate destruction rarely develops in children. It is possible that posterior joint ankylosis "protects" the anterior intervertebral joints.[87,92]

Differential Diagnosis.—Rheumatic fever with polyarthritis is often a consideration in differential diagnosis. Subperiosteal bone apposition in the vicinity of involved joints virtually never occurs in rheumatic fever. *Chronic infectious arthritis*,[170] such as tuberculosis, must often be ruled out in cases of monarticular rheumatoid arthritis. Extensive bone destruction in such cases strongly favors infectious arthritis for it is unusual to have bone destruction in monarticular rheumatoid arthritis. *Hemophilic*[69,171] and rheumatoid arthritis may be difficult to distinguish particularly when observations are confined to one joint such as the knee (Fig. 7–15). Enlargement of the femoral and tibial epiphyses and patella may occur in either condition. Although irregular widening of the femoral intercondylar notch, probably due to erosion, is frequent in hemophilia,[112] it may occasionally be observed in rheumatoid arthritis. Generalized polyarthritis is rare in hemophilia but selective involvement of the elbow[162] with secondary dysplasia of the radial head is common. Secondary degenerative joint disease often occurs in children and young adults with *epiphyseal dysplasia* and may simulate a late stage in rheumatoid arthritis.[20,163]

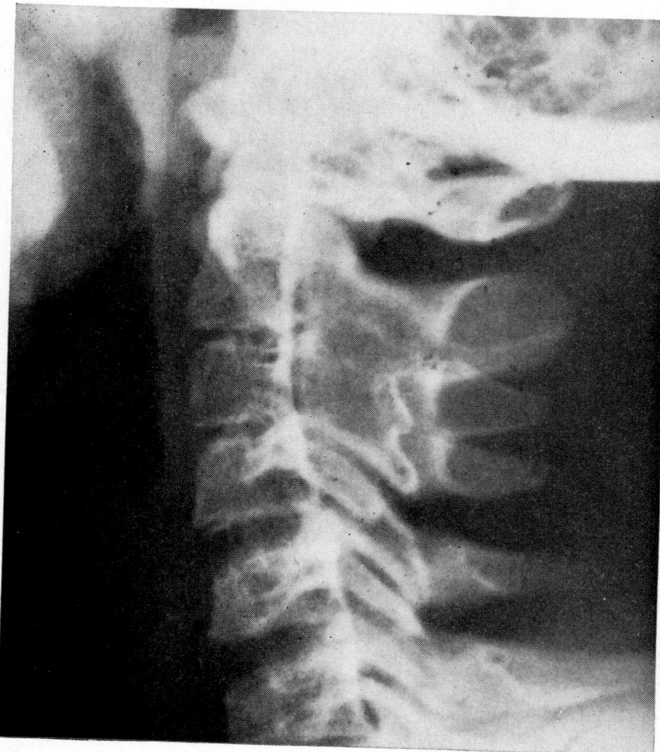

FIG. 7–14.—Cervical spondylitis in juvenile rheumatoid arthritis. The intervertebral discs and vertebrae are small at C_{2-3} and C_{3-4} where the apophyseal joints are ankylosed but approach more normal proportions at those levels where fusion has not occurred.

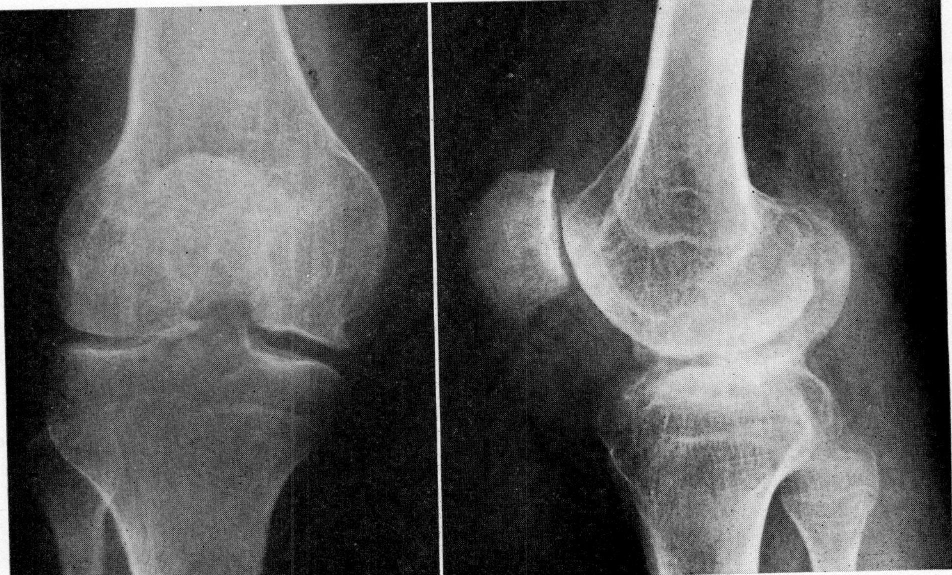

FIG. 7–15.—Chronic arthritis secondary to hemophilia. The ends of the bones appear "ballooned" and the patella has a "square" configuration. There is irregular widening of the femoral intercondylar notch.

The symmetry of the joint lesions and the discrepancy between joint involvement and skeletal deformity are clues to the diagnosis. *Mucopolysaccharidoses*[169] may also be confused with juvenile rheumatoid arthritis but a skeletal radiologic survey will usually indicate that the joint lesions are secondary. *Torticollis* in children may be confused with atlanto-axial subluxation. This commonly occurs as a nonspecific sequel to pharyngeal, cervical or mastoid infections. In some instances a true atlanto-axial subluxation develops[166] and should not be confused with the atlanto-axial subluxation of rheumatoid arthritis. The latter rarely occurs early in the disease without simultaneous arthritis in the extremities. Spontaneous atlanto-axial subluxation has also been described in *Down's syndrome*.[100,105,138] Finally, the distinction between a *congenital skeletal malformation* and one secondary to juvenile rheumatoid arthritis may be raised inasmuch as the latter often begins in the first few years of life.[103] Radiologic examination of other parts of the skeleton in such instances may serve to differentiate these conditions.

ANKYLOSING SPONDYLITIS

Ankylosing spondylitis[11,24,49,108,123,129] is primarily a disease of the spine although the rhizomelic and anterior thoracic joints are often affected. Synovial joints may be involved but, unlike rheumatoid arthritis, there is an outstanding predilection for ligamentous attachments and fibrocartilaginous joints such as the symphysis pubis, intervertebral and sternomanubrial joints. (*See also* Chapter 41.) The term *rheumatoid spondylitis* as a synonym for ankylosing spondylitis is unfortunate for it implies that this is the spinal equivalent of rheumatoid arthritis. There is a spinal form of rheumatoid arthritis, as noted above, and its pattern is quite different from ankylosing spondylitis. Not only are there clinical, therapeutic and prognostic differences between these two diseases, but the radiologic manifestations also differ significantly both in the spine and extremities.

Spine.—The bone erosions in this disease, whether in the spinal or extraspinal joints, are usually *superficial* and associated with reactive sclerosis, bone proliferation and bony ankylosis. Deep erosions with large osteolytic, cyst-like lesions, as occur in rheumatoid arthritis, are distinctly uncommon and the erosions are often overshadowed by bone production. In addition the pattern of joint involvement is distinctive.

The sacroiliac joints are invariably affected at the time the earliest lesions are evident in the spine (Fig. 7–16). Early sacroiliac changes may be subtle, consisting of an indistinctness or blurring of the subchondral bony margins. This is accompanied by an adjacent reactive sclerosis which may be quite marked, obliterating the subchondral margins, or, depending on the stage of the disease and individual variation, it may be quite minimal. Both sacroiliac joints are involved simultaneously although, initially, this may be somewhat asymmetrical. Eventually, the sacroiliac arthritis is quite symmetrical in the overwhelming majority of cases. Although it is axiomatic that the presence of normal sacroiliac joints is virtually incompatible with the diagnosis, it should be emphasized that early sacroiliac arthritis may be subtle and further radiologic examination may be indicated after several months if the disease is suspected. It is desirable to obtain stereoscopic views of the sacroiliac joints with the patient supine and central ray angled cephalad 20 degrees. The interosseous sacroiliac cartilage spaces become narrowed and finally obliterated and solid bony ankylosis ensues. A thin dense line may denote the site of the previous joint or there may be no vestige of the joint. Reactive sclerosis disappears as ankylosis supervenes and osteoporosis usually develops.

Superficial erosions of the pelvic bones occur at ligamentous attachments and these are usually associated with reactive sclerosis and marginal bone production. These sites include the attachments of the sacroiliac ligaments, above the joints, femoral trochanters, and iliac and ischial margins, particularly the latter. These lesions are usually bilateral but may persist unilaterally. The symphysis pubis

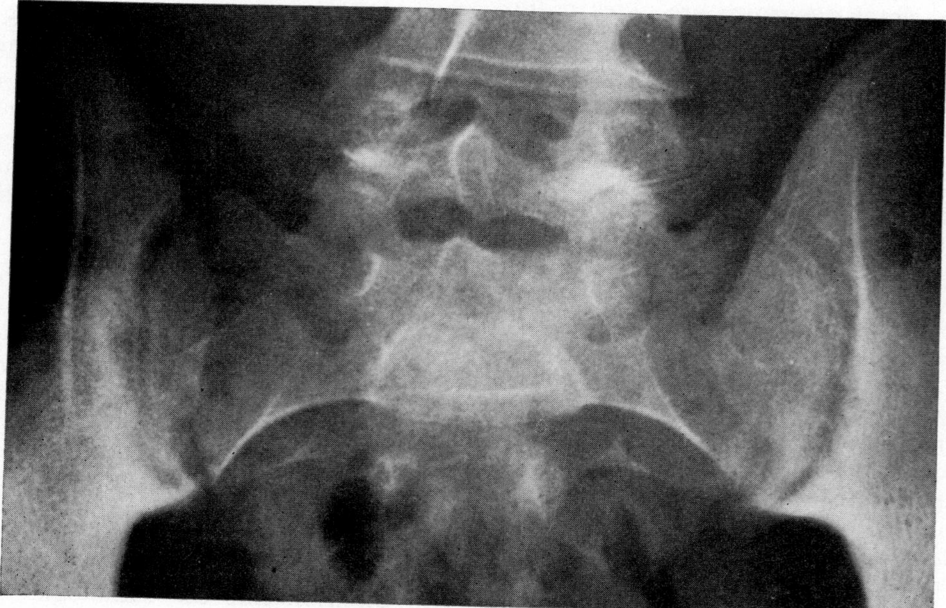

Fig. 7–16.—Bilateral sacroiliac arthritis in an adolescent boy with ankylosing spondylitis. The subchondral margins are irregular and indistinct and there is characteristic reactive sclerosis bilaterally.

is frequently affected in a manner analogous to that seen in the sacroiliac joints.

The concept of an ascending and descending form of the disease in the spine is misleading. The vertebrae and spinal joints are affected in a characteristic manner with the changes tending to develop first at the spinal flexures, particularly the dorsolumbar junction and, to a lesser degree, the lumbosacral junction. The lumbar spine is most frequently affected but the dorsal spine may be involved simultaneously. Cervical spondylitis may develop subsequently or at the time the dorsolumbar segment is affected but it is unusual for the cervical region and sacroiliac joints to be extensively involved with sparing of the rest of the spine.

Superficial erosions develop at the superior and inferior anterior corners of the vertebral bodies giving a "planed down" or "squared" appearance in the lateral projection (Fig. 7–17). This is particularly evident in the lumbar vertebrae which normally have a pronounced anterior concavity. Only one corner of a vertebral body, usually the superior one, may be affected. The reactive sclerosis which develops near the erosions is the basis for the so-called "shining corner." In addition, typical paravertebral ossifi-

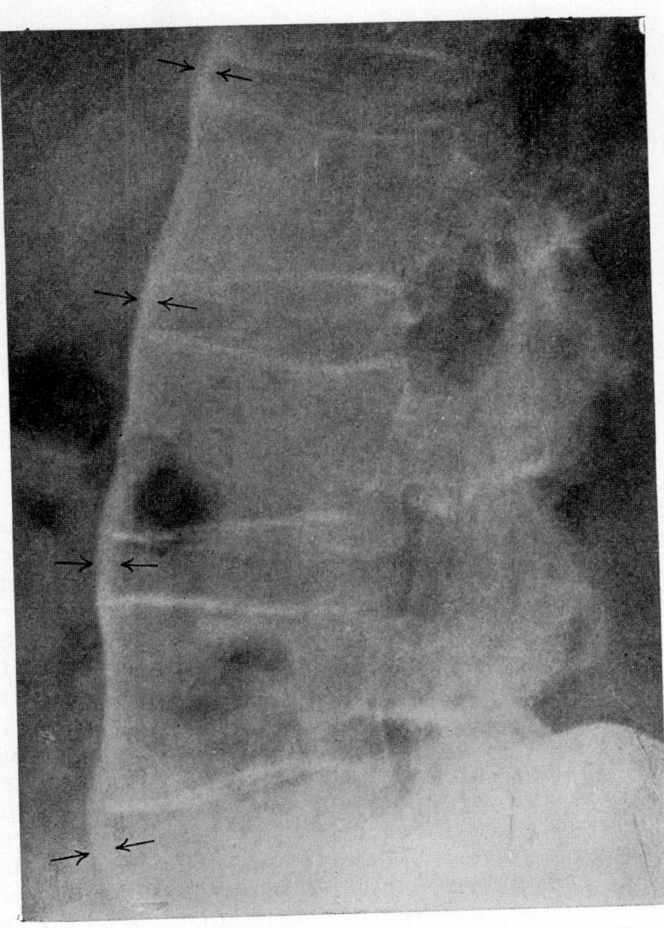

Fig. 7–17.—Advanced ankylosing spondylitis, lumbar spine. There is ossification (arrows) along the anterior longitudinal ligament with loss of the normal concavity of the lumbar vertebrae giving a "squared" appearance. The apophyseal and sacroiliac joints are fused. Note osteoporosis.

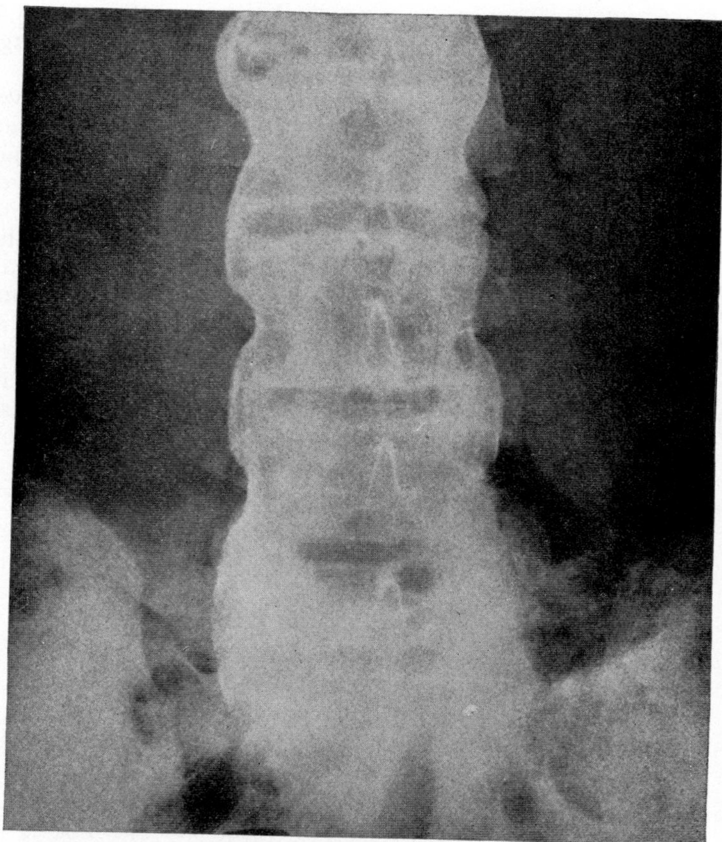

FIG. 7–18.—Advanced ankylosing spondylitis, lumbar spine. There is generalized symmetrical osseous bridging between vertebrae (syndesmophytes). The apophyseal and sacroiliac joints are fused.

cations, *syndesmophytes*, develop near the erosions and extend vertically, bridging adjacent vertebrae. The syndesmophytes develop between the spinal ligament and vertebrae and may appear delicate and indistinct. They are often seen near the spinal flexures but can occur at any level. As the disease advances they become generalized, bilateral and well-defined, causing the "bamboo spine" appearance (Fig. 7–18). Erosions also occur at the disco-vertebral junctions, particularly anteriorly, often at multiple levels. These develop during the active phase of the disease and tend to be self-limited, progressing to bony ankylosis. The apophyseal and costovertebral joints are often affected early but it is difficult to detect minimal arthritis in these joints. The apophyseal joints can be evaluated in the frontal projection in the lumbar segment, in oblique projections in the dorsal spine and in the lateral view in the cervical spine. The interosseous spaces of the apophyseal joints become narrow, often in association with subchondral reactive sclerosis, and eventually fuse. As these joints ankylose, the vertebrae become osteoporotic[52] and the intervertebral disc spaces narrow. The spine may become straightened with complete loss of the normal curvatures or there may be an exaggerated dorsal kyphosis. Cervical vertebral ankylosis tends to become generalized and complete (Fig. 7–19) and, in advanced cases, may

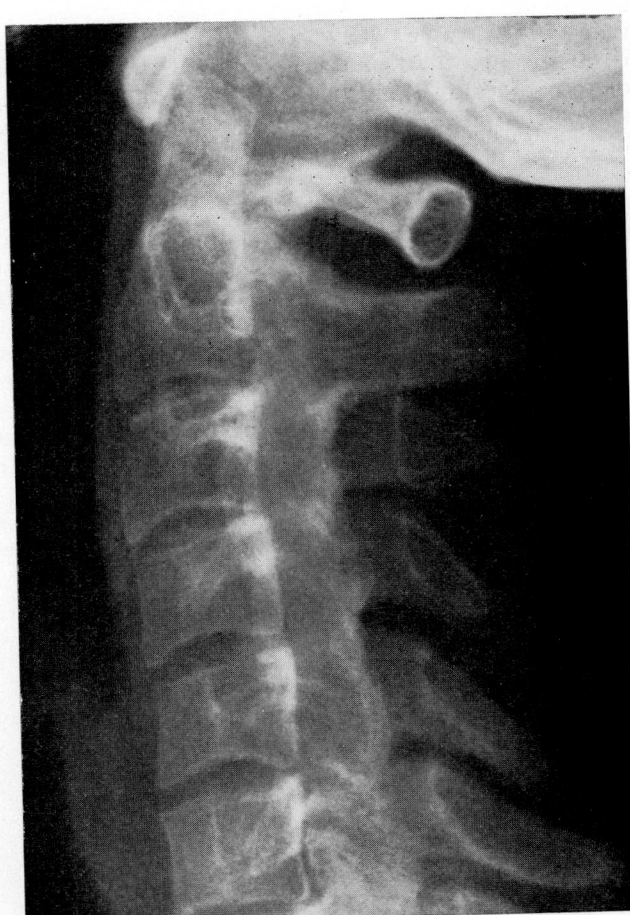

FIG. 7-19.—Advanced ankylosing spondylitis, cervical spine. The apophyseal joints are fused and there is a somewhat "squared" appearance to the vertebral bodies with minimal reactive sclerosis along the antero-inferior margin of C_3. Note the osteoporosis, narrowed intervertebral disc at C_{2-3} and loss of cervical lordosis. The dorsolumbar spine and sacroiliac joints were involved.

be complicated by a pathologic fracture.[81] Superficial surface erosions of the spinous processes, causing them to have a "sharpened" appearance, are particularly evident in the lower cervical and upper dorsal region;[88] the resulting deformities are similar to those of rheumatoid arthritis.

A lesion characteristic of the late stage of the disease which mimics infectious spondylitis consists of destruction of an intervertebral disc and adjacent vertebrae often leaving smooth sclerotic margins.[128,167] Such lesions probably represent pseudoarthroses and are usually associated with unrecognized fractures through previously ankylosed posterior joints. These lesions progress slowly, for months or years, occur at a single level and develop in a spine that is almost always extensively ankylosed both above and below the lesion. They usually develop in the lower dorsal or upper lumbar segments. Another finding late in the disease is extensive bone resorption from the anterior surface of the lower cervical spine.[104] This is invariably associated with complete ankylosis of the cervical spine and extreme dorsal kyphosis. This abnormality should not be confused with the cervical growth disturbance of juvenile rheumatoid arthritis. In the latter there is a generalized reduction in the size of the cervical vertebral bodies whereas in ankylosing spondylitis it is primarily the anteroposterior diameters that are reduced.

Extremities.—The extraspinal arthritis

is often associated with a disability that is far greater than one expects from the degree of joint destruction. As in the spine, the erosions are generally superficial and severe bone loss, "arthritis mutilans" as seen in rheumatoid arthritis, is quite rare. Large discrete, osteolytic lesions, "pseudocysts," are virtually never observed, even in severely affected joints.

Arthritis is said to develop in the extremities in approximately 50% of cases, usually affecting the shoulders and hips; the anterior thoracic joints are also frequently involved.[129] Transient synovitis may occur in the hands, wrists or feet, usually leaving no residual deformity, but progressive destructive arthritis is relatively uncommon. When it does occur in these joints, the involvement is characteristically nonuniform, with some joints being markedly deformed and others hardly at all. There may be minimal to moderate subperiosteal bone apposition adjacent to involved joints. Calcaneal erosions[23] are not rare and occur at the same sites as in rheumatoid arthritis but are more superficial and associated with reactive sclerosis.

As in other chronic inflammatory diseases, the cartilage space is uniformly narrowed whether it be in the hip, shoulder or other joints. Symptoms of arthritis may precede narrowing of the interosseous space, particularly in the hip. In such cases traction on the hip during the roentgenographic exposure may disclose the presence of free fluid. This recently described technique[97] for

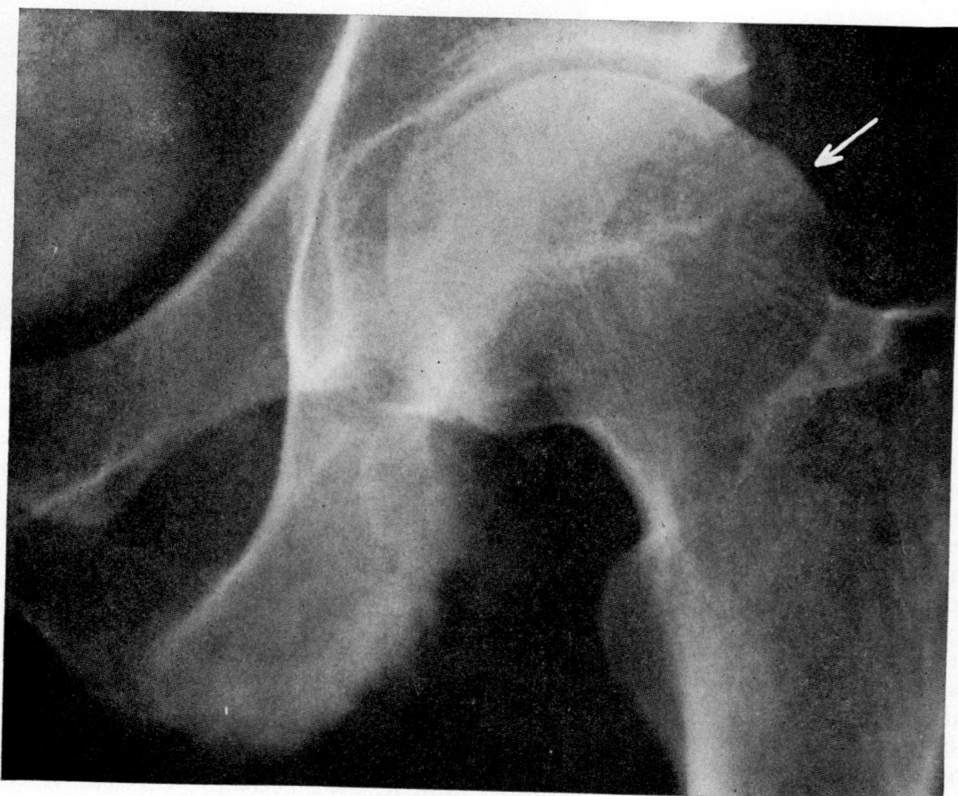

FIG. 7–20.—Ankylosing spondylitis. There is a large bony protuberance at the margin of the articular cartilage (arrow) which is associated with reactive sclerosis in the femoral head. The interosseous space is not narrowed in this case. Note the irregular bone formation and sclerosis at the ischial margin and the absence of buttressing at the inferior aspect of the femoral neck.

evaluating fluid in the hip lends itself to other diseases as well and often provides a method for evaluating the articular cartilage without resorting to conventional arthrography. As the disease progresses, a delicate bony spur forms at the superior aspect of the junction of the femoral head and neck. Eventually this may develop as a ridge of osteophytes around the femoral head, not unlike that seen in osteoarthritis (Fig. 7–20). However, in spondylitis the osteophytes tend to be absent or minimal at the acetabular margins and lateral subluxation of the femoral head does not occur. "Buttressing" or thickening of the inferior cortex of the femoral neck is quite rare but is very common in osteoarthritis. Inward protrusion of the acetabulum may be observed but is usually minimal or moderate whereas in rheumatoid arthritis this is often severe. Bony ankylosis occasionally develops. Arthritis of the glenohumeral, acromioclavicular and sternoclavicular joints is in many ways analogous to that seen in the hips in that the erosions tend to be superficial and reactive sclerosis and bone apposition are frequent. Sternomanubrial arthritis, leading to bony ankylosis, is common.

Juvenile Ankylosing Spondylitis.—Ankylosing spondylitis is not rare in adolescence and occasionally develops in childhood. In such cases extraspinal arthritis may be the presenting feature and outstanding manifestation for years. The diagnosis should be suspected in male children who have symptoms referable to the sacroiliac joints, lumbodorsal spine or hip beginning late in childhood or adolescence. Such children may have transient arthritis of a few peripheral joints. Significant features in distinguishing these patients from those with juvenile rheumatoid arthritis are the relative sparing of the hands and wrists even after years, sacroiliac arthritis, remittent oligoarthritis and relatively late onset in childhood.[77] In addition, tests for rheumatoid factors and antinuclear antibodies are consistently negative. The normal indistinctness of the subchondral margins of the sacroiliac joints in childhood makes radiologic evaluation difficult. However, the presence of reactive sclerosis of the subchondral bone, particularly when associated with narrowing of the interosseous spaces, justifies the diagnosis of sacroiliac arthritis.

Differential Diagnosis.—Some of the conditions to be included in the differential diagnosis of ankylosing spondylitis will be considered briefly.[136] *Infectious disease* must be ruled out in cases of unilateral sacroiliac arthritis; the latter has also been observed in psoriasis and Reiter's disease.[101,139] Persistent unilateral sacroiliac arthritis is virtually never due to ankylosing spondylitis. A transient peripheral arthritis which clinically simulates rheumatoid arthritis often develops in *regional enteritis* and *ulcerative colitis.* These cases are characterized by an absence of cartilage and bone erosion and residual joint deformity. Some patients with enterocolitis, however, exhibit a spondylitis[83,141,176] which resembles ankylosing spondylitis, although sometimes the features suggest Reiter's disease. Workers in the polyvinyl chloride industry may develop a chemical *acro-osteolysis*[37,53,168] associated with bilateral sacroiliac arthritis similar to that seen in ankylosing spondylitis. Other spinal changes characteristic of ankylosing spondylitis have not been described in this condition. Bilateral erasure of the sacroiliac subchondral cortices, simulating arthritis, may also be observed in hyperparathyroidism. Ankylosis of the sacroiliac joints occurs in *paraplegia*[1] but there is no evidence that this is a consequence of arthritis; it may represent atrophy rather than destruction of the cartilage. Sclerosis of the iliac bones adjacent to the sacroiliac joints is characteristic of *osteitis condensans ilii.*[119,134] This usually occurs in females, often after childbirth and may be unilateral or bilateral. It is usually easily differentiated from sacroiliac arthritis in that the subchondral plate is not eroded, sclerosis is limited to the ilium and the interosseous space is normal (Fig. 7–21).

Osteophytes in *degenerative spondylosis*[151] are often confused with the syndesmophytes of ankylosing spondylitis. The former grow as a response to a bulging annulus fibrosus affected by degenerative changes. Hence, osteophytes are oriented horizontally although they may, as they become larger, grow vertically. Furthermore, osteophytes are broad-based and usually quite well defined. Syndesmophytes, on the other hand, are oriented vertically and are often poorly defined when small. *Senile ankylosing hyperostosis*[45] is a condition of the elderly which is generally a coincidental radiologic finding characterized by ossification of the anterior longitudinal ligament (Fig. 7–22). This appears like a thick, often irregular ribbon of bone extending along the anterior aspect of the vertebral bodies. It represents ossification of the anterior ligament itself and in the lateral roentgenogram appears to undulate along the normal concavities of the dorsal and lumbar vertebrae. A relative "clear space" is often seen at some points between the ossified ligament and vertebral body. In ankylosing spondylitis, however, the anterior ossification permits no such clear space and is quite straight, exhibiting no undulation in the lateral projection. Dorsal kyphosis may be present in senile ankylosing hyperostosis but the apophyseal and sacroiliac joints are characteristically not fused.

PSORIATIC ARTHRITIS AND REITER'S SYNDROME

Patients with psoriasis or Reiter's syndrome often exhibit an arthritis, both

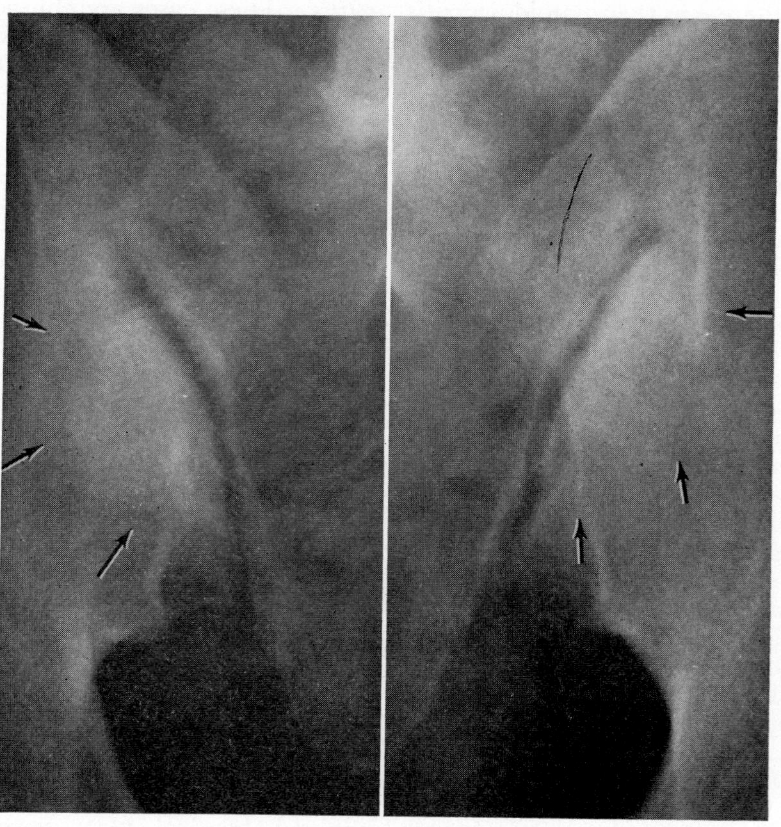

Fig. 7–21.—Bilateral osteitis condensans ilii, more marked on the right. The sclerosis involves the ilium (arrows) and is characteristically adjacent to the sacroiliac joint. The subchondral cortex is sharply defined and the interosseous space is preserved.

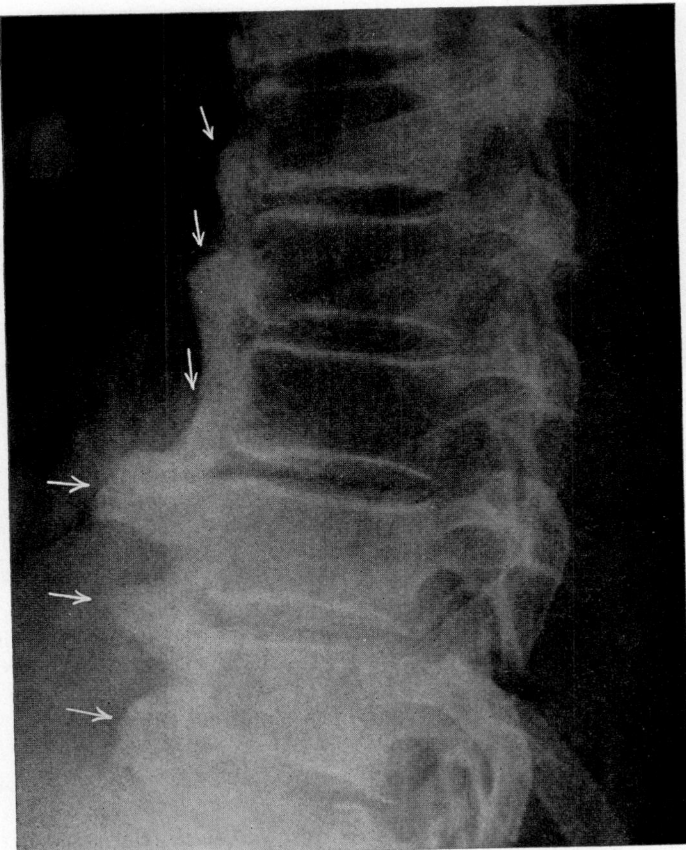

Fig. 7–22.—Senile ossification of the anterior longitudinal ligament. There is a thick, irregular, undulating ribbon of bone (arrows) extending along the anterior aspect of the dorsal spine. The delineation of the anterior surface of some of the vertebral bodies indicates a non-ossified plane between the ossified ligament and the vertebrae. Compare with Figure 7–17.

in the spine and extremities, which is radiologically distinctive. Although the radiologic manifestations of these two conditions differ in certain respects, they have much in common[125] and, therefore, will be considered together. The spondylitis has often been confused with ankylosing spondylitis and the peripheral arthritis with infectious or rheumatoid disease. It is worth emphasizing that the skin lesions in psoriasis may develop *after* the arthritis (*see also* Chapter 42) and those in Reiter's disease (*see also* Chapter 65) may be severe and indistinguishable both clinically and histologically from pustular psoriasis. Furthermore, it is conceivable that some patients with psoriatic-like lesions may have had clinically undetected urethritis, diarrhea or conjunctivitis. However, recent studies of carefully selected patients indicate that the apparent over-lap in radiologic manifestations does not merely reflect an inability to clinically distinguish these diseases. Nevertheless, depending on the joints involved, it may be easier to differentiate these conditions from ankylosing spondylitis, on the one hand, and rheumatoid arthritis on the other, than from one another. However, differences between them are significant and merit emphasis.

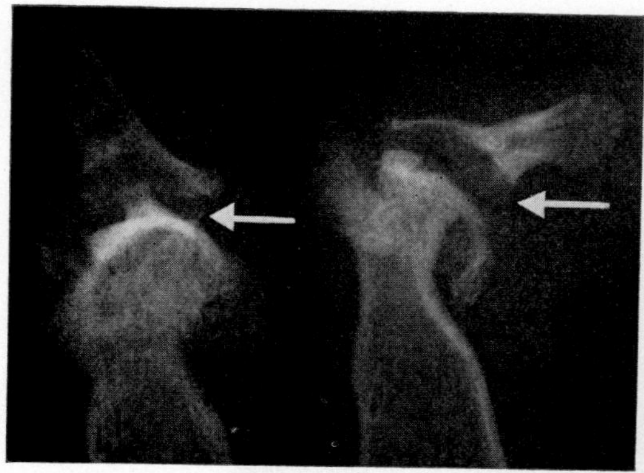

FIG. 7–23.—Terminal interphalangeal joints in psoriatic arthritis. There is extensive resorption of the subchondral bone on both sides of the joints (arrows). The joint on the right appears to have an "overhanging edge" but the distribution of involved joints and absence of a tophus distinguish this from gout. Compare with Figure 7–36.

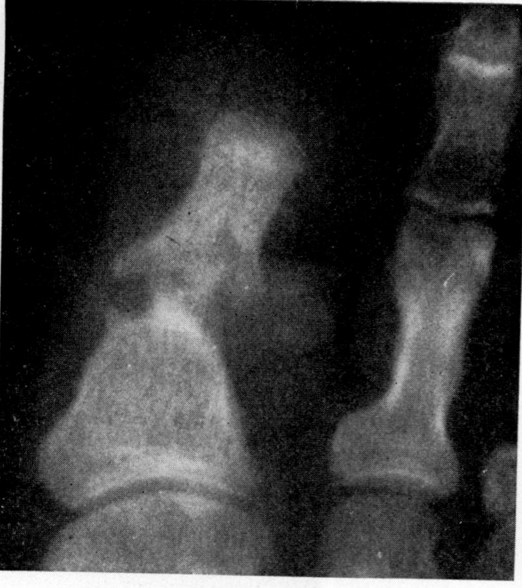

FIG. 7–24.—Psoriatic arthritis. There is extensive destruction of the interphalangeal joint of the great toe with resorption of the terminal tuft. Note lack of osteoporosis. A similar appearance may be observed in Reiter's syndrome.

Extremities.—The joints affected in rheumatoid arthritis may also be involved in these diseases but the *pattern* of joint involvement differs.[172] In psoriasis there is a characteristic predilection for the terminal interphalangeal joints, particularly in the hands[7] (Fig. 7–23). Involvement of these joints in Reiter's syndrome is uncommon and virtually never selective. In both conditions there is a pronounced tendency to involve the interphalangeal joint of the great toe, often with resorption of the terminal tuft[7,101,139] (Fig. 7–24). Resorption of the terminal tufts of the fingers is occasionally found with terminal interphalangeal arthritis in psoriasis and should not be confused with scleroderma. Instead of terminal interphalangeal arthritis, some psoriatic patients develop generalized arthritis of the hands and wrists which is often asymmetric and may progress to "arthritis mutilans." Although asymmetric arthritis occurs in Reiter's syndrome, *widespread* arthritis in the hands and wrists is distinctly rare; furthermore, proximal interphalangeal arthritis is common, usually affecting one or two joints, but metacarpophalangeal arthritis is relatively unusual. In fact, there is an outstanding predilection for the knees, ankles and feet in this syndrome and relative sparing of the upper extremities is characteristic.[44,139,165] Sparing of the latter may be conspicuous in the presence of persistent polyarthritis of the lower extremities with severe destruction of the pedal joints. It is noteworthy that the hips are not commonly affected. Calcaneal erosions are frequent in both conditions.[101,139]

Articular soft tissue swelling in these diseases resembles that seen in rheumatoid arthritis but osteoporosis is often absent despite extensive bone destruction. Uniform narrowing of the interosseous space is characteristic although in many cases bone destruction is so severe as to leave a widened space, containing fluid and soft tissues, between the eroded bone ends. Bone erosions may develop at the "marginal sites," typical of rheumatoid arthritis, but more often there is extensive destruction relatively early in the course of the disease with little selectivity for the marginal areas (Fig. 7–25). The erosions may extend far along the shaft beyond the capsular attachment in continuity with the articular erosion, causing a "pencil-like" tapering of the bone. While this is often observed, it is not pathognomonic of these conditions. A similar deformity occasionally occurs in other diseases associated with *severe* joint destruction including rheumatoid arthritis. However, a major distinction between these conditions and rheumatoid arthritis is the presence of subperiosteal bone apposition which is often exuberant (Fig. 7–26). This was noted in the peripheral joints in 9 of 14 patients with psoriatic arthritis and in 19 of 26 cases of Reiter's syndrome.[101] It may be linear, particularly in the metacarpals and metatarsals, but it is more often fluffy and arises near involved joints. The irregularity and poor definition of these bone formations suggest that it may be secondary to peri-

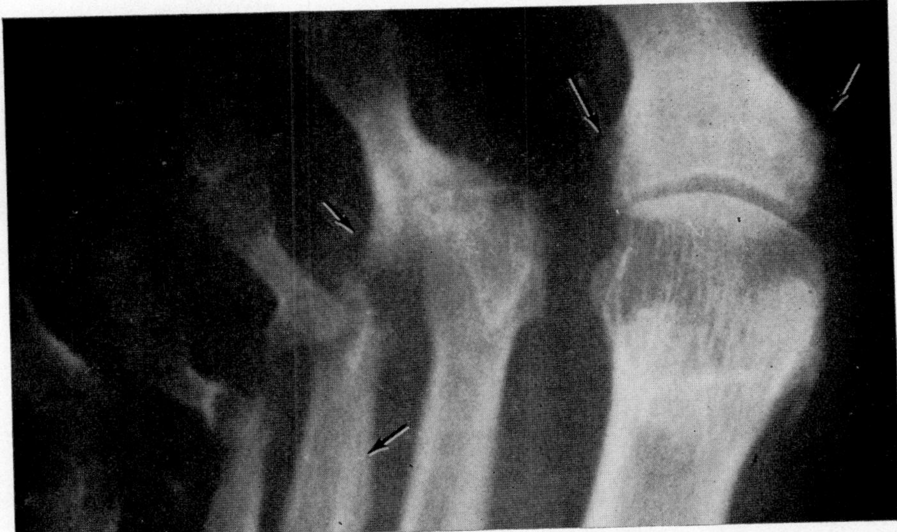

Fig. 7–25.—Extensive destruction of the metatarsophalangeal joints in psoriatic arthritis. Note subperiosteal bone apposition (arrows) and minimal erosions in the interphalangeal joint of the great toe.

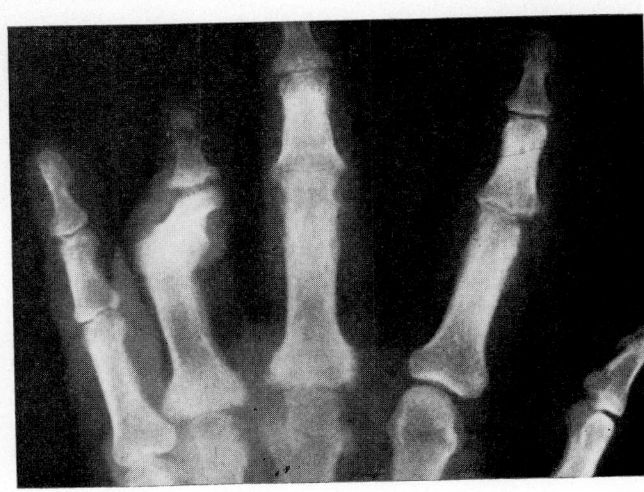

Fig. 7–26.—Psoriatic arthritis. Extensive involvement of several joints in the left hand characterized by flexion contractures and fluffy subperiosteal bone apposition. Note involvement of the terminal interphalangeal joints of the third and fourth digits and absence of osteoporosis.

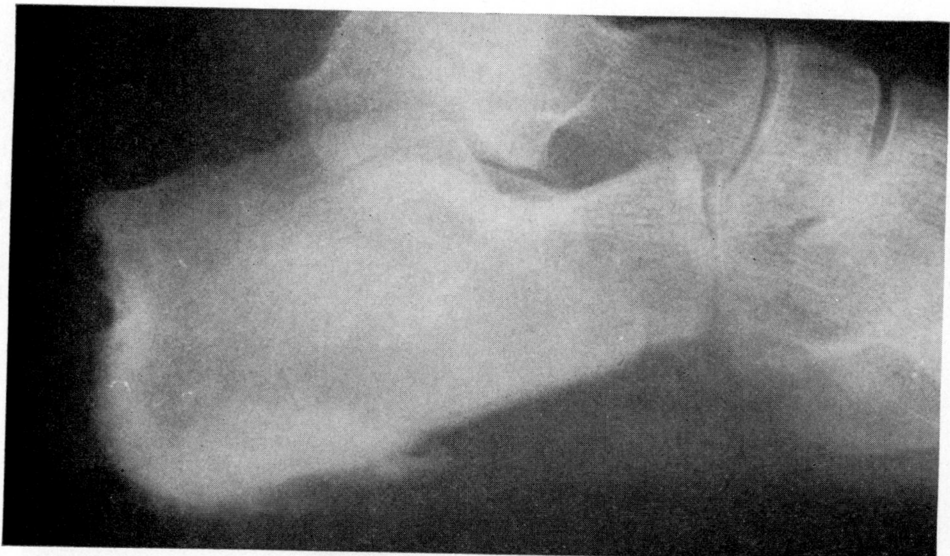

Fig. 7–27.—Reiter's syndrome with calcaneal erosions, extensive sclerosis and fluffy subperiosteal bone apposition. An identical appearance may be observed in psoriatic arthritis.

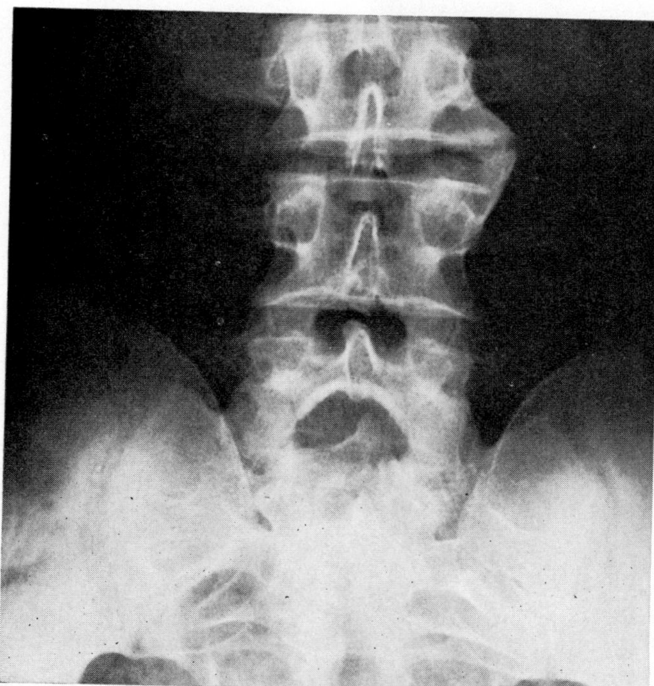

Fig. 7–28.—Reiter's syndrome. There is a large ossification which bridges L_3–L_4 on the left side associated with bilateral sacroiliac arthritis. The latter is characterized by subchondral erosions and reactive sclerosis similar to that seen in ankylosing spondylitis. Similar asymmetric "syndesmophytes" may also be observed in psoriatic arthritis.

ostitis. Bone apposition may cause widening of the end of a bone and, should the opposing bone be tapered, the so-called "pencil-in-cup" deformity results.[7] The calcaneal lesions in psoriatic arthritis and Reiter's syndrome are identical (Fig. 7–27). Bone formation is often outstanding and diffuse. It is usually fluffy, poorly marginated and tends to develop at the postero-inferior margins, associated with cortical erosions.

Spine.—Spondylitis[135,165] is common and is characteristically associated with peripheral joint involvement. This association is helpful in differentiating it from ankylosing spondylitis in which destructive lesions in the joints of the hands and feet are relatively uncommon. However, the spondylitis itself often exhibits distinguishing radiologic features. The frequency of spinal involvement will depend on case selection but it appears to be quite common in patients with destructive peripheral arthritis. In one series, comparing Reiter's syndrome with psoriatic arthritis, spondylitis was noted in approximately 80% of cases in each category.[101]

Bilateral, symmetrical sacroiliac arthritis is common and may be indistinguishable from that seen in ankylosing spondylitis (Fig. 7–28). Blurred, irregular subchondral margins, reactive sclerosis, and narrowing of the interosseous spaces are characteristic features which may progress to bony ankylosis. There is often unilateral or markedly asymmetric involvement of the sacroiliac joints and this asymmetry may persist for years; it may be observed both in Reiter's syndrome and psoriatic arthritis[101,136,139] (Fig. 7–29). Occasionally, in Reiter's syndrome there is patchy sclerosis of both sacral and iliac subchondral margins, involving only a portion of the joint and associated with narrowing of the interosseous space. This is not to be confused with osteitis condensans ilii.

Sacroiliac arthritis may develop without lesions elsewhere in the spine. However, in both conditions one commonly finds paraspinal ossifications bridging adjacent vertebral bodies which are distinctive in that they develop asymmetrically, do not usually become generalized and are often quite large (Fig. 7–28). They resemble large syndesmophytes and are frequent in the upper lumbar and lower dorsal spine; when solitary they may be confused with a post-traumatic condition. Although "squaring" of the vertebral bodies does occur, one often finds these large asymmetric bone formations with relative

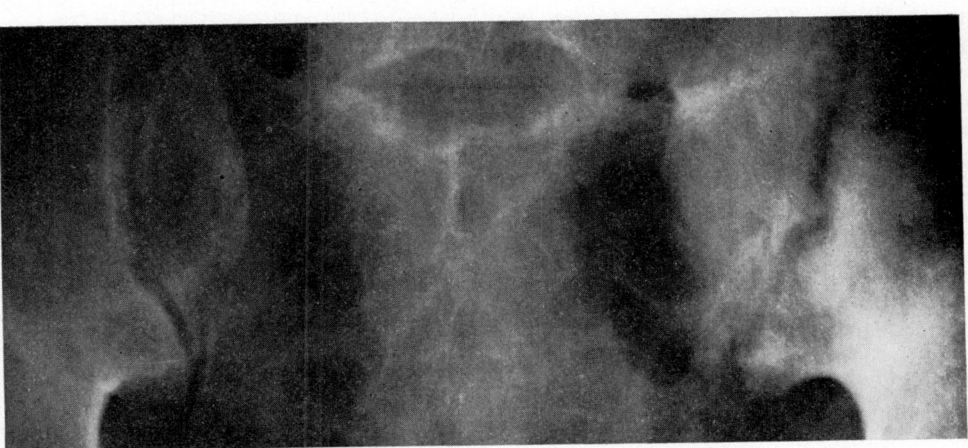

Fig. 7–29.—Unilateral sacroiliac arthritis in psoriatic arthritis. The unilaterality was persistent for several years and associated with extensive arthritis in the joints of the extremities. Unilateral involvement of the sacroiliac joints also occurs in Reiter's syndrome.

absence of "squaring." Attention has recently been called to a peculiar, fluffy paravertebral ossification in psoriatic arthritis apparently along the lateral longitudinal ligaments.[21] Apophyseal or costovertebral arthritis may occur in either condition but generalized involvement of these articulations is probably unusual in Reiter's syndrome. Cervical involvement is also probably much more common in psoriatic arthritis than in Reiter's syndrome. Spontaneous atlanto-axial subluxation and fracture dislocation of the ankylosed cervical spine may develop.[96]

It should be emphasized that not all patients with psoriatic arthritis or Reiter's syndrome progress to joint destruction. In many cases the arthritis is transient appearing to leave no joint damage but careful radiologic evaluation will often disclose minimal residua of previous arthritis. This may consist of a focal area of sclerosis or cortical thickening secondary to earlier erosion or peri-articular periostitis.

OSTEOARTHRITIS

Osteoarthritis may occur as a primary idiopathic disease or as a secondary condition which is a late sequel to acute and chronic disease or trauma.[40] (*See also* Chapter 56.) The joints affected in secondary osteoarthritis will depend on the pre-existing disease; usually, not many joints are affected unless the latter is itself widespread or systemic (e.g. Wilson's disease,[111] epiphyseal dysplasias,[163] ochronosis,[35,71] mucopolysaccharidoses[169]). In primary disease, however, the affected joints are usually more widely distributed. Once the cartilage degenerates, whatever the cause, a characteristic sequence of pathologic changes ensues.[147] Hence, with some exceptions, the radiologic manifestations are generally similar with respect to individual joints.

Degeneration and erosion of the articular cartilage usually develop first in the nonpressure, peripheral areas of a joint.[54,155] Cartilage hyperplasia develops at the margins of the articular cartilage; the most notable example of such hyperplasia is the Heberden's node. Focal invasion of the marginal hypertrophic cartilage by a vascular granulation tissue follows with resultant bone formation giving rise to the characteristic osteophyte. As the effective joint surface diminishes, a high cone of pressure is exerted on the remaining part of the articular cartilage and is particularly deleterious in weight-bearing joints such as the hip. This excessive pressure over a prolonged period causes further fibrillation and disintegration of the remaining cartilage with ingrowth of granulation tissue into the subchondral bone. This leads to further bone formation which is reflected radiologically as sclerosis of the subchondral plate. The presence of osteophytes generally indicates degenerative change in the articular cartilage and subchondral sclerosis denotes more advanced cartilage destruction. The degree of cartilage degeneration may best be appreciated in lower extremity joints, such as the knee, by obtaining roentgenograms with weight-bearing.[3] Virtually all of the articular cartilage may eventually degenerate leaving bone to bone contact at the joint surfaces. This is analogous to the situation in advanced rheumatoid arthritis except that in osteoarthritis there is no inhibition of reparative osteogenesis; this manifests itself as osteophyte formation and subchondral sclerosis. Microfractures and *focal* areas of ischemic necrosis may develop and could be related to the pathogenesis of characteristic subchondral cyst-like rarefactions.[54,59,64] The latter may also be due to an ingrowth of granulation tissue via defects in the articular cartilage or to areas of subchondral metaplasia. These rarefactions occasionally present as rounded, discrete lesions but are always marginated by thickened trabeculae which are seen radiologically as a thin or thick sclerotic line (Fig. 7–30*A*). They are typically found beneath the weight-bearing portion of a joint but at times

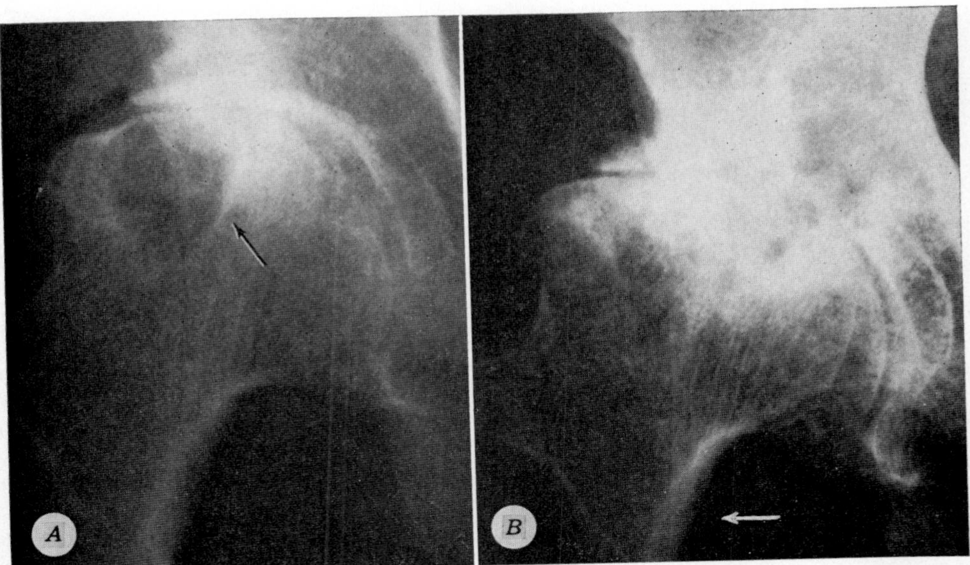

FIG. 7–30.—Osteoarthritis. *A*. Showing subchondral cyst-like rarefaction with thin sclerotic margins (arrow). *B*. Five years later. Deformity of the articular surface associated with collapse of the subchondral lesion. Note double contour of acetabulum due to marginal osteophyte formation, osteophytes at the lateral margin of the femoral head and buttressing of the inferior aspect of the femoral neck (arrow). The femoral head is slightly subluxed laterally and the interosseous space is narrowed nonuniformly. Compare with Figure 7–8.

near the periphery. Similar lucencies develop near the attachment of the joint capsule, particularly in certain joints such as the shoulder. It is possible that the various lucencies associated with degenerative disease, loosely designated as "osteoarthritic cysts," do not have the same pathogenesis. Rarely, solitary subchondral lucencies develop prior to radiologically demonstrable alterations in the cartilage space, particularly the hip. Whether these in fact have the same derivation as "osteoarthritic cysts" is not clear. These lesions, which contain fluid or fibrous tissue, may collapse, particularly in weight-bearing joints, causing marked deformity of the articular surfaces (Fig. 7–30*B*). In later stages there may be minimal to moderate malalignment and slight subluxation, a consequence of nonuniform narrowing of the articular cartilage, osteophyte production, collapse of the subchondral bone and remodeling of the articular surfaces.

Extremities.—There is a predilection for the interphalangeal joints of the hands,[150] particularly the terminal joints and for the joints between the first metacarpal and greater multangular and between the latter and the navicular (Fig. 7–31). One does not see *diffuse* involvement of the intracarpal joints, a feature of rheumatoid arthritis, nor are the radiocarpal and distal radioulnar joints affected in primary osteoarthritis. Metacarpophalangeal joint involvement is rare, minimal and usually associated with the more obvious interphalangeal changes. However, a form of osteoarthritis has been described, primarily in the elderly, in which there is a predilection for the metacarpophalangeal joints often with sparing of the interphalangeal joints.[107] This may be observed in idiopathic pseudogout as well as in pseudogout associated with hemochromatosis.[6,46,130]

Osteoarthritis is common in the *first*

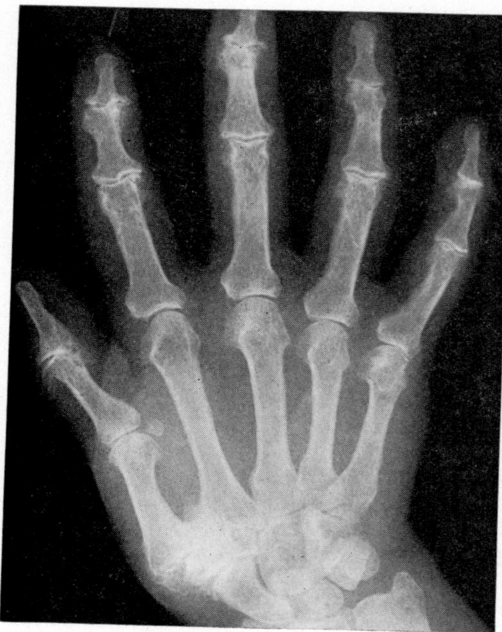

Fig. 7–31.—Osteoarthritis involving the interphalangeal joints and the joints between the first metacarpal and greater multangular and between the latter and the navicular. Note subchondral sclerosis and osteophytes in these joints. There is uniform narrowing of the interosseous spaces of the metacarpophalangeal joints but erosions of the metacarpal heads are conspicuously absent.

metatarsophalangeal joint but very rare in the others (Fig. 7–32). The first tarsometatarsal and talonavicular joints may be involved but uniform involvement of the tarsal joints, as is seen in rheumatoid arthritis, is distinctly uncommon. The hips, knees, glenohumeral and acromioclavicular joints are commonly affected.

Soft tissue swelling and joint effusion may occasionally be observed, particularly in the fingers, but it does not usually involve multiple joints simultaneously. It may be due to trauma superimposed on the osteoarthritic process but it is conceivable that *minimal* inflammation is part of the early pathologic process in some forms of osteoarthritis. Osteoporosis and soft tissue atrophy are not features but may occasionally be present as manifestations of aging. Linear subperiosteal bone apposition does not occur but on rare occasion it may be observed in the fingers in association with articular soft tissue swelling. Thickening of the inferior cortex of the femoral neck or "buttressing" is common in osteoarthritis of the hip[115] (Fig. 7–30).

Narrowing of the interosseous space is characteristically *non*-uniform with occasional exceptions, such as the small joints of the hands, where the cartilage is markedly destroyed. The medial cartilages in the knee are more often destroyed than the lateral ones, resulting in a varus deformity. There may be isolated retropatellar cartilage involvement or the latter may occur in association with erosion of the medial cartilages. Occasionally the cartilage of the lateral compartment is affected but it is unusual for the cartilage spaces of all three compartments to narrow uniformly. Acetabular protrusion is quite rare and usually minimal when it does occur.

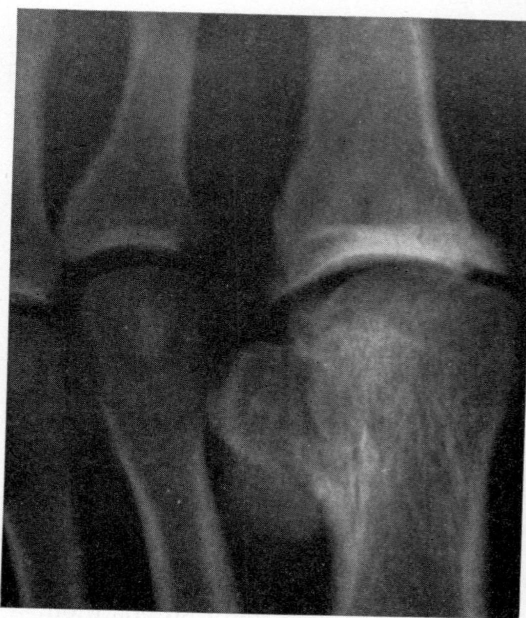

Fig. 7–32.—Osteoarthritis of the first metatarsophalangeal joint. Note subchondral sclerosis, osteophyte formation and non-uniform narrowing of the interosseous space. (Courtesy of J.A.M.A.)

Slight lateral subluxation of the femoral head is frequent in advanced disease and is associated with marked osteophyte formation (Fig. 7–30). Hallux valgus is typical and the fingers generally exhibit moderate medial or lateral deviation (Fig. 7–31).

In interphalangeal osteoarthritis the subchondral cortex may become irregular secondary to erosion following cartilage destruction but its accentuation due to sclerosis helps distinguish it from rheumatoid arthritis. One may observe tiny foci of para-articular ossification within zones of cartilage hyperplasia at the joint margins. Bony ankylosis of the interphalangeal joints is not rare.

Osteoarthritis is usually slowly progressive with radiographic changes developing gradually over years; the diagnosis should be questioned if lesions develop within weeks or even months. An exception to this generalization may be found in the interphalangeal joints of elderly patients. One or a few such joints exhibiting painful soft tissue swelling and extensive subchondral erosion may deteriorate over several months. Rarely, there is minimal subperiosteal bone apposition adjacent to such a joint. The term "*erosive osteoarthritis*" has been used to describe this condition[31,72,124] which may be confused, both clinically and radiologically, with rheumatoid or psoriatic arthritis (Fig. 7–33). The pattern of joint involvement in the hands and feet, the sites of bone erosion and the usual absence of subperiosteal bone apposition are clues to the diagnosis. In some cases of erosive osteoarthritis the changes are limited largely to the interphalangeal joints of the hands and the first metatarsophalangeal joint of the foot but in other patients it appears to be part of generalized osteoarthritis. In patients with interphalangeal osteoarthritis, there often is generalized narrowing of the interosseous spaces of the metacarpophalangeal joints which is usually quite uniform and may be unassociated with subchondral sclerosis or osteophyte formation. This feature is not widely recognized and may be the basis for confusion with rheumatoid arthritis. The characteristic absence of marginal erosions despite cartilage space narrowing is important, particularly in these joints, in differentiating these conditions.

Spine.—Degenerative disease of the spine may be manifested as an osteoarthritis when it involves the synovial joints[43] or as "degenerative spondylosis" when it affects the intervertebral fibrocartilaginous joints.[18,62] These two types

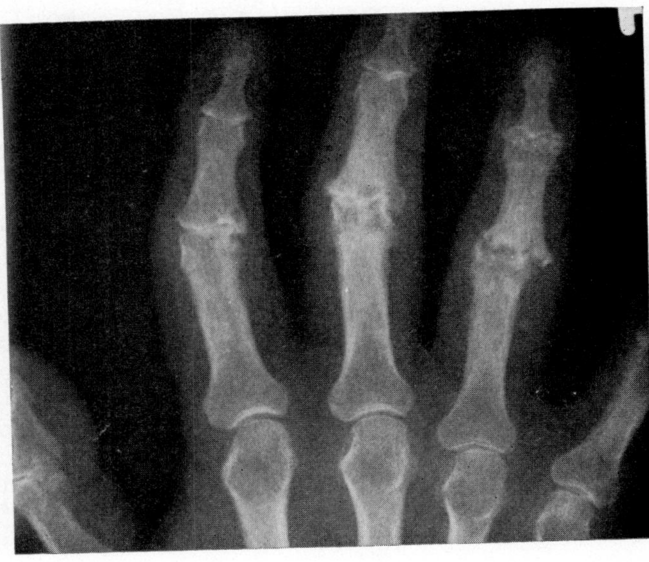

Fig. 7–33.—Erosive osteoarthritis There is severe subchondral erosion in the interphalangeal joints, particularly the proximal joints of the third and fourth digits. The pattern of involvement and subchondral sclerosis are consistent with osteoarthritis. The absence of subperiosteal bone apposition is significant. Compare with Figure 7–26. Uniform narrowing of the metacarpophalangeal interosseous spaces should not be confused with rheumatoid arthritis. Similar changes were present in the opposite hand.

of lesions differ in their pathogenesis and, although they often coexist, may be independent of one another. Degenerative spondylosis is independent of osteoarthritis in the joints of the extremities but significant osteoarthritis of the spine is usually part of primary generalized osteoarthritis. These lesions may occur anywhere in the spine but those in the cervical region are more often associated with clinical manifestations. Intervertebral disc degeneration is considered to be part of the aging process; the average age of patients with cervical disc degeneration is approximately ten years more than that of patients with cervical apophyseal osteoarthritis. Degenerative changes of apophyseal joints and intervertebral discs usually take years to develop. Among autopsied patients there is a ten year average age difference between cases showing mild disc degeneration and those with severe changes.[62] Cervical spondylosis primarily affects the lower intervertebral discs whereas osteoarthritis tends to involve the mid and upper cervical apophyseal joints.[62] Severe thinning of an intervertebral disc may result in telescoping of the posterior articulations which may cause secondary osteoarthritis.

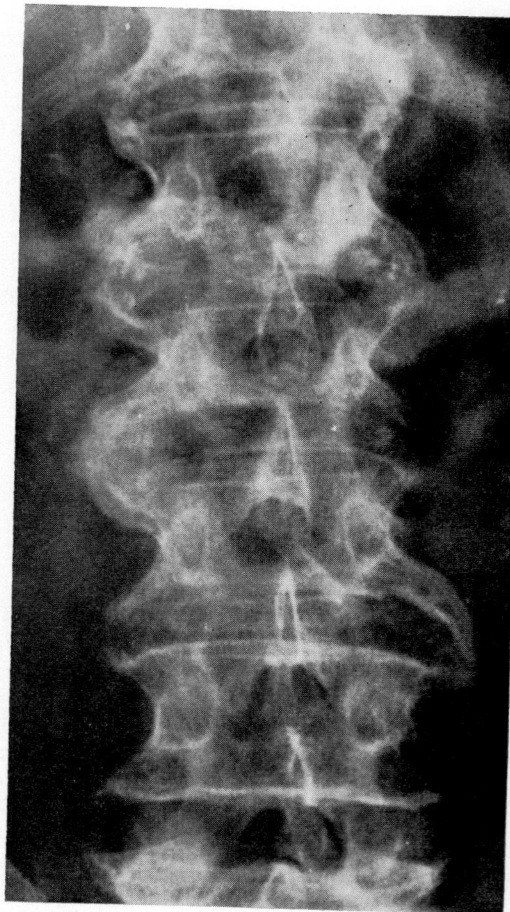

Fig. 7–34.—Degenerative spondylosis, lumbar spine. Although some of the osteophytes "turn vertically," they are, for the most part, oriented horizontally at their "take off" from the vertebral bodies. The apophyseal and sacroiliac joints were not ankylosed. Compare with Figure 7–18.

The radiologic manifestations of cervical apophyseal osteoarthritis are analogous to those seen in the extremities. As an intervertebral disc degenerates, the intervertebral space narrows, not necessarily uniformly, and the disc spreads outwards, stripping the periosteum from the bone and causing osteophytes to form on the adjacent lips of the vertebral bodies (Fig. 7–34). The horizontal orientation of these osteophytes reflect their development along the bulging annulus fibrosus; they may form anteriorly, laterally, or posterolaterally. Posterolateral osteophytes may impinge upon the spinal cord or posterior nerve roots as they emerge from their foramina. There is poor correlation between the radiologic changes of cervical spondylosis and symptoms of cord or nerve root compression. Radicular compression by osteophytes may be aggravated by the telescoping effect of vertebrae, inasmuch as this will cause further narrowing of the intervertebral foramina. It is not uncommon to have radiologic changes of severe disc degeneration with normal nerve roots but it is relatively uncommon to have damaged nerve roots due to degenerative intervertebral disc disease without any radiologic manifestation of the latter.[18,62] The narrowest anteroposterior diameter of the spinal canal is probably the most important single finding in correlating degenerative spondylosis with cervical myelopathy.[63]

Osteoarthritis is commonly present in the sacroiliac joints, even in middle-aged individuals, though it is not easily identified radiologically. There is usually little problem in differentiating these lesions from ankylosing spondylitis. Instead of erasure and obliteration of the subchondral cortex typical of the latter, there is an accentuation and sclerosis of the subchondral bone. Secondary "osteoarthritis" may develop in gout and after severe trauma, with partial obliteration of the interosseous space.

GOUT

Gout primarily affects the synovial joints of the extremities, particularly the hands and feet. (*See also* Chapter 59.) Spinal involvement is unusual but, on rare occasions, tophi with bone erosion have been demonstrated in the sacroiliac joints. Although there is a well-known predilection for the first metatarsophalangeal joint, arthritis of other joints often occurs without involvement of the latter. The lesions are not usually symmetrical and many joints may be affected simultaneously. Joint effusion may occur both in the acute and chronic stages. Tophi are a manifestation of chronic disease and usually develop after years of intermittent episodic arthritis. Tophi may develop in virtually any location but show affinity for certain sites such as the dorsum of the foot and ankle and various bursae, particularly the olecranon bursa. Erosions may develop in joints which show surprisingly little interosseous space narrowing but in the later stages such narrowing is common and often *uniform*, particularly in the ankle, wrist, knee and small joints of the hands and feet (Fig.

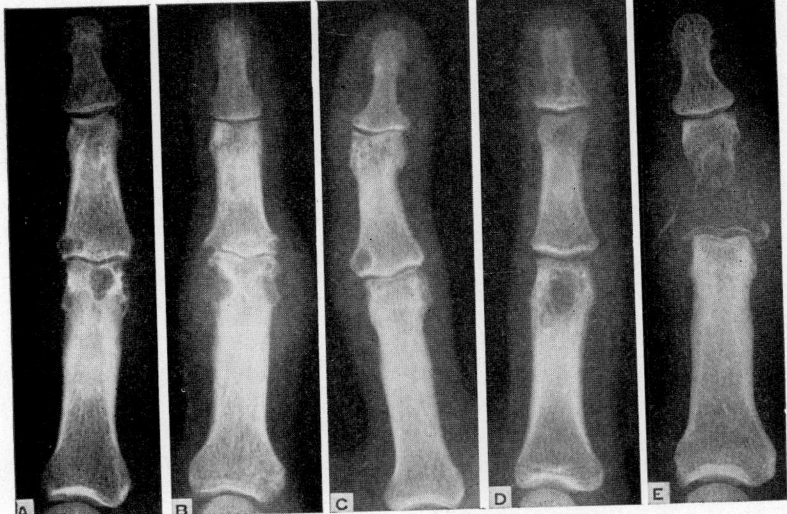

FIG. 7–35.—Differential diagnosis of "erosions" in the interphalangeal joints. *A*. Rheumatoid arthritis. *B*. Gout. *C*. Osteoarthritis. *D*. Sarcoidosis. *E*. Metastatic bronchogenic carcinoma. The erosions in rheumatoid arthritis have a characteristic marginal distribution and in addition there is probably a small central subchondral pseudocyst. The erosions in this example of gout follow the pattern in rheumatoid arthritis but there is a suggestion of small overhanging margins. The lesion in osteoarthritis is characteristically bounded by cortex precluding its being projected as a "marginal erosion"; note its sclerotic margin. The lesion in sarcoidosis is centrally located within the bone and does not involve the joint. In *E*, the irregular, poorly marginated destruction of the middle phalanx associated with discontinuity and displacement of the cortex indicates an aggressive, rapidly growing lesion. The relative preservation of the subchondral plate suggests that this is primarily a lesion of the bone rather than of the joint. The interosseous spaces are narrowed in *A*, *B* and *C* but not in *D* or *E*.

7–35). This feature may be responsible for a mistaken radiologic diagnosis of rheumatoid arthritis.

The intra-articular erosions of bone occasionally follow the pattern of marginal erosions in rheumatoid arthritis (Fig. 7–35*B*). This is consistent with the concept that such erosions may develop as a consequence of chronic synovitis. It is much more common and characteristic, however, to find bone erosions in relation to tophi and, consequently, they may be para-articular, intra-articular, or unrelated to the joint. The erosions of gout have been characterized as being sharply marginated or "punched-out." Such erosions occur in a number of diseases, including rheumatoid arthritis, making this an unreliable feature in terms of differential diagnosis. In about 40% of patients with bone erosion due to gout one may expect a characteristic *over-hanging margin* at the site of the erosion, a segment of eroded cortex extending over the tophus, elevated and displaced from the normal bone contour[91] (Figs. 7–36 and 7–37). This displacement which may be likened to a small "blow-out deformity" helps distinguish these lesions from the pocketed erosions of rheumatoid arthritis. In the latter there is no displacement of the eroded cortex away from the bone contour. This con-

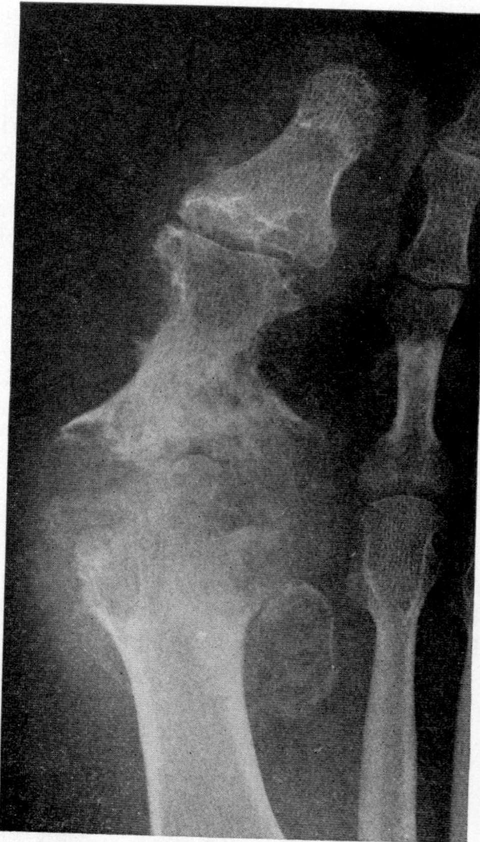

Fig. 7–37.—Gout. Advanced destructive changes in the metatarsophalangeal and interphalangeal joints of the great toe with large tophaceous deposits and "over-hanging margins." Note relative absence of osteoporosis.

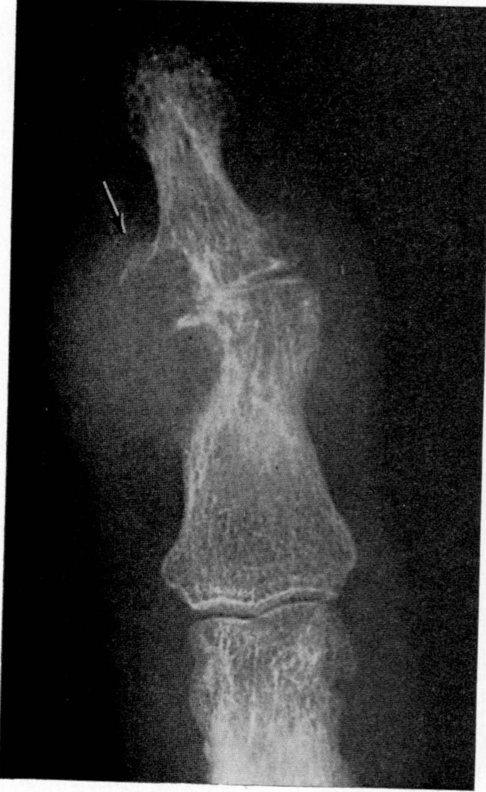

Fig. 7–36.—Gout. There is a tophus at the ulnar aspect of the fifth finger with a characteristic overhanging margin of bone (arrow). There is also an erosion at the radial aspect of the distal phalanx. Note high radiographic density of the tophus. (Courtesy of J.A.M.A.)

figuration may derive from the relationship of the erosion to the bone-tophus interface; as the tophus increases in size, causing erosion, there is concomitant bone apposition at the outer aspect of the cortex. This may be observed in metacarpals, metatarsals and phalanges and is significant in that it is rare in rheumatoid arthritis. Although it is characteristic of gout, it is not pathognomonic and has occasionally been observed in other conditions, such as psoriatic arthritis and villonodular synovitis. Large osteolytic lesions of the tarsal or carpal joints often develop in association with tophi at the dorsal aspects of these areas. Rheumatoid erosions in these joints are usually small and generalized and large osteolytic lesions are uncommon. Tophaceous joint destruction may occasionally be observed in unusual sites, such as the acromioclavicular and sacroiliac joints. Intraosseous tophi usually develop near a joint, in the patella for example, and often have characteristic multilocular or scalloped margins; they may also be solitary and rounded.

Subperiosteal bone apposition is not a conspicuous feature but may occasionally be noted as a minimal finding in the hands and feet, adjacent to an obvious tophus. Joint destruction may lead to bony ankylosis. Neither osteoporosis nor soft tissue atrophy are part of the picture of gout but regional osteoporosis may occur in patients with extensive inflammation and severe bone destruction. Joint malalignment and subluxation are not characteristic but may be caused by large, intra-articular tophi or, in late stages, by secondary osteoarthritis. The latter may be secondary to intra-articular urate deposition and chronic inflammation but osteoarthritis may also be a coincidental finding in older patients.

Cartilage calcification (chondrocalcinosis) is sometimes seen in patients with gout[36,50] but it primarily involves fibrocartilaginous structures such as the menisci of the knee and triangular fibrocartilage of the wrist and less commonly, hyaline cartilage; it is often poorly defined and subtle in the latter. *Generalized* chondrocalcinosis, commonly observed in pseudogout, is probably rare. However, para-articular calcification may be observed and, as in pseudogout, may involve joint capsules, tendons or bursae. Whether its chemical composition is calcium urate is not clear. It is probable that on occasion gout and pseudogout may coexist.

PSEUDOGOUT SYNDROME

Pseudogout[82,114,140] is a condition characterized by acute episodes of arthritis resembling those of gout but tophi never develop, serum urate is usually not elevated, the fluid from affected joints contains calcium pyrophosphate rather than sodium urate crystals, and chondrocalcinosis is usually detectable roentgenologically (Fig. 7–38). (*See also* Chapter 60.) Such calcification involves fibrocartilages, particularly the menisci in the knee, triangular cartilage of the wrist, acetabular and glenoid labra, symphysis pubis and intervertebral discs. The calcification also involves hyaline articular cartilage, usually appearing finely linear. When it occurs in fibrocartilage, it is more often coarse and floccular. It is bilateral in most cases, whether in hyaline or fibrocartilage. Although chondrocalcinosis is characteristic, it is not pathognomonic of this syndrome. It has been observed in rheumatoid arthritis,[114] gout,[36] and in elderly people[13] who may have no significant joint symptoms at the time chondrocalcinosis is detected. Chondrocalcinosis in these situations tends to be restricted to a few joints, particularly the knees and wrists, and mainly involves the fibrocartilages. Although chondrocalcinosis may be localized to one or two joints in the pseudogout syndrome, it more often involves several groups of joints.[107] Pseudogout is probably not a disease but a *syndrome* which may be associated with a number of different conditions among which are diabetes mellitus, hemochromatosis,[6] idiopathic familial arthropathy[175] and hyperparathyroidism. Chondrocal-

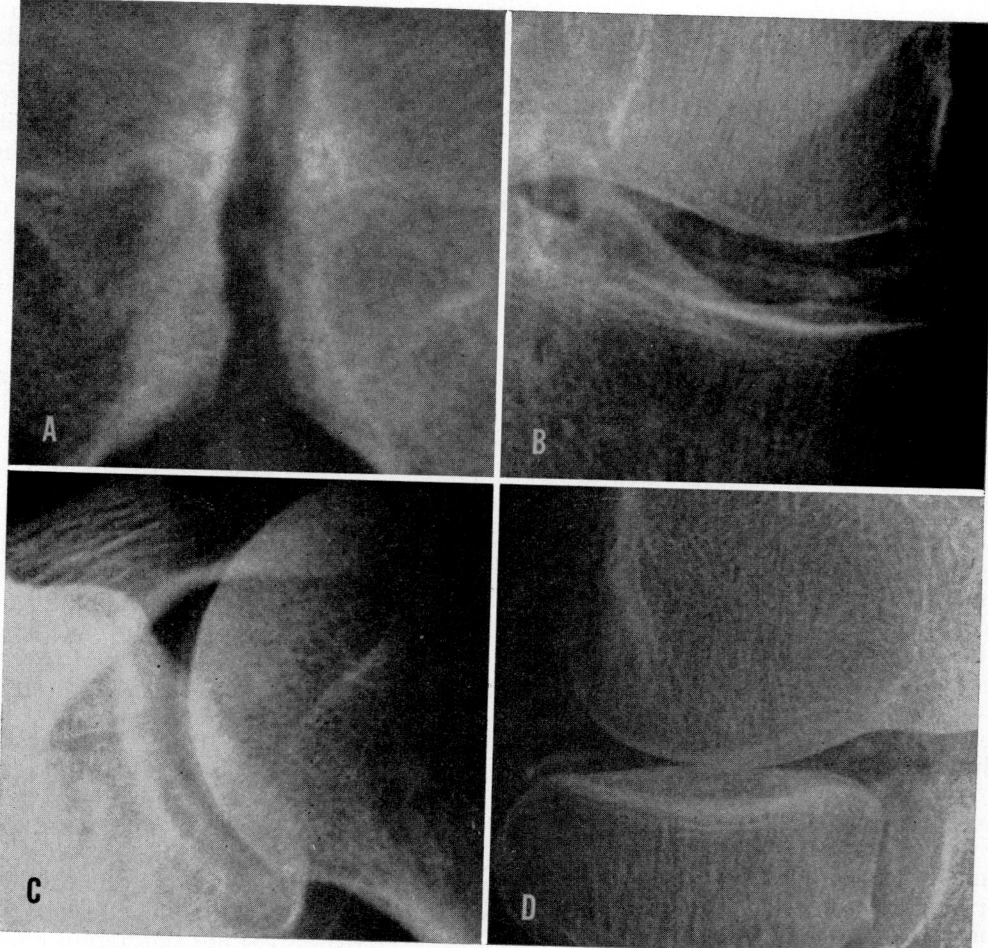

FIG. 7–38.—Chondrocalcinosis in a patient with pseudogout. *A.* Symphysis pubis. *B.* Medial side of the knee. *C.* Shoulder. *D.* Radiohumeral joint. Calcification within fibrocartilage tends to be coarse or floccular whereas it is usually more linear and delicate in hyaline cartilage.

cinosis may be the only skeletal manifestation of the latter. Chondrocalcinosis has also been described in a number of conditions including Wilson's disease,[15] acromegaly,[79] and hypophosphatasia.[120] Calcification in pseudogout is not limited to cartilage but may also be seen in the articular and para-articular soft tissues. The latter should be distinguished from capsular calcification occurring primarily in the interphalangeal joints in patients with chronic renal failure following hemodialysis;[25,121] in these cases the calcium exists as hydroxyapatite crystals and chondrocalcinosis is typically absent. In addition, patients with chronic renal failure from any cause may develop periarticular "tumoral calcinosis."[121]

A roentgenologically distinctive arthropathy, consistent with "osteoarthritis," has recently been described among patients with the pseudogout syndrome.[107] It is often severe and shows a predilection for the elbows, wrists, ankles, knees and, in particular, the metacarpophalangeal joints (Fig. 7–39). Discrete subchondral rarefactions representing so-called "osteoarthritic cysts" are conspicuous and may

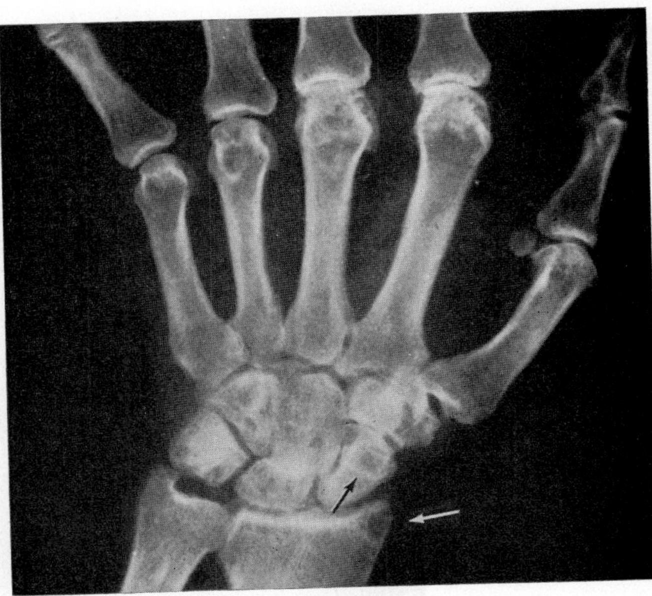

FIG. 7–39.—Metacarpophalangeal arthritis in a patient with pseudogout (idiopathic). An identical appearance may be observed in patients with hemochromatosis who have chondrocalcinosis and pseudogout. Note para-articular calcification adjacent to 3rd metacarpal head and multiple subchondral lucencies (arrows). There is minimal calcification in the triangular cartilage (small arrow).

develop prior to radiologically apparent cartilage degeneration or calcification. The possibility of pseudogout should be considered and chondrocalcinosis searched for in elderly patients who have episodic acute arthritis with this type of "osteoarthritis." Such patients are often misdiagnosed as atypical rheumatoid arthritis because of the selective changes in the metacarpophalangeal joints. Chondrocalcinosis may not be evident in joints in which the articular cartilage is severely destroyed. For example, calcification may appear to involve only the lateral meniscus of the knee if the medial cartilage is eroded. Furthermore, the cartilage calcification may be quite subtle and should be carefully sought for utilizing special roentgenographic techniques.

NEUROPATHIC JOINT DISEASE

Neuropathic joint disease (*see also* Chapter 72) is a progressive degenerative arthropathy, a complication of a number of disorders among which are: tabes dorsalis, diabetes mellitus, syringomyelia, myelodysplasia and peripheral nerve lesions.[160] All of these conditions have in common a loss of protective proprioception in the affected joints.[41] The disease may be monarticular but polyarticular disease is quite common.[10] The pattern of joint involvement is generally related to the underlying cause. Thus, upper extremity joints are involved in syringomyelia (Fig. 7–40) whereas the lower extremities are more commonly affected in tabes dorsalis (Fig. 7–41) and diabetes mellitus. There is a well-known predilection for the ankle and tarsal joints in diabetes mellitus but involvement of upper extremity joints has recently been described.[42,133] The spine may sometimes be affected in tabes dorsalis, usually involving the lower dorsal and lumbar segments; it may resemble severe degenerative spondylosis or there may be vertebral fragmentation. Myelodysplasia is a frequent cause of neuropathic joints in children and characteristically involves the lower extremities. Congenital insensitivity to pain[2] and Charcot-Marie-Tooth disease[19] are rare cases of neuropathic joints in children and young adults, respectively.

An early manifestation is soft tissue swelling, often massive, due to persistent or recurrent joint effusion. Minimal subluxation, narrowing of the articular

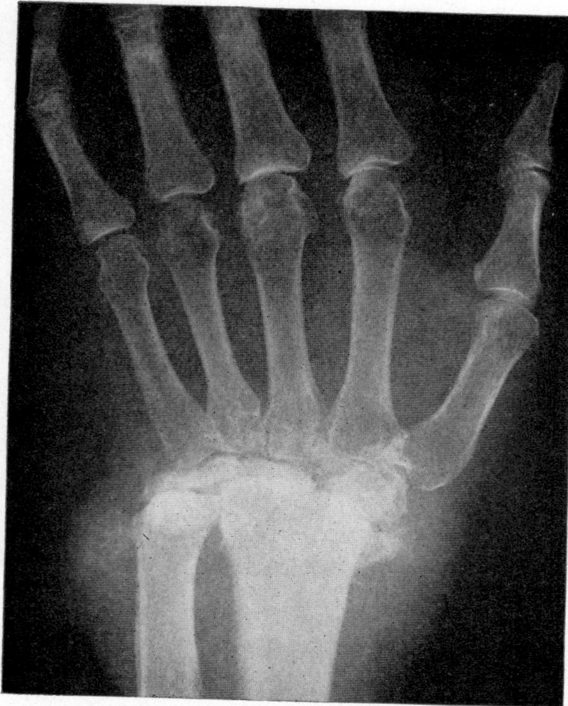

Fig. 7–40.—Neuropathic joint in a 76 year old man with syringomyelia. Note extensive destruction of the bones of the wrist with complete disorganization of joint structure. Sclerosis and bone fragmentation are characteristic. Note subperiosteal bone apposition in the ulna.

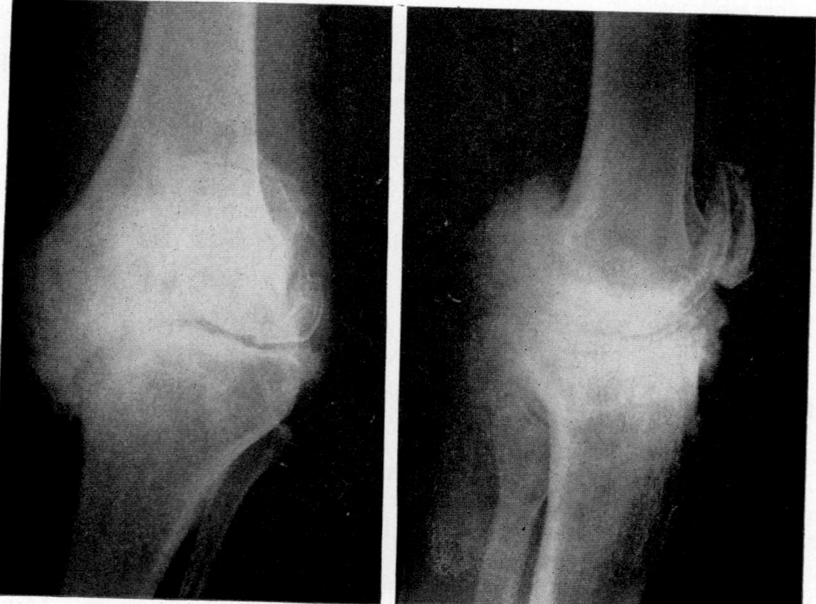

Fig. 7–41.—Charcot joint (tabes dorsalis). There is extensive destruction of the articular cartilage associated with sclerosis, subluxation, and bone fragmentation at the articular margins.

cartilage and calcific or bony fragments embedded in the articular and para-articular soft tissues are often evident early in the disease. The arthropathy usually progresses slowly but it may also do so within several weeks.[117] Rarely, joint destruction will proceed so rapidly as to simulate infectious arthritis. In later stages there is more obvious subluxation which may progress to gross structural disorganization. Extensive subchondral sclerosis and osteophyte formation associated with denudation of articular cartilage supervenes. Marginal fractures are responsible for the bone fragments in the para-articular soft tissues; gross epiphyseal and metaphyseal fractures may also be observed.[68] Subperiosteal bone apposition, possibly due to trauma with subperiosteal hemorrhage, may be conspicuous. In some cases there is dramatic resorption of the bone ends. Whether bone production or resorption predominates does not appear to be related to the underlying disease. Resorption may be a salient feature in one joint and bone production in another in the same individual. The neurologic effect on vessels supplying the bone may be an important factor.

The lack of osteoporosis is an important and fairly constant feature of neuropathic joints regardless of cause. It has particular diagnostic significance in the presence of fracture and persistent effusion. Joint instability and the lack of pain and adequate immobilization contribute to poor quality in the newly-formed bone which is prone to refracture and fragmentation. The bone margins may be fuzzy or indistinct due to microfractures and calcified callus. Sometimes progressive destruction in a previously normal joint seems to be triggered by relatively insignificant trauma with or without a demonstrable fracture.

ARTHROPATHY SECONDARY TO ISCHEMIC NECROSIS

Ischemic necrosis may involve the metadiaphyseal or intra-articular portions of long bones.[66] When the latter is affected, a secondary arthropathy develops which is nonspecific clinically but often distinctive radiologically. The hip and shoulder are the most commonly affected joints, particularly the former, secondary to necrosis in the femoral and humeral head. Other joints may be affected including the knee, ankle and elbow and are associated with necrosis of the femoral condyles, talus and distal humerus, respectively.

The lesion may be post-traumatic, usually following fracture or subluxation, but occasionally in the absence of either. *Osteonecrosis* may also occur as a complication of a number of systemic conditions[14,67] including sickle cell disease, decompression sickness, Gaucher's disease, alcoholism, pancreatitis,[48] lupus erythematosus[38] and hypercortisonism.[57] The pathogenesis of these lesions is essentially the same regardless of the underlying cause with the exception that secondary structural failure may be especially common in corticosteroid-induced necrosis.

Roentgenograms are usually diagnostic when joint symptoms develop. The manifestations will depend on the stage of the disease, extent of the lesion and rapidity with which bone death takes place. They are due to a combination of hyperemic demineralization of the non-necrotic adjacent bone, varying degrees of fragmentation, compression and resorption of dead bone and revascularization with bone production. The latter may develop diffusely on the scaffold of the necrotic bone trabeculae or it may take place by "creeping substitution" at the margins of partially resorbed necrotic bone. Calcification of necrotic marrow may be visualized, particularly in the metadiaphyseal areas. The zone of necrosis is almost always subchondral when intra-articular bone is affected and certain areas are characteristically affected, depending on the vascular supply to the end of the bone. For example, in the femoral head the antero lateral zone is often selectively involved.

A loss of sharpness of the subchondral

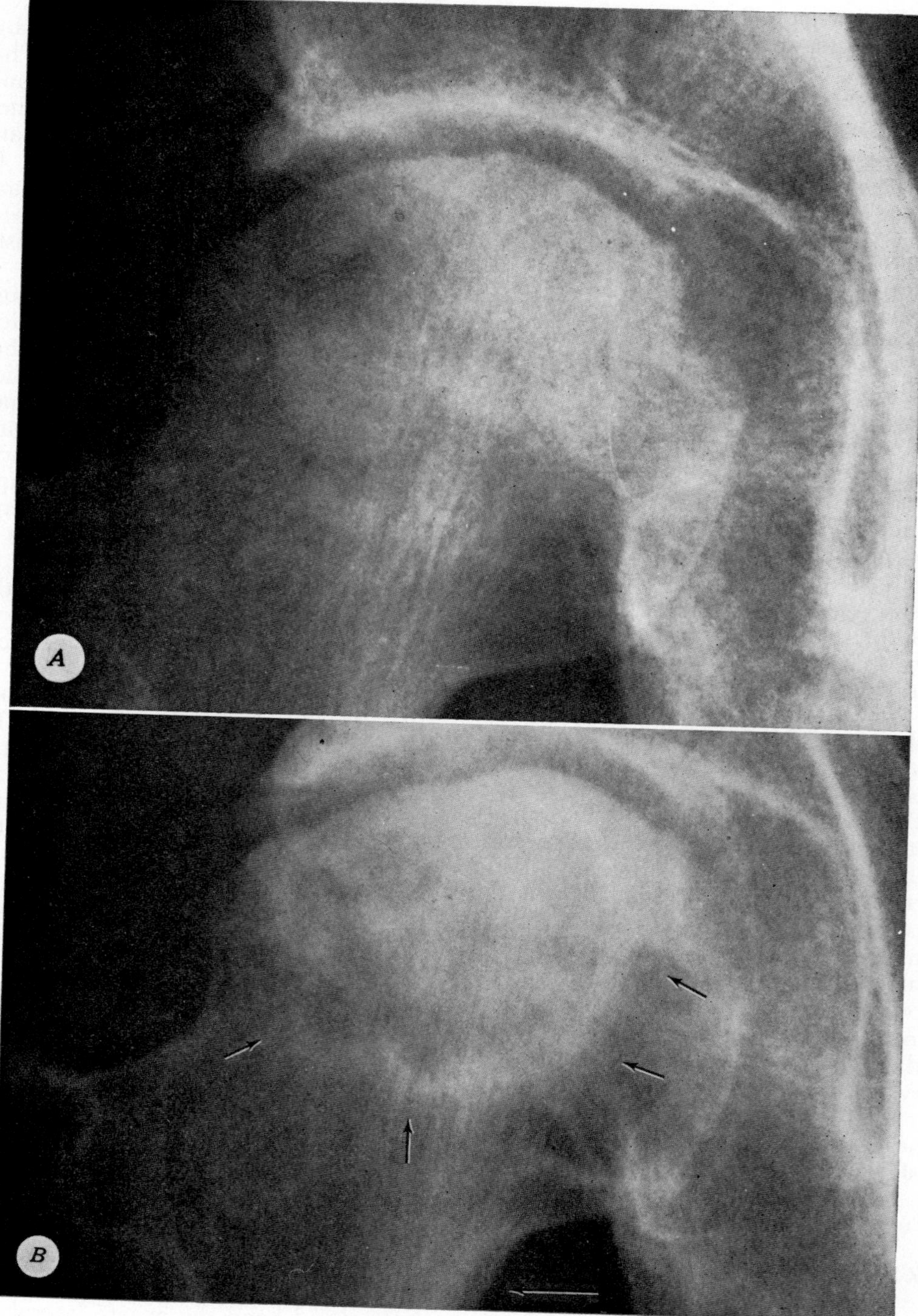

FIG. 7–42.—Ischemic necrosis of the femoral head. *A.* Early. *B.* Several months later. Note the mottling of the trabecular pattern and subsequent collapse of the subchondral bone associated with a large irregular rarefaction bounded by fuzzy sclerosis (arrows). The interosseous space is relatively maintained and there is buttressing of the femoral neck (large arrow).

cortex is an early finding. There may be diffuse mottling of trabecular pattern, or a discrete subchondral rarefaction with irregular margins, surrounded by coarse, fuzzy sclerosis (Fig. 7–42). One may find a diffuse increase in the density of the end of the bone or only a patch of sclerosis, often ill-defined, adjacent to small areas of rarefaction. A pathognomonic finding in the femoral head, both in Legg-Perthe's disease[161] and adults with osteonecrosis,[116] is a radiolucent crescent line which parallels the subchondral surface. This represents a zone of separation or fracture within the necrotic subchondral cortex. It separates the articular cartilage and rim of necrotic cortex from the remainder of the necrotic bone and is best seen in abduction. The extreme radiolucency of this line has suggested that it may be due to a vacuum effect within the zone of separation.[98] Traction of the hip during the radiographic exposure may accentuate this line, helping to confirm the diagnosis. Similar subchondral lucent lines may be observed in other joints involved by osteonecrosis. Secondary synovitis with joint effusion is commonly present. It may be detected in the hip by the traction technique. An important finding is the relative preservation of the cartilage space despite extensive changes in the underlying bone.

Structural failure of the necrotic bone commonly supervenes.[99] At first there is focal depression of the subchondral cortex which progresses to flattening of the articular surface (Fig. 7–42*B*). As the condition goes unrecognized, particularly in weight-bearing joints, generalized intra-articular fragmentation may develop associated with extensive bone resorption. Bone apposition at the inferior aspect of the femoral neck frequently accompanies advanced necrosis of the head. This is similar to the buttressing that occurs in osteoarthritis, and may be caused by remodeling secondary to mechanical alterations at the articular surface, changes in the joint capsule, or coexisting synovitis.

The most severe articular changes in this condition develop in association with hypercortisonism.[99] The mechanism by which the latter induces ischemic necrosis is not clear but there is fairly convincing evidence that a causal relationship exists. Steroids, in addition, inhibit osteogenesis preventing the bone replacement which would ordinarily take place following infarction. Consequently, structural failures in such joints might be expected more often than in necrosis caused by other conditions. The term "Charcot-like arthropathy"[152] refers to a crumbling and resorption of the intra-articular portion of bone associated with steroid therapy. It is likely that many such cases actually represent examples of unrecognized ischemic necrosis. In these cases fragments of bone and calcium within the soft tissues are not uncommon and easily confused with what one observes histologically in true neuropathic joints.

If the condition is allowed to progress, secondary degenerative changes will eventually develop with some hypertrophic bone formation and narrowing of the interosseous space due to cartilage degeneration. Roentgenograms obtained at this time may erroneously be interpreted as "osteoarthritis" without recognizing that the underlying condition is bone necrosis.[99] In osteonecrosis sufficiently advanced to simulate osteoarthritis much of the femoral head is involved rather than only the subchondral portion as in osteoarthritis. In addition the bone changes usually precede the cartilage space narrowing whereas the converse is true in osteoarthritis. The cortex of the upper margin of the femoral head is usually well defined in osteoarthritis but tends to be vague and poorly marginated in necrosis. Furthermore, the areas of rarefaction in the latter tend to be irregular and poorly defined with fuzzy, sclerotic margins whereas in osteoarthritis the sclerotic margins are often thin and sharply defined. Although some compression of the subchondral bone develops in osteoarthritis, generalized crumbling, collapse and large "bite-like" subchondral defects, as occur in osteonecrosis, are distinctly unusual.

INFECTIOUS ARTHRITIS

Infectious arthritis is probably more common in children than adults and is often observed in aged and debilitated individuals. (*See also* Chapter 68.) The infecting organisms are usually disseminated hematogenously to the joint tissues, probably lodging preferentially in the synovial membrane. Sometimes infection involves the joint secondarily as an extension of osteomyelitis. The disease is usually monarticular although occasionally more than one joint will be affected particularly when associated with a systemic condition. Infection may complicate pre-existing arthritis and is particularly common in neuropathic joints. It may occur in other arthropathies, such as rheumatoid arthritis, and should be suspected where intra-articular injections have been given. Joint alterations due to a pre-existing condition may mask changes due to infection. In rheumatoid polyarthritis, however, the possibility of this complication should be considered when the joint in question appears to be deteriorating rapidly, as judged radiologically, while other involved joints remain unchanged. The radiologic manifestations of infectious arthritis will depend on the age of the patient and the infecting organism, the particular joint involved, duration of disease and whether there has been antibiotic therapy. The latter, particularly when incomplete, may modify the natural course of the disease and mask typical radiological features.

Extremities.—Large joints such as the knee are affected more often than the small peripheral joints. Pyogenic arthritis is typified by a sudden onset of soft tissue swelling, generally associated with obvious clinical signs of inflammation. There is rapid destruction of cartilage and bone associated with extensive subperiosteal bone formation and sequestrum formation, particularly if untreated. Structural alterations do not usually develop until 8 to 10 days after the onset of symptoms. This timing is an important diagnostic feature; normal roentgenograms obtained within several days after symptoms develop do not exclude the diagnosis. Osteoporosis may be absent at the very outset but generally becomes evident rapidly especially when joint destruction is present. The advanced radiologic picture of suppurative arthritis is rare since the advent of antibiotics. If the disease is allowed to continue untreated, however, and progresses to cartilage destruction, bony ankylosis may eventually be expected. A variety of pathogenic bacteria have been incriminated in suppurative arthritis. Streptococcus is often the responsible organism early in infancy and staphylococcus is more common in older children and adults.

The radiologic manifestations of nonsuppurative arthritis, tuberculosis being a notable example (*see also* Chapter 66), differ significantly from those of pyogenic infection (Fig. 7–43). As in suppurative arthritis, the large joints are more frequently affected than the small ones but the onset of the disease is usually insidious and soft tissue swelling is often less marked and may be minimal. Regional osteoporosis is usually present. Early, the cartilage tends to be preserved, even when there are bone erosions, but it too becomes destroyed late in the disease. Unlike pyogenic arthritis in which there is early destruction of the subchondral bone, tuberculous arthritis shows a predilection for the marginal or nonweight-bearing portions of the joint and in this respect resembles rheumatoid arthritis. Sequestra may develop but are relatively small and, unlike pyogenic arthritis, subperiosteal bone apposition is characteristically minimal or moderate. The disease tends to be more indolent than suppurative arthritis and weeks may elapse before radiologic changes are evident. Bony ankylosis may result as an end stage. Rarely, a tendon sheath or bursa is the site of tuberculous infection. Brucellosis

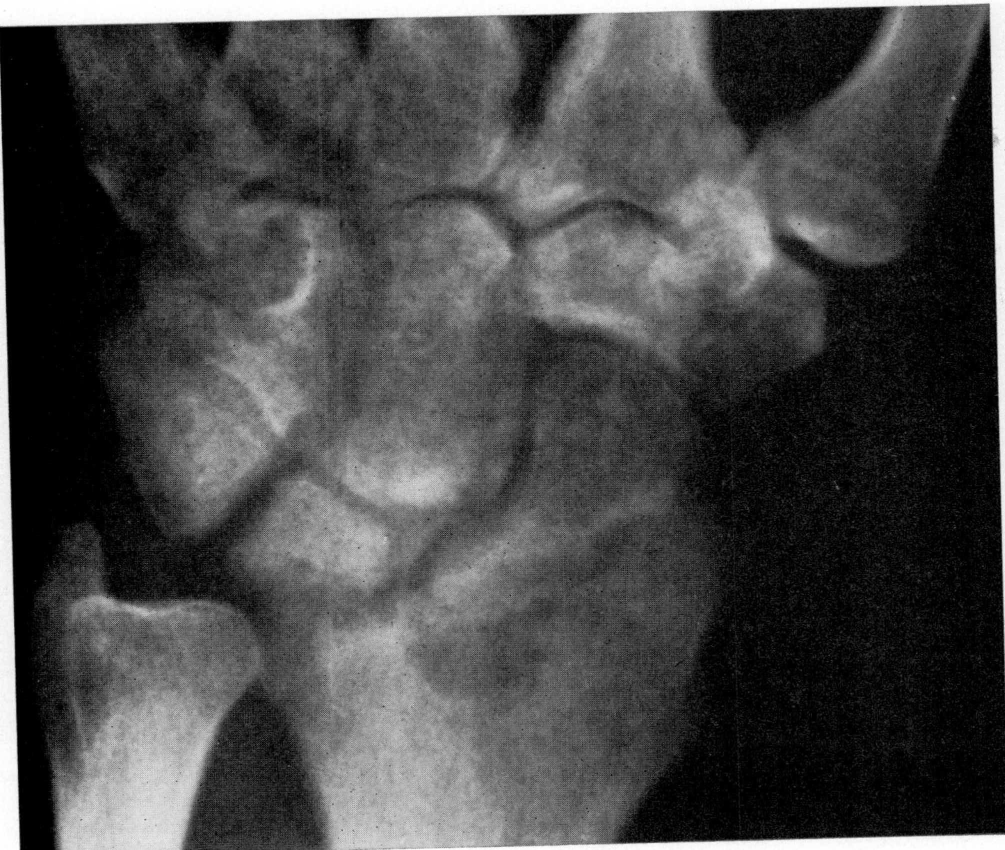

Fig. 7–43.—Tuberculous arthritis. There is extensive destruction of the radiocarpal joint and joints between the proximal carpal bones. The pattern of bone destruction differs from that observed in rheumatoid arthritis. Compare with Figure 7–1.

may mimic tuberculous arthritis and occasionally a fungus is responsible. (*See also* Chapter 68.)

Spine.—Infections of the spine usually involve the vertebral bodies and discs but, on rare occasions, the apophyseal joints and neural arches have been affected. Lesions of the lumbar spine are common but any spinal segment may be involved. The earliest lesion often consists of an area of rarefaction or cortical indistinctness at the superior or inferior aspect of a vertebral body, adjacent to the disc. The adjacent intervertebral disc space is almost always narrowed, sometimes only slightly, at the time a defect is evident in the adjacent bone (Fig. 7–44). As the lesion progresses, the narrowing becomes more marked, either due to extension of the infection or herniation of disc material secondary to weakening of the end-plate. A soft tissue paraspinal mass may be evident and extensive reactive sclerosis and spur formation eventually develop, particularly in suppurative arthritis. In the late stages there may be complete bony fusion of the adjacent vertebral bodies with obliteration of the disc interspace.

As in the extremity joints, tuberculosis of the spine progresses more slowly than pyogenic infection and a paravertebral soft tissue mass which may contain calcium is often present. Bone destruction may extend along the anterior surface of

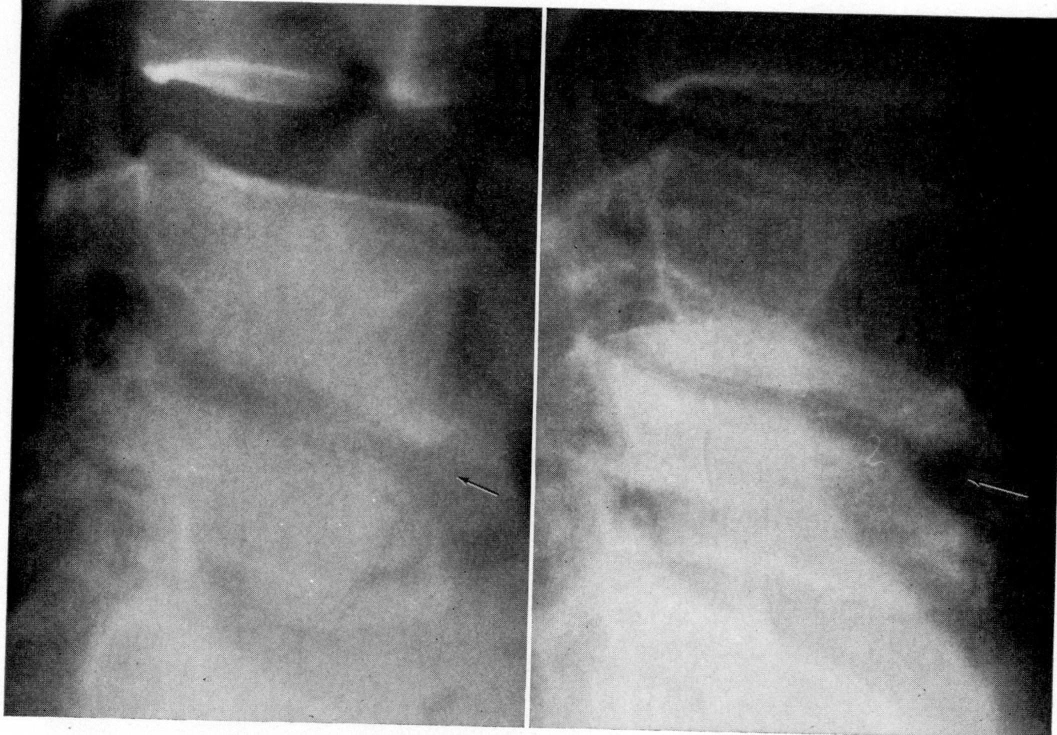

FIG. 7–44.—Staphylococcal spondylitis. *A.* Lateral roentgenogram, lumbar spine. *B.* One year later. There is narrowing of the disc space at L_{4-5} (arrow) with destruction of the vertebral margins. Later film shows further narrowing and sclerosis causing better definition of the intervertebral margins. This eventually progressed to bony ankylosis.

the spine and more than one level may be involved. Bone formation and sclerosis tend to be less marked than in pyogenic arthritis but this is a less reliable point in differentiation than is the temporal factor. A psoas abscess may develop. Mycotic infections of the spine are relatively uncommon but should be considered in the differential diagnosis of spondylitis particularly when there are multiple lesions, sinus tracts and large soft tissue masses.

MISCELLANEOUS CONDITIONS

Pigmented villonodular synovitis (*see also* Chapter 75) is an inflammatory disease of unknown etiology which primarily affects young adults although it has been described in children and older individuals. It may involve synovial tissue in joints or tendon sheaths (giant cell tumor of tendon sheath) and is almost always monarticular; rarely, two joints have been affected simultaneously.[47] An insidious onset of joint or soft tissue swelling and discomfort are characteristic. Roentgenograms generally disclose soft tissue swelling within the joint or a discrete soft tissue mass when a tendon sheath is affected.[17,143] Soft tissue calcification is virtually never observed and osteoporosis is often absent, particularly if joint destruction is minimal. Characteristically, the interosseous space is relatively preserved until late in the disease and malalignment and subluxation are absent. Bone erosions develop as cortical irregularities or discrete rarefactions which may be cyst-like in appearance (Fig. 7–45).

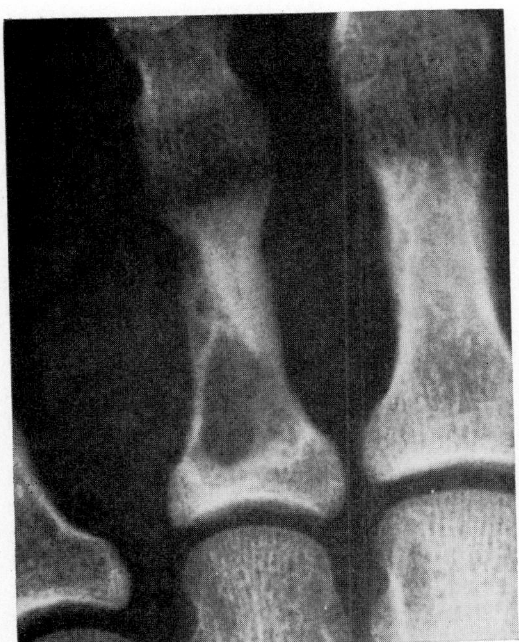

Fig. 7–45.—Giant cell tumor of tendon sheath (pigmented villonodular synovitis) involving the proximal phalanx of the fourth toe. Note preservation of bone density and phalangeal separation due to the soft tissue mass. (Courtesy of D. W. MacEwan, M.D., University of Manitoba.)

Scleroderma (*see also* Chapter 54).—A common, early radiologic manifestation of scleroderma is resorption of the terminal tufts of the distal phalanges in the hands[132,173] (Fig. 7–46). Calcification within the adjacent soft tissues is often present and may be found in periarticular soft tissues as well[156] (Fig. 7–47). Occlusive changes in the digital arteries are common. Arthritis does not generally occur, although rarely joint changes in the hands and wrists, simulating rheumatoid arthritis, may develop.[126] It is conceivable that some patients have both rheumatoid arthritis and scleroderma. These joint manifestations often develop in patients with severe, longstanding contracture deformities and it is also possible that the latter somehow alter the articular cartilage leading to these destructive

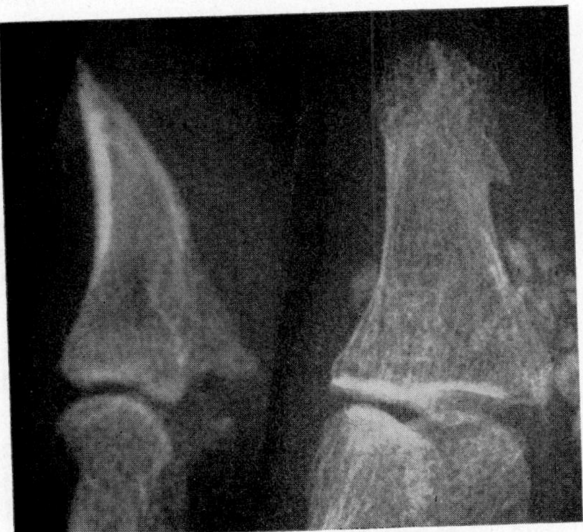

Fig. 7–46.—Scleroderma. (Left) Severe resorption of the terminal tuft of the thumb giving a tapered appearance. Note soft tissue calcification at the volar aspect of the joint. (Right) Moderate resorption of the terminal tuft of the thumb with adjacent soft tissue calcification. Calcific deposits are often present in the tips of the fingers.

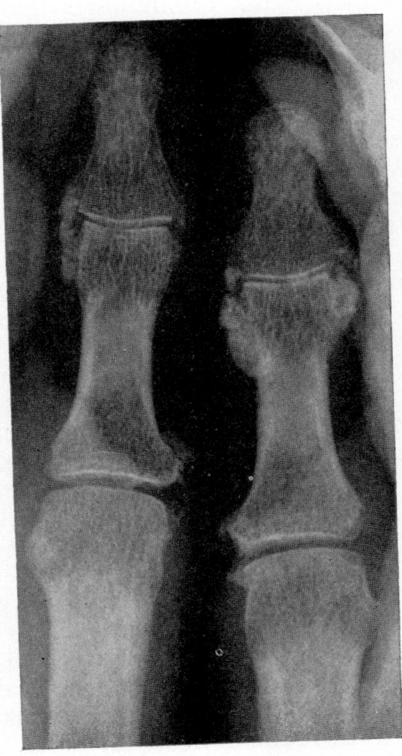

Fig. 7–47.—Scleroderma. Periarticular calcification in the vicinity of the metacarpophalangeal and interphalangeal joints of both thumbs. Note osteoporosis.

changes. Rarely, there are severe rib erosions. Thickening of the periodontal membrane has been described[149] but the usefulness of this sign and its frequency are uncertain. Diffuse interstitial fibrosis of the lungs is common and may lead to bronchiolar ectasia and bronchiectasis. Unlike rheumatoid arthritis, pleural effusion is uncommon and discrete pulmonary and pleural nodules do not occur. Motility disturbances[156] in the esophagus and both small and large intestine are frequent, secondary to replacement of muscle by fibrous tissue. Dilatation of the esophagus with stasis of the barium with the patient in the horizontal position is characteristic. Peptic esophagitis frequently supervenes. The esophageal dilatation is usually due to loss of smooth muscle but it may be secondary to a peptic stricture in the lower esophagus. Small bowel dilatation and delay in transit are common and are usually associated with esophageal involvement. The colon may show "pseudodiverticular pouches" which differ from diverticula in that they involve the entire thickness of the bowel wall and have wide openings.

Dermatomyositis (*see also* Chapter 53).—In dermatomyositis one often finds pronounced muscular atrophy and calcification,[58] either around joints or along muscle planes. Disturbance in muscular activity may be reflected in the pharynx and cervical esophagus by inability to swallow or retention of barium in the pharynx following deglutition. General motility disturbances in the esophagus and bowel have been described but these are probably uncommon.

Jaccoud's syndrome.—Jaccoud or post-rheumatic fever syndrome[157] is an uncommon condition characterized by flexion deformities of the metacarpophalangeal joints with ulnar deviation but, unlike rheumatoid arthritis, the malalignment is not rigid. It may be the result of periarticular, fascial and tendon fibrosis rather than synovitis. Bone changes are absent or minimal although there is evidence that metacarpal erosions may develop in some cases.

Disseminated lupus erythematosus (*see also* Chapter 51).—Articular soft tissue swelling and osteoporosis are often present.[26,39,76,126] Joint destruction as in rheumatoid arthritis is relatively uncommon and tends to be minimal and slowly progressive when it does occur. Rarely, severe joint changes simulating rheumatoid arthritis are demonstrated and, in such cases, it is not clear whether the patient has two diseases[70] or whether there is an overlap in clinical or radiologic manifestations. Plate-like areas of atelectasis may be observed in the lower lung but diffuse pulmonary parenchymal changes are uncommon. Several cases have been reported in which ischemic necrosis of the femoral head developed prior to the administration of steroid therapy. Ischemic necrosis of joints is common and probably reflects widespread, prolonged steroid therapy in most cases. Ulnar deviation of the metacarpophalangeal joints without bone erosion, simulating the findings in Jaccoud's syndrome, has been described.[76]

Sarcoidosis (*see also* Chapter 70).—Some patients with sarcoidosis develop transient arthritis which characteristically leaves no residual joint deformity and roentgenograms show no bone or cartilage erosion.[118,148] In a few cases, perhaps 1 or 2 per cent, and not necessarily those who had arthritis, discrete lytic lesions develop, particularly in the ends of the phalanges, metacarpals and metatarsals[61] (Fig. 7–35*D*). These are centrally located, virtually never involve the margins, and often have a reticulated configuration. Joint destruction is rare and usually an extension of adjacent bone destruction; in such cases there are usually skin lesions of sarcoidosis and large para-articular tissue masses.

Ochronosis (*see also* Chapter 61).—The most frequently and severely affected joints in ochronosis are shoulders, hips, knees and intervertebral joints of the spine[35,74] (Fig. 7–48). The intervertebral discs are universally narrowed with

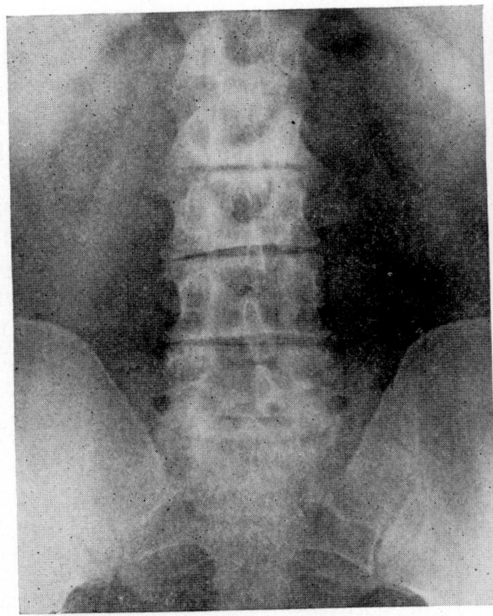
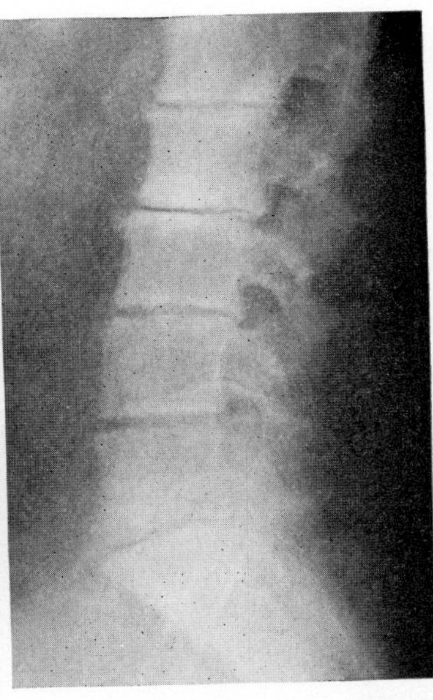

FIG. 7–48.—Ochronosis. There is severe, generalized narrowing of the intervertebral discs with small osteophytes and subchondral sclerosis. Intervertebral disc calcification is faintly evident in the frontal projection at L_{3-4} and L_{4-5}. A streak-like horizontal lucency within the disc, seen in the lateral projection at L_{2-3}, represents a "vacuum phenomenon" within the degenerated fibrocartilage.

calcification of the annulus fibrosus. The calcification may be partially obscured because the cartilages are so markedly degenerated. Such degeneration is reflected by a "vacuum phenomenon" presumably within fissures in the fibrocartilage. Although intervertebral disc calcification may be observed in patients with pseudogout, such marked, uniform and universal narrowing of the discs virtually never develops. Severe "osteoarthritis-like" changes of large joints with relative sparing of the small peripheral joints occurring in young adults should raise the possibility of ochronosis. The arthropathy in the extremity joints may be so severe as to simulate neuropathic joints.

Calcific tendinitis and bursitis.—Calcific tendinitis and bursitis are common causes of shoulder pain. (*See also* Chapter 80.) It may involve any of the tendons which comprise the rotator cuff (supraspinatus, infraspinatus and teres minor) and subscapularis.[159] The most common site is the supraspinatus tendon which forms the floor of the subdeltoid bursa. Calcific debris may rupture from the supraspinatus tendon into the latter (Fig. 7–49). The supraspinatus tendon inserts just above the junction of the greater tuberosity and humeral head whereas the other three tendons are located slightly lower. Precise localization of calcific deposits will require rotational views of the shoulder. Calcification may be completely obscured in certain views and clearly demonstrated in others. Calcific tendinitis in the hands and feet and occasionally other sites may be confused with acute arthritis.[56,153,154]

Neoplasms and Associated Conditions (*see also* Chapter 75).—Some tumors, either primary or metastatic, may arise within a joint, causing secondary synovitis which mimics primary joint disease. Malignant tumors such as plasma cell myeloma, metastatic carcinoma, lymphoma, and malignancies originating in the joint tissues may more commonly induce such synovitis because of their infiltrative tendency. Neoplastic metastases are generally uncommon distal to the elbows and knees but there are many exceptions including various malignant tumors in children and certain tumors in adults. Bronchogenic carcinoma is among the latter and it not infrequently metastasizes to the small bones of the hands, simulating primary arthritis if the end of a bone is involved (Fig. 7–35*E*). Bronchogenic carcinoma may also cause hypertrophic osteoarthropathy. In such cases there is pain and soft tissue swelling, particularly about the ankles and wrists. Roentgenograms show linear, subperiosteal bone apposition which is primarily metaphyseal in the early stages and characteristically symmetrical. It often involves the metatarsal, metacarpals and phalanges and sometimes the diaphyses of long bones. *Osteoid osteoma* often develops intra-articularly,[84] particularly in the hips and elbows, where it typically

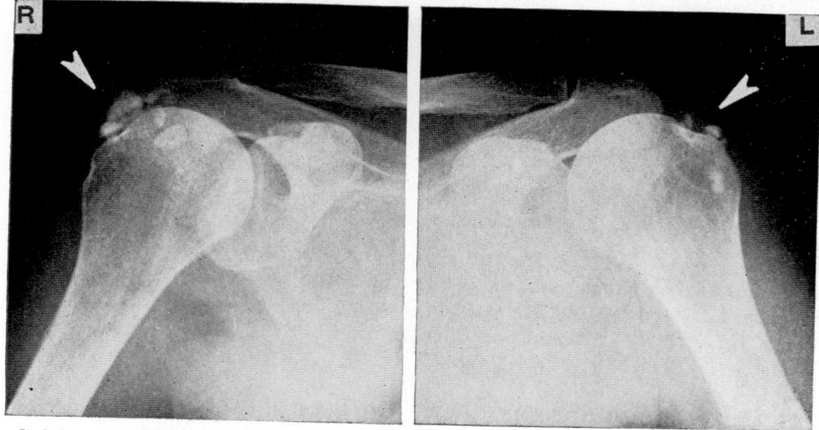

Fig. 7–49.—Calcific tendinitis and bursitis. The distribution of the calcific deposits suggests that they are in the supraspinatus tendons and subdeltoid bursae.

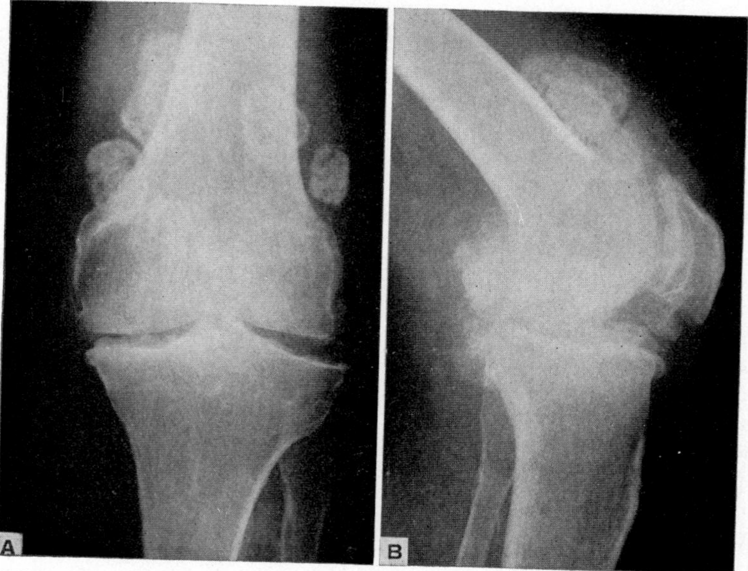

Fig. 7–50.—Multiple calcific lesions within the knee joint probably representing synovial chondromatosis. Osteoarthritis is also present.

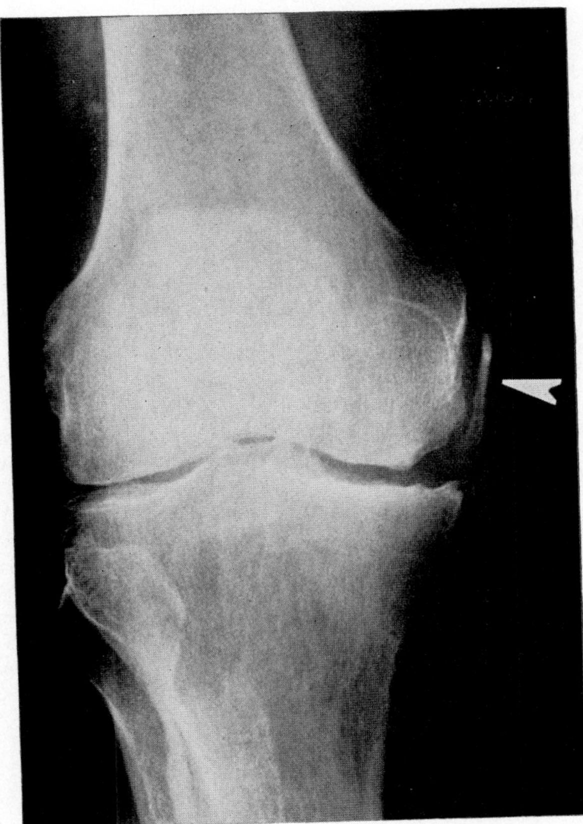

Fig. 7–51.—A para-articular soft tissue density (arrow), probably representing localized heterotopic bone formation in a characteristic site (adjacent to the adductor tubercle). In most cases this is post-traumatic in origin.

causes a synovitis easily confused with rheumatoid arthritis both clinically and histologically.[85] *Synovial sarcoma* may occur within a joint but more often develops *near* a joint, especially in the lower extremities. The soft tissue mass of these tumors is likely to be ill-defined and often contains focal calcification; bone erosion is often minimal even when the tumor is in a juxta-cortical or juxta-articular location. Other intra-articular masses which may contain focal calcification include: hemangioma,[80] chondroma, chondrosarcoma, and synovial chondromatosis (Fig. 7–50). Para-articular ossification unassociated with neoplasm may be observed following acute and chronic trauma (Fig. 7–51), burns and paraplegia among other conditions (*see also* Chapter 76). Amyloidosis (*see also* Chapter 69), often associated with myeloma, may cause thickening of the articular and periarticular tissues with destruction of cartilage and bone which often simulates rheumatoid arthritis.[122] Subluxation of large joints, such as the hip and shoulder, frequently occurs as a consequence of ligamentous destruction and large intra-articular deposits of amyloid.[164]

BIBLIOGRAPHY

1. Abel, M. S.: Radiology, *55*, 235, 1950.
2. Abell, J. M. and Hayes, J. T.: J. Bone & Joint Surg., *46A*, 1287, 1964.

3. AHLBÄCK, S.: Acta Radiol., Suppl. 277, 1968.
4. ANSELL, B. M. and BYWATERS, E. G. L.: Bull. Rheum. Dis., *9*, 189, 1959.
5. ARKLESS, R.: Radiology, *88*, 543, 1967.
6. ATKINS, C. J., McIVOR, J., SMITH, P. M., HAMILTON, E., and WILLIAMS, R.: Quart. J. Med., *39*, 71, 1970.
7. AVILA, R., RUGH, D. C., SLOCUMB, C. H. and WINKELMANN, R. K.: Radiology, *75*, 691, 1960.
8. BÄCKDAHL, M.: Acta Rheumat. Scand. Suppl., 5, 1963.
9. BADLEY, B. W. D. and ANSELL, B. M.: Ann. Rheum. Dis., *19*, 135, 1960.
10. BEETHAM, W. P., JR., KAYE, R. L. and POLLEY, H. F.: Ann. Intern. Med., *58*, 1003, 1963.
11. BERENS, D. L.: Clin. Orthop., *74*, 20, 1971.
12. BERENS, D. L., LOCKIE, M., RU-KAN LIN and NORCROSS, B. M.: Radiology, *82*, 645, 1964.
13. BOCHER, J., MANKIN, H. J., BERK, R. N., and RODNAN, G. P.: New Engl. Jour. Med., *272*, 1093, 1965.
14. BOETTCHER, W. G., BONFIGLIO, M., HAMILTON, H. H., SHEETS, R. F., and SMITH, K.: J. Bone & Joint Surg., *52A*, 312, 1970.
15. BOUDIN, C., PÉPIN, B., and HUBAULT, A.: Rev. Rhum. *31*, 594, 1964.
16. BRATTSTRÖM, M.: Acta Rheum. Scand., *9*, 102, 1963.
17. BREIMER, C. W. and FREIBERGER, R. H.: Amer. J. Roentgenol., *79*, 4, 1958.
18. BROOKER, A. E. W. and BARTER, R. W.: Brain, *88*, 925, 1965.
19. BRUCKNER, F. E. and KENDALL, B. E.: Ann. Rheum. Dis., *28*, 577, 1969.
20. BRULAND, H.: Acta Rheum. Scand., *6*, 209, 1960.
21. BYWATERS, E. G. L.: Ann. Rheum. Dis., *24*, 313, 1965.
22. ————: Bull. Rheum. Dis., *11*, 231, 1960.
23. CALABRO, J. J.: Arth. & Rheum., *5*, 19, 1962.
24. CALABRO, J. J. and MALTZ, B. A.: New Engl. Jour. Med., *282*, 606, 1970.
25. CANER, J. E. Z. and DECKER, J. L.: Amer. J. Med., *36*, 571, 1964.
26. CARPENTER, R. R. and STURGILL, B. C.: J. Chron. Dis., *19*, 117, 1966.
27. CARTER, M. E., ed., *Proc. Internat. Symposium: Radiological Aspects of Rheumatoid Arthritis.* Amsterdam, Excerpta Medica Foundation, International Study Centre for Rheumatic Diseases, 1963.
28. CASSIDY, J. T., BRODY, G. L., and MARTEL, W.: J. Pediat., *70*, 867, 1967.
29. CASTILLO, B. A., EL SALLAB, R. A., and SCOTT, J. T.: Ann. Rheum. Dis. *24*, 522, 1965.
30. CORRIGAN, A. B.: Austral. Radiol., *13*, 370, 1969.
31. CRAIN, D. C.: J.A.M.A., *175*, 1049, 1961.
32. CRUICKSHANK, B.: Clin. Orthop., *74*, 43, 1971.
33. CRUICKSHANK, B., MACLEOD, J. G. and SHEARER, W. S.: J. Fac. Radiologists, *5*, 218, 1954.
34. DESEZE, S., DEBEYRE, N., MANUEL, R.: In *Proc. Internat. Symposium: Radiological Aspects of Rheumatoid Arthritis*, ed. Mary E. Carter, Amsterdam, Excerpta Medica Foundation, International Study Centre for Rheumatic Diseases, 1963, p. 147.
35. DETENBECK, L. C., YOUNG, H. and UNDERDAHL, L. O.: Arch. Surg., *100*, 215, 1970.
36. DODDS, W. J. and STEINBACH, H. I.: New Engl. Jour. Med., *275*, 745, 1966.
37. DODSON, V. N., DINMAN, B. D., WHITEHOUSE, W. M., NASR, A. N. M., and MAGNUSON, H. J.: Arch. Environ. Health, *22*, 83, 1971.
38. DUBOIS, E. L. and COZEN, L.: J.A.M.A., *174*, 966, 1970.
39. DUBOIS, E. L. and TUFFANELLI, D. L.: J.A.M.A., *190*, 104, 1964.
40. ELLIS, R., SHORT, J. G., and SIMONDS, B. D.: Radiology, *93*, 857, 1969.
41. ELOESSER, L.: Amer. Surg., *66*, 201, 1917.
42. FELDMAN, M. J., BECKER, K. L., REEFE, W. E., and LONGO, A.: J.A.M.A., *209*, 1690, 1969.
43. FIELDING, J. W., JR.: J. Bone & Joint Surg., *46A*, 1779, 1964.
44. FORD, D. K.: Bull. Rheum. Dis., *20*, 588, 1970.
45. FORESTIER, J. and LAGIER, R.: Clin. Orthop., *74*, 65, 1971.
46. FRANCON, F., EPINEY, J., BLANCHARD, H., JOLY, L., VISNIKS, E. and DIAZ, R.: Presse Med., *76*, 1809, 1968.
47. GEHWEILER, J. A. and WILSON, J. W.: Radiology, *93*, 845, 1969.
48. GERLE, R. D., WALKER, L. A., ACHORD, J. L. and WEENS, H. S.: Radiology, *85*, 330, 1965.
49. GIBSON, H. J.: J. Fac. Radiol., *8*, 193, 1957.
50. GOOD, A. E. and RAPP, R.: New Engl. Jour. Med., *277*, 286, 1967.
51. GROKOEST, A. W., SNYDER, A. I. and SCHLAEGER, R.: Juvenile Rheumatoid Arthritis, Boston, Little, Brown & Co., 1962.
52. HANSON, C. A., SHAGRIN, J. W., and DUNCAN, H.: Clin. Orthop., *74*, 59, 1971.

53. Harris, D. K. and Adams, W. G. F.: Brit. M. J., *3*, 712, 1967.
54. Harrison, M. H. M., Schajowicz, F. and Trueta, J.: J. Bone & Joint Surg., *35B*, 598, 1953.
55. Harrison, M. O., Ranawat, C. S., and Freiberger, R. H.: Arthropathy in the Rheumatoid Wrist. Amer. J. Roentgenol., *112*, 480, 1971.
56. Hauptman, H. A.: N.Y. State J. Med., *70*, 955, 1970.
57. Heimann, W. G. and Freiberger, R. H.: New Engl. Jour. Med., *263*, 672, 1960.
58. Herd, J. D. and Vaughan, J. H.: Arth. & Rheum., *7*, 259, 1964.
59. Hermodsson, I.: Acta Orthop. Scandinav., *41*, 169, 1970.
60. Hinck, V. C. and Hopkins, C. E.: Amer. J. Roentgenol., *84*, 945, 1960.
61. Holt, J. F. and Owens, W. I.: Radiology, *53*, 11, 1949.
62. Holt, S. and Yates, P. O.: J. Bone & Joint Surg., *48B*, 407, 1966.
63. Hughes, J. T. and Brownell, B.: Riv. Pat. Nerv. Ment., *86*, 196, 1965.
64. Jacobs, P.: Brit. J. Radiol., *36*, 129, 1963.
65. Jacqueline, F., Boujot, A. and Canet, L.: Rheumatism, *4*, 500, 1961.
66. Jaffe, H. L.: Med. Radiography and Photography, Eastman Kodak Co., Rochester, New York, *45*, 58, 1969.
67. Jeremy, R.: Med. J. Austral., *1*, 323, 1967.
68. Johnson, J. T. H.: J. Bone & Joint Surg., *49A*, 1, 1967.
69. Jordan, J. H.: *Hemophilic Arthropathies*, Springfield, Charles C Thomas, 1958.
70. Kantor, G. L., Bickel, Y. B. and Barnett, E. V.: Amer. J. Med., *47*, 433, 1969.
71. Katz, I., Rabinowitz, J. G. and Dziadiw, R.: Amer. J. Roentgenol., *86*, 965, 1961.
72. Kidd, K. L. and Peter, J. B.: Radiology, *86*, 640, 1966.
73. Kiss, J., Martin, J. R., McConnell, F., and Wlodek, G.: J. Canad. A. Radiologists, *19*, 19, 1968.
74. Kolář, J. and Křížek, V. L.: Fortschr.a.d. Geb. d. Röntgenstrahlen, *109*, 203, 1968.
75. Kramer, L. S., *et al.*: Arth. & Rheum., *13*, 329, 1970.
76. Labowitz, R. and Schumacher, H. R.: Arth. & Rheum., *13*, 330, 1970.
77. Ladd, J. R., Cassidy, J. T. and Martel, W.: Juvenile Ankylosing Spondylitis. Accepted for publication in Arth. & Rheum., 1971.
78. Laine, V. A. I., Vaino, K. J. and Pekanmäki, K.: Ann. Rheum. Dis., *13*, 157, 1954.
79. Lamotte, M., Segrestaa, J. M., and Krassinine, G.: Sem. Hôp. Paris, *42*, 2420, 1966.
80. Larsen, I. J. and Landry, R. M.: J. Bone & Joint Surg., *51A*, 1210, 1969.
81. Lemmen, L. J. and Laing, P. G.: J. Neurosurg., *16*, 542, 1959.
82. McCarty, D. J. and Haskin, M. E.: Amer. J. Roentgenol., *90*, 1248, 1963.
83. McEwen, C., Lingg, C., Kirsner, J. B. and Spencer, J. A.: Amer. J. Med., *33*, 923, 1962.
84. Marcove, R. C. and Frieberger, R. H.: J. Bone & Joint Surg., *48A*, 1185, 1966.
85. Martel, W.: Personal Observation.
86. ———: *Proc. Internat. Symposium Radiological Aspects of Rheumatoid Arthritis*, ed. Mary E. Carter, Amsterdam, Excerpta Medica Foundation, International Study Centre for Rheumatic Diseases, May 1963, p. 189.
87. ———: Amer. J. Med., *44*, 441, 1968.
88. ———: Amer. J. Roentgenol., *86*, 223, 1961.
89. ———: Radiol. Clin. North America, *2*, 221, 1964.
90. ———: Med. Clin. North America, *52*, 655, 1968.
91. ———: Radiology, *91*, 755, 1968.
92. ———: Univ. of Mich. Med. Ctr. J., Special Arthritis Issue, 269, 1968.
93. Martel, W. and Abell, M. R.: Arth. & Rheum., *6*, 224, 1963.
94. Martel, W. and Bole, G. G.: Radiology, *90*, 948, 1968.
95. Martel, W. and Duff, I. F.: Radiology, *77*, 744, 1961.
96. Martel, W. and Page, J. W.: Arth. & Rheum., *3*, 546, 1960.
97. Martel, W. and Poznanski, A. K.: Radiology, *94*, 497, 1970.
98. ———: Radiology, *94*, 505, 1970.
99. Martel, W. and Sitterley, B. H.: Amer. J. Roentgenol., *106*, 509, 1969.
100. Martel, W. and Tishler, J. M.: Amer. J. Roentgenol., *3*, 630, 1966.
101. Martel, W., Griffin, P. E., and Good, A. E.: A Comparison of the Radiologic Manifestations of Reiter's Disease and Psoriatic Arthritis. Presented at the 54th Annual Meeting of the Radiological Society of North America, Chicago, Illinois, December, 1968.
102. Martel, W., Hayes, J. T., and Duff, I. F.: Radiology, *84*, 204, 1965.
103. Martel, W., Holt, J. F., and Cassidy, J. T.: Amer. J. Roentgenol., *88*, 400, 1962.

104. Martel, W., Holt, J. F., and Robinson, W. D.: Ann. Rheum. Dis., *21*, 199, 1962.
105. Martel, W., Uyham, R., and Stimson, C. W.: Radiology, *93*, 839, 1969.
106. Martel, W., Abell, M. R., Mikkelsen, W. M., and Whitehouse, W. M.: Radiology, *90*, 641, 1968.
107. Martel, W., Champion, C. K., Thompson, G., and Carter, T.: Amer. J. Roentgenol., *109*, 587, 1970.
108. Middlemiss, J. H.: J. Fac. Radiologists, *7*, 155, 1956.
109. ———: Proc. Royal Soc. Med., *44*, 805, 1951.
110. Miller, W. T. and Restifo, R. A.: Radiology, *86*, 652, 1966.
111. Mindelzun, R., Elkin, M., Scheinberg, I. H. and Sternlieb, I.: Radiology, *94*, 127, 1970.
112. Moseley, J. E.: *Bone Changes in Hematologic Disorders* (*Roentgen Aspects*), New York, Grune & Stratton, 1963.
113. ———: J. Mt. Sinai Hosp., *29*, 5, 1962.
114. Moskowitz, R. W. and Katz, D.: Amer. J. Med., *43*, 322, 1967.
115. Murray, R. O.: Brit. J. Radiol., *38*, 810, 1965.
116. Norman, A. and Bullough, P.: Bull. Hosp. Jt. Dis. XXIV.
117. Norman, A., Robbins, H. and Milgram, J. E.: Radiology, *90*, 1159, 1968.
118. North, A. F., Jr., *et al.*: Amer. J. Med., *48*, 449, 1970.
119. Numaguchi, Y.: Radiology, *98*, 1, 1971.
120. O'Duffy, J. D.: Arth. & Rheum., *13*, 381, 1970.
121. Parfitt, A. M.: Arch. Intern. Med., *124*, 544, 1969.
122. Pear, B. L.: Amer. J. Roentgenol., *111*, 821, 1971.
123. Perry, C. B.: J. Fac. Radiol., *7*, 11, 1956.
124. Peter, J. B., Pearson, C. M. and Marmor, L.: Arth. & Rheum., *9*, 365, 1966.
125. Peterson, C. C., Jr. and Silbiger, M. L.: Amer. J. Roentgenol., *101*, 860, 1967.
126. Phocas, E., Andriotakis, C., Kaklamanis, P., *et al.*: Acta Rheum. Scand., *13*, 137, 1967.
127. Poznanski, A. K. and Holt, J. F.: Amer. J. Roentgenol., *112*, 443, 1971.
128. Rivelis, M. and Freiberger, R. H.: Radiology, *93*, 251, 1969.
129. Romanus, R. and Ydén, S.: *Pelvo-Spondylitis Ossificans*, Chicago, The Yearbook Medical Publishers, Inc., 1955.
130. Ross, P. and Wood, B.: Amer. J. Roentgenol., *109*, 575, 1970.
131. Sairanen, O.: Acta Rheum. Scand., Suppl., 2, 1958.
132. Scharer, L. and Smith, D. W.: Arth. & Rheum., *12*, 51, 1969.
133. Schwarz, G. S., Berenyi, M. R., and Siegel, M. W.: Amer. J. Roentgenol., *106*, 523, 1969.
134. Segal, G. and Kellogg, D. S.: Amer. J. Roentgenol., *71*, 643, 1954.
135. Sharp, J.: Bull. Rheum. Dis., *7*, 125, 1957.
136. ———: J. Proc. Roy. Soc. Med., *59*, 453, 1966.
137. Sharp, J. and Purser, D. W.: Ann. Rheum. Dis., *20*, 47, 1961.
138. Sherk, H. H. and Nicholson, J. T.: J. Bone & Joint Surg., *51A*, 957, 1969.
139. Sholkoff, S. D., Glickman, M. G. and Steinbach, H. L.: Radiology, *97*, 497, 1970.
140. Skinner, M. and Cohen, A. S.: Arch. Intern. Med., *123*, 636, 1969.
141. Skinner, M. and Fernandez-Herlihy, L.: Med. Clin. North America, *50*, 417, 1966.
142. Smith, E. M., Pearson, J. R., Bender, L. F. and Juvinall, R. E.: Arth. & Rheum., *7*, 467, 1964.
143. Smith, J. H. and Pugh, D. G.: Amer. J. Roentgenol., *87*, 1146, 1962.
144. Soila, P.: Acta Rheum. Scand., *3*, 328, 1957.
145. ———: Acta Rheum. Scand., Suppl. 1, 1, 1958.
146. ———: Acta Rheum. Scand, *4*, Suppl. 1, 1958.
147. Sokoloff, L.: *The Biology of Degenerative Joint Disease*, Chicago, The University of Chicago Press, 1969.
148. Spilberg, I., Siltzbach, L. E. and McEwen, C.: Arth. & Rheum., *12*, 126, 1969.
149. Stafne, E. C.: *Oral Roentgenographic Diagnosis*, Philadelphia, W. B. Saunders Company, 112, 1963.
150. Stecher, R. M.: Ann. Rheum. Dis., *14*, 1, 1955.
151. ———: Geriatrics, *16*, 167, 1961.
152. Steinberg, C. L., Duthie, R. B. and Piva, A. E.: J.A.M.A., *181*, 145, 1962.
153. Swannell, A. J., Underwood, F. A. and Dixon, A. St J.: Ann. Rheum. Dis., *29*, 380, 1970.
154. Thompson, G. R., Ting, Y. M., Riggs, G. A., Fenn, M. E. and Denning, R. M.: J.A.M.A., *203*, 122, 1968.
155. Trueta, J.: Clin. Orthopaedics, *31*, 7, 1963.
156. Tuffanelli, D. L. and Winkelman, R. K.: Arch. Derm., *84*, 359, 1961.

157. TWIGG, H. L. and SMITH, B. F.: Radiology, *80*, 417, 1963.
158. VAINIO, K.: Ann. Chir. et Gynaec. Fenniae, *45*, Suppl. 1, 1956.
159. VIGARIO, G. D. and KEATS, T. E.: Amer. J. Roentgenol., *108*, 806, 1970.
160. WALBOM-JØRGENSEN, S.: Clin. Radiol., *17*, 365, 1966.
161. WALDENSTRÖM, HENNING: J. Bone & Joint Surg., *20*, 559, 1938.
162. WEBB, J. B. and DIXON, A. St. John: Ann. Rheum. Dis., *19*, 143, 1960.
163. WEINFELD, A., ROSS, M. W. and SARASOHN, S. H.: Amer. J. Roentgenol., *101*, 851, 1967.
164. WEINFELD, A., STERN, M. H. and MARX, L. H.: Amer. J. Roentgenol., *108*, 799, 1970.
165. WELDON, W. V. and SCALETTAR, R.: Amer. J. Roentgenol., *86*, 344, 1961.
166. WERNE, SVEN: Acta Orthoped. Scand., Suppl. 23, 1957.
167. WHOLEY, M. H., PUGH, D. G. and BICKEL, W. H.: Radiology, *74*, 54, 1960.
168. WILSON, R. H., MCCORMICK, W. E., TATUM, C. F., and CREECH, J. L.: J.A.M.A., *201*, 577, 1967.
169. WINCHESTER, P., GROSSMAN, H., LIM, W. N. and DANES, B. S.: Amer. J. Roentgenol., *106*, 121, 1969.
170. WOLFSON, J. J., QUIE, P. G., LAXDAL, S. D., and GOOD, R. A.: Radiology, *91*, 37, 1968.
171. WOOD, K., OMER, A., and SHAW, M. T.: Brit. J. Radiol., *42*, 498, 1969.
172. WRIGHT, V. and MOLL, J. M. H.: Bull. Rheum. Dis., *21*, 627, 1971.
173. YUNE, H. Y., VIX, V. A. and KLATTE, E. C.: J.A.M.A., *215*, 1113, 1971.
174. ZIFF, M., GRIBETZ, H. F., and LOSPALLUTO, J.: J. Clin. Invest., *39*, 405, 1960.
175. ZITNAN, D. and SIT'AJ, S.: Ann. Rheum. Dis., *22*, 142, 1963.
176. ZVAIFLER, N. J. and MARTEL, W.: Arth. & Rheum., *3*, 76, 1960.

Chapter 8

The Acute Inflammatory Response

By K. Frank Austen, M.D.

The inflammatory response can be viewed as a biological mechanism, organized and staged to protect man from a hostile microbiological environment with minimal injury to his own tissues. Inherent to this view is that distinct reaction pathways are designed to deal with particular groups of microorganisms or with the same microorganism in an orderly sequence. When the composite reactions constituting the inflammatory response are activated simultaneously, as in acute gouty arthritis, or without limitation due to misdirection as in rheumatoid arthritis, the result is self-destruction by those very mechanisms which are more usually coordinated to be protective.

There are innumerable symposia and reviews[89,156,163] on the general subject of inflammation emphasizing microcirculatory alterations, increased local blood flow, and enhanced vascular permeability. The microcirculatory alterations and in turn their clinical expression—heat, redness, swelling, and pain—are consequences of the activation of mediator systems acting directly upon the microvasculature through chemical substances or indirectly by attraction and/or activation of certain cellular elements of the host. Although it is not yet possibile to interrelate fully the diverse ingredients of the inflammatory response, it is now possible to identify some of the discrete reaction pathways and to indicate a number of points of interaction. The effector systems of the acute inflammatory response to be considered include: the complement system, the kinin-forming sequence, certain aspects of the clotting system, and the secretion of the amine(s) and slow-reacting substance of anaphylaxis (SRS-A) from tissue mast cells. The attraction and/or activation of cells such as polymorphonuclear neutrophilic or eosinophilic leukocytes, macrophages, lymphocytes, and platelets will be considered only in relation to the above-mentioned primary mediator systems.

THE COMPLEMENT SYSTEM

The complement system consists of a group of nine distinct serum proteins which interact sequentially to mediate certain effects of antigen-antibody interactions. The schematic presentation of the complement reaction sequence depicted in Figure 8–1 employs the nomenclature agreed upon under the auspices of the World Health Organization.[3] The immune hemolytic sequence shown in Figure 8–1 uses sheep erythrocytes (E) as the target cell, although similar reactions have been shown with other cell systems,[167] bacteria,[56] and for soluble antigens.[48] The union of IgG or IgM immunoglobulins with their corresponding antigen activates the complement system; in immune hemolysis the fixation and activation of C1 to $C\bar{1}$* usually requires either a doublet of IgG molecules or a single IgM molecule. The first component, C1, is an inactive complex of three subunits, C1q, C1r, and C1s.[94,113] The subunit C1q carries the binding site which physically combines

* A line over a component signifies its activated state.

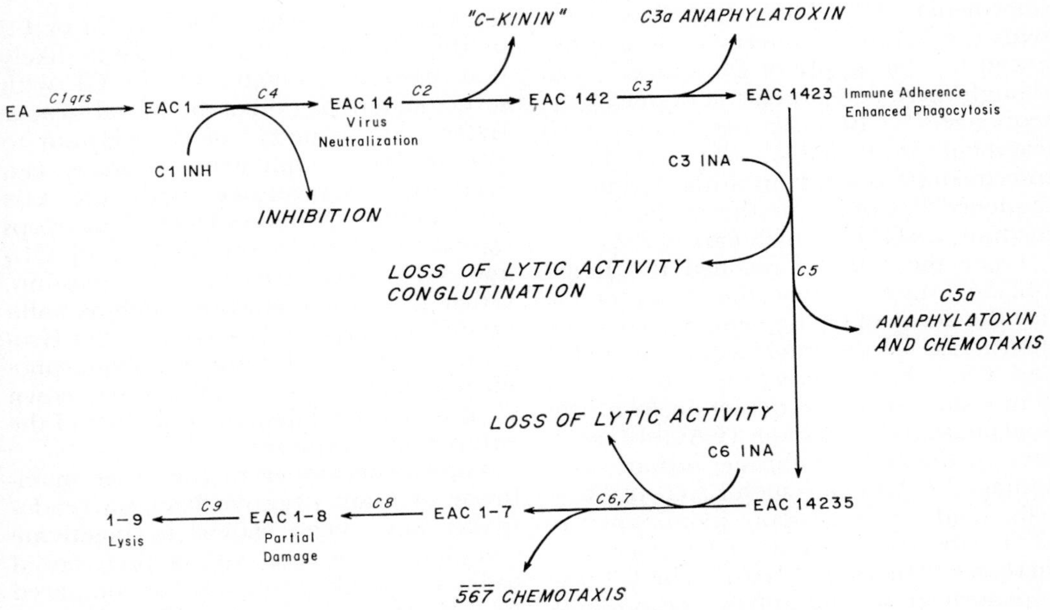

FIG. 8–1.—The complement sequence.

with the immunoglobulin, thereby activating C1r,[114] which in turn activates C1s to C$\bar{1}$s. The C$\bar{1}$s subunit alone or in the C$\bar{1}$s portion of the C$\bar{1}$ molecule demonstrates esterolytic activity on the synthetic substrates such as p-toluene sulfonyl L-arginine methyl ester (TAMe), N-acetyl L-arginine methyl ester (AAMe), N-acetyl L-tyrosine methyl ester (ATMe) or ethyl ester (ATEe)[87] and splits C4 into at least two portions.[109] The major product, C4b, either is bound to the cell membrane forming the cellular intermediate EAC14,[178] or remains in the fluid phase as a hemolytically inactive product, C4i.

It has long been appreciated that C4 precedes C2 in the hemolytic sequence even though both are natural substrates of the C$\bar{1}$s subunit.[93] The basis of this order of reaction has only recently become apparent[52,53] with the finding that the activity of C$\bar{1}$ upon C2 is markedly enhanced by the prior interaction of C$\bar{1}$, free in the fluid phase or cell-bound (EAC1), with C4. It has been postulated that the C$\bar{1}$–C4 interaction alters the configuration of the C$\bar{1}$ molecule, exposing the enzymatic site responsible for C2 utilization. The action of the C$\overline{14}$ enzyme on C2 leads to the physical uptake of the major fragment, C2a, by the EAC14 intermediate to generate the EAC142 complex,[104,105] which decays to release C2a[d] into the fluid phase, thereby reverting to the original EAC14 state.[14] This intermediate is able to interact again with native C2 to regenerate the EAC142 intermediate. Major fragments not immediately taken up by the EAC142 complex become hemolytically inactive and are designated C2i. The assembly of the major fragments of C4 and C2 yields a new enzymatic activity, C$\overline{42}$, termed C3 convertase, which cleaves C3 into C3a and C3b. The major fragment, C3b, remains on the intermediate, EAC1423, or appears in the fluid phase as the hemolytically inactive byproduct, C3i. The lesser fragment, C3a, appears only in the fluid phase.[110,112]

The interaction of the intermediate EAC1423 with C5 releases a lesser fragment of C5, C5a, into the fluid phase and binds the major fragment, C5b, to the intermediate.[149] The interaction of C5 with the EAC1423 intermediate is influenced by the supply of C6 and C7 even though these components act later in the sequence.[116] Because the bound C5b fragment is unstable, the EAC14235 intermediate is a rate-limiting step in the sequence[150] similar to the earlier intermediate EAC142, which carries C2a.

Once the cell has reached the EAC-1423567 state, neither the decay of C2 nor the decay of C5 prevents the effective interaction of the intermediate with C8 and C9. The interaction with C8, as demonstrated by C8 depletion from the fluid phase and formation of EAC14235678 sites on the cell membrane, initiates cell damage.[158] Although such EAC14235678 cells tend to lyse upon incubation at 37° C, the introduction of C9 markedly increases their rate of lysis. The C9 disappears from the fluid phase and is found specifically bound to the cells.[61] Electron microscopic studies have revealed the appearance of the characteristic ultrastructural alterations on the cell membrane following C9 action;[15,67] similar alterations have recently been reported to occur in cells in the EAC14235 state.[132]

Alternative Mechanisms or Pathways of Activation of the Complement System

The complement system can be activated by mechanisms or pathways which apparently differ from the classical immunological mechanism of activation described above. These include: direct activation of C1 by other serum enzyme systems; interaction of certain factors with the complement sequence in a manner which achieves relative sparing of C1, C4, and C2 and intense utilization of C3 and the other terminal components; and a complete bypass of C1, C4, and C2 through direct activation of C3 followed by utilization of the subsequent component proteins.

The addition of streptokinase to human serum activates plasminogen to plasmin and depletes the serum of C4 and C2; since plasmin has no effect on C4 or C2 in the absence of Cl,[130] it seems likely that plasmin activates C1 to $C\bar{1}$ with subsequent depletion of the $C\bar{1}$ substrates. Indeed, the capacity of the plasmin to initiate the complement sequence can even be demonstrated with the $C\bar{1}s$ moiety of the $C\bar{1}$ molecule which develops esterase activity in the absence of C1q and C1r when treated with plasmin. Other proteolytic enzymes such as kallikrein[38] or trypsin[114] as well as the lysosomal enzymes of human polymorphonuclear leukocytes[161] can also be shown to initiate the sequential activation of the complement sequence.

Polysaccharides from the outer membrane of gram negative bacteria (endotoxin) have been shown to inactivate complement *in vitro* with a preferential utilization of C3 through C9 as compared to the early components.[48,131] Human serum contains a β-globulin, termed C3 proactivator, which complexes with a cobra venom factor to activate directly C3;[34,111] the same protein is apparently split upon endotoxin[58] treatment of serum to yield a major fragment with gamma mobility, termed C3 activator, which directly activates C3[30] and thereby the subsequent complement proteins. Although this bypass mechanism may represent an extremely important route to recruitment of the terminal complement components for the inflammatory response, it is not unlikely that endotoxin also interacts with natural antibody to initiate the more conventional mechanism of sequence activation. Support for the latter view comes from the observation that sera from individuals genetically deficient in C2[85] or the C1r subunit[128] inactivate the late components in the presence of endotoxin less efficiently than do normal sera.[49]

Recently a fragment, apparently derived from kallikrein, has been shown to modify fully active C1 to diminish its C4 and C2 utilizing capacity, while increasing markedly the ability of the C4 and C2 so treated to inactivate C3.[55] Thus, under circumstances where there is simultaneous activation of the complement and kinin-forming systems, an apparent bypass of early components could result, merely reflecting the highly efficient formation of 42 convertase.

Control Mechanisms of the Complement System

The sequential interaction of the complement proteins is limited by both inherent and external influences. The rapid decay in terms of function of the C2a fragment,[14,105,151] in C3 convertase and of the C5b[150] fragment represents intrinsic controls of the reaction mechanism. Extrinsic retardation is the result of natural inhibitors or inactivators which combine with or destroy activated forms of certain complement proteins essential to the progression of the reaction.

The inhibitor of $C\bar{1}$ ($C\bar{1}$INH), an $\alpha 2$ globulin in human serum,[95] inhibits the esterolytic and hemolytic[51,95] activities of $C\bar{1}$s and $C\bar{1}$ either in the fluid phase or bound to a cell. $C\bar{1}$INH also inhibits the activation of C1s by $C\bar{1}$r and the esterolytic activity of the $C\bar{1}$r subunit.[114] In addition, $C\bar{1}$INH of human origin can effectively inhibit the action of kallikrein[54] either on its natural substrate, kininogen, or on synthetic substrates; this interaction, like that with $C\bar{1}$, is stoichiometric. Plasmin also has been shown to be inhibited by $C\bar{1}$INH; however, as a result of this interaction the inhibitor is enzymatically degraded.[63] Further, the functional activity of activated Hageman factor and prothrombin antecedent (PTA) is blocked by $C\bar{1}$INH.[136] $C\bar{1}$ and plasma kallikrein are the only two enzymes for which a stoichiometric inhibition by $C\bar{1}$INH has been demonstrated in the presence of the natural substrates, C4 and C2, and kininogen, respectively, at approximately physiologic concentrations of all reactants. Nonetheless, the demonstrated effects of $C\bar{1}$INH on $C\bar{1}$r to interfere with complement activation, on activated Hageman factor and PTA, and on plasmin indicate a central role in the control of the inflammatory response.

The action of C3 convertase upon C3 to yield C3b bound to the complex and a fluid phase C3a fragment with anaphylatoxin activity is counteracted by natural inactivators of both fragments. An inactivator of the C3b fragment, C3bINA, has been described in man[143] and other species;[160] C3bINA destroys the hemolytic, immune adherence, and phagocytosis-enhancing activities[50] associated with the cell-bound C3b fragment of the cellular intermediate EAC1423. The action of C3bINA is time- and temperature-dependent and is accompanied by the release of a protein fragment C3c into the fluid phase leaving C3d on the cellular intermediate.[144] The data available suggest that C3bINA is an enzyme identical with the conglutininogen activating factor.[90] An inactivator of anaphylatoxin, C3aINA,[13] has been characterized as an α globulin of human serum with a molecular weight of approximately 310,000. C3aINA removes the C-terminal arginine residue from C3a, from an additional reaction fragment C5a with anaphylatoxic and chemotactic activity, and from the nonapeptide bradykinin. The action of C3aINA, a carboxypeptidase, which inactivates both the anaphylatoxic byproducts of the complement component interaction and bradykinin, which also has a C-terminal arginine residue and is the product of the kinin-forming sequence, represents another control point shared by these two plasma protein systems.

An inactivator of the sixth component of complement is present in rabbit, guinea pig and human serum.[160] As with C3bINA, C6INA acts on cell-bound C6 destroying the hemolytic activity of the cellular intermediate EAC142356.

Contributions of the Complement System to the Inflammatory Response

The products and byproducts of the complement reaction sequence depicted in Figure 8–1 have all been demonstrated by *in vitro* techniques, and conclusions as to their *in vivo* significance are only speculative. Nonetheless, it is reasonable to point out that the potential biologic meaning of the system is no longer only in terms of completion of the whole sequence with consequent death of some antigen-carrying cells, but also includes the elaboration of various ingredients of the inflammatory response.

Under certain conditions, antisera against herpes simplex virus produces little or no neutralization unless complement is present. The mechanism by which complement adds to the action of γ globulin suggests that the presence of $C\bar{1}$ and C4 on the sensitized virus results in neutralization by more extensive coverage of the surface of the virus. Although $C\bar{1}$ and C4 are sufficient to enhance virus neutralization, under certain circumstances C2 and C3 can further augment the reaction.[33] No effect of the later components has yet been demonstrable.

A vasoactive peptide distinguishable from bradykinin has been isolated from the plasma of patients with angioedema of the hereditary type.[39] This material may represent a previously unrecognized split product of C2, and has been temporarily termed C-kinin; it differs from the known kinins in being susceptible to inactivation by trypsin as well as chymotrypsin and in producing a pressor effect in the rat. The major fragments resulting from the sequential action of $C\bar{1}$ on C4 and C2 generate C3 convertase;[112] through the action of this enzyme a small fragment of the C3 molecule, C3a, is released into the fluid phase; this fragment anaphylatoxin causes a local wheal when injected intracutaneously into man, releases histamine *in vitro* from rat peritoneal mast cells, and causes the isolated guinea pig ileum to contract.[36] C3b, the major fragment of C3, either is bound to the cellular intermediate EAC-1423, or remains free in the fluid phase as the hemolytically inactive C3i. The presence of C3b on the cell confers upon it the ability to participate in the immune adherence phenomenon, a reaction in which the C3b-coated cell binds to a specific receptor site on erythrocytes, polymorphonuclear leukocytes, or platelets.[115] This phenomenon enhances phagocytosis by polymorphonuclear leukocytes.[50]

The interaction of the EAC1423 intermediate with C5 liberates a small molecular weight fragment C5a with anaphylatoxin properties[25] and chemotactic activity for polymorphonuclear leukocytes.[171]

In the course of the formation of EAC1–7 an additional chemotactic factor for polymorphonuclear leukocytes[169] is generated. This activity resides in a high molecular weight complex formed by the interaction of C5, C6 and C7. The activation of the complement sequence is associated with the appearance of characteristic membrane discontinuity which has been observed by electron microscopic studies of negatively stained membranes from lysed erythrocytes and other target cells.[15,67,132]

Whether the immunologic activation of the complement sequence is considered beneficial or detrimental to the host depends at least in part on the location of the antigens against which the mediating antibody is directed. Antibodies directed against a soluble foreign protein result in the deposition of aggregates in vessel walls and activation of the complement system with a local increase in vascular permeability, the elaboration of principles chemotactic for polymorphonuclear leukocytes, and enhanced phagocytosis of the aggregates; the latter results in the release of lysosomal enzymes with secondary focal necrosis of the vessel wall. This detrimental hypersensitivity reaction is termed the Arthus reaction.[23] In contrast, the same non-cytotoxic reaction sequence directed against an invading pyogenic bacterium with resultant enhanced phagocytosis would be considered a beneficial aspect of the immune response. Similarly, when the complete sequence is activated to yield a cytotoxic reaction directed against the host's own red cells or those received by transfusion, the event is considered hypersensitivity;

whereas if the target cell were a gram negative bacterium the bactericidal reaction would be considered immunity.

The possible immunobiological significance of the complement system has recently been extended by several additional observations. The report that target cells carrying the first four reacting components undergo enhanced ingestion by macrophages, while those carrying the first seven components experience accelerated damage upon exposure to a suspension of purified lymphocytes introduces a role for complement in reactions predominating in mononuclear cells.[127]

Further, the appreciation that a trimolecular complex of activated C5, C6, and C7 can interact with an unsensitized bystander cell to yield an intermediate susceptible to cytolytic destruction by C8 and C9 broadens the potential consequences of specific activation of the system.[57,164] Possible solid tissue effects of activation of the complement system are also in the early stages of recognition, including mitogenesis of lymphocytes in response to immune complexes[11,84] and activation of tissue lysosomal activity[37,91] with attendant implications for the development of immunologically competent cells and tissue necrosis, respectively.

THE KININ SYSTEM

In 1930, Kraut, Frey, and Werle[88] demonstrated that the intravenous injection of pancreatic extract into dogs produced hypotension and termed the active principle kallikrein. *In vitro* experiments revealed that kallikrein reacted with an α-globulin in plasma to form a smooth muscle-stimulating principle, kallidin.[175] During the same period, Rocha e Silva *et al.*[141] reported that trypsin and some snake venoms also released from an α-globulin in plasma a hypotensive, smooth muscle-stimulating principle referred to as bradykinin. Bradykinin was subsequently shown to be a nonapeptide by degradation studies,[41] while kallidin was identified as a decapeptide differing only in the presence of an N-terminal lysine.[129] Synthesis of the nonapeptide,[12] bradykinin or kallidin I, and the decapeptide, kallidin II, has now been accomplished. Glandular kallikrein, salivary or pancreatic, and urinary kallikrein produce kallidin II, which is converted to kallidin I by an aminopeptidase in plasma, whereas plasma kallikrein yields kallidin I directly.[129,173] The kallidins are rapidly inactivated in human plasma by at least two kininases—a carboxypeptidase N which cleaves the C-terminal arginine[43] and a peptidase which splits off a C-terminal dipeptide (phenylalanine-arginine).[180] The kallidins and related polypeptides have been grouped under the generic term, plasma kinins.[42] The α-globulin from which the kinins are formed by the action of kallikreins is termed kininogen.

Five pharmacological activities of bradykinin have been reported:[40] smooth muscle stimulation, vasodilatation, increase in capillary permeability, attraction of leukocytes, and stimulation of pain fibers. The decapeptide, kallidin II, has similar pharmacological activity which differs in degree depending on the assay.[173] On intravenous administration, both kallidin I and II increase the resistance of the lungs of the anesthetized guinea pig to inflation;[28] this bronchoconstrictor activity is antagonized by analgesic antipyretics, such as acetylsalicylic acid, which exhibit no antagonism against the other pharmacological activities of the kallidins.[28]

Interrelationships of the Kinin-Forming System with Clotting and Fibrinolysis

Three enzymes capable of elaborating a permeability-producing factor have been identified in plasma, i.e., plasma kallikrein, plasmin,[96] and a permeability-producing globulin activated by dilution, PF/dil.[100] Each is associated with esterase activity against p-toluene sulfonyl-L-arginine methyl ester (TAMe) and is inhibited by diisopropylfluorophosphate (DFP) or the trypsin inhibitor from soy beans.[172,173] Plasmin is distinguished by its marked fibrinolytic and relatively poor kinin-forming activity. The other two would seem to have been separated by chromatographic and electrophoretic differences, kallikrein being a γ-globulin and PF/dil a β-globulin.[29,74] Margolis[103] demonstrated that the surface-activated factor involved in blood clotting, Hageman factor, is required for the activation of plasma kallikrein, and it now seems likely that Hageman factor, plasmin, and the activity ascribed to PF/dil act sequentially to convert prekallikrein to kallikrein as depicted in Figure 8–3. Activated Hageman factor interacts with plasmin to yield fragments possessing the ability both to correct Hageman factor deficiency as assessed by clotting and to convert prekallikrein to kallikrein.[77,78] The prekallikrein activator[77,179] has an isoelectric point of 4.9, migrates as a pre-albumin on disc gel electrophoresis at pH 9.3, and has an approximate molecular weight of 35,000. Conversion of active Hageman factor to the pre-albumin frag-

	IN VITRO	COMPONENT REQUIRED	IN VIVO	
			HOST RESISTANCE	HYPERSENSITIVITY
NON-CYTOTOXIC REACTIONS	VIRUS NEUTRALIZATION	14	VIRUS NEUTRALIZATION	——
	IMMUNE ADHERENCE AND ENHANCED PHAGOCYTOSIS	3b (1–3)	ENHANCED INGESTION OF PYOGENIC BACTERIA	ARTHUS
	ANAPHYLATOXINS	3a (1–3) 5a (1–5)	INCREASED VASCULAR PERMEABILITY	ARTHUS
	CHEMOTACTIC FACTORS	3a (1–3) 5a (1–5) $\overline{567}$ (1–7)	LEUKOCYTE ATTRACTION	ARTHUS
CYTOTOXIC REACTION	CELL LYSIS	1–9	BACTERICIDAL REACTION	TRANSFUSION REACTION

Fig. 8–2.—Immunobiology of complement.

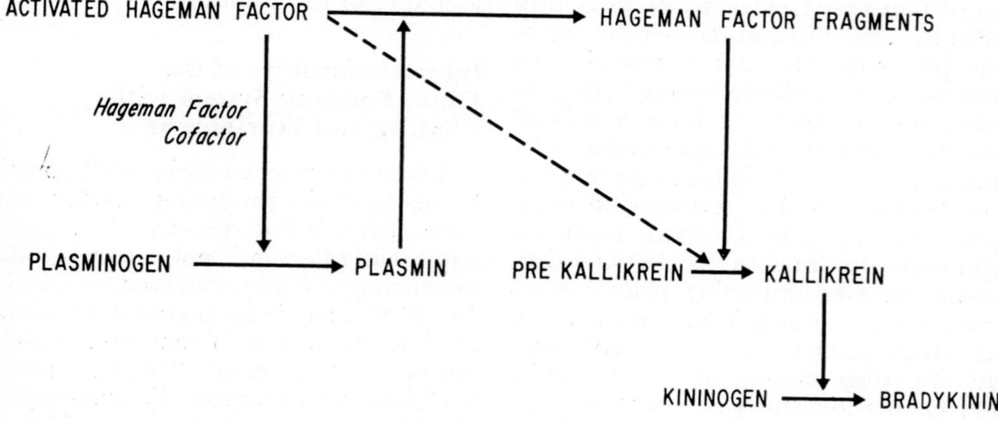

Fig. 8–3.—The kinin sequence.

ment is associated with a progressive decrease in size, increase in net negative charge, and increased prekallikrein activating ability relative to clot-promoting activity in Hageman factor-deficient plasma.[78] It thus seems that PF/dil represents a production of the interaction of active Hageman factor and plasmin; a product not yet fully converted to its final state as a prekallikrein activator.

Contributions of the Kinin-Forming System to the Inflammatory Response

The reaction scheme for bradykinin generation illustrated in Figure 8–3 is initiated by those events known to activate Hageman factor and the clotting system. However, to divert the active Hageman factor into the kinin-forming sequence, it is necessary to introduce the fibrinolytic system. It should be noted, therefore, that active Hageman factor together with a newly recognized cofactor termed "Hageman factor cofactor"[68,117] mediates conversion of plasminogen to plasmin. The plasmin so generated can activate C1 to $C\bar{1}$[114] to recruit the complement system, directly split C3 to yield anaphylatoxin,[170] or act back on the active Hageman factor to yield the prekallikrein activating fragment which converts prekallikrein to kallikrein.[78] A fragment appearing during kallikrein activation can interact with $C\bar{1}$ to shift the complement component utilization profile in favor of terminal components.[55] Kallikrein can digest kininogen to yield bradykinin and is directly chemotactic for human neutrophils.[79a] Interestingly enough, the fibrinopeptide (fibrin split products) derived from completing the clotting sequence can markedly enhance the pharmacologic effects of bradykinin.[123]

Although it was previously known that antigen-antibody aggregates could accelerate the clotting time of whole rabbit blood[140] or generate kinin from fresh guinea pig plasma,[108] the ability of soluble complexes to activate Hageman factor has only recently been noted.[79] Activation of native Hageman factor was accomplished with a complex of monoclonal human IgM antibody to human IgG; the IgM antibody reacts with a single antigenic determinant present in IgG and therefore forms only soluble complexes, binding a maximum of 5 moles of IgG per mole of IgM.

TISSUE-DERIVED MEDIATORS

Although the byproducts of the activation of humoral systems, such as the complement sequence and the kinin-forming system, afford an array of polypeptides capable of mediating the inflammatory reaction, other mediator systems already in the tissue must also be considered. These latter mediators have been most often studied in relation to immediate hypersensitivity reactions, and generally are grouped under this heading for purposes of presentation. Their importance, however, is by no means restricted to acute allergic reactions and it may well be that their ready release in tissues forms the initial phase of the inflammatory response by producing the changes in vascular permeability which activate and/or recruit the humoral systems.

Histamine

Histamine (β-imidazolylethylamine) is widely distributed in mammalian tissue,[45] but the concentration in a given organ has great species variation. Much of the tissue histamine is associated with the granules of the mast cell,[138] and the histamine content per mast cell is reasonably constant in normal tissue, ranging from 7 to 10 $\mu\mu$g in the dog,[60] 21 to 34 in the guinea pig,[16] and 10 to 59 in the rat.[66,107] The mast cells, located mainly in connective tissue in relation to blood vessels,[137] are not the only cells containing histamine. Histamine has been found in platelets[65] and in basophilic leukocytes;[59,168] it is present in high concentration in fetal liver[75] and in the mucosa of the parietal region of the stomach[45,62] even though mast cells are essentially absent. Regardless of whether or not tissue histamine is contained in mast cells, it is formed from L-histidine and degraded either by oxidative deamination or by methylation and oxidative deamination such that the principal excretion products are imidazoleacetic acid-riboside and l-methyl imidazoleacetic acid, respectively.[76,145,146,155] Schayer[146,147] has observed an increase in histidine decarboxylase activity in tissue not necessarily rich in mast cells in response to a variety of nonspecific stimuli and refers to the alleged product of this adaptive enzyme activity as induced histamine to distinguish it from that stored in mast cells.

Some of the established pharmacological actions of histamine include increase of capillary permeability, bronchiolar and other smooth muscle constriction, and stimulation of the glands of exocrine secretion. The production of leaking venules is attributed to partial disconnection of the endothelium.[32,102] The physiological role(s) of histamine is not securely established.[139] Recent studies[62] have reaffirmed the earlier view[27] that histamine is the common mediator of many gastric secretagogues, including the peptide hormone gastrin. Induced histamine, allegedly synthesized in the microvascular smooth muscle cells, is held to participate in circulatory homeostasis; and nascent histamine, also assessed in terms of histamine decarboxylase activity, is implicated as having a function in rapidly growing tissue, fetal or granulation.[21] Much of the data presented for and against a role for histamine depends on the action of antihistamines, which unfortunately are not entirely specific; antihistamines antagonize both acetylcholine and 5-hydroxytryptamine and have a local anesthetic effect.[20]

Serotonin

In mammalian tissue, serotonin (5-hydroxytryptamine) is localized primarily in the mucosal layer of the gastrointestinal tract, and to a lesser extent in brain tissue and platelets.[44,153] Carcinoid tissue, a tumor derived from the enterochromaffin cells of the gastrointestinal tract of man, contains 1 to 2 mg serotonin per g, which is about 1,000 times the normal gastrointestinal concentration. In brain the highest concentrations, 0.5 to 1.0 μg per g, are in the hypothalamus and other primitive structures, and the lowest in the cerebellum and neocortex.[31] Normally, human blood contains about 0.1 to 0.2 μg serotonin per ml, virtually all bound to platelets.[153] Species variation in the serotonin content of organs is marked. Rat, mouse and rabbit lung contain appreciable amounts of serotonin, whereas it is virtually absent in dog, cat, guinea pig, or human lung.[126,166] Only the rat and mouse have a significant skin concentration. In the gastrointestinal tract, serotonin is presumably in the enterochromaffin cells,[9] while in the skin of the rat and mouse it is contained in the mast cells,[8] the concentration in the rat peritoneal mast cell ranging from 0.2 to 6 μμg per cell.[107] Serotonin is not present in the mast cells of dog, cat, cow, and man,[154,176] but has been identified in the platelets of most species, including horse, ox, goat, dog, guinea pig, and rabbit.[181] Serotonin is derived from the amino acid, tryptophan, by the introduction of a hydroxyl group into the 5 position and decarboxylation;[22] 5-hydroxytryptophan decarboxylase activity has been noted in the mast cells of the rat and mouse.[92] Detoxification by deamination to 5-hydroxyindoleacetic acid is accomplished by amine oxidase, an enzyme present in many tissues.[165]

The established pharmacologic effects of serotonin include smooth muscle constriction[125] and the production of leaking venules[142] due to partial disconnection of the endothelial cells;[32,102] however, the species variation in response to this amine is particularly marked.[17,126,166] The smooth muscle of the rat is very sensitive to serotonin and relatively insensitive to histamine, and thus the isolated rat colon or estrous rat uterus has been widely used in the bioassay of this material; identification is also facilitated by demonstrating inhibition with small amounts of lysergic acid.[47] The physiological role(s) of serotonin is not securely established; there is no convincing evidence that it plays a role in hemostasis,[153,181] and its possible role in central nervous system function and gastrointestinal physiology is still to be elucidated.[125,153]

Slow-Reacting Substance of Anaphylaxis (SRS-A)

The term slow-reacting substance (SRS) refers to material or materials which contract smooth muscle, usually guinea pig ileum, more slowly than histamine or acetylcholine. Feldberg and Kellaway[46] introduced this term to describe a substance obtained from guinea pig lung during perfusion with cobra venom, and a similar material was subsequently detected in the effluent collected during anaphylactic shock of the same tissue.[83] In both experiments the effluent produced a more prolonged contraction of the guinea pig ileum than was produced by histamine alone. Brocklehurst[18] used antihistamines to abolish the response of the ileum to histamine and obtain direct evidence of the anaphylactic release of a slow-reacting substance, termed SRS-A, to indicate that it appeared as a result of antigen-antibody interaction. At present, there is no way of knowing whether the SRS-A elaborated by different species is a single substance or whether it represents a family of closely related materials.

SRS-A is not extractable from sensitized tissues prior to antigen challenge and thus must be formed as well as released by antigen-antibody interaction. *In vitro* release mediated by the appropriate homologous immunoglobulin has been observed in the lungs of man, monkey, rabbit, and guinea pig;[18,69,157] in the latter species the aorta and great veins have also been shown to yield appreciable amounts of this material.[18] The chemical structure of SRS-A is not known[120] and the site of tissue origin is not definitively established. However, the finding in the rat that IgE mediates SRS-A release by a mast cell dependent pathway,[121] while IgGa mediates release by a polymorphonuclear leukocyte-complement dependent route[118] is consistent with the view that SRS-A is a byproduct, perhaps membrane-derived, of a secretory or pinocytotic reaction.[5]

SRS-A contracts only a limited number of isolated smooth muscle preparations. These include the guinea pig ileum, rabbit jejunum, fowl rectal cecum, and human bronchiole, but not the colon or uterus of the rat or bronchiole of the rabbit, dog, or cat.[18,19] The permeability-enhancing activity of SRS-A has recently been demonstrated in guinea pig skin by using a functionally pure preparation in animals pretreated with various pharmacologic antagonists.[119] Further studies must await complete isolation and perhaps chemical identification. Interest in SRS-A lies not only in its intrinsic activity and derivation from more than one type of cell but also in its remarkable capacity to potentiate the responses of smooth muscle to other well-defined chemical mediators such as histamine and bradykinin.[120]

Eosinophil Chemotactic Factor of Anaphylaxis (ECF-A)

The capacity of actively or passively sensitized guinea pig lung or passively sensitized human lung to respond to antigen challenge *in vitro*, with the release of a factor specifically chemotactic for guinea pig and human eosinophils respectively, has only recently been recognized.[81,82] In both species the release of ECF-A is accompanied by the appearance of both histamine and SRS-A. ECF-A could be separated from the other mediators and had an estimated molecular weight in the range of 500 to 1000; further, other pharmacologic agents such as histamine, serotonin, SRS-A, bradykinin, and various prostaglandins failed to attract eosinophils when examined under the same conditions by the millipore technique of Boyden. A complement-dependent byproduct, C5a, also attracts guinea pig eosinophils but is readily distinguished by a molecular weight of 15,000 to 20,000 and the conditions for formation.[80]

Control Mechanisms for the Release of These Tissue-Derived Mediators

It is now considered likely that the immunologic release of the chemical mediators of immediate hypersensitivity reactions need not be cytotoxic to the participating cells[72,97] and represents some type of secretory process.[7,98] Certain basic biochemical characteristics such as pH optimum, cation requirements, effects of ionic strength, and the need for an intact glycolytic pathway common to immunologic release of histamine have been defined in *in vitro* systems such as guinea pig lung slices, rat peritoneal cell suspensions, rabbit platelets, and human leukocytes.[1,106,124,152] Although only limited data exist on the biochemical characteristics of the release of mediators other than histamine,[1,5] it is now established that a single immunoglobulin such as human IgE may prepare tissue for the subsequent antigen-induced release of such distinctly different chemical mediators as histamine, SRS-A, and ECF-A.[69,82]

The inhibitory effect of catecholamines, now attributed to stimulation of adenyl cyclase to generate cyclic 3′, 5′-adenosine monophosphate (cyclic-AMP), on antigen-induced histamine release was observed in studies of guinea pig lung slices many years ago.[148] More recently inhibition of histamine release from human basophils prepared with IgE has been noted with a dibutyryl derivative of cyclic-AMP or methylxanthines, which protect cyclic-AMP from destruction by phosphodiesterase.[98,99] Studies with monkey or human lung fragments prepared with human IgE[70,73] contain four lines of evidence to indicate that the intracellular accumulation of cyclic-AMP suppresses not only histamine but also SRS-A formation and release: The β-adrenergic agents, isoproterenol and epinephrine, are inhibitory in a dose-response fashion, and the β-adrenergic blocker, propranolol, reverses the effect of isoproterenol; theophylline inhibits in a dose-dependent fashion; potentiation of inhibition is observed when isoproterenol and theophylline are used together; and exogenous dibutyryl cyclic-AMP is consistently inhibitory in a dose-response manner. Of additional pertinence is the finding that these drugs are not inhibitory if removed prior to antigen challenge and that tissue challenged in their presence is desensitized to repeat challenge after removal of the drugs. The inhibitory effect of cellular cyclic-AMP on the presumably enzymatic pathway, $E \rightarrow \overline{E}$, initiated by antigen-antibody interaction may be related to phosphorylation of the activated esterase ($\overline{E}$) to achieve its inactivation ($\underline{E}$) as observed by others for glycogen synthetase.[35] This possibility is particularly intriguing in view of the evidence from *in vitro* studies that the release of histamine involves an antigen-antibody activated esterase inhibitable by agents capable of phosphorylating the hydroxyl group of a serine present in the active center.[5,6,7] The capacity of the cyclic-AMP system to modulate the release of SRS-A *in vivo* in reaction pathways involving different cellular prerequisites in the rat and its ability to control the release of both histamine and SRS-A *in vitro* in monkey or human lung[70,122] require a unifying hypothesis; namely, that the release of chemical mediators from diverse cells involves "activation" of a secretory step or "reversed pinocytosis" modulated by cyclic-AMP through an effect on contractile proteins possibly via alterations in the intracellular calcium pool.[134,159]

Contributions of Tissue Mediator Systems to the Inflammatory Response

The capacity of human IgE to mediate an antigen-induced wheal and flare response in human skin,[10] suppressible by antihistamines, and the circumstantial association of IgE with an anaphylactic syndrome revealing edema, congestion, and eosinophilic infiltrates of the upper respiratory tract and lower bronchial tree[71] represent one aspect of the inflammatory response attributable to the release of histamine, SRS-A, and ECF-A. Histamine can also be released secondarily to the appearance of anaphylatoxins[36] and cationic protein derived from polymorphonuclear leukocytes.[133]

Of particular note has been the recent recognition that perhaps these tissue systems or their circulating cellular counterparts are essential to the preparation of sites for the localization of ingredients of the inflammatory response derived from plasma. The development of glomerular lesions and proteinuria in rabbits immunized to develop serum sickness correlates with the appearance of an antibody, termed homocytotropic, capable of mediating passive cutaneous anaphylaxis in a complement-depleted rabbit and platelet-dependent amine release *in vitro* from washed mixed rabbit cells.[64] Rabbits lacking the homocytotropic antibody but possessing other antibody classes as indicated by immune elimination of antigen failed to develop comparable glomerular lesions or to localize the circulating complexes to the kidneys. It had been previously shown that antagonists of the vasoactive amines suppressed localization of complexes with attendant glomerular lesions.[86] The report that the Arthus reaction in the guinea pig cannot be mediated by IgG2 interacting with antigen to activate the complement system unless another immunoglobulin, IgG1 capable of facilitating antigen-induced mediator release from mast cells,[157] is also present extends the concept of a double immunoglobulin requirement to a classical immune complex-induced tissue injury.[101]

CONCLUDING COMMENTS

A scheme interrelating some of the various ingredients of the acute inflammatory response is depicted in Figure 8–4 and represents a compilation of some of the effector systems already discussed. Such a sequence could be initiated by tissue damage of diverse types via the ready activation of the Hageman factor upon interaction with such tissue constituents as collagen[177] or basement membrane.[26] Direct immunologic activation by aggregated[108,140] or soluble[79] immune complexes could occur at either the Hageman factor or C1 level or both.

After activation the reaction scheme can be modified by internal or external factors. Examples of internal modification include the relative deviation of active Hageman factor from the clotting system to the kinin-forming sequence by plasmin;[78] or alteration of C1 by a fragment, apparently derived during kinin formation,[55] to achieve relatively intense activation of late components as compared to earlier members of the complement sequence. External modification is illustrated by the findings that certain classical immune complex-induced lesions, such as the Arthus skin reaction[101] or the nephritis of experimental serum sickness in rabbits,[64] require interaction of a non-complement fixing antibody with antigen to release vasoactive principles which in turn facilitate the localization of the soluble complexes into the target vessel wall or the glomerulus.

Perpetuation of the sequence after activation could be accomplished by the lysosomal enzymes released from polymorphonuclear leukocytes[174] attracted by complement-dependent chemotactic factors and engaging in enhanced phagocytosis because of the C3b fragment on the target complex. Lysosomal enzymes can apparently activate C1 to $C\bar{1}$[161] or directly split C5 to yield C5a with its anaphylatoxic and chemotactic properties. Further, such neutrophil cathepsins as D and E[24,26] can fragment basement membrane thereby possibly contributing to further activation of Hageman factor.

Limitation of the composite reaction at present focuses upon $C\bar{1}$INH which inhibits $C\bar{1}$ ($C\bar{1}r$ and $C\bar{1}s$), kallikrein,

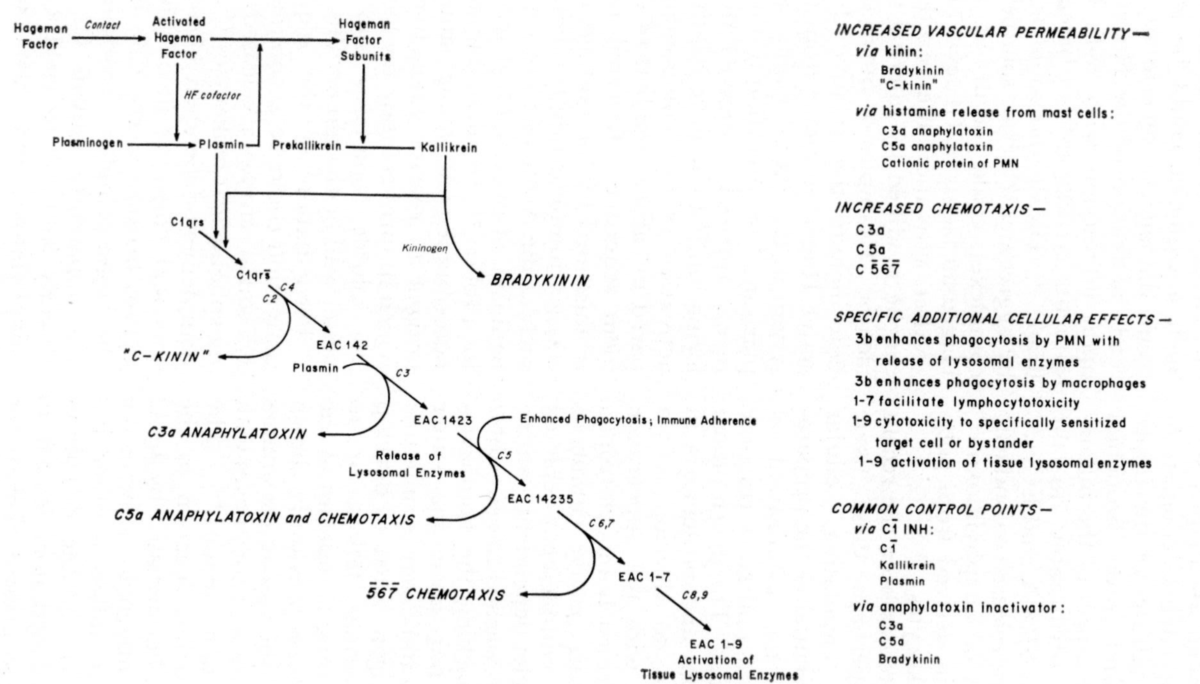

FIG. 8–4.—The acute inflammatory response.

plasmin, Hageman factor, and PTA[36,39,54,135,136] and upon C3bINA which inactivates the C3b fragment, thus limiting phagocytosis enhancement[50,143] with attendant release of lysosomal contents.

The duplication of factors with apparently similar capabilities for altering vascular permeability, contracting smooth muscle, and attracting wandering cell types in different effector systems may account for the apparent health of individuals genetically deficient in certain elements of the composite inflammatory response such as Hageman factor[136] or the C2 complement protein.[85] The interrelationships noted in Figure 8–4 do not yet focus upon related events such as: expansion of the reaction to damage bystander cells;[57,164] enhancement of solid tissue lysosomal activity;[37,91] alteration of mononuclear cell function as manifested by lymphocyte mitogenesis[11,84] or lymphocytoxicity[127] and macrophage phagocytosis;[127] or the influence of complement upon platelet-dependent aspects of clot formation.[162] Nonetheless, the scheme presented does offer the beginnings of a molecular basis of the inflammatory response in terms of activation, perpetuation, control, and deviation from one effector pathway to another; the latter is particularly important if the diverse presentations of the inflammatory response are to be unraveled. Such unraveling would permit greater understanding of the pathogenesis of the rheumatic diseases, and probably lead to more rational means for their control.

BIBLIOGRAPHY

1. Austen, K. F. and Humphrey, J. H.: Advanc. Immunol., *3*, 1, 1963.
2. Austen, K. F.: in *Immunological Diseases*, Boston, Little, Brown & Co., 1965, pp. 211–255.
3. Austen, K. F. *et al.*: Bull. Wld. Hlth. Org., *39*, 935, 1968.
4. Austen, K. F.: in *Harrison's Principles of Internal Medicine*, New York, McGraw-Hill, 1970, p. 342.
5. ———: in *VIth International Symposium on Immunopathology*, Basel, Schwabe & Co., 1971, p. 201.
6. Becker, E. L. and Austen, K. F.: J. Exp. Med., *120*, 491, 1964.
7. Becker, E. L.: in *Biochemistry of the Acute Allergic Reactions*, Oxford, Blackwell Scientific Publications, 1968, 199–211.
8. Benditt, E. P., Wong, R. L., Arase, M., and Roeper, E.: Proc. Soc. Exp. Biol. Med., *90*, 303, 1955.
9. Benditt, E. P., and Wong, R. L.: J. Exp. Med., *105*, 509, 1957.
10. Bloch, K. J.: Progr. Allergy, *10*, 84, 1967.
11. Bloch-Shtacher, N., Hirschhorn, K., and Uhr, J. W.: Clin. Exp. Immunol., *3*, 889, 1968.
12. Boissonas, R. A., Guttman, S. and Jaquenoud, P. A.: Helv. Chem. Acta, *43*, 1349, 1960.
13. Bokisch, V. A. and Müller-Eberhard, H. J.: J. Clin. Invest., *49*, 2427, 1970.
14. Borsos, T., Rapp, H. J. and Mayer, M. M.: J. Immunol., *87*, 326, 1961.
15. Borsos, T., Dourmashkin, R. R. and Humphrey, J. H.: Nature, *202*, 251, 1964.
16. Boreus, L. O. and Chakravarty, N.: Experientia, *16*, 192, 1960.
17. Brocklehurst, W. E.: in *5-Hydroxytryptamine*, New York, Pergamon Press, 1958.
18. ———: J. Physiol., *151*, 416, 1960.
19. ———: Progr. Allerg., *6*, 539, 1962.
20. ———: in *Clinical Aspects of Immunology*, Philadelphia, F. A. Davis Company, 1963.
21. Burkhalter, A.: Fed. Proc. *24*, 1341, 1965.
22. Clark, C. T., Weissbach, H., and Udenfriend, S.: J. Biol. Chem., *210*, 139, 1955.
23. Cochrane, C. G.: in *The Inflammatory Process*, New York, Academic Press, 1965, p. 613.
24. Cochrane, C. G. and Aikin, B. S.: J. Exp. Med., *124*, 733, 1966.
25. Cochrane, C. G. and Müller-Eberhard, H. J.: J. Exp. Med., *127*, 371, 1968.
26. Cochrane, C. G.: Transplantation Proc., *1*, 949, 1969.
27. Code, C. G.: Fed. Proc., *24*, 1311, 1965.
28. Collier, H. O. J.: Ann. N. Y. Acad. Sci., *104*, 290, 1963.
29. Colman, R. W., Mattler, L. and Sherry, S.: J. Clin. Invest., *48*, 11, 1969.
30. Cooper, N. R.: J. Immunol., *107*, 314, 1971 (abstract).
31. Costa, E. and Aprison, M. H.: J. Nerv. & Ment. Dis., *126*, 289, 1958.
32. Cotran, R. S. and Majno, G.: Ann. N. Y. Acad. Sci., *116*, 750, 1964.
33. Daniels, C. A., Borsos, T., Rapp, H. J., Snyderman, R. and Notkins, A. L.: Proc. Nat. Acad. Sci., *65*, 528, 1969.

34. Day, N. K. B., Gewurz, H., Johannsen, R., Finstad, J. and Good, R. A.: J. Exp. Med., *32*, 941, 1970.
35. DeWulf, H. and Hers, H. G.: Europ. J. Biochem., *6*, 558, 1968.
36. Dias da Silva, W. and Lepow, I. H.: J. Exp. Med., *125*, 921, 1967.
37. Dingle, J. T., Fell, H. B. and Coombs, R. R. A.: Int. Arch. Allergy, *31*, 283, 1967.
38. Donaldson, V. H.: J. Exp. Med., *127*, 411, 1968.
39. Donaldson, V. H., Ratnoff, O. D., Dias da Silva, W. and Rosen, F. S.: J. Clin. Invest., *48*, 642, 1969.
40. Elliot, D. F., Horton, E. W. and Lewis, G. P.: J. Physiol., *153*, 473, 1960.
41. Elliot, D. F., Lewis, G. P. and Horton, E. W.: Biochem. Biophys. Res. Commun., *3*, 87, 1960.
42. Elliot, D. F.: Ann. N. Y. Acad. Sci., *104*, 4, 1963.
43. Erdos, E. G., Renfrew, A. G., Sloane, E. M. and Wohler, J. R.: Ann. N. Y. Acad. Sci., *104*, 222, 1963.
44. Erspamer, V.: Pharmacol. Rev., *6*, 425, 1954.
45. Feldberg, W.: in *Histamine*, Boston, Little, Brown & Co., 1956.
46. Feldberg, W. and Kellaway, C. H.: J. Physiol., *94*, 187, 1938.
47. Gaddum, J. H. and Hameed, K. A.: Brit. J. Pharmacol., *9*, 240, 1954.
48. Gewurz, H., Shin, H. S. and Mergenhagen, S.: J. Exp. Med., *128*, 1049, 1968.
49. Gewurz, H.: In *Proc. Symposium on the Biological Activity of Complement*, ed. R. Ingram, in press.
50. Gigli, I. and Nelson, R. A.: Exp. Cell Research, *51*, 45, 1968.
51. Gigli, I., Ruddy, S. and Austen, K. F.: J. Immunol., *100*, 1154, 1968.
52. Gigli, I. and Austen, K. F.: J. Exp. Med., *129*, 679, 1969.
53. ———: J. Exp. Med., *130*, 833, 1969.
54. Gigli, I., Mason, J. W., Colman, R. and Austen, K. F.: J. Immunol., *104*, 574, 1970.
55. Gigli, I., Kaplan, A. and Austen, K. F.: J. Exp. Med., *134*, 1466, 1971.
56. Goldman, J., Ruddy, S., Feingold, D. and Austen, K. F.: J. Immunol., *102*, 1379, 1969.
57. Götze, O. and Müller-Eberhard, H. J.: J. Exp. Med., *132*, 898, 1970.
58. ———: J. Immunol., *107*, 313, 1971 (abstract).
59. Graham, H. T., Wheelwright, F., Parish, H. H., Marks, A. R. and Lowry, O. H.: Fed. Proc., *11*, 350, 1952, (abstract).
60. Graham, H. T., Lowry, O. H., Wahl, N. and Priebat, M. K.: J. Exp. Med., *102*, 307, 1955.
61. Hadding, U. and Müller-Eberhard, H. J.: Immunology, *16*, 719, 1969.
62. Haverback, J., Studbrin, M. I. and Dyce, B. J.: Fed. Proc., *24*, 1326, 1965.
63. Harpel, P. C.: J. Clin. Invest., *49*, 568, 1970.
64. Henson, P. M. and Cochrane, C. G.: in *Cellular and Humoral Mechanisms in Anaphylaxis and Allergy*, Basel/New York, Karger, 1969, p. 129.
65. Humphrey, J. H. and Jaques, R.: J. Physiol., *128*, 9, 1955.
66. Humphrey, J. H., Austen, K. F. and Rapp, H. J.: Immunology, *6*, 226, 1963.
67. Humphrey, H. J. and Dourmashkin, R. R.: in *Vth International Symposium in Immunopathology*, Basel, Schwabe and Co., 1965, p. 209.
68. Iatridis, S. G. and Ferguson, J. H.: J. Clin. Invest., *41*, 1277, 1962.
69. Ishizaka, T., Ishizaka, K., Orange, R. P. and Austen, K. F.: J. Immunol., *104*, 335, 1970.
70. ———: J. Immunol., *106*, 1267, 1971.
71. James, L. P., Jr. and Austen, K. F.: New Eng. J. Med., *270*, 597, 1964.
72. Johnson, A. R. and Moran, N. C.: in *Cellular and Humoral Mechanisms in Anaphylaxis and Allergy*, Basel, S. Karger, 1969, p. 122.
73. Kaliner, M. A., Orange, R. P., Koopman, W. J., Austen, K. F., and LaRaia, P. J.: Biochim. Biophys. Acta, *252*, 160, 1971.
74. Kagen, L. J., Leddy, J. P. and Becker, E. L.: J. Clin. Invest., *42*, 1353, 1963.
75. Kahlson, G.: Lancet, *1*, 67, 1960.
76. Kapeller-Adler, P.: Fed. Proc., *24*, 757, 1965.
77. Kaplan, A. P. and Austen, K. F.: J. Immunol., *105*, 802, 1970.
78. ———: J. Exp. Med., *133*, 696, 1971.
79. Kaplan, A. P., Spragg, J., and Austen, K. F.: in *Second International Symposium on the Biochemistry of the Acute Allergic Reactions*, Oxford, Blackwell Scientific Publications, in press.
79*a*. Kaplan, A. P., Kay, A. B., and Austen, K. F.: J. Exp. Med., in press.
80. Kay, A. B.: Clin. Exp. Immunol., *7*, 723, 1970.
81. Kay, A. B., Stechschulte, D. J. and Austen, K. F.: J. Exp. Med., *133*, 602, 1971.
82. Kay, A. B. and Austen, K. F.: J. Immunol., *107*, 899, 1971.
83. Kellaway, C. H. and Trethewie, E. R.: Quart. J. Exp. Physiol., *30*, 121, 1940.

84. Kinsella, T. D.: in *4th Canadian Conference on Research in the Rheumatic Diseases*, Toronto, Toronto Univ. Press, in press.
85. Klemperer, M. R., Austen, K. F. and Rosen, F. S.: J. Immunol., *98*, 72, 1967.
86. Kniker, W. T. and Cochrane, C. G.: J. Exp. Med., *127*, 119, 1968.
87. Kondo, M., Gigli, I. and Austen, K. F.: Immunology, in press.
88. Kraut, H., Frey, E. K. and Werle, E.: J. Physiol. Chem., *189*, 97, 1930.
89. Kulka, J. P.: Ann. N. Y. Acad. Sci., *116*, 1018, 1964.
90. Lachmann, P. J. and Müller-Eberhard, H. J.: J. Immunol., *100*, 691, 1968.
91. Lachmann, P. J., Coombs, R. R. A., Fell, H. B. and Dingle, J. T.: Int. Arch. Allergy, *36*, 469, 1969.
92. Lagunoff, D. and Benditt, E. P.: Amer. J. Physiol., *196*, 993, 1959.
93. Lepow, I. H., Wurz, L., Ratnoff, O. and Pillemer, L.: J. Immunol., *93*, 146, 1954.
94. Lepow, I. H., Naff, G. B., Todd, E. W., Pensky, J. and Hinz, C. F.: J. Exp. Med., *117*, 983, 1961.
95. Levy, L. R. and Lepow, I. H.: Proc. Soc. Exp. Biol. Med., *101*, 608, 1959.
96. Lewis, G. P.: J. Physiol., *140*, 285, 1958.
97. Lichtenstein, L. M. and Osler, A. G.: Proc. Soc. Exp. Biol. (N.Y.), *121*, 808, 1966.
98. Lichtenstein, L. M. and Margolis, S.: Science, *161*, 902, 1968.
99. Lichtenstein, L. M.: in *Cellular and Humoral Mechanisms in Anaphylaxis and Allergy*, Basel, Karger, 1969, pp. 176–186.
100. Mackay, M. E., Miles, A. A., Schachter, C. B. E. and Wilhelm, D. L.: Nature, *172*, 714, 1953.
101. Maillard, J. L. and Voisin, G. A.: Proc. Soc. Exp. Biol. Med., *133*, 1188, 1970.
102. Majno, G.: in *Injury, Inflammation, and Immunity*, Baltimore, Williams and Wilkins Co., 1964.
103. Margolis, J.: Ann. N. Y. Acad. Sci., *104*, 133, 1963.
104. Mayer, M. M., Levine, L., Rapp, H. J. and Marucci, A. A.: J. Immunol., *73*, 443, 1954.
105. Mayer, M. M. and Miller, J. A.: Immunochemistry, *2*, 71, 1965.
106. Mongar, J. L. and Schild, H. O.: Physiol. Rev., *42*, 226, 1962.
107. Moran, N. C., Uvnas, B. and Westerholme, B.: Acta Physiol. Scand., *56*, 26, 1962.
108. Movat, H.: J. Immunol., *103*, 875, 1969.
109. Müller-Eberhard, H. J. and Lepow, I. H.: J. Exp. Med., *121*, 819, 1965.
110. Müller-Eberhard, H. J., Dalmasso, A. P. and Calcott, M. A.: J. Exp. Med., *123*, 33, 1966.
111. Müller-Eberhard, H. J.: Fed. Proc., *26*, 744, 1967 (abstract).
112. Müller-Eberhard, H. J., Polley, M. J. and Calcott, M. A.: J. Exp. Med., *125*, 359, 1967.
113. Naff, G. B., Pensky, Y. and Lepow, I. H.: J. Exp. Med., *119*, 593, 1964.
114. Naff, G. B. and Ratnoff, O. D.: J. Exp. Med., *128*, 571, 1968.
115. Nelson, R. A.: in *The Inflammatory Process*, New York and London, Academic Press, 1965, p. 818.
116. Nilsson, U. R. and Müller-Eberhard, H. J.: Immunology, *13*, 101, 1967.
117. Ogston, D., Ogston, C. M., Ratnoff, O. D. and Forbes, C. D.: J. Clin. Invest., *48*, 1786, 1969.
118. Orange, R. P., Valentine, M. D. and Austen, K. F.: J. Exp. Med., *127*, 767, 1968.
119. Orange, R. P. and Austen, K. F.: in *Cellular and Humoral Mechanisms of Anaphylaxis*, Basel, S. Karger, 1969, p. 196.
120. ———: Adv. Immunol., *10*, 106, 1969.
121. Orange, R. P., Stechschulte, D. J. and Austen, K. F.: J. Immunol., *105*, 1087, 1970.
122. Orange, R. P., Austen, W. G., and Austen, K. F.: J. Exp. Med., *134*, 1365, 1971.
123. Osbahr, A. J., Gladner, J. A. and Laki, K.: Biochim. Biophys. Acta, *86*, 535, 1964.
124. Osler, A. G., Lichtenstein, L. M. and Levy, D. A.: Advanc. Immunol., *8*, 182, 1968.
125. Page, I. H.: Physiol. Rev., *38*, 277, 1958.
126. Parratt, J. R. and West, G. B.: J. Physiol., *137*, 169, 1957.
127. Perlmann, P., Perlmann, H., Müller-Eberhard, H. J. and Manni, J. A.: Science, *163*, 937, 1969.
128. Pickering, R. J., Naff, G. B., Stroud, R. M., Good, R. A. and Gewurz, H.: J. Exp. Med., *131*, 803, 1970.
129. Pierce, J. V. and Webster, M. E.: Biochem. Biophys. Res. Comm., *5*, 353, 1961.
130. Pillemer, L., Ratnoff, O., Blum, L. and Lepow, I. H.: J. Exp. Med., *97*, 573, 1953.
131. Pillemer, L., Schoenberg, C., Blum, L. and Wurz, L.: Science, *122*, 545, 1955.
132. Polley, M. J., Müller-Eberhard, H. J. and Feldman, J. D.: J. Exp. Med., *133*, 53, 1971.
133. Ranadive, N. S. and Cochrane, C. G.: Clin. Exp. Immunol., *6*, 905, 1970.

134. Rasmussen, H. and Tanehous, A.: Proc. Nat. Acad. Sci., *59*, 1364, 1968.
135. Ratnoff, O. D. and Naff, G. B.: J. Exp. Med., *125*, 337, 1967.
136. Ratnoff, O. D.: Adv. Immunol., *10*, 146, 1969.
137. Riley, J. F.: J. Path. Bact., *65*, 471, 1953.
138. Riley, J. F. and West, G. B.: J. Physiol., *120*, 528, 1953.
139. Riley, J. F.: Ann. N. Y. Acad. Sci., *103*, 151, 1963.
140. Robbins, J. and Stetson, C. A.: J. Exp. Med., *109*, 1, 1959.
141. Rocha e Silva, M., Beraldo, W. T. and Rosenfield, G.: Amer. J. Physiol., *156*, 261, 1949.
142. Rowley, D. A. and Benditt, E. P.: J. Exp. Med., *103*, 399, 1956.
143. Ruddy, S. and Austen, K. F.: J. Immunol., *102*, 533, 1969.
144. ———: J. Immunol., *107*, 742, 1971.
145. Schayer, R. W.: Physiol. Rev., *39*, 116, 1959.
146. ———: Ann. N. Y. Acad. Sci., *103*, 164, 1963.
147. ———: Fed. Proc., *24*, 1295, 1965.
148. Schild, H. O.: Quart. J. Exp. Physiol., *23*, 165, 1936.
149. Shin, H. S., Snyderman, R., Friedman, E. and Mergenhagen, S. E.: Fed. Proc., *28*, 485, 1969.
150. Shin, H. S., Pickering, R. J. and Mayer, M. M.: J. Immunol., *106*, 473, 1971.
151. Sitomer, G., Stroud, R. M. and Mayer, M. M.: Immunochemistry, *3*, 57, 1966.
152. Siragnian, R. P., Secchi, A. G. and Osler, A. G.: in *Biochemistry of the Acute Reactions*. Oxford, Blackwell Scientific Publications, 1968, pp. 215–228.
153. Sjoerdsma, A.: New Eng. J. Med., *261*, 181 and 231, 1959.
154. Sjoerdsma, A., Waalkes, T. P. and Weissbach, H.: Science, *125*, 1202, 1957.
155. Snyder, S. H. and Axelrod, J.: Fed. Proc., *24*, 774, 1965.
156. Spector, W. G.: Ann. N. Y. Acad. Sci., *116*, 747, 1964.
157. Stechschulte, D. J., Austen, K. F. and Bloch, K. J.: J. Exp. Med., *125*, 126, 1967.
158. Stolfi, R. L.: J. Immunol., *100*, 46, 1968.
159. Stormorken, H.: Scand. J. Haematol., *9*, 3, 1960.
160. Tamura, N. and Nelson, R. A.: J. Immunol., *94*, 582, 1967.
161. Taubman, S. B., Goldschmidt, P. R. and Lepow, I. H.: Fed. Proc., *29*, 434, 1970, (abstract).
162. Taylor, F. B. and Müller-Eberhard, H. J.: J. Clin. Invest., *49*, 2068, 1970.
163. Thomas, L., Uhr, J. W. and Grant, L.: in *Injury, Inflammation and Immunity*, Baltimore, The Williams & Wilkins Co., 1964.
164. Thompson, R. D. and Lachmann, P. J.: J. Exp. Med., *131*, 629, 1970.
165. Udenfriend, S., Titus, E., Weissbach, H. and Peterson, R. E.: J. Biol. Chem., *219*, 335, 1956.
166. Udenfriend, S. and Waalkes, T. P.: in *Mechanisms of Hypersensitivity*, Boston, Little, Brown & Co., 1959.
167. Valentine, M. D., Bloch, K. J. and Austen, K. F.: J. Immunol., *99*, 98, 1967.
168. VanArsdel, P. P., Middleton, E., Sherman, W. B. and Buchwald, H.: J. Allergy, *29*, 429, 1958.
169. Ward, P. A., Cochrane, C. G. and Müller-Eberhard, H. J.: Immunology, *11*, 141, 1966.
170. Ward, P. A.: J. Exp. Med., *126*, 189, 1967.
171. Ward, P. A. and Newman, L. J.: J. Immunol., *102*, 93, 1969.
172. Webster, M. E. and Pierce, J. V.: Proc. Soc. Exp. Biol. Med., *107*, 186, 1961.
173. ———: Ann. N. Y. Acad. Sci., *104*, 91, 1963.
174. Weissmann, G., Duker, P. and Sessa, G.: in *Immunopathology of Inflammation*, Excerpta Medica, in press.
175. Werle, E.: in *Polypeptides which Stimulate Plain Muscle*, Edinburgh, E. & S. Livingstone, Ltd., 1955.
176. West, G. B.: J. Pharm. Pharmacol., *11*, 513, 1959.
177. Wilner, G. D., Nossel, H. L. and LeRoy, E. C.: J. Clin. Invest., *47*, 2608, 1968.
178. Willoughby, W. F. and Mayer, M. M.: Science, *150*, 907, 1965.
179. Wuepper, K. D., Tucker, E. S., III and Cochrane, C. G.: J. Immunol., *105*, 1307, 1970.
180. Yang, H. Y. T. and Erdos, E. G.: Nature, *215*, 1402, 1967.
181. Zucker, M. B.: Progr. Hemat., *2*, 206, 1959.

Chapter 9

The Rheumatoid Factors

By John H. Vaughan, M.D.

The sera of patients with rheumatoid arthritis contain anti-gamma-globulin antibodies. These anti-gamma-globulins are commonly called rheumatoid factors. Rheumatoid factors are not peculiarly or uniquely a characteristic of rheumatoid arthritis. Nevertheless, most patients seen in hospitals and clinics with rheumatoid arthritis exhibit them. Intensive study of rheumatoid factors has been pursued in the hope of opening the way to a better understanding of the disease. The profits of this research have been enormous not only in rheumatology, but also in the field of genetic control of gamma globulins.

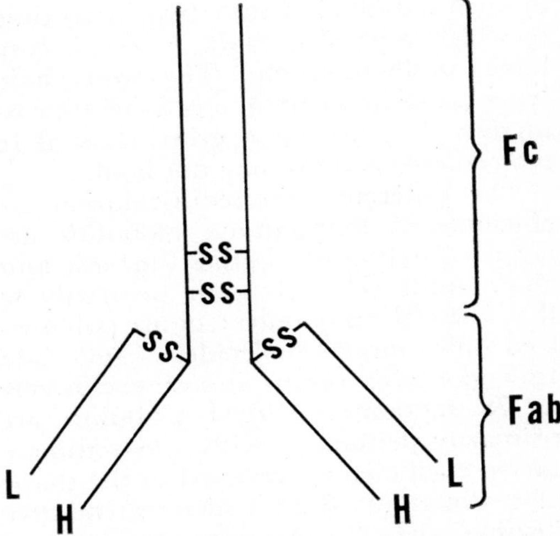

Fig. 9–1.—Schematic representation of a gamma globulin molecule.

GAMMA GLOBULINS

A discussion of the rheumatoid factors requires some understanding of gamma globulins in general.[44] The bulk of the protein in the gamma globulin peak in serum electrophoresis consists of IgG molecules. Each of these is composed of four polypeptide chains, two of which are heavier and two of which are lighter in ultracentrifugal analysis.[39,86] Edelman called these H and L chains, respectively. A schematic representation of the ways in which these chains are related to each other in IgG globulins is presented in Figure 9–1. The Y-shaped structure has been demonstrated by electron microscopy.[109]

The ability of a gamma globulin molecule to bind antigen—and thus exhibit its unique antibody property—appears to depend upon surface configurations in the areas of the molecule where the H and L chains are in close apposition, the two Fab pieces. Upon combining with antigen, the molecule appears to undergo a conformational change in which the Fab portions of the molecule assume a 180° angle in respect to each other, rather than the acute angle illustrated in the figure.

Other properties of IgG molecules, such as complement-fixing activity, ability to cross the placenta, or capacity to fix to skin in cutaneous anaphylaxis, appear to be related to configurations on the portions of the H chains distant from the L chains, i.e., the Fc piece.

Five major classes of gamma globulins are now recognized. These classes differ from each other in the types of H chains they contain (Table 9–1). Each class is

TABLE 9–1.—CHARACTERISTICS OF GAMMA GLOBULINS

Class	*Sedimentation Coefficient*	*Chains H*	*Chains L*	*Approximate Proportions in Serum*
IgG	7S	γ	κ or λ	84%
IgA	8S–15S	α	κ or λ	10%
IgM	19S	μ	κ or λ	5%
IgD	7S	δ	κ or λ	1%
IgE	8S	ϵ	κ or λ	0.02%

in turn subdivided into two, according to which type of L chain, κ or γ, is contained in the molecule. The two L chain types occur in serum in a ratio of approximately 2:1, but for a given class of Ig molecules this ratio may not hold.

The differences in sedimentation coefficients of the gamma globulins are largely a matter of whether the basic four chain units (H_2 L_2) occur primarily in that form (the monomer), or are polymerized into larger molecules. IgG and IgD globulins occur almost exclusively as 7S monomers. IgM globulins are primarily pentamers with 19S sedimentation coefficients, arranged in the shape of a doughnut from which extend five flexible arms.[31] A monomer form of IgM has been recognized in the circulation in various pathological states, however, and this has been shown in certain instances to exhibit antibody activity.[73,90] IgA globulins may exhibit several different sedimentation coefficients, depending upon variable degrees of polymerization. The IgA that appears in exocrine secretions is combined with the secretory piece apparently added to the molecule as it passes through the gut epithelium into the lumen. The IgA of serum lacks the secretory piece, is primarily monomer in form, but also is present in significant amounts in polymer form.

Further sub-typing of each of the three major Ig classes has been made on the basis of further differences in their H chain characteristics, attributable to differences in amino acid sequences in about 10% to 20% of the chain. Four H chain sub-classes of IgG molecules are known, two sub-types of IgA molecules, and two sub-types of IgM molecules.

The importance of IgG and IgM in the body's immune defense is unquestioned. Evidence exists also that IgA may be important in developing and maintaining immunity at mucous surfaces. The role of IgD molecules is of less certainty, but antibody activity has been reported among them.[48,58] The IgE molecules compose the skin sensitizing antibodies that characterize atopic allergy and certain parasitic infestations. Whether IgE plays a role in immunity to the latter is presently unknown.

The rheumatoid factors are now known to be antibodies to IgG. They react almost exclusively with the Fc portion of the IgG molecule. They have been recognized not only among IgM, where they were first found, but also among IgA and IgG molecules.

BRIEF HISTORY

Cecil and coworkers,[30] who were interested in the possible relationship of the streptococcus to the etiology of rheumatoid arthritis, found very high agglutinating activity thought to represent large quantities of antibodies to streptococci. It is now known, however, that patients with rheumatoid arthritis have normal quantities of antibodies to streptococci, the agglutinating activity of which is enhanced in rheumatoid sera by the rheumatoid factors. Rough pneumococci and staphylococci can similarly be agglutinated in high titer by sera of patients with rheumatoid arthritis.[37] In 1948, Rose, Ragan, Pearce, and Lipman[89] called attention to agglutination of sheep cells sensitized with rabbit antibody, a finding that has provided the basis of what is now familiarly known as the "sensitized sheep cell test." Similar observations had been made in rheumatoid arthritis patients' sera by Waaler[113] in 1940 and in cirrhosis and tuberculosis by Meyer[78] in 1922. These earlier reports, however, gained little attention. It was not until 1948 that the medical world was ready to take note of the observation and to develop it further.

After 1948, numerous systems were developed to demonstrate the agglutinating activities in rheumatoid arthritis sera.[111] All of these depended upon particles coated with IgG globulins, the specific reactant with which the rheumatoid factors combine. The specificities exhibited towards IgG globulin were recognized to be like those that one would expect of antibody against IgG globulin. Rheumatoid factors have now been identified among IgG and IgA, as well as IgM molecules.

The presence of rheumatoid factors has been correlated with disease severity in rheumatoid arthritis, and they can be identified in proteins precipitated in the tissues of patients with rheumatoid arthritis. Rheumatoid factors are not, however, found only in patients with rheumatoid arthritis. Antibodies very much like rheumatoid factors can be produced experimentally in animals by hyperimmunization with bacteria, or by hyperimmunization with aggregated, autologous IgG globulins.

NATURE OF THE RHEUMATOID FACTORS

Systems for Demonstrating the Rheumatoid Factor

Many systems have been developed for coating particles with γG globulins for demonstration of rheumatoid factor agglutinating activity. Some of them are given in Table 9–2. The streptococcal agglutination reaction is of particular interest, in that it was the first agglutination reaction to be described. The relation between the streptococcal agglutination reaction in rheumatoid arthritis and the sensitized sheep cell (Waaler-Rose) test has been clarified by the studies of Lamont-Havers,[69] Wager,[114] and Thulin.[106] Rheumatoid factor activity can be separated from anti-streptococcal agglutinin activity by precipitation in distilled water. The anti-streptococcal agglutinating activity remains in the supernatant and generally is of rather low titer. The rheumatoid factors responsible for agglutinating sensitized sheep cells are in the precipitate. When the rheumatoid factor from the precipitate is recombined with the anti-streptococcal antibody in the supernatant, the typical high streptococcal agglutination titer of the original serum is restored. The strong streptococcal agglutination reaction in the sera of patients with rheumatoid arthritis thus appears to depend upon the presence of a small, and probably normal, amount of anti-streptococcal antibody which is markedly enhanced by the simultaneously present rheumatoid factor. It follows that there is no particular reason to implicate a post-streptococcal state in rheumatoid arthritis from the streptococcal agglutination reaction.

The sensitized sheep cell test employs sheep red cells sensitized with rabbit antibodies to sheep cells. The sensitizing antibody must be of the γG variety; γM antibody is ineffective. In most laboratories anti-sheep cell antibodies in the patients' sera are absorbed out of the system before the sera are exposed to the sensitized sheep cells. Agglutination can then be attributed solely to the rheumatoid factor. Wager[114] has demonstrated clearly that goat cells, ox cells, guinea pig cells, and human cells, among others, could be used with corresponding rabbit antibodies to provide sensitized cells equally susceptible to agglutination by rheumatoid sera.

Human gamma globulin has been attached to red cells by a variety of techniques and to latex and bentonite particles (Table 9–2). Human γA and γM globulins have failed to coat cells effectively for agglutination by rheumatoid factor. Denatured γG globulins provide more effective coats for these agglutination reactions than undenatured γG globulins, and inhibition of the system is more effectively brought about by denatured than undenatured γG globulin.

The most commonly used tests for the

TABLE 9–2.—TESTS FOR DETECTING RHEUMATOID FACTORS

Test	*Form of Coating Gamma Globulin*	*Type of Particle*	*Manner of Attachment of Gamma Globulin to Cell or Particle*
Bacterial Agglutination	Unaggregated Human 7S (?)	Bacterial cell	Antibody bond
Sens. Sheep Cell Agglutination	Unaggregated Rabbit 7S	Sheep Cell	Antibody bond
F II tanned cell Agglutination	Aggregated Human 7S	Tanned Sheep Cell	Adsorption
Sens. Human Cell Agglutination	Unaggregated Human 7S	Human Rh + cell	Antibody bond
Latex Flocculation	Aggregated* Human 7S	Latex	Adsorption
Bentonite Flocculation	Aggregated Human 7S	Bentonite	Adsorption

* The use of aggregated gamma globulin increases the sensitivity of the test, but unaggregated gamma globulin is satisfactory for agglutinations by many sera.

detection of rheumatoid factors are the latex and bentonite flocculation tests.[19,99] The chief values of these tests are the great sensitivities they exhibit and the ease with which they are carried out. They may be used on sera which have not been absorbed with foreign erythrocytes. Simple slide flocculation tests have been devised and are extremely useful. These tests are positive in more non-rheumatoid diseases, however, than is the sensitized sheep cell test. The major precaution is to use the serum in sufficient dilution, usually 1:20 or greater, so that prozone phenomena do not give falsely negative results. The prozone has been related to an α-globulin and some believe this to be identical with the first or second component of complement.[95] Inactivation of rheumatoid sera at 56° C. for one-half hour can abolish the prozone.

Other more complicated tests, suited more to research than ordinary clinical needs, have been developed. Franchimont and Suteanu[43] have evolved a radioimmunoassay for IgM rheumatoid factor. Torrigiani[107] has used insolubilized IgG as an immunoadsorbant, from which rheumatoid factors can be eluted and characterized. Winchester and Agnello[122] have proposed an immunodiffusion assay method. All of these methods provide better quantification and more precise information on the classes of rheumatoid factors present than can be obtained from more routine procedures.

Physicochemical Studies of the Factor

Epstein, Johnson, and Ragan[41] demonstrated that the addition of purified γG globulin (Cohn Fraction II) to sera from rheumatoid arthritis patients produces a precipitate containing rheumatoid factor. The precipitation occurs only if aggregated γG globulin is present in the added material. The shape of the curve describing the reaction resembles that produced by antigen with its precipitating antibodies.

Franklin and co-workers[45] demonstrated that rheumatoid factor activity can be differentially sedimented from some rheumatoid sera by ultracentrifugation, the factor being found in an unusually heavy fraction having a sedimentation coefficient of 22S. Such 22S peaks are dissociated into 7S and 19S components when the sera are exposed to mild acid, or other substances which are known to interfere with the interactions of antigens with antibodies. The separated components were studied independently and the agglutinating activity was found with the 19S component (Fig. 9–2). Under appropriate conditions the separated 19S agglutinating factor could be made to combine again with 7S components to re-form the 22S complex.

The strength of binding of rheumatoid factors with the 7S component (IgG) is relatively weak when compared with most hyperimmune antigen-antibody systems, but it is in line with those of early immune responses and with cross-reacting antigen-antibody systems.[82] The same is probably true of a wide variety of other autoantigen-antibody systems.

Since this early demonstration, sera have been described by Kunkel and by Chodirker and Tomasi[32] in which complexes intermediate between 7S and 19S exist. These too are dissociated by mild acid or urea in concentrations that would dissociate antigen-antibody complexes. The "intermediate complexes" reduce to 7S components. The complexes studied by Chodirker and Tomasi[32] were due to IgG rheumatoid factors of 7S size. This was made clear by fractionation studies in density gradient ultracentrifugation and DEAE cellulose chromatography, and by the failure of the agglutinating properties of this serum to be completely abolished by treatment with 2-mercaptoethanol. Rheumatoid factors of the 19S variety are completely destroyed by 2-mercaptoethanol. Schrohenloher[94] has shown anti-IgG activity to be present in the IgG molecules isolated with the intermediate complexes by taking advantage of the capacity of peptide digestion to abolish the Fc part of the IgG molecule without affecting its antibody activity.

Rheumatoid factor activity was first detected among IgA globulins by Heimer.[56] This has now been confirmed by a number of other laboratories.[1,8,107] The finding that rheumatoid factors are distributed through several classes of immunoglobulins provides further support for the belief that rheumatoid factors are antibodies, since antibodies to foreign antigens typically are found in such distribution in immunized man as well as in immunized experimental animals. Torrigiani,[107] using insolubilized IgG as an immunoadsorbant for rheumatoid factors, has been able to isolate IgA as well as IgG and IgM anti-IgG activity from a large number of rheumatoid sera. This too has been confirmed by others.

Specificities of the Rheumatoid Factors

It was first pointed out by Heller[59] that rheumatoid arthritis sera could be

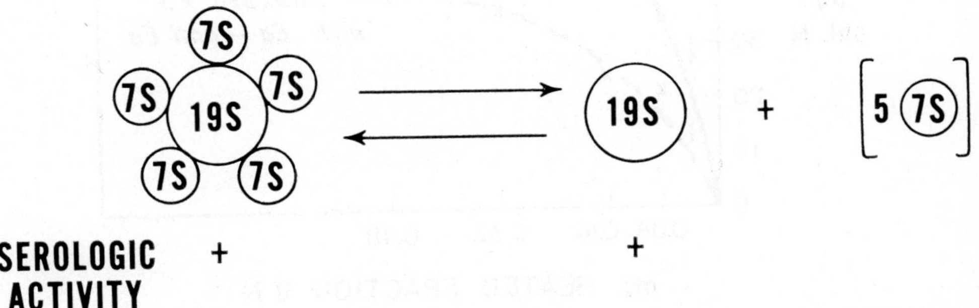

Fig. 9–2.—The reversible interaction of 19S rheumatoid (IgM) factor with 7S gamma globulin (IgG) to yield the 22S complex. (Modified from Franklin, E. C., Edelman, G. and Kunkel, H. G., in *Immunity and Virus Infection*, Najjar, V. A. (ed.), courtesy of John Wiley and Sons, Inc.)

absorbed with sheep cells coated with rabbit antibody to a point at which the sera no longer agglutinated the coated sheep cells, but still agglutinated in high titer cells coated with human IgG globulins. On the other hand, complete absorption with cells coated with human IgG globulin removed agglutinating activities for both types of coated cells. Further studies on the cross reaction thus described have been carried out by more quantitative techniques.[112] When rheumatoid sera are absorbed with aggregated rabbit IgG globulins, all of the rheumatoid factor capable of agglutinating "sensitized sheep cells" is removed and with it a considerable proportion of the factor that precipitates with aggregated human γG globulin (Fig. 9–3). The data, supplemented by other studies,[6,7,25,26,51] indicate that rheumatoid factors react, as a whole, with aggregated or denatured human IgG globulin, while only portions react with IgG globulins of other species. These findings are in keeping with the hypothesis that rheumatoid factors are antibodies to human γG globulin, cross reacting with IgG globulins of other species.

There has been considerable dispute as to whether the rheumatoid factors contain antibodies specifically directed to denatured forms of IgG. The enhanced reactivity of rheumatoid factors with the aggregated form of IgG has never been in dispute, but whether this enhanced reactivity is because of the appearance of denaturation configurations on IgG molecules, or simply because of an enhanced effective valence of IgG for rheumatoid factors when packed close together in aggregated form has been the uncertainty. In certain instances isolated rheumatoid factors have been shown clearly to react well with unaggregated IgG molecules. These studies have not ruled out, however, the possibility that some portion of the rheumatoid factors may have true specificity for denaturation configurations. The best, but not yet incontrovertible, evidence for this type of specificity has been presented by Henney,[60]

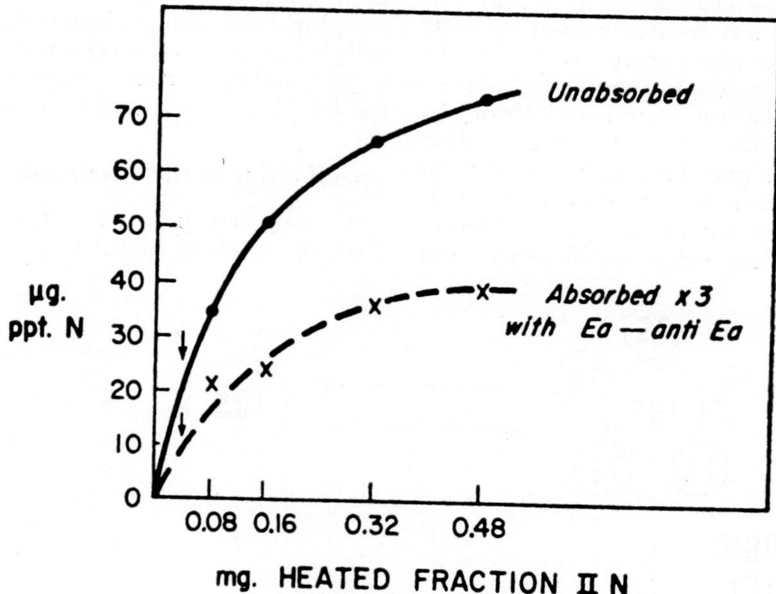

Fig. 9–3.—Precipitin curve of F II gamma globulin with untreated rheumatoid serum (top curve). Precipitin curve of same rheumatoid serum after absorption of sensitized sheep cell factor with aggregated IgG in the form of Ea-anti Ea precipitates (from reference 112).

and the demonstrations[93,117] of antibodies to "buried" determinants on IgG molecules are hard to interpret otherwise.

Chromatographic studies by LoSpalluto and Ziff[74] and by Williams and Kunkel[120] indicate, on the other hand, that rheumatoid factors having reactivity with rabbit gamma globulin may have slightly different chromatographic behavior from rheumatoid factors reactive only with human gamma globulins. Heimer[55] has described a slight difference in amino acid analysis for rheumatoid factor reacting with rabbit gamma globulin. Furthermore, the data of Milgrom and Witebsky,[80] of Williams and Kunkel,[120] and of Mellors and co-workers[76] reveal that in some systems it is possible to demonstrate anti-rabbit gamma globulin activities in preparations exhibiting little or no anti-human gamma globulin activity. At first sight, these data may seem to indicate that the anti-rabbit gamma globulin activities of the rheumatoid factors are, at least in part, completely independent of the anti-human gamma globulin activities. This in turn suggests that the anti-rabbit gamma globulins do not arise by the same means as do the anti-human gamma globulins. It may reasonably be assumed that some anti-rabbit γG globulin activities are not as easily demonstrated with human IgG globulin because they are directed to configurations present only in more denatured forms of human IgG globulins.

Most of the rheumatoid factor activity appears to be directed to configurations on the H chain portion of IgG molecules, particularly the "fast" (Fc) fragment.[52] Williams,[118] however, has presented evidence that some of the rheumatoid factor molecules may be directed to L chains. Harboe[52] has noted that activity may be directed to internal configurations in the molecule revealed only by its partial digestion. The latter type of serological reactivity has been found also in a significant number of normal sera.

Gaarder and Natvig[47a] have identified serologically seven different "antigens" on IgG molecules with which rheumatoid factors react (Table 9–3). The most frequently found specificity was for Ga, followed in order by Gm(a), non-a, and Gm(g). No one of these "antigens" is contained among all of the subclasses of IgG molecules (Table 9–3), but since all rheumatoid sera seem to contain antibodies to more than one of these "antigens," all subclasses of IgG generally can be expected to be involved in complexing with rheumatoid factors. In contrast, monoclonal anti-IgG molecules, such as may sometimes be found in mixed cryoglobulinemias,[87] may be expected to exhibit only one of these specificities and therefore one might expect that a correspondingly limited representation of IgG molecules will be in complex with the anti-IgG in those cases.

TABLE 9–3.—"ANTIGENS" ON FC PIECE OF IGG WITH WHICH RHEUMATOID FACTORS REACT.

	Portion of Fc Piece Involved	
Subclass	*N-Terminal*	*pFc*
IgG_1	Ga	a, x, "non-a"
IgG_2	Ga	non-a
IgG_3	g, b	non-a
IgG_4	Ga	

(From Gaarder and Natvig[47a])

SITES OF ORIGIN OF THE RHEUMATOID FACTORS

Studies by Mellors and co-workers[76] suggested that rheumatoid factors are produced in lymphoid tissues in a manner quite analogous to the production of antibodies. By immunofluorescent staining techniques, rheumatoid factors were demonstrated in the "large pale cells" in the germinal centers of lymph nodes and in the plasma cells surrounding the germinal centers. This same distribution was also found in lymph nodules within the synovial membrane of rheumatoid joints, together with some diffuse staining along the connective tissue bundles and staining in the round cells diffusely infiltrating this membrane.

Aggregated human gamma globulin labeled with fluorescein and rabbit gamma globulin in an immune complex labeled with rhodamine were used to differentiate sites of origin of anti-rabbit and anti-human γG globulin activities. The germinal center cells of one lymph nodule often appeared to contain one type of rheumatoid factor exclusive of the other, and a given plasma cell often contained one exclusive of the other. Other plasma cells and other lymph nodules, however, gave double staining.

Attempts have been made to demonstrate production of rheumatoid factors by lymph nodes, spleen, and synovial tissues in culture *in vitro*. Success has been achieved only in synovial tissues,[72] where the rheumatoid factors have been found to constitute an extremely small part of the total gamma globulins synthesized. The negative attempts with lymph node and spleen were done a decade ago and only informal reports of the attempts are available, so it is not possible to assess whether culture conditions or assay methods could have been more optimally constructed for the attempted demonstrations.

Bartfeld and Juliar[13] have reported that four-day cultures of peripheral blood leukocytes develop positive staining for rheumatoid factor with fluorescent labeled aggregated gamma globulins. There has been no confirmation of this report, and Kacaki, Bullock and Vaughan[64] failed to find rheumatoid factor agglutinating activity in the supernatants of similar cultures. The immunofluorescence technique is extremely susceptible to non-specific effects, especially in a system with old or dying cells, and so uncertainty still exists as to Bartfeld and Juliar's[13] report.

EXPERIMENTAL PRODUCTION OF RHEUMATOID FACTOR-LIKE SUBSTANCES

Further support for the belief in the antibody nature of the rheumatoid factors comes from the success which several laboratories have had in inducing antibodies which are like rheumatoid factors in experimental animals. Milgrom first accomplished this by injecting rabbits repeatedly with streptococci. The appearance of an "anti-antibody" was thought to be due to development of new surface configurations on antibody molecules complexed with antigen with consequent development of an antibody response to these new configurations. To support the idea that quite gentle forces exerted on gamma globulins were sufficient to create such new antigenicity, Milgrom[80] precipitated the gamma globulins of rabbit serum with ammonium sulfate, redissolved this in saline solution, and after freezing and thawing, reinjected this fraction back into the original animals. Anti-gamma globulin activity again was encountered.

These studies have been confirmed and extended by several other laboratories. Christian[33] has shown that rheumatoid factor-like activity which develops in rabbits hyperimmunized with E. coli is 19S in its ultracentrifugal sedimentation, reacts better with human γG globulin than rabbit γG globulin, and reacts better with denatured rabbit γG globulin than undenatured rabbit γG globulin. Catsoulis, *et al.*[29] have found that the anti-γG globulin developed in rabbits injected with alkali-denatured autogenous γG globulins is a 7S protein which fails to cross react with the animals' own undenatured γG globulins. Williams[119] has observed the development of anti-γG globulins in animals injected with ferritin. The anti-gamma globulin antibodies disappear rapidly after the immunization is stopped.

The stimulus for the production of rheumatoid factors in rheumatoid arthritis appears to be some unknown process which causes a change in the patient's own IgG to make it auto-immunogenic. Chronic infections can induce rheumatoid factor synthesis, presumably because of immunization by IgG that has reacted with antigen and is thereby in antigen-antibody complex. If rheumatoid arthritis were a chronic infection, a ready explanation for rheumatoid factors would exist. Two additional possibilities should be considered: that there is some acquired intrinsic abnormality in the IgG synthesized in rheumatoid arthritis, causing it to aggregate spontaneously and thus to become auto-immunogenic; or there is a protein-catabolizing mechanism in rheumatoid arthritis which yields abnormal IgG fragments which are auto-immunogenic. There is as yet no good evidence to make us favor or reject either of these latter notions. It seems unlikely that rheumatoid factors are products of an abnormal machinery for synthesizing antibodies.

THE Gm AND InV SYSTEMS

Reactions of Rheumatoid Factors with Anti-Rh Antibodies

The ability of sera from patients with rheumatoid arthritis to agglutinate Rh positive human red cells sensitized with non-agglutinating anti-Rh antibody was pointed out in 1956. Certain anti-Rh antibodies were effective in sensitizing cells for this agglutination by rheumatoid arthritis sera, while others were not.[50,116] The capacity to be a good sensitizer does not depend upon quantity of anti-Rh antibody. Some qualitative difference in the anti-Rh antibody and some selective specificity of the anti-γG globulins in the rheumatoid arthritis sera must be implied. Two anti-Rh sera in particular, those from the donors Ri and Mu,[47,116] have been unusually good in sensitizing for agglutination reactions for a wide variety of rheumatoid arthritis sera. Aho and co-workers[4] note that heavy sensitization by the serum Ri probably allows a type of close packing of gamma globulin molecules on the cell surface that is essential both for complement fixation and for rheumatoid factor attachment.

Gm Specificities[100]

Using other anti-Rh sera, Grubb and Laurell[50] recognized that only a small proportion of rheumatoid arthritis sera induce agglutination of sensitized cells, and that the agglutination in these instances is inhibited by the gamma globulins of some normal sera but not by others. The inhibition reaction was shown to be a genetically determined property of serum both in family studies and in general population studies. This inhibition is independent of the absolute amount of gamma globulins in the serum and therefore it describes a qualitative characteristic. Grubb referred to this characteristic as the Gm (gamma) characteristic and named the gene responsible for it the Gm^a gene.

Harboe[53] identified the next Gm factor using combinations of other rheumatoid arthritis sera with other anti-Rh antibodies and showed it also to be a genetic marker. He named the newly defined gene Gm^b. The number of identified genetic markers has expanded considerably since then, at least 24 being known. Each of the IgG H chain subtypes have been recognized[67,101] to have at least one marker. All but two of the markers are on the Fc portions of the H chains.

Genetically determined gamma globulin subtypes analogous to the Gm subtypes in man have been recognized in rabbits. They are referred to as allotypes. It is probable that similar genetically determined differences in gamma globulins occur within many species. Primates have been examined to see whether their gamma globulins have Gm characteristics. Only the chimpanzee has shown them; gibbons and several species of monkeys lack Gm specificities.[20]

Anti-Gm Antibodies

Anti-Gm antibodies in sera of rheumatoid arthritis patients are highly specific components in a much more extensive array of anti-IgG globulin antibodies composing the rheumatoid factors (Table 9–3). However, anti-Gm antibodies have also been found in certain normal sera, and these anti-Gm antibodies exist alone, without the concomitant array of other anti-IgG antibodies of rheumatoid factor. The sensitized sheep cell and latex agglutination reactions are negative in these normal sera. The antibody activities in the normal sera are thus much more highly selective than those present in the sera of rheumatoid patients.

The presence of anti-Gm antibodies in normal sera appears to depend on a previous transfusion of plasma containing a γG globulin of a different Gm type from the recipient, or else upon the individual having had a mother with a Gm type different from his own.[102] In the latter instance the placental transfer of maternal γG globulin apparently constitutes the transfusion of incompatible gamma globulin which is prerequisite to the development of the anti-Gm antibody. In all normal sera studied, the anti-Gm activity has had allospecific* characteristics, never being directed to the Gm type of the person's own γG globulins. Antisera which define the InV specificites have been found exclusively among such normal sera.

The relation between the anti-Gm specificities in sera of patients with rheumatoid arthritis and the Gm types of the patient's own γG globulins has been extensively studied.[47,51,52,77,100] Although the majority of rheumatoid arthritis sera examined have had anti-Gm antibodies corresponding to the Gm types in the patient's own γG globulins, which indicates that the anti-Gm antibodies in these instances are autospecific, other sera have anti-Gm antibodies which are directed to Gm specificities not contained in the patient's own γG globulins.[47,52] Rheumatoid arthritis sera have also been described in which autospecific and allospecific anti-Gm activities have been identified within the same serum.

The existence of allospecificity in the anti-Gm activities in rheumatoid arthritis sera has raised a serious question about whether rheumatoid factor in these instances can be considered to be an autoantibody to IgG globulin. Vaughan[110] isolated autogenous IgG globulins from such a serum and showed that, although it failed to inhibit its own anti-Gm (a+) activity in its originally isolated form, it did so after appropriate denaturation. This observation is consistent with Steinberg's earlier observation[100] that IgG globulin which behaves as though it is Gm (a—) with rheumatoid arthritis sera behaves as though it were Gm (a+) after denaturation. On the other hand, this apparent shift from Gm (a—) to Gm (a+) is not seen, if anti-Gm antibody from a normal serum is used rather than anti-Gm in a rheumatoid serum. The presence of antibodies to denatured IgG in rheumatoid arthritis sera and their absence from normal sera could explain these findings.

BIOLOGIC ACTIVITIES OF THE RHEUMATOID FACTORS

Protective Role

It has been suggested that rheumatoid factors may have a protective role in the body's economy. This is an attractive hypothesis, appealing to teleologic reasoning and the sensibleness of nature. The ability of rheumatoid factors to combine with soluble antigen-antibody complexes and thereby render them less soluble and more easily cleared by the reticuloendothelial system is an example whereby the patient may be protected from serum sickness-like phenomena in chronic infections.

Gough and Davis,[49] noting that rheumatoid factor is capable of blocking the ability of antigen-antibody aggregates to fix guinea pig complement, have set up a parallel demonstration *in vivo*. Human IgG injected intraperitoneally into rats failed to lower the rat serum complement titer when rheumatoid factor serum was also injected into the peritoneum. The concept was presented by these investigators that, in its ability to help prevent

* Also called "isospecific," a term which has led to confusion since in experimental animals isospecificity refers to different animals within an inbred strain; in man, an outbred animal, the proper term would be allospecific.

complement fixation by antigen-antibody complexes, rheumatoid factor may provide a means of protection against serum sickness-like reactions.

Schmid and Roitt[92] showed that rheumatoid factors can prevent complement-fixing immune injury to thyroid cells *in vitro*. Davis and Bollet[35] showed inhibition of a complement-mediated immune injury to mitochondria. Romeyn and Bowman[88] showed inhibition of immune lysis of red cells. Thus rheumatoid factors in model systems can indeed protect target cells from a directly destructive effect of complement-fixing antibody.

On the other hand, Messner and co-workers[77] have indicated that rheumatoid factors are able to interfere with the opsonic activity of 7S-IgG antibodies obtained from patients with subacute bacterial endocarditis. When rheumatoid factor was present in the system, the opsonization of bacteria coated with antibody was not as great as it was when the rheumatoid factor was absent from the system From these data it could be argued that rheumatoid factor enhances patients' susceptibility to infection. Clinically, patients with rheumatoid arthritis do in fact have an increased susceptibility to infection.

Effects on Immunoglobulin Metabolism

Studies by Harris and Vaughan[54] and Gordon, Eisen, and Vaughan[48a] have indicated that the presence of rheumatoid factors in high titers in serums of individuals may be attended by no gross change in overall immunoglobulin metabolism. Catsoulis et al.[29] failed to find increased disappearance of normal IgG in rabbits immunized with autologous denatured gamma globulin with resultant production of rheumatoid factor-like activity. On the other hand, Davis and Torrigiani[36] noted increased breakdown of aggregated IgG, or of thyroglobulin (Tg) given as a Tg-anti-Tg complex, when rheumatoid factor was present. Bluestone et al.,[17] studying the catabolism and synovial transport of a labeled rheumatoid factor isolated from a cryoprecipitating IgG-anti-IgG complex, presented evidence suggesting that rheumatoid factors of high-binding avidity may be capable of reacting with IgG to produce *in vivo* precipitates and rapid clearance from the body fluids, while low avidity rheumatoid factors cannot. The existence of, or effects of, such high avidity interactions, whether based on the aggregated IgG reacting with "normal" rheumatoid factors or "normal" IgG reacting with high avidity rheumatoid factors, might have been missed in the earlier studies cited above, if the proportion of IgG rapidly cleared by the interaction were small relative to the total quantity of circulating IgG.

The observations of Waldmann, Johnson and Talal[114a] provide additional evidence that rheumatoid factor can influence immunoglobulin metabolism. They studied a patient with Sjögren's syndrome who had a high serum concentration of monoclonal IgM with rheumatoid factor activity which formed soluble IgM-IgG complexes at body temperature. Evidence indicated that IgM anti-IgG not only accelerated the catabolism of IgG but interfered with IgG synthesis as well.

Brown and Epstein[22] have shown that passively administered rheumatoid factors may inhibit the abilities of mouse spleens to make normal antibody responses to human IgG. Rheumatoid factor was regarded by these investigators as a "negative feed-back" to anti-IgG production in their system. King, Messner and Williams[66] have demonstrated a weak capability for rheumatoid factors to provoke mitogenic effects in lymphocytes.

Role in the Inflammatory Response

The first *in vivo* study to suggest that rheumatoid factor may be capable of producing tissue damage was that of Baum et al.[14] These workers showed that when fractions of sera enriched in rheumatoid factor were injected into the mesentery arteries of the rat vasculitis was produced. Comparable fractions of sera from patients with Waldenström's macroglobulinemia failed to induce vasculitis.

Broder and Baumal[21] have described a histamine-releasing activity in the sera of patients with rheumatoid arthritis. This could not be related to IgM rheumatoid factor. The histamine release was observed from mouse lungs perfused with macroglobulin components in rheumatoid sera. The role of this activity in rheumatoid arthritis is not clear, but the sera of those patients with more severe manifestations of disease exhibited this activity more frequently. It seems likely that the activity is due to IgG rheumatoid factor complexes.

Epstein, Tan and Melmon[42] have studied the ability of rheumatoid factor precipitates to affect the kinin system. Their demonstration that the formation of rheumatoid factor precipitates in the sera of patients with rheumatoid arthritis is capable of depleting kininogen from serum is reasonably strong evidence that the kinin system can be activated by rheumatoid factor.

McCormick et al.[75] noted that rheumatoid factors are capable of enhancing the nephrotoxicity of rabbit anti-rat kidney serum in the rat. This finding has no parallel in organ pathology in rheumatoid arthritis, but it may bear on the renal disease in lupus[3a] and in mixed cryoglobulinemic purpura.

The ability of human complement to be fixed by rheumatoid factors complexed to reduced and alkylated IgG has been very well demonstrated by Zvaifler[124] and by Tesar and Schmid.[105] Guinea pig complement is apparently not fixed. That the fixation of human complement is due to the rheumatoid factor component is attested to by the known inability of reduced and alkylated IgG by itself to fix complement. Tesar and Schmid have shown that complement-fixing activity can be found in isolated IgM rheumatoid factor. Winchester et al.[122a] have described strong reactivity of "intermediate complexes" (γG-anti γG) with the C1q component of complement.

Kaplan and Jandl[65] have noted that rheumatoid factors *in vivo* are not capable of enhancing the rate of clearance of red cells sensitized with anti-red cell antibodies. Similarly, Mongan et al.[81] have noted that there is not an increased clearance of sensitized red cells from the serums of patients containing rheumatoid factors. Kaplan and Jandl noted that the normal high level of non-complexed IgG in serum serves to inhibit the precipitation and agglutination capabilities of the rheumatoid factor with IgG and they suggested that rheumatoid factor, if it is to play a pathogenetic role in disease, is more likely to do so in tissue fluids in which there is a low protein concentration, such as the interstitial fluids.

CLINICAL OBSERVATIONS

In Population Studies

Rheumatoid factors are found in a wide variety of diseases and even in a small proportion of presumably healthy persons. Several reports show that there is an increasing incidence of these antibodies with age. The greatest incidence of positive serum latex tests has been reported in individuals residing in homes for the aged, although the sensitized sheep cell test generally gives negative results in these cases.[57,115]

Studies have been done to assess the relationship between the distribution of rheumatoid factors and rheumatoid arthritis in large populations. These have shown that factors other than the rheumatoid factor are important in the disease. In a northern England population, Lawrence and Ball[71] found a family aggregation of both seropositivity and of rheumatoid arthritis, but these did not coincide. Initially, 75 per cent of individuals who had positive reactions in the sensitized sheep cell test did not have clinically identifiable rheumatoid arthritis. Upon re-examination five years later, rheumatoid arthritis had developed in 9 of 25 individuals (36 per cent) of this group. Rheumatoid arthritis developed in only 5 of 85 individuals (8 per cent) of those who were previously healthy seronegatives.[70] The higher the titer of rheumatoid factor, the more likely the individual was to have rheumatoid arthritis. Lawrence and Ball suggested that two familial predispositions were revealed in this study. One was for the production of anti-gamma globulin antibodies and the other for the development of arthritis. When these two predispositions are superimposed, rheumatoid arthritis is more likely to occur.

Although the incidence of rheumatoid arthritis is 2 to 3 times greater in women than in men, there is no increased frequency of seropositivity among healthy women in general population studies. Seropositivity, in the English study, occurred more frequently in blood relatives of patients with rheumatoid arthritis than in the population at large. It did not occur more frequently in the patients' spouses.

Studies by several other groups[3,15,16,79] have confirmed most of the Lawrence and Ball[71] findings, although differing in detail. About 80% of Cathcart and O'Sullivan's[28] subjects who had strongly positive sera on first testing remained so three years later. Only 25% of these were designated rheumatoid arthritis on first testing, while about 35% were three years later. This conversion rate was ten times that expected from their total population.

Hospital employees at a rheumatism hospital in Finland did not have more seropositivity than controls.[68] In a number of identical twins, in whom only one has had rheumatoid arthritis, only the arthritic has been seropositive.

Survey of an Indian population has failed to reveal significant familial aggregation either of seropositivity or of overt arthritis.[24] Bennett and Burch[15] noted a very significant difference in the incidences of positive test results for rheumatoid factors in the Pima and Blackfoot Indians, and they also recognized a greater mortality for those with seropositive rheumatoid arthritis than for other groups.

In population studies in which latex tests or bentonite tests have been used to identify the rheumatoid factor, the frequency of positive test results in non-rheumatoid persons increases, and correspondingly the frequency with which positivity coincides with presence of rheumatoid arthritis decreases. Differences in frequencies of arthritis in seropositive and seronegative individuals may then become insignificant. This is less likely to occur with the sensitized sheep cell test.

In Rheumatoid Arthritis

Rheumatoid agglutination reactions are not positive in every case of rheumatoid arthritis. The original streptococcus agglutination reactions were positive in only 40 to 60 per cent of cases. The incidence of positive reactions was generally increased when sensitized red cell methods were introduced; a still higher incidence was found using redissolved euglobulin precipitates with sensitized red cells. Ziff reported that this can be accomplished without significantly increasing the number of false positives in non-rheumatoid controls. By a euglobulin agglutination-inhibition technique in the sensitized sheep cell system, Ziff reported 98 per cent of a rheumatoid population to be positive.[123] Both Clark[34] and Svartz,[103] however, reported that in their hands the agglutination-inhibition technique gave a significantly increased number of false positives in normal control populations.

There can be no doubt that some sera which test negatively for rheumatoid factors by conventional techniques do in fact have rheumatoid factors in them. The high concentration of IgG normally present in serum understandably can block demonstration of anti-IgG activities simultaneously present. This effect was well studied by Allen and Kunkel[9] and by Bluestone et al.[18] Torrigiani, Roitt, Lloyd, and Corbett[108] have reported that apparently seronegative rheumatoid sera may yield a large quantity of anti-IgG to insolubilized equine IgG, from which it can be eluted and quantified.

DeForest[38] described a small number of patients who had positive agglutination reactions during the initial manifestations of the disease and whose agglutination reactions reverted to negative following a remission from the first attack. When recrudescence of the disease occurred the test again became positive.

Aho *et al.*, in a nine-year follow-up of patients whose disease had become inactive, noted that most were serologically positive.[5] Other long-term follow-up studies have yielded similar data.

As a rule, patients who have advanced rheumatoid arthritis have positive agglutination reactions with greater frequency and these reactions exist in higher titers. Bywaters, Carter, and Scott[27] have noted that there is also a progressive increase in incidence of positive test results in patients with age. Subcutaneous nodules are almost entirely limited to patients with positive serologic reactions, although exceptions have been reported. Seropositive patients have more erosive disease visible roentgenologically and run a more relentless, progressive course.[97] Occasionally patients with very large amounts of circulating rheumatoid factors develop life-threatening hyperviscosity with impaired function of the central nervous system.[2,63,96] The development of the angiitis syndrome with peripheral neuropathy and gangrenous skin ulceration also appears to be more common among patients with extremely high titers[40,48a] (Fig. 9–4).

In juvenile rheumatoid arthritis the agglutination reactions for the rheumatoid factor are positive in only about 10 per cent of cases, although with modifications in the testing procedures, Ziff has reported much higher incidences. The families of patients with juvenile rheumatoid arthritis have been strikingly different from those of patients with adult rheumatoid arthritis in that they have a very low incidence of seropositivity in the near relatives. One interesting study[10] revealed a high incidence of spondylitis in the fathers of patients with juvenile rheumatoid arthritis and of seronegative peripheral rheumatoid arthritis in the mothers.

A mild, remittent arthritis may occur in children and adults with agammaglobulinemia. This disease has many of the characteristics of rheumatoid arthritis. It has not been possible to demonstrate significant titers of either the rheumatoid agglutinating factor or the inhibitor of rheumatoid agglutination reactions in these patients, which is consistent with the fact that the agglutinating and inhibiting substances are gamma globulins. Rotstein and Good's report[91] of patients with agammaglobulinemia and arthritis

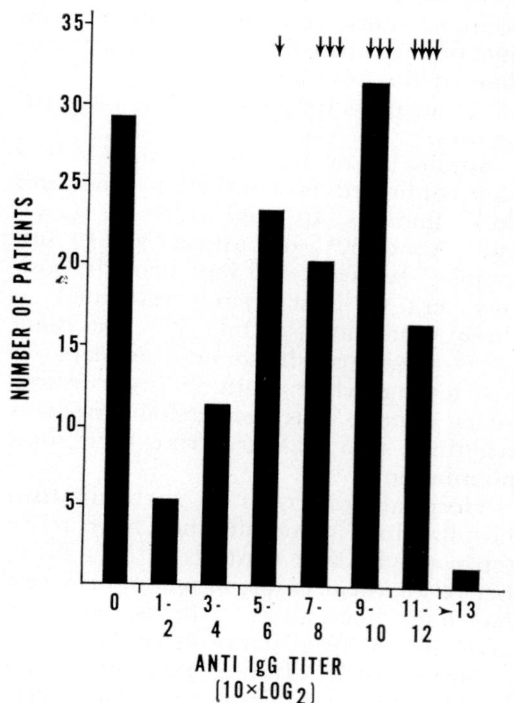

Fig. 9–4.—Incidence of angiitis (arrows) in patients with higher titers of rheumatoid factor in serum (reference 48*a*).

who also had subcutaneous nodules emphasizes the possibility that this disease may be rheumatoid arthritis, and emphasizes the need to search for factors other than the rheumatoid factors to identify fully the disease mechanism in rheumatoid arthritis. Fudenberg, German, and Kunkel's finding[46] that the sera of relatives of patients with acquired agammaglobulinemia may frequently show rheumatoid factors or other gamma globulin abnormalities has obvious implications in this regard. This familial pattern has not been seen with congenital agammaglobulinemia.

The arthritis that occurs in agammaglobulinemia is generally mild and remittent and is very low in frequency in patients adequately treated with exogenous gamma globulin. The existence of this form of arthritis does not necessarily bear on the possibility that rheumatoid factors and other antibodies in classical rheumatoid arthritis, no matter whether primary or secondary in the pathogenetic mechanisms of the disease, may have their own contribution to make to the tissue damage in the disease (see Chapter 47).

In Other Inflammatory Diseases of the Connective Tissue

The rheumatoid agglutination reaction is almost always absent from the serum of patients with rheumatic fever. Although rheumatic fever patients may show an elevated titer of anti-streptococcal agglutination, reliance is put on the anti-streptolysin O test for demonstrating that these patients' sera are in the post-streptococcal state. Patients with rheumatic fever are no different from normal control populations with regard to incidence of positive sensitized sheep cell tests.

In lupus erythematosus there is a significant incidence of positive rheumatoid agglutination reactions, in some series as high as 30 per cent. Although this is said to be more common in patients with lupus in whom there is a concomitant arthritis which is clinically indistinguishable from rheumatoid arthritis, this is not exclusively so. Since it has been reported that the sera of patients with rheumatoid arthritis exhibit a higher than normal incidence of positive L.E. reactions and of antinuclear antibodies, there exists a serological counterpart to the recognized clinical overlapping of these two disease entities.

In Sjögren's syndrome, with or without arthritis, Bunim[23] has found positive agglutination reactions in 100 per cent of cases. His series was probably highly selective for severe disease, however, so the true incidence of serological abnormality is probably less.

Positive rheumatoid agglutination reactions have been reported in polyarteritis and scleroderma, but since clinical protocols have rarely been presented it is not clear that all would agree on the diagnoses in these instances. "Polyangiitis" is a well-known complication of rheumatoid arthritis in the late stages and this may have accounted for positive test results in many patients diagnosed as having polyarteritis nodosum. Under any circumstance, the frequency of positive reactions among these patients is no greater than 20 per cent.

In Other Diseases[11,12,84,85,98]

In ankylosing spondylitis without peripheral joint involvement, dermatomyositis, palindromic rheumatism, psoriatic arthritis, Reiter's syndrome, osteoarthritis, specific infectious arthritis, gout, and the arthritis of ulcerative colitis, the serological agglutination test results are usually negative.

Positive agglutination reactions in high titer were recognized early in patients with hyperglobulinemia associated with liver disease, kala-azar, sarcoidosis, and syphilis. Generally, these positive reactions occurred in about 10 to 15 per cent of the respective patient populations. The strong agglutination reactions in these non-rheumatoid diseases appeared to be more frequently demonstrable with latex agglutination and human γG precipitation reactions. The sensitized sheep cell test result was usually negative. The factor responsible for the agglutinating activity in sera from sarcoid patients has been shown to be associated with a 22S complex similar to that observed in patients with rheumatoid arthritis. Differential adsorption studies in positive sera from syphilitic patients have demonstrated that the rheumatoid factor is distinct from the Wassermann antibody. The clinical picture of rheumatoid arthritis was present in none of these patients.

There has been a steady expansion in the list of diseases[61,62,104] associated with positive reactivity in the latex and bentonite systems. Leprosy, tuberculosis, schistosomiasis, yaws, and many other chronic infectious processes have been especially implicated. In some of these the sensitized sheep cell test result has also been positive. In subacute bacterial endocarditis Williams and Kunkel[121] have found a number of patients to have positive reactions to both tests during the active disease, with both reactions reverting to negative with cure. Aho and his co-workers[6] have noted the transient appearance of rheumatoid factor after especially heavy prophylactic vaccinations in army recruits. Svec and Dingle made similar observations after vaccination with influenza virus (Asian).[104]

SUMMARY

The ability of the sera of patients with rheumatoid arthritis to agglutinate bacteria or sensitized cells is due to an interaction between anti-IgG globulin antibodies in the sera of these patients and IgG globulin present as a sensitizing coat on the surface of the bacterium or red cell. When rabbit IgG globulin is used as the sensitizing material, as in the sensitized sheep cell test, only a portion of the rheumatoid factors participate in the reaction. When human IgG globulin is employed as a coating material, as in the latex or bentonite particle tests, all of the rheumatoid factors appear to participate.

Stimulus for production of rheumatoid factors is probably autoimmunization with IgG which has been converted to an immunogenic form by aggregation by antigen, or by other unknown means. This may be a consequence of chronic infection.

The results of sensitized sheep cell tests are less often positive in non-rheumatoid arthritis populations than in the bentonite or latex tests, and therefore it is more specific for rheumatoid arthritis than the other two tests.

Biologic properties of the rheumatoid factors include ability to modify phagocytosis of particles, either enhancement or inhibition being seen depending upon the system studied. Rheumatoid factors inhibit the ability of guinea pig complement to fix to antigen-antibody complexes, but can themselves weakly fix human complement. They may play an *in vivo* role in experimentally induced vasculitis and in histamine release, and in *in vitro* experiments they have been shown to affect the kininogen-kinin system. They have been reported to enhance nephrotoxic nephritis and to suppress anti-IgG production in experimental animals.

Rheumatoid agglutination reactions are not invariably found in the sera of rheumatoid arthritis patients. In general, the presence of rheumatoid agglutination activity implies a more advanced and overwhelming disease, and therefore a more reserved prognosis is indicated. Certain complications of rheumatoid arthritis such as the hyperviscosity syndrome and necrotizing vasculitis are particularly associated with high titers of rheumatoid factors. The result of the test has been found positive in a significant proportion of patients with lupus erythematosus and to a lesser degree in other inflammatory diseases of the connective tissues. In certain other types of diseases agglutinating reactions closely resembling the rheumatoid agglutination reactions can also be seen. This has been most extensively described in patients with sarcoidosis, in syphilis, and other chronic infections.

Acknowledgement:

The author wishes to express his sincere appreciation to Dr. Thomas F. Disney and Miss Mary Zorn for their considerable help in assembling this revised chapter.

BIBLIOGRAPHY

1. Abraham, G. N., Clark, R. A., Kacaki, J. and Vaughan, J. H.: Arth. & Rheum., *13*, 300, 1970.
2. Abruzzo, J. L., Heimer, R. and Martinez, J.: Arth. & Rheum., *12*, 653, 1969.
3. Adler, E., Abramson, J. H., Goldberg, R., Elkan, Z. and Ben Hador, S.: Amer. J. Epidemiol., *85*, 378, 1966.
3*a*. Agnello, V., Koffler, D., Eisenberg, J. W., Winchester, R. J. and Kunkel, H. G.: J. Exp. Med., *134*, 228s, 1971.
4. Aho, K., Harboe, M. and Leikola, J.: Immunol., *7*, 403, 1964.
5. Aho, K., Kirpila, J. and Wager, O.: Ann. Med. Exp. Fenn., *37*, 377, 1959.
6. Aho, K., Konttinen, A., Rajasaline, M. and Wager, O.: Acta Path. Microbiol. Scand., *56*, 478, 1962.
7. Aho, K., Ripatti, N., Saris, N. E. and Wager, O.: Ann. Med. Exp. Fenn., *40*, 481, 1962.
8. Allen, J. C.. J. Clin. Invest., *45*, 981, 1966.
9. Allen, J. C. and Kunkel, H. G.: Arth. & Rheum., *9*, 758, 1966.
10. Ansell, B. M., Bywaters, E. G. L. and Lawrence, J. S.: Ann. Rheum. Dis., *21*, 243, 1962.
11. Bartfeld, H.: Ann. Intern. Med., *52*, 1059, 1960.
12. ————: N. Y. Acad. Sci., *168*, Art. 1, 30, 1969.
13. Bartfeld, H. and Juliar, J. F.: Lancet, *2*, 767, 1964.
14. Baum, J., Stastny, P. and Ziff, M.: J. Immunol., *93*, 985, 1964.
15. Bennett, P. H. and Burch, T. A.: in *Population Studies of the Rheumatic Diseases*, P. H. Bennett and P. H. N. Wood, Eds., Excerpta Medica Fndn., Amsterdam/N.Y., *27*, 192, 1968.
16. Bennett, P. H. and Wood, P. H. N.: *Population Studies of the Rheumatic Diseases*, Excerpta Medica Fndn., Amsterdam/N.Y., 1968.
17. Bluestone, R., Cracchiolo, A., Goldberg, L. S. and Pearson, C. M.: Ann. Rheum. Dis., *29*, No. 1, 47, 1970.
18. Bluestone, R., Goldberg, L. S. and Cracchiolo, A.: Lancet, *2*, 878, 1969.
19. Boizecevish, J., Bunim, J., Freund, J. and Ward, S. B.: Proc. Soc. Exp. Biol. Med., *97*, 180, 1958.
20. Boyer, S. H. and Young, W. J.: Science, *133*, 583, 1961.
21. Broder, I., Baumal, R., Gordon, D. and Bell, D.: N.Y. Acad. Sci., *168*, 126, 1969.
22. Brown, J. C. and Epstein, W. V.: Arth. & Rheum., *12*, 1, 1969.
23. Bunim, J. J.: Ann. Intern. Med., *61*, 509, 1964.
24. Burch, T. A., O'Brien, W. M. and Bunim, J. J.: Amer. J. Publ. Health, *54*, 1184, 1964.
25. Butler, V. P., Jr. and Vaughan, J. H.: Immunol., *8*, 144, 1965.
26. ————: Proc. Soc. Exp. Biol. Med., *116*, 585, 1964.
27. Bywaters, E. G. L., Carter, M. E. and Scott, F. E. T.: Ann. Rheum. Dis., *18*, 233, 1959.
28. Cathcart, E. S. and O'Sullivan, J. B.: N. Y. Acad. Sci., *168*, 41, 1969.
29. Catsoulis, E. A., Rothschild, M. A., Oratz, M. and Franklin, E. C.: Arth. & Rheum., *8*, 39, 1965.
30. Cecil, R. L., Nichols, E. E. and Stainsby, W. J.: Amer. J. Med. Sci., *181*, 12, 1931.
31. Chesebro, B., Bloth, B. and Svehag, S. E.: J. Exper. Med., *127*, 399, 1968.
32. Chodirker, W. B. and Tomasi, T. B., Jr.: J. Clin. Invest., *42*, 876, 1963.
33. Christian, C. L.: J. Exper. Med., *118*, 827, 1963.
34. Clark, W. S.: in *Serological Reactions of Rheumatoid Arthritis: Summary of First Conference*, Arthritis and Rheumatism Foundation, January 1957.
35. Davis, J. S. and Bollet, A. J.: J. Immunol., *92*, 139, 1964.
36. Davis, J. S. and Torrigiani, G.: Proc. Soc. Exp. Biol. & Med., *125*, 772, 1967.
37. Dawson, M. H., Olmstead, M. and Boots, R. H.: J. Immunol., *23*, 187, 1932.
38. deForest, G. K., Mucci, M. B. and Biosvert, P. L.: Arth. & Rheum., *1*, 387, 1958.
39. Edelman, G. M. and Benaceraff, B.: Proc. N.A.S., *48*, 1035, 1962.

40. Epstein, W. V. and Engelman, E. P.: Arth. & Rheum., *2*, 250, 1959.
41. Epstein, W., Johnson, A. M. and Ragan, C.: Proc. Soc. Exp. Biol. Med., *91*, 235, 1956.
42. Epstein, W. V., Tan, M. and Melmon, K. L.: N. Y. Acad. Sci., *168*, 173, 1969.
43. Franchimont, P. and Suteanu, S.: Arth. & Rheum., *12*, 483, 1969.
44. Franklin, E. C.: Ann. Rev. Med., *20*, 155, 1969.
45. Franklin, E. C., Holman, H. R., Müller-Eberhard, H. J. and Kunkel, H. G.: J. Exper. Med., *105*, 425, 1957.
46. Fudenberg, H., German, J. L., III and Kunkel, H. G.: Arth. & Rheum., *5*, 565, 1962.
47. Fudenberg, H. and Kunkel, H. G.: J. Exper. Med., *114*, 257, 1961.
47*a*. Gaarder, P. I. and Natvig, J. B.: J. Immunol., *105*, 928, 1970.
48. Gleich, G. J., Bieger, R. C. and Stankievic, R.: Science, *165*, 606, 1969.
48*a*. Gordon, D. A., Eisen, A. Z., and Vaughan, J. H.: Trans. Assn. Amer. Phys., *76*, 222, 1963.
49. Gough, W. W. and Davis, J. S.: Arth. & Rheum., *9*, 555, 1966.
50. Grubb, R. and Laurell, A. B.: Acta Path. Microbiol. Scand., *39*, 390, 1956.
51. Harboe, M.: Ann. Rheum. Dis., *20*, 363, 1961.
52. ———: Arth. & Rheum., *6*, 427, 1963.
53. ———: Nature, *183*, 1468, 1959.
54. Harris, J. and Vaughan, J. H.: Arth. & Rheum., *4*, 47, 1961.
55. Heimer, R., Federico, O. M. and Freyberg, R. H.: Proc. Soc. Exp. Biol. Med., *99*, 381, 1958.
56. Heimer, R. and Levine, F. M.: Arth. & Rheum., *7*, 738, 1964.
57. Heimer, R., Levine, F. M. and Rudd, E.: Amer. J. Med., *35*, 175, 1963.
58. Heiner, D. C., Saha, A. and Rose, B.: Fed. Proc., *28*, 766, 1969.
59. Heller, G., Jacobson, A. S., Kolodny, M. H. and Kammerer, W. H.: J. Immunol., *72*, 66, 1954.
60. Henney, C. S.: N. Y. Acad. Sci., *168*, Art. 1, 52, 1969.
61. Houba, V. and Allison, A. C.: Lancet, *1*, 848, 1966.
62. Huntley, C., Costan, M. C., Williams, R. C., Lyerly, A. and Watson, R. D.: J.A.M.A., *197*, 552, 1966.
63. Jasin, H. E., LoSpalluto, J. and Ziff, M.: Arth. & Rheum., *12*, 304, 1969.
64. Kacaki, J. N., Bullock, W. E. and Vaughan, J. H.: Lancet, *1*, 1289, 1969.
65. Kaplan, M. E. and Jandl, J. H.: J. Exp. Med., *117*, 105, 1963.
66. King, R. A., Messner, R. P. and Williams, R. C., Jr.: Arth. & Rheum., *12*, 597, 1969.
67. Kunkel, H. G., Joslin, F. G., Penn, G. M. and Natvig, J. B.: J. Exper. Med., *132*, 508, 1970.
68. Laine, V., Sievers, K., Wager, O. and Aho, K.: Acta Rheum. Scand., *8*, 229, 1962.
69. Lamont-Havers, R. W.: Proc. Soc. Exp. Biol. Med., *88*, 35, 1955.
70. Lawrence, J. S.: Arth. & Rheum., *6*, 166, 1963.
71. Lawrence, J. S. and Ball, J.: Ann. Rheum. Dis., *17*, 160, 1958.
72. Lochead, J. A., Smiley, J. D. and Ziff, M.: Arth. & Rheum., *14*, 171, 1971.
73. LoSpalluto, J.: Arth. & Rheum., *11*, 831, 1968.
74. LoSpalluto, J. and Ziff, M.: J. Exper. Med., *110*, 169, 1959.
75. McCormick, J. N., Day, J., Morris, C. J. and Hill, A. G. S.: Clin. Exper. Immunol., *4*, 17, 1969.
76. Mellors, R. C., Nowoslawski, A. and Korngold, L.: Amer. J. Path., *39*, 533, 1961.
77. Messner, R. P., Caperton, E. M., Jr., King, R. A. and Williams, R. C., Jr.: N. Y. Acad. Sci., *168*, 93, 1969.
78. Meyer, K.: Ztschr. J. Immun., *34*, 229, 1922.
79. Mikkelsen, W. M., Dodge, H. J., Duff, I. F., Epstein, F. H. and Napier, J. A.: in *Epidemiology of Chronic Rheumatism*, J. H. Kellgren, M. R. Jeffry and J. Ball, Eds., Oxford, Eng., Blackwell Sci. Pub., *1*, 1963, p. 239.
80. Milgrom, F. and Witebsky, E.: J.A.M.A., *174*, 56, 1960.
81. Mongan, E. S., Leddy, J. P., Atwater, E. C. and Barnett, E. V.: Arth. & Rheum., *10*, 502, 1967.
82. Normansell, D. E.: Immunochem., *7*, 878, 1970.
83. Oker-Blom, N.: Nord. Med., *41*, 74, 1949.
84. Pinto, L. and Barbieri, G.: G. Mal. infett., *16*, 456, 1964.
85. Polish, E. and Muschel, L. H.: Amer. J. Digest. Dis., *7*, 677, 1962.
86. Porter, R. R.: in *Symposium on Basic Problems in Neoplastic Disease*, New York, Columbia University Press, 1962, p. 177.
87. Potter, M.: New Eng. J. Med., *284*, 831, 1971.

88. Romeyn, J. A. and Bowman, D. M.: Nature (Lond.), *216*, 180, 1967.
89. Rose, H. W., Ragan, C., Pearce, E. and Lipman, M. O.: Proc. Soc. Exp. Biol. Med., *68*, 1, 1948.
90. Rothfield, N. F., Frangione, B. and Franklin, E. C.: J. Clin. Invest., *44*, 62, 1965.
91. Rotstein, J. and Good, R. A.: Ann. Rheum. Dis., *21*, 202, 1962.
92. Schmid, F. R. and Roitt, I. M.: J. Lab. and Clin. Med., *66*, 1019, 1965.
93. Schoenfeld, L. and Epstein, W.: Vox Sang., *10*, 482, 1965.
94. Schrohenloher, R. C.: J. Clin. Invest., *45*, 501, 1966.
95. Schubart, A. F., Cohen, A. S. and Calkins, E.: New Eng. J. Med., *261*, 363, 1959.
96. Shearn, M., Epstein, W. and Engleman, E. P.: Arch. Intern. Med., *112*, 684, 1963.
97. Sievers, K.: Acta Rheum. Scand., *9*, 1, 1965.
98. Singer, J. M.: Amer. J. Med., *31*, 766, 1961.
99. Singer, J. M. and Plotz, C. M.: Amer. J. Med., *21*, 888, 1956.
100. Steinberg, A. G.: in *Progress in Medical Genetics*, New York, Grune and Stratton, 1962, (Vol. 2), p. 1.
101. Steinberg, A. G.: Ann. Rev. Genetics, *3*, 25, 1969.
102. Steinberg, A. G. and Wilson, J. A.: Science, *140*, 303, 1963.
103. Svartz, N.: Ann. Rheum. Dis., *16*, 441, 1957.
104. Svec, K. H. and Dingle, J. H.: Arth. & Rheum., *8*, 524, 1965.
105. Tesar, J. T. and Schmid, F. R.: J. Immunol., *105*, 1206, 1970.
106. Thulin, K. E.: Acta Rheum. Scand., *1*, 22, 1955.
107. Torrigiani, G. and Roitt, I. M.: Ann. Rheum. Dis., *26*, 334, 1967.
108. Torrigiani, G., Roitt, I. M., Lloyd, K. N. and Corbett, M.: Lancet, *1*, 14, 1970.
109. Valentine, R. C. and Green, M.: J. Mol. Biol., *27*, 615, 1967.
110. Vaughan, J. H.: Arth. & Rheum., *6*, 437, 1963.
111. Vaughan, J. H. and Butler, V. P., Jr.: Ann. Intern. Med., *56*, 1, 1962.
112. Vaughan, J. H., Ellis, P. J. and Marshall, H.: J. Immunol., *81*, 261, 1958.
113. Waaler, E.: Acta Path. Microbiol. Scand., *17*, 172, 1940.
114. Wager, O.: Ann. Med. Exp. Biol. Fenn., (suppl. 8), *28*, 1, 1950.
114*a*. Waldmann, T. A., Johnson, J. S. and Talal, N.: J. Clin. Invest., *50*, 951, 1971.
115. Waller, M., Toone, E. C. and Vaughan, E. V.: Arth. & Rheum., *7*, 513, 1964.
116. Waller, M. V. and Vaughan, J. H.: Proc. Soc. Exp. Biol. Med., *92*, 198, 1956.
117. Williams, R. C., Jr.: Arth. & Rheum., *6*, 798, 1963.
118. ———: Arth. & Rheum., *7*, 368, 1964.
119. ———: in *Conference on the Immunologic Aspects of Rheumatoid Arthritis and Systemic Lupus Erythematosus*, New York, Grune and Stratton, 1963, p. 404.
120. Williams, R. C., Jr. and Kunkel, H. G.: Arth. & Rheum., *6*, 665, 1963.
121. ———: J. Clin. Invest., *41*, 666, 1962.
122. Winchester, R. J. and Agnello, V.: Pan Am. Congr. Rheum., Uruguay, Dec. 1970.
122*a*. Winchester, R. J., Agnello, V. and Kunkel, H. G.: Clin. Exp. Immunol., *6*, 689, 1970.
123. Ziff, M.: J. Chron. Dis., *5*, 644, 1957.
124. Zvaifler, N. J.: N. Y. Acad. Sci., *168*, 146, 1969.

Chapter 10

The L.E. Cell Phenomenon and Antinuclear Antibodies

By GEORGE J. FRIOU, M.D.

One of the most provocative observations in our knowledge of systemic lupus erythematosus (SLE) was made by Hargraves and his associates when they described the L.E. cell phenomenon in heparinized, incubated bone marrow from several patients with the disease.[59] This observation was confirmed,[66] and opened a field of investigation that attracted many other workers. An appreciation of the clinical significance of the L.E. cell phenomenon developed rapidly through a large number of reports which soon appeared in the literature. Curiosity about the mechanism of L.E. cell formation led to expanding knowledge of the immunologic nature of the phenomenon. We are now aware that the L.E. cell factor has the properties of an antibody to deoxyribonucleoprotein, and is one of a family of autoantibodies, occasionally found in human serums, which are directed against antigens of cell nuclei. The antinuclear antibody responsible for L.E. cell formation has not itself been clearly implicated in pathogenesis of lupus, although the possibility has not been excluded. The prevailing concept of the major cause of death in SLE, glomerulonephritis, is that it results from interaction and deposition of complexes of another of these antinuclear antibodies, anti-DNA, its antigen, and complement in the glomerulus. This development is attributable in large part to study of the L.E. cell phenomenon.

Steps in L.E. Cell Induction

The events following the additions of serum containing the L.E. cell factor to leukocytes have been studied in some detail.[50,57,117,120,121,135] In the initial phase of the reaction the factor must first gain contact with nucleoprotein of cell nuclei present in the preparation. The normal cell wall and nuclear membrane appear to be impervious to the gamma globulin factor, but when the cell is injured by physical, chemical, or mechanical means, antinucleoprotein may penetrate through to the nuclear material. Within a few seconds, the nucleus changes in appearance and the normal chromatin pattern of the nucleus is lost. Subsequently the mass takes a pale homogeneous purple staining property identical with that of the L.E. cell inclusion body. It has been shown by supravital stains, phase microscopy and the immunofluorescent technique[44,46,73] that gamma globulin is added to the nuclear material, and that the actual mass of the nucleus is increased.[117] As the damaged cell deteriorates the lobes of the nucleus are extruded to become free-lying, purplish, homogeneous masses. It has recently been shown that if complement is excluded from the reaction L.E. cells will still not be formed even though the serum factor is present. In the presence of complement the nuclear material,[51] previously coated with serum factor, is then phagocytized by an adjacent viable leukocyte to form the characteristic L.E. cell. None of these events or properties are exhibited following incubation of leukocytes with normal gamma globulin.

Nature of the L.E. Cell Inclusion

Both the hematoxylin body, found in the tissues of SLE patients, and the L.E. cell inclusion, have been shown to exhibit a positive Feulgen reagent staining reaction typical of DNA.[21,55,57,83,121,132] Both have other similarities indicating origin from nuclear material, and they are generally considered to be similar in origin. Both have been studied in attempting to expand our understanding of the L.E. cell phenomenon. On the basis of a loss of affinity for methyl-green staining of the hematoxylin body in the presence of a strongly positive Feulgen reaction, it was concluded by early workers that the DNA in the hematoxylin body was depolymerized.[55] Further studies[49,50] indicated that these staining reactions were due to a competition of the basic amino groups of the protein present with the methyl-green dye for binding sites on the DNA. Preliminary acetylation of the proteins restored the normal DNA staining reactions. Thus, it seems clear that depolymerization of DNA plays no essential role in the production of a hematoxylin body. It has been found that the hematoxylin body fails to stain with alkaline fast green, suggesting that the histone moiety of the nucleoprotein is either degraded, lost or masked in the process of hematoxylin body formation.[49,50] Other chemical analyses of the hematoxylin body indicate that it does not contain glycogen, lipids, acid or alkaline phosphatase.[28] Ultrastructural studies have been consistent with these observations, revealing the L.E. cell inclusion as densely homogeneous without recognizable internal structure,[95] surrounded by a single layered membrane.[143] All of these chemical and histological data are consistent with the concept that the L.E. cell inclusion material is deoxyribonucleoprotein and that the serum factor is an antibody to it.

Nature of the L.E. Cell Factor

In the performance of any of the tests for the presence of the L.E. factor, the only contribution that must be made by the patient is the specific serum factor. The factor has all the properties of an autoantibody directed against the deoxyribonucleoprotein component of cell nuclei. Various physical, chemical and immunologic techniques have clearly demonstrated the gamma globulin nature of the factor.[65,90] Absorption studies and the use of specific anti-gamma globulin immunofluorescent reagents have confirmed these observations.[46] Thus, absorption of L.E. serum with suspensions of cell nuclei resulted in removal of L.E. cell activity from the serum.[47,103] It has been shown that nuclei and nucleoprotein extracts from calf, rabbit, and other species are as effective as human cell nuclei[47,49] in absorbing L.E. factor from serum.

Specific immunological methods have demonstrated that in the formation of L.E. cells gamma globulin becomes bound to the nucleoprotein and fixation of complement (C) occurs.[47,72,73,127] Rapid formation of L.E. cells soon after blood is drawn is ample evidence that the factor can react with an individual's own nucleoprotein prior to any substantial degradation. This has also been demonstrated by the immunofluorescent technique. Thus, it is evident that this antibody to nucleoprotein behaves as an autoantibody. Although the species specificity possessed by classical artificially induced antibody is lacking, specificity based on chemical structure is present, and this is the nature of specificity common to all antibodies. When a foreign protein is introduced into an animal, the parts of the molecule recognizable by the recipient animal as different are structural details possessed only by the donor species, and antibody is therefore specific for those structures. Species differences in structure are not important in the origin of an autoantibody but other parts of the structure serve as specific antigenic determinants. The similarities of the L.E. cell factor to an autoantibody against nucleoprotein are, therefore, well substantiated.

L.E. factor has been identified in urine of patients with proteinuria,[80] pleural fluid,[152] and synovial fluid,[70] and can be transmitted across the placental barrier.[10,18] This distribution corresponds with that of an immunoglobulin of the IgG class. Earlier immunochemical studies indicated that the L.E. cell factor may have differences of structure[64] distinguishing it from other gamma globulins, but this has subsequently been shown not to be the case.[72,158] Study with the L.E. cell test technique revealed that the factor sediments along with the 7S gamma fraction (IgG) when examined in the ultracentrifuge,[39,73,158] and in a corresponding fraction after the use of column chromatography.[41,158] Most studies with immunological techniques for demonstration of antinulcear antibodies have confirmed the observation that the antibody is principally in the IgG class in most sera, but like most antibodies, antinucleoprotein as well as other antinuclear antibodies can also be of the IgM or IgA classes.[5,54] These antibodies are among the few to have been demonstrated in the IgD class.[119] There is some evidence[7] that antinuclear antibodies present in rheumatoid arthritis may more often be of the IgM class, the same immunoglobulin class in which the rheumatoid factors are principally found, whereas those in SLE are mainly IgG. Others have reported little correlation between immunoglobulin class of ANA and the clinical findings. Induction of L.E. cells has been shown to be inhibited by bacterial contamination, heating to 65° C., para-aminobenzoic acid,[61] excessive heparin,[62] atabrine,[34] and cold,[140] but it apparently is not influenced by cortisone, testosterone, estradiol, or progesterone.[61] Most of these substances appear to alter the part played by leukocytes in the reaction, rather than acting on the serum antibody itself.

Role of Complement (C) in L.E. Cell Induction

Accessory factors necessary for the L.E. phenomenon have been investigated. The importance of complement (C) in formation of L.E. cells has been documented in recent studies after earlier conflicting results.[1,42,55,90] Not all sera that contain antinucleoprotein antibody induce L.E. cells. It has been shown that those with antibody high in complement-fixing activity produce L.E. cells readily, while others with antibody low in complement-fixing activity do so less well.[111] Certain sera containing antinucleoprotein antibody fail to induce L.E. cells, but instead yield "globs" of extracellular material (ECM) which resemble the L.E. cell inclusions, but have not been phagocytized.[3,134] Study of circumstances leading to this phenomenon revealed that sera which produce L.E cells in the presence of C yield only ECM when all traces of C activity are carefully eliminated.[51] Thus, presence of C is necessary for the phagocytic step in formation of L.E. cells. IgM antibody to nucleoprotein does not activate C, and produces ECM without L.E cells. IgG antibody to nucleoprotein yields L.E. cells except when present in low concentration. Presumably at low concentrations of the nucleoprotein antigen activation of C does not take place. This finding is consistent with other studies showing that two closely spaced molecules of IgG reacted with antigen are necessary to initiate C activation. Reaction of the L.E. cell factor with nucleoprotein, and subsequent phagocytosis of the antibody-coated material by leukocytes, are therefore analogous to the sensitization of bacteria to phagocytosis by addition of C after reaction with them of specific antibody.

The observation that fixation of C occurs when the L.E. factor becomes associated with whole nuclei or with nucleoprotein[127] serves as a basis for one of the serological methods for the detection of antibody to nucleoprotein,[71,152] and provides further support for the view that the combination of L.E. factor and nucleoprotein is an antigen-antibody reaction.

Earlier unconfirmed experiments raised the possibility that there may be a substance associated with platelets which is necessary for the production of the L.E. cell phenomenon,[91] and that this substance may be related to thromboplastin-like activity. It is a common clinical observation, however, that individuals with SLE and marked thrombocytopenia may have a strongly positive L.E cell phenomenon.[29] The possible role of anticoagulants is of some importance. A positive L.E. preparation can be obtained with defibrinated[4] as well as clotted blood,[122,132] or in the presence of anticoagulants. Use of excessive amounts of anticoagulant is to be avoided, however, since this may inhibit the L.E. phenomenon.[72] In one large series,[60] there were no positive test results using clotted blood when the tests were not also positive with heparinized blood.

Technical Aspects of L.E. Cell Tests

Since the original descriptions of the L.E. cell,[59,66] a number of variations and modifications of the L.E. cell test have appeared (Table 10–1). The two most commonly used are the clot method[58,94,161] and the rotary glass bead method.[162] In a recent comparison between these techniques the rotary method was found to be of good sensitivity and suitability for a clinical screening test, yielding better cytology than the two hour clot test.[35] Regardless of the method used, the most important feature is a thorough and systematic search for typical phagocytic cells, paying strict attention to the characteristic morphology of the inclusion bodies. There is no doubt that meticulous care in carrying out the test, and examination of the test by an experienced observer result in a higher yield from patients known to have antinucleoprotein antibody present. Most hospital laboratories do not expend such a substantial effort, however.

Early observations on the demonstration of L.E. cells directly from the bone marrow and peripheral blood were not confirmed. Since that time, with rare exceptions,[159] it has been thought that L.E. cell formation is a phenomenon occurring only after at least a brief period of in-vitro incubation. The use of heparinized, incubated bone marrow samples to demonstrate L.E. cells proved to be an inconvenient method. It was soon determined that the nucleoprotein required as substrate for the

TABLE 10–1.—METHODS FOR THE DETECTION OF CIRCULATING L.E. CELL FACTOR BY PHAGOCYTIC TECHNIQUES

Author	*Nucleoprotein substrate*	*Anticoagulant*	*Source L.E. factor*	*Remarks*
Lee[89]	Patient leukocytes	Heparin	Pt. venous blood	Simple cell sedimentation technique
Hargraves[58]	Patient leukocytes	Clotted blood	Pt. venous blood	Clot passed through wire screen
Snapper[132]	Normal blood	Clotted blood	Finger tip or ear lobe	Ringed clot technique
Conley[162]	Patient leukocytes	Heparin	Pt. venous blood	Rotate with glass beads
Davis[31]	Normal blood	Heparin	Pt. venous blood	Cover slip technique
Teague[147]	Mouse leukocytes	Clotted blood	Mouse venous blood	Capillary micromethod

L.E. factor activity could be obtained from sources other than the patient's bone marrow. The patient's circulating blood, leukemic leukocytes, tumor cells and even bone marrow and peripheral blood cells from other species were found to contain satisfactory substrates.[4,13,40,52,66,88,105,107,141] Similarly, the source of viable phagocytes to complete the L.E. cell formation may be provided not only by other individuals, but by the peripheral blood and bone marrow of other species.

Since nucleoprotein must be made available for the action of the L.E cell factor, several methods have been devised to increase the amount of substrate present by inducing cell injury (see Table 10–1). This may be done by permitting heparinized blood to stand at room temperature,[87] by passing clotted blood through a wire screen,[132] rotation of heparinized blood with glass beads[162] or simply by permitting air drying of a smear of concentrated leukocytes.[31] Whatever the method of injury, the number of typical L.E cells is apt to be increased when a large amount of substrate is provided, and such methods have proven to be more effective. At the same time, with increased cell injury there is an increase in the number of bizarre cells in various stages of disintegration,[44] as well as the appearance of large amounts of extracellular material.

Some of the morphologic difficulty in identifying a true L.E. cell results from a number of commonly observed nonspecific cellular reactions to injury. Along with the initial description of the L.E. cell,[59] a somewhat similar phagocytizing histiocyte was observed called the "tart cell." Phagocytosis of nuclei, erythrocytes and platelets has been seen in a wide variety of illnesses, especially in allergic disorders.[100] Extracellular material may be seen in an L.E. cell preparation either as a consequence of cell disruption or as a result of spontaneously precipitating material in patients with abnormal serum proteins. The extracellular material may resemble free-lying hematoxylin bodies or, if phagocytized, a fully developed L.E. cell. In a true L.E. body, stain with the Feulgen reagent reveals the presence of DNA.[153]

As a result of our increased understanding of the process of L.E. cell formation, emanating from immunological studies, increased emphasis can be placed on the formation of masses of extracellular material having the morphological characteristics and staining reaction of the L.E. cell inclusion, even when phagocytosis has not occurred. Finding of such material may be interpreted as indicating presence of the specific antibody even when L.E. cells in such preparations result from failure of complement activation and consequent absence of phagocytosis. ECM alone may occur in SLE when the titer of antibody is low, as after treatment with large doses of corticosteroids.[134] It is observed most commonly when antinucleoprotein is present in other conditions, as in rheumatoid arthritis, and probably reflects differences in complement-fixing activity, or immunoglobulin class, as well as the low titers usually present in such patients. L.E.-like cells have been seen after treatment of leukocytes with heparin and with polyvinyl alcohol polysulfonic acid ester, but the preparations are actually artifacts unrelated to presence of any specific gamma globulin factor.

Introduction to the Immunofluorescent Technique[45]

In addition to the L.E. cell test a variety of serologic techniques have been used to detect antinuclear antibodies. Indirect immunofluorescence is the most widely utilized method for detection of antinuclear antibodies in clinical practice. There are also a number of other applications of the method in rheumatology. A description of the main features of this method is appropriate. In principle the method utilizes a fluorescent dye chemically linked to a specific antibody which reacts with, and thus marks the location of specific antigen in the substrate of tissue, a smear of cellular material, or a spot of purified material.

In the "indirect" technique for antinuclear antibodies the substrate is first flooded with the serum to be tested. Antinuclear antibodies, if present, bind to antigen in the cell nuclei. After washing, fluorescent anti-globulin is applied. If antinuclear antibodies were present in the serum, the antibody globulin already reacted with the cell nuclei then binds the fluorescent anti-globulin reagent and can be seen as bright nuclear fluorescence when examined under ultraviolet light with appropriate optics. A schematic representation of the steps in the procedure is shown in Figure 10–1.

The indirect immunofluorescent technique is applied in detection of a variety of anti-tissue antibodies. The direct technique is often applied in immunopathology to detect presence of deposited gamma globulin and complement in tissue.[76,99] In the direct technique a fluorescent-labeled antibody to gamma globulin or complement is applied directly to tissue, after preliminary washing to remove free serum proteins.

In all fluorescent antibody work, satisfactory results are obtained if proper attention is paid to the quality of the immunofluorescent reagents, particularly regarding specificity and titer of the antibody, and the amount of fluorescent label per protein molecule. Excessive fluorescent labeling results in preparations which are very nonspecific in their reactions. Use of proper controls, thorough washing, and an effective optical system are important. Results of tests for antinuclear antibodies can only be compared with other laboratories if careful attention has been given to standardization of technique. The author recommends preparations of cell nuclei which have been widely evaluated, such as sections of rat or mouse liver, smears of human peripheral blood leukocytes, or

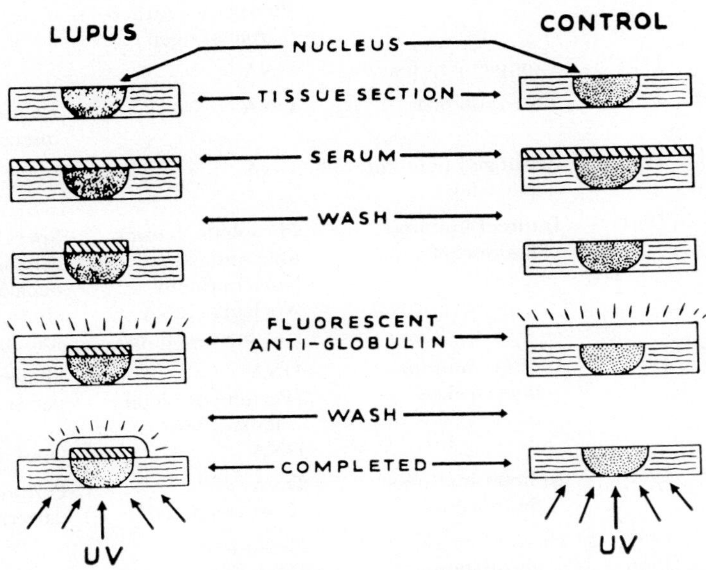

Fig. 10–1.—Principle of Indirect Immunofluorescent Tests for Antinuclear Antibodies. Steps in the procedure move sequentially downward in the figure. Antinuclear antibody, present in serum from an SLE patient, binds to nuclei in section, left, leaving an immunoglobulin coating. After thorough washing the preparation is incubated with fluorescent anti-human globulin which binds only where the antinuclear antibody had bound on incubation with serum. As a result, nuclei that had been exposed to the SLE serum fluoresce on examination under the fluorescence microscope while those incubated with the control (negative) serum do not.

spots of purified deoxyribonucleoprotein or DNA.[45]

Serologic Detection of the Various Antinuclear Antibodies

Discussion of the L.E. cell factor and antinuclear antibodies would not be complete without consideration of the diversity of serum antibodies which react with antigens of cell nuclei (see Table 10–2). Antinucleoprotein and anti-DNA both react with nuclear antigens containing DNA. A third rather commonly occurring factor reacts with a glycoprotein component of the cell nucleus not containing DNA.[71] The antigen is easily extractable from nuclei by saline or phosphate buffer, and by ultracentrifugation is a molecule of about 2.0 to 3.5 S. Ability of nuclei to bind this antibody in immunofluorescent tests is unaffected by

TABLE 10–2.—SEROLOGIC METHODS FOR DETECTION OF ANTINUCLEAR ANTIBODIES

Author	*Year*	*Procedure*	*Antigen*	*Comments*
Miescher[102]	1957	Antiglobulin consumption	Whole nuclei Nucleoprotein	
Friou[46,48]	1957	Indirect immunofluorescence	Whole nuclei Nucleoprotein	Nucleoprotein spot test
Holman[72]	1957	Complement fixation	Whole nuclei DNA Nucleoprotein Histone Phosphate extractable antigen	
Seligmann[127]	1958	Complement fixation	DNA	
Deicher[32]	1959	Precipitin test	DNA	Relatively insensitive
Bozicevich[16]	1960	Sensitized bentonite particles	DNA	
Beck,[8] Lachmann[84]	1961	Indirect immunofluorescence	Phosphate extractable antigen Nucleoprotein Nucleolar RNA (rat liver sections)	Speckled, homogeneous and nucleolar patterns of nuclear staining
Casals[23]	1963	Indirect immunofluorescence	DNA (Peripheral blood leukocytes) DNA	Shaggy nuclear pattern. DNA spot test
Gonzales[53]	1966	Indirect immunofluorescence	DNA (Liver sections)	Peripheral nuclear pattern
Levi,[92] Koffler[77]	1965 1966	Passive hemagglutination	Denatured DNA	
Wold[160]	1968	Ammonium sulfate method	Native DNA	
Benson[12]	1970	Horseradish peroxidase labelled antibody	Whole nuclei	Similar principle to indirect immunofluorescence

deoxyribonuclease or ribonuclease but is abolished by periodate treatment. The antibody has been detected by immunofluorescence and complement-fixation techniques. It occurs very regularly in serum of patients with SLE, along with antinucleoprotein. Recently the possibility has been raised that this type of antibody, as detected in a hemagglutination test may play a protective rather than a pathogenic role.[131] It has been reported most often without concomitant antinucleoprotein in serum from patients with various diseases, especially rheumatoid arthritis, Sjögren's syndrome, liver disease and ulcerative colitis.[9,84] The antibody does not react with nucleoprotein or DNA in serological tests, and is not absorbed from serum by these substances. Sera containing this antibody alone do not cause L.E. cell formation, even when present in high titer, as is often the case. In serum of SLE patients, simultaneous presence of antinucleoprotein often obscures the detection of this factor in immunofluorescent tests, except at higher dilutions.

Information on the nature of this antigen has been slow to appear. Initially it was referred to as the "phosphate extractable antigen."[72] Later an antigen with somewhat similar properties was described which has been referred to as Sm antigen.[146a] It has been realized for some time that there is a relationship between "phosphate extractable antigen," Sm antigen, and the antigen responsible for the speckled pattern of staining in indirect immunofluorescent tests for antinuclear antibodies. Quite recently characterization of this antigen has again been pursued, and the term "ENA" introduced to refer to a soluble nuclear antigen, which is related to the other extractable antigens referred to above[131] (antibody has been detected using antigen coated on tanned erythrocytes). Most recently ENA has been shown to consist of two distinct components, both causing speckled immunofluorescent staining,[108a] but separable by analysis in radial immunodiffusion. One is the Sm antigen, previously described, which appears to contain neither DNA nor RNA. Antibody is found chiefly in patients with systemic lupus erythematosus. The other antigen appears to be nuclear ribonucleoprotein (RNP). Antibodies to RNP appear in earliest reports to be especially associated with "mixed connective tissue diseases" and scleroderma, rather than more typical cases of systemic lupus with nephritis.[131a]

When the immunofluorescent technique is used to detect antinuclear antibodies, different patterns of binding fluorescent antiglobulin are seen with different sera, representing the several different antinuclear factors bound in the *in vitro* test to specific antigens in different patterns of localization in the nucleus (Figure 10–2). Different antibodies can, therefore, be distinguished by a careful observer when present separately.[8,48] Antinucleoprotein yields a characteristic "homogeneous" pattern, anti-DNA a pattern described as "shaggy," while a third factor yields a "speckled" pattern. The term "peripheral" has also been introduced to describe the pattern produced by anti-DNA.[53] The difference between "shaggy" and "peripheral" is attributable to differing substrates, the former term introduced in relation to preparations made with human peripheral blood leukocytes and the latter using sections of rat or mouse liver. A fourth factor detectable with the immunofluorescent technique reacts with a component localized in nucleoli. This factor is far less common than the others and has been reported to be especially associated with diffuse systemic sclerosis. An additional fifth factor, detected by complement fixation with histone, has been detected occasionally in SLE as well as serum from other types of patients.[73] This factor has not been shown to yield a recognizable pattern by the immunofluorescent technique. It has been shown that a pattern of immunofluorescent nuclear staining similar to that yielded by anti-DNA may also be produced by an antibody to a distinct soluble fraction

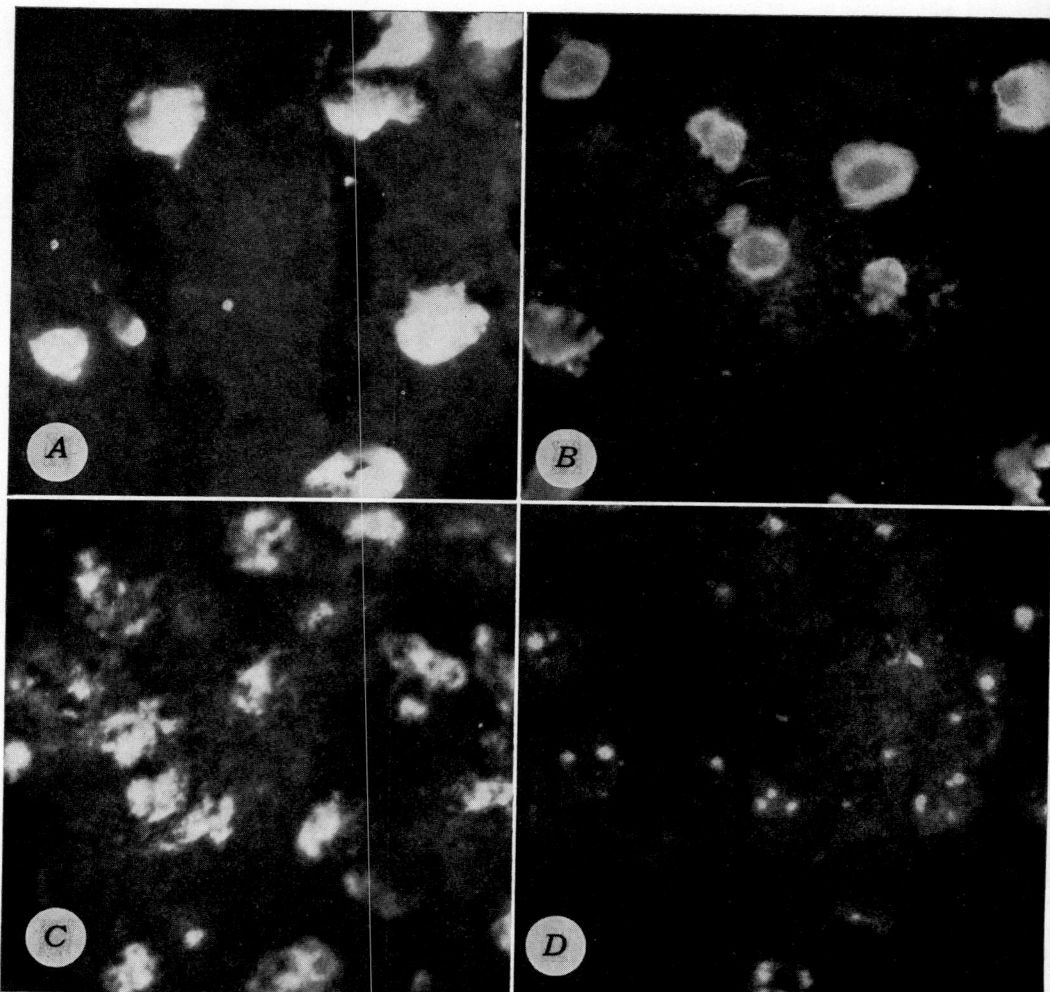

FIG. 10–2.—Patterns of immunofluorescent staining of nuclei produced by antinuclear antibodies (*A*) Homogeneous, (*B*) "peripheral or "shaggy, (*C*) "speckled, (*D*) nucleolar. Preparations consist of sections of rat liver processed in standard indirect immunofluorescent technique, using sera with antibodies of different reactivity. Identical magnifications. See text p. 179.

of desoxyribonucleoprotein (sNP antigen).[146b]

In most instances workers with the immunofluorescent technique have not distinguished the factors reacting with different nuclear antigens, reporting all observed nuclear fluorescence as simply indicating "antinuclear antibodies" or ANA. I have used the term "total ANA" to refer to such methods. Under these conditions, results of the immunofluorescent method yield the highest incidence of positive results in diseases other than SLE, since results include all of the different factors. Reports of occurrence of antinuclear antibodies in up to 50 per cent of patients with rheumatoid arthritis as well as a comparable per cent of patients with ulcerative colitis and other diseases are accounted for by this type of technique. Such reports do not reflect a correct relationship of antinuclear antibodies to L.E. cells, since some of the factors detected do not produce L.E. cells.

Reports have appeared indicating the occurrence of antinuclear antibodies in normal individuals.[118] When present such antibodies are usually detected in low titer. With the immunofluorescent technique as carried out with whole cell nuclei ("total ANA") the sensitivity is such that non-specific results may be obtained with apparent positive tests not always due to actual presence of antibody. Although reported results may be high there is no doubt that antinuclear antibodies do occur in some normal individuals. Other workers have reported an increasing incidence of antinuclear antibodies in the aged.[142] In my personal experience these antibodies in normal individuals and in the aged are directed against the so-called phosphate extractable antigen, rather than deoxyribonucleoprotein or DNA. Some normal relatives of patients with SLE do have antinucleoprotein antibody in their serum (Table 10–3).

An attempt can be made to distinguish the characteristic patterns of the different factors, but this may be difficult since several may be present simultaneously in a single serum. Immunofluorescent spot tests, using purified antigens, have been developed for detection of antinucleoprotein[44] and anti-DNA,[23] but a spot test is not available to detect antibody against the "speckled" or other antigens. Purified antigens have also been used in several other types of serologic tests (Table 10–2), including complement fixation,[71,127,152] antiglobulin consumption using nucleoprotein,[101] precipitin tests with DNA,[32] DNA coated bentonite particles,[16] passive hemagglutination, and ammonium sulfate precipitation.[20,77,92,160] A technique utilizing latex particles coated with an extract of nucleoprotein has not been adequately sensitive for satisfactory use as a diagnostic method. In interpreting results of studies of antinuclear antibodies an evaluation of the specificity and sensitivity of the method used is of paramount importance. Recently the use of horseradish peroxidase as an antibody label has been advocated as a substitute for fluorescein.[12] This label has the potential advantage of the use of an ordinary microscope instead of special fluorescence equipment. A substantial amount of work will be needed to evaluate such questions as sensitivity, and other important characteristics, in comparison with immunofluorescence. It appears likely that problems of nonspecific reactions and other details of the two methods may be similar.

TABLE 10–3.—RESULTS OF IMMUNOFLUORESCENT SPOT TEST FOR ANTINUCLEOPROTEIN ANTIBODY IN 493 PATIENTS

Diagnosis	*No. Tested*	*Positive*	*Per Cent Positive*	*High Titer*	*Low Titer*
SLE	53	52	98	42	10
Rheumatoid Arthritis	92	13	14	3	10
Acute Drug Hypersensitivity	19	3	16	0	3
Active Chronic Hepatitis	10	4	40	1	3
Dermatomyositis and Scleroderma	10	3	30	1	2
Necrotizing Vasculitis	8	2	25	0	2
Infections	87	4*	5	0	4
Healthy Relatives of SLE Patients	66	2	3	0	2
Glomerulonephritis	30	0	0	0	0
Acute Rheumatic Fever	16	0	0	0	0
Other Medical Patients	294	3†	1	0	3

* Two cases each of primary atypical pneumonia and active tuberculosis.
† One case of anaplastic carcinoma, two lymphoma.

CLINICAL SIGNIFICANCE OF L.E. CELLS AND ANTIBODY TO NUCLEOPROTEIN

Although most patients with SLE develop a positive result to an L.E. cell test at some time during the course of their disease, it is not uncommon to find a negative test result in an individual with otherwise well-documented disease. In such cases antibody to nucleoprotein is detectable in the serum by other methods. L.E. cells may be demonstrable for some time before other features of the disease become apparent. With increasing awareness of the natural history of SLE, it has become obvious that a single negative test result for L.E. cells is of no particular significance. There is only a very general relationship between the severity of the disease manifestations, the response to therapy employed, and the presence or absence of L.E cells.[123]

When the test result has been found to be negative, it has been the practice to repeat it frequently if the clinical situation warrants, because the technique may fail under conditions when it should obviously be positive. In accordance with our present knowledge, a better practice in such a patient would be to test the serum for antinucleoprotein by one of the serological methods, and thus make a definite determination of the presence or absence of the antibody.[23,44,124,152] Standard L.E. cell techniques are simpler than serological techniques, but the serological tests have the advantage of consistency because the antibody titer changes slowly and is seldom negative in active SLE. In the patient with a negative result of an L.E. cell test and otherwise well documented SLE, a serologic test would confirm the presence of antibody.

In most series of cases studied, the incidence of positive test results among patients with SLE varies up to about 80 per cent when using a standard L.E. cell test method. Serologic tests reveal that antinucleoprotein is almost invariably present in the serum in active SLE, and test results of this type are, therefore, almost invariably positive. During periods of remission antinucleoprotein antibody tends to be lower in titer, or may rarely be absent, while during increased clinical activity titers tend to be higher. During corticosteroid therapy with large doses, titers usually fall, and the results may become negative at such times.[23] There are considerable individual differences in these correlations, however, and the relationship of titer to clinical activity is not sufficient to suggest that antinucleoprotein plays any direct role in causation of the acute manifestations of the disease.[23,44,152] The occurrence of a negative L.E. cell test result in SLE may be due to absence of the serum factor when this occurs after a few weeks of treatment with corticosteroids, but otherwise negative L.E. cell test results in acute SLE are unexplained, although impaired phagocytic activity has been reported and could explain the failure of L.E. cell formation at such times.

Among the sporadic case reports describing a positive L.E. cell preparation in patients thought not to have SLE are individuals with rheumatoid arthritis, other connective tissue diseases, allergic disorders,[100,110] skin disease,[96] hepatitis[14] or hematologic diseases. In general, antinucleoprotein antibody has been demonstrated in all clinical situations in which bona fide L.E. cells have been reported. Observations on the occurrence of antinucleoprotein in medical patients are summarized in Table 10–3. In each case the incidence has been significantly higher than the reported incidence of positive L.E. cells. This may be explained by the observation that when antinucleoprotein occurs in these other conditions it is most often of low titer, or of low complement-fixing activity, and therefore less likely to yield positive L.E. cell preparations. Antinucleoprotein antibody is rarely seen in other types of medical patients. For this reason, coupled with its almost universal occurrence in SLE, demonstration of the absence of this factor in an untreated patient where SLE is suspected constitutes strong evidence against SLE. Since negative L.E. test results can occur when antinucleoprotein is present, a negative result of L.E. cell test does not exclude the presence of antibody nor the diagnosis of SLE.

Interpretation of serologic studies in conditions other than SLE have been complicated by the use in many studies of methods which detect, without distinction, several different antinuclear antibodies simultaneously. This is true when preparations containing whole cell nuclei are used in immunofluorescent tests or other methods, and no attempt is made to distinguish antibodies to different nuclear antigens. Antibody to a phosphate-extractable antigen of nuclei occurs commonly in a variety of situations and when no attempt is made to distinguish different activities, a high incidence of antinuclear antibodies is observed. This factor as well as others have quite different implications, and, where possible, a distinction should be made. This is especially true when consideration is being given to the possibility of an immunological overlap with SLE, since antinucleoprotein is characteristic of lupus and only this antibody has been demonstrated to participate in L.E. cell formation.

One of the more common situations in which L.E. cell tests are found, associated with a condition other than SLE, is in patients with rheumatoid arthritis. Sera of these patients have been studied with immunofluorescence and other serological tests, and antinucleoprotein antibody has been found, usually in low titer. Antinucleoprotein is also seen in serum of some patients with dermatomyositis and scleroderma. In rheumatoid arthritis the occurrence of L.E. cells, or of antinucleoprotein antibody in low titer, seen in about 15 per cent of cases, does not usually seem to correlate with any other features, such as severity of the disease or occurrence of complications, nor does it serve to predict their future occurrence with regularity.[44,69,151,154] On the other hand, a few patients are seen who show arthritis indistinguishable from rheumatoid arthritis, high titers of antinucleoprotein, and findings indistinguishable from SLE.[81] Demonstration of this serological overlap between SLE, rheumatoid arthritis[68] and certain other "connective tissue" diseases, tends to confirm the earlier descriptions of overlapping clinical findings and point to a fundamental relationship between these conditions.

Similarly, in liver disease, the earlier reports of positive L.E. cell test results have been followed by demonstration of the presence of antinucleoprotein in the serum. This has been seen especially in young females, who also may have coincidental ulcerative colitis, high levels of serum gamma globulin, abundance of plasma cells in the hepatic tissue, a high incidence of arthralgia and arthritis, and other features also seen in SLE. Patients with this syndrome of "lupoid hepatitis" have been considered by some to show a true clinical overlap with SLE.[93] Most workers, while not denying a possible role of immunologic mechanisms in progressive liver disease, take the view that occurrence of L.E. cells, or antinucleoprotein antibody, in these cases does not imply a close relationship to systemic lupus.[74] Occasional patients with acute infectious hepatitis also have antinucleoprotein in their serum.

Antinuclear antibodies specific for the nucleoprotein of polymorphonuclear leukocytes have been identified especially in the serum of patients with rheumatoid arthritis.[37a] This is a unique type of antinuclear antibody, since others are lacking in organ or tissue specificity. Recently, antibodies of this type have been demonstrated in lysates of leukocytes from synovial effusions of subjects with inflammatory arthritis, especially rheumatoid arthritis.[163] Antibodies were sometimes present in synovial fluid when absent from the serum. It has also been observed that synovial fluid of patients with rheumatoid arthritis may contain small amounts of soluble nucleoprotein antigen (sNP) or antibody to it.[120a] These findings suggest the possibility that complexes of antinuclear antigens and antibodies may play a role in the synovial inflammation in rheumatoid arthritis. Further evaluation of these findings is indicated.

Antinuclear Antibodies Induced by Medications

One of the most interesting instances of the occurrence of L.E. cells is among patients being treated with one of several drugs. Induction of antinuclear antibodies by drugs is of considerable interest as a potential lead to understanding the nature of the antigen active in lupus, but the mechanism is not yet understood. Drug-induced L.E. cells and antinuclear antibodies were first reported in patients with hypertension receiving high dosages of hydralazine.[37,102,112] In some instances a clinical picture similar to that of SLE may develop (*see* drug-induced lupus, Chapter 51). The clinical symptoms and the positive L.E. preparation subside following withdrawal, except in occasional cases where pre-existing lupus appears to have been activated by the drug. This observation led to a more extensive testing of patients receiving hydralazine therapy and individuals were found who had a positive L.E. cell preparation at a time when they were without symptoms.[37,108] A single autopsied human case of delayed hydralazine toxicity showed histologic findings compatible with SLE.[30] Antinucleoprotein has been demonstrated in serum of such cases.[44] Early reports of reproduction of this phenomenon in animals have not been substantiated.[17,30]

Another example of drug-induced antinuclear antibodies is those which occur in patients receiving procainamide for cardiac arrhythmias.[15] Up to 75 per cent of such patients develop antibodies to nucleoprotein, and a substantial number of these also have antibodies to DNA.[106] These antibodies are low in complement-fixing activity when compared with those in lupus nephritis,[150] and there is evidence that the anti-DNA antibodies are mainly against denatured DNA.[116] Very few of these patients develop lupus-like symptoms, those that do rarely manifest renal involvement (*see* drug-induced lupus, Chapter 51), and the serological and clinical features clear when procainamide is discontinued.

Recent reports have added oral contraceptive drugs to the list of medications inducing antinuclear antibodies.[75,125] This is an observation of considerable potential importance in view of the widespread use of these agents. In my laboratory antinucleoprotein and anti-DNA were not observed to occur.[36] Induction of SLE has not been reported, but the full significance of these observations remains to be more fully evaluated.

Occurrence of positive L.E. cells and antinucleoprotein antibody in patients with acute hypersensitive reactions to drugs is of interest because such reactions are known to serve as the event precipitating the onset of SLE. In most patients with drug reactions that have been studied, the antibody has appeared as a transient event during a notably severe reaction, and clears with recovery.[44]

Characteristics of Antibody to DNA

An antinuclear antibody of particular importance in SLE is an autoantibody to deoxyribonucleic acid (DNA) rather than deoxyribonucleoprotein. This is of special theoretical interest because DNA was long thought to be non-antigenic. The DNA used in the reaction may be prepared from calf thymus, fish sperm, bacteriophage, bacteria, or human nuclei. *In vitro* precipitation, complement fixation, immunofluorescent, passive hemagglutination, and other immunological reactions have been observed,[20,23,73,77,92,127,160] between DNA and SLE sera. Typical lines of precipitate are seen in immunodiffusion experiments with highly purified DNA. Quantitative precipitin curves similar to those obtained with other antigen-antibody systems can be prepared.[32,128]

Passive cutaneous anaphylaxis can be demonstrated.[33] In this test, tiny amounts of antibody injected into guinea pig skin sensitize the area. When small amounts of DNA are injected intravenously along with Evans blue dye, localized increase in vascular permeability in a positive test result causes blue staining around the injection site in the skin. Demonstration that anti-DNA can induce passive cutaneous anaphlyaxis is important because the reaction is a classic immunological method and the observation, therefore, provides strong support for the antibody nature of the anti-DNA factor. Anti-DNA has been shown to be capable of reacting with a patient's own DNA.[23] It is absorbed from serum along with antinucleoprotein when exposed to nucleoprotein, but when DNA is added to serum, anti-DNA activity is inhibited whereas antinucleoprotein remains.[22,32] Anti-DNA exhibits negligible or no capacity to induce L.E. cells and DNA has no inhibitory action on L.E. cell formation by antinucleoprotein.[73,127] DNAase digestion prevents the reaction of both factors.

The overall conclusion reached from these absorption and inhibition studies is that anti-DNA reacts with DNA whether free or combined with protein, whereas antinucleoprotein reacts with DNA only when in combination with histone, possibly because certain specific sites on the DNA molecule are exposed only under such conditions. Critical investigation of the specificity of the reaction of lupus sera with DNA has revealed that some sera react with native (double stranded) DNA only, some with both native and denatured DNA, and some with denatured DNA (single stranded) only.[2,128,129,130,136] Antibodies to denatured DNA exhibit considerable heterogeneity in reactivity against specific determinants in the single stranded DNA molecule.[137,138,139] In at least some sera a single antibody is apparently reactive against both single and double stranded material since a line of identity between them is seen in immunodiffusion experiments.[144]

Many patients with SLE do not exhibit anti-DNA in their serum, and therefore, tests for it have little value in excluding the diagnosis. On the other hand, it is seldom seen in rheumatoid arthritis and other conditions and is, therefore, highly specific for SLE when it does occur. More recently, newer techniques have revealed that antibody to denatured DNA does occur with some regularity in other conditions, but antibody to native DNA is restricted to SLE. Impressive correlations between antibody to native DNA and acute SLE are seen, and this factor is seldom absent from the serum during acute exacerbations.[23,128]

Detailed clinical studies have revealed striking correlations between appearance of anti-DNA in the serum, reductions in the serum complement value[152] and occurrence of active lupus with nephritis. Determinations of anti-DNA and serum complement have now become established as guides in management of the disease and the response to corticosteroid therapy.[126]

Pathogenic Significance of Antibodies to DNA

Investigators studying antinuclear antibodies, including anti-DNA, have generally considered two possible types of mechanisms whereby these antibodies might contribute to pathogenesis of tissue damage. One possibility was that the antibodies were in themselves directly cytotoxic, or implicated by some other direct mechanism; however, antinuclear antibodies fail to cross cell membrane barriers, and appear incapable of reaching the location of the nuclear antigen within the cell.[155] Serum containing these factors fails to affect the growth of cells in tissue culture.[155] Further evidence against direct action was the fact that newborn infants of mothers with SLE are usually unaffected even though the L.E. factor is demonstrable in their blood.[10,18] Transfer of SLE serum to healthy recipients has not transmitted the disease.[11] Actually, only a very general correlation exists between levels of antibody to nucleoprotein and disease activity, and patients may have high titers of this antibody without evidence of acute disease.[44,152] These observations caused some to view antinuclear antibodies as phenomena of purely secondary significance in SLE.

Considerable evidence has now accumulated in support of an alternative mechanism of involvement of antinuclear antibodies, especially DNA, in immune tissue damage. It is felt that immune complexes of DNA, anti-DNA and complement, deposit in the glomerulus and in small vessels, and cause damage through mechanisms involving complement activation.[78] Early observers had noted a similarity between some of the clinical features of SLE and human serum sickness. Following elucidation of the immunological aspects of foreign protein disease in rabbits,[97] the experimental counterpart of human serum sickness, evidence developed that there were further parallels between this condition and SLE. In addition to the association of occurrence of anti-DNA with acute SLE and active nephritis,[23,128,152] DNA was also demonstrated in the serum at such times.[145] Especially significant was the demonstration by immunofluorescence of deposits of gamma globulin and complement components in renal glomeruli affected by lupus nephritis,[76,99] and small vessels in which changes of lupus vasculitis were present.[99] DNA has also been demonstrated to be present in the same location.[19] In addition, by electron microscopy presence of amorphous masses of material was demonstrable along the basement membrane of glomerular capillaries.[26,27] All of these changes are strikingly similar to the electron microscopic and immunofluorescent findings in the experimental disease in rabbits. Using immunochemical methods which had succeeded in the animal model, several workers have recovered gamma globulin from the kidneys of patients dying of SLE and have shown that it consisted in large part of antinuclear antibodies, chiefly anti-DNA.[43,79,82]

The evidence cited above appears to clearly implicate complexes of DNA-anti-DNA in lupus nephritis, but their exact role remains unclear. The evidence is so far indirect, and one may only say that presence of DNA in the serum is associated with active renal disease and presence of complexes in the kidney. Actual complexes of DNA with anti-DNA have not been demonstrated in the serum. Furthermore, in addition to anti-DNA, antibodies to several other antinuclear and antitissue antibodies have been eluted from the kidney,[79,82] and none of these have been demonstrated in the serum as complexes. Finally, there is a type of complex, the mixed cryoglobulins, which contain immunoglobulins and complement and which regularly occur in serum during the acute SLE. Although some have reported presence of anti-DNA in these complexes, most workers feel that they do not contain anti-DNA.[6,56,133] This failure to demonstrate complexes in the serum causes one to consider the possibility that the autoantibodies which can be eluted from the kidney did not arrive there as preformed complexes from the serum but have been trapped there on reacting with antigens of degenerating leukocytes, already in the kidney as a result of a more primary pathogenic process. The DNA-anti-DNA complexes formed might be unimportant, or they could markedly accentuate the earlier inflammatory process through an "Arthus" type of immune mechanism.

Origin of Antinuclear Antibodies

A great deal of interest and effort has been devoted to the question of the nature and origin of the antinuclear antibodies, as well as the actual role they may play in the disease process. There was at first some hesitancy in accepting the idea that these factors are indeed true antibodies, but the accumulated information is convincing. Their autoimmune nature seems demonstrated by the capacity to react with the individual's own nuclear antigens. The nature of the original antigenic stimulus becomes an especially important consideration in resolving the question of the primary pathogenic mechanism in SLE.

One mechanism which might be proposed is that nuclear antigens lie in a sheltered location where they would not have had contact during development with the immunological "stock taking" mechanism. This possibility is hard to accept in view of the close proximity of DNA to protein synthesizing mechanisms, as well as the abundance of nuclear material which is released during cell destruction in disease as well as normal cell turnover. One might propose that a hypothetical normal clearing mechanism which prevents nuclear material from reaching immunological tissue is impaired in SLE. However, no such abnormality has been demonstrated, and the frequent occurrence of autoantibodies to other unrelated tissue substances remains unexplained by such a proposal. It has also been suggested that the disease results from appearance of a new clone of antibody-producing cells which, through mutation, fails to recognize endogenous DNA as "self," and therefore responds with an immune response as if it were an exogenous antigen. Introduction of non-tolerant cells in experimental animals results in loss of tolerance, and mutant cell lines appearing in immunological tissues might behave in a similar fashion. This concept, like that above, fails to explain the multitude of autoantibodies seen in SLE. One might attempt to explain this feature by proposing that a whole series of mutations were taking place, but this is biologically very unlikely. Furthermore, the heterogeneity of the antinuclear antibodies is not consistent with this possibility. A single mutant clone would produce an antibody population uniform in its antigen specificity and immunoglobulin class, and possessing light chains of a single type, kappa or lambda. Study of antinuclear antibodies has found them to be polyclonal in origin by each of these criteria.

Some autoantibodies seem to result because the particular antigenic component did not appear until after the critical period of early immunological "stock taking" had passed. Antigens not present during this early period would be reacted to as if foreign when encountered later in life. This mechanism could obviously only apply to DNA if changes were to occur in somatic DNA structure during life which would cause it to be recognized as foreign to the immune tissue. This could occur as a result of mutation, the result of introduction of viral genome, degradation, denaturation or other changes in the molecule. Particularly interesting, in view of the longstanding clinical observation of exacerbation of SLE by sun exposure, is the demonstration that ultraviolet irradiation causes structural changes in DNA which are antigenic in animals.[146]

Such antibody would at first be reactive chiefly with the new antigenic structures. This interesting concept finds some support from studies on the termination of artificially induced immunological tolerance.[112] It is also consistent with experimental attempts to produce antinuclear antibodies in which guinea pigs,[77] or rabbits[20] were immunized with various antigens, all containing nucleoprotein or DNA from one source or another. Following hyperimmunization of rabbits with *B. subtilis*, with injection of organisms several times per week for many months, anti-DNA appeared in the serum. In sequence in these animals there appeared first agglutinating antibodies to *B. subtilis*, then antibody to denatured gamma globulin indistinguishable from rheumatoid factor, and finally antibodies to denatured DNA.[25] The association of anti-DNA with another autoantibody (rheumatoid factor) is somewhat parallel with the occurrence of a variety of other autoantibodies in SLE, as well as the spontaneous occurrence of antibodies to denatured tissue antigens in experimental animals.[157] Other investigators demonstrated that antibodies to denatured DNA could be induced rather readily under appropriate conditions.[115] In these experiments DNA was considered as a "hapten." This immunological term refers to a substance which only elicits antibodies when given bound to a foreign "carrier" protein molecule. When DNA was bound to methylated bovine serum albumin, rabbits readily made antibody to it, whereas when given alone the DNA was a poor antigen. The antibody formed was reactive with denatured, but not native, DNA. As indicated earlier, antibodies to both native and denatured DNA occur in SLE, but recently antibody to denatured DNA has been demonstrated to occur relatively often in a variety of chronic inflammatory diseases. The high frequency of occurrence of antinuclear antibodies, as well as antibody to DNA in patients receiving procainamide, is very relevant to these considerations. One third of these individuals developed antibody to DNA.[106] This was directed against denatured DNA in those investigated.[116] This clearly revealed that many, or perhaps all, individuals are capable of producing this type of antibody. On the basis of these clinical and experimental observations, antibody to denatured DNA can be viewed as relatively easily induced by a variety of stimuli, such as long continued inflammatory states where DNA degradation may be occurring, including SLE.

Antibody to native DNA has not been induced experimentally by hyperimmunization nor does it occur in human diseases other than SLE. This suggests that some other mechanism may exist whereby native DNA becomes immunogenic in SLE. The mechanism involved may well be that of "antigenic cross reaction." It is a fundamental immunological principle that antibody produced initially reacts to specific portions of a molecule, such as might be exposed in denatured DNA, or to viral DNA. With continued immunization, antibody of wider reactivity appears with specificity for additional, adjacent portions of the molecule. It is established that genetic control of the response to certain antigens is linked to genes controlling histocompatibility antigens in animals.[97a] Reports of association of HL-A W15 histocompatibility antigen with SLE suggest a possible genetically determined immune variation in that disease.[54a] Conceivably many humans produce antibody to alterations in DNA structure, but only a small portion of the population, possibly as a result of genetic predisposition, makes antibody which cross reacts with adjacent portions of the native DNA molecule. Appearance of antibody reactive with native DNA in this way could provide the basis for the serologic findings and immune complex nephritis and vasculitis of SLE. This concept would require that the SLE patient have a primary source of some type of altered DNA plus some type of difference in immune responsiveness.

An inbred strain of mice (NZB) has been reported which spontaneously develops autoimmune hemolytic anemia with high frequency. When these animals are crossed with the NZW strain the F_1 generation develops a disease which bears a striking relationship to human SLE.[67] Antinuclear antibodies, including DNA, appear, and the animals develop fatal glomerulonephritis (Figure 10-3). During the course of the nephritis serum complement levels are low, study of the kidneys reveals deposition of gamma globulin, complement and DNA, and anti-DNA can be eluted from renal tissue by methods similar to those used in human SLE.[85,48a] An interesting additional finding has been the demonstration of a chronic viral infection in these animals.[98] It has been reported that antibody to viral capsid antigens appears in serum at about the same time as anti-DNA, and recovery of antiviral antibody from the kidney has been reported.[33a] Relationship of the viral infection to the lupus-like disease has not been clarified, but the suspicion that a latent or hidden virus mechanism is a primary process in human SLE is increased by these obser-

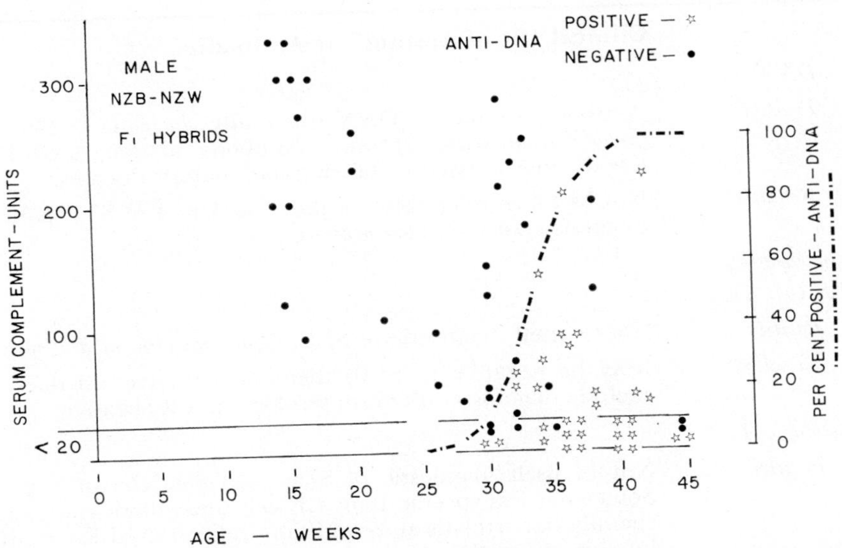

FIG. 10–3.—Anti-DNA in NZB/NZW mice, an experimental model for SLE. Relationship of age, presence of anti-DNA, and serum hemolytic complement values. Each point represents a single anti-DNA determination (●-positive, ✶-negative), and its vertical position indicates complement value on that day. Broken line represents cumulative per cent of positive anti-DNA tests according to age. Deaths from glomerulonephritis begin to occur soon after anti-DNA appears in serum. The immunological features of these animals bear a striking resemblance to human SLE. See text p. 188.

vations. Recent findings in SLE have further stirred this interest. On examination of renal glomeruli by electron microscopy, peculiar intracellular filamentous structures have been seen in endothelial cells which have been thought by some to resemble viral inclusions.[109] Considerable caution in interpreting this finding is indicated since there is no direct evidence indicating the viral nature of the inclusions, and there are many other possible explanations. Because of the possible resemblance of these inclusions to myxovirus, one group of workers compared titers of anti-measles antibodies in patients with SLE and controls and found significantly higher titers in the former.[113] Subsequently, SLE sera have been reported to have higher titers to several viruses when compared with controls.[38] In addition it has been shown that anti-measles antibody titers of both groups are more closely related to total gamma globulin levels than to diagnosis.[114] Thus the data, while raising the suspicions initially of chronic viral infection, now appear to raise again the question of underlying immunologic abnormality.

Certain other strains of inbred mice, including the A/J strain, develop antinuclear antibodies with increasing frequency with age.[147] Although the occurrence is relatively benign, since the animals seldom develop nephritis, the cause of the occurrence of the antibodies is of considerable interest. Thymic function appears to play a significant role, since the antibodies appear at an earlier age after thymectomy,[149] and appearance is delayed by introducing thymic cells from very young animals of the same inbred strain of animals.[148] Thus there is the suggestion that the immunologic function of the thymus may be a significant factor in determining the appearance of the antibodies. It has recently been suggested that increased susceptibility to viral infection resulting from deficiency of cell-mediated immunity of thymus

Clinical Use of Antinuclear Antibodies

Anti-DNA[1]	
Positive	Antibody to native DNA essentially *diagnostic.* Indicates *probability of active nephritis.* Antibody to denatured DNA less diagnostic, seen in other inflammatory diseases.
Negative	Not useful in diagnosis—negative in ½ to ⅓ of SLE patients. Suggests *absence of active nephritis.*
Antinucleoprotein	
LE Cell Test	
Positive	Not in itself diagnostic of SLE. *Confirms clinical diagnosis.*
Negative	May be negative in SLE, therefore negative test does not exclude diagnosis. Perform serologic test if negative.
Serologic Test[2]	
Positive	Not in itself diagnostic of SLE. *Confirms clinical diagnosis.* Somewhat less specific than LE cell test – more common in rheumatoid arthritis and conditions related to SLE. Positives infrequent in other medical conditions.
Negative	Rarely if ever negative except after long high dose steroids. *Negative result strongly against SLE diagnosis.* Repeat only if laboratory error suspected.
Total ANA[3]	
Positive	Not strongly confirmatory. Positives relatively common in variety of chronic diseases and in the aged.
Negative	Rarely if ever negative except after long high dose steroids. *Negative result strongly against SLE diagnosis.* Repeat only if laboratory error suspected.

1 Tests using pure DNA as antigen; also shaggy or peripheral immunofluorescent patterns.
2 Tests using deoxyribonucleoprotein as antigen; also homogeneous immunofluorescent pattern.
3 Tests using whole nuclei without distinguishing antigens or patterns.

origin allows added exposure to viral antigens[86] and consequent antigenic stimulation.

In considering the evidence on the origin of anti-DNA in SLE there appear to be two main themes whose exact roles are so far unresolved. Evidence is indirect, but there is a suggestion that a chronic or latent infection, possibly viral, might be the primary process and source of the antigenic stimulus for auto-antibody production. There are also recurring hints that some type of immunologic variable or abnormality may be involved, possibly determined by genetic factors. A derangement of early cellular mechanisms of the immune response might initiate a chronic inflammatory state which could also provide the necessary antigenic stimulus. Presence of a chronic viral infection in itself might be a result of an immunologic abnormality. Obviously further studies will be needed to fully resolve these interesting and important questions.

(*The assistance of Dr. Francisco Quismorio in the preparation of this chapter is gratefully acknowledged.*)

BIBLIOGRAPHY

1. Aisenberg, A. C.: J. Clin. Invest., *38*, 325, 1959.
2. Arana, R. and Seligmann, M.: J. Clin. Invest., *46*, 1867, 1967.
3. Arterberry, J. D., Drexler, E. and Dubois, E. L.: J.A.M.A., *187*, 389, 1964.
4. Barnes, S. S., Moffatt, T. W. and Weiss, R. S.: J. Invest., Dermat., *14*, 397, 1950.
5. Barnett, E. V., Condemi, J. J., Leddy, J. R. and Vaughan, J. H.: J. Clin. Invest., *43*, 1104, 1964.
6. Barnett, E. V., Kantor, G., Bickel, Y., Forsen, R. and Gonick, H. C.: Calif. Med., *111*, 467, 1969.
7. Baum, J. and Ziff, M.: Arth. and Rheum., *5*, 636, 1962 (abstract).
8. Beck, J. S.: Lancet, *1*, 1203, 1961.
9. Beck, J. S., Anderson, J. R., Bloch, K. J., Bunim, J. J. and Buchanan, W. W.: Ann. Rheum. Dis., *24*, 16, 1965.
10. Beck, J. S. and Rowell, N. R.: Lancet, *1*, 134, 1963.
11. Bencze, G., Cserhati, S., Kovacs, J. and Tiboldi, T.: Ann. Rheum. Dis., *17*, 426, 1958.
12. Benson, M. D. and Cohen, A. S.: Ann. Intern. Med., *73*, 943, 1970.
13. Berman, L., Axelrod, A. R., Goodman, H. L. and McClaughry, R. I.: Amer. J. Clin. Path., *20*, 403, 1950.
14. Bettley, F. R.: Lancet, *2*, 269, 1955.
15. Blomgren, S. E., Condemi, J. J., Bignall, M. C., and Vaughan, J. H.: New Engl. J. Med., *281*, 64, 1969.
16. Bozicevich, J., Nasov, J. P. and Kahoe, D. E.: Proc. Soc. Exper. Biol. Med., *103*, 636, 1960.
17. Braverman, I. M. and Lerner, A. B.: J. Invest. Derm., *30*, 317, 1962.
18. Bridge, R. G. and Foley, F. E.: Amer. J. Med. Sci., *227*, 1, 1954.
19. Browne, J. T., Hutt, M. P., Regers, J. F. and Smith, S. W.: Arth. & Rheum., *6*, 599, 1963.
20. Burns, R. M. and Rheins, M. S.: Proc. Soc. Exp. Biol. Med., *122*, 714, 1966.
21. Carrera, A. E., Swid, M. V. and Kurnick, N. B.: Blood, *9*, 1165, 1954.
22. Casals, S. P., Friou, G. J. and Teague, P. O.: J. Lab. Clin. Med., *62*, 625, 1963.
23. Casals, S. P., Friou, G. J. and Myers, L. L.: Arth. and Rheum., *7*, 379, 1964.
24. Christian, C. L., DeSimone, A. R. and Abruzzo, J. L.: Arth. and Rheum., *6*, 766, 1963.
25. Christian, C. L., DeSimone, A. R. and Abruzzo, J. L.: J. Exp. Med., *121*, 309, 1965.
26. Churg, J., Mautner, W., Grishman, E. and Eisner, G. M.: Arch. Intern. Med., *109*, 97, 1962.
27. Comerford, F. R. and Cohen, A. S.: Medicine, *46*, 425, 1967.
28. Damashek, W. and Bloom, M. L.: Blood, *5*, 101, 1950.
29. Dameshek, W., Rubio, F., Mahoney, J. P., Reeves, W. H. and Burgin, L. A.: J.A.M.A., *166*, 1805, 1958.
30. Dammin, G. J., Nora, J. R. and Reardan, J. B.: J. Lab. Clin. Med., *46*, 806, 1955.
31. Davis, B. J., and Eisenstein, R. J.: J. Mt. Sinai Hosp., *24*, 580, 1957.
32. Deicher, H., Holman, H. R. and Kunkel, H. G.: J. Exp. Med., *109*, 97, 1959.
33. Deicher, H., Holman, H. R., Kunkel, H. G. and Ovary, Z.: J. Immunol., *84*, 106, 1960.

33*a*. Dixon, F. J., Oldstone, M. B. A. and Tonietti, G.: J.E.M., *6*, 65s, 1971.

34. DuBois, E. L.: Arch. Dermat. & Syph., *71*, 570, 1955.
35. DuBois, E. L.: *Lupus Erythematosus*. New York, McGraw-Hill Book Co., 1966, p. 302.
36. DuBois, E. L., Strain, L., Ehn, M., Bernstein, G. and Friou, G. J.: Lancet, *2*, 679, 1968.
37. Dustan, H. P., Taylor, R. D., Corcoran, A. C. and Page, I. H.: J.A.M.A., *154*, 23, 1954.

37*a*. Elling, P.: Ann. Rheum. Dis., *27*, 406, 1968.

38. Evans, A. S., Niederman, J. C. and Rothfield, N. F.: Arth. and Rheum., *14*, 160, 1971 (abstract).
39. Fallet, G. H., Lospalluto, J. and Ziff, M.: Arth. and Rheum., *1*, 419, 1958.
40. Finch, S. C., Ross, J. F. and Ebaugh, F. G.: J. Lab. Clin. Med., *42*, 555, 1953.
41. Fisher, G. S. and Moyer, J. B.: Bull. Detroit, Mich. Grace Hosp., *28*, 3, 1950.
42. Formijne, P. and Van Soeren, F.: Lancet, *2*, 1206, 1958.
43. Freedman, P. and Markowitz, A. S.: Brit. Med. J., *1*, 1175, 1962.
44. Friou, G. J.: Ann. Intern. Med., *49*, 866, 1958.
45. Friou, G. J.: The LE Cell Factor and Antinuclear Antibodies, in *Laboratory Diagnostic Procedures in the Rheumatic Diseases*, edited by Alan S. Cohen, Boston, Little, Brown and Company, 1967, p. 114.

46. Friou, G. J., Finch, S. C. and Detre, K. D.: Fed. Proc., *16*, 413, 1957.
47. Friou, G. J.: J. Immun., *80*, 476, 1958.
48. ———: Arth. and Rheum., *7*, 161, 1964.
48*a*.———: in *Atypical Virus Infections—Possible Relevance To Animal Models and Rheumatic Disease*, New York, The Arthritis Foundation, 1971, p. 71.
49. Godman, G. C., Deitch, A. D. and Klemperer, P.: Am. J. Path., *32*, 616, 1956.
50. Godman, G. C. and Deitch, A. D.: J. Exp. Med., *106*, 575, 1957.
51. Golden, H. E. and McDuffie, F. C.: Ann. Intern. Med., *67*, 780, 1967.
52. Gonyea, L. M., Kallsen, R. A. and Marlow, A. A.: J. Invest. Dermat., *15*, 11, 1950.
53. Gonzales, E. N. and Rothfield, N. F.: New Engl. J. Med., *274*, 1333, 1966.
54. Goodman, H. C., Fahey, J. L. and Malmgren, R. A.: J. Clin. Invest., *39*, 1595, 1960.
54*a*. Grumet, F. C., Coukell, A., Bodmer, J. G., Bodmer, W. F. and McDevitt, H. O.: New Engl. J. Med., *285*, 193, 1971.
55. Gueft, B.: Arch. Derm. & Syph., *61*, 892, 1950.
56. Hanauer, L. B. and Christian, C. L.: J. Clin. Invest., *46*, 400, 1967.
57. Hargraves, M. M.: Proc. Staff Meet. Mayo Clin., *24*, 234, 1949.
58. Hargraves, M. M.: Postgrad. Med., *16*, 163, 1954.
59. Hargraves, M. M., Richmond, H. and Morton, R.: Proc. Staff Meet. Mayo Clin., *23*, 25, 1948.
60. Harvey, A. M., Shulman, L. E., Tumulty, P. A., Conley, C. L. and Schoenrich, E. H.: Medicine, *33*, 291, 1954.
61. Haserick, J. R.: Arch. Derm. Syph., *61*, 889, 1950.
62. ———: Ann. Intern. Med., *44*, 497, 1956.
63. Haserick, J. R. and Bortz, D. W.: J. Invest. Dermat., *13*, 47, 1949.
64. Haserick, J. R. and Lewis, L. A.: Blood, *5*, 718, 1950.
65. Haserick, J. R., Lewis, L. A. and Bortz, D. W.: Amer. J. Med. Sci., *219*, 660, 1950.
66. Haserick, J. R. and Sundberg, R. D.: J. Invest. Dermat., *11*, 209, 1948.
67. Helyer, B. J. and Howie, J. B.: Nature, *197*, 197, 1963.
68. Hijmans, W., Doniach, D., Roitt, I. M. and Holborow, E. J.: Brit. Med. J., *2*, 909, 1961.
69. Hijmans, W., Kievits, J. H. and Schutt, H. R. E.: Acta Med. Scand., *161*, 341, 1958.
70. Hollander, J. L., Reginato, A. and Torralba, T. P.: Med. Clin. N. Amer., *50*, 1281, 1966.
71. Holman, H. R., Deicher, H. R. G. and Kunkel, H. G.: Bull. N. Y. Acad. Med., *35*, 409, 1959.
72. Holman, H. R. and Kunkel, H. G.: Science, *126*, 125, 1957.
73. Holman, H. R., Robbins, W. C., Deicher, H. and Kunkel, H. G.: Science, *126*, 1232, 1957.
74. Jones, W. A. and Castleman, B.: Amer. J. Path., *40*, 315, 1962.
75. Kay, D. R., Bole, C. C., Jr. and Ledger, W. J.: Arth. and Rheum., *14*, 239, 1971.
76. Koffler, D., Agnello, V., Carr, R. I. and Kunkel, H. G.: Amer. J. Path., *56*, 305, 1969.
77. Koffler, D., Carr, R. I., Agnello, V., Frezi, T. and Kunkel, H. G.: Science, *166*, 1648, 1969.
78. Koffler, D. and Kunkel, H. G.: Amer. J. of Med., *45*, 165, 1968.
79. Koffler, D., Schur, P. H. and Kunkel, H. G.: J. Exp. Med., *126*, 607, 1967.
80. Korting, G. W. and Schnitz, R.: Urin. Derm. Wchnschr., *125*, 174, 1952.
81. Kramer, L. S., Ruderman, J. L., DuBois, E. L., and Friou, G. J.: Arth. & Rheum., *13*, 3:329, 1970 (abstract).
82. Krishnan, C. and Kaplan, M. H.: J. Clin. Invest., *46*, 569, 1967.
83. Kurnich, N. B., Schwartz, L. I., Pariser, S. and Lee, S. L.: J. Clin. Invest., *32*, 193, 1953.
84. Lachmann, P. J. and Kunkel, H. G.: Lancet, *2*, 436, 1961.
85. Lambert, P. H. and Dixon, F. J.: Jour. of Exp. Med., *127*, 507, 1968.
86. ———: Clin. & Exp. Immunol., *6*, 829, 1970.
87. Lee, S. L.: Amer. J. Clin. Path., *31*, 492, 1951.
88. ———: J. Mt. Sinai Hosp., *22*, 74, 1955.
89. ———: Clin. Res. Proc., *3*, 98, 1955.
90. Lee, S. L., Michael, S. R. and Vural, I. L.: Amer. J. Med., *10*, 446, 1951.
91. Lee, S. L., Schwartz, L. I. and Pariser, S.: Blood, *9*, 965, 1954.
92. Levi, M. L. and Poverenny, A. M.: J. Hyg. Epidem., *9*, 465, 1965.
93. Mackay, I. R., Taft, L. I. and Cowling, D. C.: Lancet, *2*, 1323, 1956.
94. Magath, T. B. and Winkle, V.: Amer. J. Clin. Path., *22*, 586, 1952.
95. Maldonado, J. E., Alarcon-Segovia, D., Pease, G. and Brown, A. L., Jr.: Proc. Mayo. Clin., *38*, 219, 1963.

96. Marmont, A.: Acta Haemat., *13*, 257, 1955.
97. McCluskey, R. T., Benacerraf, F., Potter, J. L. and Miller, F.: J. Exper. Med., *3*, 181, 1959.
97*a*. McDevitt, H. O. and Benacerraf, B.: Advan. Immunol., *11*, 31, 1969.
98. Mellors, R. C. and Huang, C. Y.: J. Exp. Med., *124*, 1031, 1966.
99. Mellors, R. C., Ortega, L. G. and Holman, H. R.: J. Exp. Med., *106*, 191, 1957.
100. Meyler, L.: Acta Med. Scand., *150*, 33, 1954.
101. Miescher, P. A.: Arth. & Rheum., *6*, 524, 1963.
102. Miescher, P. A., Cooper, N. S. and Benacerraf, F.: J. Immunol., *85*, 27, 1960.
103. Miescher, P. A. and Fauconnet, M.: Experientia, *10*, 252, 1954.
104. Miescher, P. A. and Strassle, R.: Vox Sanguinis, *2*, 283, 1957.
105. Moffatt, T. W., Barnes, S. S. and Weiss, R. S.: J. Invest. Derm., *14*, 153, 1950.
106. Molina, J., DuBois, E. L., Bilitch, M., Bland, S. L. and Friou, G. J.: Arth. & Rheum., *12*, 6:608, 1969.
107. Moyer, J. B. and Fisher, G. S.: Amer. J. Clin. Path., *20*, 1011, 1950.
108. Muller, J. C., Rast, C. L., Jr., Pryor, W. W. and Orgain, E. S.: J.A.M.A., *157*, 894, 1955.
108*a*. Northway, J. D. and Tan, E. M.: Arth. & Rheum., *15*, 130, 1972.
109. Norton, W. L.: J. of Lab. & Clin. Med., *73*, 369, 1969.
110. Pascher, F., Borota, A. and Davis, B.: J. Invest. Derm., *24*, 311, 1955.
111. Peltier, A. P.: Path. Biol. (Paris), *16*, 439, 1968.
112. Perry, H. M., Jr. and Schroeder, H. A.: J.A.M.A., *154*, 670, 1954.
113. Phillips, P. E. and Christian, C. L.: Science, *168*, 982, 1970.
114. ————: Arth. & Rheum., *14*, 180, 1971 (abstract).
115. Plescia, O. J. and Braun, W.: Adv. in Immunol., *6*, 231, 1967.
116. Quismorio, F. P. and Friou, G. J.: Unpublished observations.
117. Rifkind, R. A. and Godman, G. C.: J. Exp. Med., *106*, 607, 1957.
118. Ritchie, R. F.: Arth. & Rheum., *10*, 544, 1967.
119. ————: Arth. & Rheum., *11*, 506, 1968.
120. Robineaux, R.: in *Mechanisms of Hypersensitivity*, Boston, Little, Brown & Co., 1959, Chapter 24.
120*a*. Robitaille, P. and Tan, E. M.: Arth. & Rheum., *15*, 126, 1972.
121. Rohn, R. J. and Bond, W. H.: Amer. J. Med., *12*, 422, 1952.
122. Rosenfeld, S., Swiller, A. I. and Morrison, M.: J.A.M.A., *155*, 568, 1954.
123. Rothfield, N. F. and Page, N.: New Engl. J. Med., *266*, 535, 1962.
124. Rothfield, N. F., Phythyon, J. M., McEwen, C. and Miescher, P.: Arth. & Rheum., *4*, 223, 1961.
125. Schleicher, E.: Lancet, *1*, 821, 1968.
126. Schur, P. H. and Sandson, J.: New Engl. J. Med., *278*, 533, 1968.
127. Seligmann, M.: Rev. Francais d'Etudes Clin. et Biol. *3*, 558, 1958.
128. ————: Arth. and Rheum., *6*, 542, 1963.
129. Seligmann, M. and Arana, R.: in *Nucleic Acids in Immunology*, O. J. Plescia and W. Braun, editors. New York, Springer Verlag, 1968, p. 98.
130. Seligmann, M., Arana, R. and Cannat, A.: in *Rheumatic Diseases*, J. J. R. Duthie and W. R. M. Alexander, editors, Baltimore, Williams & Wilkins Company, 1968, p. 211.
131. Sharp, C. C., Irvin, W. S., LaRoque, C. V., Daly, V., Kaiser, A. D. and Holman, H. R.: Jour. Clin. Invest., *50*, 350, 1971.
131*a*. Sharp, G. C., Irvin, W. S., Northway, J. D. and Tan, E. M.: Arth. & Rheum., *15*, 125, 1972.
132. Snapper, I. and Nathan, D. J.: Blood, *10*, 718, 1955.
133. Stasny, P. and Ziff, M.: New Engl. J. Med., *280*, 1376, 1969.
134. Stevens, M. B., Abbey, H. and Shulman, L. E.: New Engl. J. Med., *268*, 976, 1963.
135. Stich, M. H., Feldman, F. and Morrison, M.: Arch. Derm. and Syph., *65*, 581, 1952.
136. Stollar, D. and Levine, L.: J. Immunol., *87*, 477, 1961.
137. ————: Arch. Biochem., *101*, 335, 1963.
138. ————: Arch. Biochem., *101*, 417, 1963.
139. Stollar, D., Levine, L., Lehrer, H. I. and Van Vunakis, H.: Proc. Nat. Acad. Sci., U.S.A., *48*, 874, 1962.
140. Suksta, A. and Conley, C. L.: J. Lab. & Clin. Med., *37*, 597, 1951.
141. Sundberg, R. D. and Lick, N. B.: J. Invest. Derm., *12*, 83, 1949.
142. Svec, K. H. and Veit, B. C.: Arth. & Rheum., *10*, 509, 1967.
143. Takahashi, T., Lee, C. L., Biava, C. and Davidsohn, I.: Nature, *207*, 1071, 1965.
144. Tan, E. M., Schur, P. H., Carr, R. I. and Kunkel, H. G.: J. Clin. Invest., *45*, 1732, 1966.

145. Tan, E. M., Schur, P. H. and Kunkel, H. G.: 57th Annual Meeting Amer. Soc. Clin. Invest., *44*, 1104, 1965.
146. Tan, E. M. and Stroughton, R. B.: Proc. Nat. Acad. Sci., *62*, 708, 1969.
146*a*. Tan, E. M. and Kunkel, H. G.: J. Immunol., *96*, 464, 1966.
146*b*. Tan, E. M.: J. Lab. Clin. Med., *70*, 800, 1967.
147. Teague, P. O. and Friou, G. J.: Science, *143*, 1333, 1964.
148. ———: Arth. & Rheum., *8*, 474, 1965.
149. Teague, P. O., Yunis, E. J., Rodey, G., Fish, A., Stutman, O. and Good, R. A.: Lab. Invest., *22*, 121, 1970.
150. Tojo, T. and Friou, G. J.: Science, *161*, 904, 1968.
151. Toone, E. C., Irby, R. and Pierce, E. L.: Amer. J. Med. Sci., *240*, 599, 1960.
152. Townes, A. S., Stewart, C. R. and Osler, A.: Bull. Johns Hopkins Hosp., *112*, 183, 1963.
153. Van Doormaal, T. A. J. and Schreuder, J. T. R.: Dermatologica, *101*, 167, 1950.
154. Ward, D. J., Johnson, G. D. and Holborow, E. J.: Ann. Rheum. Dis., *23*, 306, 1964.
155. Ward, J. R., Cloud, R. S., and Turner, L. M.: Ann. Rheum. Dis., *23*, 381, 1964.
156. Weigle, W. O.: Immunol., *7*, 239, 1964.
157. Weir, D. M. and Elson, C. J.: Arth. and Rheum., *12*, 254, 1969.
158. Willkens, R. F., Dreschler, M. and Larsen, D. L.: Proc. Soc. Exp. Biol. & Med., *99*, 645, 1958.
159. Wilson, R. M., Abbott, R. R. and Miller, D. K.: Amer. J. Med. Sci., *241*, 73/31, 1961.
160. Wold, R. T., Young, F. E., Tan, E. M. and Farr, R. S.: Science, *161*, 806, 1968.
161. Zimmer, F. E. and Hargraves, M. M.: Proc. Staff Meet. Mayo Clin., *27*, 424, 1952.
162. Zinkham, W. H. and Conley, C. L.: Bull. Johns Hopkins Hosp., *98*, 102, 1956.
163. Zvaifler, N. J. and Martinez, M. M.: Clin. Exp. Immunol., *8*, 271, 1971.

Chapter 11

Arthritis in Animals

By Carl M. Pearson, M.D.

Arthritis of various types occurs in both wild and domesticated animals, and most of these conditions are either inherited dysplasias, infectious in origin or degenerative in nature. Many resemble fairly closely analogous ones which occur in man. However, with respect to their importance in the overall problem of human arthritis they have not so far contributed a great deal to our basic understanding or management of articular disorders. On the other hand, they are of great interest to the veterinarian both as research challenges and as major economic and husbandry problems, especially in marketable stock.

So far as is known, there are no ideal non-human models for rheumatoid arthritis, ankylosing spondylitis, Reiter's syndrome, psoriasis with arthritis and other related diseases whose etiology still remains obscure. However, a chronic arthritis in swine, due to infectious organisms, has some histological resemblances to rheumatoid arthritis. Also adjuvant arthritis, a disease inducible in rats by injection of Freund's adjuvant, has some features which suggest either Reiter's syndrome or rheumatoid arthritis.

In addition, certain animal models, not necessarily purely articular but apparently related to human connective tissue diseases, are either being discovered or created in the laboratory. A number of these are quite similar to the connective tissue diseases that are seen in the clinic. In this category can be included: (a) homologous disease,[56] an inducible disorder in the rat, which is due to aggressive action by foreign but immunologically competent lymphocytes which are placed into a homologous (non-identical) host. (b) Various models of necrotizing or non-necrotizing hypersensitivity angiitis or arteritis, which closely resemble polyarteritis nodosa and which can be initiated by serially timed injections of foreign protein substances[20] or antigen-antibody complexes[13] into any of several species. (c) A naturally occurring counterpart of polyarteritis called Aleutian mink disease which occurs in conjunction with glomerulonephritis, hypergammaglobulinemia and plasma cell proliferation in certain hereditary strains.[29] This disease has

General Introduction

Experimental Production of Arthritis
- A. Adjuvant Arthritis
  - 1. Clinical Features
  - 2. Pathology
  - 3. Investigative Observations
  - 4. Comparison with Human Disease

Infectious Animal Diseases Associated with Arthritis
- A. Erysipelas Arthritis in Swine
- B. Mycoplasmal
- C. Glasser's Disease
- D. Arthritic Disease of Sheep
- E. Other Infections

6-Sulfanilamidoindazole-Induced Arthritis in Rats

Degenerative Joint Diseases in Animals

Miscellaneous Arthritides

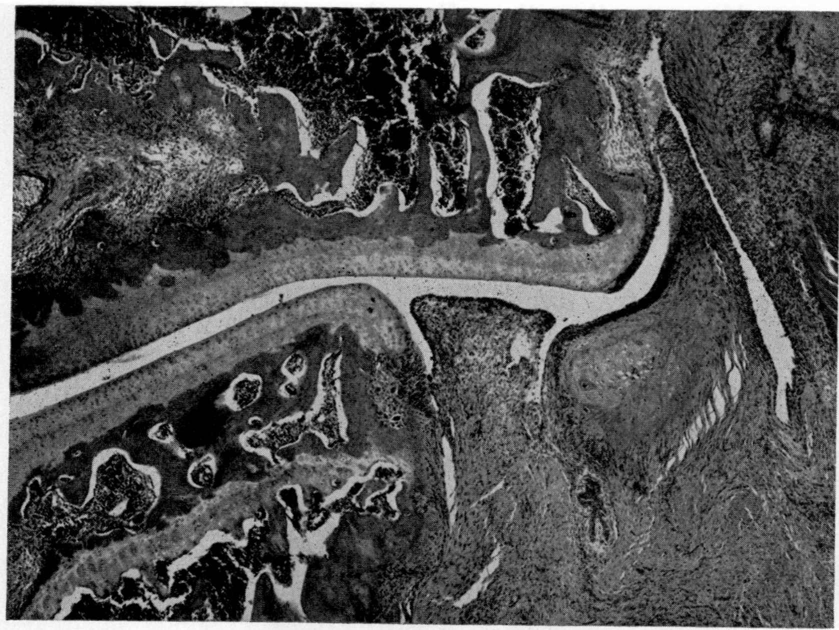

Fig. 11–2.—Ten days after acute onset of adjuvant arthritis in a tarsal joint there is extensive inflammatory granulation tissue (pannus) invading the subchondral bone in at least three zones. HE × 53

Investigative Observations.—Following the initial outline of the disease syndrome and its pathological characteristics a great amount of investigation has gone into: (*a*) attempts to delineate the mechanisms involved in the production of the disease, especially during the latent period, (*b*) to determine the role played by lymphocytes and lymph nodes in the genesis of the disease, (*c*) to vary the incidence and severity of the disease process by experimental manipulations, including its complete inhibition, and (*d*) to utilize adjuvant arthritis as a model of an inflammatory reaction in search for therapeutically effective anti-inflammatory drugs. These lines of approach, especially the first three, will be very helpful in an eventual understanding of the mechanisms which underlie this disorder. Such mechanisms may be reasonably similar to those which operate in comparable human articular and connective tissue disease.

When the disease was originally observed, it was thought to be likely that a latent infection of some sort was being activated in the rat. However, as other experimental results were obtained this possibility seemed less and less likely until now it is almost certainly excluded. Evidence which has been helpful in ruling out infection includes: (*a*) inability to consistently or even occasionally culture a bacteria or PPLO from affected tissues,[48] (*b*) ineffectiveness of penicillin or broad-spectrum antibiotics, (*c*) the ease with which "germ-free" rats develop the entire syndrome,[44] (*d*) inability to transfer the disease by contact between involved and healthy rats or by inoculations of serum or affected articular tissues into normal controls, (*e*) success in transferring the disease when viable sensitized lymphocytes, obtained either from lymph nodes and spleen or through thoracic duct drainage, are passed from previously inoculated animals into highly inbred controls[42,62,63] and failure to achieve transfer if disrupted (by freezing) lymphoid tissue cells are used.

Nearly all of the evidence now seems

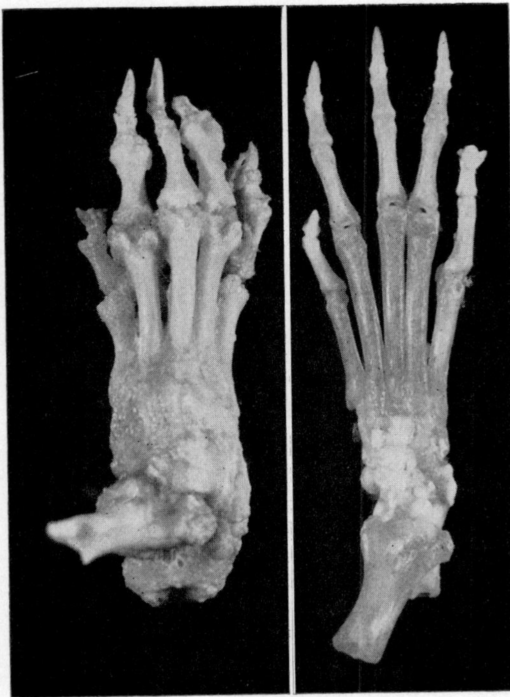

FIG. 11–3.—Skeletal preparation revealing marked periosteal and bony proliferation, especially adjacent to joints, forming bony ankylosis in adjuvant arthritis about fifty days after onset of acute disease in one hind paw. The normal specimen on the right is for comparison.

to point to adjuvant arthritis as being an immunologic disease, probably due to delayed hypersensitivity, or some variant of it. Until now the precise sensitizing "antigen" has not been identified, although it may be some component of the acid-fast bacillus such as one of the wax fractions which in almost pure form, free of all detectable protein including tuberculoprotein, can still readily induce the disease. Observations which favor a hypersensitivity reaction include: (1) the lymphocyte transfer experiments as mentioned above; (2) the ability to curtail completely the development of disease if all of the lymph nodes which drain the site of inoculation are resected within five days;[36] (3) the invariable latency period of at least ten days between the time of inoculation and the onset of disease; (4) the suppressive effect of whole body irradiation when given immediately before adjuvant inoculation; (5) the ability to induce a refractory state akin to immune tolerance when the animals are exposed early in life to adjuvant, or when more than 100 mcg. of dead tubercle bacilli were given in suspension during the incubation period after adjuvant inoculation;[10] (6) tuberculin (PPD) in doses of from 4 to 100 mcg. accentuated the lesions if the PPD was given during the incubation;[10] (7) suppression of the disease by simultaneous administration of heterologous anti-lymphocyte globulin;[11] and (8) the disease can only be transferred by sensitized lymphocytes between the seventh and eleventh post-inoculation day, when these cells must then be competent. Earlier they apparently lacked full competence and, hence, need a lymph node environment in which to develop further. Later (after the eleventh day) they apparently were released to the circulation and out into the tissues since the lymph nodes at that time became small, pale and hypocellular.

A number of other miscellaneous observations have been made in this interesting model. These include anti-inflammatory effects, much the same as noted in man, of corticosteroids, salicylates, phenylbutazone,[5] gold (aurothiomalate), 6-mercaptopurine, and indomethacin.[35] Many compounds (such as some barbiturates and promazine derivatives) have a measure of anti-inflammatory activity in models like the induced granuloma pouch in animals, but these compounds do not significantly affect inflammation in man. Such compounds similarly lack anti-inflammatory actions in adjuvant arthritis. A number of relatively unrelated compounds also appear to have inhibitory effects in adjuvant disease. Thus several so-called immunosuppressive agents such as cyclophosphamide clearly inhibited the disease,[5] whereas the interferon-inducing agent pyran copolymer also inhibited the disease even though it appeared not to have any anti-inflammatory action.[27] Observations such as this leave the question open concerning the role of a virus or a virus-like microorganism in the pathogenesis of adjuvant disease.

Because of the various pharmacological actions as described above, adjuvant arthritis appears, so far, to be the best experimental form of arthritis with which to screen compounds for their effects on inflammation. This is particularly notable since the parallelism of drug effects appears to be quite close to the actions as observed in human disease, especially in rheumatoid arthritis.

Various serum protein changes, as determined by electrophoresis on starch gel, can be noted within a few hours after adjuvant inoculation.[21,32] There is a prompt fall in the albumin and prealbumin, followed in three days by a rise and then another fall at the time of onset of arthritis. With the latter several new pre- and post-albumin bands appear as well as a slow $\alpha 2$ globulin. The majority of the changes in electrophoretic pattern seem to be results of inflammation, although a few are found early even in animals which do not come down with any clinically recognizable disease. The level of glycoprotein rises in both the $\alpha 1$ and β globulin when arthritis is active. Fractions comparable to the human rheumatoid factor, the L.E. substance or antinuclear factor have not been found in adjuvant disease.

For induction of the disease, killed tubercle bacilli or some fraction of it, especially the Wax D fraction, is necessary. However, the acid-fast organism Nocardia has shown an arthritis-inducing capacity,[16] as has the heat-killed organism *Corynebacterium rubrum.*[37] One or another of these substances must be incorporated into a mineral oil base before injection. Intracutaneous inoculations have proved effective, as have injections into a foot pad or the base of the tail. It has recently been shown that injection into an external ear is more effective in smaller quantities than in any other site. Apparently all of these locations possess a rich lymphatic supply to regional lymph nodes, and such are necessary in order to set the machinery in operation for subsequent development of arthritis.

Other continuing observations on adjuvant arthritis[43] are providing more information about this model which seem to be leading to a fuller understanding of the mechanisms involved in its production and propagation. The observations include:

(1) Quantification of the response to Wax D and oil, using the sensitive external ear route for injection. By this method, in one strain, it has been found that as little as 0.01 mgm. of Wax D possesses arthritogenic properties in nearly all animals.

(2) Slight chemical alteration of Wax D, such as by acetylation, renders it incapable of inducing arthritis.[3,43] On the other hand, prior injections of acetylated wax, or even of some chemical fractions of the wax, especially if they contain certain critical amino acids such as alanine, D-glutamic acid, and diaminopimelic acid, can protect the animals against development of arthritis by later injections of complete Wax D adjuvant.

(3) Prior injection of certain bacterial lipopolysaccharides in oil, such as those from some gram-negative bacteria, can also protect against subsequent attempts to induce adjuvant arthritis.

(4) The incorporation of certain protein antigens such as hen egg albumin or bovine gamma globulin into complete adjuvant can inhibit the development of arthritis, apparently by providing the animals with a stronger antigenic or immunologic stimulus (i.e. antigenic competition) than that provided by adjuvant alone.[64] Thus it is thought that the available immunologically competent cells are utilized by this potent stimulus and a few or none remain to react against the joints. These animals become highly sensitized to the incorporated protein and show anaphylactic reactions to subsequent intravenous injections of the specific protein.

Comparison with Human Articular Diseases

It is not unreasonable to attempt to compare adjuvant arthritis with certain human articular diseases, and this has already been done.[39] There are some remarkable similarities, considering the species differences, and, of course, a number of discrepancies. The basic mechanisms might be somewhat similar. The closest parallels are with Reiter's syndrome or rheumatoid arthritis. The similar and dissimilar features of several conditions are tabulated in Table 11–1.

INFECTIOUS ANIMAL DISEASES ASSOCIATED WITH ARTHRITIS

A variety of infectious agents have at one time or another been associated with inflammatory mono- or polyarthritis in either wild or domesticated animals. Much more is known about the latter and it has been established that various bacteria, Mycoplasma (PPLO), and perhaps viruses are responsible for some epidemics or the endemic persistence of animal arthritis. Some of the arthritides are acute and suppurative, whereas many more are insidious in onset and chronic in their course. In some respects the latter resemble human rheumatoid arthritis. They often present grave economic problems to the breeder and farmer. A few of these disorders are described briefly in the following sections.

Erysipelas Arthritis of Swine

In 1940 the British workers Collins and Goldie[8] described a chronic polyarthritis

TABLE 11–1.—COMPARISON OF ADJUVANT DISEASE WITH CERTAIN HUMAN DISORDERS (from Pearson[39])

	Adjuvant disease	*Reiter's disease*	*Rheumatoid arthritis*	*Ankylosing spondylitis*	*Psoriasis and arthritis*	*Erythema nodosum*
Clinical						
Acute and recurrent arthritis						
Peripheral joints	++	++	++	+	++	+
Spinal joints	+	+	0	++	+	0
Chronic deforming arthritis	++	+	++	++	+	0
Skin lesions	+	+	0	0	++	++
Genital lesions	++±	++±	0	0	+±	0
Eye lesions	+	++	+	+	0	+
Progressive and destructive joint disease	++	+	++	++	+	0
Skin and subcutaneous nodules						
Rheumatoid nodules	0	0	++	0	0	0
Vasculitis only	+	0	0	0	0	++
Pathologic						
Acute and subacute synovitis	++	++	++	+	+	+
Primarily mononuclear cell response	++	+	++	++	+	0
Invasion of bone and joint space by pannus	++	+	++	+	+	0
Bursitis and tendinitis	++	+	++	+	0	+
Osteitis and periostitis						
Ankylosis						
Fibrous	++	+	+	+	0	0
Bony	+	0	+	++	0	0

0 = almost never
\+ = rarely
++ = commonly
± = in males

of pigs which could be induced experimentally by the organism *Erysipelothrix rhusiopathiae* (now usually called *E. insidiosa*). They demonstrated that the arthritis was not preceded by signs of acute or subacute swine erysipelas, but only by minor skin or febrile responses. The authors also isolated this organism from blood or joints in some field cases. Subsequent to that time, especially within the past twenty years, ample confirmation of the occurrence of *E. insidiosa* as the etiologic factor of this chronic polyarticular disease has been confirmed,[18,50] and a number of interesting additional features have been described. The disease produces lameness, poor performance, weight loss and chronically swollen and sometimes deformed joints of the extremities and also of the spine. Histopathologically an intense synovitis is found with perivascular foci of lymphocytes, plasma cells and other mononuclears, in conjunction with vascular congestion and some proliferative vascular changes. In advanced cases, in addition to the proliferative changes in the synovial membrane, are found granulation tissue extensions out over the articular cartilages (pannus formation) of the joint capsule and invasion of the subchondral bone and the epiphyseal plate cartilage.

One will immediately recognize that such changes are quite similar to those which are found in rheumatoid arthritis, and this has been commented upon repeatedly.[50] Moreover, in a number of the chronically affected joints no organisms can be cultured, even though the animals were originally experimentally injected with *E. insidiosa*. This has led to the speculation that the chronic form of polyarthritis is due to a low-grade hypersensitivity reaction to products of the organism, perhaps lodged in the synovium, rather than to continued propagation of *E. insidiosa* in the joint tissues proper. A number of observations seem to support this view, including: (*a*) induction of arthritis by multiple injections of non-viable *E. insidiosa*, (*b*) enhanced severity of arthritis in animals vaccinated against swine erysipelas which are then given an injection of viable organisms, (*c*) the appearance of serum protein alterations in affected pigs, including higher level of gamma and beta-2 globulins and even in some animals a positive sheep cell agglutination test, (*d*) the development of an agglutinating factor which could be eluted with 5 per cent Dextran from erythrocytes of swine which have the infection.[51] Apparently the human latex fixation test, done on blood serum of arthritic swine, was also positive in most animals, and (*e*) the ability to sensitize swine passively with sterile filtered immune serum and then induce synovial lesions by intra-articular inoculation of sterile erysipelothrix antigen.

In some fairly recent studies when the organism *E. insidiosa* was injected intravenously into rabbits, a subacute generalized arthritis was produced.[1] The arthritic rabbits exhibited several serological manifestations which are considered to be characteristic of human rheumatoid arthritis. Pathologically there was hyperplasia of the synovial cells and hypertrophy of the villi, with infiltration by lymphocytes and plasma cells. This rabbit model had a number of anatomical similarities to human rheumatoid arthritis.

All of these features make erysipelas arthritis of swine a most interesting tool for continued study, especially because of the apparent interplay between infection and immunologic response and the implications that this may have in some possibly analogous human arthritides.

Mycoplasmal Arthritis in Swine

Switzer[59] in 1953 first demonstrated that a pleuropneumonia (PPLO) organism, now called *M. hyorhinis*, was capable of producing polyserositis and polyarthritis in pigs. This organism is commonly present in the nasal passages and pneumonic lungs of swine. It is responsible for significant economic losses in the swine industry.

The polyarthritis appears in from five to twelve days after an intraperitoneal inoculation of a viable culture of organisms and may persist after the acute stage in a chronic or subacute form for weeks or months. The mortality from this infection is low but the morbidity rate is high.

Pathologically the synovium is hypertrophied, hyperemic, and loaded with chronic inflammatory cells. The pathologic changes are quite similar to those described in swine erysipelas. Lesions of periarticular bone are somewhat less prominent than in the latter condition, but occur in a few animals.[47] The fine ultrastructure of changes in the synovial tissues of swine experimentally infected with M. hyorhinis revealed accumulations of lymphocyte and plasma cells about the capillaries and a particular increase in Type A cells in the synovium.[14] Mycoplasmal organisms could not be identified with certainty in the synovium in these ultrastructural studies. Other acute lesions include a pleuritis, peritonitis and pericarditis.

By use of proper cultural techniques, *M. hyorhinis* can be recultured from nearly all of the involved joints, even after a lengthy interval. Hence, this disease seems to be due to the direct propagation of and persistence of the implicated organism in the affected joint tissues themselves.

Glasser's Disease

This condition is a fibrinous polyserositis and polyarthritis which affects pigs, especially in Europe and Australia. It has been reported to be due to the organism *Hemophilus influenzae suis.*[23] The mortality rate is high. The synovial pathology resembles quite closely that observed in infection by *M. hyorhinis.*

Arthritic Disease of Sheep ("Stiff Lamb Disease")

Sheep men have annually reported heavy economic losses from a chronic clinical condition occurring in their sheep, especially in the western half of the United States. Clinically, the disease is characterized by varying degrees of stiffness, lameness, fever, anorexia, weight loss, depression, reluctance to move, and a high morbidity rate with a low mortality rate. Pathologically, the condition is found to be a polyarthritis, with proliferative inflammatory reactions involving especially the synovial membranes, tendon sheaths, joint capsules, tendons, ligaments, periarticular tissues and muscles. In the visceral organs of the body there may be varying degrees of inflammatory alteration. The disease is contagious, occurring during certain seasons, especially during the summer, late summer and fall months of each year. It is caused by an agent which appears to be a member of the psittacosis-lymphogranuloma venereum group.[49] In affected animals this agent can be regularly isolated from joint fluid and various other body fluids and tissues as well as from fecal samples.

Other Infectious Arthritides

A large number of other forms of diffuse infectious synovitis have been described in various species. Many of these are due to Mycoplasma (PPLO) species especially in goats[9] and in poultry,[30] or the L-phase bacterial form in chickens and turkeys.[46] Mycoplasma species may occasionally induce an acute or a chronic form of arthritis in rats and mice,[2] although these organisms do not seem to be involved in adjuvant-induced arthritis in rats. A chronic low grade but destructive form of synovitis and arthritis has also appeared several months after parenteral injections of certain strains of nonchromogenic or atypical Mycobacteria into various animals.[28]

An infectious arthritis has been described fairly frequently in cattle, primarily in weight-bearing joints. The organism responsible for these septic arthritides is primarily *Corynebacterium pyogenes.*[60] The lesions produced visible effusion and distention of the joint capsule, periarticular edema and fibrosis and lameness. Analysis of the synovial effusion revealed it to be characteristic of a septic, infectious arthritis.

6-SULFANILAMIDOINDAZOLE-INDUCED ARTHRITIS IN RATS

In 1964 Mielens and Rozitis[33] described an inflammatory reaction confined to joints and periarticular connective tissue of the hind paws of older rats medicated orally with 6-sulfanilamidoindazole (6-SAI). The inflammation usually appeared between days five and ten of drug administration, reached maximum intensity two to three days later and then resolved slowly despite continued medication. Using blind passage techniques, Mycoplasma were occasionally isolated from cardiac blood and from certain tissues, including periarticular tissues.[7] However, certain animals did not reveal Mycoplasmas and the general consensus now is that 6-SAI is an oral, active phlogistic agent that induces joint inflammation in experimental animals.[34]

6-SAI regularly induced arthritis in adult rats, and the lesions were primarily confined to the hind paws. The incidence of arthritis in orally medicated rats was related, in part, to the body weight of the animals at the time of the initial feeding. Histologically, the lesions were nonsuppurative and proliferative. Lymphocytes were present in all stages of the inflammation preceding the appearance of fibroblasts, which were the most consistent and the most striking cellular components. The inflammation of the joints was not associated with anemia, elevation of serum uric acid or other findings.

The site and mode of action of this sulfonamide on the vascular system, which leads to edema formation in the paws, mononuclear cell infiltration and fibroplasia, remain to be established. Neither immediate nor delayed types of hypersensitivity reactions appear to be implicated since both gross and microscopic tissue lesions appear as early as three days after the initiation of 6-SAI feedings. This latency period would seem to be too short in duration for synthesis and release of a humoral antibody. Furthermore there is no evidence to suggest the development of kinin formation through activation of the Hageman factor or from any other known mechanism. The fact that the animals are generally either adult or elderly before they can develop the disease suggests the gradual appearance of some type of phlogistic agent or the lack of resistance to the release of such an agent in these animals. This arthritis model is a very interesting one for continued study.

DEGENERATIVE JOINT DISEASE IN ANIMALS

Degenerative joint disease, or osteoarthritis (also called osteoarthrosis), has been known for many years to occur frequently in large bulky animals. Hence, arthritis is perhaps the most ancient of known diseases, probably having existed almost since vertebrate life began. Such information can be obtained from examining museum specimens which are several million years old, as well as from a study of the more readily available wild and domesticated animals. Most of the articular changes which are seen in these specimens are those of degenerative arthritis and there is little doubt that this kind of disorder is the one which existed in the majority of these cases, although such a disease would be better preserved because of its involvement of the bony skeleton, especially the periarticular areas. Disorders such as rheumatoid arthritis, which predominantly involve soft tissues would be difficult to recognize in the bone specimens of ancient times, unless destructive changes of advanced disease occurred, which apparently was not the case. The most authoritative discussions of this facet of articular disease have been given by Fox[17] as well as a more recent discussion by Dawson.[12]

It has generally been assumed that the pathologic changes of osteoarthritis, which redominantly occur in bulky mammals s well as in man, have a distribution which is correlated with weight-bearing nd other mechanical influences on ar-icular surfaces. With this view, it is widely held that osteoarthritis is a trau-natic or destructive lesion rather than a legenerative one. Careful examination f affected animals, and man, disclose hat the lesion is not a generalized one out is more prone to occur in certain por-ions of certain joints for some reason that s as yet not fully explained. Pathologists eel that the earliest gross changes of os-eoarthritis consist of small, localized reas of splitting of the articular cartilage along its fibrillary planes. This is found n conjunction with (*a*) local prolifera-ion of chondrocytes; (*b*) local necrosis of chondrocytes, and (*c*) alteration of chro-nophilic properties of the intercellular natrix.

There are various clues that perhaps osteoarthritis may be more than traumat-c in origin, and in fact, may have a genetic basis. In man this appears to be uggested by the apparent hereditary nature of Heberden's nodes.[57] A very significant advance in this direction was nade in the observation by Silberberg and Silberberg[52] that osteoarthritis of nicroscopic proportion does indeed oc-cur in mice under certain conditions. These laboratory rodents are susceptible not only to inbreeding and outbreeding experiments in osteoarthritis, but also to careful histological and histochemical studies. Such studies have been con-ducted by the above-mentioned authors as well as by Sokoloff[54,55] in a large num-ber of such mice.

It has been found that: (*a*) The de-generative joint disease in the mouse shares a number of basic anatomical similarities with the lesion which occurs in man. Hence, it originates in focal areas of abrasion and degeneration of articular cartilage and extensive detach-ment of the articular cartilage ensues. Eventually the erosion results in a de-formity of the contours of the articulating surfaces, and the development of a re-active sclerosis. The disease almost in-variably occurs in older animals; (*b*) The individual histologic changes are quite similar to those found in the human and consist of localized necrosis of chondro-cytes and the loss of metachromatic material from the matrix. These changes along with hypertrophy and hyperplasia of the articular chondrocytes can be found in this genetic mouse disease or osteoarthritis induced by mechanical means; (*c*) Since the epiphyses rarely close until very late in the life of the mouse, if they close at all, it was thought possible that a degree of fusion of the epiphyses could be responsible for the development of osteoarthritis. However, in careful studies no correlation could be established between the development of osteoarthritis and skeletal aging as mea-sured by epiphyseal union; (*d*) Various experimental procedures have been util-ized to intensify or minimize the degree of joint disease which occurs in these mice. Hence, a diet high in certain food oils such as cottonseed oil enhanced the appearance of osteoarthritis. Two strains of mice which developed obesity on a very high vegetable fat diet also demon-strated an increased amount of degenera-tive joint disease, and (*e*) Certain hor-mones exert a deleterious effect upon joint cartilage. Strains of mice that are susceptible to osteoarthritis have an accelerated appearance of it under the influence of somatotrophic hormone or from implantation of isografts of the an-terior hypophyses.

MISCELLANEOUS ARTHRITIDES

Dumonde and Glynn[15] have induced delayed hypersensitivity to autologous or heterologous fibrin in rabbits by injec-tions of fibrin in Freund's adjuvant. A subsequent injection of fibrin into the knee joints of sensitized rabbits produced a chronic arthritis, the histology of which bore a number of resemblances to human rheumatoid arthritis.

Most normal rabbits have a spon-taneously occurring auto-antibody, known as homoreactant, which combines specifically with the Fab fragment of rabbit IgG, but not with the intact IgG molecule. Two groups of rabbits were studied[45] in one of whom the autoantibody was present and in the other it was lacking. Those animals containing the serum homoreactant developed synovitis which had many resemblances to human rheumatoid arthritis.[45] When rabbits which initially had no serum homoreactant were given three times weekly injections of the Fab fragment, an acute synovial reaction developed which was again characteristic of an immunologically-induced synovitis. It is proposed that there is considerable analogy between this model and human rheumatoid arthritis and that this experimental system might serve as a model for future investigations of human rheumatoid disease.

A detailed treatise on the comparative pathology of a wide variety of induced and naturally occurring forms of arthritis in many species was published in 1960.[4]

BIBLIOGRAPHY

1. Astorga, G. P.: Arth & Rheum., *12*, 589, 1969.
2. Barden, J. A. and Tully, J. G.: J. Bact., *100*, 5, 1969.
3. Bonhomme, F., Boucheron, C., Migliore, D. and Jolles, P.: Internat. Arch. Allergy, *36*, 317, 1969.
4. Brandly, C. A. and Jungherr, E. L.: *Advances in Veterinary Science*, Vol. 6 New York, Academic Press, 1960.
5. Brown, J. H., Schwartz, N. L., Mackey, H. K. and Murray, H. L.: Arch. Internat. Pharmacol., *183*, 1, 1970.
6. Burstein, N. A. and Waksman, B. H.: Yale J. Biol. Med., *37*, 177, 1964.
7. Cole, B. C., Miller, M. L. and Ward, J. R.: Proc. Soc. Exper. Biol. Med., *130*, 994, 1969.
8. Collins, D. H. and Goldie, W.: J. Path. Bact., *50*, 323, 1940.
9. Cordy, D. R. and Adler, H. E.: Ann. N.Y. Acad. Sci., *79*, 686, 1960.
10. Currey, H. L. F.: Ann. Rheum. Dis., *29*, 314, 1970.
11. Currey H. L. F. and Ziff, M.: J. Exper. Med., *127*, 185, 1968.
12. Dawson, J. E.: Ann. Phys. Med., *5*, 16? 1960.
13. Dixon, F. J.: In *Mechanisms of Cells and Tissu Damage Produced by Immune Reaction*, Ed. b Graber, P. and Miescher, P., New York Grune and Stratton, 1961, p. 71.
14. Duncan, J. R. and Ross, R. F.: Amer. J Path., *57*, 171, 1969.
15. Dumonde, D. C. and Glynn, L. E.: Brit. J Exper. Path., *43*, 373, 1962.
16. Flax, M. H. and Waksman, B. H.: Internat Arch. Allergy, *23*, 331, 1963.
17. Fox, H.: Tr. Amer. Phil. Soc., *31*, 73, 1939
18. Freeman, M. J., Segre, D., and Berman, D. T.: Amer. J. Vet. Res., *24*, 135, 1964.
19. Gardner, D. L.: Ann. Rheum. Dis., *19*, 297, 1960.
20. Germuth, F. G. and Heptinstall, R. H.: Bull. Johns Hopkins Hosp., *100*, 58, 1957.
21. Glenn, E. M., Gray, J. and Kooyers, W.: Amer. J. Vet. Res., *26*, 1195, 1965.
22. Gorham, J. R., Leader, R. W., and Henson, J. B.: J. Infect. Dis., *114*, 341, 1964.
23. Hjarre, A. and Wramby, G. M.: Skand. Vet.-tidskr., *32*, 257, 1942.
24. Holmes, M. C. and Burnet, F.: Ann. Intern. Med., *59*, 265, 1963.
25. Jones, R. S. and Ward, J. R.: Arth. & Rheum., *6*, 23, 1963.
26. Jones, T. C.: Lab. Invest., *8*, 1471, 1959.
27. Kapusta, M. A. and Mendelson, J.: Arth. & Rheum., *12*, 463, 1969.
28. Kubin, M., Druml, J. and Janku, A.: Acta Tuber. Penum. Scand., *44*, 160, 1964.
29. Leader, R. W., Wagner, B. M., Henson, J. B. and Gorham, J. R.: Amer. J. Path., *43*, 33, 1963.
30. Leece, J. G., Sperling, F. G., Hayflick, L. and Stinebring, W.: J. Exper. Med., *102*, 489, 1955.
31. Lewis, R. M., Schwartz, R. and Henry, W. B.: Blood, *25*, 143, 1965.
32. Lowe, J. S.: Biochem. Pharmacol., *13*, 633, 1964.
33. Mielens, Z. E. and Rozitis, J.: Proc. Soc. Exper. Biol. Med., *117*, 751, 1964.
34. Miller, M. L., Ward, J. R., Cole, B. C. and Swinyard, E. A.: Arth. & Rheum., *13*, 222, 1970.
35. Newbould, B. B.: Brit. J. Pharmacol., *21*, 127, 1963.
36. ———: Ann. Rheum. Dis., *23*, 392, 1964.
37. Paronetto, F.: Proc. Soc. Exper. Biol. & Med., *133*, 296, 1970.
38. Pearson, C. M.: Proc. Soc. Exper. Biol. Med., *91*, 95, 1956.
39. ———: J. Chronic Dis., *16*, 863, 1963.

40. Pearson, C. M., Waksman, B. H. and Sharp, J. T.: J. Exper. Med., *113*, 485, 1961.
41. Pearson, C. M. and Wood, F. D.: Amer. J. Path., *42*, 73, 1963.
42. ————: J. Exper. Med., *120*, 547, 1964.
43. Pearson, C. M. and Wood, F. D.: Immunology, *16*, 157, 1969.
44. Pearson, C. M., Wood, F. D., McDaniel, E. G. and Doft, F. S.: Proc. Soc. Exp. Biol. Med., *112*, 91, 1963.
45. Rawson, A. J., Quismorio, F. P. and Abelson, N. M.: Amer. J. Path., *54*, 95, 1969.
46. Roberts, D. H.: Res. Vet. Sci., *5*, 441, 1964.
47. Roberts, E. D., Switzer, W. P. and Ramsey, F. K.: Amer. J. Vet. Res., *24*, 19, 1963.
48. Sharp, J. T., Waksman, B. H., Pearson, C. M. and Madoff, S.: Arth. & Rheum., *4*, 169, 1961.
49. Shupe, J. L. and Storz, J.: Amer. J. Vet. Res., *25*, 943, 1964.
50. Sikes, D.: Rheumatism, *17*, 19, 1961.
51. Sikes, D., Fletcher, O. J. and Jones, T. J.: Amer. J. Vet. Res., *31*, 2191, 1970.
52. Silberberg, M. and Silberberg, R.: Amer. J. Anat., *68*, 69, 1941.
53. ————: Arch. Path., *77*, 519, 1964.
54. Sokoloff, L.: A.M.A. Arch. Path., *62*, 118, 1956.
55. Sokoloff, L. and Jay, G. E.: A.M.A. Arch. Path., *52*, 129, 1956.
56. Stastny, P., Stembridge, V. A. and Ziff, M.: Arth. & Rheum., *6*, 64, 1963.
57. Stecher, R. M.: Ann. Rheum. Dis., *14*, 1, 1955.
58. Stoerck, H. C., Bielinski, T. C. and Budzilovich, T.: Amer. J. Path., *30*, 616, 1954.
59. Switzer, W. P.: J. Amer. Vet. Med. Assoc., *123*, 45, 1953.
60. Van Pelt, R. W.: J. Amer. Vet. Med. Assoc., 156, 457, 1970.
61. Waksman, B. H. and Bullington, S. J.: Arch. Ophthal., *64*, 751, 1960.
62. Waksman, B. H. and Wennersten, C.: Internat. Arch. Allergy, *23*, 129, 1963.
63. Whitehouse, D. J., Whitehouse, M. W. and Pearson, C. M.: Nature, *224*, 1322, 1969.
64. Wood, F. D., Pearson, C. M. and Tanaka, A.: Internat. Arch. Allergy, *35*, 456, 1969.
65. Zahiri, H., Gagnon, J., Ayotte, R. and Laurin, C. A.: Canad. Med. Assoc. J. *101*, 269, 1969.

PART II

Factors Influencing the Onset or Course of the Rheumatic Diseases

Section Editor: William D. Robinson, M.D.

Chapter 12

The Epidemiology of Rheumatic Diseases

By W. M. Mikkelsen, M.D.

Classic epidemiology has been based on the study of populations or groups rather than individuals in order to gain information regarding the etiology of a disease so that preventive measures can be devised. This approach has produced great successes in the fields of infectious and nutritional disease. It is only in recent decades that these techniques have been applied to the study of chronic diseases, which have assumed increasing importance with the control of many infectious diseases and the increase in numbers of older persons. It has become apparent that the epidemiologic problems posed by chronic disorders such as rheumatoid arthritis, coronary heart disease, cancer, and hypertension differ in many respects from those of most acute disorders. Epidemiologic studies have been of great value in increasing our knowledge regarding risk factors for coronary heart disease and more limited results have been achieved in the cancer field, most notably with Burkitt's lymphoma. This chapter will attempt to summarize achievements to date in the epidemiologic study of rheumatoid arthritis.

METHODOLOGY

Early epidemiologic studies relied on gross estimates of morbidity or mortality. Such studies were adequate to establish the magnitude of the public health problem presented by the rheumatic diseases, but were too crude and inaccurate to permit comparison of prevalence rates in different geographic areas or meaningful correlation with other observed characteristics of the population. For this reason emphasis shifted to studies in which possible association between disease and other characteristics are analyzed on the basis of detailed personal examination of the study population. This type of study is difficult and costly, but essential if an adequate degree of precision is to be obtained. Carefully planned longitudinal studies of this sort afford greater promise of yielding clues to the etiology of the disease and evaluation of genetic and/or environmental factors associated with the disease. They also provide a unique background in which to study the natural history and manifestations of the disease.

There are many problems in the planning and performance of epidemiologic studies of rheumatoid arthritis. Some are common to all population studies, among them the selection of a representative community or population sample, attainment of a high response rate, maintenance of cooperation in longitudinal studies, selection of appropriate control groups, effect of observer variation, high expense in terms of time and money, and the unavailability in many geographic areas of adequate personnel or medical facilities. (For more complete discussion of methods and principles see refs. 36 and 74.) The characteristics of the disease present some additional problems. Diagnosis of early or atypical cases may be difficult or impossible in a single determination in a field situation. The more sophisticated diagnostic procedures, such as aspiration of synovial fluid and biopsy of synovial tissue or subcutaneous nodules, are generally not possible. Advanced or severe cases may not be able to attend an examination clinic and may be missed unless home visits are made. The relative infrequency of the disease means that a large population group is required if an adequate number of cases for meaningful statistical analysis is to be obtained. Although clinical experience suggests that rheumatoid arthritis is most often a persistent disease and complete remissions rare, Beall and Cobb[14,27] have presented evidence to suggest that in the general population it may be intermittent in a higher proportion of cases and that as a result significant numbers of cases may escape detection in a single examination. They have emphasized that a single examination measures "point prevalence" and have estimated that "annual prevalence," defined as persons with at least one attack per year, may be approximately twice as great. The demonstration of a "point prevalence" of 3 per cent could thus reflect a population in which 3 per cent were afflicted with the disease 100 per cent of the time, or one in which 15 per cent were afflicted 20 per cent of the time. These authors have suggested that it would be desirable in geographic studies to determine the frequency distribution of persons according to "proportion of time in episode" as well as overall prevalence. A one year period prevalence study in a rural population of the Netherlands in which subjects were examined monthly revealed that of 16 with evidence of rheumatoid arthritis on one or more occasions only 3 suffered from the disease throughout the year.[107] The number of cases per month (essentially a measure of point prevalence) varied from 4 in the summer to a maximum of 9 in October and could not be attributed to observer variance, which was evaluated. Such observations are also influenced by the many nonrheumatoid types of polyarthritis occurring in a general population.

Diagnostic Criteria

Diagnostic criteria are an essential requirement for meaningful and comparable clinical or epidemiologic studies. Lacking knowledge of the etiology, the diagnostic criteria proposed by a committee of the American Rheumatism Association constitute the most satisfactory definition of rheumatoid arthritis for most purposes.[90,91] They have contributed greatly to both clinical and epidemiologic investigation of rheumatoid arthritis. (*See* also Chapter 25.) These criteria will be reviewed briefly from the standpoint of their utility in population studies.

1. "Morning stiffness"

   Although this symptom is generally prominent in active rheumatoid arthritis, it has the disadvantages of subjectivity, nonspecificity and the fact that it is generally absent in inactive cases. In several population studies, assessment of morning stiffness has been shown to be of low reliability,[1] impracticable because of semantic or conceptual problems,[41] and of limited value in promoting recognition of rheumatoid arthritis.[23,58,62] It has been suggested that this criterion might be strengthened by requiring that morning stiffness be of at least ten minutes duration,[23] and in the most recent modification of this criterion a duration of not less than 15 minutes is specified.[15]
2. "Pain on motion or tenderness in at least one joint."
3. "Swelling in at least one joint."
4. "Swelling in at least one other joint."
5. "Symmetrical joint swelling."

   Criteria 2–5, like morning stiffness, can be employed in any population study. Joint pain or tenderness is to some extent subjective. Minimal degrees of joint swelling are difficult to detect and subject to a high degree of inter- and intra-observer error. It may be difficult to differentiate soft tissue swelling from bony enlargement. In field surveys it is obviously difficult to establish that the duration of joint swelling is at least 6 weeks, or that any symptom-free period between episodes of joint swelling is not greater than 3 months.

6. "Subcutaneous nodules . . ."

Although highly specific and valuable diagnostic signs when present, rheumatoid nodules are frequently difficult to distinguish clinically from other subcutaneous nodular lesions and have been sufficiently rare in population studies as to be of little value in case detection.[58]

7. "X-ray changes typical of rheumatoid arthritis (which must include at least bony decalcification localized to or greatest around the involved joints) . . ."

For epidemiological purposes this criterion is too vaguely worded. It requires for minimal fulfillment only the presence of juxta-articular demineralization of bone, a finding very difficult to recognize or assess. Population studies have suggested that osteoporosis, unless clearly confined to the joint area, is most often due to nonrheumatoid causes. British investigators have therefore tended to place greater emphasis on the presence of bone erosions.[63,71,78] Even these, when mild in degree, have often shown little evidence of association with rheumatoid arthritis in population studies. Their high frequency in foot films in several tropical populations where shoes are not customarily worn suggests that trauma may play a role in their development.[70,84] It has been stated that radiographs provide the evidence which constitute the most important source of information on differences between populations.[70] Inter- and intraobserver variability have been found to be significant, however, with the greatest disagreement in the area of doubtful to mild abnormality.[56,59] In comparing films from several surveys interpretation and grading should ideally be carried out by a single observer employing a set of standard reference films. *The Atlas of Standard Radiographs of Arthritis*, currently being revised, is valuable for this purpose.[57]

8. "Positive agglutination test."

There are a number of modifications of serologic tests for rheumatoid factor which satisfy the requirement of not more than 5 per cent positive results in nonrheumatoid controls. In population studies a major problem, especially if results of different investigators are to be compared, is the standardization of test procedures. This problem has been met in some studies by exchange of sera, or by examination of all speciments in a single laboratory. The use of standard sera and reference laboratories has been recommended as an aid to quality control of rheumatoid factor test procedures.[50] In a comparative study of 9 different serologic tests for rheumatoid factor employing 74 selected blood samples it was found that the sensitized sheep cell test was most specific and the F II tanned cell test most sensitive.[109] However, it was suggested that "when time and skill are considerations" the latex test was the most suitable titration test; suggestions were offered for its standardization.

9. "Poor mucin precipitate from synovial fluid . . ."
10. "Characteristic histologic changes in synovial membrane . . ."
11. "Characteristic histologic changes in nodules . . ."

Criteria 9, 10 and 11 are seldom practicable in epidemiologic studies.

A diagnosis of classical rheumatoid arthritis required 7 of the 11 criteria, definite 5, and probable 3. Possible rheumatoid arthritis was based on two or more of the following: morning stiffness, tenderness or pain on motion, joint swelling, subcutaneous nodules, elevated sedimentation rate or C-reactive protein, and iritis.

Proposed diagnostic criteria for population studies. Because of difficulties in applying the American Rheumatism Association criteria to epidemiologic studies, certain revisions were proposed at the 1961 Rome symposium on *Population Studies in Relation to Chronic Rheumatic Diseases.*[53] The requirements that joint swelling be of at least 6 weeks duration and that any symptom-free period between episodes of joint swelling be not greater than 3 months were dropped. Because it was recognized that criteria 9, 10 and 11 were inapplicable to population studies, only criteria 1–8 were retained as criteria for active rheumatoid arthritis. The "possible" diagnostic category was eliminated as being too nonspecific. Ankylosing spondylitis was added to the list of exclusions (which still fail to include rheumatic syndromes clearly related to trauma, physical activity, or occupation, which are commonly encountered in many population groups). It was proposed that the "full gradient of disease" be evaluated by listing the proportion of individuals fulfilling 1, 2, 3 etc. criteria. In addition, a second set of criteria was proposed for inactive rheumatoid arthritis: (1) "a past history of polyarthritis"; (2) "symmetrical deformity of peripheral joints consisting of ankylosis or irreducible subluxation especially of the lateral metatarsophalangeal or metacarpophalangeal joints; there must be some involvement of the hand or foot; involvement limited to large joints such as the elbows or knees does not satisfy this criterion;" (3) "X-ray changes of rheumatoid arthritis of grade 2 or more"; (4) "positive serological test for rheumatoid factor." A "definite" diagnosis was to be based on fulfillment of 3 or 4 criteria and a "probable" diagnosis on fulfillment of 2.

Further modifications of the diagnostic criteria were proposed at the *Third International Symposium on Population Studies in the Rheumatic Diseases* in New York in 1966.[15] Criteria 1 through 5 were proposed for active polyarthritis, apparently in recognition of the fact that much of the disease identified by their application in population studies is nonrheumatoid. It was specified that morning stiffness be not less than 15 minutes in duration. The earlier criteria for inactive rheumatoid arthritis were modified with the goal of identifying those cases acceptable as rheumatoid arthritis to a clinical rheumatologist. In addition, the use of a "joint score" was proposed in order to quantify the extent of involvement.

Future modifications of diagnostic criteria. It has been suggested that the diagnostic criteria might be improved by weighting them on the basis of their discriminatory value[1] or their estimated "relative health value."[23] It seems improbable, however, that further revision or regrouping of the existing criteria will significantly improve their value in population studies. The urgent need is for a more precise definition of rheumatoid arthritis based on knowledge of etiology or pathogenesis.

Field Methods

Most investigators engaged in population studies of rheumatoid arthritis have employed the following procedures, with varying modifications:

(1) inquiry by personal interview or questionnaire regarding rheumatic symptoms,
(2) physical examination,
(3) serologic tests for rheumatoid factor, and
(4) radiologic examination, often of hands and wrists, feet, and cervical spine.

In some instances attempts have been made to use the interview and/or physical examination to screen subjects for more thorough evaluation. Rubin, Rosenbaum, and Cobb[93] suggested that a positive "index of rheumatoid arthritis," defined as "yes" replies to questions regarding a history of arthritis or rheumaism, joint swelling, and morning stiffness or aching in the joints or muscles, could be used as a screening procedure. They reported a positive index in 65 per cent of clinically diagnosed cases of rheumatoid arthritis, and in 5 per cent of subjects who were clinically nonrheumatoid. Experience with these 3 questions in the Tecumseh study was quite similar.[80] Of the more than 7,000 Tecumseh respondents, 281 or 4 per cent had a positive index; of these almost 60 per cent had no supporting evidence for a diagnosis of rheumatoid arthritis. Of the 28 respondents classified as "definite" rheumatoid arthritis, 75 per cent had a positive index, and of the 61 classified as "probable," 34 per cent. Of all respondents 34.8 per cent answered "yes" to one or more of the questions. Of the 65.2 per cent who answered all the questions "no," 99.6 per cent presented no evidence of rheumatoid arthritis. Very similar findings were reported from Hiroshima-Nagasaki[52] and Jerusalem.[3] It would appear that this degree of sensitivity and specificity is not sufficiently precise for most investigative purposes and may be quite misleading if used as a basis for comparison of populations with differing language and cultural background.[2] Cobb, Hunt, and Harburg[28] have recently described a more detailed interview measure of rheumatoid arthritis which appears to have greater validity.

Even the combination of interview and physical examination may be insufficient for screening purposes, since it has been shown that some subjects without prior clinical evidence of rheumatoid arthritis may have radiologic evidence of the disease.[58] In addition, all studies to date have suggested that a high proportion of positive serologic tests for rheumatoid factor occur in subjects without clinical evidence of the disease. Therefore, it seems essential that the study population, either a total defined population or a random sample thereof, be subjected to complete examinations if valid and comparable results are to be obtained.

Extensive or repeated radiologic examination of apparently healthy subjects can be objected to on the grounds of unnecessary exposure to ionizing radiation. Certainly, if such examinations are to be included, the equipment and technique should be such that exposure is kept to a minimum. Examination of the sacroiliac joints is probably indefensible in premenopausal females and should not be undertaken in males without proper gonadal shielding. On these grounds it might be questioned whether radiologic examination of the joints should not be restricted to subjects presenting clinical evidence of past or present arthritis. Although there is some evidence to suggest that some cases of rheumatoid arthritis might escape detection if this were done, it must be questioned whether certain of the radiologic changes observed in clinically nonrheumatoid subjects are not due to other causes.

RESULTS OF POPULATION STUDIES OF RHEUMATOID ARTHRITIS

Prevalence Estimates of Rheumatoid Arthritis

Prevalence estimates of rheumatoid arthritis are now available for a number of population groups throughout the world (Table 12–1). Direct comparison of the prevalence data from various studies is difficult, however, because of differences in methodology. A summary of some of the results of such studies follows.

Sex.—Population studies are in general agreement with clinical experience in indicating a prevalence of rheumatoid arthritis 2 to 3 times greater in females than males. However, for reasons not yet apparent, most studies have indicated an approximately equal prevalence of rheumatoid factor seropositivity and erosive x-ray changes in the two sexes.

Age.—Most studies also agree in indicating that rheumatoid arthritis in the general population is very rare in children and young adults, but shows an in-

TABLE 12–1. GEOGRAPHIC DISTRIBUTION OF POPULATION STUDIES OF THE PREVALENCE OF RHEUMATOID ARTHRITIS

Population	*Age*	"*Definite*" *plus* "*Probable*" *RA*			"*Definite*" *RA*		
		Males	*Females*	*Both*	*Males*	*Females*	*Both*
Europe							
Wensleydale-Leigh[63]	15+	2.5	6.0	4.3	0.47	1.6	1.07
Wales[78]							
Rhonda Fach	15+	1.1	1.8	1.4	0.7	0.6	0.75
Vale of Glamorgan	15+	2.7	5.6	4.15	1.0	1.1	1.0
Marken, Netherlands[104]	15+	0.6	3.5	2.1			
Heinola, Finland[62]	15+	3.9	10.1	7.5	1.3	4.2	3.0
Sweden[49]	15+			3.1 *			
Stockholm, Sweden[8]	31–74			2.7 ±			
Piestany, Czechoslovakia[101]	15+	0.7	1.2	1.0	0.3	0.5	0.4
Sofia, Bulgaria[106]	15+	0.9	4.0	2.9	0.2	1.2	0.9
Rotterdam, Netherlands[35]	15+	0.9	2.4		0.5	1.2	
United States and Canada							
Pittsburgh, Pa.[30]	15+	0.6	4.7	2.7			0.7
Tecumseh, Mich.[80]	15+	0.7	2.6	1.6	0.3	0.7	0.5
Framingham, Mass.[43]	35+	1.4	4.4				
Sudbury, Mass.[25]	15+	1.3	3.8				0.84
American Indian[20]							
Blackfeet	30+			4.1			
Pima	30+			5.4			
Haida Indian[39]	15+	1.7	2.0	1.8	0.4	1.5	0.9
U.S. Health Exam. Survey[85]	18–79	1.7	4.6	3.2			0.96
Caribbean							
Guaynabo, Puerto Rico[75]	15+	0.32	1.2	0.92	0.16	0.4	0.34
Jamaica[68]				11.0			1.7
Africa and West Asia							
Jerusalem, Israel[4]	20+	0.5	2.0		0.0	0.4	
Nigeria-Liberia[84]							
Igbo-Ora	15+			0.8			
Isheri	15+			1.6			
Cavalla	15+			2.8			
Pacific and Orient							
Japan							
Toyonaka-Tojo-Iwata[96]	20+			0.3			
Hiroshima-Nagasaki[52]	20+				0.4	0.7	0.55
Rotorua, New Zealand[92]							
Europeans				12.3			6.5
Maoris				3.2			1.6

± Figure given for "crude prevalence" of RA
* Figure given for classical, definite, probable, and possible RA

creasing prevalence with advancing age beginning in middle life.[25,80,85] In many studies this increasing prevalence continues into the oldest age groups, as would be expected of a chronic disease without marked effect on longevity. In some there has been an apparent decrease in disease frequency after age 65, but in many populations relatively few subjects in the older age groups are included. In addition, there is the possibility that those with rheumatoid arthritis may have died at an earlier age as a result of some other disease with a higher prevalence and a high or higher mortality ratio. Because of these age trends comparison of prevalence rates between populations of different age composition may be quite misleading unless appropriate age corrections are made.

Geography and climate.—To date no meaningful geographic differences in the prevalence of rheumatoid arthritis have been demonstrated. When attempts have been made to ensure uniformity of methodology prevalence rates have generally proved to be quite similar for different population groups. For example, comparison of data from 6 communities in the United Kingdom, Finland, and the Netherlands disclosed no regional differences in disease prevalence[71] and rates for Hiroshima-Nagasaki, Japan[52,112] and Tecumseh, Michigan[80] were quite similar.

The early suggestion that the disease might be less frequent in the tropics has not been confirmed, prevalence rates for Guaynabo, Puerto Rico, for example, being very close to those reported from Hiroshima-Nagasaki[112] and Tecumseh, Michigan.[80] Probable rheumatoid arthritis was significantly more prevalent in Jamaica than in several North American and European population groups, but definite disease was not.[68] No relationship between disease prevalence and latitude was observed in this study. Investigation of two tribes of American Indians living under sharply contrasting climatic conditions revealed no significant difference in disease prevalence.[20]

Ethnic factors.—All ethnic and racial groups appear to share susceptibility to rheumatoid arthritis. In the U.S. Health Examination Survey[85] the prevalence of rheumatoid arthritis was the same in white and black adults. Jamaican blacks had more "probable" disease, but a prevalence of "definite" rheumatoid arthritis that was not significantly different from that of several North American Indian and European Caucasian groups.[68] The prevalence of "probable" and "definite" rheumatoid arthritis in 3 African localities was not significantly different from that observed in Leigh and Wensleydale, although "definite" disease was rare.[84] The prevalence of rheumatoid arthritis in Japan was similar to that reported from Western population groups.[112]

Although their significance is obscure, several observations of ethnic differences in disease prevalence have been made. In Jerusalem women immigrants, but not men, of European origin had more rheumatoid arthritis than those from North Africa or Asia.[4] In Rotorua, New Zealand rheumatoid arthritis was more prevalent among Europeans than Maoris.[92]

Social, psychological, and economic factors.—The U.S. National Health Survey indicated a higher prevalence of rheumatoid arthritis in adults of either sex with less than 5 years of education.[85] For males rates decreased as years of education increased. Men in the professional, technical, and managerial fields had relatively low rates. In Leigh, England, however, there appeared to be no correlation of rheumatoid arthritis with occupation (comparing miners, laborers, tradesmen, and business and professional groups) and none with injuries, conditions of cold or dampness at home or work, or type of housing.[60]

In the National Health Survey prevalence rates were somewhat higher for males with less than $2,000 family income, but not for females, suggesting that this might be a reflection of decreased earning power as a result of disease disability.[85] In this study metropolitan areas with populations of 0.5 to 3 million had somewhat lower prevalence rates, a finding compatible with the earlier report that in the Netherlands the lowest rates were observed in the largest towns.[34] Studies in the United Kingdom failed to reveal significant urban-rural differences in the prevalence or severity of clinical or radiologic evidence of the disease, although the presence of rheumatoid factor positivity was significantly greater in urban samples.[10]

Cobb and his associates have pioneered in the investigation of the relationships between social stress and rheumatoid arthritis. In their most recent study they report a number of associations between rheumatoid arthritis and certain social and psychological variables including marital hostility, parental status stress, recalled parent-child relationships, self-esteem, etc., different for men and women.[29] The National Health Survey indicated that widowed men, unmarried females, and females over age 45 without children had significantly less rheumatoid arthritis. While several studies have suggested that rheumatoid arthritis is more frequent among sibs from large families,[16,26] the Manchester[66] and National Health Surveys[85] failed to confirm such a relationship. An earlier report[61] that rheumatoid arthritis was more frequent among mothers of 4 or more children was likewise not confirmed by the National Health Survey.

Extensive reviews of the social[96] and personality[82] factors associated with rheumatoid arthritis have appeared.

Incidence of rheumatoid arthritis.—Most population studies of rheumatoid arthritis have provided estimates of point prevalence of the disease. It would be expected that measures of incidence rates (the number of *new* cases appearing during a specified time period among a specified unit of population) would be more valuable for comparing different population groups for possible clues to the etiology of the disease. Such estimates are available for Hiroshima-Nagasaki (0.097 per cent),[52] Tojo, Japan (0. per cent),[97] Sudbury, Mass. (0.29 pe cent),[24] and Rotterdam (0.86 per cent).[3 In view of the relative rarity of rheuma toid arthritis in the general population the fluctuating severity of the disease, an the less than satisfactory reproducibilit of the diagnostic criteria in populatio studies, it remains to be determine whether the potentially greater value o incidence data can be realized. Longi tudinal studies in which members of representative population are examine on 2 or more occasions not only permi estimates of disease incidence, but als provide a unique opportunity to stud the spectrum and natural history of disease manifestations.

Etiologic hypotheses.—Thus far, epidemi ologic studies of rheumatoid arthriti have provided a great deal of descriptiv data, but only negative information relat ing to etiology. Most studies that hav been designed to test a specific etiologic hypothesis have focused on genetic factors or possible geographic or climatic variations in disease prevalence. The Adult Health Study conducted by the Atomic Bomb Casualty Commission in Hiroshima-Nagasaki provided a unique opportunity to investigate the relationship between radiation and disease prevalence.[112] No such association was found, providing strong evidence against an earlier suggestion that rheumatoid arthritis might be the result of somatic mutation.[21]

"Benign Polyarthritis"

In the survey of subjects age 55 to 64 in Leigh, England 36 of the total 380 persons examined gave a past history of transient attacks of polyarthritis.[58] On extending the study to include subjects from age 15 on, a past history of polyarthritis was encountered in 5 per cent of males and 7 per cent of females.[69] Similar figures were obtained in the Wensleydale and South Wales studies. This condition, which the authors termed benign polyarthritis, was characterized by painful swelling of joints lasting for 2 to 3 months and followed by complete recovery. It occurred at all ages, but was common between ages 5 and 24. Clinical residua of joint disease were encountered at an earlier age and were 5 times more common in those with a past history of polyarthritis than in those without. Radiologic changes in the cervical spine were also somewhat more common, but sheep cell agglutination test positivity did not differ in the two groups. In a few such subjects cardiac or rheumatoid residua suggested the likelihood that the earlier episode of polyarthritis was rheumatic fever or juvenile rheumatoid arthritis. Clinical evidence suggested that these were not examples of Jaccoud's arthritis, palindromic rheumatism, or peripheral arthritis associated with spondylitis. The possible relationship to rubella, measles, infections, hepatitis, or respiratory infection was considered, although such histories were usually not obtained. On the basis of the similarity in seasonal onset with that reported by Short, Bauer, and Reynolds[99] for exacerbations of rheumatoid arthritis, it was suggested that viral or other infections might be the inciting event in both conditions. The authors concluded that such cases might be "related to" the seronegative type of inflammatory polyarthritis, thought to pursue a relatively benign course. Kellgren has recently questioned whether this syndrome should be regarded as a mild attack of rheumatoid arthritis, noting that it is infrequent in the past history of patients with classical rheumatoid arthritis.[54] He has observed that if it is not rheumatoid arthritis it will seriously interfere with epidemiologic studies of that disease since it usually fulfills the 5 clinical diagnostic criteria and is relatively common.

The same problem exists in relationship to other recognized nonrheumatoid forms of polyarthritis. A number of viral agents have been associated with clinical polyarthritis.[102] Rubella has been most frequently reported in this regard, but arthritis has also been described as a manifestation of mumps, smallpox, erythema infectiosum, and, less commonly, other of the common viral infections. In most of these conditions arthritis has been more frequent in adults. In Australia an epidemic polyarthritis associated with rash has been observed with Group A arbovirus infections. In Africa Chikungunya and O'nyong-nyong fever, also regarded as Group A arbovirus infections, have been associated with prominent rheumatic manifestations. The relationship of these relatively well-defined conditions to other African disorders reported as "acute nonspecific arthritis in the African"[38] and "acute tropical polyarthritis"[42] is unclear. Reports of arthritis and arthralgia with urticaria in association with viral hepatitis have recently rekindled interest in this area.[9,37] The inability in most epidemiologic studies to correctly identify these various forms of polyarthritis and distinguish them from rheumatoid arthritis creates a dilemma which is recognized, but not resolved, by proposing diagnostic criteria for polyarthritis.

Serologic Tests for Rheumatoid Factor

The various serologic tests for rheumatoid factor have been generally accepted as worthwhile diagnostic procedures in clinical practice although their nonspecificity is well recognized. In established rheumatoid arthritis, test positivity has ranged from 60 to 90 per cent, or more. In apparently healthy, normal controls the rate of seropositivity with most procedures has been less than 5 per cent, the figure specified in the A.R.A. diagnostic criteria. Apparently false positive results have been reported with greater frequency in a variety of other disease states, many of which share the common feature of hypergammaglobulinemia. Rheumatoid-like factors have been induced in experimental animals in response to intense antigenic stimulation, suggesting that their appearance in man might reflect similar prolonged immunologic stimulation.

These serologic tests have been employed in a number of population studies in which sizable numbers of subjects from a wide span of ages were included (Tab e 12–2). These studies are in general agreement on the following points:

1. The prevalence of seropositivity is approximately equal in males and females.[5,10,24,52,78,80,111]
2. The prevalence of seropositivity increases with age.[6,10,24,52,71,80,111]
3. These tests have proved to be inefficient as case detection tools for rheumatoid arthritis. In most studies only a minority of seropositive subjects, 20 per cent in the experience of Ball and Lawrence[10] and 33 per cent in the Tecumseh study,[80] has presented other evidence of rheumatoid arthritis. Seropositivity has shown a tendency to persist on retesting in some studies,[24,111] while in others[5,79] 65 to 75 per cent of seropositive subjects have reverted to seronegativity, suggesting that many of the initial results may have been transient false positive reactions associated with intercurrent infectious diseases. The many infectious and noninfectious diseases which may be associated with positive rheumatoid factor tests have recently been reviewed.[13]
4. Among subjects found to have evidence for rheumatoid arthritis the rate of seropositivity has generally been significantly lower than that reported from clinic or hospital series.[5,6,24,63,80,108] This discrepancy is doubtless due in large part to the fact that patients with more severe and more persistent disease, who are more likely to present themselves to clinics or hospitals, are also more likely to be seropositive. It is likewise compatible with the view that rheumatoid arthritis as it exists in the general population is more often a milder, more benign disease than would be suspected from hospital experience.
5. In most population studies the prevalence of positivity has been less than 5 per cent and variations in prevalence have probably reflected in part variations in technical aspects of serological testing. Several studies have attempted to overcome this problem of standardization of serologic procedures by

TABLE 12–2. POPULATION STUDIES OF THE PREVALENCE OF RHEUMATOID FACTOR TEST POSITIVITY

Population Studied	*Age Range*	*Test Employed*	*Per Cent Positivity*		
			Males	*Females*	*Both*
Leigh-Wensleydale[63]	15 years and over	Sheep cell agglut.	4.0	5.0	
Seven European communities[71]	15 years and over	Sheep cell agglut.	3.7	4.4	
		Bentonite flocc.	4.0	4.0	4.0
Tecumseh, Mich.[80]	6 years and over	Latex fixation	3.4	3.3	3.35
Haida Indians[39]	15 years and over	Sheep cell agglut.	1.2	3.5	2.2
Sudbury, Mass.[24]	15 years and over	Sheep cell agglut.	0.82	0.93	0.88
		Bentonite flocc.	1.55	1.27	1.4
Jerusalem, Israel[5]	20 years and over	Human erythrocyte agglut.	0.8	1.2	1.0
		Latex fixation	4.4	4.5	4.4
Hiroshima, Japan[52]	15 years and over	Latex fixation	8.7	8.9	
USA (NHS)[85]	18–79	Bentonite flocculation			2.6*

* of respondents without RA

having all sera tested in a central laboratory. In one such study seropositivity was more frequent in urban (5.1 per cent) than in rural (2.4 per cent) areas, but was not accompanied by a proportionate difference in prevalence of rheumatoid arthritis.[5] High rates of seropositivity in certain populations, especially in tropical regions, have been attributed to the greater frequency of acute and chronic infectious diseases. It has been suggested that the increased prevalence of seropositivity in the aged and that observed in certain geographic areas may have a common etiology, reflecting "an antibody response to differing rates of antigenic experience, that in the aged occurring as a function of increased exposure to disease with time, and that in different areas resulting from geographic variations in disease exposure."[83]

6. Although not emphasized in most reports, there is a serious problem of the reproducibility of rheumatoid factor tests in longitudinal studies. Despite careful attempts at standardization, much of the variability of test results can be explained reasonably only by variation in technical factors.

Not yet adequately answered is the important question as to whether or not positive serologic tests for rheumatoid factor in otherwise healthy individuals identify those with an increased risk of subsequent development of rheumatoid arthritis. Suggesting that they do was the early study of Ball and Lawrence[11] who found on reexamination after 5 years of 19 seropositive subjects who originally had no clinical or radiological evidence of rheumatoid arthritis that 7 had developed evidence of the disease, as compared with 5 of 57 seronegative subjects similarly followed. More recently, in the Sudbury, Mass. study it was reported that on reexamination after 3 years the incidence of rheumatoid arthritis (employing the New York criteria) among subjects initially positive with the bentonite flocculation test was 1.1 per cent;[24] the corresponding figure for those positive with the sensitized sheep cell agglutination test was 1.9 per cent. Incidence rates for a positive history of an episode of polyarthritis in these two groups were 2.8 and 3.3 per cent respectively. These figures contrasted with an annual incidence rate of rheumatoid arthritis in a random sample of the Sudbury population, including seropositive as well as seronegative subjects, of 0.29 ± 0.16 per cent.[88] In this population it was noted that all persons who were positive for rheumatoid arthritis by both history and physical examination were over 45 years of age and that relatively few seropositive subjects over age 45 had no evidence for rheumatoid arthritis.[24] Burch and Bennett[22] in a 2 to 6 year followup of seropositive and seronegative Pima Indians reported that the risk of development of probable or definite rheumatoid arthritis was 6.25 times greater in the seropositive group. Of the 19 individuals out of 5127 subjects followed for up to 20 years in the Framingham, Mass. study, who converted their latex fixation test from negative to positive in a titer of 1:80 or more, 4 developed probable or definite rheumatoid arthritis, 6 had bone or joint complaints which were difficult to assess, 1 posed a diagnostic problem between gout and rheumatoid arthritis, 2 had nonrheumatoid conditions possibly related to their latex positivity (hyperglobulinemic purpura, granulomatous mesenteritis), and 8 had no apparent associated abnormality."[44]

Several other investigations show less evidence for the emergence of clinical rheumatoid arthritis in seropositive but otherwise healthy subjects. Finnish investigators, reexamining a small group of 7 subjects with apparently false positive sheep cell agglutination tests after a 9-year interval, found that none had developed rheumatoid arthritis and that only 3 remained seropositive.[7] Waller and Toone[110] reported that evaluation of

included in such an investigation. This potential bias can be overcome if the rheumatoid and control index cases are selected in the course of examination of a total population or random sample thereof. In several studies this has been accomplished. Miall[77] reported evidence by history and/or examination of rheumatoid arthritis in 3.1 per cent of 354 parents and siblings of 59 index cases, as compared to 0.6 per cent of 502 relatives of 89 index control subjects. Lawrence and Ball[67] found clinical evidence of rheumatoid arthritis on personal examination in 9 per cent of relatives of pro-

in the controls. Radiologic and serologic evidence of the disease did not occur more frequently in the seronegative families than in the controls, although clinical rheumatoid arthritis was somewhat more frequent. In a similar investigation Bremner, Alexander, and Duthie[18] found the prevalence of clinical, radiologic and serologic evidence of the disease to be the same (4.4 per cent) in families of seropositive probands, while in the seronegative families clinical disease (5.5 per cent) was more frequent than radiologic (2.7 per cent) or serologic (1.8 per cent) manifestations. DeBlecourt, Boerma,

3 normal individuals with high titer of rheumatoid factors followed for 6 to 9 years revealed no evidence of disease. However, they later reported in a brief communication that 1 of these 3 persons had developed probable systemic lupus erythematosus.[105] Reexamination after an average interval of 4 years of 105 subjects in the Tecumseh, Michigan study who had initially had positive latex fixation tests revealed that 46.7 per cent remained seropositive but presented no other evidence for rheumatoid arthritis, 7.6 per cent presented evidence for questionable or possible and 1.9 per cent for

There is also reason to suspect that erosive x-ray changes in the hands and feet may be due to nonrheumatoid changes in a significant number of cases. In comparing radiographs from 8 different populations erosive changes were observed more frequently in Jamaicans than in North American Indians, and more frequently in the latter than in Caucasians.[68] The greater prevalence in males in the Indian populations suggested spondylitis or Reiter's disease as a possible cause. The high prevalence of minimal changes in the Jamaicans, most

TABLE 12–4. STUDIES OF RELATIVES OF SEROPOSITIVE AND SERONEGATIVE PROPOSITI WITH RHEUMATOID ARTHRITIS

Reference	*Number of Propositi*	*Number of Relatives*	*Per Cent with Clinical R.A.*	*Per Cent with Rheumatoid Factor*	*Per Cent with X-ray Findings*
Lawrence and Ball[67]	64	183	9.0	13.0	7.0
Seropositive	35	95	16.0	20.0	12.0
Seronegative	29	88	8.0	6.0	1.2
Controls		183	2.0	5.0	3.0
Bremner, Alexander, and Duthie[18]	63				
Seropositive	28	92	4.4	4.4	4.4
Seronegative	35	110	5.5	1.8	2.7
DeBlecourt, Boerma, and Vorenkamp[32]	62				
Seropositive	31	226	2.2	6.6	
Seronegative	31	233	0.45	0.9	
Lawrence[64]					
Seropositive		345	9.6		11.7
Seronegative		300	5.3		3.0
Seroneg., excl. psoriasis		237	4.6		
Bunim, Burch, and O'Brien[20]					
Seropositive	22	71	2.8	1.4	
Seronegative	20	63	3.2	6.3	
Controls		211	5.6	4.3	

and Vorenkamp[32] in an investigation of relatives of probands with definite or classical rheumatoid arthritis, found clinical rheumatoid arthritis (2.2 per cent) and seropositivity (6.6 per cent) to be more frequent in the seropositive families than in the seronegative (0.45 and 0.9 per cent respectively). Only the difference in seropositivity was significant at the 5 per cent level of confidence, however. The authors concluded that their data suggested a slight hereditary trend for the seropositive form of rheumatoid arthritis, but not for the seronegative variety. In their investigations of the Pima and Blackfeet Indians, Bunim, and O'Brien[20] found no familial aggregation of rheumatoid arthritis, or of positive rheumatoid factor tests. Using a statistical analytic method employing the estimated gene frequency in these populations, they found that their data were incompatible with either a dominant or recessive mode of inheritance but agreed closely with the values expected on the basis of random distribution. In a recent investigation in 3 regions of Sweden in which virtually all residents over age 7 were examined no significantly higher frequencies of rheumatoid arthritis were found among relatives of rheumatoid arthritics than among matched relatives of matched controls.[48] Schull and Cobb,[95] utilizing a "Rheumatoid Arthritis Measure" based on a detailed interview, likewise failed to find evidence that heredity was an important feature of the etiology of rheumatoid arthritis. These authors suggest possible mechanisms by which earlier studies might have suggested familial aggregation of disease when, in fact, none existed. Despite these negative reports, Lawrence[66] has suggested that genetic predisposition, while playing little part in the etiology of seronegative rheumatoid arthritis, may be important in the more severe seropositive disease.

The occurrence of rheumatoid arthritis among spouses of index cases is of considerable interest since they share a common environment to a large degree but have a dissimilar genetic background. While some studies have failed to show an increased frequency of clinical disease or seropositivity in spouses as compared with control groups,[16,31,32,47,67] others have indicated an increased prevalence of disease, thus suggesting that environmental factors may be of some importance.[40,45,51,93,94]

A few twin studies have been undertaken in attempt to clarify the role of heredity in rheumatoid arthritis. If hereditary influences are great one would expect a significantly higher rate of concordance in monozygotic as compared with dizygotic twins. In reviewing reported experience on arthritis in monozygous twins, Meyerowitz, Jacox and Hess[76] observed that 25 of the 28 twin pairs had been discordant. In 4 of the 5 adult twin sets studied by the authors psychological stress had appeared to play a role in initiation of the disease. Several groups of investigators have attempted the systematic identification of twins prior to their examination for rheumatoid arthritis in order to avoid the bias toward reporting concordant twin pairs. A study of Danish twins born during the period 1870 to 1910 indicated that 16 of 47 monozygous pairs with rheumatoid arthritis were concordant as compared with 10 of 141 dizygous pairs.[46] Investigation in Great Britain revealed no appreciable difference in concordance for rheumatoid arthritis between monozygous and dizygous twin pairs.[64] Similarly, study of 145 twin pairs in Scotland revealed no appreciable difference in concordance for rheumatoid factor, or any of 4 other autoantibodies, when monozygotic and dizygotic twins of either sex were compared, suggesting that in healthy persons formation of these antibodies was governed mainly by environmental influences.[19] Such observations provide little support for a strong role for genetic factors in the production of clinical rheumatoid arthritis or rheumatoid factor. The potential value of discordant monozygous twins, all of whom presumably share whatever genetic predisposition exists, in the search for environmental etiologic factors has been emphasized.[66,86]

For more detailed discussion of methodology and results of genetic studies of rheumatoid arthritis the reader is referred to reviews by Blumberg,[17] O'Brien,[87] and Lawrence.[66]

FUTURE STUDIES

The major emphasis in future epidemiologic studies of rheumatoid arthritis should be on the detection of etiologic and pathogenetic factors. Specific areas in which carefully conducted longitudinal studies can contribute importantly include: the significance of positive rheumatoid factor tests in otherwise healthy subjects, the origin of erosive radiologic changes in clinically nonrheumatoid subjects, the spectrum and natural history of rheumatoid arthritis in the general population as opposed to hospital or clinic, the various etiologies of "benign polyarthritis" and its relationship to rheumatoid arthritis, the possible role of genetic factors in the seropositive form of the disease, and the relationship of various social and psychological factors to rheumatoid arthritis. To be most fruitful epidemiologic studies should be as closely linked as possible to current clinical and laboratory investigations of rheumatoid arthritis. They provide a means of testing etiologic hypotheses arising from more basic investigations.

There are important obstacles to successful continuation of epidemiologic investigations of rheumatoid arthritis. A major problem is the relative rarity of the disease in the general population. Also critical is our lack of a suitable definition of the disease. Kellgren[55] has commented that in hospital patients with rheumatoid arthritis there is reasonable concordance between the clinical, serologic, and radiologic manifestations of the disease, which tends in this setting to be progressive and accompanied often by nodules and occasionally by evidence of vasculitis. In population studies the degree of concordance has been much less and the interpretation of results uncertain and often speculative. There is also grave doubt at the present time as to whether society acting through its elected representatives is willing to invest the substantial amounts required to continue epidemiologic as well as basic research. Despite the need for more adequate delivery of the best available medical care to all segments of society, there can be no quarrel with the need for more fundamental knowledge regarding rheumatoid arthritis and the other rheumatic diseases, and it seems inevitable that the necessary investment will be made—eventually, if not now. When it is made, the epidemiologist, the clinical rheumatologist, and the basic researcher can profitably combine their talents in the quest for knowledge of the etiology of the disease.

BIBLIOGRAPHY

1. Abramson, J. H.: J. Chronic Dis., *20*, 275, 1967.
2. Abramson, J. H., Adler, E., Hader, S. B., Elkan, Z., Gabriel, K. R. and Wahl, M.: Arth. & Rheum., *7*, 153, 1964.
3. Adler, E. and Abramson, J. H.: Israel J. Med. Sci., *4*, 210, 1968.
4. Adler, E., Abramson, J. H., Elkan, Z., Ben Hador, S. and Goldberg, R.: Am. J. Epid., *85*, 365, 1967.
5. Adler, E., Abramson, J. H., Goldberg, R., Elkan, Z. and Ben Hador, S.: Am. J. Epid., *85*, 378, 1967.
6. Aho, K., Julkunen, H., Laine, V., Ripatti, N. and Wager, O.: Acta Rheum. Scand., *7*, 201, 1961.
7. Aho, K., Kirpila, J. and Wager, O.: Ann. Med. Exp. Fenn., *37*, 377, 1959.
8. Allander, E.: Acta Rheum. Scand., *16*, Suppl. 15, 1970.
9. Alpert, E., Costen, R. L. and Schur, P. H.: Arth. & Rheum., *13*, 303, 1970 (abstract).
10. Ball, J. and Lawrence, J. S.: Ann. Rheum. Dis., *20*, 235, 1961.
11. Ball, J. and Lawrence, J. S.: Ann. Rheum. Dis., *22*, 311, 1963.
12. Barter, R. W.: Ann. Rheum. Dis., *11*, 39, 1952.
13. Bartfeld, H.: Ann. N.Y. Acad. Sci., *168*, Art. 1, 30, 1969.
14. Beall, G. and Cobb, S.: J. Chron. Dis., *14*, 291, 1961.
15. Bennett, P. H. and Burch, T. A.: Bull. Rheum. Dis., *17*, 453, 1967.
16. Bennett, P. H. and Burch, T. A.: in *Population Studies of the Rheumatic Diseases*, Amsterdam, Excerpta Medica Foundation, 1968, p. 136.
17. Blumberg, B. S.: Arth. & Rheum., *3*, 178, 1960.
18. Bremner, J. M., Alexander, W. R. M. and Duthie, J. J. R.: Ann. Rheum. Dis., *18*, 279, 1959.
19. Buchanan, W. W., Boyle, J. A., Greig, W. R., McAndrew, R., Barr, M., Anderson, J. R. and Goudie, R. B.: Ann Rheum. Dis., *25*, 463, 1966.
20. Bunim, J. J., Burch, T. A. and O'Brien, W. M.: Bull. Rheum. Dis., *15*, 349, 1964.
21. Burch, P. R. J.: Lancet, *1*, 1253, 1963.
22. Burch, T. A. and Bennett, P. H.: V Panamerican Congress of Rheumatology, Punta del Este, Uruguay, 1970, p. 43.
23. Burch, T. A. and O'Brien, W. M.: Milbank Memorial Fund Quarterly, *43*, 161, 1965.
24. Cathcart, E. S. and O'Sullivan, J. B.: Ann. N.Y. Acad. Sci., *168*, 41, 1969.
25. Cathcart, E. S. and O'Sullivan, J. B.: New Engl. J. Med., *282*, 421, 1970.
26. Chen, E. and Cobb, S.: J. Chron. Dis., *12*, 544, 1960.
27. Cobb, S.: Amer. J. Pub. Health, *52*, 1119, 1962.
28. Cobb, S., Hunt, P. and Harburg, E.: J. Chron. Dis., *22*, 203, 1969.
29. Cobb, S., Schull, W. J., Harburg, E. and Kasl, S. V.: J. Chron. Dis., *22*, 295, 1969.
30. Cobb, S., Warren, J. E., Merchant, W. R. and Thompson, D. J.: J. Chron. Dis., *5*, 636, 1957.
31. Dalakos, T. G., McSween, R. N. M., Whaley, K., Dick, W. C., Boyle, J. A., Jasani, M. K., Wilson, E., Buchanan, W.W., and Goudie, R. B.: Ann. Rheum. Dis., *28*, 329, 1969.
32. DeBlecourt, J. J., Boerma, F. W. and Vorenkamp, E. O.: Ann. Rheum. Dis., *21*, 339, 1962.
33. DeBlecourt, J. J., Polman, A. and DeBlecourt-Meindersma, T.: Ann. Rheum. Dis., *20*, 215, 1961.
34. DeGraaff, R.: in *Proceedings of the ISRA Symposium on the Social Aspect of Chronic Rheumatic Joint Affections Especially Rheumatoid Arthritis*, Amsterdam, Excerpta Medica Foundation, 1960, p. 7.

35. Den Oudsten, S. A., Planten, O and Postuma, E. P. S.: in *Population Studies of the Rheumatic Diseases,* Amsterdam, Excerpta Medica Foundation, 1968, p. 99.
36. Doll, R., editor: *Methods of Geographic Pathology,* Oxford, Blackwell Scientific Publications, 1959.
37. Fernandez, R. and McCarty, D. J.: Ann. Intern. Med., *74,* 207, 1971.
38. Gelfand, M.: Cent. Afr. J. Med., *9,* 276, 1963.
39. Gofton, J. P., Robinson, H. S. and Price, G. E.: Ann. Rheum. Dis., *23,* 364, 1964.
40. Goldenberg, A., Singer, J. M. and Plotz, C. M.: J. Mount Sinai Hosp., *27,* 480, 1960.
41. Greenwood, B. M.: Ann. Rheum. Dis., *28,* 488, 1969.
42. Greenwood, B. M.: Quart. J. Med., *38,* 295, 1969.
43. Hall, A. P.: Personal Communication, Quoted by Adler, E., *et al.*: Am. J. Epid., *85,* 365, 1967.
44. Hall, A. P.: Arth. & Rheum., *12,* 301, 1969 (abstract).
45. Hartmann, F., Behrend, T., Deicher, H., Fricke, R., Manecke, H. and Walpurger, G.: in *The Epidemiology of Chronic Rheumatism.* Oxford, Blackwell Scientific Publications, and Philadelphia, F. A. Davis Co., 1963, p. 277.
46. Harvald, B. and Hauge, M.: in *Genetics and the Epidemiology of Chronic Diseases,* Washington, D.C., U. S. Government Printing Office, 1965, p. 61.
47. Hellgren, L.: Acta Rheum. Scand., *15,* 135, 1969.
48. Hellgren, L.: Acta Rheum. Scand., *16,* 211, 1970.
49. Hellgren, L.: Acta Rheum. Scand., *16,* 293, 1970.
50. Hijmans, W.: in *Population Studies of the Rheumatic Diseases,* Amsterdam, Excerpta Medica Foundation, 1968, p. 222.
51. Holsti, O. and Rantasalo, V.: Acta Med. Scand., *88,* 180, 1936.
52. Kato, H., Duff, I. F., Russell, W. J., Uda, Y., Hamilton, H. B., Kawamoto, S. and Johnson, K. G.: J. Chron. Dis., *23,* 659, 1971.
53. Kellgren, J. H.: Bull. Rheum. Dis., *13,* 291, 1962.
54. Kellgren, J. H.: Arth. & Rheum., *9,* 658, 1966.
55. Kellgren, J. H.: in *Population Studies of the Rheumatic Diseases,* Amsterdam, Excerpta Medica Foundation, 1968, p. 151.
56. Kellgren, J. H. and Bier, F.: Ann. Rheum. Dis., *15,* 55, 1956.
57. Kellgren, J. H., Jeffrey, M. R. and Ball, J., eds.: *The Epidemiology of Chronic Rheumatism,* Oxford, Blackwell Scientific Publications, and Philadelphia, F. A. Davis Co., 1963, 2 vols.
58. Kellgren, J. H. and Lawrence, J. S.: Ann. Rheum. Dis., *15,* 1, 1956.
59. Kellgren, J. H. and Lawrence, J. S.: Ann. Rheum. Dis., *16,* 485, 1957.
60. Kellgren, J. H., Lawrence, J. S. and Aitken-Swan, J.: Ann. Rheum. Dis., *12,* 5, 1953.
61. King, S. H. and Cobb, S.: J. Chron. Dis., *7,* 466, 1958.
62. Laine, V. A. I.: Acta Rheum. Scand., *8,* 81, 1962.
63. Lawrence, J. S.: Ann. Rheum. Dis., *20,* 11, 1961.
64. Lawrence, J. S.: Clin. Exp. Immunol., *2,* 769, 1967.
65. Lawrence, J. S.: Rheumatology, *2,* 1, 1969.
66. Lawrence, J. S.: Ann. Rheum. Dis., *29,* 357, 1970.
67. Lawrence, J. S. and Ball, J.: Ann. Rheum. Dis., *17,* 160, 1958.
68. Lawrence, J. S., Behrend, T., Bennett, P. H., Bremner, J. M., Burch, T. A., Gofton, J., O'brien, W., and Robinson, H.: Ann. Rheum. Dis., *25,* 425, 1966.
69. Lawrence, J. S. and Bennett, P. H.: Ann. Rheum. Dis., *19,* 20, 1960.
70. Lawrence, J. S., Bremner, J. M., Ball, J. and Burch, T. A.: Ann. Rheum. Dis., *25,* 59, 1966.
71. Lawrence, J. S., Laine, V. A. I. and DeGraaff, R.: Proc. Royal Soc. Med., *54,* 454, 1961.
72. Lawrence, J. S., Valkenburg, H. A., Bremner, J. M. and Ball, J.: Ann. Rheum. Dis., *29,* 269, 1970.
73. Lewis-Faning, E.: Ann. Rheum. Dis., *9,* suppl., 1950.
74. Masi, A. T.: Annual Review of Medicine, *18,* 185, 1967.
75. Mendez-Bryan, R., Gonsalez-Alcover, R. and Roger, L.: Arth. & Rheum., *7,* 171, 1964.
76. Meyerowitz, S., Jacox, R. F. and Hess, D. W.: Arth. & Rheum., *11,* 1, 1968.
77. Miall, W. E.: Ann. Rheum. Dis., *14,* 150, 1955.
78. Miall, W. E., Ball, J. and Kellgren, J. H.: Ann. Rheum. Dis., *17,* 263, 1958.

79. MIKKELSEN, W. M. and DODGE, H. J.: Arth. & Rheum., *12*, 87, 1969.
80. MIKKELSEN, W. M., DODGE, H. J., DUFF, I. F. and KATO, H.: J. Chron. Dis., *20*, 351, 1967.
81. MIKKELSEN, W. M., DUFF, I. F. and DODGE, H. J.: J. Chron. Dis., *23*, 151, 1970.
82. MOOS, R. H.: J. Chron. Dis., *17*, 41, 1964.
83. MOSKOWITZ, R. W., BENEDICT, K. J. and STAUFFER, R.: J. Chron. Dis., *30*, 291, 1967.
84. MULLER, A. S.: *Population Studies on the Prevalence of Rheumatic Diseases in Liberia and Nigeria*, The Hague, J. H. Pasmans, 1970.
85. National Center for Health Statistics: P.H.S. Publication No. 1000, Series 11, No. 17, U.S. Government Printing Office, Washington, D.C., Sept. 1966.
86. O'BRIEN, W. M.: Arth. & Rheum., *11*, 81, 1968.
87. O'BRIEN, W. M.: Clin. Exp. Immunol., *2*, 785, 1967.
88. O'SULLIVAN, J. B., CATHCART, E. S. an BOLZAN, J. A.: in *Population Studies of the Rheumatic Diseases*, Amsterdam, Excerpta Medica Foundation, 1968, p. 109.
89. ROBECCHI, A. and DANEO, V.: Acta Rheum. Scand., *5*, 245, 1959.
90. ROPES, M. W., BENNETT, G. A., COBB, S., JACOX, R. F. and JESSAR, R. A.: Bull. Rheum. Dis., *7*, 121, 1956.
91. ROPES, M. W., BENNETT, G. A., COBB, S., JACOX, R. F. and JESSAR, R. A.: Bull. Rheum. Dis., *9*, 175, 1958.
92. ROSE, B. S. and ISDALE, I. C.: in *Epidemiology of Chronic Rheumatism*, Oxford, Blackwell Scientific Publications, and Philadelphia, F. A. Davis Co., 1963, p. 156.
93. RUBIN, T., ROSENBAUM, J. and COBB, S.: J. Chron. Dis., *4*, 253, 1956.
94. SCHMID, F. R. and SLATIS, H.: Arth. & Rheum., *5*, 319, 1962 (abstract).
95. SCHULL, W. J. and COBB, S.: J. Chron. Dis., *22*, 217, 1969.
96. SCOTCH, N. A. and GEIGER, H. J.: J. Chron. Dis., *15*, 1037, 1062.
97. SHICHIKAWA, K.: in *Population Studies of the Rheumatic Diseases*, Amsterdam, Excerpta Medica Foundation, 1968, p. 55.
98. SHORT, C. L., ABRAMS, N. R. and SARTWELL, P. E.: in *Rheumatic Diseases*, Philadelphia, W. B. Saunders Co., 1952, p. 47.
99. SHORT, C. L., BAUER, W. and REYNOLDS, W. E.: *Rheumatoid Arthritis*, Cambridge, Mass., Harvard University Press, 1957.
100. SIEGEL, M., LEE, S. L., WIDELOCK, D., GWON, N. V. and KRAVITZ, H.: New Engl. J. Med., *273*, 893, 1965.
101. SIT'AJ, S. and SEBO, M.: in *Population Studies of the Rheumatic Diseases*, Amsterdam Excerpta Medica Foundation, 1968, p. 64.
102. SMITH, J. W. and SANFORD, J. P.: Ann. Intern. Med., *67*, 651, 1967.
103. STECHER, R. M., HERSH, A. H., SOLOMON, W. M. and WOLPAW, R.: Amer. J. Hum. Genetics, *5*, 118, 1953.
104. STEINER, F. J. F., WESTENDORG-BOERMA, F., DEBLECOURT, J. J. and VALKENBURG, H. A.: in *Population Studies of the Rheumatic Diseases*, Amsterdam, Excerpta Medica Foundation, 1968, p. 67.
105. TOONE, E. and WALLER, M.: Arth. & Rheum., *11*, 460, 1968.
106. TZONCHEV, V. T., PILOSSOFF, J. and KANEV, K.: in *Population Studies of the Rheumatic Diseases*, Amsterdam, Excerpta Medica Foundation, 1968, p. 60.
107. VALKENBURG, H. A.: in *Population Studies of the Rheumatic Diseases*, Amsterdam, Excerpta Medica Foundation, 1968, p. 93.
108. WAGER, O., RIPATTI, N., LAINE, V., JULKUNEN, H. and AHO, K.: Acta Rheum. Scand., *7*, 209, 1961.
109. WALLER, M.: Ann. N.Y. Acad. Sci., *169*, 5, 1969.
110. WALLER, M. and TOONE, E. C.: Arth. & Rheum., *11*, 50, 1968.
111. WALLER, M., TOONE, E. C., VAUGHAN, E. and CURRY, N.: Arth. & Rheum., *7*, 513, 1964.
112. WOOD, J. W., KATO, H., JOHNSON, K. G., UDA, Y., RUSSELL, W. J. and DUFF, I. F.: Arth. & Rheum., *10*, 21, 1967.
113. ZIFF, M., SCHMID, F. R., LEWIS, A. J. and TANNER, M.: Arth. & Rheum., *1*, 392, 1958.

Chapter 13

Psychogenic Factors in Rheumatic Diseases

By Theodore B. Bayles, M.D.

As early as 1890 Garrod[9] was interested in the precipitating events of rheumatoid arthritis and among them psychic factors. In the intervening years psychic factors in rheumatic conditions have continued to attract attention. In general, the inquiry has been in two main directions: (1) attempts to determine whether personality patterns and emotional states play significant parts in the etiology and clinical course of rheumatoid arthritis, (2) investigations of large groups of cases with ill-defined musculoskeletal disabilities characterized by subjective complaints and in whom there are no significant objective findings, *i.e.* fibrositis.

PSYCHOGENIC FACTORS IN RHEUMATOID ARTHRITIS

There are many theories concerning the cause of rheumatoid arthritis.[6] None of these can be fully accepted because each lacks proof (*see* Chapter 18, p. 297). Failure to distinguish sharply between specific cause and contributing or precipitating factors has fostered many erroneous theories. While the specific cause of rheumatoid arthritis is not known, there is reason to believe that many factors including infections, physical exposure, local joint trauma, debilitating states and emotional disturbances may precipitate or aggravate the disease. If these statements could be proved to be true, it would be of great importance in our understanding of the development of this disease and might help in the prevention and treatment of patients with rheumatoid arthritis. Cobb, Bauer and Whiting[7] have recorded examples of rheumatoid arthritis developing immediately following emotional shock and showed the clinical course may be influenced by anxiety, worry and other psychologic factors. Direct temporal relationships between the onset of arthritic symptoms and emotional crises are repeatedly observed by physicians who care for these patients. Sometimes exacerbations and remissions may run parallel to changes in the environmental stress. Cobb, Bauer and Whiting[7] studied the psychiatric and social factors in 50 patients with rheumatoid arthritis, a life chart being used to synchronize these factors with the clinical course of the disease. They found that a close temporal relationship existed between life stress and exacerbation in 31 (62 per cent) of the 50 cases. In a "control" group, hospitalized because of varicose ulcers, only 12 per cent showed similar relationship. The conclusion was drawn that environmental stress, especially poverty, grief and family worry, bore more than a chance relationship to the onset and exacerbation of the disease. Among the male patients, financial worries or lack of work constituted the most common stress. Among female patients the major burden was also financial, often because of the husband's inability to find work or because of other sustained stress, such as illness in the family and other economic adversities. Family worries, loss of a parent or a spouse, marital unfaithfulness, living with in-laws and marital discord also played important roles in some.

One wonders whether in some instances the financial and psychic adversities were not founded on more basic psychologic problems.

A more recent summary of the precipitating factors by Short, Bauer and Reynolds[22] showed that strain—mental, physical or both—was the most common type of precipitant. Of 293 patients, 144 (49 per cent) had one or more possible precipitants. Strain—mental, physical or both—had occurred in 27.3 per cent of the patients, in contrast to 16 per cent after infection, 10 per cent after exposure to cold or dampness, 5 per cent after surgical operations and 5 per cent after trauma. These workers concluded that the strain in males was occupational; and they implied that females had occupational strain, usually their own housework plus an outside job and/or the worry and care of a sick relative. They also noted that strain was the more common precipitating factor in women whose disease began after forty than in the group with an earlier onset. In males the frequency of strain as a precipitant was not related to age at onset of the arthritis. Short, Bauer and Reynolds[22] reviewed a number of series of patients who had been studied for precipitants, and pointed out that in earlier publications strain was found in only 9 per cent of 1033 patients, but in more recent papers 28 per cent of 437 patients were found to have strain as a precipitant. The highest figures, approaching 50 per cent, were obtained in two small series compiled by physicians especially interested in the psychosomatic aspects of the disease.[12,19]

Patterson and associates[19] found in half of 25 cases that emotional factors were related to rheumatoid arthritis. Discussion of the emotional problems caused a drop in the patient's skin temperature, indicating a change in peripheral circulation. They concluded that emotional factors could produce exacerbation and affect the course of the disease. Swaim[23] believed there was emotional instability prior to the onset of arthritis. He felt that patients who discussed these problems and then cultivated mature faith and belief in a superbeing reacted with less fear and anger under emotional stress. Hence their health would be better and the rheumatoid arthritis improved. Halliday[11] was quite willing to classify rheumatoid arthritis as a psychosomatic disease. He felt that patients had a particular personality pattern of marked emotional inhibition and dependency. He pictured patients with rheumatoid arthritis as "quite a decent lot" with a poverty of facial expression; they hide and repress their inner emotional life. He stated that they had been shy and retiring in childhood and in later life were "home birds" and demonstrated obsessional trends, being meticulous, orderly and tidy. Some were overconscientious, slaves to routine, and demonstrated an excessively developed sense of duty.[13] Halliday[12] found that in 9 of 20 rheumatoid arthritics there was a definite upsetting event antecedent to or connected with the first symptoms. External events precipitated recurrence in 7 patients. The events were manifold and included shock following acute danger, anxiety over finances, misbehavior of relatives, fear of loss of an object, resentment concerning superiors, frustration of being jilted, etc. These patients, he said, tend to "bottle up." In 1969, from Finland, Rimon[20] more recently reported 100 female outpatients admitted to an ambulatory clinic with definite or classical rheumatoid arthritis. Importantly, they were *consecutive* cases and the controls for part of the study were patients in a general medical clinic matched for age, sex, marital status and duration of somatic illness. Seventeen patients had psychiatric disturbances prior to the rheumatoid arthritis and 7 patients developed psychiatric symptoms after its onset. Twenty-five patients showed a distinct mild or moderate depressive reaction and 4 were severe; 2 patients had clear clinical evidence of possible occult depression. In 55 patients there was a correlation between important conflict situations and the first joint symptoms, while 12 patients had "parallel conflicts" which were less significant and considered coincidental. Finally, 33 patients showed *no* correlation between psychodynamic factors and the first rheumatoid symptoms. Rimon suggests that the physician should be alert to psychodynamic factors and psychiatric symptoms in the early stages of rheumatoid disease, as anxious and depressed patients seem to respond less well to medical regimens. In selected early cases he advises psychotherapeutic treatment consisting of supportive psychotherapy and also anxiolytic or antidepressive drugs to "save the patient" from "advancing disability and psychic depression."

Despite the hazards of twin studies,[18] a thorough study by Meyerowitz, Jacox and Hess[16] of 8 sets of monozygotic twins discordant for rheumatoid arthritis concluded that psychosocial data obtained from 4 of the 5 adult twins (80%) revealed that a period of psychological stress preceded the disease onset. Of the 3 younger sets of twins less clear psychological stress was found in 2. In all pairs the unaffected twin had no comparable experience of stress.

Observations on the apparent lack of rheumatoid arthritis in overtly psychotic individuals have been made by Gregg[10] and Nissen and Spencer.[17]

It is fair to say that at the present time this extreme view that rheumatoid arthritis represents a psychosomatic illness offers interesting speculation. We can conclude from this that the final word has not been published on the effect of mental or physical strain on the onset and course of rheumatoid arthritis. There is no careful statistical and modern study of rheumatoid arthritic patients in numbers sufficient to allow us to draw safe conclusions. The psychophysiologic effects of chronic mental or physical strain are just beginning to be measured in a few areas and it will take some years before the exact effect of these factors in rheumatoid arthritis can be determined. It would seem fair to think of this subject as Short, Bauer and Reynolds[22] have, in that psychogenic influences may be one of several precipitating factors, but certainly in many instances the disease "falls out of the sky." Much of the difficulty revolves around the definition of psychosomatic disease. A reasonable concept could hold that in these diseases causative factors are multiple, but, among these, psychologic factors have considerable importance. We abandon the cart and horse concept, but rather appreciate that in the development of a pure physical state the physiologic consequences of emotional states in vulnerable people play a great part in the ultimate development of evident structural disability. It is conceivable that the emotional state is merely a psychological reflection of the tremendous physiologic forces at play at that moment. These physiologic forces continuing unabated can then produce structural change. Finally, the organic disability can produce further stress which functions as a "feedback" mechanism to alter the personality further.[8]

In rheumatoid arthritis the simple primitive responses of defense of the individual are threatened. In addition to this, there is the hovering cloud or threat of worsening of the general condition. Finally, the retrospective studies on the type of personality in rheumatoid arthritis are largely historical and anecdotal and very few can study the patient prior to the catastrophic disease, rheumatoid arthritis. Long-term prospective population studies are badly needed to unravel these difficulties.

THE PHYSICIAN'S ROLE WITH RHEUMATOID ARTHRITIC PATIENTS

The physician dealing with patients with rheumatoid arthritis needs to communicate a sense of security to the patient in the treatment situation.[15] He must at times act as a crutch on whom the patient may lean with confidence. He will wisely allow the patient to vent hostility at the many inhibiting factors and unhappy situations in his disease and life. Otherwise, the emotional tension may be dammed up into the sick organism and give rise to various problems of psychophysiologic nature. He should help the patient express his fears about his disease and discuss them frankly with an honest, but optimistic, point of view. The physician learns to anticipate some of the questions that perplex his patients when doubts arise as to the efficacy and wisdom of what is being done. Patients deserve a thorough explanation of what is being done, and why, also the chances of success and, most important, the reasons for being faithful to the program. The physician attempts to reassure his patient concerning the future, and provides other simple psychological support. Such moral support for the patient can be brought to bear at an appropriate time when there is need for him to assume increased activity or responsibility. Compulsive drives, physical overactivity and rebellion against physical limitation during the course of treatment, which may be used by the patient as a defense against his dependent attitudes, must be handled with understanding and sympathy. This outlet for aggression should be encouraged within reasonable limits. The facilities and skills of the physical therapist and occupational therapist are of great assistance here.

PSYCHOGENIC FACTORS IN FIBROSITIS

The term "fibrositis" has been used to cover a multitude of diagnoses varying from prodromal rheumatoid arthritis to vague, long-term musculoskeletal symptoms unaccompanied by objective changes in the joints. In some of these latter patients the anxieties and tensions of their psychoneurosis are demonstrated in the musculoskeletal system as the end-organ. These have been incorrectly diagnosed "fibrositis." Because both fibrositis and functional musculoskeletal disorders usually present only subjective symptoms without objective findings, differential diagnosis may be difficult or impossible at times. According to Hench and Boland[14] psychogenic rheumatism and fibrositis can be separated clinically. According to them, fibrositis places its victims at the mercy of changes in external environment: weather, heat, cold, humidity, rest, exercise, etc., characteristically influence most of them for better or worse. On the other hand, the psychogenic musculoskeletal disorder generally puts its victims at the mercy of changes in internal environment: thus their symptoms may vary with mood or psyche, pleasure, excitement, mental distraction, vacation, trips, depression, worry or fatigue. Patients with psychogenic rheumatism have days of complete freedom from symptoms depending on their specific daily activities or interests, as opposed to the patients with prodromal rheumatoid arthritis or "fibrositis" who more often have daily symptoms regardless of their psychic status.

Fibrositis is a term, not a diagnosis, employed to describe the symptoms of aching muscles, soreness and stiffness, local tenderness and trigger points in fascial planes, sheaths of muscles and nerves, ligaments, tendons, periosteum, and subcutaneous tissues. The causes of the symptoms have been said to be rheumatic, traumatic, infectious, toxic, endocrine, psychogenic, etc.[1]

One might well ask, "Is there such a condition as fibrositis?" The answer is not at hand, and certainly many patients suspected of this diagnosis may be classified later as having psychogenic rheumatism, rheumatoid arthritis, degenerative joint disease or the rarer "collagen" group disorders. I prefer to consider these patients as having symptoms referable to the connective tissue and musculoskeletal system, but avoid too early diagnosis and classification. Those rheumatologists with an orderly mind may feel compelled to "pigeonhole" these patients, and consequently erudite descriptions and classifications of fibrositis appear in the medical literature. It is probable that fibrositis or connective tissue discomfort is the result of many different insults which are not always diagnosable.

Fibrositis has been classified *anatomically*, *i.e.*, "Where does the patient hurt?" It has been clinically classified as: (1) *primary*, *i.e.*, not related or due to any recognized mental or physical disorder, and (2) *secondary*, concomitant with or as a sequel of: (*a*) infection; (*b*) one of the recognized rheumatic states as rheumatic fever, rheumatoid arthritis, gout, etc.; (*c*) exposure to inclement weather; (*d*) strain or trauma, acute or chronic; (*e*) occupation; (*f*) structural abnormalities; (*g*) anxiety or tension states or other psychiatric difficulties, such as hysteria. I have yet to make the first clinical diagnosis of primary fibrositis, while symptoms which could be called secondary fibrositis are seen very frequently.

PSYCHOGENIC RHEUMATISM (Psychoneurotic Musculoskeletal Complaints)

Most physicians are familiar with the fact that functional disorders or symptom complexes may be expressed in various systems, including disabilities of the locomotor system. Functional musculoskeletal symptoms are too often mislabeled as arthritis or some other organic disease. The tense, anxious patient with a few bony spurs seen on radiologic study of the lumbar spine has frequently been labeled osteoarthritic rather than psychogenic rheumatic. Unfortunately by treating for arthritis the patient who really has psychogenic rheumatism, the disability is encouraged rather than alleviated. An entirely satisfactory diagnosis has not yet been suggested to describe the musculoskeletal disabilities which result from psychoneurosis. The term, "psychogenic rheumatism," is objected to by some rheumatologists and psychiatrists because it is claimed that "rheumatism" is too vague and already surrounded by enough approbrium without linking the word "psychogenic" to it. Others contend that functional muscle and joint complaints also are often vague, and that the word "psychogenic" at least points to the origin of symptoms. Psychiatric diagnoses based on underlying psychological mechanisms are preferred by psychiatrists: such terms as anxiety, depressive state, conversion hysteria, hypochondriasis, (type), as manifested by musculoskeletal symptoms. For the internist or orthopedist not trained as a psychiatrist, the diagnosis of functional disease starts by recognizing that the complaints and findings do not conform to any syndrome of organic disease with which he is familiar. In practice, therefore, the qualitative characteristics of the bodily complaints should be studied with a simultaneous exploration of the psychologic mechanisms. If its limitations are understood, "psychogenic rheumatism" may serve as a useful term. Psychogenic rheumatism may be defined as the musculoskeletal expression of functional nervous disorders, tension states or psychoneurosis. It implies that such symptoms as pain, stiffness, subjective sense of swelling or limitation of motion in muscles and joints may be caused, intensified or perpetuated by emotional influence. It does not mean that an organic joint or muscle disease has resulted from emotional stress.[4] The term should be restricted to those cases in which the actual disability results from functional symptoms, and implies that this is not a prodrome of an organic syndrome. It should not include minor emotional reactions which develop in patients with rheumatoid arthritis or other organic diseases.

Incidence

Psychogenic rheumatism is one of the common causes of rheumatic complaints, along with osteoarthritis, rheumatoid arthritis, rheumatic fever, "fibrositis," etc.[2] In a 1948 study of 500 consecutive civilian patients with rheumatic disease, the diagnosis of psychogenic rheumatism was made in 13.4 per cent of cases, while osteoarthritis was diagnosed in 25 per cent, rheumatoid arthritis in 20.4 per cent and primary fibrositis in 18.2 per cent.[2] During World War II, in one army hospital 34 per cent of the 450 soldiers admitted for rheumatic complaints had psychogenic rheumatism.[3] All soldiers in this 34 per cent had received organic diagnoses, usually arthritis, in other army medical installations.[3] In an army hospital located overseas, Short[21] found that 16.5 per cent of soldiers with articular complaints were incapacitated because of psychogenic rheumatism. This incidence was equal to that of osteoarthritis, and exceeded only by that of rheumatoid arthritis. The overall experience in United States Army rheumatism centers during World War II indicated that 1 out of every 7 soldiers diagnosed "arthritis" was disabled because of psychogenic rheumatism.[14]

There are in general three requisites for the development of any psychogenic disorder: (1) a psychoneurotic predisposition, (2) an inciting emotional conflict and (3) restriction of outward expression of the conflict. Regardless of whether they are normal or psychoneurotic, all persons seek flight from the mental sufferings occasioned by disturbing life problems. If emotional tension is dissipated by outward expression, muscular or verbal, all is well: a person feels better by taking some form of action or doing something about it, thereby "getting it off his chest." However, if there is constant restriction of emotions, the tension gradually mounts and, in a psychoneurotic type of individual especially, the eventual outlet takes form in somatic complaints. When bodily symptoms emerge, the psychoneurotic individual tends to focus his attention on them and thereby obtains some degree of relief from his inner mental tension. Not fully understood, but undoubtedly complex, are the psychophysiologic mechanisms by which psychic disturbances are displaced into physical symptoms. Recently it has been suggested that *emotions may affect the autonomic nervous system*, either directly or *through the medium* of the endocrine system, and thereby produce increased muscle tension, vasospasm, or metabolic changes in various organs and structures (*see also* Chapter 16).

"Smoldering resentment" is regarded by Weiss as the common basic psychopathology in psychogenic rheumatism.[24] He pictures resentment as breeding feelings of discontent and rebellion. For one reason or another the outward display of rebellion is inhibited, and this creates a continuous sense of hostility which prevents the patient from relaxing. A state of constant muscle tension is created which leads to symptoms of aching, tenseness, stiffness and muscular fatigue. Although the underlying psychologic mechanisms are open to question, the somatic effect of chronic muscle spasm appears probable.

Diagnosis and Clinical Picture

Diagnosis depends on (1) the absence of organic disease or insufficient disease to account for the disability, (2) the functional characteristics of the presenting complaints (*see* above), and (3) the positive diagnosis of psychopathology. The mere exclusion of objective evidence of organic disease is not enough.

Absence of Organic Disease or Insufficient Diseases to Account for the Disability

There are varying degrees of psychogenic rheumatism: (1) Pure—when there is a total lack of clinical, laboratory and roentgenographic evidence of organic joint or muscle disease; (2) Superimposed—that is when incapacitating psychogenic symptoms are associated with nondisabling organic joint or muscle disease (functional overlay); (3) Residual—when an organic joint disease has been present but has totally subsided and yet the disability is perpetuated because of functional symptoms (functional prolongation). This is sometimes seen after rheumatic fever. Boland[5] reported that nong 1021 cases of psychogenic rheu-atism, observed at an army rheumatism nter during World War II, the relative equency of these categories was as llows: pure 41.6 per cent, super-nposed 39.5 per cent, and residual 18.9 r cent. It seems that among civilian tients the pure type is less common.

The less serious rheumatic diseases, pecially so-called fibrositis and osteo-thritis, diseases which of themselves ually have only nuisance value, can be mmonly associated with superimposed sabling functional complaints. Minimal costoses in the knees or lumbar spine, or eberden's nodes may be accompanied y persistent and marked disability far it of proportion to that usually seen ith such changes. This is especially marked if the patient is aware of the roentgenographic changes and develops an anxiety reaction to them. Thus, an emotionally unstable person may elevate a minor organic discomfort to the status of a major disability. The experienced physician is able to detect incongruities between the severity of the symptoms and the structural changes present. Authoritative reassurance, simple psychic support and safe therapeutic advice are often very helpful to the patient. This can be properly provided by the intelligent physician who is aware of these relationships.

Residual psychogenic rheumatism may often follow trauma to the musculoskeletal system. Recovery sometimes fails to result even after prolonged bed rest or

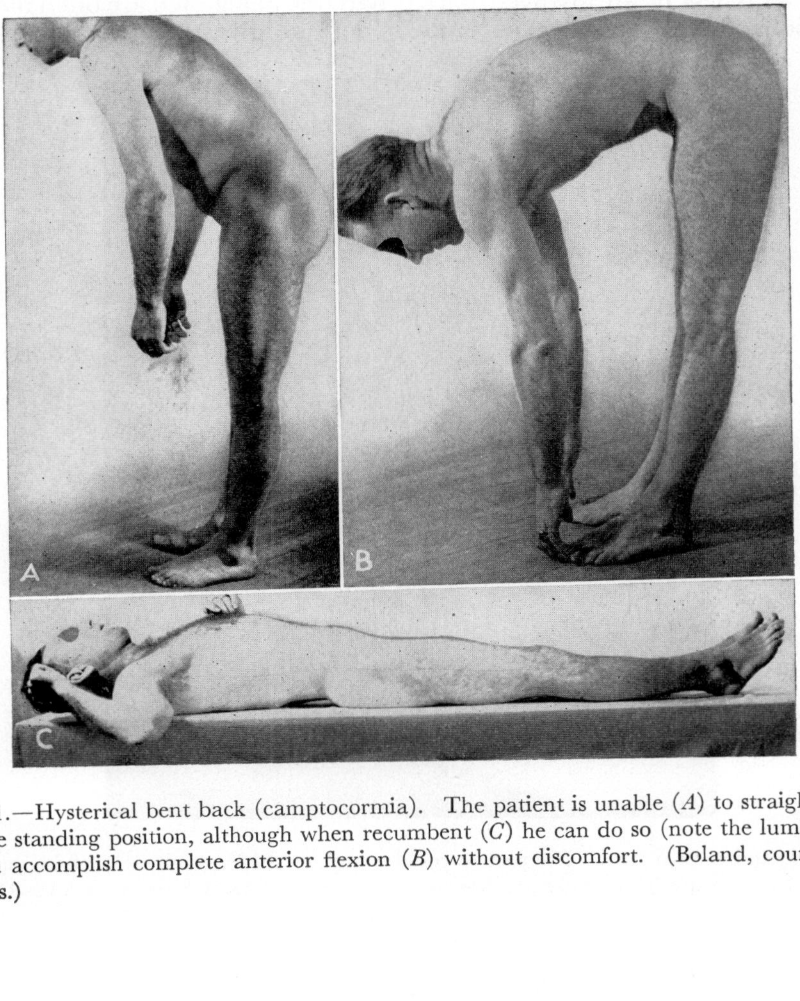

Fig. 13-1.—Hysterical bent back (camptocormia). The patient is unable (*A*) to straighten his back while in the standing position, although when recumbent (*C*) he can do so (note the lumbar lordosis), and he can accomplish complete anterior flexion (*B*) without discomfort. (Boland, courtesy of Ann. Rheum. Dis.)

immobilization. Characteristically, a gradual change in the quality of the symptoms develops as the psychogenic factors usurp command of the disability. The initial symptoms may be typical of organic disease, but eventually the complaints change their colors and assume obvious functional characteristics.

Qualitative Functional Characteristics of the Disability

The complaints may be generalized, "all over," may predominate in one region or they are sometimes vague in quality and location and the patient has difficulty in describing them. The most common symptoms consist of pain and tenderness, stiffness, limitation of motion, a subjective sense of swelling, muscle fatigue or weakness of an involved part. Exacerbations follow episodes of emotional stress, mental or physical fatigu Mental distractions, such as vacations, good movie, football game or soci gathering, may give temporary relie depending upon the circumstances of tl social or sporting event. The patien however, usually states that he has *pai* The sensations are those of weaknes fatigue, prickly feeling, numbness, ti gling, deadness, burning, fullness an pressure, but these are interpreted a pain by the patient. It is often felt tha the patient has paresthesias rather tha pain. It may be constant—"bad all th time," "present day and night"—or may be fleeting, lasting for only a fe seconds. Local heat and various physic therapeutic measures frequently fail t give relief or make the symptoms eve worse. Salicylates, even cortisone an narcotic analgesics, are often ineffective— "nothing gives me relief." Usually th

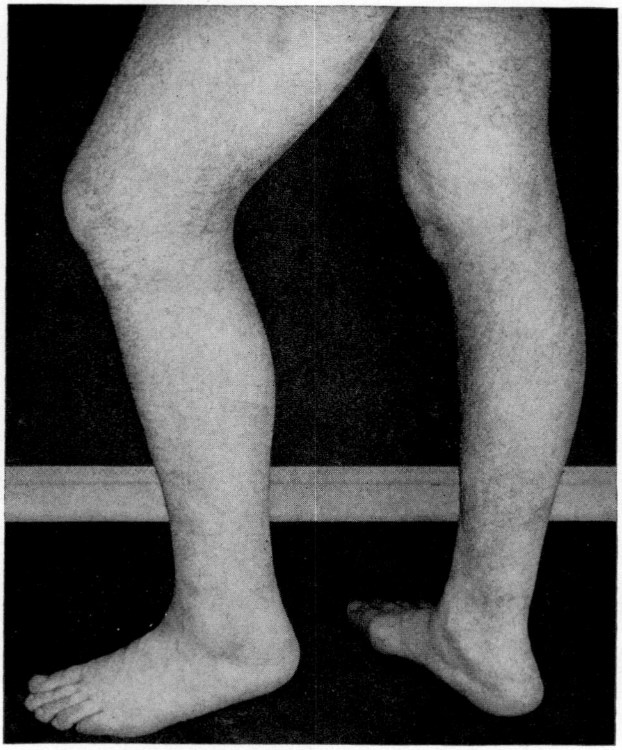

FIG. 13–2.—Hysterical bent knee. The patient could straighten the knee fully while lying but not whil standing. He had a bizarre gait, semi-squatting with each step. (Boland, courtesy of Ann. Rheum. Dis.)

ain is not anatomical. It may skip ere and there with disregard for anatomy, nstead of being located in or about ursae, tendons or joints. As stated arlier, usually rest does not cause in-rease in aching or stiffness.

In general, psychogenic rheumatism uts its victims at the mercy of their nternal environment, the symptoms vary-ng with mood or psyche, pressure, excite-nent, mental distraction, worry or fatigue. Varying degrees of apparent muscle pasm may be found on physical exam-nation, mostly those of defense and, vhen marked, there may be limitation of oint motion. The patient's attitude is tense, anxious, defensive or antagonistic. Now and then a patient appears who outwardly does not manifest any of these attitudes, but rather smiles in a Mona Lisa fashion and describes in great detail the excruciating pain that he or she is suffering. In general, however, there is fear or resistance to examination. The patient cries out with pain on palpation or motion of the joint and he may over-react, jump, grimace or groan on slight palpation of some muscle group. Over-dramatization, lack of consistency of painful motions are characteristic. Some-times, by distracting the patient's atten-tion, the joint can be examined indirectly

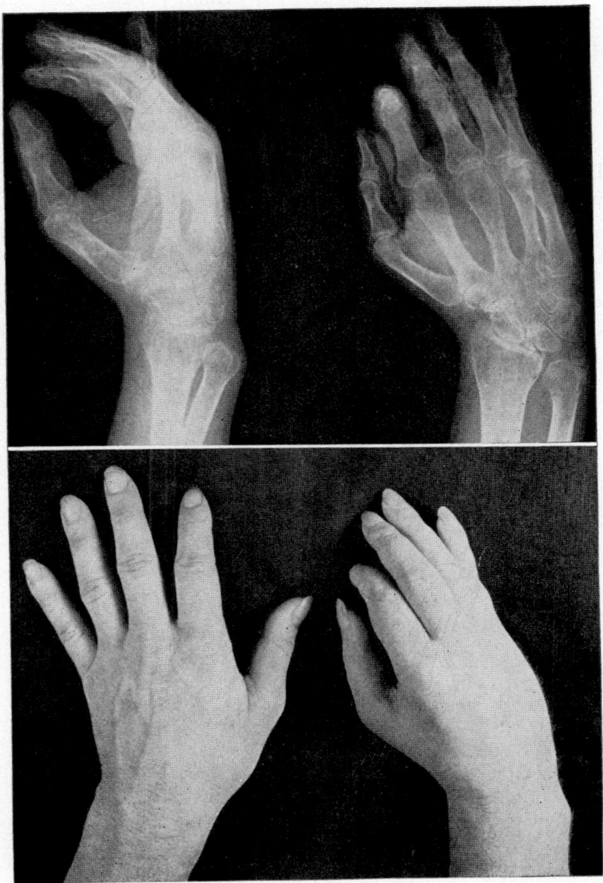

Fig. 13-3.—Hysterical deformity of the right hand of eleven months' duration. Roentgenograms of the involved hand show marked diffuse secondary bone atrophy from disuse. (Boland, courtesy of Ann. Rheum. Dis.)

and the psychogenic aspects of the joint disease determined. He may protest to being hurt by grasping the examiner's hand, a "touch-me-not" reaction. Some patients reciprocate more vigorously by grasping the physician's body, neck or wrist to illustrate the pain, and at times this can be disconcerting. There are, of course, major hysterical conversions, such as develop in compensation or military cases, manifested by intractable back pain, bizarre limps, gaits, posture or hysterical contractures (Figs. 32–1 to 3). These cases are infrequent, are usually seen in special situations, and are referred to the psychiatrists promptly and properly.

BIBLIOGRAPHY

1. Bayles, T. B.: Med. Clin. North America, *39*, 1483, 1955.
2. Boland, E. W.: Calif. Med., *26*, 273, 1948.
3. ———: Calif. & West. Med., *40*, 7, 1944.
4. Boland, E. W. and Corr, W. P.: J.A.M.A., *123*, 805, 1943.
5. Boland, E. W., Stephens, C. A. L. and Hench, P. S.: *Arthritis*, 6th Ed., Hollander, J. L., Ed., Philadelphia, Lea & Febiger, 1960.
6. Christian, C. L.: Arth. and Rheum., *7*, 455, 1964.
7. Cobb, S., Bauer, W. and Whiting, I J.A.M.A., *113*, 668, 1939.
8. Feldman, T.: Personal communication, 196
9. Garrod, A. E.: *A Treatise on Rheumatism an Rheumatoid Arthritis*, London, Griffin, C., 189
10. Gregg, D.: Amer. J. Psychiat., *95*, 853, 193
11. Halliday, J. L.: Practitioner, *150*, 6, 194
12. ———: Proc. Roy. Soc. Med., *35*, 45 1941.
13. ———: Lancet, *2*, 692, 1943.
14. Hench, P. S. and Boland, E. W.: Ann. Int Med., *24*, 808, 1946.
15. Margolis, H. M.: *Progress in Rheumatoi Arthritis*, Talbott, J. H. and Lockie, L. M. Eds., New York, Grune & Stratton, 1958.
16. Meyerowitz, S., Jacox, R. F. and Hess D. W.: Arth. & Rheum., *11*, 1–21, 1968.
17. Nissen, H. A. and Spencer, K. A.: Nev Engl. J. Med., *214*, 576, 1936.
18. O'Brien, W. M.: Arth. & Rheum., *11*, 81–86, 1968.
19. Patterson, R. M., Craig, J. B., Waggoner, R. W. and Freyberg, R. H.: Amer. J. Psychiat., *99*, 775, 1943.
20. Rimon, R.: Acta Rheum. Scand., Suppl. 13, 1969.
21. Short, C. L.: New Engl. J. Med., *236*, 383, 1947.
22. Short, C. L., Bauer, W. and Reynolds, W. E.: *Rheumatoid Arthritis*, Cambridge, Harvard University Press, 1957.
23. Swaim, L. T.: Ann. Int. Med., *19*, 118, 1943.
24. Weiss, E.: Ann. Int. Med., *26*, 890, 1947.

Chapter 14

Infectious and Immunological Considerations in Rheumatic Diseases

By John H. Vaughan, M.D.

Rheumatoid arthritis, systemic lupus erythematosus, and polyarteritis have long been recognized to be a triad of diseases which, although distinct from one another in their classical presentations, nevertheless may often be difficult to differentiate. Rheumatoid arthritis stands at the center of the triad. Although rheumatoid arthritis is a chronic inflammatory disease involving predominantly the synovial membranes, it has a tendency to generalized vasculitis which sometimes can be severe. In its exaggerated form this vasculitis is indistinguishable from that of classical polyarteritis nodosum, with vascular occlusions, peripheral neuropathy, digital gangrene, and infarctions of the viscera. In other instances rheumatoid arthritis is accompanied by pleuritis, pericarditis, and many other vasculitic and serologic features which are indistinguishable from those of systemic lupus erythematosus. All three of these rheumatic diseases are inflammatory diseases of the connective tissues and have sometimes been called collagen-vascular diseases. No organ or tissue is invariably and uniquely affected by the diseases, unless it be the connective tissues or the blood vessels themselves.

None of these diseases have yet been shown to be due to infection, although in all three there have been repeatedly documented instances in which infection has initiated the first overt expression of the disease. No organisms have been consistently identified in cultures of tissues or fluids from the diseases.

Whether these three diseases are "immunological diseases" in the sense of their being attributable only to the immunological disorders characterizing them, or whether they are diseases of some other nature in which immunological events are provoked secondarily, is not known. That immunological events take place in them is no longer to be seriously doubted; and, increasingly, evidence is mounting that these events may, at least in certain instances, constitute important pathogenetic factors in the diseases. This chapter will review the basis for belief in these pathogenetic factors. Probable mechanisms involved will be emphasized, together with corresponding implications for therapy.

MODELS IN EXPERIMENTAL ANIMALS

A number of experimental diseases have been described which bear striking resemblances to rheumatic diseases. Some are non-infectious in nature; others are caused by viruses or other microorganisms. None of them can be considered exact equivalents of the rheumatic diseases, but they provide in the aggregate an impressive framework for our current thinking about rheumatic diseases.

Experimental Serum Sickness

The prime model of immunological disease in animals is serum sickness, and in many ways rheumatoid arthritis, lupus erythematosus, and polyarteritis can be fitted into this model. The characteristic feature of experimental serum sickness is the deposition of antigen-antibody complexes in the walls of the blood vessels and in the glomeruli of the kidney.[31] After a large dose of antigen, the lesions of serum sickness appear just at the time at which antigen begins to disappear rapidly from the circulation. The disease process is terminated when an excess of antibody appears. Serum complement levels are lowered during the acute phase, due to fixation by the complexes. Immunofluorescence studies have demonstrated antigen, antibody and complement components in the vascular and glomerular lesions.

The studies of Cochrane, *et al.*,[26] have indicated that polymorphonuclear leukocytes are an essential component in the Arthus reaction. If animals are depleted of these leukocytes, antigen-antibody precipitates in the vascular wall cause little or no vasculitis. Phagocytosed antigen-antibody complexes have been shown to induce disruption of leukocytic lysosomes resulting in a release of enzymes and pyrogens. It is generally believed that much of the tissue damage in immunologically induced inflammation may be mediated through this mechanism.

Serum sickness is associated with the development of large amounts of precipitating antibody. Both γG (7S) and γM (19S) antibodies are usually present, but the γG variety predominates. Whether antibodies of the two classes are equally effective in provoking the vasculitis of serum sickness is not known, but from quantitative considerations alone γG globulins would appear to be the more important of the two. In man, serum sickness often occurs without the detection of any γM antibody.[12]

Experimental "Autoimmune" Disease

There are a number of organ diseases in experimental animals which have been provoked by immunization with the animal's own organ antigens in complet Freund's adjuvant.[133] Experimental al lergic encephalomyelitis serves as a protc type and thyroiditis, adrenalitis, an aspermatogenesis are other examples. I each of these, it is clear that the develop ment of an immune response to th specific organ antigen results in diseas in the organ containing the antigen Transfer of the disease can be achieved b injecting normal animals with livin lymphoid cells from diseased animals These diseases have therefore been though to be due to "cellular" hypersensitivity These "autoimmune" diseases exhibi strict organ or tissue specificity cor responding to that of the immunizin antigen, rather than diffuse disease such as is seen in rheumatoid arthritis, sys temic lupus erythematosus, and poly arteritis.

"Graft vs. Host" Disease

In animals that have been injectec neonatally or prenatally with large numbers of immunologically competent lymphoid cells from homologous donors, it has been found that a "runting syndrome" may develop.[20,116] This syndrome is essentially a "graft-versus-host" response, in which the ingrafted lymphoid cells develop an immunological response against their host's. Coombs positive hemolytic disease has been noted. Splenic enlargement is marked. Eventually an agammaglobulinemic state supervenes, due to the death of the lymphoid cells of both host and donor.

Stastny and co-workers[118] have extensively studied a closely related experimental model in adult animals. In this case homologous cells are grafted into adults rendered tolerant in the neonatal period. The "graft vs. host" reaction in this case is called "homologous disease." During an early phase the animals exhibit polyarthritis, dermatitis, and visceral inflammatory reactions resembling those of the rheumatic diseases; afterwards these signs of inflammation are replaced by the agammaglobulinemic tate. Some features of scleroderma and ermatomyositis have also been noted in he early acute phase of the disease.

Naturally Occurring "Lupus" in Animals

A strain of New Zealand mice (NZB) has been described[53] which regularly xhibits Coomb's positive hemolytic disease in adulthood and occasionally also nephritis. When crossed with another nbred mouse strain, hybrids (NZB/W) esult which invariably exhibit nephritis, out little hemolytic disease is produced. n all cases, the animals are born healthy, out develop disease as they pass into adulthood. L.E. cells are occasionally een in the original NZB animal, but are much more commonly seen in the hybrid.

A number of inbred strains of mice have been more recently described in his country in which antinuclear antibodies without evident disease have been noted. Since the antibodies have been confined to certain strains of mice, they have appeared to be the expression of a genetic factor in the strain. The animals are born free of the antibodies, but develop them as they age. A report by Shulman has indicated that an environmental factor may contribute to the development of these antibodies.[115]

The onset of disease in the NZB/W mice corresponds in time with the development of antibodies to a murine leukemia-like virus present in the B/W mice since birth.[84] This same virus is present in many other laboratory mouse strains but is tolerated by these other strains for life with no immune response and no evidence of lupus or hemolytic disease. Acceleration of the time of onset of disease in the NZB/W strains can be brought about by injection of splenic extracts of sick animals containing the murine leukemia-like virus into young NZB/W animals. It can also be accelerated in onset by injection of young NZB/W animals with viruses other than the murine leukemia-like virus, such as that responsible for lymphocytic choriomeningitis (LCM).[125] The nephritis that develops appears to be due not only to deposits in the glomeruli of virus-antibody immune complexes but also host DNA-anti-DNA immune complexes.

Talal[120] has provided evidence that NZB/W mice have a poorly developed ability to maintain immune tolerance to a number of immunogens, microbial and otherwise, and has attributed this to deficient thymic function. He has argued that the genetic predisposition to lupus in these mice can be equated to the thymic defect, which in turn results in an overproduction of antibodies, to various microbial agents, some cross reacting with normal tissue constituents and yielding auto-reactive antibodies. This interpretation finds a close parallel in our current thinking about systemic lupus erythematosus in man (*v. infra*).

"Lupus" has also been noted as a spontaneously occurring disease in dogs.[78] L.E. cell preparations are positive and antinuclear antibodies are present by immunofluorescence. The clinical picture is that of polyarthritis, dermatitis, and nephritis.

Experimental Forms of Arthritis

One important experimental model of arthritis is "adjuvant disease," studied intensively by Pearson.[97] The disease is provoked by the injection of complete Freund's adjuvant into rats and is characterized by a proliferative synovitis and perisynovitis that can progress to cause cartilaginous erosions. This disease depends upon the presence of mycobacteria in the adjuvant, or a suitable microbial substitute. Dissemination of the microbial antigen throughout the tissues of the injected animal occurs. Waksman[133] believes that the arthritis depends upon the phagocytic activity of synovial cells, permitting concentration of antigen in this area. Animals can be protected from the development of the disease by drugs which suppress the immunological response.

An arthritis very closely resembling

rheumatoid arthritis has been produced in rabbits by injecting heterologous fibrin into the joint space.[32] Along with an immunological response to the foreign fibrin there develops a round cell infiltration of the synovial membrane, a pannus, and a polymorphonuclear leukocytic synovial effusion.

Rawson, Quismorio, and Abelson[105] have taken advantage of the observation by Mandy[80] that some rabbits have a naturally occurring antibody (homoreactant) to gamma globulin (anti Fab) in their sera to test the ability of this antibody to provoke arthritis when Fab is injected intra-articularly. These workers reported that homoreactant-positive rabbits develop arthritis and homoreactant-negative animals do not, when Fab is injected.

An arthritic disease in swine caused by erysipelothrix has been studied by Collins.[27] Following injection of the bacteria intravenously, inflammatory joint disease develops due to local deposit of the organisms. The arthritis, however, persists after the disappearance of demonstrable bacteria from the joint fluid and synovial tissues. Rheumatoid factor-like globulins have been noted to develop in the sera of affected animals.[5] This model is intriguing to those who suspect that rheumatic disease may be initiated by infection, but maintained by other factors.

PPLO infection of rats and other animals also is marked by polyarthritis.[2,30] The organisms are readily cultivated from the joints, however; and the gross appearance of the joint disease is more nearly like that of acute septic arthritis than the chronic, persistent arthritis seen in rheumatoid disease.

Grayzel, Janis and Haberman[45] have described a chronic arthritis that can be produced by the injection of rubella virus intra-articularly in rabbits. They noted that they could not grow synovial cells in tissue culture from the rubella-injected animals.

Weissmann[134] has injected streptolysin-S into joints. Streptolysin-S is known to disrupt lysosomes and to release the products stored therein. After repeate injections of streptolysin-S, animals d velop a chronic infiltrative synovi that also very much resembles rheum toid arthritis. This demonstration su gests that any system capable of chro ically disrupting lysosomes and liberatir their products can lead to an arthrit with characteristics of rheumatoid a thritis in humans. Polymyxin, filipi and other polyene disruptors of cell mem branes do the same thing.[135]

Polyarteritis in Animals

Vasculitic diseases due to viral infe tions have been described in deer, mic and in horses.[67,82] In all of these, ep demic disease is seen, and, in this respec and in their acuteness, these diseases d not resemble the rheumatic disease Nevertheless, lesions in equine viral arter tis are in the media of the arteries an strikingly resemble those of polyarteriti nodosum in man.

An even more intriguing infectiou vasculitis is Aleutian mink disease.[55] Thi disease has been seen in a mutant strai of mink prized for its blue fur, which i inherited as a homozygous recessiv trait. Such animals frequently develo an intense plasma cell infiltration of th kidneys and liver, a glomerulonephritis a generalized vasculitis, and a marke hypergammaglobulinemia. The diseas can be transmitted from affected t unaffected animals of the same strain b suspensions of spleen or other tissues Other mink are resistant to the disease The vascular pathology is limited t medium-sized muscular arteries. Anti nuclear factors have been described b Barnett *et al.*[14] The disease is obviousl of interest in that it appears to be ar arteritis that can be transmitted from affected animals only into a peculiarl susceptible host. Whether the vascula lesions are attributable to the virus itsel or to the host's developing hypersensi tivity to the virus (as occurs in the NZB disease discussed above, and in murine mphocytic choriomeningitis) is not ıown.

PATHOLOGICAL FEATURES

Lymph nodes from patients with ıeumatoid arthritis, systemic lupus ythematosus and polyarteritis may khibit a high degree of cellular reacvity.[89,90,92] One often finds increased umbers of plasma cells, prominent llicles, and occasionally sufficient cellur activity to produce marked distortion f the normal architecture of the nodes. Iypergammaglobulinemia is frequent.

By fluorescent staining it has been emonstrated that gamma globulin and omplement are bound in the vasculitic nd glomerulitic lesions of lupus and olyarteritis and the synovial lesions of heumatoid arthritis.[35,75,76,108,132] These ndings resemble those of experimental erum sickness. By hematoxylin and osin stains, edema, degeneration, fibrioid change, inflammation, necrosis, and yperplasia are seen.

The meaning of the presence of "bound" amma globulin in fibrinoid lesions has ften been challenged. Any exudative esion, whether or not produced by mmunological mechanisms, can be exected to contain some gamma globulin long with other serum proteins. Such amma globulins, however, should be eadily washed out of the tissue section y the washing procedures ordinarily ısed. The finding that complement comonents are present along with the bound amma globulins in the rheumatic diseases favors an immunological interpretation in these instances. Moreover, many other inflammatory diseases have been described in which gamma globulins are not significantly found in the lesions. The Schwartzman reaction and thrombotic thrombocytopenic purpura are good examples.

ETIOLOGIC CONSIDERATIONS

A number of events have been recognized to provoke the rheumatic diseases. Fatigue, physical or emotional trauma, exposure to cold, infection, and drug reactions are among the events that have been cited. The diversity of the list bespeaks our ignorance of fundamental etiologies, but at the same time it introduces certain intriguing concepts of pathogenesis.

Infection

There is a long tradition for emphasizing a role for infection in the precipitation of *rheumatoid arthritis*, but the days of belief in "focal infection" are gone. There is now general agreement with the statement in the 1949 Primer on Rheumatic Diseases: "No one now believes that the removal of an infected focus will alter the course of rheumatoid arthritis, and extraction of teeth, tonsils, gallbladders, and pelvic organs is to be condemned unless they are so diseased that they should be removed for their own sake."

Nor is the streptococcus any longer regarded in this country as playing a particular role in the development of rheumatoid arthritis, as it does in rheumatic fever. The streptococcal agglutination reaction, which occurs in high titer in a large number of patients with rheumatoid arthritis, is now understood in terms of activity of antigammaglobulin antibodies composing the rheumatoid factors. High agglutination titers against bacteria other than streptococci are also seen. Early reports of the isolation of streptococci from the tissues of patients infected with rheumatoid arthritis are now regarded as having been due to contamination of the specimens in their handling. Antibody levels to streptococcal products such as the antistreptolysin O antibody are not elevated in rheumatoid arthritis patients, nor in any of the other rheumatic diseases aside from rheumatic fever.

Students of rheumatoid arthritis nevertheless continue to be intrigued by certain recurring themes that suggest relationships between infections and joint disease. Gonorrhea, for instance, is capable not only of producing typical gonorrheal arthritis (*see* Chapter 64), but also of occasionally introducing a chronic arthritis which evolves into typical rheumatoid arthritis. No statistics are available on the incidence with which this occurs, so one cannot know how much to stress the relationship. Tonsillitis or pharyngitis may also be followed by a polyarthritis, which at first appears to be rheumatic fever, but which evolves into rheumatoid arthritis. Acute viral infections, especially rubella in young women, may be followed by persistent polyarthritides involving small joints as well as large; these arthritides generally run a several-month course of persisting joint disease resembling rheumatoid arthritis before gradually subsiding.

Pleuropneumonia organisms have attracted considerable attention as possible causes of rheumatoid arthritis. Numerous attempts to isolate mycoplasma have been made, but success has generally been limited. Jansson and Wager,[64] for instance, could isolate mycoplasma from only 2 of 28 specimens of synovial tissues or fluids; Barnett, Balduzzi, and Vaughan[9] from none of 17; and Sharp[113] from none of 8.

In view of all those negative findings, the reports of Bartholomew[15] and of Williams[136] of positive isolates of mycoplasma in high percentages of their patients with rheumatoid arthritis are both puzzling and intriguing. Williams, Brostoff, and Roitt[137] more recently have reported that *M. fermentans* inhibits the migration of leukocytes from patients with rheumatoid arthritis like PPD does the leukocytes of persons with tuberculin hypersensitivity. Ford[36] has commented upon circumstances that can falsely lead to isolation of mycoplasma from cultures of specimens that are really sterile. It is not clear whether any of these circumstances applied to the Bartholomew and Williams studies.

The possibility that rheumatoid arthritis may be associated with an active, virus-carrier state is offered by the finding[44] that the rubella virus will not infect cultures of synovial cells from patien with rheumatoid arthritis. Rubella capable, however, of infecting synovi cells from non-rheumatoid arthritide One of the known mechanisms for block ing the infectivity of a tissue for one viru is to induce a prior infection of it b another virus. Nevertheless, numerou laboratories have failed to obtain b virus isolation any direct evidence for virus infection in rheumatoid arthriti and serum antibody studies have nc yielded any suggestive evidence for it.[6

While chronic infection by an unknow agent remains a popular presumption fo the etiology of rheumatoid arthritis, n hard data exist to support the presump tion. Some students of the disease sus pect that if infection is a factor it may nc be infection by any specific type of micrc organism, but rather infection by a wid variety of banal microorganisms with a altered host response generated by th infections responsible for the disease.

In the case of systemic lupus erythema tosus a great deal of provocative data tc suggest virus infection has been brough forth. Like rheumatoid arthritis, SLE can apparently be ushered in by acute infection, and this has always beer cause for some thought. The identifica tion[38,43,48,62,71,94] of virus-like inclusion in the cytoplasms of endothelial cells ir the glomeruli of patients with SLE se off an intensive effort by numerou laboratories to pinpoint the issue. With time it has become evident that the inclusions described can be found in a wide variety of diseases[94] and that tissues containing the inclusions fail to yield viral growth when used to inoculate a variety of tissue cultures in standard isolation techniques.[34]

Serologic studies were undertaken and they early revealed[101] that patients with SLE have significantly elevated titers of antibodies to para-influenza-1 and measles viruses. The initial encouragement to the belief that these higher titers indicated chronic myxovirus infections in SLE has been dulled by the finding of high antibody titers for yet other viruses,[58] nd especially high titers for the E. B. irus.[110] A particularly difficult aspect of nese findings is that the cytoplasmic nicrotubules that have been described n the endothelial cells in lupus do not natch in size the known dimensions of he myxoviruses[102] or the E. B. virus.[126] The interpretation may be preferred that he higher antibody titers in SLE reflect he known disposition of SLE patients to produce excessive antibody responses to wide variety or immunogens (*v. infra*) and that no specific or singular chronic nfection is the cause of SLE. The finding of Pincus, *et al.*,[102] that the glomeruli of patients with lupus nephritis may stain pecifically with fluoresceinated hyperimmune antisera to several viruses and hat individual kidneys behaved differently with the various antisera suggests again that any of several viruses may be nvolved in lupus.

Like rheumatoid arthritis and lupus, *polyarteritis nodosa* can also be ushered in by nfection. Rose[109] particularly emphasized respiratory infections as a cause of that form of polyarteritis which exhibits pulmonary infiltrates and eosinophilia. Recently Gocke *et al.*[40] reported that they found circulating Australia (Au) antigen in 4/11 patients with polyarteritis, in three of whom this antigen appeared to be present in immune complex with antibody. In one patient Au antigen was also demonstrated along with immunoglobulin and complement in the vasculitic lesion of the arterial wall. It can be expected that other viruses besides Au will in the future be added to a growing list of viruses associated with polyarteritis.

Drug Reactions

Drugs have often been incriminated in the onset of systemic lupus erythematosus and of polyarteritis. Sulfonamides and gold were particularly well-recognized inciting agents two decades ago. Penicillin, anti-convulsants, phenylbutazone, procainamide, and hydralazine have been frequent offenders more recently.

It is difficult to know whether any of these drugs can initiate the diseases *de novo*. In some instances one can, by careful questioning, elicit from patients a history suggestive of rheumatic disease antedating the use of an inciting drug. A report from the Mayo Clinic[4] emphasized this point in the development of the lupus syndrome following large doses of hydralazine. Persistence of minor symptoms and serological abnormalities long after the hydralazine has been stopped has also been noted. Prospective studies have now been carried out with procainamide[23] which indicate that induction of manifestations of lupus occurs far more frequently than would be expected if the induction depended simply upon unveiling "idiopathic" lupus in a population of people peculiarly predisposed to that disease. The maximum age-related prevalence of SLE in Rochester, Minnesota was reported by Nobrega *et al.*[93] to be about 1 per 1000, and in most series values significantly lower than that are found. By contrast, Blomgren, Condemi, Bignall, and Vaughan[23] found that half the patients they examined in their prospective study developed antinuclear antibodies and a quarter of these developed symptoms. Perry *et al.*[100] had figures of 31/57 and 12/57 for appearance of antinuclear antibodies and of symptoms in a non-prospective study of hydralazine, and numerous other studies of drug induced lupus are consistent with the magnitudes of these figures. It thus seems likely from these differences in magnitude that drugs elicit a lupus-like syndrome independent of any underlying predisposition to idiopathic lupus. It is nevertheless also clear that these same drugs should be regarded as dangerous for patients with idiopathic lupus and that they probably do elicit the initial expression of the disease in some of them.

Familial Factors

It has long been suspected that some genetic predisposition to develop rheumatic diseases exists in the families of patients with lupus. Several family studies have been brought forth to support this view (*cf.* Holman[60]). An extensive and carefully pursued study by Leonhardt in southern Sweden has confirmed the earlier claims. Leonhardt[77] examined the blood relatives of patients with lupus and used their spouses as controls. The blood relatives exhibited twice the incidence of rheumatoid arthritis as did the controls. There was also a higher incidence of symptoms such as Raynaud's phenomenon, arthralgias, and skin rashes in the blood relatives, along with hypergammaglobulinemia, an increased incidence of antinuclear factors, an increased incidence of rheumatoid factors, and some increase in the levels of ASO and other antibodies. These findings were more common among the females than among the males.

Two other studies, if substantiated by others, lend further support to the probability of a genetic factor in lupus. Strejcek, Herzog, and Bielicky[119] have reported that by Gm serotyping the Gm^a gene appears to be represented in lupus more commonly than normally. Grumet *et al.*[47] have found the HLA histocompatibility antigen to be present in lupus patients more commonly than normally.

Aggregation of cases of rheumatoid arthritis in certain families has been repeatedly noted. Bennett and Burch[19] examined this in Pima Indians, however, and concluded that this did not occur on a genetic basis. They thought environmental factors were probably determinant.

IMMUNOLOGICAL RESPONSIVENESS

Immunization Studies

A number of instances have been noted in which an inordinate number of antibodies to unusual red blood cell antigens have developed after transfusion in the serums of patients with lupus.[59] Immunization studies have confirmed that lupus patients are hyper-responsive. Immunization studies with A and B blood group substance have been followed not only with an exaggerated isoagglutinin response, but also by the appearance of anti-tissue antibodies and anti-coagulant globulins.[139]

Patients with rheumatoid arthritis have also been studied in various immunization programs. Using brucella vaccine Meiselas and co-workers[83] found a slightly enhanced production of agglutinins, and Greenwood[46] reported a slightly enhanced antibody production to pneumococcal polysaccharides. Vaughan and Butler,[130] however, immunizing with soluble tetanus toxoid, found no enhanced antibody production by rheumatoid arthritis patients. Houba and collaborators,[61] studying a skin test response to streptococcal antigens (streptokinase-dornase), found an enhanced rise in serum anti-streptokinase antibody. Rawson and co-workers[104] found reduced isoagglutinin titers in group O patients. The differences noted by these various investigators in immunological responsiveness in their patient groups may have been related to differences in the antigens employed, or to differences in the clinical status of the patients studied. In none of these series were the latter well described. Under any circumstance, the degree of enhanced antibody responsiveness claimed to exist among rheumatoid arthritis patients is certainly less than that exhibited by patients with lupus.

Two reports have concentrated their attention specifically on the IgM antibody responses in SLE[16] and rheumatoid arthritis.[17] In both reports there was suggestion that the IgM component of the immune response was deficient. Nothing is known about the antibody responsiveness of patients with polyarteritis.

Autoantibodies

It is of note that the three diseases, systemic lupus erythematosus, rheumatoid arthritis, and polyarteritis, can be anked according to their tendencies to xhibit autoantibodies. Among patients vith systemic lupus, antinuclear anti-odies are almost invariably seen in the cute phase of the disease. Anti-thyroid ntibodies, anti-cytoplasmic antibodies, nti-gamma globulin antibodies, Wasser-nan antibodies, and other autoantibodies re also frequently reported. In rheuma-oid arthritis, this tendency exists, but is enerally less striking; antinuclear anti-odies (*see* Chapter 10) are found less requently and the other autoantibodies ar less frequently. Anti-gamma globu-ins (rheumatoid factors), however, are ommon. In polyarteritis, both anti-γ-globulin antibodies and antinuclear anti-odies have been described, but they are robably not present in more than about 20 per cent of cases. The degree of hypergammaglobulinemia exhibited in the three diseases parallels the frequency of occurrence of autoantibodies.

Barnett and co-workers[11] have taken advantage of the immunofluorescence technique for study of antinuclear antibodies to show that these antibodies are contained in the three major classes of immunoglobulins (*see* Chapter 10) and in both L-chain types of immunoglobulins. In patients with juvenile rheumatoid arthritis, their evidence suggested that the antinuclear antibodies develop as a late manifestation of the disease and may appear in the IgM class of immunoglobulins before they appear in the other classes. The antibodies in rheumatoid arthritis differed in no qualitative respect from those in lupus erythematosus. There was less IgG antinuclear antibody in the patients with rheumatoid arthritis than there was in the patients with lupus.

In the above respects, the antinuclear antibodies in these diseases resemble normal antibodies. The distribution of the antibodies through the immunoglobulins is diffuse, not sharply restricted in "clonal" patterns such as are seen in the paraproteinemias of multiple myeloma. If an abnormality in the control of antibody production exists in lupus or rheumatoid arthritis, therefore, it would seem likely to be at a level of general control of plasma cell function, rather than at a peculiarly clonal level.

Cellular Immune Mechanisms

Block *et al.*[22] have reported that by skin tests to common antigens patients with systemic lupus erythematosus or rheumatoid arthritis have normal reactivity. Skin tested to DNA, normal[22] or abnormal (tuberculin-like)[41,66] responses have been described in SLE. Lymphocytes from SLE patients have shown weak mitogenic responses[41,96] *in vitro* to DNA. One report[21] claims that SLE patients selected during the period of acute onset of their disease are deficient in function both by skin test and by lymphocyte response *in vitro*.

When patients with rheumatoid arthritis were skin tested with aggregated IgG, they showed reactions which differed in no way from normals,[25] and their lymphocytes *in vitro* failed to show a mitogenic response.[69] Rheumatoid lymphocytes were found by Astorga and Williams[7] to exhibit a diminished mitogenic response when exposed to the lymphocytes of other rheumatoid patients as compared to normals. The effect was such as to suggest that rheumatoid lymphocytes are more similar to each other antigenically than they are to normal lymphocytes.

"Aggressive," cytotoxic activities of the peripheral blood lymphocytes of patients with SLE[128] and to the joint fluid leukocytes of patients with rheumatoid arthritis[51] for standard cells in tissue cultures have been described. The nature of this activity is not well understood. It may be seen with cells from patients with illnesses other than SLE or rheumatoid arthritis.

In the absence of good means of measuring the function or integrity of the thymus in man, little is known of its possible malfunction in the rheumatic diseases. It has been of interest to note such reports, therefore, as that of Singh[117] on a patient with a thymoma and the

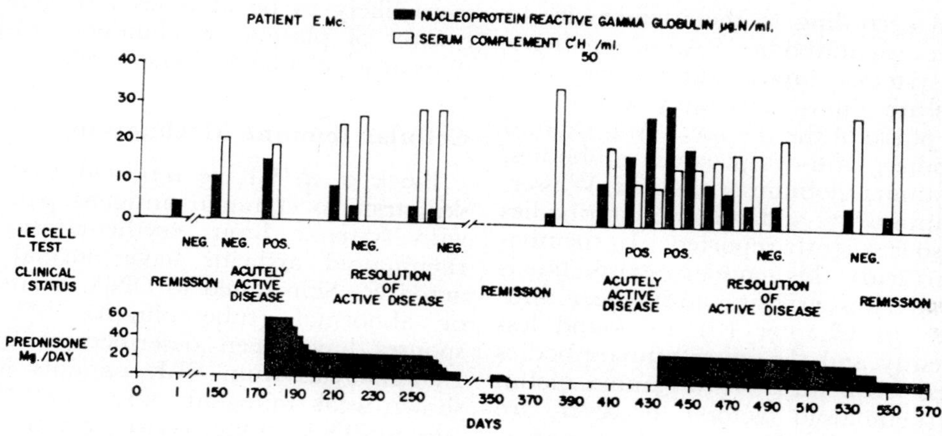

Fig. 14–1.—Relation between complement titers and antinuclear antibodies in a patient with lupus. (Townes, courtesy of Arthritis and Rheumatism.)

lupus syndrome. Ordinarily, however, SLE is apparently characterized by a smaller than normal thymus,[50] which histologically exhibits cortical atrophy, disorganization of the medulla with cystic Hassell's corpuscles, and germinal centers.[42,79] These changes have been interpreted as indicating deficient thymic function,[79] or as the effects of an auto-aggressive event with the thymus as the target organ.[42] Thymectomy has failed to produce striking clinical changes.[86]

The thymus in rheumatoid arthritis[79] may resemble that seen in lupus, and thymectomy has produced no clear-cut benefits in two patients.

PATHOGENETIC CONSIDERATIONS

Factors capable of precipitating rheumatic diseases include infections and reactions to drugs, and these factors may therefore be important in etiological considerations. Autoantibodies are almost invariably demonstrable in systemic lupus erythematosus, however, and usually are demonstrable in rheumatoid arthritis. While we are not yet certain why the autoantibodies develop, we can nevertheless now accept that they do contribute in pathogenesis.

In Systemic Lupus Erythematosus

There were a number of reasons for doubting, after their first demonstration, that the autoantibodies in the serums of patients with lupus contributed in pathogenesis. Discrepancies were noted in the degree of activity of clinical disease and the titers of given autoantibodies. Transfusion experiments[81] were carried out with plasmas of patients with lupus, and observations were made on the newborn of mothers with lupus,[18] which demonstrated that the circulating autoantibodies responsible for the L.E. cell phenomenon did not transmit any overt expression of disease in the recipient. In tissue culture experiments,[75] antinuclear antibodies exhibited no toxic effect on healthy, intact cells.

It has subsequently been demonstrated, however, that the selfsame antibodies that apparently were non-pathogenic in the above circumstances could assume a pathogenetic role when combined with antigen in the form of circulating immune complexes. The evidences for this are as follows: (1) The vascular and glomerular lesions in lupus contain gamma globulins and among these are specific antibodies to nuclear antigens.[37] (2) The vascular and glomerular lesions in lupus contain DNA shown by Feulgen stainng.[73] (3) Lesions in the glomeruli have een shown to contain native DNA by specific staining with fluorescein-labeled antiody to native DNA.[74] (4) Complement xation in the lesions has been demontrated by immunofluorescence.[76] (5) erum levels of hemolytic complement re lowered in acute lupus, especially vith concomitant active nephritis.[91,127,29] (6) Lowered serum complement iters have been closely correlated with he presence of circulating, complementixing immune complexes.[3] (7) Native DNA has occasionally been seen in the irculation in hyperacute lupus, producng a temporary state of "antigen excess" vith disappearance of demonstrable anti-DNA.[122] The vasculitis and glomerulitis of systemic lupus erythematosus have, herefore, the form of "serum sickness" lue to circulating and precipitating utoantigen-antibody complexes, espeially native DNA-anti-DNA.

A further pathogenetic potential for antinuclear antibodies exists. Though these antibodies may be non-pathogenetic for healthy cells, they may conceivably pose a threat to sick cells. Tan and Kunkel[121] made the observation that in biopsies of skin lesions in lupus the nuclei of some of the cells in the areas of inflammation may stain directly for gamma globulins, indicating that antinuclear antibodies had gained access to the nuclei in those instances. Hench *et al.*[54] have found the same phenomenon in kidney biopsies, and Tonietti *et al.*[125] have made comparable observations in the kidneys of NZB/W animals. It remains for future investigations to determine whether such ingress of antinuclear antibodies compromises the cell's ability to remain in, or to recover, good health.

There are certain obvious circumstances in which other autoantibodies in lupus do have a direct and occasionally striking role in pathogenesis in lupus. The cytopenias are examples. Autoantibodies to red blood cells are well documented and their contribution to hemolytic disease reasonably established. Antiplatelet antibodies have been clearly described and are responsible for some cases of thrombocytopenia. It can be assumed that the leukopenia that so often characterizes lupus is also immunologically mediated, possibly by the antibodies recently described in lupus in the HLA histocompatibility groups.[13,87] Antibodies to proteins in the coagulation system may lead to problems in hemorrhage and purpura.

Cellular hypersensitivity to DNA has been reported.[39,95] Skin tests may be positive with tuberculin-type reactions, and lymphocyte transformation occurs *in vitro* with DNA. The contribution made by this hypersensitivity in pathogenesis in lupus is not known.

In Rheumatoid Arthritis

It has been repeatedly observed that the usual serological tests in rheumatoid arthritis are negative in some patients who seem by all other criteria to have the disease. Transfusion studies using high-titered sera from rheumatoid arthritis patients have failed to induce the disease in recipients.[130] Some persons, who are presumably healthy, may exhibit the serological reactions without exhibiting the disease. On these accounts, it has been thought that the autoantibodies in rheumatoid arthritis may have little pathogenetic meaning.

Hollander, McCarty, and co-workers[57,103,106] reported, however, that *the leukocytes in synovial effusions* in rheumatoid arthritis patients have cytoplasmic inclusions containing γ-globulins. They called these "R.A. cells." The cells resemble the "glitter" cells of the urines of patients with pyelonephritis, and are the same as the *ragocyte*, or "raisin cell," described by Delbarre and collaborators.[29] Rawson *et al.*[103] demonstrated that the inclusions were nearly always composed of both IgG and IgM globulins, and in a number of experiments latex flocculating activity was recovered from the washed leukocytes after ultrasonic disruption.

Hollander and co-workers postulated

that the "R.A. cell" is a cell filled with ingested rheumatoid factor-gamma globulin complexes (IgG-anti IgG) and that the joint inflammation in rheumatoid disease was attributable to this ingestion. To test this, heat aggregated (and in one instance unaggregated) IgG isolated by DEAE chromatography was injected intra-articularly into rheumatoid arthritis patients and into a number of non-rheumatoid patients.[106] Five of 6 rheumatoid arthritis patients experienced marked inflammatory reactions from their own IgG, while 6 of 7 experienced no reactions from IgG isolated from normal persons or from other rheumatoid arthritis patients. With the induced arthritis, "R.A. cells" appeared or increased in numbers in those affected. None of 4 patients with osteoarthritis injected with rheumatoid IgG experienced arthritis. In further studies,[56] ability of IgG to provoke arthritis was thought to be related to whether it had Gm types appropriate to the anti Gm activity in the rheumatoid factor of the recipient.

While other investigators have had difficulty in repeating the provocation experiments, many have confirmed and elaborated upon the "R.A. cell." Vaughan *et al.*[131] not only identified rheumatoid factor in the inclusions by direct immunofluorescent staining but also showed in some that complement protein (C3) was present. There was close correlation between presence of inclusions in the leukocytes and lowered joint fluid complement titers. Ruddy and Austen[111] and Britton and Schur[2] have added evidence that the earlier complement components (C1, C2, and C4) are also fixed in the inclusions, and Ruddy, Schur, and Austen[112] have shown a lower C9 level in the joint fluid. Thus the entire sequence of activation steps in the complement cascade seems to occur in rheumatoid arthritis. Deposition of complement along with IgG and IgM in the synovial membranes indicates that the same processes occurring in the synovial fluid leukocyte occur in the membrane as well.[35,108]

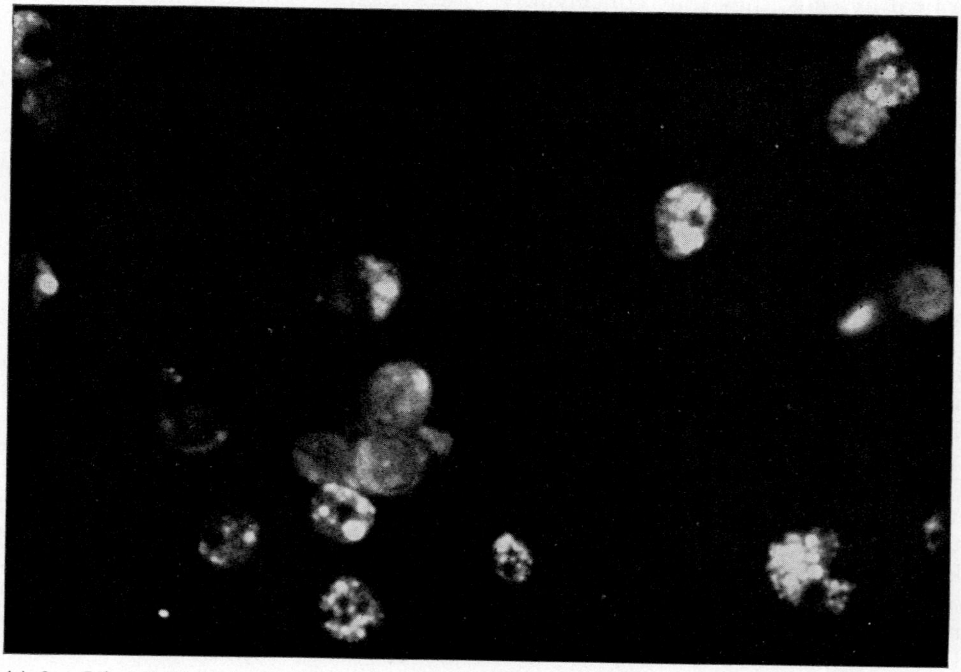

FIG. 14–2.—Joint fluid leukocytes from a patient with rheumatoid arthritis stained with fluorescein-labeled anti-gamma globulin. Numerous intracytoplasmic inclusions can be seen.

The fact that joint fluid complement titers are lowered in rheumatoid arthritis was first shown by Hedberg[52] and Pekin and Zvaifler.[98] Zvaifler[141] showed further that rheumatoid factor is itself capable of fixing human, but not guinea pig, complement after reaction with aggregated IgG. Tesar and Schmid[123] have added the demonstration that this occurs with 19S rheumatoid factor.

More recently Hannestad[49] and Winchester *et al.*[138] have described IgG-IgG complexes in the joint fluids of patients with seronegative rheumatoid arthritis. These complexes are capable of fixing complement. They can also react with 19S rheumatoid factor to produce precipitates that can be phagocytosed by leukocytes to produce typical "R.A. cells."[63] It is possible that IgG-IgG complexes will provide a molecular common denominator between seronegative and seropositive rheumatoid arthritis.[72]

Aggregates or precipitates other than rheumatoid factor precipitates may also play a role in formation of "R.A. cells." Evidence has been presented to implicate both fibrin[107,140] and DNA-anti DNA[10,28] in some cases.

The "R.A. cell" is not entirely specific for rheumatoid arthritis—*e.g.*, patients with Reiter's syndrome, tuberculous arthritis, polymyositis, pseudogout and postoperative effusion have been reported positive.[29] Still the vast majority of patients with "R.A. cells" in synovial effusions have had rheumatoid arthritis.

Astorga and Bollet[6] have reported that rheumatoid factor precipitated with aggregated gamma globulin can release lysosomal enzymes from leukocytes; and Weissmann has shown that repeated injections of joints of experimental animals with an agent (streptolysin S) capable of disrupting lysosomes can lead to a chronic arthritis histologically indistinguishable from rheumatoid arthritis. These observations give support to Hollander's speculation that leukocytic ingestion of rheumatoid factor complex may lead to tissue damage by released lysosomal products. Kaplan and Jandl's suggestion[70] that rheumatoid factors may be more predisposed to precipitate from the interstitial fluids of joint tissues than from the peripheral blood is pertinent.

Some evidences exist that *gamma globulin complexes in the circulating blood* may contribute to disease.[33] There is a tendency for patients with very high titers of rheumatoid factors to exhibit severe vasculitis characterized by skin ulcers, gangrene, and peripheral neuropathy. It has been suggested that these complications occur because of precipitation of complexes intravascularly. Tomasi *et al.*[124] called attention to pulmonary fibrosis complicating rheumatoid arthritis in patients with "intermediate complexes" (*see* Chapter 9). Ball[8] has noted in extracts of skin, tendon, synovial membrane and nodules higher titers of rheumatoid factor activity than would be expected from the amounts of blood in these tissues, but this was not seen in liver extracts. Pernis[99] has reported from immunofluorescence studies that rheumatoid factor is deposited in the vessel walls in biopsy specimens of vasculitic lesions in rheumatoids, and Mellors and co-workers[85] have noted rheumatoid factor in amyloid lesions accompanying rheumatoid arthritis.

Cerebral hypoxia and delirium have occurred in some patient with very high serum viscosities due to extremely large quantities of rheumatoid factors with intermediate complexes in the circulation.[1,88,114]

In Polyarteritis

A number of different diseases may be indicated by the diagnosis polyarteritis. Generally, the diagnosis refers to an inflammatory vasculitis, especially but not exclusively on the arterial side of the circulation, and involving vessels in all parts of the body. Gamma globulin and complement are deposited in the lesions. Usually the glomeruli are involved, or eventually become involved. It is generally assumed that, as in serum sickness, vascular damage is due to immune complexes.

There are three clinical conditions which seem to predispose to the onset of polyarteritis: (1) drug reactions, (2) respiratory infections and (3) rheumatoid arthritis. In many cases the disease arises idiopathically, no such antecedent or association being recognized. As noted above Gocke *et al.*[40] have found Australia (Au) antigen-antibody complexes in the serums of some patients with polyarteritis and evidence of deposition in the arteritic lesions of one. Presumably other antigens will be found in other patients with polyarteritis, possibly with characteristic antigens for each of the main forms of polyarteritis.

TREATMENT

The management of infections in rheumatoid diseases should differ in no way from the management of infections in any other clinical setting, save the need of avoiding drugs known to exacerbate the particular patient's disease. Foci of infection should be given no particular place in one's thinking; they should be treated only as indicated by the local condition itself.

Suppression of patients' inflammatory and immunological responses by drugs is now widely practiced. The agents used vary from salicylates, through chloroquin and penicillamine to corticosteroids and antimetabolites, the last being still on an experimental basis. The mechanisms of action of these various agents is not entirely clear. Suppression of immunological responsiveness may be effected by corticosteroids and antimetabolites in high dosage, but both these drugs also have direct anti-inflammatory effects independent of their abilities to suppress the immune response. Chloroquin and corticosteroids have the interesting capacity of stabilizing lysosomes and making the release of lysosomal enzymes by agents such as vitamin A and ultraviolet irradiation more difficult to achieve. Specific dose schedules, and recommended sequences in use of these drugs, will be dealt with in other chapters.

CONCLUSIONS

The three rheumatic diseases, systemic lupus erythematosus, rheumatoid arthritis, and polyarteritis, have certain overlapping clinical and immunological features. All three diseases are characterized by deposition of gamma globulins and complement in the tissue lesions. All may exhibit hypergammaglobulinemia. Autoantibodies are most common in lupus and least common in polyarteritis.

Both drugs and infections have been incriminated in the precipitation of these diseases, but each disease may last long after direct evidences of such precipitating events have disappeared.

That some inherited immunological hyperresponsiveness exists in rheumatoid arthritis and lupus erythematosus is suggested by family studies, which indicate that there is a predisposition among these patients' families to develop hypergammaglobulinemia, certain autoantibodies and clinical expressions suggestive of rheumatic disease are also seen. Possible specific pathways by which immunological events may contribute to the pathology of the diseases have been discussed.

Acknowledgement:

The author wishes to express his sincere appreciation to Dr. Thomas F. Disney and Miss Mary Zorn for their considerable help in assembling this revised chapter.

BIBLIOGRAPHY

1. Abruzzo, J. L., Heimer, R. and Martinez, J.: Arth. & Rheum., *12*, 653, 1969.
2. Adler, H. E.: Lab. Invest., *8*, 1394, 1959.
3. Agnello, V., Winchester, R. J., and Kunkel, H. G.: Immunol., *19*, 909, 1970.
4. Alarcon-Segovia, D., Worthington, J., Ward, E. L. and Watkim, K. G.: New Engl. J. Med., *272*, 462, 1965.

5. ASTORGA, G. P.: Arth. & Rheum., *12*, 589, 1969.
6. ASTORGA, G. P. and BOLLET, A. J.: Arth. & Rheum., *8*, 511, 1965.
7. ASTORGA, G. P. and WILLIAMS, R. C., JR.: Arth. & Rheum., *12*, 547, 1969.
8. BALL, J.: Ann. Rheum. Dis., *21*, 272, 1962.
9. BARNETT, E. V., BALDUZZI, P. C., VAUGHAN, J. H. and MORGAN, H. R.: Arth. & Rheum., *9*, 720, 1966.
10. BARNETT, E. V., BIENENSTOCK, J. and BLOCH, K. J.: J.A.M.A., *198*, 143, 1966.
11. BARNETT, E. V., NORTH, A. F., JR., CONDEMI, J. J., JACOX, R. F. and VAUGHAN, J. H.: Ann Intern. Med., *63*, 1, 1965.
12. BARNETT, E. V., STONE, G., SWISHER, S. N., and VAUGHAN, J. H.: Amer. J. Med., *35*, 113, 1963.
13. BARNETT, E. V. and TERASAKI, P. I.: Arth. & Rheum., *14*, 149, 1971.
14. BARNETT, E. V., WILLIAMS, R. C., JR., KENYON, A. J. and HENSON, J. E.: Immunology, *16*, 241, 1969.
15. BARTHOLOMEW, L. E.: Arth. & Rheum., *8*, 376, 1965.
16. BAUDILLA, K. K., PITTS, N. C. and MCDUFFIE, F. C.: Arth. & Rheum., *13*, 214, 1970.
17. BAUM, J. and ZIFF, M.: J. Clin. Invest., *48*, 758, 1969.
18. BECK, J. S. and ROWELL, N. R.: Lancet, *1*, 134, 1963.
19. BENNETT, P. H. and BURCH, T. A.: in *Population Studies of the Rheumatic Diseases*, (P. H. Bennett and P. H. N. Woods, Eds.). Amsterdam, Excerpta Medica Fdn., 1968, p. 136.
20. BILLINGHAM, R. E., BRENT, L. and MEDAWAR, P. B.: Transplantation Bull., *5*, 377, 1958.
21. BITTER, T., BITTER, F., SILBERSCHMIDT, R., and DUBOIS, E. L.: Arth. & Rheum., *14*, 152, 1971 (Abst.).
22. BLOCK, S. R., GIBBS, C. B., STEVENS, M. B. and SHULMAN, L. E.: Ann. Rheum. Dis., *27*, 311, 1968.
23. BLOMGREN, S. E., CONDEMI, J. J., BIGNALL, M. C. and VAUGHAN, J. H.: New Engl. J. Med., *281*, 64, 1969.
24. BRITTON, M. C. and SCHUR, P. H.: Arth. & Rheum., *14*, 87, 1971.
25. CHAMBERLAIN, M. A., SHAPLAND, C. G. and ROITT, I. M.: Ann. Rheum. Dis., *29*, 173, 1970.
26. COCHRANE, C. G., WEIGLE, W. C., DIXON, F. J.: J. Exp. Med., *110*, 481, 1959.
27. COLLINS, D. H. and GOLDIE, W., JR.: J. Path. Bact., *50*, 323, 1940.
28. CRACCHIOLO, A. and GOLDBERG, L.: Arth. & Rheum., *14*, 157, 1971 (Abst.).
29. DELBARRE, F., KAHAN, A., AMOR, B. and KRASSININE, G.: Presse Med., *72*, 2129, 1964.
30. DERINGER, M. K.: Lab. Invest., *8*, 1461, 1959.
31. DIXON, F. J., VAZQUEZ, J. J., WEIGLE, W. D. and COCHRANE, C. G.: in *Cellular and Humoral Aspects of the Hypersensitive States*, New York, Paul B. Hoeber, Inc., 1959.
32. DUMONDE, E. C. and GLYNN, L. E.: Brit. J. Exp. Path., *43*, 373, 1962.
33. EPSTEIN, W. V. and ENGLEMAN, E. P.: Arth. & Rheum., *2*, 250, 1959.
34. FEORINO, P. M., HIERHOLZER, J. C. and NORTON, W. L.: Arth. & Rheum., *13*, 378, 1970.
35. FISH, A. J., MICHAEL, A. F., GEWURZ, H. and GOOD, R. A.: Arth. & Rheum., *9*, 267, 1966.
36. FORD, D. K.: Med. Clin. N. Amer., *52*, 673, 1968.
37. FREEDMAN, P. and MARKOWITZ, A. S.: Brit. Med. J., *1*, 1175, 1962.
38. FRESCO, R.: Fedn. Proc., *27*, 246, 1968.
39. FRIEDMAN, E. A., BARDAWIL, J. P. and HANAU, C.: New Engl. J. Med., *262*, 486, 1960.
40. GOCKE, D. J., HSU, C., MORGAN, C., BOMBARDIERI, S., LOCKSHIN, M. and CHRISTIAN, C. L.: Lancet, *2*, 1149, 1970.
41. GOLDMAN, J. A., ADAMS, L. E., KRUEGER, R. C., LITWIN, A. and HESS, E. V.: Arth. & Rheum., *14*, 163, 1971.
42. GOLDSTEIN, G.: Brit. Med. J., *2*, 475, 1967.
43. GRAUSZ, H., EARLEY, L. E., STEPHENS, B. G., LEE, J. C., and HOPPER, J., JR.: New Engl. J. Med., *283*, 506, 1970.
44. GRAYZEL, A. I. and BECK, C.: J. Exper. Med., *131*, 367, 1970.
45. GRAYZEL, A. I., JANIS, R. and HABERMAN, E.: Arth. & Rheum., *14*, 164, 1971.
46. GREENWOOD, R. and BARR, M.: Ann. Phys. Med., *5*, 258, 1960.
47. GRUMET, F. C., CONKELL, A., BODMER, J. G., BODMER, W. F. and MCDEVITT, H. O.: New Engl. J. Med., in press.
48. GYORKEY, F., MIN, K. W., SINCOVICS, J. G. and GYORKEY, P.: New Engl. J. Med., *280*, 333, 1969.
49. HANNESTAD, K.: Clin. Exp. Immunol., *2*, 511, 1967.
50. HARE, W. S. and MACKAY, I. R.: Arch. Intern. Med., *124*, 60, 1969.
51. HEDBERG, H.: Acta Med. Scand., Suppl. 479, 1967.

52. ———: Acta Rheum. Scand., *10*, 109, 1964.
53. Helyer, B. J. and Howie, J. B.: Brit. J. Haemat., *9*, 119, 1963.
54. Hench, P. K., Tan, E. M. and Wilson, C. B.: Arth. & Rheum., *12*, 668, 1969 (Abst.).
55. Henson, J. B., Gorham, J. R., Leader, R. R. and Wagner, B. M.: J. Exp. Med., *116*, 357, 1962.
56. Hollander, J. L., Fudenberg, H. H., Rawson, A. J., Abelson, N. M. and Torralba, T. P.: Arth. & Rheum., *9*, 675, 1966.
57. Hollander, J. L., McCarty, D. J., Jr., Astorga, G. and Castro-Murillo, E.: Ann. Intern. Med., *62*, 271, 1965.
58. Hollinger, F. B., Sharp, J. T., Lidsky, M. D. and Rawls, W. E.: Arth. & Rheum., *14*, 1, 1971.
59. Holman, H. R.: Amer. J. Med., *27*, 525, 1959.
60. ———: Arth. & Rheum., *6*, 513, 1963.
61. Houba, V., Adam, M., Malecek, J. and Tesarek, B.: Experientia (Basel), *20*, 522, 1964.
62. Hurd, E. R., Eigenbrodt, E., Ziff, M., and Strunk, S. W.: Arth. & Rheum., *12*, 541, 1969.
63. Hurd, E. R., LoSpalluto, J. and Ziff, M.: Arth. & Rheum., *13*, 724, 1970.
64. Jansson, E. and Wager, O.: N.Y. Acad. Sci., *143*, 535, 1967.
65. Jasin, H. E., LoSpalluto, J. and Ziff M.: Arth. & Rheum., *12*, 304, 1969.
66. Jones, H. E., Derbes, V. J., Gum, O. B. and Azoury, F. J.: Arch. Derm., *95*, 559, 1967.
67. Jones, T. C.: Lab. Invest., *8*, 1471, 1959.
68. Kacaki, J N., Balduzzi, P. C. and Vaughan, J. H.: Clin. Exp. Immunol., *6*, 885, 1970.
69. Kacaki, J. N., Bullock, W. E. and Vaughan, J. H.: Lancet, *1*, 1289, 1969.
70. Kaplan, M. E. and Jandl, J. H.: J. Exp. Med., *117*, 105, 1963.
71. Kawano, K., Miller, L., Kimmelstiel, P.: New Engl. J. Med., *281*, 1228, 1969.
72. Kinsella, T. D., Baum, J., and Ziff, M.: Arth. & Rheum., *13*, 734, 1970.
73. Klemperer, P.: in *Progress in Fundamental Medicine* (J. F. A. McManus, Ed.) Philadelphia, Lea & Febiger, 1952.
74. Koffler, D., Schur, P. H. and Kunkel, H. G.: J. Exp. Med., *126*, 607, 1967.
75. Lachmann, P. J.: Immunology, *4*, 153, 1961.
76. ———: J. Exp. Med., *115*, 63, 1962.
77. Leonhardt, T.: Acta Med. Scand., *176*, Suppl. 416, 1964.
78. Lewis, R. M., Schwartz, R. and Henry, W. B., Jr.: Blood, *25*, 143, 1965.
79. MacSween, R. N. M., Anderson, J. R. and Milne, J. A.: J. Path. Bact., *93*, 611, 1967.
80. Mandy, W. J. and Kormeier, L. C.: Science, *154*, 651, 1966.
81. Marmont, A., Negrini, A., Damasio, E.: Comp't. rend. Soc. Biol. (Paris), *156*, 1012, 1962.
82. McNutt, S. H.: Lab. Invest., *8*, 1427, 1959.
83. Meiselas, L., Zingale, S. B., Lee, S. L., Richman, S. and Siegel, M.: J. Clin. Invest., *40*, 1872, 1961.
84. Mellors, R. C., Aorki, T. and Huebner, R. J.: J. Exper. Med., *129*, 1045, 1968.
85. Mellors, R. C., Nowoslawski, A., Korngold, L. and Sengson, B. L.: J. Exp. Med., *113*, 475, 1961.
86. Milne, J. A., Anderson, J. R., MacSween, R. N., Fraser, K., Short, I., Stevens, J., Shaw, G. B. and Tankel, H. I.: Brit. Med. J., *1*, 461, 1967.
87. Mittal, K. K., Rosen, R. D., Butler, W. T., Sharp, J. T. and Lidsky, M. D.: Arth. & Rheum., *13*, 338, 1970 (Abst.).
88. Mongan, E. S., Cass, R. M., Jacox, R. F. and Vaughan, J. H.: Amer. J. Med., *47*, 23, 1969.
89. Moore, R. D., Weisberger, A. S. and Bowerfind, E. S.: Arch. Path., *62*, 472, 1956.
90. More, R. H. and Movat, H. Z.: J. Path. Bact., *75*, 127, 1958.
91. Morse, J. H., Muller-Eberhard, H. J. and Kunkel, H. G.: Bull. N.Y. Acad. Med., *38*, 641, 1962.
92. Motulsky, A. C., Weinberg, S., Shaphir, O. and Rosenberg, E.: Arch. Int. Med., *90*, 660, 1952.
93. Nobrega, F. T., Ferguson, R. H., Kurland, L. T. and Hargraves, M. M.: in *Population Studies of the Rheumatic Diseases*, (P. H. Bennett and P. H. N. Wood, Eds.) Amsterdam, Excerpta Medica Fdn., p. 259, 1968.
94. Norton, W. L.: J. Lab. Clin. Med., *74*, 369, 1969.
95. Ores, R. O. and Lange, K.: Amer. J. Med. Sci., *248*, 562, 1964.
96. Patrucco, A., Rothfield, N. F. and Hirschhorn, K.: Arth. & Rheum., *10*, 32, 1967.
97. Pearson, C. M., Waksman, B. H. and Sharp, J. T.: J. Exp. Med., *113*, 485, 1961.
98. Pekin, T. J. and Zvaifler, N. J.: J. Clin. Invest., *43*, 1372, 1964.
99. Pernis, B.: Reumatismo, *15*, 187, 1963.
100. Perry, H. M., Jr., Tan, E. M., Carmody, S. and Sakamoto, A.: J. Lab. Clin. Med., *76*, 114, 1970.
101. Phillips, P. E. and Christian, C. L.: Science, *168*, 982, 1970.

102. Pincus, T., Blacklow, N. R., Grimley, P. M. and Bellanti, J. A.: Lancet, *2*, 1058, 1970.
103. Rawson, A. J., Abelson, N. M. and Hollander, J. L.: Ann. Intern. Med., *62*, 281, 1965.
104. Rawson, A. J., Abelson, N. M. and McCarty, D. J.: Arth. & Rheum., *4*, 463, 1961.
105. Rawson, A. J., Quismorio, F. P. and Abelson, N. M.: Amer. J. Path., *54*, 95, 1969.
106. Restifo, R. A., Lussier, A. J., Rawson, A. J., Rockey, J. H. and Hollander, J. L.: Ann. Intern. Med., *62*, 285, 1965.
107. Riddle, J. M., Bluhm, G. B. and Barnhart, M. I.: Arth. & Rheum., *8*, 463, 1965.
108. Rodman, W. S., Williams, R. C., Jr., Bilka, P. J. and Muller-Eberhard, H. J.: J. Lab. and Clin. Med., *69*, 141, 1967.
109. Rose, G. A. and Spencer, H.: Quart. J. Med., *26*, 43, 1957.
110. Rothfield, N. and Niederman, J. C.: Lancet, *1*, 167, 1971.
111. Ruddy, S. and Austen, K. F.: Arth. & Rheum., *13*, 713, 1970.
112. Ruddy, S., Schur, P. H. and Austen, K. F.: Arth. & Rheum., *13*, 346, 1970 (Abst.).
113. Sharp, J. T.: Arth. & Rheum., *13*, 263, 1970.
114. Shearn, M. A., Epstein, W. V., Engleman, E. P., Taylor, W. F.: J. Lab. Clin. Med., *61*, 677, 1963.
115. Shulman, L. E., Gumpel, J. M., D'Angelo, W. A., Souhami, R. L., Stevens, M. B., Townes, A. S. and Masi, A. T.: Arth. & Rheum., 7, 753, 1964 (Abst.).
116. Simonsen, M.: Acta Path. Microbiol. Scand., *40*, 480, 1957.
117. Singh, B. N.: Aust. Ann. Med., *18*, 55, 1969.
118. Stastny, P., Stembridge, V. A. and Ziff, M.: Arth. & Rheum., *6*, 64, 1963.
119. Strejcek, J., Herzog, P. and Bielicky, T.: Int. Arch. Allergy, *31*, 145, 1967.
120. Talal, N.: Arth. & Rheum., *13*, 887, 1970.
121. Tan, E. M. and Kunkel, H. G.: Arth. & Rheum., *7*, 348, 1964 (Abst.).
122. Tan, E. M., Schur, P. H., Carr, R. I. and Kunkel, H. G.: J. Clin. Invest., *45*, 1732, 1966.
123. Tesar, J. T. and Schmid, F. R.: J. Immunol., *105*, 1206, 1970.
124. Tomasi, T. B., Jr., Fudenberg, H. H. and Finby, N.: Amer. J. Med., *33*, 243, 1962.
125. Tonietti, G., Oldstone, M. B. A. and Dixon, F. J.: J. Exper. Med., *132*, 89, 1970.
126. Toplin, I. and Schidlovsky, G.: Science, *152*, 1084, 1966.
127. Townes, A. S., Stewart, C. R., Jr. and Osler, A. G.: Bull. Johns Hopkins Hosp., *112*, 183, 1963.
128. Trayanova, T., Sura, V. and Svet-Moldavsky, G.: Lancet, *1*, 452, 1966.
129. Vaughan, J. H., Bayles, T. B. and Favour, C. B.: J. Lab. Clin. Med., *37*, 698, 1951.
130. Vaughan, J. H. and Butler, V. P., Jr.: Ann. Intern. Med., *56*, 1, 1962.
131. Vaughan, J. H. and Jacox, R. F.: Arth. & Rheum., *11*, 135, 1968.
132. Vazquez, J. J. and Dixon, F. J.: Lab. Invest., *6*, 205, 1957.
133. Waksman, R. B.: Medicine, *41*, 93, 1962.
134. Weissmann, G., Becher, B., Wiedermann, G. and Bernheimer, A. W.: Amer. J. Path., *46*, 129, 1965.
135. Weissmann, G. Pras, M. and Rosenberg, L.: Arth. & Rheum., *10*, 325, 1967.
136. Williams, M. H.: in *Pfizer Medical Monograph*, No. 3 (J. J. R. Duthrie and W. R. M. Alexander, Eds.), Edinburgh, 1968.
137. Williams, M. H., Brostoff, J. and Roitt, I. M.: Lancet, *2*, 277, 1970.
138. Winchester, R. J., Agnello, V. and Kunkel, H. G.: J. Exp. Immunol., *6*, 689, 1970.
139. Zingale, S. B., Avalos, J. C. S., Andrada, J. A., Stringa, S. G. and Manni, J. A.: Arth. & Rheum., *6*, 581, 1963.
140. Zucker-Franklin, D.: Arth. & Rheum., *9*, 24, 1966.
141. Zvaifler, N. J.: N.Y. Acad. Sci., *168*, 146, 1969.

Chapter 15

Climate and Arthritis

By Donald F. Hill, M.D.

Climate is usually described as being cold or warm, dry or wet. Casual appraisal gives little recognition to the contributing weather factors which make up average climate. Dordick[4] referred to these important components when he reported: "The well-known change in symptoms experienced by many on the approach of weather changes cannot be attributed to pressure change alone, since the total weather change includes other variations as well." Specifically, all components of climate, the average of "total weather," are: temperature, humidity, barometric pressure, ionization, air movements, solar radiation, gases and particles, and now smog—the effluent of civilization.[13a]

All variables of weather and climate, considered comprehensively, present a difficult combination to reduce to predictable, measurable terms. Correlating these variables in terms of effect on the already complex picture in arthritis constitutes a formidable challenge. A large number of clinical studies have been reported over many years which appear to substantiate a worsening effect of climatic changes on arthritis.[8,16] Almost all such studies have been made on an empirical basis, either depending on a diary kept by each patient on the weather and the condition of the arthritis, or on a similar type record on hospitalized arthritic patients. Another empirical type of study consists of notations by each

Definitions

Climate:

The average condition of the atmosphere being affected by temperature, moisture, wind, barometric pressure, ionization, particles and bases, and variations of these factors over a period of time.

Weather:

Denotes a single occurrence or event in the series of conditions which make up climate.

Weather Sensitivity:

Reports have estimated that approximately 80 to 90 per cent of patients will observe worsening of their symptoms and even exhibit objective signs with changes in weather, *e.g.* falling barometer and rising humidity.

Lansbury's Clinical Index:

Evaluation of the activity of arthritis by assigning numerical values to five parameters of arthritis: duration of stiffness, number of aspirin needed for pain relief, strength of hand grip, walking time, and the articular index (joint count). (*See* Chapter 26.)

patient who moves from one climate to another, such as from New York to Arizona.

Neither of these methods of study can be accurate, since they are based on completely subjective data, cannot be controlled, and ignore the other stresses, such as emotional, dietary, or physical factors which vary tremendously, as well as the occurrence of infections, poor sleep, etc. The human organism includes so many variables that even the most carefully organized and controlled studies are often suspect because of unknown variables, such as suggestibility in short-term observations.

Fairly critical observations have been made by Hill and Holbrook,[6] L. Hill,[7] and, more recently, by Nava and Seda.[15] All such careful studies have concluded that climatic changes influence the course and symptomatology of various types of arthritis, but there has been no consistent pattern of the type of change which causes such effect. Most studies conclude that the periods immediately preceding a rainfall or storm are most painful for the arthritic,[15] and that seasonal changes near the times of equinox may also be important. The monograph by Peterson[16] represents the most detailed and thorough of the empirical mass studies on effect of climate on the patient and his disease. Some of his conclusions would appear to be valid as a result of subsequent studies.[11] Search of the literature reveals that with the notable exception of the Climatron research, there has been no recent controlled investigation of climate effects *per se*.

THE CLIMATE CHAMBER

More than 25 years ago Edström[5] reported on studies on rheumatoid arthritic patients confined for long periods in a constant warm, dry "microclimate." The patients were housed in an insulated room with an entrance vestibule preventing outside air from entering. The temperature was kept constant at about 84° F., and the humidity at about 35 per cent. After periods of up to three months in this first arthritis climate chamber, most of the patients seemed improved by decrease in pain, stiffness and swelling of joints, decreased numbers of pathogenic bacteria in throat culture, etc., but they usually relapsed when returned to their original home environment. These were the first experimental studies on the effect of climate on arthritis.

Stimulated both by the studies of Edström, and the somewhat controversial conclusions of Peterson,[16] Hollander conceived and arranged the construction of a "Controlled Climate Chamber" or "Climatron,"[9] in which to study climatic effects on rheumatoid arthritic patients, and those with other forms of rheumatic disease under completely controlled conditions. This was designed, like Edström's chamber, for long-term inhabitation by arthritic patients, with all the usual comforts and facilities of a two-bed hospital room and bath, with all nursing and other services brought in to the patients. Climatic changes could be made "blind" to the patients by controls invisible to them outside the room. The purpose was to study the effects of constant environment, the effect of variation of single weather parameters, and the effect of combinations of weather variables under completely controlled and reproducible conditions.

The Climatron was developed and constructed at the University of Pennsylvania Hospital, and was completed in 1961. Patients are comfortably accommodated for protracted periods with continuous control of five separate climatic factors: temperature, humidity, barometric pressure, airflow, and ionization.

The Climatron chamber is a 15 feet square room, built with 10 inch thick, reinforced concrete walls to withstand pressure variations. It is entered by an air lock vestibule. Much thought was given to psychological aspects as well as to physical comfort.[9] The conditioned air is pumped into the chamber through multiple tiny perforations in the false ceiling, and exhausted through a duct near the floor. Automatic recording instruments on the control panel outside the chamber write a continuous record of temperature, dew point temperature, barometric pressure, rate of air movement, amount of fresh air taken into the system and change in concentrations of ions in the air. Controls for the desired changes in temperature, humidity, and barometric pressure are also placed on the control panels as well as alarm mechanisms to signal any deviation from the prescribed course. Ionization of the room air is generated by coronal discharge of high voltage from three small needle-ionizing heads in the ceiling, powered by the generator in the control panel. Controls keep all variables constant in the chamber and can vary them singly, or in combination, at predetermined rates, completely without knowledge of the patients.

The patients have regular attention of doctors, nurses, physical therapists, occupational therapists, and are allowed visitors.

Most of the rheumatoid arthritic patients and all of the osteoarthritic patients tested were "weather sensitive," *i.e.*, they claimed that climatic changes worsened their arthritic symptoms.[10,11]

Of equal importance, the condition of their arthritis was numerically computed by the method of Lansbury.[12] The numerical value of this "Clinical Index" was derived from Lansbury's tables, using duration of stiffness, number of aspirin needed for pain relief, strength of hand grip, walking time, and the articular index (joint count) as the five parameters (*see* Chapter 26). In addition to these objective measurements were the patients' own reports of symptoms from their daily diaries.

Four times daily, each patient noted on a diary sheet his body weight, intake and output of fluids, oral temperature, the time of onset, location, severity and duration of joint stiffness or pain, the number of analgesic tablets for pain relief and any changes in environmental conditions, or his own well being detectable to him.

At least twice each day, clinical observations were made of the strength of hand grip, time required by patient to rise from chair, walk across chamber and reseat himself, blood pressure, pulse, and general condition. Particularly important was a "joint count," for which each joint of the body was checked for tenderness, swelling, and/or pain on motion. These dual data were transposed to a continuous "running data sheet."

For the first five to seven days of each experiment, all five climatic factors were kept completely constant. This allowed adjustment of the patients to the change of living, and the duties and observations expected.

In a subsequent series of studies, air flow was kept constant at 1000 cubic feet per minute, dry bulb temperature was kept constant at 76° F., and ionization was kept at "background count" (positive ions 400/ml. air, negative 300/ml. air) throughout the study. Humidity at "standard" level was 30 per cent and "standard" barometric pressure was 30 inches of mercury absolute.

After the five- to seven-day control period, and without the patients' knowledge, the pressure was first increased over a two-hour period to 31.5 inches, then decreased over a four-hour period to 28.5 inches, then returned to 30 inches. This cycle was programmed over a twelve-hour period.

A day or two later, a similar humidity change cycle was instituted with rise of humidity from 30 to 80 per cent, and down again over a twelve-hour period.

Within the following day or two, the same changes in pressure and humidity were carried out *simultaneously*. This combined change was repeated at random intervals. In some experiments, the programming clocks were stopped in the cycle to compare the effects of prolonged, stable high humidity-low barometric pressure with effects of continually changing conditions.

In Figure 15–1, the linear representa-

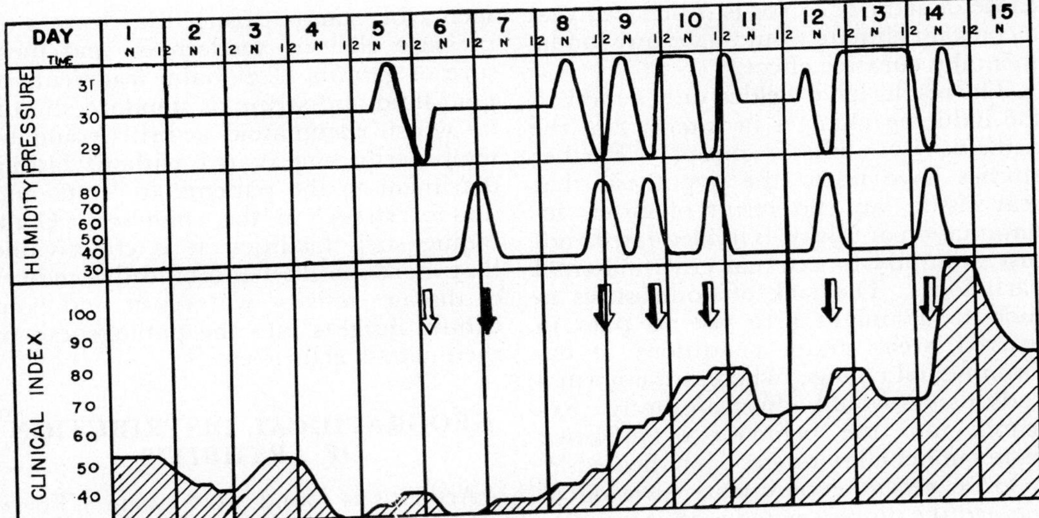

FIG. 15–1.—Course of patient with rheumatoid arthritis subjected to barometric change and humidity change cycles, at first single, then in combination. Conditions of arthritis below.

tions of barometric pressure and humidity changes are shown with the Clinical Index of the patient below. A white arrow shows the time of onset of the pressure variation cycle (falling). The black arrow shows the time of onset of humidity (rising). White and black arrows mark the onset of *simultaneous* pressure drop with humidity rise.

In plotting the Clinical Index, the onset of fluctuations corresponds with the start of subjective complaints, and the height of each peak or plateau is the actual value of the arthritic activity at the time of the next examination. Changes in the Clinical Index were regarded as significant only if the probability of coincidence, as compared with the control period mean value, was less than 1 per hundred by T-test analysis ($P = < .01$).

Table 15–1 summarizes the results of such experiments on 8 patients with rheumatoid arthritis. In 7 of the 8 there was significant worsening of arthritis within a few hours after onset of combined humidity rise and barometric fall in 29 of 46 exposures to the combined cycle.

TABLE 15–1

Patient	Total trials	Increased arthritis	Per cent
B. B.	7	4	57
F. F.	11	8	73
D. M.	6	4	67
E. L.	6	0	0
R. M.	5	3	60
D. N.	3	2	67
L. L.	3	3	100
E. A.	5	5	100
Total	46	29	63

From these studies, Hollander and Yeostros[11] concluded: "It would appear that at least one combination of changing weather factors—rising humidity with falling barometric pressure—fairly consistently exerts a detrimental effect on arthritic symptoms and signs." It would also appear that *the changing conditions*, rather than the high humidity or low barometric pressure, are responsible. It now seems reasonable to conclude that weather effect on arthritis is a definite phenomenon, and not just another old wives' tale. It is not implied that climatic changes have any direct bearing on the cause of arthritis. Nor is it believed that a constant climate would have any fundamentally curative effect.

The results have yielded only a method for inducing changes in intensity of the arthritis by climatic means. Further studies have tested the hypothesis that scar tissue, an end result of either inflammation or injury, is inadequate to adjust promptly to external environmental variations. The lack of homeostasis in such tissue might give rise to pain in scarred areas under conditions of environmental change, whereas the normal body tissues would adjust promptly. Research into the behavior of inflamed tissues under climatic stress is indicated.[10a]

More recent experiments have documented the diuresis noted with increasing humidity and decreasing barometric pressure, and fluid retention which occurs with rising barometric pressure and decreasing humidity in rheumatoid and non-rheumatoid subjects. These shifts of fluid are believed to represent the homeostatic process of maintenance of cellular structure in a changing external total water-vapor pressure.

The hypothesized mechanism by which pain is increased under conditions of falling barometer and rising humidity (as before a storm) is as follows: Normal tissues adjust to the decreasing pressure by extrusion of intracellular fluid into the blood stream. Diseased tissue is not so permeable, holds fluid, and therefore maintains a relatively higher intracellular pressure than the surrounding normal tissue. This gradient in pressure leads to increased pain and swelling of the diseased part. *In vitro* studies of normal and inflamed tissue permeability have been made, as well as *in vivo* studies on tissue pressure, blood flow, and intra-articular pressure.[10a]

Studies augmenting the Climatron series have developed several foci for urgent pursuit. Hollander suggests three main targets: more objective assessment of the intensity of rheumatoid inflammation such as joint temperature measurement; intra-articular pressure measurement for standardizing the degrees of pressure eliciting tenderness; and measure of gamma G globulin fragments in joint fluid and serum as standard stimuli by which rheumatoid arthritis could be temporarily aggravated without lasting detriment to the patients at "rest" and under "stress" in the chamber. Combining such facilities, it is conceivable that more sensitive and objective indices of disease activity will result and contribute insights into the pathogenesis of rheumatoid arthritis.

GEOGRAPHICAL DISTRIBUTION OF ARTHRITIS

Arthritis is found world-wide. There are many reports in the medical literature of population studies, either ethnically or geographically oriented (*see* Chapter 12), which involved single or multiple clinical indices. As yet, none of these has demonstrated that climatic factors have any important influence on the development of any type of arthritis. Some excellent comparative studies, using the criteria of the American Rheumatism Association[17] have been contributed. Cobb *et al.*[2] and Cobb and Lawrence[3] report variations in comparable case incidence of rheumatoid arthritis between Pittsburgh, Pennsylvania and Leigh in Northwest England. However, the authors caution that since there exist geographic variations *within* countries this may not be generalized into a comparison between England and the United States. Arthritis in Alaskan Eskimos was reported by Blumberg *et al.*[1] as occurring in 1 per cent of the population.

Short and his colleagues[18] compared country of origin of arthritics at Massachusetts General Hospital. This revealed that a disproportionately large number of Scandinavians were arthritics and very few patients came from Italy or Southern Europe.

Lawrence *et al.*,[13] from a comprehensive, multicountry sampling and examination of more than 6000 persons, concluded that no relationship to latitude was discovered in the incidence of rheumatoid arthritis.

Mendez-Bryan, Roger, and Gonzalez-Alcover report[14] from Puerto Rico that the total population (age fifteen and over) in Guaynabo was screened by clinical, radiological and serological means in a study under the auspices of the Puerto Rico Medical School and NIAMD. Criteria of the A.R.A. were employed. Results indicate a significantly lower prevalence of rheumatoid arthritis when compared to reports from studies in the temperate zones, and represent the lowest prevalence rates yet reported for this disease.

These are interesting studies and would have greater significance if they could be incorporated into a world-wide survey. Up to the present time three main difficulties militate against conclusive evidence: lack of uniform criteria employed for diagnosis; no standardization of methods for sampling populations; and lack of statistically significant numbers and spread of studies (*see also* Chapter 12).

Geographical areas with various climates also must be considered in relation to the effect on *treatment* or *management* of arthritis. Moens,[14a] interested in Hollander's data from the climate chamber studies, recorded weather effects in Brussels over a 2-year period: "We compared a number of patients attending a rheumatology clinic with the variations in barometric pressure and the degree of humidity. There was a correlation between the two values."

With no substantial objective data available in the past, physicians and patients have thought dryness and warmth to be the most important factors. As a result, increasing numbers of patients are visiting or migrating to the southwestern desert in the United States.

The desert climate is dry with low average humidity often below 10 per cent. The days are warm but nights are cool. In winter months, diurnal fluctuations of temperature occur up to 50°. Barometric pressure changes are of a lower degree and lesser frequency than in the north central United States, or the coastal areas. The sun shines the year around and heat becomes uncomfortable only when the humidity rises in July and August, during the summer rainy season.

Now the observations made in the Climatron confirm the clinical impression that "weather sensitive" patients, or "weather prophets" suffer more with changes in weather, *i.e.* the falling barometric pressure—rising humidity that precede a storm. There is some evidence that the patient's reaction may be proportionate to the magnitude of fluctuation in barometric pressure and humidity, as well as the rate and frequency of change. Because of this, the relatively dry, warm and fairly stable climate of the Southwestern United States might produce less "weather stress" to the rheumatoid arthritic patient.

CLIMATOTHERAPY

From clinical observations, patients' experiences, and now the documented observations in the Climatron, there is sufficient evidence to say that climate does have an effect on arthritis. Though objective data are limited, it is reported that 80 to 90 per cent of the arthritic patients are weather sensitive, while apparently 10 to 20 per cent are not affected.[6,8,19] Many, as we know, can predict weather changes long before they occur. This sensitivity applies to osteoarthritis as well as rheumatoid arthritis and varies from minimal to maximal. A few appear to have definite exacerbations and remissions with weather changes. With the considerable increase in travel of patients from one climate to another, as well as by repeated visits and migration, these clinical observations assume more meaning.

Determining which patients might be benefited is difficult. Conspicuously absent is any single test or yardstick for measuring weather sensitivity and patient response. Patients who are obvious reactors and readily predict weather

Summary

1. Climatic factors and symptoms of established arthritis have been proved interactive in a preliminary controlled study. As shown by continued experiments, arthritic patients are affected by the change incident to combined falling barometric pressure and rising humidity.
2. This interaction cannot be construed as either causing or curing arthritis.
3. Incidence of arthritis is world-wide. Insufficient data are available to claim higher prevalence for one part of the world over another.
4. Warm, dry climates may have some benefit in the overall management of arthritis, but a sound medical program is still needed. Thorough consideration of economic, social and psychological factors should be included before recommending a change of climate to the arthritic patient.

changes are probably more likely to be benefited by climatotherapy.

In prescribing a change of climate, several factors in addition to weather sensitivity should be considered. Economics are important. Patients must eat, have adequate medical care and nursing, proper housing, and freedom from financial worry. Separation from family and friends can be detrimental, if not disastrous, for some. Others may be much improved by removal from the pressure and frustrations of home and business. Patients should not be advised to go to a certain climate and "bake in the sun." This is patent oversimplification, and bad advice. Too much sun can be toxic and debilitating and the possibilities should always be kept in mind of lupus erythematosus and the photosensitizing capacity of some drugs. In concentrating on sun, patients often neglect the most basic essentials of rehabilitation. For patients who do well, or even go into remission with a change in climate, there is unfortunately no assurance that they will remain well on their return to a less favorable environment.

Climate is not a cure for arthritis, although there may be an occasional dramatic remission. In general, for patients on a good medical program, the addition of a change to a mild, dry climate may be beneficial.

BIBLIOGRAPHY

1. Blumberg, B. S., Bloch, K. J., Black, R. L., and Dotter, C.: Arth. and Rheum., *4*, 325, 1961.
2. Cobb, S., Warren, J. E., Merchant, W. R., and Thompson, D. J.: J. Chron. Dis., *5*, 636, 1957.
3. Cobb, S. and Lawrence, J. S.: Bull. Rheum. Dis., *7*, 133, 1957.
4. Dordick, I.: Weather, *13*, 359, 1958.
5. Edström, G.: Ann. Rheum. Dis., *7*, 76, 1948.
6. Hill, D. F. and Holbrook, W. P.: Clinics, *1*, 577, 1942.
7. Hill, L.: British Med. J., *2*, 276, 1939.
8. Holbrook, W. P.: in *Arthritis and Allied Conditions*, Hollander, J. L., Ed., Philadelphia, Lea & Febiger, 1960, pp. 577–581.
9. Hollander, J. L.: Trans. New York Acad. Sci., *24*, 167, 1961.
10. ———: Arch. Environ. Health, *6*, 89, 1963.

10*a*.———: Personal communication, 1970.

11. Hollander, J. L. and Yeostros, S. J.: Bull. Amer. Meteorological Soc., *44*, 489, 1963.
12. Lansbury, J.: Arth. and Rheum., *1*, 505, 1958.
13. Lawrence, J. S., Behrend, T., Bennett, P. H., Bremner, J. M., Burch, T. A., Gofton, J., O Brien, W. and Robinson, H.: Ann. Rheum. Dis., *25*, 425, 1966.

13*a*.Licht, S. (ed.): *Medical Climatology*, New Haven, E. Licht, 1964.

14. Mendez-Bryan, R., Roger, N. L., and Gonzalez-Alcover, R.: Arth. and Rheum., *7*, 171, 1964.

14*a*.Moens, C.: Rev. rhum., *34*, 578, 1967.

15. Nava, P. and Seda, H.: Brasil-Medico, *78*, 71, 1964.
16. Peterson, W. F.: *The Patient and the Weather*, Ann Arbor, Edwards Brothers, 1936.
17. Ropes, M. W., Bennett, G. A., Cobb, S., Jacox, R. and Jessar, R. A: Ann. Rheum. Dis., *18*, 48, 1958.
18. Short, C. L., Bauer, W., and Reynolds, W. E.: *Rheumatoid Arthritis*, Cambridge, Harvard University Press, 1957.
19. Thompson, H. E.: Arizona Med., *8*, 31, 1951.

Chapter 16

The Endocrinology of the Rheumatic Diseases

By S. Richardson Hill, Jr., M.D., and Howard L. Holley, M.D.

The formulation of the general adaptation syndrome[69] and the discovery of the dramatic therapeutic effect obtained in patients with rheumatic diseases by the administration of C_{21} 11-17-oxygenated corticosteroids and corticotropin[29,79] were followed by many medical research studies designed to delineate the possible role of the endocrine glands in the pathogenesis of rheumatoid arthritis and other rheumatic diseases. Although numerous investigations of this subject have been reported there has been, as yet, no consistent, unique or specific abnormality of endocrine function found in patients with rheumatic diseases. That a clinical relationship does exist between certain rheumatic diseases and differences in endocrine function is well established. The remissions in rheumatoid arthritis during pregnancy, the preponderance of ankylosing spondylitis and gout in males and of disseminated lupus erythematosus in females are examples of such a clinical relationship. However, based on experimental evidence available thus far, it would seem that if endocrine factors are basically related to rheumatic diseases, they play a permissive[37] or conditioning[73] role rather than a direct etiologic one (*vide infra*). It is apparent that the benefit obtained from the adrenal cortical steroids in such diseases is not related to a gross deficiency of these steroids; and that they do not alter the fundamental disease process, but rather act through a non-specific anti-inflammatory mechanism.

THE PITUITARY GLAND

The hormones from the anterior pituitary act in part by way of target endocrine glands and in part directly on end-organ tissues themselves. No attempt will be made to discuss separately the possible actions of the cerebral cortex or hypothalamus on the anterior pituitary (*see* Chapter 17).

Polyarticular lesions have been reported in rats following prolonged treatment with lyophilized whole anterior pituitary extract.[70] Other workers have noted improvement in subjects with rheumatoid arthritis in whom calf and hog anterior pituitary glands have been implanted.[18] Still other investigators have noted improvement from posterior lobe pituitary extracts,[54] and from pitressin.[27] These studies still await confirmation. Luteotropic hormone (LTH) or prolactin has been shown to act synergistically with growth hormone in producing polyarthritis in the adrenalectomized, desoxycorticosterone-maintained and in the hypophysectomized rat.[40] Prolactin appears to play a greater role than does growth hormone in the production of these arthropathies. There is no clear relationship between the other gonadotropins and the rheumatic diseases.

Growth Hormone

The physiologic effects of growth hormone are to increase the rate of skeletal growth, enhance the storage of nitrogen, phosphorus, and calcium, and to inhibit the action of insulin. Experimentally the administration of growth hormone has induced changes suggesting hypertrophic polyarthritis in rats,[62,66] and has stimulated fibroblastic proliferation,[76] and collagen production by fibroblasts in rats.[68]

The arthritis of acromegaly was described by Marie in 1886.[51] The kyphosis and spondylitis of acromegaly are related to the laying down of new periosteal bone on all borders of the vertebral bodies and to severe osteoporosis late in the course of the disease. There is no increased incidence of rheumatoid arthritis in patients with acromegaly, but synovial thickening and recurrent effusions have been seen in acromegalic patients. Treatment of this disease consists of irradiation or surgical removal of the eosinophilic adenoma which is undertaken for the general manifestations of the disease and not specifically for the arthritis and osteoporosis which are usually only incidental findings.

THE ADRENAL CORTEX

The concept of the diseases of adaptation and the remarkable clinical effect obtained by the administration of the C_{21} 11-17-oxygenated corticosteroids to patients with rheumatic diseases promptly led to numerous attempts to link the pathogenesis of these diseases with a disturbance in adrenal cortical secretory activity. Such studies have been carried out predominantly in patients with rheumatoid arthritis, and the majority suggest that while gross adrenal cortical secretory activity is apparently within normal limits, subtle, but perhaps significant, deviations from normal may occur. It is possible, though unproven, that such small changes might provide a favorable environment in susceptible individuals for rheumatic diseases to manifest themselves by some entirely independent process.

Again there is no obvious clinical relationship between overt hyper- or hypoadrenocorticism and the rheumatic diseases. There is no increase or decrease in the incidence of rheumatic diseases in patients with Addison's disease, in which the adrenal cortex is destroyed; in patients with Cushing's syndrome, in which there is hypersecretion of glucocorticoids; in patients with the adrenogenital syndrome, in which there is hypersecretion of adrenal androgens; or in patients with primary hyperaldosteronism.

Although certain clinical characteristics of rheumatoid arthritis, such as profound muscle weakness, lassitude, frequent attacks of stiffness, and occasional skin pigmentation, resemble some characteristics of Addison's disease, they are in general non-specific, and represent the body's reaction to the disease rather than the disease itself. At present it seems certain that the adrenal glucocorticoids act by a non-specific suppression of inflammatory responses, rather than by an alteration of the fundamental disease process.

STRESS AND RHEUMATIC DISEASES: THE CONCEPT OF DISEASES OF ADAPTATION

More than three decades have elapsed since it was first postulated that certain maladies are "diseases of adaptation" in which a derailment of physiologic adaptive reactions plays a decisive etiologic role.[69]

Several early experimental observations led Selye to the belief that some diseases that are not primarily due to an increased or insufficient corticoid secretion may, nevertheless, be attributed to hypo- or hypercorticism, respectively.[72] For example, a decreased resistance to infections may be regarded as being due (at least in part) to an increase in glucocorticoids (*e.g.*, during stress), since an excess of exogenous or endogenous ACTH and cortisone does, in fact, diminish resistance to infections. Conversely, a diminished activity of prophlogistic hormones (*e.g.*, an STH growth hormone) may have the same effect, as judged by the observation that, in animals, injections of STH are highly effective in restoring towards normal the decreased resistance to infection that can be induced by antiphlogistic hormones. Furthermore, acute gastric ulcers—such as are characteristic of the alarm reaction—can be produced with an excess of glucocorticoids both in experimental animals and in man. This finding suggested the possibility that spontaneous gastroduodenal ulcers may likewise partly depend upon an increased antiphlogistic hormone activity. If this concept is correct, we should then consider certain maladies that tend to develop during stress as "diseases of adaptation"; maladies due not only to the actions of the apparent pathogen, but also to changes in disease susceptibility induced by inadequate hormonal reactions to stress.

Disease is a dynamic process, a fight between the pathogen and the affected organism. The latter defends itself against the producer of the disease by adaptive phenomena. Hence, adaptation is an integral element of all disease. In some maladies, the direct actions of pathogens, in others, the failure of adaptive phenomena are of the greatest importance; only in the latter case do we speak of diseases of adaptation.

In the supposed diseases of adaptation of man, marked changes in the blood level or urinary elimination of hormones can rarely be observed. The finding that this is true as regards the rheumatic diseases also led many investigators to the conclusion that endocrine factors do *not* play a decisive role in the pathogenesis of such maladies.

However, the theory of the diseases of adaptation does not postulate an absolute increase or decrease in hormone production, but rather a change in hormone activity. The latter may be due to faulty "conditioning," and, hence, need not be reflected by any absolute change in hormonal levels. Thus, a nearly "normal" glucocorticoid level such as suffices to maintain homeostasis at rest, is grossly insufficient to maintain the life of an adrenalectomized animal exposed to stress. Such a "normal" secretion also fails to prevent inflammation in the presence of an irritant (*e.g.*, formalin in experimental "arthritis," or ovalbumin in anaphylactoid inflammation). Here, the pathogenic factor would be precisely the maintenance of the normal hormone level when the situation calls for a considerable increase. Selye[71] has reported to have observed that in many of his experiments, ordinarily well-tolerated amounts of desoxycorticosterone (DOC) or growth hormone (STH) can assume severe pathogenic potencies, owing to changes in the metabolic conditions that determine susceptibility to their toxic effects. Therefore, an increase in corticoid activity does not necessarily represent an increase in corticoid hormone secretion.

Selye postulated that no disease is due exclusively to a "derailment" of adaptive phenomena, nor is there any malady in which the adaptive phenomena do not play a role to some extent. He observed that in order to produce disease there always must exist some direct, purely aggressive and nonadaptive action of a pathogen. On the other hand, he concluded that there exists virtually no pathogenic action that does not elicit some adaptive phenomena. Such an overlap between groups does not minimize the practical value of the principle of classification. He argued that nearly every disease could be properly included in several of the classic categories of pathology. Thus, rheumatic fever is undoubtedly a disease of the joints, but it is also a cardiac disease, a connective tissue disease and probably an infectious disease. In this concept, although the subjects of the natural sciences cannot be separated into water-tight, non-overlapping compartments, this does not alter the fact that without classification there is no science. Therefore, if we now consider rheumatic fever as a disease of adaptation, we do not further complicate the above classification, but rather, by this generalization, the pathogenesis of the disease can be analyzed from a new viewpoint.

In a narrower sense, Selye considers as diseases of adaptation those pathologic processes predominantly due to stress and often mediated by a pathogenic hormonal activity. In this sense, he distinguishes, at least in principle, the following main groups of diseases of adaptation:

1. Disease due to an absolute excess or deficiency in the secretion of adaptive hormones (for example, corticoids, ACTH and STH).
2. Disease due to variations in the absolute blood level of adaptive hormones, resulting from a stress-induced derangement of hormone metabolism rather than from increased or decreased secretion.
3. Disease due to a derangement in the normal balance between antagonistic adaptive hormones, *e.g.*, between ACTH and antiphlogistic corticoids on the one hand and STH and prophlogistic corticoids on the other. Such disease can result from a disproportion in the secretion or detoxication of these hormones during stress.
4. Disease due to stress-produced derangements that alter the response of target organs to the adaptive hormones through the phenomenon of conditioning.
5. Finally, although hormones play a prominent role in the general adaptation syndrome, stress-induced derangements of nonendocrine organs, *e.g.*, the nervous system, liver and kidney, may also cause diseases of adaptation.

The regulation of tissue reactivity, for instance through corticoids, often determines whether the body succumbs to disease or resists a potential pathogen by means of adaptation. Thus, the effects of non-specific therapeutic procedures (*e.g.*, of climatotherapy and hydrotherapy, so often used in rheumatology) and particularly those of the adaptive hormones, largely depend upon "conditioning factors," some of which are external (diet, temperature, light), others internal (heredity, constitution, previous exposure, etc.). A state of stress is produced in the body through multiple pathways, its effect always being modified by the variable specific actions of the eliciting agents, and by the conditioning factors (the "constitution" or "terrain") that differ in every individual and, indeed, in every part of the individual. These factors can affect the various targets and pathways selectively and thereby vary the manifestations of what, in essence, is but a single stress response. A more unified concept of pathology may be established, in which the most varied manifestations of diseases (and especially those of the diseases of adaptation) would be considered to have a tripartite pathogenesis consisting of: (1) the direct actions of exogenous agents; (2) endogenous factors that inhibit this action; and (3) endogenous factors that facilitate this action. Selye and Bajusz[74] state that if this concept is used as a guide in analyzing the pathogenesis of diseases, we must always consider each of these three components, because it is now evident that nonspecific adaptive reactions can act both as defensive (or even therapeutic) and as disease-producing agents, depending upon conditioning circumstances. Pathogenicity may depend upon genetic factors, the portal of entry, the previous weakening of resistance through malnutrition or cold, etc. That is why it is often difficult to decide which among the many factors in the pathogen is necessary for the production of disease, which is the conditioning factor, and which is useful in the prevention of disease; usually the full pathogenic situation must be realized before the malady can become manifest.

The experimental analysis of conditioning influences may help us to recognize some factors in the mechanism particularly of such maladies as the collagen diseases, in which the search for a single pathogen has been fruitless; these maladies may be due to "pathogenic constellations," *i.e.*, interactions of conditioning influences.[74]

THE ADRENAL CORTEX AND RHEUMATIC DISEASE

The influence of the mineralocorticoids including aldosterone and desoxycorticosterone on mesenchymal tissues is, in general, to stimulate the formation of foreign body granuloma, the proliferation and activity of fibroblasts in connective tissue and the formation of granulation tissue.[58,59] Experimental arthritis and cardiovascular lesions have occasionally been produced in specially prepared rats by these substances.[70]

The effects of the glucocorticoids on connective tissue are entirely different from and, in some respects, counteract those of the mineralocorticoids. Cortisol and cortisone have been demonstrated to inhibit the growth and migration of fibroblasts by some workers, to inhibit the fibroblastic production of collagen, to inhibit the migration of polymorphonuclear leukocytes and macrophages in inflammation, to decrease the intercellular content of acid mucopolysaccharide and hexosamine, and to reduce the relative amount of ground substance.[2,3,24,61]

ADRENAL CORTICAL HORMONES AND ARTHRITIS IN MAN

Adrenocortical secretory activity in patients with rheumatoid arthritis has generally been evaluated by studying the urinary excretion of hormone metabolites and the blood levels of these hormones.

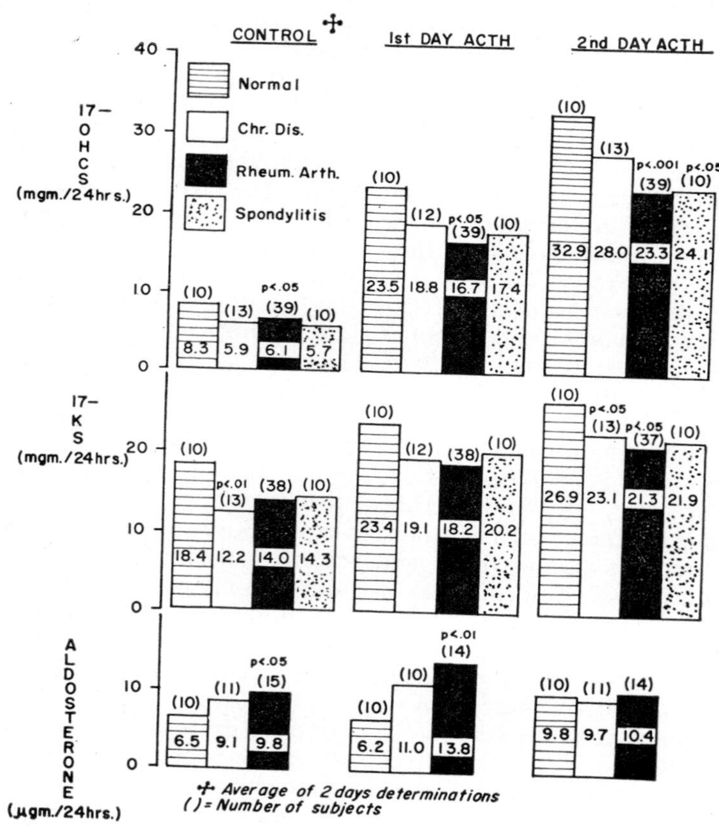

FIG. 16–1.—The mean urinary 17-hydroxycorticosteroid, 17-ketosteroid and aldosterone levels in response to 25 units of ACTH administered intravenously over 8 hours on two consecutive days to normal subjects and patients with non-rheumatoid chronic disease, rheumatoid arthritis and ankylosing spondylitis.[35]

Although numerous investigations of the subject have been reported, there is as yet no general agreement on whether adrenal cortical function is normal, decreased or increased in patients with rheumatoid arthritis.[17,32] Most of these studies have utilized changes in urinary 17-ketosteroid, 17-ketogenic steroid, or total 17-hydroxycorticosteroid levels as indicators of adrenal cortical activity. In addition studies of the free plasma corticoids and urinary aldosterone levels have also been made. Although great variation has been noted in these indices, it seems clear that there is no gross deficiency or excess of any of these steroids in patients with rheumatoid arthritis.[34,35,36,42,43] Although, in general, the levels of adrenal cortical hormones fall within the normal range, several studies have indicated qualitative and quantitative variations from normal in patients with rheumatoid arthritis.[14,16,34,35,36,42,43] Unfortunately these findings have not proved to be unique for patients with rheumatoid arthritis. Abnormalities have been suggested in the diurnal rhythm of adrenal cortical activity but these have not been significantly different from those noted in patients with non-rheumatic chronic diseases.[32]

Figure 16–1 illustrates the mean twenty-four hour urinary 17-hydroxycorticosteroid, 17-ketosteroid, and aldosterone levels on control days and in response to ACTH administered on two consecutive days to normal subjects and to patients with non-rheumatoid chronic disease, rheumatoid arthritis, and ankylosing spondylitis.[35] This study which confirms and extends previous ones[32] demonstrates that mean urinary 17-hydroxycorticosteroid control-day levels and their response to corticotropin administration were less than those observed in normal subjects. The urinary 17-ketosteroids varied in the same direction but their differences were less pronounced. In contrast, urinary aldosterone levels under similar circumstances were higher than those observed in normal subjects. These changes appear to be a manifestation of nonspecific chronic disease rather than a unique abnormality of rheumatic disease. The fate of radioactively labeled corticoids in patients with rheumatoid arthritis also appears to be normal.[57]

Some studies on adrenal steroid patterns and metabolites in patients with rheumatic disease suggest a slight relative decrease in 11-beta- and 17-hydroxylating activity with a consequent increase in the levels of corticosterone and 11-desoxycorticosterone and their metabolites.[34,42] In addition patients with rheumatoid arthritis have a relative suppression of 11-beta dehydrogenase activity resulting in a preponderance of cortisol and its metabolites over cortisone; and a relative decrease in 5-alpha reductase activity resulting in a relative increase in 5-beta steroid metabolites such as etiocholanolone.[34] Again, all of these changes are similar to those seen in patients with a great variety of chronic and stressful diseases.

It seems clear from evidence available thus far that the adrenal cortical steroids do not play a major role in the etiology of the rheumatic diseases. It is equally clear that variations in the amounts of these steroids may modify, at least temporarily, various rheumatic disease states. The mechanism of this action remains obscure.

THE THYROID GLAND AND ARTHRITIS

The thyroid hormones, thyroxine and 3,5,3′ triiodothyronine, normally regulate the rate of cellular oxidative processes throughout the body, but the exact mechanism by which they act is not completely understood. An excess of hormone induces a significant rise in basal oxygen consumption of the tissues (hypermetabolism). Insufficiency of thyroid hormone is followed by a reduction in the rate of oxidative reactions and a decrease in basal oxygen consumption (hypometabolism). There is a reciprocal relationship between the anterior pituitary thyroid-stimulating hormone and the circulating level of thyroxine and triiodothyronine. A reduction in the quantity of circulating thyroid hormone stimulates the output of TSH, which in turn increases the secretory activity of the thyroid gland. Conversely, increased levels of circulating thyroid hormone tend to depress the secretion of TSH and so, in turn, reduce thyroid activity. Thus, the thyroid hormone in animals acts to inhibit the typical thyrotropin effects noted previously.[2,38] The thyroid hormones, therefore, decrease the content of acid mucopolysaccharides, hyaluronic acid and hexosamine in ground substance. In addition the formation of collagen fibers is also decreased in growing connective tissue.[38]

There is no overt clinical relationship between hyper- or hypothyroidism and the rheumatic disease states. Although rare, rheumatoid arthritis does occur in patients with hyperthyroidism; it is somewhat more common in patients with hypothyroidism. There are vague muscular and articular pains which occur in myxedema, presumably as a result of the infiltration of connective tissue with mucopolysaccharide material. Indeed some patients with hypothyroidism seek medical advice as a result of these muscular and articular pains, and consequently, myxedema, masquerading as "arthritis," should always be considered. The pains in hypothyroidism are usually associated with stiffness and coldness and are diffuse in location, and are generally more apt to be confused with fibrositis than with rheumatoid arthritis. As these symptoms are readily abolished by the oral administration of thyroactive substances, the recognition of hypothyroidism is of great importance. It is of interest to note that, following thyroidectomy in patients with rheumatoid arthritis a large percentage have a clinical exacerbation of their arthritis.[49]

Several reports have indicated that hypertrophic pulmonary osteoarthropathy may develop in patients with postoperative myxedema.[12,65,78]

It should be borne in mind that prolonged therapy with adrenal cortical glucocorticoids may result in inhibition of the thyroid gland.[33] The relationship of this phenomenon to the exacerbation of rheumatoid arthritis following cortisone withdrawal or the exacerbation seen during hypercortisonism is unknown. If hypothyroidism does develop, however, the steroid should either be withdrawn or replacement thyroid therapy should be administered.

THE GONADAL HORMONES

Studies on gonadal hormone metabolites in the urine of patients with rheumatic diseases have revealed no specific abnormality. Numerous attempts at therapy of rheumatoid arthritis with estrogens, androgens, progesterone, and related steroids have not been successful in carefully controlled studies and have shed no light on the underlying disease process. Further actions of the gonadal hormones are discussed in the section on pregnancy and arthritis, *vide infra*.

MENOPAUSE

The female climacteric or menopause is a type of physiologic primary ovarian insufficiency. In keeping with a gradual decrease in estrogen, there is a gradual rise in urinary gonadotropin excretion during this period. This state has its onset, in the majority of instances, between the ages of forty-five and fifty-five years. Along with the gradual disappearance of menstruation there is a more gradual regressive change in the uterus, vagina, and breasts. Pubic and axillary hair tend to become somewhat sparse and eventually osteoporosis may become evident. Certain vasomotor and nervous symptoms may accompany the changes just described; these include periodic feelings of warmth in the face, neck, and upper thorax, and less frequently sudden surges of heat involving the whole body, and accompanied by drenching sweat. There may be nervousness, irritability, fatigability, and lassitude. While these symptoms appear in most women, they are of marked degree or long duration in only a small proportion of women. After a few months or years the symptoms gradually disappear. Occasionally emotional instability may become severe at this period and, aside from producing psychoneurotic symptoms, it may be one of the trigger mechanisms which leads to rheumatoid arthritis. (*See* chapter on psychogenic factors in rheumatic diseases.) Arthritis not uncommonly begins at the time of menopause, and one study has reported the onset of 9.7 per cent rheumatoid and 18 per cent osteoarthritis at the time of menopause in a series of approximately 250 cases of each.[20]

Menopausal Arthralgia

Diffuse aches, pains, and stiffness in muscles and joints are common during the first two years following cessation of menstruation. When there are no objective signs of true arthritis, such as joint swelling, heat, redness, tenderness or crepitus, and no increase in the sedimentation rate, the term menopausal arthralgia has been used to describe this state. The same picture may follow castration in young women. The symptoms are readily controlled by estrogens. There is no proof that these pains are directly due to the hormonal changes occurring at this time. Although some authors favor this view,[56] others would explain the symptoms on the basis of generally increased awareness of bodily sensations during the menopause.

Postmenopausal Osteoporosis (*see also* Chapter 62)

Women are prone to develop osteoporosis on an average of ten years after the physiologic menopause. The early studies of Albright which demonstrated that osteoporosis may be related to a failure of the osteoblasts to maintain normal protein osteoid matrix for the deposition of calcium and phosphorus salts are now under question (*see* Chapter 62). Other factors which are of importance in this type of osteoporosis are general senescence, disuse, and possibly faulty diet. It has been demonstrated[64] that rarefaction of bone is normally progressive from about age 20 onward, although the rate of progress increases with advancing years. In postmenopausal osteoporosis, the spine and pelvic bones are chiefly involved and, in addition, the long bones are involved in severe cases, but the skull is spared. This is an aid in distinguishing the decreased density of the bones seen in hyperparathyroidism where the skull is affected early in the disease. In addition to osteoporosis there are signs of general tissue aging with thinning of the skin and fragility of the blood vessels. Affected patients may have no complaint until a compression fracture of the spine occurs following trivial trauma, after which pain is felt at the site of the fracture. About 30 per cent of the patients complain of pain in the lower thoracic and lumbar spine with perhaps some stiffness and weakness of the back, which is relieved by lying down. Physical findings are not remarkable. There may be muscle spasm, shortening of the spine and kyphosis in severe, far-advanced cases. The diagnosis is usually made by x-ray examination which shows varying degrees of rarefaction of the vertebral bodies. There may be fractured or crushed vertebrae, or biconcavity of the vertebral bodies due to expansion of the intervertebral discs (fish vertebrae) and herniation of the nucleus pulposus through end plates of these bodies. Serum calcium and phosphorus levels are normal although there may be increased calcium excretion early in the disease. There are no clear-cut differences between postmenopausal osteoporosis and senile osteoporosis (*see* Chapter 62 for details).

The administration of estrogens has been shown to induce at least a temporary positive calcium balance and to relieve the pain in some patients with postmenopausal osteoporosis.[1,33] In general the x-ray picture does not change significantly following long-term treatment. There may be some advantage to giving small doses of androgens, as well as estrogens, to patients with this type of osteoporosis.[33] A convenient form of long-acting estrogen and androgen has been developed in the form of estradiol valerate and testosterone enanthate which are effective for about one month. The usual suggested monthly intramuscular dose is 1 ml. of the combined material containing 90 mg. of testosterone enanthate and 4 mg. of estradiol valerate.[1,33] Patients with postmenopausal osteoporosis should also be advised to eat a diet high in protein, and to avoid excessive immobilization. Unquestionably, an increase in intake of calcium is indicated.[35]

Some authors have suggested that estrogen therapy may be of benefit in many rheumatic diseases arising at the time of menopause.[12] Diethylstilbestrol, a synthetic estrogen, may be effective, and is usually given orally in doses of 0.1 to 0.5 mg. daily.

PARATHYROID GLANDS

There is no known relationship between abnormal parathyroid function and arthritis, calcinosis or scleroderma. Rheumatoid arthritis has been observed in both hyper- and hypoparathyroidism. In addition the parathyroid glands have been histologically normal in patients with "chronic rheumatism."[11] Occasionally the bone lesions of hyperparathyroidism may cause bone pain and arthralgias with limitation of motion, and so may be confused with arthritis. There is no relationship between parathyroid disease and the osteoporosis of rheumatoid arthritis or of postmenopausal or senile osteoporosis.

THE PROSTATE GLAND

There is no evidence to suggest that ankylosing spondylitis is related to a disturbed production of phosphatase by the prostate, as has been suggested. In a carefully controlled study no significant deviation from normal was found in 24 patients with ankylosing spondylitis.[5]

EFFECT OF PREGNANCY

It is now well established that during pregnancy there may occur a suppression of the manifestations of a number of diseases. This effect has been noted in migraine, asthma, angioneurotic edema, primary fibrositis, intermittent hydrarthrosis, psoriatic arthritis, rheumatoid arthritis and ankylosing spondylitis. A similar suppressive effect in rheumatoid arthritis and several others of the diseases listed may occur in the course of hepatitis and jaundice. As is now well known, these suppressive effects of both pregnancy and jaundice were the basis from which Hench successfully reasoned his way to the discovery of the anti-rheumatic action of cortisone.[30]

The naturally occurring suppressions of the rheumatic and allergic diseases are of importance because they suggested a new approach to the therapy of arthritis through the use of hormones, and because a fuller understanding of the mechanisms involved may throw some light on the fundamental nature of rheumatic diseases.

Clinical Aspects of the Pregnancy Effect

In 20 of 22 cases of pregnancy occurring in young rheumatoid arthritics a notable suppression of arthritic activity was reported by Hench.[28] Luchessi[50] observed great amelioration in 14 of 18 pregnancies occurring in 8 patients, 6 of whom had peripheral rheumatoid arthritis and 2 ankylosing spondylitis. If relief has been attained in one pregnancy, subsequent pregnancies generally, but not always, cause similar relief. Occasionally arthritis may undergo an exacerbation during pregnancy, or may even have its onset during gestation. Similar variations in the effect of pregnancy on allergy are observed.

Relief of arthritic pain may begin as

early as the end of the first month of gestation but in some cases does not appear until the last trimester. In general the character of the relief is similar to that obtained from ACTH and cortisone with varying degrees of lessening of pain, swelling, and stiffness, recovery of joint and muscle function and an increase in feeling of well-being. The average duration of relief in Hench's series was 9.4 months, relapse generally occurring in the first month after delivery although in rare instances persisting for several months. The return of symptoms may be insidious or sudden and bears no constant relationship to the return of menstruation or the termination of lactation.

Mechanism of the Pregnancy Effect

Although the mechanism of the beneficial effect of pregnancy on the rheumatic diseases is not entirely solved, it now appears that elevated plasma 17-hydroxycorticosteroid levels may account for much of this effect. Markedly increased plasma and moderately elevated urinary 17-hydroxycorticosteroid levels have been repeatedly demonstrated during pregnancy.[9,11,23,45,63,82,83] This is partially explained by studies which show that the adrenal glands are hyper-responsive to ACTH;[9,11] and that there is a decreased clearance of infused cortisol, suggesting a delayed inactivation, during pregnancy.[11] It has also been shown that the increased plasma cortisol levels of pregnancy are dependent upon a functioning adrenal cortex.[10] Furthermore, it has been demonstrated that estrogens will elevate the level of free plasma 17-hydroxycorticosteroids as a result of increased protein binding (transcorten) of hydrocortisone.[85] There are also unidentified substances of extra-adrenal origin in the plasma during pregnancy which will, by certain assay procedures, be measured as 17-hydroxycorticosteroids, but which are found not to be cortisol or one of its metabolites upon careful analysis.[10] One investigator felt that since the elevated plasma corticoid levels dropped to normal within six days after delivery, they could not account for the prolonged beneficial effects of pregnancy on rheumatoid arthritis.[23] However, other studies indicate that, although the elevated plasma corticoid levels tend to fall after delivery, they may remain elevated in many patients for as long as six to nine weeks postpartum, and therefore could account for the beneficial effect of pregnancy on arthritis.[63]

It is clear, however, that the effect of estrogens alone on plasma cortisol levels cannot explain the beneficial effects of pregnancy on arthritis, as numerous attempts at therapy with estrogens have not been universally successful.

Several other possible mechanisms of the pregnancy effect have been investigated as noted below:

1. *The Fetal Adrenals.*—These are not developed until the third month of gestation at which time the cortex is made up of a temporary structure, presumably representing the innermost zone, which in adults is believed to be the source of androgenic steroids, and which involutes rapidly after birth. Since the pregnancy effect may begin before this fetal adrenal cortex is histologically identifiable, it seems unlikely to be the source of the antirheumatic factor. The favorable effect on rheumatoid arthritis (as yet unconfirmed) of injections of umbilical cord serum[81] does not prove that the effective factor is of fetal adrenal origin.

2. *The Corpus Luteum.*—Progesterone from the corpus luteum is secreted very early in pregnancy and could therefore theoretically be a factor in the antirheumatic effect noted in the first few weeks of gestation. Attempts to reproduce the pregnancy effect by intramuscular administration of progesterone[44,47,60,84] must on the whole be regarded as unsuccessful. Nevertheless, there is some evidence of a suppressive effect even though this is erratic and unpredictable. One may conclude that, although progesterone may be a contributing factor

to the pregnancy effect, it is certainly not the main or only factor. Sommerville *et al.*[75] noted that patients suffering from rheumatoid arthritis excrete an abnormally high proportion (19 to 36 per cent) of parenterally injected progesterone. They suggest that this indicates that there is an abnormal metabolism of steroids in the disease.

3. *Relaxin.*—Relaxin is an ovarian hormone, probably secreted by the corpus luteum, which has a relaxing effect on the sacroiliac ligaments and symphysis pubis. Relaxin extracted from the ovaries of pregnant sows has been administered by Lansbury[48] to one case of typical ankylosing spondylitis and one case of typical peripheral rheumatoid arthritis. The patients were "primed" by 5 mgm. of estrone intramuscularly for three days and then given relaxin, 1 mg. hypodermically every six hours for nine successive days. No change, beyond the expected variations of the disease, was observed.[48]

4. *The Placenta.*—The placenta produces numerous substances any one of which, or any group of which, might conceivably be the factor causing suppression of rheumatic activity. Theoretically this action might be a direct one on the tissues of the mother, or it might be indirect through an influence on the mother's adrenal cortex, pituitary or other glands. Both adrenal cortex and anterior pituitary glands are known to undergo hypertrophy during pregnancy. Attempts to identify the anti-rheumatic placental factor are briefly noted below.

Placental Adrenocorticotropins.—Jailer and Knowlton[39] found adrenocorticotropic activity in acetone-dried human placentas which was not destroyed by boiling—a procedure which does destroy gonadotropic and posterior pituitary hormones. Tarantino[80] identified a corticotropic substance in the chorion but not in the decidua of bovine placentas. Opsahl, Long and Fry[54] demonstrated a hyaluronidase-inhibiting substance in the urine of pregnant women which was apparently distinct from chorionic gonadotropin, and later, Opsahl and Long[55] obtained fractions from fresh placental tissue with corticotropic activity comparable to that of commercial preparations of ACTH.

Chorionic Gonadotropins.—Opsahl, Long and Fry[54] found corticotropic activity in chorionic gonadotropins prepared from the urine of pregnant women (presumed to be of placental origin). The activity remained after destroying the gonadotropic activity by heat thus indicating that corticotropic and gonadotropic factors are separate entities. It appears that gonadotropins per se have no corticotropic action.[31] Attempts to treat rheumatoid arthritis with gonadotropin, which will be discussed later, confirm their lack of anti-rheumatic activity.

Placental Steroids.—The status of progesterone has already been discussed under the heading of the Corpus Luteum. Salhanick *et al.*[67] have recently isolated progesterone from the human placenta, thus confirming previous beliefs as to its presence there. Johnson and Haines[41] have demonstrated adrenal corticoid activity in the human placenta (as judged by glycogen deposition) in concentrations equivalent to 0.29 mg. of hydrocortisone per kilogram.

Commercial estrogens from various sources, placental or otherwise, have long since been discounted as effective anti-arthritic agents. Dobriner[15] noted a tremendous excretion in pregnancy of *pregnanolone* and *pregnanediol*, which are metabolites of progesterone, and a great increase in estrogens. Also he found a pronounced decrease in the excretion of *androsterone*, *11-hydroxyandrosterone* and of *etiocholanolone*.

Altered Serum Constituents in Pregnancy

Pregnancy is associated with widespread bodily changes. Among these, alterations in blood lipids, proteins and amino acids have been studied in a search for the mechanism whereby pregnancy suppresses rheumatic activity.

During gestation there is a marked increase in plasma neutral fat and later on in cholesterol and phospholipids. This occurs equally during pregnancy in normal and rheumatoid women.[4] In postpartum plasma the cholesterol content is low.[26] Serum lipolecithin is unchanged in normals, in jaundice, in pregnancy and in rheumatoid arthritis.[35] The blood of rheumatoid arthritics is not deficient in serum lipids, phospholipids or cholesterol.[60] Various serum lipids are increased during ACTH and cortisone administration. This elevation occurs gradually and is preceded by the anti-rheumatic effect.

Although changes in serum lipids occur during the anti-rheumatic effect of jaundice, pregnancy and cortisone or ACTH administration, the relationship between these lipid changes and the anti-rheumatic effect, if any, is at present unknown.

During normal gestation there is a general lowering of total serum proteins due to steadily increasing hydremia; there is also a relative decrease in albumin, an increase of alpha and especially beta globulin but no change in gamma globulins.[53] Borden *et al.*[6] found similar alterations in amino-acid metabolism in cases of rheumatoid arthritis during remissions caused by pregnancy, jaundice, and ACTH or cortisone administration. The fibrinogen is increased despite the lowering of the total serum proteins. Granirer[25] has reported an average total plasma protein of 4.35 gm. per cent with albumin 2.15 per cent and globulin 2.2 per cent (A/G ratio 0.9) in postpartum plasma used by him as an anti-rheumatic agent. It would therefore seem that any virtue which may exist in the proteins of pregnancy blood is unlikely to be due to its albumin content. Brown *et al.*[8] have reported a striking but temporary benefit from intravenous administration of small amounts of human serum albumin in typical rheumatoid arthritis.

Reviewing all of the above studies, we must conclude that the mechanism producing the ameliorating effect of pregnancy is probably related in some manner to the increased plasma 17-hydroxycorticosteroid level. The increased responsiveness of the adrenal cortex may be related to continued stimulation by placental corticotropins. Just how long the adrenal cortex remains in a state of increased responsiveness to the action of corticotropin is unknown but it may be on an individual basis. This factor may offer some explanation of the finding of elevated plasma levels of 17-hydroxycorticoids in postpartum patients for varying lengths of time. It is entirely possible, however, that in addition to the increased plasma corticoids other factors may also play a role in the pregnancy effect.

THERAPEUTIC ATTEMPTS WITH PREGNANCY PRODUCTS

Attempts to reproduce the pregnancy effect in the management of arthritis by transfusions of pregnancy blood, postpartum pregnancy plasma, umbilical cord blood, progesterone, relaxin, immune placental globulins, chorionic gonadotropins, various estrogens and placental corticotropins have so far *failed to prove these agents as an established treatment of rheumatoid arthritis* despite the fact that a small degree of antirheumatic activity is demonstrated by several of them. The adrenal corticoids reproduce the effect of pregnancy on rheumatoid arthritis more closely than any other compounds which have been studied thus far.

ADVISABILITY OF PREGNANCY IN THE ARTHRITIC

This is a decision of the greatest importance which requires wise and mature clinical judgment in which the total life situation of the patient and her husband, their emotional needs, their financial resources and an accurate appraisal of the activity, extent and prognosis of the arthritis must all be carefully weighed. The possible harmful effects on the fetus of steroids and other substances used in the treatment of rheumatoid arthritis should also be carefully considered in a decision concerning the advisability of pregnancy.

If the disease is active or far advanced so that the patient has difficulty in caring for herself and her house, obviously a pregnancy could be considered only if the patient has the full-time services of a nurse and a maid, or members of the family who can really be counted on to perform these functions. If the disease is mild with little functional impairment, pregnancy may be advised since, of itself, it seldom aggravates arthritis. The main problem is, then, the postpartum relapse which occurs at a time when the care of the baby plus the regular household duties constitute an increase in total stress which often precipitates a serious and sometimes permanent worsening of the disease.

THE AMELIORATING EFFECT OF JAUNDICE

As already mentioned, spontaneous jaundice may cause a remission in rheumatoid arthritis and periarticular fibrositis. This effect was first carefully studied and its importance realized by Hench.[28] He also observed relief of pain in psoriatic arthritis, osteoarthritis and intrapelvic protrusion of the hips, but the pain of gout, neuralgia and neuritis was not benefited, perhaps because the degree of jaundice was too slight. (Remissions in hay fever and migraine have also occurred during spontaneous jaundice but these effects have not been intensively studied.) It would thus seem that the jaundice effect is of a general nature and not specific for rheumatoid arthritis. Almost any kind of obstructive or intrahepatic jaundice can produce the effect, but hemolytic jaundice apparently does not do so.

The anti-rheumatic action of jaundice appears to be constant if the jaundice is sufficient to cause a serum bilirubin of 8 to 10 mg. per cent, although milder degrees may also produce the effect.

Character of the Remission

Suppression of arthritic manifestations usually occurs by the time jaundice is noted and possibly earlier. The duration of the remission is not directly related to the depth and duration of jaundice in all cases. In contrast to the rapid relapse of arthritis after pregnancy, a remission due to jaundice may persist for several months, and in exceptional instances for two or three years. In a few cases, the disease has recurred in a milder form.

The Mechanism of Action

Careful studies of the metabolism of corticoids in patients with liver disease have revealed subnormal levels of conjugated 17-hydroxycorticosteroids in the plasma,[5] and a delay in the removal of cortisol but not of tetrahydrocortisol from the plasma.[7,19] Thus, the apparent impairment of 17-hydroxycorticosteroid conjugation in patients with liver disease was not observed following the infusion of tetrahydrocortisol. It appears, therefore, that there is no detectable impairment of glucuronide conjugation, provided the proper substrate for conjugation is supplied. The delay is in the enzymatic transformation of cortisol to reduced 17-hydroxycorticosteroids, which are then readily conjugated.[19] As the non-reduced hormones are active biologically, whereas the reduced forms are inactive, it is possible that this might explain, in part, the anti-rheumatic effect of liver disease. Studies of liver function in patients with rheumatoid arthritis have been normal or inconclusive. Thus far, none of the bile constituents have been found to be responsible for the anti-rheumatic effect of jaundice.

Attempts to Reproduce the Jaundice Phenomenon

Efforts at therapy by reproducing the jaundice effect fall into two main categories; first, the administration of bile products. These include bile salts, both natural and synthetic, diluted ox bile and human bile, blood transfusions from jaundiced patients, and a combination of bile salts and bilirubin. *None of these ingenious attempts has produced a satisfactory treatment* or indeed any serious claim to any anti-rheumatic effect.

In the second category are attempts to reproduce the anti-rheumatic effect by hepatotoxic agents. Synthetic compounds such as toluylene diamine and also lactophenin are capable of being administered in doses sufficient to cause a moderate hepatitis and jaundice with some anti-rheumatic effect but are potentially dangerous and have never come into practical use. Good remissions have been produced by infecting rheumatoid patients with the secretions of patients with infectious hepatitis. MacCallum *et al.*[22,52] produced hepatitis in about 10 per cent of inoculated volunteers and noted a satisfactory remission, averaging about forty days, in 25 of 32 of these patients. The method, however, cannot be recommended because of its inherent danger and because it can at best produce a temporary remission (*see also* Chapter 46).

BIBLIOGRAPHY

1. Albright, F. and Reifenstein, E. C.: *The Parathyroid Glands and Metabolic Bone Disease*, Baltimore, The Williams & Wilkins Co., 1948.
2. Asboe-Hansen, G.: Amer. J. Med., *26*, 470, 1959.
3. Barker, B. L. and Abrams, G. D.: Ann. Rev. Physiol., *17*, 61, 1955.
4. Bayles, T. B. and Riddell, C. B.: Amer. J. Med. Sci., *208*, 343, 1944.
5. Bongiovanni, A. M., Eberlein, W. R., Grumbach, M. M. and Van Wyk, J. J.: Proc. Soc. Exper. Biol. & Med., *87*, 282, 1954.
6. Borden, A. L. *et al.*: J. Clin. Invest., *31*, 375, 1952.
7. Brown, H., Willardson, D. G., Samuels, L. T. and Tyler, F. H.: J. Clin. Invest., *33*, 1524, 1954.
8. Brown, T. McP., Wichelhausen, R. H., Merchant, W. R. and Robinson, L. B.: Amer. J. Med. Sci., *221*, 618, 1951.
9. Christy, N. P., Wallace, E. Z. and Jailer, J. W.: J. Clin. Invest., *34*, 899, 1955.
10. Christy, N. P. and Jailer, J. W.: J. Clin. Endocrinol. & Metab., *19*, 263, 1959.
11. Cohen, M., Stiefel, M., Reddy, W. J. and Laidlaw, J. C.: J. Clin. Endocrinol. & Metab., *18*, 1076, 1958.
12. Cushing, E. H.: Internat. Clin., *2*, 200, 1937.
13. Desmarais, M. H. L.: Ann. Rheum. Dis., *7*, 105, 1948.
14. Denis, R.: Ann. Endocrinol., *12*, 451, 1951.
15. Dobriner, K.: Bull. Rheum. Dis., *2*, 3, 1951.
16. Dobriner, K.: in *Symposium on Steroids*, Philadelphia, The Blakiston Co., 130, 1951.
17. Dresner, E.: J. Chron. Dis., *5*, 612, 1959.
18. Edström, G. and Thune, S.: Ann. Rheum. Dis., *10*, 163, 1951.
19. Englert, E., Jr., Brown, H., Wallach, S. and Simons, E. L.: J. Clin. Endocrinol. & Metab., *17*, 1395, 1957.
20. Fletcher, E.: *Medical Disorders of the Locomotor System Including the Rheumatic Diseases*, Baltimore, The Williams and Wilkins Co., 1947.
21. Freyberg, R. H..: J.A.M.A., *119*, 1165, 1942.
22. Gardner, F., Stewart, A. and MacCallum, F. O.: Brit. Med. J., *2*, 677, 1945.
23. Gemzell, C. A.: J. Clin. Endocrinol. & Metab., *12*, 519, 1952.
24. Gerarde, H. W. and Jones, M.: J. Biol. Chem., *201*, 553, 1953.
25. Granirer, L. W.: Science, *111*, 204, 1950.
26. Granirer, L. W.: Surg., Gynec. & Obst., *91*, 591, 1950.
27. Haydu, G. G. and Haydu, B. W.: Amer. J. Med. Sci., *223*, 1, 1952.
28. Hench, P. S.: Proc. Staff Meet. Mayo Clin., *13*, 161, 1938.
29. Hench, P. S., Kendall, E. C., Slocumb, C. H. and Polley, H. F.: Proc. Staff Meet. Mayo Clin., *24*, 181, 1949.
30. Hench, P. S., Kendall, E. C., Slocumb, C. H. and Polley, H. F.: Ann. Rheum. Dis., *8*, 97, 1949.
31. Hibbett, L. L., Starnes, W. R. and Hill, S. R., Jr.: J. Clin. Endocrinol. & Metab., *18*, 1315, 1958.
32. Hill, S. R., Jr., Holley, H. L., Ulloa, A., Starnes, W. R. and McNeil, J. H.: Arth. & Rheum., *2*, 114, 1959.
33. Hill, S. R., Jr., Reiss, R. S., Forsham, P. H. and Thorn, G. W.: J. Clin. Endocrinol. & Metab., *10*, 1375, 1950.
34. Hill, S. R., Jr., and Dempsey, H.: in *Inflammation and Diseases of Connective Tissue*, Mills, L. C. and Moyer, J. H., Eds., Philadelphia, W. B. Saunders Co., 1961, pp. 529–538.
35. Hill, S. R., Jr., Ulloa, A., Starnes, W. R. and Holley, H. L.: Arch. Intern. Med., *112*, 603, 1963.

36. Hughes, E. R., Ely, R. S. and Kelley, V. C.: Amer. J. Dis. Children, *104*, 610, 1962.
37. Ingle, D. J.: Acta Endocrinol., *17*, 172, 1954.
38. Iverson, K.: in *Connective Tissue in Health and Disease*, Asboe-Hansen, G., Ed., Copenhagen, Munksgaard, 1954, p. 130.
39. Jailer, J. W. and Knowlton, A. I.: J. Clin. Invest., *29*, 1430, 1950.
40. Jasmin, G. and Bois, P.: Endocrinol., *65*, 494, 1959.
41. Johnson, R. H. and Haines, W. J.: Science, *116*, 456, 1952.
42. Kelley, V. C. and Ely, R. S.: Ann. N.Y. Acad. Sci., *86*, 1115, 1960.
43. Kelley, V. C.: in *Inflammation and Disease of Connective Tissue*, Mills, L. C. and Moyer, J. H., Eds., Philadelphia, W. B. Saunders Co., 1961, pp. 575–580.
44. Kling, D. H.: Ann. West. Med. & Surg., *4*, 378, 1950.
45. Knowlton, A. I., Mudge, G. H. and Jailer, J. W.: J. Clin. Endocrinol., *9*, 514, 1949.
46. Kuzell, W. C. and Davison, R. A.: J. Lab. & Clin. Med., *31*, 1223, 1946.
47. Kyle, L. H. and Crain, D. C.: Ann. Intern. Med., *32*, 878, 1950.
48. Lansbury, J.: Unpublished data.
49. Lowe, J. A. I.: Ann. Rheum. Dis., *13*, 250, 1954.
50. Luchessi, O.Y.M.: El Dia Medico, *18*, 333, 1946.
51. Marie, P.: Rev. de Med., *6*, 297, 1886.
52. MacCallum, F. O. and Bradley, W. H.: Lancet, *2*, 228, 1944.
53. Moore, D. H., Martin, DuP. R. and Buxton, C. L.: Amer. J. Obst. & Gynec., *57*, 312, 1949.
54. Opsahl, J. C., Long, C. N. H. and Fry, E. G.: Yale J. Biol. & Med., *23*, 399, 1951.
55. Opsahl, J. C. and Long, C. N. H.: Yale J. Biol. & Med., *24*, 199, 1951.
56. Osgood, R. B.: Amer. J. Med. Sci., *200*, 429, 1940.
57. Peterson, R. E., Wyngaarden, J. B., Guerra, S. L., Brodie, B. B. and Bunim, J. J.: J. Clin. Invest., *34*, 1779, 1955.
58. Pirani, C. L., Stepto, R. C. and Sutherland, K.: J. Exper. Med., *93*, 217, 1951.
59. Ragan, C., Holmes, E. L., Plotz, C. M., Meyer, K., Blunt, J. W. and Lattes, R.: Bull. N.Y. Acad. Med., *26*, 251, 1950.
60. Reich, N. E.: Amer. Practitioner, *4*, 1, 1949.
61. Reifenstein, E. C., Jr. and Howard, R. P.: Metabolism, *7*, 364, 1958.
62. Reinhart, W. O. and Li, C. H.: Science, *117*, 295, 1953.
63. Robinson, H. J., Bernhard, W. G. *et al.*: J. Clin. Endocrinol. & Metab., *15*, 317, 1955.
64. Rose, A. R.: Clin. Orthoped., *55*, 17, 1967.
65. Rynearson, E. H. and Sacasa, C. F.: Proc. Staff Meet. Mayo Clin., *16*, 353, 1941.
66. Salgado, E.: Ann. Rheum. Dis., *14*, 73, 1955.
67. Salhanick, H. A., Noall, M. W., Zarrow, M. X. and Samuels, L. T.: Science, *115*, 708, 1952.
68. Scow, R. O.: Endocrinology, *49*, 641, 1951.
69. Selye, H.: *Stress. The Physiology and Pathology of Exposure to Stress.* Montreal, Acta, Inc., 1950.
70. Selye, H.: Amer. J. Med., *10*, 549, 1951.
71. Selye, H.: *The Story of the Adaptation Syndrome*, Montreal, Acta, Inc., 1952.
72. Selye, H., Horava, A. and Heuser, G.: *Annual Reports on Stress*, 1st-5th, Montreal, Acta, Inc., 1952.
73. Selye, H. and Bajusz, E.: Acta Endocrinol., *30*, 183, 1959.
74. Selye, H. and Bajusz, E.: in *Arthritis and Allied Conditions*, 7th ed., Hollander, J. L., Ed., Philadelphia, Lea & Febiger, 1966, pp. 618–630.
75. Sommerville, I. F., Marrian, G. E., Duthie, J. J. R. and Sinclair, R. J.: Lancet, *1*, 116, 1950.
76. Taubenhaus, M. and Amromin, G. D.: J. Lab. & Clin. Med., *36*, 7, 1950.
77. Taubenhaus, M., Taylor, B. and Morton, J. V.: Endocrinology, *51*, 183, 1952.
78. Thomas, H. M., Jr.: Arch. Intern. Med., *51*, 571, 1938.
79. Thorn, G. W., Bayles, T. B., Massel, B. F., Forsham, P. H., Hill, S. R., Jr., Smith, S. and Warren, J. E.: New Engl. J. Med., *241*, 529, 1949.
80. Torantino, C.: Folia Endocrinol., *4*, 197, 1951.
81. Tufts, M., Pessin, S. B. and Greenwalt, T.: Staff Meet., St. Mary's Hosp., Milwaukee, Wis., 1950.
82. Venning, E. H.: Endocrinology, *39*, 203, 1946.
83. Venning, E. H., Dyrenfurth, I., Lowenstein, L. and Beck, J.: J. Clin. Endocrinol. & Metab., *19*, 403, 1959.
84. Vignos, P. T., Jr. and Dorfman, R. I.: Amer. J. Med. Sci., *222*, 29, 1951.
85. Wallace, E. Z. and Carter, A. C.: Unpublished data.

Chapter 17

Corticotropin and Corticosteroids: Chemistry, Physiology and Metabolic Effects

By Clifton K. Meador, M.D., and S. Richardson Hill, M.D.

Revised by Howard L. Holley, M.D.

An impressive body of scientific knowledge has been acquired during the first two decades of the corticosteroid era in clinical medicine. As in many scientific ventures, these advances have been brought about through the coordinated efforts and imagination of many investigators in organic chemistry, biochemistry, physiology and clinical investigation. The benefits of the modern union of fundamental sciences with bedside medicine are nowhere better illustrated than in the advances brought about in the corticosteroid field.

This new knowledge has given us a clearer insight into the mechanisms that regulate corticotropin secretion, the pathways of biosynthesis of the major active endogenous adrenocortical hormones, the exquisite relationship between molecular structure and biological activity of the synthetic corticosteroids, the physiologic disposition and metabolic fate of these compounds and factors which regulate the form and rate of excretion of these hormones. A considerable amount of information is available concerning the effects of these corticosteroids on carbohydrate, protein and electrolyte metabolism, and on processes of tissue reaction to injury and host defense. These advances will be reviewed briefly in this chapter.

CORTICOTROPIN

Regulation of Secretion

Corticotropin (ACTH) is secreted by the adenohypophysis (pituitary) and its secretion is regulated by the hypothalamus. The hypothalamus has extensive anatomic connections with the cerebral cortex, temporal lobe ganglia, thalamus, midbrain and the sensory afferent pathways. The neurophysiological function of these connections, however, is not precisely known. The special anatomical arrangement of a portal system arising from a network of capillaries in the hypothalamus provides an intimate vascular connection between the median eminence and the adenohypophysis. It was such anatomical observations of Harris which laid the foundation to the theory of the neurohumoral control of the hypothalamus over the anterior pituitary.[12]

Nuclei in or near the median eminence of the hypothalamus elaborate a neurohumoral substance(s) called *corticotropin releasing factor* (CRF), which is carried by the portal system to the anterior pituitary where it acts specifically to release ACTH. The exact chemical nature of CRF has not been precisely elucidated nor has any general agreement been reached as to whether or not there is only one specific CRF.[31] There is evidence for the existence of several polypeptides in hypothalamic tissue which possess CRF activity. Furthermore, the problem of biologic specificity is complicated by the finding of polypeptides of hypothalamic origin which have direct ACTH activity in hypophysectomized animals or which may themselves serve as biosynthetic precursors of ACTH. An amino acid analysis of the most potent CRF (designated Beta CRF) reveals that it contains all of the amino acids of lysine vasopressin plus serine and histidine. A provisional amino acid sequence of Beta CRF reveals the N-terminus of Alpha-MSH and the C-terminus of lysine vasopressin.[31] The finding of many pharmacologically active compounds in hypothalamic extracts is indeed exciting. The continued investigative focus on that part of the diencephalon hopefully will lead to a coherent pattern of the neurohumoral control of the adenohypophysis in the near future.

ACTH secretion, although mediated ultimately by the hypothalamus, occurs as a consequence of stimulatory and inhibitory stimuli arising from afferent CNS pathways and similar stimuli which arise from the well-known negative feedback relationship between ACTH secretion and the level of plasma cortisol (hydrocortisone). Kendall identified the locus of the steroid feedback receptor as being distant from the anterior pituitary and direct microimplantations of steroids into the hypothalamus will inhibit ACTH secretion.[5a,16] The precise role of the servomechanism in regulating endogenous ACTH secretion is not clear. Under certain conditions a negative feedback relationship cannot be demonstrated. For example, with severe surgical stress in man, the restraining action of circulating cortisol, even with infusions of very large doses of cortisol, is no longer effective in suppressing ACTH output and ACTH secretion occurs regardless of the degree of elevation of plasma cortisol.[7] Perhaps under less stressful physiologic conditions the servomechanism serves as a modulator or restrainer of basal ACTH secretion.

Physiological Effects

The major physiological activity of ACTH is stimulation of the cells of the adrenal cortex to synthesize and secrete adrenocortical steroids into the circulation. A variety of extra-adrenal actions of ACTH have been described; however, the exact physiologic significance of these actions is yet to be determined.[6] The suggestion by Engel that tropic hormones act in a common fashion by stimulating general "growth and energy metabolism" is indeed intriguing. In such a scheme, specificity of tropic hormones would relate to their high affinity for their target glands and to the unique functional capacity of each tissue (hormone synthesis and secretion) rather than to each tropic hormone's unique mechanism of action.[6]

A great variety of adrenocortical steroids are secreted in response to ACTH stimulation. The physiologic activity of these steroids is also quite varied and for many is either nil or not yet identified. While it is true that androgens, estrogens and mineralocorticoids are all secreted by the adrenal cortex, cortisol is the major biologically active steroid released in response to ACTH and its effects predominate. Clinically, the results from administration of corticotropin are in most respects similar to those produced by cortisol alone.

Chemical Structure

ACTH was first isolated from the adenohypophysis in 1943 by Li and Sayers.[17,30] The past twenty years have seen the identification of the molecular weight, characterization of the amino acid composition and sequence, and finally the successful synthesis of polypeptides with full ACTH activity by Li and by Hofman.[13,18] Native pituitary ACTH is a polypeptide with 39 amino acids containing N-terminal serine and C-terminal phenylalanine and has a biologic activity of 400 international units per mg.

Direct Measurements of Plasma ACTH

Preparations of ACTH vary in potency, mg. for mg., so that all preparations must be subjected to bioassay. The U.S.P. assay is based on adrenal ascorbic acid depletion in the hypophysectomized rat. One U.S.P. unit is the biological activity present in 1 mg. of the U.S.P. standard.

A sensitive and specific bioassay based on adrenal vein steroid secretion in the hypophysectomized rat combined with plasma extraction techniques allowed more precise studies of ACTH secretion and regulation in man.[20] Direct assays of plasma ACTH levels have provided a clearer insight into pituitary-adrenal dynamics. The normal plasma ACTH level in man at 6 A.M. is 0.25 (range 0.1 to 0.59) milliunits per 100 ml. plasma and is 0.11 (range 0.04 to 0.25) milliunits per 100 ml. plasma at 6 P.M.[22] This diurnal variation in plasma ACTH is not merely a reflection of the diurnal pattern of plasma cortisol, since diurnal decreases in plasma ACTH levels are still demonstrable in the Addisonian patient receiving constant infusions of physiologic amounts of exogenous cortisol.[10] The circadian rhythm of the pituitary-adrenal

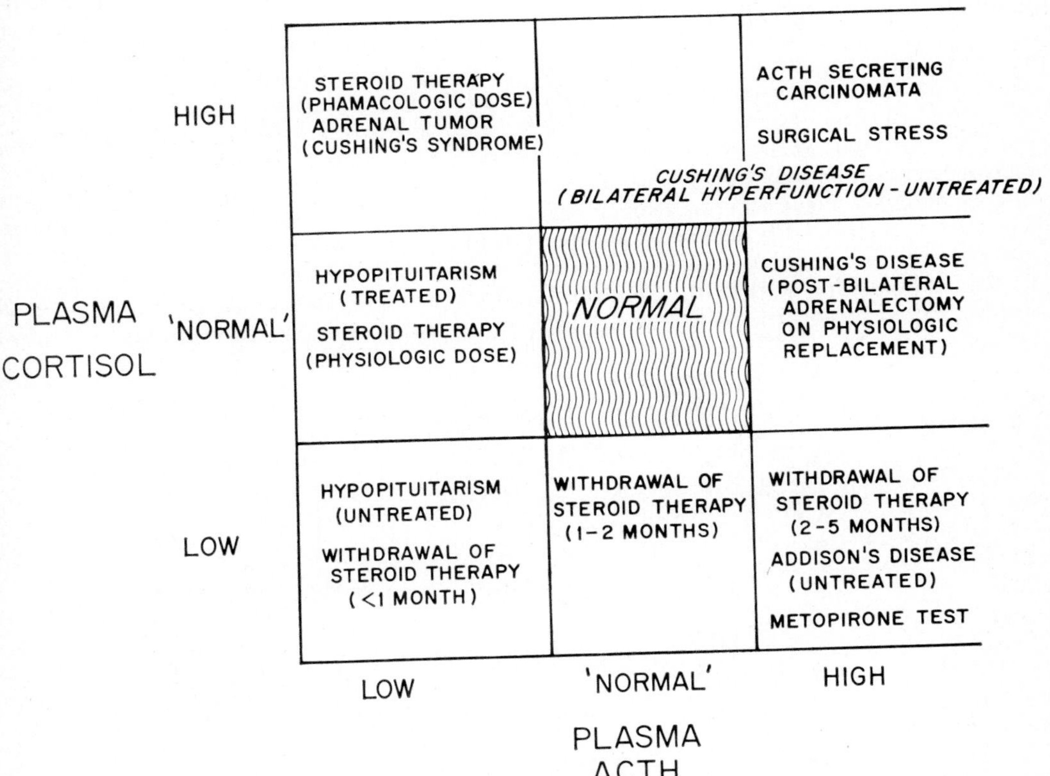

Fig. 17–1.—Schematic relationship of plasma cortisol to plasma ACTH. The range of "normal" relates to values obtained in normal individuals between 6 A.M. and 8 A.M. For purposes of emphasis, only typical relationships are shown; overlapping values have been omitted. Note the rising ACTH values with continued low plasma cortisol levels following withdrawal of steroid therapy (bottom row and see text).

axis then resides either in the pituitary gland itself or more likely in the central nervous system. Direct bioassays of ACTH in human plasma have confirmed the previously mentioned negative feedback relationship between plasma cortisol levels and ACTH secretion—an observation made as early as 1938 by Ingle using less refined methods.[14] Assays of plasma ACTH levels under stress or with graded intravenous infusions of ACTH suggest that a level of about 3 milliunits per 100 ml. plasma is sufficient to invoke maximal adrenocortical response.[22] It has been estimated that the anterior pituitary secretes less than 1.0 unit per day in normal man.[5] Disappearance studies in humans indicate that plasma ACTH is rapidly inactivated with an estimated plasma half-life of ten minutes.

Plasma ACTH levels can be interpreted to be high, low or normal only when they are viewed simultaneously with the plasma cortisol level. For example, an ACTH level which would ordinarily be normal, but which exists with an elevated plasma cortisol level, indicates disordered homeostasis; such a combination has been observed preoperatively in Cushing's disease (bilateral adrenocortical hyperfunction). In actual fact, the "normal" ACTH level under such conditions is high since one would ordinarily expect to find undetectable ACTH levels when plasma cortisol is elevated. An ACTH level therefore which is high, low or "normal" must be evaluated in terms of whether the simultaneously determined cortisol level is high, low or normal. Figure 17–1 depicts such relationships under a variety of conditions.[7,10,11,20]

CORTICOSTEROIDS

Major Adrenocortical Hormones

Four major groups of steroids are secreted by the adrenal cortex and possess glucocorticoid, mineralocorticoid, androgenic or estrogenic activity. For the purposes of this chapter, only the steroids with mineralocorticoid and/or glucocorticoid activity will be discussed. Cortisol (hydrocortisone or Compound F), corticosterone (Compound B) and aldosterone are now established as the three major adrenocortical hormones of biological importance secreted by the adrenal cortex. Cortisol exerts principally glucocorticoid effects and aldosterone principally mineralocorticoid effects. Three

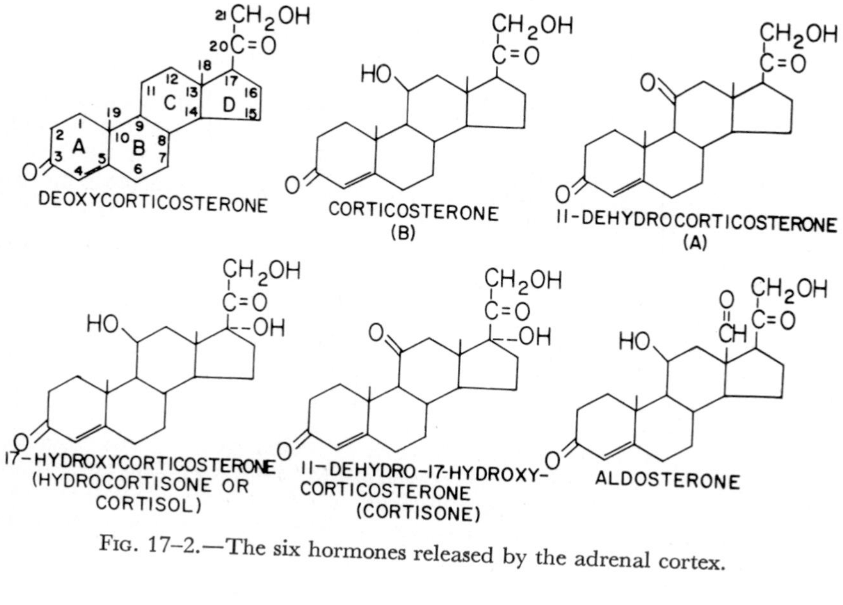

DEOXYCORTICOSTERONE
CORTICOSTERONE (B)
11-DEHYDROCORTICOSTERONE (A)
17-HYDROXYCORTICOSTERONE (HYDROCORTISONE OR CORTISOL)
11-DEHYDRO-17-HYDROXY-CORTICOSTERONE (CORTISONE)
ALDOSTERONE

FIG. 17–2.—The six hormones released by the adrenal cortex.

minor endogenous corticosteroids that exhibit physiological activity are deoxycorticosterone, 11-dehydrocorticosterone (Compound A), and cortisone (Compound E), (Fig. 17–2). In all, more than 46 crystalline steroids have been isolated from the adrenal cortex but many are intermediates and most do not possess biological activity.

In man, the adrenal cortex normally secretes, in twenty-four hours, 10 to 30 mg. of cortisol, 2 to 4 mg. of corticosterone and 50 to 200 micrograms of aldosterone. In humans, adrenal venous blood concentration of cortisol is about 240 micrograms and of corticosterone is about 80 micrograms per 100 ml. of blood.[25] The diurnal variation in the rate of cortisol secretion is parallel to the diurnal variation in ACTH secretion. Maximal values are achieved between 6 and 9 A.M., when the average plasma (arm vein) concentration of cortisol is 13.3 micrograms per 100 ml. (range = 6–25).[26] The secretory rate slowly declines and reaches minimal values between midnight and 4 A.M.[26] Upon maximal stimulation by exogenous corticotropin, endogenous secretion of cortisol increases seven- to ten-fold.

Chemical Structure—Biologic Function Relationships

All six biologically active corticosteroids (Fig. 17–2) consist of a four-ring phenanthrene nucleus (rings, A, B, C, and D), ketone radicals at C-3 and C-20, a double-bond between C-4 and C-5 and a two carbon side chain (C-20 and C-21) attached to C-17.

Steroids referred to as "glucocorticoids" or which act as anti-inflammatory agents may also possess slight mineralocorticoid activity; however, the effects on organic metabolism predominate. All of the steroids which have been demonstrated to affect organic metabolism and inhibit inflammation possess the basic structure of Δ^4-pregnene-11βol-3,20-dione and *two* or more additional components (Fig. 17–3*A*). Enhancement of this activity is achieved by the addition of the following components: Δ^1, 9α-halogen, 16-methyl, 17α-hydroxyl, and 21-hydroxyl. Attenuation of organic effects is achieved by the presence of Δ^6, 14α-hydroxyl, and 16α-hydroxyl components.[19]

Corticosteroids which principally affect mineral (sodium and potassium)

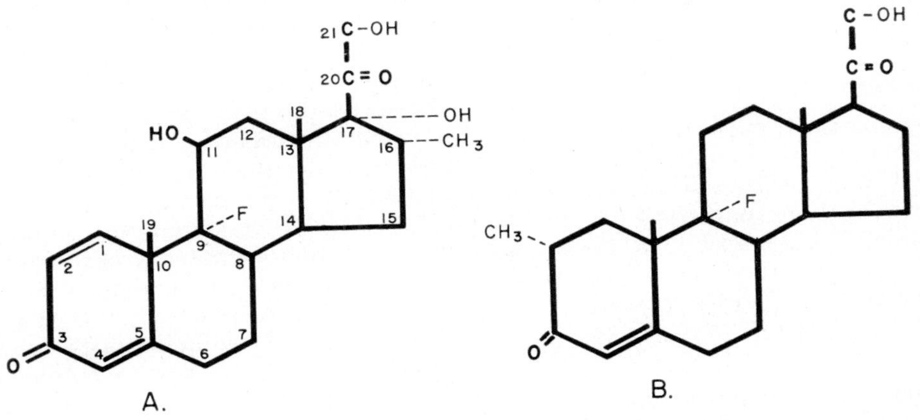

A. Δ^4-Pregnene-11β-ol-3,20-dione

B. Δ^4-Pregnene-3,20-dione

FIG. 17–3.—Structural formulas basic to the biologic activity of (*A*) anti-inflammatory steroids and (*B*) mineralocorticoids are drawn in bold lines. Components which potentiate activity are represented by lighter lines. Two or more additional substituents are required for biologic activity of *A* and one or more for biologic activity of *B*.

metabolism have had the basic structure Δ^4-pregnene-3,20-dione and *one* or more potentiating substituents (Fig. 17–3*B*). Electrolyte-regulating activity is enhanced by the presence of the following structural components: 2α-methyl (if 11β-hydroxyl is present), 9α-halogen, and 21-hydroxyl. Mineralocorticoid activity is attenuated by the presence of 16α-hydroxyl, 16-methyl and 17α-hydroxyl components.[19]

Conversion of Cortisone to Cortisol

There is abundant experimental evidence that cortisone is converted to cortisol by the liver. Exogenous cortisone administered orally or intramuscularly is rapidly metabolized to cortisol. It is quite likely that most, if not all, of the physiologic activity of administered cortisone could be accounted for by that fraction that is transformed to cortisol. This phenomenon probably explains why cortisol is about 1.25 times more potent than cortisone as an anti-inflammatory agent. Cortisone esters injected into inflamed joints produce no improvement, whereas cortisol esters are quite effective. This is because synovial tissues are unable to convert cortisone to cortisol.[27]

Biosynthesis

Adrenocortical steroids may be synthesized *in vivo* from either cholesterol or acetate. It is believed that one of the major biosynthetic pathways for cortisol is as follows: cholesterol → Δ^5-pregnenolone → progesterone → 17α-hydroxyprogesterone → 11-desoxycortisol (Compound S) → cortisol.

Absorption and Distribution

Corticosteroids are rapidly and completely absorbed from the gastrointestinal tract. For example, when a single dose of 200 mgm. of cortisol is given orally to a normal subject, maximal plasma concentration is attained in one or two hours and is about 200 μg per 100 ml.; at eight hours the level is about 25 per cent of peak value and in twelve hours the plasma concentration returns to normal.[28] With newer preparations (such as cortisol hemisuccinate), intramuscular absorption is quite rapid and the plasma levels differ very little from orally administered cortisol. Certain preparations (particularly cortisol acetate), however, are so slowly absorbed from an intramuscular injection site that little or no biologic activity is observed over a period of several days; the same preparations given orally are rapidly absorbed and quickly effective. In contrast, aldosterone is quite active biologically when administered intramuscularly but physiologically inert when given by mouth, presumably because of rapid inactivation on its initial passage through the liver.[3] Different routes of administration may well account for some of the discrepancies in biologic activity of a steroid when animal assays are compared to assays in humans.

The rate at which corticosteroids administered intravenously disappear from the plasma (biologic half-time) varies considerably from one compound to another and is appreciably altered in certain disease states (Table 17–1).[3,19,26] The rate of removal of a given steroid is governed by the rate at which it is transformed by the liver rather than the rate of urinary excretion. Less than 1 per cent of endogenous cortisol is excreted unchanged in the urine and none in the feces. It will be noted that enhanced anti-inflammatory potency of the various compounds cannot be explained entirely on the basis of the plasma half-time alone, (Table 17–1). Dexamethasone is approximately 25 to 30 times more potent than cortisol, but its rate of disappearance from the plasma as compared to cortisol is delayed only by a factor of two. Differences in distribution in body fluids, cell permeability and affinity to binding proteins are other possible factors which may govern biologic potency of the various steroids.

Table 17-1.—Biologic Half-Times (Minutes) of Plasma Steroids[3,26] and Anti-Inflammatory Potency (Cortisol as 1)[19]

	Half-Time (Min.)		
	Normal Subjects	*Cirrhosis*	*Anti-Inflammatory Potency*
Cortisone	30	35	0.8
Prednisone	60	–	3–4
Cortisol	110	300	1
Prednisolone	200	240	4
9α-Fluorocortisol	90	95	10
9α-Fluoroprednisolone	100	100	20
Dexamethasone	200	–	25–30
Aldosterone	34	63	nil

Metabolic Fate and Excretion

The chief metabolic pathway of cortisol and cortisone in man consists of reductive reactions involving ring A. These reactions occur primarily in the liver and are impaired in the presence of liver disease and hypothyroidism. First, the double bond between carbon 4 and 5 and the ketone group at carbon 3 are reduced, resulting in "tetrahydro" derivatives (four hydrogen atoms having been added).[33,34] Tetrahydrocortisol and tetrahydrocortisone, the reduced forms of cortisol and cortisone, are biologically inactive. Following reduction, the tetrahydro metabolites are conjugated with glucuronic acid, again principally in the liver.[15] Glucuronide conjugates of cortisol usually account for one-fourth to one-third of the endogenously secreted cortisol in normal individuals. Additional reduction products and conjugates (sulphates) of cortisol and cortisone are also present in urine. Alternate metabolic pathways, perhaps as 6β-hydroxylation, predominate with certain drugs or diseases and may lead to low urinary values for 17-Hydroxycorticosteroids (17 OHCS) if one examines only the urinary glucuronide conjugates.[21] Determinations of plasma 17 OHCS levels and cortisol secretion rates are often necessary to define adrenocortical function under such conditions.

Biologic Activity of Adrenocortical Steroids

There are few physiologic processes which are not influenced by corticosteroids. The search for a single fundamental mechanism of action, however, has not been successful and one must still describe effects in rather general terms. While not necessarily implying a separation in mode of action for the steroids, it is convenient to group the physiologic and clinical consequences of these hormones into four classes: (1) effects on organic metabolism; (2) effects on inorganic (mineral) metabolism; (3) effects on inflammatory processes, tissue reactivity and host defense; and (4) suppression of pituitary corticotropin secretion.

Effects on Organic Metabolism

Carbohydrate Metabolism (Table 17–2).—The effect of cortisol on carbohydrate metabolism is at least two-fold: gluconeogenesis from protein is stimulated and the action of insulin in transporting glucose across the cell membranes is opposed. In man, impairment of carbohydrate tolerance resulting from steroid administration will depend on the dosage of the compound and on the subject's capacity to increase insulin secretion when challenged with a glucose load. Presumably, the functional reserve of the islet cells of the pancreas is so abundant that almost all but the diabetic or latent diabetic can tolerate prolonged corticosteroid administration without developing glycosuria or hyperglycemia or a requirement for exogenous insulin.[9]

In fact, impairment of glucose tolerance detected during the initial days of steroid administration will disappear in most non-diabetic patients because of compensatory increase in insulin production. After prolonged administration, the beta cells may become exhausted and the glucose tolerance test again gives abnormal results.

The diabetic state due to glucocorticoid excess is usually mild and differs from diabetes mellitus in that steroid diabetes: (1) is resistant to insulin; (2) is not ketoacidosis prone; (3) is readily controllable with diet, adequate insulin dosage, or both; (4) shows evidence of greater protein loss; (5) is characterized by an increase in liver glycogen; and (6), unlike diabetes mellitus, is usually reversible.[9]

Table 17-2.—Laboratory Changes Induced by Corticosteroids

Carbohydrate Metabolism
Gluconeogenesis increased
Glycogen deposition in liver increased
Glucose tolerance reduced
Glycosuria
Protein Metabolism
Gluconeogenesis increased
Amino acid nitrogen in serum and urine increased
Uric acid excretion increased
Creatine excretion increased
Electrolyte Metabolism (variable depending on steroid used)
Renal potassium wasting
Hypokalemia
Alkalosis
Renal sodium retention
Circulating Blood Cells
Eosinophils reduced
Lymphocytes reduced
Neutrophils increased
Erythrocytes increased

Protein Metabolism (Table 17–2).—Perhaps the best-documented action of the corticosteroids is that of increasing gluconeogenesis from protein. Following cortisol administration there is a rise in serum amino acid nitrogen and a concomitant increase in urinary excretion of a number of amino acids; total urinary nitrogen excretion is increased; and if the dosage is large enough a negative nitrogen balance is produced. Concomitantly, hepatic sugar production and output may increase by a factor of 7 or 8.[35]

The clinical consequences of this protein wasting are well known. Wasting of the subcutaneous tissues and an increase in capillary fragility result in cutaneous striae and ecchymoses. Wound healing is impaired and peptic ulcers may heal with difficulty.

It is also known that corticosteroids impair linear growth in children. This effect is seen not only in children with juvenile rheumatoid arthritis (in whom growth is impaired even without steroid therapy, as a result of disease activity), but also in those receiving steroids for asthma or rheumatic fever.[1] This inhibition of growth is reversible and, in fact, a compensatory growth spurt occurs when the steroid dosage is reduced to low levels or is discontinued. The potential adult stature is not altered even after prolonged corticosteroid administration. There are at least two well-documented actions of steroids which can explain the growth retardation. The above-mentioned catabolic or protein wasting effect is certainly of principal importance. In addition, Frantz and Rabkin recently have demonstrated a direct suppression of growth hormone secretion with corticosteroids.[8] Inadequate growth hormone and the intense nitrogen wasting produced by steroid therapy present a rather vicious catabolic combination and presumably are the major factors in inhibiting growth.

Effects on Mineral Metabolism

Electrolyte and Water Metabolism.—One of the most brilliant achievements of the steroid chemists has been the synthesis of steroids which lack sodium-retaining and potassium-losing effects but which retain the effects on organic metabolism. This dissociation in function produced by molecular alteration has been clearly documented in the synthetic steroids, in some more than others, but it appears to be also dose dependent. The success of such chemical manipulation offers some hope that other clinically undesirable effects can be dissociated from the therapeutically desirable anti-inflammatory effects.

It will be recalled that Na^+, the principal cation of extracellular fluid, is filtered by the glomerulus and then partially reabsorbed in the proximal renal tubule. A portion of the remaining tubular Na^+ is reabsorbed in the distal tubule, presumably under the influence of corticosteroids (primarily aldosterone) by means of a cation-exchange process in which K^+ and H^+ egress from the tubular cell to tubular urine. Hence, steroids which possess mineralocorticoid activity promote Na^+ and Cl^- retention and an increase in excretion of K^+ and H^+.

The net effect of a given steroid on sodium excretion will vary directly with the degree to which it increases glomerular filtration rate (GFR) and inversely with the extent to which it enhances tubular reabsorption. Another factor which determines the quantitative response to a given steroid is the dietary sodium intake. In the face of dietary Na^+ restriction, eventually very little Na^+ reaches the distal tubule; under such conditions, exogenously administered mineralocorticoids will exert little or no effect on Na^+ retention or net K^+ excretion. Conversely, Na^+ loading produces a large distal tubular Na^+ load and exogenous mineralocorticoid administration under this circumstance promotes a large Na^+ retention and K^+ excretion.[32]

The naturally occurring corticosteroids, cortisone and cortisol, when given in large doses, increase tubular reabsorption of Na^+ to a greater extent than GFR and usually induce sodium retention and potassium loss. Prednisone and prednisolone, on the other hand, increase GFR to a greater degree and, therefore, in therapeutic doses do not lead to the electrolyte imbalance observed with the natural steroids. Thus, the double bond between carbons 1 and 2 (see Fig. 17–3) potentiates the organic effects and slightly attenuates the mineralocorticoid effects of cortisol. A fluorine atom attached to carbon 9 of cortisol or even of the prednisolone nucleus, in contrast, enhances the electrolyte effect and the resulting compounds cause marked retention of sodium and loss of potassium. Further, when carbon 16 of the 9α-fluoroprednisolone molecule is either hydroxylated (triamcinolone) or methylated (dexamethasone), its aldosterone-like effect on tubular reabsorption of Na^+ is markedly, if not completely, reduced. Triamcinolone and dexamethasone produce a slight increase in sodium excretion, apparently as a result of increased GFR.[19]

Bunim and his associates, in a well-designed experiment, demonstrated that the homeostatic control of aldosterone secretion is not altered by exogenous synthetic glucocorticoids.[2] Interplay of sodium restriction, urinary sodium loss, aldosterone secretion and exogenous corticosteroid administration and their net effect on homeostasis are illustrated by their experiment depicted in Figure 17–4. Urinary aldosterone excretion in a normal subject on a constant sodium intake of 87.0 mEq. and potassium intake of 150 mEq. was found to be 12 μg. per 24 hours. When sodium intake was restricted to 8.7 mEq. daily (potassium intake held constant at 150 mEq.) an initial loss of sodium occurred and aldosterone excretion increased to 32 μg., at which time positive Na^+ balance was restored. Dexamethasone was then given in daily doses of 6 mg. for twelve days. A negative sodium balance developed, aldosterone increased further to 58 μg. per twenty-four hours and sodium conservation and a positive balance were again established. Five days after discontinuing dexamethasone but maintaining sodium restriction, urinary aldosterone excretion reached 70 μg. per day. The results of this experiment demonstrate that aldosterone production unlike cortisol (low plasma 17 OHCS in Figure 17–4) is independent of anterior pituitary suppression by dexamethasone, that dexamethasone and aldosterone are not mutually antagonistic, and that dexamethasone failed to interfere with normal aldosterone secretion and responsiveness to dietary sodium restriction or urinary sodium loss.

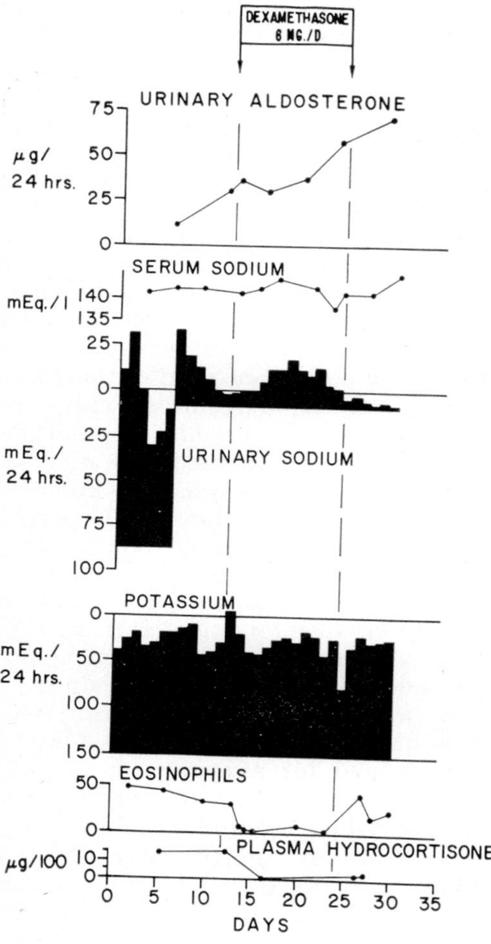

FIG. 17–4.—Aldosterone responsiveness to restriction of dietary sodium beginning on day 6 (reduced from 87 to 8.7 mEq. per twenty-four hours) and again to sodium loss temporarily induced by dexamethasone administration (6.0 mg. daily). Effects of dexamethasone on urinary potassium excretion (note first day of drug administration and withdrawal), on serum sodium (during sodium deprivation and loss), on circulating eosinophils and on concentration of plasma hydrocortisone are also demonstrated (see text for further details).

A large body of experimental data now supports the contention that control of aldosterone secretion is independent of the anterior pituitary and is mediated by the kidney. Through a reduction of some functional component of the arterial tree, the kidney is stimulated to release renin which is then converted to angiotensin. Angiotensin in turn stimulates the adrenal cortex to secrete aldosterone.[4]

Calcium and Bone Metabolism.—The effects of corticosteroids on calcium and bone metabolism in man and their role in the pathogenesis of osteoporosis remain poorly understood. It is widely believed that the protein-wasting effects of excessive glucocorticoids lead to osteoporosis chiefly by impairing deposition of osteoid matrix in bone and not by interfering directly with calcium metabolism. This postulate holds that, with the loss of protein matrix, calcium salts cannot be deposited at the bone surface and consequently the quantity of calcium excreted is increased. This view has now been challenged.

Following this line of reasoning, one might expect to observe a parallel relationship between nitrogen and calcium loss, or retention, upon administration of glucocorticoids or androgens, respectively. However, when complete (fecal and urinary) nitrogen, calcium, and phosphorus balance studies were done on patients to whom these steroids were given, no such relationship could be consistently established.[37] Furthermore, although increased *urinary* excretion of calcium following administration of glucocorticoids has been reported, *complete* balance studies done by Whedon and associates on patients receiving corticosteroids for thirty days or longer revealed no consistent change. Some patients showed calcium storage, others no change in calcium balance and several, calcium loss, depending principally upon changes in fecal calcium excretion.

An example of the apparently complex relationships of glucocorticoids and gonadal steroids is given in the balance data of a fifty-six-year-old woman with active rheumatoid arthritis and osteoporosis of the spine (Fig. 17–5).[37] When prednisolone, in a dosage of 30 mg. per day, was administered, the expected nitrogen loss was observed but calcium was retained and a positive mineral balance resulted. When methyl testosterone and estrone sulphate were supplemented, calcium storage was not enhanced although the nitrogen balance became positive. When prednisolone was discontinued and gonadal steroids alone continued, calcium retention was accentuated. It should be emphasized that a positive calcium balance was achieved throughout the experiment and that the patient was maintained at an intake level of 1300 mg. of calcium daily.

A consideration of the quantitative

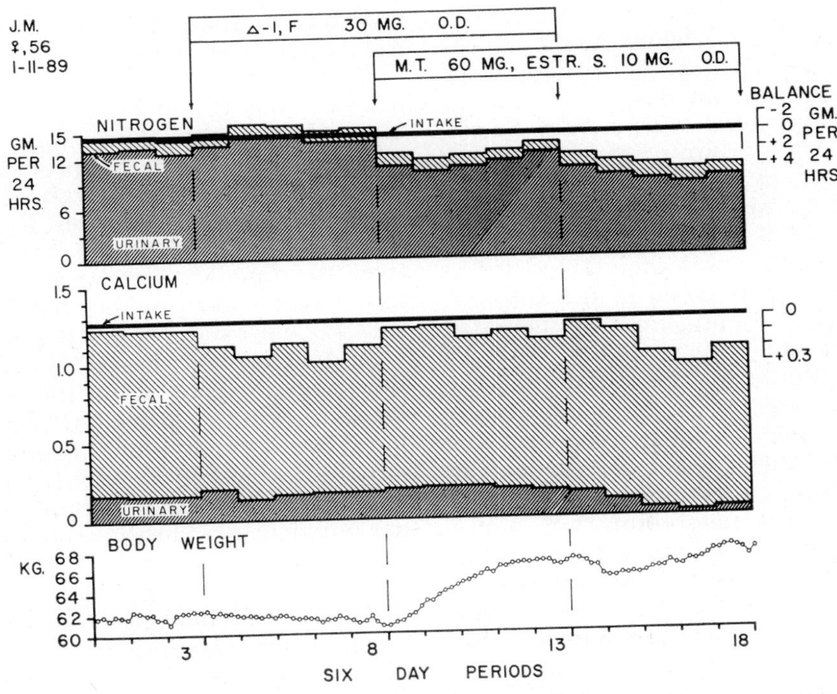

FIG. 17–5.—Nitrogen and calcium balances and changes in body weight in a fifty-six-year-old woman with active rheumatoid arthritis and osteoporosis of the spine. Over the time periods indicated, the patient was maintained on calcium intake of 1270 mg. daily and received prednisolone (30 mg. daily orally), then methyl testosterone (60 mg. daily orally) and estrone sulphate (10 mg. daily orally). In this metabolic balance graph, when urinary and fecal outputs together rise above the base line, negative balance or loss of the element is occurring; when the summed urinary and fecal outputs fall below the base line, positive balance or storage is taking place (Whedon[37]). Δ-1,F = prednisolone. O.D. = daily dose. M.T. = methyl testosterone. Estr. S. = estrone sulphate.

relationship between calcium and protein in bone illustrates the difficulty in establishing or refuting, by conventional balance techniques, the thesis that faulty matrix is the exclusive defect in osteoporosis. From data on the chemical composition of the adult human body, Whedon has calculated that the amount of nitrogen in bone is 0.275 gm. per gm. of calcium.[36] Assuming that stored protein will be generally distributed to all tissues, 1.4 gm. of nitrogen would be required to store 1 gm. of calcium.[36] Alteration in calcium balance rarely exceeds 0.5 gm. daily, which would require the storing of only 0.7 gm. of nitrogen in the whole body—a value of doubtful significance by conventional balance techniques.

Other studies by Whedon *et al.* and Nordin have demonstrated the favorable influence of high calcium intake on calcium balance in patients with osteoporosis, both of the spontaneous variety and of the type associated with steroid administration.[24,38] Positive calcium balance with vaues of +500 mgm./day was produced by raising the calcium intake to 1600 to 2400 mgm./day. The positive calciuml balance was maintained for as long as a year in some of the subjects. These observed influences of increased calcium intake on calcium balance introduce doubt to the belief that the etiology of osteoporosis is related purely to an interference with synthesis of tissue protein and suggest that it is, at least in part, related to a disturbance in calcium and phosphorus metabolism.[23,38]

Effects on Inflammatory Process, Tissue Reactivity and Host Defense.—Liddle has pointed out that it is somewhat ironical that the anti-inflammatory action of steroids is the one most widely used therapeutically in clinical medicine.[19] This is particularly true when one considers that the major actions of endogenously secreted adrenocortical glucocorticoids are directed at organic metabolism and that the quantity of steroids normally secreted exerts very little effect on inflammation. In most therapeutic applications, the undesirable changes in organic metabolism which have been labeled "side effects" are in actual fact exaggerated normal effects. Clinical pharmacology finds itself in the unusual position of attempting to design steroid molecules which hopefully will lack these physiologic functions but which will retain the pharmacologic anti-inflammatory activity. It should be emphasized that the anti-inflammatory effect is not discriminating. Corticosteroids in large doses not only inhibit "undesirable" inflammation (such as that associated with connective tissue disorders), but also suppress "desirable" inflammation which is so vital in host defense against a variety of infectious agents. The latter action of suppressing host defenses is perhaps the most hazardous of the clinically undesirable effects of the anti-inflammatory steroids.

Effects on Connective Tissue.—In experimental animals and in cultures of fibroblasts, large doses of cortisone suppress reproduction, growth and proliferation of connective tissue cells and also genesis of fibrils and ground substances. Ragan and his associates demonstrated that cortisone given to animals in very large dosages delays wound healing by retarding fibroplasia, vascularization and deposition of ground substances; however, only slight interference with epithelization was observed.[29] Finally, protein depletion produced by starvation facilitates interference with wound healing by cortisone and, conversely, cortisone administration accentuates impairment of healing due to protein depletion.

Effects on Tissue Inflammatory Responses (Table 17–3).—Biologically active glucocorticoids will promptly suppress inflammation regardless of the causative agent, whether it be microbial, chemical or physical irritant, foreign protein, hypersensitivity reaction or when the causative agent is unknown as in the connective tissue diseases (such as rheumatoid arthritis).

The observed anti-inflammatory effects of corticosteroids consist of preservation

Table 17-3.—Effect of Corticosteroids on Inflammation

Vascular "tone" preserved
Integrity of endothelium preserved
Enhanced capillary permeability reversed
Exudation of inflammatory cells suppressed
Destruction of fibroblasts inhibited
Reparative process and granulation tissue proliferation suppressed
ESR reduced
CRP reduced
Clinical signs of inflammation and "toxemia" subside
Causative agent unaffected

Table 17-4.—Effect of Corticosteroids on Immunity

Production of humoral antibodies (in man) not affected
Antigen-antibody union not inhibited
Release of histamine-like substances not suppressed
"Immediate" skin reactions not altered
"Delayed" skin reactions (tuberculin) suppressed
Reactivity of tissue to antigen-antibody union suppressed

of integrity of the endothelium, reversal of enhanced permeability associated with inflammation, marked suppression of diapedesis of inflammatory cells and inhibition of fibroblast destruction. Systemic signs and laboratory indices of inflammation, such as fever, elevated erythrocyte sedimentation rate, presence of C-reactive protein and "toxicity," subside. The signs of the process are obliterated but the causative agent is not eradicated or even altered. Microorganisms, if originally present, not only remain but increase in number and the infectious process may spread with ease.[15a]

Effects on Host Defense and Immune Responses (Table 17–4).—Studies by many workers on the influence of corticosteroids on antibody responses, while conflicting in several instances, have led to agreement on many important conclusions. Many experiments utilizing diverse types of antigens, wide ranges of dosages, and varied temporal relationships between institution of steroid therapy and administration of antigens have been performed. There is general agreement that cortisone, in man, does not significantly affect production of humoral antibodies in response to specific antigens, nor does it alter the antibody titer already present. (However, in a few specific disorders, such as acquired hemolytic anemia, antibody inhibition can be demonstrated.) Steroids also are unable to inhibit union of antibody and antigen nor do they suppress the capacity of tissues to release histamine-like substances. Delayed local skin reactions (*e.g.* to tuberculin) are significantly modified by corticosteroids administered prior to challenge, but "immediate" skin reactions associated with release of histamine-like substances are not so altered. It has been concluded that although the steroids do not interfere with antigen-antibody union, they do suppress the reaction of tissues to this event.[15a]

Suppression of Pituitary Corticotropin Secretion.—One of the major problems which attends the administration of anti-inflammatory steroids is suppression of ACTH secretion and the resulting adrenocortical atrophy. These effects of the steroids have important clinical implications for they account for the catastrophic adrenocortical insufficiency that occasionally follows surgery, trauma or infection in patients who had been receiving exogenous hormones prior to these stresses but who had not been prepared with adequate amounts of steroids during such events.

Recently the natural history of the recovery of pituitary adrenal function following cessation of long-term steroid therapy has been defined. Graber and his associates determined in the first month following withdrawal of corticosteroids that *both* plasma ACTH and 17-Hydroxycorticosteroids (17 OHCS) levels (determined at 6 A.M.) are subnormal; from two to five months plasma ACTH rises to levels which are supernormal but plasma 17 OHCS levels remain low; finally, from five to nine months following withdrawal, both plasma ACTH and 17 OHCS levels return to normal (see Fig. 17–1).[11] It was also observed from two to five months following withdrawal of steroids that plasma ACTH levels at 6 P.M. were low or undetectable at a time when the 6 A.M. values were elevated, indicating a persistence of the normal diurnal pattern of ACTH secretion. These results indicate that the anterior pituitary is capable of secreting ACTH even in supraphysiologic amounts within two months after cessation of chronic steroid therapy and that the recovery of normal adrenocortical function followed the recovery of the anterior pituitary. Persistence of the diurnal pattern of ACTH secretion (low plasma ACTH levels in the evening) is a contributory factor in the prolonged recovery of the total system. Small doses of exogenous ACTH might facilitate the return of the system to normal. Such a study has been recently reported which demonstrated that there is less risk of severe depression of the system after appropriately timed long-term ACTH therapy than after continuous oral corticosteroids.[1a]

Considerable misunderstanding about the indications for ACTH administration exists among some clinicians. It should be emphasized that the above studies pertain only to the period following withdrawal of long-term steroid therapy. During periods of stress in patients still receiving exogenous steroids, ACTH administration has no rationale as an emergency treatment; reliance on exogenous ACTH to produce sufficient cortisol secretion to cover the stress is hazardous. Administration of adequate doses of parenteral cortisol remains the only reliable means of preventing adrenocortical insufficiency in the emergency situation.

BIBLIOGRAPHY

1. Ansell, B. M. and Bywaters, E. G. L.: Ann. Rheum. Dis., *15*, 295, 1956.

1a. Bacon, P. A., Daley, J. R., Myles, A. B., and Savage, O.: Ann. Rheum. Dis., *27*, 7, 1968.

2. Bunim, J. J., Black, R. L., Lutwak, L., Peterson, R. E., and Whedon, G. D.: Arth. and Rheum., *1*, 313, 1958.

3. Coppage, W. S., Jr., Island, D. P., Cooner, A. E., and Liddle, G. W.: J. Clin. Invest., *41*, 1672, 1962.

4. Davis, J. O., Hartroft, P. M., Titus, E. O., Carpenter, C. C. J., Ayers, C. R., and Spiegel, H. E.: J. Clin. Invest., *41*, 378, 1962.

5. Di Raimondo, C., Orr, R. H., Island, D. P., and Forsham, P. H.: J. Clin. Invest., *34*, 930, 1955.

5a. Endroczi, E., Lissak, K., and Tekeres, M.: Acta. Physiol. Acad. Sci. Hung., *18*, 291, 1961.

6. Engel, F. L.: Vitamins Hormones, *19*, 189, 1961.

7. Estep, H. L., Island, D. P., Ney, R. L., and Liddle, G. W.: J. Clin. Endocrinol., *23*, 419 1963.

8. Frantz, A. G. and Rabkin, M. T.: New Engl. J. Med., *271*, 1375, 1964.

9. Frawley, T. F., Kistler, H., and Shelley, T.: Ann. Acad. Sci., *82*, 868, 1959.

10. Givens, J. R., Ney, R. L., Nicholson, W. E., Graber, A. L., and Liddle, G. W.: Clin. Res., *12*, 267, 1964.

11. Graber, A. L., Ney, R. L., Nicholson, W. E., Island, D. P., and Liddle, G. W.: Trans. Assn. Amer. Physicians, *77*, 296, 1964.

12. Harris, G. W.: *Neural Control of the Pituitary Gland.* London, Edward Arnold, 1955.

13. Hofmann, K. and Yajima, H.: Recent Progr. Hormone Res., *18*, 41, 1962.

14. Ingle, D. J., Higgins, G. M., and Kendall, E. C.: Anat. Rec., *71*, 363, 1938.

15. Isselbacher, K. J.: Recent Progr. Hormone Res., *12*, 134, 1956.

15a. Kass, E. H. and Finland, M.: Ann. Rev. Microbiol., *7*, 361, 1953.

16. Kendall, J. W., Jr.: Endocrinology, *71*, 452, 1962.

17. Li, C. H., Evans, H. M., and Simpson, M. E.: J. Biol. Chem., *149*, 413, 1943.

18. Li, C. H.: Recent Progr. Hormone Res., *18*, 1, 1962.

19. Liddle, G. W.: Clin. Pharmacol. Ther., *2*, 615, 1961.

20. LIDDLE, G. W., ISLAND, D. P., and MEADOR, C. K.: Recent Progr. Hormone Res., *18*, 125, 1962.
21. NEY, R. L., COPPAGE, W. S., JR., SHIMIZU, N., ISLAND, D. P., ZUKOSKI, C. F., and LIDDLE, G. W.: J. Clin. Endocrinol., *22*, 1057, 1962.
22. NEY, R. L., SHIMIZU, N., NICHOLSON, W. E., ISLAND, D. P., and LIDDLE, G. W.: J. Clin. Invest., *42*, 1669, 1963.
23. NORDIN, B. E. C.: In Astwood, E. B., Ed., *Clinical Endocrinology I.* New York, Grune & Stratton, 1960, p. 233.
24. NORDIN, B. E. C.: Proc. Lankenau Research Conference, *Bone as a Tissue*, New York, McGraw-Hill, 1960.
25. NUGENT, C. A., EIK-NES, K., SAMUELS, L. T., and TYLER, F. H.: J. Clin. Endocr., *19*, 334, 1959.
26. PETERSON, R. E.: Ann. N.Y. Acad. Sci., *82*, 846, 1959.
27. PETERSON, R. E., BLACK, R. L., and BUNIM, J. J.: Arth. and Rheum., *2*, 433, 1959.
28. PETERSON, R. E., WYNGAARDEN, J. B., GUERRA, S. L., BRODIE, B. B., and BUNIM, J. J.: J. Clin. Invest., *34*, 1779, 1955.
29. RAGAN, C.: Ann. Rev. Physiol., *14*, 51, 1952.
30. SAYERS, G., WHITE, A., and LONG, C. N. H.: J. Biol. Chem., *149*, 425, 1943.
31. SCHALLY, A. V., BOWERS, C. Y., and LOCKE. W.: Amer. J. Med. Sci., *248*, 79, 1964.
32. SELDIN, D. W., WELT, L. G.. and CORT, J.: J. Clin. Invest., *30*, 673, 1951.
33. TOMKINS, G. M.: J. Biol. Chem., *225*, 13, 1957.
34. TOMKINS, G. M.: Ann. Acad. Sci., *82*, 836, 1959.
35. WELT, I. D., STETTEN, DE W., JR., INGLE, D. J., and MORLEY, E. H.: J. Biol. Chem., *197*, 57, 1952.
36. WHEDON, G. D.: In Engle, E. T., Ed., *Hormones and the Aging Process.* New York, Academic Press, Inc., 1956, p. 221.
37. WHEDON, G. D.: Proc. Fourth Congress Internat. Gerontol. Assoc., Fidenza, Italy, Tipografia Tito Mattioli, 1959, p. 615.
38. WHEDON, G. D.: Am. Inst. Nutrition Symp., April 14, 1959, Fed. Proc., *18*, 1112, 1959.
39. WHITE, A., HANDLER, P., SMITH, E., and STETTEN, D.: *Principles of Biochemistry*, 2nd Ed., New York, McGraw-Hill, 1959.

PART III

The Study of Rheumatoid Arthritis

Editor: Edward W. Boland, M.D.

Chapter 18

The Etiology of Rheumatoid Arthritis

By William D. Robinson, M.D.

The etiology of rheumatoid arthritis is unknown. Intensive efforts have failed to establish that it is caused by a specific infectious agent, by nutritional excess or deficiency, by metabolic aberrations, by faulty or unbalanced endocrine secretions, or by a well-defined mechanism involving dysfunction of the autonomic nervous system or the somatic reflection of emotional or personality disorders. Impressive evidence is accumulating to suggest the importance of an immunologic mechanism in the pathogenesis of the disease, although the initiating events still remain obscure. Statistical considerations suggest an hereditary influence, but no clear-cut genetic pattern has emerged. Hypotheses as to the cause of rheumatoid arthritis usually attempt to explain certain epidemiologic, clinical, pathological or laboratory findings characteristic of the disease, or derive from evaluation of factors which appear to influence its course. Generally accepted facts regarding the disease include: its predilection for women and for "temperate" climates, its peak of onset between the ages of twenty to fifty, the constitutional nature of the disease, the almost ubiquitous distribution of the inflammatory lesions in connective tissue, the self-perpetuating nature of the synovial inflammation, the tendency toward symmetrical distribution of the joint involvement, and the unpredictable course which the disease may follow in an individual patient, including exacerbations and remissions without apparent rhyme or reason. A number of studies have called attention to the high incidence of vasomotor disturbances which may accompany the disease, and to the frequency with which onsets or recurrences are related to emotional shocks and acute illnesses, but only rarely has the influence of these factors been compared to an appropriate control group.[10]

Is Rheumatoid Arthritis an Infectious Disease?

The inflammatory features and constitutional manifestations of rheumatoid arthritis—the synovitis and granulomatous lesions, the fever, tachycardia, leukocytosis, lymphadenopathy and occasional splenomegaly, the accelerated erythrocyte sedimentation rate and other changes in "acute phase reactants"—are all compatible with an infectious process. But such features suggesting an infectious origin are seen in diseases of non-infectious etiology such as metabolic and hypersensitivity disorders and in neoplasia. Competent and repeated bacteriologic studies have failed to recover consistently an infectious agent from the blood, synovial fluid, synovial tissues or subcutaneous nodules.[1] Attempts to transmit the disease by injecting joint fluid from patients with rheumatoid arthritis into the joints of other human subjects have been unsuccessful.[9] Subcutaneous nodules have failed to survive following homologous transplantation.[2]

"The overwhelming negative results of bacteriologic studies suggest that rheumatoid arthritis is not the work of an easily culturable or characterized bacterium."[3] The search for microorganisms with more elusive properties is discussed in Chapter 14.

An infectious process may appear to precipitate the onset of rheumatoid arthritis in a significant number of patients, and may exert a deleterious influence on the course of the disease when it has already been established. There is some statistical evidence to support this clinical impression,[10] but the same can be said of non-infectious and traumatic incidents. The previously widely accepted theory that rheumatoid arthritis is associated with "focal infection" has failed to stand the test of careful clinical and laboratory investigation (*see also* Chapter 14).

Many attempts have been made to produce a disease in animals similar to rheumatoid arthritis. While a variety of bacteria can produce arthritis in animals, they fail to reproduce the clinical and pathologic features of rheumatoid arthritis, particularly the self-perpetuating character of the proliferative arthritis. Arthritis bearing some semblance to the human disease has been produced in mice by pleuro-pneumonia-like organisms[17] and in swine by Erysipelothrix rhusiopathiae.[18] The concept that these organisms may initiate a hypersensitivity mechanism has been postulated.[18] (See Chapter 11.)

Is Rheumatoid Arthritis an "Auto-immune" Disease?

Many workers have suspected that an immunologic mechanism is somehow concerned with the production of rheumatoid arthritis. The demonstration that the sera of many patients with this disease contained a macroglobulin (rheumatoid factor) with an unusual affinity for gamma globulin of smaller molecular size (7S) has led many to classify rheumatoid arthritis among the "diseases of autoimmunity."

The brilliant investigative work which defined and characterized rheumatoid factor (*see* Chapter 9) did not immediately lead to clarification of the etiology and pathogenesis of rheumatoid arthritis. A high agglutinating titer was maintained passively for six weeks by transfusing rheumatoid plasma into non-arthritic subjects without provoking manifestations of the disease.[21] Attention was called to the fact that not all macroglobulins are antibodies and that, in some pathologic conditions, large protein molecules may "issue from cells whose synthetic apparatus has been subverted by the disease to the production of apparently functionless material."[5]

In the past decade several lines of investigation clearly implicate an immunologic mechanism in the pathogenesis of joint inflammation in rheumatoid arthritis. Evidence supports the concept that, in the rheumatoid joint, the combination of antigen and antibody activates the complement sequence, with generation of biologically active materials which initiate and perpetuate the inflammatory process. (*See* Chapter 19.)

Nevertheless, several steps remain obscure in the elucidation of a completely satisfying immunologic explanation of rheumatoid arthritis. If rheumatoid factor is an antibody, presumably 7S gamma globulin must be the antigen.[8,15] Several observations suggest that some alteration in the 7S gamma globulin molecule may be required to provide such antigenic properties.[8,15] There are few clues as to the nature of such alterations or the factors which could cause them. The role of the immune response in the mediation of tissue injury does not preclude a possible genetic basis for a predisposition to rheumatoid arthritis or the potential of microorganisms in provoking an antigenic challenge.[3]

Is Rheumatoid Arthritis a Nutritional or Metabolic Disease?

Intensive search has been made in an effort to uncover a nutritional or metabolic fault in rheumatoid arthritis. Patients with the disease usually lose weight and often they present evidences of nutritional deficiency. However, careful studies of carbohydrate, fat, and protein metabolism have shown no abnormalities that can be considered etiologically significant. Minor delays in carbohydrate utilization may be detected in some patients but usually these deviations in the glucose tolerance curve can be corrected by feeding a high-carbohydrate diet for a few days prior to testing. In its active stages, the disease is not necessarily accompanied by protein wastage; positive nitrogen balance can be established if the intake of calories and proteins is adequate.

Some years ago, careful studies yielded no evidence of significant abnormalities of sulfur, calcium or phosphorus metabolism in patients with rheumatoid arthritis. Patients with this disease have been found to excrete abnormally large amounts of tryptophane metabolites[14] and of tyrosine precursors.[12] The specificity and significance of these findings remain obscure.

At one time it appeared that advances in knowledge of vitamins might solve some of the problems of rheumatoid arthritis. Since the primary pathology of the disease is in the connective tissue, ascorbic acid was particularly implicated because of its importance in the formation of the fibrillar components of intercellular tissue. Although low concentrations of ascorbic acid were found in the plasma of many patients with this disease, the clinical course of the arthritis was unaffected by correction of the biochemical deficiency. More recently, the gap between such biochemical evidence of lack of saturation of body stores with a particular vitamin and a clinically significant impairment of body function due to the deficiency has been more widely appreciated. In a somewhat similar fashion, the occasional borderline deficiency, or even frank deficiency, of the vitamin B complex which may accompany the disease has been accepted as consequence of a chronic constitutional disease rather than as its cause.[16]

Despite these failures to demonstrate any etiological role of nutritional deficiencies or metabolic errors in rheumatoid arthritis, attention to the nutritional state of the individual patient is often an important aspect in the management of this disease. Sound dietary practices, common to the management of any chronic systemic disease, are necessary to restore caloric balance, provide favorable conditions for the rebuilding of muscle, and correct any specific deficiencies that may be present. A diet liberal in calories and protein and high in vitamin and mineral content is usually indicated.

Is Rheumatoid Arthritis an Endocrine Disease?

The higher incidence of rheumatoid arthritis in women and the striking amelioration of the disease which may occur during pregnancy are observations which have suggested a possible disturbance of gonadal function. But direct attempts to produce or influence the disease with sex hormones have met with failure. Relationship of the onset of rheumatoid arthritis to the menopause is quite clearly a matter of chance[10] and has no significant bearing on etiology (*see also* Chapter 16).

The discovery of the remarkable ability of adrenocorticosteroids to suppress the inflammatory manifestations of rheumatoid arthritis stimulated an intensive search for an abnormality of adrenal or pituitary function. As rapid strides in endocrine physiology and steroid analytic techniques permitted precise evaluation of the function of these glands, a host of studies attest to the fact that adrenal cortical and anterior pituitary functions in patients with rheumatoid arthritis do not differ significantly from those in normal subjects.

The hypothesis that an imbalance between hormones secreted by the adrenal cortex or by the pituitary gland was responsible for several human diseases, including rheumatoid arthritis, has not been supported either by clinical investigation or experimental studies.

It has long been apparent that the suppressive effects of adrenocortical steroids are by no means restricted to rheumatic diseases. But the way in which these agents exert their ameliorating effects has remained a mystery. If the clinical improvement could be consistently correlated with some of the many alterations in total body metabolism which follow the administration of adrenocorticosteroids, it was reasonable to hope that such observations might lead to a better understanding of etiology. But none of the many changes in body chemistry which have been measured appears to be specifically related to the clinical effect of these agents in the rheumatic diseases, and the metabolic changes which occur in patients with rheumatoid arthritis do not differ significantly from those in normal subjects given adrenocorticosteroids or corticotropin. The demonstration that these agents are effective by local application (for example, by intra-articular injection) has tended to shift the search for a biochemical explanation of their mode of action from the area of total body chemistry to the level of the connective tissue itself.

Are the Pathologic Lesions of Rheumatoid Arthritis a Clue to Etiology?

For many years indirect evidence has suggested that the initial lesion of rheumatoid arthritis involves the intercellular component of connective tissue, particularly the interfibrillar ground substance. Attention has focused on the carbohydrate-containing components of the amorphous ground substance, and the concept that an alteration in their physical or chemical state may be responsible for the initial lesion. Evidence that the initial lesion involves the ground substance has been obtained almost entirely by methods which are incapable of distinguishing whether the changes arise *de novo* or reflect alterations derived from the blood stream. Since the cause of these alterations is completely unknown, they are of little help in uncovering the etiology of the disease.

In studies of synovial cells in tissue culture, several workers have found persistent differences in the characteristics of cells derived from normal and rheumatoid synovium—differences which are propagated in successive subcultures throughout the culture life of the cells. It has been suggested that this persistent alteration in metabolic activity may result from persistent infection of the rheumatoid cell with a "slow" virus which can escape detection by standard techniques.[19]

Is Rheumatoid Arthritis a Psychosomatic Disease?

There is widespread speculation concerning the role of predisposing personality structure and of emotional trauma in the initiation and maintenance of this disease. Personality traits and psychologic mechanisms in patients with rheumatoid arthritis have been described as similar to schizophrenia,[6] characterized by repressed aggressiveness and hostility[11] and by a unique body image resulting from parental influences.[4,7] Rarely has it been possible to separate the emotional factors secondary to the chronic disease from those which were present prior to its onset. Results in one study suggested that the psychosocial variables studied might be related to the development of severe disease, but probably were not related to the development of mild disease.[7] When 532 patients with rheumatoid arthritis were questioned, more than half of them considered worry, shock, other illness, chills or trauma to be related to the onset of their disease. Yet the frequency of such precipitating factors, especially those occurrences likely to produce mental stress, was no greater among these patients than in a carefully matched control group who did not have rheumatoid arthritis. From this it was concluded that any difference between sufferers and non-sufferers resides in some feature of the individual himself rather than in any difference of stress experience[10] (*see also* Chapter 13).

The way in which abnormal personality traits can produce pathologic changes in the tissues remains unexplained. But clinical experience certainly supports the concept that in certain patients the course of the disease appears to be influenced by emotional and personality factors. An understanding attitude on the part of the physician, directing care to the patient as a whole rather than to isolated segments of either anatomy or psyche, is essential.

Is Rheumatoid Arthritis an Hereditary Disease?

The possibility that rheumatoid arthritis occurs in persons who have a genetically predisposed constitution or susceptibility is supported by several studies. In one of the most extensive, the disease was present in 3.1 per cent of 1,677 relatives of patients with rheumatoid arthritis as compared to an incidence of 0.58 per cent of 2,759 control subjects.[20] It was estimated that approximately one-half of persons with the proper genetic constitution actually developed the disease. Evidence from twin studies favors the existence of a weak but definite genetic influence.[13]

It should be noted that the genetically determined constitution predisposing to the development of rheumatoid arthritis has never been sharply delineated.

SUMMARY

In any disease of unknown and possibly complex etiology, it is necessary to consider the soil, or background, of constitutional and environmental factors which permit the disease to develop, as well as the seed, or postulated noxious agent, which actually starts the disease process on its way. Continued exploration of both avenues of approach can be expected to be fruitful.

BIBLIOGRAPHY

1. Angevine, D. M., Rothbard, S. and Cecil, R. L.: J.A.M.A., *115*, 2112, 1940.
2. Bauer, W., Clark, W. S. and Dienes, L.: The Practitioner, *166*, 5, 1951.
3. Christian, C. L.: Arth. & Rheum., *7*, 455, 1964.
4. Cleveland, S. E. and Fisher, S.: Psychosom. Med., *16*, 327, 1954.
5. Heimer, R.: Arth. & Rheum., *2*, 266, 1959.
6. King, S. H.: J. Chronic Dis., *2*, 287, 1955.
7. King, S. H. and Cobb, S.: Arth. & Rheum., *2*, 322, 1959.
8. Kunkel, H. G., Franklin, E. C. and Muller-Eberhard, H. J.: J. Clin. Invest., *38*, 424, 1959.
9. Levinsky, W. J. and Lansbury, J.: Proc. Soc. Exper. Biol. & Med., *78*, 325, 1951.
10. Lewis-Faning, E.: Ann. Rheum. Dis., Suppl., 9, 1950.
11. Ludwig, A. O.: Med. Clin. North America, *39*, 447, 1955.
12. McCann, D. S., Mitchell, J. G., Keech, M. K. *et al.*: J. Chronic Dis., *20*, 781, 1967.
13. O'Brien, W. M.: Arth. & Rheum., *11*, 81, 1968.
14. Pinals, R. S.: Arth. & Rheum., *7*, 662, 1964.
15. Restifo, R. A., Lussier, A. J., Rawson, A. J., Rockey, J. H. and Hollander, J. L.: Ann. Intern. Med., *63*, 285, 1965.
16. Robinson, W. D.: J.A.M.A., *166*, 253, 1958.
17. Sabin, A. B.: Science, *89*, 228, 1939.
18. Sikes, D., Neher, G. M. and Doyle, L. P.: Amer. J. Vet. Res., *16*, 367, 1955.
19. Smith, C. and Hamerman, D.: Arth. & Rheum., *12*, 639, 1969.
20. Stecher, R. M., Hersh, A. H., Solomon, W. M. and Wolpaw, R.: Amer. J. Human Genetics, *5*, 118, 1953.
21. Vaughan, J. H. and Harris, J.: Arth. & Rheum., *2*, 51, 1959.
22. Zvaifler, N. J.: Arth. & Rheum., *13*, 895, 1970.

Chapter 19

Pathogenetic Mechanisms in Rheumatoid Arthritis

By Nathan J. Zvaifler, M.D.

The ancient Greeks thought that rheumatism, the affliction of the joints, was due to abnormal substances moving through the body cavities. Two thousand years later, employing the sophisticated techniques of immunology and biochemistry, medical scientists returned to the study of rheumatoid arthritis. Currently, rheumatoid arthritis remains a disease of unknown cause, but knowledge gained from investigations of the inflammatory process, in general, and the phlogistic properties of antigen-antibody complexes, in particular, has provided new insights into the pathogenesis of rheumatoid joint inflammation.

In the 1950's and into the 60's, the majority of investigations of rheumatoid arthritis focused upon serologic reactions in serum. Two findings, however, redirected attention to the articular cavity. The first was the observation that despite relatively normal serum concentrations of hemolytic complement, there was a disproportionate lowering of complement, compared to other joint fluid proteins, in rheumatoid synovial fluids.[16,29] The other was the demonstration that synovial fluid leukocytes contain intracytoplasmic particulate complexes consisting of 19S and 7S immunoglobulins.[10,19] From these studies it was inferred that complement was being fixed, presumably by immune complexes present in the synovial membrane or fluid. Subsequent studies have reinforced this view. The accumulating evidence favors the idea that, in the rheumatoid joint, antigen(s) combining with antibody(s) activates the complement sequence, generating a variety of biologically active materials, including some with potent chemotactic properties. These bring polymorphonuclear leukocytes into the articular cavity, where they are attracted to and ingest the immune complexes. After phagocytosis the neutrophils discharge from their lysosomal granules a variety of hydrolytic enzymes. It is these substances that appear to play a central role in the proliferative and destructive changes characteristic of rheumatoid arthritis. This chapter will summarize the evidence supporting this pathogenetic concept. The headings chosen define the constituent parts of the sequence of reactions, but are artificial designations since they are interdependent and not mutually exclusive.

COMPLEMENT AND COMPLEMENT COMPONENTS

The extensive information on the chemical structure and reaction mechanisms of the various components of complement has been reviewed by Muller-Eberhard[28] and in Chapter 8. The complement system is comprised of a group of 12 proteins, nine components and at least three inhibitors. The interaction of these proteins in a prescribed sequence results in a variety of biologic phenomena, which include the release of vasoactive peptides, the attraction of polymorphonuclear leukocytes, the enhancement of phagocytosis, and the production of defects in cell membranes. The decrease in synovial fluid total hemolytic complement activity observed in rheumatoid effusions could result from one of several mechanisms: selective destruction of a single component, an increase in activity of an inhibitor of complement, or consumption of the late acting components of the complement sequence by activation through an alternate pathway (see Chapter 8). Therefore, the overall pattern of complement depletion has been determined. C1, C4, C2, and C3 are all depressed, and depressed proportionately.[33,53] Rheumatoid fluids also show evidence of the presence of C3 convertase[51] and the trimolecular complex of C5, C6, and C7.[42] These results are most consistent with immune activation of the complement sequence.

The remarkable accumulation of neutrophils in rheumatoid synovial effusions, the knowledge that small molecular weight proteins derived from C3 and C5 have chemotactic activity,[41] and the finding of breakdown products of C3 in some rheumatoid joint fluids,[51] suggested that synovial fluids should be analyzed for chemotactic activity. These efforts were rewarded by the demonstration of two distinct substances with chemotactic properties for neutrophils in the majority of rheumatoid joint fluid studied. One, a heavy molecular weight protein, seems identical to the activated trimolecular complex (C567) of the complement sequence. The other, a lightweight material, is a cleavage product of human C5.[42] In addition, about half of the rheumatoid effusions studied contained an enzyme that produces a small molecular weight chemotactic factor from isolated human C5. A similar, if not identical, enzyme has also been found in the leukocytes from rheumatoid joint fluids.[42]

ANTIGEN, ANTIBODY AND COMPLEXES

While it is recognized that certain proteolytic enzymes, such as plasmin, can activate C1 and thus initiate the complement sequence, the bulk of evidence (cited above) favors the concept that complement depletion in rheumatoid joint fluids is caused by immune complexes or their equivalents. This is further supported by the observation of Broder and his associates that a factor resembling a soluble antigen-antibody complex is detectable in three-quarters of rheumatoid synovial fluids. These fluids, perfused into intact guinea pig lungs, cause the release of histamine.[3]

The intra-articular injection of an antigen into a previously hyperimmunized animal results in an arthritis with many of the histologic features of rheumatoid arthritis. Similar findings can be induced by repeated introduction of immune complexes into the articular cavity.[30] Experimental synovitis has been produced by the injection of autologous intact IgG or the Fc or Fab fractions into the uninvolved knee joints of patients with seropositive rheumatoid arthritis.[18,31] However, several papers have challenged the hypothesis that rheumatoid subjects are unusually sensitive to autologous IgG.[34,35]

Complement-fixation, histamine-release and experimental synovitis are all indirect indicators of antigen-antibody reactions. More recent investigations have actually demonstrated immune complexes in some rheumatoid effusions. Hannestad used an IgM rheumatoid factor to precipitate complexes from some rheumatoid joint fluids.[14] Winchester *et al.* detected similar complexes by ultracentrifugal analysis, and demonstrated that they were composed of IgG and a 7S anti-IgG.[47] The complexes did not contain proteins other than immunoglobulins. They noted a direct relationship between the amount of complexes and the depression of complement activity of the joint fluid. The complexes could also be demonstrated by direct precipitation with isolated C1q.[1] Cryoprecipitable complexes containing varying proportions of IgG, IgM, DNA and antinuclear factors have been detected regularly in fluids from seropositive rheumatoid patients but not in companion serum samples.[2,26]

It has been proposed that the perpetuation of rheumatoid joint inflammation depends, at least in part, on the development of an autoimmune response to antigens which are a constant by-product of the inflammatory reaction. This would be independent of the specific initiating event, or cause, of rheumatoid arthritis. Glynn suggested that fibrin might be such an antigen, since a chronic arthritis follows even a single intra-articular injection in a previously sensitized animal.[13] Nucleoprotein, released from degenerating leukocytes, reacting with antinuclear antibodies might serve as an immune complex perpetuating rheumatoid inflammation.[49] Both DNA and nucleoprotein are regularly found as particulate material in the cytoplasm of leukocytes in rheumatoid synovial effusions.[7,25] The demonstration of denatured DNA and antinuclear activity in cryoprecipitates from rheumatoid synovial effusion also supports this view, as do several other observations: granulocyte-specific antinuclear antibodies are found with greatest frequency in rheumatoid arthritis and more often in rheumatoid effusions than in the corresponding serum;[11] antinuclear antibodies are present in greater concentrations in synovial leukocytes than in the surrounding fluid.[52]

The rheumatoid synovial membrane contains most of the immunoreactants demonstrated in synovial fluid leukocytes. Immunofluorescent studies have shown that IgG and complement components usually occur together as small discrete deposits or as large amorphous collections in the interstitial tissues.[7,12,32] Anti-γ-globulins and IgM are detected most often in the walls of blood vessels or as perivascular deposits in synovial tissue from seropositive (rheumatoid factor) patients.[6,7,12] Fibrin deposits are common and particulate complexes containing nucleoprotein have been identified in interstitial areas and in the cytoplasm of synovial lining cells.[7] Isolated lining cells can be obtained by trypsin digestion of biopsy samples. A diffuse immunofluorescent staining for IgG and C3 was a regular finding in cells from rheumatoid subjects, but not from other joint diseases studied. In addition, cells from patients with rheumatoid factor had large cytoplasmic inclusions staining for IgM or anti-γ-globulins.[23,40]

RHEUMATOID FACTORS (ANTI-γ-GLOBULINS)

Those patients with rheumatoid arthritis and positive test results for theumatoid factor have a more severe form of the disease. No explanation for this altered prognosis has been provided by studies of circulating anti-γ-globulins. On the other hand, anti-γ-globulins appear to be intimately associated with rheumatoid joint inflammation. Conventional IgM rheumatoid factors have been demonstrated within synovial leukocytes,[10,19,39] and their presence in either cells or fluid can be related to the degree of depression of hemolytic complement[17,33,40] or the conversion of C3.[51] These observations prompted a reassessment of the ability of IgM rheumatoid factor to fix complement, since prior evidence suggested it fixed complement poorly, if at all.[50] A technical problem was the anti-complementary nature of aggregated IgG. This was overcome by reduction and alkylation of the gamma globulin prior to aggregation. In this way complement fixation by IgM rheumatoid factor could be demonstrated.[54] These findings have been confirmed with other antigen-antibody systems.[9,38]

As noted above, complexes of IgG and 7S anti-IgG fix complement. The addition of IgM rheumatoid factor to synovial fluid containing such complexes results in more complement fixation than occurs with the complexes alone.[47] IgM rheumatoid factor can convert soluble immune complexes to complement fixing aggregates.[38] This may explain the observation that while normal white blood cells suspended in joint fluid from subjects with seronegative rheumatoid arthritis seldom form leukocyte inclusions, the addition of purified IgM rheumatoid factor yields IgG, IgM, and C3 staining inclusions in more than half of the seronegative fluids studied.[20] Thus, rheumatoid factors may exaggerate the phlogistic properties of altered γ-globulin either by augmenting complement fixation, or by changing the size or solubility of the complexes, thereby enhancing their phagocytosis by leukocytes.

NEUTROPHILS AND LYSOSOMES

Rheumatoid synovial fluids contain large numbers of blood cells, predominantly neutrophilic leukocytes. The magnitude of this cellular response is not sufficiently appreciated until one considers that a knee joint with a 10 cc. effusion and 10,000 neutrophils/cu. mm. actually contains 100 million neutrophils. These cells have a 3 to 4 hr. half-life in the rheu-

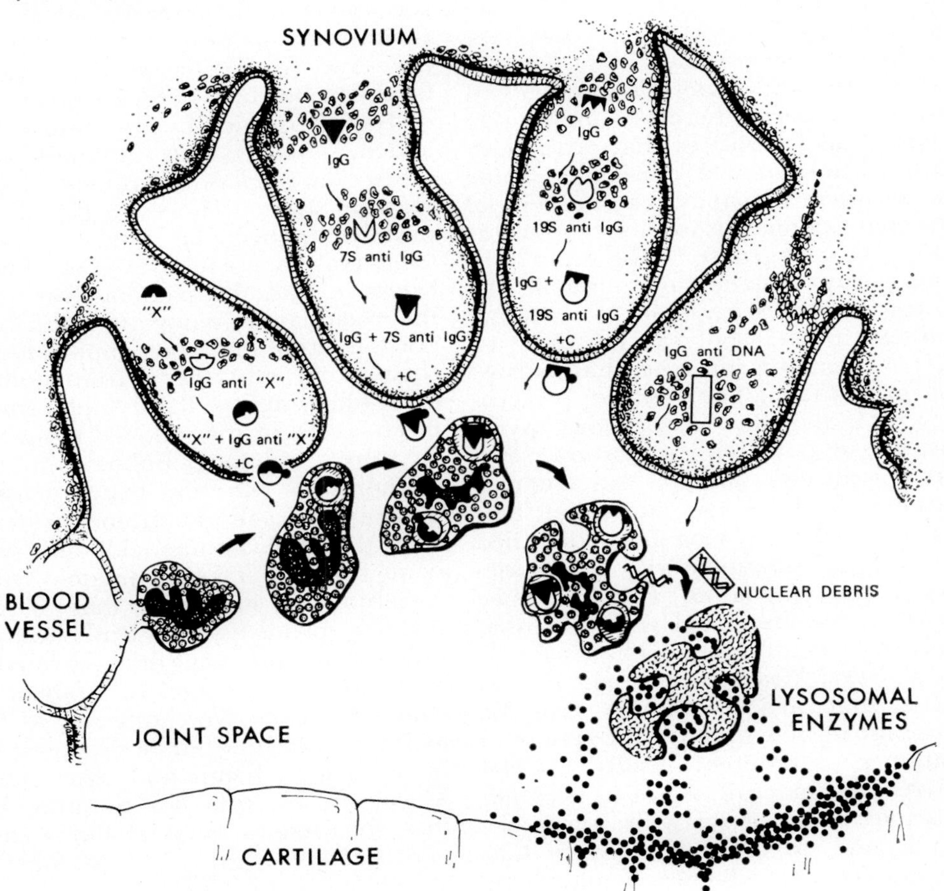

Fig. 19–1.—A schematic representation of some of the events in the pathogenesis of rheumatoid joint inflammation. Antibodies produced by lymphocytes and plasma cells of the synovial membrane are shown combining with antigens in the synovium *e.g.* locally produced IgG (▼), (▩) or an unknown antigen "x" (▲) or with antigens from the synovial fluid *e.g.* DNA (▲). Some or all of these complexes may fix and activate complement (●) causing the generation of a number of phlogistic and chemotactic substances. Ingestion of the complexes by polymorphonuclear leukocytes leads to vacuole formation, release of lysosomal constituents and cell death. The enzymes released from lysosomes can injure articular cartilage, and enhance pannus formation.

matoid joint.[4] Thus, in the example outlined, 50 million neutrophils would be entering the articular cavity six times daily to participate in the inflammatory response.

Tissue injury in experimental immune complex diseases is accomplished by the lysosomal enzymes discharged from polymorphonuclear leukocytes.[8] The release of hydrolytic enzymes is presumed to follow the phagocytosis of particulate material or immune complexes. There is abundant morphologic,[46] histochemical,[25] immunofluorescent,[19,39] and electron microscopic evidence[48] that the cells in rheumatoid effusions contain ingested matter. Similarly, there is a long catalog of lysosomal hydrolases that have been identified in synovial effusions. Some are of interest mainly as markers of lysosomal enzyme release; others, such as white cell collagenase,[24] the cathepsins which disrupt basement membranes,[8] the neutral proteases capable of cleaving cartilage protein-polysaccharide[44] or C5,[42] the cationic proteins that disrupt mast cells and induce vascular permeability,[21,44] and the endogenous pyrogens,[5] are all potentially important mediators of joint inflammation and articular destruction. It is not surprising that these same enzymes have been identified in a variety of inflammatory joint diseases other than rheumatoid arthritis, since almost all are associated with increased numbers of neutrophils. The *final common pathway hypothesis of joint diseases* implies that articular injury can be accomplished by lysosomes in response to a number of different insults.[43] The relative importance of lysosomal enzymes in various forms of synovitis will probably depend on the factors controlling their release, the influence of inhibitors, and the availability of appropriate substrates.

INTERRELATIONSHIP OF SYNOVIAL FLUID AND SYNOVIAL MEMBRANE

Despite an increasing appreciation of the variety of immunologic phenomena demonstrable in the effusions of patients with rheumatoid arthritis, there are some investigators who are still reluctant to ascribe profound significance to them. One view holds that, at best, immunologic reactions can only explain the joint inflammation in rheumatoid arthritis, but not the tissue destruction. A less charitable opinion is that the joint fluid is only a mirror reflecting the more important events occurring in the synovial membrane. Neither view gives sufficient cognizance to the interdependence of the rheumatoid pannus and the inflammatory exudate. For instance, normal joint fluid can be considered a simple plasma dialysate to which hyaluronate has been added. As articular inflammation increases more plasma proteins enter the synovial space. However, not all of the proteins in synovial fluid are derived from plasma. There is now abundant evidence that the mononuclear cells of the rheumatoid synovium contribute a portion of the immunoglobulins found in rheumatoid effusions. Immunofluorescent studies suggest that lymphocytes and plasma cells in the synovial villus make, or store, immunoglobulins and anti-γ-globulins.[6,27] *In vitro* experiments employing radiolabeled amino acids indicate that the immunoglobulin synthesizing capacity of the rheumatoid synovial membrane is similar to that of lymph nodes or splenic tissue.[37] Radioisotope dilution techniques have demonstrated that 12 to 24% of the IgG in synovial fluid comes from the synovium and as much as 100 mg. of IgG can be produced daily in a single rheumatoid knee joint.[36] Moreover, Kinsella has recently shown that rheumatoid synovial fluids can be blastogenic for, and cause transformation of, human lymphocytes.[22]

The data showing an effect of the inflammatory exudate on the synovial membrane are less direct, but nonetheless provocative. Weissmann and his coworkers produced all the classic morphologic changes of rheumatoid arthritis, *i.e.* hypertrophy and hyperplasia of synovial lining cells, round cell infiltration, pannus formation and cartilage degradation, in rabbit knee joints by the chronic intra-articular injection of lysates prepared from granules of rabbit heterophil leukocytes.[45] These authors have also speculated that lysosomal neutral proteases might act to hydrolyze repressor proteins present in the nuclei of synovial lining cells or fibroblasts. This would lead to augmented RNA and protein synthesis, and increased DNA synthesis and cell division. Extrapolating specifically to the collagenase which is found in small amounts in normal synovium, and is probably produced in synovial cells of mesenchymal origin,[15] it is possible to see how proteases in the inflammatory exudate might induce the formation of large amounts of this potentially important enzyme in the rheumatoid synovium.

The material summarized in this chapter clearly shows that antigen-antibody complexes are a regular feature of rheumatoid joint inflammation. Therefore, it is reasonable to propose that rheumatoid arthritis be added to the list of human "immune complex diseases." Information about the manner in which such complexes produce tissue injury is becoming quite definitive but knowledge of the antigens participating in their formation is limited. The detection of viral material in the lesions of certain types of human vasculitis (*see* Chapters 14 and 52) and of DNA-anti-DNA complexes in systemic lupus erythematosus (*see* Chapters 10 and 51) represents significant advances. Hopefully, the antigen (or antigens) which initiates the rheumatoid inflammatory reaction will soon be identified, thus opening the way to preventing or manipulating this disabling disease.

BIBLIOGRAPHY

1. Agnello, V., Winchester, R. J. and Kunkel, H. G.: Immunol., *19*, 909, 1970.
2. Barnett, E. V., Bluestone, R., Cracchiolo, A. *et al.*: Ann. Intern Med., *73*, 95, 1970.
3. Baumal, R. and Broder, T.: J. Clin. Exp. Immun., *3*, 555, 1968.
4. Bertino, J. R., Hollingsworth, J. W. and Cashmore, A. R.: Trans. Assoc. Amer. Physicians, *76*, 63, 1963.
5. Bodel, P. T. and Hollingsworth, J. W.: Brit. J. Exp. Path., *49*, 11, 1968.
6. Bonomo, L., Tursi, A., and Gillardi, U.: Ann. Rheum. Dis., *27*, 122, 1968.
7. Brandt, K. D., Cathcart, E. S., and Cohen, A. S.: J. Lab. Clin. Med., *72*, 631, 1968.
8. Cochrane, C. G.: Advances Immunol., *9*, 97, 1968.
9. Davis, J. S. and Noell, P.: Clin. Res., *18*, 82, 1970.
10. Delbarre, F., Kahan, A., Amor, B. *et al.*: Path. Biol. (Paris) *14*, 796, 1966.
11. Elling, P.: Ann. Rheum. Dis., *27*, 225, 1968.
12. Fish, A. J., Michael, R. F., Gewurz, H. *et al.*: Arth. & Rheum., *9*, 267, 1966.
13. Glynn, L. E.: Ann. Rheum. Dis., *27*, 105, 1968.
14. Hannestad, K.: Clin. Exp. Immun., *2*, 511, 1967.
15. Harris, E. D., Evanson, J. M., DiBona, D. R. *et al.*: Arth. & Rheum., *13*, 83, 1970.
16. Hedberg, H.: Acta Rheum. Scand., *10*, 109, 1964.
17. ———: Acta Med. Scand. (Suppl.), 479, 1967.
18. Hollander, J. L., Fudenberg, H. H., Rawson, A. J. *et al.*: Arth. & Rheum., *9*, 675, 1966.
19. Hollander, J. L., McCarty, D. J., Astorga, G. *et al.*: Ann. Intern. Med., *62*, 271, 1965.
20. Hurd, E. R., LoSpalluto, J. and Ziff, M.: Arth. & Rheum., *13*, 724, 1970.
21. Janoff, A., Schaeffer, S., Scherer, J. *et al.*: J. Exp. Med., *122*, 841, 1965.
22. Kinsella, T. D.: Arth. & Rheum., *13*, 328, 1970.
23. Kinsella, T. D., Baum, J. and Ziff, M.: Arth. & Rheum., *13*, 734, 1970.
24. Lazarus, G. S., Daniels, J. R., Brown, R. S. *et al.*: J. Clin. Invest., *47*, 2622, 1968.
25. Malinin, T. I., Pekin, T. J. and Zvaifler, N. J.: Amer. J. Clin. Path., *47*, 203, 1967.
26. Marcus, R. L. and Townes, A. S.: J. Clin. Invest., *50*, 282, 1971.
27. Mellors, R. C., Heimer, R., Corcos, J. *et al.*: J. Exp. Med., *110*, 875, 1959.
28. Muller-Eberhard, H.: Advances Immun., *8*, 1, 1967.
29. Pekin, T. J. and Zvaifler, N. J.: J. Clin. Invest., *43*, 1372, 1964.
30. Rawson, A. J. and Torralba, T. P.: Arth. & Rheum., *10*, 44, 1967.
31. Restifo, R. A., Lussier, A. J., Rawson, A. J. *et al.*: Ann. Intern. Med., *62*, 285, 1965.

32. Rodman, W. S., Williams, R. C., Bilka, P. J. *et al.*: J. Lab. Clin. Med., *69*, 141, 1967.
33. Ruddy, S. and Austen, K. F.: Arth. & Rheum., *13*, 713, 1970.
34. Runge, L. A. and Mills, J. A.: Arth. & Rheum., *12*, 694, 1969.
35. Sliwinski, A. J. and Zvfailer, N. J.: Arth. & Rheum., *12*, 504, 1969.
36. Sliwinski, A. J. and Zvaifler, N. J.: J. Lab. Clin. Med., *76*, 304, 1970.
37. Smiley, J. D., Sachs, C. and Ziff, M.: J. Clin. Invest., *47*, 624, 1968.
38. Tesar, J. T. and Schmid, F. R.: J. Immunol., *105*, 1206, 1970.
39. Vaughan, J. H., Barnett, E. V., Sobel, M. V. *et al.*: Arth. & Rheum., *11*, 125, 1968.
40. Vaughan, J. H., Jacox, R. F. and Noell, P.: Arth. & Rheum., *11*, 135, 1968.
41. Ward, P. A.: Arth. & Rheum., *13*, 181, 1970.
42. Ward, P. A. and Zvaifler, N. J.: J. Clin. Invest., *50*, 606, 1971.
43. Weissmann, G.: Arth. & Rheum., *9*, 834, 1966.
44. Weissmann, G. and Spilberg, I.: Arth. & Rheum., *11*, 162, 1968.
45. Weissmann, G., Spilberg, I. and Krakauer, K.: Arth. & Rheum., *12*, 103, 1969.
46. Williamson, N. and Ling, N. R.: Ann. Rheum. Dis., *24*, 513, 1965.
47. Winchester, R. J., Agnello, V. and Kunkel, H. G.: Ann. N. Y. Acad. Sci., *168*, 195, 1969.
48. Zucker-Franklin, D.: Arth. & Rheum., *9*, 24, 1966.
49. Zvaifler, N. J.: Arth. & Rheum., *8*, 289, 1965.
50. ———: Ann. N. Y. Acad. Sci., *168*, 146, 1969.
51. ———: J. Clin. Invest., *48*, 1532, 1969.
52. Zvaifler, N. J. and Martinez, M. M.: Clin. Exp. Immun., *8*, 271, 1970.
53. Zvaifler, N. J. and Pekin, T. J.: Clin. Res., *11*, 180, 1963.
54. Zvaifler, N. J. and Schur, P.: Arth. & Rheum., *11*, 523, 1968.

Chapter 20

The Pathology of Rheumatoid Arthritis and Allied Disorders

By Leon Sokoloff, M.D.

INTRODUCTION

The principal lesions of rheumatoid arthritis are found in the diarthrodial joints and, to a lesser extent, the related tissues—tendons and their sheaths, bursae and periarticular subcutaneous tissue. Systemic manifestations have been the subject of much study during the past two decades. The name "rheumatoid disease" rather than "rheumatoid arthritis" has sometimes been recommended to take account of these. While extra-articular lesions undoubtedly occur, they should not be exaggerated; they are far less frequent and severe than in the articular tissues.

Several excellent descriptions of the long-standing joint changes have been published.[22] Our knowledge of the morbid anatomy of rheumatoid arthritis is limited by a number of factors. The chronicity of the disease in most cases makes tissue available for study only in its late stages. The lesions often lack histologic specificity and vary from site to site within the joints.[24] The structures principally affected are frequently not accessible to the pathologist. For these reasons, intensive study of biopsy material obtained early in the course of the illness has provided certain insights into the histogenesis of the lesions that have not been possible on postmortem examination.

ARTICULAR LESIONS OF RHEUMATOID ARTHRITIS

All present evidence indicates that the joint changes have their inception in the synovial tissue. Despite similarities in the character of the synovitis to that of infectious conditions, and also despite the fact that subchondral involvement of the bone may be prominent in rheumatoid arthritis, there is no basis for believing that the synovial inflammation follows an initial seeding of the adjacent bone marrow as it commonly does in hematogenous, infectious arthritis.

Synovitis

The microscopic appearance of the synovial tissue is highly variable, depending on the location, duration and recurrent character of the inflammation. Three pathologic elements, although integrally related and continuous, should be distinguished:

1. *Exudation.*—Congestion and edema are most marked at the internal surface of the synovium, particularly close to margins of the articular cartilage (circulus vasculosus), and have their counterpart in effusion into the joint space. In focal areas of desquamation of synovial lining cells and of necrosis of the superficial synovial tissue, compact fibrin exudes onto the surface and, to an extent, into the swollen tissues.

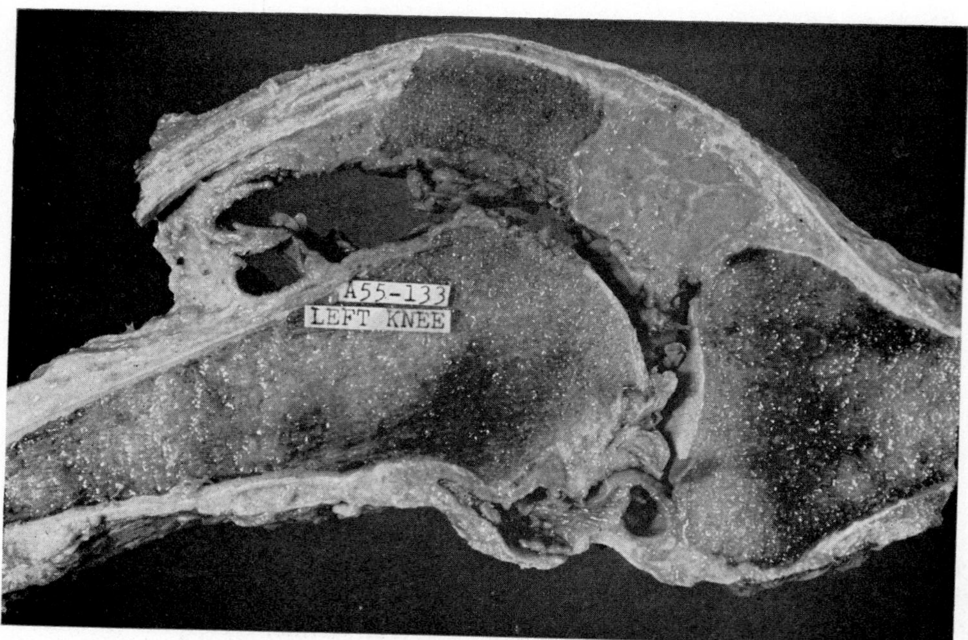

Fig. 20–1.—Sagittal section of knee, rheumatoid arthritis. Markedly thickened, villous synovial tissue is seen in the suprapatellar pouch. A small Baker's cyst protrudes from the popliteal surface. A papillary pannus has completely replaced the articular cartilage of the patella and smaller segments on the femur and tibia. The dark portions of the marrow of the femur and tibia are areas of congestion and osteitis.

2. *Cellular Infiltration.*—Small numbers of polymorphonuclear leukocytes emigrate with edema fluid. Foci of necrosis and purulent exudation are seen at times in older lesions, and secondary infection need not be invoked on this score.

The principal infiltrating cell, particularly in early lesions, is a small lymphocyte. It is distributed in two patterns in the superficial portions of the synovium: diffusely and in small, nodular aggregates. These cells may or may not be arranged about small blood vessels. The nodular aggregates, sometimes called Allison-Ghormley nodules, characteristically lack the reticular framework of lymphoid nodules. In long-standing lesions, however, true lymphoid follicles, with germinal centers, are not rare (Fig. 20–2).

In late cases, a large proportion or majority of the infiltrating cells are plasma cells. When aggregated gamma globulin is labeled with fluorescent dye and used to stain the synovial tissue by the Coons immunochemical technique, it is found principally in the cytoplasm of the plasma cells. This indicates that these cells are the site of production of the rheumatoid factor.[54,55,69] Rheumatoid factor may be preserved in formalin-fixed tissues provided that low melting point paraffin is used for embedding,[11] but fresh frozen blocks are preferable. By doubly labeling the antibody with ferritin as well as fluorescein, rheumatoid factors can also be identified in electron-microscopic preparations.[18] Areas of old hemorrhage are quite common in synovectomy specimens, as evidenced by deposition of hemosiderin[64] and, sometimes, by the presence of foam cells.

Multinucleated giant cells are not common, but two types are seen at times.[37] One is an ovoid pleomorphic cell, close to the synovial lining. It has 3 to 8 peripheral nuclei and a somewhat baso-

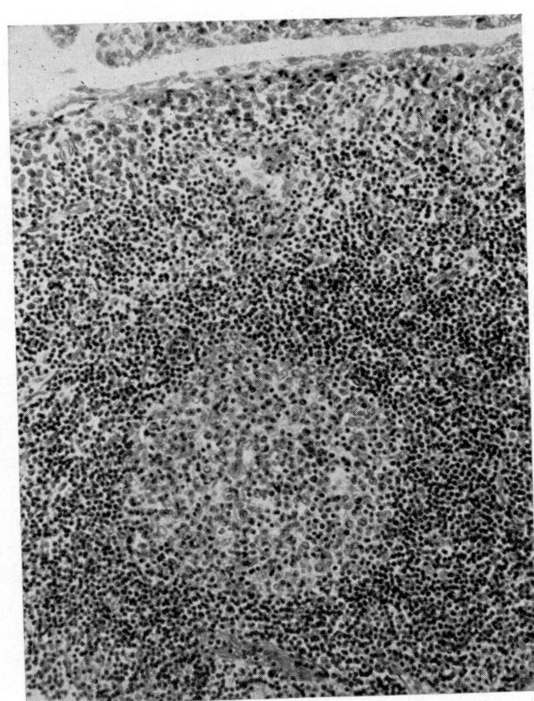

FIG. 20–2.—Chronic synovitis, long-standing rheumatoid arthritis. In addition to the usual diffuse infiltration of chronic inflammatory cells into the synovial tissue, a true lymphoid follicle with a germinal center is present. The larger cells, subjacent to the swollen synovial lining, are plasma cells. (Hematoxylin and eosin, × 182.)

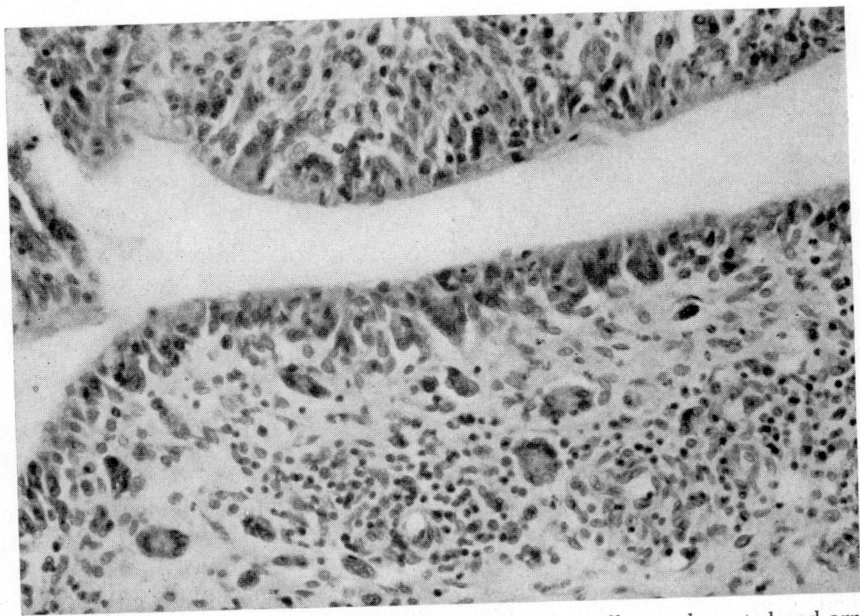

FIG. 20–3.—Synovitis in rheumatoid arthritis. Synovial lining cells are elongated and arranged in a palisade radial to the surface. Some of the lining cells appear multinucleated and similar giant cells are located at a slight distance from them. (Hematoxylin and eosin, × 234.)

philic cytoplasm similar to those of synovial lining cells (Fig. 20–3). The other type of multinucleated cell is a foreign body phagocyte related to bone and cartilage detritus.

3. *Granulation Tissue.*—Proliferation of blood vessels and of synovial fibroblasts is most marked in areas of cellular infiltration. This is accompanied by multiplication and enlargement of synovial lining cells. In places, the lining cells become markedly elongated and are oriented in a closely arranged palisade perpendicular to the surface.

As a result of these three processes, the synovial tissue becomes grossly thickened. The hypertrophy has a villous character that is most marked near the joint cartilages. The papillary fronds may reach an inch in height and are approximately 1 to 2 mm. in diameter (Fig. 20–1). They may or may not adhere to each other. The oxygen uptake, glucose utilization and lactate production of the tissue are greatly increased as a result of the proliferation of granulation tissue and also the infiltration of inflammatory cells.[27,28] The high metabolic activity has, presumably, as its morphologic counterpart, several increased histochemical diaphorase activities located in the proliferating lining cells.[38] The electronmicroscopic appearance and the enlargement of the ergastoplasm of these cells also may be interpreted as evidence of increased synthetic activity.[5,38]

It should be emphasized that these changes, although typically present in rheumatoid arthritis, are lacking in histologic specificity. Indistinguishable changes may be seen in unrelated disorders in man[86] and other species.[89]

Subchondral Bone

An inflammatory reaction is commonly found in the epiphyseal bone. Its histologic character is quite similar to that in synovial tissue, although numbers of osteoclasts are sometimes present. The subchondral granulation tissue is continuous with that in the synovium, through defects in the cortex of the bone near the joint. These defects are presumed to have originally been normal vascular foramina, but are greatly enlarged by osteitis. Grossly, the marrow appears congested in these areas. The bone undergoes irregular osteolysis and this accounts for the loss of radio-opacity in the para-articular tissues. In juveniles, the osteitis may extend into the epiphyseal plate; in such instances bone growth is retarded (*rheumatic dwarfism*). Sizable cyst-like areas of bone destruction may be present (Fig. 20–4). The articular cortex also is involved by the osteolysis. Side by side with the osteolysis, new bone formation occurs and remodeling of the bone progresses under the direction of mechanical forces acting on the joint. In phalanges, "periostitis" is frequently described as part of rheumatoid arthritis. This is not, strictly speaking, accurate. The synovial recesses in the phalanges are frequently large and extend for a long distance proximally on the bone shafts. In such instances, the synovitis may evoke new bone formation in the immediately adjacent cortex. Nevertheless, periostitis, unrelated to synovitis, is not characteristic of rheumatoid arthritis and thereby distinguishes it from Reiter's disease and from infectious arthritides.

Articular Cartilage

The articular cartilage is relatively resistant to inflammatory lysis. Its surface is involved by extension of the inflammatory process from the adjacent synovium; the granulation tissue that forms a covering mantle is known as a *pannus* (Fig. 20–1). Like the hypertrophic synovitis, pannus formation is not a specific feature of rheumatoid arthritis. Concurrent with the ingrowth of the pannus and the subchondral granulation tissue, the articular cartilage disappears. The precise mechanism for this is unknown. Immediately adjacent chondrocytes may be necrotic. Whether granulations *per se* cause the cartilage destruc-

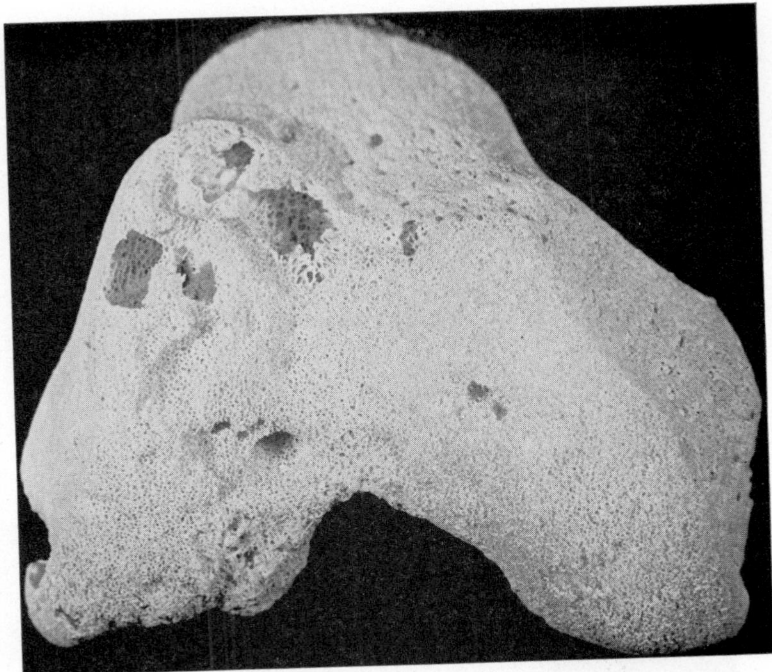

Fig. 20–4.—Advanced destruction of articular cortex of distal femur, rheumatoid arthritis. What appear to be cystic spaces and pores in this macerated preparation are occupied *in vivo* by granulation tissue in the subchondral marrow and adhesions in the joint cavity.

tion or represent a concomitant to an exudative, chondrolytic inflammation is unknown. The vascularity, it has been suggested, may allow leaching out of cartilage matrix that normally retains its integrity by being avascular. Other views are that the pannus may impede the normal, nourishing percolation of interstitial fluid in the tissue. Several different enzymatic mechanisms have been proposed for chondrolysis. These include a protease derived from polymorphonuclear leukocytes,[104] plasmin[47] and cathepsins, accompanying acid phosphatase produced in synovial lining cells.[5] Pannus formation is most marked at the vascular margins of the joint surfaces. In joints which retain active use, pannus is not usually well preserved, presumably be-because of abrasion. Indeed, secondary osteoarthritic changes are commonly seen in long-standing lesions of this sort.

Ankylosis

The granulation tissue may form adhesions and undergo cicatrization. The newly formed articular connective tissue has a pluripotential capacity for maturation. It may variously undergo metaplasia into synovial tissue, fibrous or hyaline cartilage or bone; the adhesive bands may thereby cause fibrous, cartilaginous or bony ankylosis (Fig. 20–5).

Joint Deformities

Several factors contribute to the deformities of the joints in rheumatoid arthritis. Most important of these is the inflammatory destruction and remodeling of the articulating surfaces under the influence of the mechanical forces of muscle pull. These may lead to subluxation (Fig. 20–7). Weakening of capsular and ligamentous supports by

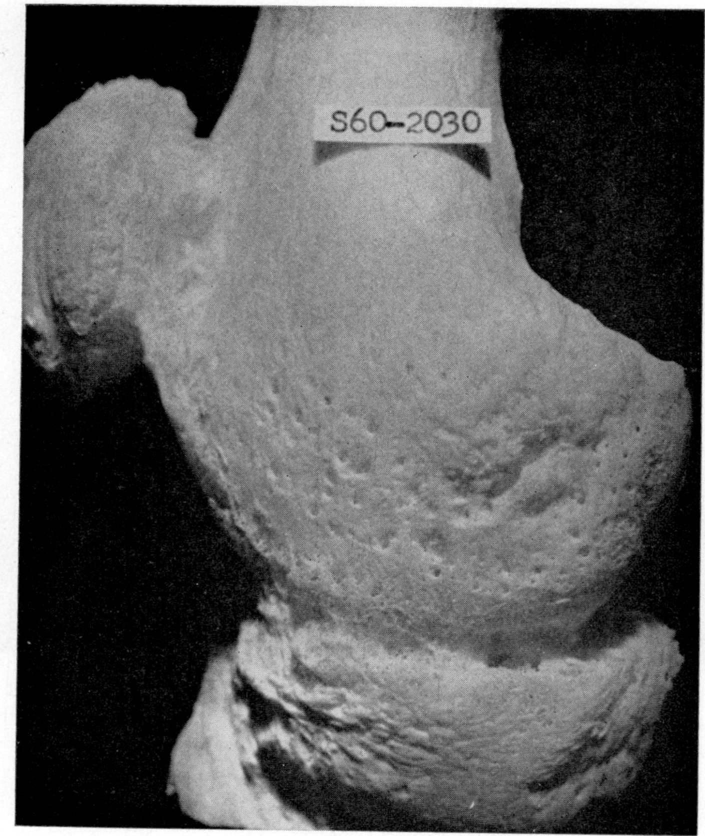

Fig. 20–5.—Bony ankylosis of knee, rheumatoid arthritis. A bridge of bone unites the patella to the femur, and the condyles of the femur and tibial plateau to each other.

the inflammation may be of considerable importance, particularly in small joints where these tissues are in close proximity to the synovium.[95] Tendon contractures and ruptures also are an important element in finger and toe deformities (Fig. 20–6).

VERTEBRAL LESIONS

In rheumatoid arthritis, involvement of cervical vertebrae has been recognized increasingly.[12] Both the diarthrodial (apophyseal) joints and intervertebral discs have been affected; sometimes there has been extensive destruction of spinal ligaments as well. Ball[10] observed the destruction of the annulus fibrosus to proceed with formation of granulation tissue from synovitis of the neurocentral (Luschka) joints in 17 of 18 unselected cases. Instances of cervical rheumatoid arthritis with little or no peripheral joint involvement have been reported. The inflammatory changes have been like those described below in the tendons and ligaments of the peripheral joints.[2] They result in subluxation at times, and may lead to neurological defects or occasionally sudden death. Apophyseal joint involvement in rheumatoid arthritis also occurs in the lumbar region, but is less frequent and severe than in the cervical region.[48]

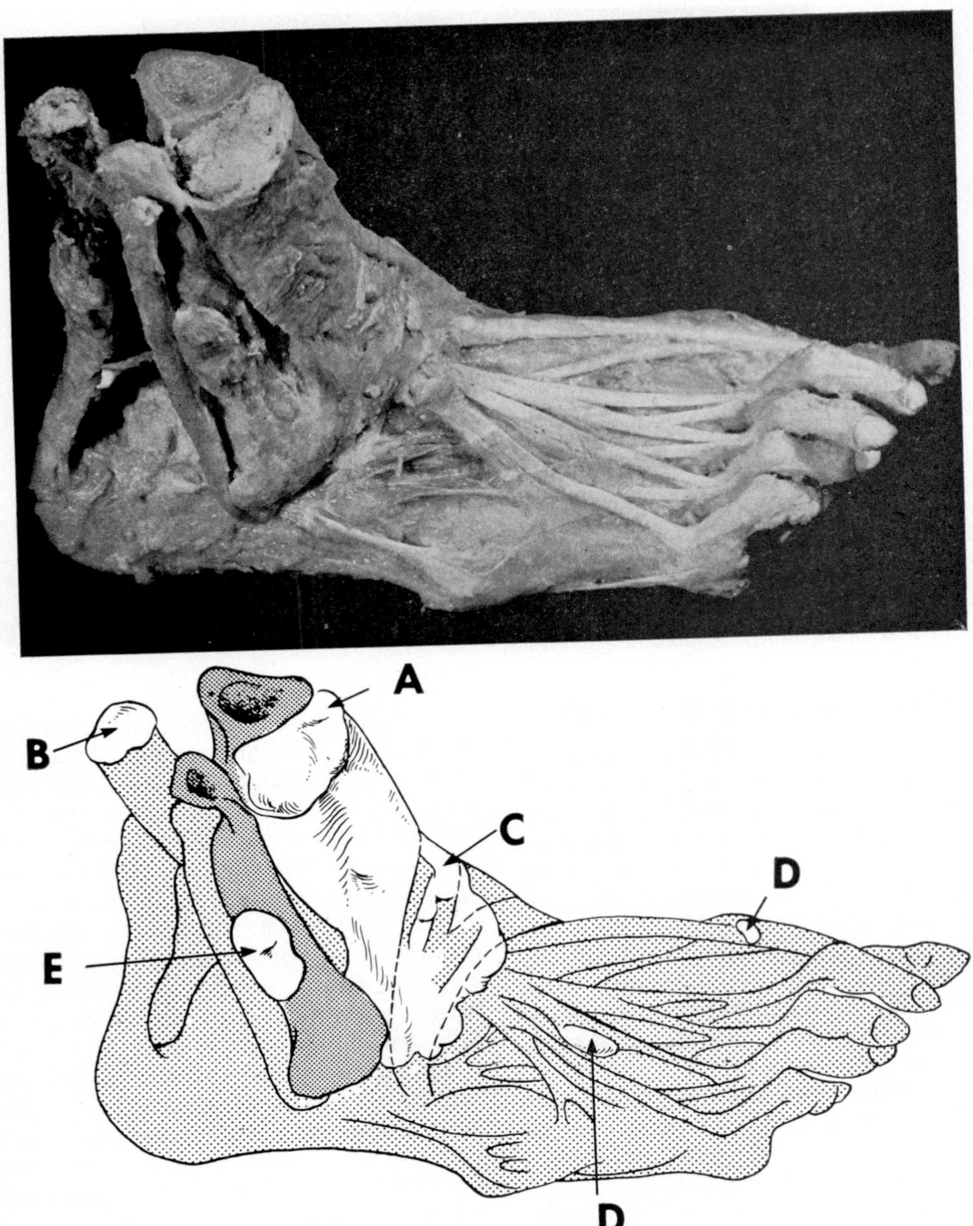

Fig. 20–6.—Tendon and tendon sheath involvement in rheumatoid arthritis. White grumous exudate occupies the substance and sheaths of the anterior tibial and extensor digitorum tendons (*A*), and the Achilles tendon (*B*). The inferior extensor retinaculum (*C*) is irregularly infiltrated and nodules are also present in the extensor tendons of the foot (*D*). The surface of the tendons is irregular and dull because of inflammatory adhesions. The changes are responsible for the cock-up deformities of the toes. A subcutaneous nodule (*E*) adheres to the periosteum of the fibula immediately anterior to the peroneus longus tendon.

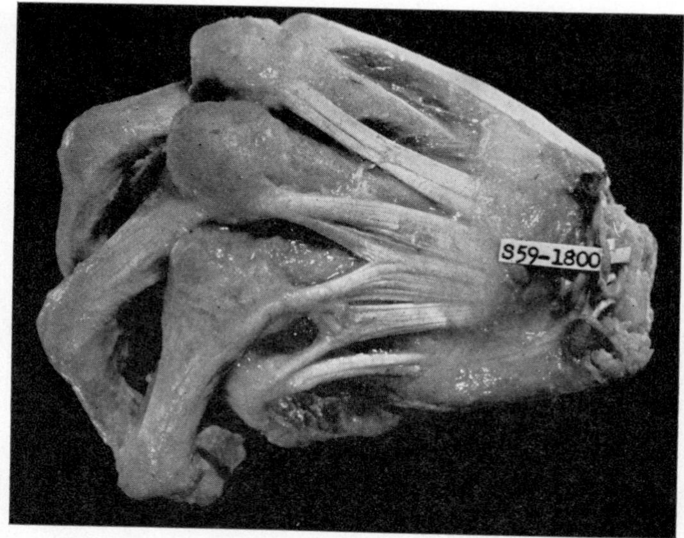

Fig. 20–7.—Characteristic knuckle deformities, rheumatoid arthritis. The proximal phalanges are subluxated beneath the metacarpal heads. The tendons are displaced from their normal position over the center of the joint in association with the ulnar deviation of the fingers. There is, however, no gross inflammatory change in the tendons, unlike Figure 20–6.

SUBCUTANEOUS NODULES

In approximately 1 of 5 patients with peripheral rheumatoid arthritis, chronic inflammatory nodules develop in para-articular subcutaneous tissue. They are most common over the olecranon process of the ulna. Less frequently they are found on the extensor aspects of the finger joints. Foot involvement is still less frequent, but the subcutaneous tissue may be affected in many areas subject to mechanical pressure, including the occipital region.

Subcutaneous nodules in rheumatoid arthritis are usually larger than in rheumatic fever and may achieve a diameter of several centimeters. Large nodules are tough, lobulated and multicentric. They are not encapsulated and cannot be sharply dissected from underlying articular tissue, bursa or periosteum. Geographic areas of necrosis are recognized by their yellow color because lipochrome pigments accompany large amounts of lipid (neutral fat, cholesterol and phospholipids) in the necrotic material.

The histologic appearance of a well-developed subcutaneous nodule is quite characteristic. It resembles many infectious or foreign body granulomata in having three distinct zones: central areas of necrosis of subcutaneous fibrous and granulation tissue; a palisade of elongated, connective tissue cells arranged radially in a corona about the necrotic zone; and an enveloping granulation tissue in which chronic inflammatory cells are distributed (Fig. 20–8).

The necrotic centers have, to a varying extent, a "*fibrinoid*" appearance. This term should not be understood to indicate a specific compound, a single pathogenetic significance, or identity with pathologic materials in other rheumatic or non-rheumatic disorders. It is a histologic term, and simply describes the necrotic material as being oxyphilic, somewhat refractive and reacting as fibrin does rather than as collagen does with certain stains, *viz.* Van Gieson, Masson, phosphotungstic acid-hematoxylin and Gram stains. The composition of the necrotic material in the rheumatoid nodule varies

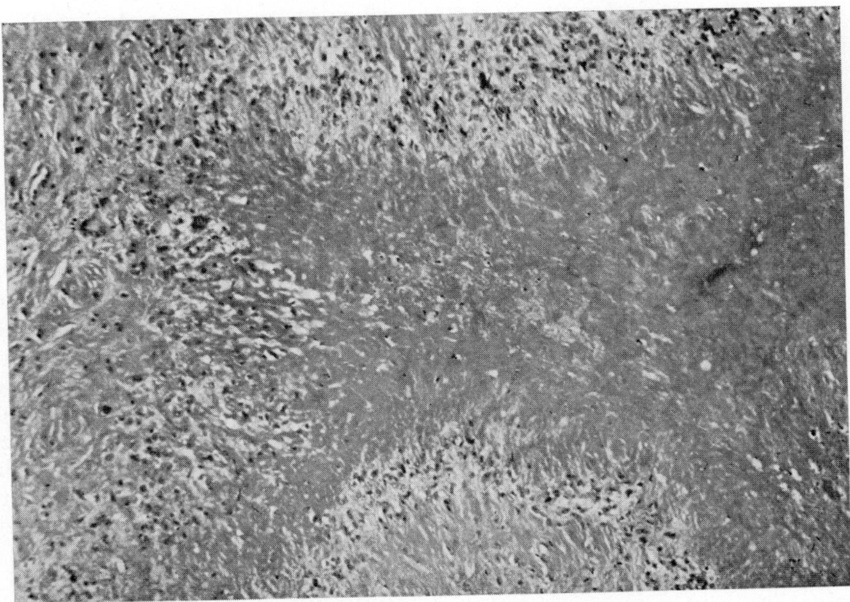

FIG. 20–8.—Subcutaneous nodule of rheumatoid arthritis. Although this is a long-standing lesion, the presence of nuclear fragments in the "fibrinoid" central zone is presumptive evidence of recent necrosis. (Hematoxylin and eosin, × 95.)

as the lesion progresses or burns out. It contains collagen, lipids, nucleoproteins, acid mucopolysaccharides, serum proteins, including immunoglobulins,[34,70] and, in certain active states, material that probably is fibrin.[21,62,63] The fibrin-like component is most prominent in active or youthful lesions. The lipid material may persist in an otherwise semifluid center of the nodule, converting it to a bursa-like or cystic structure. Unlike many types of persistent, lipid-rich necrotic debris, calcification of rheumatoid nodules is rare.

The precise nature of the cells in the marginal palisade has not been established.[21,33] Although the cells to a certain degree resemble and sometimes are called epithelioid cells (as in tuberculoid granulomas), cytologic studies[65] have failed to demonstrate the phagocytic activity against neutral red characteristic of such cells. Electron microscopically, however, studies[67] show that there are macrophage-like cells, capable of taking up colloidal gold, both in the palisades and proliferating granulation tissue of the subcutaneous nodule and also in the synovial lining. Histochemically, lysosome activity, as demonstrated by acid-phosphatase stains, and indicative of a histiocytic nature, has been demonstrated in them. Stain for aminopeptidase has demonstrated proteolytic enzyme activity in relation to areas of fibrinoid exudation.[35] Cytoplasmic fat droplets may abound in the palisaded cells and also be present in the adjacent necrotic tissue. Whether the droplets reflect the phagocytosis of lipid, derived from the blood stream or ground substance, or are products of the cells has not been established. Multinucleated giant cells, occasionally seen in such areas, however, are usually of Touton type and presumably are lipophages. The cells assume their radial arrangement because their axes are oriented against the fibers entering the zones of necrosis.

The enveloping granulation tissue is highly vascular in its early stages, and ultimately cicatrizes. Lymphocytes and smaller numbers of plasma cells are disposed about some of the peripheral venules. In the proliferating areas of vascularity, the perivascular cells are primarily plump fibroblasts and mononuclear cells. Scattered eosinophils may be present in the earliest lesions.

This granuloma-like appearance of the subcutaneous nodule of rheumatoid arthritis is quite different from that described in the joints. Making due allowance for the fact that such nodules can at times be confused diagnostically with tuberculous and other lesions such as necrobiosis lipoidica and granuloma annulare[103] and also for the fact that nodules may appear in advance of the articular manifestations of the disease, it remains true that para-articular lesions of this sort occur at times in individuals who have no evidence of any rheumatic disease. These idiopathic subcutaneous nodules present a spectrum of appearances, including some which resemble those of rheumatic fever; some, rheumatoid arthritis and some, granuloma annulare.[50,56]

In the early phases of its development, the appearance of the subcutaneous nodule is quite different from that seen in the older lesion. This is discussed more fully in the section on pathology and pathogenesis.

TENDONS AND LIGAMENTS

The tendons and articular ligaments are involved pathologically with considerable, though undetermined, frequency. The inflammatory process may be of non-specific sort in which lymphocytes, mononuclear and a few plasma cells infiltrate the bundles of collagen.[42] In severe instances, however, focal areas of "fibrinoid" necrosis develop and the lesion may be identical to that of the subcutaneous nodule. The nodular areas are at times palpable grossly (Fig. 20–6). Ruptures may take place in such areas of necrosis.[30] Where the tendons lie in sheaths, the tendinitis is accompanied by tenosynovitis. The ruptures and adhesions of the tendons to each other and adjacent tissue are an integral part of the development of joint deformities in many instances.

STRIATED MUSCLE

The skeletal muscle in severe cases of rheumatoid arthritis frequently has the histologic appearances of disuse atrophy. There is an irregular diminution in the circumference of the fibers, and a corresponding condensation of sarcolemmal nuclei. In approximately two of every three cases, scattered focal compact aggregates of chronic inflammatory cells, principally lymphocytes, are seen about venules in endomysium or perimysium. The lesion is lacking in diagnostic specificity, but is more frequent in rheumatoid arthritis and its variants than in non-rheumatic disorders.[94] Unlike dermatomyositis, necrosis and regenerative activity are not conspicuous in the muscle in rheumatoid arthritis.

PERIPHERAL NERVES

Perivascular aggregates of lymphocytes and mononuclear cells, comparable to those of striated muscle, are also present in the endoneurium and perineurium of peripheral nerves. Myelin and axon changes are not present unless there is complicating arterial disease. Other than minute perivascular cellular infiltrates, lesions have not been seen in conventional sections of the sympathetic ganglia.

ARTERIES

Arterial lesions of varying severity and character have been recognized in numerous studies of rheumatoid arthritis; there is no unanimity as to their significance.[91] Several anatomic facts appear reasonably agreed upon: the arteritis affects principally small segments of terminal arteries, 35 to 40 microns in external diameter; the lesions are chronic and lack distinctive histologic characteristics; and, although they may occur in many areas, the principal sites of involvement are the peripheral nerves and skeletal muscle. At one end of the spectrum of vascular lesions is the non-necrotizing, segmental arteritis of striated muscle that can be detected only after extensive serial sections have been made. This has been demonstrated in approximately 10 per cent of unselected cases. At the other, is a fulminant systemic disease that is difficult to distinguish from polyarteritis nodosa (PAN), either on clinical or on anatomic grounds. The latter is by far less usual.

Among the hypotheses entertained about the nature of the arteritis is that it results from treatment of rheumatoid arthritis with corticosteroid hormones. This view is based on the greater frequency with which peripheral neuropathy and cutaneous gangrene are now observed than in past years, and by the greater number of instances of arteritis seen at autopsy. It also is predicated in part on the experimental demonstration that several types of vascular damage are potentiated by the hormonal preparations. Corticosteroid therapy of other than rheumatic disorders has on rare occasions also been reported complicated by necrotizing arteritis.[88] Arteritis unquestionably is seen at times in patients with rheumatoid arthritis who have never received such compounds. There is a widespread belief that this therapy has increased the development of these changes. Inasmuch as this mode of therapy is so widely employed and tissues are not readily available for histological examination in asymptomatic cases, the magnitude of the increased frequency is difficult to estimate.

Another view is that the arteritis is a form of PAN, that reflects anaphylactic hypersensitivity sometimes postulated to underlie the development of rheumatoid arthritis.[80] There are, however, several important differences between the usual vascular lesions of rheumatoid arthritis and those of PAN. In rheumatoid arthritis, the lesions are usually mild, few and affect minute vessels. In PAN, the arteritis is a widespread lesion, in which medium-sized arteries, rather than small ones, are involved. Obliteration of the lumen or ectasia and rupture are characteristic of PAN. The prognosis of PAN is ominous, whereas the vascular lesions of rheumatoid arthritis have been known to exist for many years without causing detectable symptoms. In PAN, cutaneous gangrene of the extremities is most unusual, whereas it is relatively frequent in rheumatoid arthritis when corticosteroid therapy has been employed. Parenthetically, it should be pointed out that the nosologic status of PAN is also uncertain. Whether it is a single disorder or always the result of anaphylactic hypersensitivity appears questionable to some authorities.

The most satisfactory concept to this reviewer is that the vasculitis is a specific manifestation of rheumatoid arthritis, sharing etiologic or pathogenetic factors with the joint disease and mediating the development of the latter. This view is based on the observation that vasculitis is an intrinsic part of the development of the granuloma-like subcutaneous nodules. In the early nodule, the important histologic processes are exudation of fibrin-rich edema fluid into subcutaneous fibrous tissue, formation of highly vascular granulation tissue[33,91] that is soon accompanied by proliferation of plump fibroblasts (and apparently also macrophages[67]), and by necrosis of small arteries and more minute blood vessels.[21] The exudation and necrosis proceed centrifugally about the nodular buds of granulation tissue. These foci eventually coalesce to form the characteristic necrotic centers of the mature nodules. Kulka has emphasized the venular rather than terminal arterial disturbances in the genesis of the lesions.[44,45]

Clinically manifest arteritis is frequently associated with high titers of rheumatoid factor and also with the presence of subcutaneous nodules. The arteritis in peripheral nerves is the usual cause of the peripheral neuropathy that sometimes complicates rheumatoid arthritis.

HEART

Most clinical studies of heart disease in rheumatoid arthritis have noted cardiac abnormalities to be uncommon; anatomic investigations, by contrast, have demonstrated frequent lesions of several sorts.

Rheumatic Heart Disease

Although rheumatic heart disease was reported in many older postmortem studies to occur in from 21 to 66 per cent of patients, most recent papers have placed the figure, exclusive of calcareous aortic stenosis, at 6 to 10 per cent. There are several reasons for the lack of consistency in the findings. The anatomic criteria for the differential diagnosis of rheumatic heart disease are imprecise in part; in addition, complicated statistical biases have been hidden in the specimen material available for such studies.[52]

Calcareous Aortic Stenosis

Whether all instances of this condition are the result of rheumatic inflammation has not been resolved to the satisfaction of all students. As in the acceptable rheumatic valvular lesions, the frequency of this abnormality also was greater in several studies of rheumatoid arthritis patients than in controls.

Rheumatoid Heart Disease

Lesions that resemble the granuloma-like process of the subcutaneous nodules to a greater or lesser extent occur at times in the valve leaflets, valve rings, myocardium or epicardium in patients with peripheral rheumatoid arthritis. Although there is considerable variation in the histologic appearance, the active lesions differ from those of infectious or rheumatic carditis.[3] Their frequency is difficult to estimate, but has been reported in various series as 2 of 19, 7 of 36, 5 of 100 and 10 of 43 necropsies.[92] They appear to have been confined to the left side of the heart. Clinically, some have been silent; others have produced valvular insufficiency, heart block, Adams-Stokes syndrome and congestive heart failure. The granuloma-like lesions may co-exist with pericarditis, coronary arteritis and interstitial myocarditis—three other frequent findings that may individually be morphologically nonspecific, but lacking in other explanations than the rheumatoid disease. In the pathological diagnosis of any given case, co-existing systemic lupus erythematosus may loom as a possibility. The end result of burned-out lesions may be similar to those of rheumatic heart disease and thereby account for some of the high frequency of rheumatic heart disease sometimes reported in rheumatoid arthritis.

Idiopathic Pericarditis

Virtually all necropsy studies have demonstrated remote or sometimes active pericarditis in approximately 40 per cent of cases of rheumatoid arthritis. Usually, this has been manifested by fibrous obliteration of the pericardial cavity. Infrequently, the lesion has had a granuloma-like character resembling that of the rheumatoid nodule or synovial lesion. It is only the frequency of the association with the arthritis that supports the rheumatoid nature of the process. Significant clinical consequences are recognized only infrequently.[43] They may include pericardial constriction that may respond to pericardiotomy, fatal hemopericardium and pericardial effusion.

Interstitial Myocarditis

In addition to the occasional granuloma-like nodules already noted in the myocardium, small infarcts secondary to coronary arteritis have been observed on rare occasions, some surrounded by a palisade of elongated cells, and some not. More often, however, focal idiopathic, non-specific interstitial myocarditis is seen. When extensive, the process is indistinguishable from Fiedler's myocarditis. In some instances, the leukocytic infiltrate included many eosinophils. Whether allergic or other drug toxicity or viral infection complicating corticosteroid therapy may have been the etiological basis of some cases of the myocarditis, rather than the rheumatoid disease, cannot be ascertained in the absence of appropriate differential diagnostic tests.

Coronary Arteritis

Coronary arteritis, affecting scattered small vessels, is an occasional finding by this reviewer; it has been more frequent in the experience of others. It has been associated with disseminated arteritis in other sites—splanchnic and extremities. As in the case of the peripheral arteritis, it is conceivable that some of the variation in the amount of coronary involvement in different laboratories may be influenced by the different therapeutic regimens employed.

Aortic Insufficiency

In ankylosing spondylitis, an apparently specific form of aortic valve insufficiency has been recorded. This lesion has gross similarities to those of syphilis insofar as the principal changes are related to the gross destruction of the elastic tissue of the root of the aorta and the adjacent aortic valve ring. They differ from syphilitic aortitis in being confined to the root and not affecting the ascending portion of the aorta. The commissures of the valve are separated and the edges of the leaflets rolled toward the ventricular cavity as a result of the regurgitation. This lesion does not occur in peripheral rheumatoid arthritis, although rheumatoid valvulitis may occasionally involve and make incompetent the aortic valve.

Miscellaneous Lesions

Although it has been stated on a number of occasions that hypertension and myocardial infarction are less frequent in patients with rheumatoid arthritis than in the general population, the validity of this statement has not been clearly established by several recent studies.[92] Myocardial infarction and fibrosis secondary to coronary arteriosclerosis probably account for most of the clinical cardiac dysfunction encountered in patients with rheumatoid arthritis. Secondary amyloidosis, that may complicate rheumatoid arthritis, infrequently affects the myocardium. Aortic insufficiency has been reported as an occasional finding in ankylosing spondylitis associated with psoriatic arthritis and Reiter's disease. It has been proposed[101] that a chronic form of rheumatic fever may lead to deformities (so-called *Jaccoud's disease*) of the joints as well as the heart valves. The existence of such a category has not been generally accepted by American rheumatologists. Takayasu's disease is not generally regarded as a rheumatic condition, but isolated instances of aortic arch syndrome have been reported in rheumatoid arthritis.[31]

PULMONARY LESIONS

Three patterns of chronic pulmonary disease have been proposed as occasional manifestations of rheumatoid arthritis.

1. *Caplan's syndrome* refers to a type of unusually large, silicotic nodule formation seen in anthracite coal miners who are afflicted with rheumatoid arthritis. With the exception of their large size, their appearance is that of a silicotic lesion.[36] It has been suggested that the exuberant character of these nodules is due to an altered tissue reactivity to the silica particles. Although the lesion appears relatively frequently in Great Britain, it has not been common in the United States.[77]

2. Granulomatous lesions, resembling subcutaneous nodules of rheumatoid arthritis, are infrequent findings. It may be difficult to distinguish them from infectious granulomata.

3. Whether idiopathic interstitial pneumonia or diffuse interstitial fibrosis of the

lungs is a fortuitous finding or a true manifestation of rheumatoid arthritis has been debated in a number of papers. The lesions described have not had anatomic characteristics that would distinguish them from the pulmonary fibrosis observed in systemic scleroderma or the Hamman-Rich syndrome.[25,84] Although Brannan[13] observed 27 of 13,598 patients with rheumatoid arthritis to have extensive bilateral pulmonary disease otherwise unexplained, Aronoff and co-workers found no more chest disease than in control populations.[1] Extensive pleural adhesions and fibrinous pleurisy are sometimes associated with pericardial disease in rheumatoid arthritis.

SPLEEN, LYMPHOID TISSUES AND BONE MARROW

Enlargement of the regional lymph nodes draining affected joints is fairly frequent in rheumatoid arthritis Although there are some reports to the contrary,[58] generalized lymphadenopathy involving the deeper chains is infrequent.[81] The enlargement is caused by a non-specific hyperplasia associated with formation of prominent germinal centers. Plasma cells are usually few; rheumatoid factor has been demonstrated in them.[54,55] Numerous reticulum cells may be found in the sinuses. The hypertrophy of the nodes at times reaches dimensions sufficient to raise a suspicion of malignant lymphoma; the histologic picture has too often been confused with Brill-Symmers' giant follicular lymphoma.[61,68]

Distinctive changes are not present in the spleen. In the splenomegaly of *Felty's syndrome*, enlargement of the white pulp may be seen.[26] Thymic hypertrophy is not characteristically present. The proportion of plasma cells is increased in the bone marrow.

ENDOCRINE GLANDS

Because of the dramatic clinical response of rheumatoid arthritis to the administration of corticotropin and adrenocortical steroids, a number of studies have been carried out on the state of the adrenal cortex and the pituitary gland. The adrenal cortex has no morphologic changes that distinguish it from the adrenal cortex in non-rheumatic diseases, and it responds to the administration of therapeutic compounds as it does in various other disorders.[93] Pearse described a significant degree of degranulation of beta cells of the anterior pituitary lobe that was regarded as evidence of a distinct endocrine abnormality.[74] This observation did not correspond to the experience of others.[8]

Lymphocytic thyroiditis, sometimes sufficiently severe as to resemble Hashimoto's struma, has been reported in some studies to occur in as many as 17 per cent of patients with rheumatoid arthritis.[7,14] Others[53] have, however, not found it more frequent than in a control population.

OCULAR LESIONS

The episcleritis, sometimes seen in rheumatoid arthritis, has its inception in focal, chronic inflammatory cell infiltration and necrosis of the sclera. When these foci become larger and chronic, they may resemble the subcutaneous nodules of rheumatoid arthritis. In instances in which the scleral necrosis is sufficient to result in softening of the wall of the eye, uveal tissue may herniate through the scleral defect, a condition known as *scleromalacia perforans*. The latter condition sometimes occurs in patients with no evidence of rheumatoid arthritis.[99]

The *uveitis* (iridocyclitis) of Still's disease and ankylosing spondylitis does not have distinctive clinical characteristics. The pathologic anatomy has apparently not been documented. *Band-shaped keratopathy*, a characteristic equatorial corneal opacity, due to fibrosis of the cornea, apparently is a sequela of the iridocyclitis, and in children is most often, if not always, associated with the arthritic condition.

Posterior subcapsular cataracts have been observed in up to 42 per cent of patients with rheumatoid arthritis and other rheumatic diseases during the course of corticosteroid therapy. Whether they result from this medication has been argued both ways. Little is known of their pathologic anatomy. In one well-studied, relatively early (nine months' duration) case, preservation of lens epithelium and the architecture of the lens bow distinguished the lesion from that of the usual senile cataract. Another surgically removed lens, however, had changes indistinguishable from the senile lesion.[71]

Keratoconjunctivitis sicca, associated with diminished lacrimation, is discussed more fully in the section on Sjøgren's syndrome.

SJØGREN'S SYNDROME

Although the cardinal symptoms of this syndrome are referable to diminished secretion by the lacrimal and salivary glands, it is related to rheumatic diseases as evidenced by the consistent presence of various rheumatic serological factors. In approximately one third of cases, classical peripheral rheumatoid arthritis is present. The bizarre association of the lesions in the lacrimal and salivary tissues and those in the joints lacks any attractive hypothetical explanation at present.

A considerable variation is found in the salivary lesions. Four principal patterns are found. (1) Most often, the predominant finding is like that described in *Mikulicz's disease*. Two different histologic elements are distingushed in this.[59] One is a peculiar metaplastic change in the epithelium of the striated ducts. These cells proliferate and assume a stratified, polymorphous appearance rather than a normal columnar one. Their cytoplasm loses its normal oxyphilia. Because of the resemblance of the cells to the myoepithelial cells that normally lie subjacent to the duct epithelium, the ducts showing solid, heaped-up cells of this sort have been referred to as "epimyoepithelial" islands. Duct-like metaplasia of acini, with irregular ectasia and attenuation, also occurs with this and acini undergo variable atrophy. The other principal component in this lesion is infiltration of lymphocytes about the intralobular ducts. At times, germinal centers appear in the lymphoid aggregates, and acini may be obliterated by the infiltrate. Nevertheless, the lobular limits are characteristically respected by the infiltrate. (2) In a few instances a localized area of lymphoid infiltration associated with duct metaplasia of the sort just noted reaches tumor-like proportions—benign lymphoepithelial lesion of Godwin. These may present histologic difficulties in differential diagnosis from malignant lymphomas of the salivary glands. (3) Occasionally the cellular infiltration is so mild and the duct unchanged, so that the appearance cannot be distinguished from a control population. (4) After many years, the parenchymal lobules show extreme atrophy and replacement by adipose tissue, even though lymphocytic infiltration and duct metaplasia no longer are present. Minor salivary and labial glands also are often infiltrated with lymphocytes and may thus be suitable for biopsy. Intralobular aggregates of lymphocytes also are seen in the lacrimal glands, but they are smaller than in salivary glands and only rarely accompanied by epimyoepithelial islands.[32] Other glandular tissues, including the pancreas, failed to disclose a comparable pattern.

The pathologic ramifications of Sjøgren's syndrome are more complicated than this account suggests. Localized tumor-like nodules of infiltrating lymphoid tissue ("pseudolymphoma") have been observed in lymph nodes and lung.[96] Indeed, in rare instances, unequivocal malignant lymphomas—principally reticulum cell sarcomas—have developed. Isolated instances of Waldenström's macroglobulinemia, small cell lymphosarcoma and Hodkgin's disease also have been observed. The obverse of this situation, *viz.* lymphomas causing Mikulicz syndrome through lacrimal and salivary invasion, has not resulted in Sjøgren's syndrome or its serological abnormalities.

STILL'S DISEASE

This disorder is generally considered as the juvenile form of rheumatoid arthritis, although it differs in several respects from the adult counterpart: in the infrequent occurrence of circulating serologic rheumatoid factors; in a more frequent picture of ankylosing spondylitis; a greater frequency of iritis and band-shaped keratopathy; in the lower frequency of subcutaneous nodules; and in frequently having an erythematous skin eruption (*see also* Chapter 24).

Articular Lesions

The pathologic changes in the peripheral joints are comparable to those described in the adult disease, with the exception that the subchondral inflammatory process may arrest or distort epiphyseal bone growth and thereby lead to so-called rheumatic dwarfism. Monarticular involvement is more frequently seen in the childhood than the adult disease.

Subcutaneous Nodules

The histologic appearance differs both from those of the adult rheumatoid nodule and from the nodule of rheumatic fever.[15] In material available to this reviewer, the nodules consisted largely of fibrous tissue containing irregularly disposed aggregates of proliferating fibroblasts in relatively small numbers, and irregular areas of fibrinous exudation. Neither geographic areas of necrosis nor palisade formation were evident. In one early lesion, proliferation of blood vessels and focal vasculitis were present.

Ocular Changes

Iridocyclitis and subsequent band-shaped keratopathy are far more frequent in Still's disease than in adult rheumatoid arthritis (see above).

Spondylitis

The spinal changes are similar to those of Marie-Strumpell disease.[85] In the minds of some, such lesions may represent juvenile forms of ankylosing spondylitis rather than of rheumatoid arthritis. According to this view, the term "Still's disease" is preferable to "juvenile rheumatoid arthritis" insofar as it encompasses two distinct entities.

Cardiac Lesions

Pericardial involvement occurs in the juvenile form approximately as frequently as in adult rheumatoid arthritis,[49] although it may be detected clinically with some greater frequency.

Skin Eruptions

The erythema is of transient form. Histologically, only mild perivascular aggregation of mononuclear cells in the superficial dermis has been observed.[41]

ETIOLOGY AND PATHOGENESIS OF RHEUMATOID ARTHRITIS

The following considerations are oriented toward the pathologic findings in rheumatoid arthritis. A systematic treatment of the topic appears in Chapters 18 and 19.

The histologic appearance of the articular tissues has in the past suggested that rheumatoid arthritis is an infectious disease—indeed, the condition is still called chronic infectious arthritis in many parts of the world. Many types of spontaneous or induced infectious polyarthritis in species other than man have similar histologic appearances. Arthritis caused by the enteric erysipeloid organism (*Erysipelothrix insidiosa*) in swine, for example, is one of the leading causes of pork condemnation in federally inspected meat plants in the United States. It closely resembles rheumatoid arthritis histologically.[89] Rather similar, though generally less chronic, synovitides occur in poultry and in pigs with species-specific types of *Mycoplasma*. These are minute, filtrable bacteria, the so-called pleuro-pneumonia-like organisms or PPLO. Another type of filtrable agent causing disease in other species is the large or psittacosis-lymphogranuloma type of "virus" (*Bedsonia*) of lambs. Subcutaneous nodules of the sort seen in rheumatoid arthritis have not been found in these infectious diseases, however, and serologic tests for rheumatoid factor are generally negative.

The affinity for joints and frequency of occurrence of arthritis in bacteremias in these species have prompted many microbiologic studies. Most of these, including some utilizing demanding tissue culture methods for viruses,[19,20,97] have failed to disclose infectious agents in rheumatoid arthritis. A preliminary report by one reliable laboratory, however, described recovery of pleuro-pneumonia-like organism from synovial fluid in 6 of 7 cases of rheumatoid arthritis.[6] The investigators were aware of the possibility of contamination of cultured tissue by *Mycoplasma;* control material was free of them. These findings have not been confirmed.

In the absence of demonstrable infectious agents, the principal hypotheses entertained relate rheumatoid arthritis to one form or another of hypersensitivity.[4,29,80,98] Among the types of evidence adduced for these are: (1) the failure to demonstrate an infectious origin; (2) the similarity of the "fibrinoid" necrotic material in the subcutaneous nodules to changes seen in acute allergic inflammation; (3) the resemblance of the vascular lesions to polyarteritis nodosa, as well as experimentally induced serum sickness;[80] (4) the elevated gamma globulin content of the serum; and (5) the antibody-like nature of the serological rheumatoid factors. The latter, by reacting with gamma globulin, a normal body component, have some features of an autoantibody. Of particular interest is the report that heat-aggregated serum gamma globulin of rheumatoid patients, injected into the knee joint of the *same* individuals, evoked an acute synovitis.[79]

From what has already been pointed out, the first three arguments have in themselves little compelling force. Whether the rheumatoid factor exerts a pathogenic effect or, in manner analogous to the Wassermann reagin in syphilis, is primarily a byproduct of the inflammation has not yet been established.[46] Among the arguments against the hypersensitivity hypotheses are: (1) the development of an arthritis, resembling rheumatoid arthritis, in patients who have deficient immunoglobulin - producing mechanisms and no rheumatoid factor;[83] (2) failure of transfusion of large amounts of high-titer sera to cause rheumatoid arthritis in human recipients;[39] and (3) the increasing recognition of rheumatoid type of serological factors in many other experimental and clinical states characterized by hypergamma-globulinemia, *viz.* sarcoidosis and syphilis.[73]

Little of contemporary thinking about the nature of this disease will stand rigorous tests of validity. Suitable experimental models do not exist; indeed, there are few definitive criteria by which one could even judge the validity of such a model were it to be found.

Concerning the histogenesis of the disease, certain speculations may be offered. One of the peculiarities of the morbid anatomy of the disease is that the synovial lesions, as described, are morphologically non-specific, while the subcutaneous nodules look quite different and are relatively specific. If there were no common histogenetic sequence of events in the nodules and the joints, it would be difficult to understand how a common pathogenetic mechanism would produce both lesions. The following hypothesis may be offered to account for this: that the nodular type of reaction does at times occur in joints, particularly in the compact fibrous parts. The necrosis noted in superficial portions of the synovial tissue may be compared to the central zones in the nodules. At their base, an ingrowth of fibroblasts and palisades of synovial lining or elongated cells also closely resembles those of subcutaneous nodules. Their appearance is indistinguishable from that of subcutaneous nodules that have undergone central softening with formation of bursa-like cavities. Collins[22] referred to the latter as pseudosynovial spaces. The simplest explanation for the difference between such synovial foci and the subcutaneous nodules is that, in the latter, the necrotic material is circumscribed by firm cicatrix, while in the synovial location, the necrotic debris is cast off into the joint space and may appear as a *rice body*. In the joint, the inflammation would thus become dissipated in the articular cavity and give rise to the more diffuse, non-specific components of the synovitis that may also be seen in the granulation tissue about the nodules.

In the earliest days or weeks of their development, the subcutaneous nodules consist largely of vascular granulation tissue, in which the processes of necrosis and exudation proceed centrifugally about inflamed small arteries or islands of newly formed capillary or sinusoidal vessels.[33,44,60,62,63,91] It is only later that coalescence of the areas of necrosis is followed by the granuloma-like appearance that characterizes the mature subcutaneous nodule. Aside from this intrinsic association between the inflammatory process and the vasculitis, a principal reason for believing that the blood vessels play a role in the development of the nodules is that, in the same patients, arteritis is frequent in other tissues as well. Accordingly, it may be proposed that disseminated arteritis is an integral manifestation of rheumatoid arthritis, and that the development of the nodular and synovial lesions is in some manner mediated through the affected arteries to the terminal vascular bed of the affected tissues. This hypothesis does not have universal acceptance, but it has the virtue of being based on rather unique specimen material and provides a unitary concept of the histogenesis of the disorder.[91]

ANKYLOSING SPONDYLITIS

Although classified as rheumatoid spondylitis by the American Rheumatism Association for many years, many American as well as European rheumatologists consider this disorder a different entity than rheumatoid arthritis (*see also* Chapter 41).

In the diarthrodial joints of the spine, the sacroiliac and peripheral joints, the pathologic processes are quite like those of peripheral rheumatoid arthritis, except that bony ankylosis is more prominent in ankylosing spondylitis.[23] The initial events in the changes of the intervertebral discs have not been well documented histologically, although it seems quite clear, by roentgenographic studies, that osteolytic resorption of the margins of the vertebral bodies to which the annulus fibrosis is attached occurs early.[82] Whether there is an inflammatory infiltrate in the bone or disc tissue at this time is not known. There occurs, however, a metaplastic ossification of the annulus fibrosus, penetrating from the margin of the vertebral bodies into the annulus. It should be emphasized that, although commonly referred to as ossification of the spinal ligaments, the principal changes do not affect the ligaments so much as they do the annulus fibrosus (Fig. 20–9). This is quite apparent when one simply observes the ankylotic bridges existing, in anteroposterior roentgenographic projections, on the lateral aspects of the vertebral bodies. It will be recalled that the longitudinal spinal ligaments are anterolateral and posterior, but not lateral. When extensive, the bony bridges replace not only the annulus fibrosus, but also parts of the nucleus pulposus. The ossific tissue in time is remodeled to form a continuous structure.

Although this picture is not observed characteristically in the vertebral involvement of rheumatoid arthritis, quite similar

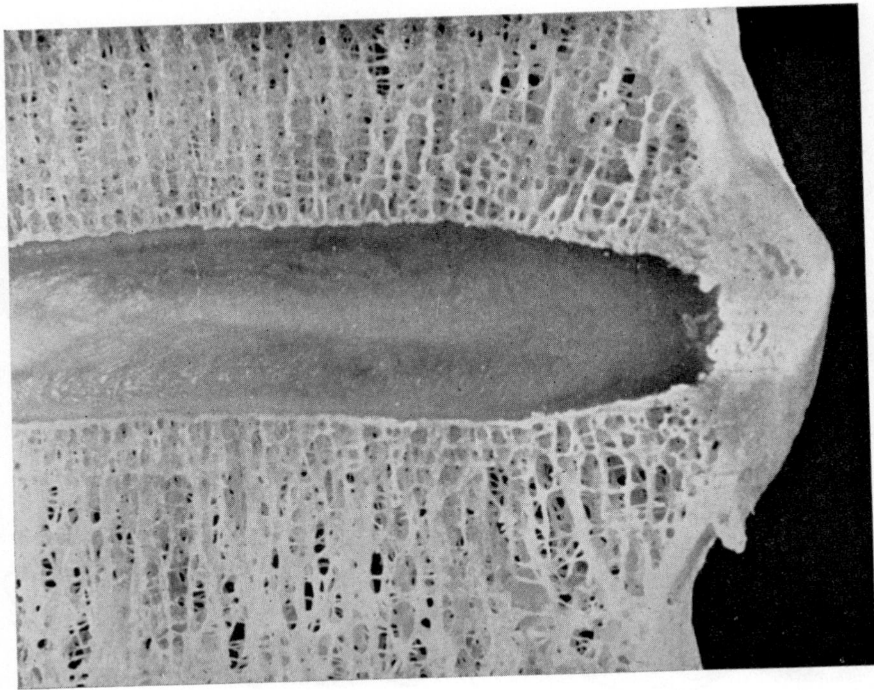

FIG. 20–9.—Ankylosing spondylitis. Trabecular and cortical bone occupy the position of the annulus fibrosus. (Photograph, courtesy of Dr. Roger Terry.)

patterns are found at times in Still's disease, psoriatic arthritis and in Reiter's disease. Unlike rheumatoid arthritis, subcutaneous nodules and vascular lesions are exceedingly rare. Cardiac disease is, however, significant and is discussed more fully in the sections dealing with the heart in rheumatoid arthritis. The systemic nature of ankylosing spondylitis is further indicated by the ocular lesions already described.

PSORIATIC ARTHRITIS

The histologic changes in the joints in this condition are similar to those of rheumatoid arthritis, but differ in two respects: (1) the structures affected are principally the most distal rather than proximal joints (Fig. 20–10), and (2) more extensive destruction occurs in articular and adjacent bone.[9,87] The osteolysis is effected by a granulation tissue in which osteoclasts are present. As a result of this resorption, the bone may "telescope" within the skin of the extremity, and give rise to the so-called *opera-glass deformity*. Aside from these changes, a bulbous swelling of the periarticular soft tissue may result from proliferation of fibrous tissue in which thick-walled blood vessels are present.

The changes in the skin in psoriasis are fairly characteristic. The papillary element of the epidermis is hypertrophied and forms coarse, club-shaped appendages while the non-papillary portion is attenuated. The latter is, however, covered by a thick parakeratotic and keratotic scale. The superficial portions of the subjacent dermis are chronically inflamed and infiltrated with large numbers of lymphocytes. A direct continuity between the dermal inflammation and the periarthritis or arthritis in psoriasis has not been established (*see also* Chapter 42).

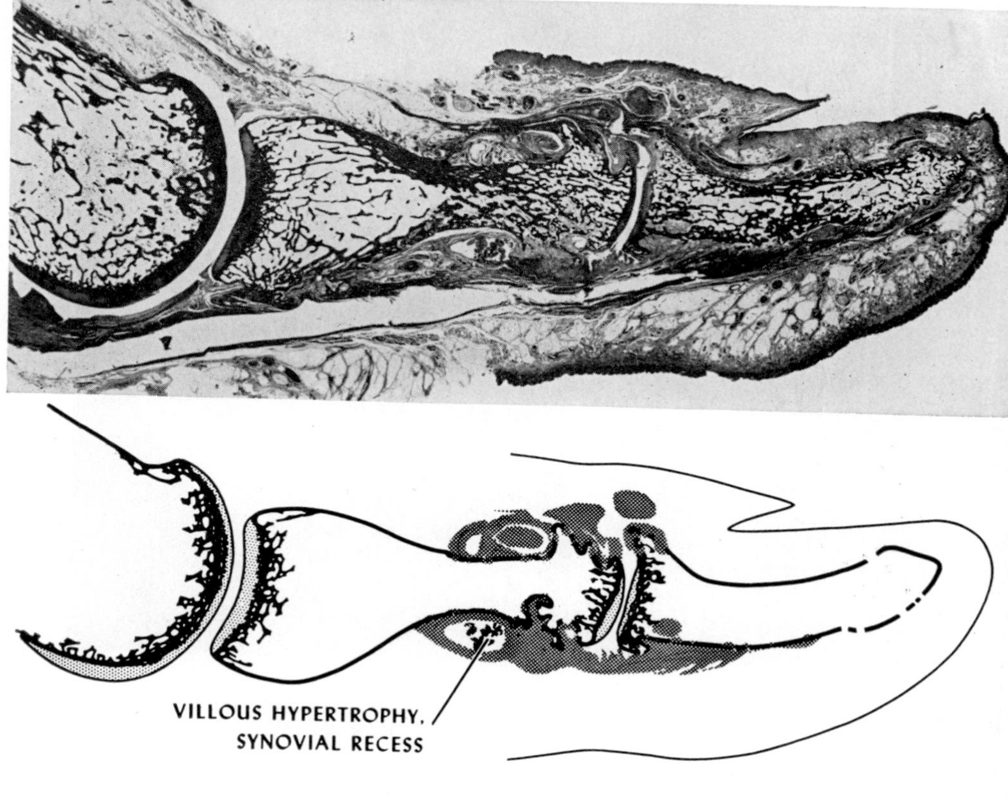

Fig. 20–10.—Psoriatic arthritis, great toe. The extensive periarticular inflammation and destruction of bone about the distal interphalangeal joint are quite characteristic of this disorder. The metatarsophalangeal joint is spared. (Masson's trichrome, × 2.5.)

REITER'S DISEASE

The synovitis is quite similar to that of rheumatoid arthritis, although in the early phases of the disease, it has a more purulent character.[100] The long-standing changes also are quite similar, but periosteal involvement, with new bone formation in attached tendons and ligaments, is characteristic of Reiter's disease rather than rheumatoid arthritis. In this respect, the joint lesions are reminiscent of infectious arthritis.

The cutaneous lesions are histologically indistinguishable from those of pustular psoriasis; *i.e.*, psoriatic lesions, like those described above except that focal purulent infiltration of the epidermis is present (*see also* Chapter 65).

ARTHRITIS ASSOCIATED WITH WHIPPLE'S DISEASE, REGIONAL ENTERITIS AND ULCERATIVE COLITIS

A relationship between chronic enteritic disorders and deforming arthritis exists not only in Reiter's disease, which may be initiated by episodes of dysentery at times, but also in other entities. The synovium, in the arthritis accompanying ulcerative colitis, has non-specific inflammatory changes.[15,66] So far as is known, the peculiar macrophages that characterize the intestinal and lymph node lesions of Whipple's disease have not been observed in synovial tissue in this condition[17] (*see also* Chapter 46).

ARTHRITIS ASSOCIATED WITH AGAMMAGLOBULINEMIA

In approximately 25 per cent of patients with congenital or acquired agammaglobulinemia or hypogammaglobulinemia, rheumatic symptoms develop. Most conspicuous among these is chronic synovitis, that resembles rheumatoid arthritis in several respects. The arthritis usually affects fewer joints than does rheumatoid arthritis, and more often spares the small joints. Histologically, the pattern of synovitis is non-specific; it is like that seen in rheumatoid arthritis with the exception that plasma cells characteristically are absent.[83]

Subcutaneous nodules have been reported on several occasions; the few sections seen by this reviewer have disclosed a less characteristic appearance than the subcutaneous nodules of rheumatoid arthritis. Somewhat lobulated areas of proliferating fibroblasts and ill-defined palisades suggested more the appearance of subcutaneous nodules seen in Still's disease. Vascular lesions of several sorts have also been described in rare instances (*see also* Chapter 47).

AMYLOIDOSIS

Secondary amyloidosis complicates rheumatoid arthritis, Still's disease and ankylosing spondylitis in approximately 20 per cent of severe cases. It has no features that distinguish it from amyloidosis complicating other chronic inflammatory diseases.[57] Amyloid infiltration represents the principal cause of renal dysfunction in rheumatoid arthritis, except when the joint disease co-exists with systemic lupus erythematosus[75] (*see also* Chapter 69).

BIOPSY AS AN AID IN DIAGNOSIS

Joint Tissues

From what has already been stated, it is apparent that synovial biopsy has no place in the differential diagnosis of the several conditions discussed in this chapter. It is, however, distinctly useful in distinguishing rheumatoid arthritis from gout and from infectious arthritides at times. Closed and open biopsy techniques are available. Two sorts of punch biopsy needles have been specifically designed for this purpose.[72,76] Open biopsy, carried out under local anesthesia, may be preferable because it provides more adequate samples of tissue and causes no more appreciable discomfort to the patient. In distinguishing the arthritis from gout, precautions should be taken to preserve any urate crystals present by fixation of the specimen in absolute alcohol rather than aqueous fixatives. When infection is suspected, synovial tissue rather than fluid should be subjected to microbiologic study.[90]

Skeletal Muscle

The principal indication for muscle biopsy in this group of disorders is the demonstration of arteritis. Because of the focal nature of this lesion, it is necessary to have adequate amounts of tissue examined. On the part of the surgeon, this requires that the specimen be of sufficient size; $2 \times 1 \times 1$ cms. are realistic dimensions. Because of the ease with which contracture of the muscle fiber can be induced by the surgical manipulation, the tissue should be grasped only at one edge. Fixation, for the same resaon, should be delayed for a half hour or so after excision. Bouin's solution is a useful fixative for this tissue. In most cases, serial sections are necessary. Making 100 sections, each fifth slide stained, as routine procedure, has yielded four times as many positive diagnoses of arteritis as has isolated, random sections.

Subcutaneous Nodules

In the differential diagnosis from a tophus, fixation of the nodule in absolute alcohol may serve the same useful purpose suggested in synovial biopsy. Epidermoid cysts in the olecranon region occasionally simulate rheumatoid nodules, and biopsy may be indicated when sufficient diagnostic weight is placed on them.[102]

Lymph Nodes

The principal indications for lymph node biopsy are (1) the differential diagnosis from specific infectious arthritides, in which case the tissue should also be cultured; and (2) the differential diagnosis from malignant lymphomas.

Amyloidosis

Needle punch biopsies of liver, spleen and kidney offer no difficulties to the pathologist, but apparently have occasionally resulted in serious visceral hemorrhages. Gingival or buccal mucosal biopsies have at times established the presence of amyloid deposits in the walls of minute blood vessels in rheumatoid arthritis, as in other types of secondary amyloidosis. Rectal biopsy has been recommended for similar purposes. In each of these procedures, the diagnosis is valid only when positive and not excluded when negative for amyloid material.

SUMMARY

Each of the deforming arthritides discussed in this chapter has certain similarities and common pathologic features with the others. The inflammatory reactions in the joints, while inherently quite indistinguishable from each other, are at the same time nonspecific as a type reaction. Overlapping serologic reactions with the "collagen diseases"; histologic similarities in the subcutaneous nodules; common patterns of vertebral bridges in ankylosing spondylitis, Still's disease, psoriatic arthritis and Reiter's disease; and of ocular lesions in Still's disease and ankylosing spondylitis; of cutaneous lesions in Reiter's disease and pustular psoriasis; and also of joint disease complicating the several sorts of chronic enteritis—all defy a rigid nosologic concept. Whether they are truly variants of rheumatoid arthritis, as often described, or independent diseases, or non-specific reaction patterns remains an unanswerable question at the present time.

BIBLIOGRAPHY

1. Aronoff, A., Bywaters, E. G. L. and Fearnley, G. R.: Brit. Med. J., *2*, 228, 1955.
2. Baggenstoss, A. H., Bickel, W. H. and Ward, L. E.: J. Bone Joint Surg., *34A*, 601, 1952.
3. Baggenstoss, A. H. and Rosenberg, E. F.: Arch. Path., *37*, 54, 1944.
4. Banerjee, S. K. and Glynn, L. E.: Ann. N.Y. Acad. Sci., *86*, 1064, 1960.
5. Barland, P., Novikoff, A. A. and Hamerman, D.: Amer. J. Path., *44*, 853, 1964.
6. Bartholomew, L. E.: Arth. and Rheum., *8*, 376, 1965.
7. Becker, K. L., Titus, J. L., Woolner, L. B. and Ferguson, R. H.: Proc. Staff Meet. Mayo Clin., *38*, 125, 1963.
8. Bennett, W. A.: J. Bone Joint Surg., *36A*, 867, 1954.
9. Biressi, P. C., di Vittorio, S. and Marrazzi, G.: Reumatismo (Milan), *13*, 92, 1961.
10. Ball, J.: Lancet, *1*, 86, 1958 (Abstract).
11. Ball, J., Bahgat, N. E. D. and Taylor, G.: J. Histochem., *12*, 737, 1964.
12. Bland, J. H., Davis, P. H., London, M. G., Van Buskirk, F. W. and Duarte, D. G.: Arch. Int. Med., *112*, 892, 1963.
13. Brannan, H. N.: *Mesenchymal Reactions in the Lungs in Patients with Rheumatoid Arthritis.* Thesis, University of Minnesota, April, 1963.
14. Buchanan, W. W., Crooks, J., Alexander, W. D., Koutras, D. A., Wayne, E. J. and Gray, K. G.: Lancet, *1*, 245, 1961.
15. Bywaters, E. G. L. and Ansell, B. M.: Ann. Rheumat. Dis., *17*, 169, 1958.
16. Bywaters, E. G. L., Glynn, L. E. and Zeldis, A.: Ann. Rheumat. Dis., *17*, 278, 1958.
17. Caughey, D. E. and Bywaters, E. G. L.: Ann. Rheumat. Dis., *22*, 327, 1963.

18. Chapman, J. A., and Taylor, G.: J. Roy. Microscop. Soc., *85*, 455, 1966.
19. Clark, S. K. R.: Ann. Rheumat. Dis., *17*, 51, 1958.
20. Clause, G., McEwen, C., Brunner, T. and Tsamparlis, G.: Brit. J. Ven. Dis., *40*, 170, 1964.
21. Cochrane, W., Davies, D. V., Dorling, J. and Bywaters, E. G. L.: Ann. Rheumat. Dis., *23*, 345, 1964.
22. Collins, D. H.: *The Pathology of Articular and Spinal Diseases*. Baltimore, The Williams & Wilkins Co., 1949.
23. Cruickshank, B.: Ann. Rheumat. Dis., *10*, 393, 1951.
24. ————: Ann. Rheumat. Dis., *11*, 137, 1952.
25. ————: Brit. J. Dis. Chest, *53*, 226, 1959.
26. Denko, C. W. and Zumpft, C. W.: Arth. and Rheum., *5*, 478, 1962.
27. Dingle, J. T.: Proc. Roy. Soc. Med., *55*, 109, 1962.
28. Dingle, J. T. and Page Thomas, D. P.: Brit. J. Exper. Path., *37*, 318, 1956.
29. Dumonde, D. C. and Glynn, L. E.: Brit. J. Exper. Path., *43*, 373, 1962.
30. Ehrlich, G. E., Peterson, L. T., Sokoloff, L. and Bunim, J. J.: Arth. and Rheum., *2*, 332, 1959.
31. Falicov, R. and Cooney, D. F.: Arch. Int. Med., *114*, 594, 1964.
32. Font, R. L., Yanoff, M. and Zimmerman, L. E.: Amer. J. Clin. Path., *48*, 365, 1967.
33. Gieseking, R., Bäumer, A. and Backmann, L.: Z. Rheumaforsch., *28*, 163, 1969.
34. Gitlin, D., Craig, J. M. and Janeway, C. A.: Amer. J. Path., *33*, 55, 1957.
35. Glenner, G. G., Burstone, M. S. and Meyer, D. B.: J. Nat. Cancer Inst., *23*, 857, 1959.
36. Gough, J., Rivers, D. and Seal, R. M. E.: Thorax., *10*, 9, 1955.
37. Grimley, P. M., and Sokoloff, L.: Amer. J. Path., *49*, 931, 1966.
38. Hamerman, D., Barland, P. and Stephens, M.: In *Inflammation and Diseases of Connective Tissue* (Mills, L. C. and Moyer, J. H., eds.). Philadelphia, W. B. Saunders Co., 1961, p. 158.
39. Harris, J. and Vaughan, J. H.: Arth. and Rheum., *4*, 47, 1961.
40. Hendry, N. G. C. and Carr, A. J.: Nature (London), *199*, 392, 1963.
41. Isdale, I. C. and Bywaters, E. G. L.: Quart. J. Med., *25*, 377, 1956.
42. Kellgren, J. H. and Ball, J.: Ann. Rheum. Dis., *9*, 48, 1950.
43. Kirk, J. and Cosh, J.: Quart. J. Med., *38*, 397, 1969.
44. Kulka, J. P.: J. Chron. Dis., *10*, 388, 1959.
45. ————: Ann. N. Y. Acad. Sci., *116*, 1018, 1964.
46. Kunkel, H. G. and Williams, R. C.: Ann. Rev. Med., *15*, 37, 1964.
47. Lack, C. H.: J. Bone Joint Surg. (Brit.), *41B*, 384, 1959.
48. Lawrence, J. S., Sharp, J., Ball, J. and Bier, F.: Ann. Rheumat. Dis., *23*, 205, 1964.
49. Lietman, P. S. and Bywaters, E. G. L.: Pediatrics, *32*, 855, 1963.
50. Lowney, E. D. and Simons, H. M.: Arch. Derm., *88*, 853, 1963.
51. Luscombe, M.: Nature (London), *197*, 1010, 1963.
52. Mainland, D.: Amer. Heart J., *45*, 644, 1953.
53. Masi, A. T., Hartmann, W. H., Hannahs, B. Y., Abbey, H. and Shulman, L. E.: Arth. and Rheum., *7*, 328, 1964 (Abstract).
54. McCormick, J. N.: Ann. Rheumat. Dis., *22*, 1, 1963.
55. Mellors, R. C., Heimer, R., Corcos, J. and Korngold, L.: J. Exper. Med., *110*, 875, 1959.
56. Mesara, B. W., Brody, G. L. and Oberman, H. A.: Amer. J. Clin. Path., *45*, 684, 1966.
57. Missen, G. A. K. and Taylor, J. D.: J. Path. Bact., *71*, 179, 1956.
58. Morandi, G. A., Marini, G., Pelù, G. and Frosecchi, M.: Nunt. Radiol., *34*, 357, 1968.
59. Morgan, W. S.: New Engl. J. Med., *251*, 5, 1954.
60. Mori, R.: Riv. Patol. Clin. Sperim. (Padova), *4*, 1, 1964.
61. Motulsky, A. G., Weinberg, S., Saphir, O. and Rosenberg, E.: Arch. Int. Med., *90*, 660, 1952.
62. Movat, H. Z.: Virchows Arch. path. Anat., *330*, 425, 1957.
63. Movat, H. Z. and More, R. H.: Amer. J. Clin. Path., *28*, 331, 1957.
64. Muirden, K. D., and Senator, G. B.: Ann. Rheum. Dis., *27*, 38, 1968.
65. McEwen, C.: Arch. Path., *25*, 303, 1938.
66. McEwen, C., Lingg, C., Kirsner, J. B. and Spencer, J. A.: Amer. J. Med., *33*, 923, 1962.
67. Norton, W. L. and Ziff, M.: Arth. and Rheum., *9*, 589, 1966.
68. Nosanchuk, J. S., and Schnitzer, B.: Cancer *24*, 343, 1969.
69. Nowaslawski, A., and Brzosko, W. J.: Path. Europ., *2*, 198, 1967.

70. Nowaslawski, A., and Brzosko, W. J.: Path. Europ., *2*, 302, 1967.
71. Oglesby, R. B., Black, R. L., von Sallman, L. and Bunim, J. J.: Arch. Ophthal., *66*, 625, 1961.
72. Parker, R. H. and Pearson, C. M.: Arth. and Rheum., *6*, 172, 1963.
73. Peltier, A. and Christian, C. L.: Arth. and Rheum., *2*, 1, 1959.
74. Pearse, A. G. E.: Lancet, *1*, 954, 1950.
75. Pollak, V. E., Pirani, C. L. and Kark, R. M.: Arth. and Rheum., *5*, 1, 1962.
76. Polley, H. F. and Bickel, W. H.: Ann. Rheumat. Dis., *10*, 277, 1951.
77. Ramirez, R. J., Lopez-Majano, V. and Schultze, G.: Amer. J. Med., *37*, 643, 1964.
78. Rawson, A. J., Abelson, N. M. and Hollander, J. L.: Ann. Int. Med., *62*, 281, 1965.
79. Restifo, R. A., Lussier, A. J., Rawson, A. J., Rockey, J. H. and Hollander, J. L.: Ann. Int. Med., *62*, 285, 1965.
80. Rich, A. R.: Harvey Lect., *42*, 106, 1946–7.
81. Robertson, M. D. J., Hart, F. D., White, W. F., Nuki, G. and Boardman, P. L.: Ann. Rheum. Dis., *27*, 253, 1968.
82. Romanus, P. and Yden, S.: *Pelvo-Spondylitis Ossificans*. Copenhagen, Munksgaard, 1955.
83. Rötstein, J. and Good, R. A.: Ann. Rheumat. Dis., *21*, 202, 1962.
84. Rubin, E. H.: Amer. J. Med., *19*, 569, 1955.
85. Sharp, J.: Brit. Med. J., *1*, 975, 1957.
86. Sherman, M. S.: Bull. Hosp. Joint Dis., *12*, 110, 1951.
87. ————: J. Bone Joint Surg., *34A*, 831, 1952.
88. Skoog, W. A. and Adams, W. S.: Amer. J. Med., *34*, 417, 1963.
89. Sokoloff, L.: Advances Vet. Sci., *6*, 193, 1960.
90. ————: Med. Clin. North America, *45*, 1171, 1961.
91. ————: In *The Peripheral Blood Vessels* (Orbison, J. L. and Smith, D. E., eds.). Baltimore, The Williams & Wilkins Co., pp. 297–325, 1963.
92. ————: Mod. Concepts Cardiovasc. Dis., *33*, 847, 1964.
93. Sokoloff, L., Sharp, J. T. and Kaufman, E. H.: Arch. Int. Med., *88*, 267, 1964.
94. Sokoloff, L., Wilens, S. L., Bunim, J. J. and McEwen, C.: Amer. J. Med. Sci., *219*, 174, 1950.
95. Straub, L. R.: Bull. Hosp. Joint Dis., *21*, 322, 1960.
96. Talal, N., Sokoloff, L. and Barth, W.: Amer. J. Med., *43*, 50, 1967.
97. Utz, J. P., Phelps, E. T. and Smith, L. G.: Bull. Georgetown U. Med. Center, *12*, 198, 1959.
98. Vaughan, J. H.: Amer. J. Med., *26*, 596, 1959.
99. Walter, J. R. and Boldt, H. A.: Amer. J. Ophthal., *55*, 922, 1963.
100. Weinberger, H. J., Ropes, M. W., Kulka, J. P. and Bauer, W.: Medicine, *41*, 35, 1962.
101. Weintraub, A. M. and Zvaifler, N. J.: Amer. J. Med., *35*, 145, 1963.
102. Wilson, J. T., and Sokoloff, L.: J.A.M.A., *214*, 593, 1970.
103. Wood, M. G. and Beerman, H.: J. Invest. Derm., *34*, 139, 1960.
104. Ziff, M., Gribetz, H. J. and LoSpalluto, J.: J. Clin. Invest., *39*, 405, 1960.

Chapter 21

The Clinical Picture of Rheumatoid Arthritis

By Charles Ragan, M.D.

Since Garrod[2] coined the name "Rheumatoid Arthritis," the clinical picture of the classical disease has changed very little. Confusion about early, mild or atypical forms of the disease may lead to difficulties in diagnosis, and some disagreement. Clinicians must be aware of the possibility that a multitude of diseases may be included under one label—a possibility substantiated, perhaps, by the variegated end-result. Before the clinical picture of the disease can be described, a few of the difficulties which face the student of rheumatoid arthritis and which apparently are not familiar to the medical world in general should be mentioned.

The Sample

In a description of this disease, almost every phrase has to be qualified (*see* Chapter 25). It is particularly important to state the source of a group of patients with rheumatoid arthritis since this may greatly influence its clinical characteristics including the average age, age at onset, course, severity, prognosis, number of patients with nodules, etc. A group taken from an outpatient clinic in a general hospital, for example, will differ markedly from one derived from a special hospital for arthritis or from a chronic disease hospital. In the latter, more severe disease will be seen with greater frequency as a result of selection. In contrast, the total population studies carried out in England[6] have uncovered patients with typical disease who have never sought medical care and who would not be included in a clinic sample.

"Activity" of the Disease

We talk glibly about activity of the disease but this is not easily measured (*see* Chapter 26). There are objective signs of activity—fever, minimal leukocytosis, the presence of acute phase reactants, an elevated erythrocyte sedimentation rate, anemia, local heat, swelling which can be measured by tape measure or rings, and weakness evident as changes in grip strength measured by dynamometer or folded blood pressure cuff. Actually, much subjective evidence has to be included in an assessment of activity: the so-called "morning stiffness," pain, fatigue and malaise. Factors which involve the patient's motivation such as his work record and even his activities in daily living must also be included in such an assessment. The extent to which a physician may be influenced by subjective and motivational factors in his total assessment of activity can easily lead to great differences in conclusions of individuals conducting even the same study (*see also* Chapter 26).

Historical and Geographical Distribution

No accurate data exist concerning the worldwide distribution of this disease. Historically, there is no evidence that the disease existed before modern times.

Skeletal remains from ossaria provide little knowledge since a distinction between rheumatoid arthritis and infectious arthritis or degenerative joint disease is difficult from study of the bones alone. The disease has not been found in mummies. The high frequency with which it appears after the age of 50 in total population studies would tend to result in a lower prevalence in populations with a short life span. This would apply to the populations in the period before the industrial revolution in western Europe and in underdeveloped areas in the world today. Various world travelers have reported seeing typical instances of rheumatoid arthritis in subtropical India, Central America and the Mediterranean countries. It is seen in Puerto Rico in prevalence probably somewhat below that seen in temperate climates. Historically, before the mid-nineteenth century, an analysis of the disease was difficult because of diagnostic confusion with gout, rheumatic fever, and degenerative joint disease. The classic Greek tendency to portray only the ideal would militate against a statue of a person with a deformity, and none portraying a patient with rheumatoid arthritis exists to our knowledge. Copeman[5] has carefully reviewed the history of rheumatoid arthritis and suggests that Hippocrates described the disease and that it was mentioned in writings from the second century A.D. He also notes certain important people who probably suffered from rheumatoid arthritis, including Columbus, Mary Queen of Scots, and President James Madison. These comments do not imply that rheumatoid arthritis is necessarily a disease of modern times with its stresses and aging populations. They are mentioned solely to point out that no accurate historical analysis of the disease is feasible and that no worldwide geographical study of validity has been made.

Body Habitus and Personality Type

Rheumatoid arthritis leads to wasting, and the average patient with far-advanced disease presents a malnourished appearance. Before the development of the disease, however, no anthropomorphic type seems to predominate.

Considerable comment has been made in psychosomatic circles about the personality pattern of the patient in whom rheumatoid arthritis is likely to develop. It has been stated that the aggressive female of the tomboy type with a strong subconscious dislike for her mother is prone to develop the disease. This has not been our experience. We feel that the patient with rheumatoid arthritis displays no characteristic pattern but has deep-seated anxieties which are difficult to express. This may be the result of severe chronic disease. It seems difficult to believe that this wearing disease, which can beat down the most stout-hearted individual, might not warp one's psychic outlook. For this reason, retrospective studies—of the patient after the disease has put in its appearance—might be meaningless. No forward-looking studies of the personality of patients who develop rheumatoid arthritis have been made *before* the disease makes its appearance. The role played by genetic influences is discussed in Chapter 12.

The Clinical Picture

In clinic studies, the onset of the disease is seen most commonly between the ages of twenty and sixty, with two peaks at thirty-five and forty-five, but it may begin at any age from the first year of life to the ninth decade. In clinic populations, women are affected more frequently than men, *i.e.*, 2 or 3 females to 1 male. In the epidemiologic study of total populations carried out by Kellgren and Lawrence,[6] however, there was an equal distribution of the sexes in classical rheumatoid arthritis, whereas, if one included all joint symptoms without restriction to classical disease, a preponderance of females was noted.

"Precipitating" causes are myriad and can apparently represent any type of traumatic episode (stress) whether it be

Symptoms of Rheumatoid Arthritis

Sex incidence—clinic population: 2 to 3 females to 1 male. Total population studies: equal distribution in classical disease.
Race—no particular predisposition.
Geography—more reported from temperate zones but data incomplete.
Climate—no adequate data.
Season—onset probably more frequent in the spring.
Anthropomorphic type—no definite type.
Personality pattern—no particular one.
Age of onset—any age, peaks at thirty-five and forty-five.
Prodromes—fatigue, malaise occasionally; frequently none.
Onset—usually insidious, but may be sudden or episodic.
Frequency of joint involvement—proximal interphalangeal, metacarpophalangeal, toes, wrist, knee, elbow, ankle, shoulder, hip, temporomandibular joint.
Joint swelling—fusiform, spindle-shaped.
Stiffness—common after inactivity; its duration in morning used as index of activity.
Fever—usually negligible except during steroid withdrawal.
Tachycardia—may be present.
Loss of weight—may be present.
Subcutaneous nodules—in 20 to 25 per cent of classical rheumatoid arthritics at some time during the disease.
Muscular atrophy—marked and out of proportion to the activity of disease.
Anemia—normocytic, normochromic with an element of aplasia or hemolysis, or both. Fails to respond to iron.
Skin changes—atrophy, bronzing, "liver palms" cold, moist extremities.

physical, psychic, infectious, or exposure. The majority of patients have an insidious onset but it may occasionally be acute and fulminating. The existence of prodromal symptoms is a matter of debate since the fatigue or malaise occasionally seen is considered by many to represent an integral part of the disease. Occasionally, actual joint involvement may be preceded by general malaise and fatigue with paresthesias of the extremities but, by and large, joint pain and/or stiffness is the most common first symptom. The usual onset is manifested by spotty joint involvement but an acute onset of symmetrical polyarthritis may be noted. There is evidence that a significantly large number of patients put the date of the onset of their disease in the spring—particularly in the month of March. The significance of this is unknown.

It cannot be too strongly emphasized that rheumatoid arthritis is a generalized disease. The disorder affects chiefly the joints and muscles but there is generalized systemic involvement if one looks for it (*see* Chapters 20 and 22). This is manifested symptomatically in the feeling of *general malaise* and *fatigue* from which these people suffer. The fatigue is totally nonspecific but constitutes a major part of the patient's complaints. It can serve as a good indicator of the amount of physical activity which can be performed and when this is exceeded and fatigue increases, an exacerbation may develop. As the disease develops, the patient's complaints are of *joint pain*, more evident on motion but also present at rest, *swelling*, *stiffness after inactivity* (gelling) and *limitation of motion* due to pain and stiffness. The typical joint presents a spindle-shaped appearance with thickening of the periarticular structures (*soft tissue swelling*) and atrophy of the contiguous muscles.

In classical disease, joint involvement

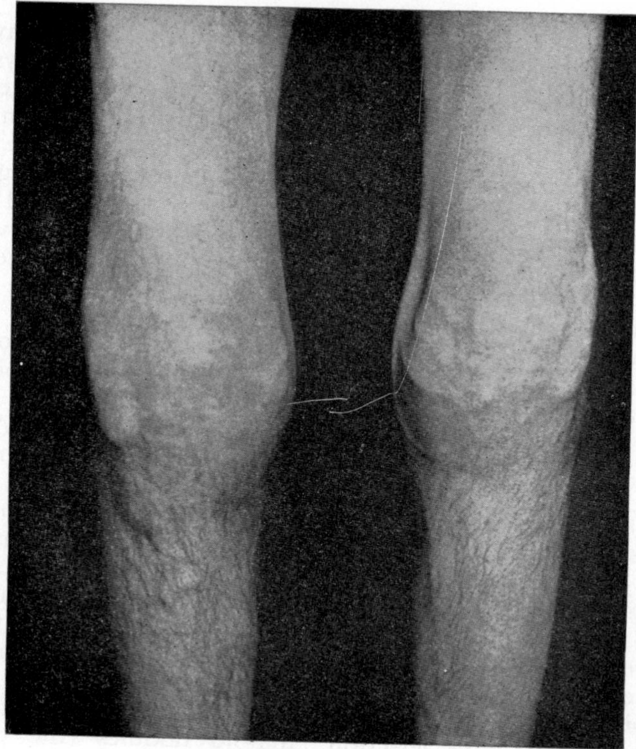

Fig. 21–4.—Rheumatoid arthritis of the knees in a middle-aged male.

Generalized lymph node enlargement will appear in about one-half the patients at some point in the course of their disease and splenomegaly in about 15 per cent. *Vasomotor instability* seems to represent a part of the disease and is manifested principally by cold, clammy hands and feet, with increased sweating. Perhaps related to this are the so-called "liver palms"—erythema of the thenar and hypothenar eminences—which appear almost as often in rheumatoid arthritis as in Laennec's cirrhosis whence they derive their name. There may be *atrophy of the skin*, at times, with increased pigmentation and bronzing. The association with psoriasis is discussed in Chapter 42. Inflammatory lesions of the uveal tract are seen sometimes in severe disease but less frequently than in ankylosing (rheumatoid) spondylitis. A very destructive lesion of the eye is seen in *scleromalacia perforans* where rheumatoid nodules develop in the sclera. These may undergo softening with perforation of the globe and extrusion of its contents; unless this can be arrested promptly, the eye is lost.

The crippling process which interferes most markedly with function is the *flexion contracture*. This is so designated because in most diarthrodial joints the flexor group of muscles is the stronger. Presumably there is involuntary splinting in an inflamed painful joint and the stronger group of muscles prevails, leading to the phenomenon of the flexion contracture. At the outset, the contracture is maintained solely by muscular components with probably some tendinous shortening. Ultimately, with progression of the disease, the scarring process in the cartilage continues and there is actual fibrous ankylosis in the flexed position. In weight-bearing joints

-such as knees or hips—the flexion eformity leads to great difficulty in ostural and functional dynamics. Flexion ontractures should be avoided, if at all ossible, by the proper application of ntiphlogistic drugs, active exercises gainst resistance, and the use of appropriate splinting. In joints other than the veight-bearing ones, flexion contractures nay lead to less functional impairment. 'or example, an elbow flexed at 90 egrees is much more useful than one vith reduced flexion. The ulnar deviaion seen in the hands is presumed to be lue to the displaced extensor tendons oulling to the ulnar side.

This brief explanation of the theory by vhich flexion contractures develop should oe accepted as theory only and not absolute fact. It does not imply continuous muscle contraction of the flexor groups which is physiologically unlikely, out intermittent contraction, possibly combined with an element of tendon hortening, must play a prominent role. This is in keeping with the concept of endon sheath involvement as a major accompaniment of the synovial inflamnation seen in this disease.

Sharpe[4] has pointed out that neck nvolvement may accompany peripheral oint rheumatoid arthritis and the Manchester group[6] feel it is rather characterstic. In their study, the most common symptom was painful limitation of movement of the neck. Radiologically the intervertebral discs were narrowed without much osteophytosis. Narrowing, erosion or even ankylosis of the zygapophyseal joints was observed. Vertebral subluxation—usually forward—was seen and on several occasions was accompanied by signs of long-tract compression.

Laboratory findings include the presence of acute phase reactants, most commonly measured by the sedimentation rate which is usually elevated during the active phase of the disease (*see* Chapter 23). Roentgen findings and the rheumatoid factor are discussed in Chapters 7 and 9, respectively. The anemia is normocytic and normochromic, usually fails to respond to iron and on investigation has, in some instances, the characteristics of an aplastic type and in others a hemolytic component. It is variable in degree, being most pronounced in severe and active disease. If the hematocrit is below 30 per cent, some other cause for the anemia should be suspected.

Course of the Disease

At the onset of rheumatoid arthritis, it is almost impossible to predict the course the disease will follow. In general, it follows one of two types—the *episodic* or the *sustained*. Frequently the disease will begin in episodes and ultimately become sustained.

An episode may be short-lived and a period of less than a year has been considered brief. During an episode, the rheumatoid process produces a certain amount of irreparable damage. In general, the time interval through which this process acts accounts for the amount of damage found, since none takes place during periods of remission. The amount of joint destruction and the degree of muscle wasting are related roughly to the length of time the disease is active. Since these two effects impair function, the "amount" of functional impairment is also related to the period of time the disease remains active. The terms—episodic and sustained—can only be used in retrospect and a major need at this time is for a sure way to predict the type of course the disease might be expected to follow. Its importance in ultimate prognosis and even in the type of management cannot be overemphasized. As an example, if one could predict that a given individual would have an episode lasting six months or a year, there would be no point in exposing him to the dangers of chrysotherapy but there might be good reason to expose him for that period of time to fairly heavy-dose steroid therapy to achieve the maximal suppression during the episode. Unfortunately, our ability to prophesy as to achievement of these ends is far from perfect. In our experience, no clinical feature of the disease serves as a prognostic index. In the great majority of patients who have the rheumatoid factor in their serum, the disease is sustained.[1,3] Disease starting early in adulthood also has a poor prognosis.[3] Forward-looking studies have yet to be carefully documented regarding the prognostic significance of a high-titered serum early in the disease. It has, however, been amply demonstrated that a positive rheumatoid serology does carry a poor prognosis on a statistical basis.

It was formerly said that rheumatoid arthritis never killed a patient and that the life expectancy of a patient with this disease was decreased somewhat — by approximately five years—probably because of debility and consequent increased susceptibility to intercurrent infections. In recent years, the development of a necrotizing arteritis as the final episode in the course of rheumatoid arthritis has been observed in many clinics throughout this country. It seems clear that these patients have no evidence of systemic lupus erythematosus which may also appear in the course of rheumatoid arthritis and which is another reason for premature death. The development of systemic lupus erythematosus has also been observed country-wide and has led to much discussion regarding the similarities between the two diseases. It seems only fair to state that such coexistence undoubtedly occurs, but at this time no hypotheses concerning pathogenesis can be substantiated. When a patient with rheumatoid arthritis develops multiple system involvement—renal, serosal, or pulmonary parenchymal involvement—these two eventualities—necrotizing arteritis or systemic lupus erythematosus—must be kept in mind as well as the possibility of secondary amyloid. Without a positive L.E. preparation or a positive biopsy, a definite diagnosis cannot be reached. There are, however, certain findings which make one consider primarily either necrotizing arteritis or systemic lupus. Peripheral neuritis, both motor and sensory, leg ulcers, and digital gangrene have, in our experience, been associated with a necrotizing arteritis whereas hematuria and particularly the nephrotic syndrome have been associated with systemic lupus erythematosus. Pericarditis, cardiac arrhythmias and the development of mitral or aortic murmurs have not necessarily been associated with either arteritis or lupus but have been observed when careful pathological study showed no lesion other than rheumatoid arthritis.

The association of the conversion of rheumatoid arthritis into systemic lupus erythematosus with the prior administration of chrysotherapy has been suggested but is far from proved. The association of the conversion of rheumatoid arthritis into necrotizing arteritis with the use of steroids has also been suggested. One may only say that this latter development was seen prior to the advent of steroids but *has been observed much more frequently* since their use.

Prognosis

In terms of the individual, prognosis can seldom be very accurate. It is fair to say we worry when the rheumatoid factor is present in the serum, particularly in high titer, early in the course of the disease. Regardless of the type of management utilized, when the patients with rheumatoid arthritis are studied as a group, the numbers doing poorly increase with time. Individuals will enter long remissions but the number doing badly will be greater at ten years than at five and increase even more at fifteen years than at ten. The complete incapacitation of a bed and chair existence develops only in a relatively small number who enter this category by ten and fifteen years. The likelihood of a complete remission of any duration is extremely slight after three years of sustained disease activity.[1,3]

It seems a truism, but must be emphasized, that patients who accept their limitations and live within them do better than those who are unable to do so, and better than those who refuse to help themselves.

The reader who desires a more comprehensive description and study of the symptomatology and course of rheumatoid arthritis is referred to the excellent monograph of Short, Bauer, and Reynolds[7] on this subject.

BIBLIOGRAPHY

1. Duthie, J. J. R., Brown, P. E., Knox, J. D. E. and Thompson, M.: Ann. Rheumat. Dis., *16*, 411, 1957.
2. Garrod, A. B.: *A Treatise on Gout and Rheumatic Gout.* 3rd Ed., London, Longman Green and Co., 1876. (Proposed in 1st Ed., 1858.)
3. Ragan, C. and Farrington, E.: J.A.M.A., *181*, 663, 1962.
4. Sharpe, J.: Brit. Med. J., *1*, 975, 1957.
5. Copeman, W. S. C.: *A Short History of the Gout and the Rheumatic Diseases.* Berkeley and Los Angeles, University California Press, 1964.
6. Lawrence, J. C., in Kellgren, J. H. (ed.): *Population Studies in Rheumatoid Arthritis,* Arth. and Rheum. Fdn. and Nat. Inst. of Arth. and Metabol. Dis., U.S.P.H.S., New York, p. 13, 1958.
7. Short, C. L., Bauer, W. and Reynolds, W. E.: *Rheumatoid Arthritis,* Cambridge, Harvard University Press, 1957.

Chapter 22

Extra-Articular Rheumatoid Disease

By John L. Decker, M.D.

"Rheumatoid disease" is often suggested as a name to be preferred over "rheumatoid arthritis." The extraordinary range of manifestations and features, regarded as part and parcel of the disease but without apparent direct relationship to its synovitis, is cited as justifying such a preference. The disease is, of course, primarily a chronic polyarthritis and most of the ill health suffered is due to joint inflammation and dysfunction. Nevertheless systemic manifestations, visceral features, and extra-articular findings are common. The extra-articular manifestations are not usually overwhelming and commonly contribute only to the backdrop while joint inflammation is at center stage. On other occasions, however, the threat of death due to rheumatoid arteritis or the nearness of blindness due to scleromalacia perforans can dominate the clinical foreground. Death due solely to rheumatoid arthritis is rare indeed; when it occurs it is due to the extra-articular manifestations.

It is today inappropriate to regard such findings as pleural effusions, splenomegaly, or sensory neuropathy as "complications"; rather, they are part of the disease. Two major disease patterns, Sjögren's syndrome and amyloidosis, are regularly associated with rheumatoid arthritis and should be regarded as "concomitants." They are described in detail elsewhere in this volume (*see* Chapters 47 and 69), but need consideration when one is evaluating such findings as purpura, neuropathy or pulmonary infiltrates. Most extensive descriptions of the extra-articular manifestations of rheumatoid arthritis do not exclude or detail patients with Sjögren's syndrome; in view of its prevalence, the inclusion of individuals with the sicca syndrome may very well be distorting what is taken to be data on rheumatoid arthritis. "Complications" would include such events as fractures of osteopenic bone due to minimal trauma or pyogenic infections of joints already damaged by rheumatoid arthritis.

The notable effects of various drugs will not be discussed here. Nevertheless, neuromyopathy and retinal degeneration due to antimalarials, rashes and marrow effects of gold salt administration, major problems of peptic ulceration associated with many drugs, and posterior subcapsular cataracts and purpura due to adrenal corticosteroids are examples of drug-related phenomena which must be remembered and considered in the management of patients with rheumatoid arthritis.

The extra-articular manifestations of the rheumatic diseases in general are of significance in diagnostic work because they tend to display more variety than does the joint disease. Under these circumstances, it must be clear at the outset that this material deals with adult, usually seropositive, rheumatoid arthritis. The extra-articular manifestations of, for example, juvenile rheumatoid arthritis or ankylosing spondylitis are often different in kind, prevalence and implication. It is unhappily true that in many good studies of, for example, ocular disease in arthritis, the distinctions specified above are not honored and thus the exact pertinence of the findings to the several confusable entities may remain unclear. Nevertheless the effort below is oriented to the patient with adult rheumatoid arthritis of seropositive type. It is, perhaps, suitable to note that most of the extra-articular manifestations tend to be: (1) more frequent as the prevalence of seropositivity increases in a group of patients and (2) more frequent in patients with higher titers of rheumatoid factor than in those with lower.

ANEMIA

Moderate normocytic normochromic anemia is the most common extra-articular manifestation of rheumatoid arthritis and is probably present at times in virtually all patients with the disease. In women there is more of a tendency to hypochromia and microcytosis. The degree of anemia is clearly related to disease activity and recedes as the disease is brought under control.[96] It is uncommonly sufficiently profound to cause symptoms save in patients who have suffered major, acute hemorrhages.

The mechanisms resulting in the anemia have engaged the attention of numerous investigators over many years[68,70] and a considerable number of facts are clear. Chronic blood loss, due perhaps primarily to salicylates, does not seem to be a major factor[5] since the anemia is not that of iron deficiency. Serum iron levels are low but the serum iron-binding globulin is also low or normal rather than elevated as is the case in iron deficiency. The uptake of oral iron is mildly reduced to levels below that seen in comparable degrees of iron deficiency anemia. Increased destruction of red cells due to extracorpuscular factors does occur in Felty's syndrome and cell life spans are shortened to some degree in most patients with active rheumatoid arthritis. Nevertheless the six- to eight-fold increase in erythrocyte production of which the normal marrow is capable should easily compensate for the shortened half life in most patients. Expanded plasma volume with secondary hemodilution may play a small role.

In the normal state, the iron utilized is derived primarily from the breakdown of senescent red cells; the release of this iron may be diminished in rheumatoid arthritis.[73] Intravenously administered iron is rapidly cleared from the plasma and the low baseline levels are re-established. An iron chelating agent, desferrioxamine B, results in greater iron excretion from rheumatoid arthritic patients suggesting that their stores of iron are increased above normal. Taken together, these studies suggest that the major defect rests in an increased uptake or diminished release of iron from a site where it is unavailable for erythropoiesis. The avidity of the site appears to vary rapidly with disease activity. With acute inflammatory suppression induced by ACTH, iron clearance returns to normal[69] and, in the absence of iron supplements, serum and marrow iron promptly rise which is subsequently mirrored in a rising hemoglobin concentration.

Current evidence suggests that lymph nodes[71] and synovial tissues[69] contribute to the iron sequestration. In both sites erythrophagocytosis has been observed and, in the synovium at least, could readily account for the increased iron content observed. It has not yet been demonstrated, however, that these tissues are responsible for the observed rapid plasma iron clearance.

The hypothesis does accord with the clinical fact that the anemia of rheumatoid arthritis is best relieved, not by hematinics, but by bringing the disease activity under control.

RHEUMATOID NODULES

These familiar lesions, typically subcutaneous in location, are the hallmark of seropositive rheumatoid arthritis and, especially when multiple, serve to warn the clinician that his patient has a more guarded prognosis for joint function and a greater chance to develop features of systemic rheumatoid disease than does the patient without nodules.

The superficial lesions are rare in the

dermis, common in the subcutaneous tissue, and may involve all manner of deeper connective tissue structures such as bursae, periosteum, tendon sheaths, and tendons. They vary in size from seed-like to enormous, confluent masses of nodular tissue overlying the olecranon process. They are remarkably asymptomatic and are likely to cause only cosmetic complaints.

They tend to appear insidiously, often first being noted by the physician, usually in association with increasing symptoms of synovitis but they are notably capricious in time of onset. As they mysteriously increase in size over one or several months, just so mysteriously do they gradually disappear in a like time period. In other patients they may persist indefinitely. It is not rare to witness the development of a new nodule at a time when the patient feels well and is supposed by the physician to be in remission.

They are clearly more likely to appear in areas subjected to repeated microtrauma—over the olecranon, over the ischial tuberosity, over the Achilles tendon at the point where ill-fitting shoes impinge, or on the bridge of the nose where spectacles are supported. They also appear in areas where no trauma is recognized, for example, overlying the helix of the ear in patients who are ambulatory. In hemiplegic individuals only the non-paralyzed limbs develop nodules.[8]

By far the most important complication is breakdown of the overlying skin and discharge of the central core of the necrobiotic granuloma—"fistulous rheumatism." Such lesions are painful, heal poorly, and almost invariably become infected. They present a particularly difficult problem in a bedridden patient when they develop over the sacrum or over the ischial tuberosity.

Excision is the only useful treatment and is usually at least temporarily successful for the uncomplicated nodule; recurrences are very common, often in the original wound scar. When spontaneous drainage has occurred, wide excision is sometimes successful; skin grafting may be required where adequate closure cannot be achieved.

There are a multitude of nodular lesions which, upon clinical examination, can be mistaken for a rheumatoid nodule; gouty tophi, sebaceous cysts, basal cell carcinoma, ganglions of the hand or wrist, xanthomatous tendon lesions, and the nodules of multicentric reticulohistiocytosis are examples. For the vast majority of patients, there is, unfortunately, little doubt as to the nature of the lesion in the setting of seropositive polyarthritis. Nevertheless excision biopsy should be performed if there are unusual or suspicious features; bearing the gouty tophus in mind, a portion of the nodular tissue removed should always be fixed in a nonaqueous fixative.

LYMPHADENOPATHY

Lymph node enlargement is common in rheumatoid arthritis. However, the definition of adenopathy varies widely, as illustrated by comparing two studies; one group found enlargement in 29 per cent of patients and 9 per cent of controls while in another adenopathy was recorded in 82 per cent of patients and 52 per cent of controls.[79,87] Males showed the higher prevalence among both patients and controls. Enlargement is more common in rheumatoid factor positive patients and in those with active disease.

Clinical examination and lymphangiography indicate that the nodes immediately proximal to joints exhibiting synovitis are more likely to be enlarged than more remote nodes although this is certainly not invariable. The nodes are not tender or inflamed, show no tendency to mat, and are firm and rubbery.

In dealing with suspicious or unexpected lymphadenopathy, temporization is probably justified. The probability that the enlargement will recede is good. Enthusiasm for diagnostic biopsy must be restrained by the fact that virtually all series of node biopsies in rheumatoid arthritis include one or several cases who received radiation or cancer chemotherapy because the lesion was interpreted as malignant, a finding not justified by the subsequent course.[23,67,72] Lymphomas do, however, occur.

OCULAR MANIFESTATIONS

Historically rheumatoid arthritis was regarded as causing inflammation of two portions of the eye—the sclera and the anterior uveal tract composed of the iris and the ciliary body. In the latter process many terms are used referring to the area of most intense involvement— iritis, iridocyclitis when ciliary involvement is prominent, anterior uveitis when all the structures are involved save the choroid which constitutes the posterior element of the uveal tract. The process is said to be non-granulomatous when diffuse exudative phenomena are most apparent on examination and dense, nodular infiltrates are not identified. The latter lesion, a cardinal feature of granulomatous iridocyclitis, is the usual feature of sarcoidosis and such chronic infections as tuberculosis or brucellosis.

Within the last 10 or 15 years it has become apparent that anterior uveitis is no more common than in the general population; that corneal and conjunctival manifestations of the sicca syndrome of Sjögren are the most common ophthalmological feature of rheumatoid arthritis; that disease of the sclera is a rare but characteristic manifestation; and that many of the drugs used in the management of the disease may affect the eye.[90] Gold deposition in the cornea as a result of chrysotherapy, posterior subcapsular cataracts due to adrenal corticosteroids, and corneal and retinal changes related to anti-malarial therapy are the principal offenders in the latter group.

Non-granulomatous anterior uveitis is a typical feature of ankylosing spondylitis and juvenile rheumatoid arthritis and actually serves in part to distinguish these processes from rheumatoid arthritis.[50] In one large experience uveitis was regarded as a feature of ankylosing spondylitis in men and in women of a distinctive disease pattern characterized as a seronegative, asymmetrical polyarthritis with minimal radiologic findings; it showed a predilection for the joints of the lower extremity, especially those of the feet.[99]

The sclera, an opaque, avascular, and relatively acellular tunic of collagen, envelops the eye and is continuous with the transparent cornea. Superficial to the sclera and loosely connected to Tenon's capsule and the conjunctiva, lies the episclera, an ill-defined layer of highly vascular, loosely organized connective tissue. Rheumatoid disease affects both the episclera and the sclera.

Episcleritis appears over the anterior sclera anywhere from the extraocular muscle insertions to the cornea but is most frequent within a few millimeters of the limbus. It may be localized ("nodular") or more diffuse.[59] Typically it appears rather acutely as a raised lesion a few millimeters across, cream colored to violaceous and surrounded by intense hyperemia which is darker purple in the deeper vessels as compared to the bright red of conjunctival hyperemia. Discomfort is common but pain is not. The lesions may be transient but are often persistent over weeks or months despite the use of topical corticosteroids. They rarely ulcerate and tend to remain superficial. Transient lesions, healing without residua, are seen; in the more chronic form the conjunctiva tends to become bound down in a slate-colored scar.

The lesions may involve one or both eyes, are sometimes multiple, and seem to be more prevalent in women. They are common in patients who show manifestations of rheumatoid arteritis. The specificity of the lesion is established by its histological features, typical of a rheumatoid nodule.[31]

Scleritis (Figure 22–1*A*) is a rarer and more serious problem which may present as a painful, highly inflammatory condition with widespread necrosis (necrotiz-

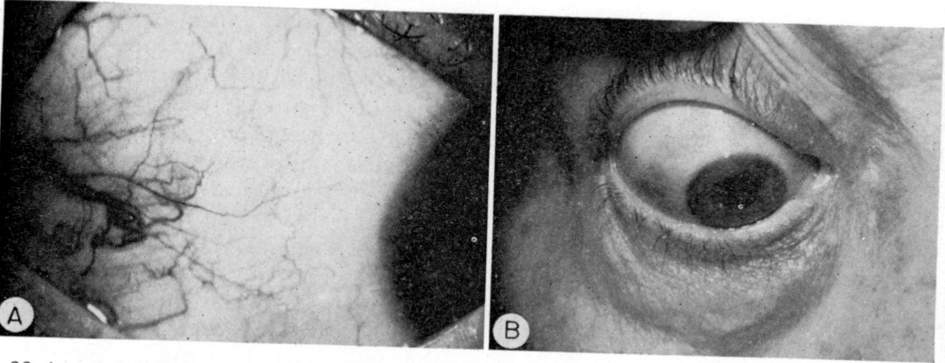

FIG. 22–1.—*A*. Medial sclera showing vascularity overlying nodular scleritis in a 52-year-old woman with 18 years of seropositive rheumatoid arthritis. Subcutaneous nodules had first appeared 5 years before and scleromalacia perforans developed in the opposite eye 2 years earlier (Courtesy Dr. Vernon Wong). *B*. This patient was 67 years old; rheumatoid arthritis had been apparent since about age 35. The darkening of the lateral sclera had the distinctly bluish hue of choroidal pigmentation, seen because of scleral thinning due to previous scleritis. The destruction had occurred in three episodes over a year's time, the last ending a year earlier (Courtesy Dr. Werner Barth).

ing nodular sclerosis); more commonly an indolent, slowly progressive, asymptomatic nodular destruction of the sclera (*scleromalacia perforans*) takes place. The incidence is greatest 10 or 15 years after the onset of rheumatoid arthritis appearing usually in patients more than 50 years of age; the reported cases include twice as many females as males presumably corresponding to the prevalence of the underlying process in the two sexes.[86]

There is some evidence that the more hectic process is associated with arteritis while the more indolent is usually due to a typical nodule. Thus the two related processes—arteritis and rheumatoid nodule formation—are regarded as alternate causes of the scleral necrosis.

The lesions are most likely to appear superiorly in the sclera of the anterior eye as raised, yellow nodules with the degree of hyperemia varying with their acuteness. The sclera at the site may become thinned and transparent revealing the dark blue of the choroid (Figure 22–1*B*) within or the nodule may slough out leaving patches of choroid exposed. The distinction between episcleritis and scleritis may be difficult but is ultimately based upon whether or not thinning of the sclera develops. In contrast to episcleritis, ophthalmological complications of scleritis are common and threatening to vision. They include uveitis (including choroiditis with retinal detachment), sclerosing keratitis (extension to the cornea), cataracts, secondary glaucoma, and perforation.

Treatment is not satisfactory. Topical steroids reduce the acute inflammation and may prevent some of the necrosis but do not effect closure of the scleral holes. These have occasionally been successfully treated by grafting.

LARYNGEAL MANIFESTATIONS

Since most authors ascribe this condition to typical rheumatoid arthritis appearing in the synovial membrane of the diarthrodial crico-arytenoid joints, it might be excluded from material on extra-articular manifestations; nevertheless consideration is justified on the grounds that the region is rarely included in the typical joint examination, that potentially reversible disease can be swiftly lethal, and that some feel the symptoms to be due not to arthritis but to arteritis of the vasa nervorum of the laryngeal nerves with abductor paralysis.[109]

Crico-arytenoid joint disease is found at autopsy in rheumatoid arthritis with a frequency approaching half the cases.[7,37] Detailed assessment in life of series of patients with generalized disease suggests that symptoms or findings will be found in something over a quarter of the patients.[58] Nonetheless, clinically manifest problems are rare.

Acute and chronic symptoms are described. Pain or difficulty with swallowing, fullness or tension in the throat, hoarseness, dyspnea on exertion, and stridulous respirations may be noted acutely. With the exception of pain, the symptoms may be persistent over extended periods. The number of patients with laryngeal disease who do not suffer hoarseness or voice changes is remarkable. In some instances dyspnea and stridor are believed to be absent simply because advanced arthritis limits exertion. The laryngeal symptoms may be so mild as to be overlooked without specific questioning; on occasion, they have been regarded as hysterical.

Indirect laryngoscopic examinations may show acute redness and swelling overlying the arytenoids but the more common finding is immobilized crico-arytenoid joints with either one or both vocal processes, and with them the cords, adducted to the midline (Fig 22–2). If the adduction is symmetrical, the airway may be reduced to a chink and the cords can be seen to bow outward on inspiration due to the pull of the internal thyroarytenoid muscle. Joint pain can often be demonstrated by an attempt to move the arytenoid cartilage with a spatula.

In the chronic situation with fixation in adduction superimposed respiratory infection of any kind can put the patient at substantial risk because of laryngeal and cord edema. Emergency tracheotomy may be required.[77] After the recession of the acute superinfection, arytenoidectomy is usually advised in preference to a permanent tracheotomy. Surgical intervention is often not needed if the joint fixation on either side is in a position other than adduction. The possible presence of compromised crico-arytenoid motion should be borne in mind when intubation is needed.

PLEUROPULMONARY MANIFESTATIONS

The pleuropulmonary lesions of rheumatoid arthritis are diverse and relatively uncommon. At the bedside or in the office one is much more likely to find that pulmonary symptoms or findings can be ascribed to common causes such as

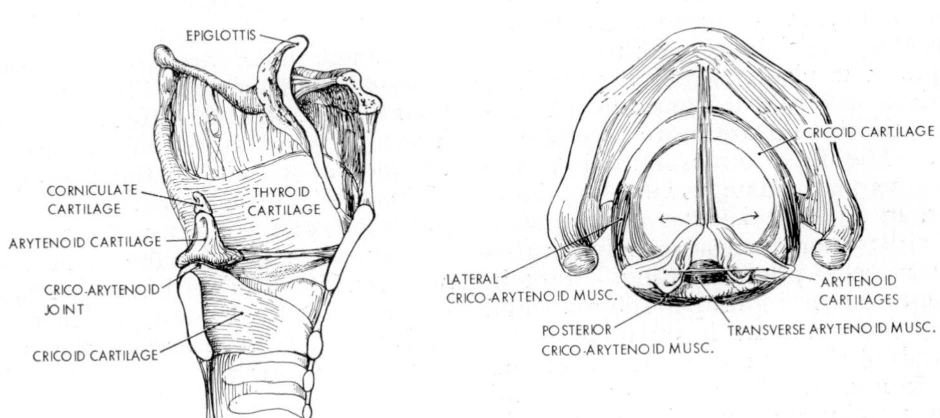

Fig. 22–2.—The cartilaginous skeleton of the larynx in lateral section and from above. The cords and vocal processes are shown adducted by the action of the lateral crico-arytenoids. The arrows are toward abduction, the position produced by the action of the posterior crico-arytenoid muscle.

pulmonary tuberculosis, bronchiectasis, or emphysema than to any of the more specific processes which have been related to rheumatoid arthritis, itself a common disease. Studies have shown such lesions as old apical scarring, bronchitis, and bronchiectasis to be more prevalent than in age- and sex-matched hospital patients without rheumatoid arthritis.[3,100] Nevertheless pleural, nodular, pneumoconiotic and diffuse interstitial fibrotic processes may be found in association with rheumatoid arthritis or with rheumatoid factor in the absence of arthritis.

Pleural Manifestations

Rheumatoid pleural disease is most likely to exhibit itself as asymptomatic pleural effusion, as notable pleural thickening at the bases by x-ray,[88] or as widespread and prominent pleural adhesions at autopsy.[89] Symptomatic pleurisy in brief episodes, usually in association with increases in disease activity but sometimes before the diagnosis of rheumatoid arthritis is apparent, does occur at a rate approximately double that seen in nonrheumatoid patients; the incidence is higher in men than in women.[101]

Pleural effusions usually appear painlessly and may be an incidental finding although in some instances the collections can become so massive as to impair respiratory exchange. Effusions, like symptomatic pleurisy, may substantially antedate or herald the onset of rheumatoid arthritis and are more common in men. The fluid on examination is a typical serous exudate, usually containing less than 5,000 leukocytes per cu. mm. with either mononuclear or polymorphonuclear cells predominating. Protein content exceeds 3 gms. per 100 ml. while the glucose content is often (but not invariably)[102] reduced to levels of less than 15 mg. per 100 ml.[14] Rheumatoid factor activity may exceed that found in simultaneous serum samples, complement values are low, and intracellular gamma globulin inclusions have been demonstrated with indirect immunofluorescent staining.

The course of such effusions tends to be chronic, in a good proportion persisting for more than a year. Extensive reactive fibrosis may appear in the long persistent case even producing restrictive ventilatory defects requiring decortication. Pleural biopsies have usually failed to recover tissue which could be definitely regarded as of rheumatoid origin; chronic, low grade inflammation with fibrosis is the usual finding.

Biopsies do, of course, help to exclude other diagnoses such as tuberculosis and since the diagnosis of rheumatoid pleurisy is essentially one of exclusion, the procedure is useful. Many other entities need to be considered and excluded with care; pulmonary embolism is an example. Empyema may also be of concern, either as the entire explanation for an effusion or as a superimposed infection of a previously diseased space as is seen with the rheumatoid joint. It is also to be noted that rheumatoid pericardial effusion (*see* Cardiac Manifestations) is more likely to accompany a pleural effusion than to appear in a patient without other evidence of serosal involvement.

While the exact role of rheumatoid disease in the above forms of nonspecific pleural disease may be debated, there also exist patients with rheumatoid nodules, histologically defined, appearing in the lungs; these are often subpleural, plaque-like structures. They may also be found in the parietal pleura. From both locations the nodules may ulcerate into the pleural space with the development of pleural effusions or, more rarely, pneumothorax. Under these circumstances, the nature of the pleural space fluid exactly parallels that which appears without nodules, lending credence to the notion that both processes are part of rheumatoid disease.

Nodular Pulmonary Disease

Although rheumatoid nodules of the lungs are often so peripheral as to involve the visceral pleura, they may develop singly or multiply, within the parenchyma itself. They appear as round shadows, 0.5 to 3 cm. in size, and usually in an asymptomatic male patient with seropositive rheumatoid arthritis; the lesions are less prone to occur in females. Like the subcutaneous nodule itself, the pulmonary nodule appears and disappears without a close relationship to synovial disease activity. It may persist for years without change or may slowly enlarge to an enormous size.

Nodular parenchymal disease in the absence of pleural findings is, however, exceptionally rare and thorough study, probably including thoracotomy, is justified to exclude other causes; this is particularly true of the single coin lesion. Spontaneous cavitation with little pericavitary inflammation has been reported; indeed some patients have presented a cavity as the first sign, only subsequently to develop other nodules.

Rheumatoid Pneumoconiosis (Caplan's Syndrome)

If pneumoconiotic exposure is a part of the rheumatoid patient's background, however, parenchymal nodules are routine findings. In these circumstances, they constitute one of the elements of a larger picture referred to as rheumatoid pneumoconiosis or Caplan's syndrome.[12] Welsh miners, exposed primarily to soft coal dust, were found to exhibit chest roentgenographic patterns which differed from ordinary pneumoconiosis if the individual had rheumatoid arthritis; about 35 per cent of rheumatoid miners show the condition.[66] In some instances the pattern appears years before the development of overt rheumatoid arthritis.

The "classical" roentgenogram shows multiple, well-defined round opacities greater than 1 cm. in diameter distributed through all lung fields especially peripherally (Fig. 22–3). Cavitation is often a feature. More commonly patients show discrete nodular shadows varying from 0.3 to 1 cm. in diameter. These smaller nodules may be few and confined to the upper zones or they may present a "snowstorm" appearance widely distributed throughout the chest. Other patients show scattered irregular opacities, often with evidence of cavitation, but with little simple pneumoconiosis in

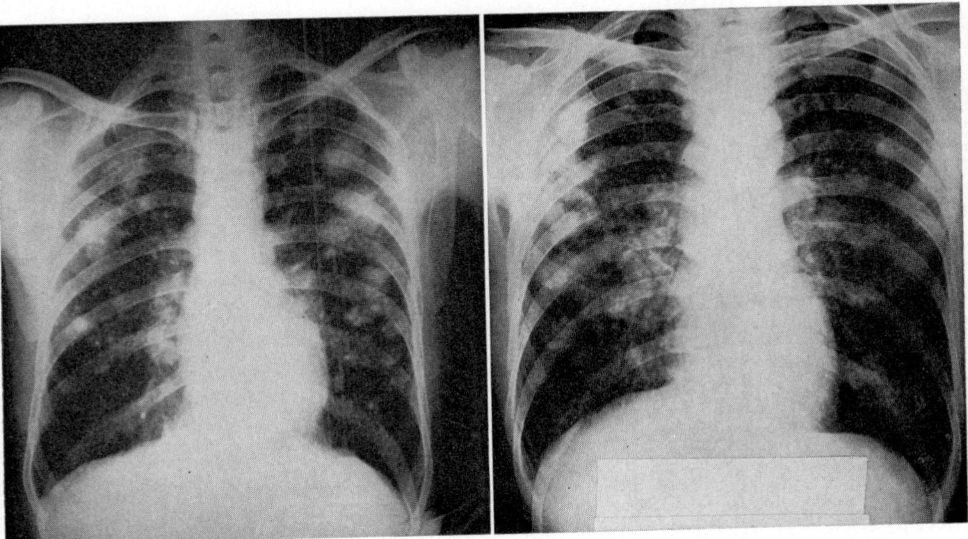

Fig. 22–3.—Two examples of rheumatoid pneumoconiosis in the classical form (Courtesy Dr. A. Caplan).

the background. Two-thirds of patients with the "classical" picture have definite rheumatoid arthritis. Rheumatoid factor activity has been found in the serum of more than 80 per cent of the miners presenting these roentgenographic changes.[13]

Pathological study of the lesions has shown non-specific inflammation about necrotic granulation tissue. The three classical zones of the rheumatoid nodule are usually well defined although interpretation of the pathological material is made more complex by the background of simple pneumoconiosis. Central calcification is occasionally noted.[35] The epidemiological, clinical and pathological picture justify the name, rheumatoid pneumoconiosis, and suggest that the tissue responses to dust of the rheumatoid or pre-rheumatoid individual differ from those of the general population.

There is abundant evidence that the syndrome is not confined to soft coal miners; it has been identified in workers with asbestos, abrasives, foundries and silica although in some of these cases the x-rays are not identical to those described for the miners.

Diffuse Interstitial Fibrosis

The term "rheumatoid disease" was coined in 1948 in a report describing the first recognized association of diffuse interstitial fibrosis and rheumatoid arthritis.[26] Since that time scattered descriptions of the pulmonary lesion have appeared under several names including chronic pulmonary fibrosis, fibrosing pneumonitis, and fibrosing alveolitis.

Dyspnea on exertion, cough with scanty sputum, and clubbing are typical manifestations of the syndrome. Diffuse or, more often, basilar crepitant rales are found. The effective lung size and compliance are both reduced, producing a restrictive ventilatory defect. Defects in gas transfer may be observed and are ascribed to wide variations in ventilation: perfusion ratios.[82]

By x-ray early disease may appear as soft fluffy patches or fine reticulonodular shadowing almost always most prominent at the bases. Subsequently diffuse mottling and "harder" pulmonary fibrosis gradually appear with cysts and fibrotic "honeycombing" being typical of end stage disease. This whole picture can evolve within a year, but a five- to ten-year course is more common. The essential histological features are thickening of the alveolar walls with cells and fibrosis and the presence of large mononuclear cells, presumably of alveolar origin, within the alveolar spaces. Neither the radiological nor histological examination provides an unequivocal link to rheumatoid arthritis; they are non-specific. In the great majority, rheumatoid arthritis precedes the pulmonary fibrosis by years but the pulmonary process can begin first.

Approximately 100 cases of rheumatoid arthritis and diffuse interstitial fibrosis have been reported, the majority in males. Many sizable groups of patients with rheumatoid arthritis have been surveyed without detecting even a single case of diffuse interstitial fibrosis; eight cases were recently identified in a study of 516 rheumatoid arthritis patients.[103] Looked at from the chest physician's vantage point, however, 15 to 20 per cent of all patients with diffuse interstitial fibrosis have rheumatoid arthritis, a proportion unlikely to be due to random coincidence.

The relationship of the pulmonary process to rheumatoid factor also tends to link the two processes. In one series pulmonary fibrosis, diagnosed by x-ray only, was found in 32 per cent of 66 individuals with high factor titers and in 12 and 8 per cent, respectively, of patients with more modest or negative titers.[76] Almost half of 52 patients with fibrosis but without rheumatoid arthritis had circulating rheumatoid factor.[97,98] The pulmonary capillary circulation would presumably be the first capillary bed met by newly formed antigen-antibody complexes in the circulation. On the other hand, it can be argued that the mononuclear cell infiltrates found in the lungs may be the source of much of the circulating factor.

In summary, specific pulmonary disease associated with rheumatoid arthritis is rare while non-life-threatening pleural disease is substantially more common. All of the pleuropulmonary processes are curiously more common in males and are relatable to rheumatoid factor. Two patterns, rheumatoid nodules of the lung and rheumatoid pneumoconiosis, are unequivocally part of rheumatoid arthritis while the other two, nonspecific pleural inflammation and diffuse interstitial fibrosis, bear a somewhat more uncertain relationship to the underlying disease. Both rheumatoid pneumoconiosis and diffuse interstitial fibrosis do cause death. The diversity of the processes discussed does not encourage the use of the loose phrase "*rheumatoid lung*."

CARDIAC MANIFESTATIONS

The variety and extent of cardiac lesions described in postmortem studies of rheumatoid arthritis never cease to amaze the clinician who is usually able to recall only a handful of patients who exhibited cardiological findings which he related to their rheumatoid arthritis. The autopsy findings should, however, spur him to more careful and frequent evaluation of the heart since such efforts do reveal unexpected changes.[51] Nevertheless the man at the bedside is probably correct in believing that most such autopsy findings are not clinically manifest, that some are detectable but not of importance to his patient, and that a very few are the cause of significant functional impairment of the heart.

Pericarditis

Clinical pericarditis was identified in 10 of 100 consecutive patients with rheumatoid arthritis of sufficient severity to require hospitalization for articular problems. All patients as well as an equal number of age- and sex-matched controls were examined on at least three occasions and all had chest films and electrocardiograms. Pericardial friction rubs were detected in all 10, only one had chest pain, and seven were entirely asymptomatic; pericarditis was identified in a single control subject.[51]

The process is generally benign and self-limited, rarely causing significant symptoms although numerous cases of pericardial tamponade and constrictive pericarditis requiring pericardiectomy have been reported.[56,80] When the process is active, low grade fever is usual and the electrocardiogram often shows ST or T wave changes although the classical features of pericarditis are uncommon.[9,51] The inflammation may appear early in the course of the disease, especially in men, but the median duration of rheumatoid arthritis to clinical pericarditis is 8 to 10 years. In a series based upon postmortem examinations, it was noted that a substantially larger proportion of those with pericardial involvement were disabled by their joint disease (Class IV) than were those without pericarditis.[9]

As with pleural disease, the pathological findings—fibrinous pericarditis when acute and pericardial fibrosis when chronic—are not usually pathognomonic of rheumatoid arthritis although rarely typical rheumatoid granulomata may be seen. Evidence of past or present pericarditis has been found in about 40 per cent of rheumatoid patients coming to autopsy.[15]

Adrenal corticosteroid therapy has been successful in resolving life-threatening pericardial disease especially when administered for that indication.[32]

Myocardium

Myocardial insufficiency and death due to congestive heart failure are frequent in rheumatoid arthritis but how frequently is this due to rheumatoid arthritis? Probably not often. "A patient with a severe debilitating disorder such as rheumatoid disease dies, as it were, by inches. Cardiac deaths are common in such a group of extremely ill patients. Very good pathological evidence must therefore be found at necropsy before the diagnosis of rheumatoid heart disease is justified."[39] Thus the role of interstitial foci of mononuclear cells found in the myocardium is of uncertain significance[91] although its appearance and severity may match that of Fiedler's myocarditis. Diffuse myocarditis with frank necrosis of muscle is also seen.[54]

Coronary artery disease plays a major role despite the fact that coronary atherosclerosis appears to be somewhat less common than in control autopsy material;[9] myocardial infarction due to atherosclerosis is a common cause of death. Rheumatoid arteritis seems rarely to involve the large vessels of the heart and rarely to produce myocardial ischemia and infarction[47] as occurs in polyarteritis nodosa but subacute inflammation, sometimes with vessel wall necrosis, does involve the small arteries or arterioles[22] especially in patients exhibiting clinical rheumatoid arteritis.

Endocardium

No way to distinguish the endocardial lesions of inactive rheumatic fever from the fibrosed and nodular valve leaves that are found post mortem in rheumatoid arthritis has yet come to light. The exact criteria used become of importance when one attempts to assess pathological reports which describe such lesions in 25 to 60 per cent of rheumatoid patients.[91] Reports on gross examination revealed "thickening" in about half of both seropositive patients and a control series.[9]

In any event valvular disease of this type is not of clinical significance from a hemodynamic point of view. Stenotic lesions virtually never occur and systolic murmurs are equally common whether or not leaf thickening is subsequently observed.

Granulomatous Lesions

Areas of fibrinoid necrosis, often surrounded by palisaded histiocytes and chronic mononuclear inflammatory cells, are considered to be specifically rheumatoid in nature. They involve all layers of the heart and may be nodular or more diffuse in appearance. They occur in 5 to 10 per cent of all seropositive patients coming to autopsy[24] and may be associated with any of the more nonspecific changes described above.

As endocardial lesions they are most likely to affect the valves, usually of the left side of the heart and away from the free edges nearer the base of the leaflet. At this location they may involve the valve rings or "skeleton of the heart."

In contrast to the purely fibrous endocardial lesions, the granulomata are often associated with severe, symptomatic heart disease. Stenosis is similarly uncommon but valvular incompetence may result. The process may be so intense as to cause necrosis and perforation. In addition to valve leaf damage, involvement of the valve ring may produce loss of structural integrity permitting dilatation of the ring with resulting valvular insufficiency.

The aortic valve annulus lies in proximity to the atrioventricular node and the bundle of His and these structures may be compromised. Such disease has produced complete atrioventricular block and sudden death.[36,38] The pathological process at the root of the aorta in ankylosing spondylitis may have the same clinical effects in terms of conduction difficulties and aortic insufficiency but shows patchy destruction of the media of the aortic root and intimal fibrosis of the regional arterioles, a very different histological pattern.

NEUROMUSCULAR MANIFESTATIONS

The evaluation of neuromuscular features of rheumatoid arthritis is a time-consuming and difficult task. Patients with pain, stiffness, and weakness associated with active polyarthritis may not mention symptoms which would suggest neuropathy to the examiner. The physician will recognize myasthenia but is usually unable to exclude arthritic disease as its primary cause. Nevertheless one often sees patients who will report that "something fresh, new, and unpleasant has happened to their feet which feel different and are painful in a different way."[40] Likewise there is no mistaking the abrupt onset of foot drop in the ambulatory patient. These problems and others, all manifestations of rheumatoid arthritis, occur in about 10 per cent of patients with the disease and deserve careful evaluation because of therapeutic and prognostic implications.

The classification of the neurological lesions of rheumatoid arthritis varies widely. Diffuse distal neuropathy will be considered first and then a few specific lesions, both central and peripheral, which may have neurological manifestations. Finally some of the features of the myopathy will be mentioned.

Diffuse Neuropathy

The diffuse distal neuropathy, in its most common form, presents with numbness of the feet, usually symmetrical and usually stocking like in distribution. Hypesthesia, electric shock sensations, or burning pain do occur. Examination reveals a loss of vibration sensation in most together with altered appreciation of light touch and pinprick. Position sense is usually retained. The findings may not follow exactly the symptomatic areas. Neither the symptoms nor the findings usually correspond to the distribution of a major nerve. In some patients relatively minor motor changes are also detectable with muscle wasting. The achilles reflex, particularly, may be lost. Electrophysiological studies may be normal but gross slowing of motor conduction in the affected limb is also observed.[17] Similar lesions are seen in the hands where clumsiness may be a complaint; in the great majority of those with involved hands, foot symptoms are also present. Careful assessment of the fingers has been particularly telling in bringing out numbness of the tips or hypesthesia along one side of a digit.[75]

The above patterns are typically seen in elderly seropositive patients with disease of 10 to 15 years' duration. Subcutaneous nodules have been found in about half of them. The prognosis is generally good with partial or complete recovery in most. In some the findings remain static while in a few progression over weeks or months can lead to more widespread findings.

Patients with severe motor impairment based on peripheral nerve disease present a somewhat different pattern and seem to be, in large part, a separate group. While they may, either at onset or in course, have sensory deficits, the usual picture is one of rapid change in and progressive deterioration of motor function. Early the abruptly developing foot or wrist drops often represent a *mononeuritis multiplex* (motor and sensory impairment in the distribution of two or more peripheral nerves); this tends to evolve into a severe sensorimotor neuropathy with complete paralysis of several extremities and dense sensory loss.[75]

The prognosis for life is bad and the more widespread the neuropathy, the worse it becomes.[30] Many of these patients have died and virtually all have shown arteritis, in many instances involving the vasa nervorum. This swift pattern occurs most commonly in males, invariably with nodules and high titers of rheumatoid factor (see Rheumatoid Arteritis).

Whether or not arteritis should be regarded as the cause of all diffuse neuropathy is unclear. Cases with obvious disease have been found to be free of arteritis related to peripheral nerve after exhaustive postmortem search.[40] The symmetrical distribution and the many patients with sensory lesions only are not readily explained by vascular inflammation. It is conceivable that the impairment, more common in the patient taking too much corticosteroid or changing doses too rapidly, has some other basis; perhaps it is more of a "rheumatoid" neuropathy than is known.

The recognized specific lesions due to

rheumatoid arthritis are all associated with pressure on neural tissue and include pressure on the spinal cord as a manifestation of cervical subluxations, the several syndromes of peripheral nerve entrapment, and manifestations resulting from rheumatoid nodules impinging on the central nervous system.

Cervical Myelopathy

Neurological manifestations of cervical spine disease are recognized with only modest frequency when one considers the prevalence of radiological abnormalities of the area. In one study of 333 patients, requiring hospitalization for active physiotherapy and rehabilitation, a single lateral view of the cervical spine in *full flexion* was made. *Atlanto-axial subluxation* (defined as a distance of greater than 2.5 mm. in women and 3.0 mm. in males between the posterior aspect of the anterior arch of the atlas and the anterior surface of the odontoid process) was found in 84 and serial subluxation of other cervical vertebrae in 23.[19] Destruction of the transverse ligament of the atlas and the anterior atlanto-axial ligament by rheumatoid arthritis permit the dens to move posteriorly into the spinal canal; cord compression is, however, uncommon perhaps primarily because of the generous size of the canal at this level (Fig. 22–4*A*). Cervical spine pain is more frequent and compression findings less frequent with atlanto-axial disease than with subluxation of lower cervical vertebrae, most common at C3–C4, where pain is often absent and the signs of cord compression may be overwhelming; at the lower level, the canal is less capacious (Fig. 22–4*B*).

Cervical cord compression is most

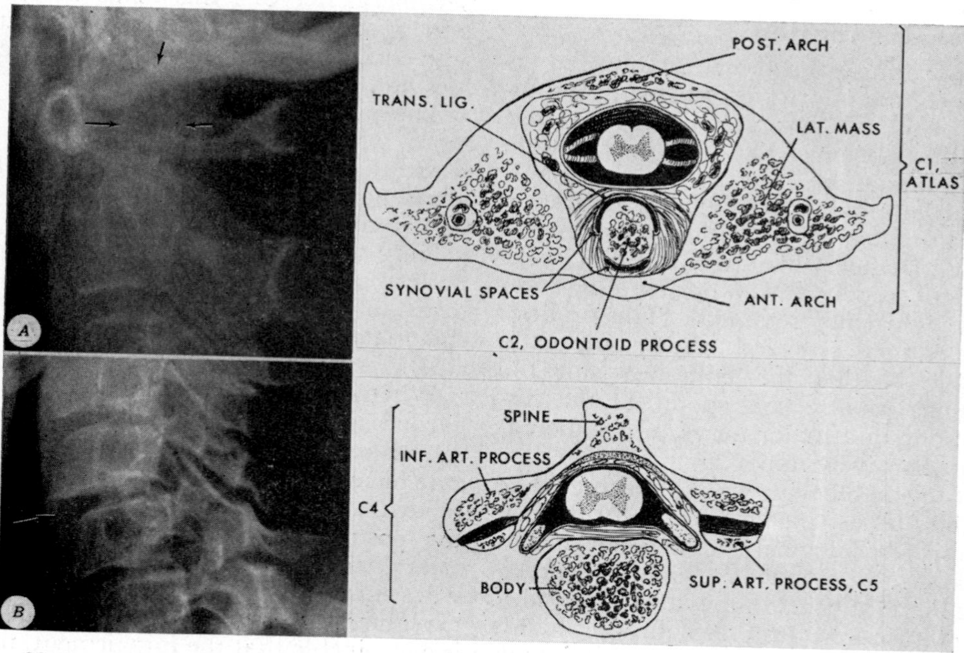

FIG. 22–4.—*A*. Flexion films of the upper cervical spine with the odontoid process of C2 outlined by arrows. The dislocation measured 7 mm. The patient, a 59-year-old woman, had had seropositive rheumatoid arthritis with nodules for 17 years. She had severe deformities with finger extensor tendon destruction. She had had posterior cervical pain but there were neither symptoms nor findings of neural compression. *B*. Mild subluxation of C4 on C5 in longstanding rheumatoid arthritis. This less common change can be, but here was not, accompanied by findings of cord compression (Courtesy Dr. John Bland).

likely to develop in those patients in whom it is most difficult to detect, that is, those with longstanding, seropositive, deforming rheumatoid arthritis with extensive erosive disease, much joint instability, and tendon rupture.[19,64,74] Cervical spine pain is occasionally entirely absent. The radiological finding of atlanto-axial subluxation can be supplemented by actual palpation of the joint through the posterior pharyngeal wall. Upper motor neuron signs, such as weakness, unexplained "giving way" of the knee, flexor spasm, positive Babinski sign, and increased deep tendon reflexes, may be identified. Bowel and bladder dysfunction occurs. In view of the many musculoskeletal problems in the typical patient, sensory examination is important. Position sense and two point discrimination are lost early. The findings range from barely detectable to full-blown tetraplegia as in cord transection. Death has resulted not only due to cord compression but due to vertebral artery thrombosis induced by kinking secondary to excess motion of the axis.[62,104,106] Traumas of various types—automobile accidents, intubation, extreme head positions under anesthesia—are dangerous for these patients.

A variety of surgical procedures are available for immobilizing the cervical spine and offer a very substantial chance for return to active life even in severe cases.[20,21] Complete reduction of the subluxation is not necessary for good results and traction should be used with care. Gentle collar immobilization is the best choice for conservative management; unless this promptly reverses the neurological manifestations, operative intervention should be undertaken.

Pressure Neuropathy

The entrapment or pressure neuropathies in rheumatoid arthritis are caused by inflammation or edema at a point, usually juxta-articular, where non-distensible structures restrain the peripheral nerve involved. The symptoms tend to subside if the local inflammation recedes consequent to rest, local corticosteroid injection, or adequate systemic therapy. Surgical intervention is dramatically successful in virtually all instances. Compression neuropathies may occur at any stage of the disease and, in a number of instances, appear to have been the first detectable manifestation of rheumatoid arthritis.

Median nerve compression in the carpal tunnel is by far the most common and rheumatoid arthritis is its most common systemic cause.[110] The ulnar nerve can be affected at elbow or wrist. The radial or posterior interosseous nerve is less often involved at the elbow as it passes anterior to the lateral epicondyle.[61] Anterior tibial nerve palsy with foot drop can be associated with popliteal space compression or the external compression of braces or casts as the nerve rounds the fibular head. The posterior tibial nerve can be compressed in the tarsal tunnel beneath the flexor retinaculum distal to the medial malleolus; it is there accompanied by the tendons of the long flexors and their sheaths.[18,57]

Rheumatoid Nodules

There are only scattered case reports of rheumatoid nodules impinging on the central nervous system. Over the cranium these have been found to involve primarily the dura mater or the leptomeninges.[27,95] The neural tissue is uninvolved save for occasional vasculitis. The lesions have not been clearly related to symptoms although one patient had "what appeared to be Jacksonian fits."[27] Extradural rheumatoid nodules involve the spinal canal and occasionally produce nerve root compression.[34,35]

Muscle Disorders

Weakness and atrophy of skeletal muscle are among the earliest and most pervasive manifestations of rheumatoid arthritis. They are evident virtually throughout the disease course and contribute very significantly to the total disability of the process. They affect small muscles as well as large. Muscle pain and stiffness are common symptoms. The weakness and wasting can, of course, be a sequel to neurological dysfunction, described earlier, but more frequently appear in the absence of discernible neurological impairment. While perhaps more common in muscles acting across painful and damaged joints, they appear in areas remote from synovial inflammation. The course is irregular in that dramatic muscle weakness may occur over 3 to 6 months while in extended periods both before and after the episode weakness may not be prominent. Occasionally corticosteroid therapy seems to be a major causative factor.

In essence, however, the weakness is unexplained. Striking elevations of muscle-related enzymes are not observed[60,105] but serum creatine-creatinine ratios are increased, consistent with diminished muscle mass.[105] Electromyographic analysis has found "myositis" and "myopathy," as variously defined, to be present but the findings are poorly related to clinically observed weakness and wasting and to neighboring joint activity.[60,94] Myositis, characterized by nodular or diffuse infiltrates of lymphocytes and plasma cells with muscle necrosis, and muscle cachexia, characterized by a reduction in muscle-cell bulk with both diminution in caliber and an accumulation of nuclei, are the dominant findings on biopsy; neither change is specific for rheumatoid arthritis.[41] Current histochemical studies distinguish two types of fibers one of which has been found to be selectively atrophic;[41,46] this atrophy, also seen in other conditions, has been ascribed to limitation of muscle activity.[10]

RHEUMATOID ARTERITIS

Histological terms such as "arteritis" or "vasculitis" are often used in describing the appearance of vascular lesions found in the tissues of patients with rheumatoid arthritis. Experience has shown that the presence of such lesions does not connote a single, easily distinguishable clinical syndrome but rather reflects a pathogenetic mechanism responsible for a host of clinical manifestations of the disease. Indeed, inflammatory change in arterioles and venules has been reported to be the earliest detectable change in the two cardinal lesions—synovitis and subcutaneous nodules.[52,92] There is good reason to believe, in fact, that arterial inflammation is detectable in something more than a fourth of rheumatoid arthritis patients coming to autopsy, the prevalence being proportional to the diligence of the search and the exact morphological criteria used.

In recent years the contributions of many students of the disease have, however, built a *clinical picture* which is properly called "rheumatoid arteritis."[1,28,45,48] It is characterized primarily by polyneuropathy, skin infarction and ulceration, digital gangrene, and evidence of visceral ischemia most notable in the form of intestinal infarction. The prognosis for life is poor when advanced neuropathic findings[30,75] and digital gangrene occur and the term "*malignant rheumatoid arthritis*"[6] has been applied by some when such manifestations are present.

The clinical syndrome of rheumatoid arteritis is exceedingly rare, appearing in far less than 1 per cent of patients who seek medical advice for rheumatoid arthritis. Although the point has been under continuing debate, it seems likely that the syndrome was more prevalent in the early steroid era—1950 to 1960. With the smaller and more carefully regulated adrenal steroid dosage in general use today, the syndrome is again becoming less frequent.[39]

The severe form of the process seems to be more common in men. It may appear, rather abruptly, after years of seropositive, erosive rheumatoid arthritis with subcutaneous nodules. Most (but not all) patients have been on steroid therapy, show Cushingoid changes, and give a history of erratic, widely swinging

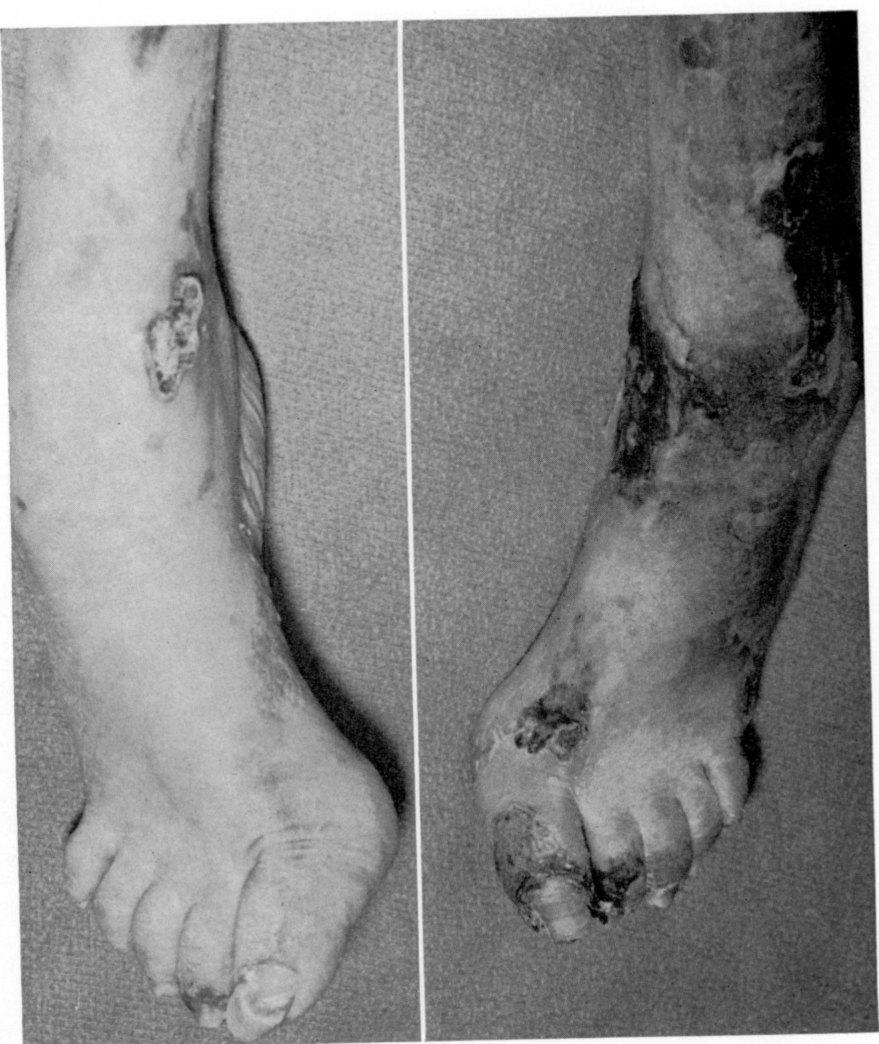

Fig. 22–5.—The feet of a 69-year-old woman with 10 years of rheumatoid arthritis, heavily steroid treated. She had high titers of rheumatoid factor, abundant joint erosion by x-ray, and biopsy demonstrated active and healed arteritis with arterial wall necrosis. The ankle inversion of bilateral foot drop, extensive necrotic skin ulceration about the left ankle, and multiple cyanotic or gangrenous toe tips are all features of rheumatoid arteritis.

doses in the recent past. Synovitis is usually not prominent. At its worst, peripheral neuropathy may involve three or four limbs, with foot and wrist drop often being the most obvious change (Fig. 22–5). Then fingers or toes turn blue and may later develop frank dry gangrene with autoamputation (Fig. 22–6). Malleolar or tibial skin necrosis is common and ulcerations may become extensive and create serious problems. The patient is commonly febrile with temperatures mounting to 104° F. or higher. Polymorphonuclear leukocytosis is frequent. Episcleritis, pleuritis, pericarditis and myocarditis are often detected or these may have antedated the onset of neural and cutaneous changes.

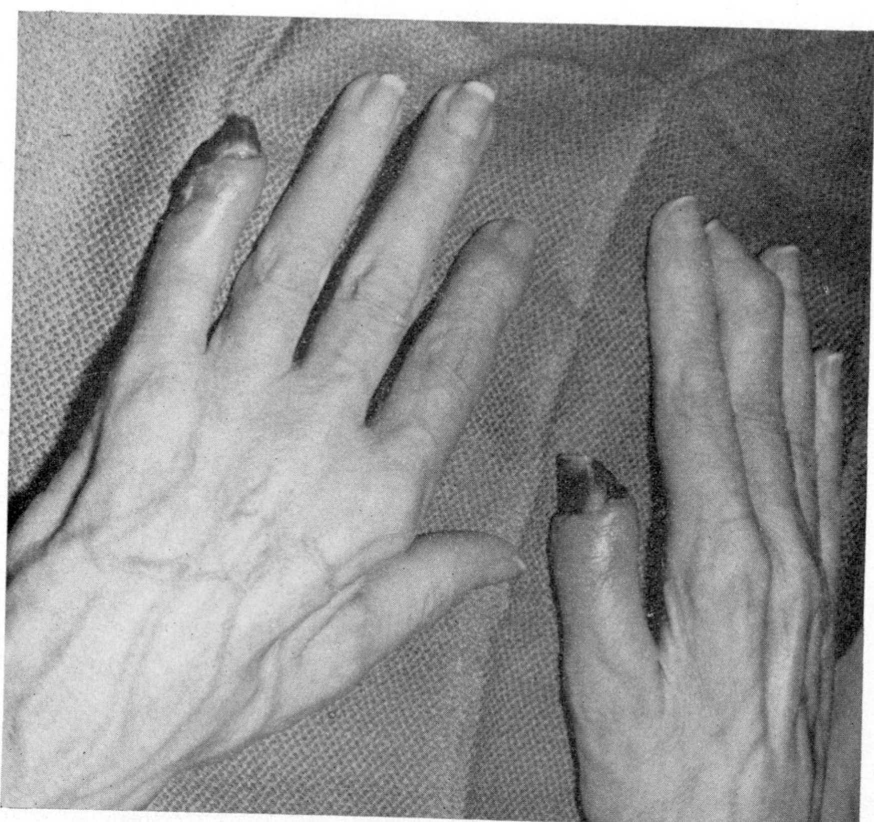

FIG. 22–6.—Gangrenous fingertips of the same patient as in Figure 22–5. The necrotic fingers showed their first cyanosis 5 weeks before this picture was made.

At times, but not frequently, central nervous system involvement and renal disease contribute to the downhill course. The blood pressure is usually consistent with iatrogenic Cushing's and malignant hypertension is uncommon. The terminal picture may be extremely complex with infection, malnutrition, gastrointestinal bleeding, and congestive heart failure often playing roles. In this setting, mesenteric thrombosis with bowel gangrene may constitute the final insult.

Such a pattern usually evolves over a period of three to six months but each of the events may appear singly over a period of years and at widely scattered intervals. Pathological examination shows widespread, severe necrotizing arteritis of small to medium-sized arteries morphologically indistinguishable from those of polyarteritis nodosa save for certain features. For example, the digital arteries usually show a bland, concentric intimal thickening and fibrosis with a generally intact elastic lamina—obliterative endarteritis. In the visceral vasculature this bland intimal fibrosis may be present in some vessels, while in the same area or organ other arteries will show fibrinoid necrosis of the entire wall, complete thrombosis, and an intense polymorphonuclear response.[85]

Two features of the arterial lesions are clinically pertinent. It is a "nodose" lesion in that the severe inflammation may be localized to short segments of an artery, extending for less than 100 mμ, with both proximal and distal segments of the vessel anatomically undisturbed. Thus assessment of serial sections is important in the study of biopsy material. Secondly, at autopsy the overall picture is usually notably asynchronous with healing and recanalization apparent in one section and fresh, severe arteritis in another. The healed lesions imply that the acute process is, in some measure, reversible, thus compounding the prognostic uncertainties.

The pathogenesis of the clinical syndrome of rheumatoid arteritis is unclear. It is usually considered to be a phase of rheumatoid arthritis, fortunately rare. There are excellent grounds for believing it to be more common in the steroid-treated patient. It is virtually confined to patients with high titers of rheumatoid factor. In addition LE cell preparations may be positive[83] and antinuclear factor is usually demonstrable by fluorescence methods. There is, however, no adequate explanation of the origin of the vascular necrosis. Preliminary reports indicate that, in contrast to "regular" rheumatoid arthritis, serum complement levels are reduced in the patient exhibiting manifestations of arteritis.[33] Since the progression of the syndrome is usually sufficiently slow to permit the hope of therapeutic reversal, the mechanisms producing the lesions are of crucial import in selecting appropriate therapy.

The management of these rare cases has not been subjected to systematic study and has varied widely. Despite the fact that corticosteroids are believed to play a role in inducing the process, they should not be withdrawn in a febrile phase with evolving neuropathy or progressive cutaneous lesions. Under such circumstances the dosage should probably be raised to the range of 30 to 60 mg. prednisone equivalents daily and kept there, unaltered, for a time period extending into months. If the process comes under control, a slow decrease would then be justified. If manifestations of life-threatening arteritis appear in a patient not on corticosteroids, the medication should be begun. There is, however, the possibility that neither raising nor beginning corticosteroids will have a substantial effect on the process.

Various forms of cytotoxic therapy with purine analogues, such as azathioprine, or alkylating agents, such as chlorambucil or cyclophosphamide, have been used. Penicillamine appears to have reversed several cases.[44] Anticoagulation has been suggested despite the obvious attendant risks. In the full-blown picture, the prognosis is sufficiently grave to warrant exceptional measures but, because of the irregular progression of the syndrome, the same cannot be said for the management of isolated lesions such as episcleritis, chronic leg ulcers, or the identification of arteritis by muscle biopsy which may or may not herald the full syndrome.

This is especially true of the minor digital skin lesions ("*digital arteritis*") which often do precede clinical rheumatoid arteritis but are also seen in patients

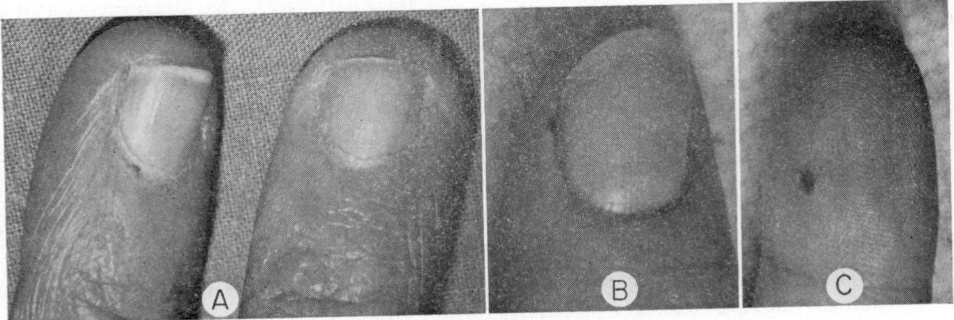

Fig. 22–7.—*A.* Prominent nail fold arterioles, *B.* nail edge infarction, and *C.* volar finger pulp brown spot all in rheumatoid arthritis.

who have little or no other evidence of vascular inflammation (Fig. 22–7). These include small, often tender, nodules of the volar pads especially over the terminal phalanges. These may heal leaving a transient brown scar or, in other instances, a depressed lesion with tissue loss. Infarction of the nail edges results in a sharply localized black lesion, usually asymptomatic; within weeks the black scale flakes off leaving unscarred normal nail edges. These lesions are said to appear in as many as 8 per cent of hospitalized patients with rheumatoid arthritis. They are more common in males, twice as prevalent in those on corticosteroid therapy,[25] and are usually accompanied by rheumatoid and antinuclear factor in the serum.[16] *Gangrenous change* may involve entire digits, or indeed a whole hand, but is more common in only one or two terminal phalangeal areas. Previously observed Raynaud's phenomenon is by no means a prerequisite. Arteriographic studies in life and post mortem have revealed extensive insufficiency of digital arteries both in the presence and the absence of overt clinical findings.[84]

The degree to which these findings are likely to be accompanied or followed by polyneuropathy or the full picture of rheumatoid arteritis with visceral infarction is not clear. Bywaters and Scott noted such lesions in 34 patients; 10 deaths occurred in the group, 4 of them due to visceral infarction.[11]

FELTY'S SYNDROME

Felty observed and reported 5 middle-aged patients with deforming rheumatoid arthritis who showed weight loss, pigmentation of exposed skin surfaces, splenomegaly and leukopenia. The white cell counts ranged from 1,000 to 4,200 per cu. mm. Differential counts in 3 cases showed less than 50 per cent polymorphonuclear leukocytes in two.[29]

The syndrome is now recognized as a variant of rheumatoid arthritis appearing in rather less than 5 per cent of cases coming to medical attention.[102] The basic disease is usually deforming in nature, accompanied by subcutaneous nodules, and characterized by the presence of rheumatoid factor in the serum at higher titers than is seen in patients without splenomegaly. The arthritis has its onset many years before the detection of the splenomegaly which usually occurs between 45 and 65 years of age. It is not uncommon to find the patient severely crippled but with only modestly active joint disease. The spleen ranges from barely palpable to very large and is not usually tender although splenic infarcts and traumatic rupture do occur. Slowly progressive size changes, either an increase or decrease, may be detected as the patient is followed. Other manifestations of systemic rheumatoid disease such as pericarditis, episcleritis, and peripheral neuropathy are often present.

Total white blood cell counts, in the presence of splenomegaly, vary but the vast majority of patients show regular counts below 4,500 cells per cu. mm. and counts as low as 500 have been observed. The greatest part of the reduction is in the neutrophilic leukocytes which rarely constitute more than 40 per cent of the cells and have been totally absent in a few patients. There is also often a reduction in lymphocytes but to a lesser degree. Monocytes and eosinophils are said not to be reduced and one does occasionally see a relative eosinophilia. Marrow examinations are reported as varying from hypoplastic to hyperplastic although the usual picture is one of modest hyperplasia of all elements save for a deficiency of mature neutrophils, "maturation arrest." The anemia is hypochromic, as is usual in rheumatoid arthritis, but in addition accelerated red cell destruction may be detected. After administration of chromium-labeled cells, the degree of splenic uptake suggested that the anemia would be alleviated by splenectomy and this proved to be the case.[43] Increased platelet destruction has also been observed but rarely produces purpuric manifestations.

The cause of the leukopenia is unknown. Possible explanations might include accelerated destruction, reduced production, some form of selective sequestration in a pool other than that reflected in peripheral venous samples, or any combination of these factors. The marrow findings are not suggestive of decreased production. The peripheral count and marrow suggest a new steady state with both accelerated production and destruction. However the leukocytosis which follows splenectomy occurs so swiftly (within one to two hours) as to suggest that accelerated production can hardly explain it. A granulocyte reserve, sequestered in venules or capillaries, may contribute to the sharp rise[42] but studies of the granulocyte reserve by adrenalin, endotoxin or etiocholanolone testing have shown it to be markedly deficient.

The granulocytosis found 12 to 18 hours after the intramuscular injection of etiocholanolone is a measure of marrow reserve. In contrast to normals and other patients with rheumatoid arthritis who increase their resting granulocyte count by at least 2,600 cells per cu. mm., six patients with Felty's syndrome responded inadequately with a mean of approximately 800 cells per cu. mm. A single patient was found to revert to a normal granulocyte response 6 months after splenectomy. When autologous plasma, obtained prior to splenectomy, was infused, there was no change in the baseline granulocyte count but etiocholanolone dramatically failed to induce granulocytosis. Five days after plasma infusion her responsiveness had returned to normal. Plasma obtained at a time when the stimulation test was normal and infused 8 months later did not alter the response. Thus circulating factors, perhaps of splenic origin, seem to have effects on the patient's ability to respond to a granulocyte stimulus.[108]

Whether or not the eponym should be applied to patients with splenomegaly but without leukopenia or to those who have only leukopenia is uncertain. Suffice it to say that in individuals both the degree of splenic enlargement and of white count reduction can vary substantially from month to month without apparent relationship to each other. Leukopenia and neutropenia often recur after splenectomy (*vide infra*).

Two notable features seem to be related to the neutropenia or to the splenomegaly—chronic leg ulcers and an increase in bacterial infections. These were reported in 41 and 52 per cent, respectively, of 27 patients studied.[81]

Indolent ulcerations overlying the tibia or the ankles have frequently been described in patients with Felty's syndrome. The lesions tend to be deep, painful and chronically infected with a mixed flora typical of uninvolved skin surfaces. They may be very extensive covering saucer-sized areas or only 2 to 4 cm. in diameter. It is common to find fresh ulcers developing in the scars left by earlier lesions (Fig. 22–8). Some cases have had arterial and others venous insufficiency of the lower extremity but neither loss of pulses nor marked edema is usual. Draining rheumatoid nodules can appear. *Pyoderma gangrenosum*, usually associated with chronic ulcerative colitis, should be excluded. After all the known causes of such lesions are considered, there remains a group of rather elderly patients with leukopenia, deforming rheumatoid arthritis, and chronic leg ulcers. The ulcers begin as a hemorrhagic papule surrounded by a pale zone. The central area forms an eschar and eventually sloughs out leaving an ulcer which slowly spreads. Regional biopsies have shown arteritis with fibrinoid necrosis and low grade inflammation sufficient to cause occlusion of small vessels.[53] Thus both clinical and biopsy findings are consistent with ischemic disease in an area of poor collateral circulation.

In one study six of eight cases showing this type of ulceration had either splenomegaly or leukopenia or both.[107] In one instance leg ulcers first appeared with the leukopenia which had developed progressively after an initially successful splenectomy. Upon comparison of small groups of patients, one with leg ulcers

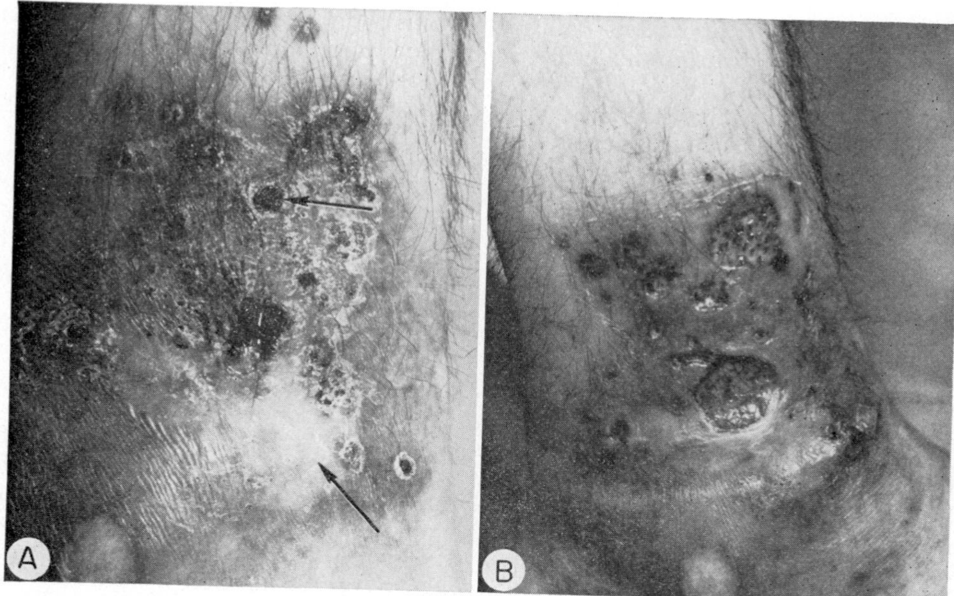

FIG. 22–8.—Proximal to the right lateral malleolus in a young man with Felty's syndrome and recurrent leg ulcers. *A*. Here abundant scar tissue (lower arrow) of earlier ulcers abruptly developed dark red and later black spots (*e.g.* at upper arrow). *B*. Two weeks later, sharply marginated multiple ulcers have appeared, exactly reflecting the points of earlier infarction (Courtesy Dr. Robert Willkens).

and one without, but both showing splenomegaly and leukopenia, those with leg ulcers had disease of longer duration, smaller spleens by palpation, and a higher prevalence of positive direct LE cell preparations. Rheumatoid factor titers are high and antinuclear factors, usually including those of IgM type, are invariably present. Conversely when 50 LE cell positive patients with rheumatoid arthritis were compared to 100 consecutive cases of LE cell negative rheumatoid arthritis, splenomegaly was present in 6 of the former and 1 of the latter.[49] Some have ascribed the condition to systemic lupus erythematosus[2] while others speak of the two diseases as "*overlapping*." In view of the widespread and often severe erosive joint changes, the high titers (and not just presence) of rheumatoid factor, and the almost complete freedom from central nervous system and renal disease, it seems best to classify these patients under the heading of rheumatoid arthritis and the variant, Felty's syndrome.

Chronic, recurrent bacterial infections of various sorts and often severe are seen, although one is also impressed with patients who carry on for years with striking neutropenia and no apparent tendency to bacterial complications. Ruderman *et al*. divided their series into those with more or less than 500 granulocytes per cu. mm.; the frequency of infection was identical in both groups.[81] The infections seen included furunculosis, recurrent pulmonary disease, and urinary tract infections with typical bacterial pathogens. Patients usually respond to acute infections with some increase in granulocytes but rarely manage a leukocytosis. Infections are a common cause of death even in the antibiotic era and secondary infections, resistant to antibiotics, are regularly seen.

Treatment

Adrenal corticosteroid therapy at tolerable dose levels does not alleviate the leukopenia and would have to be regarded as a poor approach to the infection problem although some have found them to have a favorable effect on the indolent ulcers. Most physicians consider the indications for splenectomy to be limited to patients presenting with recurrent infections. The effect of splenectomy on the ulcer is irregular, at best. The procedure does not have any recognized long-lasting effects on the polyarthritis and is rarely justified by the low grades of hemolytic anemia seen.

The results of splenectomy are difficult to assess because of the tendency to report favorable results and because the followup period is often short. A prompt and major granulocytosis is usually observed and current acute infections usually improve or disappear but this latter outcome is by no means assured. In Ruderman's series nine splenectomies were done. The recurrent infection problem tended to persist in those who had exhibited it preoperatively and those patients, initially free of infections, continued free postoperatively. It is clear that approximately a third of patients undergoing splenectomy suffer a gradual reappearance of their neutropenia so that within 2 or 3 years of operation, they are back to baseline values again. In some cases accessory splenic tissue has been identified and removed with a good response. On balance, splenectomy is justified for recurrent or chronic infections of significance but one cannot make such a decision with any feeling of certainty.

The leukopenic patient is always of concern when one believes chrysotherapy or cytotoxic therapy to be indicated by the polyarthritis. The potential role of splenectomy in permitting such therapy is dubious indeed. Chrysotherapy may be permissible if administered under strict control; cytotoxic agents which are expected to produce leukopenia should not, in the current state of knowledge, be used.

MISCELLANEOUS MANIFESTATIONS

Finally, mention should be made of a few other common extra-synovial features of rheumatoid arthritis, the problem of peptic disease, and several organ systems which are rarely significantly involved. Each of these aspects is deserving of more detailed analysis than can be presented here.

Common Features

Low grade fever is often noted and night sweating can be a problem. Shaking chills are unusual but do occur, accompanied by high fever, in the arteritic. *Raynaud's phenomenon* precedes or accompanies the disease in perhaps 10 per cent[87] and sweaty, soft palms, thenar and hypothenar erythema, and atrophic skin are cited as the result of vasomotor instability.

The *psychiatric manifestations of rheumatoid arthritis* have been extensively studied.[78] The key questions have revolved around the premorbid personality and premorbid psychotrauma in an effort to understand why one person develops the disease while another does not.[65] Whatever the findings before disease onset, however, the impact of the disease on the emotional life of the patient can be devastating and constitutes beyond question its most important extra-articular manifestation when conceived in terms of the *quality* of life with the disease.

Osteoporosis, regularly juxta-articular in location but often much more widespread, is presumed to have a number of causes including locally increased blood flow, disuse, postmenopausal status, and, commonly, the therapeutic use of adrenal corticosteroids. Fracture, resulting from the most minor trauma, is often the final, painful straw which reduces the patient to permanent bed confinement. No prophylactic program is of demonstrated value but the osteopenia constitutes a compelling argument for trying to keep the patient up and moving.

Doubtful Features

Since virtually all drugs administered in rheumatoid arthritis, including aspirin, which has often been used before the first visit to a physician, are considered by most (but not all) to be "ulcerogenic," it has not been possible to establish beyond reasonable doubt that *peptic ulcer* is more prevalent in its victims because they have the disease. The pathological tissue does not usually demonstrate a rheumatoid lesion although it is clear that rheumatoid arteritis may involve any part of the enteric vasculature.

However, the important practical point remains—patients with treated rheumatoid arthritis manifest a high incidence of peptic ulcers and are subject to the usual complications.[4] Gross bleeding and perforation are relatively more common than are obstructive symptoms perhaps because gastric ulcers are relatively more frequent in rheumatoid arthritis than in uncomplicated peptic ulcer patients.

The therapeutic problem is a most difficult one. Some of the most severely crippled patients seen on rheumatic disease services are those from whom aspirin and corticosteroids have been rather abruptly withdrawn for the very good reason that hematemesis or perforation supervened while the patients were taking those drugs. On the other hand, peptic ulceration can be shown to heal radiologically on a tightly defined antacid program while the "ulcerogenic pills" are continued. Some variation of the latter course, recognizing the risks involved, is to be preferred to the mandatory exclusion of medications upon which virtually every articular movement may depend.

Uncommon Features

No regularly recognized manifestations of the disease involve the liver, pancreas, or reproductive system. The endocrine system is likewise spared, save for a rather doubtful relationship to chronic thyroiditis.[63]

Specific rheumatoid lesions are not identified in renal tissue. Clinically significant renal disease is not common; most of it can probably be accounted for by amyloidosis, gold nephropathy and chronic pyelonephritis.[93] The nephropathy of analgesic abuse has been ascribed primarily to phenacetin; if, as has been suggested, salicylates play a similar role, the process must be exceedingly slow or the untoward effect a minimal one.

BIBLIOGRAPHY

1. Adler, R. H., Norcross, B. M. and Lockie, L. M.: J.A.M.A., *180*, 922, 1962.
2. Allison, J. H. and Bettley, F. R.: Lancet, *1*, 288, 1957.
3. Aronoff, A., Bywaters, E. G. L. and Fearnley, J. R.: Brit. Med. J., *2*, 228, 1955.
4. Atwater, E. C., Mongan, E. S., Wieche, D. R. and Jacox, R. F.: Arch. Intern. Med., *115*, 184, 1965.
5. Barager, F. D. and Duthie, J. J. R.: Brit. Med. J., *1*, 1106, 1960.
6. Bevans, M., Nadell, J., Demartini, F. and Ragan, C.: Amer. J. Med., *16*, 197, 1954.
7. Bienenstock, H., Ehrlich, G. E. and Freyberg, R. H.: Arth. & Rheum., *6*, 48, 1963.
8. Bland, J. H. and Eddy, W. M.: Arth. & Rheum., *11*, 72, 1968.
9. Bonfiglio, T. and Atwater, E. C.: Arch. Intern. Med., *124*, 714, 1969.
10. Brooke, M. H. and Engel, W. K.: Neurology, *19*, 469, 1969.
11. Bywaters, E. G. L. and Scott, J. T.: J. Chronic Dis., *16*, 905, 1963.
12. Caplan, A.: Thorax, *8*, 29, 1953.
13. Caplan, A., Payne, R. B. and Withey, J. L.: Thorax, *17*, 205, 1962.
14. Carr, D. T. and Mayne, J. G.: Amer. Rev. Resp. Dis., *85*, 345, 1962.
15. Cathcart, E. S. and Spodick, D. H.: New Engl. J. Med., *266*, 959, 1962.
16. Cats, A. and Pit, A. A.: Folia Med. Neerl., *12*, 159, 1969.
17. Chamberlain, M. A. and Bruckner, F. E.: Ann. Rheum. Dis., *29*, 609, 1970.
18. Chater, E. H.: J. Irish Med. Assoc., *61*, 326, 1968.
19. Conlon, P. W., Isdale, I. C. and Rose, B. S.: Ann. Rheum. Dis., *25*, 120, 1966.
20. Cregan, J. C. F.: Ann. Rheum. Dis., *25*, 242, 1966.
21. Crellin, R. Q., MacCabe, J. J. and Hamilton, E. B. D.: J. Bone Joint Surg., *52B*, 244, 1970.
22. Cruickshank, B.: Ann. Rheum. Dis., *13*, 136, 1954.
23. ———: Scot. Med. J., *3*, 110, 1958.

24. ————: J. Path. Bact., *76*, 223, 1958.
25. Dequeker, J. and Rosberg, G.: Acta Rheum. Scand. *13*, 299, 1967.
26. Ellman, P. and Ball, R. E.: Brit. Med. J., *2*, 816, 1948.
27. Ellman, P., Cudkowicz, L. and Elwood, J. S.: J. Clin. Path., *7*, 239, 1954.
28. Epstein, W. V. and Engleman, E. P.: Arth. & Rheum., *2*, 250, 1959.
29. Felty, A. R.: Bull. Johns Hopkins Hosp., *35*, 16, 1924.
30. Ferguson, R. H. and Slocumb, C. H.: Bull Rheum. Dis., *11*, 251, 1961.
31. Ferry, A. P.: Arch. Ophthal., *82*, 77, 1969.
32. Franco, A. E., Levine, H. and Hall, A. P.: Submitted for publication, 1972.
33. Franco, A. E. and Schur, P. H.: Arth. & Rheum., *14*, 231, 1971.
34. Friedman, H.: J. Neurosurg., *32*, 689, 1970.
35. Gough, J., Rivers, D. and Seal, R. M. E.: Thorax, *10*, 9, 1955.
36. Gowans, J. D. C.: New Engl. J. Med., *262*, 1012, 1960.
37. Grossman, A., Martin, J. R. and Root, H.: Laryngoscope, *71*, 530, 1961.
38. Handforth, C. P. and Woodbury, J. F. L.: Canad. Med. Assoc. J., *80*, 86, 1959.
39. Hart, F. D.: Brit. Med. J., *3*, 131, 1969.
40. Hart, F. D. and Golding, J. R.: Brit. Med. J., *1*, 1594, 1960.
41. Haslock, D. I., Wright, V. and Harriman, D. G. F.: Quart. J. Med., *39*, 335, 1970.
42. Hollingsworth, J. W.: *Local and Systemic Complications of Rheumatoid Arthritis*, Philadelphia, W. B. Saunders Company, 1968.
43. Hume, R., Dagg, J. H., Fraser, T. N. and Goldberg, A.: Ann. Rheum. Dis., *23*, 267, 1964.
44. Jaffe, I. A. and Smith, R. W.: Arth. & Rheum., *11*, 585, 1968.
45. Johnson, R. L., Smyth, C. J., Holt, G. W., Lubchenco, A. and Valentine, E.: Arth. & Rheum., *2*, 224, 1959.
46. Kaplan, H. and Brooke, M. H.: Arth. & Rheum., *14*, 168, 1971.
47. Karten, I.: J.A.M.A., *210*, 1717, 1969.
48. Kemper, J. W., Baggenstoss, A. H. and Slocumb, C. H.: Ann. Intern. Med., *46*, 831, 1957.
49. Kievits, J. H., Goslings, J., Schuit, H. R. E., and Hijmans, W.: Ann. Rheum. Dis., *15*, 211, 1956.
50. Kimura, S. J., Hogan, M. J., O'Connor, G. R. and Epstein, W. V.: Arch. Ophthal., *77*, 309, 1967.
51. Kirk, J. and Cosh, J.: Quart. J. Med., *38*, 397, 1969.
52. Kulka, J. P.: Bull. Rheum. Dis., *10*, 201, 1959.
53. Laine, V. A. I. and Vainio, K. J.: Acta Rheum. Scand., *1*, 113, 1955.
54. Lebowitz, W. B.: Ann. Intern. Med., *58*, 102, 1963.
55. Lindquist, P. R. and McDonnell, D. E.: J. Bone Joint Surg., *52A*, 1235, 1970.
56. Liss, J. P. and Bachman, W. T.: Arth. & Rheum., *13*, 869, 1970.
57. Lloyd, K. and Agarwal, A.: Brit. Med. J., *3*, 32, 1970.
58. Lofgren, R. H. and Montgomery, W. W.: New Engl. J. Med., *267*, 193, 1962.
59. Lyne, A. J. and Pitkeathley, D. A.: Arch. Ophthal., *80*, 171, 1968.
60. Magora, A., Wolf, E. and Gonen, B.: Acta Rheum. Scand., *16*, 280, 1970.
61. Marmor, L., Lawrence, J. F. and DuBois, E. L.: J. Bone Joint Surg., *49A*, 381, 1967.
62. Martel, W. and Abell, M. R.: Arth. & Rheum., *6*, 224, 1963.
63. Masi, A. T., Hartmann, W. H., Hahn, B. H., Abbey, H. and Shulman, L. E.: Lancet, *1*, 123, 1965.
64. Matthews, J. A.: Ann. Rheum. Dis., *28*, 260, 1969.
65. Meyerowitz, S., Jacox, R. F., and Hess, D. W.: Arth. & Rheum., *11*, 1, 1968.
66. Miall, W. E.: Ann. Rheum. Dis., *14*, 150 1955.
67. Motulsky, A. G., Weinberg, S., Saphir, O. and Rosenberg, E.: Arch. Intern. Med., *90*, 660, 1952.
68. Mowat, A. G. and Hothersall, T. E.: Ann. Rheum. Dis., *27*, 345, 1968.
69. Mowat, A. G., Hothersall, T. E. and Aitchison, W. R. C.: Ann. Rheum. Dis., *28*, 303, 1969.
70. Muirden, K. D.: Austral. Ann. Med., *2*, 97, 1970.
71. ————: Ann. Rheum. Dis., *29*, 81, 1970.
72. Nosanchuk, J. S. and Schnitzer, B.: Cancer, *24*, 343, 1969.
73. Owen, E. T. and Lawson, A. A. H.: Ann. Rheum. Dis., *25*, 547, 1966.
74. Page, J. W.: J. Mich. State Med. Soc., *60*, 888, 1961.
75. Pallis, C. A. and Scott, J. T.: Brit. Med. J., *1*, 1141, 1965.
76. Pearsall, H. R., Wilske, K. R., Morgan, E. H., Taylor, W. J., Curtis, V. L. and Beggs, D.: Bull. Mason Clinic, *21*, 151, 1967.
77. Polisar, I. A., Burbank, B., Levitt, L. M., Katz, H. M. and Morrione, T. G.: J.A.M.A., *172*, 901, 1960.

78. Rimon, R.: Acta. Rheum. Scand., Supp. 13, pp. 154, 1969.
79. Robertson, M. D. J., Hart, F. D., White, W. F., Nuki, G., and Boardman, P. L.: Ann. Rheum. Dis., *27*, 253, 1968.
80. Romanoff, H., Rozin, R. and Zlotnick, A.: Arth. & Rheum., *13*, 426, 1970.
81. Ruderman, M., Miller, L. M. and Pinals, R. S.: Arth. & Rheum., *11*, 377, 1968.
82. Scadding, J. G.: Proc. Roy. Soc. Med., *62*, 227, 1969.
83. Schmid, F. R., Cooper, N. S., Ziff, M. and McEwen, C.: Amer. J. Med., *30*, 56, 1961.
84. Scott, J. T., El Sallab, R. A., and Laws, J. W.: Brit. J. Radiol., *40*, 748, 1967.
85. Scott, J. T., Hourihane, D. O., Doyle, F. H., Steiner, R. E., Laws, J. W., Dixon, A. St. J., and Bywaters, E. G. L.: Ann. Rheum. Dis., *20*, 224, 1961.
86. Sevel, D.: Trans. Ophthal. Soc. U. K., *85*, 357, 1965.
87. Short, C. L., Bauer, W. and Reynolds, W. E.: *Rheumatoid Arthritis*, Cambridge, Harvard Univ. Press, 1957.
88. Sievers, K., Aho, K., Hurri, L. and Perttala, Y.: Acta Tuberc. Scand., *45*, 21, 1964.
89. Sinclair, R. J. G. and Cruickshank, B.: Quart. J. Med., *25*, 313, 1956.
90. Smiley, W. K.: Ann. Phys. Med., *10*, 157, 1969.
91. Sokoloff, L.: Mod. Conc. Cardiovasc. Dis., *33*, 847, 1964.
92. Sokoloff, L., McCluskey. R. T. and Bunim, J. J.: A.M.A. Arch. Path., *55*, 475, 1953.
93. Sorensen, A. W. S.: *The Kidney in Rheumatoid Arthritis and the Effect of Drugs on Renal Function*, Copenhagen, Munksgaard, 1966.
94. Steinberg, V. L. and Parry, C. B.: Brit. Med. J., *1*, 630, 1961.
95. Steiner, J. W. and Gelbloom, A. J.: Arth. & Rheum. *2*, 537, 1959.
96. Strandberg, O.: Acta Med. Scand., *180*, 1, 1966.
97. Tomasi, T. B., Jr., Fudenberg, H. H. and Finby, N.: Amer. J. Med., *33*, 243, 1962.
98. Turner-Warwick, M. and Doniach, D.: Brit. Med. J., *1*, 886, 1965.
99. Van Metre, T. E., Brown, W. H., Knox, D. L. and Maumenee, A. E.: J. All., *36*, 158, 1965.
100. Walker, W. C.: Quart. J. Med., *36*, 239, 1967.
101. Walker, W. C. and Wright, V.: Ann. Rheum. Dis., *26*, 467, 1967.
102. ————: Medicine, *47*. 501, 1968.
103. ————: Ann. Rheum. Dis., *28*, 252, 1969.
104. Webb, F. W. S., Hickman, J. A. and Brew, D. St. J.: Brit. Med. J., *2*, 537, 1968.
105. Wegelius, O., Pasternack, A. and Kuhlback, B.: Acta Rheum. Scand., *15*, 257, 1969.
106. Whaley, K. and Dick, W. C.: Brit. Med. J., *2*, 31, 1968.
107. Willkens, R. F. and Decker, J. L.: Arth. & Rheum., *6*, 720, 1963.
108. Wolff, S. M., Kimball, H. R., Talal, N., Plotz, P. H., and Decker, J. L.: Clinical Research, *16*, 326, 1968.
109. Wolman, L., Darke, C. S. and Young, A.: J. Laryng. Otol., *79*, 403, 1965.
110. Yamaguchi, D. M., Lipscomb, P. R. and Soule, E. H.: Minn. Med., *48*, 22, 1965.

Chapter 23

Laboratory Findings in Rheumatoid Arthritis

By Morris Ziff, M.D., and John Baum, M.D.

The laboratory findings in rheumatoid arthritis are those of a chronic inflammatory disease. There is no truly specific laboratory test for the disease. Yet, there is a constellation of laboratory findings which the experienced clinician can examine with great advantage in arriving at a diagnosis and in the management of therapy.

HEMATOLOGY

Erythrocytes

A recalcitrant normochromic or hypochromic normocytic anemia, usually moderate in degree, is common in rheumatoid arthritis.[125] Among Danish women with active disease, 22.7 per cent had less than 10 grams per cent of hemoglobin; among men, 11.5 per cent had less than 11 grams. In children, anemia is usually present,[85,174] especially in the systemic or "Still's" form of the disease. In the series of Toumbis and co-workers,[174] 64 per cent of children had less than 10 grams of hemoglobin.

The anemia of rheumatoid arthritis is the type seen in chronic inflammation. It has been intensively studied in relation to a number of possible contributory factors.

The influence of hemolysis has been examined in detail. Early studies using the Ashby selective agglutination technique[2,56,57,118] indicated a reduction in the survival of erythrocytes transfused from normal donors to patients with rheumatoid arthritis. More recent investigations have utilized chromium-51 to label the patient's own erythrocytes for similar studies. Though Ebaugh and co-workers[42] and Weinstein[181] have found evidence of some degree of hemolysis, it was emphasized by the latter that the magnitude of the red cell destruction could not account for the development of anemia in the presence of adequate bone marrow compensation. Three recent studies[102,139,144] using chromium-51 have confirmed these earlier reports, disclosing only a mild hemolytic tendency of an extracorpuscular type, insufficient to explain the associated anemia.

The plasma volume in rheumatoid patients has been found by a number of investigators to be greater than normal.[38,83,86,142] The basis for this increase is not well understood. Increase in plasma volume in compensation for a reduced corpuscular volume[64,83] is probably one factor. In addition, the fact that the lean body mass tends to constitute a larger percentage of the weight of the rheumatoid patient than of controls probably leads to calculation of a spuriously high value for the plasma volume as per cent of body weight relative to controls.

The serum iron is usually moderately and sometimes markedly decreased.[22,42,57,82,125,144,148] Transferrin concentrations, however, are normal or near normal, and the utilization of intravenously injected tracer doses of iron for hemoglobin synthesis has also been found to be normal.[57,144] Although Roberts and co-workers[144] have noted a reduced capacity to absorb iron in patients with active rheumatoid arthritis and mild anemia, other studies[148,181] have found this function to be normal in most patients.

Although absent or decreased marrow iron stores are present in at least one-third of patients,[117,140] no correlation has been demonstrated between the amount of iron demonstrable in the marrow and the hemoglobin level or erythrocyte count. The refractoriness to oral iron therapy of the anemia of most cases of rheumatoid arthritis is in accord with this observation since absorption of iron appears to be normal in most patients.

To explain the low plasma iron, which is the most constant characteristic of the anemia of inflammation, Freireich and co-workers[57] have proposed an impairment of release of iron from the reticuloendothelial tissues. In the presence of normal utilization of transferrin-bound iron, such an impairment would account for the low iron concentration in the plasma. This suggestion is based on the observations that (*a*) amounts of iron which exceed the plasma-binding capacity tend to be deposited in the tissues and thus be poorly utilized in patients with inflammation;[50] (*b*) iron injected intravenously into animals with an inflammatory reaction is diverted from normal hemoglobin formation and deposited in storage sites;[25] and (*c*) the re-utilization of iron from senescent cells is reduced in animals with an inflammatory reaction. Freireich and co-workers have assumed that the reticuloendothelial system is the site at which iron is stored in non-releasable form. Insufficient release would result in the low plasma iron concentration which is presumably responsible for the impaired capacity of the bone marrow to produce erythrocytes. This subject has been well reviewed by Cartwright.[24a] Mowat and Hothersall[120a] measured the iron content of synovial tissue. They found significantly increased iron levels in synovial tissue from patients with rheumatoid arthritis and concluded that the amount of iron retained could contribute to the low serum iron and anemia of active rheumatoid arthritis.

Since most patients with rheumatoid arthritis receive salicylate therapy, the role of salicylates in the production of anemia must be considered. Occult blood in the feces has been observed in many patients who receive this drug.[39,131] This loss, although usually of minor importance, may be the cause in some patients of an anemia which responds to iron therapy. Another factor in the anemia may be an erythropoietin deficiency since serum levels in rheumatoid arthritis were lower than in patients with a comparable degree of iron-deficiency anemia.[179a]

White Blood Cell Count

Though white cell counts are usually in the normal range or only slightly elevated, Short, Bauer and Reynolds[157] have reported that about 25 per cent of their patients had counts above 10,000 per mm.^{3}. Leukocytosis was generally not associated with increased activity of the disease. It was noted with the acute and severe type of onset and with acute exacerbation of this disease.

Although counts in the 12,000 to 20,000 range are sometimes observed without other cause,[35] the occurrence of counts above 14,000 should raise a suspicion of factors other than the disease itself. Patients receiving steroid therapy may show counts above 20,000 because of the stimulating effect of steroids on the bone marrow.[146,165] Leukocytosis is common in juvenile rheumatoid arthritis.[85,104,152,174] In the series of Toumbis and co-workers,[174] 38 per cent of juvenile patients had counts between 11,000 and 16,000. When this condition is associated with marked systemic features, a leukemoid reaction may be seen with counts as high as 100,000 per mm.^{3} and marked shift to the left.[85]

Leukopenia is rare in rheumatoid arthritis;[157] when present it is more likely to be observed in the chronic stage of the disease. Rare cases of leukopenia with arthritis and splenomegaly, long referred to as Felty's syndrome,[49] appear to be instances of rheumatoid arthritis with a selective neutropenia due to hypersplenism.

The differential white cell count is usually within normal limits, but an increase in polymorphonuclear leukocytes may occur in more acute cases.[35] Short and co-workers[157] have, however, observed a number of patients in whom the occurrence of neutrophil counts above 90 per cent was unrelated to the activity, severity, or duration of the arthritis. In a few patients, the neutrophils were decreased below 50 per cent in association with a lymphocytosis. This change was also unassociated with unusual features. Eosinophilia was present in 12.6 per cent of patients, and this was, likewise, not associated with unusual clinical findings.

The chromosomal complement of the leukocytes of the blood has been reported to be normal.[11]

ACUTE PHASE INDICES

A relatively large group of substances of diverse origin reflect, by their concentration in the plasma, the presence and degree of inflammatory activity in the body. These substances, which have been called acute phase reactants, appear to be proteins in all cases. When they are conjugated proteins, tests for individual acute phase reactants may be directed at the non-protein moiety of the conjugated protein, as for example, serum hexosamine in serum glycoprotein.

Measurement of acute phase reactants is helpful in diagnosis and treatment. Although non-specific in their response, they aid in the diagnosis of rheumatoid arthritis in patients who present vague or borderline symptomatology. Since their concentration tends to reflect the activity of the disease, they are useful in management. There is often a discrepancy, however, between the clinical appearance of the patient and the magnitude of the acute phase response. For this reason, change in the level of an acute phase reactant is often of greater significance in guiding therapy than the actual level itself.

ERYTHROCYTE SEDIMENTATION RATE

The erythrocyte sedimentation rate (ESR) is the single, most important laboratory test of inflammatory activity in the connective tissue diseases. Although the increased rate of settling of erythrocytes in the blood of patients with inflammatory diseases was known for many years, it was first measured by Fahreus[45] in 1918. In seeking an early test for pregnancy, Fahreus noted that the speed of sedimentation was increased not only in pregnancy, but in many other conditions.[46,47] Measurement of the ESR was first applied to the study of acute and chronic rheumatism by Hermann in 1924.[78]

The Nature of the Sedimentation Phenomenon

The sedimentation of erythrocytes is related to rouleaux formation. In general, the ESR increases in proportion to the size of the erythrocyte aggregates.[73,81] The size of the aggregates, in turn, is dependent upon the properties of the blood plasma rather than the cells themselves. Rouleaux formation is enhanced by large asymmetric molecules. The plasma components which influence the sedimentation rate most are the fibrinogen and the alpha and gamma globulins.

It is well established that there is an increase of the plasma fibrinogen as a result of increased synthesis by the liver in the presence of inflammation elsewhere in the body. The elevation is rapid, usually being detectable on the day after onset of inflammation. It usually subsides within ten days after cessation of the inflammatory process.[98]

The early observation that the plasma fibrinogen was usually increased when the ESR was accelerated led to the assumption that the sedimentation rate was related to the concentration of fibrinogen in the plasma.[65,73] There is, in fact, a linear correlation between the sedimentation rate and fibrinogen level when patients with serum globulin levels over 2.5 grams per cent are excluded, the coefficient of correlation being 0.90.[53] In patients in whom the serum globulin is over 2.5 grams per cent, however, the correlation is only 0.60. Under circumstances in which plasma fibrinogen is low,[73] as in liver disease, close correlation between plasma globulin concentration and the ESR has been observed.

Addition of serum fractions to defibrinated blood has confirmed that the ESR is almost entirely dependent[43,75] on the concentration of such asymmetric molecules as fibrinogen and alpha-2 and gamma globulins. The relative effect on the ESR of these proteins, when added in equal concentration, was in the ratio, 10:5:2.

Westergren Method

This is the most dependable of the methods currently in use.[184] In this procedure four volumes of venous blood are mixed with one volume of 3.8 per cent sodium citrate. The blood is drawn to the 200 mm. mark in a 1 ml. glass tube having an internal diameter of 2.5 mm. and the distance in mm., which the red blood cell column has sedimented, is read at the end of an hour. Normal values given by Westergren were a fall of 1 to 3 mm. in one hour for males and 4 to 7 mm. for females.

The upper limit of normal was found to rise slowly with age.[79] While a fall of 7 mm. was regarded as normal in males in the eighteen- to thirty-year age group (Table 23–1), 13 mm. was considered normal above age sixty. In the female, the upper limits were 10 and 20 mm. respectively in the same age groups. A more recent study[18a] of a large number of normal individuals has arrived at the following normal limits (mm. per hour): below age fifty, 15 for men and 25 for women; above age fifty, 20 for men and 30 for women.

Table 23–1.—Upper Limits of Normal in Westergren ESR
(Mean ± 2 S.D.)

Age (Years)	*Males (mm. in 1 hour)*	*Females (mm. in 1 hour)*
18–30	7	10
31–40	8	11
41–50	10	13
51–60	12	18
60+	13	20

(From Hilder, F. M. and Gunz, F. W.: J. Clin. Path., *17*, 292, 1964.)

Wintrobe Method

The method of Wintrobe[187] uses less than 1 ml. of blood for the measurement, which is performed in a hematocrit tube. A mixture of powdered potassium and ammonium oxalate is used as the anticoagulant. Correction for anemia is no longer recommended.[186] An advantage of this method is that it permits the determination of the hematocrit on the same blood sample. Normal values range from 0 to 6.5 mm. in healthy young males, and 0 to 16 mm. in healthy young females.

A number of workers[43,62,66,67] have pointed out the occasional failure of the Wintrobe method to reflect the presence of active disease under circumstances in which the Westergren ESR is elevated. Parallel determinations with the Westergren method have frequently produced widely divergent results.[43] When this occurred, the ESR was usually elevated by the Westergren method and in the normal range by the Wintrobe. When a high Westergren and low Wintrobe ESR occurred together, the clinical evidence suggested that the latter was in error.

Factors in the Measurement of the ESR

(1) *Erythrocyte Concentration.*—The settling of erythrocytes results in upward displacement of the medium. The upward current causes the apparent settling velocity of the erythrocytes to be less than the actual velocity of fall. The greater the concentration of erythrocytes, the greater is the volume of plasma displaced, and consequently, the greater the retardation of the apparent settling velocity. This is probably the major mechanism underlying the variation in the ESR produced by alteration of the red blood cell count. Since undiluted blood samples are used in the Wintrobe method,[43,154] the incidence of erroneous results increases rapidly as the hematocrit level rises above 40 per cent. Dilution of the red blood cells by anticoagulant in the Westergren method diminishes the effect of red cell concentration in retarding the ESR.

(2) *Plasma Viscosity.*—Frictional resistance to the movement of cells and plasma occurs at the cell-plasma and plasma-glass wall interfaces. With plasma of high viscosity, the frictional resistance between the plasma and the wall of the tube becomes a limiting factor in the downward movement of the cells and upward displacement of the plasma. Since the frictional resistance offered by the tube wall to the upward movement of plasma at any viscosity level is inversely proportional to the fourth power of the radius of the tube, the internal diameter of the tube becomes increasingly important at high viscosity. In view of the fact that there is no dilution of the plasma by the dry anticoagulant used in the Wintrobe method, the 2.5 mm. bore of the Wintrobe tube leads to anomalous results when plasma viscosity is high.[43,154] The same diameter does not create difficulty in the Westergren method because of the dilution afforded by the citrate anticoagulant solution.

(3) *Tube Length.*—Tube length is also a factor of significance in the measurement of the ESR. Studies by Cutler[31] have shown that erythrocyte sedimentation occurs in three phases: (*a*) a phase of aggregation and acceleration of the particles; (*b*) a phase of constant velocity of fall, which is the portion most susceptible to precise measurement; and (*c*) a phase of packing or marked deceleration caused by the piling up of erythrocytes at the bottom of the tube. For methods like the Westergren and Wintrobe, in which a single observation is made at the end of one hour, a long tube length is a distinct advantage, since it permits greater acceleration of the settling velocity and also allows a greater period of constant fall. In this way it provides a wider range of abnormal values. The Westergren column length of 200 mm., therefore, has a definite advantage over the 100-mm. Wintrobe column in this regard.

The long tube utilized in the Westergren method decreases the influence of erythrocyte packing; and dilution of the red blood cells with anticoagulant diminishes the effect of red cell concentration in retarding the ESR. For these reasons, the Westergren ESR is less likely to be increased in the presence of anemia than the Wintrobe. Nevertheless, the Westergren ESR is significantly increased by marked anemia and decreased by polycythemia.[123]

Other Methods for Measurement of the ESR

In the Rourke-Ernstene[147] and Cutler methods,[31] the ESR is measured by taking readings at five-minute intervals in wide bore tubes and plotting a rate curve. From this curve the ESR may be determined during the phase of constant fall. The usefulness of these methods is reduced, however, by the necessity to make the frequent observations required to plot a sedimentation curve.

Miscellaneous Factors

Deviation of the sedimentation tube by only a few degrees from the vertical causes a striking acceleration of the sedimentation rate.[73] When the tube is not vertical, plasma streams rapidly along the upper side of the tube, and the erythrocytes are thus subjected to less hindrance from the upward displacement current, as in the familiar example of the angle centrifuge.

The type of anticoagulant employed may have a significant influence on the ESR. Heparin has been observed to accelerate the rate.[73] The dry ammonium-potassium oxalate mixture affects the red cells, so that when this anticoagulant is used, the ESR must be measured within two or three hours after the blood is drawn. When the potassium salt of ethylenediamine tetra-acetic acid (EDTA) is used, however,[61,119] there is only minimum alteration of the ESR after twenty-four hours. Dilution of four parts of EDTA blood with one part of diluent is considered necessary to obtain reproducible results. For the influence of storage of the blood and of temperature on the ESR, the review of Ham and Curtis[73] should be consulted.

ESR IN DISEASE

Rheumatoid Arthritis

In active cases the ESR is usually markedly elevated and tends to parallel the activity of the disease. Increased values were found in 85 per cent of cases of mild severity, and in 95 per cent of cases of moderate to severe involvement.[158] In the series of Richardson,[137] only 11.5 per cent of cases in the total group had Westergren sedimentation rates under 10 mm. per hour.

Exacerbations are usually accompanied by an increase and remissions by a decrease in the ESR. In the complete Grade I remission, the values tend to become normal. Nevertheless, continuously elevated values may be observed in patients who have shown considerable decrease in joint inflammation, reflecting presumably the continued elevation of the serum globulin after clinical activity has subsided. In this circumstance, frequently repeated measurement of the ESR is usually unrewarding, although the elevated values no doubt signify underlying activity of the rheumatoid process. Conversely, clinically active cases may have normal sedimentation rates. This occurred in 7.3 per cent of the series of Dawson, Sia, and Boots[34] and approximately 5 per cent of the series of Richardson.[137]

Osteoarthritis

The sedimentation rate in primary osteoarthritis is usually normal. Nevertheless, values above 30 mm. were noted in 9.6 per cent of patients by Dawson and co-workers.[34] It is not uncommon to observe mild elevation of the Westergren ESR in the middle-aged woman with osteoarthritis. Thus, if the history and physical examination are consistent with the diagnosis of osteoarthritis, it should not be excluded on the basis of the ESR.

Fibrositis

Measurement of the ESR is of value in distinguishing fibrositis[36] from rheumatoid arthritis, since the ESR is normal in fibrositis. However, in the condition known as polymyalgia rheumatica,[68] which has features in common with both fibrositis and rheumatoid arthritis, the ESR is usually moderately to markedly elevated.

Unexplained Elevation

In some individuals, the sedimentation rate may be persistently elevated without obvious cause. In a group of 35 of such patients observed by Olhagen and Liljestrand,[103,127] 14 were eventually demonstrated to have one of the following: asymptomatic pulmonary tuberculosis, macroglobulinemia of Waldenstrom, hepatic cirrhosis, multiple myeloma and systemic lupus erythematosus. The remaining 21 patients, however, continued to have persistently elevated sedimentation rates for periods of three to twenty years with an otherwise benign course. In 9, this was associated with an increased gamma globulin level. The rest had unexplained elevations of either the beta lipoprotein or fibrinogen, or showed the presence of paraproteins of the myeloma type on electrophoresis of their serum. Ansell and Bywaters[7] found evidence of serious illness on follow-up of 20 of 31 cases of unexplained elevation of the ESR. Thus, the presence of an elevated ESR as the sole abnormality should lead to careful investigation of the patient, although it is not necessarily associated with a poor prognosis.

The ESR is elevated in the majority of patients with malignancy.[118a] Often this is a result of secondary infection or tumor necrosis. Extreme elevation with malignancy is associated with skeletal metastasis.[130] Very marked elevation of the sedimentation rate occurs in multiple myeloma.[40] In this condition, the elevation is due mainly to the high concentration of paraprotein in the blood. The ESR can be significantly elevated in women taking oral contraceptives.[22b] Finally, unexplained elevated levels have also been found in a hospitalized elderly population.[21a]

ESR and Congestive Heart Failure

Congestive heart failure is believed to lower the ESR, especially in young individuals with rheumatic carditis,[129,151,190] as a result of a decrease in the synthesis of fibrinogen in the passively congested liver. This widely accepted conclusion has recently been denied on the basis of an extensive analysis of the ESR in congestive heart failure occurring in patients with rheumatic heart disease.[163] Numerous exceptions to the conclusion that heart failure reduces the ESR are also to be found in the data of Sanghvi.[150] The latter commonly noted elevation rather than depression of the ESR in patients with heart failure as a result of either the rheumatic activity, respiratory infection, or myocardial damage usually associated with the failure. Nevertheless, the available evidence suggests[129,151,190] that the effect of hepatic congestion *per se* in congestive heart failure is to retard the ESR, though the net effect of all factors appears more often to result in elevated values.

C-REACTIVE PROTEIN TEST

In a study of pneumococcal pneumonia, Tillett and Francis in 1930[172] reported that addition of the C-polysaccharide of the pneumococcus to the serum of acutely ill patients resulted in precipitation. No reaction occurred with the serum of the same patients during convalescence. The substance which precipitated, subsequently called the C-reactive protein (CRP), was also noted in a number of other infectious diseases, as well as rheumatic fever. It was later found to occur in non-infectious conditions like myocardial infarction and a group of miscellaneous diseases.[76,106] MacLeod and Avery, in 1941,[109,110] isolated the CRP and produced a specific antiserum against it. Detection of the CRP by incubation of the antiserum with the patient's serum in a capillary tube proved more sensitive than the C-polysaccharide precipitation method. In 1947, the CRP was crystallized from empyema and ascites fluid of patients with infection,[113] and these fluids have been the source of this protein for the production of antiserum in recent years.

The occurrence of the CRP in various disease states has been summarized in detail by Hedlund.[77] The elaboration of the CRP, like the ESR, is a nonspecific response to inflammation. Nevertheless, most cases of acute upper respiratory infection, and about 50 per cent of cases of acute appendicitis have shown negative tests. An important advantage of the CRP reaction is its resistance to the influence of three factors which tend to influence the ESR, *i.e.* anemia, congestive heart failure, and the hyperglobulinemia which may persist after the subsidence of inflammation.

In rheumatoid arthritis, the CRP is

present in practically all patients with clinical evidence of disease activity.[114] It tends to parallel the ESR closely. Unlike the situation in rheumatic fever, salicylate and hormone therapy do not readily depress the CRP, or for that matter the ESR, in patients with rheumatoid arthritis. Measurement of the CRP does not appear to offer any special advantage over the ESR in the management of this disease.

In spite of the non-specificity of the response, Anderson and McCarty[6] have concluded that the presence of CRP in the blood is probably the most sensitive available indicator of activity in rheumatic fever. However, the CRP tends to revert to normal in patients with rheumatic fever sooner than the ESR and at a time when inflammation appears to be continuing.[51]

SERUM PROTEINS

Electrophoretic Studies

Electrophoresis of the serum proteins has permitted detailed examination of their concentration in disease. Increases in alpha-2 globulin and fibrinogen occur non-specifically in the presence of inflammation. A rise in the gamma globulin level in inflammatory disease is presumptive evidence of a response to antigenic stimulation, even though the identity of the antigen is often not known.

The electrophoretic pattern in rheumatoid arthritis is not specific and is frequently within normal limits. Its most significant features have been a low serum albumin concentration and elevation of the mean concentrations of the alpha-2 and gamma globulin.[126,169,170,185] Alpha-1 globulin and beta-globulin were not significantly changed. Albumin levels were significantly lower and gamma globulin levels higher in stages III and IV of the disease.[170] The alpha-2 globulin level was correlated with disease activity.[126] The highest levels of this fraction were seen early in the course of the disease and frequently persisted as the only abnormality after years of illness. Elevation of the gamma globulin was also associated with disease activity.[21]

The mechanism of the hypoalbuminemia in rheumatoid arthritis has recently been studied[84a] using I^{131} labeled albumin for determination of pool sizes and breakdown rates in 7 patients.[185a] Increased albumin breakdown, as a part of the general hypermetabolic state, was demonstrated in 5 patients, in proportion to the activity of the rheumatoid arthritis.

The electrophoretic pattern in systemic lupus erythematosus (SLE) resembles that seen in rheumatoid arthritis although the gamma globulin elevation is usually more pronounced. Similar, though perhaps less marked changes, are seen in the other connective tissue diseases.[126]

With the development of the radial diffusion technique for the determination of immunoglobulin levels, several studies have shown increased levels of IgM and IgA in patients with rheumatoid arthritis.[9a,136a] There was little apparent correlation between the elevation of immunoglobulin levels and duration of activity or rheumatoid factor titers. Seropositive patients have also shown increased levels of IgG.[178a]

Serum Protein-Bound Carbohydrate

Using the terminology of Winzler,[189] two groups of compounds contain both carbohydrate and protein: the glycoproteins and the mucoproteins.

The glycoproteins are made up of protein linked to carbohydrate by a stable covalent bond. Since all of the serum globulins contain carbohydrate, they may be classed as glycoproteins. Because the alpha-1 and alpha-2 globulins rise during inflammation, one may detect an increase in protein-bound carbohydrate in the serum. This has led to the determination of serum glycoprotein as a measure of inflammatory activity.[143] The serum glycoproteins may be determined[188] as protein-bound hexose (galactose, mannose), protein-bound hexosamine (glucosamine, galactosamine), or protein-bound sialic acid.

The seromucoid fraction of the glycoprotein may also be followed as an index of inflammatory activity. This fraction represents a more soluble group of carbohydrate-containing proteins which are not precipitable either by heat or by ordinary concentrations of perchloric acid. The carbohydrate portion comprises a relatively large part of the molecule.[19] The seromucoid fraction is analyzed[188] by precipitating first with perchloric acid to remove the major bulk of serum proteins and then with phosphotungstic acid to obtain the seromucoid fraction itself.

The serum mucoproteins are a class of proteins which contain mucopolysaccharide linked to protein usually by a hydrogen bond or salt linkage.[188] In contrast to the glycoproteins, the mucoproteins are present in the serum in very low concentrations, *i.e.* in microgram rather than milligram quantities per 100 ml. The mucopolysaccharides which they contain appear to be of the chondroitin sulfate type[20] and are localized in the euglobulin fraction.[8] The serum mucoprotein fraction has been found to be significantly elevated in patients with rheumatoid arthritis.[8] This elevation was attributed to an increase in the amount of euglobulin.

Serum glycoprotein, analyzed as protein-bound hexose and hexosamine, has been noted to be consistently elevated in patients with rheumatoid arthritis[155] and active rheumatic fever,[89,90,156] usually paralleling the ESR. Shetlar and coworkers[155] have also found the ratio of protein-bound hexose to protein in the serum to be a useful index of inflammatory activity.

Boettiger, Malmquist, and Olhagen,[17,18] have made a detailed study of the serum glycoprotein levels (seromucoid and protein-bound carbohydrate) in patients with various rheumatic disorders. The normal variation of the seromucoid fraction was found to be quite large and the differentiating capacity of this determination, therefore, limited. Protein-bound hexose, hexosamine, and sialic acid, however, which tended to vary together, showed a smaller range of normal variation than the seromucoid. The levels in inflammatory states correlated well with the ESR. However, it was the conclusion of the authors that determination of serum glycoprotein offered no advantage over the ESR in terms of precise differentiation of normal from abnormal findings.

Mucopolysaccharide Excretion

This has been studied in patients with connective tissue diseases.[37,105,171] The polysaccharides in the urine appear to be a mixture of chondroitin sulfates and possibly some hyaluronic acid. Excretion is elevated in active, untreated adult patients with rheumatoid arthritis and also other inflammatory conditions. It was unexpectedly decreased in patients with juvenile rheumatoid arthritis, however, when compared with excretion in control children.[105] This was attributed to the decreased skeletal growth in this condition.

Haptoglobins

Haptoglobin levels are increased in rheumatoid arthritis, probably as a non-specific response to inflammation. The increase is not related to the titer of the rheumatoid factor,[4] nor is occurrence of rheumatoid arthritis related to any particular genetic pattern of the haptoglobin.

Cryoglobulins

These have been occasionally demonstrated in rheumatoid sera.[141]

Urinary Gamma Globulin

Gordon, Eisen and Vaughan[67b] found that the quantity of urinary γ-globulins excreted was higher in rheumatoid arthritis than in controls. These were composed of L chains, 7S gamma globulin and traces of gamma A globulin. It was concluded that there is an increased protein excretion in rheumatoid arthritis. The mechanism for this is unknown.

AMINO ACIDS

Analysis of serum amino acid levels in rheumatoid arthritis[122] has demonstrated lowered concentrations of arginine, tyrosine, and histidine. Glutamic acid was increased in concentration. Total urinary amino acid excretion was in the normal range.[149]

Hydroxyproline peptide excretion was found to be normal in patients with rheumatoid arthritis and other connective tissue diseases.[194] Rodnan and Cammarata[145] have reported the excretion of this amino acid to be elevated in active cases of scleroderma.

An abnormally large decline in the concentration of serum glycine has been observed following administration of sodium benzoate to patients with rheumatoid arthritis.[101] A similar change was seen in patients with SLE and active rheumatic fever but not in patients with degenerative joint disease.

Tryptophane Metabolism

Elevated amounts of tryptophane metabolites have been found in the urine of patients with rheumatoid arthritis and the other collagen diseases, especially scleroderma. Significantly increased amounts of the tryptophane metabolite 3-hydroxy anthranilic acid (HAA) were excreted in 24 to 74 per cent of rheumatoid patients.[116,132,164] Controls were patients with other diseases. Increased excretion of kynurenine, another metabolite, has also been reported.[15]

Following a tryptophane load, excretion of kynurenine and hydroxykynurenine, but not of HAA, was found to be significantly elevated in patients with rheumatoid arthritis and other collagen diseases when compared with normal controls.[14,15,54,132] When controls were patients with other diseases, the excretion of hydroxykynurenine but not kynurenine was significantly increased.[132] Two authors (Spiera,[164a] Bett[15a]), studying tryptophane metabolites, have both concluded that elevated excretion of tryptophane metabolites is not specific for rheumatoid arthritis since the same defect was found in other diseases.

Most workers have observed no correlation between the elevated excretion of tryptophane metabolites in rheumatoid arthritis and any particular clinical or laboratory parameter, though one investigator has found some relation between hydroxykynurenine and kynurenine excretion and the sedimentation rate.[132] Abnormalities of tryptophane metabolism have also been observed in porphyria, pregnancy, cancer, pulmonary tuberculosis, Hodgkins' disease, hypoplastic anemia, leukemia and diabetes. This phenomenon is, therefore, not specific for the connective tissue diseases.

In view of the critical relationship of pyridoxal phosphate to the metabolism of tryptophane, the excretion of 4-pyridoxic acid, a metabolite of pyridoxine, has been measured in rheumatoid patients as an index of possible pyridoxine deficiency. The excretion of this metabolite was not decreased in rheumatoid patients indicating that the intake of pyridoxine was probably adequate.[54] However, administration of supplemental pyridoxine decreased the abnormally elevated excretion levels of the tryptophane metabolites observed after tryptophane loading. This has suggested a functional pyridoxine deficiency in these patients which is demonstrable, at least with respect to excretion of kynurenine and its hydroxy derivative, only after loading.

SEROLOGIC REACTIONS

Non-Specific Serologic Reactions

Biologic false-positive Wassermann reactions have been reported in 6.3 to 11.6 per cent of patients with rheumatoid arthritis.[93,179] Kievits and co-workers[93] have noted a relationship between the false-positive Wassermann reaction and the occurrence of positive L.E. cell tests in this disease. Of 27 patients who had positive L.E. tests, 8 had positive Wassermann reactions, while none of 42 with negative L.E. cell preparations gave this reaction.

Properdin assays by the zymosan technique in 24 patients with rheumatoid arthritis gave low values in 8 and prozone phenomena in 5.[96]

Rheumatoid Factors

Since an immune response appears to play a major role in the development of rheumatoid inflammation, it is not surprising that a number of laboratory findings are observed which reflect this response. Among them is the elaboration of a group of macroglobulins known as rheumatoid factors.[177,193] Although rheumatoid factor-like proteins are present in a variety of chronic inflammatory states, presumably as a consequence of chronic antigenic stimulation, they reach their highest titers in patients with rheumatoid arthritis. Since they are usually not detectable in significant titer in the serum of patients with other arthritides, they offer a relatively specific test for rheumatoid disease. In addition, a number of studies[41,91,135] have demonstrated that there is a relationship between the presence of rheumatoid factor in the serum and the progression of the rheumatoid process. Thus, the presence of this abnormal protein appears to have prognostic as well as diagnostic significance (see Chapter 9 for a full discussion of this subject).

L.E. Phenomenon

This reaction has been reported to be positive in from 8 to 27 per cent of patients with rheumatoid arthritis in most recent studies. Friedman and co-workers[58] found an increased incidence of subcutaneous nodules, Felty's syndrome, and elevation of the gamma globulin in rheumatoid patients who showed positive L.E. cell tests. However, pathognomonic features of SLE were not observed. The increased incidence of subcutaneous nodules was confirmed by Parr and co-workers.[128] The only significant features found in another well-controlled study[67a] of patients with positive L.E. preparations were a more frequent occurrence of leukopenia and, as above, a higher mean serum gamma globulin level. Kievits and co-workers[93] have observed a higher frequency of splenomegaly, anemia, false-positive Wassermann reactions, abnormalities of the urinary sediment, and elevated ESR in the group with positive L.E. cell tests.

Of 11 cases of rheumatoid arthritis with positive L.E. cell test studied by Toone, Irby and Pierce,[173] four with disease of many years' duration later developed multisystem involvement of a type seen in SLE, suggesting at least in this small group, the coexistence of the two diseases. The latter observation has, however, been unusual. Though rheumatoid patients with a positive L.E. cell test have tended, as a group, to have more pronounced systemic involvement, they have not shown pathognomonic features of SLE, and appear to merit, in most cases, no other diagnosis than that of rheumatoid arthritis (*see also* Chapter 10).

Antinuclear Factors

Gamma globulins capable of reacting with nuclear constituents have been referred to as antinuclear factors. Reaction between these factors and the nucleus is usually demonstrated by the fluorescent antibody technique, although other methods have been utilized.[175] The antinuclear reaction is observed most commonly in patients with SLE, but is seen with varying incidence in the other connective tissue diseases. It is a more sensitive reaction than the L.E. cell phenomenon. In a group of 710 patients with rheumatoid arthritis collected from the literature by Pollak,[133] 24 per cent had positive antinuclear tests. In the series reported by Weir,[182] in which only 3 per cent showed positive L.E. tests, the antinuclear reaction was positive in 14 per cent. It is of interest that the antinuclear factor is present mainly as a macroglobulin (IgM) in rheumatoid sera, and mainly as a 7S or light gamma globulin (IgG) in SLE sera.[13]

Studies on the significance of positive antinuclear tests in patients with rheumatoid arthritis were carried out by two groups.[29a,132a] Both concluded that such patients had more severe disease. Although one group showed a higher frequency of vasculitis in the antinuclear positive group,[132a] this was not confirmed in the other study.[29a] Also, antinuclear positivity appeared significantly more frequently in those patients who were rheumatoid factor positive.

The occurrence in rheumatoid serum of the abnormal factors discussed above is presumably secondary to a more fundamental process which is responsible for the initiation of the disease. Rheumatoid factors, antinuclear factors and biologic false Wassermann antibody have all been found in other conditions associated with chronic inflammation. Experimentally, prolonged hyperimmunization of rabbits with formalin-killed bacteria has resulted in the development of "rheumatoid-like" factors[1] and even anti-DNA factors,[28] indicating the relationship of these proteins to prolonged antigenic stimulation (*see also* Chapter 10).

Isohemagglutinins and Blood Groups

A deficiency of anti-A and anti-B isohemagglutinins in blood group O individuals with rheumatoid arthritis has been reported.[136] In Japan the frequency of the AB blood type in rheumatoid arthritis was significantly higher than the others in the ABO system.[189a] This disease was also said to be characterized by a significant absence of the Rh antigen D and the N antigen but this result could not be confirmed in two subsequent studies[13a,71a] which found a normal distribution. No correlation was found with the antigens of the ABO, C or E blood groups.[29]

SERUM COMPLEMENT

The serum complement level in rheumatoid arthritis is usually either normal or somewhat elevated.[44,97,176] In contrast, the level of complement is reduced in most patients with SLE, especially in the presence of active disease.[44,95] Practically all lupus erythematosus patients with renal disease have been observed to have lowered levels. The striking difference in complement level between rheumatoid arthritis and SLE suggests that antigen-antibody complexes play a prominent role in the latter disease. In rheumatoid arthritis, where complement levels are not decreased, such complexes are presumably not formed in quantity. However, it has been demonstrated by Mongan and co-workers[119a] that serum complement activity was significantly reduced in patients with vasculitis. In addition, the complement levels of seropositive patients were lower than those of seronegative patients.

In rheumatic fever, Fischel, Pauli, and Lesh[52] found elevated complement levels in 45 of 50 patients at some time in the course of the attack. The increase was particularly marked early in the illness. The complement level appeared to be correlated with the course of the rheumatic fever episode, behaving in this respect like an acute phase reactant.

Immunoconglutinin, believed to be an autoantibody to complement fixed in the body, usually appears in the serum in response to antigenic stimulation. It is a gamma$_{1M}$ (IgM) immunoglobulin with properties reminiscent of the rheumatoid factor in the sense that it is a macroglobulin believed to be produced by an autoimmune response to a serum component. High levels are found in conditions where immune reactions are thought to occur.[30] Elevated levels of immunoconglutinin have been found in rheumatoid arthritis,[26,30] but this is not a specific finding since immunoconglutinin is also elevated in other rheumatic diseases.

LIVER FUNCTION

Mild to moderate abnormalities of liver function have been reported in rheumatoid arthritis but these have been confined mainly to tests of liver function which reflect serum protein synthesis, *i.e.*, albumin-globulin ratios and the cephalin flocculation and thymol turbidity tests.[32,99,149] Histologic changes, though found in up to 25 per cent of biopsies, have been minimal[99,120] and not correlated with the chemical abnormalities noted. They have consisted of slight to moderate fatty infiltration, slight evidence of fibrosis and, rarely, infiltration of portal areas with a few mononuclear cells. Clinical or biochemical evidence of liver disease was found[184a] in 0.7 per cent of 997 patients with rheumatoid arthritis.

Serum alkaline phosphatase levels[100] have been in the normal range. Serum glutamic-oxalacetic transaminase[10,112] and serum glutamic-pyruvic transaminase levels[112] have also been normal, though 15 per cent of patients did show some elevation of serum ornithine-carbamoyl transferase.[112] Serum bilirubin and urine urobilinogen were within normal limits.[32] Urine coproporphyrin excretion, however, was significantly elevated. Though Castenters and co-workers[27] observed decreased bromsulphalein excretion in more than 90 per cent of patients and Darby[32] in 23 per cent, Roy and co-workers[149] found no significant incidence of abnormal dye retention.

RENAL FUNCTION AND ELECTROLYTES

Urinary abnormalities are relatively uncommon in rheumatoid arthritis. More than a faint trace of albumin was found in the urine of only 7.2 per cent of patients of the Massachusetts General Hospital series.[157] This figure does not include patients with albuminuria associated with pyuria; however, urinary tract infection was not found to be increased in patients with rheumatoid arthritis.[120a] Fearnley and Lachner observed persistent proteinuria in 24 of 183 of their patients.[48] When they investigated 20 patients of this group, the proteinuria was explainable on the basis of unrelated renal disease in 12; in the remaining 8, evidence of amyloidosis was demonstrated. Similar results were obtained by Pollak and co-workers on renal biopsy of 13 rheumatoid patients with persistent proteinuria.[134] The biopsies disclosed normal kidneys in 3, arteriosclerosis or nephrosclerosis in 4, lupus nephritis in 2, and amyloidosis in 4. It is of interest, in view of these findings, that the incidence of amyloidosis in autopsied cases of rheumatoid arthritis in the Massachusetts General Hospital series was as high as 26 per cent.[23] Other studies have given similar results. Persistent, unexplained proteinuria in rheumatoid arthritis should, therefore, lead to a search for amyloid disease.

The blood non-protein nitrogen was elevated in only 1.7 per cent of rheumatoid patients.[157] A series of Scandinavian studies[3,159–161] have, however, reported a small to moderate decrease in the creatinine clearance in rheumatoid patients. The average reduction was 36 per cent.[160] Impairment of glomerular filtration was observed to be related to the stage and duration of the disease as well as to the presence of rheumatoid factor. It was unrelated to past history of drug intake, including phenacetin. Thus, though the occurrence of occasional proteinuria and the reduction of the creatinine clearance in some patients have been suggestive of a renal abnormality in rheumatoid arthritis, histologic studies, except for certain early reports,[9,60] have not disclosed evidence of a specific renal abnormality other than the well-established complication of amyloidosis.

Serum sodium levels have been normal in rheumatoid patients, but a significant small elevation in serum potassium has been claimed.[87] The sweat Na/K ratio was found to be increased in about half of the patients in one series,[71] though information about previous steroid therapy was not given in this study.

Increased serum copper[84,124] and decreased levels of serum albumin[124] have been reported. It should be remembered that increased copper levels, which are associated with increase in the alpha-2 globulin, ceruloplasmin, are a nonspecific feature of inflammatory disease. The increased levels were, in fact, correlated with the ESR but not with the presence of rheumatoid factor or with the stage of the disease.[111] Zinc levels are normal.[132b]

ADRENAL FUNCTION

Adrenal cortical function has been evaluated on the basis of the excretion of 17-OH corticosteroid, 17-ketosteroid[80] and other adrenal cortical metabolites.[167] Except for a decrease in excretion of 17-hydroxycorticosteroids in the early morning hours, the adrenal corticosteroid excretion pattern in rheumatoid arthritis was similar to that seen in other chronic diseases. Normal secretion rates of cortisol have also been found.[127a] Adrenal medullary function, as measured by the urinary excretion of epinephrine and norepinephrine, has been found to be within normal limits.[59,162]

MISCELLANEOUS

Uric Acid

Occasional studies have reported elevated levels of serum uric acid in patients with arthritides other than gout. Grayzel, Liddle, and Seegmiller,[70] who found elevated levels in 10 of 57 males with rheumatoid arthritis, ascribed this finding to retention of uric acid induced by low doses of salicylate. In other studies,[157,180] the levels of uric acid in rheumatoid arthritis were considered to be in the normal range.

Serum Cholesterol and Plasma Lipids

In rheumatoid arthritis, as in other inflammatory arthritides, the total cholesterol level tends to be reduced.[107] The mean reduction in rheumatoid factor-positive patients was 53.7 per cent. The decrease was related to the severity and activity of the disease and was not affected by steroid therapy. Plasma lipid levels have been reported to be within normal limits.[16,92]

Vitamin Levels

Blood levels of the vitamins are commonly decreased in patients with rheumatoid arthritis. Blood concentrations of ascorbic acid are usually low.[55] Serum levels of thiamine and cocarboxylase are also decreased.[94] Blood pantothenic acid has been found to be markedly decreased. The amount of decrease was correlated with the activity of the disease[12] and with a significantly increased excretion of this vitamin.[88] Riboflavin, thiamine, and occasionally nicotinic acid levels were also diminished;[88] however, folate levels were not significantly different.[24b] An observed increase in imidazole excretion was believed to be related to increased reticuloendothelial tissue activity.[179b] Pyridoxin excretion has been found to be significantly depressed.[115]

Gastric Acidity

This has been studied in several large series of rheumatoid patients, and the findings summarized by Short and coworkers.[157] Following histamine stimulation, these authors found an increased frequency of anacidity in patients under forty, which was unassociated with any particular feature of the disease. This tendency was not present in patients over forty.

Electromyography

Electromyographic findings in rheumatoid arthritis are not specific. There is, however, an increased frequency of abnormal findings. Polyphasic potentials of short and long duration are fre-

Table 23-2.—Laboratory Findings in Rheumatoid Arthritis

Blood Elements

Erythrocytes—Moderate normochromic or hypochromic, normocytic anemia; low plasma iron; moderately decreased marrow iron stores; normal utilization of plasma iron; slightly decreased erythrocyte survival time; inadequate release of iron from tissue stores.

Leukocytes—Normal or slightly elevated in most adult cases. Leukopenia rare; eosinophilia occasional. Leukocytosis with left shift common in juvenile disease.

Acute Phase Phenomena

Erythrocyte Sedimentation Rate—Moderately to markedly increased in most cases.
C-Reactive Protein—Positive reaction in most cases.
Serum Proteins—Alpha-2 globulin, fibrinogen, and gamma globulin usually increased; alpha-1 globulin may be increased. Albumin usually decreased and beta globulin unchanged.
Seromucoid, Protein-Bound Hexose and Haptoglobins—Usually increased.
Mucopolysaccharide Excretion—Usually elevated in adults and decreased in children.

Immune Factors

L.E. Factor—Present in about 10 per cent.
Antinuclear Factor—Present in about 25 per cent.
Rheumatoid Factor—Present in majority of adult cases.
Biologic False-Positive Wassermann Reaction—Present in 5 to 10 per cent.
Complement—Usually normal or somewhat elevated.
Immunoconglutinin—Usually elevated.

Liver Function

Cephalin Flocculation—Often positive.
Thymol Turbidity—Often increased.
Alkaline Phosphatase, SGOT and SGPT—Usually normal.

Renal Function

Proteinuria—May be present due to amyloidosis or unrelated renal disease.
NPN—Rarely elevated.
Creatinine Clearance—Often shows some decrease.

Miscellaneous Findings

Urinary Amino Acid and Hydroxyproline Excretion—In normal range.
3-Hydroxyanthranilic Acid (HAA) and Kynurenine Excretion—Often increased.
Serum Uric Acid—Usually normal.
Blood Cholesterol—Often reduced.
Plasma Lipid—Usually normal.
Blood Vitamin Levels—Usually decreased.
Serum Ceruloplasmin and Serum Copper—Usually elevated.
Gastric Acidity—Often reduced in patients under forty.

quently seen.[33,69,166] Fibrillation potentials have been reported by some authors,[33,69,191] but not by others.[5,121,166,192] Daughety and co-workers noted the presence of complicating factors such as polyneuropathy, terminal bronchopulmonary disease, and recent surgery in all of their patients who showed fibrillation potentials.[33] Electrophysiological studies of nerve conduction time in rheumatoid patients have shown these to be normal.[183]

Pleural Fluid

A distinctive finding in rheumatoid arthritis has been the extremely low glucose concentration of pleural effusions in this disease. Carr and Mayne[24] found glucose levels between less than 5 mg. per cent and 17 mg. per cent in 10 of 11 such effusions. Schools and Mikkelsen[153] found values of 3, 0, and 0 mg. per cent respectively in three effusions proved by pleural biopsy to be of rheumatoid etiology. The cause of this low concentration is not known. Oral[24b] or intravenous[39a] administration of glucose failed to raise the glucose level in the effusions. (For a discussion of the synovial fluid, see Chapter 6.)

Other Findings

Serum sulfhydryl levels have been reported to be low in rheumatoid arthritis, especially in the presence of vasculitis.[108] Ceruloplasmin levels were increased, non-specifically reflecting inflammatory activity.[138,168] Although Neidermeier[124] found markedly raised concentrations of copper in synovial fluid from patients with rheumatoid arthritis (75 per cent of this was present as ceruloplasmin), the mean serum copper and ceruloplasmin concentrations were no different in patients with rheumatoid arthritis than in controls. Gerber[63] found increased amounts of copper-binding substances in half of rheumatoid patients. The exact nature of these substances has not been determined. Adenosine triphosphatase[72] and total serum lactic dehydrogenase[178] activities were within normal limits. Serum cholinesterase levels have been variable.[74] Kinogen plasma levels and erythrocyte kininase levels have been normal, but plasma kininase levels have been significantly decreased.[22a] Serum plasmin activity has been shown to be correlated with the activity of the disease.[5a]

BIBLIOGRAPHY

1. Abruzzo, J. L. and Christian, C. L.: J. Exp. Med., *114*, 791, 1961.
2. Alexander, W. R. M., Richmond, J., Roy, L. M. H. and Duthie, J. J. R.: Ann. Rheum. Dis., *15*, 12, 1956.
3. Allander, E., Bucht, H., Lofgren, O. and Wehle, B.: Acta Rheum. Scand., *9*, 116, 1963.
4. Allison, A. C. and Blumberg, B. S.: Arth. and Rheum., *1*, 239, 1958.
5. Amick, L. D.: Arth. and Rheum., *3*, 54, 1960.

5*a*. Andersen, R. B., and Winther, O.: Acta Rheum. Scand. *15*, 178, 169.

6. Anderson, H. C. and McCarty, M.: J. Exp. Med., *93*, 25, 1951.
7. Ansell, B. and Bywaters, E. G. L.: Brit. Med. J., *1*, 372, 1958.
8. Badin, J., Schubert, M. and Vouras, M.: J. Clin. Invest., *34*, 1317, 1955.
9. Bagenstoss, A. H. and Rosenberg, E. F.: Arch. Path., *35*, 503, 1943.

9*a*. Barden, J., Mullinax, F., and Waller, M.: Arth. and Rheum. *10*, 228, 1967.

10. Barr, J. H., Jr., Stolzer, B. L., Eisenberg, C. H., Jr., Kurtz, J. E. and Margolis, H. M.: Arth. and Rheum., *1*, 147, 1958.
11. Bartfeld, H.: New Engl. J. Med., *267*, 551, 1962.
12. Barton-Wright, E. C. and Elliot, W. A.: Lancet, *2*, 862, 1963.
13. Baum, J. and Ziff, M.: Arth. and Rheum., *5*, 636, 1962.

13*a*. Baxter, A., Izaff, M. M., Jasani, M. K., and McAndrew, R.: Acta Rheum. Scand., *14*, 79, 1968.

14. Beetham, W., Jr., Fischer, S. and Schrohenloher, R.: Proc. Soc. Exp. Med. Biol., *117*, 756, 1964.
15. Bett, I. M.: Ann. Rheum. Dis., *21*, 63, 1962.

15*a*. ———: Ann. Rheum. Dis., *25*, 556, 1966.

16. Block, W. D., Buchanan, O. H. and Freyberg, R. H.: Arch. Int. Med., *68*, 18, 1941.

17. Boettiger, L. E., Malmquist, E. and Olhagen, B.: Ann. Rheum. Dis., *23*, 489, 1964.
18. ————: Ibid., *23*, 495, 1964.
18*a*. Böttinger, L. E. and Svedberg, C. A.: Brit. Med. J., *2*, 85, 1967.
19. Bollet, A. J.: Arch. Int. Med., *104*, 152, 1959.
20. Bollet, A. J., Jerayderian, M. W. and Simpson, W. F.: J. Clin. Invest., *36*, 1328, 1957.
21. Bonomo, L.: Ann. Rheum. Dis., *16*, 340, 1957.
21*a*. Boyd, R. V., and Hoffbrand, B. I.: Brit. Med. J., *1*, 901, 1966.
22. Brandstrup, P.: Acta Med. Scand., *146*, 384, 1953.
22*a*. Breseid, K., Dyrud, O. and Rinvik, S.: Acta Pharmacol., *24*, 179, 1966.
22*b*. Burton, J. L.: Brit. Med. J., *3*, 214, 1967.
23. Calkins, E. and Cohen, A. S.: Bull. Rheum. Dis., *10*, 215, 1960.
24. Carr, D. T. and Mayne, J. G.: Am. Rev. Resp. Dis., *85*, 345, 1962.
24*a*. Cartwright, G. E.: Seminars in Hematology, *3*, 351, 1966.
24*b*. Carr, D. T., and McGuckin, W. F.: Am. Rev. Resp. Dis., *97*, 302, 1968.
25. Cartwright, G. E. and Wintrobe, M. M.: *Modern Trends in Blood Diseases*, New York, Paul B. Hoeber, Inc., 1955, p. 183.
26. Caspary, E. A. and Ball, E. J.: Brit. Med. J., *2*, 1514, 1962.
27. Castenters, H., Hultman, E. and Lofgren, O.: Acta Rheum. Scand., *10*, 128, 1964.
28. Christian, C. L., DeSimone, A. R. and Abruzzo, J. L.: Arth. and Rheum., *6*, 766, 1963.
29. Cohen, A. S., Boyd, W. C., Goldwasser, S. and Cathcart, E. S.: Nature, *200*, 1215, 1963.
29*a*. Condemi, J. J., Barnett, E. V., Atwater, E. C., Jacox, R. F., Mongan, E. S. and Vaughan, J. H.: Arth. & Rheum., *8*, 1080, 1965.
30. Coombs, R. R. A., Coombs, A. M. and Ingram, D. G.: *The Serology of Conglutination, and Its Relation to Disease*, Springfield, Charles C Thomas, 1961, p. 137.
31. Cutler, J.: Am. Rev. Tuberc., *19*, 544, 1929.
32. Darby, P. W.: J. Clin. Path., *6*, 331, 1953.
33. Daughety, J. S., Baum, J. and Krusen, U.: Arch. Phys. Med. & Rehabil., *45*, 224, 1964.
34. Dawson, M. H., Sia, R. H. P. and Boots, R. H.: J. Lab. Clin. Med., *15*, 1065, 1930.
35. Dawson, M. H. (Revised by C. Ragan): *Loose Leaf Medicine*, Thos. Nelson & Sons, V, 1946, p. 605.
36. Decker, J. L., Bollet, A. J., Duff, I. F., Shulman, L. E. and Stollerman, G., eds.: Primer on Rheumatic Diseases, J.A.M.A., *190*, 509, 1964.
37. DiFerrante, N.: J. Clin. Invest., *36*, 1516, 1957.
38. Dixon, A. St. J., Ramarchau, S. and Ropes, M. W.: Ann. Rheum. Dis., *14*, 51, 1955.
39. Dixon, A. St. J., Scott, J. T. and Harvey-Smith, E. A.: Brit. Med. J., *1*, 1425, 1960.
39*a*. Dodson, W. H. and Hollingsworth, J. W.: New Engl. J. Med., *275*, 1337, 1966.
40. Drusholm, A.: Acta Med. Scand., *176*, 609, 1964.
41. Duthie, J. J. R., Brown, P. E., Knox, J. D. E. and Thompson, M.: Ann. Rheum. Dis., *16*, 411, 1957.
42. Ebaugh, F. G., Peterson, R. E., Rodnan, G. P. and Bunim, J. J.: Med. Clin. North America, *39*, 489, 1955.
43. Editorial: Brit. Med. J., *1*, 1717, 1960.
44. Ellis, H. A. and Felix-Davies, D.: Ann. Rheum. Dis., *18*, 215, 1959.
45. Fahreus, R.: Biochem. Ztschr., *89*, 335, 1918.
46. ————: Acta Med. Scand., *55*, 1, 1921.
47. ————: Physiol. Rev., *9*, 241, 1929.
48. Fearnley, G. R. and Lachner, R.: Brit. Med. J., *1*, 1129, 1955.
49. Felty, A. R.: Bull. Johns Hopkins Hospital *35*, 16, 1924.
50. Finch, C. A., Gibson, J. G., Peacock, W. C. and Fluharty, R. G.: Blood, *4*, 905, 1949.
51. Fischel, E. E.: Med. Clin. N. Amer., *41*, 685, 1957.
52. Fischel, E. E., Pauli, R. H. and Lesh, J.: J. Clin. Invest., *28*, 1172, 1949.
53. Fletcher, A. A., Dauphinee, J. A. and Ogryzlo, M. A.: J. Clin. Invest., *31*, 561, 1952.
54. Flinn, J. H., Price, J. M., Yess, N. and Brown, R. R.: Arth. and Rheum., *7*, 201, 1964.
55. Forster, J. E. and Engleman, E. P.: Arth. and Rheum., *4*, 418, 1961.
56. Freireich, E. J., Ross, J. F., Bayles, T. B., Emerson, C. P. and Finch, S. C.: Ann. Rheum. Dis., *13*, 365, 1954.
57. ————: J. Clin. Invest., *36*, 1043, 1957.
58. Friedman, I. A., Sickley, J. F., Poske, R. M., Black, A., Bronsky, D., Hartz, W. H., Feldhake, C., Reeder, P. S. and Katz, E. M.: Ann. Int. Med., *46*, 1113, 1957.

59. Fruehan, A. E. and Frawley, T. F.: Arth. and Rheum., *6*, 698, 1963.
60. Fugerman, D. L. and Andrum, F. C.: Ann. Rheum. Dis., *3*, 168, 1943.
61. Gambino, S. R., Dike, J. J., Monteleone, M. and Budd, D. C.: Tech. Bull. Reg. Med. Technol., *35*, 1, 1965.
62. Gelman, D. and Sykes, A. J.: Brit. Med. J., *2*, 4196, 1951.
63. Gerber, D. A.: Arth. and Rheum., *9*, 795, 1966.
64. Gibson, J. G., Harris, A. W. and Swigert, V. W.: J. Clin. Invest., *18*, 621, 1939.
65. Gilligan, D. R. and Ernstine, A. C.: Amer. Jour. Med. Sci., *187*, 552, 1934.
66. Goldberg, A. and Conway, H.: Brit. Med. J., *2*, 315, 1952.
67. Goldberg, S., Glynn, L. E. and Bywaters, E. G. L.: Brit. Med. J., *1*, 202, 1962.
67*a*. Goldfine, L. J., Stevens, M. B., Masi, A. T., and Shulman, L. E.: Ann. Rheum. Dis., *24*, 153, 1965.
67*b*. Gordon, D. A., Eisen, A. Z., and Vaughan, J.: Arth. & Rheum., *9*, 575, 1966.
68. Gordon, I., Rennie, A. M. and Branwood, A. W.: Ann. Rheum. Dis., *23*, 447, 1964.
69. Graudal, H. and Huid, N.: Acta Rheum. Scand., *5*, 34, 1959.
70. Grayzel, A. I., Liddle, L. and Seegmiller, J. E.: New Engl. J. Med., *265*, 763, 1961.
71. Gronboek, P.: Acta Rheum. Scand., *6*, 102, 1960.
71*a*. Grönvik, A. M., Kornstad, L., and Guldberg, D.: Nature, *206*, 836, 1965.
72. Gyorki, J. and Sandell, B. M.: Acta Rheum. Scand., *7*, 127, 1961.
73. Ham, T. H. and Curtis, F. C.: Medicine, *17*, 447, 1938.
74. Hammersten, G., Jonsson, E., Lindgren, G. and Nettelbladt, E.: Acta Rheum. Scand., *5*, 42, 1959.
75. Hardwick, H. and Squire, J. R.: Clin. Sci., *11*, 333, 1952.
76. Hedlund, P.: Acta Med. Scand., Suppl., *196*, 579, 1947.
77. ———: Acta Med. Scand., *169* (Suppl. 361), 35, 1961.
78. Hermann, H.: Munchen. Med. Wochnschr., *71*, 1714, 1924.
79. Hilder, F. M. and Gunz, F. W.: J. Clin. Path., *17*, 292, 1964.
80. Hill, S. R., Jr., Holley, H. L., Ulloa, A., Starnes, W. R., Hibbett, L. L. and McNeil, J. H.: Arth. and Rheum., *2*, 114, 1959.
81. Hollinger, N. F. and Robinson, S. J.: Pediatrics, *42*, 304, 1953.
82. Jeffrey, J. R.: Blood, *8*, 502, 1953.
83. Jeffrey, M. R.: Ann. Rheum. Dis., *15*, 151, 1956.
84. Jeffrey, M. R. and Watson, D.: Acta Haemat., *12*, 169, 1954.
84*a*. Jeremy, R. and Wilkinson, P.: Arth. and Rheum., *7*, 740, 1964.
85. Johnson, N. J. and Dodd, K.: Med. Clin. North America, *39*, 459, 1955.
86. Kalliomaki, J. L., Kirpila, J., Koskinen, H. M. and Laine, V. A. L.: Acta Rheum. Scand., *4*, 79, 1958.
87. Kalliomaki, J. L. and Kosunen, A.: Ann. Med. Int. Fen., *44*, 141, 1955.
88. Kalliomaki, J. L., Laine, V. A. and Markkonen, T. K.: Acta Med. Scand., *166*, 275, 1960.
89. Kelley, V. C.: J. Ped., *40*, 405, 1952.
90. ———: J. Ped., *40*, 413, 1952.
91. Kellgren, J. H. and Ball, J.: Brit. Med. J., *1*, 523, 1959.
92. Kelly, H. G., Hill, J. G. and Boyd, E. M.: Canad. Med. Assoc. J., *70*, 660, 1954.
93. Kievits, J. H., Goslings, J., Schuit, H. R. E. and Hijmans, W.: Ann. Rheum. Dis., *15*, 211, 1956.
94. Kodama, T.: Acta Med. Okayama, *13*, 137, 1959.
95. Lange, K., Wasserman, E., Wedgewood, R. J. and Janeway, C. A.: Pediatrics, *11*, 569, 1963.
96. Laurell, A. B. and Grubb, R.: Acta Path. et Microbiol. Scand., *43*, 310, 1958.
97. ———: Ibid., *43*, 1372, 1964.
98. Lawrence, J. S. and Glynn, L. E., eds.: Bull. Rheum. Dis., *14*, 323, 1963.
99. Lefkovits, A. M. and Farrow, I. J.: Ann. Rheum. Dis., *14*, 162, 1955.
100. Lehman, M. A., Kream, J. and Brugua, D.: J. Bone Joint Surg., *46A*, 1732, 1964.
101. Lemon, H. H., Chasen, W. H. and Looney, J. M.: J. Clin. Invest., *31*, 993, 1952.
102. Lewis, S. M. and Porter, I. H.: Ann. Rheum. Dis., *19*, 54, 1960.
103. Liljestrand, A. and Olhagen, B.: Acta Med. Scand., *151*, 425, 1955.
104. Lindjberg, I. F.: Arch. Dis. Childhood, *39*, 576, 1964.
105. Loewi, G.: Ann. Rheum. Dis., *18*, 239, 1959.
106. Lofstrom, G.: Brit. J. Exp. Path., *25*, 21, 1944.
107. London, M. G., Muirden, K. D. and Hewitt, J. V.: Brit. Med. J., *1*, 1380, 1963.
108. Lorber, A., Pearson, C. M., Meredith, W. L. and Gantz-Mandell, L. E.: Ann. Int. Med., *61*, 423, 1964.

109. MacLeod, C. M. and Avery, O. T.: J. Exp. Med., *73*, 183, 1941.
110. ————: Ibid., *73*, 191, 1941.
111. Mäkisara, P., Ruutsalo, H. M., Nissila, M., Ruotsi, A., Mäkisara, G. L.: Ann. Med. Exp. Biol. Fenn., *46*, 177, 1968.
112. Malmquist, E. and Reichard, H.: Acta Rheum. Scand., *8*, 170, 1962.
113. McCarty, M.: J. Exp. Med., *85*, 491, 1947.
114. McEwen, C. and Ziff, M.: Med. Clin. North America, *39*, 765, 1955.
115. McKusick, A. B., Sherwin, R. W., Jones, L. G. and Hsu, J. M.: Arth. and Rheum., *7*, 636, 1964.
116. McMillan, M.: J. Clin. Path., *13*, 140, 1960.
117. McRae, P.: Ann. Rheum. Dis., *17*, 89, 1958.
118. McCrea, P. C.: Lancet, *1*, 402, 1957.
118*a*. Mead, J., and Lerson, D. L.: J. Amer. Geriat. Soc., *18*, 489, 1970.
119. Melville, I. D. and Rifkind, B. M.: Brit. Med. J., *1*, 107, 1960.
119*a*. Mongan, E. S., Cass, R. M., Jacox, R. F., and Vaughan, J. H.: Amer. J. Med., *47*, 23, 1969.
120. Movitt, E. R. and Davis, A. E.: Amer. J. Med. Sci., *226*, 516, 1963.
120*a*. Mowat, A. G., and Hothersall, T. E.: Ann. Rheum. Dis., *27*, 345, 1968.
121. Mueller, E. E. and Mead, S.: Amer. J. Phys. Med., *31*, 67, 1952.
121*a*. Muirden, K. D.: Austral. Ann. Med., *19*, 97, 1970.
122. Nettelbladt, E. and Sandell, B. M.: Ann. Rheum. Dis., *22*, 269, 1963.
123. Newman, T. H. and Waterfield, R. L.: Guy's Hosp. Reports, *110*, 128, 1961.
124. Niedermeier, W., Creitz, E. C. and Holley, H. L.: Arth. and Rheum., *6*, 653, 1962.
125. Nilsson, F.: Acta Med. Scand., Suppl., *210*, 1, 1948.
126. Ogryzlo, M. A., Maclachan, M., Dauphinee, J. A. and Fletcher, A. A.: J. Clin. Invest., *27*, 596, 1959.
127. Olhagen, B. and Liljestrand, A.: Acta Med. Scand., *151*, 441, 1955.
127*a*. Pal, S. B.: Clin. Chim. Acta, *29*, 129, 1970.
128. Parr, L. J. A., Shipton, E. A., Benjamin, P. and White, P. H. H.: Med. J. Australia, *1*, 900, 1957.
129. Payne, W. W. and Schlesinger, B.: Arch. Dis. Childhood, *10*, 403, 1935.
130. Peyman, M. A.: Brit. J. Cancer, *16*, 56, 1962.
131. Pierson, R. N., Holt, P. R., Watson, R. M. and Keating, R. P.: Amer. J. Med., *31*, 259, 1961.
132. Pinals, R. S.: Arth. and Rheum., *7*, 662, 1964.
132*a*. Pitkeathly, D. A., and Taylor, G.: Ann. Rheum. Dis., *26*, 1, 1967.
132*b*. Plantin, L. D., and Straaberg, P. O.: Acta Rheum. Scand., *11*, 30, 1965.
133. Pollak, V. E.: New Engl. J. Med., *271*, 165, 1964.
134. Pollak, V. E., Pirani, C. L., Steck, I. E., and Kark, R. M.: Arth. and Rheum., *5*, 1962.
135. Ragan, C. and Farrington, E.: J.A.M.A., *181*, 663, 1962.
136. Rawson, A. J. and Abelson, N. M.: Arth. and Rheum., *7*, 391, 1964.
136*a*. Rhodes, K., Scott, A., Markham, R. L., and Monk-Jones, M. E.: Ann. Rheum. Dis., *28*, 104, 1969.
137. Richardson, A. T.: Proc. Roy. Soc. Med., *50*, 466, 1957.
138. Rice, E. W.: Clin. Chim. Acta, *6*, 652, 1961.
139. Richmond, J., Alexander, W. R. M., Potter, J. L. and Duthie, J. J. R.: Ann. Rheum. Dis., *20*, 133, 1961.
140. Richmond, J., Gardner, D. L., Roy, L. M. H. and Duthie, J. J. R.: Ann. Rheum. Dis., *15*, 217, 1956.
141. Ritzmann, S. E., Thurm, R. H., Truax, W. E. and Levin, W. C.: Arch. Int. Med., *105*, 939, 1960.
142. Robinson, G. L.: Ann. Rheum. Dis., *3*, 207, 1943.
143. Robinson, W. D. and Roseman, S.: Bull. Rheum. Dis., *7*, S-31, 1957.
144. Roberts, F. D., Hagedorn, A. B., Slocumb, C. H. and Owen, C. A.: Blood, *21*, 470, 1963.
145. Rodnan, G. P. and Cammarata, R. J.: Clin. Res. *11*, 179, 1963.
146. Ross, J. F. and Bayles, T. B.: Blood, *6*, 1034, 1951.
147. Rourke, M. D. and Ernstene, A. C.: J. Clin. Invest., *8*, 545, 1930.
148. Roy, L. M. H., Alexander, W. R. M. and Duthie, J. J. R.: Ann. Rheum. Dis., *14*, 63, 1955.
149. Roy, L. M. H., Wigzell, F. W., Demers, R., Sinclair, R. J. G., Duthie, J. J. R., Atherdon, S. M. and Marrian, G. F.: Ann. Rheum. Dis., *14*, 183, 1955.
150. Sanghvi, L. M.: Geriatrics, *18*, 382, 1963.
151. Schlesinger, B.: Practitioner, *157*, 38, 1946.

152. Schlesinger, B. E., Forsyth, C. C., White, R. H. R., Smellie, J. M. and Stroud, C. E.: Arch. Dis. Childhood, *36*, 65, 1961.
153. Schools, G. S. and Mikkelsen, W. M.: Arth. and Rheum., *5*, 369, 1962.
154. Shannon, F. T. and Bywaters, E. G. L.: Brit. Med. J., *2*, 1405, 1957.
155. Shetlar, M. R., Payne, R. W., Padron, J., Felton, F. and Ishmael, W. K.: J. Lab. Clin. Med., *48*, 194, 1956.
156. Shetlar, M. R., Schmidt, H. L., Lincoln, R. B., DeVore, J. K., Bullock, J. A. and Hellbaum, A. A.: J. Lab. Clin. Med., *39*, 372, 1952.
157. Short, C. L., Bauer, W. and Reynolds, W. E.: *Rheumatoid Arthritis*, Cambridge, Harvard University Press, 1957, pp. 353, 357–361.
158. Short, C. L., Dienes, L. and Bauer, W.: J.A.M.A., *108*, 2087, 1937.
159. Sørenson, A. W. S.: Acta Rheum. Scand., *6*, 115, 1960.
160. ————: Ibid., *7*, 138, 1961.
161. ————: Ibid., *7*, 304, 1961.
162. Smyth, C. J. and Staub, A.: Arth. and Rheum., *7*, 687, 1964.
163. Spagnuolo, M. and Feinstein, A. R.: Pediatrics, *33*, 653, 1964.
164. Spiera, H.: Arth. and Rheum., *6*, 363, 1963.
164*a*.————: Arth. & Rheum., *9*, 318, 1966.
165. Sprague, R. G., Frick, S. C. and Crockett, C. L.: Arch. Int. Med., *85*, 199, 1950.
166. Steinberg, V. L. and Wynn-Parry, C. B.: Brit. Med. J., *1*, 630, 1961.
167. Stuart, F. S., Starnes, W. R., Partlow, T. and Hill, S. R., Jr.: Clin. Res., *10*, 237, 1962.
168. Sullivan, J. F. and Hart, K. T.: J. Lab. Clin. Med., *55*, 260, 1960.
169. Sunderman, F. W., Jr.: Amer. J. Clin. Path., *42*, 1, 1964.
170. Sydnes, O. A.: Acta Rheum. Scand., *9*, 237, 1963.
171. Thompson, G. R. and Castor, C. W.: J. Lab. Clin. Med., *68*, 617, 1966.
172. Tillett, W. S. and Francis, T., Jr.: J. Exp. Med., *52*, 561, 1930.
173. Toone, E. C., Irby, R. and Pierce, E. L.: Amer. J. Med. Sci., *240*, 101, 1960.
174. Toumbis, A., Franklin, E. C., McEwen, C. and Kuttner, A. G.: J. Ped., *62*, 463, 1963.
175. Townes, A. S., Stewart, C. R. and Osler, A. G.: *Mechanisms of Cell and Tissue Damage Produced by Immune Reactions*, 2nd Int'l Symp. on Immunopath., Basel, Benno Schwabe, 1961, p. 315.
176. Vaughan, J. H., Bayles, T. B. and Favour, C. B.: Amer. J. Med. Sci., *222*, 186, 1951.
177. Vaughan, J. H. and Butler, V. P., Jr.: Ann. Int. Med., *56*, 1, 1962.
178. Vesell, E. S., Ostedard, K. C., Bearn, A. G. and Kunkel, H. G.: J. Clin. Invest., *41*, 2012, 1962.
178*a*.Veys, E. M. and Claessens, H. E.: Ann. Rheum. Dis., *27*, 431, 1968.
179. Waldenstrom, J. and Winblad, S.: Acta Rheum. Scand., *4*, 2, 1958.
179*a*.Ward, H. P., Gorden, B., and Pickett, J. C.: J. Lab. Clin. Med., *74*, 93, 1969.
179*b*.Wardle, E. N.: Ann. Rheum. Dis., *28*, 310, 1969.
180. Weaver, W. F. and Smyth, C. J.: Arth. and Rheum., *6*, 373, 1963.
181. Weinstein, I. M.: Blood, *14*, 950, 1959.
182. Weir, D. M., Holborow, E. J. and Johnson, G. D.: Brit. J. Med., *1*, 933, 1961.
183. Wells, R. M. and Johnson, E. W.: Arch. Phys. Med., *43*, 244, 1962.
184. Westergren, A.: Acta Med. Scand., *54*, 247, 1920.
184*a*.Whaley, K., Goudie, R. B., Williamson, J., Nuki, G., Dick, W. C., Buchanan, W. W.: Lancet, *1*, 861, 1970.
185. Wilkinson, M. and Jones, B. S.: Ann. Rheum. Dis., *21*, 51, 1962.
185*a*.Wilkinson, P., Jeremy, R., Brooks, F. P. and Hollander, J. L.: Ann. Intern. Med., *63*, 109, 1965.
186. Wintrobe, M. M.: *Clinical Hematology*, 5th Ed. Philadelphia, Lea & Febiger, 1961, p. 331.
187. Wintrobe, M. M. and Landsberg, J. W.: Amer. J. Med. Sci., *189*, 102, 1935.
188. Winzler, R. J.: *Methods of Biochemical Analysis*, Vol. II, New York, Interscience Publishers, 1955, p. 279.
189. Winzler, R. J.: *Ciba Foundation Symposium on Chemistry and Biology of Mucopolysaccharides*, ed. by G. Wolstenholme, Boston, Little, Brown & Co., 1958, p. 245.
189*a*.Wood, J. W., Kato, H., Johnson, K. G., Uda, Y., Russel, W. J., and Duff, I. F.: Arth. & Rheum., *10*, 21, 1967.
190. Wood, P.: Quart. J. Med., *5*, 1, 1936.
191. Wramner, T.: Acta Med. Scand. Suppl., *242*, 18, 1950.
192. Yates, D. A. H.: Ann. Rheum. Dis., *22*, 342, 1963.
193. Ziff, M.: J. Chron. Dis., *5*, 644, 1947.
194. Ziff, M., Kibrick, A., Dresner, E. and Gribetz, H. J.: J. Clin. Invest., *35*, 579, 1956.

Chapter 24

Juvenile Rheumatoid Arthritis

By John J. Calabro, M.D.

In any account of this disease, it is important to appreciate that there are many features peculiar to juvenile rheumatoid arthritis that distinguish it clinically from its adult counterpart. Moreover, rheumatoid arthritis may have different modes of onset in children, and while the diagnosis may be apparent in those with obvious polyarthritis, it may be vexing when the disorder begins only with systemic features or with monarticular arthritis. Laboratory findings are highly variable and nonspecific, and diagnosis may depend on repeated and careful observations or histopathologic documentation. Finally, a program of management should permit the child an optimal growth and development despite the persistence of active disease.

HISTORY

Juvenile rheumatoid arthritis was first described by Cornil[23] in 1864. In 1890, Diamentberger,[24] on the basis of 35 published cases and 3 cases of his own, suggested that most are first observed in the large joints, that the onset is often acute and the course remittent, that disturbances of growth are frequent, and that the prognosis is better in children than in adults. In 1897, George Frederick Still[69] described additional features, including high fever, pericarditis, lymphadenopathy, and splenomegaly. In fact, this acute form of the illness is sometimes referred to as Still's disease, although this eponym is also used for juvenile rheumatoid arthritis in general.

EPIDEMIOLOGY AND ETIOLOGY

Juvenile rheumatoid arthritis is a systemic rheumatic disorder beginning before puberty with protean clinical manifestations.[18] It rarely begins before six months of age, and is slightly more common in girls than in boys.[5,64a,74] The incidence of rheumatoid arthritis in American children is estimated at 175,000.[17c]

While rheumatoid arthritis is in many respects similar in both children and adults, there are certain differentiating features (Table 24–1).[16a] Among these may be mentioned the more frequent occurrence in children of high fever, rash, leukocytosis, uveitis, failure to grow, monarticular disease, less joint pain, and the infrequency in the child of subcutaneous nodules and rheumatoid factor. The tendency of children to manifest more vivid systemic reactions to disease may explain some of these differences.

The etiology is unknown. The roles of infectious, traumatic, psychologic, immunologic, and hereditary factors are uncertain. Upper respiratory infection[48,59] and, to a lesser extent, trauma[27,64a] are often cited as precipitating factors, but these are difficult to assess. Psychologic stresses appear to be linked to the onset and to exacerbations. Grokoest and co-workers[37] suggest a well-masked anxiety state among patients, and family members seem prone to illnesses and emotional disturbances.

The role of heredity has not been clarified. In a study[5] of 6 pairs of

Table 24-1.—Features Characterizing Juvenile Rheumatoid Arthritis as Contrasted with Adult Rheumatoid Disease.

Feature	Juvenile	Adult
Systemic		
High Fever	25%[17b,59]	1%[66]
Evanescent rash	30%[15,44]	1–6%[15,44]
Chronic iridocyclitis	5–15%[18c,64e]	1%[66]
Articular		
Absence of joint pain	25%[37]	Unusual[50]
*Monarticular onset	30%[27,37]	8%[66]
Nonarticular		
Subcutaneous nodules	6%[5]	20%[66]
Abnormalities in growth and development	50%[1]	Notapplicable
Laboratory		
Leukocytosis, above 12,000 cells	45–50%[48,64a]	25%[66]
†Rheumatoid factor	10–20%[14,10a]	65–85%[14,16a]

*Defined as involvement of one joint for a minimum of one month.
†By direct agglutination.

homozygous twins, 2 were concordant for juvenile rheumatoid arthritis, whereas no concordance was noted in 4 heterozygous pairs. On vertical starch gel electrophoresis a significant number of children had haptoglobin 1–1, suggesting a possible genetic linkage.[43]

In a study[7] relating familial association of juvenile rheumatoid arthritis with other connective tissue diseases, Ansell and colleagues noted that male relatives had more spondylitis and sacro-iliitis, and females more peripheral polyarthritis, than a random sample of similar age and sex, although the sheep-cell agglutination incidence was not greater than among controls.[2] But this study has to be reexamined, since 7 of the 91 patients with juvenile rheumatoid arthritis have subsequently been reclassified after ankylosing spondylitis developed.

CLINICAL FEATURES

Onset

In about 20 per cent of children, usually boys under age seven, the onset is acute or fulminating, primarily with systemic manifestations but often *without arthritis*.[17e] Recognition may be difficult when high fever, rash, pericarditis, pneumonitis, splenomegaly, or failure to thrive are the presenting cardinal features. Eventually, however, arthritis becomes manifest and the diagnosis more evident (Fig. 24–1). In one-half of children, the onset is polyarticular (adult type), with abrupt or insidious arthritis of four or more joints. In 30 per cent of patients arthritis begins with involvement of one joint (monarticular)[18d,27,37] or a few joints (oligoarticular),[15a,36] often asymmetrical, and except for chronic iridocyclitis, few or no systemic manifestations.

Joints

Children with systemic manifestations initially may have few or no signs of arthritis, although transitory arthralgia may be present. About one-quarter of juvenile patients have few or no complaints of joint pain,[37] and arthritis is often first suggested by swelling, a limp, or guarding of joints. In a comparative study,[50] it was disclosed that children suffer less discomfort in affected joints than adults, perhaps because children react differently to pain. Occasionally, joint pain may be severe, especially with hip involvement.[45]

Knees, wrists, ankles, and neck are common *initial* sites, especially in young children. Involved joints are usually warm, swollen, and restricted in motion, while tenderness and redness may or may not be present. Depending upon the amount of inflammatory exudate, arthritis may be divided into wet and dry types. Effusion may offer joint cartilage some protection from erosion and adhesion, provided capsular stretching does not permit subluxation. Early morning stiffness is difficult to assess in the young.[37]

Older children usually first manifest arthritis of small joints. Symmetrical involvement of proximal interphalangeal and metacarpophalangeal articulations is usual, while distal interphalangeal joints may be affected in about 15 per

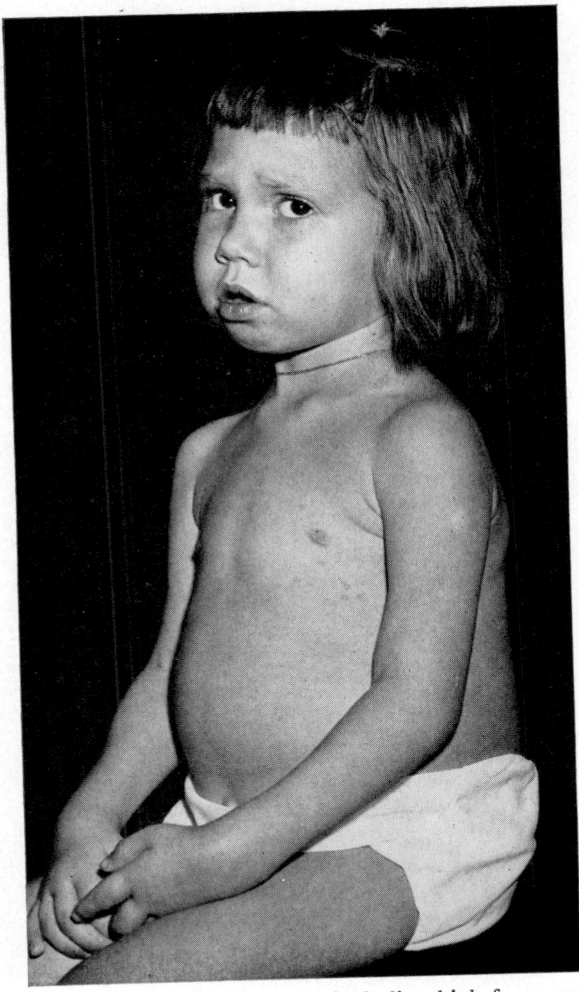

Fig. 24-1.—A five-year-old child with acute onset, including high fever, rash, hepatosplenomegaly, and lymphadenopathy, demonstrating anxious appearance, guarding of joints, and discrete macules on chest. Despite swelling of fingers (fusiform), wrists, elbows, and sternoclavicular joints, she complained of pain only on cervical rotation.

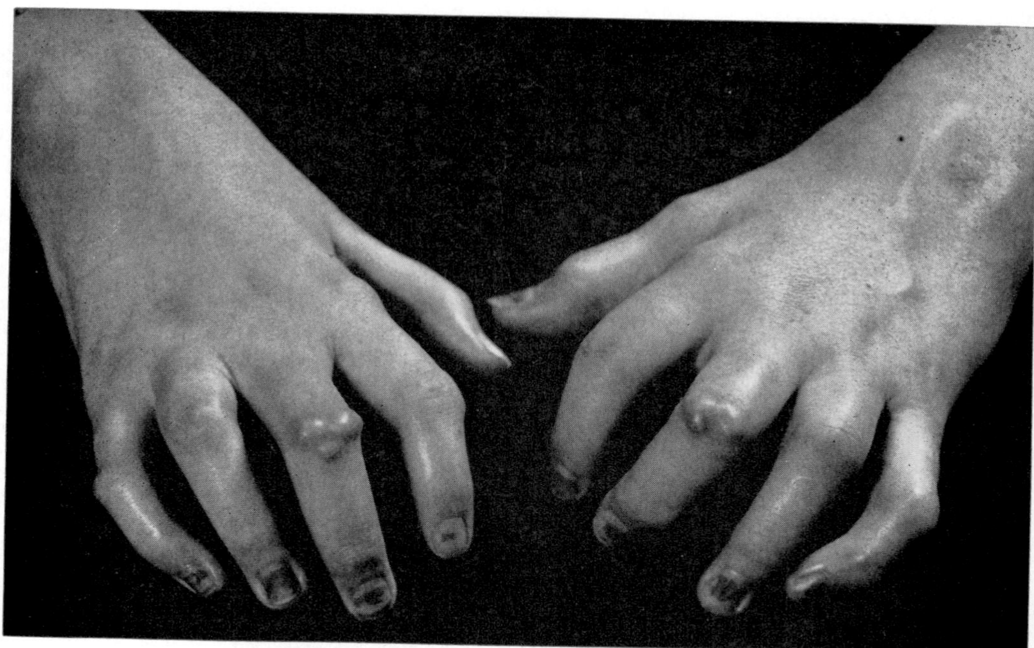

Fig. 24–2.—Hands of a seventeen-year-old girl with juvenile onset at age twelve, with typical rheumatoid changes, including subcutaneous nodules over middle proximal interphalangeal joints, except for radial (rather than ulnar) deviation. Hard dorsolateral proliferations at distal and proximal interphalangeal joints, especially in fifth fingers, are similar to Heberden's and Bouchard's nodes, respectively.

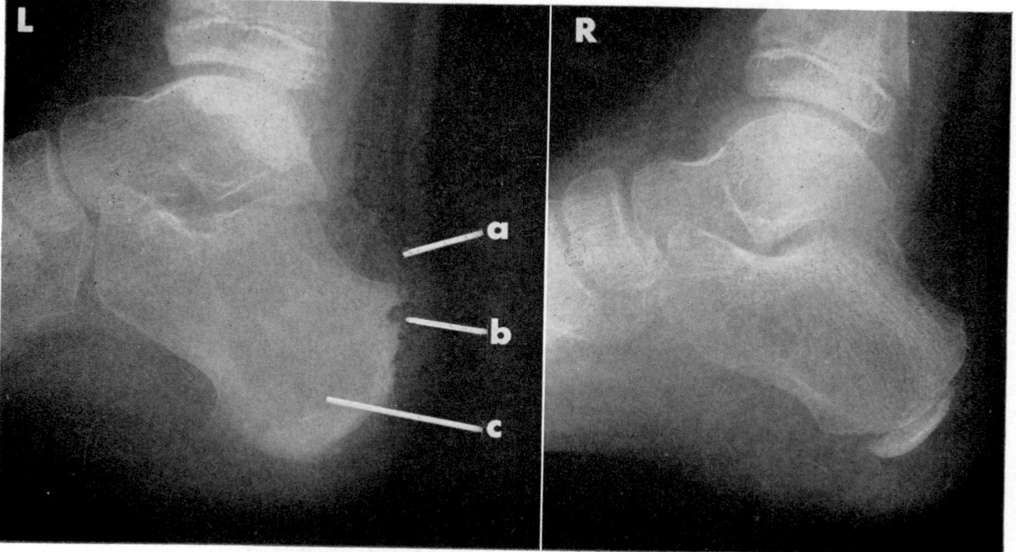

Fig. 24–3.—Lateral heel x-rays with weight-bearing of an eleven-year-old boy, after six years of recurrent disease chiefly in left heel, with tenderness and swelling. Observe (*a*) soft tissue radiodensity of achillobursitis, (*b*) calcaneal erosion and minute spurs, and (*c*) early fusion of left apophysis. Note left calcaneal overgrowth and loss of fine trabecular pattern.

cent of patients[5] (Fig. 24–2). In children, radial deviation appears to be more common than ulnar (Fig. 24–2). Forefoot deformities include progressive hallux valgus, hammer toes, and prominence of metatarsal heads. Rheumatoid achillobursitis and achillotendinitis may cause tender, swollen heels, and on x-ray, calcaneal erosions, minute spur formation, and early apophyseal closure (Fig. 24–3).[16]

Transient temporomandibular complaints are frequent, while ankylosis is a rare but difficult problem.[8,12] Cervical involvement is reported in about one-half of children.[3,11] The result may be loss of cervical extension and rotation (Fig. 24–4) and in a young child failure of vertebral growth and apophyseal ankylosis. Roentgenographic findings[3,29,37,54] may include loss of cervical lordosis; narrowing and irregularity of apophyseal joints, chiefly at C_2–C_3; failure of development of vertebral bodies; atlanto-axial subluxation; disc space narrowing; and, rarely, fusion between vertebral bodies

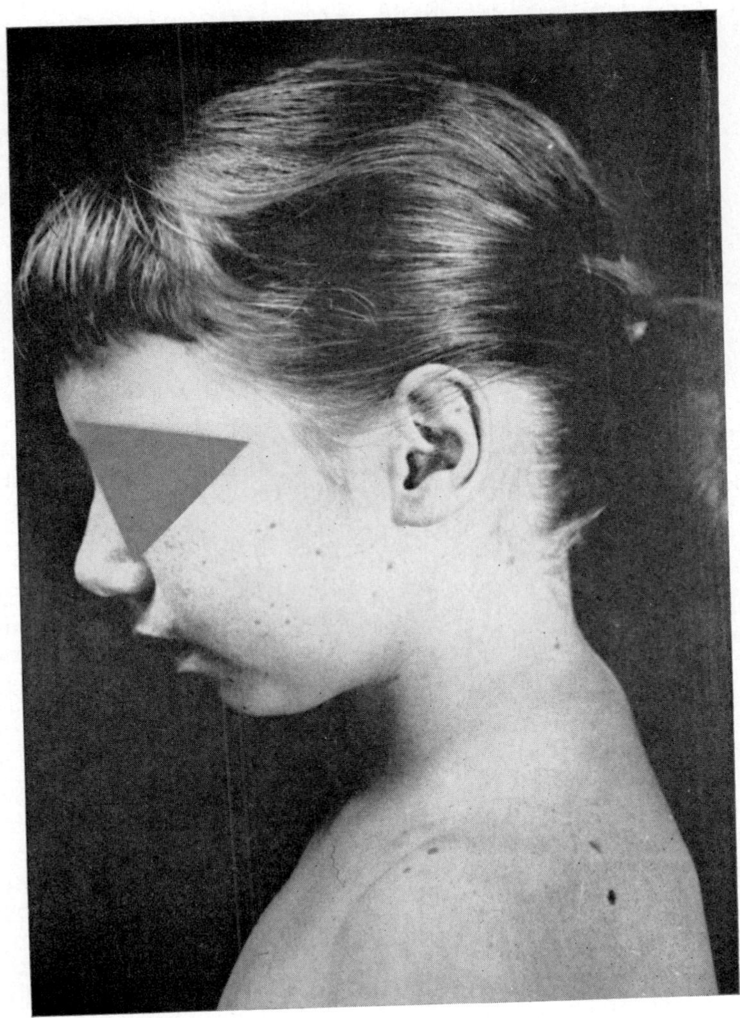

FIG. 24–4.—A twelve-year-old girl, with disease onset at age four. Typical posture due to cervical involvement portrays fixed forward flexion of head and neck. Note mandibular recession as well.

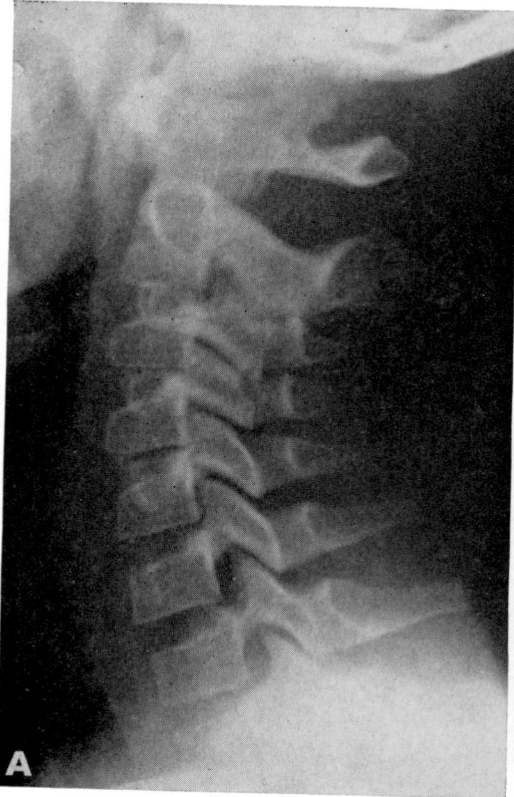

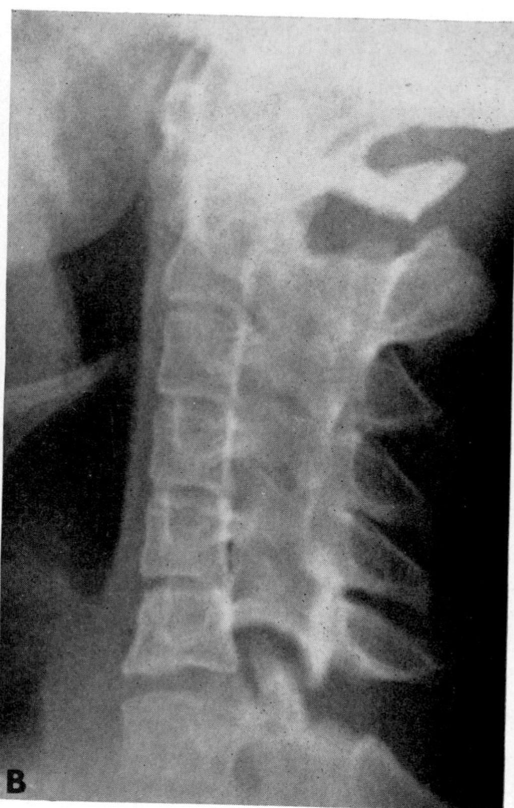

FIG. 24–5.—Serial lateral cervical x-rays of child in Figure 24–4, (*a*) at age twelve, showing loss of the sharp margin of apophyseal joint at C_2–C_3, and (*b*) at age sixteen, demonstrating progression to apophyseal fusion from C_2–C_6 and failure of development of vertebrae 2–6.

(Fig. 24–5). Unlike adults, juveniles seldom show subluxation of other cervical vertebrae. Sacro-iliitis occurs in 45 per cent of children with neck involvement, yet cervical changes, seen on x-ray, may occasionally be the sole sequela.[3]

Asymptomatic sacro-iliitis is a roentgenographic finding in about 24 per cent of patients.[20] Sacro-iliitis may even be present on postmortem examination without radiologic evidence during life.[21] It appears to correlate with disease onset after ten years of age, hip involvement, and presence of rheumatoid factor.[20] Though sacro-iliitis has been reported as more common in children than in adults,[20] recent surveys[25,65] support a comparable prevalence. Despite this frequency of cervical and sacro-iliac involvement in juvenile rheumatoid arthritis, few patients develop typical ankylosing spondylitis;[4,29,78] those that do are usually older boys with arthritis mostly of hips, knees, and feet.[18a,64b]

Fever and Rash

Fever is observed in the majority of children; low-grade in most cases, but high in approximately 20 per cent.[17e,72] Low-grade pyrexia (to 102° F. or 38.9° C. rectally) is intermittent in character and is common among patients with a polyarticular onset.

High fever, present in only 1 per cent of adults,[66] is often a prominent feature among children who initially have principally systemic manifestations.[32] The febrile pattern is generally intermittent with midday or early evening spikes up to 105° F. (40.5° C.) rectally and wide diurnal swings (Fig. 24–6), but is occasionally remitting, relapsing, or even periodic. The child may be extremely ill with anorexia, weight loss, and malaise, or other systemic manifestations, but may have few or no articular complaints (Fig. 24–1). Yet, paradoxically, some children appear well, even at the height of fever spikes. Hyperpyrexia frequently *precedes* articular findings by weeks, months, or years, usually labeled as "fever of unknown origin." The child is often subject to exhaustive diagnostic studies, trials of antibiotics, and even exploratory laparotomy (Fig. 24–6).[17b]

Approximately 30 per cent of patients with juvenile rheumatoid arthritis manifest a characteristic erythematous rash, a finding seen in only 1 to 6 per cent of adults.[15,44,17d] The eruption, which is rarely pruritic, usually consists of discrete

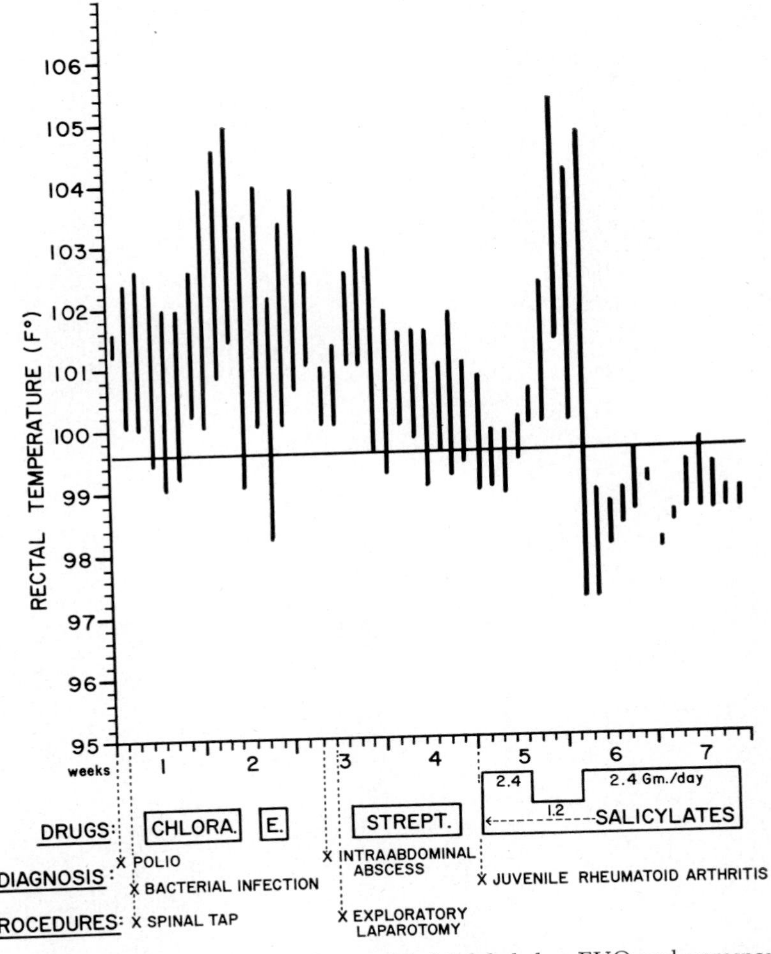

FIG. 24–6.—Pattern of high fever in a seven-year-old girl, labeled as FUO and unresponsive to antibiotics, including chloramphenicol, erythromycin, and streptomycin. Cervical stiffness was thought to be due to poliomyelitis, until results of spinal tap proved to be normal. An intra-abdominal abscess was suspected because of abdominal pain, but laparotomy disclosed only mesenteric adenopathy. Fever responded to regular administration of 60 mg./lb./day of aspirin. Weight of patient was 40 lb.

macular or maculopapular lesions, but occasionally may be confluent (Figs. 24–1 and 24–7). Macules are rarely larger than 5 mm. in diameter, and large ones may exhibit central fading. Though distribution is chiefly on the limbs and trunk, it may be widespread, including the face, palms, and soles. The eruption tends to be evanescent, appearing toward evening and concomitantly with high fever spikes, and may be migratory from day to day. The degree of erythema may be variable. Faint outcroppings may be intensified by massage, scratching, or heat.

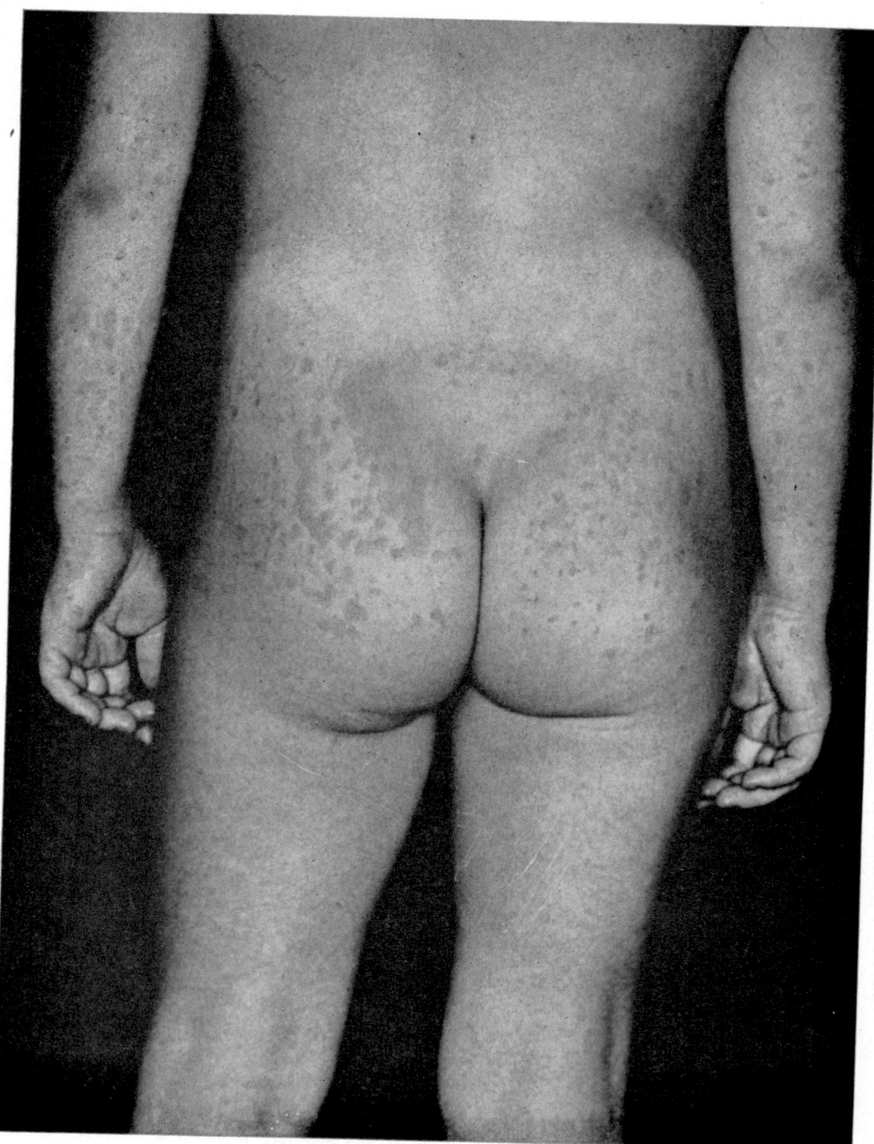

Fig. 24–7.—Rash of juvenile rheumatoid arthritis in child whose febrile pattern is depicted in Figure 24–6. Rash lasted nine months; distribution, which varied remarkably from day to day, was usually prominent over the trunk, limbs and palms. Papules are predominantly discrete, but occasionally confluent.

Rash is frequently observed in conjunction with high fever, lymphadenopathy, and other systemic features prior to arthritis. It is variable in duration, from weeks to months and even years, and tends to recur, but usually in the presence of other systemic or articular manifestations. Transient recurrences of the eruption may be precipitated by emotional, infectious, or surgical trauma.[17]

Heart and Lungs

Carditis, rarely an initial manifestation, is reported clinically in 10 per cent of children. Myocarditis may produce cardiac enlargement and failure. Endocarditis does not occur, and though murmurs may be present during acute episodes, they are probably functional.[73] Except for the studies of Sury,[70] chronic valvular lesions are not reported.

Pericarditis is detected clinically in only 7 per cent of patients, but observed in approximately 45 per cent of those with postmortem examination.[52] It usually follows, but may occur before or concomitantly with, the onset of arthritis. An attack may be accompanied by precordial pain or dyspnea. Yet, pericarditis is more often insidious, perhaps overshadowed by other systemic features, and escapes clinical recognition.[64a] It should be suspected in patients with high fever, rash, lymphadenopathy, and leukocytosis, and the child should be checked regularly for friction rub and ECG changes.[52] Pericarditis tends to recur, but rarely causes cardiac dysfunction or constrictive pericarditis.

Pneumonitis and pleuritis are uncommon but may occur in patients initially having primarily systemic manifestations. Chronic rheumatoid disease of the lung, however, is rarely reported.[47]

Other Systemic Manifestations

The ocular lesions of juvenile rheumatoid arthritis include iridocyclitis, from which band keratopathy and cataract may develop.[26,64c] Iridocyclitis occurs in 5 to 15 per cent of cases, mostly in those with a monarticular onset.[18d,22] Rarely preceding arthritis, it usually occurs during the course of active disease, but can persist or recur long after arthritis becomes quiescent.[18c,68] Characteristically, iridocyclitis smolders quietly for weeks or months until vision fails from adhesions (synechiae), glaucoma, or other complications, unless averted by periodic slit-lamp examinations—the only means of early iridocyclitis detection.[18c]

Generalized lymphadenopathy, often marked, indicates prominence of systemic rather than articular disease, and bears no regional relationship to the joints affected. Adenopathy appears to be most prominent in axillary, epitrochlear, and cervical sites. Enlargement of mesenteric nodes may cause abdominal pain, simulating an acute surgical abdomen at times, a circumstance which may lead to surgical exploration (Fig. 24–6).[17b] Splenomegaly is seen in about one-quarter of patients, while hepatomegaly is slightly less common.[5]

Vasculitis and encephalitis have been reported rarely.[27] Amyloidosis is uncommon, usually developing after many years of progressive disease, but may occur as early as one year after onset.[5]

Subcutaneous Nodules

Nodules are comparatively less common in children than in adults, being reported in about 6 per cent of children[5] and 20 per cent of adults,[66] but appear to share the same distribution in both groups. Histologically, nodules in children generally more closely resemble those of rheumatic fever than the adult subcutaneous nodule.[14] Moreover, nodules histologically indistinguishable from those observed in rheumatic fever or rheumatoid arthritis may occur in otherwise healthy children.[71]

Disturbances of Growth and Development

Impairment of general growth and development occurs in about half of the children,[1] and may be related to active disease, as well as to prolonged administration of corticosteroids.[1,10,26a] Growth is often resumed and the child may reach normal proportions rapidly when the disease becomes inactive. When the disease is actively prolonged, premature closure of epiphyses will prevent further growth, while the development of secondary sex characteristics may be retarded as well.[1]

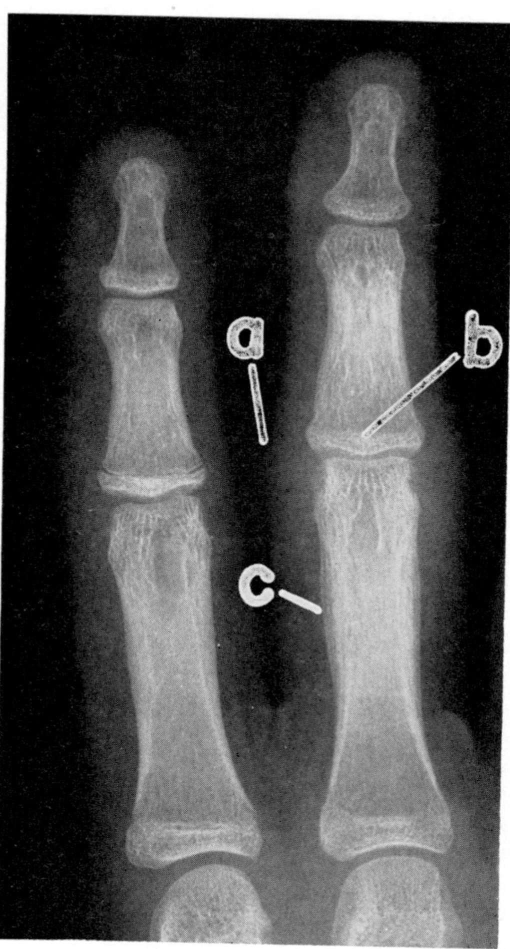

Fig. 24–8.—X-ray of hand of twelve-year-old girl with oligoarticular disease of four months, with asymmetrical involvement of right knee and right third proximal interphalangeal joints. X-ray features include (*a*) soft tissue swelling, (*b*) early closure of epiphysis, and (*c*) periosteal new-bone along shaft of proximal phalanx.

Local growth abnormalities in the areas of affected joints are probably due to alteration in blood supply, and perhaps to prolonged steroid administration.[8] The most common are premature appearance of epiphyses in the young and premature fusion in the older child (Fig. 24–8). This is particularly common in the metacarpals and metatarsals, causing abnormally small digits, and in the mandible, producing micrognathia (Fig. 24–4). Occasionally, particularly in oligoarticular disease, overgrowth of epiphyses and metaphyses may occur (Fig. 24–3).[15a,36]

LABORATORY FINDINGS

Laboratory studies are of limited value for diagnosis because findings are variable and lack specificity. Segmented neutrophilic *leukocytosis* is found frequently in children,[48,64a] especially among those with acute or fulminating disease. Counts are generally in the range of 15,000 to 25,000, and rarely exceed 50,000. Leukopenia has been reported in 15 per cent of children.[48] A moderate normocytic, hypochromic anemia, with hemoglobin values in the range of 8 to 11 gm./100 ml., is common. Leukocytosis and anemia are more likely to occur in patients with active disease. The erythrocyte sedimentation rate (ESR) and C-reactive protein (CRP) are usually abnormal during active disease, but are sometimes normal, particularly in oligoarticular arthritis.[36,37] Except for febrile proteinuria, the routine analysis of urine is unremarkable. In patients with prolonged activity of the disease, the development of proteinuria may signify secondary amyloidosis. Beta-hemolytic streptococci have been cultured from the throats of about one-third of patients whose disease was preceded by an upper respiratory infection.[48,59] Moreover, the antistreptolysin-O (ASO) titer is elevated in 30 to 50 per cent of patients with juvenile rheumatoid arthritis,[51,53,63,67,70] making the differentiation from rheumatic fever difficult at times.

Rheumatoid factor, as observed by

direct agglutination techniques, is present much less frequently in juvenile rheumatoid arthritis (10 to 20 per cent) than in adult rheumatoid subjects (65 to 85 per cent).[14,67] The prevalence of rheumatoid factor appears to exceed 20 per cent when other techniques are employed, such as immunofluorescence of leukocytes[41,60] and the euglobulin inhibition test.[72] Antinuclear antibody has been observed in the sera of 13 per cent of children.[5] Positive L.E. preparations occur rarely.[5] Serum protein abnormalities are comparable to those seen in adult patients, Elevated levels of IgG, IgA and IgM antigammaglobulins are found when disease is active.[9a]

X-RAY FEATURES

Roentgenographic findings of juxta-articular demineralization, erosions, and narrowing of joint space are generally late developments, while cervical zygapophyseal fusion, most prominent at C_2–C_3 (Fig. 24–5*A*), periosteal bone apposition (Fig. 24–8) and premature epiphyseal closure (Figs. 24–3 and 24–8) occur early and are more characteristic of rheumatoid arthritis in children.[37,56] Abnormal periosteal bone accretion occurs at all ages early in the course of the disease, but may undergo resorption in spite of continuous disease activity.[1] Not infrequently osseous overgrowth of the terminal and proximal interphalangeal joints of the hand may occur, bearing a striking resemblance to the x-ray configuration of Heberden's and Bouchard's nodes, respectively.[1]

DIAGNOSIS

In the absence of specific laboratory tests, diagnosis depends on clinical judgment and awareness of the highly protean manifestations. The proposed diagnostic criteria[62] of the American Rheumatism Association for adult rheumatoid arthritis are difficult to apply to children, and separate criteria are currently being devised. Several authors[4,37,38,40,70] have proposed other guides for diagnosis. Errors in diagnosis are common, being reported in one-half of referrals in a recent survey.[38]

In diagnosing juvenile rheumatoid arthritis *sine* arthritis, many other causes of fever of unknown origin must be excluded. Careful and repeated examinations are important for detecting the typical rash and minimal signs of asymptomatic joint involvement. Monarticular rheumatoid disease may be mistaken for septic, tuberculous and even traumatic arthritis.[58] Joint fluid analysis is most helpful, but closed synovial biopsy or arthrotomy may be required. Except for synovial complement activity which tends to be less suppressed,[39] synovial fluid analysis is similar to that of adults.[42,61] The histopathology of involved joints discloses nonspecific synovitis with synovial hypertrophy, increased vascularity, and round cell infiltration. With nonspecific articular derangements, such as osteochondritis, epiphysitis, or meniscus tear, distinctive clinical and x-ray signs may be helpful. In "transient synovitis of the hip," pain is minimal, while laboratory and x-ray studies are normal.

Rheumatic fever offers the greatest difficulty in differential diagnosis, especially in the early course of the disease. Early features that suggest juvenile rheumatoid arthritis rather than rheumatic fever include (1) onset under age five, (2) nonmigratory, symmetrical polyarthritis, especially of small joints, (3) monarticular disease, (4) cervical involvement, (5) a poor mucin clot on synovial fluid analysis, (6) typical rash, (7) hyperpyrexia, (8) hepatosplenomegaly in the absence of cardiac failure, and (9) marked leukocytosis. Findings that offer confusion since they may be present in both disorders are (1) asymmetrical polyarthritis, (2) low-grade fever, (3) pneumonitis and pleuritis, (4) abdominal pain, (5) elevated ASO titers, (6) pericarditis, and (7) response to aspirin and other antirheumatic agents. Joint manifestations lasting less than twelve weeks are uncommon in juvenile rheumatoid arthritis but are usual in rheumatic fever.[4] Moreover, joint sequelae are unusual in rheumatic fever.[16c]

The diagnosis of childhood systemic lupus erythematosus, polyarteritis, scleroderma, or dermatomyositis may be difficult to establish, particularly when the manifestations are atypical.[38a] Yet in this group renal and gastrointestinal lesions, as well as hypertension, are common while arthritis is less pronounced and joint x-ray changes are rare. Serum complement is decreased in systemic lupus erythematosus, but elevated in childhood rheumatoid arthritis.[76,9a]

In childhood leukemia and related disorders, which share many juvenile rheumatoid features, including high fever, lymphadenopathy, and joint pain, profound anemia occurs early.[16b,16f] Serum sickness and Schönlein-Henoch syndrome may be distinguished by urticarial skin eruptions. Patients with hypogammaglobulinemia frequently have diffuse connective tissue diseases, most often a chronic polyarthritis.[35] Since the arthritis of the congenital type, limited to males, becomes apparent in childhood, patients with juvenile rheumatic disorders should be screened for decreased immunoglobulins.

MANAGEMENT

The protean manifestations of juvenile rheumatoid arthritis pose problems no individual physician can completely master. While the child and family need, over the years, *one* doctor to be responsible for over-all management, the pediatrician, rheumatologist, orthopedist, ophthalmologist, psychiatrist, physical therapist, social worker, and others may be required in the child's optimal care. The goals of treatment are to achieve a state wherein the child can live at home like other children, attend an ordinary or special school, and remain free of contractures and gross deformities.[5] The principles of management include basic supportive measures, and a limited number of anti-inflammatory drugs.[16d]

Basic Supportive Measures

The first step is to educate family members on the nature of the disease and their role in treatment. Regardless of the course of the disease, the psychological, social, and educational needs of the child deserve thoughtful attention. The child needs a well-balanced diet, while supplemental vitamins may be added for those who are not eating properly. Infections should be promptly cared for, since these often precipitate exacerbations of the rheumatoid disease.[13] Every child should receive periodic slit-lamp examination in order to achieve early detection of iridocyclitis.

While the disease is in an active stage, the child should have adequate rest, properly balanced with physical measures. Exercise is the most rewarding form of physical therapy, and rather than relying on a formal hospital program, it is preferable for parents to be educated to carry this out regularly in the home. Heat helps in the relief of joint pain and stiffness and is useful prior to exercise. Loss of joint function may be prevented by splints worn at night or by other means to keep involved joints in proper alignment. Deformities may be corrected by serial splinting (day and night), and specific exercises. The prolonged use of cylindrical plaster casts may produce fibrous ankylosis and marked muscular atrophy, while wedging circular casts may result in fracture.[37] Early synovectomy may be useful in selected patients.[29a,29b] Physical and orthopedic measures, described and illustrated in Chapters 34 to 40, may be more beneficial than drugs, especially for patients with oligoarticular disease, or those with inactive disease having residual deformity.[17]

Anti-inflammatory Agents

Table 24–2 lists the drugs employed in the management of juvenile rheumatoid arthritis, along with toxic effects peculiar to the child. Once active disease is suppressed, the drug should be

Table 24-2.—Drugs Employed in the Management of Juvenile Rheumatoid Arthritis with Maintenance and Side-Effects Specifically Seen in Children.

Agent	Maintenance	Reactions Peculiar to Children
Aspirin	90–130 mg. per kg. daily	Chronic toxicity (lethargy, episodic hyperpnea) difficult to detect. Acute toxicity produces metabolic acidosis in infants, but respiratory alkalosis in older children.
Corticosteroids	0.1–0.4 mg. per kg. daily of prednisone or its equivalent	Decrease in statural growth and skeletal maturation. Pseudotumor cerebri.
I.M. Gold	1 mg. per kg. monthly	Rash, nephritis, and blood dyscrasias occur more frequently in children under 6 years.
Chloroquine	62.5–250 mg. daily	Rapid cardiorespiratory arrest with as little as 1 gm.
Phenylbutazone	50–200 mg. daily	Hepatitis, thrombocytopenia, and agranulocytosis occur more often in children.

maintained for weeks to months before withdrawal, being cautiously tapered and never stopped abruptly.

Aspirin is a most satisfactory suppressive agent,[6,17,37] and most children can be maintained on moderately large doses for prolonged periods. The majority of children require about 40 mg. per pound body weight (90 mg. per kg.) of aspirin divided into 5 or 6 doses daily. Since tinnitus is difficult to assess in the young, and correlation with serum salicylate levels often unreliable, one may judge best by individual parameters, such as low-grade fever, arthritis, or systemic manifestations.

In children with marked systemic features, especially hyperpyrexia, 60 mg. per pound (130 mg. per kg.) daily, divided into four hourly doses, may be required. Failure to suppress hyperpyrexia with aspirin is usually, but not invariably, due to inadequate dosage[17,57] (Fig. 24–6). Unlike the dramatic salicylate effect in rheumatic fever, the high fever of juvenile rheumatoid arthritis more often subsides gradually over three to four days, and may require as long as three or four weeks.[17] As severe systemic features may be short-lived, there should be periodic attempts to decrease aspirin to a maintenance dosage of 40 mg./lb./day, in order to avoid chronic salicylate intoxication.

Early signs of chronic salicylism, chiefly drowsiness and brief bouts of hyperpnea, are easily overlooked, especially in the preverbal child. Aspirin should be stopped for twenty-four hours or until all side-effects disappear, and then reinstituted at a lower dosage. With acute toxicity, age appears to condition the type of disturbance. Infants show intense ketosis and acidosis, whereas older children (and adults) usually develop respiratory alkalosis.[77]

Corticosteroids can initially produce remarkable symptom suppression, but do not seem to influence the natural remission rate or ultimate prognosis.[5,28,33] Systemic corticosteroids should be used when the disease is life-threatening, as in the patient with cardiac decompensation. With eye involvement, prolonged

39. Hedberg, H.: Acta Rheum. Scand., *10*, 109, 1964.
40. Hellström, B.: Acta Ped., *50*, 529, 1961.
41. Hess, E. and Ziff, M.: Arth. and Rheum., *4*, 574, 1961.
42. Hollander, J. L., Jessar, R. A. and McCarty, D. J.: Bull. Rheum. Dis., *12*, 263, 1961.
43. Howard, A. and Ansell, B. M.: Ann. Rheum. Dis., *23*, 232, 1964.
44. Isdale, I. C. and Bywaters, E. G. L.: Quart. J. Med., *25*, 377, 1956.
45. Jacqueline, F., Boujot, A. and Canet, L.: Arth. and Rheum., *4*, 500, 1961.
46. Jeremy, R., Schaller, J., Arkless, R., Wedgwood, R. J. and Healey, L. A.: Amer. J. Med., *45*, 419, 1968.
47. Jordan, J. D. and Snyder, C. H.: Amer. J. Dis. Child., *108*, 174, 1964.
48. Kelley, V. C.: Ped. Clin. North America, *7*, 435, 1960.
49. Kelley, V. C. and Limbeck, G. A.: Mod. Treatment, *1*, 1270, 1964.
49*a*. Kelsey, W. M. and Scharyj, M.: J.A.M.A., *199*, 586, 1967.
49*b*. Laaksonen, A-L.: Acta Rheum. Scand. (Suppl.), *166*, 1, 1966
50 Laaksonen, A-L. and Laine, V.: Ann. Rheum. Dis., *20*, 386, 1961.
51. Laurin, C. A. and Favreau, J. C.: Canad. Med. Ass. J., *89*, 288, 1963.
52. Lietman, P. S. and Bywaters, E. G. L.: Ped., *32*, 855, 1963.
53. Lindbjerg, I. F.: Arch. Dis. Child., *39*, 576, 1964.
54. Lucchesi, M. and Lucchesi, O.: Rheum., *13*, 88, 1957.
55. Markowitz, H. A. and McGinley, J. M.: J.A.M.A., *189*, 950, 1964.
56. Martel, W., Holt, J. F. and Cassidy, J. T.: Amer. J. Roentg., *88*, 400, 1962.
57. McMinn, F. J. and Bywaters, E. G. L.: Ann. Rheum. Dis., *18*, 293, 1959.
58. Miller, D. S.: Med. Clin. North America, *49*, 33, 1965.
59. Norcross, B. M., Lockie, L. M. and MacLeod, C. C.: In *Progress in Arthritis*, Ed. by Talbott, J. H. and Lockie, L. M., New York, Grune & Stratton, 1958, p. 57–85.
60. Rawson, A. J., Abelson, N. M. and Hollander, J. L.: Ann. Int. Med., *62*, 281, 1965.
61. Ropes, M. W. and Bauer, W.: *Synovial Fluid Changes in Joint Disease*, Cambridge, Harvard University Press, 1953.
62. Ropes, M. W., Bennett, G. A., Cobb, S., Jacox, R. and Jessar, R. A.: Bull. Rheum. Dis., *9*, 175, 1958.
63. Roy, S. B., Sturgis, G. P. and Massell, B. F.: New Engl. J. Med., *254*, 95, 1956.
64. Sairanen, E. and Laaksonen, A-L.: Ann. Paediat. Fenn., *8*, 105, 1962.
64*a*. Schlesinger, B. E., Forsyth, C. C., White, R. H. R., Smellie, J. M. and Stroud, C. E.: Arch. Dis. Child., *36*, 65, 1961.
64*b*. Schaller, J., Bitnum, S. and Wedgwood, R. J.: J. Ped., *74*, 505, 1969.
64*c*. Schaller, J., Kupfer, C. and Wedgwood, R. J.: Ped., *44*, 92, 1969.
65. Sharp, J. T., Calkins, E., Cohen, A. S., Schubart, A. F. and Calabro, J. J.: Med., *43*, 41, 1964.
66. Short, C. L., Bauer, W. and Reynolds, W. E.: *Rheumatoid Arthritis*, Cambridge, Harvard University Press, 1957.
67. Sievers, K., Ahvonen, P., Aho, K. and Wager, O.: Rheum., *19*, 88, 1963.
68. Smiley, W. K., May, E. and Bywaters, E. G. L.: Ann. Rheum. Dis., *16*, 371, 1957.
69. Still, G. F.: Med. Chir. Trans., *80*, 47, 1897.
70. Sury, B.: *Rheumatoid Arthritis in Children*, Copenhagen, Munksgaard, 1952.
71. Taranta, A.: New Engl. J. Med., *266*, 13, 1962.
72. Toumbis, A., Franklin, E. C., McEwen, C. and Kuttner, A. G.: J. Ped., *62*, 463, 1963.
73. Vanace, P. W. and Tuncali, M.: Arth. and Rheum., *5*, 326, 1962.
74. Walsh, H.: Med. J. Australia, *49*, 507, 1962.
75. Walker, A. E. and Adamkiewicz, J. J.: J.A.M.A., *188*, 779, 1964.
76. Wedgewood, R. J. P. and Janeway, C. A.: Ped., *11*, 569, 1953.
77. Winter, R. W.: In *Salicylates: An International Symposium*, Ed. by Dixon, A. St. J., Martin, B. K., Smith, M. J. H., and Wood, P. H. N., London, Little, Brown and Co., 1963, p. 270–280.
78. Ziff, M., Contreras, V. and McEwen, C.: Ann. Rheum. Dis., *15*, 40, 1956.

Chapter 25

The Diagnosis and Differential Diagnosis of Rheumatoid Arthritis

By CURRIER MCEWEN, M.D.

THE diagnosis of rheumatoid arthritis, like that of most diseases, can be made with ease in some instances but with great difficulty and uncertainty in others, depending on the presence or absence of the characteristic features. Among the most typical of these features are: slowly progressive polyarthritis with great tendency for symmetrical joint involvement; fusiform, soft tissue swelling during the first few years of disease; morning stiffness; characteristic rheumatoid subcutaneous nodules; the development of typical deformities such as ulnar deviation of the fingers in the later years; and a positive test for rheumatoid factor. In a patient presenting all or most of these features, the diagnosis can hardly be missed. Yet in other cases the clinical features and course of disease during the early months or even years may be so atypical that the diagnosis can be no more than suspected.

Because of these difficulties a committee was appointed by the American Rheumatism Association to draw up criteria for the diagnosis of rheumatoid arthritis. These criteria[8] are summarized here with the permission of the Committee. It must be emphasized that the criteria are subject to change as new information dictates from time to time.

The Committee suggests that, depending on the definiteness of the features presented by the individual patient, four grades of diagnosis be made: classical, definite, probable or possible rheumatoid arthritis. Any one of the features listed under "Exclusions" will exclude a patient from all of these categories.

Classical Rheumatoid Arthritis is to be diagnosed only if at least seven of the following eleven criteria are present and if the total duration of joint symptoms including swelling has been continuous for at least six weeks:

1. Morning stiffness (1 hour or more).
2. Pain on motion or tenderness in at least one joint.

Important Diagnostic Features of Rheumatoid Arthritis
1. Slowly progressive polyarthritis with great tendency for symmetrical joint involvement. 2. Fusiform, soft tissue type of joint swelling during the early years of disease. 3. Prolonged early morning stiffness. 4. Development of typical deformities such as ulnar deviation of the fingers in later years. 5. Typical rheumatoid subcutaneous nodules. 6. Positive test for rheumatoid factor.

3. Swelling (soft tissue thickening or fluid—not bony overgrowth alone) in at least one joint continuously for not less than six weeks.
4. Swelling of at least one other joint (any interval free of joint symptoms between the two joint involvements may not be more than three months).
5. Symmetrical joint swelling with simultaneous involvement of the same joint on both sides of the body (bilateral involvement of proximal interphalangeal, metacarpophalangeal or metatarsophalangeal joints is acceptable without absolute symmetry). Distal interphalangeal joint involvement will not satisfy this criterion.
6. Subcutaneous nodules over bony prominences, on extensor surfaces or in juxta-articular regions.
7. X-ray changes typical of rheumatoid arthritis (which must include at least bony decalcification localized to, or greatest around, the involved joints and not just degenerative changes). However, degenerative changes do not exclude the diagnosis of rheumatoid arthritis.
8. Positive sheep cell agglutination test. (Any modification will suffice that does not give more than 5 per cent of positive results in non-rheumatoid control subjects.)
9. Poor mucin precipitate from synovial fluid (with shreds and cloudy solution).
10. Characteristic histologic changes in synovial membrane with three or more of the following: marked villous hypertrophy; proliferation of superficial synovial cells often with palisading; marked infiltration of chronic inflammatory cells (lymphocytes or plasma cells predominating) with tendency to form "lymphoid nodules"; deposition of compact fibrin, either on the surface or interstitially; foci of cell necrosis.
11. Characteristic histologic changes in nodules showing granulomatous foci with central zones of cell necrosis, surrounded by proliferated fixed cells, and peripheral fibrosis and chronic inflammatory cell infiltration, predominantly perivascular.

Definite Rheumatoid Arthritis.—This diagnosis calls for at least five of the above criteria with a total duration of joint symptoms including swelling for a continuous period of at least six weeks.

Probable Rheumatoid Arthritis. — This diagnosis requires at least three of the above criteria and a total duration of joint symptoms of at least four weeks.

Possible Rheumatoid Arthritis.—This diagnosis requires two of the following criteria and total duration of joint symptoms of at least three weeks:

1. Morning stiffness.
2. Tenderness or pain on motion with history of recurrence or persistence for three weeks.
3. History or observation of joint swelling.
4. Subcutaneous nodules.
5. Elevated sedimentation rate or C-reactive protein.
6. Iritis.

Exclusions.—The presence of any of the following excludes the diagnosis of rheumatoid arthritis:

1. The typical rash of systemic lupus erythematosus.
2. High concentration of lupus erythematosus cells (four or more in two smears). However, because of the frequent finding of L.E. cells in patients with clinically typical rheumatoid arthritis, the Committee suggests that such patients be listed separately.
3. Histologic evidence of polyarteritis nodosa with segmented necrosis of arteries associated with nodular leukocytic infiltration extending perivascularly and tending to include many eosinophils.*
4 Weakness of neck, trunk and pharyngeal muscles or persistent muscle swelling of dermatomyositis.
5. Definite scleroderma (not limited to the fingers).

* Because of the occurrence of arteritis of this type during the course of typical rheumatoid arthritis it would appear well to list such patients separately also.

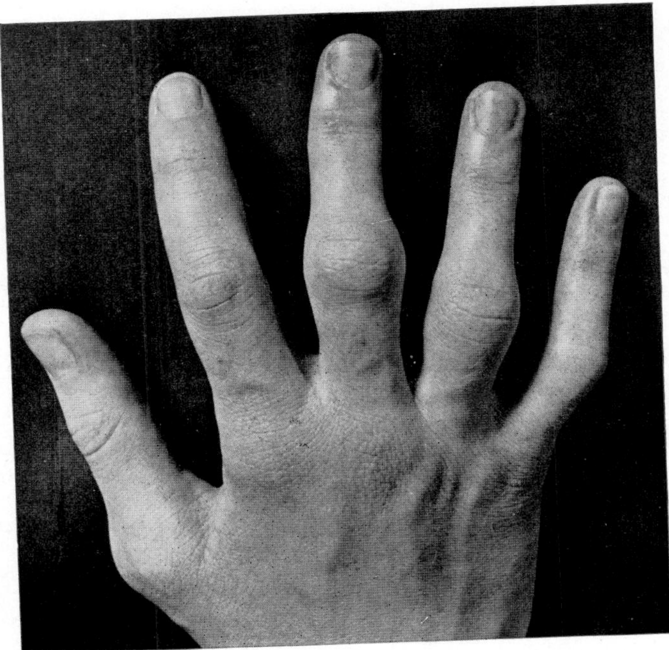

FIG. 25–1.—Rheumatoid arthritis. Note the fusiform swellings and deformities in the proximal interphalangeal joints and swelling of the first three metacarpophalangeal joints of this young woman.

6. A clinical picture characteristic of rheumatic fever with migratory joint involvement and evidence of endocarditis, especially if accompanied by subcutaneous nodules or erythema marginatum or chorea. (An elevated antistreptolysin titer will not rule out the diagnosis of rheumatoid arthritis.)
7. A clinical picture characteristic of gouty arthritis with acute attacks of swelling, redness and pain in one or more joints, especially if relieved by colchicine.
8. Tophi.
9. A clinical picture characteristic of acute infectious arthritis of bacterial or viral origin with: an acute focus of infection or in close association with a disease of known infectious origin; chills; fever; and an acute joint involvement, usually migratory initially (especially if there are organisms in the joint fluid or response to antibiotic therapy).
10. Tubercle bacilli in joints or histological evidence of joint tuberculosis.
11. A clinical picture characteristic of Reiter's syndrome with urethritis and conjunctivitis associated with acute joint involvement, usually migratory initially.
12. A clinical picture characteristic of the shoulder-hand syndrome with unilateral involvement of shoulder and hand, with diffuse swelling of the hand followed by atrophy and contractures.
13. A clinical picture characteristic of hypertrophic osteoarthropathy with clubbing of fingers and/or hypertrophic periostitis along the shafts of the long bones especially if an intrapulmonary lesion is present.
14. A clinical picture characteristic of neuroarthropathy with condensation and destruction of bones of involved joints and with associated neurological findings.
15. Homogentisic acid in the urine detectable grossly with alkalinization.
16. Histological evidence of sarcoid or positive Kveim test.
17. Multiple myeloma as evidenced by marked increase in plasma cells in the bone marrow, or Bence Jones protein in the urine.

18. Characteristic skin lesions of erythema nodosum.
19. Leukemia or lymphoma with characteristic cells in peripheral blood, bone marrow or tissues.

In December 1963 a revised classification of arthritis was adopted by the American Rheumatism Association,[1] in which spondylitis of the Marie-Strumpell type is no longer called rheumatoid spondylitis, but ankylosing spondylitis, and in which the forms of arthritis accompanying psoriasis and ulcerative colitis also are considered to be distinct from rheumatoid arthritis. At the time this edition went to press, the American Rheumatism Association's committee on diagnostic criteria had not revised the list of exclusions. However, in conformity with the new classification it can be assumed that at least three new exclusions will be added to the above list, namely "a clinical picture characteristic of ankylosing spondylitis, of psoriasis and of ulcerative colitis or regional enteritis."

Diseases Requiring Differentiation from Various Forms and Stages of Rheumatoid Arthritis

1. Arthritis with chronic or subacute involvement of multiple joints without deformities other than swelling:
   - Systemic lupus erythematosus
   - Subacute gouty arthritis
   - Reiter's disease
   - Tuberculous arthritis
   - Hypertrophic osteoarthropathy
   - Viral arthritis
   - Sarcoidosis
   - Ankylosing spondylitis
   - Psoriatic arthritis
   - Arthritis of ulcerative colitis
   - Osteoarthritis
2. Arthritis with chronic involvement of multiple joints with advanced deformities:
   - Chronic gouty arthritis
   - Systemic lupus erythematosus
   - Psoriatic arthritis
   - Reiter's disease
   - Ankylosing spondylitis
   - Arthritis of ulcerative colitis
   - Osteoarthritis
   - Sarcoidosis
3. Arthritis with acute onset:
   - Rheumatic fever
   - Acute gouty arthritis
   - Pyogenic arthritis
   - Reiter's disease
   - Systemic lupus erythematosus
   - Psoriatic arthritis
   - Palindromic rheumatism and intermittent hydrarthrosis
   - Leukemia
   - Foreign protein reaction
   - Pseudogout
   - Arthritis of ulcerative colitis
4. Monarticular arthritis:
   - Tuberculous arthritis
   - Gout
   - Traumatic joint disabilities
   - Pseudogout
5. Non-arthritic cases:
   - Localized and generalized fibrositis
   - Psychogenic rheumatism
   - Polymyalgia rheumatica
6. Rheumatoid arthritis associated with features suggesting a more serious "collagen disease":
   - Systemic lupus erythematosus
   - Polyarteritis (periarteritis) nodosa
   - Dermatomyositis and polymyositis
   - Scleroderma (progressive systemic sclerosis)

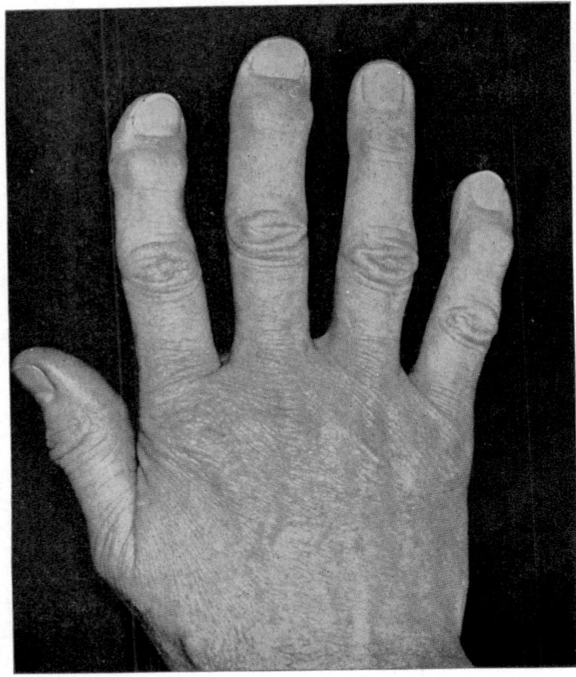

FIG. 25–2.—Degenerative joint disease of the hand. Heberden's nodes seen at the distal interphalangeal joints.

Differential Diagnosis of Rheumatoid Arthritis

In general, six types of differential diagnostic problems may arise in rheumatoid arthritis depending on whether the disease is: (1) chronic or subacute and in an early, non-deforming stage; (2) chronic and in a deforming stage; (3) acute in onset; (4) monarticular; (5) non-arthritic; or (6) associated with features suggesting a more serious form of collagen disease.

1. **Arthritis with chronic or subacute involvement of multiple joints without deformities other than swelling:** In such cases the differential diagnosis customarily lies between rheumatoid arthritis and: (*a*) systemic lupus erythematosus; (*b*) gouty arthritis; (*c*) Reiter's disease; (*d*) tuberculous arthritis; (*e*) hypertrophic osteoarthropathy; (*f*) sarcoidosis; (*g*) osteoarthritis; (*h*) ankylosing spondylitis with peripheral joint involvement; (*i*) psoriatic arthritis; (*j*) arthritis accompanying ulcerative colitis and (*k*) viral arthritis and (*l*) osteoarthritis.

(*a*) *Systemic lupus erythematosus:* Pain and swelling in peripheral joints are one of the most common manifestations of systemic lupus erythematosus; indeed in some series they have been the most common feature.[4] Hence, in many patients with early rheumatoid arthritis the presence of fever and other evidences of systemic disease may suggest lupus. Furthermore, from 12 to 20 per cent of randomly selected patients with rheumatoid arthritis show a positive L.E. test[3] and this finding also can confuse the issue. In the light of current knowledge, the diagnosis of systemic lupus is not warranted unless other features of that disease such as high fever, renal disease, pleuritis or pneumonitis, hemolytic anemia or repeatedly strongly positive L.E. tests and antinuclear antibody tests are present. Nevertheless, the finding of L.E. cells in a patient thought to have rheumatoid arthritis demands particular observation of the patient over a period of months and years. This is discussed further at the end of the chapter.

(*b*) *Gouty arthritis:* Attacks of gouty arthritis can sometimes be relatively mild and persist for several weeks, especially when the disease is in transition between the acute and chronic stages. However, the story of previous, more acute attacks subsiding without residual disability points to the correct diagnosis, which can be substantiated by the presence of a high serum uric acid level and urate crystals in the synovial fluid.

(*c*) *Reiter's disease*: The characteristic combination of urethritis, eye lesions and arthritis with or without balanitis, diarrhea and keratosis blennorrhagica usually makes the diagnosis of Reiter's disease simple. When, however, eye and skin lesions are lacking, and especially when urethritis is mild and transient, diagnosis may be difficult. In such cases, asymmetrical joint involvement and negative tests for rheumatoid factors help in excluding the diagnosis of rheumatoid arthritis. The true nature of the disease may remain obscure, however, unless balanitis or eye or skin lesions subsequently develop.

(*d*) *Tuberculous arthritis:* This usually involves only one to two joints and seldom

Rheumatoid Arthritis vs. Osteoarthritis

Synonyms	Atrophic; chronic infectious; proliferative	Hypertrophic; degenerative joint disease; degenerative arthritis
Age of onset	Usually between 20–45 years	Most often after forty years
Involvement of hands	Especially proximal interphalangeal and metacarpophalangeal joints; distal interphalangeals very rarely involved	Especially terminal interphalangeal joints (Heberden's nodes), but proximal interphalangeals also in 20% of those with Heberden's nodes
Other joints commonly involved	Any joints may be effected	Knees, lumbar spine, sacroiliac, lower cervical spine, hips
No. of joints involved	Usually many	Usually few
Symmetry of joint involvement	Most often symmetrical	Often asymmetrical
Type of onset	Usually insidious; may be abrupt	Insidious
Constitutional symptoms	Fever, loss of weight, anemia, tachycardia; often enlargement of lymph nodes and spleen	Usually none
Type of joint swelling	Usually fusiform or spindle shaped	Usually irregular or knobby
Muscular atrophy	Usually present and may be marked	Not frequent; not marked
Skin changes	Cold, clammy hands; smooth, shiny skin in extremities	None except those of age

Rheumatoid Arthritis vs. Osteoarthritis *(Continued)*		
Joint effusion	Usually present; may be marked	Usually little unless trauma superimposed
Subcutaneous nodules	Present in 15 per cent	Absent
Sedimentation rate	Usually rapid	Usually normal
X-ray findings	Early: fusiform periarticular soft tissue swelling; rarefaction of trabeculated ends of bones and systemic decalcification Later: decrease of joint space, lipping and osteophytes, punched-out areas of bone at articular margins, and possibly ankylosis, subluxations, etc.	Early: narrowing of the joint space due to destruction of cartilage; formation of osteophytes and lipping Later: cysts at ends of bone, deformities from pressure and traction; no ankylosis except rarely in fingers
Ankylosis	Common in later stages	(See above)
Primary pathological changes	Synovitis	Degeneration of hyaline articular cartilage; no inflammatory changes
Test for rheumatoid factor	Usually positive after several months of illness	Negative
Progress of the disease	Marked tendency to progression despite treatment	Slow progress
Prognosis	Very doubtful; 10 per cent progress to some degree of invalidism despite good therapy	Usually good as regards function; usually no crippling unless hips involved

is difficult to distinguish from the usual type of rheumatoid arthritis now under discussion. Occasionally, however, multiple joint involvement can suggest rheumatoid arthritis. The negative tests for rheumatoid factors and the clinical features should suggest the correct diagnosis which can be confirmed by bacteriological culture of synovial fluid and synovial biopsy. The administration of corticosteroids either systemically or intra-articularly can of course cause serious aggravation of tuberculous arthritis and such therapy must be avoided so long as the diagnosis remains in doubt.

(*e*) *Hypertrophic osteoarthropathy:* Customarily this causes aching chiefly in the long bones between the joints, and less often true arthralgia. Often, however, obvious swelling of several joints may be present as well as pain. The correct diagnosis is immediately suggested by the periosteal changes of hypertrophic osteoarthropathy on x-ray. Frequently, also, x-ray examination of the chest will reveal pulmonary neoplasm.

(*f*) *Sarcoidosis:* This is another relatively rare cause of confusion in the diagnosis of rheumatoid arthritis. Usually other manifestations of the disease, such as skin or pulmonary lesions, point to the true nature of the process, which may then be confirmed by biopsy and by a positive Kveim test.

(*g*) *Osteoarthritis:* The bony character of the joint swelling, the benign course, and the lack of evidence of inflammation make this seldom a cause of confusion.

However, many patients with degenerative joint disease also have mild to moderate intra-articular inflammation, probably from mechanical irritation of the synovial membrane, with resultant local warmth and increase in erythrocyte sedimentation rate. In such cases considerable relief may be given by salicylates which further suggests a primarily inflammatory process. However, the diagnosis usually soon becomes clear as the course of disease is followed.

(*h*) *Ankylosing spondylitis:* This disease was designated "rheumatoid spondylitis" in the classification of the American Rheumatism Association up to December 1963 when the new classification was adopted listing it as a separate entity. In ankylosing spondylitis involvement of the sacroiliac joints occurs early and is bilateral, and involvement of the spine occurs first in the lumbar region and only later in the dorsal and cervical areas.[2] In contrast, involvement of sacroiliac joints occurs late in rheumatoid arthritis and then in only approximately 25 per cent of cases; and in roughly half of these cases it is unilateral. Furthermore, spinal involvement in rheumatoid arthritis is predominantly in the cervical region. Hip and shoulder involvement is common in both diseases. In ankylosing spondylitis, involvement of these joints, like that of sacroiliacs and spine, is progressive and leads to permanent damage. Involvement of more peripheral joints is relatively uncommon, except for the knees, and usually is transient, leaving little or no residual disability.[2] Occasionally, however, progressive and permanent damage does occur and may lead to an erroneous diagnosis of rheumatoid arthritis. Examination of the sacroiliac joints and spine will usually indicate the correct diagnosis.

(*i*) *Psoriatic arthritis:* In arthritis accompanying psoriasis the cutaneous lesions immediately call attention to the underlying disease. This, plus arthritic involvement of the distal interphalangeal joints, which are less often affected in rheumatoid arthritis (except through more proximal rupture of extensor tendons), makes the diagnosis readily apparent. In approximately one-third of cases the distal interphalangeal joints are not involved. In such patients, however, the joint disease tends to be asymmetrical, subcutaneous nodules are lacking, and tests for rheumatoid factors are negative just as in the case of those with typical involvement of the distal interphalangeal joints.[7] Most difficult to differentiate are those cases in which arthritis precedes cutaneous lesions. In such patients a careful examination of the nails may reveal pitting or other psoriatic changes and suggest the correct diagnosis.

(*j*) *Arthritis of ulcerative colitis:* Arthritis of peripheral joints accompanying ulcerative colitis differs from rheumatoid arthritis chiefly in the absence of subcutaneous nodules, negative test for rheumatoid factor, and especially the tendency to transient attacks clearing in a few weeks to a few months leaving little or no residual joint disability. A smaller percentage of patients with ulcerative colitis develop sacroiliac disease and spondylitis of a sort that appears clinically and radiographically to be the same as ankylosing spondylitis.[6]

(*k*) *Viral arthritis:* Subacute polyarthritis with swelling and moderate pain and tenderness is not rare during and after various viral diseases. It has been noted especially accompanying rubella and vaccination against that disease, and early in the course of hepatitis. At onset it may be indistinguishable from early rheumatoid arthritis but the course is usually transient. That feature plus the underlying disease makes the diagnosis clear. The more persistent but also non-destructive polyarthritis accompanying lymphogranuloma venereum is distinguished from rheumatoid arthritis by the presence of the venereal disease and its response to sulfonamides.

2. **Arthritis with chronic involvement of multiple joints with advanced deformities:** In these cases the most important diagnoses to differentiate from rheumatoid arthritis are: (*a*) chronic

gouty arthritis, (*b*) systemic lupus erythematosus, (*c*) sarcoidosis, (*d*) osteoarthritis (*e*)psoriatic arthritis,(*f*) Reiter's disease, (*g*) ankylosing spondylitis and (*h*) arthritis of ulcerative colitis.

(*a*) *Chronic gouty arthritis:* The arthritis of gout can mimic advanced rheumatoid arthritis strikingly with the production of even such characteristic deformities as ulnar deviation of the fingers. When these are combined with the presence of tophi just distal to the olecranon processes the clinical resemblance can be great. Even on x-ray examination the confusion may continue because punched-out areas in bone are common in rheumatoid arthritis as well as in gout, and only if soft tissue shadows of tophi are seen can the x-ray diagnosis of gout be certain. Nevertheless, the correct diagnosis should be obvious from the history of repeated attacks of acute arthritis clearing with no residual disability over a period of many years prior to the gradual development of chronic deforming changes. Once suspected, the presence of gout can be readily confirmed by a high serum uric acid level, by the demonstration of urate crystals in the synovial fluid, and by suitable biopsy of a gouty tophus. In the latter connection it must be remembered that the well-known murexide test is not completely reliable; and also that if urates are to be sought in microscopic sections, special fixative must be used which does not dissolve the crystals.

(*b*) *Systemic lupus erythematosus:* This will be discussed at the end of this chapter.

(*c*) *Sarcoidosis* can simulate the deforming stage of rheumatoid arthritis just as it can in earlier phases of the disease.

(*d*) *Osteoarthritis* rarely causes deformities suggesting advanced rheumatoid arthritis except for swelling of the proximal interphalangeal joints of the fingers. The hard, knobby character of this enlargement differs sharply from the fluctuant, fusiform swelling of early rheumatoid arthritis, but occasionally fluctuation may be present also. A common diagnostic question is whether knobby proximal interphalangeal enlargement is due to primary osteoarthritis of those joints or to secondary osteoarthritis superimposed on old rheumatoid arthritic damage. Of course there is no problem if characteristic rheumatoid arthritic changes are present elsewhere. X-ray study may help, also, by revealing osteoporosis suggesting the existence of underlying rheumatoid arthritis. A positive test for rheumatoid factors will help confirm the latter, but a negative test does not rule out that diagnosis.

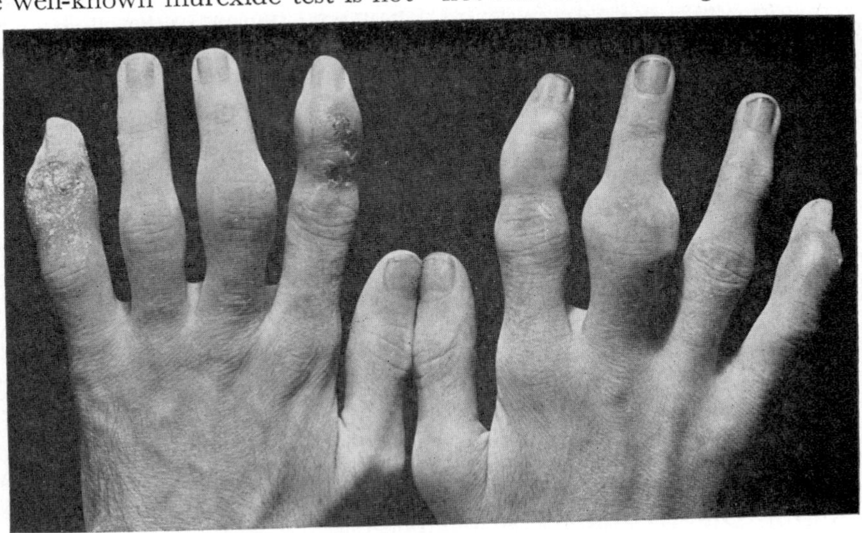

FIG. 25–3.—Gout. Note asymmetrical swellings and drainage from ulcerated tophi.

(*e*) *Psoriatic arthritis* frequently mimics the deforming stage of rheumatoid arthritis; especially when distal interphalangeal joints are spared. Differentiation is as discussed in 1(*i*) above.

(*f*) *Reiter's disease* ordinarily does not progress to a chronic and deforming stage. In those instances in which it does, a history of other features which characterize Reiter's disease—urethritis, conjunctivitis, keratodermia blennorrhagica, balanitis and diarrhea—will make the true nature of the illness apparent.

(*g*) *Ankylosing spondylitis* should seldom be misinterpreted because by the time peripheral joints have become deformed, the spinal involvement is striking and characteristic.

(*h*) *Peripheral arthritis accompanying ulcerative colitis and regional enteritis* is usually transient and non-deforming. Occasionally, however, progressive and deforming changes do occur. The obvious disease of the intestine makes the correct diagnosis clear.

3. **Arthritis with acute onset:** Although rheumatoid arthritis usually begins insidiously or subacutely, onsets with fever of 103° F. or higher and acute joint involvement are far from rare and can lead to confusion with other forms of acute polyarthritis such as: (*a*) rheumatic fever, (*b*) acute gouty arthritis, and (*c*) pyogenic arthritis. Other forms of arthritis which may start acutely are those of (*d*) Reiter's disease, (*e*) systemic lupus erythematosus, (*f*) palindromic rheumatism and intermittent hydrarthrosis, (*g*) leukemia, (*h*) foreign protein reaction, (*i*) psoriatic arthritis, (*j*) pseudogout, and (*k*) arthritis of ulcerative colitis.

(*a*) *Rheumatic fever:* This disease can be strikingly mimicked by acute rheumatoid arthritis; indeed it may be impossible to distinguish between the two during the first week or two of illness. Not only can the fever and the character of polyarthritis be the same, but also the therapeutic response to salicylates can be equally dramatic in the two diseases. In rheumatoid arthritis, however, the course of disease differs and after the initial week or two the joint pain and swelling gradually reappear. Laboratory features which may be helpful are a high antistreptolysin-O titer in rheumatic fever, and positive test for the rheumatoid factor in rheumatoid arthritis, although the latter test is often negative early in the disease.

(*b*) *Acute gout:* In contrast to the chronic deforming stage of gouty arthritis which can simulate advanced rheumatoid arthritis, the acute attack of gout sometimes is mistaken for acute rheumatoid arthritis. This is a mistake which should not be made, however, if the possibility of gout is kept in mind. Rheumatoid arthritis, even when acute, rarely causes the brawny type of inflammation so frequent in gout. Furthermore, a classical response to colchicine and a high serum uric acid level should promptly make the diagnosis clear. Most important of all in establishing the diagnosis is the presence of urate crystals in aspirated synovial fluid from the inflamed joint.

(*c*) *Pyogenic arthritis:* Pyogenic arthritis seldom presents a problem in differential diagnosis for more than the first day or two of observation. Following transient pain in several joints the inflammation tends to settle seriously in one or two and assume an indurated character. Demonstration of the causative bacteria in aspirated synovial fluid makes the definitive diagnosis. Prompt clearing after suitable antibiotics, and failure to respond significantly to salicylates strongly support the diagnosis even in the absence of bacteriological proof.

(*d*) *Reiter's disease:* This disease when starting acutely in the absence of obvious urethritis can simulate the acute form of rheumatoid arthritis just as it can the more customary form.

(*e*) *Systemic lupus erythematosus:* This disease when starting with acute joint involvement can be mistaken for acute rheumatoid arthritis. Its differentiation has already been discussed.

(*f*) *Palindromic rheumatism and intermittent hydrarthrosis:* These differ from the usual acute form of rheumatoid arthritis chiefly in their relatively short duration and

	Rheumatoid Arthritis	Gout
Sex	2 or 3 females to each male	95 per cent of cases are males
Onset	Usually insidious	Attacks usually appear suddenly
Age of onset	Usually between twenty to forty-five years	Usually after thirty-five years
Frequency of attacks	Onset usually insidious; recurrent attacks occasionally early in the disease	Varying from several months to several years
Freedom from symptoms	Symptoms usually continue for months or years without marked intermissions	Usually complete freedom from symptoms between attacks in early stage
Relief of symptoms by full dose of colchicine	None	Usually prompt
Serum uric acid	Usually normal	Usually elevated
Tophi	None; but subcutaneous nodules may resemble them	Present in 50 per cent of cases in later stages of disease
Involvement of big toe	Not characteristic	Occurs in 70 per cent in initial attack and sooner or later in 90 per cent
Generalized osteoporosis by x-ray	Usually seen	Not a feature
Joint swellings	Usually symmetrical	May be symmetrical
Sudden development of joint symptoms in minutes or hours	Does not occur this suddenly	Common
Associated olecranon bursitis	Not common	Common
Subcutaneous nodules	In 15 per cent	Not found, but tophi may mimic them
Muscular atrophy	Usually present and may be marked	Usually none except terminal stages
Ankylosis	May occur	Rare
Test for rheumatoid factor	Often positive after some months of illness	Negative
Family history of gout	Usually negative	Often positive
No. of joints involved	Usually multiple	First attack is usually monarticular
Pain	Usually mild, relieved by rest	Often excruciating; relieved by adequate doses of colchicine
Urate crystals	Not found	Present in synovial fluid and in biopsies of synovial membrane

	Rheumatoid Arthritis	Rheumatic Fever	Pyogenic Arthritis
Age at onset	90 per cent of cases after age of fifteen	First attack under fifteen years in 70 per cent	May occur at any age
Preceding sore throat	Rare	Clinically evident in 60 or more per cent	In about 10 per cent
Roentgen-ray study of joints	Characteristic: may be negative early; later generalized osteoporosis, etc.	Negative except for soft tissue swelling	May show rapid bony destruction after fourteen days
Permanent joint damage	May occur after 6 months	None	May be marked
Subcutaneous nodules	Present in about 15 per cent of cases; may persist for months to years; relatively large	Present in about 15 per cent of cases; may persist for weeks to months; small	Absent
Response to salicylates	Temporary relief, but no dramatic response in usual case; but may be dramatic in cases with acute onset	Usually dramatic with complete relief of pain and return of temperature to normal if adequate doses are used	Not dramatic; slight relief of pain and some reduction of temperature
Response to specific antibiotics	None	None	Excellent within twenty-four to seventy-two hours
Tests for rheumatoid factor	Strongly positive in most cases of some months' duration	Negative	Negative
Antistreptolysin-O titer	Normal	Increased	Normal unless bacterial agent is hemolytic streptococcus
Synovial fluid	Sterile	Sterile	Bacteria demonstrable by smear or culture
Electrocardiogram	Negative	Often evidence of cardiac involvement	Usually negative

numerous brief recurrences. The problem of their differentiation is made greater by the fact that some instances of both types of intermittent joint disease ultimately assume the character of straight-forward rheumatoid arthritis. In this situation tests for rheumatoid factors may be informative.

(*g*) *Leukemia:* Especially in children, leukemia may cause joint pain and swelling suggesting acute rheumatoid arthritis. Suitable examination of the blood, of course, makes the correct diagnosis clear.

(*h*) *Foreign protein reaction:* The polyarthritis following foreign protein administration, such as serum sickness and penicillin reactions, can be readily distinguished when accompanied by urticaria, but may present a difficult diagnostic problem when urticaria is lacking. Both rheumatoid arthritis and foreign protein arthritis respond equally well to salicylates and corticosteroids. In the absence of a positive test for rheumatoid factor, a definite diagnosis may be possible only after observing the course of disease for several weeks.

(*i*) *Psoriatic arthritis* can also have an acute onset simulating acute rheumatoid arthritis or even gout. In the latter connection it must be remembered that the serum uric acid level is frequently elevated in psoriasis.

(*j*) *Pseudogout:* This acute form of articular chondrocalcinosis resembles acute gout clinically but is differentiated by the presence in the synovial fluid of crystals of calcium pyrophosphate dihydrate instead of urate.

(*k*) *Arthritis of ulcerative colitis* not infrequently begins sufficiently acutely to suggest an acute onset of rheumatoid arthritis or rheumatic fever. As in cases with the more usual type of onset the correct diagnosis is immediately suggested by the colitis.

4. **Monarticular arthritis:** Monarticular attacks of rheumatoid arthritis, while not common, occur sufficiently frequently to be sometimes confused with (*a*) tuberculous arthritis, (*b*) traumatic disability of a joint, (*c*) gout, and (*d*) pseudogout.

(*a*) *Tuberculous arthritis:* As noted earlier, the differentiation between tuberculous arthritis and monarticular rheumatoid arthritis is especially important because of the serious effects which might follow intra-articular injection of corticosteroid in the case of the former. It may be impossible to be sure of the diagnosis on clinical grounds, but tests for the rheumatoid factor may be of aid. Definitive diagnosis demands bacteriologic proof of tuberculosis on culture of the synovial fluid or evidence for or against that disease on the basis of synovial biopsy. Positive evidence of tuberculosis from study of a "needle biopsy" is sufficient, but if negative it is not safe to assume that tuberculosis is absent unless confirmed by a more adequate specimen obtained by open biopsy.

(*b*) *Traumatic arthritis:* This diagnosis is suggested by a history of recent trauma, although we have seen instances of rheumatoid arthritis apparently first manifesting itself after local injury. Synovial fluid of normal viscosity, lack of osteoporosis on x-ray, and essentially normal

Roentgen Differentiation of Rheumatoid Arthritis from Gout

Punched-out areas may occur in both rheumatoid arthritis and gout.
When overlaid by a sharply circumscribed swelling in the soft tissues (tophus), these punched-out areas are typical of gout.
Gout rarely shows bony ankylosis.
Gout shows no systemic decalcification, less frequent thinning of cartilage and a more asymmetrical distribution of joint swelling.
Bony cysts are usually larger in gout than in rheumatoid arthritis.

erythrocyte sedimentation rate all suggest a traumatic etiology; but sometimes one can be sure of the diagnosis only after weeks of observation.

(*c*) *Gouty arthritis:* As noted above, gout is often confused with other forms of acute arthritis. Since the attacks may be subacute, and particularly since the condition is monarticular in the earlier stages of the disease, it is also mentioned here. If the possibility of gout is kept in mind, there should be little confusion. The serum uric acid level is usually elevated, the synovial fluid examination will show crystals of sodium urate (*see* Chapter 6), the brawny swelling with marked tenderness of the joint is suggestive, and the response to colchicine is usually rapid and dramatic (*see* Chapter 59 for details).

(*d*) *Chondrocalcinosis articularis* (*Pseudogout*)*:* In older patients, often having osteoarthritis, acute attacks of arthritis in a single joint may be caused by the deposition of calcium pyrophosphate crystals in the joint leading to acute inflammation in a previously mildly painful or inactive articulation. Diagnosis depends on the finding of the weakly positively birefringent crystals in the aspirated synovial fluid, and on calcium deposits in the menisci and articular cartilage on x-ray (*see also* Chapter 60). The latter may also indidate the correct diagnosis in older patients with subacute or chronic pain with or without swelling in one or two joints.

5. **Non-arthritic cases:** Not infrequently obvious rheumatoid arthritis may be preceded by episodes of vague

Differential Diagnosis of Fibrositis from Rheumatoid Arthritis

	Fibrositis	*Rheumatoid arthritis*
Joint pain	Pain is periarticular; usually worse on awakening; improved following gentle exercise	Definite joint pain; improved following gentle exercise; improved by rest but worse on motion after rest
Joint swelling	No synovial exudate or effusion	Synovial exudate frequent
Joint tenderness	Absent or very mild	May be marked
Stiffness of joints	Rarely objective; usually subjective only	Commonly subjective and objective
Loss of weight	Rare	Frequent
Muscular atrophy	Absent	Common
Remissions	Frequent	Less common
Constitutional phenomena	Usually absent	Fever, tachycardia, loss of weight, etc.
Sedimentation rate	Normal; occasionally elevated	Markedly elevated in most cases
Tests for rheumatoid factor	Negative	Usually negative in early cases
Anemia	Rare	Common
Roentgen-rays of joints	Normal	May be normal early but abnormal later
Prognosis	Good, from the standpoint of the joints; recurrences are frequent	Very uncertain; often poor
Response to therapy	Very variable; occasionally prompt	Slow, except for relief of pain and stiffness by corticosteroids

arthralgias or aching pain in soft tissue in various parts of the body. When true arthritic changes appear the diagnosis becomes clear. Meanwhile, however, the complaints suggest localized or generalized fibrositis or psychogenic rheumatism. Increased erythrocyte sedimentation rate or other acute phase reactants tend to exclude these and indicate the early stage of some form of musculoskeletal disease associated with inflammation. In these cases rheumatoid arthritis can be no more than suspected. However, if there is a positive test for rheumatoid factor the suspicion becomes stronger. Unfortunately false positive tests for rheumatoid factor occur and the usual techniques rarely give a positive result early in the disease.

Polymyalgia rheumatica can suggest early rheumatoid arthritis. The correct diagnosis is suggested early by the high erythrocyte sedimentation rate, out of proportion to arthralgia, in a patient over 50 years of age. The failure of arthritis to develop with passing time, the severe proximal muscle aching and the occurrence of giant cell arteritis, if present, confirm the diagnosis of polymyalgia (*see also* Chapter 50).

6. **Rheumatoid arthritis associated with features suggesting a more serious "collagen disease":** Reference has already been made to features of rheumatoid arthritis and systemic lupus erythematosus coexisting in the same patient. Similarly, necrotizing arteritis having the histological features of polyarteritis nodosa may also occur in patients with rheumatoid arthritis[9] and evidences of dermatomyositis and of scleroderma (progressive systemic sclerosis) may rarely be found.

In recent years attention has been directed especially to overlapping manifestations of systemic lupus and rheumatoid arthritis; and they can serve for a consideration of the general problem presented by all the collagen diseases. It has been shown that not only clinical, but also pathologic and laboratory features of both diseases coexist.[5] Positive L.E. tests can be demonstrated in 12 to 20 per cent of patients with clinically classical rheumatoid arthritis and, conversely, patients with clinically evident systemic lupus have been shown to give a positive test for rheumatoid factor in about 25 per cent of cases. The latter has been found, however, only in patients with chronic joint disease, especially in the presence of deformities of rheumatoid character.[10]

In the face of such overlapping manifestations it probably is not feasible today to lay down hard and fast criteria for deciding when such cases should be considered rheumatoid arthritis and when lupus. Until information is available to permit better understanding of the relationship of these diseases when they occur together, it would appear reasonable to list both diagnoses when clear clinical features of both exist. The same is true in the case of polyarteritis occurring during the course of otherwise definite rheumatoid arthritis. A more difficult question is posed by the rheumatoid arthritic patient with no evidence of lupus except for a positive L.E. test. The American Rheumatism Association's Committee on Diagnostic Criteria for Rheumatoid Arthritis has suggested that systemic lupus erythematosus be listed if four or more L.E. cells are found in two smears prepared from heparinized blood incubated not over two hours, but that if fewer cells are found the diagnosis of rheumatoid arthritis alone be made.[8] If systemic manifestations of lupus erythematosus are also present, the decision is, of course, obvious.

BIBLIOGRAPHY

1. Blumberg, B. S., Bunim, J. J., Calkins, E., Pirani, C. L. and Zvaifler, N. J.: Arth. and Rheum., *7*, 93, 1964.
2. Dilsen, N., McEwen, C., Poppel, M., Gersh, W. J., Ditata, D. and Carmel, P.: Arth. and Rheum., *5*, 341, 1962.
3. Hall, A. P., Bardawil, W. A., Bayles, T. B., Mednis, A. D. and Galins, N.: New Engl. J. Med., *263*, 769, 1960.
4. Harvey, A. M., Shulman, L. E., Tumulty, P. A., Conley, C. L. and Schoenrich, E. H.: Medicine, *33*, 291, 1954.

5. McEwen, C.: Maryland State Med. J., *8*, 143, 1959.
6. McEwen, C., Lingg, C., Kirsner, J. B. and Spencer, J. A.: Amer. J. Med., *33*, 923, 1962.
7. McEwen, C., Ziff, M., Carmel, P., Ditata, D. and Tanner, M.: Arth. and Rheum., *1*, 481, 1958.
8. Ropes, M. W., Bennett, G. A., Cobb, S., Jacox, R. F. and Jessar, R. A.: Bull. Rheum. Dis., *7*, 121, 1956; Ibid., *9*, 175, 1958.
9. Schmid, F., Cooper, N., Ziff, M. and McEwen, C.: Amer. J. Med., *30*, 56, 1961.
10. Ziff, M., Esserman, P. and McEwen, C.: Arth. and Rheum., *1*, 332, 1958.

Chapter 26

Methods for Evaluating Rheumatoid Arthritis

Revised by DANIEL J. MCCARTY, M.D.

SUPERFICIALLY, the evaluation of activity and progression of rheumatoid arthritis appears deceptively easy. Actually, it remains a baffling problem because of our lack of knowledge concerning the true nature of the disease. Attempts to determine the intensity of the rheumatoid process by evaluating clinically obvious signs, can, at best, be no more than indirect estimations, yet the clinician must have as accurate an estimate as possible in order to determine whether the treatment he administers is actually producing a significant improvement in his patient's condition. Also, in therapeutic trials where numerous observers are involved, the grading of rheumatoid activity needs to be done in an accurate and uniform manner.

In this chapter we plan to outline the fundamental principles of evaluation; to consider those features of the disease which can be used for assessing joint inflammation, the amount of structural damage and impairment of function. We shall also outline the main schemes for evaluation that have been proposed.

Within certain limits it is possible for both patient and doctor to say whether the arthritis is better or worse. But, if we ask "Better or worse than what?" no answer is forthcoming because no comparative, standard base line has been established, and we actually refer merely to a vague memory of a "clinical impression" at the time of the last visit. The inadequacy of such statements becomes painfully apparent, if on reviewing a clinical record we find that, a year ago, the patient had "improved" or was "quite a bit better." Such statements are meaningless in retrospect.

Even experienced rheumatologists may judge the activity of rheumatoid arthritis by quite different criteria, and often there is little agreement even as to what constitutes a clinical remission, much less as to moderate changes in the activity of the disease. There is probably some agreement as to very severe and very mild disease, but the area in between these two extremes, where most of the variations in the disease occur, is still largely undefined and continues to present a challenge to all those who are interested in assessing the course of the disease and its responses to drug therapy. Since the introduction of gold therapy in 1929, and again following the introduction of corticosteroids in 1949, a growing number of methods of evaluation have been reported. The trend toward more sophisticated controlled trials involving many observers and multiple clinics makes a certain agreement about criteria necessary for evaluation.

Review of Attempted Solutions

The numerous systems of evaluation which have been proposed fall into three main categories and were initiated in the following order: (1) The Pictorial Method exemplified by Jansen's Ciphers in 1930 (Fig. 26–1);[16,17] (2) The Matching Description Method of Taylor in 1937;[37]

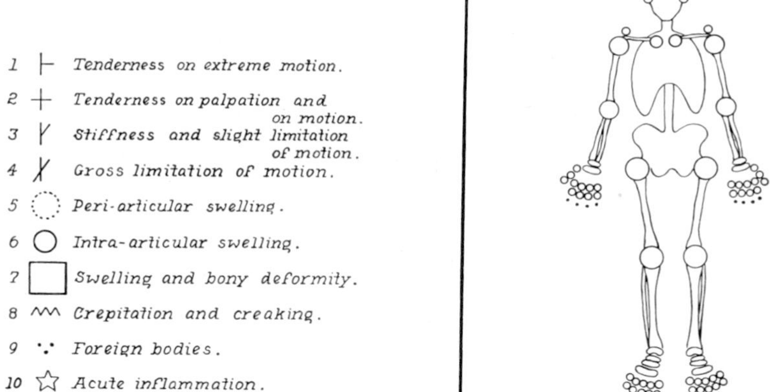

FIG. 26–1.—Two pictorial ways in which the "spread" of joint involvement may be used to indicate the status of rheumatoid arthritis.

and (3) The Numerical Method of Steinbrocker and Blazer in 1946.[35] These three approaches have fared somewhat as follows:

Pictorial methods still survive on printed forms in arthritis clinics but otherwise are little used. The Matching Description Method culminated in the American Rheumatism Association's "Recommendations for Uniform Therapeutic Criteria"[36] in 1949. In this scheme Taylor's two categories were increased to three by forming a separate Functional Class (which had been part of his more general "activity" category). The three new categories of Anatomic Stage, Functional Class and Therapeutic Grade proved of seminal importance and have been universally accepted; indeed, their permanence seems assured. However the feasibility of grading each category by trying to match the patient's findings to one of the three or four descriptive slots is still in doubt. No studies of interobserver reliability have been published and only minor changes in grading have been suggested since the method was brought out in 1949. Thus, although the three great categories have been accepted, the Matching Descriptive Method itself seems to have reached a dead end and so is unlikely to become a springboard for inventing improved solutions.

Numerical Methods, first suggested by Steinbrocker and Blazer,[35] have been refined and elaborated, in turn, by the Committee for Evaluation of New Therapeutic Agents[19] and the Committee on Diagnostic and Therapeutic Criteria.[5] All these numerical systems necessitate measuring various facets of the disease, and currently, more importance is probably being attached to the selection of these facets and methods for measuring them than to the proposed numerical methods for summing up their combined data. Indeed, a fourth method of evaluation has been suggested which consists of simply recording a half dozen or so measurable criteria without attempting to formally summate their combined information. (Any summing up which is done will be done by intuition—the very thing we are trying to get away from in devising methods of evaluation!)

In addition to the above main-stream efforts, numerous independent schemes have been reported. Those interested in the history of the subject are referred to the publications of Bayles and Hall (1942),[1] Holmdahl and Inglemark (1946),[15] Mandel (1956),[26] Savage (1958)[30] and Smyth *et al.* (1958).[33] In addition, schemes for evaluating disease activity have been devised for the purpose of calibrating certain serum protein findings by Shetlar *et al.* (1956),[31] by Decker *et al.* (1960)[10] and by Smukler *et al.* (1964).[32] Also noteworthy are devices for increasing the precision of individual measurements such as the Davis Bag for recording grip strength,[30] the jeweler's rings introduced by Hart (1951),[13] and volumetric determinations by Eccles (1956)[11] with important refinements by Smyth *et al.* (1964);[34] the arthrograph devised by Wright and Johns (1960)[40] to measure stiffness, also Hollander's Palpameter described in 1963[14] and McCarty's Dolorimeter[27a,27b] (1965) both of which represent refinements and certain advantages over Steinbrocker's Palpometer[34a] introduced in 1949 to standardize measurement of joint tenderness. The Dolorimeter has been standardized; the inter- and intraobserver errors are known. It has been used to provide data that permit mathematical analysis of joint inflammation.[27]

The Nature of the Problem

Because the nature of the rheumatoid process is still poorly understood and cannot be observed directly, we are forced to rely on indirect clinical and laboratory observations in order to measure its intensity. These constitute the "host response" and fall into two great categories: (1) Inflammatory manifestations which are reversible and which may be either articular or systemic in nature, and which taken together constitute the "activity" of the disease, and (2) Structural changes which are only partly reversible and are often permanent, such as cartilage erosion.

If we accept the view that rheumatoid arthritis is primarily an inflammatory disease and that the structural changes are the result of the inflammation, it would be theoretically possible, with ideal methods of evaluation, to reduce the whole process to the formula: "Average inflammatory activity × duration of disease = stage of structural damage." However, at the cellular level, a distinction between inflammatory activity and structural changes may well be nonexistent; yet, in devising a practical scheme for evaluation, the distinction seems necessary.

If our prime therapeutic aim is to suppress, to retard, or even to abolish the inflammatory process, then quantification of the inflammatory process is of prime importance. If, on the other hand, we believe that drugs merely suppress inflammatory manifestations while the disease itself proceeds at its own pace, eventually resulting in various degrees of anatomical damage, then an assessment of structural change would be our main objective, and the interim fluctuations of inflammatory activity would be only of historic interest. This is particularly true if long-term (five to ten year) periods of observation are envisioned. Both types of evaluation are thus equally important.

Available Criteria for Clinical Evaluation

With the problem now roughly outlined and the better-known attempts at its solution listed, we are in a position to reconsider the whole matter from the ground up. Therefore, we shall first attempt to draw up a list of the more promising disease facets which can be observed and measured and to select from these the most useful ones for making assessments. (Our selection of these criteria or parameters is listed in Table 26–1.) Secondly, we shall review the numerical methods now available for putting together the information furnished by these criteria.

A study of Table 26–1 brings out certain important facts: (1) No single item can be relied on, by itself, to reflect adequately the total picture of disease activity; (2) All items are subject to various degrees of observational error, so that we must accept the fact that there is *no such thing* as a perfect criterion; (3)

Table 26-1.—Observable Manifestations of Rheumatoid Arthritis

Category A.	*Quantifiable Items Found in Nearly All Gradations of Rheumatoid Activity.* Joint inflammation and dysfunction; muscle weakness; sedimentation rate; morning stiffness; pain; fatigue.
Category B.	*Similar Items Which Are Not Always Present in Active Disease.* Anemia, weight loss, fever, leukocytosis, deviations in serum albumin and globulin, non-specific tests for inflammation. Serologic tests for rheumatoid factor.
Category C.	*Qualitative Items of Dubious Value in Assessing Rheumatoid Activity.* Anorexia, depression of mood, achlorhydria, hydremia, paresthesias, vasomotor changes, muscle twitching and spasm, and lowered basal metabolism.
Category D.	*Items Indicating Anatomic Changes Caused by Disease Activity.* Muscle atrophy, tenosynovitis, tendon rupture, joint contractures, fibrous ankylosis, osteoporosis, cartilage or bone erosion, bony ankylosis, nodules, vasculitis, pneumonitis, valvulitis, nephritis, neuritis, lymphadenopathy, splenomegaly, episcleritis amyloidosis.

Since evaluation must be based on a battery of these criteria, some method for expressing the combined information would be helpful.

VIRTUES AND DEFECTS OF VARIOUS CRITERIA

We shall now take up a detailed analysis of all the available criteria in the order in which they are listed in Table 26–1, at the same time making references to the more important studies concerning them.

(1) *Joint Inflammation.*—Joint findings occupy a prominent place in all methods of assessment, often to the neglect of the more general, systemic manifestations of the disease. On the surface, it would seem that grading inflammation by means of such obvious parameters as tenderness, pain, swelling, warmth, redness and range of motion should be easy and highly objective. That this plausible concept is deceptive has been shown by numerous meticulous studies, mainly by British observers, which have been summarized by Mandel[26] in an article which is well worth consulting. The present consensus in Britain, as expressed by Savage[30] and Copeman,[9] is that tenderness is the most reliable parameter. Goniometric determinations of range of motion are considered either too insensitive or too inaccurate to reflect moderate changes in activity, although some attention is still given to range of finger-motion (making a fist), also to rest pain as opposed to motion pain. Attempts to measure swelling of joints are exemplified by Hart's measurement of knuckle swelling with jeweler's rings.[13] We have found a jeweler's tape an extremely precise, rapid way to measure swelling of small joints (±1 mm. reproducibility). Smyth *et al.*[34] have shown that measures of hand and foot volume by water displacement (based on the original work of Eccles[11]), are reproducible with an error of about 1 per cent.

It seems to us that it *is* possible to distinguish between the *extremes* of all these criteria, also to decide whether a joint is, or is not, actively inflamed. However, we find that the great majority of affected joints present what may be considered an "average" degree of inflammation. Reliable quantification of findings in this area, where most of the changes occur, is unfortunately difficult, if not impossible. Even if it were possible, the time required to make such evaluations of all joints renders it impracticable. Thus it seems that although most observers agree that joint evaluation is important, there is, as yet, no general agreement as to what criteria should be used, or how they should be measured and put together in a standardized manner.

Apart from the difficulty of quantifying these criteria, another difficulty, which is only now beginning to be appreciated, is that the most accurate appraisal of inflammation in one joint, let us say the knee, does *not* tell us what is going on in other joints such as the elbow, wrist or ankle. Perhaps a little information about *all* the joints is better than a lot of information about a few joints.

Estimating Total Joint Inflammation.—The idea of taking into account the "spread" of the disease, the total amount, or pool, of active arthritis, dates from the work of Jansen[16,17] (Fig. 26–1*A*). His marks were designed to indicate conveniently ten observable joint abnormalities and were inscribed at the appropriate places on the outline of a human form. The great merit of his method was, as he put it, to present a "summary survey" of *all* the patient's joints.

In addition to the crude "visual" summation which Figure 26–1 permits, we may take a further step by simply adding up the total number of involved joints. The numerical values so obtained are probably valid in multi-center drug trials, since, in a large series of cases, the number of large, medium-sized and small joints will, on the average, probably be about the same in both groups of patients. But, in following individual patients from month to month, we have found it necessary to take the size of joints into consideration, for, obviously, if we are trying to summate the total amount of active arthritis, a small joint, such as a knuckle, cannot possibly contribute as much to the totality of inflammation as can a large joint, such as a knee.[19,21] The *Articular Index* is the sum of the values based on relative size of joints times the number of joints involved (Fig. 26–3), *e.g.*, each knee = 24, each knuckle = 1, times number of each involved.

Using pain and tenderness as end-points, a review of our cases shows that, as patients improve, these disappear *serially*, one joint after another becoming free of frank inflammatory signs. Thus, the process of recovery is the mirror image of the familiar process of *successive* involvement of new joints during worsening of the disease. Because the Articular Index automatically records both expansion and contraction of the total pool of arthritic involvement, it provides a method for assessment of rheumatoid activity insofar as it relates to the joints themselves. Trends of activity during periods of worsening and improvement are shown in Figure 26–2.

It should be emphasized that counts of affected joints, or the Articular Index, are, in essence, *methods of summation* which are applied to clinical findings. The result can only be as good as are the findings. Detection of tenderness and pain on passive motion have a superficial air of objectivity, but a subjective element is also present. Thus, the degree of pressure applied to each joint by the examiner will vary considerably, and, on the other hand, the point at which the examinee will register pain will also vary from patient to patient. The inexperienced examiner generally fails to exert sufficient pressure over the joints. We have used the Articular Index for over ten years and have found it very helpful in recording the progress of rheumatoid arthritis patients.

(2) *Joint Dysfunction.*—Restoration of joint function to normal may be thought of as the ultimate goal of any kind of management, whether it be physical, pharmacological or even psychological. However, as a therapeutic criterion, we must remember that impaired function may be due either to current joint and

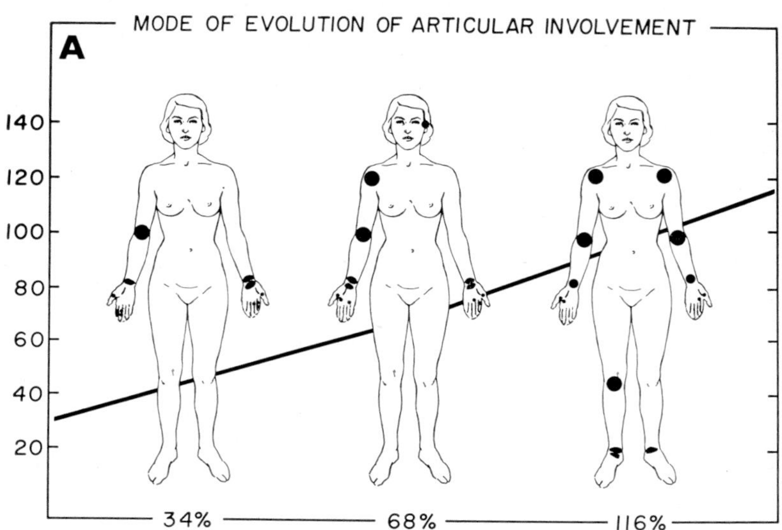

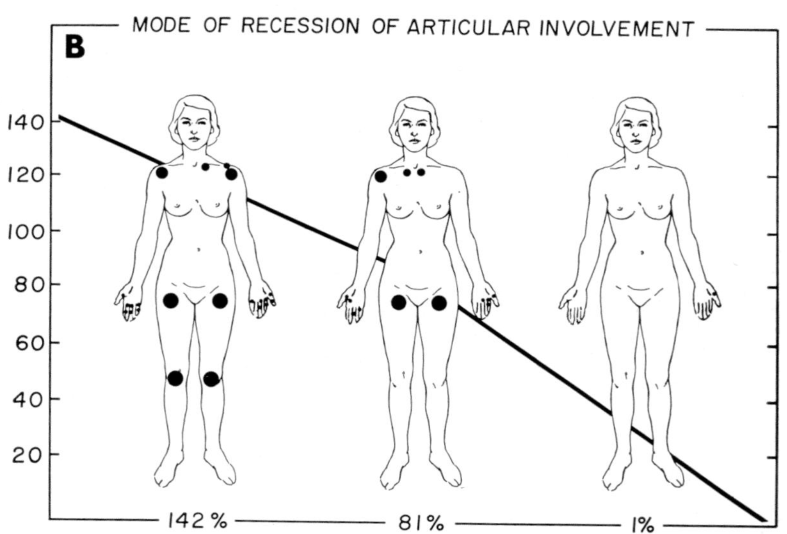

FIG. 26–2.—*A* and *B* demonstrate the changing pattern of joint involvement (judged by pain and tenderness) observed in two patients over a period of months. *A* shows the familiar spread to new joints as the patient gets worse. *B* shows just the reverse—a serial clearing of joint inflammation as the patient improves. The Articular Index percentages are proportional to the total amount or pool of joint involvement as judged by the size of the articulating surfaces.

Table 26–2.—A. R. A. Functional Class[36]

Class	
I	Complete Ability to carry on all usual duties without handicaps
II	Adequate for normal activities Despite handicap of discomfort or limited motion at one or more joints
III	Limited Only to little or none of duties of usual occupation or self-care
IV	Incapacitated, largely or wholly Bedridden or confined to wheelchair; little or no self-care

muscle inflammation, which is reversible, or to permanent structural changes which are irreversible, or to a combination of both. Since evaluations of range of motion, *per se*, cannot distinguish between these, its value in assessing responses to drug therapy is limited to cases where reversibility of structural change can be expected.

Functional Classifications.—It appears that Taylor in 1937,[37] was first to include overall functional impairment in his four categories; "slight, moderate, severe, and extreme." In 1949, Steinbrocker's committee[36] put forward criteria for these grades which were more sharply defined. These are given in Table 26–2 and have been used by the British with a rewording of the definitions.[30] The Joint Committee of the Medical Research Council and Nuffield Foundation[28] subsequently used a 5-point scale, which may be paraphrased as follows: Grade 1—Fully employable, 2—Light or part-time work, 3—Unemployable—can do light housework, 4—Confined to house but able to care for themselves, 5—Completely bedridden.

Classifications of general functional capacity into only 4 or 5 classes have the disadvantage of being able to register only major improvements or deteriorations and are therefore too crude to detect minor responses to therapy. However, we need not limit ourselves to a restricted scale of 4 or 5 categories. Lowman[24] draws attention to a scoring system, in common use in rehabilitation centers, in which no less than 106 separate "activities of daily living" are taken into consideration. These are divided into 10 groups, each with an appropriate scale of grading. We understand that a skilled technician requires about one-half hour to complete the evaluation, so that it cannot be widely applicable, despite its greater precision. What is needed is a list of 10 to 20 representative activities which would be applicable in practically all cases. No agreement on such a list has been reached so far.

Another approach to estimating the overall functional capacity is the patient's own estimate of his per cent of "fitness." In drug trials by the Empire Rheumatism Council, the patient's own estimate was recorded on the scale of "100 per cent fit, 75 per cent, 50 per cent, 25 per cent and 1 per cent."[12] Like other functional estimates, it does not distinguish between incapacity due to activity and that due to deformity, but is still capable of registering improvement if it occurs. In multi-clinic trials, a statement by the patient would be of confirmatory value, even though its quantitative value seems dubious.

In addition to these appraisals of general functional ability, numerous functional tests have been devised, mostly by British workers. These include maneuvers and set tasks, such as: tying knots, picking up pins, arm flailing, rising from a recumbent position to an erect position, climbing on to a chair, rising from a sitting to a standing position, ascending and descending steps, kneeling, hopping and standing on toes.

Copeman,[9] after long experience with such tests, has discarded them because they are too much influenced by the "learning curve," and, on constant repetition, become quite boring to both patient and examiner. Of all the "set tasks" only a timed walk of 50 feet has won general acceptance. We have found that it gives fairly repeatable results, but it has the disadvantage of being rather unsuitable for private office practice.

Range of Motion.—The shortcomings of measures of range of motion as a measure of disease activity have already been mentioned. Nevertheless, they are capable of registering major changes in function and extent of deformity. To be really effective, a quick method for summing up *total impairment* of range of motion is needed. This will be discussed under the heading of structural changes.

(3) *Muscle Weakness.*—We found weakness of the hand grips in 98 of 100 consecutive cases of rheumatoid arthritis as measured by the patient's ability to compress an inflated sphygmomanometer cuff under standard conditions. Average values in 150 unselected cases were 120 mm. of mercury for men and 80 for women.[2] There is general agreement that, with reasonably careful techniques, the readings are reliable and repeatable with minimal interobserver error.[28,39] A standard bag was designed for this purpose by Davis[30] which eliminates variations in folding the ordinary cuff. Our experience over ten years gives convincing proof that even small changes in rheumatoid activity are registered by this technique *provided* deformities, muscle fibrosis and atrophy are not sufficient to interfere. Even in the presence of considerable muscle wasting, grip strength may eventually return to normal after the patient attains a true remission.

Nevertheless, it must not be forgotten that the information which the grip test supplies is generally composite and, only under certain conditions, a true measure of muscle strength. Thus, hyperextension deformities of the proximal interphalangeal joints may give a totally false low reading; on the other hand, normal grip strength may coexist with well-marked ulnar deviation. Grip strength is also considerably affected by joint pain, by effusions into tendon sheaths, and even by acute arthritis of the elbow or shoulder without any involvement of the distal joints. Occasionally we have seen weak grips where the arthritis is confined to the lower extremities, but, on the other hand, some patients maintain normal grip strength despite obvious involvement of the hands. In drug trials[3,8] where patients with far-advanced disease are included, grip strength may be a relatively insensitive index of improvement. Wright[39] has demonstrated a marked diurnal variation in grip strength, even in normal hands. Repeated evaluations of grip are best made at the same time of day. However, despite these drawbacks, we believe that a properly conducted test of grip strength deserves to be incorporated into any scheme of evaluation.

(4) *The Sedimentation Rate.*—The sedimentation rate is accepted by nearly all observers as one of the most reliable and objective criteria of disease activity, but in short-term drug trials it has not always provided statistically significant information.[8,33] In rare instances it may remain exceedingly rapid despite clinical evidence that the disease is relatively inactive. In such cases the abnormally rapid rate may be looked on as a fixed, irreversible "serologic deformity." In the great majority of our cases it varies quite consistently with other measures of disease activity, and is almost universally increased in the presence of demonstrably active disease.

Of the various methods, we prefer the maximum 5-minute fall by the Cutler method, although the Westergren method is less laborious and most widely accepted. The Wintrobe method, as performed routinely, has been less satisfactory in our experience though quite accurate when performed under rigid supervision. For further details, the reader is referred to Chapter 23.

(5) *Morning Stiffness and Gelling.*—Since we first drew attention in 1956 to the possibility of quantifying morning stiffness, there has been a growing awareness of its value as an index of rheumatoid activity. An analysis of our records of duration of morning stiffness, going back as far as 1942, indicates that it is almost universally (97 per cent) present in active rheumatoid arthritis. Its average duration after rising is three and one-half hours in *untreated* cases. Furthermore, as patients go into remission, the duration of morning stiffness steadily declines. Estimations of morning stiffness have proved worthwhile in several drug trials[3,8,38] also in mass surveys for rheumatoid disease.[7]

Clinicians seeking "objective" measures of rheumatoid activity are naturally disconcerted by the introduction of what seems to be an "entirely subjective" parameter. We agree that answers to such direct questions as "How bad is your pain?" or "How stiff are you?" are generally worthless. However, our long experience in inquiring as to the *duration* of morning stiffness, rather than its *severity* convinces us that the vast majority of patients are *unconcerned* regarding the time element and so give an accurate, emotion-free account of its duration. This may require a little cross-questioning on the part of the doctor, but no more than he would cheerfully undertake in eliciting time factors in duration of anginal pain or the pain of a peptic ulcer. We have no hesitation in recommending duration of morning stiffness for inclusion in any system of evaluation.

(6) *Quantification of Pain.*—We have already noted that direct questions as to the severity of pain are unreliable. Nevertheless, valid distinctions can be made between pain felt only on motion and pain felt at rest; also between pain which is severe enough to prevent sleep; or pain which is, or is not, controlled by salicylates. These distinctions, however, are qualitative, and distinguish only between extreme and average degrees of pain.

Several authors have reported on a count of aspirin, or other analgesic tablets, needed per day, as a measure of pain. We have found a daily "aspirin tablet count" much more helpful than we had originally anticipated, and we now have a multitude of records in which, as the patient improved, his aspirin intake was spontaneously lowered, and vice versa. Although the measure is a rough one compared, for instance, with the scale of the sedimentation rate, and although extreme degrees of pain may not always be registered, the daily aspirin count *does* give reliable quantitative information *just where we need it most*, that is, in the zone of average or moderate disease activity. We therefore recommend it as a useful parameter. Its chief limitation is that it depends on an intelligent, cooperative patient. We have found it to be insensitive in the case of most city hospital clinic patients. In a certain sense, a count of inflamed joints, or the Articular Index, may also be considered as a measure of pain provided we use pain and tenderness as our end-points. Again, as has been demonstrated for stiffness and grip strength, pain, as measured by quantification of pain threshold with a standardized instrument (Dolorimeter), has been shown to vary diurnally. It is most severe (greatest tenderness) in the morning.[27a] Hence, the patient should be examined at the same time of day in order to control this variable.

(7) *Quantification of Fatigue.*—Fatigue is a cardinal manifestation of active rheumatoid disease, and may even precede the appearance of joint inflammation in early cases. We found it to be present in 74 per cent of untreated cases. If

present, it gradually subsides as the patient improves, and increases as he gets worse. On the average, fatigue is noted about 4 hours after rising so that the elapsed time after rising in the morning and the onset of fatigue can be used as a parameter, although considerable cross-questioning may be required to establish this point. The time of its onset may also be influenced by the patient's activity during this period. Despite these difficulties, we feel that it should be considered in schemes of evaluation because it is a cardinal feature of the disease, and because it is present through all gradations of activity, and because, when present, it is one of the most sensitive criteria. Nevertheless, we would welcome an improved method for quantitating it.

(8) *Anemia as a Criterion.*—Hemoglobin values have been incorporated into several schemes for evaluation on the assumption that they are "objective" and therefore accurate. However, in our experience, variations of plus or minus 1 gm. are quite frequent. The value of anemia as a measure of rheumatoid activity is also lessened by the fact that it is present in less than half of the cases with active disease. Nevertheless, when present, it gradually returns to normal as patients go into remission, even though no hematinics are given. Hemoglobin values may also be decreased on account of hydremia induced by drugs (such as corticosteroids, phenylbutazone) as well as from silent intestinal bleeding attributable to chronic ingestion of aspirin.

(9) *Body Weight as a Criterion.*—Over long periods of time, changes in weight may reflect variations in the trend of disease activity. However, weight gain under corticosteroid administration, due either to water retention or to an artificially stimulated appetite, may vitiate these data. Conversely, weight loss due to anorexia associated with the administration of antimalarials may also occur in the face of obvious improvements in the activity of the disease, and therefore also give false information. For these and other reasons, we doubt the value of body weight as an indicator of activity, and do not recommend it as a criterion.

(10) *Fever as a Measure of Disease Activity.*—Many patients with severely active rheumatoid arthritis and some with moderate activity may be febrile. A review of 76 hospital admissions indicated that in active rheumatoid arthritis the temperature was elevated on one or more occasions in 22 per cent of patients studied. The average degree of fever was 99.4° F. (37.5° C). Because of this low incidence of fever, we feel that it would be of little or no value as a criterion. In our clinic (which takes place in the morning) only 2 per cent of patients showed a rise of temperature above 98.3° F.

(11) *The Leukocyte Count as a Guide to Activity.*—This has been recorded in some schemes of evaluation, but its relation to disease activity, if any, has not been well studied. Severely ill patients may have a leukocytosis, a leukopenia or a normal count. Leukocytosis may diminish as the patient improves, but we doubt if this occurs with sufficient regularity to recommend the leukocyte count as a measure of activity.

(12) *Serum Proteins as a Guide to Rheumatoid Activity.*—Lowering of serum albumin and/or elevation of serum globulins are intimately associated with the activity, and possibly with the stage of the disease. However, little work has been done to clarify this relationship and no opinion, therefore, can be expressed as to the value of serum protein levels for our present purposes.

The Role of Other Laboratory Tests

Under this heading we mention the following tests: C-Reactive Protein, Formolgel Reaction, the Sheep-Cell Agglutination Test and its modifications, the Latex and Bentonite Fixation Tests, the Mucopolysaccharide-protein Ratio and the Sialic Acid Test. Few of these have been adequately studied in relation to disease activity over sufficiently long periods of time to permit an authoritative opinion as to their value as measurements of rheumatoid activity. However, it is quite possible that some of them may turn out to be valuable criteria.

This completes a review of the items listed in Table 26–1 under Categories A and B. (Those under Category C will not be considered because they are not quantifiable and are often uncommon or rare manifestations of the disease.) It will be seen that only a few of the observable manifestations can be measured with reasonable accuracy. Because of this, and in order to get an adequate sample, we shall have to accept subjective as well as objective criteria (Table 26–3).

Basis for Numerical Systems of Evaluation

Once we have agreed to take half a dozen or so measurable facets of the disease as indicators of its activity, we must find some way of putting them together again if we wish to identify the intensity of the whole process. Indeed, we cannot escape from some form of summation because all observers, reviewing the data before them, will form an opinion as to the severity of disease activity. This may be a plausible guess, a crude estimate of "zero, slight, moderate" or "severe" or a numerically exact, standardized procedure. In any case, it is a form of summation. In constructing a numerical system we merely aim to find a regular rather than a haphazard way of doing this.

The pioneer numerical systems[26,35] provided methods for summing up their intuitive estimates of the severity of various disease facets. However, to illustrate the numerical method, we shall take the Activity Index as our model because it is

Table 26-3.—Quantifiable Objective and Subjective Criteria

*Fully Objective**

1. Joint Swelling (measured by ring-size, water displacement).
2. Ankylosis, Subluxation, Muscle Atrophy, Rheumatoid Nodules.
3. Oral Temperature, Body Weight.
4. X-ray Findings (Cartilage Erosion, Osteoporosis, etc.).
5. Laboratory: ESR, Hemoglobin, Serum Proteins, Rheumatoid Factor, etc.

Partly Objective

1. Joint Tenderness and/or Pain on Passive Motion. (Tenderness may be measured by Steinbrocker's Palpometer, Hollander's Palpameter or McCarty's Dolorimeter.)
2. Goniometric determinations of limitation of Range of Motion.
3. Functional tests, such as Grip Strengths determined by Davis Bag, or Time to walk a standard distance, such as 50 feet.
4. Stiffness, as measured by the Arthrograph of Johns and Wright.

Purely Subjective

1. American Rheumatism Association Functional Class.
2. Percentage of Fitness (British Scheme).
3. Duration of Morning Stiffness, Time of onset of Fatigue, Aspirin need for control of pain (as used in the Indexes).

* Fully objective criteria are those which cannot be interfered with by poor patient-cooperation. It must not be assumed that because of this they are free from observer error. Subjective criteria are obviously more prone to error, but this is not sufficient to prevent their usefulness.

Table 26-4.—Some Requisites for Items of Evaluation

1. They should be simple, requiring no special apparatus and capable of being carried out by any competent clinician.
2. They should require no more than 5 or 10 minutes to do.
3. They should be applicable to the great majority of cases of rheumatoid arthritis.
4. They should measure either Disease Activity, Functional Status or Structural Changes in pure form and not a mixture of these.
5. They should be based on actual measurements, avoiding vague clinical impressions and guesswork grades of 0–1–2–3, etc.
6. The various items to be observed must be sufficiently numerous to constitute an adequate sample of the total clinical picture.
7. For practical reasons the items should be mainly clinical and laboratory determinations should be few or absent.

the only entirely quantitative system and because it has been extensively studied and frequently used over the last decade.

The Activity Index

The "Activity Index" was made to the specifications listed in Table 26–4 and is a combination of the earlier Systemic and Articular Indexes.[19] As will be seen from Table 26–5 and Figure 26–3 and the protocol on page 431, it is based on six fully reversible and quantifiable items, as follows: First, three subjective or interview items: Duration of morning stiffness; Hours after rising when fatigue begins and the Daily number of aspirin tablets needed for pain: then, three semi-objective items: Grip Strength, Articular Index and Westergren sedimentation rate. (Grips should not be included if deformities prevent them from being fully reversible. They should properly be classed as a functional test.)

The Percentage Equivalents given in Table 26–5 were arrived at by assigning the figure 100 to the average value found (in 1954) for each item in a series of over 100 cases before "specific" therapy had been instituted. A scale was then constructed from zero (remission) values to 100 and extrapolated beyond to 200. A subsequent study on 150 patients seen between the years 1954 to 1964 has shown average values within 10 per cent of the original values, except in the case of aspirin consumption, which was greater, and the Articular Index, which was 20 per cent less. Thus, in general, the two series confirm each other and suggest that these percentage equivalents express the relation of each item to the others with sufficient accuracy for practical use.

Since the introduction of the indexes in 1956, enough experience has accumulated to indicate their virtues and limitations and to identify those roles where they are most useful. Three main uses have been suggested for them:

(1) To indicate and identify for other physicians the degree of rheumatoid activity in a given patient. For this purpose it is also well to include the data from each item (as in the rubber stamp) because the same numerical value may not mean quite the same thing for each patient and may, indeed, result from a profile having considerably different values for its component items.

Methods for Evaluating Rheumatoid Arthritis

Directions for eliciting data for the **Activity Index**

(In eliciting the first three items, try to get an average value for the preceding few days rather than the value for a given day.)

1. **Duration of Morning Stiffness.**—Note the time at which patient usually rises. Ask if he is stiff. If so, ask by what time the stiffness wears off or when he "limbers up." Estimate the duration of his stiffness and write down the percentage value for this as indicated in the table. If the stiffness wears off slowly over a period of an hour or so, take the time of beginning of the change as the end-point. Beware of the patient who says he is "stiff all day." Usually he only means that, all day long, after resting he is again stiff for a few minutes.
2. **Time of Onset of Fatigue.**—Using the same type of questioning, ascertain the number of hours after rising, before he gets tired or exhausted, and write down the percentage equivalent from the table. (If patient is tired on waking due to poor sleep, do not count this as fatigue at zero hours, but find out when true fatigue comes on later in the day. If he takes a scheduled afternoon nap, ask him to observe his fatigue on a day (such as Sunday) when the nap is omitted. Be sure not to confuse the need to "get off one's feet because of foot pain" with fatigue.) Also, do not write down "0" for "NO fatigue," because "0" means fatigue at zero hours, *i.e.*, at rest.
3. **Aspirin Need.**—Note the average daily number of aspirin tablets (or other salicylate), write down its percentage value from the table. (If patient does not take aspirin have him try a prescribed dose of 8 to 12 tablets a day for a few days but record only the amount taken thereafter on an "ad lib" basis. Be sure it is being taken for pain and not from habit, and not as a prescribed dose or as a sedative on retiring.)
4. **Grip Strength.**—An ordinary sphygmomanometer, registering to 260 mm. Hg, is preferred. The valve at the top of the mercury column must be open. The rubber part of the cuff is folded exactly twice, and the cotton flap rolled not too tightly around it. The system is inflated to 20 mm. Hg. With the mercury column in full view and with his arm unsupported, the patient squeezes the cuff as hard as possible. Three tries are allowed for each hand, and the average of the highest reading for each hand is noted. Its percentage value (from the table) is recorded.
5. **Joint Count (Spread, or Articular Index).**—To estimate the total "amount" of active joint inflammation, all the peripheral joints are examined for tenderness on pressure or pain on passive motion. (Pay no attention to swelling, fluid, heat, or restricted motion.) Elicit tenderness by squeezing the knuckles, by pressing directly with the thumbs on the carpal mosaics, the sternoclavicular joints, acromioclavicular joints and tarsal mosaics. Put the other joints through a full range of passive motion. To elicit jaw pain, ask the patient to bite firmly. PAIN is the end-point. Tick each 'positive' joint on chart (Fig. 26–1 or 26–3) and add up all values. Find the percentage equivalent for this total from the Table under "Joint Count."
6. **Sedimentation Rate.**—Either the Westergren or Cutler technique may be used. (In the case of the Cutler method, record the maximum fall in any one five-minute period. Tables for this can be supplied.) Record the percentage value of the reading. (Wintrobe values not acceptable.)

For following cases from month to month it is very helpful to graph the data so that one can see at a glance trends in disease activity and therapeutic responses which would not be obvious from inspecting a simple sequence of numbers.

Table 26-5.—The Rheumatoid Activity Index
Table for Converting Observed Values into Their Percentage Equivalents

Subjective Items						*Objective Items*					
Morning Stiffness		*Fatigue After*		*Aspirin /Day*		*Grips*		*Joint Count*		*Westergren ESR*	
Hrs.	%	*Hrs.*	%	*Tabs.*	%	*mm.*	%		%	*mm.*	%
1/6	1	12.0	0	1	2	260	0	5	1	10	0
1/3	2	11.0	2	2	5	250	1	10	2	15	2
1/2	3	10.0	4	3	7	240	2	15	3	20	3
3/4	4	9.0	7	4	10	230	3	20	4	25	5
1.0	6	8.0	10	5	12	220	4	25	5	30	5
1.5	9	7.0	13	6	15	210	6	30	6	35	8
2.0	11	6.0	16	7	17	200	7	35	7	40	10
2.5	14	5.0	18	8	20	190	8	40	8	45	12
3.0	17	4.5	20	9	22	180	9	45	9	50	13
3.5	20	4.0	21	10	25	170	11	50	10	55	15
4.0	23	3.5	23	11	27	160	12	55	11	60	17
4.5	26	3.0	24	12	30	150	13	60	12	65	18
5.0	29	2.5	26	13	32	140	15	65	13	70	20
5.5	31	2.0	27	14	35	130	16	70	14	75	22
6.0	34	1.5	28	15	37	120	17	75	15	80	23
6.5	37	1.0	30	16	40	110	19	80	16	85	25
7.0	40	0.5	31	17	42	100	20	90	18	90	27
7.5	43	0	32	18	45	90	21	100	20	95	28
8.0	46			19	47	80	22	110	22	100	30
				20	50	70	23	120	24	105	32
						60	24	130	26	110	33
						50	25	140	28	115	35
						40	26	150	30	120	37
						30	27	160	32	125	38
						20	28	170	34	130	40
						10	29	180	36	135	42
						0	30	190	38	140	43
								200	40	145	45

The above percentage values are given at one fifth of their full value so that, for following patients in practice, a sum of the first five items constitutes the "Clinical Index." For a full Activity Index, the ESR values are added and the whole multiplied by 5/6 to bring the Index to scale. The full Activity Index is used for drug trials. (In practice, the ESR may be substituted for any item which cannot be elicited, such as fatigue or grip strengths.)

(2) To follow the response of patients to treatment. We have no doubt whatsoever as to the value of the Indexes for this purpose. Over the last ten years we have recorded many hundreds of Index figures and have found their charted curves from month to month an unfailing aid to directing therapy. Since in this situation we are measuring changes peculiar to the profile of a given patient, attention to the individual items seems less necessary, although these are always available and may be referred to in case of unexpected changes in the Index.

(3) To follow the course of patients in drug trials. Here, if the test and control groups are well apportioned, the total "amount" of stiffness, fatigue, etc. should, theoretically, be about the same for each group, so that an Index alone would probably provide adequate information as to overall improvement. In addition,

	R	L		R	L			%
JAW 2			HI 24			ST		
ACR 1			KN 24			FA		
STE 4			ANK 8			AS		
SH 12			AST 4			GR		
EL 12			CHO 4			JO		
WRI 4			TAR 8			ES		
CAR 4			BUN 2					
KNU ※			TOE ※			INDEX		

Observations at the time of each visit can be made by means of the rubber stamp shown on the left. Joints which are painful on pressure or motion are ticked and their values added up. Percentage values for this and the other items are listed and their sum is the Index.

(Abbreviations for the names of joints signify the following from above down: Jaw, Acromioclavicular, Sternoclavicular, Shoulder, Elbow, Wrist, Carpal Bones, Knuckles, and Hip, Knee, Ankle, Astragalar, Chopart's, Tarsus, Bunions and Toes. Abbreviation in the right-hand column are for: Stiffness, Fatigue, Aspirin, Grips, Joint Count and Sedimentation Rate.)

Fig. 26–3.—Rubber stamp for recording data on patient's chart.

as was shown by Mainland and Sutcliffe,[25] an Index combining the information provided by each item may prove statistically more significant than were any of its component items. Nevertheless, in drug trials each item should also be separately recorded and evaluated, as was done by Mainland and Sutcliffe[25] and by Clark and Mills,[6] since a trial drug might affect certain items more than others.

Although an index as described here has proved empirically useful in the management of an individual patient, where serial findings are always referable to the initial "baseline" findings, it is not the most sensitive way to handle such data in therapeutic trials. Mainland has clarified this point in a recent editorial.[25a] Rather than the fixed system of weighting of items described here, he advocates the use of the "discriminant function" of Fisher, where items that best discriminate between drug and placebo, or between two drugs, are weighted more heavily than those that do not. This statistical method can easily be employed using a desk calculator for up to 3 items. For summation of more than 3 items he advocated the use of a computer.

As evidence of the reliability of the indices, a comparison of 80 pairs of simultaneously obtained readings of the Systemic and Articular Indexes which are based on entirely different kinds of observation showed a good correlation ($r = .78$, $P < 0.01$);[20] also, serial records of both Indexes charted for many months showed a striking degree of parallelism in 75 per cent of cases.[19] In addition, a study of intra- and inter-observer error among experienced clinicians indicated coefficients of 0.11[22] and 0.13[23] respectively (Fig. 26–4).

In sum, both a numerical Index and its component items are useful. But they are never mutually exclusive. In certain situations, one may be more useful than the other.

Prospects for Agreement on Methodology

There is probably no good reason for universal acceptance of any "system" of evaluation, for this implies near-perfection of such a system. The accompanying rigidity might make further progress more difficult. Agreement by various observers and clinics on methodology for evaluation in a given trial using a given therapy is, of course, essential.

Certain criteria seem to have gained wide acceptance, and will probably be used for a long time. The duration of morning stiffness, grip strength, number

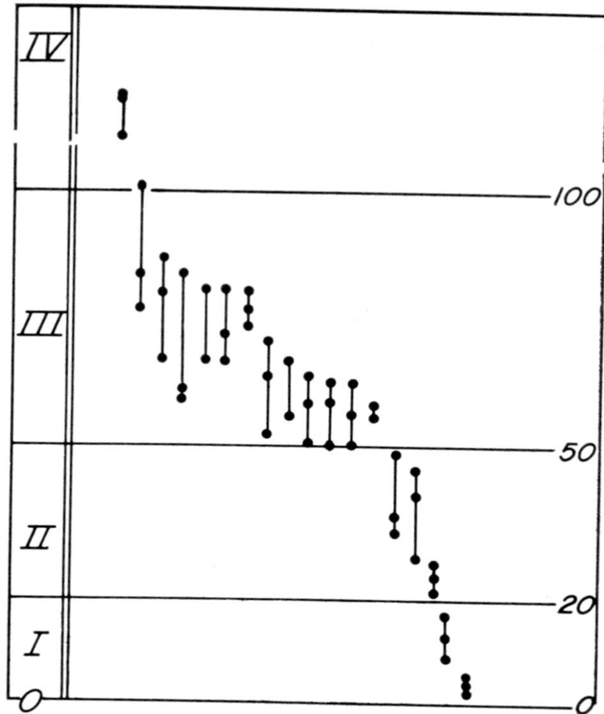

Fig. 26–4.—A study of interobserver variations with the activity index. The above chart shows the degree of interobserver variation found when three expert observers examined each of 18 patients at intervals of one week. The vertical lines join three points, each of which represents the Activity Index as determined by a different observer. The length of the vertical lines indicates the degree of variation which is due partly to observer error and partly to weekly fluctuations in rheumatoid activity. The variations must be viewed as segments on a scale of 0 to 150 or more points or as Grades 0-I-II-III-IV.

of tender joints, time to walk 50 feet, sedimentation rate, and serial roentgenograms seem to be employed in most trials. My personal bias would add measurement of circumference of proximal interphalangeal joints using a jewelers tape graduated in millimeters, and quantitative pain threshold measurements.

Marked discrepancies between criteria do occur, such as that noted between sedimentation rate and radiologic evidence of progression in the recent controlled trial of cyclophosphamide conducted by the ARA combined clinics.[8b] Here, the sedimentation rate responded little to treatment but the development of new erosions was strikingly reduced. One is forced to the conclusion that with an effective drug, evaluation in a controlled trial is relatively easy using ordinary criteria and looking at them separately; conversely, evaluation of the effectiveness of weakly potent drugs is difficult to determine because of the high natural "background" fluctuation in disease activity. Thus the effects of indomethacin, salicylate and placebo could not be distinguished even when the most sensitive technique of summing up all available data, *i.e.*, the Fisher discriminant functions analysis, was used.[8a]

Another point worth noting is the length of time that a patient or group of patients needs be followed on treatment with a given drug in order to determine efficacy depends on the nature of the drug itself. Thus efficacy can be seen with aspirin or adrenocorticosteroids within one week, whereas gold, antimalarials, and cytotoxic drugs require many weeks or months before clearly detectable effects are manifest.

Value of Serial Roentgenograms

Although radiograms are not often helpful in early diagnosis of rheumatoid arthritis, they do represent an easily obtainable, easily standardized, permanent record of destructive joint changes. Chapter 7 contains a detailed discussion of criteria for radiologic evaluation. This examination is an important one, because retardation, or even reversal, of bony erosions and joint space narrowing is good evidence that a given therapeutic agent is effective. Such evidence was particularly striking in the recently reported ARA cooperating clinics trials of cyclophosphamide.[8b] The effect of the drug in preventing radiologic progression was more striking than was its effect on the clinical parameters measured.

STAGE OF STRUCTURAL OR ANATOMICAL DAMAGE

Until now we have devoted all our attention to methods for evaluating the inflammatory *activity* of rheumatoid arthritis. We now turn to consider means for recording the structural damage caused by, or associated with, this activity. In so doing, we enter a comparatively tranquil field where changes in opinion occur slowly, if at all, and concerning which there is already considerable agreement and far less controversy. However, with an increasing awareness of the importance of long-range studies on the course of the disease, the need for accurate reporting of structural changes is becoming more apparent. Also, agreement on grading anatomical change is desirable for categorizing groups of cases to be used in therapeutic trials.

A review of items listed under Category D in Table 26–1 will indicate that the problem is not a simple one. Up to now attention has been mainly confined to a consideration of anatomical changes in the musculoskeletal system and scant attention has been paid to lesions in other systems. It will be seen that many of these are important, particularly vascular lesions as seen in the malignant phase of rheumatoid arthritis, as well as ocular and renal lesions or general disturbances, such as amyloidosis. However, granting the importance of these extra-articular lesions, from a practical clinical point of view, we must have some measure of crippling or impairment of musculoskeletal structures. The only scheme which has attained any measure of acceptance for the categorization of the anatomical stage of the disease is that put forward by Steinbrocker, Traeger and Batterman[36] where it forms the first part of their system. Their criteria for the four stages are given in Table 26–6.

The wide acceptance which this scheme has attained testifies to its utility. However, recent studies on interobserver agreement have turned up an unexpected degree of error. Since the scheme relied heavily on x-ray findings, Kellgren's studies[18] on interobserver error in judging roentgenograms must also be taken into consideration. However, the main difficulty is that cases are classified according to the status of the worst joint, which is, by definition, not representative of the other joints. We see no way out of this dilemma because it would be impractical to x-ray all the involved joints.

Some attempts have been made to sum up the total impairment of range of motion in all affected joints. Here goniometry (measurement of angles of greatest flexion, extension, etc.) is satisfactory, although its usefulness in judging minor changes in activity has been seriously questioned. However, the greatest obstacle to the widespread use of goniometry is not its lack of accuracy but the large amount of time required to assay the range of motion of all joints. Even an expertly trained physiotherapist needs a full half hour for this procedure, and, obviously, a busy clinician cannot fit this extra procedure into his routine.

Table 26-6.—A. R. A. Anatomical Stages[36]

Stage I, Early
- *1. No destructive changes roentgenologically.
- 2. Roentgenologic evidence of osteoporosis may be present.

Stage II, Moderate
- *1. Roentgenologic evidence of osteoporosis, with or without slight bone destruction; slight cartilage destruction may be present.
- *2. No joint deformities, although limitation of joint mobility may be present.
- 3. Adjacent muscle atrophy.
- 4. Extra-articular soft tissue lesions, such as nodules and tenovaginitis, may be present.

Stage III, Severe
- *1. Roentgenologic evidence of cartilage and bone destruction, in addition to osteoporosis.
- *2. Joint deformity, such as subluxation, ulnar deviation or hyperextension, without fibrous or bony ankylosis.
- 3. Extensive muscle atrophy.
- 4. Extra-articular soft tissue lesions, such as nodules and tenovaginitis, may be present.

Stage IV, Terminal
- *1. Fibrous or bony ankylosis.
- 2. Criteria of stage III.

* The criteria prefaced by an asterisk are those which must be present to permit classification of a patient in any particular stage or grade.

If facilities are available for goniometry, a numerical method is available for summing up the findings. At the National Institute for Arthritis and Metabolic Diseases an "Index of Range of Motion" is used which has been found to give satisfactorily repeatable results.[4] The motion in all planes of peripheral joints is recorded, but, for practical reasons, finger and toe motions are omitted. Joint size is not taken into consideration. The observed range of motion, in degrees, is then added up and expressed as a percentage of normal range of motion. The resulting Index is therefore a deficit percentage so that the figure decreases with improvement of joint function.

Detailed methods for evaluation of structural and functional status of the rheumatoid hand have been proposed by Flatt[12a] and by Swanson, Mays and Yamuchi;[36a] a less detailed rapid method with standardization by a vigorous item-by-item statistical analysis has been described recently by Treuhaft, Lewis, and McCarty.[37a] The advantages of this method in addition to speed (about 20 minutes are needed per patient), are that the inter- and intraobserver errors are known. Similar methods for structural and functional evaluation are needed for other areas of the body such as forefoot and knee, that are both commonly afflicted by the disease and commonly subjected to surgery. The proof of any method ultimately rests on its (1) utility (will people use it?), (2) sensitivity (does it discriminate?), (3) reliability (is it reproducible?), and validity (does what it measures really matter?).

A Look at the Future of Clinical Estimation of Rheumatic Activity

It may be possible that the era of the "automated" drug trial is dawning. Nuclides that result in visualization of inflamed joints such as technetium^{99m} provide a totally objective method of evaluation. Dick *et al.* have compared the peak count rate per minute over an inflamed knee after injection of a standard dose of ^{99m}Tc obtained when the patient was on indomethacin, salicylate and placebo. Even this relatively crude quantification of nuclide localization provided data that were as discriminatory as such clinical measurements as grip strength, joint size, and articular index.[10a] While data such as these may be expensive to obtain, they will be a bargain if they are free of subjective bias on the part of both observer and patient.

In the future, the work of evaluating both Activity and Structural Damage will no doubt be carried forward and present-day methods will be further refined and standardized. To potential workers in this field we point out that making a plausible suggestion is easy, but to put the suggestion on a solid basis of proved utility is usually the work of years.

BIBLIOGRAPHY

1. Bayles, T. B. and Hall, M. G.: New Engl. J. Med., *228*, 418, 1942.
2. Bepler, C. R.: Unpublished study.
3. Bepler, C. R. *et al.*: Arth. and Rheum., *2*, 403, 1959.
4. Black, R. L. *et al.*: Arth. and Rheum., *3*, 112, 1960.
5. Calkins, E.: Committee report to A. R. A. Membership June 1962. (Unpublished.)
6. Clark, G. M. and Mills, D.: Arth. and Rheum., *5*, 156, 1962.
7. Cobb, S. *et al.*: Penna. Med. J., *57*, 37, 1954.
8. Cohen, A. S. and Calkins, E.: Arth. and Rheum., *1*, 297, 1958.

8*a*. Cooperating Clinics Committee of Amer. Rheum. Assoc.: Clin. Pharmacol. & Therapeut., *8*, 11, 1967.

8*b*. ———: New Engl. J. Med., *283*, 883, 1970.

9. Copeman, W. S. C.: Personal communication.
10. Decker, B. *et al.*: Arth. and Rheum. *3*, 49, 1960.

10*a*. Dick, W. C., Grayson, M. F., Woodburn, A., Nuki, G. and Buchanan, W. W.: Ann. Rheum. Dis., *29*, 643, 1970.

11. Eccles, M. V.: Brit. J. Phys. Med., *19*, 5, 1956.
12. Empire Rheumatism Council: Ann. Rheum. Dis., *14*, 353, 1957.

12*a*. Flatt, A. E.: *Rheumatoid Hand Research Project* (Booklets), Iowa City, Univ. of Iowa Dept. Orthopedics, 1963.

13. Hart, F. D. and Clark, C. J. M.: Lancet, *1*, 775, 1951.
14. Hollander, J. L. and Young, D. G.: Arth. and Rheum., *6*, 277, 1963.
15. Holmdahl, D. E. and Ingelmark, B. E.: Acta. Med. Scand., Suppl., *170*, 568, 1946.
16. Jansen, H.: Acta Rheum., *2*, 22, 1930.
17. ———: Acta Med. Scand., *74*, 353, 1931.
18. Kellgren, J. H. and Lawrence, J. S.: Ann. Rheum. Dis., *16*, 485, 1957.
19. Lansbury, J.: Arth. and Rheum., *1*, 505, 1958.
20. Lansbury, J. and Free, S. M., Jr.: Amer. J. Med. Sci., *233*, 375, 1957.
21. Lansbury, J. and Haut, D. D.: Amer. J. Med. Sci., *232*, 150, 1956.
22. Lansbury, J. and Menduke, H.: Arth. and Rheum., *6*, 353, 1963.
23. Lansbury, J. *et al.*: Arth. and Rheum., *5*, 445, 1962.
24. Lowman, E. W.: Arth. and Rheum., *1*, 38, 1958.
25. Mainland, D. and Sutcliffe, M. I.: Bulletin of Rheum. Dis., *13*, 287, 1962.

25*a*. Mainland, D.: Arth. & Rheum., *10*, 71, 1967.

26. Mandel, L.: Can. Med. Assoc. J., *74*, 515, 1956.
27. McCarty, D. J. and Gatter, R. A.: Arth. & Rheum., *9*, 325, 1966.

27*a*. McCarty, D. J., Gatter, R. A. and Phelps, P.: Arth. and Rheum., *8*, 551, 1965.

27*b*. McCarty, D. J., Gatter, R. A. and Steele, A. D.: Arth. & Rheum., *11*, 696, 1968.

28. Med. Res. Council and Nuffield Foundn.: Brit. Med. J., *1*, 1223, 1954.
29. Mikkelsen, W. M.: Unpublished study.
30. Savage, O.: *A Symposium on Clinical Trials*, Pfizer Ltd., p. 34, Apl. 25, 1958.
31. Shetlar, M. R. *et al.*: J. Lab. Clin. Med., *48*, 194, 1956.
32. Smukler, N. M. *et al.*: Arth. and Rheum., *7*, 344, 1964.
33. Smyth, C. J. *et al.*: Exhibit at 107th Ann. Meeting, of A. M. A., 1958.

34. Smyth, C. J., Velayos, E. E. and Hlad, C. J.: Acta. Rheum. Scand., *9*, 293, 1963.

34*a*. Steinbrocker, O.: Arch. Phys. Med., *30*, 289, 1949.

35. Steinbrocker, O. and Blazer, A.: New Engl. J. Med., *235*, 501, 1946.

36. Steinbrocker, O., Traeger, C. H. and Batterman, R. C.: J.A.M.A., *140*, 659, 1949.

36*a*. Swanson, A. B., Mays, J. D. and Yamuchi, Y.: Surg. Clin. North America, *48*, 1003, 1968.

37. Taylor, D.: Can. Med. Assoc. J., *36*, 608, 1937.

37*a*. Treuhaft, P. S., Lewis, M. R., McCarty, D. J.: Arth. & Rheum., *14*, 75, 1971.

38. Vaughn, P. R., Howell, D. S. and Keim, I. M.: Arth. and Rheum., *2*, 213, 1959.

39. Wright, V.: Clin. Sci., *18*, 17, 1959.

40. Wright, V. and Johns, R. J.: Arth. and Rheum., *3*, 328, 1960.

PART IV

Basic and Drug Treatment of Rheumatoid Arthritis

Editor: RICHARD H. FREYBERG, M.D.

Preface to Parts IV and V

These sections deal with the treatment of rheumatoid arthritis. In the separate chapters the opinion of experts concerning each form of treatment is set forth and should be helpful as a guide in using these individual treatment procedures. The practicing physician, however, has an *additional* important problem of *combining* many modalities and factors of treatment into a complete management program. He needs to select from the assortment of available analgesic and suppressive agents the ones best suited for his patient. He must have definite objectives of treatment in mind. Long-range management for rheumatoid arthritis often can be best accomplished by *teamwork* of experts in various medical and paramedical specialties as outlined below, whenever indicated and available.

Chapter 27

Conservative Management of Rheumatoid Arthritis

BY EPHRAIM P. ENGLEMAN, M.D.

CHOICE of treatment for rheumatoid arthritis is a particular challenge to the physician. The unknown etiology of the disease and the multiplicity of its manifestations have given rise to modes of therapy as numerous and diverse as the concepts of its pathogenesis. The disease is characterized by spontaneous remissions and exacerbations, making evaluation of treatment extremely difficult. So-called specific agents may be effective in reducing the symptoms and signs of rheumatoid arthritis, sometimes to a dramatic and deceiving degree. Unfortunately, the risks are often great and the eventual course of the disease probably unaltered by their use. All evidence to date indicates that conservative management offers a long-term prognosis at least no worse than that of more spectacular measures. Because none of these latter measures is in any way curative, a conservative approach should be the method of first choice.

Once the diagnosis of rheumatoid arthritis has been established, every thought is directed toward maximal control of the disease at minimal risk. The primary objectives are to reduce inflammation and pain, preserve function, and prevent deformity. To effect this, a simple regimen, comprised of rest, physical therapy, and salicylates would appear to afford the soundest basis for rehabilitating the patient without trading existing problems for others which may be even more devastating. In any event, these measures are so basically necessary as to warrant their continuation even when more heroic steps must be taken. In other words, this simple regimen to be outlined is considered the "basic program" of treatment, to which other treatment is *added*, if necessary.

Often, the patient's own attitude is the strongest deterrent to conservative care, for he may resist all suggestions that are based on time and waiting. He has read about the latest "cures"—or he knows someone whose arthritis "disappeared after three injections"—and he obviously expects his doctor to dispense the magic medicine without further ado. In an era of medical miracles, this attitude is an increasing threat to intelligent treatment of chronic disease. The physician must, despite all importuning, disabuse the patient of "sure cure" credence. In special circumstances, however, the physician may eventually elect to employ steps to provide more immediate symptomatic relief. A man whose job is in jeopardy because of his illness, or a woman whose household is in complete and uncontrollable disruption because of her disability, may require more definitive measures; potent therapeutic agents, with all their attending threats, can hold no terror akin to that of economic and domestic disaster. Fortunately, most persons can manage to resolve their socioeconomic situation long enough to give the conservative program a fair trial.

BASIC PROGRAM

The conservative management of rheumatoid arthritis includes the following major therapeutic considerations: systemic and emotional rest, articular rest including orthopedic supports, physical therapy, analgesic drugs, and proper nutrition.

Systemic Rest

As indicated previously, the unpredictable features of rheumatoid arthritis make it extremely difficult to appraise the true effect of any given therapy. However, there is a preponderance of empirical evidence for the benefits of systemic rest.[13] The term "arthritis" is somewhat of a misnomer implying involvement limited to the joints. That rheumatoid arthritis is a systemic disease with widely divergent manifestations is well established. Rest can certainly be considered the common therapeutic denominator being without contraindications, treating as it does the person as a whole. It behooves the physician, therefore, to institute rest, in some measure, immediately upon diagnosis of active disease, regardless of manifestations. Additional treatment is dependent upon the type and severity of these manifestations.

The amount of daily rest must be decided for each patient. Complete bed rest, without even lavatory privileges, may be desirable and even imperative, particularly in patients with profound systemic and articular involvement. This is usually unnecessary, however.[7a] In mild disease, two to four hours of rest each day may suffice, allowing the patient to continue his work by restricting only his avocational activities. The feeling of stiffness which may follow a rest period ("gelling") should not influence the amount of rest, being more apparent at the beginning, but diminishing with the continuation of the rest program. (The equally important, concomitant exercise program is referred to later.) A patient often becomes discouraged and apprehensive when rest leaves him "stiff in every joint"; unless the physician stresses the transient nature of this and the vital importance of rest, the patient may begin to "cheat" and surreptitiously push activity despite pain and fatigue, lest he become "permanently stiff."

The duration of the rest program naturally depends upon the patient's course. In general, the prescribed rest should be continued until remission has occurred or until significant subjective and objective improvement has become stabilized. After improvement has become sustained for at least two weeks, the regimen may be liberalized; however, the process of restoring physical activity must proceed gradually and with appropriate support for any involved weight-bearing joints (see below). Recrudescence or increase in signs of active disease should serve as warning to retard the rate of physical restoration.

A conservative program of any magnitude immediately poses the problem of where it can best be carried out. If adequate facilities for care are available, and if the atmosphere is tranquil and the family cooperative, the patient may do quite well at home. However, the disadvantages may be great and the demands sometimes insurmountable if the patient is on complete bed rest. Such a person, invalided in the midst of well people, may exhaust himself in his efforts to carry on socially, from his bed, with family and visitors. The frustrations and tensions he becomes prey to can seriously deter his recovery. He may become too dependent or he may become hostile to all help. The advantages of hospitalization are self-evident, particularly as regards a regimen requiring much supervision and attention. Improvement often occurs after admission to the hospital even though the basic program is unaltered. Freed of extraneous problems, the patient may enjoy some immediate subjective improvement and be more receptive to the realities of his disease. When he is perforce removed from his environment, he is more apt to be honest with the doctor, especially in matters that might otherwise have precipitated decisions he was not prepared to face, such as taking time off work and curtailing activities. Nevertheless, the choice between home and hospital must be tempered by circumstances. Financial consideration usually must come first and is reason enough for electing home care. Also, few hospitals are geared to care for arthritics on a long-term basis. (Regrettably, there is virtually no sanatorium care available in the United States for patients with rheumatoid arthritis.) Regardless of the considerations involved, however, it is incumbent upon the physician to stress the importance of systemic rest.

From the *pros* and *cons* of hospital and home management has evolved a very satisfactory system of intermittent hospitalization for patients with severe disease.[3] The patient is hospitalized initially and given the benefit of a rigid regimen for a week or two. If he does well, he is released to his home to carry out the program in which he has been instructed. Provided he continues to improve, or sustains his improvement, and if the home situation is tenable for all concerned, he does not return to the hospital until the physician deems it time to reappraise his status. Relatively short periods of hospitalization, alternated with longer ones of home care, have proved very effective both physically and emotionally.

Emotional Rest

The importance of emotional factors in rheumatoid arthritis and the need for psychologic support cannot be overemphasized, yet, formal psychiatric management is rarely necessary or even successful. In a disease that can be an emotional as well as physical crisis, with each militating against the other, a good rapport between the patient and his own doctor is the ideal situation. In this, the doctor must be prepared to go more than half way, for it is a rare patient who fully understands himself in relation to his illness. It falls to the physician to steer him between the Scylla of unrealistic hope and the Charybdis of unwarranted despair.

Emotional rest is only one of the many facets of therapy, but it must be supervised as constantly and judiciously as any measures for physical support; motivation can sag easily if not propped with continual reassurance, and it is so important to appreciate that without the patient's will to improve the program is doomed to failure. An understanding of the patient's personality and his emotional reactions to his illness (and to all the exigencies of his life) allows the doctor to guide him in his present problems and to anticipate many others. A physician arms both himself and his patient when he takes the time to explain candidly, and in lay terms, the nature of the disease, its treatment, limitations, and prognosis.[10] Complete honesty, unshakable equanimity, unremitting patience in answering questions, and obvious willingness to keep his patient completely informed not only inspire confidence, but do much to rout the "misunderstood" feeling which so often leads to doctor-shopping.

If tenseness and emotional unrest are real problems in a patient's management, and particularly if insomnia results, the prudent use of phenobarbital or other barbiturate may be indicated. The newer tranquilizers and "muscle relaxants" are prescribed these days with an alarming abandon and such drugs as meprobamate, phenothiazines and others have been widely touted by the pharmaceutical firms. However, there is no convincing clinical evidence that any of these has any specific beneficial action on rheumatoid arthritis, nor any advantage over the time-tested barbiturates, properly administered.

Articular Rest

Experience dictates that decrease of articular inflammation may be expedited by adequate rest. Articular rest is accomplished by bed rest (in the case of weight-bearing joints) and may be further enhanced by appropriate, simple orthopedic supports or splints.[12] Splints are of particular value in the presence of deformity, whether such deformity be due to the flexor muscle spasm and pain resulting from inflammation, as in early, acute disease, or from the soft-tissue contractures of subacute or chronic disease. The purpose of splints is not only to provide rest for inflamed joints, but also to relieve spasm and thus pain, and to prevent deformities or to reduce deformities already present. Such supports include plaster splints or shells for the hands and wrists, knees, and ankles; sling with or without a swathe for shoulders; and Russell-type suspension for hips (*see* Chapter 37).

Usually the best splints are simple ones which may be made by the physician from readily available plaster of Paris. Certain general rules may be helpful in their preparation and use. When flexion deformity resulting from muscle spasm of acute disease is present, the initial shape of the cast or brace should be such as to allow the extremity to be in a position of comfort and, if need be, deformity. Forceful extension will only aggravate flexor muscle spasm and pain. As muscle spasm and flexion deformity decrease, the shape of the splint is altered (usually once every week or two) so as to improve the position of the joint. The use of adjustable casts or braces obviates the necessity of making new supports as the deformity subsides (Figs. 27–1 and 27–2). In chronic disease where soft-tissue contractures have already occurred, correction is obtained (without trauma) by taking up the slack which occurs after ligaments and muscles have been held for a week or so at their limit of extensibility without tension. Here again, one should avoid forceful pressure against tight structures, for this will cause pain and resistive muscle spasm.

These orthopedic supports must be removable to permit daily motion and exercise of the affected extremities (*see* below). Casts should be bivalved; solid casts are contraindicated. Exclusive of the daily periods of exercise (which will increase in duration and frequency as the activity of the disease decreases), splints should be worn as much as possible and especially during the sleeping hours when unguarded motion may be painful and involuntary flexion tends to increase.

When ambulation is started, care must be taken to avoid such weight-bearing as will aggravate the flexion deformities. This can be accomplished with the aid of supports such as crutches and braces until the tendency to contracture has subsided. It is important that the brace or a light plaster shell be worn at night during the early stages of ambulation. Foot pads made of sponge rubber and leather, and metatarsal bars may be the source of much symptomatic relief if ample and properly-fitted shoes are worn (*see also* Chapter 78 for details).

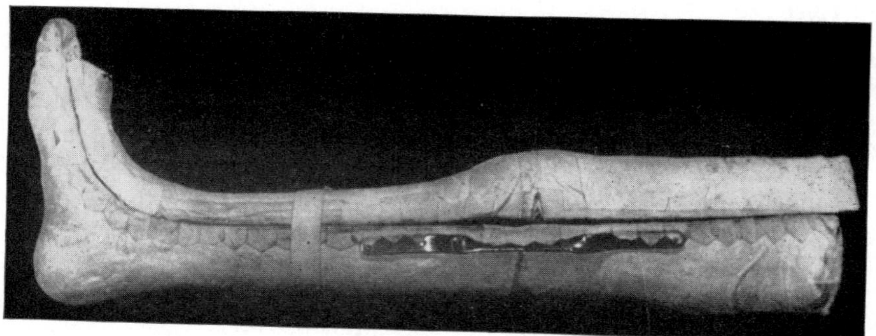

Fig. 27–1.—Anterior and posterior shells of leg cast with bendable strip "hinges" in position of optimal correction. (Rhinelander and Ropes, courtesy of Jour. Bone and Joint Surg.)

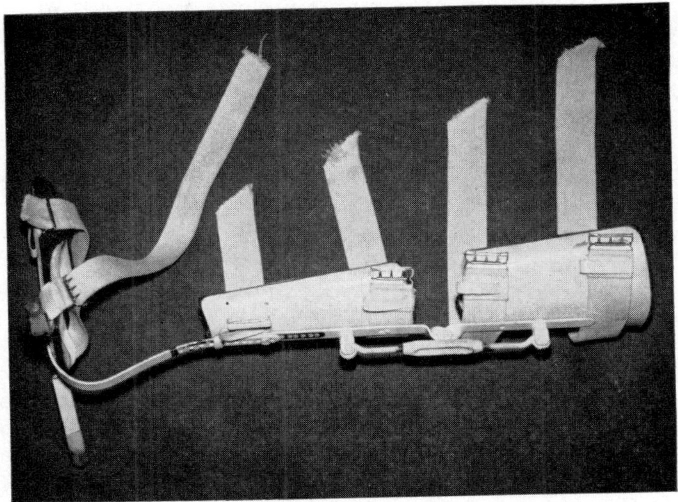

FIG. 27–2.—Relaxing Knee Brace: designed for the conservative treatment of knee flexion contracture. The degree of flexion or extension is controlled behind the knee. The thigh and calf cuffs, and foot plate, support the extremity. Length is adjustable. An outrigger on the foot plate prevents rotation of the leg. (Courtesy of William S. Cappeller.)

Physical Therapy

The most important modality in the physical therapy of rheumatoid arthritis is exercise.[16] *Indeed, the conservative program is based on the concomitant administration of rest and therapeutic exercise, always in proper balance* (*see also* Chapter 34).

Therapeutic exercises are designed to preserve joint motion, muscular strength and endurance. Most effective in the maintenance or improvement of range of motion are exercises of the active-assistive variety. These should be performed, within the limits of pain, from the very beginning of management. The duration and frequency of such exercises should be limited not by an increase of pain experienced during, but that persisting after the completion of, the exercises. Pain lasting more than an hour or two after exercise usually indicates that the exercise was too vigorous and should be decreased in amount, but *not* discontinued. As tolerance for exercise is increased, and as the activity of the disease subsides, progressive resistive exercises are most effective in the improvement of muscular function. The exercise program should be part of the patient's daily activities, whether in the hospital or at home, until muscular and joint function have recovered and remission of the disease has occurred.

Another useful modality is heat, which is used primarily for its muscle-relaxing and analgesic effects. Luminous or moist heat is generally most satisfactory; the ambulatory patient will find warm tub baths most convenient. Exercise may be better performed after exposure to heat (*see* Chapter 34 for details). A most helpful guide to physical therapy will be found in "Home Care in Rheumatoid Arthritis," a booklet published by The Arthritis Foundation, 1212 Avenue of the Americas, New York City.

Analgesic Drugs

Successful management of patients with rheumatoid arthritis depends, among other things, upon relief of pain. That certain general measures and physical support of joints contribute to the comfort of the patient has been iterated above. But the most effective measure in the relief of pain is the judicious use of analgesic drugs of which the salicylic acid derivatives—acetyl salicylic acid (aspirin) and sodium salicylate—are the choice.[4] If there is universal agreement concerning the usefulness of any therapeutic measure in rheumatoid arthritis it is in the efficacy of these drugs. Relatively free of undesirable effects and inexpensive, they provide many patients with excellent relief of pain and stiffness. There is evidence, furthermore, that salicylates exert an anti-inflammatory effect on the synovitis of rheumatoid arthritis[5a] (*see* Chapter 28 for fuller discussion of aspirin therapy).

It may be helpful to supplement salicylates with still other analgesic drugs, such as dextro-propoxyphene (Darvon) or ethoheptazine citrate (Zactirin). Codeine in a bedtime dose of 30 mg. ($\frac{1}{2}$ grain) should be reserved for patients with severe nocturnal pain. Other narcotics should not be used. If such analgesics are not effective in making pain at least tolerable, more potent agents as outlined in Chapter 30 or 31 may be indicated.

Adequate Nutrition

The diet for the rheumatoid arthritic patient should be well balanced and adjusted to meet each individual's requirements There is no specific food known to be contraindicated and, provided the dietary intake is normal, there is usually no need to use supplemental vitamins. Although patients with rheumatoid arthritis require only an optimal or ideal diet, it is often of considerable practical importance to see that the patient is actually given such a diet and eats it. Practical dietary guidelines will be found in "Diet and Arthritis," another handbook for patients published by The Arthritis Foundation.

The anemia of rheumatoid arthritis does not respond to hematinic agents. Whole-blood transfusions are indicated for patients with marked anemia, despite the hazard of homologous serum jaundice. Significant iron deficiency is not unusual following long-term loss of microscopic amounts of blood per rectum associated with the prolonged use of salicylates. Iron salts given orally are helpful in such cases.

RESULTS

Faith in the long-term results of conservative management has been instilled largely by the observations of Bauer and his associates at the Massachusetts General Hospital. In one of their reports,[15] a series of 250 unselected patients receiving this type of care were observed for periods ranging from six months to sixteen years (average, 9.6 years).[15] At the time of this report, improvement was observed in 133 patients (53 per cent), 38 of whom were in complete remission (15 per cent of the total group). The disease was stationary in 32 (13 per cent) and worse in 85 (34 per cent). In a similar series of 374 patients followed by Ragan from five to twenty years (average, eleven years), 48 per cent were in remission or markedly improved.[11] Duthie observed the status of 282 patients observed for a shorter interval (average, two years) and reported 71 per cent improved.[2] Such results compare favorably with the so-called definitive agents, gold and corticoids.[1,5,7,8,9,14] Conservative management, or any other therapy, may not alter the course of the disease. Difficulties in early diagnosis of rheumatoid arthritis, the lack of untreated controls, and, as heretofore mentioned, the unpredictable spontaneous variations in the course of the disease make evaluation of any mode of therapy difficult. The comparable percentages of patients showing improvement under a disparate variety of treatment could be no more than an expression of the natural course of the disease.

Conclusion

In the welter of conflicting ideas concerning the management of rheumatoid arthritis, one cogent point can give both physician and patient pause before resorting to measures over and above those dictated by conservatism: there is no definite evidence that the natural progression of the disease is altered by *any* of the available types of therapy. However, much can be done to reduce pain, preserve function, and deter and even prevent deformities. *Those measures*, then, *which accomplish* this and allow *maximal alleviation at minimal risk are most desirable.* The physician's own acceptance of this *credo* is a necessary factor to its success, for it is he who, more than any family member or friend, inspires the patient's cooperation. *His* faith is his patient's courage. It is not surprising that results of the simple, conservative regimen appear to be best in those patients whose physicians, steadfastly convinced of the efficacy of such management, are bulwarks of strength, both medically and emotionally, to their patients.

BIBLIOGRAPHY

1. Bunim, J. J., Ziff, M. and McEwen, C.: Bull. Rheumat. Dis., *5*, 73, 1954.
2. Duthie, J. J. R., Thompson, M., Weir, M. M. and Fletcher, W. R.: Ann. Rheumat. Dis., *14*, 133, 1955.
3. Engleman, E. P.: Unpublished data.
4. Engleman, E. P., Weinberger, H. J., Sacasa, C. F., Headley, N. E., Davison, R., Mettier, S. R. and Rhinelander, F. W.: Calif. Med., *82*, 367, 1955.
5. Engleman, E. P., Krupp, M. A., Saunders, W. W., Wilson, L. E. and Fredell, E. W.: Calif. Med., *80*, 369, 1954.

5a. Fremont-Smith, K. and Bayles, T. B.: Arth. and Rheum., **7**, 309, 1964.

6. Goodman, L. S. and Gilman, A.: *The Pharmacological Basis of Therapeutics*, 2nd Ed., New York, Macmillan Company, 1955, p. 285.
7. Howell, D. and Ragan, C.: Medicine, *35* 83, 1956.

7a. Mills, J. A., Pinals, R. S., Ropes, M. W., Short, C. L. and Sutcliffe, J.: New Engl. J. Med., *284*, 453, 1971.

8. Ragan, C. and Tyson, T. L.: Am. J. Med., *1*, 252, 1946.
9. Ragan, C.: Bull. New York Acad. Med., *27*, 63, 1951.
10. ———: J. Chronic Dis., *1*, 253, 1955.
11. ———: J.A.M.A., *141*, 124, 1949.
12. Rhinelander, F. W.: Arth. and Rheum., *2*, 270, 1959.
13. Ropes, M. W.: J. Chronic Dis., *5*, 697, 1957.
14. Short, C. L., Beckman, W. W., and Bauer, W.: New Engl. J. Med., *253*, 404, 1955.
15. Short, C. L. and Bauer, W.: New Engl. J. Med., *238*, 142, 1948.
16. Smyth, C. J., *et al.*: Ann. Int. Med., *50*, 366, 1959; *50*, 634, 1959.

Chapter 28

Salicylate Therapy for Rheumatoid Arthritis

By Theodore B. Bayles, M.D.

Since the days of Hippocrates, Celsus, Pliny, and Galen bitter material, used medicinally, has been extracted from the barks and roots of various bushes and trees. The medicinal value of the bark of the willow (Latin, *Salix*) was first noted in 1763 by the Reverend Edward Stone in a communication to the Royal Society. He revealed that the bark of the willow was useful, particularly "where agues chiefly abound," and concluded that extract of willow bark was useful in the treatment of human ills such as agues, fevers, abscesses and fluxes. Thereafter, the willow bark was used primarily as an antipyretic and only by accident in rheumatism. Even in these early years in England the willow bark had to compete with the poplar bark and the Peruvian or Jesuits' bark which yielded quinine. As Copeman[5] has stated, "The barks of the willow and the poplar trees were found to yield a substance which was an antipyretic and useful as a bitter—and bitters were popular in those days for medicinal purposes. (Until the world-shattering invention of angostura bitters, during the last century, the poplar bark was also used for flavoring drinks, salicin being the active principle—as quinine is, I believe, of its successor)." In 1876 MacLagan of Glasgow first described in *Lancet* the definitive use of salicylates in rheumatic diseases. He used salicin extracted from the bark of the willow and invoked the Doctrine of Signatures which would suggest that plants and trees which grew in damp areas would be the logical source of a cure for complaints which were made worse by dampness and cold. After MacLagan's excellent description of the clinical treatment of rheumatic fever with salicin, salicylates have been used for rheumatic conditions. Synthetic acetylsalicylic acid (hereinafter aspirin) was introduced to medicine in 1899 and has been with us since. Approximately 30 tons are used in the United States every day, so that it behooves physicians to be knowledgeable about this analgesic, anti-inflammatory and antinociceptive medicament.

CHEMISTRY

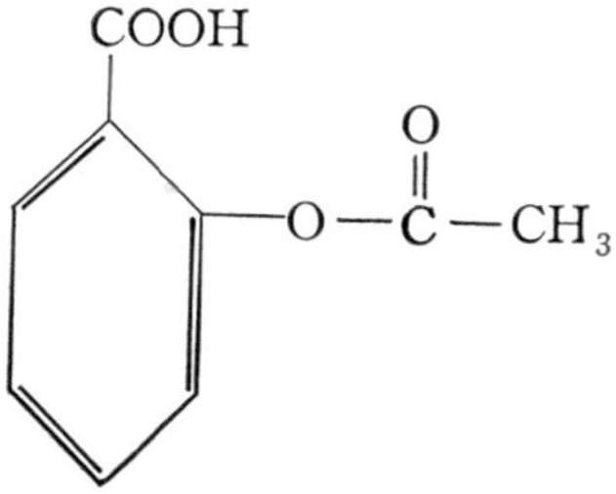

COOH

O—C(=O)—CH_3

Fig. 28–1.—Acetylsalicylic acid (aspirin).[12]

The salicylates now being used in medicine are produced almost exclusively by synthesis; the most common forms are acetylsalicylic acid and sodium salicylate. Aspirin is stable in dry air, but hydrolyzes in moist air to salicylic and acetic acids. The efficacy of the different salicylates depends partially on the amount of salicylic ion liberated in the body.

PHARMACOLOGY

Antipyresis.—Salicylates lower the body temperature in febrile patients, but rarely affect the temperature in a person who does not have fever. The salicylates act on the hypothalamic nuclei and regulate the peripheral mechanisms concerned with the production and loss of body heat. Heat dissipation results from increased peripheral blood flow and sweating in the presence of fever.

Analgesia.—Certain types of pain are alleviated by the action of salicylates on the central nervous system; the mechanism is not known, but the action in the central nervous system is thought to be subcortical. In addition, there is a blocking effect in the peripheral chemoreceptors. In rheumatic diseases and certainly in rheumatoid arthritis, the anti-inflammatory effect is important because the alleviation of the inflammation removes the irritation of the pain receptors. Salicylates are particularly useful in myalgia, arthralgia and musculoskeletal structures. In careful studies Beecher[3] found that 325 mg. of aspirin was equivalent to 32 mg. of codeine. Confusion, dizziness, tinnitus, high-tone deafness, delirium and coma may occur with high dosages. When more modest doses are used there may be hearing loss in decibels which is completely reversible in two or three days after withdrawal of the drug.[14] The nausea and vomiting caused by salicylate are largely of central origin, although there may be some gastric irritation of mucosal receptors. The nausea and vomiting of central nervous system origin usually develop at a plasma salicylate level of about 30 mg. per cent; local gastric irritation can occur at much lower levels of therapy.

Respiration.—Full therapeutic doses of salicylates increase oxygen consumption and CO_2 production in experimental animals and man.[16] This is primarily the result of salicylate-induced uncoupling of oxidative phosphorylation in skeletal muscles. When salicylate reaches the medulla, it directly stimulates the respiratory center and produces marked hyperventilation with an increase in depth and a pronounced increase in rate. Respiratory alkalosis ensues. Hyperventilation in man develops between 35 mg. per cent and 50 mg. per cent plasma salicylate levels. The response to respiratory alkalosis is renal excretion of bicarbonate accompanied by sodium and potassium. Plasma bicarbonate is lowered and the blood pH returns toward normal. As respiratory alkalosis continues, metabolic acidosis is produced at the same time. This occurs when respiratory depression from toxic doses of salicylates supervenes. Metabolic acidosis is caused by (1) the salicylic acid derivatives dissociating in blood; (2) the vasomotor depression causing lowering of renal function with accumulation of sulfuric and phosphoric acids and finally, (3) organic acids accumulating secondary to salicylate-induced derangement of carbohydrate metabolism, notably pyruvic, lactic and acetoacetic acids. A detailed description of these changes can be found in a symposium published in 1963.[19]

The Cardiovascular System.—Ordinary doses of salicylates have no important effect on cardiovascular action. However, the peripheral vessels tend to dilate after large doses due to direct effect on the smooth muscle. We have been able to demonstrate this directly in normal individuals; this increased peripheral blood flow may be beneficial in the treatment of rheumatic disease.[17] While salicylates are not injurious to the normal heart, large doses in the presence of rheumatic carditis can precipitate pulmonary edema and congestive heart failure by increasing cardiac output and work of the heart.[4]

Gastrointestinal Effects.—Originally it was assumed that salicylic acid was liberated from sodium salicylate by the acid in the stomach and that the liberated acid in turn irritated the mucous membrane of the stomach, but when *in vitro* experiments showed that suspensions of aspirin hydrolyzed *very slowly* in acidic conditions such as found in the stomach, it was suggested that aspirin was superior to sodium salicylate for this reason. Now it is known that aspirin is absorbed largely in the stomach and small intestine as intact aspirin and, while there are esterases in the plasma and other tissues capable of rapidly hydrolyzing the aspirin, appreciable quantities of aspirin (up to 25 per cent of the total salicylate) are found in the blood five to 15 minutes after a single oral dose.

In about 70 per cent of patients on maintenance salicylate therapy there is an average blood loss of about 4.3 ml. per day due to the direct irritating effect on the gastric mucosa;[10,18] in relatively rare instances acute intestinal hemorrhage has been associated with salicylate therapy.[1] In one group of 175 patients[9] and in another of 244 patients[2] with rheumatoid arthritis on prolonged salicylate therapy studies failed to support the idea that salicylate actually caused the anemia of rheumatoid arthritis. While Gibberd[9] showed that iron deficiency may play a role in the severe anemia of rheumatoid arthritis, it is well known that other mechanisms are involved in the usual anemia of rheumatoid arthritis.[6]

Kidney.—Serum uric acid levels are lowered by *large* doses of salicylates (4.0 gm. or more per day) because of interference with tubular resorption of uric acid; however, small doses of salicylates have been reported to increase serum uric acid levels.

Platelets and Bleeding.—For some years it has been thought that use of aspirin causes bleeding, but the effect on prothrombin time has not been consistent or significant. Recent work[3a] suggests that aspirin's effect on bleeding time and on hemostasis may be a direct action on platelet function. Platelet clumping is probably the first step in hemostasis, and can be induced by adenosine diphosphate (ADP). Aspirin blocks the release of platelet ADP, and aggregation is inhibited. Also, the ability of collagen particles to induce platelet aggregation is impaired by aspirin (and several other drugs). This action of aspirin is not shared by sodium salicylate.

Significantly lower than normal levels of ascorbic acid in platelets were found in rheumatoid arthritic patients on high doses of aspirin.[14a] It was felt that platelet levels of ascorbic acid were more accurate in reflecting depleted tissue stores than serum ascorbic acid levels, and aspirin seems to block uptake of ascorbic acid by platelets, so that patients receiving large doses of aspirin should have supplemental vitamin C.

A third group of studies showing effects of aspirin on platelets[18a] suggests that the drug inhibits the ability of platelets to produce prostaglandin, and inhibits the release of prostaglandin from the spleen. Such prostaglandins are implicated in the production of fever and inflammation, so it is suggested that this inhibition by aspirin could explain its anti-inflammatory activity.

METABOLISM OF SALICYLATES

The maximum blood level of combined free and protein-bound salicylate occurs about two and a half hours after the oral dose, and a 600 mg. dose can be detected in the blood for as long as 8 to 12 hours in the normal person. It should be noted, however, that after 48 hours no salicylate metabolites are found in the urine regardless of the longevity of prior salicylate therapy; this shows that aspirin is relatively quickly metabolized and excreted. As Levy[11] has pointed out, various mechanisms regulating salicylate blood levels after the administration of salicylate combinations are: "(1) dissolution rate, (2) gastric emptying time, (3) intrinsic absorption rate, (4) serum protein binding, (5) rate and extent of biotransformations, and (6) excretion rate." The aspirin blood level remains very low and does not ordinarily exceed 2 mg. per 100 millimeters at ordinary therapeutic doses, so while aspirin may provide analgesia for headache, there is no evidence that aspirin is more anti-inflammatory than non-acetylated salicylate.

The physician interested in treating rheumatic diseases is concerned with total blood levels and with the highest blood and tissue levels following administration of salicylate, and schedule of dosage which will maintain such significant levels. The most important factor in therapy presumably is the level of *free* salicylate (not bound to protein) at the site of inflammation or pain. Studies conducted in our clinic indicate that the lower concentration of albumin in blood of patients with rheumatoid arthritis binds quantitatively less salicylate, but it binds as well qualitatively as does plasma albumin of normal individuals. The three chief metabolic products of salicylate are the conjugates with glycine to form salicyluric acid and with glucuronic acid to produce the ether or phenolic glucuronide and the ester of acyl-glucuronide. In addition, a small amount is oxidized to gentisic acid and traces of di- or trihydroxybenzoic acids. Fremont-Smith[7] in our clinic, using a spectrophotometric method, has found that the urinary excretion of salicylate and its metabolites by patients with active rheumatoid arthritis does not differ qualitatively or quantitatively from that of control subjects under the same conditions of physical activity and urinary acidity. In clinical practice and investigation of salicylate excretion, it is important to remember that the excretion is little influenced by changes in the urinary pH on the acid side, but on the alkaline side, at pH 8.0, the mean clearance is about four times more than at pH 7.0. Therefore, sodium bicarbonate should not be prescribed with salicylate if one wants to maintain adequate therapeutic levels of salicylate in the patient under treatment.

Mode of Action of Salicylates.—During the 90 years since the introduction of synthetic preparations of salicylates, a voluminous literature has accumulated. Nevertheless, it is not possible to delineate a precise formulation as to mode of action for therapeutic benefit or for toxicity. For further information concerning basic studies of the metabolism, biochemical and immunological parameters, anti-inflammatory and other effects of salicylates, the proceedings of the international symposium held in London in 1962 is highly recommended.[5]

Toxicity.—The physiologic abnormalities of salicylate toxicity in infants and children have been reported by Segar and Halliday.[15] A summary of complications and toxicity associated with various levels of salicylate administration is presented herein (Figure 28–2).[13]

Many allergic manifestations, including asthmas most commonly, angioneurotic edema rarely, and very uncommonly anaphylactic shock, rhinorrhea, urticaria, and purpura, have been caused by aspirin sensitivity. The clinical history seems to be the only satisfactory method of diagnosing aspirin allergy, and it is unknown why these patients are not sensitive to other salicylate-containing compounds.

Anti-inflammatory Effect of Salicylates on Rheumatoid Arthritis.—Salicylates are the most universally used therapeutic agent in rheumatoid arthritis. The fact that they are analgesic and also antiphlogistic, or anti-inflammatory, has been widely accepted by experienced clinicians for many decades. A recent review of the literature failed to reveal a significant documentation, by objective means, of the anti-inflammatory effect of salicylates in patients with rheumatoid arthritis. This led to the recent important and conclusive experiments by Fremont-Smith[8] in which he showed by objective measurements that 21 of 25 patients with active rheumatoid arthritis had less measurable evidence of joint inflammation when on full dosage of aspirin and objectively worsened when aspirin was discontinued.

PLAN OF TREATMENT

All patients with active rheumatoid arthritis, mild to severe, should receive salicylates regularly in the largest tolerated dosage excluding only those with proven adverse gastrointestinal symptoms or bleeding, peptic ulcer, or allergic

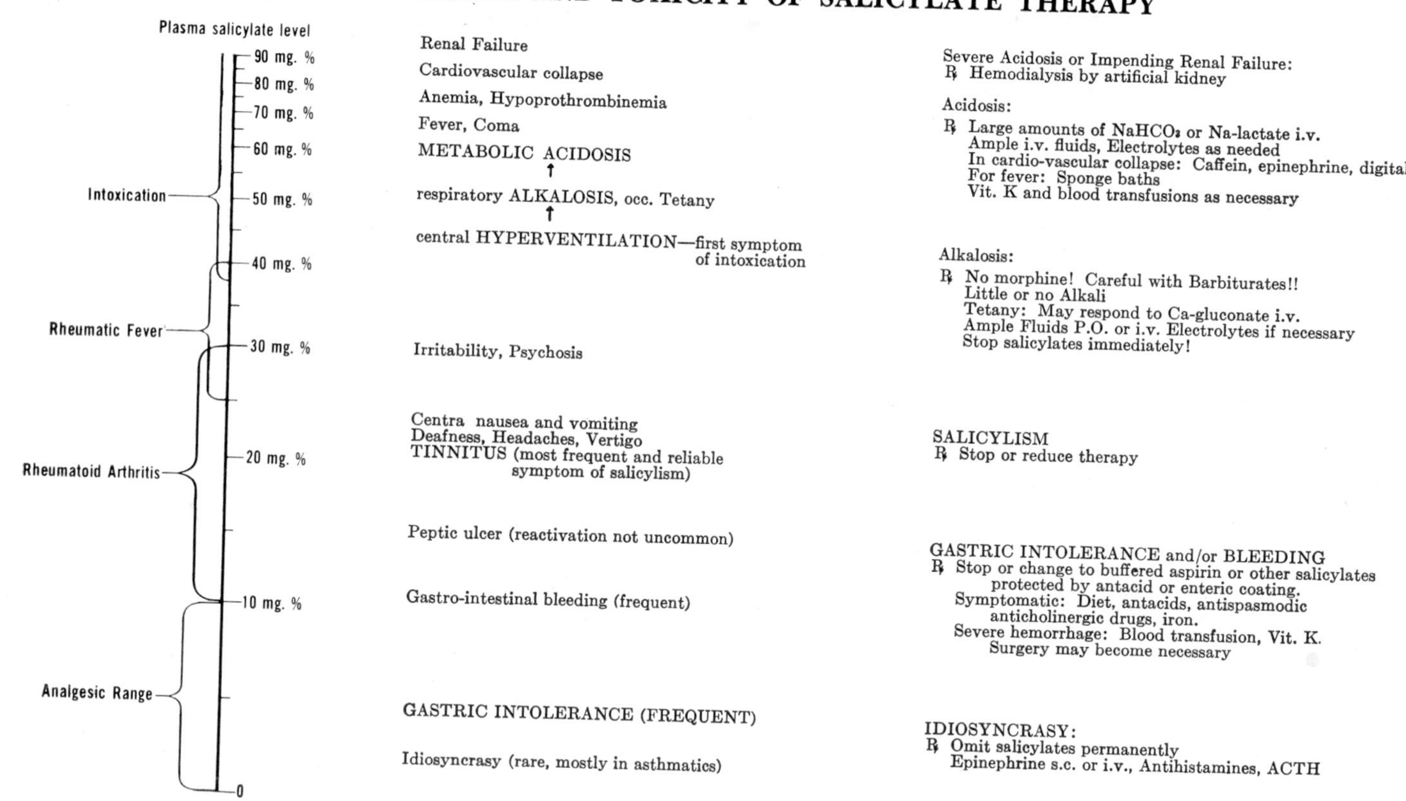

FIG. 28–2.—(Courtesy of Bayles and Tenckhoff, Exhibit Amer. Med. Assn., Dec. 1958.)

manifestations due to salicylates. Other drugs which may affect the symptoms or course of rheumatoid arthritis should be used regularly *with* salicylates and not instead of them. (*See also* under indomethacin, Chapter 30.)

With the knowledge of these facts, what are the practical considerations in salicylate therapy in rheumatoid arthritis? The primary goal would seem to be to administer salicylates in adequate and sufficient dosage to produce maximally effective plasma levels and, more important, tissue levels with the least toxicity. On continuous salicylate administration at a high level, gastric intolerance is the first toxic effect. This can be mitigated by using enteric coated, buffered or liquid preparations of salicylate. The absorption of enteric coated preparations is the least predictable. The administration of salicylates with food, milk or antacids is helpful in reducing gastric mucosal irritation.

Dosage Schedule.—If no gastric intolerance develops on two 300 mg. tablets of aspirin every four hours, the dosage is increased by two tablets every two days up to 5 to 6 gm. daily or until salicylism occurs. The first sign of salicylism is usually tinnitus; when this occurs the dose is reduced to the amount immediately below that which will cause salicylism (often a decrease of 300 or 600 mg.) and is then maintained at this level.

Many investigators have sought the proper, or "ideal," blood level of salicylates in the treatment of rheumatoid arthritis, but as gastric intolerance and salicylism vary greatly in different patients, no hard and fast rule as to what that level should be can be stated. In general, we try to maintain a fairly constant blood level of salicylates in adults at *circa* 20 mg. per cent, and this can be difficult or essentially impossible in the very sick patient with low plasma albumin. Children tolerate *higher* (30 mg. or more) blood levels without salicylism, but should be carefully monitored for toxicity.

Joint damage is the most difficult manifestation of rheumatoid arthritis to control because pathologic changes in the joint structures and crippling cannot be prevented by any drug or other medical therapeutic program. Therefore, any agent which will reduce the inflammation contributes importantly to the prevention or postponement of these structural changes—the most worrisome aspect of rheumatoid arthritis. In this respect the anti-inflammatory effect of salicylates is of greater importance in the treatment of rheumatoid arthritis than the concomitant analgesic effect.

BIBLIOGRAPHY

1. Alvarez, A. S. and Summerskill, W. H. J.: Lancet, *2*, 920, 1958.
2. Baragar, F. D. and Duthie, J. J.: Brit. Med. J., *1*, 1106, 1960.
3. Beecher, H. K.: Pharmac. Rev., *9*, 59, 1957.

3a. Bowie, E. J. W. and Owen, C. A.: Circulation, *40*, 757, 1969.

4. Bywaters, E. G. L. and Thomas, G. T.: Brit. Med. J., *1*, 1628, 1961.
5. Copeman, W. S. C.: In *Salicylates: An International Symposium*, Dixon, A. S., Martin, B. K., Smith, M. J. and Wood, P. H. N., eds. Boston, Little, Brown & Co., 1963.
6. Freireich, E. J., Ross, J. F., Bayles, T. B., Emerson, C. P., Finch, S. C. and MacDonald, C.: J. Clin. Invest., *36*, 1043, 1957.
7. Fremont-Smith, K.: Personal Communication.
8. Fremont-Smith, K. and Bayles, T. B.: J.A.M.A., *192*, 1133, 1965.
9. Gibberd, F. B.: Acta Scand. Rheumat., *12*, 122, 1966.
10. Holt, P. R.: J. Lab. Clin. Med., *56*, 717, 1960.
11. Levy, G.: In *Salicylates: An International Symposium*, Ed. by Dixon, A. S., Martin, B. K., Smith, M. J. and Wood, P. H. N., Boston, Little, Brown & Co., 1963, p. 9.
12. Lockie, L. M. and Norcross, B. M.: In *Arthritis and Allied Conditions*, Ed. by Hollander, J. L., Philadelphia, Lea & Febiger, 1966, 7th ed., p. 334.
13. ————: Ibid, p. 337.
14. Myers, E. N., Bernstein, J. M. and Fostiropolous, G.: New Engl. J. Med., *273*, 587, 1965.

14a. Sahud, M. A. and Cohen, R. J.: Lancet, *1*, 937, 1971.

15. Segar, W. E. and Halliday, M. A.: New Engl. J. Med., *259*, 1191, 1958.
16. Smith, M. J. H.: J. Pharm. Pharmac., *11*, 705, 1959.
17. Strom, E. A. and Bayles, T. B.: Arth. and Rheum., *9*, 544, 1966.
18. Stubbe, L. T.: Brit. Med. J., *2*, 1062, 1958.
18*a*. Vane, J., Smith, J. B., *et al.*: Science News, *100*, 38, 1971.
19. Winters, R. W.: In *Salicylates: An International Symposium*, Ed. by Dixon, A. S., Martin, B. K., Smith, M. J. and Wood, P. H. N., Boston, Little, Brown & Co., 1963, p. 270.

Chapter 29

Gold Therapy for Rheumatoid Arthritis

By Richard H. Freyberg, M.D.

Revised by Morris Ziff, M.D., and John Baum, M.D.

Gold compounds have been used for the treatment of rheumatoid arthritis for approximately forty years. Even though the manner in which these preparations produce their effects is not known, and although other agents have been found which help to suppress rheumatoid disease, gold continues to have a favored place in the therapeutic program for rheumatoid arthritis in many circumstances. Recent investigation and added experience of the past decade have provided a basis for more security in the use of chrysotherapy and better understanding of the problems and limitations of this form of treatment.

History of Gold Therapy

The first reported use of gold for the treatment of rheumatoid arthritis was that of Lande[43] who, in 1927, reported benefit from the use of gold thioglucose in 14 patients. In the same year Pick[56] reported two failures with gold used to treat arthritis. The greatest stimulus to interest in chrysotherapy for arthritis was Forestier's report[22] in 1929 that gold therapy benefited many patients who had rheumatoid arthritis. His use of this form of therapy was based on the knowledge that gold could inhibit growth of tubercle bacilli *in vitro*, and that benefit was reported in tuberculous patients treated with gold; because of some clinical similarities between rheumatoid arthritis and tuberculosis, to him it seemed reasonable that gold might help rheumatoid patients. Thus, this therapy for rheumatoid arthritis had its inception on quite an empirical basis. In 1934 Forestier discussed this subject at several treatment centers in the United States and in the following year a summary of Forestier's six years' experience with gold therapy for rheumatoid arthritis appeared.[23] The earliest American reports on chrysotherapy appeared in 1936.[38,50,55] Since then numerous investigations of gold therapy have been reported; most of these reports indicate benefit from the use of gold for rheumatoid arthritis, although definite shortcomings and hindrances are recognized and discussed.

LABORATORY INVESTIGATIONS OF GOLD THERAPY

The early clinical trials of chrysotherapy were made with little knowledge of the behavior of gold when injected into the animal body. Since then, much has been learned regarding the effects of gold by carefully conducted laboratory research.

Effects of Gold in Experimentally Produced Arthritis in Laboratory Animals

Polyarthritis can be consistently produced by the injection of pleuropneumonia-like organisms into mice and rats.[20,66] The pathology and the clinical course of this experimental arthritis are in some ways different from rheumatoid arthritis, but many features of this type of laboratory arthritis are similar to the human disease. Fusiform joint swelling develops, often symmetrically. Proliferation of the synovium and extension of the inflammatory tissue damage the articular cartilage and subchondral bone. New joints become involved several weeks after the animal has been infected.

Sabin and Warren[67] showed that this type of experimental arthritis could be completely cured when suitable gold compounds were injected early in the course of the disease. Others[57] confirmed these results and showed further that the arthritis could be prevented if the gold was injected within a few days of infection. Sabin found that the therapeutic effectiveness of soluble gold depended upon the concentration of gold in the compounds. Gold chloride was therapeutically effective but quite toxic. The more effective and less toxic gold compounds contained sulfur. Salts identical with therapeutically effective gold compounds except that they contained no gold were ineffective therapeutically and prophylactically for this experimental arthritis.[57] The therapeutically effective gold compounds included several soluble organic formulations, such as gold sodium thiomalate and gold thioglucose; the insoluble organic compound, gold calcium thiomalate and soluble inorganic materials, such as gold sodium thiosulfate and gold chloride. Most of these same compounds have been reported to be beneficial in rheumatoid arthritis. The gold compounds which were effective therapeutically exhibited no antimicrobial action *in vitro* against the same strain of pleuropneumonia-like organisms which caused the arthritis.

Rothbard, Angevine and Cecil[65] reported that gold compounds prevented hemolytic streptococcal arthritis in rats, but did not cure the arthritis once it was established. Jasmin[39] found gold sodium thiomalate to be effective in preventing and remedying experimental arthritis that occurred in rats injected with Murphy rat sarcoma both in the intact animal and in adrenalectomized rats. The effect of gold compounds on adjuvant arthritis is unclear. Although Newbould[49a] claimed that gold sodium thiomalate could inhibit the development of the induced arthritis, Jessop and Currey,[40] using a larger series of animals and higher doses, were unable to show any suppression. Recently, it was reported that formalin-induced arthritis could be modified by gold therapy.[68a]

Investigations have been conducted to learn the distribution of gold through the different tissues after gold compounds were injected into laboratory animals, and to study the nature of the tissue damage that might result.[4] Different groups of rats and mice were injected daily with a variety of gold compounds; after fourteen days the animals were killed and the organs studied for their gold content and histopathology. In the animals injected with soluble gold the highest tissue concentration of gold was found in the kidneys. The excretion of gold occurred chiefly in the urine, and the kidneys were the only organs which showed important changes. There was congestion in the glomeruli; extensive degeneration and necrosis occurred in the tubules and the urine contained much albumin. Large aggregates of precipitated gold or gold compounds were found in the convoluted tubules. The renal pathology was proportional to the amount of gold administered. It should be emphasized that in these studies of toxicity in animals the amount of gold injected was always much greater than the amount used therapeutically in humans. In these animals the liver contained a considerable amount of gold but less than was found in kidney; no cellular damage was seen in the liver.

Classic chemical procedures for analysis of gold have been very laborious. Recently, the techniques of neutron activation analysis[76a] and atomic absorption analysis[47b] have greatly facilitated the detection of heavy metals such as gold in biological fluids. Because of the necessity for costly equipment, neutron activation analysis does not lend itself readily to clinical application. In atomic absorption analysis, the element being measured is incinerated at 3000° K and determined spectrophotometrically. This method has provided a rapid and accurate method of analysis of gold in serum, urine and synovial fluids. The availability of these techniques has stimulated new attempts to relate therapeutic dosage to plasma levels.[42,47a,71] Good therapeutic effects have been thought to be correlated with more elevated plasma gold levels. However, satisfactory data relating plasma gold levels to therapeutic response are not yet available.

The recent studies of Sliwinski and associates[71] using the neutron activation analysis have added much information regarding the distribution of gold and its excretion in rats. These investigators showed that the carrier, that is the complex in which gold is incorporated when it is injected intramuscularly, is an important determinant of the distribution and excretion of the metal; that enhanced urinary excretion increases the amount of gold concentrated in kidney tissue and thus increases the danger of renal toxicity; and that under certain circumstances excretion of gold is greater in feces than in urine. Further pursuit of such studies should be very helpful to provide better understanding of pharmacologic effects of gold compounds.

THE METABOLISM OF GOLD IN HUMANS

Investigations of the absorption, circulation and excretion of gold have been conducted during treatment of patients with different preparations of gold;[25] knowledge gained from such studies has provided a basis for a more intelligent therapeutic use of gold compounds.

In these metabolism studies gold-containing preparations commonly used for therapy, and representative of classes of compounds which possess different chemical and physical characteristics, were employed (Table 29–1). Since the effects of all gold compounds depend upon the amount of gold they contain, comparison of different preparations required the use of doses of the different preparations containing equivalent amounts of gold.

Using a sensitive chemical method developed by Block and Buchanan,[2,3] determinations of the gold content of plasma, urine and feces were made over long periods during and after repeated injections of the different gold compounds, usually at weekly intervals. Graphic representations of the type of study and the results observed appear in Figures 29–1 and 29–2. Blood cells were found to contain insignificant traces of gold; all of the circulating gold was in the protein fraction of plasma. Clemmeson[13] has reported that circulating gold is

Table 29–1.—Preparations Representing Gold Compounds Possessing Different Chemical and Physical Characteristics

Gold Compound	*Proprietary Name*	*Solubility in Water*	*Physical State*	*Gold Content of Compound (Per Cent)*
Gold Sodium Thiosulfate	Sanochrysine Crisalbine Sanocrysin	Yes	Aqueous solution	37
Gold Sodium Thiomalate	Myochrysine	Yes	Aqueous solution	50
Gold Thioglucose	Solganol	Yes	Oil Suspension	50
Gold Thioglucoanalide	Lauron	No	Oil Suspension	54

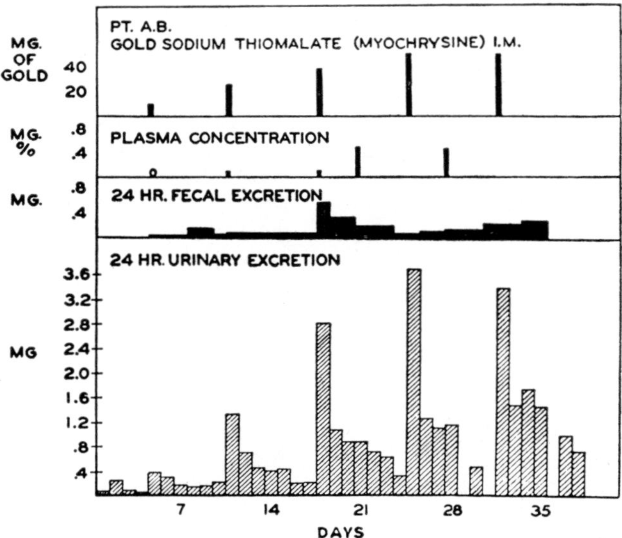

FIG. 29–1.—Plasma concentration and excretion of gold in a patient with rheumatoid arthritis treated with gold sodium thiomalate injected intramuscularly in increasing doses. (Courtesy of *Clinics*, J. B. Lippincott Company.)

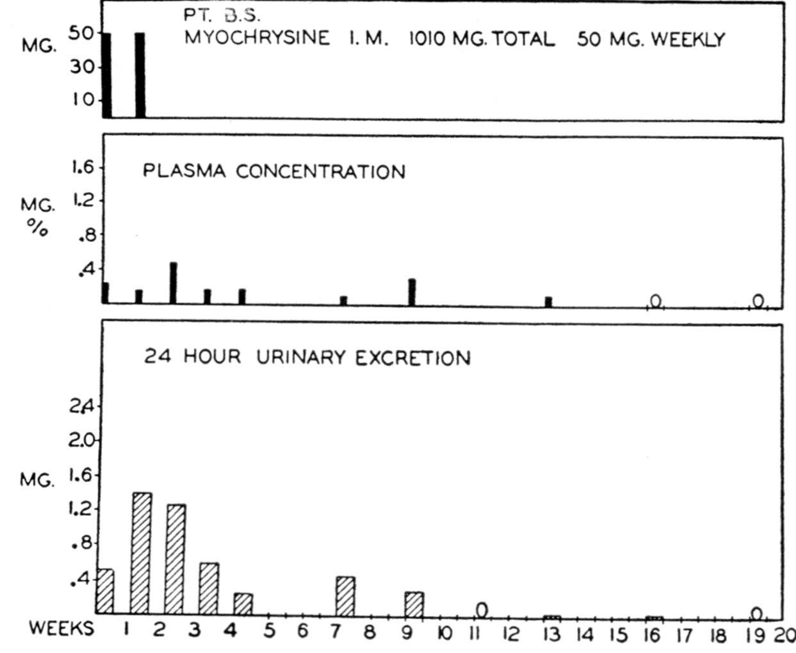

FIG. 29–2.—Plasma and urine content of gold observed for many months after discontinuing injections of gold sodium thiomalate which had been given at weekly intervals until a total of 1010 mgm. of the compound (505 mgm. of gold) had been injected. The last two injections and corresponding plasma and urine values for gold are shown. (Courtesy of J. Clin. Investigation.)

loosely bound to alpha$_1$ globulin in the plasma, as a gold-protein complex. The chemical state of gold in urine and feces has not been established.

When aqueous solutions of crystalline gold compounds, organic or inorganic, are injected in increasing dose, there is a step-like increase in plasma gold content corresponding to the increase in dosage. The plasma concentration of gold thus depends upon the size of the dose; however, gold does not accumulate in the blood with continued treatment employing weekly doses of the same amount of gold. When injected in soluble form, gold is excreted chiefly in the urine; larger amounts of gold were eliminated on the day of injection. The larger amount of gold found consistently in the urine on days of injection did not apparently arise from higher plasma concentrations for, between injections, content of gold in the plasma remained relatively constant. The rather sharp decrease in urinary excretion of gold after the day of injection suggests that, soon after injection, gold is absorbed into the blood and circulates through the kidneys in a state that will be eliminated readily in the urine, and that after several hours less gold remains circulating in this readily excretable form. Fecal excretion was small and irregular; slightly larger amounts of gold were found in the feces when larger amounts were injected.*

Figure 29–1 shows that large amounts of gold are retained in the body during the period of its administration. This feature of the metabolism of gold was found to be true in whatever form it is administered. From Figure 29–1, for instance, it can be calculated that during the seven days after the injection of 40 mgm. of gold (80 mgm. of the compound) made on the eighteenth day, only 7.5 mgm. of gold were excreted in the urine and 2 mgm. in the feces, so that if one disregards the gold injected previously, it is found that 76 per cent of the gold injected on the eighteenth day was retained in the body. With continued injections the gold retained in the body increases. Since the excretion of gold does not increase significantly when constant weekly doses are employed, it can readily be appreciated that the magnitude of the retention during treatment becomes great. The amount of gold retained during a period of thirty-nine days of continuous observation was found to be 81 and 86 per cent of the amount injected in two different patients.

After treatment is stopped, gold is found in the blood and is excreted for long periods of time; the duration depends chiefly on the size of the weekly dose. In patients who received weekly injections of 50 mgm. of gold, gold continued to circulate and be excreted in decreasing amounts for many months (observed up to fifteen months). After weekly doses of 25 mgm. of gold were administered to a comparable total amount, gold was eliminated for a shorter period of time, often no longer than three or four months. Following weekly injections of 12.5 mgm. of gold, the urine usually contained no gold after two or three months following cessation of treatment.

Lawrence found that when sodium aurothiomalate labeled with radioactive gold was injected into rheumatoid patients, there was up to $2\frac{1}{2}$ times as much gold in painful (inflamed) joints as was found in symptomless (non-inflamed) joints. When gold sodium thiosulfate, an inorganic aqueous soluble gold compound, was injected in comparable doses intramuscularly, essentially the same metabolic findings were observed as with gold sodium thiomalate.

A distinctly different picture was observed when the insoluble gold calcium thiomalate was injected intramuscularly in oil. The plasma gold concentration was very small in most patients; there was considerable variation from time to time in the same patient during

* Reinvestigation, in current studies still in progress, indicates that in some patients as much as 50% of the gold excretion is in the feces. Fecal excretion cannot be ignored in complete metabolism studies.[48a]

a prolonged period when a constant weekly dose was injected, and the plasma gold level varied considerably in different patients treated similarly. The urine content of gold was much smaller than obtained when comparable doses of gold were given in solution, and on many days no gold was found in the urine. These findings clearly indicate that absorption of insoluble gold is sharply retarded; consequently, there is to be expected a greater retention than when soluble gold is used. Gold was found in the plasma, urine and feces long after treatment was discontinued.

Colloidal gold and colloidal gold sulfide behave quite differently in the human body than do the soluble gold compounds. After intramuscular injections of these colloidal preparations, gold was rarely found in more than traces in the plasma. Intravenously administered colloidal radioactive gold in humans localizes primarily in the reticuloendothelial system, most of it in the liver.[63] Ganz and Brucer[28] found in dogs that intravenously administered radioactive colloidal gold was taken up quickly by the reticuloendothelial system; 94 per cent of the injected dose was found in the liver. Gilg and Vraa-Jensen[32] reported that gold injected for the treatment of rheumatoid arthritis does not cross the blood-brain barrier.

MANNER OF ACTION OF GOLD

The way in which gold produces a therapeutic effect is not known, in spite of extensive research aimed to elucidate this. It has already been noted that gold has a prophylactic and therapeutic effect on the experimental arthritis produced by pleuropneumonia-like organisms in mice and rats and that it prevents the development of arthritis that is usually caused by infection of rats by hemolytic streptococci. Hartung and Cotter[37] found serum of patients treated with gold to be bactericidal against hemolytic streptococci. Although gold has a marked chemotherapeutic effect against hemolytic streptococci, tubercle bacilli and some other bacteria,[37,57,65,67] it is unlikely that the effect of gold in rheumatoid arthritis is due to effects on bacterial organisms since there is no evidence that rheumatoid arthritis is caused by a microbe.

Bollett[7] also reported that amounts of gold in patients with rheumatoid arthritis were sufficient to suppress the synthesis of glucosamine-6-phosphate through enzyme inhibition *in vitro*, and in albino rats administration of gold results in decreased enzyme activity in connective tissue. These observations lend support to the concept that gold may favorably alter enzyme function in patients with rheumatoid arthritis. There is evidence from the work of Persellin, Hess and Ziff[53a] that gold does not act to modify an immune response. These authors found no effect of gold sodium thiomalate on the delayed hypersensitivity response, serum antibody formation and on the levels of a rheumatoid factor-like protein induced in hyperimmunized rabbits. Nevertheless, it should be pointed out that chrysotherapy has effected the reduction of rheumatoid factor to a significant degree.[17]

Research recently reported by Persellin and Ziff[54] suggests a possible mechanism whereby gold may exert a therapeutic effect. Gold thiomalate was shown to inhibit the lysosomal enzymes, acid phosphatase and beta glucuronidase. When guinea pig peritoneal macrophages were incubated with gold sodium thiomalate, there was a significant decrease in acid phosphatase and beta glucuronidase content in the lysosomes of the macrophage, suggesting an active transport of the gold compound into the macrophage. Because lysosomal enzymes have been postulated as agents in the development of inflammation, these observations may lead to clarification of the manner of action of gold compounds in rheumatoid arthritis. The lysosomal inhibition mechanism proposed is consistent with the repeated observation that gold accumulates at sites of inflammation. Measurements of tissue gold concentrations required to inhibit lysosomal enzymes are reached in some tissues.[33a] Norton, Lewis and Ziff[49c] have demonstrated electron dense deposits in the lysosomes of the rheumatoid synovium following both systemic and intra-articular injection of gold sodium thiomalate. A number of other recent reports[18a,37a,51a] deal with the effects of gold compounds on lysosomal enzymes.

It has been suggested that gold in the tissues may compete for the SH radical in such a way as to alter the cellular metabolism in a manner favorable to the patient with active rheumatoid arthritis. Studies of Gerber[30] have shown that gold thiomalate reacts with the mercaptide anion (ionized sulfhydryl group) and inhibits the sulfhydryl disulfide interchange reaction that ordinarily occurs when bovine serum albumin is denatured by heat. The concentration of gold thiomalate required for an effect on denaturation is less than that commonly existing in plasma of gold-treated patients. In later studies[31] it was shown that rheumatoid serum protein may be characterized by increased disulfide interchange. These biochemical studies provide more possibilities to explain the manner of action of gold in the treatment of rheumatoid arthritis.

Because striking improvement in arthritis often attends a severe toxic reaction, some physicians[52] have considered the action of gold to be that of mild shock therapy oftentimes prolonged in duration. That toxic reactions are not required for benefit from gold therapy in rheumatoid arthritis is a fact which does not support this theory.

Evidence to be discussed later clearly indicates that, no matter what the mechanism, the only benefit gold may have in the rheumatoid arthritic is to suppress activity of the rheumatoid process—an anti-inflammatory effect.

Although some theories that have been proposed to explain the manner of action of gold are attractive and reasonable, the manner of action of gold in the treatment of rheumatoid arthritis is not known.

CLINICAL EXPERIENCES WITH GOLD THERAPY

Among the many difficult clinical problems in modern medicine none is harder than the accurate evaluation of some forms of treatment for rheumatoid arthritis. At the top of this list is the problem of assaying gold therapy. It is readily understandable that there will be differences of opinion and uncertainty when one appreciates the many factors which need to be considered. Although the disease is usually characterized by remissions and relapses, it is one of protean nature and has an unpredictable course in every patient. The gold compounds employed for treatment are numerous and vary greatly in chemical and physical nature; the manner of treatment and dosage have been decidedly different; and the severity of illness and stage in which treatment is employed differ among many physicians. To these factors must be added the difficulty in allocating the true portion of change attributable to gold salts when they have been employed simultaneously with other treatments. However, most of the clinicians who have had experience with this form of treatment, or who have made special investigations concerning it, have a firm conviction as to its efficacy. It is instructive, therefore, to review clinical reports concerning gold therapy, many of which are summarized in Table 29–2. Not included in this table are some controlled studies which will be discussed separately. This tabulation is presented, not for the purpose of a total summation of clinical results, but to show the trend of the results and for ready reference. It should be noted from these reports that the majority of these nearly 7700 patients were considered to be significantly improved as the result of gold therapy. In approximately one-third of all trials manifestations considered to be indicative of gold intoxication occurred,

TABLE 29–2.—RESULTS IN 7,693 PATIENTS WITH RHEUMATOID ARTHRITIS TREATED WITH GOLD REPORTED BETWEEN 1935 AND 1958

Investigator	*Year of Report*	*No. of Cases*	*Period of Observation (Years)*	*Arrested or Greatly Improved (Per Cent)*	*Moderately Improved (Per Cent)*	*Slightly Improved (Per Cent)*	*Duration of Improvement (Years)*	*Relapsed* after Treatment was Stopped (Per Cent)*	*Toxicity† (Per Cent)*
Forestier[23]	1935	550	6	75.			2 to 3		
Hartfall, Garland & Goldie[35]	1937	690		66.7	13.	6.2		20.9	40.0
Sashin, Spanbock & Kling[68]	1939	80	1 to 5	43.7	38.7			10.4	23.7
Goldie[33]	1939	400	½ to 4	76.	10.5	4.		18.5	17.0
Logefeil & Hoffman[47]	1941	139	1 to 5	56.8	24.5	14.	1.8	13.7	12.9
Smyth & Freyberg[73]	1941	80		61.			½ or more		33.0
Dawson, Boots & Tyson[15]	1941	100		51.	25.	9.	½ to 2	12.	50.
Gardner[29]	1941	250		40.	40.			12.	8.4
Cecil, Kammerer & de Prume[12]	1942	245	1 to 5	66.	20.		½ to 5	40.	42.
Price & Leichtentritt[58]	1943	101	1 to 3	60.		12.	1	55.	38.
Hartung[36]	1943	264		54.				21.	
Graham & Fletcher[34]	1943	95	1 to 3	67.	20.				51.5

Rawls *et al.*[61]	1944	100	1 to 4	53.	21.	12.			42.
Robinson[62]	1944	200	1 to 5	50.		25.			
Oren[51]	1946	250		84.5			1 (median)	7.2	4.6
Ragan & Tyson[60]	1946	142	3 to 6½	50.	39			75.	30.
Rose[64]	1947	91	½ to 1	73.	11.	5.5			20.
Waine, Baker & Mettier[81]	1947	58	3	20.7	36.2	24.1			50.
Browning *et al.*[8]	1947	47	1½ to 6	23.				4.	62.
Sundelin[78]	1948	2441	1 to 12		—90—‡				50.
Cohen, Dubbs & Goldman[14]	1948	475		68.3		21.1			21.
Adams & Cecil[1]	1950	106	1½ to 5	70.8	17.			26.1	48.6
Cecil & Kammerer[11]	1951	49	1 to 10	68.		12.			25.
Snorrason[74]	1952	295§	4	72.			‖		
Schwartz, Blain, Geiger & Hartung[69]	1954	56	3	3.6	37.5	32.			14.
Lockie & Riordan[46]	1958	369¶	¼ to 25	8.	49.	35.			
Total		7693						24.3	32.2

* Up to 80 per cent improved again on further therapy.
† Includes mild toxicity not requiring cessation of therapy; only 4.5 per cent of reactions were severe.
‡ Degree of improvement not reported, "90 per cent were objectively and subjectively improved."
§ Includes Stage I and II disease only; total number of patients, 368.
‖ After ten years, 2 per cent of men, 16 per cent of women still showed arrested disease.
¶ Includes only those patients receiving more than 300 mg. of gold salt.

although these were severe in only 4.5 per cent of instances. Relapses were frequent.

Controlled Evaluation of Therapeutic Effect of Gold Compounds

The first report of a controlled clinical trial of gold therapy is that of Ellman, Lawrence and Thorold,[16] summarized in Table 29–3. All patients had active disease. Half of the patients who received gold were injected with 200 mgm. of gold thioglucose in oil weekly, and half were given 100 mgm. weekly. The authors report that among those persons receiving larger doses of the gold compound, there was a tendency toward greater improvement, but also increased toxicity. Fraser[21] reported a study of 110 patients in which he controlled the study of gold therapy by the now well-known double blind method. All patients were suffering from active disease which had existed from two to five years. Approximately half of the patients received injections of a placebo.

Evaluation was carefully made, but the patients were observed for only one year. The results are summarized in Table 29–4. Benefit from gold therapy is evident from these data. Fraser states that after treatment with gold, 17 of 19 formerly incapacitated patients were able to resume employment; of the controls, only 4 of 14 could return to work. There was a greater decrease in the erythrocyte sedimentation rate in the gold-treated group. Treatment was stopped in four of the gold-treated group and three of the control group because of "toxicity" of the injected material. (The "toxicity" considered to exist in patients who received no gold will receive further comment.) Fraser prudently points out that the better results claimed for gold therapy

TABLE 29–3.—SUMMARY OF CONTROLLED STUDY OF GOLD THERAPY FOR RHEUMATOID ARTHRITIS BY ELLMAN, LAWRENCE AND THOROLD

Patients	*Gold Used*	*Asymptomatic and E.S.R. Returned to Normal (Per Cent)*	*Some Degree of Improvement (Per Cent)*
60	Gold Thioglucose	37	94*
30	Placebo (sterile oil)	3	76

* Improvement was greater than in controls.

TABLE 29–4.—SUMMARY OF THERAPEUTIC EFFECT OF THE CONTROLLED STUDY OF GOLD THERAPY BY FRASER

	Patients			
Improvement	*Treated with Gold (Number)*	*Treated with Placebo (Number)*	*Treated with Gold (Per Cent)*	*Treated with Placebo (Per Cent)*
Great	24	4	42	8
Moderate	12	6	21	13
Slight	11	11	19	24
None	5	10	9	22
Worse	5	15	9	33
Total	57	46		

by the majority of other physicians are unjustifiably high because of the lack of adequate control observations (a criticism which applies to the published reports of nearly all evaluations of separate forms of treatment for rheumatoid arthritis).

Another controlled study of chrysotherapy in rheumatoid arthritis is that of Waine, Baker and Mettier[81] who studied 120 patients with active rheumatoid arthritis. A control series consisting of 62 consecutively admitted patients were treated with limitation of physical activity, dietary regulation, salicylates and physical therapy. The average duration of treatment and observation was three years. Injections of gold sodium thiosulfate or gold sodium thiomalate were given to 58 patients. The average period of treatment and observation was 2.9 years. The average dose of gold was 25 mgm. given weekly, biweekly, or monthly varying with the activity of the disease. The total dose averaged 1.6 grams of gold; none received less than 0.5 gram. Results of this study, summarized in Table 29–5, show definite benefit from gold. Of the 10 patients who were unimproved when managed for an average of 2.7 years without gold and later were treated with gold, 5 were "markedly improved" and 3 were "improved."

The study that has been most convincing that gold therapy is beneficial for rheumatoid arthritis is the "double blind" controlled trial conducted by the research subcommittee of the Empire Rheumatism Council.[17,18] This extensive study was conducted simultaneously in 24 rheumatism centers in Great Britain. One hundred patients with rheumatoid arthritis were given 1 gram of gold sodium thiomalate over twenty weeks by intramuscular injection of 50 mg. at weekly intervals. A comparable group of control patients were given .01 mg. of gold sodium thiomalate over twenty weeks by injection of 0.5 microgram at weekly intervals—an infinitesimal amount. Assessments were made at the start and at one, three, six, twelve and eighteen months. As assessed by functional capacity (judged by physicians), subjective fitness, joint involvement, grip strength, number of analgesic tablets taken daily, sensitized sheep cell agglutination titre, hemoglobin and erythrocyte sedimentation rate, the gold-treated patients improved to a greater degree than the controls from the third month onwards. The improvement was still apparent twelve months after the last injection although it was reduced in degree. No such advantage was shown by roentgenographic studies. Dangerous toxicity was uncommon. It was concluded that "gold therapy undoubtedly improved the average clinical condition of the majority of patients in the gold-treated group over a period of eighteen months." Thereafter a reverse trend was noted, so that by the thirtieth month after beginning the gold therapy (twenty-five months after the last injection), most of the advantage

TABLE 29–5.—SUMMARY OF THERAPEUTIC RESULTS IN THE CONTROLLED STUDY OF GOLD THERAPY BY WAINE, BAKER AND METTIER

State of Disease at End of Observation	*Treated with Gold (Number)*	*Treated without Gold (Number)*	*Treated with Gold (Per Cent)*	*Treated without Gold (Per Cent)*
Arrested	12	6	20.7	9.7
Markedly improved	21	12	36.2	19.4
Improved	14	17	24.1	27.4
Unimproved	11	27	19	43
Total	58	62		

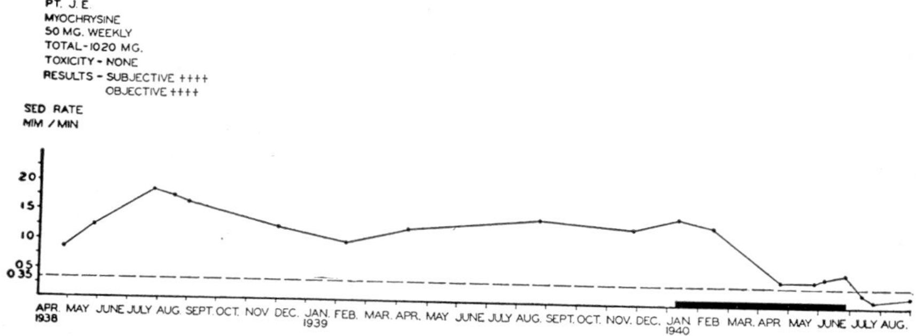

Fig. 29–3.—The erythrocyte sedimentation rate of a patient with classical rheumatoid arthritis before, during and for a short period after treatment with weekly intramuscular injections of 50 mgm. of gold sodium thiomalate (25 mgm. of gold). The broken line represents the upper limit of normal. The period of gold administration is shown by the heavy bar at the base line. (Courtesy of *Clinics*, J. B. Lippincott Company.)

seen at the eighteenth month had disappeared. (This relapsing trend is quite as would be expected, knowing the metabolism and excretion of gold, and as had been observed by others after cessation of a "course" of gold therapy. This observation further emphasizes that benefits of gold therapy cannot be expected to continue after gold is no longer retained in the patient—a problem to be considered further on.) Patients who did not improve with the first course of treatment, failed to respond to a second course of injections given in the same manner as had been done in the first course of treatment.

The Cooperating Clinics Committee of the American Rheumatism Association recently sponsored a double-blind trial of gold therapy to reassess the results of the Empire Rheumatism Council trial with additional clinical and laboratory measurements. Preliminary results (supplied through the courtesy of Dr. John L. Decker, Chairman, Cooperating Clinics Committee) are as follows: The differences between gold- and placebo-treated patients over a 27-week period were not marked, although the gold-treated patients did do better. Although the improvement reported was slight, rheumatoid factor-positive patients appeared to do somewhat better than factor-negative patients. The most marked difference between the treated and control groups was in the fall in the sedimentation rate observed in the treated patients.

Many investigators have shown that not infrequently with the use of gold added to generally good treatment, remission or substantial improvement can be obtained in a few months that, without gold therapy, would require much longer. When a result such as is shown graphically in Figure 29–3 is observed, one cannot help but be impressed with the potential value of this form of treatment. The patient, whose erythrocyte sedimentation rate is shown in this graph, was incapacitated by rheumatoid arthritis for two years while different forms of treatment were employed with little or no benefit. The change in sedimentation rate was paralleled by clinical improvement until the disease became completely arrested and the patient returned to work.

Despite these many convincing reports, there are many clinicians who consider gold therapy undependable, of too small a degree of benefit, or too toxic to use or advocate its use. However, the majority of investigators who have studied this form of therapy are convinced that it has merit and the bulk of reported data supports this conviction.

The usefulness of chrysotherapy in palindromic rheumatism has recently been pointed out.[48b]

Lewis and Ziff[45] have recently studied the effect of intra-articular injection of gold sodium thiomalate in the knee joints of patients with rheumatoid arthritis. The majority of patients showed evidence of significant local response in the treated knees with decrease in swelling, increase in range of motion, fall in synovial fluid leukocyte count and rise in joint fluid viscosity. While the authors did not consider their evidence sufficient to recommend intra-articular gold salt administration as a routine therapeutic measure, the data obtained indicated that these agents exert a beneficial local action upon the rheumatoid inflammatory process.

Effect on Laboratory Parameters

Gold therapy has been reported to return elevated blood glycoproteins to normal.[77b] Plasma fibrinogen, α_2 globulins and the erythrocyte sedimentation rate also fell.[1c,48c]

Selection of Patients for Treatment

The selection of patients suitable for gold therapy is an important consideration and one about which there should be little or no debate if decision is based upon a knowledge of (1) metabolism and pharmacology of gold, and (2) the nature of the disease. It should be emphasized that gold can be helpful to patients with rheumatoid arthritis in only one way, by suppressing the activity of the disease. This is the only therapeutic effect that gold can contribute; it does not repair damaged cartilages or bones, nor does it restore deformed and ankylosed joints. Therefore, benefit from gold can be expected only when employed during the active stage of the disease. If the arthritis can be arrested in an early stage before irreparable damages have occurred, the patient will be spared crippling and incapacitation that these destructive changes frequently cause. It is, therefore, in this early active stage of rheumatoid arthritis that gold can be of most benefit. In a later stage of the disease, when cartilage and bone damage have occurred, the only contribution gold therapy can make is to check progression and prevent further structural damage to joints. Anatomic changes already present will not be improved. Although patients in a late stage of rheumatoid arthritis may benefit from the use of gold compounds by suppressing continuing inflammation, the physician and the patient should realize the limitations of gold therapy in such circumstances. The patient who suffers only from crippling and whose arthritis is no longer active cannot be rehabilitated by gold therapy; in such instances gold should not be used. Most benefit from the proper use of gold has occurred[1,36,41] in early stages of rheumatoid arthritis, although in some long-standing chronic cases with active inflammation results are gratifying.

No firm rules can be laid down for the institution of gold therapy. Because of potential toxicity, the decision to employ this treatment should be made only after careful considerations of all circumstances and with seasoned judgment. It is unwise to decide upon the use of gold therapy at the first contact with a patient who appears to have rheumatoid arthritis. The diagnosis should be substantially established and sometimes this cannot be done until the course of the disease has been observed for several months. Furthermore, in many instances, rheumatoid arthritis is not severe but may be quite mild, and a good program of treatment without the use of gold salts may be rewarded with excellent results. Hence it seems reasonable to institute a satisfactory program of treatment which does not include gold therapy and carefully evaluate progress at monthly intervals; if gratifying improvement occurs, gold therapy should be withheld. If the disease is observed steadily to advance and involve joints not previously affected, it seems correct to consider seriously one of the special forms of suppressive treatment, including gold.

When to use gold therapy in preference to corticosteroids is not easy to determine. Investigators are generally agreed that corticosteroids are more potent therapeutic agents. However, they may produce more serious undesirable side effects. It seems reasonable therefore that if the disease is becoming progressively more severe and spreading, gold therapy might be tried. If it is effective and well tolerated, the problems of hormone and metabolic side effects of corticosteroids need not be risked. In patients who have active peptic ulcer, diabetes, tuberculosis, or other complications which prevent or militate against the use of corticosteroids, gold is the choice, and in some patients who have received corticosteroids for a prolonged period and have "side effects" making it desirable to discontinue steroid therapy, gold may prove beneficial even though not as potent as the corticosteroids. (See also discussion related to selection of patients for cortisone or corticotropin in Chapter 31.)

Gold therapy should not be used unless the physician and the patient know what can be expected of it therapeutically, and appreciate the possibilities of toxicity. When, without its use, the arthritis is progressing, and one knows of the serious consequences of the continuing active disease, certainly there is wisdom in using a form of treatment that may arrest or suppress the activity of the process, even though the treatment has potential toxicity. If decided against, the question should be reconsidered at intervals of two or three months unless the disease is abating. In the last analysis, the decision for the use of gold therapy should be made jointly by the physician and the patient after carefully evaluating the potential and relative advantages of the drug against the risks of its toxicity.

Special Forms of Rheumatoid Arthritis

In juvenile rheumatoid arthritis (Still's disease), gold compounds have been found to have the same potentialities for benefit as in adults. Recent reports on the use of gold in juvenile rheumatoid arthritis have been favorable.[67a,1b,82] However, no controlled trials have been performed as in adult arthritis. As with adults, the results of therapy are better the earlier in the course the drug is given. A significant fall in rheumatoid factor titer was observed in 22 of 75 patients.[82]

The dosage for children is usually half the adult dose.[49b,7a] After an initial test dose of 10 mg of gold sodium thiomalate, 25 mg. are given at weekly intervals for 20 weeks, then followed by 25 mg. every 2 to 4 weeks. Others[67a] recommend that gold be given on an age basis: up to age 6, 10 mg. weekly for 10 to 20 injections, then at 2 to 4 week intervals; over age 6, 30 mg. weekly for 10 to 20 injections, then at 2 to 4 week intervals.

In patients with psoriasis who have rheumatoid arthritis, the problem is the same as in the person with uncomplicated rheumatoid arthritis; psoriasis is not a contraindication to the use of gold.[25] Results of gold treatment for ankylosing spondylitis have usually been unsatisfactory. Moreover, in patients with this type of arthritis, toxicity is more frequently encountered; for these reasons and because other treatment is usually quite effective, gold is not advised for spondylitis.

TOXICITY OF GOLD

The toxic potentialities justify hesitancy in selecting this form of treatment, but the risk of toxicity is similar and may even be greater with other special forms of treatment. Antidotes for and treatment of gold toxicity are now very good—so that fear of this form of treatment is not justified. Even so, everyone who contemplates using gold therapy should be thoroughly acquainted with its toxicity.

In humans the toxic effects of gold may affect many organs and systems. Cutaneous manifestations are by far the most common.

Dermatitis

With few exceptions the eruption is preceded by pruritus for several days or even weeks. Itching may be mild or intense and may be generalized or localized to the sites of dermatitis. It is the rule that pruritus accompanies gold dermatitis; hence it is a valuable symptom to aid in the diagnosis of cutaneous toxicity. Without pruritus it is unlikely that dermatitis occurring during treatment is caused by the gold.

Dermatitis caused by gold may be of many different forms. Erythema or a fine morbiliform rash on the arms, neck and thighs may occur after the first two or three injections of a gold compound. This type of dermatitis usually disappears within a few days, and subsequently injections may be tolerated well. Dermatitis, as is true with other forms of toxicity, usually does not appear until 300 or 400 mgm. of gold have been injected. A common form of skin eruption is at the outset localized at the neck, axillae, groin, intercrural regions, the chest and back, where the lesions are discrete, oval and rosaceous, resembling pityriasis rosea. The lesions have a thin, wrinkled epidermal surface. This form of rash usually persists many weeks, and is very pruritic. The lesions may slowly fade during desquamation of a fine branny scale and then disappear leaving either depigmented atrophic scars, or pigmented slightly thickened scars; or the eruption may spread and the lesions may coalesce so that the dermatitis takes on characteristics of a generalized exfoliative dermatitis. Localized itching and eczematoid dermatitis may occur about the ears, eyes and scalp, may be very stubborn to treatment and slow in resolution. Vesicles may develop on the palms and soles and soon be followed by generalized exfoliative dermatitis. Discrete lesions resembling lichen planus may appear on a few parts of the body or may be quite generalized. Such an eruption usually persists several months and heals slowly. Lesions resembling lichen planus may appear during the recrudescence of generalized dermatitis. Purpura has occasionally developed over the arms, legs and trunk due to thrombocytopenia or to endothelial damage. Pre-existing tinea or seborrheic dermatitis may become aggravated during the course of treatment with gold.

Because of the variety of dermatitides which may develop due to gold toxicity, any eruption, especially if it is pruritic, which develops during gold therapy should be considered with suspicion until its nature becomes clarified. Gold dermatitis usually becomes progressively worse if gold therapy is continued. Exposure of the skin to sunlight may accentuate gold dermatitis.

The most serious form of eruption that might arise as a toxic manifestation is generalized exfoliative dermatitis. Although it may be frightening, it can be quickly suppressed by corticosteroid treatment. Skin appendages may be damaged and complete alopecia occasionally is seen; usually there is regrowth of hair after a few months; but alopecia may persist for two or three years.

Mouth Lesions

Oftentimes stomatitis accompanies dermatitis; it may appear without skin eruption. A "metallic taste" may precede stomatitis. Discrete inflammatory lesions develop in the oral mucous membranes; these may develop into ulcerative stomatitis, glossitis or gingivitis. Like gold dermatitis, mucous membrane lesions tend to be chronic unless effective treatment is instituted.

Gastrointestinal Toxicity

Although mentioned among the forms of toxicity, disturbances of the digestive system seldom are seen as a result of gold intolerance. Nausea, anorexia, diarrhea and abdominal cramps have frequently been ascribed to use of gold. A few cases of severe ulcerative entero-colitis, rarely with fatal termination, have been reported.[1a] Hepatitis and acute yellow atrophy have been reported, but if they occur as a result of gold toxicity these lesions are indeed rare. One of the authors (R.H.F.) has not seen an instance of important digestive disorder or liver disease in thirty years of experience with gold therapy in over 2000 cases.

Nephritis

Toxic nephritis may be caused by gold. Slight transient albuminuria may occur during gold therapy, and have no relationship to treatment. Significant amounts of proteinuria occur in 1 to 3 per cent of patients.[71a] Frequently albuminuria indicates existence of toxic nephritis, usually tubular degeneration but glomerular lesions may occur with hematuria. Nephrotic syndrome was noted in 2 of 75 patients treated.[71a] Light and electron microscopic studies[44] of renal biopsy material from three rheumatoid patients treated with gold showed lipoid nephrosis in one instance and in the other two, membranous glomerulonephritis. The nephritis may be trivial and of short duration, or more severe and pass through a subacute phase with elevated blood pressure, retinitis, and systemic effects before it subsides months after onset.

In two patients with gold nephrotoxicity, Strunk and Ziff[76b] noted deposits in the peripheral capillary wall of the glomerulus resembling the deposits seen in immune complex disease. These differed in appearance from gold inclusions seen in the lysosomes of the glomerular epithelial and endothelial cells in these patients and in rats injected with gold thiomalate. Silverberg and coworkers[71a] observed no difference in blood and urine gold levels between two patients who developed nephrotoxic syndrome and 25 patients who did not. These authors and Vaamonde and Hunt[80a] have reviewed the subject of gold nephrotoxicity.

Hematologic Disorders

Blood dyscrasia due to gold toxicity rarely occurs but when it does, it may be serious unless promptly and effectively treated. Thrombocytopenic purpura,[15,70,77,80] hypoplastic or aplastic anemia,[59] granulopenia and secondary anemia have been reported. Occasional fatalities have been ascribed to subdural or cerebral hemorrhage.[58] Eosinophilia frequently precedes or accompanies gold toxicity, especially dermatitis, hence its presence suggests impending or existing toxicity. However, eosinophilia may develop in arthritic patients who are receiving no special treatment, so it cannot be relied upon as an indication of toxicity.

The mechanism of the depressive effect of gold on the bone marrow and blood elements is still unclear. Gold-induced purpura can occur after 46 to 450 mg. of gold, and 2 to 10 months after gold therapy is stopped.[67b] The rapid response seen after BAL, presumably due to the removal of gold from the body, has suggested an idiosyncratic effect which may be mediated by an immunological mechanism. However, a well-worked up case failed to show lytic or agglutinating antibody, complement fixation, or binding to radioactively labeled aurothiomalate.[77a] In support of the possibility that bone marrow depression was in fact due to an allergic reaction, Denman and Denman[15a] found significant lymphocyte transformation occurring when cells from 5 gold sodium thiomalate-treated patients with this toxic effect were stimulated with gold sodium thiomalate.

Miscellaneous Forms of Toxicity

Vasomotor reactions with generalized erythema, warmth, giddiness, blurred vision and vertigo may occur during the early weeks of gold therapy. Increased arthralgia sometimes is noted after the first few injections. Such symptoms usually decrease and finally disappear after five or six injections after which clinical improvement is the rule during continuing treatment. Peripheral neuritis and "gold bronchitis" have been reported.

Behrend and Rodenhauser have recently described two types of eye involvement with gold therapy.[1d] The first, a rare form, is a keratitis with inflammation and ulceration of the cornea. The second type is a subepithelial deposition of metallic gold in the cornea (chryseosis). The condition is reversible and presents no contraindication to continuation of gold therapy. It is evidently dose-dependent since it was seen in only one of 11 patients receiving less than 500 mg. of aurothioglucose and in 27 of 27 patients receiving more than 1500 mg.

Incidence of Toxicity

Toxic complications from use of gold have been reported to be as high as 55 per cent and as low as 4 per cent[51] (Table 29–2). The average incidence of all reactions in a large group of cases was 32 per cent (Table 29–2). It should be emphasized that these figures of incidence include *all* reactions, some of which are trivial, and do not require cessation of treatment; indeed, some abnormalities considered to indicate gold toxicity may not be so.[21] In recent reports the incidence of *severe* toxicity was only 4.5 per cent.

It is difficult to know in many instances when disorders occurring in a patient receiving gold therapy are caused by the gold. It has been customary to consider all abnormalities occurring during gold therapy as manifestations of gold toxicity. That this is not justified is shown by observations of Fraser[21] who found that 19 (27 per cent) of 49 patients among the control group who received placebos and no gold had what was considered by the physician, manifestations of "toxicity." These disturbances are listed as affecting the skin in 16 cases, the kidneys in 2, and oral mucous membranes in 1 case.

Toxicity from gold may occur at any time throughout the course of treatment and for several months after treatment has been discontinued. Usually, it appears after 300 to 500 mg. of gold have been injected. Toxicity is usually mild, but approximately 5 per cent of the toxic reactions represent severe disturbances which require cessation of gold and appropriate treatment. Deaths have occurred from gold-induced thrombocytopenic purpura, aplastic anemia, granulopenia or ulcerative enteritis, very rarely from severe (complicated) exfoliative dermatitis. Reported mortality was as high as 3 per cent in 1935, between 0.5 and 0.6 per cent from 1935 to 1939, and recently less than 0.4 per cent. This significant reduction in serious complications of gold toxicity is attributable to (1) employment of smaller individual doses, (2) improvement in gold compounds, (3) better understanding of the metabolism of gold and clinical response to its administration, (4) greater precautions during treatment and (5) better treatment of toxicity.

Pathogenesis of Gold Toxicity

Much research has been aimed to clarify the nature of gold toxicity, but with limited success. In animals all soluble and insoluble crystalline preparations injected caused significant parenchymal damage in the kidneys. This occurs, however, only after injections of much more gold than that used in treatment of humans, and only when an amount of gold exceeding a certain threshold is injected. Above this level the pathology is proportional to the amount of gold injected. These studies indicate that parenchymatous cell poisoning from gold may be expected in humans if large doses of gold are administered rapidly. In rats, dermatitis and mucous membrane lesions which are the most common clinical forms of toxicity have not been observed.[26]

Skin from patients with gold dermatitis contains no greater concentration of gold than skin from patients receiving comparable amounts of gold, who have no toxicity[26,27] showing that toxic dermatitis does not result from or depend upon a large amount of gold in cutaneous tissue. This form of toxicity clearly is not due to cellular poisoning from gold. There are many circumstances suggesting that gold toxicity in man is an allergic reaction: the occasional occurrence of dermatitis or blood dyscrasia after only three or four injections of gold; the development of toxicity following a single small injection of gold given after an interval of many weeks following completion of a course of injections of the same compound without intolerance; the frequent development of eosinophilia preceding and during toxicity. Efforts to elucidate the nature of such an allergic mechanism have failed. Patch and intradermal skin tests with gold compounds, used in therapy, showed no more positive reactions in patients having gold toxicity than in those who did not.[26] Neither did such tests forecast future toxicity. These observations suggest that elemental gold and the compounds used for treatment do not act unaltered as allergenic agents. Morgenstern and Kaiser[49] found support for an allergic basis for gold dermatitis (in a single patient) by demonstrating the Prausnitz-Kustner reaction in a guinea pig by skin testing and serially determined blood studies.

Because gold is transported in the protein fraction of the blood plasma, and because the urinary excretion of gold falls off sharply a few hours after injection, it is likely that a gold-protein complex develops soon after the injection of gold and that this complex, with a haptene-like linkage of protein and gold, may in some patients act as an allergen to cause the common forms of gold toxicity.

Prevention of Gold Toxicity

All gold that may have therapeutic value has toxic potentialities. Unfortunately there is no reliable method of predicting or testing to determine which persons will develop toxicity from gold as it is employed for the treatment of rheumatoid arthritis. The use of gold, therefore, resolves into a careful clinical trial using all precautions known to be of value. Knowledge of gold metabolism has taught us that the smallest amount of gold that will give satisfactory therapeutic effect should be employed, for if toxicity should develop, it may be more severe and prolonged if there is great retention of gold during treatment. Indeed it has been observed[27] that after gold toxicity develops, it frequently persists through the period of time when gold is found in plasma and urine. *It seems reasonable therefore to use the smallest amount of gold that gives satisfactory clinical benefit.* Investigations[24] have shown that gold sodium thiomalate and gold thioglucose, given in amounts equal to half the conventional doses employed in earlier days of gold therapy, give just as good therapeutic results, and considerable less toxicity, as shown in Table 29–6.

TABLE 29–6.—INCIDENCE OF TOXICITY IN 126 PATIENTS TREATED WITH DIFFERENT WEEKLY DOSES OF GOLD SODIUM THIOMALATE

Weekly Dose of Gold Compound (Mgm.)	*Patients Treated (Number)*	*Incidence of Toxicity All Forms (Per Cent)*
100	46	41
50	63	30
25	17	18

More important is the fact that the *severity* of reactions is likewise usually reduced when smaller weekly doses are employed. There is, therefore, a quantitative (but not absolutely proportional) relationship between the size of the weekly dose and the incidence and severity of toxicity.

Clinical gold toxicity has not proved to be related to plasma gold concentration or to the rate of excretion of gold. Toxic manifestations have occurred when plasma gold concentration was within the usual range, and sometimes occurred when the plasma gold was unusually low.

Much effort has been expended to improve the gold compounds with the hope that therapeutic benefit could be augmented and toxicity reduced or even eliminated. Improvements have resulted, but the major objectives have not been realized. Colloidal preparations, which have been far less toxic, have no dependable therapeutic value. All insoluble compounds including gold calcium thiomalate and gold thioglycoanilid give undependable results, and, although the incidence of toxicity is reported[62] to be less, instances of severe exfoliative dermatitis and ulcerative lesions of oral mucous membranes, with recurrences lasting more than two and one-half years have been observed.[25] The recurrences suggest that from time to time there are "auto-inoculations" from the reservoir of gold retained at the sites of injection of insoluble preparations. For these reasons insoluble gold compounds are not recommended. That large doses of insoluble gold compounds can be injected without toxicity represents no advantage as, of that injected, there is evidence that only a small amount is absorbed.

Precautions Advised During Gold Therapy

Only those physicians who know the therapeutic and toxic potentialities of gold and who are familiar with the manifestations of early toxicity should use this form of treatment. It is advised that *the physician should see the patient* at the time of each injection to interrogate concerning the occurrence of pruritus, skin eruption, purpura, sore mouth, metallic taste, indigestion or other unusual symptoms. Urine should be analyzed for protein and sediment changes weekly, until 500 mgm. of the gold compound have been injected and thereafter before each second injection. Determination of hemoglobin and total and differential leukocyte counts should be made before every second injection; if there are significant reductions of hemoglobin or cells, or symptoms which suggest toxicity, it is wise to do a complete examination of the blood. Purpura always necessitates a platelet count. Leukopenia below 4000 WBC/cmm., rapid reduction of hemoglobin, decrease in platelet count to below 75,000 per cmm., eosinophilia, albuminuria, hematuria, pruritus and stomatitis are all danger signs, though they may not be reliable signs of toxicity. Occasionally, the erythrocyte sedimentation rate falls rapidly shortly before toxicity becomes manifest. Therefore such an occurrence should lead to the suspicion of impending toxicity and treatment should be stopped until developments indicate the procedure to follow. Whenever suggestions or definite indications of toxicity appear, therapy should be promptly discontinued. As one gains experience with this form of treatment, improvement in judgment, diagnosis and management results. In doubtful situations toxicity should be considered to exist, until further studies clarify the situation.

The presence of Sjögren's syndrome in rheumatoid arthritis is a contraindication to treatment with gold since allergic reactions are frequent.[5]

The injection of large amounts of vitamins and liver extract, considered by some physicians to be prophylactic against toxicity has been found by most investigators to be of no value.

Treatment of Gold Toxicity

As soon as there is any evidence of gold toxicity, further administration should be discontinued, symptomatic and supportive care should be instituted, and appropriate corrective treatment promptly employed. Mild erythema and pruritus may disappear in a few days and are relieved by calomine lotion with phenol or corticosteroid ointment. Sedatives or tranquilizers in small doses are helpful. Treatment of severe generalized dermatitis is best done in a hospital. Colloidal baths help to relieve itching. Sunshine and ultraviolet light may aggravate the dermatitis. For stomatitis, alkaline mouthwash, non-irritating foods and sometimes triamcinolone (Kenalog) in oribase (a thick, adherent oral salve) are helpful. Constipating drugs are indicated for diarrhea. For nephritis resulting from gold toxicity, appropriate supportive treatment is required until the disease abates. Blood transfusions are advised for granulopenia, purpura and anemia. Appropriate antianemic drugs should be employed. Appropriate antibiotic is advised during granulocytopenia for prophylaxis against infection.

Dimercapto-propanol.—Two, three-dimercapto-propanol (British anti-lewisite, BAL) is effective in the treatment of gold toxicity. The earlier BAL is used after toxicity develops, the more beneficial it is; if toxicity has existed many months, it has often failed to be helpful. BAL is prepared in a 10 per cent solution of benzyl-benzoate in peanut oil for use intramuscularly. For severe intoxication, it needs to be used vigorously. In all types of gold intoxication BAL has been most effective when injected at four-hour intervals, 4 to 6 times daily during the first and second days of treatment, and twice daily, for five to eight days thereafter. If marked reduction of toxic manifestations occurs within a few days after start of BAL therapy, it may be given only once daily from the fifth to the eighth or tenth day of treatment. The dose used for each injection is the same and is calculated on the basis of body weight: 2.5 mgm. of BAL (0.025 ml. solution) per kgm. Undesirable side effects of BAL include malaise, nausea, vomiting, salivation, lacrimation, blepharospasm, paresthesia, perspiration, sensation of warmth, pain in the extremities or abdomen and commonly, headache, which may be severe. Tachycardia and mild hypertension may result from arteriolar constriction. These side effects are not serious in the doses ordinarily employed and pass off within a day after cessation of treatment. Pain and cramps in the muscles of the extremities and sometimes carpal-pedal spasms occasionally follow injections of BAL, due to lower serum calcium (and other elements). The most troublesome problems occurring with the administration of BAL are the pain and abscesses which occasionally develop at the injection site. Most abscesses have been sterile; some contain staphylococci. Because of the ease of abscess formation meticulous sterilization of skin at the site of injection is advised. Antibiotics and sometimes surgical drainage of the abscess may be required.

The therapeutic effectiveness of 3-mercapto-valine (*penicillamine*) has been demonstrated by Eyring and Engleman.[19] These investigators showed that this agent increased the excretion of gold in the urine from 50 to 4000 per cent within twenty-four hours, even when administered three months after termination of gold therapy. A marked increase in excretion of gold continued throughout three- to seven-day courses of penicillamine therapy. Successful treatment of a persistent gold dermatitis with penicillamine has been reported.[14a] This chelating agent may prove to have practical value in treating gold toxicity.

Corticotropin and Corticosteroid.—The corticosteroids dependably and quickly suppress the manifestations of gold toxicity. Dermatitis caused by gold can be quickly arrested by moderate doses of prednisone (15 to 20 mg. daily) or comparable doses of other steroids. Corticotropin-zinc or corticotropin gel in daily doses of 50 mg. intramuscularly will quickly suppress gold dermatitis. Such treatment may be needed for several weeks. Other forms of gold toxicity including thrombocytopenic purpura, hypoplastic anemia and nephritis have been successfully treated with corticosteroids. It should be appreciated that corticosteroids do not hasten the elimination of gold—nor detoxify it—so they need to be administered for quite a prolonged period until the offending heavy metal has been largely eliminated from or fixed in the body. For severe gold intoxication, BAL and corticosteroids should be used simultaneously—BAL to hasten elimination of the offending toxic material, and the steroids to suppress the symptoms of the toxicity.

Because many toxic reactions from gold may be mild and short in duration, it is not necessary to use BAL, corticosteroid or corticotropin at the first manifestation of gold intoxication. The course of the toxicity should be carefully observed and if it becomes rapidly worse and quite severe, an effective antidote should be used promptly, for best results are obtained when it is used early in the course of intoxication. If toxic manifestations recur after they have been effectively suppressed, treatment should be reinstituted.

Effect of Toxicity on Arthritis

Knowing that BAL, penicillamine, corticotropin and corticosteroids are dependable antidotes for gold toxicity, the anxiety which formerly attended the use of gold therapy has been dispelled. Even so, precaution should be exercised whenever gold is injected. When a toxic reaction from gold occurs, especially a form of dermatitis, the arthritis frequently becomes much improved and it may become completely arrested. The Empire Rheumatism Council's multiple center study, however, showed no correlation between benefits and toxicity from gold.

Reinstitution of Gold Therapy After Toxicity

The continuance or recurrence of active disease after recovery from gold toxicity sometimes prompts the consideration of reinstitution of treatment in a patient who has had toxicity. No rigid criteria can be presented to guide one in this problem. A patient who has had a severe form of intoxication should never have treatment with gold compounds thereafter, for experience has shown that serious toxicity will very likely develop again. In some patients with mild dermatitis or stomatitis, it has been possible to reinstitute gold therapy with benefit, soon after abatement of the toxicity. *In all instances*, reemployment of gold compounds should not be attempted until all signs of toxicity have disappeared, and then only with extreme caution. Small doses of gold should be used at the outset and only small increases should be made until it has been demonstrated that tolerance exists. Frequently, patients can tolerate small doses of gold indefinitely even though customary (larger) doses have caused toxicity.

RELAPSE FOLLOWING GOLD THERAPY

After cessation of treatment with gold improvement which has occurred with this therapy gives way to progress in the disease. Sometimes sharp exacerbation occurs a few months after gold treatment was discontinued; in other instances relapse occurs insidiously and with slow progression. This lack of

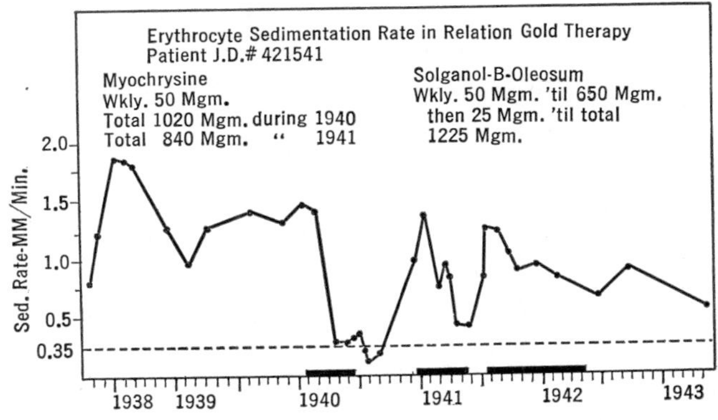

FIG. 29–4.—Continuation of the graphic representation of the erythrocyte sedimentation rate of the patient in whom the early observation is shown in Figure 29–3.

permanency of benefit from gold represents one of the important limitations of gold therapy.

Incidence of relapse has been reported variously from 4 to 75 per cent (Table 29–2). In those who had remissions, and in those who had improved greatly but in whom disease had not become completely arrested during gold therapy, 5 per cent relapsed after treatment was stopped. Ragan and Tyson[60] report the highest relapse rate; of 142 cases followed for three years, 75 per cent relapsed between six weeks and two years after cessation of treatment. The experience of Freyberg has been similar. In a small group of 21 patients, Short *et al.*[70] found 62 per cent relapsed after gold therapy was stopped.

The manner in which relapse occurs is well portrayed in the graphic curve of erythrocyte sedimentation rate shown in Figure 29–4. Notice that several months after complete arrest of the disease, a relapse occurred with sharp elevation of the sedimentation rate. The patient was unable to continue his work and normal living which he had enjoyed for the first time since the onset of arthritis several years before. Gold therapy was reinstituted and accompanied by another remission wherein the improvement was slower than was observed with the first course of gold therapy, but it did not progress to complete arrest of the disease. The patient returned to work; treatment with gold was discontinued and again there was a relapse followed by partial remission after further treatment, but with less improvement than occurred during previous treatment.

Such experiences have been observed in many patients. Fortunately, the relapse has been less severe in the majority of patients than the original disease. Fortunate also is the fact that in approximately 80 per cent of patients who relapse, gold therapy again produces benefit. The frequency of relapse after courses of gold therapy has led to maintenance treatment which has proven to be superior, as will be discussed below.

METHOD OF TREATMENT

After becoming thoroughly familiar with the nature of gold therapy, the metabolism of gold, its potential therapeutic value and toxicity, the limitations of its usefulness, and the precautions required during administration, one can more intelligently plan treatment with gold.

Choice of Gold Compound

Many gold compounds have been prepared by pharmaceutical manufacturers for treatment of rheumatoid arthritis. In the United States only the following are now available by prescription:

*Gold Sodium Thiomalate.**—This is a soluble crystalline compound prepared in aqueous solution for intramuscular injection *only*. It is 50 per cent gold.

Gold Thioglucose.†—This water-soluble organic compound is prepared as a suspension in oil for intramuscular use *only*. This compound contains 50 per cent gold. Ampules containing commonly used single doses and multiple-dose vials are available.

Gold Sodium Thiosulfate.‡—This inorganic water-soluble material contains 37 per cent gold. It can be injected intramuscularly or intravenously.

Gold Thioglycoanilid.§—This is an insoluble compound prepared in oil suspension for intramuscular injection *only*. It is 54 per cent gold.

Selection of the gold preparation for clinical use should depend chiefly upon the knowledge provided by the studies of metabolism of gold. Because colloidal particles are quickly phagocytized and held inert in the tissues, no pharmacologic effect could result. Colloidal preparations of gold or gold compounds are not recommended for treatment of rheumatoid arthritis.

* *Myochrysine*, Merck, Sharp and Dohme.
† *Solganal*, Schering.
‡ Manufactured by Searle, Inc.
§ *Lauron*, Endo Lab.

Animal investigations of Sabin[66] and others showed that the insoluble preparation (*gold calcium thiomalate*) in oil had prophylactic and therapeutic value against experimental arthritis induced by infecting the animals with pleuropneumonia-like organisms. Hence, trials of this and similar insoluble gold compounds have been made in humans with great hope that these would be effective in treatment of rheumatoid arthritis. However, results have been unpredictable, chiefly because absorption varies greatly. Moreover, toxicity in man is apparently due to factors different from those which prevail in experimental animals; toxic manifestations were frequently observed with the clinical use of insoluble gold compounds. Toxic reactions were often quite severe and prolonged, most likely because of the large reservoir of gold at the site of injection. The feature of insolubility, which prompted development of these preparations with the hope that they would be less toxic, appears to be definitely a disadvantage. In order to be therapeutically effective gold must be absorbed *in solution;* the effectiveness of such a drug, therefore, depends upon that portion which is absorbed and not upon the amount injected into the muscle.

For treatment, therefore, it is wise to select a soluble gold compound to be injected intramuscularly. There is little difference in the clinical effects of the available soluble gold preparation. Therapeutic effects are essentially the same with gold sodium thiomalate and gold thioglucose, but some investigators[10,66] have thought that the latter is slightly less toxic.

Dosage Schedule

The method of administration of gold has varied considerably and is not fully agreed upon by all investigators because smaller doses have given results frequently as good as the larger doses, and because toxicity is less frequent and less severe when smaller weekly doses of gold are injected, the following dosage schedule is recommended. For adults of average size, weekly intramuscular injections of a soluble compound containing 50 per cent gold (gold thioglucose or gold thiomalate) are given in these doses:

1st injection ....10 mg.
2nd injection ....25 mg.
3rd injection and subsequent injections
to 16th or 20th injection..........50 mg.

If the patient has shown no improvement after this amount of treatment, it is considered to be of no value and discontinued. If improvement has occurred, instead of stopping treatment for two or four months and then resuming another course of injections as was formerly customary, it is preferable to continue treatment less energetically for a prolonged period—"maintenance therapy"—in an effort to prevent relapse. Injections of 50 mg. are then spaced at two-week intervals and continued for 4 injections, after which this dose is given at three-week intervals for 4 injections, and thereafter at monthly intervals for an indefinite period, usually for several years. The time to discontinue gold therapy cannot be arbitrarily determined; it depends upon the response of each patient. Should a relapse occur when injections are given at two- to four-week intervals, resumption of weekly injections is advised for 6 or more injections, depending upon the response.

The dosage schedule for children is similar except that the amount of gold used for each injection should be in proportion to the body weight or surface area (p. 468).

That this plan of "maintenance therapy" has been superior to "course" therapy with gold has been well documented by the studies of Soler-Bechera *et al.*[76] One hundred and sixty-seven patients with rheumatoid arthritis who received such maintenance therapy for longer than one and a half years—the average duration of continuous treatment was six years—were evaluated by ARA criteria to determine how the disease state had changed and what their response to such therapy was. An evaluation was made separately for three subgroups of the 167 patients: Group 1, 71 patients treated for one and one-half to three years; Group 2, 48 patients treated three to five years; and Group 3, 48 patients treated for more than five years (average eight and one-half years). As with other forms of treatment, maintenance gold therapy never caused structural improvements of joint damage, but improvement in functional capacity of the patients was very substantial. The majority of patients *in each group* had improvement in functional capacity after prolonged treatment. This was as true for the group treated continuously for more than five years, as for those patients in Group 1 or 2, treated for shorter periods of time. For example, of the patients in Group 3, treated more than five years, 34 per cent at the end of the study were in class 1 which indicates *no limitation of function;* of Group 1, 47 per cent were in class 1. Before treatment more than 90 per cent of each group were in class 2 or 3, with moderate or marked incapacitation. Of all 167 patients, 82 per cent were in class 1 or 2 in the after-treatment evaluation. These results are quite different from those reported by the Empire Rheumatism Council Study group, and by others which show a high relapse rate after stopping treatment. Soler-Bechara's study indicates that the majority of the patients who improve during gold therapy continue to be improved during prolonged treatment—that such treatment is truly "maintenance therapy."

Another method of evaluating treatment is by applying the ARA criteria of "therapeutic response." This was done for the 167 patients. The results are shown graphically in Figure 29–5. Note that remissions had occurred and were maintained in 28, 23, and 10 per cent of patients in Groups 1, 2 and 3 respectively and that the percentage of patients with sustained major improvement was large in each group. By this means of evaluation also, the effectiveness of *maintenance* gold therapy is impressive.

Moreover, the incidence of toxicity of all types was very low in those patients who tolerated the treatment so it could be continued for prolonged periods. Maintenance treatment was discontinued in only 12 patients (7 per cent), in 4 per cent because of dermatitis, in 3 per cent because of proteinuria. Toxicity was always mild and reversible. Fear of cumulative toxicity from gold given in this form of maintenance therapy appears unjustified.

Precautions against toxicity already discussed need to continue throughout maintenance therapy. Should toxic manifestations be encountered—and they may appear *at any time* during treatment—it is necessary to stop injections of gold. If treatment is resumed, the same graded increases in dose and the same precautions should be employed when it is reinstituted as were used initially.

Smith[72] has reported better therapeutic results and less toxicity when the weekly dose is individually adjusted according to

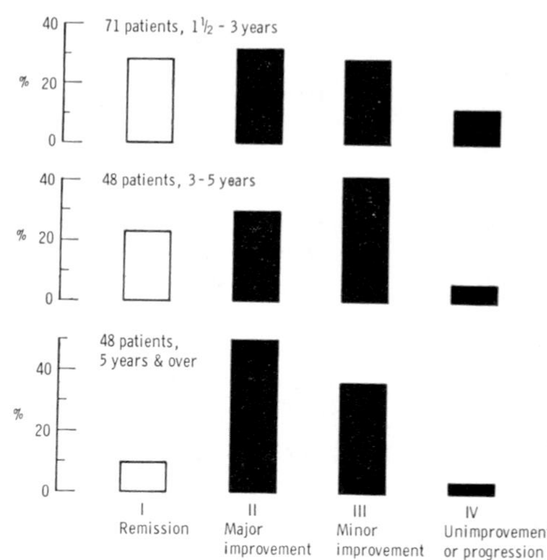

FIG. 29–5.—Graphic representation of therapeutic response of 167 patients who received "maintenance gold therapy" for 3 groups separated according to different periods of time of continuous treatment. The percentage of patients in each grade of response (I through IV) is represented by a column for patients in each group separately.

the rate of urinary excretion of gold. He explains poor therapeutic results when a fixed dose is used on the rapid elimination of gold, so that the amount retained in the body is too little for a good therapeutic effect; in such cases a larger weekly dose would accomplish superior benefits. Smith outlines a slowly increasing dose schedule and emphasizes the importance of carefully following such a schedule. Toxicity is explained on a slow excretion resulting in larger than usual amounts of gold retained in the body, exerting excessive effects. In such cases a smaller weekly dose is indicated. This theory and supporting data seem logical but more study is required before this plan of dosage can be substantially recommended.

Contraindications to Gold Therapy

The chief contraindication to the use of gold is previous, severe toxicity produced by gold or other heavy metals. Many other contraindications have been reported, but experience has demonstrated that many conditions formerly thought to prevent the use of gold actually do not. Allergic diseases have been considered to be contraindication to gold therapy by some physicians, but experience has shown that patients with asthma, hay fever or other allergic diseases usually can tolerate gold therapy quite satisfactorily. If gold is administered to persons who have other *drug* idiosyncrasies, special caution should be exercised, for in such individuals intolerance to gold may develop.

Several pregnant patients have been treated without any harmful effect on either the mother or the baby.[53] Usually, however, patients with rheumatoid arthritis are benefited by pregnancy to such an extent that gold therapy is seldom needed at this time. As with any other medicine, gold should not be given during pregnancy unless definitely needed. If congestive heart failure exists, gold therapy should not be started until effective therapy has restored good circulation. When other serious systemic illnesses exist, they should, whenever possible, be cured or controlled before the institution of gold therapy. Previous kidney or liver disease is not a contraindication to gold therapy; existing diseases of these organs contraindicate only if the functions of these organs are seriously impaired. Even then, the danger is not that toxicity is more apt to occur, but rather that, should severe toxicity occur, the summation of difficulties may produce serious consequences. Similar considerations apply if uncontrolled diabetes or severe blood dyscrasias such as thrombocytopenia, purpura, hemophilia or severe anemia exist. Granulopenia usually is caused by a drug sensitivity which should indicate great caution if gold therapy is used.

It has been thought that psoriasis is a contraindication to gold therapy, but experience has shown this is not so. If any chronic skin eruption exists, one should be particularly wary when using gold because the eruption may be aggravated. If all other considerations make it very desirable to use gold, existing dermatitis should not prevent its use unless the eruption has been caused by a heavy metal.

Age is not a contraindication to gold therapy if function of the vital organs is good.

Systemic lupus erythematosus may be made worse by gold therapy and the disease usually is not benefited even though the drug is tolerated; hence, it is wise not to use gold therapy in patients with SLE.

Mild or moderate anemia is not a contraindication to treatment.

Simultaneous Use of Gold and Corticosteroids

Patients have been treated with cortisone until the rheumatoid arthritis became substantially suppressed, then gold was begun with the hope that this form of treatment would maintain the benefits of the hormone. However, results of this manner of combined therapy have been disappointing; relapses usually follow cessation of corticosteroid therapy as they do when no gold was given. Thompson and Rowe[79] reported that concurrent administration of gold and cortisone gave an excellent basis for effecting a complete remission of arthritis, and Margolis[48] reported that simultaneous use of corticotropin and gold resulted in remission in 30 per cent of cases, which was sustained during continuing gold therapy after corticotropin was stopped. Most investigators consider that combination treatment is impractical, that if corticosteroids are needed, gold compounds administered *simultaneously* provide little or no added benefit.

BENEFITS AND LIMITATIONS OF GOLD THERAPY

Improvement from gold therapy comes about very slowly; the patient should be forewarned that weeks may pass before any benefit may be noted and that many months of treatment may be required before improvement is sufficient to decrease disability. When the therapy is effective, signs of inflammation gradually decrease, pain lessens and function improves. However, the physician should remember that this form of treatment does not help all patients and that whether or not it will be beneficial can be determined only by clinical trial.

As is true with all other forms of therapy, gold is not complete treatment for rheumatoid arthritis. Gold therapy can help only by suppressing rheumatoid inflammation and checking the progress of the disease; when used, it should be part of a well-planned program of treatment which should be carefully adjusted to the needs of each individual.

Rheumatoid arthritis is the only rheumatic disease that is helped by gold therapy (with the possible exception of palindromic rheumatism).[6,48b] This treatment should not be used for other forms of rheumatism.

BIBLIOGRAPHY

1. Adams, C. H. and Cecil, R. L.: Ann. Int. Med., *33*, 163, 1950.

1*a*. Anderson, N. L. and Palmer, W. L.: J.A.M.A., *115*, 1627, 1940.

1*b*. Anttila, R., and Laaksonen, A-L.: Acta Rheum. Scand., *15*, 99, 1969.

1*c*. Bach Andersen, R., and Winther, O.: Acta Rheum. Scand., *14*, 131, 1968.

1*d*. Behrend, T., and Rodenhauser, J. H.: Z. Rheumaforsch., *28*, 441, 1969.

2. Block, W. D. and Buchanan, O. H.: J. Biol. Chem., *136*, 379, 1940.

3. ————: J. Lab. & Clin. Med., *28*, 118, 1942.

4. Block, W. D., Buchanan, O. H. and Freyberg, R. H.: Jour. Pharmacol. & Exper. Med., *76*, 355, 1942.

5. Bloch, K. J., Buchanan, W. W., Wohl, M. J. and Bunim, J. J.: Med., *44*, 187, 1965.

6. Boland, E. F. and Headley, N. E.: Report, Annual Meeting, Amer. Rheum. Assoc., Chicago, Ill., 1948.

7. Bollett, A. J. and Shuster, A.: J. Clin. Invest., *39*, 1114, 1960.

7*a*. Brewer, E.: *Juvenile Rheumatoid Arthritis*, Philadelphia, W. B. Saunders Co., 1970.

8. Browning, J. S., Rice, R. M., Lee, W. V. and Baker, L. M.: New Engl. J. Med., *237*, 428, 1947.

9. Bruce, J. and Mackay, R.: Ann. Rheum. Dis., *11*, 206, 1952.

10. Burnett, J. A.: Brit. Med. J., *2*, 670, 1947.

11. Cecil, R. L. and Kammerer, W. H.: Amer. J. Med., *10*, 439, 1951.

12. Cecil, R. L., Kammerer, W. H. and DePrume F. J.: Ann. Int. Med., *16*, 811, 1942.

13. Clemmesen, S. M.: Acta Med. Scand. Supp., *341*, 59, 1957.

14. Cohen, A., Dubbs, A. W. and Goldman, J.: Pennsylvania M. J., *52*, 35, 1948.

14*a*. Davis, C. M.: Amer. J. Med., *46*, 472, 1969.

15. Dawson, M. H., Boots, R. H. and Tyson, T. L.: Tr. Assoc. Amer. Physicians, *56*, 330, 1941.

15*a*. Denman, E. J., and Denman, A. M.: Ann. Rheum. Dis. *27*, 582, 1968.

16. Ellman, P., Lawrence, J. S. and Thorold, G. P.: Brit. Med. J., *2*, 314, 1940.

17. Empire Rheumatism Council Subcommittee: Ann. Rheumatic Dis., *19*, 95, 1960.

18. ————: Ann. Rheum. Dis., *20*, 315, 1961.

18*a*. Ennis, R. S., Granda, J. L., and Posner, A. S.: Arth. and Rheum., *11*, 756, 1968.

19. Eyring, E. J., Bertrand, J. J. and Engleman, E. P.: Arth. and Rheum., *6*, 216, 1963.

20. Findlay, G. M., MacKenzie, R. D. and McCollum, F. O.: Brit. J. Exper. Path., *21*, 13, 1940.
21. Fraser, T. N.: Ann. Rheum. Dis., *4*, 71, 1945.
22. Forestier, J.: Bull et mem. Soc. med. d. hop. de Paris, *53*, 323, 1929.
23. ———: J. Lab. & Clin. Med., *20*, 827, 1935.
24. Freyberg, R. H.: Proc. Staff Meet. Mayo Clin., *17*, 534, 1942.
25. ———: J. Chronic Dis., *5*, 723, 1957.
26. Freyberg, R. H., Block, W. D. and Preston, W. S.: Unpublished data presented Central Soc. Clin. Research, Chicago, Ill., 1943.
27. Freyberg, R. H., Block, W. D. and Wells, G. S.: Clinics, *1*, 537, 1942.
28. Ganz, A. and Brucer, M.: J. Lab. & Clin. Med., *52*, 20, 1958.
29. Gardner, E. R.: Med. Rec., *63*, 321, 1941.
30. Gerber, D. A.: J. Pharmacol. & Exper. Med., *143*, 137, 1964.
31. Gerber, D. A., Shapiro, M. M. and Follows, J. W., Jr.: Proceedings, Eleventh Interim Scientific Session, Am. Rheum. Assoc., Bull. Rheum. Dis., *15*, 373, 1965.
32. Gilg, E. and Vraa-Jensen, G.: Acta psych. neur. Scand., *33*, 174, 1958.
33. Goldie, W.: Ann. Rheum. Dis., *1*, 319, 1939.
33*a*. Gottlieb, N. L., Smith, P. M., and Smith, E. M.: Arth. and Rheum., *14*, 164, 1971.
34. Graham, J. W. and Fletcher, A. A.: Canad. Med. Assoc. J., *49*, 483, 1943.
35. Hartfall, S. J., Garland, H. G. and Goldie, W.: Lancet, *2*, 784, 838, 1937.
36. Hartung, E. F.: Bull. New York Acad. Med., *19*, 693, 1943.
37. Hartung, E. F. and Cotter, J.: J. Lab. & Clin. Med., *26*, 1274, 1941.
37*a*. Hasebe, K.: Fukushima J. Med. Sci., *15*, 45, 1968.
38. Holbrook, W. P. and Hill, D. F.: J.A.M.A. *107*, 34, 1936.
39. Jasmin, G.: J. Pharm. Exp. Ther., *120*, 349, 1957.
40. Jessop, J. D., and Currey, H. L. F.: Ann. Rheum. Dis., *27*, 577, 1968.
41. Key, J. A., Rosenfeld, H. and Tjoflat, O. E.: J. Bone Joint Surg., *21*, 399, 1939.
42. Krusius, F.-E., Markkanen, A., and Peltola, P.: Ann. Rheum. Dis., *29*, 232, 1970.
43. Lande, K.: Munchen med. Wchschr., *74*, 1132, 1927.
44. Lee, J. C., Dushkin, M., Eyring, E. J., Engleman, E. P. and Hopper, J., Jr.: Arth. and Rheum., *8*, 1, 1965.
45. Lewis, D. C., and Ziff, M.: Arth. and Rheum., *9*, 682, 1966.
46. Lockie, L. M. and Riordan, D. J.: J.A.M.A., *167*, 1205, 1958.
47. Logefeil, R. C. and Hoffman, R. A.: Journal-Lancet, *61*, 221, 1941.
47*a*. Lorber, A., Atkins, C. J., Chang, C. C., and Starrs, J.: Arth. and Rheum., *12*, 677, 1969.
47*b*. Lorber, A., Cohen, R. L., Chang, C. C., and Anderson, H. E.: Arth. and Rheum., *11*, 170, 1968.
47*c*. Makin, M., and Robin, G. C.: J.A.M.A., *188*, 107, 1964.
48. Margolis, H. M. and Caplan, P. S.: J.A.M.A., *145*, 382, 1951.
48*a*. Mascarhenus, B., Granda, J. and Freyberg, R. H.: Unpublished studies.
48*b*. Mattingly, S.: Ann. Rheum. Dis., *25*, 307, 1966.
48*c*. Miehlke, K., Kohlhardt, I., and Wirth, B.: Z. Rheumaforsch., *27*, 445, 1968.
49. Morgenstern, A. and Kaiser, W.: Zschr. ges. inn. Med., *11*, 848, 1956.
49*a*. Newbould, B. B.: Brit. J. Pharmacol., *21*, 217, 1963.
49*b*. Niklewicz-Rodkiewiczova, J., Beisterova, A., and Znamirowska, K.: Fysiat. Reum. Vestn., *44*, 321, 1966.
49*c*. Norton, W. L., Lewis, D. C., and Ziff, M.: Arth. and Rheum., *11*, 436, 1968.
50. Oren, H.: J. Med. Soc. New Jersey, *33*, 591, 1936.
51. ———: Med. Rec., *159*, 420, 1946.
51*a*. Paltemaa, S.: Acta Rheum. Scand., *14*, 161, 1968.
52. Panel Discussion: Bull. N. Y. Acad. Med., *30*, 863, 1954.
53. Patterson, M. and Traeger, C. H.: Report, Meeting of New York Rheumat. Assn., 1951.
53*a*. Persellin, R. H., Hess, E. V., and Ziff, M.: Arth. and Rheum., *10*, 99, 1967.
54. Persellin, R. H., Smiley, J. D. and Ziff, M.: Arth. and Rheum., *6*, 787, 1963.
55. Phillips, R. T.: New Engl. J. Med., *214*, 114, 1936.
56. Pick, E.: Wien. klin. Wchnshr., *40*, 1175, 1927.
57. Preston, W. S., Block, W. D. and Freyberg, R. H.: Proc. Soc. Exper. Biol. & Med., *1*, 253, 1942.
58. Price, A. E. and Leichtentritt, B.: Ann. Int. Med., *19*, 70, 1943.
59. Prowse, R. B.: Brit. Med. J., *2*, 917, 1954.
60. Ragan, C. and Tyson, T. L.: Amer. J. Med., *1*, 252, 1946.

61. Rawls, W. B., Gruskin, B. J., Ressa, A. A., Dworzan, H. J. and Schreiber, D.: Amer. J. Med. Sci., *207*, 528, 1944.
62. Robinson, D.: Canad. Med. Assoc. J., *1*, 223, 1944.
63. Root, S. W., Andrews, G. A., Kniseley, R. M. and Tyor, M. P.: Cancer, *7*, 856, 1954.
64. Rose, P. A.: Illinois Med. J., *92*, 175, 1947.
65. Rothbard, S., Angevine, D. M. and Cecil, R. L.: J. Pharmacol. & Exper. Therap., *72*, 164, 1941.
66. Sabin, A. B.: Bact. Rev., *5*, 1, 1941.
67. Sabin, A. B. and Warren, J.: J. Bact., *40*, 823, 1940.
67*a*. Sairanen, E. and Laaksonen, A-L.: Ann. Paediat. Fenn., *10*, 274, 1964.
67*b*. Saphir, J. R. and Ney, R. G.: J.A.M.A., *195*, 782, 1966.
68. Sashin, D., Spanbock, J. and Kling, D. H.: J. Bone Joint Surg., *21*, 723, 1939.
68*a*. Scheiffarth, F., Baenkler, H. W., and Schörg, G.: Z. Rheumaforsch., *29*, 42, 1970.
69. Schwartz, S., Blain, H. R., Geiger, H. B. and Hartung, E. F.: J.A.M.A., *154*, 1263, 1954.
70. Short, C. L., Beckman, W. W. and Bauer, W.: New Engl. J. Med., *235*, 362, 1946.
71. Sliwinski, A., Zvaifler, N., and Rubin, M.: Clinical Research, *14*, 484, 1966.
71*a*. Silverberg, D. S., Kidd, E. G., Schnitka, T. K., and Ulan, R. A.: Arth. and Rheum., *13*, 812, 1970.
72. Smith, R. T., Peale, W. P., Kron, K. M., Hermann, I. F., Del Toro, R. A. and Goldman, M.: J.A.M.A., *167*, 1197, 1958.
73. Smyth, C. J. and Freyberg, R. H.: Univ. (Michigan) Hosp. Bull., *7*, 45, 1941.
74. Snorrason, E.: Acta med. Scand., *142*, 249, 1952.
75. Snyder, R. G., Traeger, C. H. and Kelly, L.: Ann. Int. Med., *12*, 1672, 1939.
76. Soler-Bechara, J., Rogoff, B., Kammerer, W. D. and Freyberg, R. H.: Unpublished observations.
76*a*. Sølvsten, S.: Scand. J. Clin. Lab. Invest., *16*, 39, 1964.
76*b*. Strunk, S. W., and Ziff, M.: Arth. and Rheum., *13*, 39, 1970,
77. Sorensen, B.: Acta med. Scand., *141*, 27, 1951.
77*a*. Stavem, P., Stromme, J., and Bull, O.: Scand. J. Haemat., *5*, 271, 1968.
77*b*. Stepan, J., and Ott, V. R.: Acta Rheum. Scand., *14*, 175, 1968.
78. Sundelin, F.: Nord. med., *37*, 303, 1948.
79. Thompson, H. E. and Rowe, H. J.: Ann. Int. Med., *36*, 992, 1952.
80. Thompson, M., Sinclair, R. J. G. and Duthie, J. J. R.: Brit. Med. J., *1*, 899, 1954.
80*a*. Vaamonde, C. A., and Hunt, F. R.: Arth. and Rheum., *13*, 826, 1970.
81. Waine, H., Baker, F. and Mettier, S. R.: Calif. Med. J., *66*, 295, 1947.
82. Zutshi, D. W., Ansell, B. W., Bywaters, E. G. L., Epstein, W. V., Holborow, E. J., and Reading, C. A.: Ann. Rheum. Dis., *28*, 541, 1969.

Chapter 30

Phenylbutazone, Indomethacin and Chloroquines in Therapy of Rheumatoid Arthritis

By L. Maxwell Lockie, M.D.

In this chapter indications for administration of each of several drugs which have been widely used in the treatment of rheumatoid arthritis during the past decade or more will be described. Phenylbutazone and indomethacin have been termed "non-steroidal anti-inflammatory agents." Others of this group in addition to the salicylates are mefenamic acid, flufenamic acid and several newer synthetic compounds which have not yet been demonstrated to have therapeutic advantage over salicylates in general use for treating rheumatoid arthritis. Acetaminophen has been widely used as a substitute for aspirin when aspirin cannot be tolerated, but has no appreciable anti-inflammatory effect. The antimalarial drugs, including the chloroquines, have been shown to have an anti-rheumatic effect but apparently not a true anti-inflammatory action.

PHENYLBUTAZONE

Phenylbutazone* and its analog, oxyphenbutazone,† have been widely used by physicians in treatment of rheumatic diseases for more than 20 years. They are more effective in the treatment of gout (*see* Chapter 59), and of ankylosing spondylitis (*see* Chapter 41) than in rheumatoid arthritis.

* Brand name: Butazolidin.

† Brand name: Tandearil

Pharmacology.—Phenylbutazone chemically is 4-butyl-1,2-diphenyl-3,5-pyrazolidinedione. This drug and its analog oxyphenbutazone have analgesic, antipyretic and anti-inflammatory activity. Absorption of either from the gastrointestinal tract is rapid and virtually complete with peak plasma concentrations obtained within two hours after administration. A therapeutic plasma level may be achieved with single or divided daily doses. Phenylbutazone can be detected in the body for as long as 21 days after last ingestion, and its half-life is 72 hours in man.[4] Glomerular filtration is not affected by the drug, but decreased excretion of water and salt results from increased renal tubular reabsorption. The intensity and duration of action of some other medications such as meperidine and morphine are increased by phenylbutazone by reducing their renal excretion rate. The drug is carried bound to albumin in the blood, and apparently displaces anticoagulants from such binding sites when administered simultaneously, thus potentiating anticoagulant effects.[25]

Phenylbutazone has no protective effect on the release of hydrolases from lysosomes,[10] nor on plasma protein binding of 11-hydroxysteroids.[34] It does not significantly alter the typical pattern of normal wound healing.[17] The drug does inhibit fixation of sulfate in cartilage.[8]

No changes were noted in synovial biopsy specimens of patients while receiving oral or intra-articular phenylbutazone.[14]

Use in Rheumatoid Arthritis.—Phenylbutazone or oxyphenbutazone may be helpful, particularly as an analgesic agent, in patients with rheumatoid arthritis who have derived little benefit from salicylates,[29] or in those who cannot tolerate aspirin or other salicylic acid derivatives.[13] In such instances a therapeutic trial of phenylbutazone or oxyphenbutazone is reasonable and justified. These drugs often produce relief of the symptoms of rheumatoid arthritis.[22,28] I share the opinion of many others that they are most effective when the articular manifestations develop rapidly.[33]

Before beginning the administration of phenylbutazone, and at regular intervals during treatment, each patient should have a physical examination, urinalysis and complete blood count. The recommended dose is 100 mg. 3 or 4 times daily, after meals or with a glass of milk. If little or no improvement has occurred after one week, the drug should be discontinued.[20] However, if the symptoms are controlled by a daily dose of 100 to 300 mg., phenylbutazone can be administered for long periods with reasonable safety, if the patient is under periodic observation by the physician.

Side Effects.—These drugs produce adverse reactions in some patients. Such reactions appeared in 22.9 to 43.8 per cent of patients in different studies.[21,26,30,31] Toxic effects are rare, however, in patients with gouty arthritis treated with high does for only a few days or in patients with ankylosing spondylitis where the effective dose is usually low.

In rheumatoid arthritis, most adverse effects occur during the first five weeks of therapy, but tolerance during this period does not preclude the possibility of a later reaction. It is noteworthy that in one group who exhibited "toxic effects," only 16 per cent experienced good relief of arthritic complaints compared with 60 per cent in the group which did not have "toxic manifestations."

Common Reactions and Management.—(1) The edema produced by the retention of sodium and chloride can be minimized by a low salt diet.[35] (2) Gastrointestinal reactions account for as much as 66 per cent of all side effects. These usually consist of epigastric distress, nausea and vomiting. Pre-existing peptic ulcer may be aggravated; only occasionally does bleeding or perforation occur. Usually the symptoms can be corrected by medication and diet. (3) Approximately 5 per cent of patients treated develop a maculopapular dermatitis accompanied by itching. Whether mild or severe, immediate discontinuation of the drug is mandatory when rash is noted. (4) Hematologic abnormalities have been reported, particularly when daily doses of more than 300 mg. per day have been taken over long periods. These have included anemia, leukopenia even to the point of agranulocytosis,[2,3,5,7,12] and thrombocytopenia. Leukemia has been reported in patients treated with phenylbutazone, and the drug was considered as a possible etiologic factor.[1,16,18,19,36] When the drug is used concomitantly with anticoagulants, the prothrombin time is prolonged and bleeding may be severe.[9,11,25] Withdrawal of the drug is indicated for any of these complications, and corticosteroid therapy may be indicated for treatment of severe problems.

Although oxyphenbutazone has appeared to be less toxic than the parent drug in most reported studies, similar precautions are indicated for its administration.[32]

Swelling of the parotid glands has been noted with administration of either phenylbutazone or oxyphenbutazone in some instances, and recurrence was noted on readministration.[15,23] In one case the thyroid gland enlarged after treatment with phenylbutazone was started and returned to normal size within a few weeks after the drug was withdrawn.[24] When a glycerine extract of thyroid was combined with phenylbutazone and this was administered to laboratory animals or to man, side effects were prevented or markedly reduced without impairing the anti-inflammatory activity of the drug.[27]

Contraindications.—Phenylbutazone or oxyphenbutazone is not recommended for treatment of rheumatoid arthritis in the presence of edema, cardiac decompensation (overt or impending), blood dyscrasias, history of drug allergy or in combination with other medication (*e.g.* gold therapy or indomethacin) which would increase the hazards of a toxic reaction. Usually the presence of, or recent history of, a peptic ulcer is a contraindication, although this opinion has been challenged.[6] In the presence of hypertension, hepatic damage, renal insufficiency, in a senile patient, or when there is a history of drug sensitivity, phenylbutazone should be administered with extreme caution and for short periods only.

Close supervision is needed at all times during treatment with phenylbutazone and oxyphenbutazone.

INDOMETHACIN*

Indomethacin was chosen as an anti-inflammatory agent from a systematic study of 300 indole acetic acid compounds, due to the antagonistic effect of such compounds on 5-hydroxy-tryptamine (serotonin) in inflammation.[13,29] Clinical trial of indomethacin began in 1961 and in 1965 it was made available on prescription in the United States as a new antirheumatic agent. For discussion of indomethacin in ankylosing spondylitis, *see* Chapter 41; for its use in gout, *see* Chapter 59; for use of indomethacin in osteoarthritis, *see* Chapter 57. It is not recommended for use in children (*see* Chapter 24).

Chemistry.—Indomethacin is 1-(p-chlorobenzoyl)-5-methoxy-2-methylindole-3-acetic acid and has the following structural formula (Fig. 30–1):

* Brand name: Indocin in U.S., Indocid, Indomee, etc. abroad.

INDOMETHACIN
1-(p-chlorobenzoyl)-5-methoxy-2-methylindole-3-acetic acid
$C_{19}H_{16}NO_4Cl$

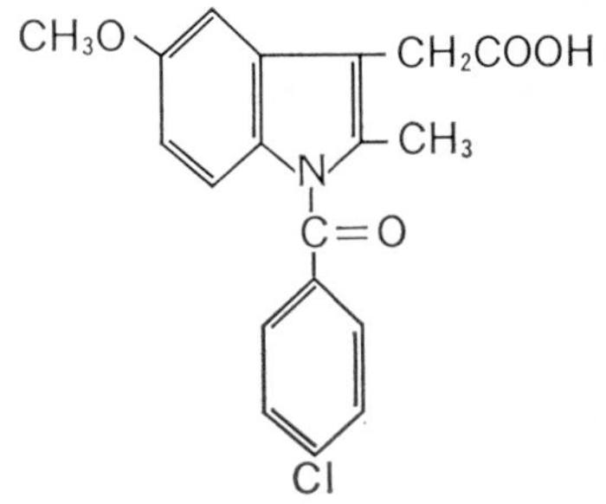

Fig. 30–1.

The molecular formula is $C_{19}H_{16}NO_4$-Cl. and the molecular weight is 357.8. The compound is relatively insoluble in water but is soluble in the common organic solvents.[29] Chemically, indomethacin has no structural relationship to other antirheumatic drugs, such as the salicylates, corticosteroids, phenylbutazone, or the chloroquines.

Pharmacology.—Indomethacin is well absorbed after oral administration in all species, including man. Peak plasma levels are reached promptly, in one-half to two hours, with a plasma half-life of approximately ninety minutes. The drug is present in plasma as the parent compound, and about 90 per cent is bound to albumin. The principal excretory pathway is via the kidney, with 60 to 75 per cent recovery as indomethacin glucuronide in the first twenty-four hours. About 25 to 30 per cent of the free drug is eliminated through the gastrointestinal tract. There has been no evidence of accumulation of indomethacin with repeated dosage, nor has there been any evidence of deacetylation, demethylation, or other metabolic breakdown of the drug in man.[3,12,15]

The anti-inflammatory and anti-pyretic effects of indomethacin have been demonstrated by standard laboratory methods. The site and mechanism of action of the drug are unknown, as they are with other anti-inflammatory drugs. Indomethacin does not require an intact pituitary-

aspirin given over a like period. In the 21 patients who completed the study, there was no significant difference in clini-

the efficacy of indomethacin in rheumatoid arthritis.[14] One said: "The drug's final role in the treatment of rheumatoid

adrenal axis for its activity, nor does it affect the function of these glands.

Extensive experimental studies have

After the insertion of rectal suppositories containing indomethacin 100 mg. in man, at the end of one hour the maxi-

arthritis has not been completely evaluated. There is no doubt it is beneficial to some patients. We need to know more about its long term side effects as against the short term effects." Another observed: "The drug has its uses, but it is not the best agent in treatment of rheumatoid arthritis. It is 'another arrow in our quiver'." Still another felt "the drug is more potent than aspirin." A fourth felt that indomethacin is useful in selected patients, and agreed with another's observation that long-term trials of any drug are essential in treating rheumatoid arthritis. A fifth rheumatologist felt the drug "is useful in a few patients only." Another emphasized that "there are a great many individual variations in response to the drug; in those who can tolerate it, the results are excellent." A seventh opinion was that "on the whole, indomethacin is not too effective in typical rheumatoid arthritis, but is excellent in those cases in whom it does work." The last observed that trials up to that time were over a relatively short term only, making it difficult to judge the efficacy of the drug on an objective basis. Such were the opinions of 8 American rheumatologists in 1967. It is probable that another survey today might reveal a similar divergence of opinions on the degree of efficacy and overall usefulness of indomethacin, but all would agree it has a place in the treatment armamentarium for rheumatoid arthritis.

In a report[6] on the assessment of drug efficacy in rheumatoid arthritis it was emphasized that trials should include serologic and radiologic evaluation over periods in excess of 6 months, during which "background therapy" must be continued, such as aspirin, physical therapy or corticosteroids. To be considered effective, a trial drug must produce measurable benefit over and above that provided by "background treatment." The same report stressed that bedside measurements, grip strength, walking time and the number of painful joints may not be truly objective as they can be influenced by both patient and examiner. Differences in methods of analysis of results and methods of reporting further complicate the effort to obtain truly reliable data in such drug trials.

Another uncontrolled variable in the above drug trials was brought out by Cata and Hazevoet[4] who followed 130 seropositive rheumatoid arthritic patients and 130 who were seronegative. Since the prognosis in seropositive patients was much worse than in the seronegative group, trials should consider results in both groups separately.

Concurrent administration of aspirin and indomethacin resulted in a decreased serum level of indomethacin in the eight patients of a recent study.[17] A decrease in urinary excretion of indomethacin was consistently noted, and 1 patient had a significant rise in fecal excretion. Decreased gastrointestinal absorption of indomethacin was postulated when the two drugs were given together. This inhibitory effect could account for the clinical observation that aspirin and indomethacin were no more beneficial than aspirin alone.

The results of many investigators reviewed in the foregoing discussion make it clear that in future trials, control patients should be matched by presence or absence of rheumatoid nodules and titer of rheumatoid factor as these are known to influence prognosis. Aspirin should not be used with indomethacin during the trial period. Finally, such drug trials should last at least 3 months before changeover to placebo or other drug to be compared for effect.

Administration and Dosage.—Indomethacin is an effective analgesic for many patients with rheumatoid arthritis. It may be prescribed provided no contraindications exist and there is no history of previous ineffective trials. The drug is best tolerated when started in a small dosage, such as 25 mg. daily and increased by one 25-mg. capsule daily at weekly intervals. The usual effective dose in rheumatoid arthritis is 25 mg. 3 to 4 times daily, always to be taken with food. Many patients are able to take 75 to 200 mg. of the drug daily for many years without obvious side effects. The medication can be discontinued and resumed at any time without evidence of reaction.[13] Aspirin is usually given with the drug, although there is evidence that this may reduce the absorption or effectiveness of indomethacin.[17]

Side Effects.—In the survey of clinical trials reviewed by O'Brien[23] there were 15 studies in which 35.6 per cent of patients noted at least one undesirable side effect, and in 14 of the reports there were 20 per cent of patients who could not tolerate indomethacin.

Gastrointestinal side effects occurred in 17.3 per cent of a total of 2487 patients tried on the drug.[25] Twelve per cent of these had nausea, 3.2 per cent noted severe abdominal pain and 2.1 per cent had symptoms of peptic ulcer. In the 60 patients in whom the site of ulceration was demonstrated, 16 were gastric, 14 duodenal and 2 ileal. Twelve ulcers perforated and in 18 instances bleeding was a significant complication. The current consensus is that patients who have a history of peptic ulcer should be studied carefully before Indocin is prescribed. Extreme caution must be exercised if the drug is given to those who have an active ulcer or a history of perforation or hemorrhage. The degree of tolerance differs greatly among individual patients; some cannot take 12.5 mg. without distress, but others can tolerate 200 mg. in capsule form for years without symptoms or bleeding. To minimize gastrointestinal intolerance, indomethacin should always be taken with food.

Indigestion is the commonest complaint; it is usually postprandial and of mild degree. So often the patient will report: "I am able to take 2 capsules all right, but when I take 3 capsules I always get indigestion." The distress may be so mild that the patient continues to take indomethacin. In those who have distress and continue medication there may develop complaints of anorexia, nausea, vomiting or abdominal pain. Diarrhea or gastrointestinal bleeding enough to produce anemia is infrequent.[1,18] Goldfarb and Smyth[11] found the incidence of peptic ulcer in 552 rheumatoid arthritic patients treated with indomethacin in doses up to 75 mg. per day was no greater than the incidence in 259 patients with various rheumatic diseases treated with other commonly used anti-inflammatory drugs (corticosteroids, gold compounds, phenylbutazone and oxyphenbutazone).

Central nervous system effects have been reported frequently from use of indomethacin. Frontal headache is common; it occurs at the onset of therapy in as many as 25 per cent of patients. Headache is less apt to occur if the drug is started at a low level, *i.e.* 25 mg. daily for the first few days, then increased as described under administration and dosage above. It is curious that the character of this side effect is of such a definite pattern; it is frontal in location and appears on awakening in the morning.[19]

Light-headedness, vertigo, mental confusion or even a sense of unreality or mental detachment may occur separately or in combination with headache. In rare instances disturbance of gait and difficulty in standing may be experienced. Errors in judgment and other psychiatric problems have been reported as side effects. Aggravation of epilepsy or parkinsonism has been noted.[25]

Ocular manifestations from use of indomethacin have been the subject of reports. Burns[2] noted decreased retinal sensitivity and reversible corneal deposits related to Indocin intake. She found no definite correlation between dosage of drug and corneal, macular or visual field changes. Deutsch and Hiatt[7] found no statistically significant changes in intraocular pressure upon use of indomethacin. Retinal sensitivity was not studied, but when corneal abnormalities were present before the drug was started they showed no progression on the agent, nor did new corneal opacities develop. Blurred vision has been reported.[18]

Infrequent complications, presumably related to indomethacin therapy include rare instances of bronchial asthma, allergy, edema and salt retention, rash or pruritus. Reports of hepatitis, uremia, pancreatitis and leukopenia on the drug are so infrequent that they may be coincidental and not caused by indomethacin. "Aspirin sensitive" patients, some with nasal polyps or asthma, may show such sensitivity to indomethacin also.

Contraindications.—Indomethacin should not be prescribed for patients with an active peptic ulcer or colitis. Great care should be taken if it is used in those with a history of a bleeding or perforated ulcer. It is *not* recommended for children under 14 years of age. It should not be used in pregnant or nursing women, in patients known to be allergic to aspirin, or in those with psychiatric disturbances, epilepsy or parkinsonism. It is not yet known whether the drug may be harmful in the patient with an active infection.

Summary.—Indomethacin is an effective anti-rheumatic drug for some patients with rheumatoid arthritis. In order to obtain a maximum therapeutic response it must be taken 2 months or longer. It is recommended as an important part of the treatment program of the rheumatoid arthritic patient who has reacted favorably to a trial of the drug. Undesirable side effects are common but rarely serious; they can be minimized by using a graduated dosage schedule starting with 25 mg. daily, with weekly increments of 25 mg. in daily dose if tolerated until 100 to 150 mg. per day are used as maintenance treatment. Early morning headache or symptoms of indigestion are signs of intolerance. This drug should be taken with food to minimize gastrointestinal side effects.

Use of indomethacin should be avoided in patients having definite contraindications, and should be used only with extreme caution in those with relative contraindication. The drug should be stopped promptly for any severe or persistent undesirable effect.

CHLOROQUINES

There have been 20 years of experience since Page's report[21] on the use of chloroquines in the treatment of rheumatoid arthritis. Of the various antimalarials tested, the chloroquines have been shown to have a definite but mild anti-rheumatic effect with relatively few side effects of a serious nature except the rarely occurring progressive retinopathy.

Hydroxychloroquine sulfate (Plaquenil) is the popular chloroquine derivative now in use. It is less toxic than, but apparently equally effective as, chloroquine phosphate (Aralen) the manufacture of which was discontinued in 1970. The antirheumatic effect is seldom noted until the drug has been used for at least 2 months. The usual dose of hydroxychloroquine is 200 mg. daily. Some physicians use 200 mg. twice daily for treatment of active rheumatoid arthritis, but reactions are more frequent with this larger dose. The drug is frequently considered for those patients with rheumatoid arthritis in whom L.E. cells have been demonstrated (*see also* Chapter 10), and in those who cannot tolerate gold therapy (*see also* Chapter 29).

Pharmacology.—Chloroquine phosphate is rapidly and completely absorbed when taken orally. The daily ingestion of 500 mg. increases the blood plasma level gradually over a period of four weeks to a maximum of 200 mcg. per liter. When it is discontinued, the blood plasma level falls to half value in five days. The concentration in the liver, spleen, kidney and lung is 400 to 700 times that in the blood plasma.[3] Parker and Irwin attribute this to affinity for nucleoproteins and nucleates.[22]

Zvaifler *et al.*[31,32] gave 150 mg. chloroquine base daily for twenty-eight days. During the first two weeks the urinary output was $\frac{1}{3}$ to $\frac{1}{2}$ the oral dose in normals. Rheumatoid patients stabilized at $\frac{1}{2}$ to $\frac{2}{3}$ and the stool chloroquine was 10 per cent of the ingested dose. Following discontinuation the urinary output dropped 50 per cent per week and after four weeks remained constant at 5 to 10 mg./twenty-four hours over a period of months. The urinary output can be decreased by taking sodium bicarbonate, and increased by ingesting ammonium chloride or by giving BAL intramuscularly. There is evidence that chloroquine can be detected in the urine five years after last ingestion.[13]

Examination of the eyes revealed the highest concentration of chloroquine to be in the choroid and pigmented epithelium. This concentration is related to total dosage and duration of treatment.[17] Rubin[25] has demonstrated that chloroquine mobilized from various tissues is either excreted in the urine or is redeposited in ocular tissue by melanin binding. He questions the wisdom of attempting to remove it by producing clinical acidosis.

Chloroquine was found to have a hypotensive effect in 22 hypertensive patients, and to induce electrocardiographic changes in 12 of 15 patients taking the drug.[10] Smooth muscle tone in the intestinal tract, arteries, trachea and ciliary bodies may be temporarily depressed during the first few weeks of treatment.[19] Chloroquine appears to inhibit the protease-induced release of peptides from incubated cartilage slices;[30] lysosomal membranes are stabilized.[28]

The action of chloroquine has been summarized by Sams[26] in the following manner: it interferes with the action of several enzymes, binds itself to melanin and deoxyribonucleic acid, stabilizes lysosomes, blocks the sulfhydryl-disulfide interchange reaction and is moderately anti-inflammatory. The drug is sometimes fatal in dosage of as little as 1 gram for a child and from 3 to 11.5 grams for an adult. No specific antidote is known, therefore *it is important to keep chloroquine out of reach of children.*[7,20]

An examination of the eyes by an ophthalmologist every 6 months during the first year of treatment, and at least every 3 to 4 months thereafter is strongly recommended to guard against the development of retinopathy. One rheumatologist,[15] who has extensive experience with the use of antimalarials in treating rheumatoid arthritis, has used chloroquine phosphate in daily doses of 125 to 250 mg. for his patients more than a decade. His opinion is that chloroquine is helpful in treating the disease and is one of the safest drugs of the antirheumatic group. The drug was discontinued in only 4 patients because of retinal pathology.

Contraindications.—The chloroquines should not be given to patients who have, in addition to rheumatoid arthritis, liver, kidney or lung disease. Psoriasis is frequently exacerbated by chloroquine therapy. Children should not receive the drug. Patients should have an ophthalmologic examination before chloroquines are started to exclude those with ocular disease which might be aggravated.

Side Effects.—Various types of toxicity may occur during the use of chloroquines over a prolonged period of time.[1,2,16,27] Maculopapular, purpuric, lichenoid and pleomorphic skin lesions may develop. They appear after several months of therapy and are usually controlled by reduction of dose. Loss of some hair, blanching in blonde or redhaired individuals, leukopenia, peripheral neuropathy,[18] neuromyopathy,[29] a generalized prickling sensation[9] and bilateral abducens paralysis[14] have been attributed to chloroquine and returned to normal after withdrawal of the drug. Chloroquine-treated patients are extremely prone to severe sunburn.

Ocular complications, including corneal deposits of the drug which may be asymptomatic or manifested by halos around lights, blurring of vision and loss of corneal sensitivity, were found to be reversible with cessation of drug.[6,11,12,28] There are reports of retinopathy in rheumatoid arthritic patients, especially those who have been on long-term therapy. This may occur during treatment with chloroquine or after therapy has been discontinued.[5] Although a rare complication, it occurs sufficiently often to require the precaution of

Chloroquine Therapy in Rheumatoid Arthritis

1. Chloroquine has a mild, long-term, anti-rheumatic effect when used in treatment of rheumatoid arthritis.
2. It is most often employed in those patients with chronic, active disease who have positive L.E. cell preparations or who have been intolerant to gold therapy.
3. Hydroxychloroquine sulfate is the form now available.
4. Maximum dosage recommended is 2 mg. per pound of body weight per day.
5. This drug may be safely used in combinations with other anti-rheumatic agents (*e.g.* salicylates, indomethacin, steroids).
6. Maximal therapeutic response is not achieved until several months after onset of treatment.
7. The drug is contraindicated in children, or in the presence of psoriasis, liver, kidney or pulmonary diseases.
8. Side effects are usually reversible and not serious, except for the development of retinopathy.
9. Patients on chloroquine therapy should wear dark glasses in sunlight or bright light, and should be examined carefully by an ophthalmologist at intervals of from 3 to 6 months.

frequent, thorough ocular examination.[24] Such retinopathy has not been reported in the thousands of persons who have received 500 mg. weekly for long periods as a malaria suppressive.[8]

Burns[4] has described the retinal abnormalities in detail. She reports one outstanding feature of chloroquine retinopathy not found in other forms of retinal degeneration, namely a peculiar ring of abnormal pigment epithelium and receptors, often with mottling, in the macular region. This is followed by the formation of a "bull's eye" with central pigmented area surrounded by atrophy of some retinal cells. If the retinopathy progresses there may be marked pigmentary changes throughout the retina.

In 1969 Percival and Behrman[23] published a 7-year study of 272 patients seen at 4-month intervals for 2 to 3 years while on and off chloroquine therapy. Included in this group were 100 control patients matched for age and sex, all healthy and with a normal retina at the start. The eyes were examined in detail. The authors described at length the various ocular findings which had been attributed to chloroquine toxicity and in many instances doubt that the change is truly due to the chloroquines. Also this report suggests that by early recognition of retinopathy and prompt discontinuation of the drug it may be possible to prevent the progression of retinopathy and the development of delayed retinal changes.

In an excellent reference article, Mackenzie[19] summarizes many observations concerning chloroquine therapy, including the mode of action and side effects. In his experience with 2000 patients, none has lost useful vision during chloroquine therapy. His guidelines for therapy are: (1) a maximum dose of 2 mg. per pound of body weight per day, (2) periodic ophthalmologic examinations using standard methods, with measurement of red-light thresholds at least at yearly intervals, and (3) when the patient is exposed to bright light, dark glasses should be worn which reduce visual wavelengths of light by about 50 per cent.

BIBLIOGRAPHY

Phenylbutazone

1. Bean, R. H. D.: Brit. Med. J., *2*, 1552, 1960.
2. Brodie, B. B. *et al.*: Amer. J. Med., *16*, 181, 1954.
3. Brownlie, B. E. W. and Strang, R. J. H.: New Zealand Med. J., *69*, 77, 1969.
4. Burns, J. J. *et al.*: J. Pharm. & Exp. Therap., *104*, 346, 1953.
5. Byron, C. S. and Orenstein, H. B.: New York J. Med., *53*, 676, 1953.
6. Carmel, P. D.: New York J. Med., *60*, 2906, 1960.

7. DENKO, C. W. *et al.*: Amer. Pract. & Digest of Treat., *6*, 1865, 1955.
8. DENKO, C. W.: J. Lab. Clin. Med., *63*, 953, 1964.
9. EISEN, M. J.: J.A.M.A., *189*, 150, 1964.
10. ENNIS, R. S. *et al.*: Arth. & Rheum., *11*, 756, 1968.
11. FOX, S. L.: J.A.M.A., *188*, 320, 1964.
12. FRAUMEIN, J. F., JR.: J.A.M.A., *201*, 828, 1967.
13. FREYBERG, R. H.: Med. Times, *95*, 724, 1967.
14. GANTNER, G. E. *et al.*: Arth. & Rheum., *6*, 711, 1963.
15. GROSS, L.: Ann. Intern. Med., *70*, 1229, 1969.
16. HART, G. D.: Brit. Med. J., *2*, 569, 1964.
17. JONES, R. F., PEACOCK, G. and JONES, R. C.: Amer. J. Surg., *115*, 759, 1968.
18. LAWRENCE, A.: Brit. Med. J., *2*, 1736, 1960.
19. LEAVESLEY, G. M. *et al.*: Med. J. Austral., *2*, 963, 1969.
20. LOCKIE, L. M.: In *Arthritis and Allied Conditions*, 6th ed., J. L. Hollander, Ed., Philadelphia, Lea & Febiger, 1960, p. 336.
21. MASON, R. M. and STEINBERG, V. L.: Brit. Med. J., *2*, 828, 1960.
22. MEANOCK, R. I. and LEWIS-FANING, E.: Ann. Rheum. Dis., *20*, 161, 1961.
23. MIRSKY, S.: Canad. Med. Assn. J., *102*, 91, 1970.
24. OPPERMANN, J. *et al.*: Dtch. Gesundh.-Wes., *22*, 2236, 1967.
25. O'REILLY, R. A. and AGGELER, P. M.: Proc. Soc. Exp. Biol. Med., *128*, 1080, 1968.
26. ROBINS, H. M. *et al.*: Amer. Pract. & Digest Treat., *8*, 1758, 1957.
27. Sarget Laboratory, Merignac-Bordeaux, France: Gazz. Med. Ital., *128*, 286, 1969.
28. SMYTH, C. J.: Ann. N. Y. Acad. Sci., *86*, 292, 1960.
29. ———: Postgrad. Med., *44*, 77, 1968.
30. SMYTH, C. J. and CLARK, G. M.: J. Chronic Dis., *5*, 734, 1957.
31. SPERLING, I. L.: Arth. & Rheum., *2*, 203, 1959.
32. ———: Lancet, *2*, 535, 1969.
33. STEINBROCKER, O. and ARGYROS, T. G.: Arth. & Rheum., *3*, 368, 1960.
34. STENLAKE, J. B. *et al.*: J. Pharmacol., *20*, 248, 1968.
35. STRANDBERG, B.: Acta Rheum. Scand., Suppl. 10, 1965.
36. WOODLIFF, H. J. and DOUGAN, L.: Brit. Med. J., *1*, 744, 1964.

Indomethacin

1. BOARDMAN, P. L. and HART, F. D.: Ann. Rheum. Dis., *26*, 127, 1967.
2. BURNS, C. A.: Am. J. Ophthalmol, *66*, 825, 1968.
3. CANTWELL, N. H. R.: Personal communication.
4. CATA, A. and HAZEVOET, H. M.: Ann. Rheum. Dis., *29*, 254, 1970.
5. Cooperating Clinics Comm.: Clin. Pharmacol. Therap., *8*, 11, 1967.
6. DECKER, J. L. and MAINLAND, D.: New Engl. J. Med., *283*, 928, 1970.
7. DEUTSCH, A. R. and HIATT, R. L.: Amer. J. Ophthalmol., *68*, 313, 1969.
8. DONNELLY, P., LLOYD, K. and CAMPBELL, H.: Brit. Med. J., *1*, 69, 1967.
9. EDLICH, R. F., NICOLOFF, D. M., BORGEN, L., BUCHIN, R. and WAGENSTEEN, O. H.: Surg. Gynec. Obstet., *130*, 789, 1970.
10. EMMERSON, B. T.: Med. J. Austral., *1*, 1078, 1967.
11. GOLDFARB, E. and SMYTH, C. J.: Arth. & Rheum., *11*, 824, 1968.
12. HARMAN, R. E., MEISINGER, M. A. P., DAVIS, G. E. and KUEHL, F. A., JR.: J. Pharmacol. & Exp. Therap., *143*, 215, 1964.
13. HEALEY, L. A.: Bull. Rheum. Dis., *4*, 483, 1967.
14. HILL, D. F., HOLLANDER, J. L., LANSBURY, J., PLOTZ, C., POLLEY, H. F., SIGLER, J. W., SMYTH, C. J. and WARD, J. R.: Med. Trib., April 10, 1967.
15. HUCKER, H. B., ZACCHEI, A. G., and COX, S. V.: Fed. Proc., *22*, 544, 1963.
16. HUSKISSON, E. C., TAYLOR, R. T., BURSTON, D., CHUTER, P. J. and HART, F. D.: Ann. Rheum. Dis., *29*, 393, 1970.
17. JEREMY, R. and TOWSON, J.: Med. J. Austral., *2*, 127, 1970.
18. LOCKIE, L. M.: Unpublished data.
19. NELSON, S. and ROBINSON, R. G.: Proc. Austral. Rheum. Congress, Sydney, 1963, p. 180.
20. NORCROSS, B. M.: Arth. & Rheum., *6*, 290, 1963.
21. ———: *Proc. Second Laurentian Conf.*, 1966, p. 60.
22. ———: Amsterdam, *Excerpta Medica Fndn.*, 1968, p. 60.
23. O'BRIEN, W. M.: Clin. Pharmacol. Therap., *9*, 94, 1968.
24. PINALS, R. S. and FRANK, S.: New Engl. J. Med., *276*, 512, 1967.
25. PITKEATHLY, D. A., BANERSEE, N. R., HARRIS, R. and SHARP, J.: Ann. Rheum. Dis., *25*, 334, 1966.
26. ROBINSON, H. J., FITZPATRICK, F. K., GRASSLE, O. E.: Fed. Amer. Soc. Exp. Biol., Atlantic City, N.J., Apr. 9–14, 1965.

27. Rothermich, N. O.: Excerpta Medica Fndn., 1968, p. 49.
28. Selye, H.: Canad. J. Physiol. Pharmacol., *47*, 981, 1969.
29. Shen, T. Y. *et al.*: J. Am. Chem. Soc., *85*, 488, 1963.
30. Smyth, C. J.: Ann. Intern. Med., *72*, 430, 1970.
31. Stentake, J. B., Davidson, A. G., Jasani, M. K. and Williams, W. D.: J. Pharm. Pharmacol., *20*, 248, 1968.
32. Struck, K.: *Internat. Symposium on Inflammation*, Freiburg, Germany, May 4–6, 1966.
33. Wright, V., Walker, W. C. and McGuire, R. J.: Ann. Rheum. Dis., *28*, 157, 1969.
34. Yesair, D. W., Remington, L., Callahan, M., and Kensler, C. J.: Biochem. Pharm., *19*, 159, 1970.

Chloroquines

1. Bagnall, A. W.: Canad. Med. Assoc. J., *77*, 182, 1957.
2. ———: Canad. Med. Assoc. J., *82*, 1167, 1960.
3. Berliner, R. W. *et al.*: J. Clin. Invest., *27*, 98, 1948.
4. Burns, C. A.: Personal communication.
5. Burns, R. P.: New Engl. J. Med., *275*, 693, 1966.
6. Calkins, L. L.: Arch. Ophthal., *60*, 981, 1958.
7. Cann, H. M. and Verhulist, H. L.: Pediatrics, *27*, 95, 1961.
8. Editorial: New Engl. J. Med., *275*, 730, 1966.
9. Ekpechi, O. L. and Okord, A. N.: Arch. Derm., *89*, 631, 1964.
10. Ghanen, M. H., Said, M. and Ezz, E.: Egyptian Rheumatologist, *4*, 30, 1967.
11. Henkind, R. and Rothfield, N. F.: Arth. & Rheum., *5*, 647, 1962.
12. Hobbs, H. E., Eadie, S. P., and Somerville, F.: Brit. J. Ophthal., *45*, 284, 1963.
13. Jailer, J., Rosenfield, H. and Shannon, J.: J. Clin. Invest., *26*, 1168, 1948.
14. Kalsbeck, F.: (quoted by Loftus) Nederl. T. Geneesk, *104*, 1414, 1960.
15. Lansbury, J.: Ann. Intern. Med., *62*, 1065, 1965.
16. La Tona, S. and Norcross, B. M.: Arth. & Rheum., *2*, 80, 1959.
17. Lawmill, T., Appleton, B. and Altstatt, L.: Amer. J. Ophthal., *65*, 530, 1968.
18. Loftus, L. R.: Canad. Med. Assoc. J., *89*, 917, 1963.
19. Mackenzie, A. H.: Arth. & Rheum., *13*, 280, 1970.
20. Markowitz, H. A. and McGinley, J. M.: J.A.M.A., *189*, 950, 1964.
21. Page, F.: Lancet, *2*, 755, 1951.
22. Parker, F. S. and Irwin, J. L.: J. Biol. Chem., *199*, 897, 1952.
23. Percival, S. P. B. and Behrman, J.: Brit. J. Ophthal., *53*, 101, 1969.
24. Rothermich, N. O.: Ann. Intern. Med., *61*, 1203, 1964.
25. Rubin, M.: Dis. Nerv. System, *29*, 67, 1968.
26. Sams, Jr., W. M.: Proc. Mayo Clin., *42*, 300, 1967.
27. Sievers, K. *et al.*: Acta Rheum. Scand., *9*, 56, 1963.
28. Von Sallman, L. and Bernstein, H. N.: Bull. Rheum. Dis., *14*, 327, 1963.
29. Whisnant, J. P. *et al.*: Proc. Mayo Clinic, *38*, 501, 1963.
30. Whitehouse, M. W. and Cowey, F. K.: Biochem. J., *98*, 118, 1966.
31. Zvaifler, N. J. *et al.*: Arth. & Rheum., *5*, 667, 1962.
32. Zvaifler, N. J. *et al.*: Arth. & Rheum., *6*, 799, 1963.

Chapter 31

Corticosteroids and Corticotropin in Therapy of Rheumatoid Arthritis

By Evelyn V. Hess, M.D., and John A. Goldman, M.D.

Few clinical discoveries in the history of medicine have had such profound influence on research in the medical sciences and on the treatment of so many different diseases as the observation by Hench, Kendall, Slocumb and Polley[74] that cortisone could suppress the inflammatory changes in rheumatoid arthritis. The number of diseases in which corticosteroids have been found useful has increased far beyond the three originally reported by Hench and his associates (rheumatoid arthritis, rheumatic fever and systemic lupus erythematosus). Cortisone, hydrocortisone (cortisol) and their synthetic analogues have revolutionized the treatment of certain diseases, prevented blindness, reduced crippling, minimized invalidism, prolonged life and reduced mortality. In many illnesses, corticosteroids are palliative but not curative. Such is the case with rheumatoid arthritis, especially in its chronic form where corticosteroids have become a popular type of therapy. A sampling survey in 1966 showed that 16% of patients being treated for rheumatoid arthritis were given systemic corticosteroids.[183] In another recent survey of over ten million patient visits to private physicians' offices for rheumatoid arthritis during 1970, oral corticosteroids were prescribed 13% of the time.[120] The extent of the clinical use of these preparations reflects the impact of these hormones on clinical practice.

The original and impressive observations of the effect of cortisone on rheumatoid arthritis, made by Hench and his co-workers in 1949, have been subjected to critical analysis and confirmed in every detail by innumerable workers. Many years of clinical experience and followup studies, however, have revealed the limitations and hazards as well as the benefits of corticosteroid therapy. Some discordance among competent investigators has developed regarding the relative merits of corticosteroids, their indications, contraindications, and ultimate value in the treatment of rheumatoid arthritis compared to other antirheumatic agents. In the pages to follow, an attempt is made, on the basis of the collective experience of many qualified investigators, to critically appraise and describe the current status of corticosteroid therapy in rheumatoid arthritis.

CLINICAL CONSIDERATIONS

Indications.—There is reasonable unanimity of opinion that corticosteroids systemically administered:

1. *Should not be the initial agent* used in the treatment of a patient with rheumatoid arthritis.
2. *Should be given only after* a conscientious and unhurried *trial of conservative measures* (*see* Chapter 27) fails to achieve satisfactory results.
3. *Should not constitute the only measure* in the treatment but should be part of a comprehensive individualized program of management.
4. *Should not be given until a careful survey* for the presence of *deterrents* and *infections* has been completed.

The patient should be informed at the outset that corticosteroid withdrawal after prolonged administration may be difficult, that risks of considerable magnitude are involved in prolonged administration and that it will be necessary to remain under a physician's care throughout the period of therapy.

The expected beneficial results from corticosteroid therapy in severe arthritis and in life-threatening conditions or fulminating diseases should outweigh the risk of serious adverse effects. In estimating expected results it should be recognized that only the active inflammatory changes in the joints and other organs can be reversed. Fibrotic and destructive changes in the joint structures cannot be repaired or halted by corticosteroid administration.

Certain comments are in order regarding some of the indications.

Three broad types of vasculitis[153] have been described in rheumatoid arthritis (*see* Chapter 22): (1) digital arteritis; (2) subacute lesions in small vessels found in skeletal and heart muscles and tendon sheaths; (3) wide-spread necrotizing arteritis indistinguishable from polyarteritis nodosa. Many of the cases with lesions of Type 1 and 2 are relatively benign but the third type of vasculitis can be devastating with severe neuritis, fever, leukocytosis and skin lesions. As the role of corticosteroids in the precipitation of vasculitis is also questioned, their use presents a therapeutic dilemma.[81] Unfortunately, vasculitis in rheumatoid arthritis is a relatively common problem but critical data on the best treatment regimens are lacking. In general, the practice is:

1. Withhold corticosteroid therapy during an episode of vasculitis unless progressive or fulminant.
2. If a patient is receiving corticosteroids, continue at the same dosage level during the acute stage and then very slowly taper the dosage when the vasculitis is remitting. Wide fluctuations in dosage should be avoided.
3. If vasculitis occurs during tapering, return to the previous corticosteroid dose.
4. If corticosteroid therapy is not helping, then other medications should be considered.

Felty's syndrome has been reported to be reversed by corticosteroid therapy but this is not the usual experience.[81] The general consensus is that patients be given a trial of such therapy prior to consideration of splenectomy.

Four types of leg ulcers are generally recognized in patients with rheumatoid arthritis:[81] (1) ulcers associated with Felty's syndrome; (2) ulcers associated with generalized vasculitis; (3) ulcers following minimal trauma in patients with iatrogenic Cushing's Syndrome; (4) "idiopathic" leg ulcers. Those with Felty's syndrome respond to correction of the leukopenia by splenectomy and those secondary to vasculitis tend to heal as the vasculitis heals (at times treated with corticosteroid therapy). Those ulcers following minimal trauma in patients with iatrogenic Cushing's syndrome should be treated vigorously at the time of the initial abrasion to prevent severe ulceration. Idiopathic lesions

Indications for Systemic Corticosteroids in Rheumatoid Arthritis:

1. Patients with severe or moderate rheumatoid arthritis which is not responding satisfactorily to a conservative program. These patients should have active and potentially reversible disease.
2. In patients threatened with inability to continue their occupational duties.
3. Severe rheumatoid vasculitis.
4. Severe hypersplenism (Felty's syndrome).
5. Rheumatoid associated leg ulcers unresponsive to other major modes of therapy.
6. Patients currently or recently receiving corticosteroids undergoing major surgery or other stress.
7. Pleurisy and pericarditis associated with rheumatoid arthritis.

seem to respond poorly to rest, local therapy and skin grafts, but this conservative therapy should be tried prior to institution of corticosteroids and may be used in conjunction with skin grafting.

Usually the pleural effusions associated with rheumatoid arthritis resolve without therapy. If there is a need to treat more vigorously, small doses of corticosteroids have been noted to be effective.[81] Those effusions that occur early in the disease are more often likely to be symptomatic. In patients with advanced disease the symptoms may be minimal and effusions relatively small in volume.

Rheumatoid pericarditis is generally benign and self-limiting,[96] but on occasion insidious development of pericardial effusion with tamponade and pericardial constriction occurs.[106] Corticosteroids have been reported to be beneficial, but most agree they have little long-term benefit.[96,181]

Temporary or short-term (several weeks to a few months) corticosteroid therapy may be useful in tiding a patient over an especially difficult or urgent period or in facilitating application of certain measures of rehabilitation. In contrast to protracted administration, when corticosteroids are given for brief periods, withdrawal may be uneventful and serious effects uncommon.

Deterrents.—Conditions which increase the likelihood that one of the serious side effects of corticosteroid therapy will develop constitute the principal deterrents. These are: peptic ulcer, osteoporosis, psychiatric conditions, thromboembolic phenomena and infections which cannot be readily controlled with antibiotic therapy. It is the masked, unrecognized infection or the type for which there is no effective antimicrobial agent that makes corticosteroid therapy hazardous. Corticosteroids, if clearly indicated, should not be withheld from a patient with rheumatoid arthritis who has active tuberculosis which could be controlled with specific chemotherapy.

Diabetes mellitus, hyperlipidemias, ocular diseases, renal insufficiency and pregnancy are not absolute contraindications. Cardiovascular disease, congestive heart failure, and hypertension require caution and careful choice of appropriate corticosteroid preparations.

General Principles of Administration and Dosage.—There are certain general considerations to be reviewed before initiation of corticosteroid or corticotropin therapy:[102,171]

The patient should have had a conscientious and unhurried trial of conservative measures (*see* Chapter 27). Corticosteroids should not be the initial agent used in the treatment program and should only be given after such a trial has failed to achieve satisfactory results.

Deterrents to Corticosteroid Therapy:

1. Peptic ulcer disease.
2. Generalized osteoporosis.
3. Certain psychiatric illnesses.
4. Thromboembolic diseases.
5. Certain infections including tuberculosis, fungal and viral diseases.
6. Diabetes mellitus.
7. Cardiovascular diseases.
8. Ocular infections and glaucoma.

Pre-Corticosteroid Questionnaire:

1. Has the patient had an adequate treatment program?
2. Has the patient had adequate trial of other medications?
3. Are other indications for corticosteroids present? (*i.e.*, vasculitis)
4. Has a careful evaluation of possible deterrents been completed?
5. What is the goal of corticosteroid therapy?
6. What will be the duration of therapy?
7. What is the anticipated effective corticosteroid dose?
8. What is the initial level of endogenous adrenal corticosteroids?
9. What is the sex and age of the patient?
10. Is the patient reliable and cooperative?

Corticosteroids certainly should not constitute the only measure in this program, but should be part of a comprehensive individualized plan for management. Consideration of other indications for corticosteroid treatment, previously mentioned, may necessitate their earlier usage. Search for the presence of deterrents is mandatory and their relevancy considered.

The proper dosage should be the least amount of medication that will moderate and keep symptoms at a minimum. As stated earlier, with a short-term course of therapy, withdrawal of corticosteroids usually is easier. If there is evidence of pituitary or adrenal insufficiency, this may suggest that an effect may be gained from replacement rather than pharmacologic dosage.[88] It also warns that withdrawal may be very difficult. If initial testing suggests a high level of adrenal corticoid activity, this suggests larger doses may be required.[171] An 8:00 A.M. blood cortisol test is the easiest way to screen for the endogenous adrenal corticosteroids.

The sex and age of the patient are of considerable importance. Men tolerate corticosteroids and adrenocorticotropic hormone (ACTH) better than women and premenopausal women better than postmenopausal women. There are individual variations within these categories. In patients with rheumatoid arthritis who generally require long-term administration, the average dose of prednisone recommended by Polley[135] is about 9 mg. a day for men, 7 mg. a day for premenopausal and 5 mg. a day for postmenopausal women.

The psychologic profile of the patient is also important. If there is a history of ready dependence on drugs, or wide mood swings, then in either case subsequent reduction in dosage may be difficult. The reliability of the patient includes not only his ability to take the medication in the prescribed dose on a daily or alternate day regimen, but also his being able to reduce medication as instructed and to contact his physician if side effects occur. It is also highly advisable that patients carry identifying information indicating they are receiving corticosteroid therapy.

Additional Studies Recommended for Patients with Rheumatoid Arthritis Prior to Starting Corticosteroid Therapy

1. Complete history and physical examination, including ophthalmologic studies.
2. Complete blood count.
3. Urinalysis.
4. 2-hour post-prandial blood sugar.
5. BUN
6. Electrolytes.
7. Chest x-ray.
8. Intradermal test for tuberculosis.

Dosage.—Another area for consideration when using corticosteroid preparations is whether to give in daily divided, once daily or alternate daily doses. It would appear that for hypothalamic-pituitary-adrenal axis (HPA) suppression the daily corticosteroid dose must exceed the physiologic range, *i.e.* about 5 mg. prednisone (20 mg. hydrocortisone).[130] To minimize the side effects associated with corticosteroid therapy, including HPA axis suppression, many regimens have been recommended:

1. Use of low dosage therapy (oral cortisone or hydrocortisone totalling 20 mg or less daily administered in divided dosage at maximal intervals of 8 hours).[88]
2. Use the lowest possible daily divided dose consistent with the desired level of suppression of the rheumatoid disease.
3. Use of a single morning dose[66,119] or at least avoidance of a night dose which suppresses endogenous ACTH secretion markedly.[123]
4. Use of an alternate day single dose regimen which usually gives uneven control of symptoms but results in a better functional status of the HPA axis[1,72] than the same total dose given in divided doses as

reflected by various functional tests, diurnal variation, response to ACTH,[72] metyrapone[47] and insulin hypoglycemia.[1,146] It is sometimes possible to convert patients from daily to alternate day corticosteroid therapy although it may take as long as 40 weeks to obtain normal responsiveness of the HPA axis.[28] Stimulation of the adrenal cortex with "booster" doses of ACTH has been suggested as a means of reducing significant hypoadrenalism. On the contrary, "booster" doses increase rather than decrease the suppressive effects of corticosteroids on the HPA axis.[27]

It would seem wisest to initiate therapy with the lowest possible dose and on an every other day basis. Starting from this point, one can evaluate the need for more drug or more frequent dosage. The initial dose will depend on the indications and the goals for corticosteroid therapy. Some physicians start with a higher dose to control symptoms as rapidly as possible and then taper the dose.

Once the arthritis has come under control, repeated and untiring efforts should be made to reduce the "maintenance" dose. The physician should never stop "bargaining" with the disease for lower dosage; even the smallest reduction is well worthwhile. Decrements should always be small (see section on corticosteroid withdrawal). The patient should be strongly warned of the dangers of increasing the dose at his own discretion. Conversely, he should be informed of the hazards of suddenly discontinuing therapy at any time, especially in the event of infection, major surgery or severe injury.

Pattern of Initial Antirheumatic Response.—In almost all cases of active rheumatoid arthritis impressive improvement, both in subjective symptoms and objective signs of joint involvement, follows soon after therapy is begun. Within hours of the first few doses, the patient reports "easing" of joint pain, diminution of stiffness and a distinct feeling of well-being. By the second day, morning stiffness is gone, joint pain is further diminished and functional capacity is increased. At this time objective improvement begins in most cases and continues to increase gradually over the next few weeks. Warmth and redness of the periarticular tissues begin to disappear within a day or two; swelling, tenderness and pain on motion diminish and range of motion increases during the first week. Joint effusions recede more slowly. The peak of improvement is generally reached in three or four weeks. Joint changes not due to active inflammation such as deformities, contractures of severe degree or long duration, subluxation, ankylosis, destruction of cartilage and bone will *not* improve as a result of corticosteroid therapy.

Systemic Response and Laboratory Changes.—There is an improvement in the general well-being of the patient with subsidence of local signs of inflammation and corresponding favorable changes in the laboratory findings. Nodules may become smaller or soften and some may disappear. New nodules have been observed to occur during therapy. Early ocular lesions frequently regress. The ESR falls appreciably and may return to normal, C-reactive protein disappears, serum globulin decreases and albumin increases, hemoglobin concentration, red blood cell count and hematocrit rise. Maximal improvement is generally attained in about four to eight weeks; thereafter, the gains made may persist or recede to some degree.

Limitations.—Unfortunately, as therapy is continued for many months, the effectiveness of corticosteroids frequently begins to diminish and in a moderate proportion of cases the degree of clinical improvement at about the end of the second year is such that the risks of objectionable side effects may no longer seem warranted. The inclination to increase dosage at this juncture should be resisted since the risk of adverse effects increases correspondingly, and sometimes without a proportionate increase in clinical improvement.

It is clear that *corticosteroids suppress but do not eliminate inflammation. They do not stop the progression of joint destruction.* Serial x-ray films of affected joints taken over a period of months or years can reveal extension of cartilage and bone destruction or new sites of osteolysis that appeared during corticosteroid administration, even though clinical and laboratory improvement had occurred.[43]

Pseudorheumatism.—"Arthritis" has been reported with corticosteroid therapy especially with triamcinolone.[133,145,178] Although the original descriptions reported this syndrome in patients with rheumatoid arthritis or systemic lupus on large doses of corticosteroids,[155] more recent reports suggest that it can occur on much lower dosage.[71] Similar symptoms have even occurred in healthy volunteers after a single 40-mg. dose of prednisone when plasma 17 hydroxycorticosteroid levels were falling but still within the normal range.[62] For rheumatoid arthritis patients, the withdrawal symptoms consist of excessive fatigability, weakness, diffuse aching in muscles, bones and joints, and emotional instability. These symptoms are cyclical, appearing as the dose is reduced and worsening with physical and mental effort. They are not relieved by aspirin, heat or physical therapy but do improve with rest. This phenomenon may be distinguished from a true flare by the absence of objective signs of synovitis. Although further increase in dosage may temporarily relieve the musculoskeletal symptoms, the emotional reaction persists. Gradual reduction of corticosteroids by small decrements—and hospitalization in more refractory cases—will fully overcome the symptoms.[75]

The pathogenesis of this pseudorheumatism is not clear. It is possibly related to a relative corticosteroid deficiency. Some patients with this complaint have had an abnormal response of plasma cortisol to synacthen (Beta 1–24 corticotropin).[71] It is possible that more than one mechanism is implicated.

Discontinuance of Corticosteroid.—Therapy may have to be stopped for many reasons: the arthritis may be well controlled with minimal symptoms and the physician may wish to determine whether a natural remission has occurred; there may be no continuing benefit from therapy and the risks of side effects do not justify an increase in the dose; serious side effects may have developed which necessitate discontinuance.

When the drug is reduced or withdrawn: (1) The signs, symptoms and laboratory changes may promptly return. The severity and completeness of a relapse vary from patient to patient. Occasionally a clinical rebound occurs and the symptoms may be even worse than before treatment; (2) In addition to a relapse, constitutional symptoms of corticosteroid withdrawal may appear within hours or days after the drug is stopped. These may consist of muscular weakness, lassitude, fatigue, exhaustion, prostration, fever, chills, anorexia, nausea, vomiting, abdominal cramps, diarrhea, diuresis, dizziness, headache, mental depression or irritability; (3) True adrenal insufficiency with hypotension and the associated biochemical changes such as hypoglycemia, hyperkalemia, hyponatremia and hypochloremia. These symptoms may appear in varying combinations and severity.[75] An overlap of these components may occur.

When the arthritis is under good control, attempts at withdrawal should be made. The availability of 1 mg. prednisone tablets makes this an easier

Reasons for Inability to Withdraw Corticosteroids:

1. Corticosteroid suppression of the HPA axis.
2. Primary insufficiency of HPA (*e.g.*, Addison's disease).
3. Relapse of the arthritis.
4. Pseudorheumatism (withdrawal syndrome).
5. Reluctance of patients to reduce their dose.

process. Patients who have been on treatment for years can be successfully withdrawn but it must be done slowly.[12] Thorn has suggested 5% of the initial dose per month[171] and in some studies, 1 mg. prednisone per month reduction has been reported.[12]

As the corticosteroid dose is reduced, the plasma cortisol steadily rises but some patients continue to show hyporesponsiveness to testing of the HPA axis.[35] It may be helpful to taper with alternate day corticosteroids. Complete withdrawal should not be contemplated until the dose has been reduced to a daily cortisone equivalent of 37½ mg. (5–7½ mg. prednisone) or an alternate day equivalent of 75 mg. (10–15 mg. prednisone) of cortisone.[171] Some authors suggest an ACTH augmentation plan[171] to aid in withdrawal but others feel it is not helpful or necessary.[12,134] Excessive ACTH may be counter to the aims of corticosteroid withdrawal as its use might increase the level of endogenous cortisol. If problems of adrenal insufficiency occur, then a program such as Thorn's is advisable to test the HPA axis.[171] The initial level of endogenous adrenal steroid secretion becomes important at this point in therapy. Symptomatic treatment and

Summary of Corticosteroid Withdrawal Program

1. Taper slowly using 1 mg. prednisone tablets or 5% of the patient's daily dose per month.
2. With higher dosage, bigger reduction increments can be attempted.
3. Be certain patient on a supportive program.
4. A concomitant anti-arthritic drug is usually required.

Suggested Corticosteroid Withdrawal Program of Thorn if Concern for Adrenal Insufficiency:[171]

1. Change steroid dose (37.5 mg. of cortisone equivalent) to dexamethasone 0.75 mg. every day or 1.5 mg. every other day.
2. Continue for 3 to 5 days. Obtain either an 8:00 A.M. blood cortisol or 24 hour urine for creatinine and 17-hydroxy steroids.
3. ACTH 50 units i.v. over an 8 hour period daily for 3 days or ACTH-gel 40 to 80 units I.M. b.i.d. for 3 days and then collect an 8:00 A.M. blood cortisol or 24 hour urinary steroid.
4. Give 40 units ACTH gel daily I.M. for 3 days—measuring blood cortisol or urinary steroids during this period.

A. If evidence of adrenal activation with: (1) increased urinary or blood steroids; (2) clinical changes such as weight gain or facial flushing, then reduce or withdraw dexamethasone.

B. If evidence of reasonably adequate adrenal response (20 mg. urinary hydroxycorticosteroid or blood cortisol greater than 25 μg %): (1) ACTH gel 20 units for 3 days followed by (2) ACTH gel 20 units every other day for 3 days and finally, (3) ACTH gel 10 units once or twice a week if necessary for 1 or more months. (Cover stress during this period with ACTH gel 10 to 40 units.) Measure blood cortisol or urinary steroids on days off ACTH.

C. If the patient is not responsive, return to maintenance dexamethasone and: (1) ACTH gel 40 to 80 units 2 times a week for 2 or 3 months and retest, or (2) Give twice the daily maintenance dose every other day for 2 or 3 months and retest.

D. If the patient still does not respond, give cortisone 20 to 37½ mg. or prednisone 5 to 7½ mg. in a single daily dose and retest in the future.

supportive measures including reassurance, salicylates and bed rest may tide the patient over this difficult period. However, in some patients, corticosteroids may have to be continued indefinitely. The possible modifying effects of various drugs on corticosteroid metabolism have been recently recognized. In particular, the barbiturates and tranquilizers have been shown to augment adrenal insufficiency.[179]

Preparation for Surgical and Other Stress.—The increase in activity of the HPA axis in stress due to infection, trauma, general anesthesia or surgery is well known. Many regimens to cover for such stress have been proposed for patients currently or recently on corticosteroids. Recently the response of the HPA axis to different surgical procedures has been investigated before, during and after surgery. Jasani *et al.*[87] have evaluated the HPA axis with synacthen, lysine 8-vasopressin, insulin hypoglycemia and metyrapone (SU4884) tests in 21 patients with rheumatoid arthritis on corticosteroids (range 3–15 mg prednisone daily) and in 20 patients not on corticosteroids. These data were correlated with the rise of plasma 11-hydroxy-corticosteroid levels during synovectomy of the knee. Patients with a subnormal response to synacthen had the smallest rise in plasma 11-hydroxycorticoids. Patients with a normal response to synacthen but a subnormal response to one of the other three tests had a greater rise. Patients with a normal response to all 4 tests had the highest mean plasma 11-hydroxycorticosteroid levels throughout surgery. Nine patients showed a subnormal response to synacthen, but only one developed hypotension. These results demonstrated the need to administer supplemental corticosteroid to patients with an abnormal synacthen test. Plumpton,[131] using the insulin hypoglycemia test, evaluated 3 groups of patients with various diseases undergoing surgery: (1) those who had never received corticosteroids; (2) those who had recently stopped corticosteroids, and (3) those currently receiving corticosteroids. Those patients with an abnormal insulin hypoglycemia test were given 20 mg prednisolone every 6 hours starting at the time of pre-medication. The results indicated that patients not receiving corticosteroids for 2 or more months did not require prophylactic coverage for surgery.

Recommended Corticosteroid Coverage for Surgery

Schedule 1

Day 1—Surgery, hydrocortisone 100 mg. I.M. at 6:00 A.M. and Solu-Medrol 30 mg. or Decadron Phosphate 6.5 mg. q. 8 hr. in I.V. fluid during surgery beginning prior to anesthesia. If signs of adrenal insufficiency—have hydrocortisone 100 mg. I.V. available.

Day 2—Solu-Medrol 15 mg. or Decadron Phosphate 3 mg. I.M. q. 8 hr.

Day 3—Solu-Medrol 10 mg. or Decadron Phosphate 2 mg. I.M. q. 8 hr.

Modified regime can be continued through Day 6 if clinical condition warrants.

Day 4—Prednisone p.o. 15 gm. 7:00 A.M. and 10 mg. 5.00 P.M.

Day 5—Prednisone p.o. 10 mg. 7:00 A.M. and 10 mg. 5:00 P.M.

Day 6—Prednisone p.o. 10 mg. 7:00 A.M. and 5 mg. 5:00 P.M.

Maintenance corticosteroid preparation given daily throughout.

Schedule 2

1. Day of surgery—hydrocortisone hemisuccinate 100 mg. I.M. every 6 hours from time of pre-medication plus the maintenance dose of corticosteroid.
2. Day 1 post-operative—hydrocortisone hemisuccinate 100 mg. I.M. every 6 hours plus maintenance dose.
3. Day 2 post-operative—the same as Day 1.
4. Day 3 post-operative—the same as Day 1.
5. Day 4 post-operative—discontinue hydrocortisone and continue with the maintenance dose.

Hydrocortisone hemisuccinate 100 mg should always be available to give i.v. immediately if signs of adrenal insufficiency occur; *i.e.*, tachycardia, hypotension, vascular collapse, respiratory failure and fever. The maintenance dose of prednisone or its equivalent should be given throughout and parenterally if the patient cannot take it orally. Any subsequent stress episodes should be treated as above.

In a practical sense, the wisest way to manage acute crises is to assume that all patients currently or within the last year on chronic corticosteroid therapy are unresponsive and treat accordingly. These principles of treatment should also be applied in severe infection and trauma. There are many schedules available—the important point is to remember that completeness of coverage and flexibility are essential. Schedule 1 is in current use at this Medical Center. Synthetic corticosteroids are used throughout to avoid electrolyte problems. Schedule 2, suggested by Plumpton,[132] uses hydrocortisone and has some experimental data to substantiate it.

PROPERTIES OF INDIVIDUAL CORTICOSTEROID PREPARATIONS

The first successful attempt at the synthesis of a compound that retained a greater anti-inflammatory property while dissociating physiological effects was reported in 1954 by Fried and Sabo[52] who introduced a fluorine atom at carbon 9 of the phenanthrene nucleus and produced 9 alpha-fluorocortisol. This alteration enhanced the anti-inflammatory

TABLE 31–1.—COMPARISON OF PREPARATIONS*

U.S.P. Name	*Structure of Synthetic Analog*	*Approx. Equivalent Dose (mg.)*	*Anti-Inflammatory Potency*	*Mineralocort. Potency*
Corticotropin IV		2 units/24 hrs. infusion	1.0	1.0
Corticotropin Gel IM		2 units/8 hrs.	1.0	1.0
Hydrocortisone (Cortisol)	—	20.0	1.0	1.0
Cortisone	—	25.0	0.8	1.0
Prednisone	Delta-1-cortisone	5.0	3.0–5.0	0.8
Prednisolone	Delta-1-cortisol	5.0	3.0–5.0	0.8
Triamcinolone	9-alpha fluoro-16-alpha-hydroxy-prednisolone	4.0	5.0	0
Dexamethasone	9-alpha-fluoro-16-alpha-methyl-prednisolone	0.75	20.0–30.0	0
Methylprednisolone	6-alpha-methyl-prednisolone	4.0	5.0	0
Fluprednisolone	6-alpha fluoro-prednisolone	1.5	15.0–20.0	0
Betamethasone	9-alpha fluoro-16-beta-methyl-prednisolone	0.6	25.0	0
Paramethasone	6-alpha fluoro-16-alpha methyl-prednisolone 21-acetate	2.0	10.0	0
Meprednisone	16-beta-methylprednisone	4.0	4.7	0

* Compiled from references 49, 63 and 166

potency tenfold that of cortisol but augmented sodium-retaining effects by a factor of 125. There soon followed in rapid succession syntheses by different chemists of numerous analogs of cortisone and cortisol. Of these, nine compounds having greater potency and less objectionable side effects than the parent steroids have been found satisfactory for clinical use as anti-inflammatory agents. The corticosteroids in common use at present are: prednisone, prednisolone, triamcinolone, 6-methylprednisolone, dexamethasone, fluprednisolone, betamethasone, paramethasone, and meprednisone. Their relative properties are listed in Table 31–1.

Figure 31–1 shows the structure of these compounds. The enhancement of anti-inflammatory activity can be influenced by various structural changes. There are still many pathways which can be explored towards decreasing unwarranted side effects while continuing or increasing the anti-inflammatory activity.[166]

Prednisone and Prednisolone.—These two compounds, which are of similar potency and physiological activity, are analogs of cortisone and cortisol respectively and differ in chemical structure from the parent steroids only in the presence of a double bond (dehydrogenation) between carbons 1 and 2. Their synthesis was a landmark since it was the first man-made corticosteroid that possessed both enhanced anti-inflammatory activity and markedly reduced propensity for retention of sodium and loss of potassium as compared to the naturally occurring corticosteroids.[76] This reduced the incidence of edema, hypokalemia, hypokalemic alkalosis, hypertension and congestive heart failure. Unfortunately, these analogs are not free of other major deleterious effects. It should be noted that prednisone has the added advantages of 1 mg tablets and low cost.

Triamcinolone.—This compound was the first halogenated corticosteroid whose chemical structure was altered by the addition of an hydroxyl group at carbon 16 to overcome the powerful sodium-retaining activity of its predecessors.[17] This compound, like prednisone, does not cause unfavorable electrolyte im-

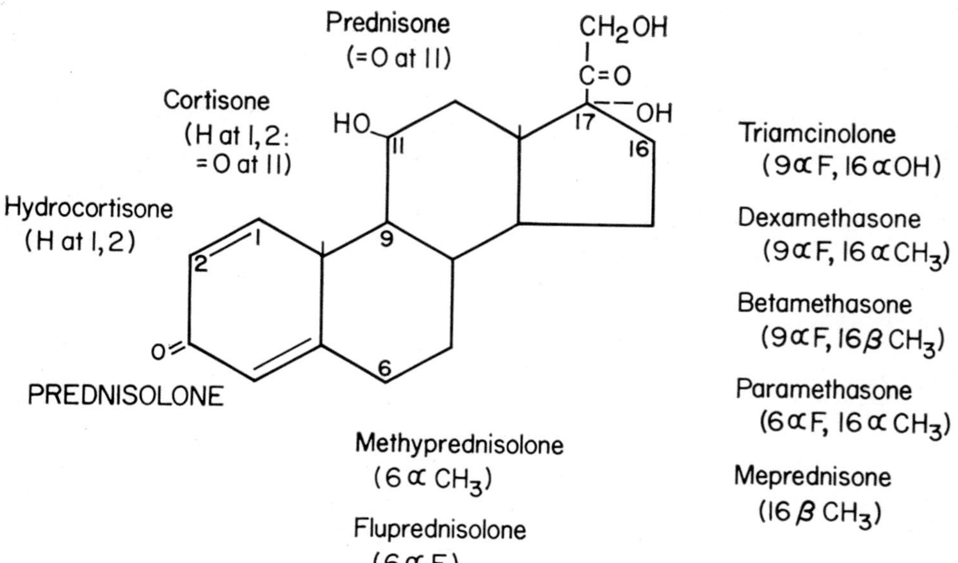

FIG. 31–1.—Structural formula of prednisolone, showing differences in formulas of cortisone analogs.[135] H. F. Polley: reprinted with permission of publisher of Trans. Amer. Acad. Ophthal. Otolaryng.

balance; in fact, it often induces sodium and water diuresis and associated weight loss. In contrast to the other corticosteroids, triamcinolone often produces anorexia, thus contributing further to weight loss. Hypertension occurs less frequently than with cortisone, cortisol or prednisone but there is disagreement as to whether psychic changes are less.[20,55,122] Myopathy has been noted in triamcinolone- and other corticosteroid-treated patients. Triamcinolone is not free from the other limitations and serious adverse effects of prolonged corticosteroid therapy.

Methylprednisolone.—This was the first of a series of nuclear methylated corticosteroids that did not cause sodium retention yet retained enhanced anti-inflammatory activity.[79,163] The anti-rheumatic activity, metabolic effects, therapeutic advantages and undesirable side effects are essentially the same as those of prednisolone.

Dexamethasone.—This compound is a halogenated methylated steroid which has reduced salt-retaining effects but in addition, has considerably increased anti-inflammatory activity.[9,126] It is the most potent anti-rheumatic steroid thus far produced. *Increased potency per milligram has no therapeutic advantage, however.* There seems to be a reduced incidence of hypertension but there is disagreement on whether the incidence of psychic changes and peptic ulcer is reduced.[19,20] A marked increase in appetite resulting in excessive weight gain occurs with this drug.

Dexamethasone allegedly produces more protracted suppression of the HPA axis, even in the alternate day regimen.[137]

Fluprednisolone, Betamethasone, Paramethasone and Meprednisone.—Fluprednisolone (6 alpha-fluoroprednisolone) was introduced in 1960.[21,80] It is twice as potent as prednisolone but has been found to have approximately the same therapeutic ratio. Side effects are the same as those produced by the other synthetic compounds except that weight gain is less likely to occur.[20]

Betamethasone (16 beta-methyl, 9 alpha-fluoroprednisolone) is similar to dexamethasone in terms of potency, therapeutic index, and side effects.[9,126]

Paramethasone (16 alpha-methyl, 6 alpha-fluoroprednisolone) has a potency similar to that of fluprednisolone, although there may be a tendency to weight gain.[20,42]

Meprednisone (16 beta-methylprednisone) is the newest synthetic corticosteroid, released in 1970.[126] The reported studies to date show an anti-inflammatory effect similar to the other synthetic preparations and, at least in short-term studies, a smaller percentage of severe side effects.[57,143]

Experience with the four newer synthetic corticosteroids has failed to reveal any striking differences in therapeutic ratios or in side effects when compared with the earlier synthetic agents.

USE OF CORTICOTROPIN (ACTH)

Corticotropin U.S.P., a purified preparation of ACTH derived from the anterior pituitary gland of animals, is available in aqueous or gelatin solution. Synthetic preparations have recently become available. The U.S.P. has adopted the Third International Standard for Corticotropin as a reference standard.[14] There is no separate standard at present for intravenous ACTH. At present, a 5 unit U.S.P. ampoule contains the equivalent of 1.5 units of the old U.S.P. intravenous assay.[63] Corticotropin is available as a lyophilized powder for intravenous or intramuscular use—and in a gelatin solution for intramuscular or subcutaneous injection. When maximal response is desired, however, aqueous corticotropin should be used intravenously by slow, continuous perfusion at the rate of 20 units per 8 hours. Larger doses do not enhance the response. Intravenous solutions of ACTH are not suitable for prolonged therapy. A long-acting highly purified corticotropin preparation, given intramuscularly once daily or several times a week, is the method of choice for maintenance therapy.

Another repository preparation, corticotropin-zinc (aqueous suspension of purified corticotropin with alpha zinc hydroxide) has also been produced. The repository substance remains active for forty-eight to seventy-two hours after a single injection; the dosage is about the same as the gelatin preparation.

Using purified corticotropin gel in daily intramuscular injections in doses sufficient to give a 24-hour urinary 17-hydroxycorticosteroid output of up to 20 mg in small adults and 30 mg in large adults, West[180] reported favorable results in the majority of 77 patients with rheumatoid arthritis who tolerated continuous treatment for one to ten years. He concluded that adrenocortical stimulation therapy was superior to oral cortisone therapy.

Savage and his associates[149,172] have reported long-term experience showing satisfactory control of rheumatoid arthritis in a large group of patients treated with corticotropin. Side effects in this group were milder than those experienced by a control group receiving corticosteroids. Carter and associates treated 14 patients with active, chronic rheumatoid arthritis with daily corticotropin in doses of 15 to 30 units daily, which, on the basis of urinary 17-hydroxy corticosteroids, were equivalent to 7.5 to 15 mgs of prednisone daily.[26] Their disease was effectively controlled and, furthermore, evaluation of the HPA function with insulin hypoglycemia and vasopressin tests showed preserved function.

ACTH VERSUS CORTICOSTEROIDS

Whether or not to use one of the synthetic oral corticosteroid preparations or corticotropin is the subject of some controversy. The advantages and disadvantages have been critically reviewed in a thought-provoking, recent article by Allander.[8] ACTH requires an intact adrenal gland while exogenous therapy does not. ACTH suppresses both hypothalamic and pituitary activity but appears to increase adrenal responsiveness, although a recent series of studies suggests that HPA responsiveness is retained.[29,34,139] Chronic corticosteroid therapy suppresses the entire HPA axis. The degree of suppression may be minimal or last up to one year.[65,82,86,107] The sequence of involvement of the HPA axis seems to be suppression of the hypothalamus first, then the pituitary and finally the adrenal.[86] Alternate day corticosteroids are associated with less[1,72] but a single dose at night with more suppression.[123] Paradoxically, "booster" doses of ACTH in patients on chronic corticosteroid therapy seem to increase rather than decrease the suppressive effects on the HPA axis.[27] Antibodies to ACTH in patients on chronic therapy have been noted.[48,53,101,112] Clinical significance has been attributed to them in so-called acquired resistance to ACTH but investigation has failed to show a correlation between antibody titer, exogenous ACTH dose, effect of exogenous ACTH, duration of treatment and function of the HPA axis.[48,53,101] Allergic reactions, sometimes severe, have been reported with ACTH; however, synthetic preparations of ACTH have reduced their incidence.[8,101] Immediate hypersensitivity reactions to corticosteroid preparations have been reported.[31,110,124] Urticaria[108] and even asthma[30] have been reported due to Tortiazine (yellow No. 5), an analine dye used as a coloring agent in Decadron (dexamethasone), paracortol (prednisone) and Deronil (dexamethasone).

ADVERSE EFFECTS OF CORTICOSTEROID THERAPY

Table 31–2 lists adverse effects of corticosteroid treatment. In general, the incidence parallels increasing doses and the duration of treatment. Almost all the objectionable effects are reversible after varying periods of time following discontinuance. Moreover, some of those listed in Table 31–2 may diminish in extent and

Factors Influencing Choice of Preparation

ACTH	*Corticosteroids*
1. Requires intact adrenal gland.	1. Do not require intact adrenal gland.
2. Suppresses hypothalamic and pituitary activity.	2. Suppress hypothalamic, pituitary and adrenal gland activity.
3. Variable dose response.	3. Less variable dose response.
4. Must be given parenterally.	4. Can be given orally.
5. In equal doses has greater mineralocorticoid effect.	5. In equal doses certain synthetic preparations have less mineralocorticoid effects.
6. Stimulates adrenal androgen secretion.	6. Inhibit adrenal androgen secretion.
7. Associated with acquired resistance.	7. Not associated with acquired resistance.
8. Associated with allergic reactions.	8. Rarely associated with allergic reactions.
9. Not useful for stress situations.	9. Indicated in stress situations.

TABLE 31–2.—ADVERSE EFFECTS OF CORTICOSTEROID THERAPY

Acne
Arteritis—necrotizing
  (neuropathy and gangrene)
Carbohydrate intolerance
Cataracts, posterior subcapsular
Ecchymosis and petechiae
Edema
Electrolyte imbalance
Fatty Deposition
  Facial rounding
  Cervical fat pads
  Supraclavicular fat pads
  Increased abdominal girth
Gastrointestinal ulceration
Glaucoma
Heart failure, arrhythmia
Hirsutism
Hyperlipidemia
Hypersensitivity reactions
Hypertension
Infections
Menopausal symptom acceleration
  (sweats and hot flashes)
Menstrual disorders
Myopathy
Ocular infections
Osteoporosis and fracture
Pancreatitis
Perspiration increase
Psychic disturbances
  Insomnia
  Restlessness, overstimulation
  Euphoria
  Depression
  Agitation
  Psychosis
Striae
Thromboembolic phenomena

severity—peptic ulcers may heal and fractures unite—even though therapy is continued. In many of these situations, decisions about continuing, tapering or stopping the corticosteroid must be made on an individual basis.

Some adverse effects occur in most patients treated for more than several weeks with any of the corticosteroids. Fortunately, the commonest effects are minor and not sufficiently troublesome to interfere with treatment. Certain adverse effects occur more commonly with some preparations than with others. The more serious ones will now be discussed in greater detail.

Peptic Ulcer.—The incidence of peptic ulceration in the general population is difficult to estimate but most studies indicate a figure of 5 to 10%.[39] Patients with rheumatoid arthritis on corticosteroid therapy have a reported incidence of peptic ulceration varying from 1 to 25% in retrospective studies.[33,97,165] Prospective studies have also shown widely varying percentages of ulceration. One study showed an incidence of 31% in patients evaluated by periodic x rays while another did not find any significant increase in a corticosteroid-treated group (23%) as compared to a non-corticosteroid-treated group (27%).[11,90] Many of the retrospective studies did not take into account certain variables such as concomitant use of salicylate, indomethacin or phenylbutazone. In fact, reports of a low incidence of peptic ulceration in other groups of patients on corticosteroids, such as pemphigus, asthma or ulcerative colitis, cast doubt on the ulcerogenicity of corticosteroids.[33,144,165] Patients with rheumatoid arthritis on larger doses (20 mg. prednisone or more) may be particularly susceptible.[164]

Usually, the ulcers are gastric (prepyloric or pyloric), relatively painless, commonly present with hemorrhage or perforation with little fibrous reaction on histologic study.[57,97] Duodenal ulcers are reported less frequently although good control data of the incidence are lacking.[60]

Patients should be questioned on every visit for digestive symptoms and have periodic hematocrits and stool guaiacs, and x rays if suspicious symptoms occur. Often the radiologist will find less than usual tenderness on palpation and less distortion of the intestine surrounding the ulcer.[77] A crater may be the only evidence of a lesion. If the diagnosis is confirmed or strongly suspected, a complete anti-ulcer regimen should be initiated and the steroid dose reduced. Some physicians prescribe antacids prophylactically to all patients receiving corticosteroids.

Pancreas.—There is an increased incidence of acute pancreatitis especially in children.[127,142] Although not always clinically apparent or misdiagnosed, Carone found a 28.5% incidence of acute pancreatitis in 54 consecutive autopsies of adult patients treated with ACTH or corticosteroids.[25] Clinical pancreatitis has been described in adults although none of these patients had rheumatoid arthritis.[121]

Other types of involvement of the gastrointestinal tract in patients on corticosteroid therapy have been reported and include esophagitis and perforation, small and large bowel ulceration and/or perforation, gallbladder rupture, liver abscesses and fatty liver.[38]

Bone Metabolism.—*Osteoporosis* is an early radiologic sign of rheumatoid arthritis. Whether the incidence is greater in patients on corticosteroid therapy is the subject of disagreement and is partly due to the difficulty of diagnosis *in vivo*.[113,150,151,175,176] Some investigators using bone biopsies have suggested that corticosteroids may inhibit new bone formation in rheumatoid arthritis.[40,98] Women over the age of 50 and immobilized patients seem the most susceptible.[151] The problems of osteoporosis are greater in the axial than in the appendicular skeleton.

Fractures occur most often in the vertebrae, ribs and pelvis and the frequency in rheumatoid arthritic patients treated with corticosteroids has been reported from 0 to 16%.[83,151] Saville and Kharmosh have reported a similar incidence of spinal compression fractures in treated and untreated rheumatoid arthritic patients. The overall incidence of osteoporosis and compression fractures is much lower under the age of 50.[151] When these adverse effects occur, it is advisable to reduce the corticosteroid to the lowest possible effective dose.

Osteonecrosis (aseptic or avascular necrosis) of bone may be a complication of corticosteroid therapy.[38,167] In rheumatoid arthritis, this occurs in patients both on and off corticosteroid therapy;[84,174] some investigators feel that corticosteroid therapy in this disease does not play a decisive role.[84,174]

Psychosis.—Many behavioral, psychological and subjective sensations occur during the administration of ACTH and corticosteroids, especially changes in appetite, sleep and motor activity.[50] Less often, severe mental disturbances have been documented, the reasons for which are not well understood.[136] Some authors feel that premorbid personality has an effect on the psychological content of the psychosis,[59] and others that the pretreatment psychic structure bears no important relationship to the effect of the drug.[64] Usually there is no correlation between the dosage, onset, duration of treatment and the type of psychosis. When it is essential to continue corticosteroids, an attempt should be made to decrease the dose. If the psychosis clears, the dosage can be readjusted as needed. Successful tolerance of previous treatment does not preclude a psychic disturbance during subsequent therapy. If treatment must be continued, ACTH or another corticosteroid preparation may be used.[78] The hazard of suicide or of protracted psychosis in the depressive reactions requires constant assessment if corticosteroids are given in these situations.

Infections.—There is a large literature showing an enhanced susceptibility to infection when laboratory animals are treated with corticosteroids[38,92] as these drugs can act on various immune mechanisms (*see* Chapter 14). Although a review of the literature suggests that infection has been recognized more frequently in rheumatoid arthritic patients,[15] especially those on high doses of corticosteroid therapy,[105] other reports have emphasized that infection rates may be comparable to controls when small doses have been used.[161] Corticosteroids may often mask symptoms of infection and prevent its recognition. It should be remembered that an increased dosage may be necessary to cover the stress of the clinical problem (*see also* Chapter 17).

Tuberculosis.—Animal studies have established the deleterious effect of corticosteroid therapy on tuberculosis[91,109] and the prophylactic value of Streptomycin[160] and Isoniazid.[185] The following recommendations are based on the guidelines provided by the Committee on Therapy of the American Thoracic Society.[23] All patients should have an intermediate (5 tuberculin unit) PPD before corticosteroid therapy. If a patient has active tuberculosis and needs corticosteroids, it is safe to continue therapy as long as effective anti-tuberculous drugs are given. If a rheumatoid arthritic patient needs corticosteroids and has a positive reaction to a tuberculin skin test, history of tuberculosis or an abnormal chest x ray is suggestive of previous tuberculosis, Isoniazid (INH) 300 mg. daily should be given. The INH should be continued for 6 weeks after discontinuing corticosteroids. If the patient is a verified untreated tuberculin converter, then Isoniazid should be continued for 12 months or longer if corticosteroid therapy is continued. Periodic chest x rays should be obtained during and for at least 12 months after discontinuation of corticosteroids. Patients on corticosteroids should not have BCG.[141]

Fungi.—Certain fungal diseases, especially moniliasis and aspergillosis, have been related to corticosteroid therapy.[38] There are no guidelines concerning institution of corticosteroid therapy in a patient with pre-existing fungal infection, a positive fungal skin test or the management of the fungal infection during therapy. Whether specific chemotherapy should be instituted is dependent on the location and severity of the fungal disease.

Viruses.—In the adult, certain viral infections including herpes zoster may complicate corticosteroid therapy.[38] In the individual situation, the available chemotherapeutic techniques, *e.g.*, antiviral drugs (Idoxuridine) and hyperimmune globulin should be used.

Patients on corticosteroid therapy should never receive live virus vaccines but can safely receive killed vaccines.[4,141]

Vasculitis.—Vasculitis occurs in patients with rheumatoid arthritis but the reported incidence is greater in patients treated with corticosteroids.[46,94,159] But corticosteroids were the principal therapy in only half of the patients with vasculitis reported up to 1961.[152] Fulminating vasculitis has rarely been reported in other rheumatic diseases treated with corticosteroids, *e.g.*, rheumatic fever and systemic sclerosis.[51,154] Vasculitis may also be part of the corticosteroid withdrawal syndrome[156] and has been reported to be more likely to occur with synthetic glucocorticoid preparations than with cortisol and cortisone.[85] If corticosteroid-induced vasculitis is suspected, an attempt at tapering the dose may be tried after the acute stage (see section on Vasculitis, page 496).

Thromboembolic Phenomena.—There is a clinical impression of increased coagulability with resultant thromboembolic events in corticosteroid-treated patients.[32,170] There are conflicting reports that these drugs may alter the coagulation time in patients taking and not taking anticoagulants.[32,45,128] The postulated hypercoagulable state has been linked with various parts of the clotting cycle including thrombocytosis, decreased prothrombin time, increased factors V and VIII and some as yet undetermined clot-promoting factors.[24,128,157,173] Interestingly, a bleeding tendency may result from prolonged corticosteroid therapy.[147]

Certainly the issue is not clear; if a patient needs corticosteroid therapy, thromboembolism is not an absolute contraindication. A patient developing pulmonary emboli should be treated in the usual manner and if surgical intervention is necessary, the appropriate corticosteroid coverage should be used.

Ocular Side Effects.—The ocular side effects of both topical and systemic corticosteroids have been reviewed in recent years.[37,73,103]

Posterior Subcapsular Cataracts (PSC).—Black and associates[18] first noted the occurrence of cataracts in rheumatoid arthritic patients taking corticosteroids; there is still dispute about the incidence.[37] Both experimental and clinical data strongly suggest a relationship between prolonged corticosteroid therapy and cataracts.[37,73,103] Earlier reports stressed that patients on higher dosages for longer periods of time were more apt to develop lesions,[125,182] but others have shown that cataracts can develop at lower dosages in shorter periods of time.[56] Such cataracts can be seen with an ophthalmoscope but are best observed by slit lamp examination. All patients receiving corticosteroids, especially high dosage, should be examined periodically. These cataracts may or may not interfere with vision. A few have had to be extracted. Spontaneous resorption in patients treated with topical ocular corticosteroids has been reported after the local therapy was stopped.[51,168]

Glaucoma.—Corticosteroids can raise intra-ocular pressure and although this is more pronounced with local administration, it can also occur with systemic therapy.[7,16,182]

Ocular Infections.—Latent ocular herpes simplex can be reactivated with corticosteroid therapy and pre-existing herpes worsened.[104] Studies have indicated that Idoxuridine (IDU) is effective with concomitant corticosteroid therapy.[93] Corticosteroids can be continued if the patient develops ocular herpes, as long as IDU therapy is given.[73,103]

Experimental Pseudomonas corneal ulcers produce much more extensive ulcerations and scarring when treated with corticosteroids.[169] Simultaneous treatment with Polymyxin B prevented extension of corneal involvement whether or not cortisone was used.[169] In man, some authors have noted the possibility that topical corticosteroids predispose to Pseudomonas infections.[69,117] Whether this is true for systemic therapy is not known.

All "red eyes" in rheumatoid arthritic patients are not related to rheumatoid eye disease and should be thoroughly investigated before institution of local or systemic corticosteroid therapy.

Myopathy.—Although the first reports of exogenously induced corticosteroid myopathy were in patients receiving triamcinolone, cases have since been reported with dexamethasone, prednisone, prednisolone and cortisone. Afifi and associates[5] have reviewed the reported cases. The syndrome is characterized by proximal muscle wasting, especially of the lower extremities. The initial complaint is usually inability to climb stairs, which progresses to inability to squat or to stand up from a sitting position. Some patients have wasting and weakness of distal muscles. Weakness and wasting solely of the upper extremities have not been reported. Muscles supplied by cranial nerves, tendon reflexes, sensory components and sphincter control are usually intact. It has occurred at any time from 1 week to several years after the start of treatment, the average time of onset being 5 months. Muscle enzyme levels are usually within normal limits. Electromyograms and muscle biopsies may show some abnormalities. The myopathy is usually reversible and has been treated by gradual withdrawal and substitution of another corticosteroid.

Effect on Glucose Tolerance.—It is well established that steroids can produce hyperglycemia, glycosuria, increased hepatic gluconeogenesis and antagonism to insulin action.[10,100] Steroid-induced diabetes is considered to be mild, stable, usually without ketosis, related to dose and duration of administration and is relatively insensitive to insulin.[70,116] Reversal usually occurs on discontinuation but may take several months.[116]

Patients with rheumatoid arthritis treated for protracted periods with corticosteroids had a higher incidence of abnormal standard glucose tolerance tests compared to a control group of rheumatoid arthritic patients.[114] However, when both groups were evaluated with standard glucose tolerance and cortisone glucose tolerance tests, there was a similar percentage (50% compared to 56%) of abnormal results. A 2-hour postprandial blood sugar and, in high-risk cases, a glucose tolerance test should be obtained before treatment. There are three basic types of patients to consider: (1) Those with overt diabetes mellitus: In general, their insulin requirements will increase by approximately 20%. (2) Those with a family history of diabetes should be watched carefully for the development of overt disease. (3) Those without a family history of diabetes. Although this group may seem at less risk, occasional patients develop ketoacidosis on treatment. Hyperglycemic, hyperosmolar non-ketotic diabetes, although uncommon in corticosteroid-treated patients, has been reported.[162] There is no need to withhold corticosteroid therapy because of the diabetes mellitus in patients who need such treatment.

Lipid Metabolism.—Corticosteroid-induced alterations of fat distribution are well recognized. There is less agreement concerning the induction of hyperlipidemia by these agents. There are conflicting reports on the effects of corticosteroids on serum lipids; further investigation is required.[2,3,13,36,54,118]

Cardiovascular Disease.—In patients with *congestive heart failure* very large doses of corticosteroids may augment fluid retention while moderate doses may help induce a diuresis.[6,67,115,140] Hypokalemia can occur with therapy although less frequently with synthetic preparations (see Table 31–1). This increases the risk of digitalis toxicity. Such patients may need potassium chloride supplementation.

The incidence of *hypertension* in patients treated with corticosteroids ranged from 4 to 25% and was related to the dose and duration of therapy, the presence of renal disease but not to pre-existing hypertension.[41,129,138,158] ACTH may demonstrate a greater tendency to increase blood pressure than prednisone.[148] If the hypertension is significant, it should be treated, bearing in mind that potassium-losing diuretics will augment the hypokalemia induced by corticosteroids.

Renal Effects.—There are many physiological effects of corticosteroids on renal function, but these do not result in significant clinical changes except for the well-known elevation of the BUN.

Vascular Effects.—Corticosteroids and ACTH have been associated with the deposition of lipids in the aortas of young patients.[44] There is also an increase in x ray evidence of vascular calcification in patients with rheumatoid arthritis taking corticosteroids as compared to controls.[89] The question of corticosteroids accelerating arteriosclerosis is unsettled,[68] and in fact they have been reported to decrease the rate of diffusion of cholesterol into the vessel wall.[49]

Pregnancy and the Fetus.—If corticosteroids are required during pregnancy, the risk to the mother is small but there is controversy concerning fetal risk.[22,177,184] Warrell[177] reports an increased incidence of fetal death, placental aging and fetal distress, while Bongiovanni and McPadden[22] found a lower fetal risk in 260 pregnancies. The possibility of fetal adrenal insufficiency has been implied,[22,111] but there are few convincing case reports and, in fact, urinary metabolites were normal in infants born of mothers receiving corticosteroids.[95,99] Data on patients with rheumatoid arthritis taking steroids during pregnancy are not available. In general, one prefers to use as few medications as possible during pregnancy, especially during the first trimester, and should weigh very carefully the indications for instituting therapy.

Acknowledgment: The authors acknowledge with appreciation the helpful comments received from Dr. Harvey C. Knowles and Dr. Emile E. Werk.

BIBLIOGRAPHY

1. Ackerman, G. L. and Nolan, C. M.: New Engl. J. Med., *278*, 405, 1968.
2. Adlersberg, D., Schaefer, L. E. and Drachman, S. R.: J.A.M.A., *144*, 909, 1950.
3. Adlersberg, D. L., Schaefer, L. E. and Drachman, S. R.: J. Clin. Endocr., *11*, 67, 1951.
4. Advisory Committee on Immunization Practices, Public Health Service. Morbidity and Mortality Weekly Report, *18*, 1, October 29, 1969.
5. Afifi, A. K., Bergman, R. A. and Harvey, J. C.: Johns Hopkins Med. J., *123*, 158, 1968.
6. Albert, R. E., Smith, W. W. and Eichna, L. W.: Circulation, *12*, 1047, 1955.
7. Alfano, J. E.: Amer. J. Ophthal., *56*, 245, 1963.
8. Allander, E.: Acta. Rheum. Scand., *15*, 277, 1969.
9. Arth, G. E., Johnston, D. B. R., Fried, J., Spooncer, W. W., Hoff, D. R. and Sarett, L. H.: J. Amer. Chem. Soc., *80*, 3160, 1958.
10. Ashmore, J. and Morgan, D.: Metabolic Effects of Adrenal Glucocorticoid Hormones in: *The Adrenal Cortex* (editor Eisenstein, A. B.) Little, Brown, Co., Boston, 1967.
11. Atwater, E. C., Mongan, E. S., Wieche, D. R. and Jacox, R. F.: Arch. Intern Med., *115*, 184, 1965.
12. Bacon, P. A., Myles, A. B., Beardwell, C. G., Daly, J. R. and Savage, O.: Lancet, *2*, 935, 1966.
13. Bagdade, J. E., Porte, D., Jr., and Bierman, E. L.: Arch. Intern. Med., *125*, 129, 1970.
14. Bangham, D. R., Mussett, M. V., and Stack-Dunne, M. P.: Bull. WHO, *27*, 395, 1962.
15. Baum, J.: Arth. & Rheum., *14*, 135, 1971.
16. Bernstein, H. N. and Schwartz, B.: Arch. Ophthal., *68*, 742, 1962.
17. Bernstein, S., Lenhard, R. H., Allen, W. S., Heller, M., Littell, R., Stolar, S. M., Feldman, L. I. and Blank, R. H.: J. Amer. Chem. Soc., *78*, 5693, 1956.
18. Black, R. L., Oglesby, R. B., Von Sallman, L. and Bunim, J. J.: J.A.M.A., *174*, 166, 1960.
19. Black, R. L., Reefe, W. E., David, J. R., Bloch, K. J., Ehrlich, G. E. and Bunim, J. J.: Arth. & Rheum., *3*, 112, 1960.
20. Boland, E. W.: Ann. Rheum. Dis., *21*, 176, 1962.
21. ———: J.A.M.A., *174*, 835, 1960.
22. Bongiovanni, A. M. and McPadden, A. J.: Fertil. & Steril., *11*, 181, 1960.
23. Busey, J. F., Fenger, E. P. K., Hepper, N. G., Kent, D. C., Kilburn, K. H. Matthews, L. W., Simpson, D. G. and Grzybowski, S.: Amer. Rev. Resp. Dis., *97*, 484, 1968.
24. Canale, V. C., Hilgartner, M. W., Smith, C. H. and Lanzkowsky, P.: J. Pediat., *71*, 878, 1967.
25. Carone, F. A. and Liebow, A. A.: New Engl. J. Med., *257*, 690, 1957.
26. Carter, M. E. and James, V. H. T.: Ann. Rheum. Dis., *29*, 73, 1970.
27. ———: Ann. Rheum. Dis., *29*, 409, 1970.
28. ———: Ann. Rheum. Dis., (Abstr.) *29*, 690, 1970.
29. ———: Ann. Rheum. Dis., *29*, 91, 1971.
30. Chafee, M.: J. Allerg., *40*, 65, 1967.

31. COMAISH, S.: Brit. J. Derm., *81*, 919, 1969.
32. COSGRIFF, S. W., DIEFENBACH, A. F. and VOGT, W.: Amer. J. Med., *9*, 752, 1950.
33. CREAN, G. P.: Vitamins & Hormones, *21*, 215, 1963.
34. DALY, J. R. and GLASS, D.: Lancet, *1*, 476, 1971.
35. DALY, J. R., MYLES, A. B., BACON, P. A., BEARDWELL, C. G. and SAVAGE, O.: Ann. Rheum. Dis., *26*, 18, 1967.
36. DANOWSKI, T. S., HEINEMAN, A. C., JR. and MOSES, C.: Metabolism, *11*, 281, 1962.
37. DAVID, D. S. and BERKOWITZ, J. S.: Lancet, *2*, 149, 1969.
38. DAVID, D. S., GRIECO, M. H. and CUSHMAN, P.: J. Chronic Dis., *22*, 637, 1970.
39. DOLL, R., JONES, F. A. and BUCKATZCH, M. M.: Med. Res. Council Spec. Rep. 276. His Majesty's Stationery Office, London, 1951.
40. DUNCAN, H.: Arth. & Rheum., *10*, 216, 1967.
41. DUSTAN, H., CORCORAN, A. C., TAYLOR, R. D. and PAGE, I. H.: Arch. Intern. Med., *87*, 627, 1951.
42. EDWARDS, J. A., RINGOLD, H. J. and DJERASSI, C.: J. Amer. Chem. Soc., *82*, 2318, 1960.
43. Empire Rheumatism Council: Ann. Rheum. Dis., *16*, 277, 1957.
44. ETHERIDGE, E. M. and HOCH-LIGETI, C.: Amer. J. Path., *28*, 315, 1952.
45. FAHEY, J. L.: Proc. Soc. Exp. Biol. Med., *77*, 491, 1951.
46. FERGUSON, R. H., and SLOCUMB, C. H.: Bull. Rheum. Dis., *11*, 251, 1961.
47. FLEISCHER, D. S. and PELLECCHIA, P.: J. Pediat., *70*, 54, 1967.
48. FLEISCHER, N., ABE, K., LIDDLE, G. W., ORTH, D. N. and NICHOLSON, W. E.: J. Clin. Invest., *46*, 196, 1967.
49. FORSHAM, P. H.: The Adrenals: in *Textbook of Endocrinology*, 4th Edition, Williams, R. H., Ed., Philadelphia, W. B. Saunders Co., 1968.
50. FOX, H. M. and GIFFORD, S.: Psychosom. Med., *15*, 614, 1953.
51. FRANDSEN, E.: Acta Ophthal., *43*, 605, 1965.
52. FRIED, J. and SABO, E. F.: J. Amer. Chem. Soc., *76*, 1455, 1954.
53. FRIEDMAN, M., and GREENWOOD, F. C.: *In* The Investigation of Hypothalamic-Pituitary, Adrenal Function, James, V. H. T. and Landon, J. (Editors). Proceedings of Symposium MEM. Soc. Endocrin. 17, Cambridge University, Press, 1968, p. 249.
54. FRIEDMAN, M., ROSENMAN, R. H., BYERS, S. O. and EPPSTEIN, S.: J. Clin. Endocr., *27*, 775, 1967.
55. FREYBERG, R. H., BERNTSEN, C. A. and HELLMAN, L.: Arth. & Rheum., *1*, 215, 1958.
56. FURST, C., SMILEY, W. K. and ANSELL, B. M.: Ann. Rheum. Dis., *25*, 364, 1966.
57. GARB, A. E., SOULE, E. H., BARTHOLOMEW, L. G. and CAIN, J. C.: Arch. Intern. Med., *116*, 899, 1965.
58. GIORDANO, M., ARA, M. and TIRRI, G.: Reumatismo, *14*, 259, 1962.
59. GLASER, G. H.: Psychosom. Med., *15*, 280, 1953.
60. GLENN, F. and GRAFE, W. R.: Ann. Surg., *165*, 1023, 1967.
61. GOOD, R. A., VERNIER, R. C. and SMITH, R. T.: Pediatrics, *19*, 272, 1957.
62. GOOD, T. A., BENTON, J. W. and KELLEY, V. C.: Arth. & Rheum., *2*, 299, 1959.
63. GOODMAN, L. S. and GILMAN, A.: The Pharmacologic Basis of Therapeutics, 4th Ed., New York, The Macmillan Co., 1970.
64. GOOLKER, P. and SCHEIN, J.: Psychosom. Med., *15*, 589, 1953.
65. GRABER, A. L., NEY, R. I., NICHOLSON, W. E., ISLAND, D. P. and LIDDLE, G. W.: J. Clin. Endocr., *25*, 11, 1965.
66. GRANT, S. D., FORSHAM, P. H. and DI-RAIMONDO, V. C.: New Engl. J. Med., *273*, 1115, 1965.
67. GREENE, M. A., GORDON, A. and BOLTAX, A. J.: Circulation, *21*, 661, 1960.
68. GROSSFELD, H.: Nature (London), *184*, 38, 1959.
69. HARBIN, T.: Amer. J. Ophthal., *58*, 670, 1964.
70. HARDWICK, C. and LESSOF, M. H.: Guys Hosp. Rep., *111*, 107, 1962.
71. HARGREAVE, F. E., MCCARTHY, D. S. and PEPYS, J.: Brit. Med. J., *1*, 443, 1969.
72. HARTER, J. G., REDDY, W. J. and THORN, G. W.: New Engl. J. Med., *269*, 591, 1963.
73. HAVENER, W. H.: Ocular Pharmacology, St. Louis, C. V. Mosby Co., 1970.
74. HENCH, P. S., KENDALL, E. C., SLOCUMB, C. H. and POLLEY, H. F.: Mayo Clin. Proc., *24*, 181, 1949.
75. HENCH, P. S. and WARD, L. E.: *In* Medical Uses of Cortisone. Lukens, F. D. W. (Editor), New York, Blakiston Co., 1954.
76. HERZOG, H. L., NOBILE, A., TOLKSDORF, S., CHARNEY, W., HERSHBERG, E. B. and PERLMAN, P. L.: Science, *121*, 176, 1955.
77. HILBISH, T. F. and BLACK, R. L.: Arch. Intern. Med., *101*, 932, 1958.
78. HOFF, E. C.: *In* Comprehensive Textbook of Psychiatry. (Freedman, A. M., Kaplan, H. I., and Kaplan, H. S., Eds.) Baltimore, Williams and Wilkins Co., 1967.

79. Hogg, J. A., Lincoln, F. H., Jackson, R. W., and Schneider, W. P.: J. Amer. Chem. Soc., *77*, 6401, 1955.
80. Hogg, J. A., Spero, G. B., Thompson, J. L., Magerlein, B. J., Schneider, W. P., Petersen, D. H., Sebek, O. K., Murray, H. C., Babcock, J. C., Pederson, R. L., and Campbell, J. A.: Chem. Industr., *77*, 1002, 1958.
81. Hollingsworth, J. W.: Local and Systemic Complications of Rheumatoid Arthritis. Philadelphia, W. B. Saunders, Co., 1968.
82. Holub, O. A., Jailer, J. W., Kitay, J. I. and Frantz, A. G.: J. Clin. Endocr., *19*, 1540, 1959.
83. Howell, D. S. and Ragan, C.: Medicine, *35*, 83, 1956.
84. Isdale, I. C.: Ann. Rheum. Dis., *21*, 23, 1962.
85. Janoski, A. H., Shaver, J. C., Cristy, N. P. and Rosenbaum, W.: On the Pharmacologic Action of 21 Hormonal Steroids (Glucocorticoids) of Adrenal Cortex in Mammals. Springer-Verlag, 1968.
86. Jasani, M. K., Boyle, J. A., Greig, W. R., Dalakos, T. G., Browning, M. C. K., Thompson, A and Buchanan, W. W.: Quart. J. Med., *36*, 261, 1967.
87. Jasani, M. K., Freeman, P. A., Boyle, J. A., Reid, A. M., Diver, N. J. and Buchanan, W. W.: Quart. J. Med., *37*, 407, 1968.
88. Jefferies, W.: Arch. Intern. Med., *119*, 265, 1967.
89. Kalbak, K.: Ugeskr. Laeg., *132*, 2115, 1970.
90. Kammerer, W. H., Freyberg, R. H. and Rivelis, A. L.: Arth. & Rheum., *1*, 122, 1958.
91. Karlson, A. G. and Gainer, J. H.: Dis. Chest, *20*, 469, 1951.
92. Kass, E. H. and Finland, M.: Advances Intern. Med., *9*, 45, 1958.
93. Kaufman, H. E., Martola, E. L. and Dohlman, C. H.: Arch. Ophthal., *69*, 468, 1963.
94. Kemper, J. W., Baggenstoss, A. H. and Slocumb, C. H.: Ann. Intern. Med., *46*, 831, 1957.
95. Kenny, F. M., Preeyasombat, C., Spaulding, J. S., Migeon, C. J., Lawrence, B. and Richards, C.: Pediatrics, *37*, 960, 1966.
96. Kirk, J., and Cash, J.: Quart. J. Med., *38*, 397, 1969.
97. Kirsner, J. B., Kassriel, R. S. and Palmer, W. L.: Advances Intern. Med., *8*, 41, 1956.
98. Klein, M., Villaneuva, A. R. and Frost, H. M.: Acta Orthop. Scand., *35*, 171, 1965.
99. Kulin, H. E., Metzl, K. and Peterson, R.: J. Pediat., *69*, 648, 1966.
100. Landau, B. R.: Vitamins & Hormones, *22*, 2, 1965.
101. Landon, J., Friedman, M. and Greenwood, F. C.: Lancet, *1*, 652, 1967.
102. Lederer, F. L., Samter, M. and Gendler, J. C.: Trans. Amer. Acad. Ophthal. Otolaryng., *71*, 262, 1967.
103. Leopold, I. H.: Trans. Amer. Acad. Ophthal. Otolaryng., *71*, 273, 1967.
104. Leopold, I. H. and Sery, T. W.: Invest. Ophthal., *2*, 498, 1963.
105. Lepper, M. H.: J. Chronic Dis., *15*, 691, 1962.
106. Liss, J. P., and Bachmann, W. T.: Arth. & Rheum., *13*, 869, 1970.
107. Livanou, T., Ferriman, D. and James, V. H. T.: Lancet, *1*, 856, 1967.
108. Lockey, S. D.: Ann. Allerg., *17*, 719, 1959.
109. Lurie, M. B., Zappasodi, P. and Dannenberg, A. M.: Fed. Proc., *10*, 414, 1951.
110. Maddin, S.: J.A.M.A., *207*, 560, 1969.
111. Margulis, R. R. and Hodgkinson, C. P.: Obstet. Gynec., *1*, 276, 1953.
112. Masaharu, M., Okumura, H., Takeda, K., Kikutani, T., Koizumi, K., Suzuki, S. and Oshima, Y.: J. Allerg., *46*, 138, 1970.
113. McConkey, B., Fraser, G. M. and Bligh, A. S.: Quart. J. Med., *31*, 419, 1962.
114. McKiddie, M. T., Jasani, M. K., Buchanan, K. D., Boyle, J. A. and Buchanan, W. W.: Metabolism, *17*, 730, 1968.
115. Mickerson, J. N. and Swale, J.: Brit. Med. J., *1*, 876, 1959.
116. Miller, S. E. P. and Nielson, J. M.: Postgrad. Med., *40*, 660, 1964.
117. Mitsui, Y. and Hanabusa, J.: Brit. J. Ophthal., *39*, 244, 1955.
118. Moses, C., Jablonski, J. R., Sunder, J. H., Greenman, J. H. and Danowski, T. S.: Metabolism, *11*, 653, 1962.
119. Myles, A. B., Bacon, P. A. and Daly, J. R.: Ann. Rheum. Dis., *30*, 149, 1971.
120. National Disease and Therapeutic Index. Ambler, Pa., 1971.
121. Nelp, W. B.: Arch. Intern. Med., *108*, 702, 1961.
122. Neustadt, D. H.: J.A.M.A., *170*, 1253, 1959.
123. Nichols, T., Nugent, C. A. and Tyler, F. H.: J. Clin. Endocr., *25*, 343, 1965.
124. O'Garra, J. A.: Brit. Med. J., *1*, 615, 1962.
125. Oglesby, R. B., Black, R. L., Von Sallmann, L. and Bunim, J. J.: Arch. Ophthal., *66*, 625, 1961.

126. Oliveto, E. P., Rausser, R., Nussbaum, A. L., Gebert, W., Hershberg, E. B., Toksdorf, S., Eisler, M., Perlman, P. L. and Pechet, M. M.: J. Amer. Chem. Soc., *80*, 4428, 1958.
127. Oppenheimer, E. H. and Boitnott, J. K.: Bull. Johns Hopkins Hosp., *107*, 297, 1960.
128. Ozsoylu, S., Strauss, H. S. and Diamond, L. K.: Nature, *195*, 1214, 1962.
129. Perera, G. A.: Proc. Soc. Expt. Biol. Med., *76*, 583, 1951.
130. Peterson, R. E. and Wyngaarden, J. B.: J. Clin. Invest., *35*, 552, 1956.
131. Plumpton, F. S., Besser, G. M. and Cole, P. V.: Anesthesia, *24*, 3, 1969.
132. ———: Anesthesia, *24*, 12, 1969.
133. Polley, H. F.: Brit. Med. J., *2*, 1253, 1956.
134. ———: Mayo Clin. Proc., *45*, 1, 1970.
135. ———: Trans. Amer. Acad. Ophthal. Otolaryng., *71*, 249, 1967.
136. Quarton, G. C., Clark, L. D., Cobb, S. and Bauer, W.: Medicine, *34*, 13, 1955.
137. Rabhan, N. B.: Ann. Intern. Med., *69*, 1141, 1968.
138. Ragan, C.: Bull. N.Y. Acad. Med., *29*, 355, 1953.
139. Reed, P. I., Clayman, C. B. and Palmar, W. L.: Ann. Intern. Med., *61*, 1, 1964.
140. Reimer, A. D.: Amer. J. Cardiol., *1*, 488, 1958.
141. Report of the Committee on Infectious Diseases. 1970, Amer. Academy of Pediatrics, Evanston, Ill., 1970.
142. Riemenschneider, T. A., Wilson, J. F. and Vernier, R. L.: Pediatrics, *41*, 428, 1968.
143. Robecchi, A., Di Vittorio, S. and Seconda, G.: Reumatismo, *14*, 150, 1962.
144. Rose, B., McGarry, E., and Knight, A.: Ann. N.Y. Acad. Sci., *82*, 913, 1959.
145. Rotstein, J.: Postgrad. Med., *31*, 459, 1962.
146. Sadeghi-Nejad, A., and Senior, B.: Pediatrics, *43*, 277, 1969.
147. Salzman, E. W. and Britten, A.: Disorders of Hemostasis *in*: Hemorrhage and Thrombosis. Boston, Little, Brown & Co., 1965.
148. Savage, O., Copeman, W. S. C., Chapman, L., Wells, M. V. and Treadwell, B. L. J.: Lancet, *1*, 232, 1962.
149. Savage, O., Davis, P. S., Chapman, L., Wickings, J., Robertson, J. D. and Copeman, W. S. C.: Ann. Rheum. Dis., *18*, 100, 1959.
150. Saville, P. D.: Arth. & Rheum., *10*, 416, 1967.
151. Saville, P. D. and Kharmosh, O.: Arth. & Rheum., *10*, 423, 1967.
152. Schmid, F. S., Cooper, N. S., Ziff, M. and McEwen, C.: Amer. J. Med., *30*, 56, 1961.
153. Scott, J. T., Hourihane, D. O., Doyle, F. H., Steiner, R. E., Laws, J. W., Dixon, A. St. J. and Bywaters, E. G. L.: Ann. Rheum. Dis., *20*, 224, 1961.
154. Sharnoff, J. G., Carideo, H. L. and Stein, I. D.: JAMA, *145*, 1230, 1951.
155. Slocumb, C. H.: Bull. Rheum. Dis., *3*, 39, 1952.
156. ———: Mayo Clin. Proc., *28*, 655, 1953.
157. Smith, R. W., Margulis, R. R., Brennen, M. J. and Monto, R. W.: Science, *112*, 295, 1950.
158. Smyllie, H. C., and Connolly, C. K.: Thorax, *23*, 571, 1968.
159. Smyth, C. J. and Gum, O. B.: Arth. & Rheum., *4*, 1, 1961.
160. Spain, D. M. and Molomut, N.: Amer. Rev. Tuberculosis, *62*, 337, 1950.
161. Sparberg, M. and Kirsner, J. B.: J.A.M.A., *188*, 680, 1964.
162. Spenny, J. G., Eure, C. A. and Kreisberg, R. A.: Diabetes, *18*, 107, 1969.
163. Spero, G. B., Thompson, J. L., Magrelein, B. J., Hanze, A. R., Murray, H. C., Sebek, O. K. and Hogg, J. A.: J. Amer. Chem. Soc., *78*, 6213, 1956.
164. Spiro, H. M.: Amer. J. Digest. Dis., *7*, 733, 1962.
165. Spiro, H. M. and Milles, S. S.: New Engl. J. Med., *263*, 286, 1960.
166. Steelman, S. L. and Hirschman, R.: *In* Adrenal Cortex (Eisenstein, A. H., Ed.). Boston, Little, Brown and Co., 1967.
167. Storey, G. O.: Proc. Roy. Soc. Med., *61*, 961, 1968.
168. Streiff, E. B.: Ophthalmologica, *147*, 143, 1964.
169. Suie, T. and Taylor, F. W.: Arch. Ophthal., *56*, 53, 1956.
170. Symchych, P. S. and Perrin, E. V.: Amer. J. Dis. Child., *110*, 636, 1965.
171. Thorn, G. W.: New Engl. J. Med., *274*, 775, 1966.
172. Treadwell, B. L. J., Sever, E. D., Savage, O. and Copeman, W. S. C.: Lancet, *1*, 1121, 1964.
173. Trieger, N. and McGovern, J. J.: New Engl. J. Med., *266*, 432, 1962.
174. Virkkunen, M., Laitinen, H., Huhmar, E. and Jokio, P.: Acta Rheum. Scand., *15*, 90, 1969.
175. Virtama, P., Helelä, T., and Kalliomäki, J. L.: Acta Rheum. Scand., *14*, 276, 1968.
176. Vose, G. P., Hoerster, S. A. and Mack, P. B.: Amer. J. Med. Electron, *3*, 181, 1964.

177. WARRELL, D. W. and TAYLOR, R.: Lancet, *1*, 117, 1968.
178. WELLS, R.: Lancet, *2*, 498, 1958.
179. WERK, E.: Med. Times, *98*, 65, 1970.
180. WEST, H. F.: Ann. Rheum. Dis., *21*, 263, 1962.
181. WILKINSON, M.: Brit. Med. J., *2*, 1723, 1962.
182. WILLIAMSON, J., PATERSON, R. W. W., McGAVIN, D. D. M., JASANI, M. K., BOYLE, J. A. and DOIG, W. M.: Brit. J. Ophthal., *53*, 361, 1969.
183. WRIGHT, I. S. and JACOBSON, W. E.: Mod. Med., *34*, 75, 1966.
184. YACKEL, D. B., KEMPERS, R. D. and McCONAHEY, W. M.: Amer. J. Obstet. Gynec., *96*, 985, 1966.
185. ZORINI, A. O.: Dis. Chest, *33*, 1, 1958.

Chapter 32

Intrasynovial Corticosteroid Therapy

By Joseph Lee Hollander, M.D.

After twenty years of trial and clinical use, the injection of hydrocortisone, or its newer derivatives, directly into an inflamed synovial space has become so widely accepted that this procedure may now be regarded as a standard adjunct for temporary palliation of a wide variety of rheumatic disorders. Since we first described this in 1951[10,13] we have administered intrasynovial injections of steroid over 250,000 times into more than 8000 patients who had inflamed joints, bursae, or tendon sheaths.[12] The generally favorable response in symptomatology resulting from the procedure has been confirmed in more than a hundred reports in the literature.[1,15,25,33] If the arthritis is limited to, or is particularly active in, only one or a few peripheral joints, it can be suppressed by repeated injections of the hormone into each, without the dangers attending *systemic* administration of cortisone or its derivatives. The techniques for use, indications and *contraindications*, *limitations*, and *precautions* for this method of local hormone therapy will be set forth in this chapter. It is emphasized at the outset that this method is only an *adjunct* in arthritis treatment, and *must be coordinated with the general plan of therapy*.

INTRODUCTION

The idea of injecting a medication directly into the joint space is not new. For many years arthritic patients have asked their physician why he could not give something "directly into the joint that hurts." The local application of heat, and the use of liniments have thus appealed to the patient because he sees and feels something is being done directly to the painful spot.

Injection of liquid petrolatum into the joint space in an effort to provide "better lubrication" was tried years ago, but failed because the oil was not miscible with joint fluid, and was soon pocketed off in one or more of the pouches of the synovial sac. Lipiodol, injected into the joint space originally for visualization of the synovial sac by roentgenogram, was later tried for treatment of arthritis, but also quickly became localized in a synovial pouch, often walled off by fibrin and the pannus of the rheumatoid arthritic process.

A solution of procaine hydrochloride has been frequently injected into the synovial cavity of inflamed joints by the physician treating a chronic synovitis produced by trauma to the joint. Such injections have been temporarily helpful, but the effect usually lasts only a few hours, and may be followed by a marked reaction after the anesthetic effect has worn off. However, injection of procaine hydrochloride solution into and around joints is still widely used for pain relief in acute sprains. Penicillin and other antibiotics also have been injected directly into the joints.

Intra-articular injections of lactic acid have been recommended by British workers[28] to "stimulate natural local tissue reactions," and evoke processes of repair in traumatized joints, but this procedure has not been generally accepted by most rheumatologists.

Shortly after the discovery of the anti-rheumatic effect of cortisone, Thorn[26] injected 10 mg. of compound F (hydrocortisone) into the knee joint of a patient with rheumatoid arthritis. The next day the injected knee was greatly improved, but there was also a coincidental general improvement in the patient's condition. He assumed the patient was very sensitive to the systemic action of the hormone, and did no further experiments along this line.

We[10,11] attempted injections of 25 mg. or more of cortisone acetate into inflamed knees of rheumatoid arthritic patients. In less than 25 per cent was there any striking subjective improvement following the injection, and objective improvement was either lacking, or minimal and transient in all. The temperature of the inflamed joint was not significantly decreased by the hormone injection. Because cortisone has such a pronounced suppressive effect on the inflammation of rheumatoid arthritis, it seemed peculiar that it had so little effect on the joints locally, particularly since topical use of cortisone was so successful in suppressing inflammation in the eye. Other workers[8] reported more success with intra-articular injections of cortisone than we had, but even to them the effect seemed too transient to be of practical value in therapy.[22]

Since evidence was accumulating to show that compound F (hydrocortisone) rather than compound E (cortisone) was probably the chief anti-inflammatory hormone secreted by the adrenal cortex,[7,18,21] we injected hydrocortisone acetate into the inflamed joints of rheumatoid arthritics as soon as it was made available by Merck and Co. in January 1951. Both by clinical observation and by joint temperature measurement the anti-inflammatory effect was striking and consistent.[13] At least partial suppression of inflammation was accomplished in 90 per cent of cases within twenty-four hours after the injection of 25 mg. of hydrocortisone into the synovial cavity. The duration of the beneficial effect has varied greatly, from two days to many weeks, with an average duration of symptomatic improvement of about six days in an active rheumatoid arthritic joint.[13] The effect was limited to the injected joint, and there were no appreciable systemic effects from the hormone injection. Successive injections had a similar effect. After the injections were discontinued, the joint gradually returned to the pretreatment state in most instances, but in none was the joint worse than before. Other investigators have confirmed these findings.[25,33]

Clinical studies of the effectiveness of the intra-articular hormone injections were then carried out in cases of osteoarthritis, where it appeared even more completely palliative for longer periods, in gouty joints, acute bursitis, traumatized joints, and even the inflamed joints of acute disseminated lupus erythematosus. The local ameliorating effect of such injections was consistent in all these conditions, demonstrating the non-specific nature of the hormone action.

EFFECTS OF INTRASYNOVIAL CORTICOSTEROID INJECTION

While the mode of action of hydrocortisone and its derivatives in suppressing inflammation is still unknown (*see* Chapter 17), the injected hormone is apparently taken up by the cells of the synovial fluid and of the synovial membrane within a few hours.[32] Wilson *et al.*[29] found the injected steroid remaining in the synovial fluid after the first two hours was nearly all hydrolyzed. Apparently the hormone held in the synovial membrane exerts the local anti-inflammatory effect, as detectable amounts of injected steroid were found in synovial biopsy specimens taken as long as two weeks following injection in our studies.[32] Any excess over the amount the synovial membrane will retain is absorbed into the systemic circulation, so the optimal amount for local injection is the maximal amount which will be held *locally*.

Symptomatic improvement in joint

symptoms usually occurs within the first twenty-four hours after intra-articular injection of corticosteroid. Improvement in pain and stiffness is sometimes dramatic, but varies greatly. Maximal relief from pain and swelling is usually attained within three days, often with complete disappearance of effusion. While the great majority of patients experience relief following local steroid injection, only about 55 per cent maintain such improvement for more than six days. The *average* duration of improvement in a rheumatoid arthritic joint injected with hydrocortisone acetate is only six days, whereas with hydrocortisone t-butyl acetate the average duration of relief is twelve days, and with prednisolone t-butyl acetate fourteen days.[11,16] We have inferred from this that the latter ester is hydrolyzed less rapidly by tissue enzymes.[32] Periods of relief following steroid injection tend to be somewhat longer in osteoarthritic joints.

Reinjection of joints may be carried out when the effect from the original injection has worn off. Such injections may be repeated every few weeks with return of the original ameliorating effect even over a hundred times, in our experience.

Many different esters and analogs of hydrocortisone have been assayed in an attempt to find more potent, longer-lasting steroids for intra-articular use.[12,15] Prednisolone acetate and t-butyl acetate, methyl-prednisolone acetate, triamcinolone acetate and acetonide, dexamethasone acetate and t-butyl acetate,[11] and many esters of hydrocortisone have been compared for local effectiveness. Aside from the substitution of t-butyl acetate for acetate, no *great* advantage in effectiveness has been evident from any of the more recently available steroids. In patients noting a decreasing effectiveness from succeeding injections the substitution of another ester or steroid has usually regained the initial degree of palliation, and it is for such instances that the wide choice of preparations is desirable.

During the past ten years we have injected triamcinolone hexacetonide into arthritic joints of more than 500 patients. In rheumatoid arthritic joints the average duration of palliation was almost twice as long as from other steroid suspensions.[12,17] Because of the potency of this new preparation, injections repeated oftener than once monthly or in excess of 20 mg. in a large joint for each injection may increase the possibility of osteoporosis of the bone ends and increasing instability of the involved joint.

The dose of newer hydrocortisone derivatives used intra-articularly is not proportional to the effective oral dose. While the reason for this is not clear, it would appear that the rate of metabolism of the newer derivatives in the joint tissues differs little from that of hydrocortisone. Cortisone and its analogues apparently cannot be converted to hydrocortisone by the synovial tissue.[22]

FAILURES AND SHORT-TERM ADVERSE REACTIONS FROM INTRA-ARTICULAR CORTICOSTEROID THERAPY

In our experience[12,14,16] the surprising fact has been that there were so few adverse effects from use of a potent hormone directly into the joint space. Nearly 90 per cent of injections have been followed by definite improvement in the local condition for at least a few days. Many of the poor results were attributable to failure in entering the joint space with the tip of the needle. This was particularly true in injections into the hip for osteoarthritis, where we noted 53 per cent failures. It is imperative that the corticosteroid suspension enter the joint space, so that it can reach the entire inflamed synovial membrane, or it will have little effect.

Following about 2 per cent of 250,000 joint injections[12,14] there was noted a local *exacerbation* of the joint inflammation. Increased pain, swelling and tenderness came on within a few hours, and persisted up to four days in a few cases. Most of these "post-injection flare-ups," however, were mild and lasted only a few hours, following which the condition of the joints improved over the pretreatment state as though there had been no exacerbation.

The incidence of these exacerbations has been unpredictable, since they have been observed after the first, or any one of a series of injections. They have seldom occurred more than once in a given joint, however, so that the occurrence of such a reaction is not a contraindication to further injections. Bacterial cultures taken at such a time have been sterile. For treatment of such flare-ups we have recommended rest, ice packs to the joint, codeine sulfate $\frac{1}{2}$ grain orally, and, when effusion is marked, aspiration of the joint for relief of tension.

McCarty and Hogan[19] have recently demonstrated that there is inflammation, with influx of leukocytes into the joint, following injection of corticosteroid crystals into normal joints. Although this is seldom evident to the patient, such "crystal-induced synovitis" is probably the explanation for some of the "post-injection flares." They suggest that some damage may occur in the cartilage from the influx of leukocytes. This reaction also indicates other reasons for injecting minimally effective doses of crystalline steroids, and reinjection no oftener than required.

Following less than 1 per cent of hydrocortisone injections into arthritic joints in our experience, there occurred a peculiar *weakness* of the extremity treated. The patient described this as a "heaviness" of the leg or arm, which persisted from one to three days. There was no instance in which this weakness persisted longer, and seldom did this occur more than once. In addition to this local feeling of weakness, 0.3 per cent of the injections were followed by a spell of generalized weakness, malaise, and vertigo which persisted for one to three days. Neither of these phenomena has as yet been satisfactorily explained, but since their occurrence has been rare, transient, and seldom recurring, they have not been particularly troublesome.

One patient developed local urticaria following injection, which was found to be due to allergy to the aqueous vehicle of the hormone suspension. Several other patients were found sensitive to procaine, and developed a local wheal following its use for local anesthesia.

Although we have made it a point to give the intra-articular corticosteroid injections as an office or clinic procedure, without using drapes, rubber gloves, or any other than routine sterile precautions, only 18 joint infections were produced by the procedure in over 250,000 injections. This low incidence of infections in our series should not mislead the physician into carelessness, however. The seriousness of such infections, and sometimes their chronicity in spite of vigorous antibiotic therapy and conservative surgical drainage, became a major problem in 7 of our 18 patients who had infected joints. Most of these, and 4 other patients referred to our Hospital for infected joints were reported in detail by Tondreau, Hodes, and Schmidt.[27] Hemolytic *Staphylococcus aureus* was the usual infecting organism. The need for careful asepsis is stressed.[8,9,16,27]

If the physician is careful to preserve surgical cleanliness in his technique he need have little fear of infection of the joint, since this has occurred *only once per 14,000 injections* in our experience.[12]

Failure to achieve palliation of joint symptoms by injection of corticosteroid into a joint may occur for several reasons. First, there are some joints which do not respond to any steroid, even though the joint has been entered, as proved by obtaining synovial fluid. Second, and most commonly, steroid injected *near* the joint space but not into it will seldom produce any effect.

Various authors have claimed that intra-articular steroid therapy is ineffective in osteoarthritis.[5,20,23c,30,31] If there is no inflammatory reaction present, there will be little or no relief. Many rheumatologists have agreed with our finding that steroid injections into painful osteoarthritic joints nearly always give relief often for a prolonged period. Trial will quickly determine whether this treatment is of value in a particular case.

A warning that indiscriminate injection of steroid into the joint can lead to cartilage destruction comes from experimental use in rabbit joints.[23b] The use of minimally effective doses and widely spaced injections is recommended.

LONG-TERM RESULTS

Although the effects of intrasynovial steroid injections are transitory and merely palliative, the increasingly widespread use of this therapeutic method during the past 20 years indicates its usefulness. Follow-up studies on more than 8000 patients treated by intra-articular corticosteroid injection in our clinic are not complete at this writing, but a thorough analysis of the first 547 patients,[2] supplemented by samplings taken at repeated intervals since the analysis was made, gives a basis for preliminary conclusions concerning long-term results after eighteen years of such treatment.[12] Accurate records have been kept of *all* adverse effects throughout the years these injections have been used.

As stated above, intra-articular steroid therapy is merely an adjunct to general therapy, making possible temporary symptomatic relief in joints which are particularly painful or disabling. This would appear futile in long-term management of a relentless disease such as rheumatoid arthritis, but coupled with adequate systemic therapy the results have been gratifying. Patients have been able to continue necessary activities throughout a period of local exacerbation in relative comfort; rehabilitation can be speeded up; and orthopedic measures can be more quickly effective when local steroid therapy is used. The disease may progress without change, but symptoms are relieved.

Of the first 200 rheumatoid arthritic patients receiving intra-articular hydrocortisone injections, nearly 40 per cent (78 patients) still receive occasional injections into joints as needed for relief of pain. Nearly half of these patients now receive prednisolone t-butyl acetate instead of hydrocortisone acetate, because of diminishing effect from the latter on successive injections.

An additional 53 patients (25 per cent) no longer receive intra-articular steroid as the rheumatoid arthritis has abated systemically or locally enough that further local treatment is not needed. The remaining 69 patients of the original series no longer receive such local therapy because of ineffectiveness (17 per cent), have been lost in follow-up (12 per cent), have transferred to other clinics or physicians (8 per cent), or have died (2.5 per cent). In none of the 5 patients who died during a twenty-year period of observation was the cause of death attributable to the intra-articular steroid therapy.

Of the original 200 patients, it is fair to estimate that the functional results in the 131 patients of the first two groups have been good. Most of these patients still have no clinical impairment of function in the treated joints, albeit with some instability developing in about 5 per cent, particularly in knees. No case of major contracture, fibrous or bony ankylosis has occurred. One patient in *this* group developed an infection in the injected joint which required surgery in the form of synovectomy and arthrodesis, however.

Radiologically, however, some progression of joint deterioration in the form of increased osteoporosis was found in 16 per cent, increased narrowing of the "joint space" (cartilage erosion) in 4 per cent, and increased cystic degeneration of subchondral bone or demonstrable degree of bone absorption in 3 per cent. These structural changes are not surprising since the treatment has no effect on the cause of the rheumatoid arthritic process.

Chandler and Wright[4] treated the knee joints of 18 patients who had rheumatoid arthritis, using intra-articular hydrocortisone. Of 25 knees treated, they were alarmed to note that 13 showed some signs of radiologic deterioration at the end of the two-month observation period, although no clinical worsening was noted. The greatest clinical improvement, paradoxically enough, was noted in those patients who showed increased x-ray deterioration of the treated knee. Reasoning from this, they concluded that clinical improvement encouraged abuse of joints which were still diseased, and pointed out that intra-articular steroid therapy was potentially dangerous since the alleviation of pain encouraged abuse.

Our own results, based on long-term observation of more than 8000 patients, show that premature wearing down of joints which have been repeatedly injected with corticosteroids occurs much less frequently.[12] In less than 1 per cent has there been noted any marked deterioration of the joint sufficient to cause instability or necessitate orthopedic correction. It is significant, however, that we have consistently injected moderate doses, repeated injections no oftener than once a month, and have always warned patients to decrease activity. The injection is given to help the patient do what he must do more comfortably, but he must never forget the joint is still arthritic and must be carefully protected from abuse.

In a later paper, Chandler, Jones, Wright, and Hartfall[3] report a "Charcot's arthropathy" developing after repeated injection of hydrocortisone into an osteoarthritic hip. Having also treated 10 patients during the past 20 years who developed what we considered to be aseptic necrosis of the femoral head, we would agree that "careful radiological supervision during such treatment" is needed, even though the incidence of such a complication is only a fraction of 1 per cent in our series.[12]

CLINICAL INDICATIONS FOR INTRA-ARTICULAR CORTICOSTEROID INJECTION

After twenty years of study, we have concluded[12] that intra-articular corticosteroid is clinically useful for local palliative therapy in the following conditions:

1. When one or only a few peripheral joints are inflamed or painful from rheumatoid arthritis, osteoarthritis, traumatic arthritis, acute or chronic gouty arthritis, or intermittent hydrarthrosis. (It may also be used with benefit in acute inflammation of the subdeltoid bursa, by injection directly into the bursal sac, but is rarely helpful in chronic or adhesive bursitis of the shoulder.) It should *never* be injected into a joint in the presence of *infection*, since the hormone appears to decrease resistance to infection in the tissues. Corticosteroids *must not be injected into a joint until a diagnosis has been established*, and specific infectious arthritis ruled out.
2. In rheumatoid or osteoarthritis particularly active in a few peripheral joints, even in the presence of more widespread low-grade joint involvement, the employment of this method as an adjunct to suppress the activity in these few worst joints is helpful.
3. In rheumatoid arthritis, intra-articular corticosteroids can be used to suppress activity in the most severely involved joints until the beneficial effects of gold therapy, or other general measures, become established.
4. In patients with rheumatoid arthritis in which gold therapy, other drug, or corticosteroid therapy is contraindicated because of cardiac failure, renal impairment, hypertension, diabetes, or other reason, the injection of corticosteroids into the most active joints may be useful.
5. When systemic corticosteroid or corticotropin therapy controls the rheumatoid arthritic activity in all but a few "resistant" joints, intra-articular injection into such joints can accomplish a more complete suppression of the process

Indications for Intra-articular Corticosteroid Injection:

1. When one or only a few peripheral joints are inflamed, provided specific infection has been excluded as the cause.
2. In a few actively inflamed joints even in the presence of more generalized low-grade involvement.
3. In rheumatoid arthritis as an adjunct to gold, or other drug therapy.
4. When systemic gold, cortisone, or other therapy is contraindicated.
5. As an adjunct to systemic cortisone or other therapy for control of "resistant" joints.
6. To assist in rehabilitation and prevention of joint deformity.
7. As an adjunct with orthopedic procedures.

on a smaller systemic (and total) dose of hormone.

6. If deformity is beginning to develop in an actively involved rheumatoid arthritic joint, a course of corticosteroid injections together with proper orthopedic measures and physical therapy can more quickly prevent the deformity, and speed the return of normal function.

7. When orthopedic correction of deformity of a certain arthritic joint is being undertaken, whether it be application of traction, wedge casts, or even arthroplasty, repeated local injections of corticosteroid into that joint can prevent the pain, and reduce the recovery period greatly.

CONTRAINDICATIONS TO USE OF INTRA-ARTICULAR CORTICOSTEROID THERAPY

In rheumatoid arthritis, other collagen diseases, and gout particularly, it must be borne in mind that the disease is systemic, and local treatment may be only a futile "placing of buckets under the worst leaks in the roof." It cannot be stressed too often that *intra-articular corticosteroid injection is a palliative, local, and temporary treatment*, even though it can be repeated apparently indefinitely. As a result of trial and error clinical use for twenty years, we conclude that the following conditions either contraindicate the use of this method, or at least render its use impractical:

1. The prime contraindication to local use of corticosteroid is the presence of infection in or about the joint. Tuberculous arthritis of an ankle, though temporarily improved after injection, became much more severe after such treatment in our experience. It is reasonable to avoid injection of a hormone, known to reduce reaction and resistance to the spread of infection, into the site of such an infection. It may be possible after considerably more research, to combine the local injection of hydrocortisone with a specific antibiotic in treating infected joints, but for the present this seems inadvisable.

2. When rheumatoid arthritis involves *many* joints actively, the injection of hydrocortisone into one or two is usually futile.

3. When severe or late osteoarthritis is secondary to a static deformity, or has itself produced severe deformity, the injection of corticosteroid can accomplish little, unless preceded by adequate corrective measures. Likewise, in joints markedly deformed by rheumatoid arthritis, intra-articular hydrocortisone or other corticosteroids can help but little.

4. In ankylosing spondylitis, or osteoarthritis of spinal joints. The joints of the spine are anatomically inaccessible to the aspirating needle, so attempts to inject any spinal joints have proved futile.

5. Arthritis in joints with no synovial space. Only the diarthroses—the joints with synovial sacs—can be successfully treated by this method. Thus arthritis in the sterno-manubrial joint, in the costochondral junctions or in the symphysis pubis is seldom amenable to such local palliation.

6. When injections of corticosteroid into a joint produce only minimal or transient benefit, on several trials, the method should be abandoned. This lack of substantial benefit occurs in about 15 per cent of patients.

7. In traumatic arthritis with a fracture into the joint, the injection of corticosteroid may impede the healing of the fracture.

8. When there is severe osteoporosis of the bones about the joint. Continued intra-articular steroid may increase local osteoporosis, and could lead to pathological fracture, or marked wearing down of bony tables at the joint.

Contraindications to Intra-articular Corticosteroid Injection:

1. Presence of infection in or near the joint.
2. Multiplicity of joint involvement in rheumatoid arthritis.
3. Severe joint destruction, or uncorrected static deformity.
4. Arthritis in spinal joints.
5. Arthritis in other than true diarthrodial (synovial) joints.
6. When trial injections have produced little or no benefit.
7. Traumatic arthritis from fracture into the joint.
8. Severe juxta-articular osteoporosis.

ADMINISTRATION AND DOSAGE

The technique for injection will be described in a subsequent section. The plan of treatment should be arranged so that no more than 2 or 3 joints are injected at one visit, in order to avoid absorption of large amounts of the hormone at one time, with resultant systemic effects. Subsequent injections into a given joint have usually been spaced according to the time of recurrence of symptoms in that joint. Thus, in a patient whose knee has become asymptomatic for a week following the injection of 25 mg. of hydrocortisone into it, the next injection is given at the end of that time when the symptoms have returned. Should the beneficial effect continue for three weeks, reinjection is usually withheld until needed. For extremely active joints, however, some workers[25] have given several injections on successive days to increase the original effect. We have given as many as 137 injections into a single joint, repeating only as often as symptoms recurred. In most patients the succeeding injections have duplicated the degree and duration of relief afforded by the first injection, but in some there has been an increasingly beneficial effect from succeeding injections. In some, a decreasing response has been noted, requiring a larger dose to maintain the suppression of inflammation. In rheumatoid arthritis the average duration of relief from each injection is about twelve days, in osteoarthritis, about two to three weeks, in traumatic arthritis and self-limited conditions subsequent injections may not be necessary. The average dose for a single joint is 25 mg. of hydrocortisone acetate suspension, less in smaller joints and more in larger joints. The dose for individual joints is given below in the description of technique for injection of each. If the suggested dose does not seem adequate, a larger dose may be tried the next time, but we have found that the response is not necessarily in proportion to the amount used, and larger doses than needed may actually decrease the benefit. Other steroids may be substituted for hydrocortisone if not effective. Prednisolone t-butyl acetate, 20 to 30 mg., has proved the most consistently effective steroid for joint injection in our experience, but triamcinolone hexacetonide, 20 mg. (for knee or hip) may palliate longer.

THE TECHNIQUE FOR INTRA-ARTICULAR INJECTION

Any arthritic peripheral joint may be injected, if indicated, and also the temporomandibular, acromioclavicular, or sternoclavicular joints. The anatomic structure and depth below the body surface of the spinal joints make local attempts to treat such articulations impractical.

An anatomical atlas, and an x-ray film of the joint being aspirated should be before the physician when he attempts to inject any joint for the first time. (No apparent harm is done when hydrocortisone is injected outside the joint space, but it is wasted because it is probably quickly dispersed into the general circulation.)

The technique for joint paracentesis and injection is fairly simple and clear-cut. The *object* is to puncture the synovial sac, aspirate excess fluid, and inject the hormone with as little pain as possible, with minimal trauma to the joint and adjacent structures, and without introducing infection into the joint cavity.

The optimum site for paracentesis is, usually, the location on the extensor surface where the synovial pouch is closest to the skin, and as remote as possible from major nerves, arteries or veins.

Materials Needed.—A small office tray with detergent, skin antiseptic, alcohol sponges, 1 per cent procaine solution, a corticosteroid suspension, two 24-gauge sterile needles 1½ inches long, two 20-gauge sterile needles 1½ to 2 inches long, a sterile 5-cc. syringe for injecting procaine, a sterile 20-cc. syringe for aspirating joint fluid, one or two sterile 2 cc.-syringes for injecting corticosteroid, a few gauze pads, and prepared small patch dressings (*e.g.*, Band-Aids) constitutes the total equipment needed. Culture tubes and a graduated glass cylinder for measuring synovial fluid may also be included. No sterile drapes or rubber gloves are necessary, but syringes and needles should be *autoclaved* before use. Disposable needles are now readily available in many sizes, and have been found excellent for intra-articular use. Disposable syringes are also recommended.

A hypospray jet injector may be used instead of syringes and needles, particularly when multiple small joints are to be treated.[1,23a]

Method.—After the optimum site for insertion of the aspirating needle has been chosen, the skin is cleansed twice with detergent, with antiseptic solution and then with alcohol. If there is marked effusion present it is seldom necessary to infiltrate the tissues with procaine, as the introduction of the needle will be quick and easy. In some individuals a brief spraying of the area with ethyl chloride solution gives sufficient anesthesia for insertion of the aspirating needle. If 1 per cent procaine infiltration is deemed advisable, a skin wheal should be made, and the subcutaneous tissue and joint capsule should be infiltrated with about 2 to 4 ml. of the solution.

The aspirating needle seldom need be larger than 20 gauge. The needle is quickly inserted through skin, subcutaneous tissue, capsule and synovial membrane. The tip of the needle is freely movable when the joint space is entered—it may even grate over the cartilage without causing pain. If excess fluid is present, it may then be aspirated.

Entrance into a distended synovial sac is as easy as puncturing an inflated balloon, but entrance into a sac not distended may be as difficult as puncturing a deflated balloon—the relaxed synovial lining may push ahead of the needle point. Folds of synovium or cellular debris may act as a flap-valve on the end of the needle, preventing easy withdrawal of fluid. When this is suspected, the needle should be moved about gently, and a little of the fluid already withdrawn reinjected to push the fold or clot away from the tip of the needle.

Aspiration may be facilitated by wrapping the joint, except for the site of paracentesis, with an elastic bandage to compress the free fluid into that portion of the sac being punctured. It is well to aspirate all readily accessible fluid at the time of paracentesis.[25]

The aspirating syringe is then detached, allowing the needle to remain in place in the joint. The desired amount of corticosteroid suspension (15 to 37.5 mg.)

is drawn into a small syringe. This syringe is then attached to the aspirating needle, still in situ. *If more than gentle pressure on the plunger is required to inject the solution, the needle is probably not free in the joint space, and should be readjusted.* Even if no fluid has been obtained, the easy movability of the needle tip, and the easy introduction of the hormone suspension can give assurance that the tip is in the joint cavity. If fluid is present, the injected suspension may be mixed with the synovial fluid by a barbotage-like repeated withdrawal and reinjection.

The needle is then withdrawn, the puncture site is wiped with an alcohol sponge, and covered with a small sterile dressing. If much fluid has been aspirated from a weight-bearing joint, it is often advisable to apply an elastic bandage to reduce the instability resulting from the now relaxed joint capsule. The patient may resume necessary activity immediately, but *he should be cautioned not to abuse the joint, even though pain and swelling disappear.*

INJECTION OF SPECIFIC JOINTS AND SUGGESTED DOSAGE

Since the technique for paracentesis of individual joints has received little attention, and includes many specific problems, a description for each of the joints frequently injected is given here.

Knee

The largest synovial cavity in the body, and a weight-bearing structure, the knee is also one of the most frequent sites of synovial inflammation. It is the easiest joint to aspirate and inject. A tightly distended knee joint can be aspirated from almost any angle without difficulty, but the following technique may be used for ready entrance into the joint space even if there is little or no excess fluid present.

The patient lies on the table with the knee fully extended. The site for puncture is on the antero-medial surface, 1 or 2 cm. medial to the inner border of the patella. The needle is inserted in a lateral and slightly posterior direction in a line aiming to slide between the posterior surface of the patella and the patellar groove of the femur. In this way the needle tip may crepitate on the undersurface of the patella, demonstrating entrance into the joint space even though no fluid can be withdrawn. Figure 32–1 shows the position of the needle. The advantages of this approach are that there are seldom folds of synovial membrane or pannus under the patella to block ready aspiration, the feel of the needle tip against cartilage is distinctive, and the medial bony margin of the patellar groove of the femur is not as prominent as the lateral margin.

If the patella is ankylosed, or there is marked flexion deformity of the knee, aspiration may be accomplished by puncture antero-posteriorly beside the inferior patellar tendon, through the fat pad into the knee joint space between the condyles of the femur. Puncture of the knee through the popliteal space is not advisable, because of the large popliteal vessels. A Baker's cyst, or posterior herniation of the knee joint capsule, may be aspirated directly, however, if it is superficial and distended. Twenty-five to 37.5 mg. of hydrocortisone suspension or 30 mg. of prednisolone t-butyl acetate are the usual doses for injection into a knee.

Ankle

As shown in the illustration (Fig. 32–2), an antero-medial approach is usual. Procaine infiltration is often advisable prior to ankle aspiration. The needle is aimed at the tibio-astragalar articulation from a point 1 cm. above, and 1 cm. lateral to the internal malleolus, just medial to the extensor pollicis tendon. The needle tip must penetrate about 3 cm. inward and slightly lateral through the ligaments of the ankle joint capsule, and then will be more freely movable between the cartilaginous surfaces of the joint. Excess fluid, if present, can then

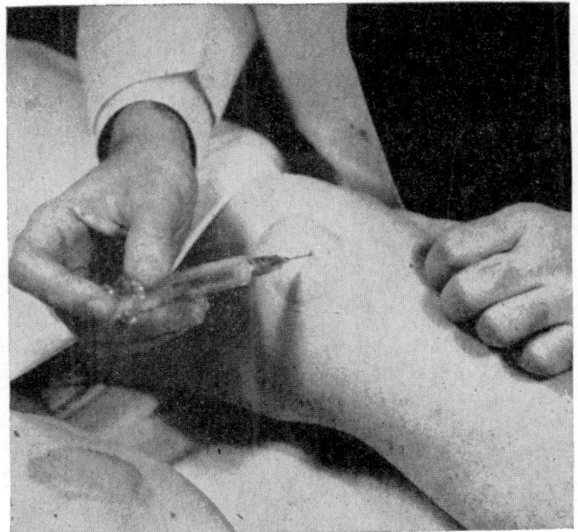

A

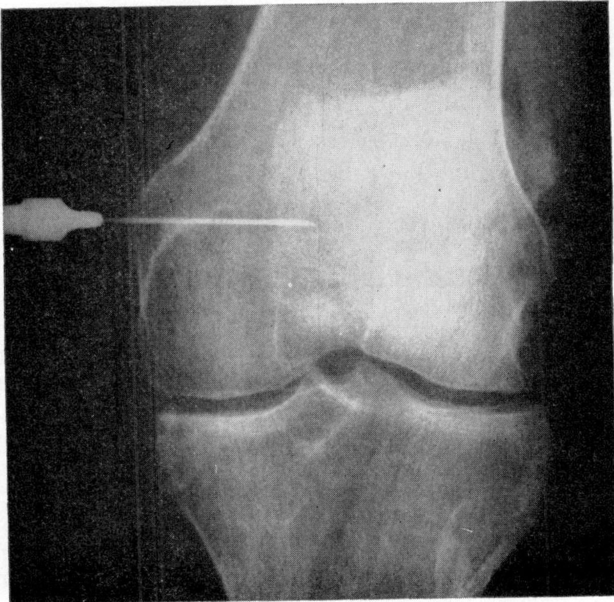

B

Fig. 32–1.—*A*, Injection into the knee. *B*, X-ray showing needle in place under medial side of patella.

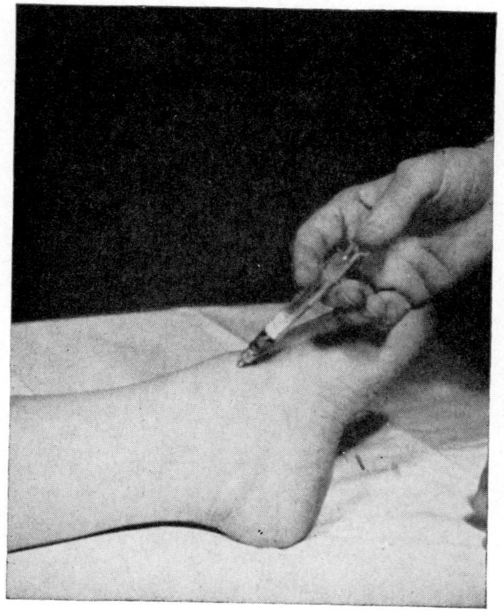

A

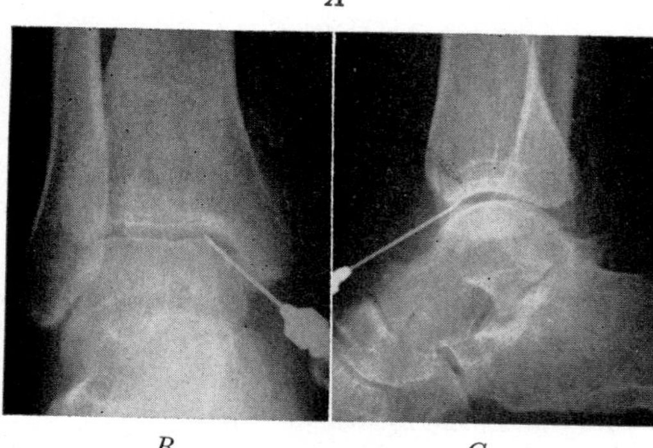

B *C*

FIG. 32–2.—*A*, Injection into left ankle—anteromedial approach. *B*, X-ray, showing A–P view of needle in place in right ankle. *C*, X-ray showing lateral view of needle in right ankle.

be aspirated. If more than gentle pressure on the plunger of the syringe is needed for injection, the needle tip is probably in ligament or cartilage. Twenty-five mg. are the usual dose of hydrocortisone used for ankle injection, or 20 mg. of prednisolone t-butyl acetate.

Tarsal Joints and Tarsometatarsal Joints

A roentgenogram of the area will help orient the operator in the location best suited for entrance into a specific space. A 22-gauge needle may be used, and procaine anesthesia is usually necessary. Because of the superficial location of the joints on the dorsum of the foot, this is the site of election, rather than the plantar surface. The needle may have to be "teased" down between the cartilages; free fluid can only rarely be aspirated. Here the freely movable needle tip, the depth of penetration, and the lack of force needed to inject the hormone suspension assure that the joint space has been entered. *Fluoroscopic guidance is very helpful when small joints are injected.* Ten to 15 mg. of hydrocortisone or prednisolone t.b.a. are the usual dose for such joints.

Toes

After procaine infiltration, a 24-gauge needle is inserted from the dorsal surface, either medially or laterally, sliding beneath the extensor tendons and between the cartilaginous surfaces, in the anatomical plane of the joint. Traction on the toe may facilitate entrance by separating the articulation. Five mg. of the hydrocortisone suspension are usually an adequate dose.

Hip

This is the most difficult joint to aspirate and inject, mainly because of the amount of soft tissue overlying it in all directions. In many cases of osteoarthritis of the hip it has been impossible to enter the joint space with certainty, even under fluoroscopic guidance, because of the flattening of the femoral head and osteophyte formation about the acetabulum. Occasionally, even in osteoarthritis, fluid may be aspirated from the hip joint, however, assuring penetration to the joint space.

The patient lies with the hip in maximal extension and internal rotation. Procaine infiltration is seldom necessary. A 20-gauge needle, $2\frac{1}{2}$ inches long, is employed for the anterior (usual) approach; 3 inches or longer for the lateral approach. The site for puncture in the anterior approach is about 2 to 3 cm below the anterior superior spine of the ilium, and 2 to 3 cm. lateral to the femoral pulse, depending on the size of the patient (*see* Fig. 32–3). The needle is inserted at an angle of 60° with the skin, pointing postero-medially, through the capsular ligaments, which are tough and thick, until bone is reached. The tip is then slightly withdrawn. Fluid occasionally can be aspirated, but in any case injection meets little resistance if the tip is in the joint space. The usual dose of hydrocortisone for the hip is 37.5 mg., or 30 mg. of prednisolone t.b.a.

The lateral approach to the hip joint is also difficult, but has the advantage that the needle "follows the bone" to the hip joint. A lumbar puncture needle is inserted just anterior to the greater trochanter, in a sagittal direction, pointed toward the middle of Poupart's ligament. The needle tip slides in anterior to the periosteum of the neck of the femur, and enters the joint space anteriorly and near the upper reflection of the synovial sac (*see* Fig. 32–3*B*).

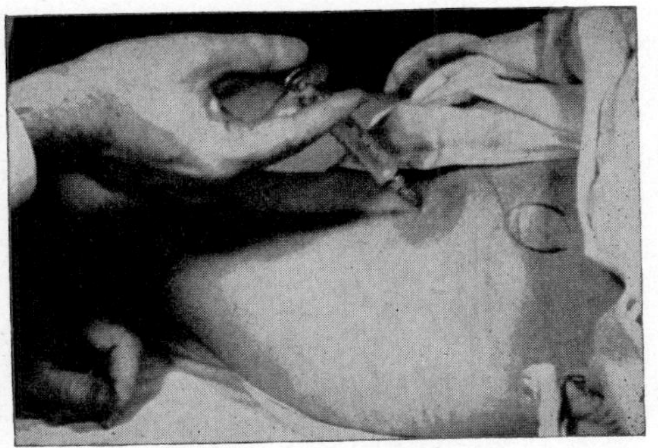

A

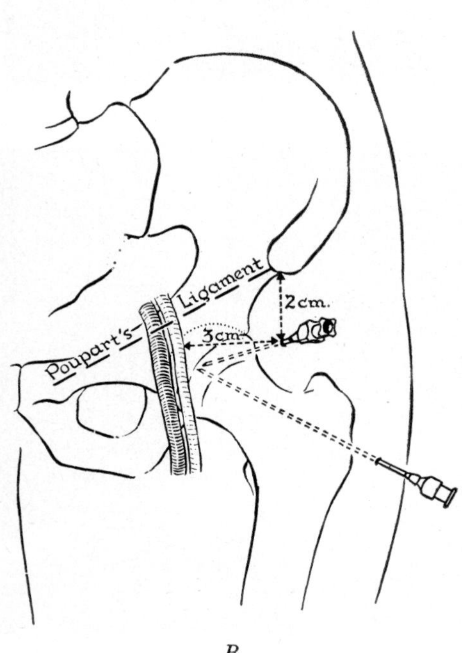

B

Fig. 32–3.—*A*, Injection of left hip. Crescent shows location of anterior superior spine of ilium; line is over Poupart's ligament. *B*, Diagram shows location of structures about left hip, and two directions of approach for injection.

Shoulder

Aspiration of the shoulder is easily accomplished by anterior puncture, inserting the needle just medial to the head of the humerus, and below the tip of the coracoid process (*see* Fig. 32–4). A lateral insertion may also be used. Effusion of the shoulder joint, though rare, nearly always bulges anteriorly. Twenty-five mg. of hydrocortisone or prednisolone t-butyl acetate are the usual dose for shoulder injection.

Acromioclavicular Joint

The plane of the joint can most easily be determined by palpation. The 22-gauge needle is inserted from above and slightly anteriorly until it is felt to slide between the joint surfaces (Fig. 32–4*B*). Fifteen mg. of hydrocortisone or prednisolone are usually sufficient.

Sternoclavicular Joint

This joint is most easily entered from a point directly anterior to the joint. Because of the fibrocartilaginous articular disc, it is a rather difficult joint to inject. Fifteen mg. of hydrocortisone are the usual injection dose.

Elbow

The elbow may either be held at 90°, or fully extended, the latter position in order to distend the capsule as tightly as possible. The bulge of synovium, when effusion is present, is noted on the extensor surface, lateral to the olecranon process of the ulna. The aspirating needle should be inserted distally just lateral to the olecranon and just below the lateral epicondyle of the humerus (Fig. 32–5). Often, particularly in in-

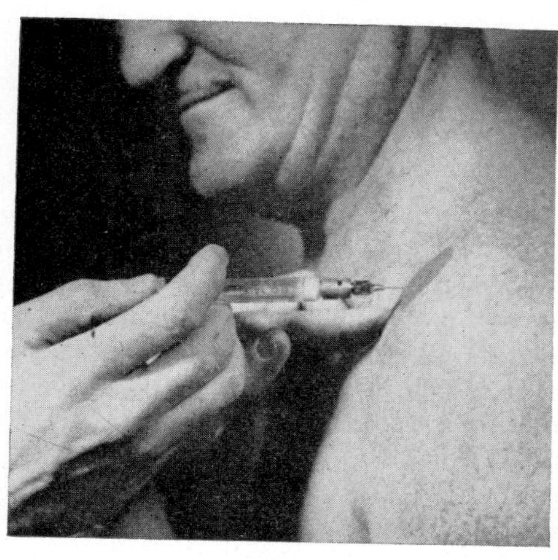

A

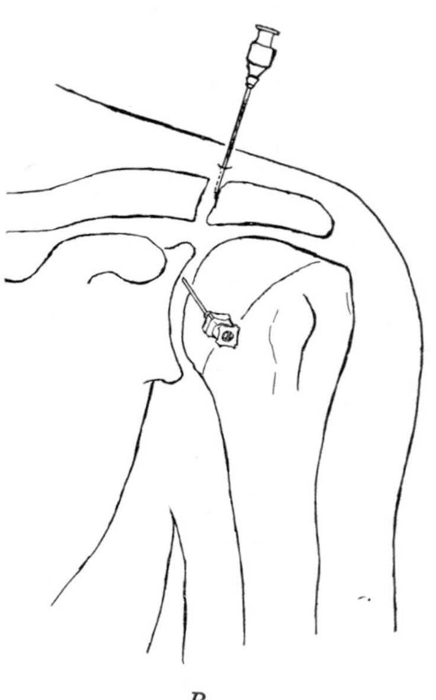

B

FIG. 32–4.—*A*, Injection of the left shoulder joint. *B*, Diagram showing position of needle for injection of shoulder joint and for acromioclavicular joint.

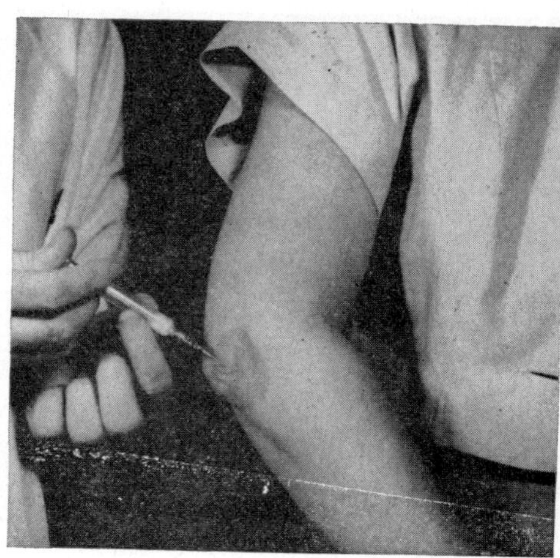

A

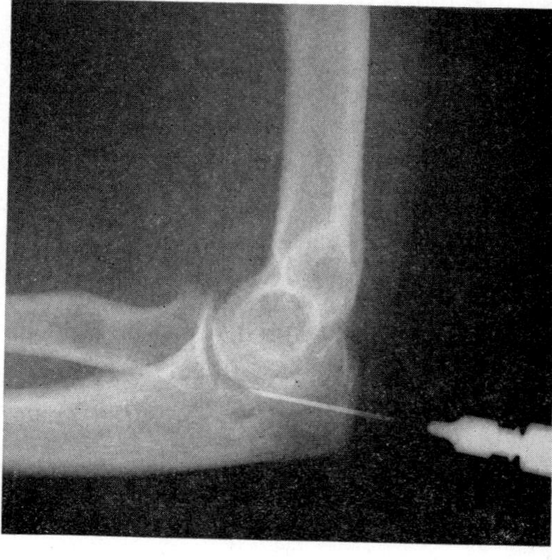

B

FIG. 32–5.—*A*, Injection of right elbow in position of maximum extension. *B*, X-ray of left elbow showing needle in place with elbow at 90°. Needle is inserted *lateral* to olecranon process of the ulna.

jecting the elbow for "tennis elbow," the lateral approach directly into the radio-humeral articulation is desirable. The needle is inserted in a medial direction at a point just distal to the lateral epicondyle (capitulum of the humerus), and just proximal to the head of the radius, to a depth of about 2 cm., when the point of the needle feels free in the joint. Aspiration of fluid from the elbow is more difficult with this latter approach. Paracentesis medial to the olecranon is inadvisable because of proximity to the ulnar nerve. The usual hydrocortisone dose in the elbow is 20 to 25 mg.

Wrist

This complex joint is most safely and easily aspirated dorsally (Fig. 32–6). The needle is inserted perpendicularly with the skin at a point just distal to the radius, and just ulnar to the "anatomic snuff box." If the needle can be easily inserted to a depth of 1 to 2 cm. and feels free, it is probably in correct position. Most of the small inter-carpal joints have connecting synovial spaces. If there is marked synovial bulging on the ulnar surface of the wrist, the joint may be entered by the insertion of the needle just distal to the ulnar styloid process, and dorsal to the pisiform bone (Fig. 32–6*B*). Fifteen to 25 mg. of hydrocortisone or prednisolone t.b.a. are usually an effective dose.

Carpometacarpal Joint of the Thumb

This small joint is frequently troublesome in osteoarthritis, and does not communicate with the other joint spaces of the wrist. It may be entered dorsally from the radial side of the hand, as shown in Figure 32–6*B*. Five to 10 mg. of hydrocortisone are usually an adequate dose.

Metacarpophalangeal and Interphalangeal Joints

These are easily punctured from the lateral or medial approach on the *dorsal*

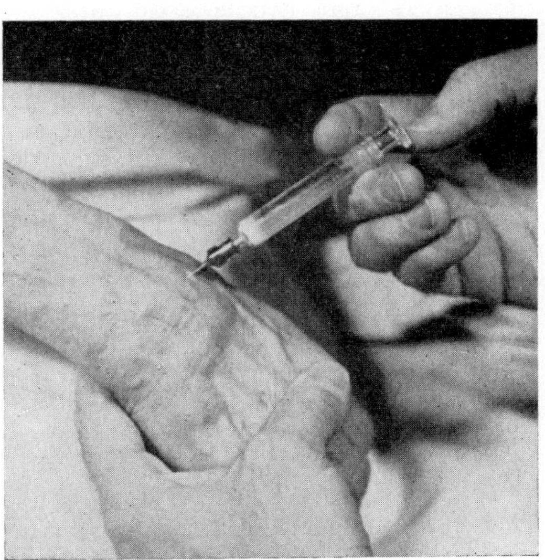

A

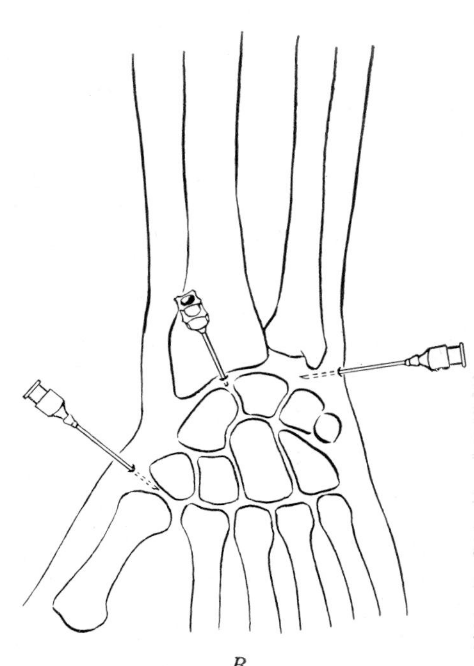

B

Fig. 32–6.—*A*, Injection into the wrist. *B*, Diagram showing location of needle for dorsal approach, ulnar approach, and for injection into carpometacarpal joint of thumb.

surface. A small needle is desirable for such injection (24 gauge) to avoid undue trauma, unless aspiration of fluid is necessary. It is frequently necessary to "tease" the needle between the cartilages, at the same time making traction on the finger to pull the joint cartilages apart. Five to 10 mg. of hydrocortisone are adequate for injection into such small joints.

Temporomandibular Joint

It is sometimes desirable to inject hydrocortisone into this joint for rheumatoid arthritic involvement, for osteoarthritis, or for "clicking jaw." A roentgenogram of the area is necessary for reference. The needle to be used for injection should be small (23 or 24 gauge). It is inserted at a point just below the zygomatic arch, about 1.3 cm. (or $\frac{1}{2}$ inch) anterior to the tragus of the ear, and carried inward, slightly backward, and upward until it has penetrated to a depth of about 1.5 cm. and feels free in the joint (*see* Fig. 32–8). Since there is a fibrocartilaginous articular disc present in the joint, it is often difficult to be sure

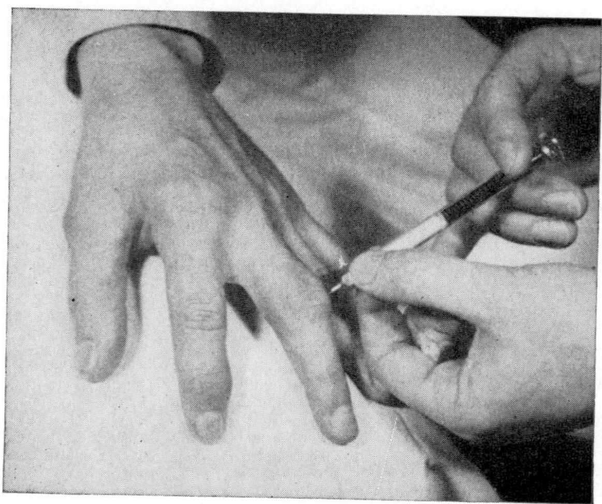

FIG. 32–7.—Injection into a proximal interphalangeal joint of finger.

Usual Effective Dose of Hydrocortisone Acetate* per Joint Injection:

Joint	*Dose*	*Joint*	*Dose*
Knee	25–37.5 mg.	Shoulder	25 mg.
Ankle	20–25 mg.	Elbow	20–25 mg.
Tarsal	10–15 mg.	Wrist	15–25 mg.
Metatarsophal.	10 mg.	Metacarpophal.	5–10 mg.
Interphal. toes	5 mg.	Interphal. fingers	5–10 mg.
Hip	37.5 mg.	Acromioclavicular	15 mg.
Temporomandibular	10–15 mg.	Sternoclavicular	15 mg.

* Equivalent amounts of other steroid preparations:

Hydrocortisone t-butyl acetate, same as above.
Prednisolone t-butyl acetate, 75 per cent of above doses.
Methylprednisolone, or triamcinolone, 75 per cent of above doses.
Dexamethasone t-butyl acetate, 10 per cent of above doses.
Triamcinolone hexacetonide 75 per cent of above doses.

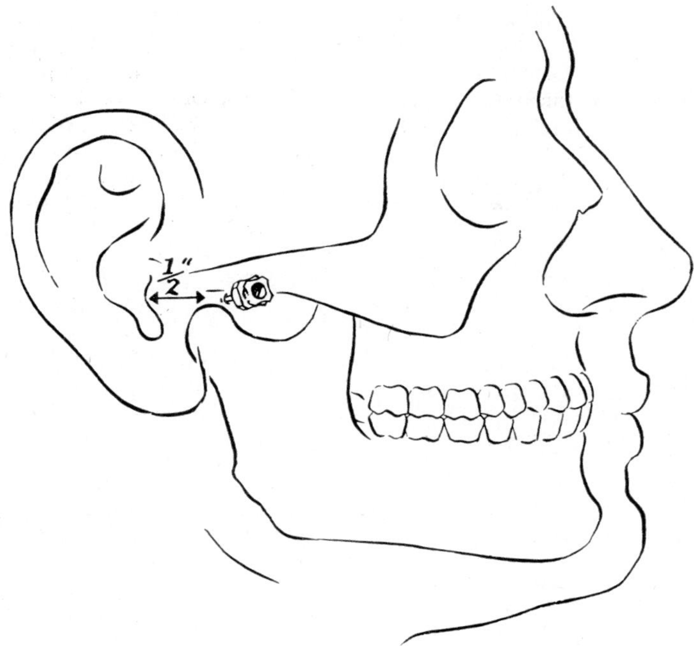

Fig. 32–8.—Diagram showing location of needle for injection of the temporomandibular joint.

the needle is properly placed. The needle is inserted well anterior to the superficial temporal artery. Ten mg. of hydrocortisone or prednisolone t.b.a. have usually proved an adequate dose. The joint space may often be more readily entered by the needle if the patient opens his mouth widely before the puncture is made.

CONCLUSION

The technique of joint paracentesis, probably because of its simplicity, is scarcely more than mentioned in most textbooks. Even textbooks on operative orthopedic surgery[6,24] do not sufficiently describe the methods for aspirating specific joints. In addition, there has grown in the minds of most physicians a fear of aspirating joints because of the possibility of thereby introducing infection. Based on the experience of performing thousands of joint aspirations for diagnosis, in research, and for corticosteroid injection into joints, we can state with confidence that there is little danger, provided careful aseptic precautions, such as observed with any intravenous injection given in a clinic or physician's office, are observed. Joint paracentesis and injection are as simple and safe a procedure as drawing blood from a vein, or injecting a solution intravenously. Just as the physician may encounter difficulty in entering an antecubital vein in some individuals, so may he also have some difficulty in aspirating or injecting a certain joint.

As skill in venipuncture is acquired by practice, it is necessary to attempt joint paracentesis often enough so that it becomes simple, quick, and painless to the patient.

Twenty years of extensive clinical trial have now established intrasynovial injection of corticosteroid as an effective method for temporary local palliation of a variety of joint, bursal, and tendon sheath inflammations. Such treatment is an adjunct to accepted general and supportive measures of therapy. It gives symptomatic relief but does not cure the condition. It is indefinitely repeatable as needed, and relatively innocuous if precautions are observed.

It is advisable to avoid injecting larger doses of corticosteroid than necessary, and not to reinject joints oftener than absolutely necessary in order to minimize the chance of joint deterioration. Activity, particularly when weight-bearing joints are involved, should be moderated or even restricted since patients may be tempted to abuse joints when pain is controlled by steroid suppression of the irritation.

BIBLIOGRAPHY

1. Baum, J., and Ziff, M.: Ann. Rheum. Dis., *26*, 143, 1967.
2. Brown, E. M., Frain, J. B., Udell, L. and Hollander, J. L.: Amer. J. Med., *15*, 656, 1953.
3. Chandler, G. N., Jones, D. T., Wright, V. and Hartfall, S. J.: Brit. Med. J., *1*, 952, 1959.
4. Chandler, G. N. and Wright, V.: Lancet, *2*, 661, 1958.
5. Chandler, G. N., Wright, V., and Hartfall, S. J.: Lancet, *2*, 659, 1958.
6. Colonna, P. C.: *Regional Orthopedic Surgery*, Philadelphia, W. B. Saunders Co., 1950.
7. Conn, J. W., Louis, L. H. and Fajans, S. S.: Science, *113*, 713, 1951.
8. Freyberg, R. H., Patterson, M., Adams, C. H., Durivage, J. and Traeger, C. H.: Ann. Rheum. Dis., *10*, 1, 1951.
9. Gowans, J. and Granieri, P.: New Engl. J. Med., *261*, 502, 1959.
10. Hollander, J. L.: Bull. Rheum. Dis., *2*, 3, 1951.
11. ————: J.A.M.A., *172*, 309, 1960.
12. ————: Maryland State Med. J., *19*, 62, 1970.
13. Hollander, J. L., Brown, E. M., Jessar, R. A. and Brown, C. Y.: J.A.M.A., *147*, 1629, 1951.
14. Hollander, J. L., Brown, E. M., Jessar, R. A., Udell, L., Bowie, M. A., Shanahan, J. R. and Stevenson, C. R.: Arch. Inter-Am. Rheum., *3*, 171, 1960.
15. Hollander, J. L., Brown, E. M., Jessar, R. A., Udell, L., Bowie, M. and Smukler, N.: Ann. Rheum. Dis., *13*, 297, 1954.
16. Hollander, J. L., Jessar, R. A. and Brown, E. M.: Bull. Rheum. Dis., *11*, 239, 1961.
17. Hollander, J. L., Jessar, R. A., Restifo, R. A. and Fort, H. J.: Arth. and Rheum., *4*, 422, 1961.
18. Mason, H. L.: *Proceedings 1st Clinical ACTH Conference*, Ed. by Mote, J. R. Philadelphia, The Blakiston Co., 1951.
19. McCarty, D. J. and Hogan, J. M.: Arth. and Rheum., *7*, 359, 1964.
20. Morison, R. A. H., Woodmansey, A. and Young, A. J.: Ann. Rheum. Dis., *20*, 179, 1961.
21. Nelson, D. H., Samuels, L. T. and Reich, H.: *Proceedings 2nd Clinical ACTH Conference*, Ed. by Mote, J. R., Philadelphia, The Blakiston Co., 1951.
22. Peterson, R. E., Black, R. B., and Bunim, J. J.: Arth. and Rheum., *2*, 433, 1959.
23*a*. Rankin, T. J. and Good, A. E.: Arth. & Rheum., *9*, 611, 1966.
23*b*. Salter, R. B., Gross, A. and Hall, J. H.: Canad. Med. Assoc. J., *97*, 374, 1967.
23*c*. Shah, K. D. and Wright, V.: Ann. Rheum. Dis., *26*, 316, 1967.
24. Speed, J. S. and Smith, H.: *Campbell's Operative Orthopedic Surgery*, St. Louis, C. V. Mosby Co., 1949.
25. Stevenson, J. R., Zuckner, J. and Freyberg, R. H.: Ann. Rheum. Dis., *11*, 112, 1952.
26. Thorn, G. W.: Personal communication.
27. Tondreau, R. L., Hodes, P. J., and Schmidt, E. R.: Amer. J. Roent., Rad. Ther. & Nuclear Med., *82*, 258, 1959.
28. Waugh, W. G.: Brit. Med. J., *1*, 873, 1945.
29. Wilson, H., Glyn, J., Scull, E., McEwen, C. and Ziff, M.: Proc. Soc. Exp. Biol. & Med., *83*, 648, 1953.
30. Wright, V.: Ann. Rheum. Dis., *23*, 389, 1964.
31. Wright, V., Chandler, G. N., Morison, R. A. H., and Hartfall, S. J.: Ann. Rheum. Dis., *20*, 179, 1960.
32. Zacco, M., Richardson, E. M., Crittenden, J. O., Hollander, J. L. and Dohan, F. C.: J. Clin. Endocrin., *14*, 711, 1954.
33. Ziff, M., Scull, E., Ford, C., and Bunim, J. J.: A.M.A. Arch. Int. Med., *90*, 774, 1952.

Chapter 33

Cytotoxic Drug Therapy in Rheumatic Diseases

By Charles L. Christian, M.D.

Cytotoxic compounds (alternatively referred to as immunosuppressive or anti-metabolite drugs) include the alkylating agents (nitrogen mustard, chlorambucil, cyclophosphamide), purine and pyrimidine antagonists (6-mercaptopurine, azathioprine, 6-thioguanine, and 5-fluorouracil) and folic acid analogs (methotrexate). In addition, actinomycin D and chloramphenicol are two antibiotics with demonstrable immunosuppressive properties. Although cytotoxic agents were developed for cancer chemotherapy, they were evaluated in the management of renal disease (including systemic lupus erythematosus)[2,7] and rheumatoid arthritis[6] more than two decades ago—before there was significant knowledge of drug immunosuppression or evidence of immunological mediation of such syndromes. This early interest in cytotoxic drug therapy of rheumatic disease ceased when corticosteroids became available.

The increasing fund of information implicating immune mechanisms in disease states such as rheumatoid arthritis and the demonstration of drug-mediated immunosuppression[17] provided stimuli for re-evaluation of cytotoxic agents in a variety of chronic rheumatic states. Although clinical impressions regarding efficacy are prevalent there is paucity of carefully controlled therapeutic observations. Accepting the premise that drugs such as cyclophosphamide and azathioprine do have roles in the management of rheumatoid arthritis and systemic lupus erythematosus, the following features of such therapy should be emphasized: 1. It is experimental—as of 1971, the U.S. Food and Drug Administration has not approved the drugs for other than malignant disease and organ transplantation. 2. Acute toxicity can be fatal. 3. Long-term effects, which are largely unknown, are potentially great. 4. Clinical remissions that ensue may be mediated more by non-specific anti-inflammatory properties of cytotoxic drugs than by immunosuppression.

Pharmacological Effects.—Although the biochemical events affected by different classes of cytotoxic drugs vary, the pharmacological effects are similar—rapidly replicating tissues are preferentially affected via alterations in cell nucleic acids.[17] With regard to immune responses, the inductive phase of primary immunization is the most sensitive to interference by cytotoxic agents. An already established immune state, which by hypothesis is involved in rheumatic disease syndromes, is relatively resistant to suppression. The quantitative aspects of drug suppression of cell-mediated (delayed hypersensitivity) events vary with different classes of cytotoxic agents but, in general, this sphere of the immune response is inhibited.

Several observers have documented non-specific anti-inflammatory properties of cytotoxic drugs.[9,10] Regardless of the character of the inflammatory stimulus, it appears that mononuclear cells involved in the exudative process of inflammation are sensitive to cytotoxic drug therapy.

Drug Toxicity.—All of the cytotoxic compounds have the potential for suppression of myeloid elements of the blood—granulocytopenia is most common. A significant percentage of patients receiving commonly utilized regimens (2 to 3 mgs/Kg of cyclophosphamide or azathioprine) will manifest myelosuppression which can be fatal if the drug is not discontinued. Infectious complications with bacterial and fungal organisms may be related to both myelosuppression and interference with the immune response.

Certain toxic features are unique to individual classes of cytotoxic compounds. A minority of patients receiving cyclophosphamide will experience reversible hair loss and hemorrhagic cystitis. Cholestatic jaundice is an infrequent complication of 6-mercaptopurine or azathioprine therapy. *Of particular importance, the drug allopurinol greatly potentiates the action of 6-mercaptopurine and azathioprine.* Either of the latter two agents, if they are given concomitantly with allopurinol, should be reduced to about 20% of the usual dose.

There is considerable concern that cytotoxic therapy may foster the emergence of primary malignant tumors,[13,15] based in part on experimental observations[3] and in part on clinical experience (40 reported cases of tumors complicating renal transplantation as of 1970).

EVALUATION OF CYTOTOXIC DRUG THERAPY IN RHEUMATOID ARTHRITIS

Several reports have summarized experience with cytotoxic drug treatment of patients with rheumatoid arthritis[8,11,12,14,16] but only one study utilized double-blind techniques and biostatistical methods of analysis.[4] The latter, a multicenter study under the auspices of the American Rheumatism Association's Cooperating Clinics Committee, compared the efficacies of two regimens of cyclophosphamide (up to 150 mgm daily versus up to 15 mgm daily) in 48 adult patients with rheumatoid arthritis. The higher dose group sustained significantly fewer new bone erosions over the period of study (32 weeks). In several studies dissociations between clinical effects and evidence of immunosuppression have been noted, suggesting that anti-inflammatory properties of cytotoxic drugs may be responsible for clinical improvement when it occurs.[1,5,19]

GUIDELINES FOR THE USE OF CYTOTOXIC DRUGS IN RHEUMATIC DISEASES

A panel of participants in an American Rheumatism Association Workshop proposed criteria for selection of patients for cytotoxic therapy.[18] They were: (1) A life-threatening or potentially serious crippling disease must be present. (2) Reversible lesions must be present. (3) Failure to respond to or intolerable side effects from conventional therapy must be demonstrated. (4) There must be no clinically active infection when treatment is started. (5) There must be no hematologic contraindication to treatment with a cytotoxic drug. (6) Meticulous follow-up, especially for signs of acute and long-term toxicity, is mandatory. (7) Methods of objective evaluation of the course of the disease by clinical and laboratory means must be used. (8) Reasons for applying such therapy and its possible hazards must be explained to each patient and his signed consent must be obtained. (9) Therapeutic protocols must be submitted to peer group review.

In the light of the above criteria and in recognition of the experimental character of cytotoxic therapy for rheumatic disease, *it is not appropriate to designate any drug regimen as "recommended."* Legally, in the United States, the use of drugs such as cyclophosphamide, azathioprine, and methotrexate is restricted to those who have been licensed by the Food and Drug

Administration through the supplier of the drug. At the present time there is no basis for concluding that any one cytotoxic agent is more efficacious than another in the management of rheumatoid arthritis. Azathioprine and cyclophosphamide are the two compounds that have had the widest use.

Since the doses and therapeutic guidelines for azathioprine and cyclophosphamide are similar, the following summarizes current practices of those who experimentally employ these agents in the management of rheumatoid arthritis: (1) The criteria for selection of patient (stated above) should be followed. (2) The dose of drug is 2 to 3 mgms per kilogram body weight in single or divided doses (or approximately 1 mgm per pound of body weight). It is common practice to give half of the above dose for the first 1 to 2 weeks of therapy. (3) Meticulous follow-up care is mandatory, including periodic blood counts (during the first few weeks of therapy complete blood counts should be performed at least weekly—those with stable blood indices should have hematologic studies at least every two weeks for as long as they remain on therapy). (4) Therapy should be discontinued at the first sign of toxicity (myelosuppression, if it develops, may worsen for a period of several days even when therapy is stopped). It is common practice to interrupt therapy if peripheral blood granulocytes fall below 2000 per mm^3. (5) If therapy is to be re-instituted after signs of toxicity have cleared, it should be given at half of the initial dose and increased cautiously if signs of toxicity do not recur. (6) Female patients in the child-bearing years should be warned of teratogenic potential of cytotoxic drugs and guided in contraceptive practices.

CONCLUSIONS

Cytotoxic drug therapy does not yet have an established role in the management of RA. As an experimental method of treatment it has some promise, especially where more conventional therapies fail or are contraindicated. Further studies of the efficacy, mode of action and toxicity of cytotoxic agents in rheumatic disease subjects are needed to indicate their place in the management of rheumatoid arthritis and related diseases.

BIBLIOGRAPHY

1. Alepa, F. P., Zvaifler, N. J. and Sliwinski, A. J.: Arth. & Rheum., *13*, 754, 1970.
2. Baldwin, D. S., McLean, P. G., Chasis, H. and Goldring, W.: Arch Intern. Med., *92*, 162, 1953.
3. Casey, T. P.: Clin. Exp. Immunol., *3*, 305, 1968.
4. Cooperating Clinics of the American Rheumatism Assoc. (Report): New Engl. J. Med., *283*, 883, 1970.
5. Denman, E. J., Denman, A. M., Greenword, B. M. *et al.*: Ann. Rheum. Dis., *29*, 220, 1970.
6. Diaz, C. J., Garcia, E. L., Merchante, A. *et al.*: J.A.M.A., *147*, 1418, 1951.
7. Dubois, E. L.: Arch. Intern. Med., *93*, 667, 1954.
8. Fosdick, W. M., Parsons, J. L. and Hill, D. F.: Arth. & Rheum., *11*, 151, 1968.
9. Hersh, E. M., Wong, V. G., and Freireich, E. J.: Blood, *27*, 38, 1966.
10. Hurd, E. R., Ziff, M.: J. Exp. Med., *128*, 785, 1968.
11. Kahn, M. F., Bedoiseau, M. and Sèze, S. de: Proc. Roy. Soc. Med., *60*, 130, 1967.
12. Mason, M., Currey, H. L. F., Barnes, C. G. *et al.*: Brit. Med. J., *1*, 420, 1969.
13. McKhann, C. F.: Transplantation, *8*, 209, 1969.
14. Möens, C. and Bracteur, J.: Acta Rheum. Scand., *11*, 212, 1965.
15. Pen, I., Howard, W., Brettschneider, L. *et al.*: Transplantation Proc., *1*, 106, 1969.
16. Renier, J., Deshayes, P., Besson, J. *et al.*: Presse Med., *75*, 2527, 1967.
17. Schwartz, R. S.: Prog. Allergy, *9*, 246, 1965.
18. Schwartz, R. S. and Gowans, J. D. C.: Arth. & Rheum., *14*, 134, 1971.
19. Swanson, M. A. and Schwartz, R. S.: New Engl. J. Med., *227*, 163, 1967.

PART V

Physical and Orthopedic Management of Rheumatoid Arthritis

EDITOR: RICHARD H. FREYBERG, M.D.

Chapter 34

Physical Therapy in Arthritis

By Morris A. Bowie, M.D.

Physical therapy is that portion of the total treatment and rehabilitation program in which physical agents are employed to relieve pain, relax muscle spasm, and increase blood flow in preparation for or to augment a therapeutic exercise program.

This concept of physical therapy requires both a patient who is motivated to help himself as much as he is able, and a physician with a thorough knowledge of the arthritis he is treating, the activity of the process, the potential reversibility of the damage therefrom, and the degree of improvement which can be expected from appropriate therapy in the patient. To utilize physical therapy adequately, safely and effectively the physician needs knowledge of the physiological effects of each of the modalities at hand and how they can be incorporated into the general plan of treatment and rehabilitation. In this chapter these measures will be discussed. In the following chapters the place of occupational therapy in treatment, and the rehabilitation program as a whole will be discussed.

Intelligent use of physical therapy is a valuable adjunct in the management of the arthritic patient. Injudicious use of physical measures may cause harm. Proper physical therapy is an important part of the basic treatment for most types of arthritis, and a "must" for rheumatoid arthritis.

The objectives of physical therapy in arthritis are to help relieve symptoms, shorten the period of disability from the disease, prevent or help correct deformities and improve function. To achieve these goals, each patient requires thorough study to determine his individual limitations and potentialities, his motivation and attitude as well as the type, activity and extensiveness of his disease. Individual prescription for physical therapy for each patient is recommended (see box summary).

Due precautions must be taken with the application of any measure, and frequent observations made, especially when any form of heat is applied. Most of the accidents are *burns caused by thermal, electrochemical or photochemical energy* although mechanical injuries and even electric shock have been reported. In older people physical medicine must be used conservatively and in small doses since they may not tolerate heat and other measures[43a] as well as younger individuals. Technicians should always be carefully supervised by the physician in charge.[141]

In order to achieve a really effective therapeutic program for the arthritic patient, *physical therapy must be carried out at home* for long periods of time. The program for each patient must be individualized and modified from time to time; the *physician should demonstrate treatment*, explain what is to be expected, and periodically re-evaluate the patient's technique and performance. Written instructions and class demonstrations have proved feasible and effective at the Mayo Clinic.[169] If *sufficiently detailed outlines are given*, a large number of these patients continue treatments at home.[53,85,151] Home care programs, under the sponsorship of hospitals and other agencies,

Prescription for Physical Therapy[58,112,119,132]

1. Specify diagnosis and indicate any special instructions or precautions for patient.
2. List the parts or area of body to be treated.
3. State *precisely the dosage* of each measure to be used.
   a. Type of heat and length of application,
   b. The kind of massage and time to be spent in massage of each part,
   c. Type of exercise and purpose (muscle strengthening, muscle re-education, coordination, or relaxation).
4. Number and frequency of treatments during the day.
5. Direct what home measures are to be employed.
   a. Technician to check patient's performance frequently.
6. Include date for re-evaluation by physician at which time he should:
   a. Ascertain that directions are carried out properly;
   b. Grade patient's performance;
   c. Add modifications, change frequency of treatments, etc.;
   d. Redetermine rest-exercise balance and coordinate total regimen;
   e. Furnish encouragement and provide support for patient's morale.

include visits by physical and occupational therapists; home care is cheaper than hospitalization.

TYPES OF PHYSICAL THERAPY EMPLOYED IN ARTHRITIS

I. Heat

The application of heat may be directed either locally or systemically. Thermal energy may be transmitted from one body to another **by conduction** (hot packs, hot water bottle, electric pads, hot air blowers or chambers, chemical heat pads, the application of hot solids or semisolids [paraffin, mud, etc.], hot tub baths, Hubbard tank, whirlpool, and therapeutic pool); **by radiation** (luminous and infrared lamps, bakers, household electric heaters); or **by conversion** (long and short wave diathermy, microwave). The physiological effects from local application of any of these measures differ very little except that penetration is least with conduction and most with conversion methods.

Among the effects to be noted by **local application of heat** are dilatation of the blood vessels, hyperemia, and local sweating. Heat relaxes muscles, improves local nutrition, and is frequently analgesic. It may cause harm if applied injudiciously, and may even act as a form of trauma. In some patients with acute arthritis, the application of heat in any form seems to aggravate the local condition; in such individuals it should be discontinued or modified. Some authorities believe that heat should not be applied to an acutely inflamed joint when the overlying skin is hot or red.[98] The incorporation of a medicinal agent, *e.g.*, hot saturated solution of magnesium sulfate, often greatly enhances the effect of local heating. It may be kept hot by repeated application or the use of a radiant lamp or hot water bottle.

Systemic application of heat is more generally used in arthritis than in most other medical conditions. Its primary effect is on the circulatory system where one of the early developments is a rise in pulse rate and a slight drop in blood pressure.[1] Maximal vasodilatation is not reached before twenty to thirty minutes.[128,167] Clearance of radiosodium is significantly increased (20 to 60 per cent) after application of radiant heat, diathermy, or exercises.[68] Pulmonary ventilation is increased, roughly paralleling the rise in body temperature, and an increased amount of water vapor is lost in the expired air. Sweating may be profuse, and large amounts of salt may be lost. Metabolism is heightened, and

Application of Heat in Rheumatoid Arthritis

1. In acute stage with red, swollen joints:
   a. Protect joints between treatments with splints, half shell casts, sandbags;
   b. Use hot fomentations for 20–60 minutes q.i.d.;
      (1) Employ hot saturated solution of magnesium sulfate for analgesic effect;
      (2) Steam packs (Hydrocollator).
   c. Radiant heat or infrared may be substituted;
   d. Diathermy and hot baths contraindicated.
2. In subacute or chronic stage:
   a. With multiple joint involvement;
      (1) Systemic heating preferable; tub bath, tank, cradle (baker).
   b. Steam packs or paraffin dips for individual joints;
   c. Infrared or radiant heat alone or with hot fomentations;
   d. Fever therapy generally ineffective.
3. Home treatments:
   a. For involvement of weight-bearing joints;
      (1) Hot compresses or steam packs 2 to 4 times daily;
      (2) Contrast baths for ankles, feet, hands;
      (3) Hot tub bath once daily.
   b. For nonweight-bearing joints;
      (1) Paraffin dips, steam packs, hot soaks;
      (2) Radiant or infrared 4 times daily.

carbon dioxide is formed in amounts larger than normal, but hyperventilation washes out more than proportional amounts of carbon dioxide. Changes in acid-base balance induce a mild alkalosis. Oxygen consumption is increased, and fluid transfer across the capillary wall is accelerated.[125] As with local heating, muscular relaxation occurs. A sedative effect on the peripheral and central nervous systems has been noted. The most obvious result of the application (to the layman) is sweating, and this has given rise to the popular idea of "elimination" as a means of therapeusis.

A. Forms of Applying Dry Heat

Heat Lamp.—The simplest type consists of a cup-shaped polished reflector and a clamp (or handle) which may be attached to a chair back or bed. A 250-watt Mazda CX bulb is connected with an ordinary electrical outlet. The part to be treated is exposed about 18 inches from the lamp. The area over which heat energy strikes the skin is rather small in this type of lamp, averaging only 8 to 10 cm. with a tungsten filament.[47] Consequently, its use is restricted to single small areas. In addition, "hot spots" are present in such lamps where heat energy is intense. Burns are more apt to occur than with lamps providing a more even distribution of heat. Similar lamps attached to an adjustable stand or with a goose neck afford more flexibility and permit perpendicular application to curved portions of the torso. The angle at which heat strikes the skin and slight changes in the distance markedly affect the amount of the energy absorbed.

Luminous Baker.—The larger types with 4 to 12 bulbs of either carbon or tungsten filament provide a uniform heat, distributed evenly over all areas beneath the reflecting surface. An inexpensive model for home use can be made by a tinsmith.[26] Details of construction are shown in the diagram. The apparatus may be covered with a sheet to prevent loss of heat.

Baking is a most comfortable way of providing systemic heat. The cradle supports should be spaced sufficiently widely so as to avoid contact with the skin. An average treatment requires about thirty minutes, and may precede daily massage. The patient should be covered with

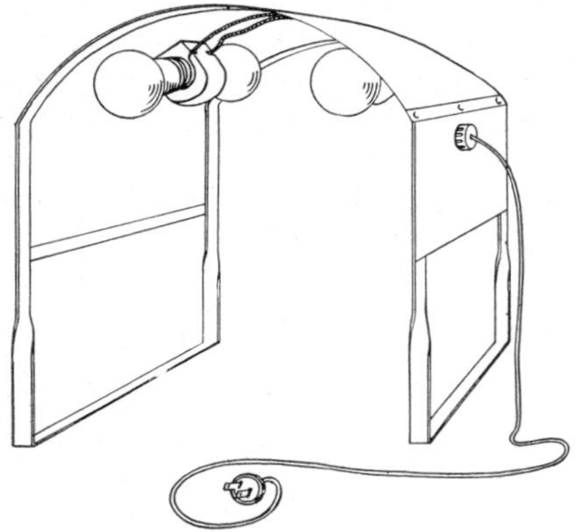

Fig. 34–1.—Homemade baker. (Council on Physical Medicine and Rehabilitation.)

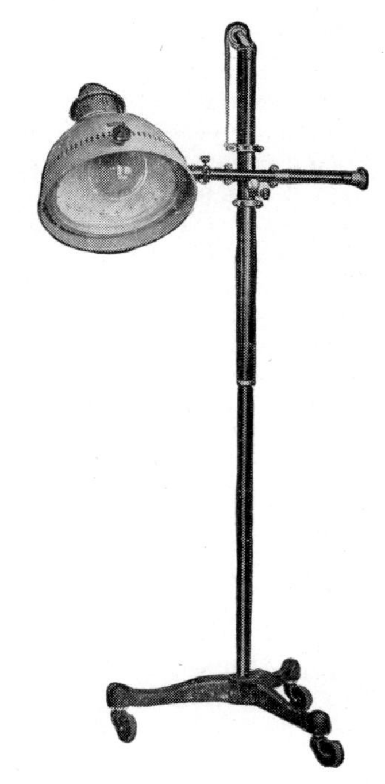

Fig. 34–2.—Large luminous heat generator on stand. (Courtesy of The Burdick Corporation.)

blankets afterward to maintain the slight hyperpyrexia.

Infrared Lamp.—Thermal radiation, with a generator producing dull red, penetrates to a distance of 10 to 1 millimeters, the depth decreasing with the wave length.[65] Heat energy from this source is concentrated in the superficial layers of the skin and is slowly dissipated by the underlying blood. Infrared radiation of short ("near") wave length (7,600 to 15,000 Angstrom units) is tolerated twice as well by the average skin as that of long ("far") wave length (15,000 to 150,000 Å). For clinical use there are advantages inherent in both types. However, the amount of radiation, even with the penetrating wave lengths, which can be tolerated is rather low.[112,153] Lamps producing a large amount of "near" infrared energy are the 250-watt CX Mazda bulb, the 250-watt carbon filament bulb, and the newer 250-watt reflector heat lamp in addition to the 500- to 1,500-watt tungsten filament bulbs. The shape of the reflector is an important item in choosing a heat lamp. The best reflectors are those coated with copper or silver. Heat from this source should be directed at right angles to the part being treated from a distance of approximately 24 inches; the distance between the generator and the patient's skin depends on the tolerance and the sensitivity of the part. Infrared lamps are the least effective means of heating the hands, forearms, and feet because loss of heat is rapid from the surfaces not directly exposed. One of the forms of hydrotherapy or a simple conductive device may be superior.

The above methods of applying dry heat all depend for their effectiveness on the emission of infrared rays. They are more economical, easier to manipulate, and less dangerous than long or short wave diathermy. Direct inspection of the part being treated is always possible.

Electric Blanket.—The commercially available electric blankets or sheets possess usefulness in preventing or ameliorating the morning stiffness of which most arthritic patients complain. Some bedridden patients with an overactive vasomotor system seem to do particularly well under an electric blanket at night or on chilly days.

Lengths and Frequencies of High Energy Waves[66,111]

Electromagnetic: Diathermy	Range: Wave length	Range: Frequency megacycles	F.C.C. Bands: Wave length	F.C.C. Bands: Frequency megacycles
Microwave	10 cm.–1 meter	300–3,000	12.2 cm.	2,450
Short wave	3-30 meters	10–100	22.0 meters	13.56
			11.0 meters	27.12
			7.3 meters	40.68
Long wave	30–3,000 meters	0.1–10	....	....
Mechanical:				
Ultrasound	0.7–1.5 mm.	0.15–3		0.8–1.0

Precautionary Measures in Application of Diathermy or Ultrasound[118]

1. Have patient assume comfortable position, either sitting or lying.
2. Use wooden table. *Do not employ chairs, tables, or beds with metal parts.* Enough heat may be generated in springs to ignite the mattress.
3. Remove clothing, wet dressings, ointments, keys, knives, money, watch, hairpins, earrings, metal buttons, dentures with metal clasps.
4. Do not allow patient to regulate current.
5. Instruct patient to inform operator of unpleasant sensations.
6. Inspect the toweling or interposed material. If this is too wet, replace.
7. In treating head, therapy must be stopped if untoward symptoms occur: drowsiness, inability to concentrate, vertigo.[153]
8. Limit duration of treatment to twenty to thirty minutes. *Set interval timer* at start.
9. *With Microwave Diathermy:*
   a. Use distance of 5 cm. from director to skin and power output of 60 to 80 watts.
   b. Duration of treatment limited to twenty to thirty minutes.
   c. Use with extreme caution over:
      (1) Any area containing metallic bodies or plates (*e.g.*, bone plate);
      (2) Ischemic areas;
      (3) Bony prominences;
      (4) Epiphyseal regions of growing bones (and children under five);
      (5) The eyes;[135]
      (6) Edematous tissue.
   d. Observe other precautions as with long or short wave diathermy.
10. *With Ultrasound:*
   a. Suggested dosage: 0.5 to 6 watts/square centimeter;
   b. Length of application: five to ten minutes;
      (1) Stop treatment if unpleasant sensation develops.
   c. Do not use over:
      (1) Brain or special organs of sense;
      (2) Reproductive organs;
      (3) Epiphysis of growing bones;
      (4) Over larger peripheral nerves;
      (5) Observe other precautions listed under microwaves.

Diathermy and Diathermy Machines.—Heat is produced when an electric current or sound wave of high frequency is passed through tissues. This action is utilized in diathermy and ultrasound machines. High frequency electrical currents or sound waves can be passed safely through the body at a sufficient intensity to raise the body temperature without stimulating the nerves or muscles.[165]

Diathermy machines approved for inclusion in "Apparatus Accepted" employ either an 11- or a 22-meter wavelength. The frequencies assigned to medical diathermy and to industry were re-allocated in 1953; tolerances on new diathermy apparatus are narrower than formerly so as to prevent interference with other frequency channels.[29] *In the selection of a machine it is suggested that "Apparatus Accepted" be consulted.*[29] The assigned wave length for microwave diathermy is 12.2 cm. (2,450 megacycles); this lies in the ultrahigh frequency band of the radio frequency spectrum.[75] Its wave length has some of the characteristics of light "in that it is apparently propagated in straight lines and can be reflected, refracted, and absorbed. Its physiological effects in some respects resemble those of diathermy but in others resemble those of radiant energy from infrared lamps. Its therapeutic effects are simply those of heat liberated in the tissues."[28] Ultrasonic waves exhibit some similarities to microwaves, and are discussed in more detail below. The fundamental reason for using currents or sound waves of high frequency is that the body temperature may be raised without injury or electrical stimulation. Because of the deep penetration of these currents, diathermy is the physical agent of choice in any condition where deep heating of the tissues is indicated.

Long wave diathermy is rarely used in arthritis.

Short wave diathermy is applied by means of an induction cable which provides an electromagnetic field and yields higher muscle temperatures than is possible with condenser pads or air-spaced electrodes; the latter produce an electrostatic field yielding high temperatures in less conductive tissues such as skin, fat, and bone. The metal electrode in the drum type is insulated with rubber or felt and may be applied directly to the skin with only one thickness of toweling

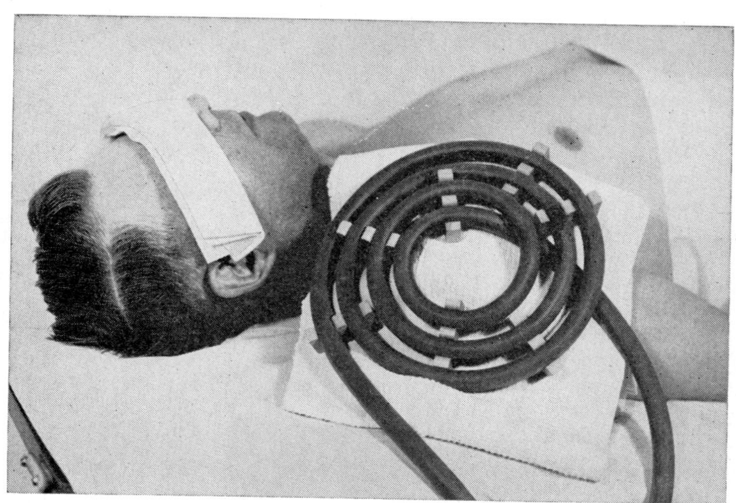

Fig. 34–3.—Short wave diathermy to the shoulder. Pancake coil technique—electromagnetic induction. (Coulter, courtesy of Med. Clin. North America.)

over the skin to absorb perspiration. Air spacing with towels or other absorbent material is necessary with the cable type. The flexible, heavily insulated cable may be wound around the part to be treated or be placed in the form of a pancake coil.

In arthritic patients with multiple joint involvement, systemic heating is usually indicated, and, for this purpose, short wave diathermy is excellent provided that the physician has adequate facilities to allow a suitable recovery period. General vasodilatation and a rise in the body temperature can be attained within thirty to forty-five minutes by insulating the patient in blankets and placing the cable over or under the patient's back.

Microwave diathermy is applied by means of hemispherical or "corner" directors which cover an area about 10 inches (25 cm.) in diameter. They are usually placed at a distance of 5 cm. from the skin and reflect the radiations directly onto the surface. An output of 60 to 80 watts has been used for most of the experimental work in both animals and man.[75,111] In order to decrease undesirable reflection from the skin, the dielectric *Mycalex* may be interposed between the director and the skin.[64] A new long director, which produces uniform heating over an area 8 by 18 inches

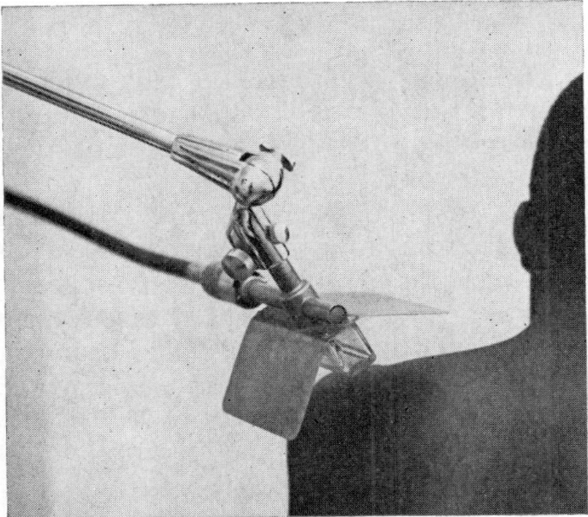

Fig. 34–4.—Application of microwave diathermy to left shoulder.

in a period of twenty to thirty minutes at a dosage of 120 to 150 ma. has extended the usefulness of microwave diathermy. Various observers have reported that only "slight elevations of skin temperature" can be detected, and that patients are aware of a pleasant sense of warmth without being conscious of the higher internal temperature.[65]

Ultrasonic radiation. — Ultrasonic waves are those acoustic frequencies between 20 and 500,000 or more kc.

European literature has contained enthusiastic accounts of the effect of ultrasonics in a variety of disease states, including many rheumatoid conditions, but much of this has been uncritical. Several general reviews may be consulted[31,66,77,97,121,122,141] and a bibliography is available.[33]

Contraindications to Local Use of Diathermy and Ultrasound[104,111,153]

1. Acute infectious arthritis and other inflammatory processes (cellulitis, thrombophlebitis, osteomyelitis, tuberculosis).
2. Over ischemic or anesthetic areas (occlusive vascular disease, nerve injuries).
3. Over metallic implants, adhesive or moist dressings.
4. Do not use through the pelvis, lower back or abdomen during pregnancy or profuse menstruation.
5. Over known or suspected malignancies or metastases.
6. Over freshly traumatized tissue, in hemorrhagic diseases, or to the back or abdomen in known peptic ulcer.
7. Do not use microwave over joints with effusion or edematous tissue. Water and other fluids absorb a high proportion of microwave energy.
8. Transcerebral applications should be done only by those familiar with the hazards involved.[153]
9. Do not use where simpler methods of applying external heat give good results.

Ultrasonic energy is applied by means of a sound head and may be used either under water or directly in light contact with the skin (a coupling medium such as mineral oil or a water pillow fitted over the sound head provide good transmission of the waves which do not pass readily through air). Ultrasound has not produced dramatic results in the treatment of arthritis.

B. Forms of Applying Moist Heat

Hot Fomentations.—These may be applied by dipping heavy Turkish towels, blankets, or woolen cloths into very hot water (about 115° F.), wringing dry, and placing over the part to be treated. One or more hot water bottles or an electric heating pad may be arranged over and around the compress, which is then covered by a dry blanket or heavy towel. A layer of cellophane or waxed paper directly over the compress prevents too rapid loss of heat, and cuts down the frequency of reapplication. The gradient between the temperature in deep muscle, subcutaneous tissue and skin is decreased in the packed area. Changes in local and peripheral temperature and in blood flow indicate that a single application for thirty to sixty minutes is as effective as more frequent changes in packs. A simple portable device, electrically heated by self-contained thermal units within a moistened pack, is available. The commercially available Hydrocollator steam packs retain heat for thirty to sixty minutes after prior immersion in hot water. These are very satisfactory for home use. The treatment period may last for fifteen to sixty minutes and three or more treatments administered daily. Hot fomentations are of great value in the treatment of acutely painful, swollen joints.

Hot Paraffin Applications.—This is an effective method of applying heat to individual joints, the back, hands, or feet. It holds heat well for some time afterward, uniformly surrounds the part, and produces good hyperemia. The protective glove or cast is left in place for thirty to sixty minutes after which it is readily peeled off. Many patients enjoy more relief from paraffin dips than from electric pads. It is also (as in the case of contrast showers) an excellent psychologic form of therapy. Paraffin applications are especially useful in the chronic stage of rheumatoid arthritis and in painful Heberden's nodes. They may be used several times daily. (See box summary for technique, p. 551.)

C. Hydrotherapy

Hot Tub Bath.—This is one of the most widely recommended of all measures for general heating in arthritis. It is particularly useful in home treatments. It is one of the most efficient means of elevating the body temperature, and because of this may become hazardous to the patient.[103] The first bath lasts only five to six minutes, primarily to test the tolerance of the patient. Subsequently, the duration of the treatments is increased up to thirty to forty-five minutes if well tolerated. There must be no undue weakness, circulatory impairment, or exacerbation of joint symptoms. The temperature of the water is gradually raised from 97° to 102° F., or in some cases to 105°, by running hot water into the tub. The temperature of the water should be determined with a bath thermometer.

The Full Wet Pack.—This type of hydrotherapy is useful in those patients with subacute or chronic arthritis who should not or cannot be moved into a tub. Muscular relaxation and relief of discomfort usually follow this procedure. It is also of aid as a preliminary measure for general or local massage. It requires no expensive equipment or special training on the part of the operator. The whole procedure can be performed by one individual. The method of application is as follows:

The room must be warm (72° F.). Rubber sheeting is placed over the entire bed, and an old blanket on top of this.

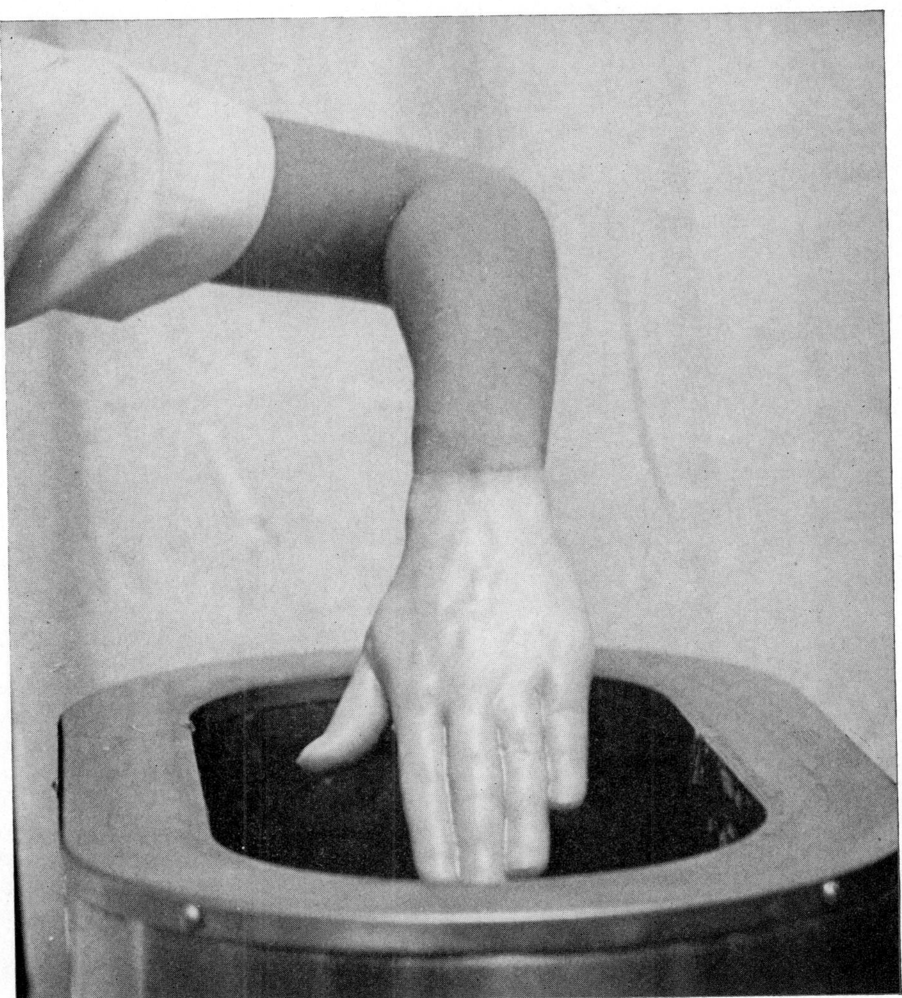

Fig. 34–5.—Warm paraffin bath. The arthritic hand is dipped briefly in melted paraffin (50°–60° C.), withdrawn, immersed again and withdrawn repeatedly until "glove" of paraffin is built up on the part.

A sheet is folded lengthwise in plait-like folds about 8 inches wide so that it may be tucked around the patient quickly.

Dip the sheet into hot water (110° F.) and wring out. Quickly spread this sheet under the nude patient. With his arms elevated, one-half of the sheet is folded about him from the neck down. The remaining half of the sheet is wrapped around him with his arms placed at the sides of the body. A layer of sheeting is arranged between the legs which are wrapped down to and including the feet. The whole sheet is tucked snugly about the patient. The underlying blanket is now brought closely around the sheet, tucking in trimly around the feet and neck. The head is the only exposed portion in the final assembly.

One or two additional blankets may be added to maintain comfort and increase the insulating effect of the covering. A layer of warm moist air collects between the patient's skin and the sheet. Rarely

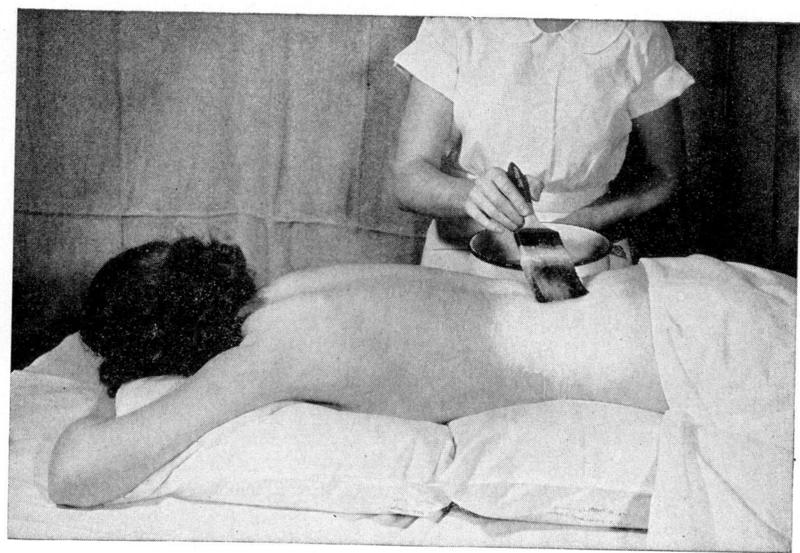

Fig. 34–6.—Method of applying hot paraffin with a paint brush. (Krusen, *Physical Therapy in Arthritis*, courtesy of P. B. Hoeber, Inc.)

is elevation of the body temperature produced. This procedure may be continued for thirty to sixty minutes several times weekly.

Contrast Baths.—Immersion of the extremities in hot and cold water alternately is often of value, especially in smoldering rheumatoid arthritis with considerable vasospasm. A spray or douche can be substituted if the patient can be moved to a tub. It is preferable to treat both upper and lower extremities simultaneously if feasible since the increase in blood flow and slight rise in mouth temperature are greater after treatment of arms and legs than after exposure of the legs or arms only. An initial ten-minute period of immersion in hot water (at 110° F.) is followed by one in cold water (at 60° F.) for one minute; the cycle is repeated, alternating in the hot and cold water for four and one minutes respectively for a half hour. Treatment should be ended by immersion in hot water.[86]

Whirlpool Bath.—This hydrotherapeutic device is an efficient means of providing heat and, at the same time, mechanical massage. It completely eliminates loss of heat from the part being treated, and is uniformly comfortable to the average patient. The water may be agitated by means of an ejector, a turbine or compressed air. Well-designed turbine agitators, which recirculate the water, are commercially available; ejector types require a thermostatic valve and pressure gauge for regulation of the temperature and force of current. Relatively large volumes of hot water may be used by the latter type. Longer models which allow immersion to the waist have recently been marketed. The initial temperature of 96° F. (35.5° C.) is gradually raised to the point of the patient's tolerance for heat (95 to 105° F. or 35 to 40.5° C.). The temperature, turbulence, and pressure in various parts of the bath will vary, depending on many factors.[74] The swirling water adds the element of gentle massage to the effect of heat; in some cases, the mechanical effect may be too traumatic. Pressures up to 4.5 atmospheres can be secured by altering the design of the jet and the pumping force, and used as a type of underwater massage.

Treatments last twenty to thirty minutes

Technique of Paraffin Application

1. Equipment:
   a. Double boiler 8 to 12 inches deep or enamel pail 10 inches in diameter.
   b. Electric hot plate or stove. Asbestos pad over gas or coal range to reduce fire hazard.
   c. Canning grade paraffin and light mineral oil in proportions of four parts paraffin to one part oil.
   d. Bath thermometer desirable. Gauze or roller bandage optional.
   e. Wax paper and flannel.
2. Heat slowly with occasional stirring.
   a. Paraffin-oil mixture melts at 120 to 140° F. (50°–60° C.).
   b. Remove from flame and allow to cool till a scum forms on top.
   c. Place receptacle on stool or chair at convenient height.
3. Protection of skin:
   a. Shave hairy parts before application.
   b. Use cold cream or other lubricant the first few times on parts to be treated.
4. For fingers, hand, and wrist:
   a. Maintain fingers and wrist in neutral position if possible with fingers separated and metacarpophalangeal joints in slight degree of flexion.
   b. Dip into melted paraffin, allow to remain a few seconds, and withdraw.
   c. When layer has hardened, repeat the immersion 8 to 10 times (or until the cast is ¼ to ½ inch thick) allowing each layer to solidify. Fingers and hand must be kept rigid to prevent cracking.
   d. Wrap in wax paper (or plastic "refrigerator" bag) and cover with flannel.
   e. Keep in place for thirty to one hundred and twenty minutes. (Glove cast can be made more rigid by incorporating gauze or roller bandage between one or more layers of paraffin.)
   f. Peel off into receptacle. Material can be used repeatedly.
   g. Hand will be red, moist and soft, and in suitable condition for massage, stretching or gentle manipulation.
5. For shoulders, elbows, knees, spine:
   a. Apply with a paint brush (8 to 10 coats) or by means of wide roller gauze impregnated with paraffin.
6. Instruct patient to use this form of heat one or more times daily.

and are administered once or twice daily. These baths are useful in circulatory, traumatic, and chronic rheumatoid conditions of the upper and lower extremities. The combined effect of the high temperature and motion of the water induces a marked stimulation to the circulation. The skin becomes red and warm and the tissues feel relaxed and supple. Exercises can be performed while undergoing treatment. The range of motion in a contracted joint can be extended either actively or with assistance while in the water; buoyancy of the latter permits a greater range of motion than would be possible for a stiff joint when out of water.

Hubbard Tank.—This type of hydrotherapy is especially valuable in arthritics with involvement of multiple joints, contractures of the joints, especially of the hips and shoulders, in many cases of spondylitis, in treatment of tendon transplants and plastic operations on the joints. Weakened muscles and joints can perform motions under water, which would be impossible out of water. The buoyancy of the water largely eliminates the force of gravity. When a body is submerged in water, it will lose as much weight as the displaced water weighs. Thus, a patient weighing 132 pounds (60 kg.) will weigh only 6 pounds (2.7 kg.) when lying in water. Muscle spasm is decreased, and the enveloping, uniform heat, which is constant throughout the period of treatment, stimulates cutaneous and venous circulation. *Passive or assistive exercises may be carried out and underwater massage may be employed.*

Hydrotherapy in a Hubbard tank or therapeutic pool should be used cautiously in acute rheumatoid arthritics because of rapid induction of fatigue. The frail patient and those with hypertension may not tolerate even a short session. Mild shock is occasionally precipitated in such patients.

In a hydrotherapeutic tank or pool, the temperature of the water is kept between 90 and 96° F. This is usually comfortable to the patient and encourages muscular relaxation. In the therapeutic tank, the temperature of the water may be changed rapidly. Some patients in the subacute or chronic stages of rheumatoid arthritis may tolerate an initial temperature of 100° F. After five minutes, if no untoward symptoms have occurred, the temperature may be gradually increased to 104 to 106° F. A rise in body temperature of 1 to 3° will be produced and may be maintained after removal from the tank by wrapping in warm blankets. It is usually best, however, to reduce the water temperature to that of the initial level before removing the patient. Passive, assistive, or active motion of the affected joints should be carried out throughout the treatment period. Treatments may be given every two or three days if no reaction occurs within twenty-four hours. The more robust patient may be treated daily.

Resistive exercises may be employed to advantage in certain cases; fins attached to a shoe or frog feet increase the load against which a weakened quadriceps operates. A similar device may be utilized for the upper extremity. Overactivity with resulting fatigue and the development of faulty movement patterns

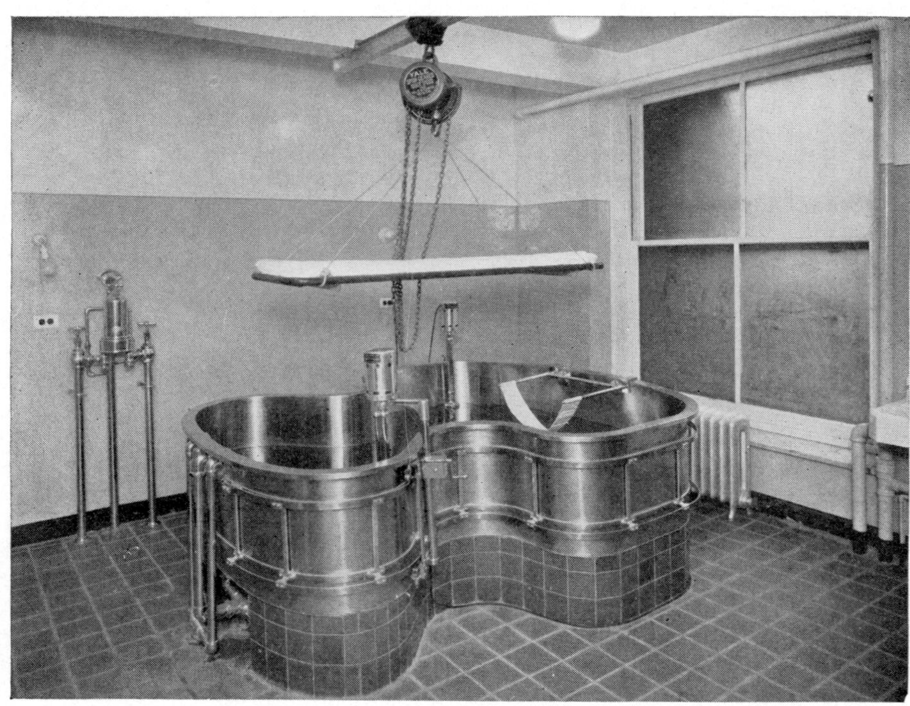

Fig. 34–7.—Modified Hubbard tank. Note overhead pulley and head rest. (Currence, courtesy of Arch. Phys. Ther.)

should be avoided; muscle incoordination may be difficult to detect under water.[88] Hospitals contemplating installation of hydrotherapy departments should consider one of the newer types of Hubbard tanks with a walking trough along one side. The Currence modification of the Hubbard tank allows complete range of motion of all joints.[32] If necessary, patients may be lowered slowly into the tank by means of a stretcher, supported by an overhead carrier. With an overhead trolley system, the patient may swim when supported under the trunk by a canvas belt. Inexpensive types of Hubbard tanks have been described for home use.[32]

Hubbard Tank Therapy in Arthritis[88,106,109,171]

1. Water temperature:
   a. Initially 96 to 98° F.
   b. Raise gradually to 101 to 104° F. during first three or four minutes. Use cold head compress if indicated.
   c. Lower slowly to initial temperature during latter part of treatment period.
2. Duration and frequency of baths:
   a. Five to ten minutes first time to test patient's reaction.
   b. Subsequently ten to twenty minutes.
   c. Use shorter periods for the frail and debilitated patient.
   d. Treat the acute case of arthritis two to three times weekly; with improvement, treat daily.
   e. After removal from tank, dry quickly and wrap in blankets for a half hour to maintain elevated temperature.
3. Underwater massage:
   a. Effleurage and gentle stroking massage may be applied above and below affected joints. Kneading may also be used.
4. Underwater exercises:
   a. Passive and assisted active exercises for subacute cases.
   b. Active exercises as soon as permissible; supervision by technician necessary to avoid faulty movement patterns.[109]
   c. Add resistive exercises (either manual or mechanical) for weakened muscle groups. Shoe fins or frog feet increase resistance.
   d. Move turbine agitators to position most favorable to aid patient in performing active exercises.

Therapeutic Pools.—These are expensive to install and to operate, but offer the advantage that a more extensive program of hydrogymnastics is possible than with a tank. Furthermore, *re-education in walking is possible.*

II. The Use of Cold in Arthritis

The manner of applying heat or cold determines whether the main effects will be mediated by local, systemic, or reflex action.[54] Locally, cold brings about cutaneous vasoconstriction, restricts exudation and bleeding, decreases cellular activity, and ameliorates pain. Chilling of the body surface as a whole induces peripheral vasoconstriction, which may also involve the deeper vessels if the exposure is long enough. The blood pressure is often elevated. Prolonged exposure may lead to necrosis of the tissues as a result of thrombosis of the deeper vessels. Considerable damage to the nerves may also result. Previously Fay and Smith[57] had developed systemic hypothermia or artificial hibernation, and this procedure has come into wide use in prolonged and complicated surgery, especially of the heart and great vessels. The anesthetic effects of local refrigeration for devitalized extremities, as originally proposed by Allen have found use in a variety of medical and surgical conditions. Intra-articular temperatures preceding and following various procedures have been determined by Horvath and Hollander.[84] In general the correlation between joint and surface temperatures was good although there were some exceptions. Surface temperature over the knees in the normal subjects ranged from 85 to 89.5° F. and corresponding intra-articular temperatures from 88.6 to 91° F. In rheumatoid arthritis a positive correlation was noted between the joint temperatures and relative clinical activity. Application of hot packs over either normal or inflamed joints induced a *drop* in the intra-articular temperature to the extent of 2.2° F. The joint temperature quickly returned to normal after cessation of the packs, and higher values were recorded within ten minutes, indicating a positive reflex effect. Cold packs, on the other hand, *raised* intra-articular temperature to a corresponding degree, and both heat and cold produced reflex effects in the opposite knee, similar to those observed in the experimental joint. The magnitude of the responses was diminished during the summer months as compared with the winter, suggesting a relation to the seasonal vascular tone in the various subjects. Apprehension, pain, alarm and smoking lowered the skin temperature and elevated that of the joint, effects similar to those noted from the application of cold. Simple passive and non-weight-bearing exercise brought about an increase of intra-articular temperature of as much as 2.5° F. In degenerative joint disease the initial temperature was somewhat higher and the cooling less rapid than in the normal or rheumatoid joint. Jones had previously demonstrated the importance of synovial fluid as a means of dissipating the heat of friction in the equine stifle joint. More prolonged application of cold than that used by the above investigators has been shown to cause a decrease of approximately 20° F. in the intramuscular temperature.

Cold Compresses.—A Turkish towel is immersed in ice water, wrung out, and applied to the part. An ice bag may be placed over the compress to accentuate the cooling effect. The very acute stage of bursitis is an indication for the use of cold, since heat may prove to be intolerable. In the acutely inflamed joints of other rheumatic conditions, especially those due to pyogenic infection, cold packs may prove beneficial. Diminution of the local metabolism and some degree of analgesia may be expected from such applications.[125] Contusions, sprains, and other types of uncomplicated trauma are benefited by several hours of cold compresses.

Contrast Baths and Scotch Douche.—The former is discussed under the section on Heat.

With the Scotch douche hot and cold water under pressure is alternately sprayed over the patient. This may be used as a tonic measure following a hot tub bath. Most patients experience a sense of well-being. A simple home spray attachment may be used, and is a fair substitute for the pressure type.

III. Massage in Arthritis

The use of massage for the relief of human suffering dates back to antiquity. Anointing parts, or all, of the body with oil was a common practice. During this procedure some stroking of the skin and deeper tissues was carried out. Often it was preceded by bathing in hot water or hot mud. Properly done, massage consists of a series of manipulations for therapeutic purposes. Best results may be expected when massage is given by trained therapists.

The physiological effects of massage are mediated through reflex and mechanical reactions. Gentle stroking massage induces muscular relaxation; rapid or deep stroking causes contraction of muscles. Reflex vasodilatation is one of the early effects. This benefits many cases of rheumatoid arthritics in whom an increased vasomotor tone is present. Massage as usually applied does not significantly increase the overall blood flow through normally innervated and spastic extremities, whereas passive stretching and electrical stimulation augment flow.[131] However, vigorous deep massage, which cannot be used on most arthritic patients, measurably increases peripheral blood flow.[163] Deep muscle temperature does not rise after massage, although that of the skin shows an abrupt increase which persists for a considerable period of time; the clearance of radioactive sodium injected into muscle prior to massage (1 to 3 microcuries Na^{24}) is not accelerated, indicating no significant increase in muscle circulation.[45] An increase in the local skin temperature occurs regularly.[45,126] Light stroking affects only the superficial vessels, whereas heavier pressure is transmitted to muscle and its blood and lymphatic vessels.

Initially, *massage stimulates both the sensory nerve endings and the deeper nerve trunks.* Reflex relaxation subsequently develops. Usually, systemic massage has a sedative influence on most patients, an effect which has led to its wide use in psychically disturbed patients. Because of the induced languor, the patient should rest or sleep following massage. The central nervous system may be influenced indirectly as judged by the amelioration of pain in many instances.

Technique of Massage

1. Pressure is applied perpendicularly to the part in the direction of the long axis.
2. *Never produce pain.*
3. Treatment should start proximally (movements directed centripetally):
   a. To empty venous and lymphatic channels.
   b. Proceed distally, massaging *toward* the trunk.
4. The patient should be completely relaxed and comfortable.
   a. Vary position of patient according to part treated.
5. Movements should be slow, gentle, and rhythmic.
6. Treatments end with rest or sleep for the patient.
7. Progress of the patient should be checked regularly, and treatment modified accordingly.

Indications for Massage in Rheumatoid Arthritis

1. In patients with extensive periarticular changes around knees, shoulders, hips, and ankles.
2. In cervical arthritis.
3. In elderly patients as a partial substitute for exercises.

The **movements used in massage** include[35,126,127] (*a*) *Stroking*, which may be superficial (effleurage), or light, medium or deep (massage proper); (*b*) *Compression*, which includes kneading, petrissage, and friction; (*c*) *Percussion* or tapotement, consisting of hacking, clapping, slapping, tapping, and beating; (*d*) *Vibration.*

Very light stroking or effleurage should be *employed at the beginning of each treatment* whether or not it is to constitute the only movement used. The masseur's hands are passed lightly over the skin in a centripetal direction.

IV. Rest and Exercise in Arthritis

Therapeutic exercise has become one of the most important agents in Physical Medicine.[47]

The **program for home treatment** of the arthritic patient should include exercise periods. Convincing the average patient to take exercises 2 to 4 times daily will require careful explanation, repeated re-evaluations of the patient's technique, and periodic check-up examinations by the physician. This is one of the most difficult prescriptions a physician is called upon to write. The first re-examination should occur shortly after institution of the program so that minor changes in the direction of progress can be shown to the patient. Improvement, which the patient can see or feel, will act as a spur to continue effort along with persistent supervision by the physician.[10,78,116,119] In any consideration of exercise it should be remembered that rest is an essential component of the process of

Aids in Establishing Proper Rest-Exercise Balance[18,129]

1. The patient must be convinced of the need for exercise.
2. He must understand that the prescription for physical medicine is an integral part of the treatment program.
3. Local corrective measures are tailored to fit the part and the patient. Muscle setting, stretching, and coordinated action through the widest possible range of motion are most important.
4. A gradual increase in amount and duration of exercise is outlined.
5. The importance of repetition at intervals each day is stressed to the patient. Undue fatigue or increased pain is to be avoided.
6. The amount of ambulatory activity allowed is inversely related to the degree of activity of arthritis in the weight-bearing joints. A decrease in the ESR and improvement in sense of well-being permit greater activity/exercise.
7. The range of motion in diseased joints is checked frequently with a goniometer (an inexpensive plastic Rulanglmeter is available commercially). Change in bulk of atrophic muscle is recorded by measuring with a tailor's tape. The average patient will be pleased to see improvement.

muscular action, as important as the contraction itself.[126] A balance must be struck for the individual patient between rest and exercise.[129]

Rest as one of the fundamentals of treatment for the arthritic patient has stood the test of time since chronic fatigue is one of the most common symptoms. To insure maximum benefit from rest it should be supervised in order to modify the time periods needed as the patient progresses. Piersol and Hollander have suggested that the "*optimum exercise-rest balance* is the ratio between the *maximum* amount of activity the patient can perform without excessive fatigue, residual increase of pain, or muscle spasm, and the *minimum* period of rest needed before the activity can be resumed in the same degree."[129] They recommend that the ratio be regarded as qualitative in relation to the type of activity and completeness of rest between, as well as quantitative.

Abuse of Rest in Bed.—Too much rest in bed is as bad for the arthritic as too little. The difference between complete immobility in bed and the avoidance of fatigue should be more widely recognized.[44,94,100] The dangers of overresting the arthritic patient are as great or greater than those of overexercise.

Therapeutic Exercise. Since two of the most important goals in the management of chronic arthritis are *to preserve or improve the range of motion* in affected joints and *to prevent muscular atrophy*, it is obvious that therapeutic exercise deserves the great prominence it has gained in the past twenty-five years. A *prescription for therapeutic exercises* should be written carefully and fitted to the patient's needs, the stage of his disease, and to any limitations he may have. The main features of such a prescription are listed in the following table.

Careful physical examination and muscle testing should precede any written prescription for exercise. Passive motion alone may need to be employed for certain joints or extremities until assistive or active motion can be undertaken. Likewise, free active motion or the ability to carry out resistive exercises will be obvious. The *prescription* to the therapist should emphasize whether the program is designed for *muscle strengthening*, *muscle reeducation*, *range of motion only*, or for *coordination and/or relaxation*. It will be possible after the first or second session to determine whether the patient is doing too little or too much.[2]

The reassessment at the time of the second visit will indicate whether the patient is doing his exercises precisely. Modifications may be necessary and

Prescription for Therapeutic Exercise[16,39,55,74,112,113,119,132,166]

1. Furnish diagnosis.
2. List precautions after thorough physical evaluation of patient:
   a. Indicate cardiovascular status and make notation of blood pressure;
   b. Describe defects of abdominal wall, herniae, etc.;
   c. Offer estimate of patient's physical reserve.
3. Signify types and purposes of exercise:
   a. Passive, assistive, free active, or resistive;
   b. Whether for muscle strengthening, reeducation, relaxation, or coordination;
   c. State which muscles are to be treated;
   d. Enumerate joints in which increased range of motion is desired;
   e. If apparatus is to be used, so indicate;
   f. Suggest supervision of ambulation with crutches, canes, or walker.
4. Designate:
   a. Daily and weekly frequency of exercise sessions;
   b. Number of sets of exercises and repetitions per set;
   c. Modifications as progress occurs;
   d. Specific list of exercises to be done;
   e. Whether to be done uni- or bilaterally;
   f. Date on which physician is to reevaluate.

these will occur to the experienced observer. In general, exercises should be performed bilaterally for the extremities, although at times one unaffected member may aid the other. It has been shown that bimanual exercise improves the work capacity of a unilaterally weak muscle group.[74] *Furthermore, the pattern of movement or "conscious proprioception" is retained by exercise involving joint motion.*

Fundamental objectives of an exercise program are (*a*) to *preserve or improve the range of motion* in affected joints; (*b*) to *prevent muscular atrophy* and to increase muscular bulk; (*c*) to *maintain a useful pattern of joint motion;* (*d*) to *maintain maximum function of the upper extremities and the ability to ambulate.*[16,67,144] The exercise program should include occupational therapy procedures; in patients confined to bed, these can be adapted to the patient's needs and aptitudes.[93] In such patients it is important that the nursing staff be instructed.

Exercise as used in Physical Medicine is of several types:

a. *Passive exercise* in which the technician moves the part and the patient does nothing except relax. It is used as a preliminary to active movement or when active contraction of muscle is contraindicated. It aids in preventing adhesions and adaptive shortening of the muscles. Its greatest utility in arthritis is in the bedfast patient.

b. *Isometric muscular contraction or "muscle setting"* does not involve joint action. It is admirably adapted to muscles encased within casts, to fractures, and to painful, swollen joints whose muscles may be contracted without moving the joint. Repeated maximal brief isometric exercises are more efficacious than those performed once a day; endurance and the amplitude of electrically induced muscle twitches can be significantly increased.[76,107,136] Isometric exercises for muscle strengthening have become popular. In some arthritic patients these may be feasible and even desirable, especially if resistive exercises are painful or contraindicated because of severe joint damage. Isometrics against maximal load may be better tolerated in such cases than *isotonic* exercises of the active or resistive type.

c. *Assistive exercise* is that type in which the patient makes an effort to move the part aided by the technician or a mechanical agent (*e.g.*, sling suspension). The latter may initiate weight lifting and gently "force" the joint beyond its range of motion from contraction of the muscle

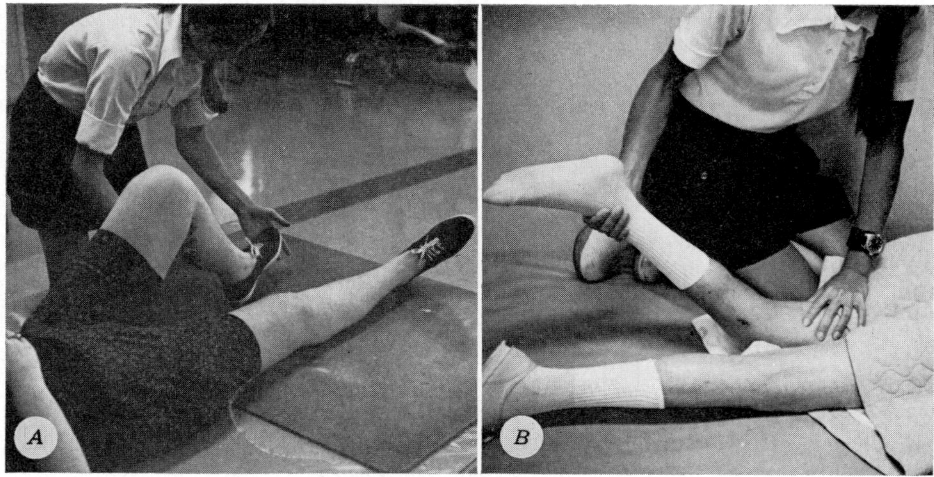

Fig. 34–8.—Assistive active exercise to increase range of motion of knee, A. with patient supine, B. with patient prone.

alone. Since most muscles in the body act as levers of the third or second power, the operator may choose to start movement for the patient, who may then continue motion in the desired range.[55] Excessive force should not be applied at the end of motion, and any discomfort produced should not persist longer than two hours.

d. *Active exercise* is movement carried out by the patient himself. It may consist in moving a joint with gravity reduced to a minimum, against gravity, or in actual gymnastics. Gravity may be reduced to a minimum by slings, smooth surfaced boards, roller skates, or by immersion in water as in tanks, tubs, and pools. Talcum powder on a large piece of cardboard may be substituted for a smooth surfaced board. In the arthritic patient who is able to do active exercises, the physician should direct special attention to the muscle groups which require strengthening or retraining in coordination.

e. *Resistive* (*active*) *exercise* is that type in which the technician resists the effort of the patient to move the part. Weights and other apparatus may substitute for manual resistance. The amount of resistance and the number of repetitions are important in relation to the rapidity with which muscle strength is restored. In some disease states there are other advantages of this type of exercise over "free" active motion: (1) single muscle groups can be made to function to an optimal degree because of an associated relaxation of the prime movers and lessened resistance; (2) there seems to be a decrease in protective spasm; and (3) the work done by the muscles can be graduated to any amount desirable.[55,94] DeLorme has thrown new light on this problem, and suggested that for relatively rapid redevelopment of muscle strength and size, high resistance-low repetition exercises are more important than low resistance-high repetition procedures (bycycle riding, lifting light weights, pulleys, sandbags).[38] He designed a special boot with an incorporated bar for the attachment of bar bells. Rose *et al.* demonstrated increased muscle strength after a maximal lift maintained for five seconds *once* daily; the increment in strength was just as great in the unexercised contralateral muscle, suggesting an improvement in the neural mechanism of muscular efficiency.[136] Other workers have not confirmed the contralateral improvement.

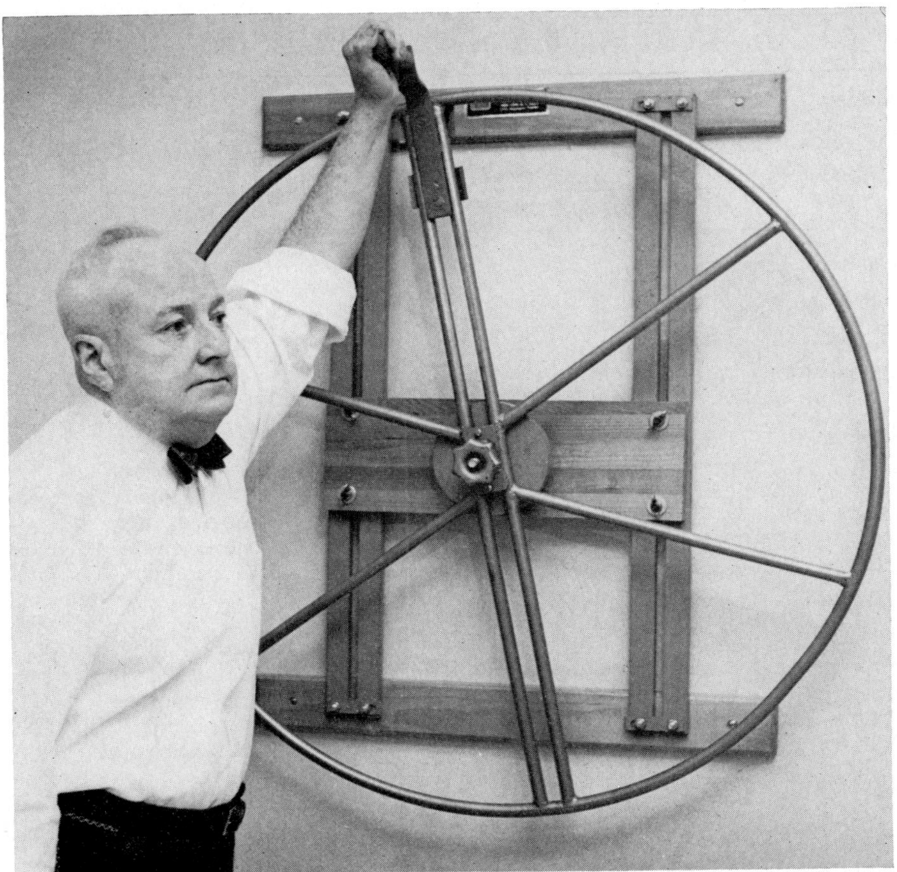

FIG. 34–9.—Active exercise to improve range of motion of shoulder using shoulder wheel.

Harris has compared the high repetition-low load regime with the low repetition-high load technique in rheumatoid patients and found little difference. However, he uses the low repetition-high load technique as a routine procedure.[67] DeLateur *et al.* have reexamined DeLorme's method in healthy young men, and could find no differences in the endurance or power attained by either variation in procedure.[37a]

f. *Hydrogymnastics* are carried out in therapeutic pools, and to a lesser extent in tanks. This is not to be confused with swimming, though swimming motions may be used. The pool should be of good size and relatively shallow (30 inches at one end to 54 inches at the other).[109] The technician should work with the patient while in the water rather than from over the side. Passive, assistive or resistive exercises can be regulated more accurately if the technician is close to the patient in the pool. The great advantages beyond that of the morale factor are that *movement is possible in all planes with the gravity load lessened* by the buoyancy of the water, and the patient with involvement of the hips and knees may walk in the water.

g. *Active exercise with the help of apparatus* frequently offers great advantages. An overhead frame to which a pulley-sling arrangement can be fitted is one of the simplest. Frequently used in surgical cases, it could profitably be employed in

Home Care Referral Form—Rehabilitation Instruction

Name____________________Sex__________M S W D S

Address____________________Phone__________Birthdate__________

Date of Onset__________Present Medication____________________

Diagnosis______________________________

Is patient Diabetic? ( ) Cardiac? ( ) Hypertensive? ( )

Bed Posture ( ) Activities Regulation ( )

Any contraindications to heat? No__________Yes__________

( ) Contrast baths ( ) Local soaks ( ) Paraffin dips

( ) Tub baths ( ) Hot compresses

Exercises:

1. ( ) Shoulder-neck routine
2. ( ) Shoulder pendulum
3. ( ) Pulleys for shoulder
4. ( ) Shoulder range of motion
5. ( ) Elbow range of motion
6. ( ) Wrist range of motion
7. ( ) Hand exercises
8. ( ) Bouncing putty
9. ( ) Back extension strengthening
10. ( ) Back flexion and abdominal strengthening
11. ( ) Hip range of motion
12. ( ) Hip stretching
13. ( ) Gluteal tensing
14. ( ) Quadriceps setting
15. ( ) Knee extension stretching with weights
16. ( ) Resistance to quadriceps
17. ( ) Hamstring stretching
18. ( ) Ankle range of motion
19. ( ) Toe mobilization
20. ( ) Crutch walking
21. ( ) Gait training
22. ( ) Spondylitis routine

Special Recommendations:

Precautions:

Date__________Physician's Signature____________________

the arthritic with hip or knee involvement. The familiar pulley weight device of the gymnasium can be used in some ambulatory patients as a form of resistive exercise for the hamstrings or quadriceps. The Kanavel table, shoulder wheel and other simple forms of apparatus may be of great aid in the redevelopment of good joint and muscle function. Scale drawings may be secured from the Council on Physical Medicine and Rehabilitation for the construction of homemade apparatus.

Manipulation or mobilization. Manipulation with or without anesthesia may be logical in some cases following the use of heat, massage and active exercise. For instance, this can be done as manual traction for the neck in cases of cervical spondyloarthrosis. It is to be done gently and with due appreciation for the fine details of anatomy of the area involved.[35, 110a] It should rarely be undertaken in the individual with marked demineralization. Relaxation on the part of the patient is necessary. The joint is "fixed" by the operator's hands or fingers. Periarticular structures are gently stretched and moved in one or more planes.[35,108a, 117] The whole procedure should *not* be very uncomfortable, and no grating, cracking, or significant discomfort should be noted by the patient.[65a,110a] This procedure should be differentiated from the bone cracking of chiropractors and/or the adjustments of the osteopath. It does not carry the hazards attached to surgical manipulation under anesthesia.

Legal action frequently follows manipulation of deformed joints. Those individuals employing mechanical apparatus for manipulations on patients with arthritis or deformed joints must realize that this is a very dangerous procedure because of the possibility of producing fractures of the weakened bones and the ankylosis which sometimes results.

Muscular exercises should be performed slowly because rapid motion fatigues muscle quickly, and sudden, rapid, jerky movements may result in further damage to arthritic joints. Muscles produce motion by causing tension between their attachments; tension is exerted on rigid skeletal levers, which increase the power and permit rotation. Muscular action regulates motion and is the *main force in stabilization of joints* by tightening the ligaments and capsule and by pulling the articular surfaces together. If this stabilizing force were not present, the joints would show many more strains and stresses, and subluxations would occur. Elasticity and extensibility are two important physical properties of muscle. When a muscle is stretched, it is capable of being extended. These properties permit smoothness of action and aid in relieving a sudden impact which might follow the inertia of load, preventing rupture of muscle fibers.[47,48,49] Contractility is a complex phenomenon; the most powerful contractions occur when the muscle is at its maximal length since its tension is greatest in this position.[48,161] Muscular tone is increased by muscular exercise. Complete muscular relaxation occurs during life only under deep anesthesia. It is the quality whereby muscle remains under sustained tension. Lack of muscular tone may add to the instability of joints and allow further injury or strain. *Muscle setting and active exercises increase muscle tone.* Reciprocal innervation and inhibition of muscles are most important in promoting coordination. *Bimanual exercise improves the work capacity of a unilaterally weak muscle group.*[74] Shortening, lengthening, and static contractions as well as the guiding action of muscles influence the degree of coordination. Contractures in rheumatoid arthritis may

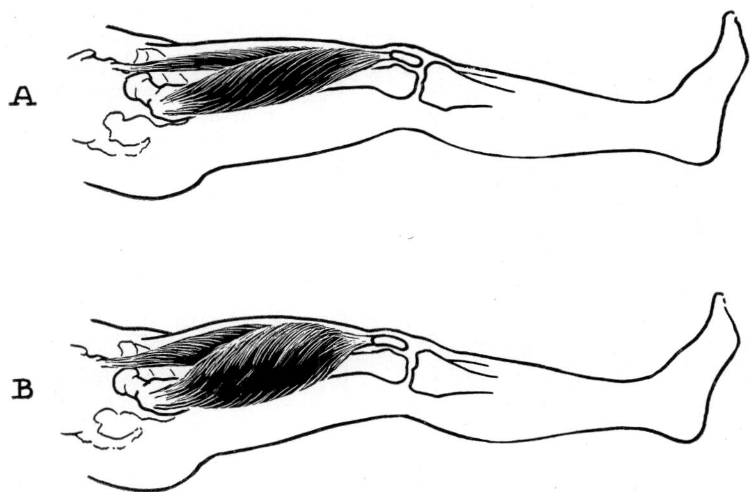

FIG. 34–10.—*Muscle setting. A* shows the quadriceps muscle at rest. *B* shows this muscle contracted (or set). This is performed with the leg extended. The position (origin and insertion) of the muscle is explained to the patient. He usually learns to "set" the quadriceps by attempting to "squeeze" the muscles of the mid-thigh. In some patients this is learned best by pushing the knee backward against the bed.

lead to disturbances of posture, especially if there is flexion of the knees or hips. Minor flexion deformities of the knees throw the center of gravity backward requiring the spinal column and trunk to compensate by assuming a more forward position.

Progressive resistance exercises can be used widely in arthritis. These are applicable to muscles of all grades of strength. For those muscles or muscle groups too weak to complete a full arc of motion against gravity the "load assisting" principle may be utilized. As strength and power improve, "load resisting" may be added. In either case, the maximal load which each muscle or muscle group can lift ten times (10-RM) is determined, and, as muscle power improves, the ten-repetition maximum is increased.[39,40,136] In load-assisting exercise, the RM means the least amount of counterbalance help necessary to permit the muscle to perform ten repetitions minimum; in the load-resisting type, RM refers to the most weight than can be lifted ten times (10 repetitions maximum). A daily session of this type exercise might include one to four sets, each to be done ten times or more; in order to allow for a "warm-up" of the muscle, one-half of the 10 RM is used for the first ten lifts in load-resisting, and twice the repetition minimum in load-assisting. Advantage can be taken of the pull exerted by gravity for weakened muscles. The average patient with rheumatoid arthritis can tolerate a program of resistance exercises without exacerbation or flare-up if judiciously handled, and especially if concurrent steroid therapy is employed. Muscle strength for such resistive exercises can be calibrated by using graduated weights.

The following list of exercises for arthritic patients has been found useful. *The Handbook on Physical Medicine and Rehabilitation*, authorized for publication by the Council on Physical Medicine and Rehabilitation, and one of the standard texts on physical medicine are recommended for supplementary use. The handbook "Home Care in Rheumatoid Arthritis" is available on request from The Arthritis Foundation, 1212 Avenue of The Americas, New York. It is to be understood that therapeutic exercises are similar to drugs in that too much or too little can be used. *Failures*

Exercises for the Arthritic Patient in Bed

1. Determine rest-exercise balance and work out time log for patient.
2. Have patient do deep breathing, abdominal retraction, and muscle setting exercises for the quadriceps, gluteals, calves, forearms 8 to 10 times hourly while awake.
3. In acutely inflamed joints precede passive exercise by use of hot fomentations or packs.
4. Emphasize exercises for upper extremities in bedridden patients and coordinate with activities of daily living.[144]
5. Start active exercises as soon as possible. Underwater and sling suspension exercises, movement with gravity eliminated, and assisted active exercise are usually tolerated early.
6. Add occupational therapy of the metric, then kinetic type, adapted to the patient's needs and aptitudes.
   a. Maintain good bed posture. Bad posture induces pain.[93]
   b. Use bivalved casts, footboard, sandbag supports.
7. Begin "free" active and resistive exercises as soon as possible.
   a. Employ suspension apparatus to gain maximum range of motion.
   b. Utilize progressive resistance techniques early. In these, heavy resistance and low repetition induce return of power and bulk of weakened muscle groups.[39,40,170]
8. Supervise ambulation via crutches, canes or walker in order to maintain a good gait or correct a faulty one.
9. Modify if overfatigue occurs or pain and stiffness persist.

Exercises for the Arthritic Patient

Instructions to the Patient

A. The exercises circled are especially indicated in your case.
B. Each exercise should be performed initially 3 to 5 times on four different occasions daily. As you progress, the number of repetitions will be increased to 10 or 20. They should not be done to the point of undue fatigue, nor should they cause pain which persists. You should report to your physician if either of these occurs.
C. The value of the exercises will be greater if you learn to resist each motion with your antagonist muscles.
D. Exercises 16, 19, 25, and 32 should be done 5 to 10 times each hour in those patients confined to bed.
E. Each exercise should be done with precision. Wiggling and purposeless movements are not effective. These exercises should accomplish several features:
   (1) They will improve the tone of your muscles and help to prevent muscular atrophy.
   (2) They will accelerate the movement of venous blood and stagnant lymph.
   (3) They will help to reduce the swelling of your joints and to reestablish normal ranges of motion.
   (4) They will make you feel better and help to relieve your aching.
F. The exercises as described are designed to be done in bed, but may be adapted to the standing position in most instances with a little reorientation of the starting position.

For the Neck and Shoulders

1. Neck hyperextended, fingers locked behind the head, elbows back.
   a. Push neck forward with hands and resist with neck. Push back with neck and resist with hands to starting position.
   b. Isometric.
      (1) Resist forward push of hands with neck muscles for five to ten seconds.
      (2) Push back of head against bed. Raise shoulders and chest off bed. Hold five seconds.
2. Head hyperextended. Rotate head toward either shoulder with sternomastoid muscle taut.
3. Head flat on bed, fingers locked behind head. Use tension. Bring arms forward till forearms are touching sides of head.
4. Arms outstretched at right angles to trunk, palms up. Touch fingertips to shoulders, return to starting position and repeat. (A small weight in either hand may be used to increase extension of the elbow when contracture is present.)
5. Arms outstretched above the body at eye level, palms outward. Bring down to bed level, repeat.
6. Arms at sides, palms toward thighs. Raise straight above head and touch thumbs to bed above head.
7. Arms at sides, palms toward thighs. Bring arms above head, keeping them lifted a few degrees off the bed.
8. Pendulum exercises: Standing position.
   a. Flex spine and allow arms to hang as pendulum.
   b. Swing forward, then backward. Come to slow stop. Elbows straight.
   c. Swing outward, then inward.
   d. Rotate clockwise, then counterclockwise, making large circles.
9. Wall climbing: Standing position.
   a. Face wall at arms' length. Crawl up wall with fingers, moving trunk forward and stretch shoulders.
   b. Stand at right angles to wall. Crawl up wall and stretch. Repeat with opposite arm.

Exercises for the Arthritic Patient (*Continued*)

For the Forearms and Hands

10. Forearms at right angles to trunk. Supinate and pronate smartly, keeping the wrists and fingers in extension. Use tension.
11. Forearms on bed, hands over the edge, palms down. Keep fingers in extension.
    a. Dorsiflex wrist, flex, and repeat.
    b. Isometric. Place fingers of opposite hand over dorsum. Resist flexion. Repeat with opposite fingers on volar surface. Resist extension.
12. Same position as 11. Close fingers into a fist, and then straighten as much as possible.
13. Same position. Invert and evert the wrist.
    a. Isometric. Resist inversion and eversion with opposite hand.
14. Same position. Approximate fingers and thumb, then spread apart.
15. Forearms on bed, hands over the edge, palms up. Repeat exercises 11, 12, 13, and 14.
    a. Isometric. Press fingers against each other with wrists dorsiflexed. Hold five to ten seconds.

For the Chest and Abdomen

16. Breathe deeply, elevating the chest as much as possible. Pull in the lower abdomen with expiration.
17. Breathe deeply and hold thorax in full inspiration. Then tighten the abdominal muscles and expire against their tension, keeping the thoracic position of inspiration as long as possible. (The use of a small pillow in both supine and prone positions is desirable when this exercise is used in spondylitis.)
18. Take a deep breath and hold. Spread the thorax by pulling up along the lower costal borders.
19. Alternately pull in and blow out the abdominal wall without relation to breathing. Lower back touches bed during "pull in."
20. Raise head and shoulders off the bed.
    a. Isometric. Flex knees, feet flat on bed. Raise head and chest off bed and flatten lower back.

For the Hips and Knees

21. Supine position, heels about 15 inches apart. Touch big toes to each other without inverting ankle. Then externally rotate thighs.
22. Raise one leg to a right angle position with the trunk. Lower slowly. Alternate.
23. Flex thigh and raise to right angle with trunk. Extend lower leg straight with thigh. Lower slowly.
24. Heel about 4 inches above the bed with knee straight. Move leg laterally and return across the other leg in a scissors fashion.
25. Leg straight. Tighten the thigh (quadriceps) muscle, relax, repeat.
26. Prone position. Raise the leg with knee straight. Lower slowly.
27. Prone position. Bend the lower leg and try to touch heel to buttocks.

For the Ankles and Feet

28. Supine position. Flex and extend the ankle, curling toes upward and downward with each motion.
29. Turn the ankle inward, then outward.
    a. Isometric. Use boot and hold in eversion or inversion five to ten seconds.
30. Rotate the ankle in a circle, curling toes upward and downward.
31. To stretch Achilles stand about 18 inches from wall; keep feet flat on floor. Flatten chest against wall. Hold five to ten seconds.

Exercises for the Arthritic Patient (*Continued*)

For the Back

Hyperextension Type

32. Prone position. Tighten buttock muscles, hold a few seconds, relax.
33. Prone position. Head and chest flat. Raise legs with knees straight.
34. Prone position. Hands on the buttocks. Raise the head and shoulders and hold two to three seconds.
35. Prone position. Combine exercises 33 and 34. This is a "jack-knife" exercise.
36. Prone position. Fingers behind the head, elbows back. Perform exercise 33.

Flexion Type

37. Supine position. Tighten buttocks and then retract abdominal muscles. This tilts the pelvis and flattens lower back.
38. Supine position. Raise one leg with knee straight to 45°. Lower slowly. Alternate.
39. Supine position. Raise both legs to 45°. Lower slowly.
40. Supine position. Raise head and shoulders (or come to a sitting position). Lower slowly.
41. Supine position. Flex thigh to 90°, clasp hands over knee and press thigh against abdominal wall. Relax, repeat. Alternate.
42. Supine position. Repeat exercise 41 with both. Attempt rocker motion.

Resistance Exercises for the Quadriceps

43. Sit over edge of table or wide window ledge. Place roll of toweling under lower thigh. Raise lower leg to extended position and hold three seconds, lower and rest five seconds. After ten lifts, add one-half maximum load (as determined by calibration) and repeat for 10 lifts. Then add full load for additional 10 lifts. Increase weight in bag by two pound increments as strength improves. Do once daily.
    a. Isometric. Same position as above. With knee extended add maximum load to foot and hold five to ten seconds. Do once daily.

may result from too short or too infrequent periods, from inadequate prescribing, from lack of supervision by the physician or technician, or from lack of cooperation on the part of the patient. A well-adjusted program of exercises, integrated into the total regimen of the patient, constitutes one of the basic measures of proved value for the arthritic patient.

When the arthritic patient is confined to bed, he should be placed on a firm, nonsagging mattress and should practice *postural exercises* three times a day. The pillow is removed from under his head and the patient lies in a horizontal position of hyperextension with the hands placed behind the neck or head, if possible, to help raise the ribs and flatten the dorsal spine. A small pillow may be placed under the chest in the beginning. Following thirty minutes in this position, the patient lies on his abdomen in the prone position for fifteen to thirty minutes, with a pillow placed under the chest and abdomen. This helps to counteract the gravitational effects on the organs. These two positions have been emphasized as the ones which give the nearest approach to complete physiologic relaxation, resulting in elevation of the diaphragm, more active circulation through the vascular channels in the abdomen, increased range of respiratory movements and a greater vital capacity. *The arthritic patient should not spend many hours sitting in a chair* as this permits the affected joints to remain for long periods in positions of the common flexion adduction deformities.

In **ankylosing spondylitis,** special emphasis must be paid to deep breathing exercises since flattening of the chest and atrophy of the thoracic muscles are regularly seen in this condition. Assistive or active hyperextension exercises should also be a part of the daily regimen. Progress can be compared by measuring the chest expansion and the distance from the floor of the fingers in the forward bending position. Older *patients with degenerative spondylitis* cannot be pushed as hard, but profit by doing exercises regularly.

In **rheumatoid** or **degenerative arthritis** of the **cervical spine,** overhead traction using a Sayre head sling affords a means of stretching supporting structures without much discomfort. This procedure should be preceded by heat and massage and followed by active exercises.[91a] The "rigid" rheumatoid neck may not tolerate traction;[15] patients with partial ankylosis may benefit considerably by wearing a felt or Stryker collar.[65a] With return of motion, resistance or tension exercises with the hands behind the head are started. The patient can then employ traction at home, using a 10 to 20 pound weight. Traction is maintained for two minutes followed by one minute of rest, and repeated for a total of ten to twenty minutes once or twice daily. The neck should be rotated slowly in each direction while stretched. Recumbent traction in bed may be used for longer periods once or oftener daily; the head of the bed should be elevated 6 inches to facilitate pull.[135]

In **degenerative joint disease affecting the cervical spine,** the pain is usually mainly mechanical with narrowing of the intervertebral spaces (through which the spinal nerves pass) and limitation of the range of motion of the neck.

In **degenerative joint disease of the lumbar spine,** exercise may aggravate the symptoms in structurally weak backs. In these individuals, it is often advisable to limit motions by curtailing such activities as golf which results in torsion strain to the lower dorsal spine and lumbar muscles. If there is marked thinning of a disc or marked hypertrophic changes, passive manipulations of the lumbar spine and straight leg raising exercises must be forbidden.

In those patients with degenerative joint disease of the lumbar spine and obesity, a high back corset or brace and fracture boards under the mattress should be prescribed. Heat and massage preceding flexion type exercises (Nos. 41 and 42 above) are beneficial in this type of patient.[8,16]

In patients with **involvement of the knees and ankles,** every step must be taken to prevent the possibility of invalidism. If these individuals are greatly overweight, this should be reduced to lessen the load upon the lower limbs. The early use of *crutches* will relieve some of the stress of weight-bearing; if the hands, wrists, elbows, or shoulders are also involved, an assistive device to the crutch may be employed. *It is often difficult to persuade patients with mild synovial irritation to use crutches, but they are extremely valuable if used early.*[36,37,41,81]

When the **hip joints** are involved in a **degenerative process,** *diathermy* often affords marked relief if it is applied directly through the hip joint. In the *early stages of degenerative hip joint disease,* the patient will usually be benefited symptomatically by a regimen of limited activity, judicious use of diathermy and massage, followed by stretching exercises. All of these patients should have daily *massage,* especially of the adductors of the thigh. Flexion and abduction exercises must be performed several times daily; passive assistance and stretching of the hip and periarticular structures afford additional protection against disability.

Relatively vigorous active exercise is *indicated in fibrositis.* In the more robust patients this should be of the resistive type. Combined with moderately deep

Schema for a Daily Exercise Program

1. Bed Patient:
   a. Firm, nonsagging mattress;
   b. Optimal position for thirty to sixty minutes t.i.d.;
      (1) Pillow under chest in supine position;
      (2) Pillow under abdomen in prone position.
   c. Muscle setting exercises q.i.d or hourly;
   d. Passive movements q.i.d to all affected joints;
   e. Active exercises, with or without apparatus, as condition permits;
   f. Emphasize exercises for upper extremities to facilitate self care.
2. Chronic stage of rheumatoid arthritis:
   a. Systemic heat (and massage locally) prior to one exercise period;
   b. Active or resistive exercises q.i.d.;
   c. Fit exercise sessions into *time log;*
   d. Tension and/or pendulum exercises for shoulders.
3. Ankylosing spondylitis:
   a. Deep breathing and rib stretching exercises 2 to 4 times daily;
   b. Postural exercises with head, shoulders, spine flattened against wall 2 to 4 times daily;
   c. Overhead cervical traction (with rotation) 1 to 2 times daily;
   d. Maintain good sitting and standing posture;
   e. Flexion exercises for the lower back twice daily.
4. Cervical arthritis:
   a. Overhead cervical traction twice daily;
   b. Tension exercises for neck and shoulders twice daily;
   c. Heat and massage to neck preceding one session;
   d. Cervical collar for night and part-time day use.
5. Arthritis of the hips:
   a. Deep heat daily or several times weekly;
   b. Massage to hip muscles (adductors especially) 1 to 2 times weekly;
   c. Flexion and abduction exercises 2 to 4 times daily;
   d. Assistive exercise and stretching once daily;
   e. Crutches for ambulation.
6. Arthritis of knees:
   a. Hot compresses or Hydrocollator steam packs twice daily;
   b. Muscle setting q.i.d.;
   c. Resistive exercises 1 to 2 times daily with maximum load;
   d. or Isometric exercise once daily;
   e. Hamstring stretching 1 to 2 times daily;
   f. Protect with braces if knees are unstable;
   g. Prescribe crutches if contractures are present.
7. Arthritis of the ankles:
   a. Flexion, extension, rotation exercises q.i.d.;
   b. Precede session with contrast bath (and massage);
   c. Manual stretching after one session;
   d. Insist on orthopedic shoes.
8. Arthritis of shoulders:
   a. Precede session by heat (infrared) or hot packs;
   b. Pendulum exercises and wall climbing q.i.d.;
   c. Overhead pulley exercises twice daily;
   d. Assistive stretching in flexion and abduction;
   e. Backward stretching with fingers behind head twice daily.

kneading and friction massage, the patient can often be kept quite comfortable.

When the **shoulders** are affected by either rheumatoid or degenerative arthritis, or by the subacute or chronic forms of calcified tendinitis, exercises are of the utmost importance in preventing atrophy of the deltoid and shoulder girdle muscles. Slight to moderate pain is not a contraindication to continued performance. *Pendulum* and wall-climbing exercises can usually be undertaken. A *pulley-weight system* (attached to a beam in the cellar or to the top of a door jamb) may allow almost complete range of motion without too much discomfort. If the patient is allowed to keep his shoulder adducted after the acute phase has subsided, adhesions form and may "freeze" the shoulder.

Medical motion pictures are available from the Film Library of the American Medical Association. The only expense incurred is that of mailing both ways. Requests should be sent to The Film Library, American Medical Association, 535 North Dearborn Street, Chicago, Illinois 60610.[4] Those of special interest to rheumatologists are "Aids in Muscle Training," "Massage," "Effects of Heat and Cold on the Circulation," "Occupational Therapy," and "Underwater Therapy." All of these mentioned are 16 mm. silent films. See the more complete listing at the end of the *Handbook of Physical Medicine and Rehabilitation.*[30]

V. Spa Therapy (Medical Hydrology)

The belief in the healing qualities of mineral waters goes back to antiquity.

A spa is a health resort where one or more mineral springs are found, or it may be a seaside watering place where saline, mud and steam baths are offered as an adjunct to the bracing effect of an ocean climate.[115,148] *Medical Hydrology* designates the science of utilizing water in all of its forms for medicinal purposes.

American spas are not well known. However, more than 40,000 patients are treated yearly at Hot Springs, Arkansas, and about 15,000 at Saratoga Springs.[6] Approximately 2000 thermal springs with claimed therapeutic benefit exist in the United States.[56] Several books on American and European spas have been published.[17,59,140] The more recently published reports by the Council on Physical Medicine and Rehabilitation[30] list American spas whose facilities met the approval of its Advisory Committee on Health Resorts. In addition to adequate physical facilities, these reports emphasize the importance of careful medical supervision of each patient; this is especially important since spas attract older people with chronic illnesses (particularly cardiovascular, hypertensive, rheumatic, and gastrointestinal). Physicians at some corporate spas request a brief *medical history from the patient's family doctor*. This would appear to be good practice for any physician who recommends spa therapy for his patients.

Private corporations or individuals own most of the large spas or health resorts in this country including Hot Springs, Virginia; Arrowhead Springs, California; Mineral Wells and Marlin, Texas; French Lick, Indiana; Glenn Springs and Sharon Springs, New York. The United States government owns the Thermal Water Reservation at Hot Springs, Arkansas, and meters the thermal waters to a government bath house as well as to hotels and private bath emporia. The springs and land of Saratoga Spa are owned by New York State. The Warm Springs Foundation of Georgia is privately operated. During World War II some of the larger spas were transferred to the jurisdiction of the War Department, and were reorganized as general hospitals.

European spas, especially those in Great Britain, France, Germany and the Soviet Union, offer rates and other information. Living accommodations in many European and American resorts center in the satellite hotels.[50] In others, sanatoria have developed, and are essentially hospitals utilizing mineral baths and stressing dietary measures. In most European countries spas are under some form of governmental supervision, and this has maintained relatively high standards.[62] Furthermore, abuses have been prevented; adequate means for care of the poor and those of moderate circumstances are provided.[61] In Europe, insurance and relief organizations have underwritten the costs for treatment of convalescents and the chronically ill among the low income brackets. At Saratoga Springs and Hot Springs, Arkansas, there are facilities for the low income classes and the indigent.[146]

Mineral waters are considered to be alkaline, alkaline-saline, saline, or acid depending on the predominating cations or anions.[59] Various gases are present in some thermal springs, chief of which are carbonic acid and hydrogen sulfide. The preferred method of classification is parts per 1,000,000 for solids and cubic centimeters per 1,000 grams at 0° C. and 760 mm. barometric pressure for gases. Among the listed thermal waters of the continental United States, the majority contain chlorides, sulfates, iron and bicarbonates as principal ingredients.[59,115] A great variety of trace elements is found, the most widely advertised of which are radium emanations. The pharmacological and physiological effects, if any, of emanations and other trace minerals have never been thoroughly substantiated though they have been called "inorganic vitamins."[9]

BIBLIOGRAPHY

1. Abramson, D. I.: Arch. Phys. Med. and Rehab., *46*, 216, 1965. (Review)
2. Allington, R. O., Baxter, M. L., Koepke, G. H., and Christopher, R. P.: Physical Therapy, *46*, 1173, 1966.
3. American Academy of Orthopaedic Surgeons: *Orthopaedic Appliances Atlas*, Vol. 1, Braces, Splints, Shoe Alterations, Ann Arbor, J. W. Edwards, 1952.
4. American Medical Association: List of Films Available through the Motion Picture Library, Chicago, 1957.
5. Anderson, T. P., Wakim, K. G., Herrick, J. F., Bennett, W. Z., and Krusen, F. H.: Arch. Phys. Med., *32*, 71, 1951.
6. Ant, H. and McClellan, W. S.: J.A.M.A. *123*, 695, 1943.
7. Aquatics for the Handicapped, New York, Swimming Pool Age, 1957–58.
8. Baker, F.: J.A.M.A., *157*, 492, 1955.
9. Baudisch, O.: J.A.M.A., *123*, 959, 1943.
10. Beaumont, W.: Practitioner, *175*, 471, 1955.
11. Beazell, W.: Report on the Spas of the Eastern United States. Report of the Saratoga Springs Commission to the Legislature, No. 70, Albany, N.Y., 1930.
12. Behrend, H. J.: Arch. Phys. Ther., *17*, 501, 1936.
13. Bergmann, L.: *Ultrasonics and Their Scientific and Technical Applications*, translated by H. S. Hatfield, New York, John Wiley and Sons, Inc., 1938.
14. Bierman, W. and Licht, S., editors: *Physical Medicine in General Practice*, 3rd ed., New York, Paul B. Hoeber, Inc., 1952.
15. Bland, J. H., Davis, P. H., London, M. G., von Buskirk, F. W., and Duarte, C. G.: Arch. Int. Med., *112*, 892, 1963.
16. Bowie, M. A.: in *Modern Treatment*, Vol. I, ed. by C. M. Pearson, New York, Paul B. Hoeber, Inc. 1964.
17. *British Health Resorts, Spa, Seaside, Inland*: Ed. by R. F. Fox, London, J. & A. Churchill, Ltd., 1937.
18. Cameron, S. H.: Physiotherapy, *50*, 89, 1964.
19. Chambers, L. A. and Florsdorf, E. W.: Proc. Soc. Exper. Biol. & Med., *34*, 631, 1936.
20. Clark, E. T. and Swenson, E. A.: Effects of Heat and Cold on the Circulation, Film Library, Chicago, American Medical Association.
21. Coblentz, W. M.: in *Handbook of Physical Medicine and Rehabilitation*, Philadelphia, The Blakiston Co., 1950.
22. Collins, W. D.: Mineral Waters in 1923, U. S. Geological Survey, Department of the Interior, p. 109.
23. Copeman, W. S. C.: *Textbook of the Rheumatic Diseases*, 4th ed., Baltimore, The Williams & Wilkins Co., 1969.
24. Coulter, J. S.: Technique of Massage, in *Handbook of Physical Medicine*, Chicago, American Medical Association, 1945.
25. Council on Physical Therapy: J.A.M.A., *113*, 40, 1939.
26. ———: Manual of Physical Therapy, War Med., *2*, 295, 1942.
27. Council on Physical Medicine: Council Article, in *Handbook on Physical Medicine*, Chicago, American Medical Association, 1945.
28. ———: Council Report, J.A.M.A., *135*, 986, 1947.

29. Council on Physical Medicine and Rehabilitation: Apparatus Accepted, Chicago, American Medical Association, 1954.
30. ———: *Handbook of Physical Medicine and Rehabilitation*, Philadelphia, The Blakiston Co., 1950.
31. Council on Physical Medicine and Rehabilitation: Ultrasonic Energy for Therapeutic Purposes, J.A.M.A., *157*, 1407, 1955.
32. Currence, J. D.: Ann. Int. Med., *32*, 682, 1950.
33. Curry, B. *et al.*: Bibliography on Supersonics or Ultrasonics, 1926 to 1949, with supplement to 1950, Stillwater, Oklahoma, Research Foundation, Oklahoma Agricultural and Mechanical College, 1951.
34. Cuthbertson, D. P.: Biochem. J., *23*, 1328, 1929.
35. Cyriax, J.: *Textbook of Orthopedic Medicine: Vol II, Treatment by Manipulation and Massage*, 7th ed., London, Balliere, Tindall, and Cassell, 1965.
36. Deaver, G. G. and Brittis, A. L.: Rehabilitation Monograph V.: Braces, Crutches, Wheelchairs—Mode of Management, New York, Institute of Physical Medicine and Rehabilitation, New York University—Bellevue Medical Center, 1953.
37. Deaver, G. G. and Brown, M.: Challenge of Crutches, Institute of Physical Medicine and Rehabilitation, New York, 1945.

37*a*. DeLateur, B. J., Lehmann, J. E., and Fordyce, W. E.: Arch. Phys. Med. and Rehab., *49*, 245, 1968.

38. DeLorme, T. L.: J. Bone Joint Surg., *27*, 645, 1945.
39. ———: in *Physical Medicine in General Practice*, ed. by W. Bierman and S. Licht, New York, Paul B. Hoeber, Inc., 1952.
40. DeLorme, T. L. and Watkins, A. L.: *Progressive Resistance Exercise: Technic and Medical Application*, New York, Appleton-Century-Crofts, Inc., 1951.
41. Dening, K. A., Deyoe, F. S., and Ellison, A. B.: *Ambulation: Physical Rehabilitation for Crutch Walkers*, New York, Funk & Wagnalls Co., 1951.
42. Physical Therapy. Essentials of a Hospital Department, American Hospital Association, Chicago, 1957.
43. Dietrick, J. E., Whedon, G. D., and Shorr, E.: Amer. J. Med., *4*, 3, 1948.

43*a*. DiTunno, J. and Ehrlich, G. E.: Geriatrics, *25*, 164, 1970.

44. Dock, W.: J.A.M.A., *125*, 1085, 1944.
45. Edel, A. and Wisham, L. H.: Arch. Phys. Med., *33*, 7, 1952.
46. Editorial: Arch. Phys. Ther., *19*, 367, 1938.
47. Elkins, E. C.: in *Physical Medicine in General Practice*, ed. by A. L. Watkins, Philadelphia, J. B. Lippincott Co., 1946.
48. ———: in *Physical Medicine and Rehabilitation for the Clinician*, ed. by F. H. Krusen, Philadelphia, W. B. Saunders Co., 1951.
49. ———: in *Handbook of Physical Medicine and Rehabilitation*, Philadelphia, The Blakiston Co., 1950.
50. Elmore, C. B. and McClellan, W. S.: J.A.M.A., *123*, 898, 1943.
51. Engel, J. P., Herrick, J. F., Wakim, K. G., Grindlay, J. H., and Krusen, F. H.: Arch. Phys. Med., *31*, 453, 1950.
52. Engel, J. P., Wakim, K. G., Ericksen, D. J., and Krusen, F. H.: Arch. Phys. Med., *31*, 135, 1950.
53. Erickson, D. J.: Postgrad. Med., *38*, 194, 1964.
54. Ewerhardt, F. H.: in *Principles and Practice of Physical Therapy*, Vol. III, Hagerstown, Maryland, W. F. Prior Co., Inc. 1940.
55. ———: Therapeutic and Remedial Exercise, in *Handbook of Physical Medicine*, Chicago. American Medical Assoc., 1945.
56. Fantus, B.: J.A.M.A., *110*, 40, 1938.
57. Fay, T. and Smith, L. W.: Ann. Int. Med. *17*, 618, 1942.
58. Fisher, A. G. T.: *Treatment by Manipulation*, 3rd ed., New York, Paul B. Hoeber, Inc., 1939.
59. Fitch, W. E.: *Mineral Waters of the United States and American Spas*, Philadelphia, Lea & Febiger, 1927.
60. Fox, R. F.: *Outlines of Medical Hydrology*, London, J. & A. Churchill, 1924.
61. Francon, F.: J. Med. Lyon., *44*, 687, 1963.
62. Francon, F. and Francon, J.: Brasil-Med., *78*, 11, 1963.
63. Fringes, H., Allen, C. H. and Rudnick, I.: J. Cell & Comp. Physiol., *31*, 339, 1948.
64. Gersten, J. W., Wakim, K. G., Herrick, J. F., and Krusen, F. H.: Arch. Phys. Med., *30*, 7, 1949.
65. Gersten, J. W., Wakim, K. G., Stow, R. W., and Krusen, F. H.: Arch. Phys. Med., *30*, 691, 1949.

65*a*. Glass, D. D.: J. Albert Einstein Med. Center, *19*, 32, 1971.

65*b*. Gordon, K. I.: Physiotherapy, *56*, 449, 1970.

66. Gregg, E. C., Jr.: Ultrasonics: Biological Effects, in *Medical Physics*, ed. by O. Glasser, Chicago, The Yearbook Publishers, Inc., 1944.

67. HARRIS, R.: in *Arthritis and Physical Medicine* ed. by S. Licht, New Haven, Elizabeth Licht, Publisher, 1969.
68. HARRIS, R.: Ann. Phys. Med., *7*, 1, 1963.
69. HARTUNG, E. H.: Arth. and Rheum., *4*, 208, 1961.
70. ————: in *Modern Treatment*, Vol. 1, ed. by C. M. Pearson, New York, Paul B. Hoeber, Inc., 1964.
71. HARTUNG, E. H. and STILLMAN, J. S.: Arth. and Rheum., *6*, 389, 1963.
72. HARVEY, E. N.: Biol. Bull., *59*, 306, 1930.
73. HELLEBRANDT, F. A., HOUTZ, S. J., and EUBANK, R. N.: Arch. Phys. Med., *32*, 17, 1951.
74. HELLEBRANDT, F. A., HOUTZ, S. J., and KRIKORIAN, A. M.: J. Appl. Physiol., *2*, 446, 1950.
75. HERRICK, J. F.: in *Physical Medicine and Rehabilitation for the Clinician*, ed. by F. H. Krusen, Philadelphia, W. B. Saunders Co., 1951.
76. HETTINGER, T. and MÜLLER, E. A.: Arbeitsphysiologie, *15*, 111, 1953.
77. HIEDEMANN, E.: *Grundlagen und Ergebnisse der Ultraschallforschung*, Berlin, W. de Gruyter & Co., 1939.
78. HILL, D. F.: Med. Clin. North America, *39*, 393, 1955.
79. HOBERMAN, M. and CINCENIA, E. F.: Occup. Therapy & Rehab., *30*, 203, 282, 377, 1951.
80. ————: Ibid., *31*, 21, 1952.
81. HOLLANDER, J. L.: Arth. and Rheum., *3*, 564, 1960.
82. ————: Arch. Environ. Health, *6*, 527, 1963.
83. HOLLANDER, J. L. and YEOSTROS, S. J.: Bull. Amer. Meteor. Soc., *44*, 489, 1963.
84. HOLLANDER, J. L. and HORVATH, S. M.: Amer. J. Med. Sci., *218*, 543, 1949.
85. HOLLEY, L. S.: J. Amer. Phys. Ther. Assn., *44*, 901, 1964.
86. HOLMES, G.: Brit. J. Phys. Med., *5*, 93, 1942.
87. HUDDLESTON, O. L.: in *Physical Medicine in General Practice,* ed. by A. L. Watkins, Philadelphia, J. B. Lippincott Company, 1946.
88. Hydrotherapy: A Symposium, Occup. Therapy, *30*, 401, 1951.
89. IMIG, C. J., THOMSON, J. D., and HINES, H. M.: Proc. Soc. Exper. Biol. & Med., *69*, 382, 1938.
90. Institute of Physical Medicine and Rehabilitation, New York University—Bellevue Medical Center: *Self Help Devices for Rehabilitation*, Dubuque, Iowa, Wm. C. Brown, 1958.
91. JARMAN, M. B.: J.A.M.A., *124*, 231, 1944.
91*a*. KAMENETZ, H. L.: in *Arthritis and Physical Medicine*, ed. by S. Licht, New Haven, Elizabeth Licht, Publisher, 1969.
92. KEMP, C. R., PAUL, W. D., and HINES, H. M.: Arch. Phys. Med., *29*, 12, 1948.
93. KENDALL, H. O., KENDALL, F. P., and BOYNTON, B. A.: *Posture and Pain*, Baltimore, The Williams & Wilkins Co., 1952.
94. KENDALL, P. H.: in *Therapeutic Exercise*, ed. by Licht, S., New Haven, Elizabeth Licht, Publisher, 1958.
95. KORNBLUEH, J. H. and PIERSOL, G. M.: Tr. Coll. Physicians of Philadelphia, Series 4, *21*, 63, 1953.
96. KRAUS, H.: *Therapeutic Exercise*, 2nd ed. Springfield, Charles C Thomas, 1963.
97. KREBS, J.: *Ultraschalltherapie*, Osnabruck, Determann, 1950.
98. KRUSEN, F. H.: *Physical Therapy in Arthritis*, New York, Paul B. Hoeber, Inc., 1937.
99. ————: *Physical Medicine*, Philadelphia, W. B. Saunders Co., 1941.
100. ————: *Concepts in Rehabilitation of the Handicapped*, Philadelphia, W. B. Saunders Co., 1964.
101. KRUSEN, F. H. and ELKINS, E. C.: in *Handbook of Physical Medicine*, Chicago, American Medical Association, 1945.
102. LARSEN, N. A.: J. Clin. Invest., *43*, 1805, 1964.
103. LAUTMAN, M. F.: South. Med. & Surg., *97*, 5, 1935.
104. LEHMANN, J. J., ERICKSON, D. J., MARTIN, G. M., and KRUSEN, F. H.: J.A.M..A, *157*, 996, 1955.
104*a*. LENOCH, F.: in *Arthritis and Physical Medicine*, ed. by Licht, S., New Haven, Elizabeth Licht, Publisher, 1969.
105. LENOCH, F., BREMOVA, A., KADLECOVA, L., KRALIK, V., and TRUHLAR, P.: Arch. Inter-Amer. Rheum., *5*, 392, 1962.
106. LE QUESNE, R. N. and GRANVILLE, M.: *Hydrotherapy*, 2nd ed., London, Cassell, 1946.
107. LIBERSON, W. T. and ASA, M. M.: Arch. Phys. Med., *40*, 330, 1959.
108. LICHT, S., ed.: *Therapeutic Electricity and Ultraviolet Radiation*, New Haven, Elizabeth Licht, Publisher, 1958.
108*a*. LICHT, S.: *Massage, Manipulation and Traction*, New Haven, Elizabeth Licht, Publisher, 1960.
109. LOWMAN, C. L.: in *Principles and Practice of Physical Therapy*, Hagerstown, Maryland, W. F. Prior Co., Inc. 1940.
110. LOWMAN, E. W.: Arth. and Rheum., *6*, 177, 1963.

110*a*. Maitland, G. D.: Physiotherapy, *56*, 14, 1970.
111. Martin, G. M. and Erickson, D. J.: in *Handbook of Physical Medicine and Rehabilitation* Philadelphia, The Blakiston Company, 1950.
112. Martin, G. M.: in *Physical Medicine and Rehabilitation for the Clinician*, ed. by F. H. Krusen, Philadelphia, W. B. Saunders Co., 1951.
113. Martin, G. M.: Arth. and Rheum., *6*, 177, 1963.
114. McClellan, W. S. and Singer, C. I.: J.A.M.A., *124*, 426, 1944.
115. McClellan, W. S. and Jung, F. T.: in *Handbook of Physical Medicine and Rehabilitation*, Council on Physical Medicine and Rehabilitation, Philadelphia, The Blakiston Co., 1950.
116. Medical and Scientific Committee: *Home Care in Rheumatoid Arthritis*, The Arthritis Foundation, New York, 1968.
117. Mennell, J. B.: *Physical Treatment by Movement, Massage and Manipulation*, 5th ed. Philadelphia, The Blakiston Co., 1945.
117*a*. Mills, J. A., Pinals, R. S., Ropes, M. W., Short, C. L., and Sutcliffe, J.: New Engl. J. Med., *284*, 453, 1971.
118. Moor, F. B.: in *Physical Medicine in General Practice*, ed. by W. Bierman and S. Licht, New York, Paul B. Hoeber, Inc., 1952.
119. ————: Postgrad. Med., *16*, 114, 1954.
120. Murphy, A. J., Paul, W. D., and Hines, H. M.: Arch. Phys. Med., *31*, 151, 1950.
121. Nelson, P. A., Herrick, J. F., and Krusen, F. H.: Ultrasonics in Medicine, Arch. Phys. Med., *37*, 6, 1950. Review.
122. Newell, J. A.: Phys. Med. Biol., *8*, 241, 1963.
123. Osborne, S. L. and Holmquest, H. J.: *Technic of Electrotherapy and Its Physical and Physiological Basis*, Springfield, Charles C Thomas, 1944.
124. Partridge, R. E. H. and Duthie, J. J. R.: Ann. Rheum. Dis., *22*, 91, 1963.
125. Pegg, S. M. H., Littler, T. R., and Littler, E. N.: Physiotherapy, *55*, 51, 1969.
126. Pemberton, R.: in *Handbook of Physical Medicine*, Chicago, American Medical Association, 1945.
127. Pemberton, R. and Scull, C. W.: Massage in *Medical Physics*, ed. by O. Glasser, Chicago, The Yearbook Publishers, Inc., 1944.
128. Piersol, G. M.: J.A.M.A., *117*, 1835, 1941.
129. Piersol, G. M. and Hollander, J. L.: Arch. Phys. Ther., *29*, 500, 1947.
130. Preston, R. L.: Arth. and Rheum., *4*, 213, 1961.
131. Randall, B. F., Imig, C. J., and Hines, H. M.: Arch. Phys. Med., *33*, 73, 1952.
132. Redford, J. B.: Northwest Med., *59*, 1399, 1960.
133. Reynolds, C. R.: J.A.M.A., *123*, 832, 1943.
134. Rhinelander, F. W. and Hollander, J. L.: Arth. and Rheum., *3*, 561–4, 1960.
135. Robinson, W. H.: Arch. Phys. Med., *32*, 346, 1951.
136. Rose, D. L., Radzyminski, S. F., and Beatty, R. R.: Arch. Phys. Med., *38*, 157, 1957.
137. Rosenthal, C.: *Die Massage und ihre wissenschaftliche Begrundung*, Berlin, 1910.
138. Rothmann, L. M. and Rogoff, G. M.: New York J. Med., *61*, 396, 1961.
139. Rusk, H.: *Rehabilitation Medicine*, 2nd ed., St. Louis, C. V. Mosby Co., 1964.
140. Schott, M.: *Health and Pleasure Resorts of Central Europe*, New York, published by the author, 120 Vermilyea Ave., 1928.
141. Schwan, H. P.: in *Therapeutic Heat and Cold*, ed. by Licht, S., New Haven, Elizabeth Licht, Publisher, 1958.
142. Schwartz, F. F.: South. M. J., *47*, 854, 1954.
143. Sherwood, K. K.: Physiotherapy Rev., *20*, 134, 1940.
144. Shotter, Lillian: in *Arthritis: General Principles. Physical Medicine and Rehabilitation*, ed. by E. W. Lowman, Boston, Little Brown & Co., 1959.
145. Sigerist, H.: Bull. Hist. Med., *11*, 133, 1942.
146. Simons, A. M.: J.A.M.A., *124*, 33, 1944.
147. Singer, C. I.: Arch. Phys. Ther., *17*, 631, 1936.
148. Singer, C. I. and Phillips, K.: J.A.M.A., *124*, 1128, 1944.
149. Smith, E. M. and Crook, B. L.: J.A.M.A., *124*, 505, 1944.
150. Smollett, Tobias: *An Essay on the Natura Use of Waters*, ed. by C. E. Jones, Bull. Institute of History of Medicine, *3*, 31, 1935.
151. Smyth, C. J. and Freyberg, R. H.: J. Michigan Med. Soc., *42*, 818, 1943.
152. Solomon, W. M.: in *Physical Medicine in General Practice*, ed. by W. Bierman and S. Licht, 3rd ed., New York, Paul B. Hoeber, Inc., 1952.
153. Stoner, E. K., and Shapiro, H.: Arch. Phys. Med., *33*, 273, 1952.
154. Taylor, H. N.: Physiological Effects of Bed Rest and Immobilization, in *Physical Medicine and Rehabilitation for the Clinician*, ed. by F. H. Krusen, Philadelphia, W. B. Saunders Co., 1951.

155. United States Department of Health, Education and Welfare: *Strike Back at Arthritis*, Washington, U. S. Government Printing Office, 1960. P.H.S. Publication 747.
156. United States War Department: *Massage in Physical Therapy*, T. B. Med., 173, Washington, Supt. of Doc., Government Printing Office, 1945.
157. Vogt, H.: *Lehrbuch der Bader- und Klimaheilkunde*, Parts 1 and 2, Berlin, Julius Springer, 1940.
158. von Werssowetz, O. F. and Painter, C. W.: Occupat. Therapy, *29*, 265, 1950.
159. Vrtiak, E., Benson, S., Kobak, D., and Carlsen, A. J.: Arch. Phys. Ther., *19*, 325, 367, 1948.
160. Waine, H.: Arth. and Rheum., *6*, 83, 1963.
161. Wakim, K. G.: in *Physical Medicine and Rehabilitation for the Clinician*, ed. by F. H. Krusen, Philadelphia, W. B. Saunders Co., 1951.
162. Wakim, K. G., Herrick, J. F., Martin, G. M. and Krusen, F. H.: J.A.M.A., *139*, 989, 1949.
163. Wakim, K. G., Martin, G. M., Terrier, J. C., Elkins, E. C., and Krusen, F. H.: Arch. Phys. Med., *30*, 135, 1949.
164. Walker, P. M. and Pointer, J. M.: Physiotherapy, *50*, 129, 1964.
165. Watkins, A. L.: *A Manual of Electrotherapy*, 2nd ed., Philadelphia, Lea & Febiger, 1962.
166. ———: Arth. and Rheum., *2*, 21, 1959.
167. Wing, H. and Leavitt, L. A.: Southern Med. J., *57*, 338, 1964.
168. Wise, C. S., Castleman, B., and Watkins, A. L.: J. Bone Joint Surg., *31-A*, 487, 1949.
169. Wright, J.: Physiother. Rev., *25*, 22, 1945.
170. Zinovieff, A. N.: Brit. J. Phys. Med., *14*, 179, 1951.
171. Zislis, J. M.: Hydrotherapy, in *Handbook of Physical Medicine and Rehabilitation*, ed. by F. H. Krusen, F. J. Kohke, and P. M. Elwood, Jr., Philadelphia, W. B. Saunders Co., 1969.

Chapter 35

Occupational Therapy in Arthritis

By Morris A. Bowie, M.D.

No part of the entire treatment of arthritis can do as much to stimulate the interest of the arthritic, boost his morale, and show him how well he can perform useful functions as can occupational therapy. Chronic arthritic patients are frequently discouraged, even depressed, by the long period of illness and inactivity, especially if they are hospitalized. Properly supervised occupational therapy can not only supply *mental and physical diversion* for such patients, but, even more important, it can begin the retraining to return to useful life from the long period of invalidism. Retraining to gain strength, cunning and range of motion in fingers, hands, wrists, elbows and shoulders by performing interesting tasks is called *functional occupational therapy.*[2,10]

Even in acute exacerbations of rheumatoid arthritis there are simple types of occupational therapy which can be utilized. A jigsaw puzzle may stimulate interest and encourage finger movements in a patient with active synovitis in finger joints without causing strain or undue fatigue. The selection of a suitable form of occupational therapy requires more than a random choice from the numerous possibilities available; it is most important that *the task be interesting to the patient.*

From his knowledge of the patient, the diagnosis, type of limitations imposed on movement, strength and endurance, the intelligence as well as morale of the patient, the physician who appreciates the potential value of occupational therapy can prescribe appropriately.[7,9,16,21] The *occupational therapist* has been trained to elicit from each patient his interests, hobbies and potential capabilities, and makes assessment of the patient's ability or disability in carrying out *activities of daily living.* Assistance to the disabled patient in ways to make easier such simple daily tasks as bathing, shaving, eating, turning doorknobs, turning faucets on and off, and many other tasks taken for granted by a healthy person can yield big dividends in improved morale and personal independence of the arthritic patient. Therapists have learned how to support weakened fingers and hands with dynamic splints which permit adequate finger motion, and many therapists have become expert at designing and making such splints. They also have at their disposal a large repertoire of forms of occupational therapy ranging from simple amusing toys, puzzles and games, to intricate arts and crafts such as ceramics, pottery, sculpture, carving, weaving, cabinet making, working with plastics, making jewelry, etc.[30] The success of the therapy, of course, depends upon choosing the right tasks for each patient.

Precautions need to be taken to be sure the activity is not painful and is neither too strenuous nor prolonged to exceed the patient's endurance. The therapist makes sure that the patient maintains good posture during therapy and is careful to adjust tables, chairs and apparatus for maximum safety, comfort and effectiveness. The element of uncertainty or fear in the patient is greatly reduced by such precautions.[18,20,23]

The psychology of progressive exer-

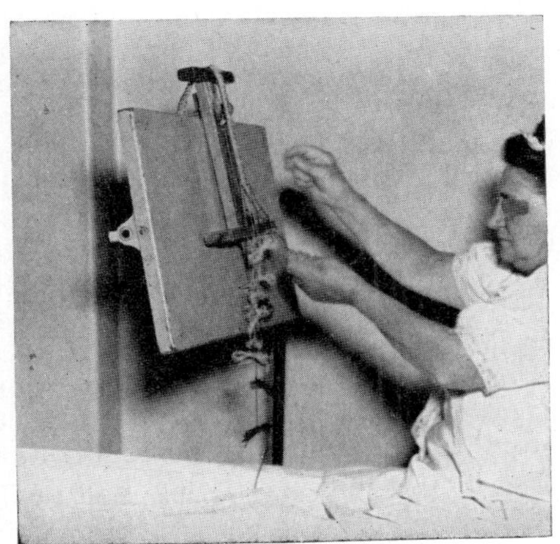

Fig. 35-1.—The patient should be comfortable and in good posture.

cise by means of an engrossing occupation stirs increasing interest.[26] To the patient, therapy becomes much more than mere exercise, it stimulates pride of accomplishment and brings out new facets of personality and means of self expression. The sight of the finished article he has made may show the patient he is again becoming a productive citizen.

Regular follow-up examinations to assess the results of occupational therapy and reports should inform the physician regarding: (*a*) the patient's progress in physical function and (*b*) the patient's emotional and psychological status as reflected by cooperation, interest and general attitude.[26] Over periods of weeks the patient's profile of capacity to work and improve is readily ascertainable.

In general, occupational therapy is more valuable in upper than lower extremity disabilities, and most useful for the hands. Since many of the items in the activities of daily living inventory involve the use of the hands, repeat evaluations will readily show change in performance.

OCCUPATIONAL THERAPY FOR SPECIFIC DISABILITIES

Hand Deformities.—The most disabling aspect of rheumatoid arthritis of the hands is the inability to flex the fingers. This is much more likely to interfere with function than the inability to extend the fingers. Severe ulnar deviation and subluxation of the finger joints may require support by splints or surgical correction (*see* Chapter 40) before occupational therapy can help restore more normal function. Functional alignment of the fingers should be maintained whenever possible. Occupational therapists have been helpful in making plastic working splints, but these must be checked by the physician to assure they are adequate. Proper support of fingers requiring it will often allow simple handiwork.

When active synovitis occurs at the wrists, splinting of these joints is very helpful especially when the forearm muscles are greatly weakened. In these patients exercises and therapeutic tasks to employ the extensors of the forearms are prescribed. Plastic splints to aid such work are easily devised and fitted. Splints may be discarded when muscle power im-

Supervision of Occupational Therapy

1. Maintain good posture.[17,19,24]
2. Avoid fatigue (one or more short periods of activity daily).
3. Avoid pain (grade resistance and speed of performance).
4. Maintain functional alignment of joints.[3,17]
5. Use splints for weakened muscle groups where necessary.[7,31]
6. Use patient's talents and previous skills.
7. Offer generous encouragement for each accomplishment.

proves. Tools with large handles can be used for sanding wood, filing, modeling, etc.[7] Knotting is a helpful task for improving supination.

Elbow Deformities.—Flexion deformities and limitation of supination are common problems in rheumatoid arthritis. These deformities may be accentuated by the efforts of the patient to pull himself up or to hold onto tables and chairs. Improperly adjusted canes or crutches may also contribute. Many patients are better off using crutches or a walker than canes which cause excess strain on both elbow and wrist. Sawing wood is a particularly useful task for such patients since the extensors of the elbow are brought into function. Reaching forward, as in weaving, is also useful (Fig. 35–1).

Shoulder Deformities.—Rheumatoid arthritis often leads to atrophy of shoulder girdle muscles, a forward droop, some internal rotation, and limitation of abduction and external rotation. The upper chest may flatten, and there is the tendency for the patient to keep his arms adducted all of the time. Weaving, carpentry, tying knots, sanding a tilted or upright board (Fig. 35–2) and the hand printing press encourage normal function. If necessary, a suspension sling may be used to support the weakened and painful arm.[6,7]

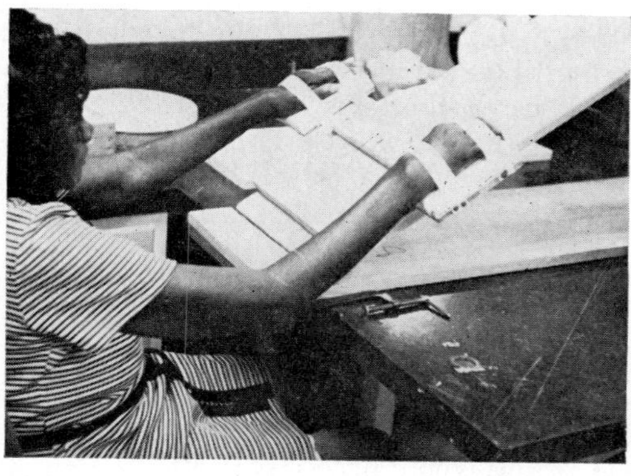

Fig. 35–2.—Patient using inclined sanding board to improve shoulder and arm function. Note straps to hold arthritic hands and wrists.

Large looms, graded for effort required in their operation, offer good exercise for the shoulders, elbows and hands. Block printing is particularly recommended for exercise of the upper extremity. Cord knotting and all of the usual carpenter's tools such as hand saws, hammers, brace and bit, planes, hand drills and the ordinary screwdriver require coordinated use of hand, wrist, elbow and shoulder, including supination and pronation, abduction and extension.

Lower Extremity Joint Deformities.—Rheumatoid arthritic involvement of hips, knees, ankles and feet is common, producing limitation of motion and extensive muscle weakness. For patients in whom weight-bearing is contraindicated, diversional therapy in bed or chair will prove helpful and will serve as a base for a more active program later. Various types of equipment can be obtained to hold or support painful and weakened parts, or to hold the materials to be worked so that the patient may devote himself wholly to the development of the craft. Functional alignment of the joints should be maintained, and postural stress should be minimized.[19,31] Colonial mat or rug weaving and cord knotting are useful starting occupations for the patient confined to bed. Other tasks are added or substituted as the skill and desire of the patient become known to the therapist. When even partial ambulation is possible, the patient is referred to the occupational therapy workshop where the cheerful atmosphere and the mingling with other handicapped individuals at work usually stimulate the patient to greater effort. Tenseness and neurotic introspection tend to disappear as he concentrates on performing the task. The therapist should guide his initial trials to insure that the exact movements prescribed are performed with the greatest economy of effort even though motion is performed against some resistance.

The pedal-driven "bicycle" jigsaw and the floor loom with its pedal controls are well adapted for hip and knee extension and flexion. Resistance may be in-

Crafts Adapted for Specific Joint Mobilization[4,30]

1. Shoulders:
   a. Elevation: knotting, braid weaving, basketry with tall spokes.
   b. Flexion: knotting, woodworking, hand printing press.
   c. Abduction: knotting, weaving, basketry, leather lacing.
   d. Rotation: winding wool, wheel weaving.
2. Elbows:
   a. Flexion: basketry, weaving, knotting, leather working, woodworking, winding yarn.
   b. Extension: hammering, braid weaving, woodwork, planing, printing press, coping saw projects.
   c. Pronation: petitpoint, crocheting, braiding, screwdriving.
   d. Supination: weave-it-squares, crocheting, needlework.
3. Wrists:
   a. Extension: block printing, pottery, wood carving, linoleum block cutting, lathe work, weaving, rug hooking, bookbinding, printing press, sanding, knitting.
   b. Flexion: basketry, carving, braid weaving, bookbinding, hooking.
4. Fingers (proximal joints):
   a. Flexion: paper cutting, puppetry, linoleum blocks, basketry, weaving, knotting, leather lacing, link belts, needlework.
   b. Extension: finger painting, block printing, pottery (coil method), braid weaving, knotting.
5. Hips:
   a. Flexion: bicycle, jigsaw, floor loom.
   b. Extension: jigsaw, floor loom, potter's wheel (kick type).
   c. Abduction: weaving on floor loom, organ playing.
   d. Adduction: weaving on floor loom.
6. Knees:
   a. Flexion: jigsaw, floor loom.
   b. Extension: jigsaw, floor loom, potter's wheel.
7. Ankles:
   a. Flexion and extension: sewing machine, foot-powered lathe, jigsaw, potter's wheel, pianola, motor-driven bicycle.

creased in either apparatus as improvement occurs. Adjustable seat and pedals are required to fit patients of different height.[6,7,23,24] At times it is useful to have straps on the pedals so that they may be pulled up as well as pushed down.

GOALS OF OCCUPATIONAL THERAPY

The effect of occupational therapy may be physical, mental, social or economic. *Physically*, it helps to improve muscle power and restore function to disabled joints. It also improves coordination. *Mentally*, occupational therapy offers encouragement to the patient, occupies his mind and eases emotional stress and restlessness.[4,6] *Socially*, the morale of the patient is improved by the association with other patients in the workshop. Often friendships are established through the common struggle to achieve. *Economically*, occupational therapy may detect skills or capabilities hitherto unknown to the patient which can assist in vocational guidance and new job training.

Periods devoted to occupational therapy should not be so prolonged as to tire the arthritic patient. Two shorter periods

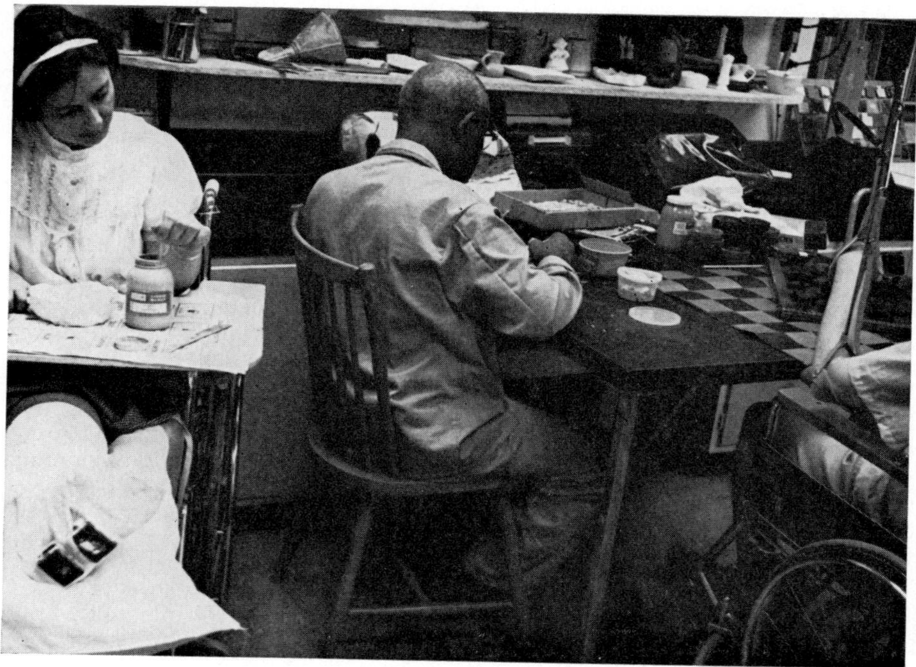

Fig. 35–3.—Typical scene in an occupational therapy workshop. Girl in wheelchair at left uses hands and arms to glaze ceramics. Man in center increases finger strength and coordination. Man in wheelchair at right uses right hand since left arm is in cast.

in each day may be more valuable than one long one. The activities should be graded and planned in an effort to prepare the patient for his return to a gainful or satisfaction-rewarding occupation. A thorough inventory of activities of daily living and former occupation at the start of therapy are helpful for this planning. The referring physician should specify to the therapist what the physical and mental limitations are for each patient, the expected length of the course of treatment, and what is hoped to be accomplished by such therapy, *e.g.*, increased range of arm motion, endurance, coordination, etc.

It is important for the occupational therapist to determine whether the patient's choice of a craft or activity should prevail over another that is less interesting but more directed toward the functional objective.[11,22] Often those activities in which the patient is most proficient may bring about the greatest improvement.[22,28,31]

In general hospitals, the utilization of the occupational therapy workshop and staff will depend upon the interest and enlightenment of the medical staff. Poor location of facilities, lack of qualified therapists and inadequate medical supervision are serious handicaps.[1,17,23,25] If adequate remedial work is performed, this form of therapy may be considered indispensable in rehabilitation, and not simply "something to pass the time" during the hospital stay. The decor of the workshop should be attractive. A background of selected music often helps tense patients feel more at ease.[12]

Manuals on administration of occupational therapy departments are available.[1,7,25] The coordination of occupational therapy with physical therapy and rehabilitation has been widely stressed.[3,8,15,19,28]

BIBLIOGRAPHY

1. Abbott, M.: *Syllabus of Occupational Therapy Procedures and Techniques as Applied to Orthopedic and Neurological Conditions*, New York, Dept. of Occupational Therapy, College of Physicians and Surgeons of Columbia University, 1957.
2. Bell, C. and Swaim, L. T.: Public Health Nursing, *32*, 243, 1940.
3. Bennett, R. L.: Amer. J. Occupat. Therapy, *5*, 94, 1951.
4. Blodgett, M. L.: in *Occupational Therapy*, ed. by Willard, H. S. and Spackman, C. S., 4th ed., Philadelphia, J. B. Lippincott Co., 1968.
5. Boeshort, L. K. and Blou, L.: Amer. J. Occupat. Therapy, *5*, 47, 1951.
6. Coulter, J. S.: in *Handbook of Physical Medicine and Rehabilitation*, Philadelphia, The Blakiston Co., 1950.
7. Council on Physical Medicine and Rehabilitation: *Manual of Occupational Therapy*, Chicago, American Medical Assn., 1947.
8. Davis, L. G.: *Occupational Therapy: One Means of Rehabilitation*, (a selected list of books and magazine articles), New York, New York Public Library, 1944.
9. Dunton, W. R. and Licht, S.: *Occupational Therapy: Principles and Practice*, 2nd ed., Springfield, Charles C Thomas, 1956.
10. Eldred, J.: Occupat. Therapy, *19*, 177, 1940.
11. Fidler, J. W., Jr.: Amer. J. Occupat. Therapy, *3*, 170, 1949.
12. Fultz, A. F.: in *Rehabilitation of the Handicapped*, ed. by Soden, W. H., New York, The Ronald Press, 1949.
13. Glass, D. D.: J. Albert Einstein Med. Center, *19*, 32, 1971.
14. Haas, L. J.: Occupat. Therapy, *25*, 1, 1946.
15. Licht, S.: in *Physical Medicine in General Practice*, ed. by W. Bierman and S. Licht, New York, Paul B. Hoeber, Inc., 1951.
16. ————: J.A.M.A., *142*, 472, 1950.
17. ————: in *Rehabilitation of the Handicapped*, ed. by W. H. Soden, New York, The Ronald Press, 1949.
18. ————: Rheumatism, *5*, 48, 1949.
19. Lowman, C. L.: Amer. J. Occupat. Therapy, *2*, 87, 1948.
20. Lyttleton, P.: Brit. J. Phys. Med., *14*, 107, 1951.
21. Martin, G. M.: in *Handbook of Physical Medicine and Rehabilitation*, ed. by F. H. Krusen, Philadelphia, W. B. Saunders, 1969.
22. Mead, S. and Harell, A.: Arch. Phys. Med., *31*, 753, 1950.
23. Molander, C. O.: Arch. Phys. Med., *31*, 757, 1950.
24. Newman, M. K.: Arch. Phys. Med., *29*, 395, 1948.
25. *Objectives and Functions of Occupational Therapy*, American Occupational Therapy Assn., New York, 1958.
26. Pattee, G.: Mod. Hosp. (No. 2), *66*, 84, 1946.
27. Pfeifer, E. J.: Amer. J. Occupat. Therapy, *3*, 227, 1949.
28. Snow, W. B. and White, H. M.: Arch. Phys. Med., *32*, 315, 1951.
29. Symposium by various authors: Occupat. Therapy, *24*, 131, 1945.
30. Willard, H. S. and Spackman, C. S.: *Principles of Occupational Therapy*, 4th ed., Philadelphia, J. B. Lippincott Co., 1968.
31. Wright, H. P.: Canad. Med. Assoc. J., *56*, 313, 1947.

Chapter 36

Rehabilitation in Arthritis

By Edward W. Lowman, M.D.

As a disease primarily involving the musculoskeletal system, arthritis poses a constant threat to efficient function. Despite the most carefully directed programs of medical, physical medical, and orthopedic care, the disease takes a considerable toll in causing deformity and physical disability. The latter to a greater or lesser degree may curtail the patient's ability to carry on normal and necessary daily activities. In addition to these physical restrictions, the factor of pain may also further impede function. Finally, it may be advisable to limit a patient's physical activity as a prophylactic measure against additional joint deterioration which in itself would jeopardize existing physical capacity.

The effects of physical incapacity ramify far beyond the area of functional independence. The patient's inability to carry on at work results in economic reverses and vocational problems. Psychologically, he is prone to exhaustion as a consequence of the frustration from the undeterred progress of the disease. His recreational as well as his vocational outlets become more and more restricted in sphere. Finally, as a result of all of these impasses, interpersonal relationships may become strained with a disruptive force of disturbing or destructive effect on his family and social milieu. In evaluating the patient chronically disabled from arthritis, it is imperative that these tangential effects be assessed and essential that measures be directed towards their compensation if the whole problem is to be met and the patient maximally benefitted. This concept of wide responsibility in the medical management of the patient is in essence *rehabilitation*.[4,7,18] This is a medical responsibility extending beyond basic diagnosis and the prescription of medical therapy. The physician thus assumes as his duty to his patient at least the direction of measures which not only will preserve life but which will preserve his patient's ability to function to the hilt of his ability despite the limits of his disability.

The importance of this concept of medical responsibility for rehabilitation is acutely accentuated in today's aging population beset as it is by chronic diseases. Rid of the threats from most acute infectious processes as the result of effective preventive health measures and the advances in specific chemotherapies, man today survives to become prey for chronic disease processes. Among these none is more devastating in its effects than arthritis. Among none is there a greater need for an understanding, appreciation, and practice of rehabilitation.[18] Because of the low mortality rate and the high morbidity effected by the arthritides, the number of disabled is steadily rising. The resultant problem is thus graver than that created by other chronic diseases wherein morbidity potentials are limited by mortality factors.

It should be emphatically pointed out that measures to prevent crippling offer the most logical and effective approach to solving the problem and need for rehabilitation. A sound program of physical therapy, as described elsewhere (Chapter 34), to maintain muscle power and joint mobility is a basic and essential part of treatment. It is when, despite these preventive measures or because of their neglect, muscle weakness and joint contracture and deformity develop, that rehabilitation becomes necessary.

The task of rehabilitating the arthritic cripple is not simple. Among many crippling diseases, such as poliomyelitis, some degree of improvement may be expected. Among others, such as transverse myelopathy, the disability is at worst a static one. On the other hand, the patient with arthritis is beset with a continuing disease process that often is a worsening one. In addition, unlike most other disabilities, the patient with arthritis must contend with pain. The problem thus can be an immensely compounded one.

In a large percentage of patients wherein the disability problem is relatively minor, the attending physician effectively can direct appropriate rehabilitation measures. It is only in the more complex disability that specialist help from a physiatrist and the special services of a rehabilitation center are needed. Treatment measures in either instance, however, are the same; the difference is that of complexity. Finally, in cases of rheumatoid arthritis where the disease process is still active, it is not necessary to wait until the disease is "burned out" before initiating rehabilitation. On the contrary, a medical, physical medical and rehabilitation regimen can and should be started as soon as possible.

EVALUATION

The over-all objective of rehabilitation must be the return of the patient to an acceptable place in society functioning to the maximum of his capability, not only physically but socially, vocationally and economically. In evaluating the patient disabled by arthritis, many kinds of information therefore are needed before a rational coordinated total program of treatment can be formulated. These data may be categorized as: (1) medical; (2) functional and (3) psychosocial.

Medical.—First in importance in setting a rehabilitation goal is the accurate assessment of the type and severity of the arthritic process. This requires a detailed general and rheumatological history and physical examination, laboratory investigations, roentgenologic studies and consultation with other specialists as may be indicated. Not only must a definitive diagnosis be established but the disease process must also be assessed in terms of its activity and prognosis for progression. In rheumatoid arthritis, for example, the success of both physical and vocational rehabilitation to a large degree depends upon how adequately this process may be stabilized by the administration of antirheumatic agents.

Functional.—Since functional independence is the major goal of a physical rehabilitation program, it is essential to have information that may modify or reinforce over-all functional objectives. Muscle power must be tested to determine the extent and location of muscle weakness; this is a standard procedure by which individual muscles are tested for strength and grades recorded on a special chart. This evaluation of muscle strength is vital, for a given joint is of limited use to a patient if the associated muscles, which are its mechanizing agents, are inadequate for its stabilization and mobilization. Further, as a result of their inability to provide adequate stability, weakness in muscles controlling arthritic joints predisposes to increased intra-articular traumatic damage and consequently added pain.

Next, joint motion must be measured. This determines both the total range of motion and the phases of the motion arcs in which limitations exist. This specific phase of limitation of motion is of considerably more significance functionally than is merely the total range of movement. A knee, for example, may have a sizable range of motion amounting to flexion through more than 90°. Yet it may be impossible to extend it fully—

Rehabilitation Evaluation	
Before a realistic treatment program and goal can be established, the *TOTAL* problem of the patient must be evaluated:	
Medically:	Medical and rheumatological history. Physical Examination. Specialist Consultations. Laboratory Examinations.
Functionally:	Muscle Test. Joint Range of Motion. Activities of Daily Living.
Psychosocially:	Psychological Testing. Social Survey. Vocational Testing.

there being perhaps 15° of flexion contracture present. This seriously hampers the mechanics of weight-bearing and predisposes to additional traumatic degeneration within the joint if ambulation is undertaken.

Finally, for his functional evaluation the patient should be tested in the actual performance of important activities. As already stated, determination of muscle power and measurement of ranges of joint motion are in themselves valuable for predicting functional capacity and potential. However, inference of such function is not always valid, for in arthritic patients pain is frequently an additional limiting factor. Patients are, therefore, tested in the practical performance of activities known to be necessary to self-sufficient living.[14] These, collectively referred to as "activities of daily living," include more than 100 acts that range from the simplest bed activities and personal hygiene functions to the performance of complex body elevation and ambulation—including travel by public transportation. The extent of functional impairment is thus directly measured and scored and, with the data recorded on the muscle power chart and the range of motion measurements, correlation of functional with physical deficiencies is made possible. This sum total indicates not only the patient's physical deficits but also reveals his physical and functional potentials upon which successful treatment may be based.

Psychosocial.—In addition to evaluating the physical effects of arthritis, disturbances in the psychologic, social, and vocational areas must be assessed and, in the over-all rehabilitation planning, positive action must be undertaken toward solution of these intimately related problems. The regulation of minutiae in these areas may prove as crucially decisive in the ultimate success of rehabilitation as any of the more obvious factors of medical management.

TOTAL TREATMENT

The sum total of medical, functional and socioeconomic data is used collectively to help set realistic rehabilitation goals. Goals as established initially must of necessity be flexible so that they can be adjusted during the course of rehabilitation in keeping with the patient's progress.

In the patient with rheumatoid arthritis, institution of therapy for the control of the rheumatoid process precedes the start of *physical* rehabilitation. Whether therapy consists of salicylates, of chrysotherapy, or of more drastic regimens such

Activities of Daily Living

(Partial list of activities on which patients are scored)

BED ACTIVITIES

Moving in bed: lying, sitting
Roll to right, to left
Turn on abdomen
Manage: pillows, blankets
Sit up
Reach objects on table
Operate signal light

WHEELCHAIR ACTIVITIES

Propel: forward, backward, turn
Open, through, close door
Up, down ramp
Bed to wheelchair
Wheelchair to bed
Wheelchair to straight chair
Wheelchair to toilet
Toilet to wheelchair
Adjust clothing
Wheelchair to tub
Tub to wheelchair
Wheelchair to shower
Shower to wheelchair

Travel:

Wheelchair to car—on curb
Car to wheelchair—on curb
Wheelchair to car—no curb
Car to wheelchair—no curb
Place wheelchair in car

SELFCARE ACTIVITIES

Hygiene:

Comb, brush hair; brush teeth
Shave (elect. razor), safety razor
Put on makeup
Turn faucet
Wash, dry hands and face
Wash, dry body, legs and arms
Take bath or shower
Use urinal, bedpan

Eating Activities:

Eat with spoon; eat with fork
Cut meat
Handle: straw, cup, glass

Dressing Activities:

Undershirt, bra; shorts, panties
Slip-over garment
Shirt, blouse; slacks, dress
Socks, stockings, (etc.)

HAND ACTIVITIES

Write name and address
Manage: watch
  match or cigarette lighter
  cigarette
  book, newspaper
  handkerchief
  lights: chain, switch, knob
  telephone: receiver, dial, coins
Handle: purse, coins, paper money

WALKING ACTIVITIES

Open, go through, and close door
Walking outside
Walking carrying

STANDING UP AND SITTING DOWN

Up from wheelchair
Down on wheelchair
Up from bed
Down on bed
Up from straight chair
Down on straight chair
Up from chair at table
Down on chair at table
Up from easy chair
Down on easy chair
Up from center of couch
Down on center of couch
Up from toilet; down on toilet
Into car, on curb, up curb
Out of car
Down on floor; up from floor

CLIMBING AND TRAVELING ACTIVITIES

Up flight of stairs with railing
  without railing
Down stairs (railing, no railing)
In and out of car, taxi
Walk one block and return
Down curb, cross street, up curb
Into bus; out of bus
Sit down, get up from bus seat

HOME SITUATION

Urban, suburban, rural
One floor, stairs
Apartment, walkup, elevator
Steps at entrance, railing, (etc.)

as those employing steroids, the maintenance levels for the drugs in terms of their antirheumatic and analgesic benefits should be established before the physical rehabilitation program is undertaken.

Physical rehabilitation should be intensive, lasting three to five hours per day, for five days each week, and must be prescribed to meet the individual needs of the patient. Treatment may include appropriate combinations of various forms of physical therapy, occupational therapy, remedial exercises, functional training in activities of daily living, training in the use of self-help devices, psychologic and psychiatric assistance, vocational testing and counseling and job retraining. The two objectives of treatment that must be given top priority are functional independence and protection of joint structures against further damage. For example, manual stretching of a knee contracted in partial flexion might be incorporated in the treatment regimen while, concurrently, the patient is being instructed to use strengthening exercises for the quadriceps muscle groups (Fig. 36–1). Obviously, both procedures are directed toward improving joint mechanics and increasing functional proficiency. Similarly, stretching of the muscles of the back may be prescribed along with abdominal muscle exercises in order to attain both the flexibility of the spine and the abdominal muscle power essential to sitting up in bed or to bending when clothing the lower extremities. Regardless of the area under treatment or the therapy employed, the objective is the same, *i.e.* function.

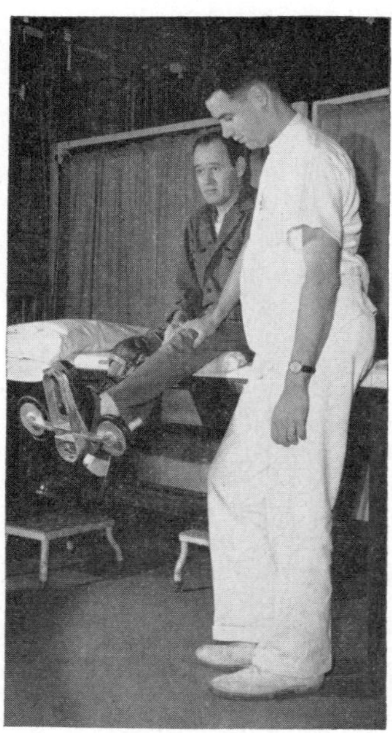

Fig. 36–1.—Quadriceps strengthening exercise.

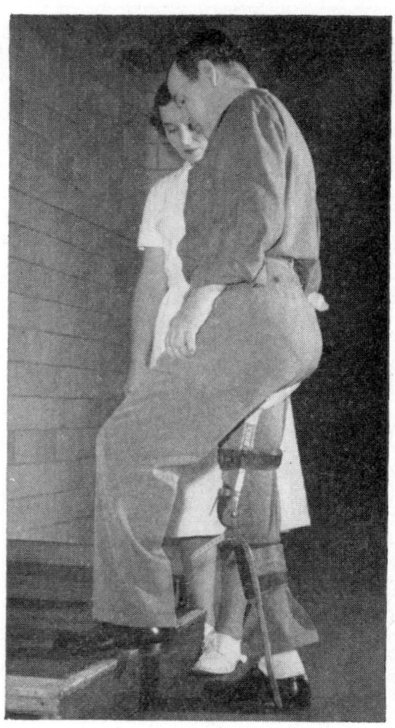

Fig. 36–2.—To enable patient to perform elevation activities.

FACTORS INFLUENCING REHABILITATION GOALS

The degree of success in the rehabilitation of the severely disabled arthritic patient can be forecast with reasonable accuracy in terms of seven major factors.[6] Cognizance of these factors is essential, not only to determine the feasibility of rehabilitation of a given patient, but also to predict the extent of rehabilitation

Factors Decisive in Rehabilitation

1. Medical Control of the Arthritis
2. Extent of Joint Damage
3. Psychologic Integrity of the Patient
4. Functional Training
5. Corrective Orthopedic Surgery
6. Self-Help Devices
7. Socioeconomic and Vocational Factors

possible for him. Harnessed positively, these seven factors will aid in the rehabilitation process; overlooked or ignored, they can negate it.

Medical Control of the Arthritic Process

It is generally agreed that, among persons crippled by rheumatoid arthritis, the best candidates for rehabilitation are those whose disease is quiescent. In such patients the arthritis has become static and control is an accomplished fact. The disability is likewise static and the worry that further progress of the disease will be followed by increasing disability is eliminated.

Unfortunately, rheumatoid arthritis sufficiently severe to produce major crippling seldom enters a phase of complete remission in the very late stages. Consequently, it is usually necessary to face the problems of active disease and accept the necessity for giving medical therapy and physical rehabilitation simultaneously. Also, crippled patients requiring intensive rehabilitation usually have already been treated without success through the whole gamut of conservative antirheumatic therapy. Such patients may require the use of steroids. This relatively more drastic therapy is needed to control the inflammatory process, and also to safeguard against further loss of already crucially impaired function. Thus, the efficacy of steroids in controlling the inflammation significantly influences the potential rehabilitation of the rheumatoid arthritic patient.

If steroid therapy is instituted in chronic cases, the therapy will probably have to continue indefinitely and without interruption. While dosage levels may vary with fluctuations of the disease, it is rarely possible to discontinue medication without a recrudescence of the arthritis. Therefore, it is essential that maintenance dosage of steroids be kept as low as possible, so as to minimize the possibility of side effects. When rheumatoid disease is so severe that adequate control cannot be achieved with low and safe dosage of steroids, it is necessary to be satisfied with partial control rather than risk the complications inherent in higher dosages. This obviously will modify the capacity of these patients to participate in a physical rehabilitation program. In attempting to alleviate the joint discomfort that attends use of mechanically impaired joints, physicians often progressively step up the dosage to much higher levels than necessary. Control of pain, the result of mechanical impairment, is best achieved by restriction of activity and by use of local palliative measures. Careful differentiation of these sources of pain, with selective and restricted use of steroids, is essential if serious manifestations of hyperadrenalism are to be avoided during long-term therapy.

In other forms of chronic arthritis, medical therapy likewise is the first step to over-all rehabilitation. Similarly, the efficacy of such therapy in stabilizing or reversing the disease process directly modifies the attainable goal.

Extent of Joint Damage

The degree of physical activity an arthritic joint can tolerate depends upon the severity of the inflammation and on the extent of mechanical damage within the joint. While inflammatory synovitis is the chief presenting sign in rheumatoid arthritis, the disease also results in chondritis, osteitis, and sterile osteomyelitis of the articular structures. These developments predispose to destructive changes in the articular cartilage and bone. Further, because of their impaired nutrition, inflamed joints cannot tolerate ordinary work loads.

The degree to which these destructive changes have taken place within the joint will directly limit the tolerance of the joint for activity, regardless of the type of arthritis. Except for those which can be modified by surgical procedures, these changes are irreversible and proportionately hamper physical rehabilitation. Accurate prediction of the amount of activity that a joint can tolerate is not always easy. Roentgenograms may be helpful but they may also be grossly misleading and are best relied upon only as confirmatory evidence. Often, patients with x-ray evidence of severe intra-articular damage can tolerate considerably more strenuous physical activity than patients with minimal roentgen signs of damage. Therefore, trial is the most reliable means of determining a patient's tolerance, and the physical goals projected should conform with demonstrated tolerance. For example, it may be apparent at the very outset of rehabilitation that weight-bearing joints cannot tolerate the demands of walking and, accordingly, treatment and training must be restricted to self-care, bed and wheelchair activities.

Destructive changes in joints of the lower extremities are considerably more restricting than are comparable changes in the upper extremities. Therefore, in terms of self-care and other self-sufficiency activities, goals may be much higher in upper extremity involvement than with lower extremity damage of comparable degree. The upper extremities, not being involved in weight-bearing, are mainly concerned with activities requiring dexterity, agility, and with specific technical functions.

Limitations of the range of joint motion and muscle weakness about the joint may modify further the tolerance of the joint for activity, thus compounding the problem already created by destructive articular changes. Tightness of the capsule and tendons about a joint, particularly a weight-bearing joint, may impose mechanical stresses that not only cause pain, but also predispose to even more extensive articular destruction.

Similarly, weakness in the supporting muscles jeopardizes the stability of the joint and invites additional trauma with consequent additional joint destruction. Vital determinants of work tolerance and efficiency are the degree to which joint contractures can be overcome to permit assumption of adequate weight-bearing positions, and the degree to which muscle strength can be restored to support the joint.

Psychologic Integrity of the Patient

More so than any other factor, the psychologic adjustment of the arthritic patient is a major influence in the success or failure of his rehabilitation.[5] Especially in a progressive disease such as rheumatoid arthritis, accompanied as it is by increasing disability and varying degrees of pain, the patient's psyche suffers from the relentlessness, the hopelessness and the frustration of the illness. Exhaustion of psychologic reserve and reversion to a passivity and dependency rarely equaled in any other chronic disease result. This reversion is not due to a predisposing "rheumatoid personality" but it is directly related in severity to the patient's psychologic soundness prior to his illness, and to the speed at which the disease is becoming worse.

Since regression to dependency is slowly cumulative, it is unreasonable to expect that reversal can be effected quickly. The reverse is true, so that refractory deep-seated dependency and passivity may more seriously restrict rehabilitation than do any other factors. Since success depends largely on active participation by the patient, strong motivation is essential. It is easy to evaluate a patient medically and physically to determine realistic goals but, *unless the patient's own ambitions equal those the physician has for him, results will fall short of objectives.*

Functional Training

While muscle power, range of joint motion, and tolerance of pain are valuable indices of the patient's potential capacity for activity, these are meaningless unless they can be translated into actual function. Therapy to increase power in weakened muscles and to enlarge the range of motion in contracted joints must be prescribed with the object of putting these gains to practical use. Thus, functional training is an integral part of rehabilitation and aims at training the patient to become as independent as possible in the activities essential to self-sufficient living.[3]

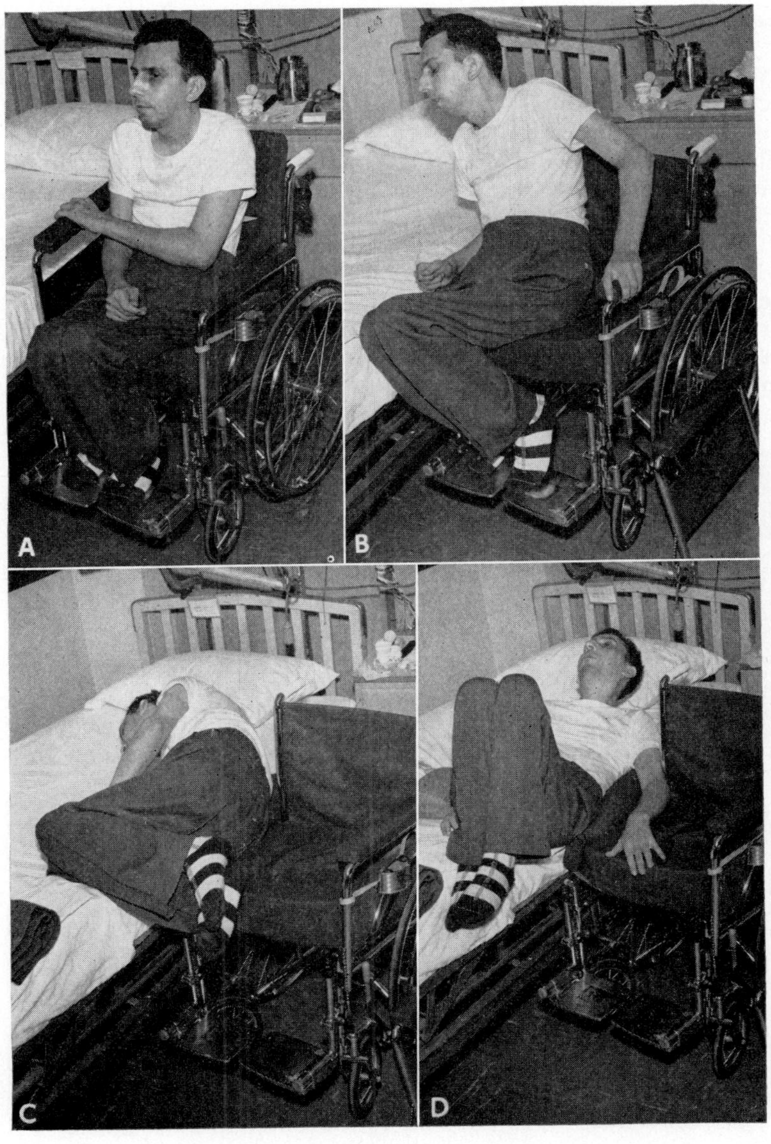

Fig. 36–3.—This patient with ankylosis of the spine and lower extremities is trained to transfer sideways from chair to bed.

For example, tight back muscles may be stretched by means of physical therapy to increase body flexibility. This, in turn, may then be utilized in functionally training the patient to bend and to dress the lower parts of his body. Similarly, the quadriceps muscles may be strengthened to provide power that will enable the patient to climb stairs, mount curbs, or get up from a toilet seat. In every instance, function is the ultimate objective.

Besides gross function, efficiency itself is an objective in functional training (Fig. 36–3). As a machine, the human body normally functions most inefficiently, the level being estimated by some at less than 25 per cent. Even in a patient with severe disabilities, this characteristically undeveloped potential provides opportunity for teaching him to attain ample efficiency to compensate for his irreversible physical deficiencies. The process may entail months of tedious training and practice but such an approach often opens the door to functional independence. This functional training is an important part of a patient's daily treatment. As he achieves proficiency in one sphere emphasis shifts to the next.

Corrective Surgical Measures

Since the advent of steroids and other drugs permitting better control of the inflammatory component of rheumatoid arthritis, patients no longer need wait for their disease to "burn out" before they seek surgical correction. Now such orthopedic procedures can be successfully undertaken while the disease is still active.[10,11] Success depends not only on good surgical technique, it also requires the diligence of the physician and therapist, with cooperation by the patient in an effective therapeutic exercise program, both preoperatively and postoperatively (*see* Chapter 34).

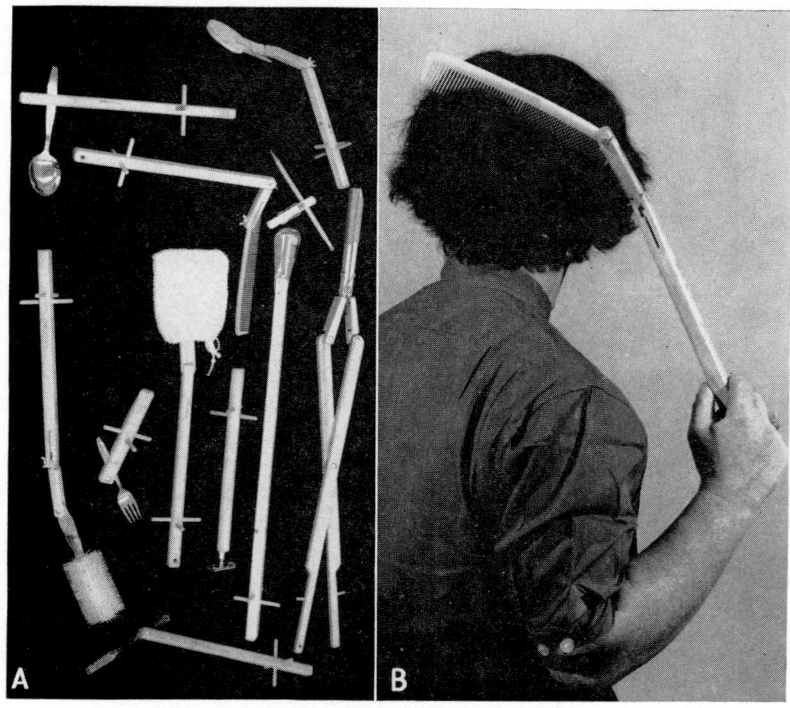

Fig. 36–4.—Elongated devices to compensate for loss in reach.

Self-Help Devices

The use of special apparatus and de-ices should be avoided unless deemed ssential to increase function or to protect mpaired joints. Only the more impor-ant devices notable for simplicity and usefulness will be described here[4,12,17] Fig. 36–4).

Devices to Aid in Dressing.—Dressing part of the body may, at times, be im-possible because of mechanical restric-ions imposed by deformities of various oints of the extremities. Zippered shoes, ong-handled shoe horns, devices for putting on socks and stockings, long-handled combs, and elastic shoe laces re often helpful. Recently attention has been focused on clothes designed espe-ially for the severely crippled patient, uch as capes instead of coats.

Devices for Feeding and Self-Care.—When deformities exist in joints of the upper xtremities, special long-handled devices or feeding, washing, toilet care and pplying cosmetics are helpful. Similarly, for patients with severe involvement of hand and wrist, special devices are available for such activities as writing, shaving and holding eating utensils.

Adapted Chairs and Toilet Seats.—Toilet seats and chairs of standard height often pose major mechanical problems for the arthritic patient with involvement of knee or hip. These seats are usually 17 or 18 inches from the floor and the patient may experience considerable pain in using them, or, if ankylosis has occurred, he may find the use of the seats mechanically impossible. However, specially built-up seats are available for temporary or permanent attachment to standard toilets. Height of chairs may be increased by lengthening their legs or by using sponge rubber seat cushions to provide extra elevation.

In patients with more generalized involvement of joints and especially in ankylosing spondylitis with peripheral joint involvement, it may be necessary to make individual modifications of chairs.

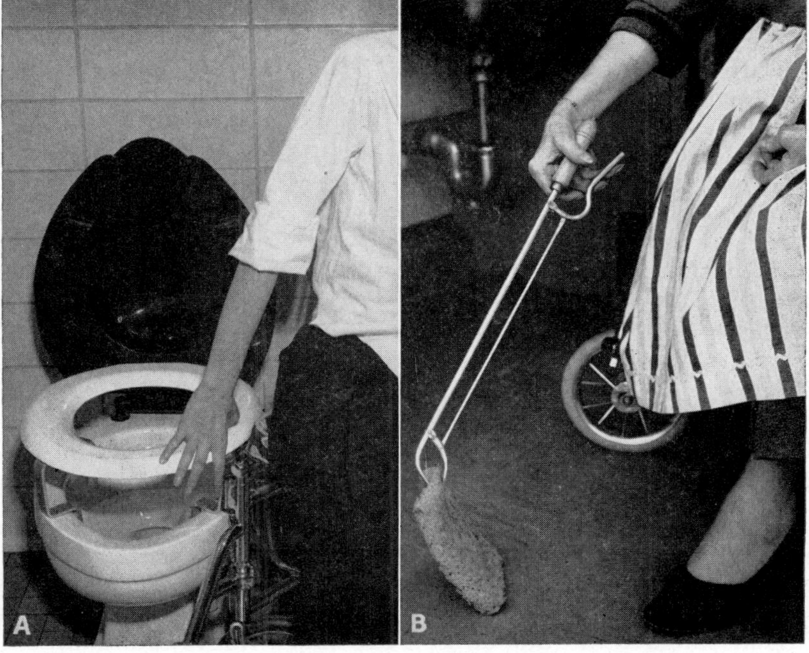

Fig. 36–5.—Self-help devices may be useful in restoring independence in many areas of living.

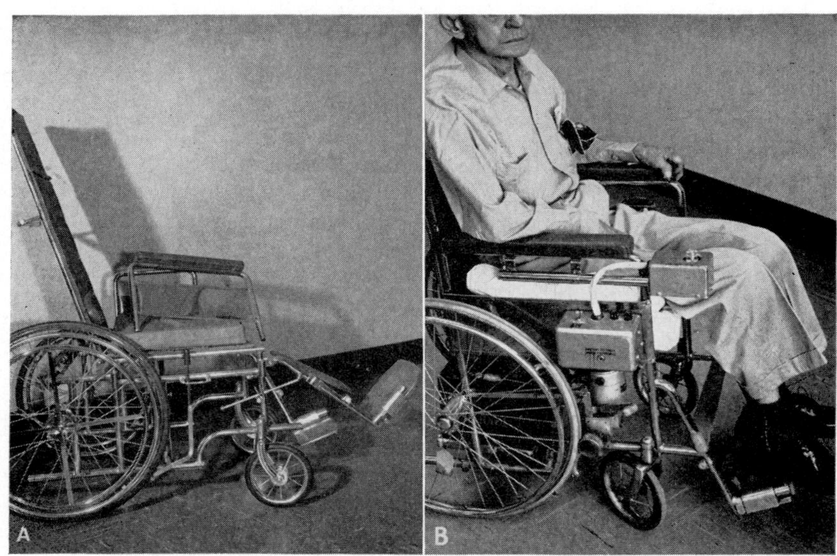

FIG. 36–6.—*A*, This demonstration wheelchair shows the various adaptations which may be prescribed according to the patient's individual needs. *B*, For the more severely crippled patient, a motorized wheelchair can be operated with ease.

This is especially true when ankylosis of the hips is present.

Wheelchairs (Fig. 36–6).—Wheelchairs must be prescribed according to the individual needs of the patient.[4] Besides various models commercially available, many different attachments are obtainable, including reclining backs, removable arms, desk arms, elongated brake handles, swinging foot rests and elevating foot pieces. Recently a motorized collapsible wheelchair, compact, serviceable, reasonable in price and easy to operate, has been developed. The control panel for this chair can be placed within range of the patient's upper extremity and even the most distorted and weakened fingers can manipulate the control buttons.

Crutches.—Because of the various combination of joint deformities that may develop in the upper extremities, "armpit" type crutches often may not suit the needs of the arthritic patient. Depending on the residual function in the upper extremity joints, crutches must be prescribed or adapted to meet the patient's special needs. The numerous types of crutches available range from the standard hand-grip type to those which permit weight-bearing at the elbows.

Energy-Saving Devices for the Home.—A woman's return to her household duties is as important to her personal dignity, her peace of mind, and her economic productivity as is the return of a man to his job. Careful planning, with reliance on such energy-saving devices as work tables on casters, adjustable ironing boards, long-handled cleaning equipment, light-weight kitchen utensils easy to manipulate, can substantially reduce the strain otherwise placed on joints by housekeeping duties.[4,13]

Socioeconomic and Vocational Factors

The optimum goal in rehabilitation of the arthritic patient is his re-establishment in a social and economic environment where he may function to his full capacity—within the limitations of his disability. Reaching this goal may require great resourcefulness and paience. Success in this sphere is commensurate with the resources of the patient himself and, probably more important, with the assistance the patient receives from the social worker, psychologist and vocational counselor.

Since chronic disease and disability affect all spheres of living, the need for dynamic assistance in readjusting to these effects is of prime importance.[4,8,9] For the patient with permanent disability, cursory social service will prove inadequate. To be worthwhile, the social services must include a detailed inquiry into the family relationships and an intimate knowledge of the living and working conditions the patient faces after his discharge from the well-organized, protective environment of the hospital. Otherwise routine details often assume crucial importance in determining the ability of the patient to function outside the hospital. The inability to negotiate a few stairsteps from house to street may spell the difference between ability and inability to travel to a job. A doorway wide enough to permit passage of a wheelchair; or a bed, chair, or toilet sufficiently high to assure the patient's independence may be the factor determining whether he can live alone in self-sufficiency or whether attendant care or a nursing home is mandatory.

In most cases, the social worker must make home visits to clarify and solve such problems. This attention is time-consuming and social workers expected to handle successfully the problem of the chronically disabled must not be given unduly large case loads. The old concept based on attention to acute illness, that one social worker could handle the patients of many clinics, is now outmoded by the increased demands of chronic disease. Success in rehabilitation is largely dependent upon awareness of this fact and the establishment of a realistic ratio of social workers to such patients.

Similarly, the psychologic complexities and vocational problems resulting from chronic disability are not transient but residual, and must be solved by the energetic efforts of informed psychologists and vocational counselors working closely together.

Job placement of the disabled arthritic is still one of the most difficult problems. Limited ability to utilize public transportation, the competitive labor market and the need for specialized placement all work to restrict employment. However, these factors can be mitigated if the approach is positive and understanding. Mawkish sympathy and preferential considerations should be avoided. If the patient's psychologic and vocational aptitudes are carefully assessed by the psychologist and the vocational counselor in collaboration with the social worker, plans for job placement or for suitable job retraining usually can be worked out.[1,2,4]

The validity of this conclusion is based upon my personal experience,[7] upon a study by the Division of Vocational Rehabilitation of the State of Georgia,[16] and on results of a "Back to Work" program[15] for patients with arthritis, conducted by the New York Chapter of the Arthritis Foundation. These experiences, especially the latter, have shown that with proper management and direction most unemployed arthritic patients can return to a wide variety of jobs in diverse industries and professions. These studies indicate that work does not necessarily aggravate the underlying disease, nor need pain, emotional factors, or physical restrictions interfere with performance. However, testing, counseling, and placement in employment must be done with intelligence, care and patient understanding, if the arthritic is to return successfully to a productive place in society.

BIBLIOGRAPHY

1. Acker, M.: J. Rehab., *22*, 6, 1956.
2. ————: Arch. Phys. Med., *37*, 743, 1956.
3. Lawton, Edith Buchwald: *Activities of Daily Living for Physical Rehabilitation*, New York, McGraw-Hill Inc., 1963.
4. Lowman, E. W. (Editor): *Arthritis, General Principles Physical Medicine and Rehabilitation*, Boston, Little, Brown, & Co., 1959.

5. Lowman, E. W., Lee, P. R., Miller, S., King, R. and Stein, H.: Arch. Phys. Med., *35*, 643, 1954.
6. Lowman, E. W.: Bull. Rheumat. Dis., *4*, 50, 1954.
7. Lowman, E. W., Lee, P. R. and Rusk, H. A.: J.A.M.A., *158*, 1335, 1955.
8. Ostrow, E. K.: The effect of arthritis on the life adjustment of a group of arthritis clinic patients and the need to extend social service in New York City arthritis clinics, The Arthritis Foundation, Inc., New York State Chapter, 221 Park Ave., New York, N. Y. 10003.
9. Out-Patient Social Service: A Demonstration and Study of Full-Time Social Work in Arthritis Clinics. The Arthritis Foundation, Inc., New York State Chapter, 221 Park Ave., New York, N.Y. 10003.
10. Preston, R. L.: New York State J. Med., *53*, 2626, 1953.
11. Preston, R. L.: *The Surgical Management of Rheumatoid Arthritis*, Philadelphia, W. B. Saunders Co., 1968.
12. Lowman, E. and Klinger, J. L.: *Aids to Independent Living, Self-Help for the Handicapped*, New York, McGraw-Hill, Inc., 1969
13. Rehabilitation Monograph VIII: A Manual for Training the Disabled Homemaker Howard A. Rusk, Edith L. Kristeller, Julia S Judson, Gladys M. Hunt, Muriel E. Zimmerman, Institute of Rehabilitation Medicine, 400 East 34 Street, New York, N. Y. 10016.
14. Rehabilitation Monograph X: A.D.L.; Activities of Daily Living, Testing, Training and Equipment. Edith Buchwald Lawton, Institute of Rehabilitation Medicine, 400 East 34th Street, New York, N.Y. 10016.
15. Manheimer, R. H. and Acker, M.: J. Chr Dis., *5*, 770, 1957.
16. Rheumatoid Arthritis Survey (Memorandum No. 283), Georgia Division of Vocational Rehabilitation, Nov. 13, 1953.
17. Rusk, H. A. and Taylor, E. J.: *Living with a Disability*, New York, Blakiston Division, McGraw-Hill, 1963.
18. Rusk, H. A.: *Rehabilitation Medicine*, 3rd Ed., St. Louis, C. V. Mosby Company, 1971.

Chapter 37

Prevention of Deformities from Arthritis

By THEODORE A. POTTER, M.D.

THE multiplicity of symptoms of rheumatoid arthritis makes it difficult for one physician to comprehend the problem intelligently and to treat it effectively. The inflammation in the joints, with the subsequent deformities and disabilities which develop, presents many problems which fall within the province of orthopedic surgery. Orthopedic principles include the methods by which deformity is prevented and the means of regaining or improving function when it is lost. The medical practitioner will help his patient greatly by learning and practicing these methods.[26] In the clinic and in the hospital the patient fares best if under the combined supervision of the rheumatologist and orthopedic surgeon.[12]

The management of patients with rheumatoid arthritis includes more than giving them drugs or physical therapy.[17] In this disease the joints are inflamed and frequently become deformed from the muscular spasm which accompanies the inflammation, and from positions which the patient assumes for comfort. In the early stages of the disease, deformities can usually be prevented by advice to the patient and by keeping the limbs in certain positions. Teaching good posture is of great value at this time, to insure good alignment of the body and prevent sprains and deformity particularly in the weight-bearing joints.

Faulty posture produces a number of changes in the function of the body.[20] The thoracic and abdominal organs work less efficiently. The spine and the weight-bearing joints will have more strain and the muscles will work less efficiently when the body is not aligned properly. The first requisite is that the patient lie in bed habitually in positions which do not encourage strain or faulty working of the thoracic and abdominal organs.

If the patient is not supervised, deformity often results from prolonged assumption of faulty positions of the trunk and limbs.[24] The bed on which the patient lies should not sag. There should be only one pillow under the head. The limbs should not be supported in a flexed position by cushions or pillows. When the patients sit in bed, a pillow should be placed under the knees to relax the hamstring muscles. For reading, the upper part of the bed can be raised or an inclined plane of pillows can be fashioned. In this position the head is raised while the entire spine remains flat. For those unable to sit or recline, such as the spondylitic, plastic prism glasses permit the patient to read comfortably while lying flat in bed with the reading material held vertically on his chest. In sitting, the feet should be placed firmly on the floor or upon the foot rest. The back of the chair should be vertical or slightly inclined. The patient sits most comfortably if the back of the chair supports the entire spine. In wheelchairs or soft chairs a pillow can be placed behind the back at the dorsolumbar junction to prevent slumping. The patient should not sit in soft chairs or wheelchairs for long periods of time.[1]

Positions

To aid in good posture and to have the patient take good positions in which

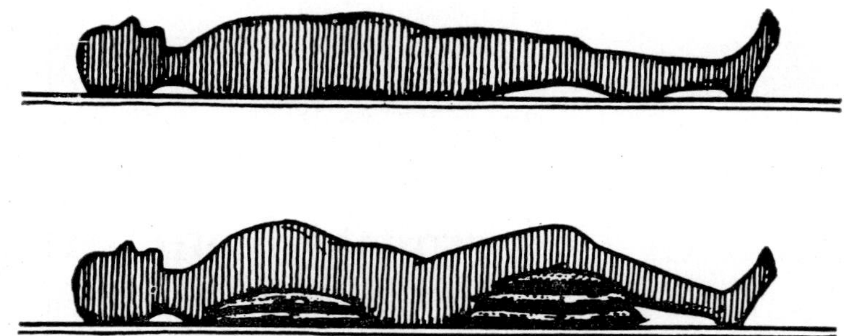

FIG. 37–1.—*Hyperextension* to expand the chest, raise the diaphragm, increase abdominal breathing and circulation and correct round shoulders. Use this position for one-half hour after meals; a pillow under dorsal spine and a pillow under the knees (to relax the muscles of the back); pillows must not be kept under the knee for long periods or contracture deformities may result.

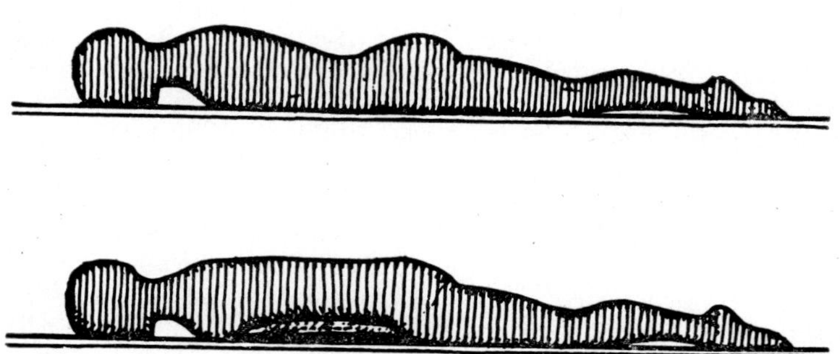

FIG. 37–2.—*Face-prone position,* support under the abdomen to flatten the lower back.

the organs will function more efficiently, the body is placed in hyperextension and in face-prone positions for one-half an hour after meals.[28] The hyperextension position is shown in Figure 37–1. On a firm bed the patient lies supine with a small pillow under the dorsal spine and a second pillow under the knees. The hands are folded under the neck. This position expands the chest, raises the diaphragm, increases abdominal breathing and circulation. It is very helpful in correcting the early deformities of ankylosing spondylitis. During the second half hour, the patient takes the face-prone position shown in Figure 37–2. The patient lies prone with a pillow under the abdomen and trunk, extending upward from the hips. The hands are placed above the head or at the sides. In this position the abdominal circulation is changed, the organs no longer press against the posterior abdominal wall.[23]

Good Posture

This is habitual good alignment of the various segments of the body. It is of importance in treating arthritis since faulty alignment in sitting and standing favors fatigue, strains, articular irritation and deformities. It also hinders proper functioning of the thoracic and abdominal organs. Posture is judged by comparison of lateral view of the body with a standard chart (Fig. 37–3) if the patient can stand. For bed patients the following criteria of habitual good posture are used:

1. There should be no increase in the anterioposterior curves of the spine. The individual should hold the spine as straight as possible.

2. The chest should be held (at rest) midway between full inspiration and full expiration. It should not be depressed at the waist line. The subcostal angle should be nearly a right angle.

3. The greatest circumference of the body should be at the xyphoid in all positions of the body.

4. The lower abdomen should be flat and the upper abdomen should be full and rounded. With this position the diaphragm can work effectively and there

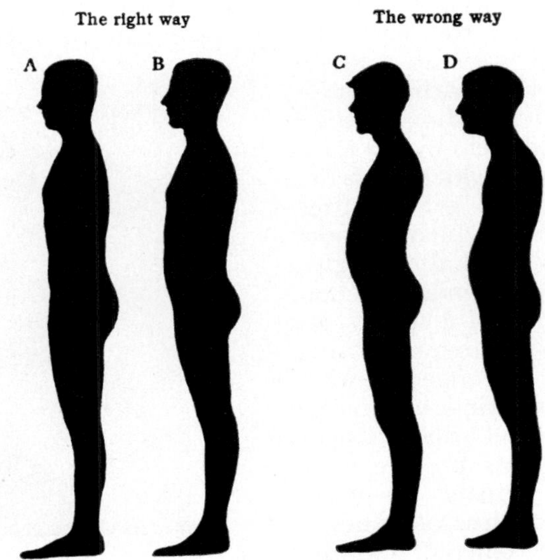

FIG. 37–3.—Chart of good and bad posture (Harvard Chart of Body Mechanics or Posture).

Positions and Exercises for Improvement of Posture of the Patient in Bed

Keep the patient on a firm bed. A fracture board should be placed under the mattress if it sags. Permit the use of only one small pillow under the head. Place a foot board or cradle at the foot of the bed.

Hyperextension position: no pillow under the head, lying on the back, pillow under the lower thoracic spine, pillow under the knees; maintain this position thirty minutes after each meal.

Prone position: lying on the abdomen, legs straight, arms placed above the head or at the side; pillow under the abdomen extending upward from the hips. Assumed for thirty minutes 3 times a day following the hyperextension position.

Exercise: lying on the back, knees flexed, hands behind the head. Breathe deeply, elevating the chest, exhale holding the lower abdomen in.

Exercise: lying on the back, knees flexed; pull the lower abdomen in; tighten the buttock muscles; flatten the lower back against the bed.

Exercise: same position. Place the hands on the lower rib margins anteriorly, breathe deeply and pull the lower rib margin upward; maintain this pull while exhaling. These exercises are performed three to ten times a day, depending upon the strength of the patient.[9]

is no pressure upon or crowding of the abdominal viscera.

Often fixed deformities in arthritis hinder or prevent the attainment of good posture. Whatever improvement is gained is reflected in more efficient functioning of the body.[20]

The usual effects of faulty posture are: increased fatigue, strain, traumatic arthritis, deformity and visceral disturbances. Fatigue is one of the earliest symptoms seen especially in standing because the parts of the body are held by the muscles. The group of muscles which holds the body against the pull of gravity tires quickly. The ligaments which support the joints of the spine and the weight-bearing extremities become overstretched when the muscles tire, and a sprain develops. With faulty alignment the surfaces of the joint are no longer parallel and greater pressure and friction come on one part. The visceral disturbances which are seen with poor posture vary greatly in different individuals. They are usually more serious in those of asthenic habitus than those of sthenic habitus. These disturbances may impair the normal excursion of the diaphragm. Through sagging and crowding of the abdominal organs digestion, assimilation and excretion may be slowed down and made less efficient.

These effects, which would be scarcely noticed by a well and active individual, assume greater importance in patients ill with arthritis. Here one wants the best possible alignment of the body. Improvement of posture is attempted throughout the treatment of rheumatoid arthritis. At first the patient may be recumbent almost all of the time, sitting up only for meals. Position, breathing and abdominal exercises are given usually twice a day. After supervision they are carried out by the patient twice a day. They are made to conform to the ability of the patient and are modified for fixed deformities. Usually two or three exercises are performed twice daily. They are performed more often and others are added as the patient's ability to perform them increases. At the same time an effort is made to correct faulty posture by special positions. As the patient improves in well-being and acquired ability in performing the exercises, sitting exercises are given. Eventually standing, foot and walking exercises are given. These are gradually discarded when good posture can be maintained habitually.

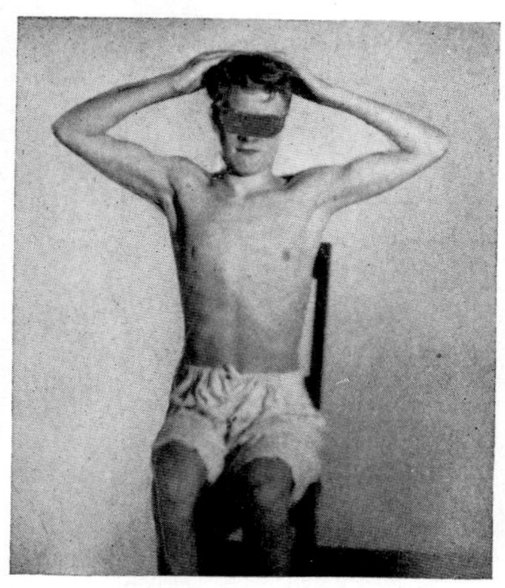

A

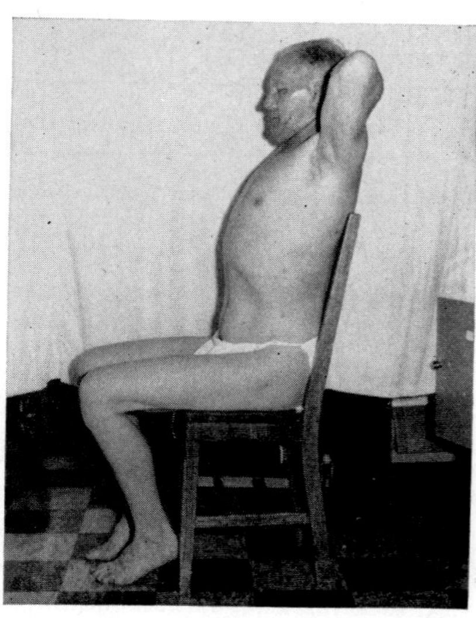

B

FIG. 37–4.—Postural exercises performed while sitting. The back is flat, the abdomen retracted. The hands are on the head or resting on the ilia.

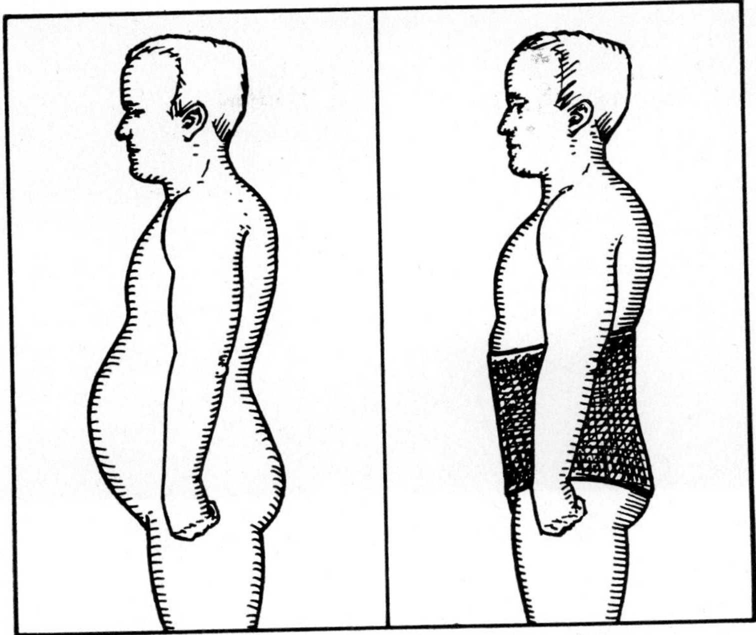

FIG. 37–5.—Aid in maintaining good posture. The chest is raised; the abdomen pulled in and up; the lumbar lordosis is decreased.

A good standing posture is one with the feet pointing forward, the weight carried on the outer side of the feet, the lower abdomen held in, the low back flat, the chest held in inspiration, the head erect with chin in.

In some patients, particularly older individuals, help must be given temporarily, sometimes permanently, to hold good alignment of the body.[4] This is accomplished by the use of spinal braces, carefully fitted to flatten the lumbar spine and to push the lower abdomen in and up. In women this can be done by wearing a properly fitting corset. Such apparatus is worn while the patient is up. It is removed for exercises and when the patient lies down. It is discarded when good posture can be held without external support.

SPLINTING OF AFFECTED JOINTS

When joints are swollen and painful on motion they should be protected.[10] The amount of protection is dependent upon the severity of the inflammation. The amount of muscular spasm determines the rigidity of the support necessary. If there is only a slight amount of swelling and little pain on motion a firm bandage about the joint may be adequate splinting.[9] The most comfortable type of bandage is an elastic cotton bandage (ACE bandage). Felt strips or sponge rubber can be applied under the elastic cotton bandage to add to its security. On small joints a bandage 2 inches wide is most effective. Wider bandages are used for the larger joints. Such bandages are effective as a temporary support during convalescence, when full recovery is expected in a few weeks. It is also used when the muscles are not quite strong enough about the joint. Bandages are not adequate support for acute, severely inflamed joints.[3]

Somewhat firmer, but still a mild form of splinting, is adhesive plaster strapping. This is used in ambulatory patients, par-

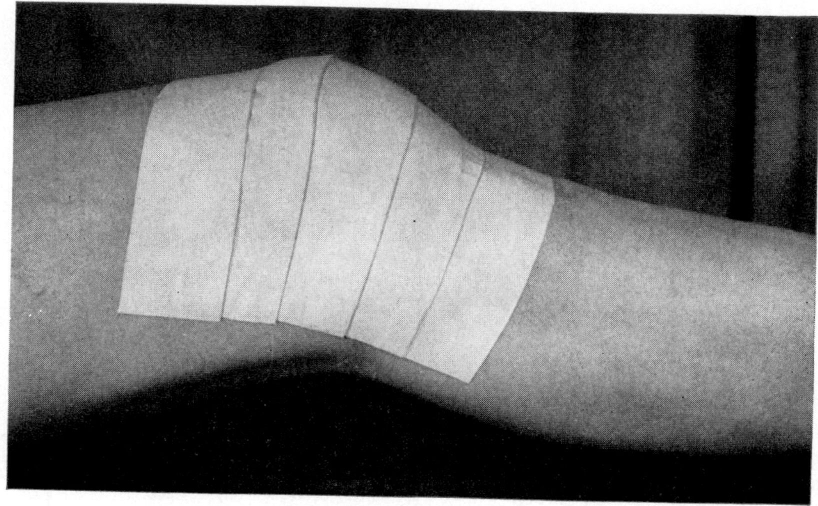

Fig. 37–6.—Adhesive strapping of inflamed knee.

ticularly for the sprains which come in joints when there is articular damage or deformity. This is common in arthritis. The joints most commonly protected are the wrist, elbow, low back, knee and ankle. Strapping never entirely encircles the joint, going about two-thirds around it. It always covers and compresses the swollen portion of the joint. Narrow strips of adhesive plaster are applied firmly, each strip overlapping the one that has been put on before. The skin is usually painted with compound tincture of benzoin before applying the adhesive plaster and a gauze bandage is put on over the adhesive strapping for twelve to twenty-four hours to prevent slipping of the adhesive. The adhesive strapping should not be immersed for long periods in water or it will loosen. Sponge baths or shower baths usually do not disturb the strapping to any serious degree. The strapping is replaced as a rule in one week. It is discontinued when the soreness and swelling subside about the joint.

A useful type of strapping, particularly about the knee, ankle, and elbow, combines adhesive dressing with pressure. This gives more support than the two previous types of bandaging. Either an elastic form of adhesive tape, or zinc gelatin paste on gauze may be used.

A somewhat more effective form of splinting of inflamed joints is *traction.*[11] This can be used both in the upper and lower extremity to relieve muscular spasm and correct mild flexion deformities. In arthritis it is used most commonly on the hip and knee joints. In the upper extremity it can be used on the elbow and finger joints, rarely at the shoulder. On the lower extremity 2-inch-wide strips of adhesive, preferably moleskin adhesive plaster, are applied to the medial and lateral sides of the leg over skin shaved and painted with tincture of benzoin. As an alternative, sponge rubber strips, applied with an elastic bandage, may be used for periods up to one week. The bony prominences about the knee and ankle are padded with felt or sheet cotton. The foot of the bed is raised about 4 inches to prevent the patient from sliding downward in bed after the traction is applied. Ten to 12 pounds of weight are applied through a rope and pulley attached to the foot of the bed. A spreader at the sole of the foot attaches the adhesive plaster strips to the traction rope. A splint or pillow

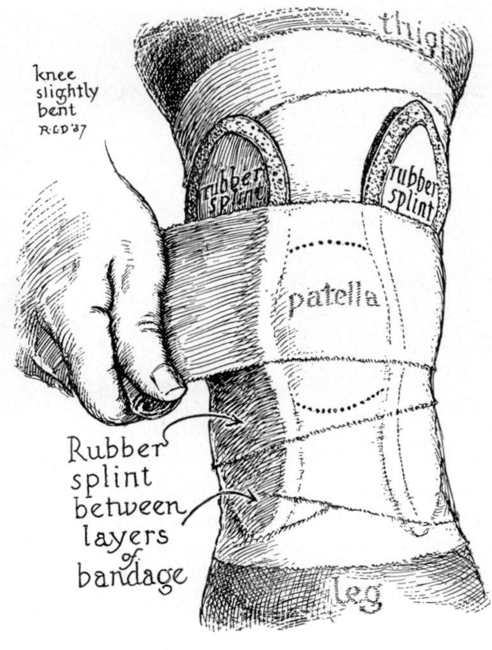

A

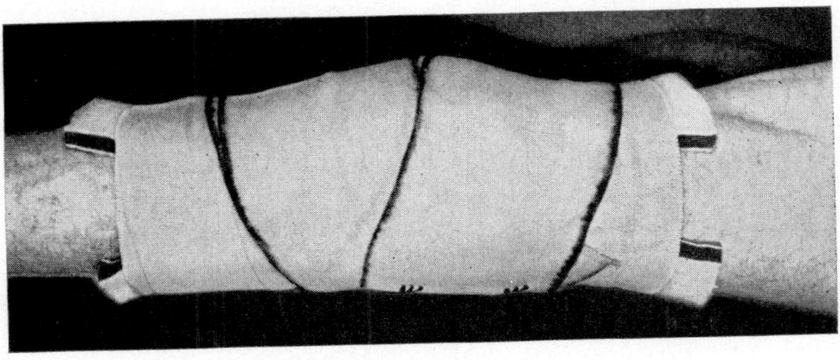

B

FIG. 37–7.—*A*, Combination *sponge rubber and elastic bandage* partly applied to the left knee, featuring the shape and position of the rubber sponge splints. To complete the support, the bandage is continued to the top edge of its inner layer. (Truslow, courtesy of J.A.M.A.) *B*, Instead of sponge rubber, strips of thick felt $1\frac{1}{2}$ inches by 8 inches can be applied to the sides of the knee joint beneath the ACE bandage.

is sometimes applied at first to secure traction in line with the deformity. To be effective, traction must be continuous. Intermittent traction gives only temporary relief of pain. A useful temporary form of traction is to apply coarsely woven cloth or strips of sponge rubber to each side of the leg and wind an elastic cotton bandage firmly about it. This will take 10 to 15 pounds of traction and can be removed from the leg quickly for other treatment simply by unwinding the bandage.

Plaster of Paris Splints

Plaster of Paris splints are commonly used as they are readily available. Effec-

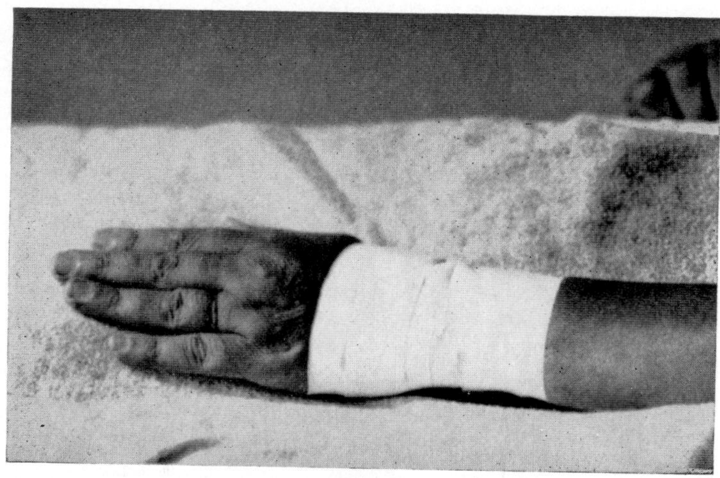

Fig. 37–8.—Strapping of the wrist joint in arthritis. The adhesive strapping is applied over tincture of benzoin. It should extend one inch beyond the joint on both sides. It does not completely encircle the wrist, leaving 2 inches uncovered on the volar surface.

tive splints can be made of metal, wire and various types of plastics. The latter have come into extensive use in the arthritis centers because they are light, durable, and waterproof. Plaster casts are applied at first over sheet cotton and usually encircle the limb.[22] On small joints a slab of plaster (about 8 layers) is applied with an elastic cotton bandage which encircles the joint.

Usually the plaster cast is kept on the limb for one or two days as a solid encasement. The plaster cast is then cut into anterior and posterior halves. This permits removal of the anterior half and later of the entire cast for short periods of the day for other treatments.[30]

When Applying Plaster:

1. Pad all sharp, bony prominences which may be covered: malleoli, anterior-superior spines, crest of the ilium, knee, etc. If the patient is thin and the spinous processes are prominent, use padding over these.
2. If all prominences are padded, additional padding elsewhere is unnecessary.
3. Avoid pressure from fingers.

For home use, strips of impregnated plaster will prove useful. These are available, already cut in various lengths which need only to be immersed in water and applied to the part involved. These are available in several different sizes—3 × 15, 4 × 15 and 5 × 30 inches, in boxes of 50 sheets each. From 7 to 10 layers (or sheets) may be needed for each splint depending upon the joint involved. It requires not more than a few seconds for the splints to become saturated in water; the plaster sets within eight to ten minutes.

When soaked in water, plaster of Paris takes up water and then crystals form and interlock rapidly.[19] Much of the ultimate strength of the plaster is derived from this tight interlocking of the crystals. The plaster must remain undisturbed during most of the setting process so that this interlocking of crystals occurs properly.

The layers will fuse to form a solid cast if plaster bandages are applied in rapid succession. When one layer of plaster-crinoline dries before another is applied, lamination of the cast occurs with non-fusion. If it is necessary to wrap fresh plaster over a dry plaster surface, one should first roughen the dry surface by

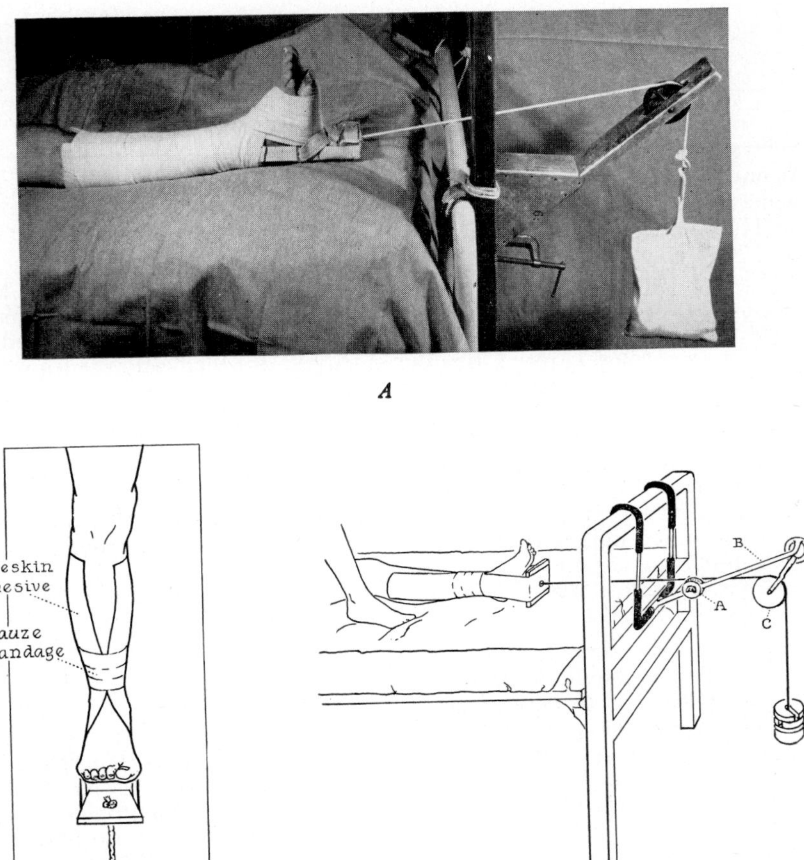

FIG. 37-9—*A*, Removable knee-traction. Sponge rubber attached to traction straps is firmly bound on each side of the lower leg with a bandage. *B*, Usual form of adhesive traction for the knee.

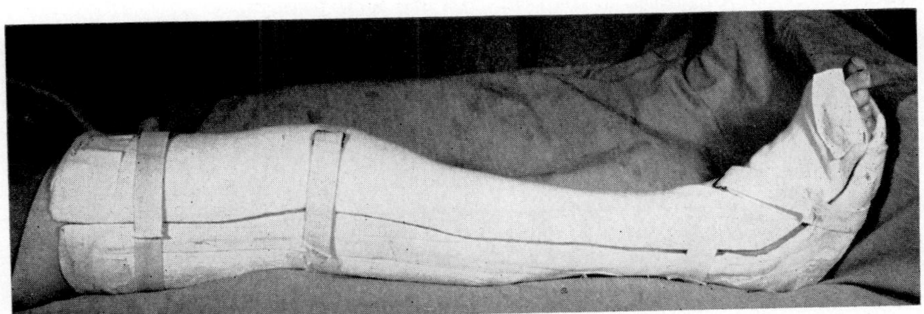

FIG. 37-10.—Resting leg cast cut into two halves to facilitate removal. This should extend from the upper thigh to the toes.

Application of Plaster Splints

A. If one desires to splint the knee joint temporarily, a simple method for the general use of the practitioner is as follows:
   1. The patient lies on his abdomen.
   2. A thin coating of petroleum jelly is applied to the thigh and leg.
   3. Plaster strips are wet and are then placed over the back of the thigh, leg and plantar surface of the foot. This may be built up until from 7 to 15 layers of plaster gauze are applied, as needed. If rolls of plaster are used, these may be cut into strips of the desired length, or rolled onto the leg wet.
   4. The plaster is molded to conform to the shape of the leg with the palm of the hand.
   5. The plaster is allowed to dry.
   6. The splint can then be lifted away easily because of the petroleum jelly coating.
   7. The splint may be placed on a radiator to dry more quickly. Splints may be made much lighter than usual if these are allowed to harden completely before using.
   8. Line the splint with felt or sheet cotton and apply to the limb with a bandage.

B. Splinting of the lower leg and ankle.
   1. The patient should lie prone (on his abdomen).
   2. The ankle may be kept at right angle.
   3. Petroleum jelly is applied to the lower leg and foot and the strips of wet plaster are then applied. Each layer is placed so that it partly overlaps the one next to it.
   4. Plaster strips may be purchased in varying sizes, or the physician may cut these from the rolls of plaster. If he desires, he may form his plaster splint by wetting the roll of plaster and rolling this back and forth on the back of the leg and sole of the foot.
   5. The plaster splint is removed when firm, padded on the inner side and is then fastened to the leg with a bandage. Such splints are only for temporary wear. They are much less effective than circular casts.

C. The technique, as described for splinting the knee joint, may also be used to make a molded posterior body shell. When a large shell is to be made, numbers of criss-cross plaster strips should be placed, especially about the hips and buttocks, where strain is to be expected. Such splints are well molded about the hips, and lower ribs are well padded.

D. For the hands and fingers, three to seven thicknesses of plaster gauze can be held against the hand and forearm which have been coated previously with petroleum jelly; these are held in the desired position until hardened. They are then lifted away and dried. In making plaster splints for the hands and fingers, the plaster is applied to the flexor aspect of the forearm and palm, usually leaving the thumb out of the splint.

scratching it with a sharp knife. In this way a broken plaster also may be patched with strips of freshly wetted plaster.

Waterproofing the splint results in a cleaner, firmer and harder splint and prevents moisture and perspiration leading to deterioration of the splint. This is of value when the splint will be worn a long time. It is not indicated if the cast will be changed to get a better position of the limb in one to two weeks.

Castex Splints

Castex splints have been used by some physicians. This material utilizes a synthetic resin. Bandages of this material (moistened with a quick-drying solvent) are supplied in various widths in 10-yard lengths; the bandages are rolled, tinted, unbleached cotton sheeting cut on the bias. The cellulose compound which is used to impregnate the cotton sheeting is pyroxylin ("airplane dope") in acetone.[9]

Fiberglass Splints

Many new materials are available for the fabrication of casts and supports for arthritic joints. One which we have found particularly useful is fiberglass. Splints have been used for the hands both to prevent deformity and after operations on the hand. The making of a fiberglass splint requires three steps—a plaster mold is made of the hand in the position one wishes it held. Three layers of fiberglass are applied over the model impregnated with ortho-bond resin. This requires about six hours to harden. It provides a light waterproof cast which can be modified by additions cemented on to hold the fingers in a special position. They are readily applied to the hand by several velcro bandages cemented to the splint.

Gelatin Casts

The gelatin or Unna boot may be applied in the conventional fashion with Unna paste and gauze. The conventional or already prepared gelatin-gauze bandages are used frequently in phlebitis and in low-grade inflammatory processes in the legs. Bandages of this type ready for use can be purchased, called Gelocast bandages. They are easily applied and dry within a short time. They are not as rigid as plaster and usually cannot be reapplied after they are removed.

RELIEF OF MUSCULAR SPASM

Numerous drugs have been used in the last twenty years to relax muscles, to block muscular spasm and lessen the deformity. However, each drug has been found wanting and none of them is used with any regularity. The drugs that have been used can be classified according to their mode of action into central sensory depressants and those which act on the myoneural junction chiefly by blocking the action of acetylcholine.

The most commonly used agents today are "Valium" (Diazepam) and "Robaxin" (Methocarbanol). Valium, a benzodiazepim derivative, acts on the thalamus and hypothalamus, inducing a calming effect. It is a useful adjunct for relief of skeletal muscle spasm due to reflexes originating from local pathology. Robaxin is a potent muscle relaxant which has an unusually selective action on the central nervous system, specially on the internuncial neurons of the spinal cord. Both of these drugs are in wide use and can be administered orally. The local action of the sensory nerves can be stopped temporarily and muscular spasm lessened by the use of novocaine, 1 or 2 per cent. The use of heat and splints is still our most effective method of relieving spasm of muscles about an inflamed joint.

PREVENTION OF DEFORMITY

It is usually much easier to prevent a deformity in arthritis than to correct one. *Deformities in most arthritic patients can be prevented.*[29]

During the early stages of an arthritis,

deformities result usually from muscular spasm with joint irritation. Such deformity is ordinarily in a position of flexion and often adduction, because this affords the patient the greatest relief from pain and because of the more powerful action of most flexor and adductor groups of muscles over the corresponding extensor and abductor groups. Other factors which favor muscular contraction and aid in the development of deformities include pressure of the bed clothes, a sagging bed, muscular strain, static influences and gravity. Several pillows under the head may force the cervical and dorsal spine into forward flexion, flexion of the hip with contraction and shortening of the powerful ilio-psoas muscles, flexion and external rotation of the knees.[30]

Resting in a chair for long periods is not advisable for arthritic patients, as the position assumed leads to flexion contractures of the spine, hips, knees, elbows and wrists with internal rotation and adduction of the shoulders and pronation of the forearms.[31]

One of the first principles in preventing deformity is to relieve muscular spasm. In cases in which there is a possibility of ankylosis, the parts should be maintained in positions which will give the patient maximum function.[10]

Deformities can be prevented if the physician has an understanding of the problem at hand and if the patient is cooperative.

Positions of Optimum Function

Knee: A few degrees of flexion (5 to 10 degrees—no more).

Ankle: The foot should be at a right angle; very slight pronation is also sometimes advisable.

Hip: Slight flexion of the hip with the leg practically straight; no rotation, abduction or adduction.

Shoulder: Not more than 45° between the humerus and the posterior border of the scapula; forward flexion (30 to 45°) and slight internal rotation of the arm (10 to 15°), so that the hand will reach the mouth.

Elbow: Depends upon the patient's occupation and wishes; in general, approximately 70 to 80° of flexion is usually best with forearm in slight supination (10 to 15°).

Wrist: About 35° of dorsiflexion and full extension if using crutches.

Hand: 30° of flexion of the fingers and metacarpophalangeal joints; slight abduction of the thumb.

Jaws: Open 1 inch at least.

Spine and Head: In good posture, head straight forward.

The Knee

The knee is the largest joint in the body and is frequently attacked by arthritis. Atrophy of the muscles about the joint may appear rapidly. Common findings include narrowing of the joint space, fixation of the patella against the femoral condyles, subluxation of the tibia on the femur, and contracture of the joint capsule, hamstring muscles and periarticular structures.

In acute arthritis involving the knee, the patient should be put to bed. No weight-bearing should be permitted.[27] If there is inability to straighten the knee a plaster cast should be applied from toes to groin with the foot at a right angle and the knee as fully extended as possible. As pain and muscular spasm subside, a new plaster cast is applied and further casts are used until the knee can be fully extended. A plaster cast is worn day and night in acute cases,[29] but is removed at least once every twenty-four hours to exercise and to permit the use of heat which aids in lessening pain and muscular spasm. Arthrocentesis with removal of joint fluid and intra-articular steroid instillation is most helpful in relieving the acute inflammatory phase and to shorten the intervals between serial cast applications. (*See also* Chapter 32.)

One of the fears of the patient with acute joint involvement is excruciating pain which may occur on slight motion of the joint. With the joint held firmly in a bivalved cast painful movement of the joint does not occur. If all movement is painful, muscle-setting exercises can be taught. These can be carried out without motion in the joint. No passive motion should be done. Following this the splints are reapplied. As long as joint pain, tenderness and swelling persist, it is advisable that splints be used for the affected joint during most of the day and night so that muscular spasm will not cause deformities.[19]

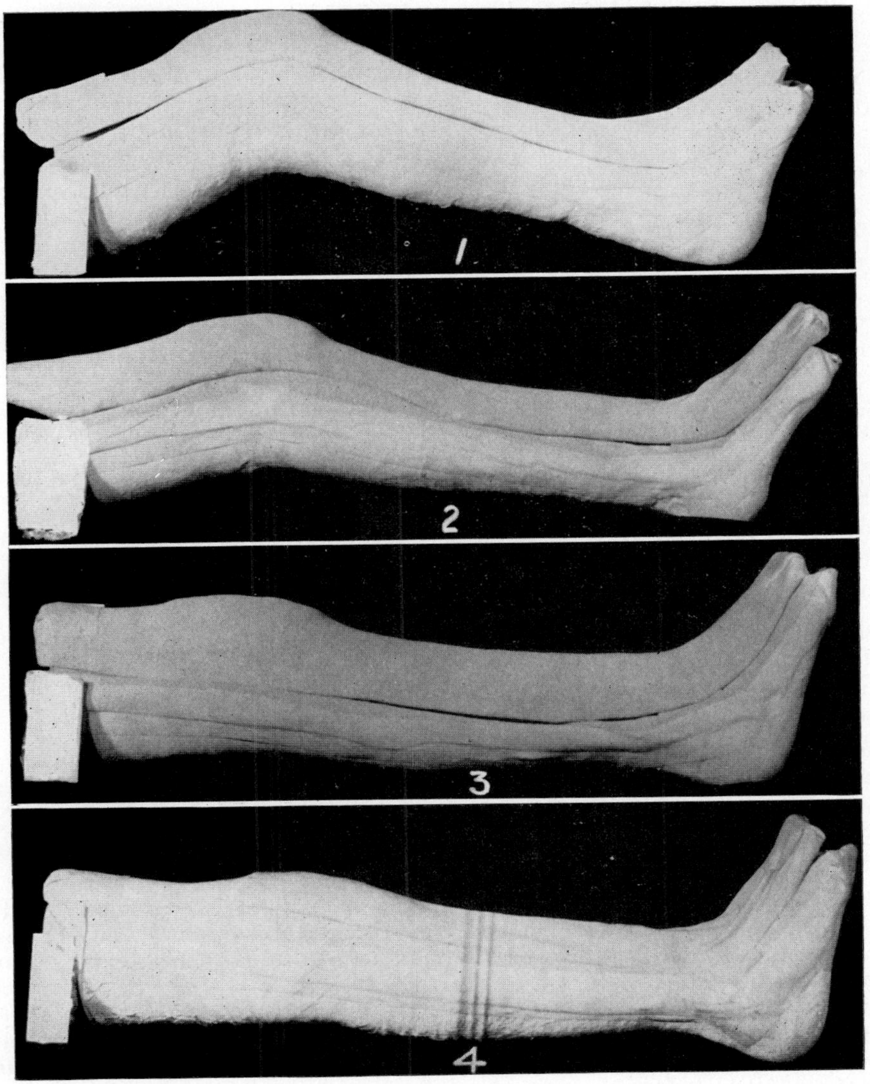

Fig. 37–11.—Gradual correction of flexion deformity of the knee by weekly changes of the plaster cast.

Prevention of Deformities in Arthritis

Physiologic rest of the involved joints in the acute stage by:

- Rest in a firm bed.
- Splinting of the affected joints (by the use of casts, splints or other apparatus) to prevent trauma and allay muscular spasm.
- Active movement of all joints through as wide a range of painless motion as possible several times a day.
- Special graded muscular exercises for each joint involved, with periods of rest following such exercise.
- Maintenance of good posture (see section on Good Posture.)

The most common deformities of the knee are flexion, subluxation and outward rotation. The cause of this flexion deformity is the desire of the patient to relieve the pain in the acute stage of the disease.[21] Flexion of the knee is the most comfortable position when swelling is present as it lessens the pull of the hamstring muscles on the posterior portion of the capsule, thus relaxing the latter, and permitting additional room for the swollen tissues of the joint. Most of these patients aid the flexion deformity by placing pillows under the knees to relieve discomfort. Other individuals bend the knees while lying on the side.[18] As the disease progresses further flexion is caused by muscular spasm. Because of this continued flexion of the knee, actual shortening occurs in the hamstring mus-

Prevention of Flexion Deformity of the Knees

Never place pillows under the knees for comfort in these patients; this is the most common cause of such a flexion deformity.[21]

Use a posterior molded splint or cast extending from the upper part of the thigh to the toes with the knee in full extension. A full cast including the foot is best.

Incorporate a wooden strip into the leg splint posteriorly at the ankle to control rotation of the hip joint and prevent outward rotation of the lower leg.

Remove the splint once daily and allow active movements.

Apply hot fomentations or other heat to the knee twenty to thirty minutes several times a day.

Employ muscle setting and non-weight-bearing exercises until the acute inflammation has subsided.

With improvement, lessen the period of splinting gradually so that within a short time, splinting may be required only at night, until inflammation has subsided.

Even in the later stages of the process, permit the splints to remain in place all night as flexion of the knees is common during sleep (unless prevented by splints).

Do not permit weight-bearing until the acute inflammation has subsided entirely and a period of exercises without weight-bearing has produced no harmful effects; the leg muscles must be in a condition to support this weight. **The patient should not walk on a flexed knee joint,** *or he will produce distortion in both lower extremities and in the trunk.* He should not be allowed to walk until he is able to hold the extended leg horizontally while sitting. During the first few weeks or months of walking, it may be advisable to use a stiff-legged brace, an elastic (ACE) bandage or a cane. A metal or wooden walker is of great assistance to these patients when they first attempt weight-bearing.[21]

cles so that the weight of the leg rests upon only the heel and the hip. This is due, at least in part, to contracture of the hamstrings. Outward rotation of the tibia on the femur usually follows within a short space of time. The prevention of such flexion deformity of the knee rests in general with the practitioner.

When correction of flexion deformity at the knee has been attained by serial plaster casts and one is ready to begin weight-bearing, support and protection must be given because of the weakened quadriceps muscles. In severe cases, it may be necessary to use metal leg caliper braces with leather support over the

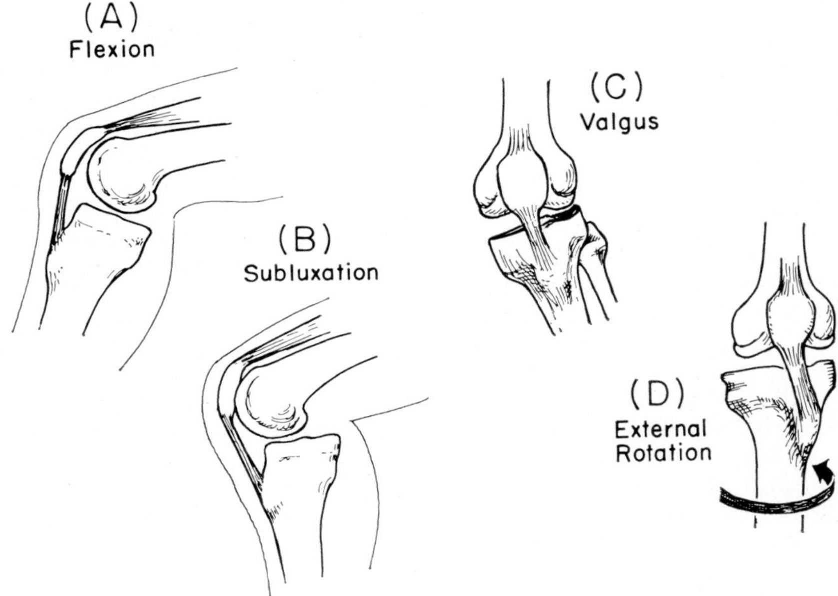

Fig. 37–12.—Schematic representation of the development of a typical deformity of the rheumatoid knee. Flexion, subluxation, valgus and external rotation components are present in varying degrees in most rheumatoid arthritic knees.[25]

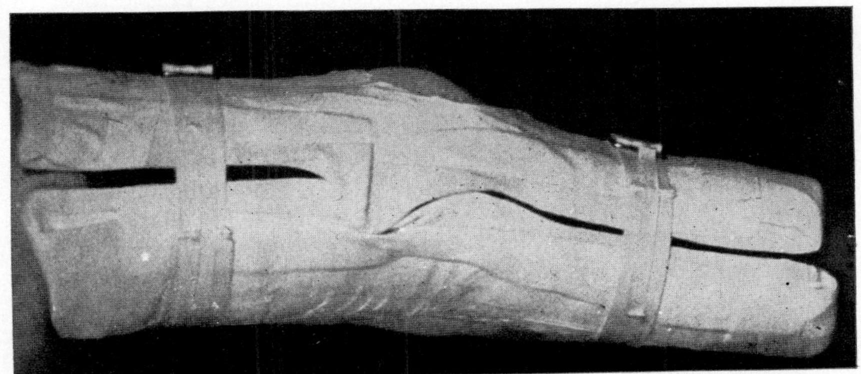

Fig. 37–13.—Plaster cylinder, bivalved, extending from upper thigh to lower third of leg. This permits walking with a straight leg when the muscles are weak.

patella, the metal uprights fitting into appropriate sockets in orthopedic shoes. Braces with hinges at the knee joint and braces of light metal may be used if they will have to be worn for a long time.

Plaster cylinders may be employed to support the knee joint until the quadriceps muscles have become stronger. If the quadriceps muscles are strong, one may employ a laced elastic knee support with or without metal hinge joints, or simply elastic bandages with a strip of felt incorporated on either side of the patella for additional support. Occupational therapy and proper exercises, heat and massage help to strengthen the atrophic muscles.[13]

Ankle and Foot

The most common deformities in arthritis involving the feet are stiff, pronated, or flat feet and deformities of the toes. Most, if not all, of the disability of the feet can be prevented by proper early treatment. With the occurrence of an arthritis involving the feet, there results a limitation of motion in the tarsal and phalangeal joints, accompanied by muscular weakness. The main factor in the progression of deformity in the feet is this muscular weakness and the added burden of weight-bearing. In bed, an equinus (plantar flexion) deformity will develop in arthritis unless a plaster cast is worn, or in the milder cases, a cradle or foot board is used.

Deformities at the hip or knee may also result in foot strain and deformity.[7] Continued flexion of the knee may cause strain and acute pain in the heads of the metatarsals. External rotation of the leg results in pronation and strain of the longitudinal arch. Long periods of confinement in bed result in relaxation of ligaments and muscles so that foot strain appears when weight-bearing is resumed.

Deformities seen in the arthritic foot include: (1) rigid valgus, (2) equinus and (3) cavus with flat anterior arch with cocked-up toes. The position of equinus, or plantar flexion, results from the pull of the strong gastrocnemius muscle, from the weight of the bed clothing and, in part, from gravity. When such patients are allowed to walk, this deformity is aggravated. Contractures of the toes are not infrequent with hyperextension at the metatarsophalangeal joints and flexion at the interphalangeal joints. Hallux valgus, subluxation and distortion at the metatarsophalangeal joints are common.

Pain in the foot in arthritis may be due to: (1) localized pressure; (2) muscular or ligamentous strain; or (3) acute or chronic inflammatory changes. The pain may be relieved temporarily by support and later by restoration and maintenance of normal function of the foot.

Pain due to excessive pressure may result from irregularities of the foot pressing against a smooth shoe or from an undue amount of weight being placed on certain bones of the foot. The most common cause of pain in the feet and legs is foot strain, a result of long hours of

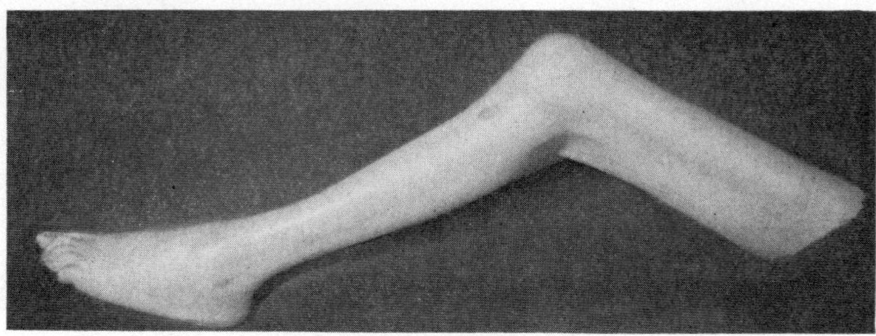

Fig. 37–14.—Foot drop with deformities at the knee, ankle and toes in neglected arthritis.

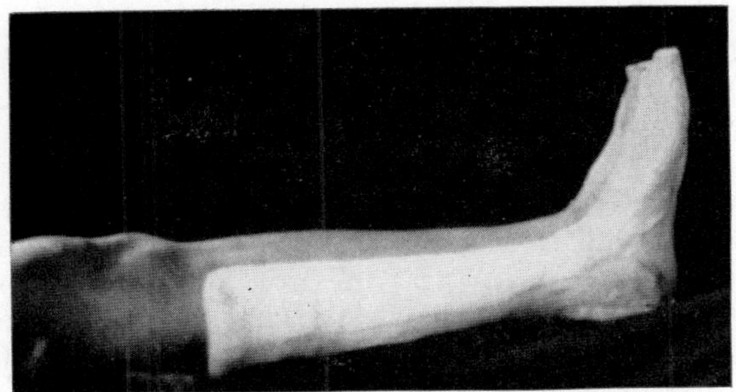

FIG. 37–15.—Short leg cast to prevent and correct deformities of the foot. Note the foot at right angles and slight varus. The arches of the foot have been molded in the plaster.

standing, excessive weight and faulty body mechanics. The foot pain may be the result of an actual inflammatory process occurring in the joints of the feet or along the ligaments or tendon sheaths.

One of the most frequent causes of deformity of the foot in the arthritic, and in other individuals, is rest in bed over long periods of time with the bed clothes tightly drawn so that the feet are pulled into a position of equinus (plantar flexion). In any patient for whom rest in bed is required, it should be a rule that the bed clothes be placed loosely over the feet, or if this cannot be done, that a cradle be placed over the feet so that the bed clothes rest upon this or upon a pillow placed under the covers at the foot of the bed rather than on the feet; otherwise, lying in bed leads to external rotation of the hips, slight flexion of the knees and mild equinus of the feet.

If there is any tendency to foot drop, the foot should be held at right angles by a posterior molded splint or cast (removed once or twice a day to permit free motion of the foot), or the head of the bed may be elevated 6 inches allowing the body to slide down somewhat in bed so that the feet may press against an upright foot board.

With the onset of rheumatoid arthritis in the ankle, muscular spasm tends to produce a valgus position of the foot, while the pull of the gastrocnemius muscle, the weight of the bed clothes and gravity lead to an equinus position of the foot. The equinovalgus which occurs

Prevention of Deformity of the Foot in Arthritis

Rest and avoidance of weight-bearing if acute inflammation is present.

Place a cradle over the feet or a pillow under the covers at the foot of the bed so that the weight of the bed clothes will not eventually produce a foot drop.

If any tendency to foot drop is seen, support the foot in a position at right angles to the leg by molded splints (to be removed daily for motion of the foot).

In arthritis involving the foot, **permit no weight-bearing until the acute stage has subsided.**

Apply hot fomentations or other forms of heat to the foot and ankle.

Prevent muscular atrophy in the foot by exercises while the patient is confined to bed.

Weak feet may be strapped in inversion for seven to ten days; later one should emphasize proper walking posture and corrective exercises and should employ proper shoes with pads, wedges or metatarsal bars or plates if necessary.

Figure-of-8 leather ankle straps may provide additional support to the longitudinal arch and prevent widening of the ankle mortise.

Hot foot baths should be given when the arthritis is acute.

When there is swelling an elastic stocking extending to the knee is helpful.

leads to depression of the metatarsal arch. With weight-bearing a spread of the forefoot follows. Later there is cocking up of the toes and in some instances hammer toes.

When the feet are involved in an arthritic process, little weight-bearing should be permitted until pain and swelling of the feet have entirely subsided, and until the foot muscles have been strengthened by non-weight-bearing exercises. *The muscles of the feet become weak and atrophied with prolonged rest in bed from any cause, unless active movements have been carried on throughout the illness.* The patient must have proper-fitting shoes and proper support to the arches of the foot before attempting to walk again.

If these procedures are carried out fully, the late changes in arthritic feet, particularly the peroneal spastic flat foot, seen so frequently in ambulatory patients, may be prevented (*see also* Chapters 39 and 78).

The Hip

The deformity which appears in arthritis at the hip joint is commonly mild flexion with adduction and external rotation.[14] If the patient walks with this deformity, flexion of the knee, knock-knee and valgus and equinus of the foot, with lateral tilting of the pelvis and increased lumbar lordosis may develop. Adjustment occurs in all parts of the limb to make walking and weight-bearing possible. In some patients the first symptom of arthritis of the hip is pain referred to the medial aspect of the knee and the anterior thigh.

Examination will disclose some muscular spasm, limitation of rotation and abduction and beginning flexion de-

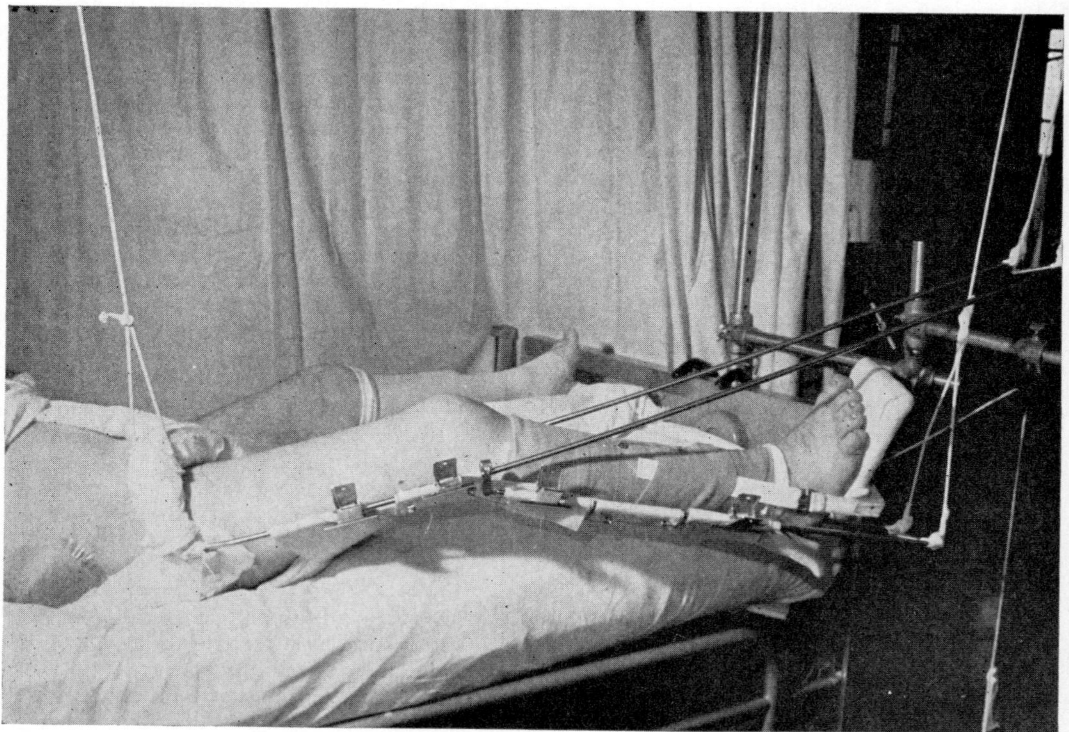

FIG. 37–16.—Hip traction: Balanced suspension with leg traction using a Thomas splint and Pearson attachment. The patient's leg can be comfortably placed in abduction and extension with 5 pounds traction. This overcomes muscle spasm and corrects the hip flexion deformity.

formity at the hip. Deformities of the hip and the spine occur at the same time. The prevention of deformities, or the correction of early deformity at the hip, depends on the vigilance of the physician in charge of the patient. Flexion and adduction deformity usually occurs before the patient complains of any discomfort at the hip joint. The patient should be flat on a firm bed. A small pillow under the buttocks for short periods of time is helpful in stretching the iliopsoas muscle. Hip-stretching exercises in extension should also be used. These can be done most easily with the patient prone. If there is muscular spasm about the hip, a plaster splint should be made, extending from the ribs to the foot, with the hip and knee in full extension. This is applied at night with an elastic bandage and is used until the muscular spasm subsides. If the muscular spasm continues, a plaster spica is applied from the ribs to foot, with the hip and knee in full extension. This is used each night with an elastic bandage and is continued until muscular spasm subsides. If the muscular spasm persists, a plaster spica extending from the ribs to the toes with the hip and knee in full extension and with the hip in 20° of abduction is applied. This plaster spica is bivalved and is removed several times a day for the application of heat to the hip area. Exercises are given particularly for extension and abduction.[15] The gluteal muscles weaken and atrophy quickly if they are not used normally. Traction of 10 pounds on the hip in the line of deformity will often bring a subsidence of muscular spasm in a few days. Balanced traction using a Thomas splint and Pearson attachment is often more comfortable and better tolerated by the patient. If applied to

Prevention of Deformity of the Hip Joint in Arthritis

Rest on a firm flat bed. If possible, the patient should lie prone for thirty minutes 3 times a day with one pillow placed lengthwise extending upward from the hip. The pillow is removed gradually as tolerated. This causes a stretching of the psoas muscle and anterior structures which permits the hip to assume a neutral position. Slight deformity at the hip may be corrected by traction of ten pounds in the line of deformity with heat applied to the hip for thirty minutes three times a day.

If there is tendency to internal rotation in adduction, hold the lower extremities in neutral position (foot pointing upward); separate the thighs to prevent shortening and contracture of the adductor muscles. Such positions can be held by sand bags or pillows placed on the inner side of the thigh. Lateral traction with a cuff around the thigh attached to a ten-pound weight on the side of the bed is helpful in overcoming adductor spasm.

If there is much pain in the hip joint it is relieved by applying a plaster spica over both hips, with the hips in full extension twenty degrees of abduction and neutral rotation. The feet should be included.

Change the patient's position frequently. The bed must have a firm mattress and a fracture-board under the mattress.

Exercises should be given as soon as tolerated. Prone exercises to strengthen the gluteal muscles are best. Permit no weight-bearing until pain, tenderness and muscle spasm have subsided. When weight-bearing is resumed, a walker and later crutches are used to lessen the weight-bearing load upon the diseased hip. A snug-fitting corset or pelvic belt is helpful about the hips. If ankylosis is inevitable the hip is held in the position of optimum function.

each leg, the adduction deformity can be stretched out by wide abduction of each balanced splint.

The Spine

If the cervical spine is involved, the tendency toward a flexion deformity (with at times rotation of the head) may be overcome by using *only one small pillow* under the head, and by lying flat in bed without a pillow several hours each night. The patient must not continually look in one direction, as this leads to a *rotation deformity* of the neck.[5]

In arthritis of the cervical spine, lateral tilting or rotation of the head may prevent normal vision and become unsightly. If there is acute muscular spasm, this can be made to relax by continuous traction applied to the cervical spine by means of a Sayre head sling attached to 5 to 10 pounds of traction at the head of the bed.

Deformity may be prevented by a Thomas collar, or by a piece of felt wrapped around the neck each night.[29] The latter should be about ⅜ inch in thickness, 1 yard long and be approximately 2½ inches in width at one end, gradually increased to a width of approximately 3½ inches at the other. This is wrapped around the neck each night beginning with the narrow end; it may be held in place by a safety pin or strip of adhesive. A medium-sized turkish towel, folded twice lengthwise, may be wrapped about the neck in a similar manner. When there is much muscular spasm, one can employ sand bags, hot fomentations, traction or plaster collars for support and muscular relaxation. Rigid collars are occasionally used in patients whose cervical spine has had rheumatoid arthritic involvement with subluxation of atlas on the axis. In severe cases a plaster head and shoulder support preventing all motion in the neck may be required.

Thoracic Spine

The thoracic spine shows deformity most often in ankylosing spondylitis, occasionally in osteoarthritis. The usual deformity is flexion with flattening of the chest anteriorly. Deformity is prevented by a firm bed, good positions of sitting and standing, and by postural exercises. If there is much soreness and muscular spasm, a molded plaster shell should be made on which the patient lies.[2] In ankylosing spondylitis, heat is applied to the back several times a day. The patient should lie prone for short periods to stretch the spine in extension. Before the patient becomes ambulatory, a plaster

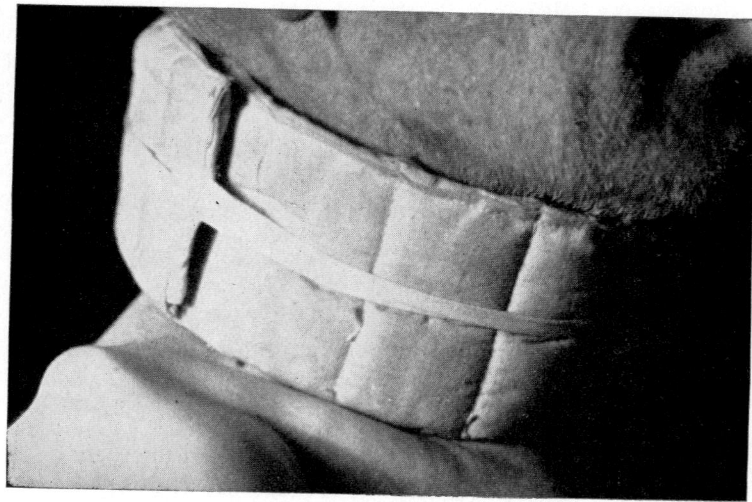

Fig. 37–17.—Padded collar worn for spasm and deformity in the cervical spine.

To Avoid Deformities of the Thoracic and Lumbar Spine:

1. Lie on a firm bed with only a small pillow. Lie on the back or abdomen most of the time.
2. The patient should lie on the back for thirty minutes after each meal, with the hands beneath the head. A pillow should be placed under the knees to flatten the lumbar spine. Later a small pillow may be used under the thoracic spine to combat forward bowing of the spine.
3. In very painful cases or those with marked muscular spasm a plaster shell is molded over the back. The patient lies in this most of the time.
4. Breathing exercises, back-stretching exercises, and later postural exercises are performed 2 or 3 times daily. These should not cause pain.
5. As soon as muscular spasm has subsided and the flexion deformity of the spine has decreased, a plaster jacket is applied over Goldthwait irons. In this the patient may be ambulatory. Another jacket is applied as soon as further correction of the spinal deformity is possible.
6. A spinal brace with shoulder straps may be used when the patient shows no further tendency to forward flexion of the spine.

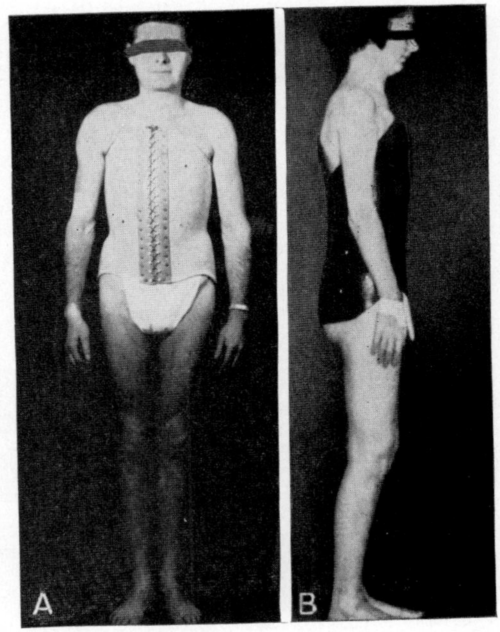

FIG. 37–18.—*A*, Celastic jacket. The jacket is cut low in back and extends to the sternal notch in front. This prevents forward bowing of the spine. Lacings or straps can be used after the jacket is cut in front for removal. *B*, Lateral view of leather jacket.

jacket is applied holding the spine in as much extension as possible. A spinal brace or firm corset is used to prevent forward bowing and sprain of the thoracic spine when convalescence is prolonged.

In the lumbar spine an increased lordosis is the usual deformity. In ankylosing spondylitis the lumbar spine may become entirely flat. A firm bed, heat to the lumbar spine, frequent changes of position, and postural exercises prevent deformities in most instances. A molded plaster shell on which the patient lies is used when the arthritis is severe. A plaster jacket fitted to hold the patient in good posture is sometimes used in ankylosing spondylitis. In other types of arthritis a back brace or firm corset is worn throughout convalescence.

The Shoulder

Pain in the shoulder region is often not due to arthritis, but to subacromial bursitis or involvement of the shoulder cuff area (which includes the muscular attachments to the tuberosities). The bursitis is often secondary to tears, hemorrhage or calcification in the supraspinatus tendon. Periarthritis and fibrositis are also common. Involvement of the acromioclavicular joint is found commonly in osteoarthritis and rheumatoid arthritis.

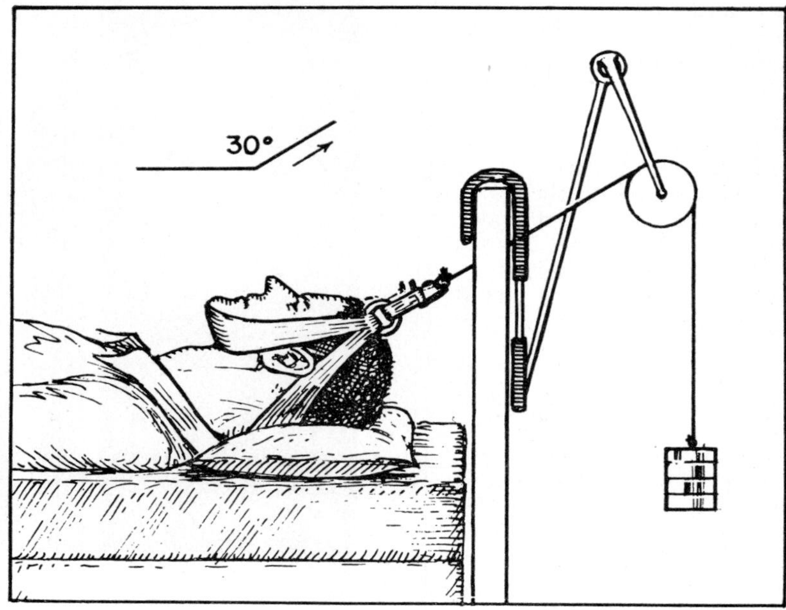

FIG. 37–19.—Head traction (5 to 10 lbs.) is applied through Sayre head sling attached to weight at head of bed. Traction applied at about 30° upward from mattress seems to be most effective.

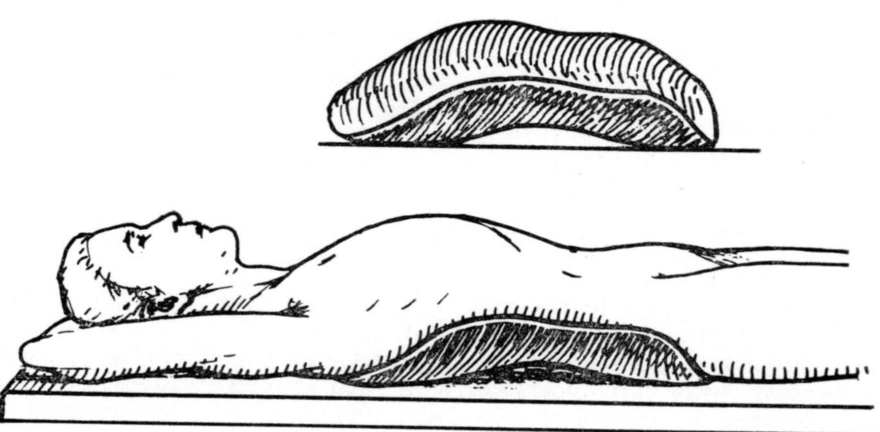

FIG. 37–20.—Back shell. This is made with the patient lying prone on a thick pillow. It is used with the patient lying supine to improve posture and to encourage better rib extension.

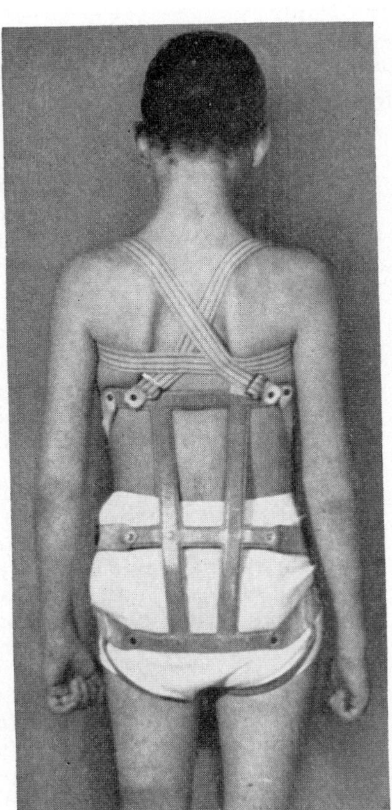

FIG. 37–21.—Spinal brace with elastic shoulder straps. This is more comfortable but gives less rigid support than a plaster jacket.

Prevention of Deformity of the Shoulder in Arthritis

In an effort to prevent deformities of the shoulders, one should avoid the use of more than one pillow beneath the head, neck or back. A firm mattress should be used. In acute arthritis rest the shoulder with the arm in 90° of abduction and about neutral rotation; this may be maintained in bed by pillows, or a removable platform splint. This will prevent the tendency to forward dropping of the shoulder with adduction and internal rotation of the arm which commonly accompanies arthritis of the shoulder.

Hot fomentations or other heat should be applied to the shoulder for thirty minutes several times a day during the acute stage of an arthritis to relax muscular spasm and relieve discomfort.

In painful, adducted shoulders, abduct the arms gradually by inserting small pillows between the arm and the chest wall. As soon as tolerated, perform exercises to maintain abduction and external rotation. Employ more vigorous physical therapy following subsidence of the acute process. When weakness or deformity has been present a long time, elastic shoulder straps attached to a brace or corset give considerable support and relief of muscular strain.

Active exercises may be encouraged by the use of pulleys or screw eyes attached

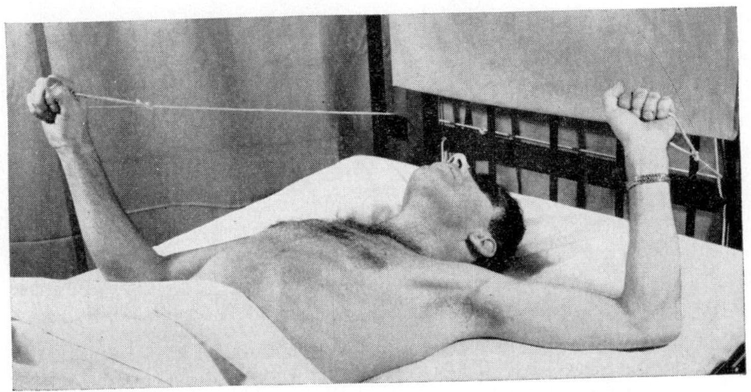

FIG. 37–22.—Rope and pulley for shoulder exercise.

to the head of the bed with a rope passing through these. The ends of the rope are held in the patient's hands and as he pulls down on one end of the rope, the other arm is pulled up and vice versa. Such traction can be used overhead when the patient becomes ambulatory. In rheumatoid arthritis of the shoulders, the patient should attempt to clasp the hands behind the head and flatten out the flexed elbows on the bed for periods of ten minutes three times a day. The reader should refer to Chapter 80 on "The Painful Shoulder" for a more detailed discussion of this subject.

The common deformities occurring in arthritis involving the shoulder joint are adduction and internal rotation of the arm; true ankylosis of the shoulder joint rarely occurs.

Prevention of Deformity at Elbow

Heat may be used to lessen muscular spasm and pain at any stage of the arthritis. Hot, moist compresses wrapped around the elbow are best.

The most common deformity at this joint is flexion with pronation of the forearm.[21] Prevent such deformity as follows:

- In acute arthritis of the elbow, a splint should be worn with the elbow at 70° including the wrist. The splint is removed at least once daily to permit several active movements of the joint.
- If ankylosis seems inevitable, the elbow is flexed to 70 to 80° and the forearm is splinted in slight supination (10 to 15°).
- Special exercises and physical therapy are instituted as soon as possible. Occupational therapy is of particular value.
- In milder forms of inflammation a firm bandage may be enough. If there is lasting damage to the elbow a laced elbow support with hinges can be worn.

The Elbow

The first deformity is slight flexion followed by limitation of full supination.[29] As the arthritis progresses, swelling develops on both sides of the olecranon. Later, severe limitation of motion and stiffness or subluxation are seen. When the elbow is involved in arthritis, it should be protected constantly by an elastic bandage. A sling is also sometimes

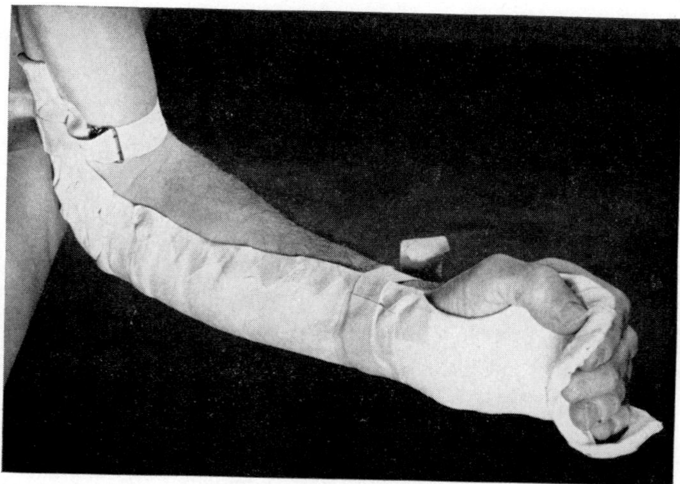

Fig. 37–23.—Resting shell for the elbow. The elbow is near right-angle flexion. The forearm is at neutral rotation.

necessary in the acute stage. Deformity is prevented by a plaster splint worn particularly at night, holding the elbow at about 70° flexion. This splint should include the forearm and wrist in about 15° of supination.

The elbow joint is often sprained by arthritic patients. It is a non-weight-bearing joint, but the arthritic individual supports himself by holding on to chairs or tables, or by using a cane if the legs are weak or deformed, thus employing the elbow as a partial weight-bearing structure. This additional trauma to the elbow joint is of importance in leading to further destruction of the joint. The customary attitude assumed by the arthritic patient in bed, with the elbow at an angle of 90° or less and the hand in pronation on the chest, assures the patient of comfort but encourages a flexion deformity. In severe arthritis a bivalved cast from axilla to fingers may be required with the elbow at 70° of the flexion and the forearm in mid rotation.

The Wrist and Hand

Palmar flexion is the common deformity of the wrist.[17] Deformity is due to the pull of the strong flexor muscles and to gravity. The flexion deformity which results decreases the normal grasping power of the hand, because the fulcrum of the flexor tendons is changed. In acute arthritis the ligaments about the distal end of the ulna become stretched by the swelling and become relaxed. Dorsal subluxation of the ulna is common. This is often followed by fraying of the extensor tendons. In late arthritis the wrist may become fused in flexion and ulnar deviation. The lower radio-ulnar joint is involved in the fusion, preventing supination and pronation.

Relaxation of the carpal ligaments, with muscle atrophy, permits flattening of the three palmar arches (proximal and distal palmar arches, and longitudinal palmar arch). This is usually brought about by weight-bearing on the outstretched hand as in getting up from a chair or bed, and leads to the "flat hand deformity of arthritis." In long-standing arthritis the carpal and metacarpal bones may become a single fused mass, or a gradual absorption of the carpal bones may occur.

The first change noted in the fingers and metacarpophalangeal joints in arthritis is swelling of these joints. This may be extensive and stretch the articular capsule, leading to instability of the joints. There is a gradual flexion in these joints. At the metacarpophalangeal joints, flexion is followed by ulnar deviation and subluxation. At the thumb, flexion occurs first at the metacarpophalangeal joint. This interferes with the grasping action of the thumb and index finger. As the distal and proximal transverse palmar arches become flattened the thumb comes to lie in the same plane as the fingers and opposition of the thumb becomes lost.[2]

In the latter stages with extensive bony atrophy, distortion and telescoping take place in the bones of the wrist and fingers. Hyperextension occurs at the proximal interphalangeal joints. At the metacarpophalangeal joints the heads of the metacarpal bones become flattened on the ulnar side. A complementary distortion occurs at the base of the first phalanx.

Prevention of Deformities at Wrist and Hand

- A cock-up splint from the upper forearm to the fingertips is applied to hold the wrist in 35° of dorsiflexion and the fingers in 10° flexion; ulnar deviation must be prevented by a flange on the ulnar side.
- Special exercises and occupational therapy for the hands are needed.
- If ankylosis is inevitable, the wrist should be held in 35° of dorsiflexion with the fingers in 30 to 40° flexion at the interphalangeal joints.[25] Paraffin wax or electric mitts are useful methods of heat application; this should be followed by active exercises.

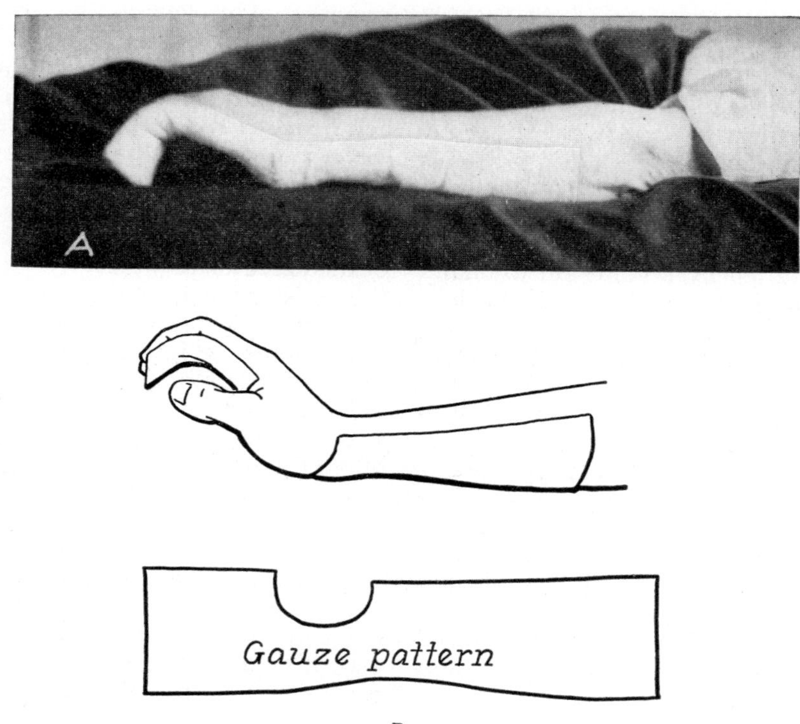

FIG. 37–24.—*A*, Resting hand cast. The fingers are slightly flexed. The wrist is dorsiflexed. The palmar arches are molded. *B*, Model for resting hand cast.

This causes permanent subluxation and ulnar displacement of the finger. The same bony disintegration involves the thumb, causing adduction and flexion of the proximal phalanx and hyperextension of the distal phalanx.

Deformities vary greatly in the hand and splinting must vary with the degree and type of deformity presented. With swelling of the interphalangeal joints and beginning flexion, a volar plaster splint should be applied extending from the upper third of the arm to the fingertips holding the wrist in 35° of dorsiflexion and the fingers in mild flexion (10°). The palmar arches are molded into the plaster. If there is beginning deformity of the thumb, the thumb should be abducted and in a position for apposition to the fingers. Such splints are worn most of the time at first. As the symptoms subside, splints are worn only at night and eventually are discarded. Mild deformities can frequently be corrected by changes of the plaster splints, each one achieving further correction of the deformity. If there is ulnar deviation, a flange is put on the ulnar side of the fingers to keep them straight. A plaster cuff, molded snugly about the metacarpophalangeal joints, is helpful in preventing ulnar deviation and subluxation at these joints. It is held by an elastic band and can be slipped on and off the hand with ease. An elastic cotton bandage or adhesive strapping makes a useful temporary support. Fixed plaster splints are used during the acute phase of arthritis and various types of spring or traction splints are used for aid in correction of deformities after the acute arthritis has subsided. Dynamic splints, using wire

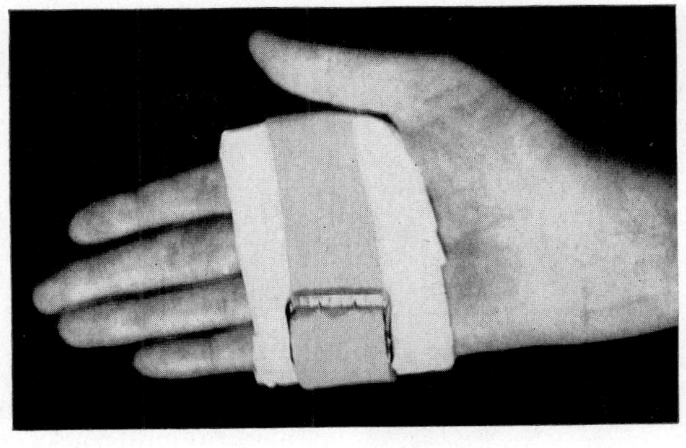

A

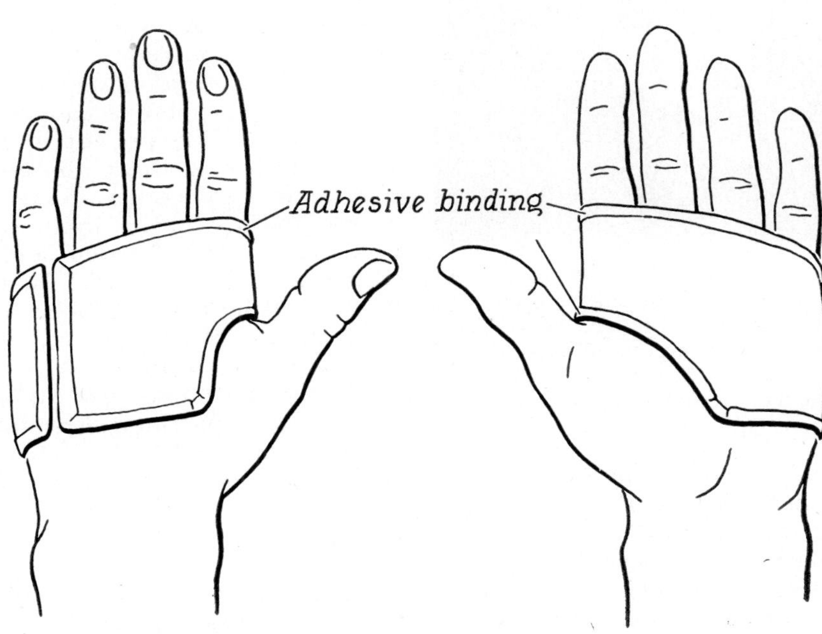

B

FIG. 37–25.—*A*, Plaster cuff to prevent metacarpophalangeal dislocation and ulnar deviation of the fingers, volar aspect. *B*, Diagram showing both dorsal and volar aspects.

loops and elastic bands, are used to gain function and correct deformity at the metacarpophalangeal joints when ulnar drift and anterior subluxation occur. They are also used pre- and postoperatively for surgery at the metacarpophalangeal joints, such as in cases of arthroplasty, synovectomy, and extensor tendon relocations (*see* Chapter 40—Hand).

The Tendon Sheaths

One of the most disabling conditions in the hand is tenosynovitis, involvement of the tendon sheaths by rheumatoid

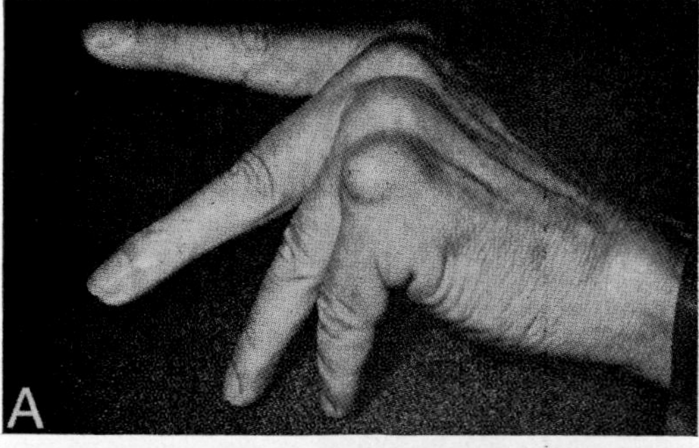

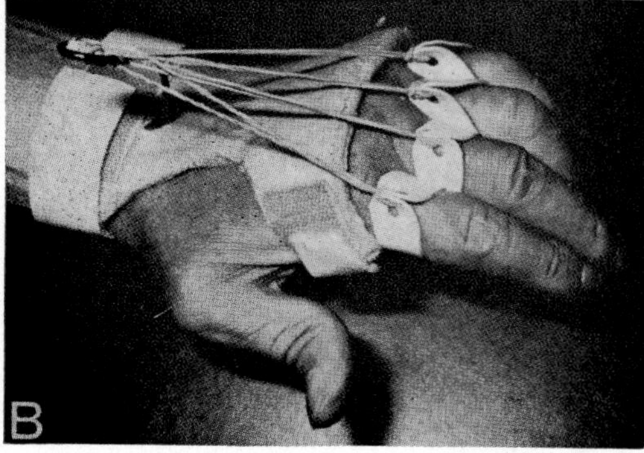

Fig. 37–26.—Dynamic splints are useful both in the preoperative and postoperative care of the rheumatoid hand. A. Patient with loss of active finger extension secondary to displacement of extensor tendons. B. Note improved postoperative posture of hand with dynamic splint.[25]

granulations. Here granulation tissue grows within the tendon sheath and upon the tendon itself. Cysts form with adhesions, degeneration and eventual rupture of the tendon. Small cysts and granulations can be excised but rarely can the pathologic lesion be removed completely. When there is extensive involvement of the tendon, suture or grafting of the tendon is often required. Often continuing degeneration leads to further disability after tendons have been repaired.

Fraying and eventual rupture of the extensor tendons at the wrist are occasionally found. These changes result from several causes. The most frequent cause is dorsal dislocation of the lower end of the ulna with subsequent pressure on the extensor tendons. Less common causes are bony overgrowth, adhesions and decreased elasticity in the tendons. Treatment is splinting of the tendon. The displaced lower end of the ulna can be excised if there is much dorsal displacement. Frayed or ruptured tendons should be repaired.

Snapping or temporary locking of one or more fingers is seen in at least a third of the hands affected by rheumatoid arthritis. This is most commonly seen in the flexor tendons in the palm of the hand. Most of these are not particularly disabling. If the locking persists, accompanied by tenderness and palpable thickening of a small portion of the tendon sheath, it can be relieved temporarily by injection of a suspension of hydrocortisone into the tendon sheath. If the lesion continues, the tendon sheath should be opened at the point of constriction. If arthritis has been present in the hand for a number of years, thickening and contracture sometimes occur in the palmar fascia. This is indistinguishable clinically and microscopically from Dupuytren's contracture. In the early stages this thickening can be helped by splinting and physiotherapy. When the palmar fascia is markedly contracted, preventing full extension of the finger, the same surgical measures are employed as are used in other cases of Dupuytren's contracture (*see also* Chapter 81).

The Jaw

The temporomandibular joint is affected in at least a fourth of the patients suffering from rheumatoid arthritis. Temporary limitation of motion is common and ankylosis of this joint is rare. Deformity, particularly shortening of the mandible, is seen most often in the juvenile form of rheumatoid arthritis. With shortening of the mandible the lower teeth come behind those of the maxilla, the receding lower jaw giving the bird-like appearance. In adults, malocclusion is more commonly seen with involvement of one temporomandibular joint. The most common deformity in both children and adults is a narrowed bite. This

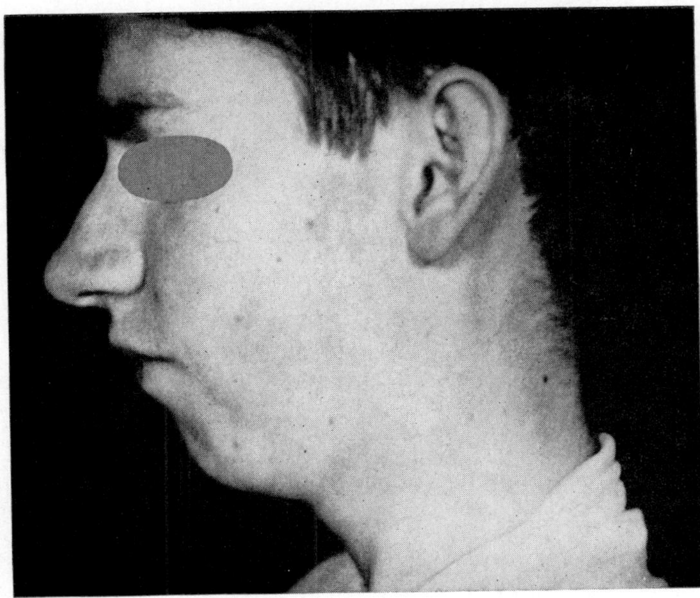

FIG. 37–27.—Shortness of the lower jaw from juvenile rheumatoid arthritis, producing "bird-like facies."

varies with the severity of the arthritis and is rarely a permanent feature. In osteoarthritis, limitation or locking in the temporomandibular joint may occur from degeneration or displacement of the fibrocartilage, occasionally from osseous proliferation about the joint.

Treatment varies with the severity of the articular inflammation. Good dental care with proper occlusion of the teeth helps to prevent inflammation. External heat over the temporomandibular joint, fifteen to thirty minutes, is applied several times a day. Rest to the jaw is obtained by the temporary use of a many-tailed bandage tied over the occiput. A liquid or soft diet which requires no chewing is helpful for a few days if all movement is painful. Injections of hydrocortisone directly into the temporomandibular joint often lead to rapid subsidence of the inflammation. If the bite is less than 1 inch wide, the jaw may be stretched by inserting tongue depressors or corks between the incisor teeth. They are later moved to the premolars and molar teeth to widen the bite. Exercises to loosen the lower jaw are prescribed.

Acute involvement of the temporomandibular joint occurs in 20 per cent of patients with rheumatoid arthritis. During the acute stage, the teeth should be in centric occlusion, barely separated, and held in this position even while eating or talking. The patient must not stretch his jaw to see how he is progressing. Mild exercises may be instituted when muscular spasm and pain have lessened considerably. Heat should be applied locally over the joint fifteen to twenty minutes several times a day. Mild gumchewing exercises may then be begun, chewing at first a soft and later a harder gum for fifteen to thirty minutes several times a day.

BIBLIOGRAPHY

1. AIDEM, H. P.: J.A.M.A., *187*, 4, 1964.
2. BAKER, L. D.: South Med. J., *36*, 180, 1943.
3. BASTOW, J.: Proc. Roy. Soc. Med., *57*, 6, 1964.

4. Dittuno, J.: Geriatrics, *25*, March 1970.
5. Gordon, K. I.: Physiotherapy, *56*, Oct. 1970.
6. Graham, D. C.: Canadian Med. Assn. J., *77*, 1128, 1957.
7. Haw, D. W.: Guy's Hospital Report, *113*, 6, 1964.
8. Hill, D. F.: Med. Clin. North America, *39*, 393, 1955.
9. Howarth, M. B.: *Textbook of Orthopedics*, Philadelphia, W. B. Saunders, 1952.
10. Joplin, R. J., and Baer, G. J.: J.A.M.A., *118*, 938, 1942.
11. Jordon, H. H.: New York State J. Med., *39*, 1823, 1939.
12. Katz, S. *et al.*: J.A.M.A., *206*, Nov. 1968.
13. Kelly, M.: New Zealand Med. J., *55*, 11, 1956.
14. ————: Med. J. Australia, *1*, 287, 1960.
15. ————: Canad. Med. Assn. J., *81*, 827, 1959.
16. Key, J. A.: West. J. Surg., *52*, 385, 1944.
17. Kuhns, J. G.: W. Virginia Med. Assn. J., *39*, 44, 1943.
18. ————: Clinics, *4*, 1463, 1946.
19. ————: Brit. J. Phys. Med., *8*, 270, 1953.
20. ————: Clin. Orthop., *25*, 60, 1962.
21. Lowman, E. W.: Public Health Reports, *72*, 1101, 1957.
22. Luck, V. L.: J.A.M.A., *124*, 23, 1944.
23. Mills, J. *et al.*: New Engl. J. Med., *284*, 9, 1971.
24. Piersol, G. M. and Hollander, J. L.: Arch. Phys. Med., *28*, 500, 1947.
25. Potter, T. A. and Nalebuff, E. A.: Surg. Clinics of North America, *49*, 4, 1969.
26. Ropes, M. R.: Med. Clin. North America, *45*, 1197, 1961.
27. Swaim, L. T.: J. Bone Joint Surg., *21*, 983, 1939.
28. Swaim, L. T.: Amer. J. Nursing, *36*, 211, 1936.
29. Swaim, L. T. and Kuhns, J. G.: J.A.M.A., *93*, 1953, 1929; *94*, 1123, 1930; *94*, 1743, 1930.
30. Taylor, D.: Canad. Med. Assn. J., *82*, 995, 1960.
31. Tegner, W.: Practitioner, *171*, 424, 1953.

Chapter 38

Synovectomy in Rheumatoid Arthritis

By John L. Sbarbaro, Jr., M.D.

The importance of the concept of removing the inflamed synovium in rheumatoid arthritis has been recognized internationally over the past decade. At a working conference held in New York City in 1963 by the American Rheumatism Association, the National Institute of Arthritis and Metabolic Diseases and the Arthritis Foundation, a group of fifty orthopedic surgeons, rheumatologists and physiatrists agreed that a number of investigations were needed, the most pressing of which was an in-depth evaluation of early synovectomy as a measure to prevent progressive joint deterioration. Further interest and emphasis were accorded this problem when an international five-day symposium was held in Amsterdam in 1967 which brought together sixty participants from twelve countries to consider "Early Synovectomy in Rheumatoid Arthritis." At the conclusion of this symposium, because the efficacy of early synovectomy was still in doubt, it was agreed to launch a controlled international multi-center five-year evaluation of early synovectomy with special interest in determining the value and limitations of this surgical procedure as a prophylactic measure. This study is now in progress.

Historical Considerations.—Early reports on synovectomy go back to the mid-19th century. However, it was not until 1900 that Mignon[11] reported its application in the treatment of rheumatoid arthritis. Sweet[16] in 1923 reported a more extensive study and claimed good results if the procedure was done early in the course of the disease. Interest was stimulated further by Key's[9] studies in 1925 which demonstrated that when the synovial membrane of rabbit joints was surgically removed, a new membrane was formed in eight weeks, and that this membrane was quite similar to the original synovium. Increasing interest was generated for a number of years but the procedure gradully went into disfavor because of conflicting reports regarding its value. Throughout this developmental period, many factors limited the application of synovectomy. Fear of exacerbation of the disease forced many surgeons to conclude that the procedure should be performed only in the late or "burned out" stages of the disease. Fear on the part of the patient for any surgical procedure and a negative attitude on the part of the physician along with poor communication to surgeons all contributed to the confusion that existed.

During the last fifteen years, there has been an expanding interest in synovectomy. This revival of interest has been in no small part due to the observation that a synovectomized joint frequently does not share in an acute rheumatoid flare-up which involves other joints in the body. The dramatic relief of pain often resulting from synovectomy has encouraged many physicians to recommend the procedure early in the course of the disease.

Many authorities on the subject have enthusiastically endorsed prophylactic synovectomy as a procedure to be carried out early, before there is any observable joint destruction. There is considerable difference of opinion as to what is ***early.***

What technique should be employed? Is synovectomy really necessary? Is it really effective? Rheumatoid arthritis is a capricious disease that in its natural course may wax and wane. The responsibility of selecting patients for synovectomy usually resides with the internist or rheumatologist who is treating the patient on a continuing basis and who is most aware of the fluctuations in rheumatoid activity. It is extremely difficult to evaluate any form of therapy, especially a surgical procedure, under these circumstances. Freyberg[5] in an excellent study of many patients demonstrated the difficulty in predicting which joints will sustain little or no damage and which joints will progress to severe destruction. Many joints will undergo spontaneous resolution of the inflammation. If these joints were among those subjected to synovectomy, the results attributable to the surgery would be falsified by this natural remission. This circumstance emphasizes the need for controlled clinical trials. The broad-based, multi-center trials now in progress in the United States and in the United Kingdom should be of great help in evaluating the efficacy of early synovectomy, especially as a prophylactic procedure.

Anatomic Considerations.—The synoviocyte is the lining cell of synovium which usually forms a thin layer that lines an articulation or envelops a tendon. Beneath these cells there is a loose fibrous stroma that is rich in mucopolysaccharides. The synovium is attached to bone at the osteochondral junction where the synovial blood supply originates. The relationship of this blood supply to bone, marrow, cartilage and synovium is an important consideration in rheumatoid arthritis. The microvascular circulation depends on long, slender vascular channels and loops with interconnecting shunts. Villous tufts are also supplied with delicate capillary loops. The synovium does not have appreciable vascular communication with the capsule. The capsule appears to be well endowed with somatic nerve fibers as demonstrated both microscopically and clinically. The synovium has scattered areas of nerve plexus whose function is obscure. The cartilage is devoid of innervation. (*See also* Chapter 4.)

Pathologic Considerations.—"Chronic nonspecific synovitis consistent with rheumatoid arthritis" is the usual diagnosis reported by the pathologist studying a synovial specimen from a rheumatoid patient. The synovial hyperplasia and stromal hypertrophy, along with lymphocytic and plasma cell infiltration, are pathologic features not limited to rheumatoid synovitis. The specific diagnosis of rheumatoid arthritis cannot be made pathologically. Branemark *et al.*[2] studied the microscopy and demonstrated that the venules had a circuitous course with variable diameter and a markedly reduced flow with stagnation of blood. Vessels in granulation tissue were seen eroding cartilage at the bone-cartilage border. These characteristics are not unique and even electron microscopy has not revealed that they are pathognomonic of rheumatoid disease.

Once initiated, the chronic synovitis tends to persist. The two characteristic findings are synovial hyperplasia and stromal hypertrophy with packing of the stromal tissues by lymphocytes and plasma cells.

Immunologic Consideration.—One cannot ignore the tremendous strides that have been made toward understanding the immunologic abnormalities of rheumatoid arthritis for these are basic to the rationale of synovectomy. Although this subject is covered in detail in Chapters 14 and 19, a brief summary is appropriate here.

An agglutinating factor,[4] later demonstrated[15] as "rheumatoid factor," was found to be present in most sera from rheumatoid arthritic patients. This was later shown in numerous studies to be a macroglobulin (IgM) which has all the characteristics of an antibody against altered gamma globulin (IgG). The etiologic agent that alters the IgG to induce its antigenicity is not known.

Cytoplasmic inclusions were noted in the polymorphonuclear leukocytes of rheumatoid arthritic synovial fluid.[6,7] These inclusions were shown to contain phagocytized IgG, IgM (presumably rheumatoid factor) and complement.[14] The hypothesis was then formulated[7] that the inflammatory reaction in the joints of rheumatoid arthritis could result from the antigen-antibody complexing of IgG with rheumatoid factor, fixing complement and attracting phagocytes by chemotaxis. As the phagocytes take up the complexes, they release their destructive lysosomal enzymes. Increased lysosomal enzyme concentrations have been demonstrated in rheumatoid synovial fluid.[1] Complement levels in rheumatoid synovial fluid are significantly decreased,[12] suggesting that it is being consumed in the reaction.

Most important here is that the rheumatoid synovium has been shown to be engorged with lymphocytes and plasma cells, which form gamma globulins in the immune reaction. The rheumatoid synovium, therefore, seems to be the source, at least in large part, of the factors which perpetuate the joint inflammation. The chain of events listed above has been largely confirmed by subsequent studies (*see* Chapter 19). It would appear rational to remove the diseased synovium and thus suppress further joint inflammation and destruction.

Clinical Considerations.—The clinical course of rheumatoid arthritis is often relentless, resulting in joint destruction and in tendon rupture when the tendon sheaths are involved. If prophylactic synovectomy can halt, or even substantially suppress, this relentless and destructive process, it is certainly justified.

To be effective, synovectomy of the rheumatoid arthritic joint must be done "early," before destructive changes result from continuing rheumatoid inflammation and while the joint appears normal by roentgenogram. If there is joint "narrowing" or marginal erosive change demonstrated by x-ray, the disease has advanced beyond the stage of soft tissue inflammation and has progressed to a destructive arthritis of the bone. It is important to realize that results of synovectomy for rheumatoid synovitis and synovectomy for arthritis involving bone would be quite different.

Another point to consider is the *adequacy* of the synovectomy. The synovium is like a sac surrounding the joint and is attached at the osteochondral junction where the marrow vessels enter the synovium. It is in this area that the synovitis is most active. Hypertrophic villi, granulation tissue and erosive changes usually spread from the osteochondral juncture. Since rheumatoid synovial tissue appears to be a "factory and storehouse" of the reacting immune globulins, most authorities agree that as much synovium should be removed as is technically possible.

The dramatic relief of pain following a synovectomy has been reported in many follow-up studies. The pain relief does not appear to be due to denervation of the joint since similar nerve endings have been demonstrated in reformed synovium by Branemark.[3] If synovectomy does interfere with the pathogenetic mechanism, the eradication of the lymphoid tissue and suppression of the inflammatory reaction probably account for the pain relief.

Normal synovium will regenerate after synovectomy in a normal joint and it has been assumed that normal synovium will regenerate in a rheumatoid joint. Concerning this there are conflicting reports and probably the studies of reformed synovium obtained by "blind" needle biopsy have added to the confusion. Indeed, normal synovium and rheumatoid synovium can be demonstrated in biopsies of the same joint lining.

Branemark[2] re-explored 12 joints which were symptom-free one year after synovectomy for verified rheumatoid arthritis and found chronic non-specific synovitis comparable to the original specimen. It is not known, however, whether the reformed synovium has the same immunologic properties as the original diseased tissue.

Ranawat *et al.*[13] also studied regenerated synovium in rheumatoid patients. The knee joints of 12 patients with rheumatoid arthritis were biopsied to study the regenerated synovium 6 months to 6 years after synovectomy. Three of the 12 patients had clinical and microscopic evidence of recurrence of rheumatoid inflammation. Specimens from the remaining 9 patients all showed mild-to-moderate synovitis. In 4 of these 9 patients who were biopsied at intervals of 3½ to 6 years after synovectomy, microscopic features of rheumatoid inflammation were quantitatively less severe than those observed in the initial specimens.

It is difficult to specify what joints in what patients should be subjected to synovectomy. There are many variables, not the least of which is the capricious nature of the disease itself, that waxes and wanes with time. The efficacy of any form of therapy must be evaluated with consideration to this irregular course of the disease activity.

It is agreed that an intensive medical program is the first line of defense against rheumatoid activity. Continued rheumatoid activity in spite of diligent medical treatment may be sufficient reason to consider synovectomy in those joints in which the procedure is technically feasible. In rapidly progressive disease, it may be prudent to consider synovectomy as early as six months following the onset of symptoms in any particular joint. In most cases the time to consider synovectomy cannot be related so much to the calendar as to the progress of synovitis which varies so greatly in speed from patient to patient as well as in different joints in the same patient.

In reviewing his experience with early synovectomy, Mason[10] referred to the dilemma that he was forced to advise synovectomy before he knew whether it was necessary or not, based on the unproven predication that continuing inflammation would surely cause irreparable joint damage; if he waited until he was certain that synovectomy was required, it would be too late.

The major indication for early synovectomy is not pain, not stiffness, but rather persistent synovitis manifested by effusion and synovial thickening. It is not the pain and it is not the stiffness that destroys a joint or tendon but rather the continuing destruction by the inflammatory process. If this cannot be controlled by appropriate medical therapy, then surgical synovectomy should be given full consideration in an attempt to abort the progressive destruction.

Special Surgical Considerations Relating to Specific Joints

Upper Extremity.—The proximal interphalangeal joints of the fingers are amenable to synovectomy. Excellent exposure is obtained through a lateral incision and detachment of the collateral ligament.

The metacarpophalangeal joints are readily approached through a dorsal transverse incision. The dorsal hood is opened with a linear incision on the radial side of the joint. The entire capsule and both collateral ligaments are excised *in toto*. In this way the volar recesses can be thoroughly explored for total synovectomy.

The flexor tendon sheaths are not amenable to routine synovectomy. Extensive postoperative adhesions usually compromise any beneficial effect from the tenosynovectomy. The flexor tendons can tolerate a considerable degree of synovitis; rupture of a flexor tendon, although possible, is rare. If a flexor tendon should rupture, formal reconstruction could be performed. (*See also* Chapter 40.)

Dorsal tenosynovitis of the wrist is quite common and is frequently associated with tendon rupture. Early synovectomy of this area is an excellent and rewarding procedure.

Synovitis of the radiocarpal and intercarpal joints is common. However, synovectomy of these joints is not practical and not advised. If disability or deformity becomes severe, stabilization or fusion of the wrist is the procedure of choice. (*See also* Chapter 40.)

Synovitis of the volar carpal canal is also common and usually presents clinically as a carpal tunnel syndrome with median nerve compression neuritis. Many of these cases can be treated successfully by intrasynovial injection of the ulnar bursa with an appropriate corticosteroid suspension. If symptoms are persistent or severe, a radical synovectomy of the volar carpal canal and palm is indicated.

Synovitis of the interphalangeal and/or metacarpophalangeal joints of the thumb can be treated by synovectomy. Great care must be taken to preserve the collateral ligaments and to secure firm fixation when they are reattached to bone.

The elbow is commonly involved in rheumatoid arthritis. Most patients develop 15 to 20 degrees of flexion contracture of this joint, but this offers very little functional impairment. For this reason, synovectomy is not indicated in most instances. If persistent florid synovitis exists, a synovectomy should be performed. This is usually done through a lateral approach together with excision of the radial head and detachment of the collateral ligament. Overhead olecranon skeletal traction relieves most of the postoperative pain and encourages early movements. The results are usually very good, even in late cases.

The shoulder is a common site of synovitis. There has been very little experience with early synovectomy of the shoulder. Most patients develop some pain and contracture; however, the disability is usually tolerable. Intractable pain and disability may require joint reconstruction with an endoprosthesis. (*See also* Chapter 40.)

Lower Extremity.—Synovectomy of the hip is technically feasible but hazardous for the capital circulation. There has been very limited experience with this procedure.

The knee has been the joint most frequently subjected to synovectomy. Usually an anterior approach is adequate but occasionally the popliteal area has to be explored for cyst excision. While it is technically difficult to remove all synovium, every effort should be made to excise as much synovium as possible. Through an anteromedial parapatellar incision, a complete anterior synovectomy is performed. The suprapatellar pouch, infrapatellar fat pad and both menisci are removed. The cruciate ligaments are debrided and a rongeur is then employed to explore and extract synovium from the posterior recesses.

The ankle and surrounding tendons have been subjected to synovectomy but relatively infrequently. The limited reports of results are encouraging. Several incisions are necessary to perform an adequate procedure.

The subtalar and mid-tarsal joints are not usually suited to synovectomy. If involvement becomes severe, triple arthrodesis will give the most serviceable foot and is considered the procedure of choice.

The forefoot is another common site of synovitis. Early synovectomy of the metatarsophalangeal joints is possible, however, the residual stiffness is undesirable. It is usually considered better to wait until deformity develops, and, if severe, proceed with a forefoot reconstruction (*see* Chapter 39).

Spine.—Synovectomy of the facets is not feasible and should not be attempted. Most involved facets will develop a fibrous ankylosis. The most critical area of synovitis is in the articulations between the odontoid of the axis and the anterior arch of the atlas. Chronic synovitis of this area leads to an attenuation of the transverse ligament. The resultant hypermobility of the atlantoaxial relationship can be lethal, if the odontoid should impinge on the cord. Synovectomy is not practical; atlantoaxial or occipitoaxial fusion is the recommended procedure.

SUMMARY

Properly performed, synovectomy can be beneficial in the majority of instances, in well-selected joints adaptable to such surgery, especially to relieve pain produced by severe progressive rheumatoid synovitis. In many patients, the joint operated upon may not exhibit recurrent inflammation for many months or years. This has led to the rationale that, if done early in the course of rheumatoid arthritis before structural damages have occurred, synovectomy may protect the joint against the cartilage, bone and tendon damage that could result from continued prolonged synovitis. Thus synovectomy could be prophylactic as well as therapeutic. However, to what extent synovectomy can be depended upon to prevent or substantially delay the development of destruction from persistent severe synovitis will require much more clinical investigation to determine. Multi-center controlled studies now under way should more clearly define the benefits and shortcomings of "early" synovectomy, and indicate its true place in the management of patients with rheumatoid arthritis. It must be remembered that each joint is only one in a system involved in progressive disease and that, at best, synovectomy is only one step—a local supplemental portion—of a treatment program. Each rheumatoid arthritic patient will continue to require adequate and sustained systemic therapy.

BIBLIOGRAPHY

1. Astorga, G. and Bollet, A. J.: Arth. & Rheum., *8*, 511, 1965.
2. Branemark, P. O., Ekholm, R., Goldie, I. and Lindstrome, J.: Acta Rheum. Scand., *13*, 161, 1967.
3. Branemark, P. O. and Goldie, I.: In *Early Synovectomy in Rheumatoid Arthritis*, Eds. Hijmans, W., Paul, W. D. and Herschel, H., Amsterdam, Excerpta Medica Fdn., 1969.
4. Cecil, R. L., Nichols, E. E. and Stainsby, W. J.: Am. J. Med. Sci., *181*, 12, 1931.
5. Freyberg, R. H.: In *Early Synovectomy in Rheumatoid Arthritis*. Eds. Hijmans, W., Paul, W. D. and Herschel, H., Amsterdam, Excerpta Medica Fdn., 1969, p. 98.
6. Hollander, J. L., Rawson, A. J., Restifo, R. A. and Lussier, A. J.: Arth. & Rheum., *7*, 314, 1964.
7. Hollander, J. L., McCarty, D. J., Astorga, G. and Castro-Murillo, E.: Ann. Intern. Med., *62*, 271, 1965.
8. Hollander, J. L., Fudenburg, H. H., Rawson, A. J., Abelson, N. M. and Torralba T. P.: Arth. & Rheum., *9*, 675, 1966.
9. Key, J. A.: J. Bone & Joint Surg., *6*, 800, 1924.
10. Mason, M. A.: In *Early Synovectomy in Rheumatoid Arthritis*. Eds. Hijmans, W., Paul, W. D. and Herschel, H. Amsterdam, Excerpta Medica Fdn., 1969, p. 50.
11. Mignon, M. A.: Bull. Soc. Clinc. Paris, *26*, 1113, 1900.
12. Pekin, T. J. and Zvaifler, N. J.: J. Clin. Invest., *43*, 1373, 1964.
13. Ranawat, C. S., Straub, L. R., Freyberg, R. H., Granda, J. L. and Rivelis, M.: Arth. & Rheum., *14*, 117, 1971.
14. Rawson, A. J., Abelson, N. M. and Hollander, J. L.: Ann. Intern. Med., *62*, 281, 1965.
15. Rose, H. W., Ragan, C., Pearce, E. and Lipman, M. D.: Proc. Soc. Exp. Biol. & Med., *68*, 1, 1948.
16. Sweet, P. P.: J. Bone & Joint Surg., *5*, 110, 1923.

Chapter 39

Correction of Arthritic Deformities

By Theodore A. Potter, M.D.

In severe rheumatoid arthritis, deformities sometimes develop despite the measures outlined in the previous chapters. Many times, also, the physician is faced with a patient who has already developed articular deformities before seeking his treatment. If these deformities are mild or early, the employment of the measures previously outlined, such as heat, exercise, physiotherapy, application of traction, use of rest splints, or even serial application of plaster casts in a position of maximum extension can correct the deformity and no more elaborate or radical procedure is needed.

When serial changes of plaster casts, traction, or corrective exercises fail to correct deformities, the following measures may be considered: skeletal traction, turnbuckles attached to Kirschner wires, manipulation of the joint under anesthesia, surgery of the juxta-articular connective tissues, or surgery of the bones and joints. In the past it was thought that the quiescence of the inflammatory process was absolutely necessary to obtain a good functional result from surgery. However, in the light of present-day thinking this is not necessary.[20] Indeed, most patients coming to surgery today have persistently elevated sedimentation rates, some anemia and many have weight loss. Most operative procedures are carried out when subacute disease is noted clinically and the microscopic appearance of most arthritic synovium has been read by experienced pathologists as showing "acute and chronic inflammation." If the surgeon waited until the arthritic process subsided before performing the planned operation, the joint would become totally destroyed and he would have fewer patients upon whom corrective surgery could be carried out. Prophylactic removal of diseased synovium has been a well-established procedure for many years and is now being utilized more and more by orthopedic surgeons as the procedure of choice to prevent joint damage in certain cases of rheumatoid arthritis of the metacarpal phalangeal joints, of the tendon sheaths and knees.[4]

Biopsy

Before considering the various corrective surgical operations, mention should be made of the important procedure of joint biopsy. When the physician has been unable to establish a specific diagnosis of the type of arthritis, when all laboratory tests and joint fluid examinations have failed to produce definitive results, biopsy may help. The procedures are carried out either by the "closed method" or open operation.

"Closed" Biopsy.—Biopsy under local anesthesia with an instrument such as the Parker-Pearson or Polley-Bickel needle is a simple procedure. Its best use is at the knee but can be employed at the hips, elbows or shoulders. The advantages of this method are the simplicity of obtaining the specimen and a relatively minor operative procedure. The disadvantages are that the procedure is blind, post-biopsy hemarthrosis may occur, and it is rarely adaptable to joint biopsy in children.

"Open" Biopsy.—This is the procedure of choice and is performed either under general or local anesthesia. The distinct advantage of this method is that the surgeon can obtain representative specimens from direct visualization. The morbidity of joint biopsy is very small.

Skeletal Traction

Skeletal traction is employed chiefly in the lower extremity for the purpose of correcting flexion deformities at the hip and knee, and subluxation at the knee. Traction of more than 15 pounds can rarely be employed. The bones are weak and the Kirschner wire will pull through the bone if too great traction is used. Skeletal traction must be supervised constantly to be effective.

Turnbuckles, attached at the sides of the deformed joint to Kirschner wires drilled through the bone and attached to stirrups above and below the joint, are a simple and effective means of correcting subluxation and flexion deformities. While this method can be used in all of the major joints, it is used most commonly about the knee. The limb is kept in balanced Russell's suspension while the stretching is progressing. The turnbuckles separate the bone ends by one or two turns each day At this rate no great pain is felt. The deformity is usually corrected in one to two weeks. When the deformity is corrected, the Kirschner wires are removed under general anesthesia and a plaster cast is applied with the deformity corrected. This cast is bivalved in two to four days when physiotherapy and exercises are begun. The joint usually shows lateral instability for one to two months but this gradually improves as the muscle power increases, especially the quadriceps.

Manipulation[33]

This is the forceful stretching of a joint under anesthesia. Manipulations are carried out for the relief of two pathological conditions: adhesions within and about the joint and contractures in the muscles and fascia. Often these can be prevented from developing or the milder ones can be corrected by casts and by exercises. If casts have been used conscientiously for several weeks without any improvement in the deformity, manipulation of the joint should be considered. This should not be done if there is acute inflammation in the joint, if roentgenograms show ankylosis, or if the bones and muscles are markedly atrophied.

As a rule, a general anesthesia is given; spinal anesthesia or brachial plexus block is occasionally used. When the patient is completely relaxed, the surgeon grasps the limb on the distal side near the joint; the bone on the proximal side is held firmly by an assistant. The joint is brought into further flexion and is then slowly and forcibly extended. The joint should be stretched only once; the limb should not be "pump-handled." With short leverage there is much less danger of fracturing the atrophic bones (a real danger in every manipulation in arthritis). There is also less danger of tearing blood vessels and nerves. Cracking noises are always heard as adhesions are freed. The stretching of contractures makes no sound. If the surgeon fears that further stretching may fracture bone or tear tissues, he should stop. A further manipulation can be undertaken in one to two weeks.

After manipulation the joint is held in the improved position with a plaster cast until soreness about the joint subsides.[6] Then physiotherapy and exercises are given. A few gentle manipulations may be required to correct a deformity completely. If no improvement follows one manipulation, further manipulations will also be useless and should not be undertaken. When manipulation brings no correction of the deformity, one must consider operation on the soft parts or upon the bones.

While manipulation is used chiefly in quiescent rheumatoid arthritis, it is occasionally a helpful measure in osteoarthritis when there is limitation of

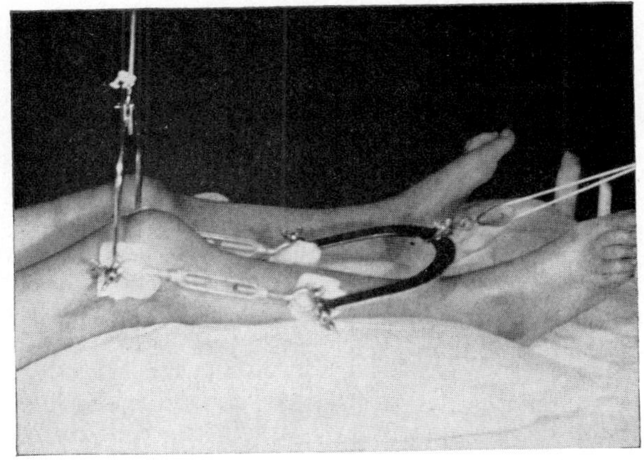

A

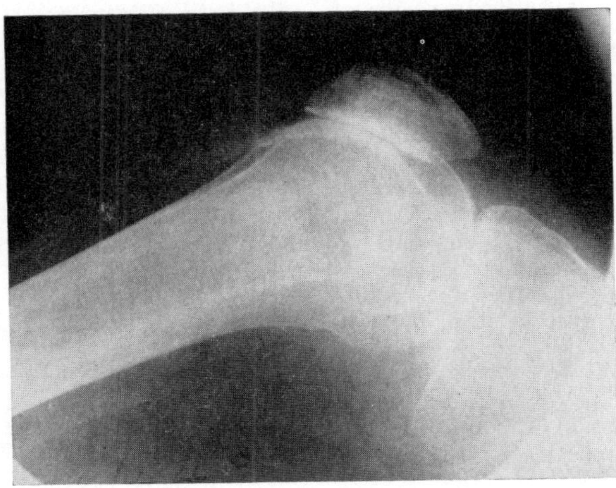

B

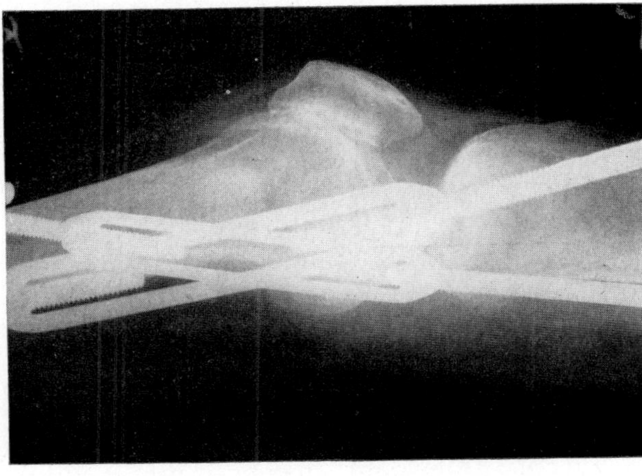

C

Fig. 39–1.—*A*, Skeletal traction with Kirschner wire applied to the knee joint. *B*, Roentgenogram of knee with flexion and subluxation before traction was applied. *C*, Roentgenogram of knee after application of traction. The flexion and subluxation have been corrected.

Manipulation of Deformed Joints:

- Should not be done during the acute stage of arthritis; when the patient is seriously ill; if roentgenograms show bony ankylosis or if there is severe atrophy of bones.
- Indicated in selected cases of deformity due mainly to adhesions within or about the joints or to muscular contractures.
- In degenerative joint disease rarely produces permanent improvement in range of motion or relief of pain; often helpful temporarily in milder cases.
- May be followed by injection of 1 per cent procaine intra-articularly, or by injecting a corticosteroid suspension, to minimize postmanipulation exacerbation of pain and spasm and the reformation of adhesions.
- Always performed under regional or preferably general anesthesia; muscular relaxation is essential for success.
- Move the limb slowly; use short leverage; stretch the limb one time only.
- Great care should be taken during the manipulation because of the possibility of producing fractures of the atrophied bones or tears of the blood vessels or nerves.
- After manipulation apply a plaster cast with the joint in the improved position. Begin exercises and physiotherapy when soreness about the joint decreases. Further manipulation to obtain more correction can be carried out in one week. If manipulation secures no correction, surgery must be considered.

motion, and roentgenograms show only minimal bony overgrowth. In the cervical spine a gentle manipulation followed by traction often relieves the stiffness and secondary irritation of the nerve roots. Manipulation into full elevation and abduction often relieves stiffness at the shoulder. At the time of manipulation of the shoulder or hip joint, a 1 per cent solution of procaine can be injected into the articular cavity. This decreases pain and makes early motion easier. Similarly, the injection of corticosteroid suspension into the joint space, just before or after manipulation, has been found to prevent the increased pain and reflex muscle spasm which may follow manipulation.[30] Manipulation should be followed by exercises to keep a full range of motion at the shoulder. At the hip joint the ability to cross the knees and to tie the shoes can often be regained by a gentle manipulation of the hip in abduction and internal rotation.[7] In these joints the greater range of motion gained is again lost in a few months if the patient does not continue to perform daily stretching exercises. Manipulation has not been found helpful in other joints in osteoarthritis. In the presence of large spurs or extensive bony deformity, manipulation is likely to cause harm.[33]

ORTHOPEDIC SURGERY IN ARTHRITIS

The importance of intensive training in muscular exercise and control for a period of at least several weeks prior to the operation is important. The patient is taught preoperatively to perform those exercises which will be required following the surgical procedure.

Surgery should always be looked upon as an adjunct in the treatment of arthritis. In quiescent or arrested cases, surgery may be required to increase the mobility of the body with a minimum expenditure of the patient's energy.

Ankylosis, per se, does not require surgery. If the ankylosis is in poor position, resulting in increased muscular fatigue, one should then employ the simplest type of osteotomy to correct the deformity. Very little surgery will be required if proper preventive orthopedics has been used early in the disease, since ankylosis, if it occurs, should be in a good position for function.

There is no hard and fast rule con-

Principles in Joint Surgery

Do not operate during the acute stage of an arthritis; joint surgery should be attempted only after a period of less than acute joint activity.

Patients who have been bedridden for years are poor operative risks. Their tissues heal slowly.

Attempt to obtain a functionally useful joint. Orthopedic surgical procedures upon the upper extremity are concerned with the use of the arms, particularly for eating, dressing and personal care, while the leg problem is concerned with the ability to stand and walk.

When both arms and legs are disabled, an attempt should be made to solve the arm problem before the leg condition.

Begin postoperative joint motion as soon as consistent with good wound healing. Hydrotherapy and muscle setting exercises are useful early measures. Later, resistive exercises should be given.

Develop surrounding muscles by exercises for several weeks prior to operation.

cerning surgery in the arthritic. One should discover whether the deformity is due to contraction of tendons or capsules or whether there is an actual bony deformity. One will then decide in that given case whether tendon lengthening, capsulotomy, osteotomy or another procedure is preferable. Usually, unless there is bony ankylosis, plaster casts and manipulation are first tried to see whether they will bring any correction in the deformity. If the deformity is resistant, surgery is next considered.

Aspiration and Arthrotomy

Aspiration for the removal of synovial fluid in a markedly swollen knee often relieves pain and may prevent persistent distention of the articular capsule. It is only temporarily helpful. As a diagnostic procedure it is frequently helpful. (*See* Chapter 6 on Synovial Fluid.) Injection of procaine solution or other analgesic into or about the joint tissues will sometimes relieve pain, but for a short period only.[23] The aspiration of fluid and intra-articular injection of corticosteroid give more lasting symptomatic and objective relief. The technique for this procedure is described in Chapter 32.

Arthrotomy (the surgical opening of a joint) is used for the removal of diseased or damaged tissue, to make a diagnosis or because of derangement in the normal mechanics of the joint. Diagnosis is sometimes difficult to establish in monarticular arthritis. Pathological examination of tissue removed from the joint is often helpful. But in most instances arthrotomy is employed when there is persistent effusion into the joint or locking of the joint. At operation a loose body, synovial fringes, osteophytes, or a degenerated cartilage may be found. After arthrotomy the joint is splinted with a plaster cast or a voluminous pressure dressing for three to five days. Then exercises are given.

Synovectomy, the partial or complete removal of the lining membrane of the joint, is performed most often at the knee but sometimes at the elbow, ankle and metacarpal joints. Synovectomy is indicated when there is persistent thickening of the synovial membrane which interferes with function. In addition there is histological evidence that the invading pannus and hypertrophic synovial lining cause destruction of articular cartilage. This is accomplished by undermining the cartilage and, more important, by direct adherence and subsequent excretion of lytic enzymes, causing gross disappearance of the cartilage. Therefore it is felt that the rationale of prophylactic surgical synovectomy is justified to prevent joint destruction. So far there have been no conclusive reports that chemical synovectomy (*i.e.* arthrocentesis with instillation of cytotoxic agents) has given any lasting effect. (*See also* Chapter 38.)

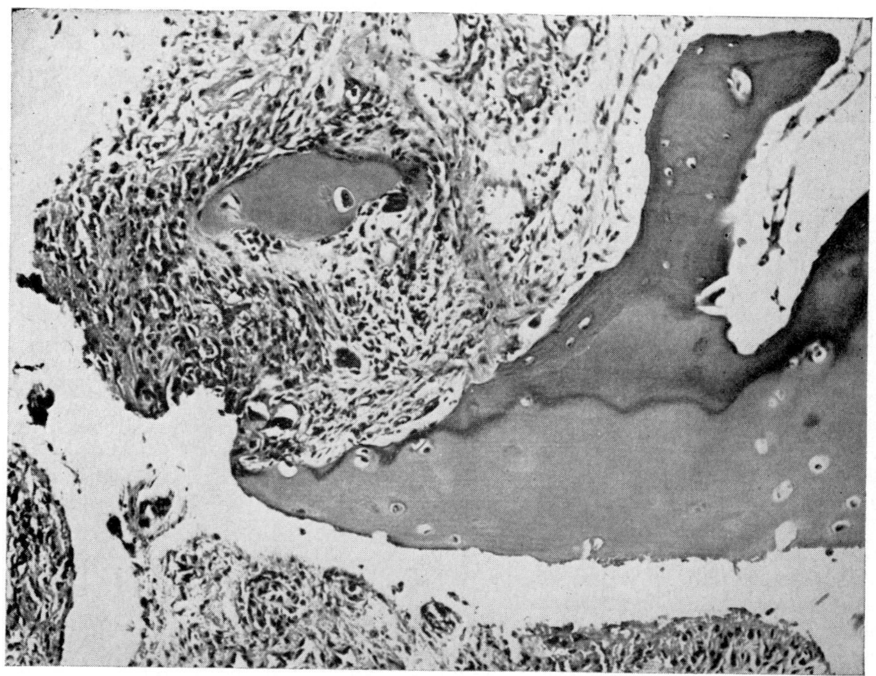

FIG. 39–2.—Histological section of tissue removed at time of synovectomy of the knee. The hyperplastic synovium has invaded the hyaline cartilage causing disintegration and ingestion of this tissue.

Synovectomy of the Knee

Hyperplastic synovial membrane, thickened and thrown into folds, may cause disability even after the arthritis is inactive. Such hyperplasia in the knee often causes chronic effusion, pain and limitation of motion on attempts to fully extend the knee. There may be tenderness around the infrapatellar fat pad, and roentgen evidence of soft tissue changes with only slight damage to the joint cartilage. The operation is most likely to succeed if performed when the damage is entirely synovial with an extensive effusion and without ulceration of cartilage.

In synovectomy of the knee the synovial tissue of the knee is removed as completely as possible; *i.e.*, dissecting out the anterior synovial membrane, the infrapatellar fat pad and the suprapatellar pouch. The semilunar cartilages are always degenerated and should be removed. Bleeding during operation is controlled by the use of the electrocautery.

Following synovectomy, large compression dressings[45] consisting of firm elastic cotton bandages over sterile sheet cotton are used for two days and active motion of the joint is begun several days postoperatively, with weight-bearing two or three weeks postoperatively.[53] If there is much pain postoperatively, a cast may be applied for four to seven days. If there has been a preceding flexion deformity, a long leg plaster cast is applied in maximum extension after the synovectomy has been performed. Early and persistent exercises must be carried out to prevent the development of painful adhesions. If the muscles are weak, walking is performed at first with plaster cylinders or calipers. (*See* Chapter 38.)

Operations for the Relief of Pain

Many surgical procedures have been attempted and are now being tried to

Selection of Patients for Synovectomy

This is used most often in cases of rheumatoid arthritis with little or no involvement of the cartilage or bone (with most of the process localized to the synovial membrane).
Synovectomy at the knee is indicated when synovial tissue and pannus have filled the anterior portion of the knee about the patella.
Patients with persistent swelling and chronic hydrops which interfere with function are often helped by synovectomy.
There should be a preceding trial of conservative therapy, including splinting, corrective and muscle setting exercises before surgery is performed.
Do not operate until an acute flare has subsided.
Patients will require prolonged post-operative physical therapy.
Synovectomy can be combined with other procedures when the joint damage is extensive.

relieve pain in severe arthritis.[32] The simplest of these are injections of anesthetic solutions into and about joints. These give only temporary relief; anesthetics of longer duration have been only slightly more helpful.[18] Injections into the nerves about the joints have also given only temporary relief. Injections of procaine into and about the sympathetic ganglia have led to prolonged warmth and improved blood flow in the arm or leg and in this way have made the patient more comfortable. Such injections are indicated particularly in the presence of trophic disturbances and when the extremity is constantly cold.

The sensory nerves supplying the articular capsule can be cut and in this way most of the pain from that joint can be relieved. Operations of this type are performed occasionally at the hip, knee and elbow. The most common of these is resection of the nerves going to the capsule of the hip, called obturator neurectomy.[49] The obturator nerve, or in exceptional cases the accessory obturator nerve, supplies the anterior capsule of the hip joint. Resection of the obturator nerve partially denervates the articular capsule of the hip. When there is pain both posteriorly and anteriorly, the branches to the posterior capsule, accompanying the nerve to the quadratus femoris, are also cut. This procedure is simple, usually non-shocking and leads to no serious sensory or motor sequelae. It is employed chiefly in debilitated patients when relief of pain is desired rather than improvement in function. Denervation has also been used to relieve pain in the elbow and knee. Although sensory nerve resection procedures have been popular in the past decade, at the present time a more aggressive approach to intra-articular surgery is utilized.

Operations on the Soft Tissues for Flexion Contractures

These are required more frequently at the knee than at any other joint. A release of contracted soft tissue is sometimes required at the toe joints, knee, hip and ankle joints.[8] In all of these areas contraction of the articular capsule on the flexor side is corrected by releasing the proximal end of the articular capsule. Shortened tendons are lengthened by a step incision which permits their re-suture in a lengthened position. Sometimes lengthening of both articular capsule and flexor tendons is required. The indications for these procedures are persistent flexion deformities which seriously interfere with function and which have not responded to splints or to manipulation.

Release of tight tendons and fascia is sometimes required about the hip. In flexion contracture the fascia lata must be cut. In severe flexion contractures the attachment of the rectus femoris tendon must be released subperiosteally from the acetabular margin and inferior iliac spine. Almost always present as a deformity of the hip is a tight and contracted iliopsoas muscle. This must be removed from the lesser trochanter, and transplanted anteriorly to the base of the neck capsule or vastus medialis muscle in order to correct the hip deformity. In severe adduction contracture, the tendons of the adductor longus and brevis must be cut at the pubic rami. Correction of adduction deformities can be accomplished by obturator neurectomies. At the ankle, the tendo Achilles must be lengthened. After cutting soft parts, the joint is fixed in full extension until the tissues have healed in the lengthened position. Then exercises are given to strengthen the extensor muscles.

At the **knee**, severe flexion contracture[33] and subluxation can often be corrected at one operation by a combined capsular release and tendon-lengthening procedure which is called a *posterior capsuloplasty.*[58] In this operation a lateral incision is made extending upward from the fibular head. The fascia lata with the intermuscular septum is cut; the tendon of the biceps femoris is lengthened. The capsule of the knee is freed from the posterior surface of the femur. In this way flexion deformity and subluxation can be corrected. The limb is then fixed in full extension in a plaster cast. Sometimes the contracture of the common peroneal nerve and popliteal artery is so severe

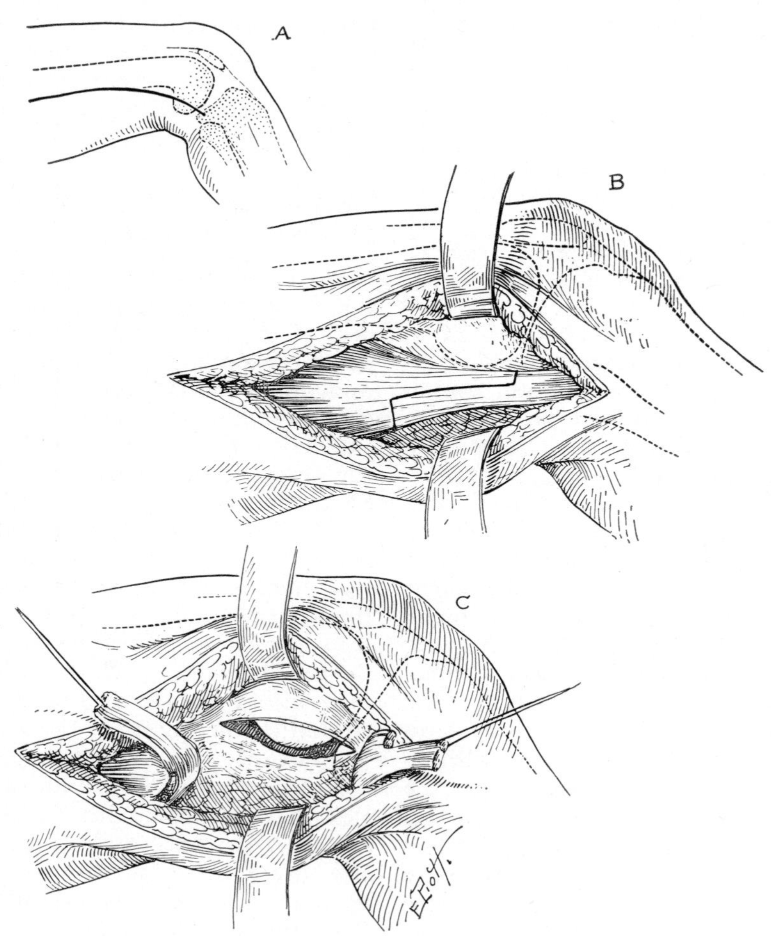

Fig. 39–3.—Posterior capsuloplasty for fixed flexion contracture of the knee.

that full extension would cause paralysis or circulatory embarassment if the knee were fully extended immediately. In such instances, gradual extension of the knee is carried out over a two-week period following the operation by several changes of plaster casts, or later manipulation.[11] Motion is begun in one week and walking with a support is permitted in two to three weeks. If there is only a narrow range of motion, but the articular surfaces are not greatly distorted, an osteotomy just above the knee, with straightening of the knee at the osteotomy site, may give a more useful extremity. A posterior capsuloplasty[48] gives a good result if the chief deformity is contracture of the soft parts and there is little destruction or distortion of the articular surfaces. If the articular surfaces are markedly eroded or destroyed, an arthroplasty or an arthrodesis are the more satisfactory procedures to consider. An analysis of our end results in cases of posterior capsulotomy of 104 knees, followed more than two years, shows that 14 joints had practically normal function and full active extension; 75 had a good result with full extension and good functional flexion of at least 70°; 9 had a fair result with recurrence of flexion deformity and limited range of motion less than 60°; and 6 had a poor result with loss of motion, recurrent flexion contracture and, in a few cases, fibrous ankylosis.

Osteotomy

Osteotomy (the cutting of a bone) is employed in chronic arthritis chiefly after a joint becomes ankylosed in a faulty position for function.

Osteotomy is used in some instances in the lumbar spine to correct ankylosis in a position of excessive forward bowing of the spine.[52] The lumbar spine is then hyperextended and a fusion is performed. This, through increased lumbar lordosis, permits the patient to look directly forward.

Spinal osteotomy has been employed less frequently in the cervical and thoracic regions. At any area of the spine, the usual indication for this procedure has been ventral flexion of the spine greater than 30°. The occupation of the patient must also be taken into consideration. The technique advocated is exposure of the spine through a posterior incision. The dissection is carried laterally beyond the articular facets. A wedge of bone is removed including the articular facets. The angle of the bony wedge is determined before operation to secure the desired correction. Care must be taken to provide adequate space for the spinal cord and nerve roots.[22] The spine is carefully extended at the osteotomy site, holding both sides of the spine firmly until both sides of the osteotomy are in contact. Then a spinal fusion is carried out across the area of the osteotomy. Thirty to 40° of correction of ventral flexion can usually be obtained. The results are chiefly cosmetic and psychological, although some functional improvement occurs in most. During the operation, and until fusion occurs, injury to the spinal cord or nerves can occur.

At the hip when ankylosis has occurred in a deforming position and the patient must stand at work, it is often better to perform an osteotomy and fix the limb in a good position for weight-bearing than to perform an arthroplasty which may leave the joint unstable and painful. The osteotomy is usually performed just below the greater trochanter. Flexion and adduction are corrected and the knee and foot face directly forward. A long plaster spica gives the most secure fixation until the osteotomy heals (twelve to twenty weeks), but fair stability and much greater comfort are given if a long blade is driven into the femoral neck with an attached plate fastened to the femoral shaft. Recently, there has been created much interest in the procedure of *sub-trochanteric osteotomy* for the relief of pain and deformity of the early osteoarthritic hip.[5] It is claimed that the procedure will stop pain, provide a smooth joint and roentgenograms will show a widened "joint space."[13,23] There are orthopedic surgeons who feel, however, that it is not sound judgment to treat one deformity by creating another.

Supracondylar–Femoral Osteotomy.—This procedure is sometimes used for correction of a fixed flexion deformity of the knee joint where other procedures would not be applicable or would end in failure.

Usually, the cases chosen for femoral osteotomy are patients with deformities of 35 to 60° in flexion, 0 to 15° in valgus, at least 30° painless range of motion, stable joints, fair muscle power, underdeveloped tibial shafts and plateaus and good hip joints. In these patients, the aim is to transfer the usable range of motion in flexion to that in full extension. The osteotomy is performed supracondylar, extra-articular, dome shaped, and fixed by a compressor plate. Earliest motion commensurate with bone healing is encouraged lest intra-articular adhesions develop. Roentgenographic appearance of the healing bone always lags behind the actual callous formation, so that by three to five weeks motion should be started. It has been our experience that one should expect at least 10 to 15 per cent loss of motion by this procedure, especially in the rheumatoid arthritic patient.

An analysis of 40 patients with supracondylar osteotomy shows that, at the end of four years all had deformities corrected, but most had varying degrees loss of motion, some as great as 50 per cent.[46] *High tibial osteotomy* for correction of angular deformity in the unilateral compartment disorder of osteoarthritis has been advocated by many authors.[17,28,56] As with osteotomies in other areas the *tibial* type re-aligns the leg such that pain in the knee joint diminishes to varying

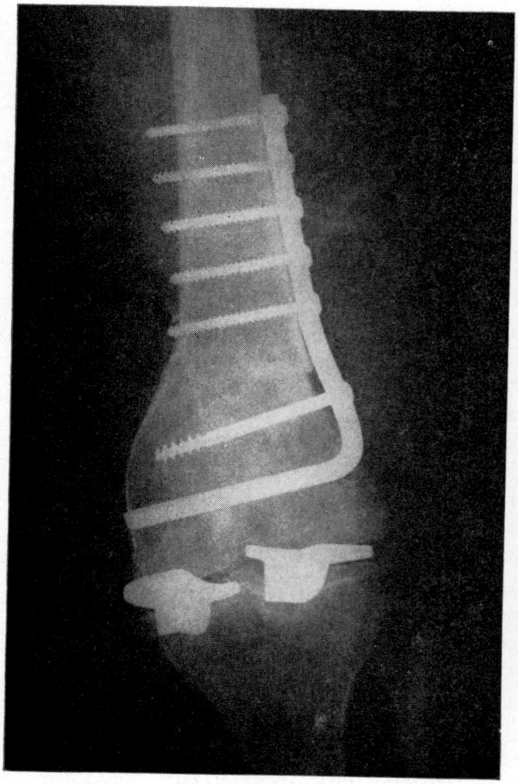

Fig. 39–4.—Corrective distal femoral osteotomy showing the compression plate and screws in place.[46]

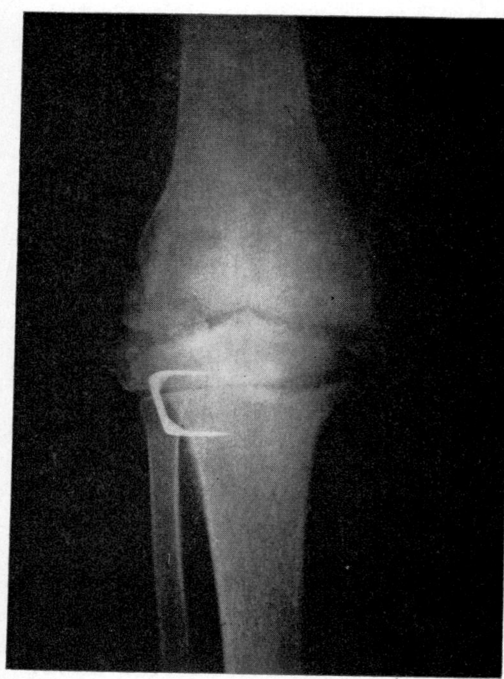

Fig. 39–5.—High *tibial osteotomy*, correcting severe medial compartment degenerative joint disease. The single metal staple holds the bone ends in place. Relief of pain has occurred in a great number of cases. (Surg. Clin. N.A., *49*: 936, 1969.)

degrees. Whether or not the joint surfaces reform and produce new fibrocartilage is open to conjecture. However, in severe cases of degenerative joint disease, the postoperative roentgenograms will show an apparent widening of the joint space.

The osteotomy site must be quite high in the tibia, above the tubercle and in the area of the old epiphyseal line.[16] After exposing the tibia an appropriate wedge is removed to correct the deformity and the bone ends are stabilized by either special staples or a compression apparatus. Stability is surprisingly good and early motion may be carried out. The results of the procedure have been reported as unusually good in osteoarthritis. It is not recommended for the rheumatoid knee.

At the foot a wedge osteotomy may be necessary when the tarsal joints are ankylosed and the foot is fixed in valgus and equinus. After operation the foot is held in a good weight-bearing position for six to eight weeks. An arch support must usually then be worn for some months longer. Exercises and physiotherapy are given after the osteotomy has healed, to obtain muscular strength and good function. Selective metatarsal neck osteotomies can be performed to relieve metatarsalgia. Usually only the 2 or 3 middle metatarsal bones can be corrected.[46]

ARTICULAR RESECTIONS

Resection of the proximal or distal portions or both sides of a joint is employed in the treatment of rheumatoid arthritis. It is particularly of value in the smaller

TIBIAL CORRECTIVE OSTEOTOMY

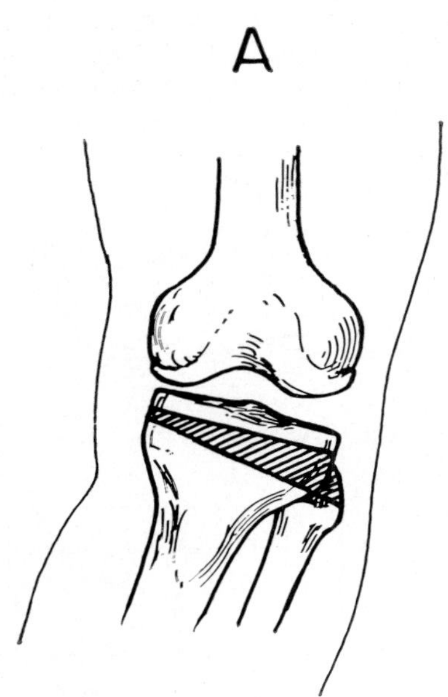

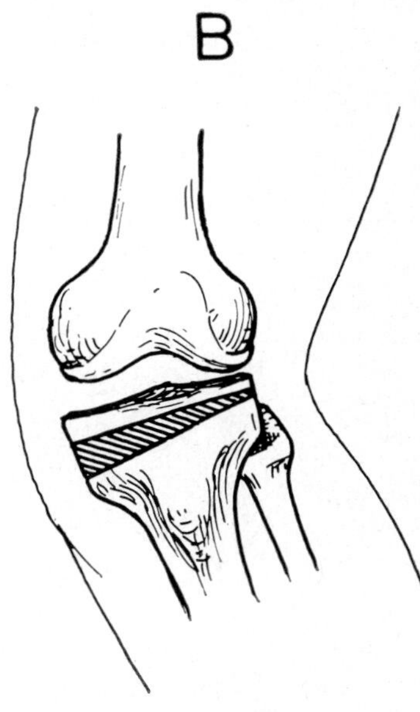

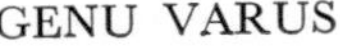

Fig. 39–6.—Diagramatic representation of the resected bone wedge, correcting valgus or varus knee deformity. The amount of bone removed is proportionate to the degree of angular correction necessary to obtain a straight leg.

joints of the hand or foot. When these joints are grossly distorted, undue pressure comes on a portion of the joint and causes pain. Articular resection is used most often in the foot, particularly at the metatarsophalangeal joints, when the forefoot is spread and a great amount of pressure comes upon the under surface of the metatarsal heads. Resection of all metatarsal heads with or without removing the base of each phalanx is an excellent method of correcting the claw toe deformity in the rheumatoid foot (*see* rheumatoid foot, p. 662).

Arthrodesis

Arthrodesis, the operative fusion of a joint in the best position for function, is performed occasionally in chronic arthritis. Arthrodesis has been advocated for severe osteoarthritis of the hips, but in light of many surgeons' experience, it has hastened the onset of arthritic symptoms in the lumbar spine and other hip joint. However, in young (aged under forty), vigorous males who must perform laborious work, arthrodesis for unilateral hip arthritis may be a procedure of choice.[35]

Arthrodesis of the knee has been a procedure of choice for many years when joint destruction has been moderate or severe. However, the indiscriminate use of this procedure in all arthritic knees is to be condemned. Arthrodesis of the knee can lead to increasing arthritis of the hip joint on the same side, to sprain of the joints of the same side, and the incidence of hip fractures is quite high from trauma following the knee fusion. Arthrodesis of both knees makes walking difficult unless one knee is flexed. Arthrodesis should, therefore, be considered only when there is severe destruction of a knee, accompanied by genu valgum, genu varum, flexion and subluxation, or when a previous procedure, such as arthroplasty, joint debridement, osteotomy, or synovectomy has failed.

In the performance of this procedure, it is essential to divide the bone ends squarely so that good contact is made and also that either intramedullary fixation or compression clamps be used to secure an early and solid fusion. This can be accomplished by either intramedullary rod fixation or an external compression clamp. If there is bilateral severe arthritis, one should consider arthrodesis of the worst side and arthro-

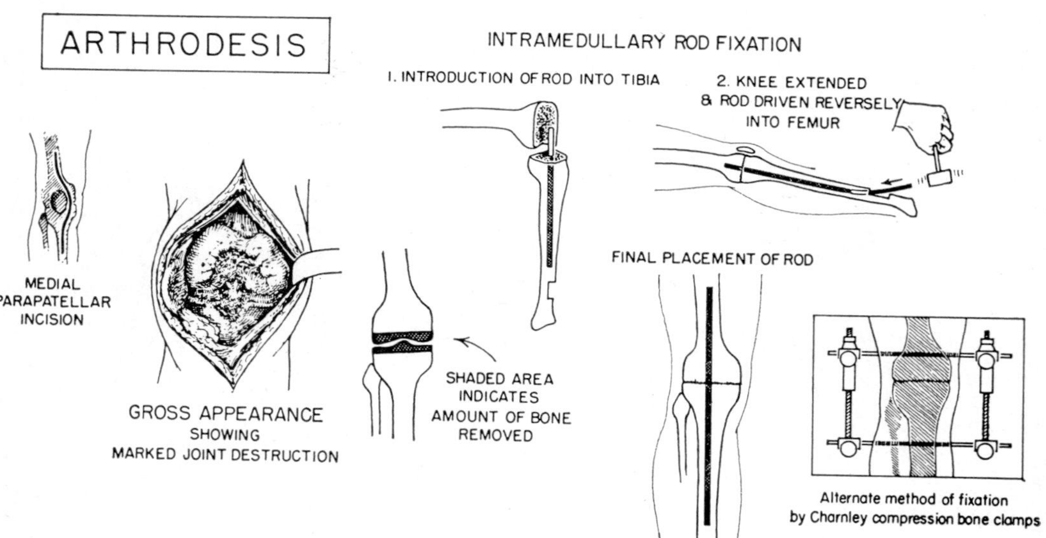

Fig. 39–7.—Arthrodesis of the knee is performed for the grossly deformed arthritic joint. After resecting the bone ends squarely, fixation is obtained either by intramedullary rod or compression clamp.

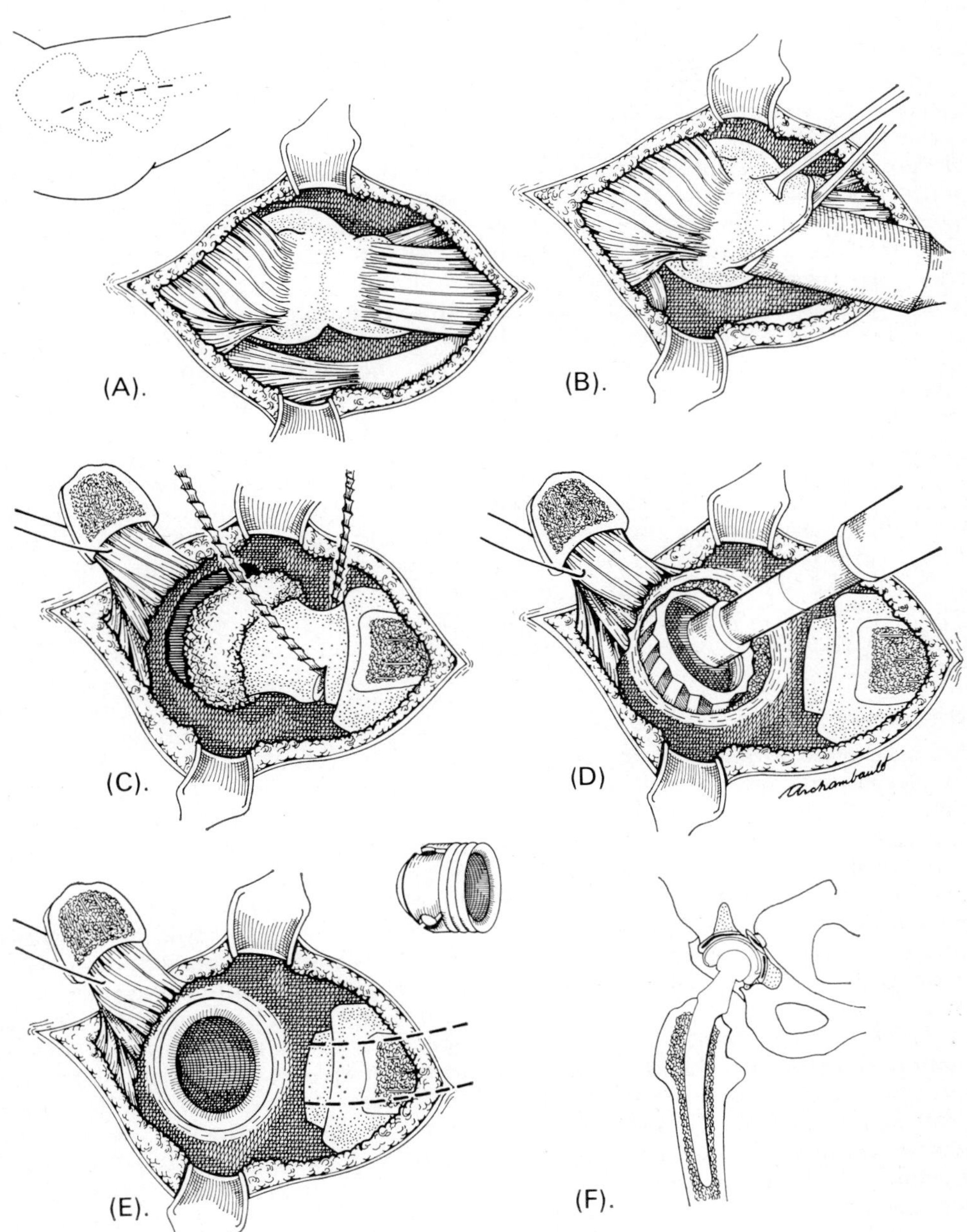

FIG. 39–8.—Diagram illustrating the major steps in total hip replacement with the Charnley-Mueller device. *A*. The postero-lateral incision of Gibson, revealing the lateral aspect of the greater trochanter. *B*. Osteotomy and removal of trochanter with chisel. *C*. After capsulotomy and dislocation of hip, resection of femoral head with Gigli saw. *D*. Deepening and widening acetabulum with power reamers. *E*. The high density polyethylene socket is anchored into the acetabulum with acrylic cement. *F*. The final fit of metallic femoral component and acetabulum with acrylic cement.

plasty of the other, since this combination gives a strong stable painless knee on the fused side and useful motion in its opposite. In our recent series of 40 patients subjected to arthrodesis, all but one secured a solid knee.[46]

Arthrodesis of the ankle is performed on a joint that has become painfully destroyed from arthritis, usually as the result of trauma, old infection or chronic sprain. In these instances fusion is desirable to permit a painless weight-bearing joint. However, in cases of multiple joint involvement such as rheumatoid arthritis, we have found that the patient maintains better knee and hip function if the ankle is *not* fused.

In the foot triple arthrodesis of the subtalar joints is done to prevent and correct the painful valgus posture.

It has been noted that the *talo-navicular area* may be the first site of arthritis in the rheumatoid foot. A talo-navicular fusion with bone graft has improved most of these cases.

Arthroplasty

An enormous amount of interest has been generated within the past two decades in the field of constructive surgery and especially in those cases requiring arthroplasty. This operation forms a new joint when ankylosis is present or when the articular surfaces have become greatly distorted. Excellent results have been obtained in the hip, knee, hand, and elbow.

In brief, the technique of such an operation is to divide the bones at the former joint line, decorticate to bleeding healthy bone, to smooth and trim the ends simulating a normal articular configuration. Then a low friction insert of either special stainless steel, plastics, or both is applied. The metal most commonly used is designated "Vitallium" (65 per cent cobalt, 30 per cent chromium, and 5 per cent molybdenum). It has been found to show the least amount of tissue reaction, and has been used successfully for many surgical implants.

Many types of *plastic joint inserts* are now in use. In *total hip replacement* the acetabular component is high density polyethylene; in the knee the same material or methylmethacylate is employed. In the finger joints silastic or a silicone rubber device has been successfully inserted. For elbow arthroplasty, fascia lata, obtained from the patient's thigh, has given a high success rate in rheumatoid arthritis.

Total joint replacement with devices that resemble but do not duplicate the original area has been performed in the hip, metacarpophalangeal, and recently the knee joint. Most implants are of two parts, expertly designed with machine fit that are anchored to the bone ends by a cold-hardening acrylic cement.

The largest number of cases recorded over the longest time have been those of Charnley with his total hip replacement.[11,12] The results of this operation in relieving pain, restoring motion, overcoming deformity have been uniformly gratifying. A strict regime of operative technique, clean and sterile air operating room environment, prophylactic antibiotics, and anticoagulants have reduced the surgical risk of complications to a minimum. This is coupled with a graduated physical therapy and exercise program to provide an orderly return of function to the extremity.

Vitallium cup or mold arthroplasty of the hip was first advocated, designed and perfected by Smith-Petersen about forty years ago.[52] His ingenuity of design opened a whole new avenue of approach to the destroyed hip. Aufranc improved the design of the cup so that hip function was increased.[2] Several advanced designs have been offered but the basic hip reconstruction procedure must be credited to these men. To date over 6,000 cup arthroplasties have been performed by this group of surgeons and the procedure has a definite place today despite the great interest in total hip replacement. Mold arthroplasty can best be applied to the monarticular arthritic young adult hip, to the very young, to the septic hip, and to many cases of rheumatoid arthritis.

Replacement of the femoral head with a metallic prosthesis, such as the Austin-Moore design, has a great deal to offer certain patients. In the light of our present-day thinking this device can best be utilized in fractures of the femoral head and neck in the aged person, avascular necrosis and tumors of the femoral head. Metallic femoral head replacement is not recommended generally in osteoarthritis when the acetabulum is involved nor rheumatoid arthritis, nor any

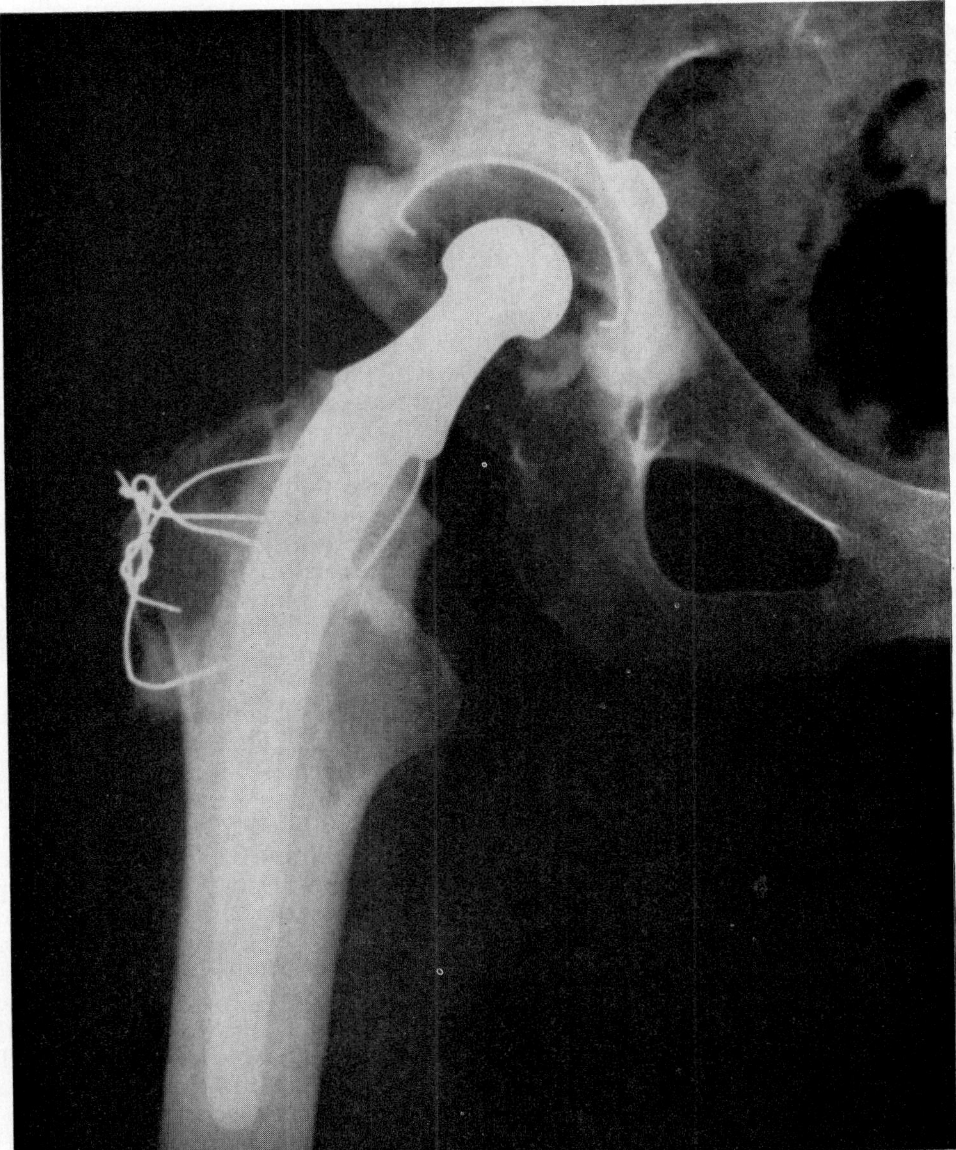

Fig. 39–9.—Roentgenogram of the Charnley Total Hip Replacement, showing the metallic femoral component—polyethylene acetabular near socket with locating wire and metal cap prevent overflow of acrylic cement into the pelvis. Two wires transfix the relocated trochanter. Barium, incorporated with the cement, defines the irregular shape necessary to produce secure union of the device to medullary bone.

other hip pathology when there is deficient or diseased hyalin cartilage at the acetabulum. The cause of the high rate of failure is sinking prosthesis, painful joint, or protrusion into the acetabulum. Our best results with the Austin-Moore femoral head replacement have been in those cases that were treated by the same postoperative regimen as we employ in hip surgery, namely a long period of partial weight-bearing and a graduated exercise program. Cementing this device into the femoral shaft has led to early protrusion of the metal ball into the acetabulum.[46]

A tremendous interest has evolved about *arthroplasty of the knee*. Originally, after a joint resection interposing materials such as fascia lata, cutis, and various plastics, such as nylon and cellophane were used. With the passage of time a more durable substance was sought and this development eventually led to knee arthroplasty, using metallic replicas of the tibial plateaus and femoral condyles. Although many designs of plateau replicas have been introduced, those of McKeever[38] and McIntosh have come into great popularity with orthopedic surgeons.[39] Many ingenious adaptations have been made, not all of which exercise sound human engineering principles.

Tibial plateau prosthesis functions best if the general contour of the joint is preserved, a reasonable range of motion is present and the femoral condyles are intact. Angular deformity can be corrected by insertion of a variable height prosthesis.

On the other hand, if the femoral side of the knee joint is destroyed, then a metallic replacement of the condylar surface by the *femoral stem prosthesis* is advised. This device, made of Vitallium, comes in many sizes to be adapted to the individual knee dimension. The implant was first advocated by Smith-Petersen, but revised and improved by Aufranc and Jones. To date over 200 of these implants have been recorded by Jones with good results.[29]

When severe or total destruction of the knee has occurred with chronic arthritis, one may consider total joint replacement, rather than arthrodesis. These *total hinge prostheses* or the newer proto-types, consisting of a plastic tibial socket and Vitallium femoral component, offer great promise. The metal hinges, as designed by Waldius and Shier, are currently in general use.[51,57] Each part of the device is inserted into its femoral and tibial shaft after resection of the knee joint to admit the hinge portion of the implant. Usually both femoral and tibial stems are cemented into place. This gives firm anchorage and prevents migration in the medullary canal.

In ankylosis of both knees, arthroplasty of one of these may be sufficient, but we have seen many satisfactory results after arthroplasties on both knees. When both hips are ankylosed, bilateral arthroplasty may be necessary to permit sitting. If both hips and both knees are ankylosed, arthroplasty is advised in both hips before the arthroplasty of the knee.

Before arthroplasty is performed, the patient is given muscle-setting and other exercises to strengthen the muscles which will later move the new joint.[31] After operation the limb is splinted with a plaster cast or sometimes with traction. Active motion is usually begun in one week. There are many types of overhead slings which can be used for exercise while the patient is still in bed. As soon as the operative wound has healed the patient is given under-water exercises in a pool or Hubbard tank. In the lower extremity, walking with crutches is permitted after arthroplasty of the hip in two to four weeks, after arthroplasty of the knee in three weeks. The joint is protected in walking with a brace or a firm bandage for about two months. In the later stages of convalescence resistive exercises are given to regain normal strength in the muscles.

Well-fitting articular surfaces can be formed easily in the major joints, but the bones do not remain as they are shaped. The osteoporotic bones and the weak, atrophied muscles are poor materials with which to work.[4] With function, the bone ends become greatly distorted, but in spite of this good function is often seen in the non-weight-bearing joints. Distortion is much less when plastic or metallic molds are fitted over the articular surfaces.

Arthroplasty of the Hip

The hip joint is an example of a true ball-and-socket joint and has wide range of motion in six directions. It is a very stable structure. Strong muscles activate the joint and propel one in walking or running with a uniform coordinated movement.[10]

In the arthritic hip, all smooth action of muscles and joint is lost, and a characteristic deformity ensues, having three components:

1. Flexion
2. Adduction
3. External rotation

Flexion is caused by the pull of the strong flexor muscles, principally the rectus and the psoas. This last muscle has great deforming action on the arthritic joint.

Adduction is caused by the pull of the strong adductor muscles.

External rotation is caused by the pull

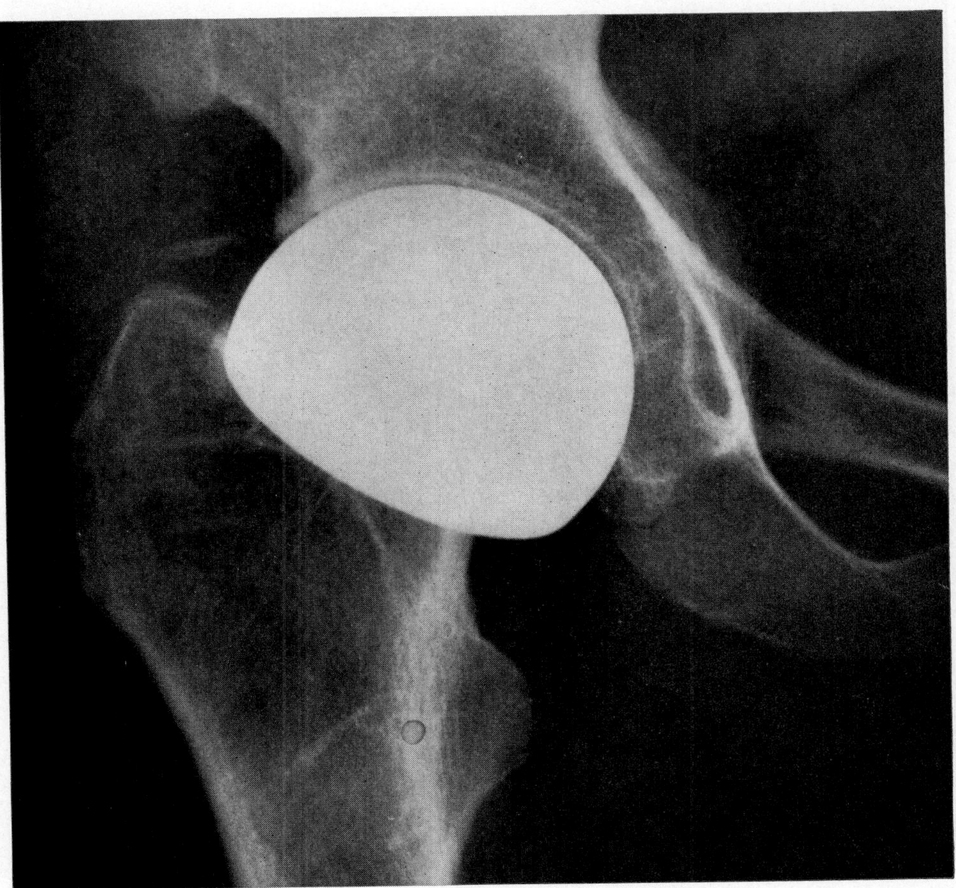

Fig. 39–10.—Roentgenogram of a successful Vitallium mold arthroplasty of the hip for osteoarthritis. This x-ray demonstrates the cup to be in good position and there has been the formation of a new "joint space." Full range of motion with no pain has afforded a normal gait.

of the gluteus muscles and the hip rotators.

Changes taking place within the joint in chronic arthritis are essentially: loss of hyaline cartilage, so that bone rubs on bone; subchondral cysts appear, may become confluent and collapse, causing a grossly distorted femoral head; overgrowth of bone occurs at the margin of the head and acetabulum, blocking motion; sloping of the acetabular roof occurs, leading to the upward subluxation of the femoral head; the capsule becomes grossly thickened and fibrotic, limiting joint motion; pannus and hypertrophic synovium are caught or pinched during joint function; and the femoral head is ground down superiorly from attrition, causing eburnated bone.[1]

Each of these pathological changes and any others must be corrected in a well-performed arthroplasty.

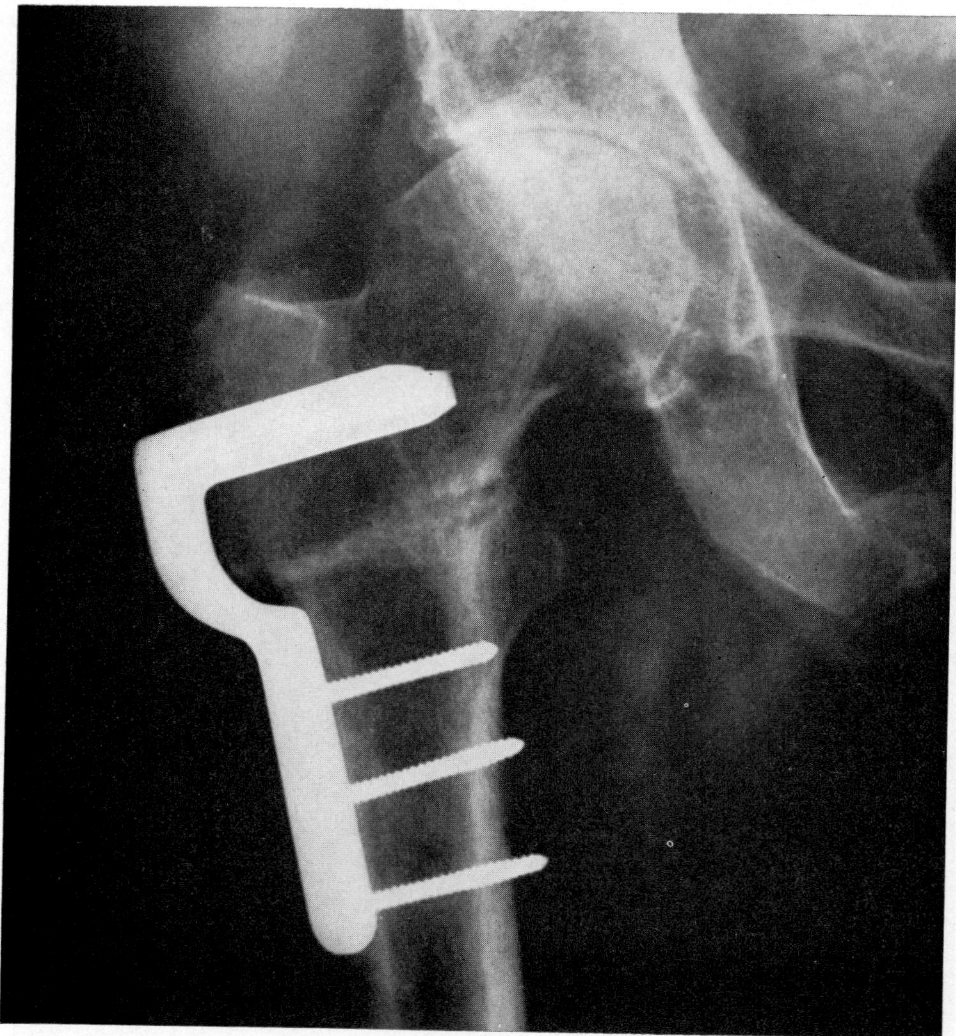

FIG. 39–11.—Subtrochanteric osteotomy for early osteoarthritis of the hip. The Harris compression plate rigidly transfixes the osteotomy site, thereby allowing early motion. Relief of hip pain has been dramatic in many cases.

The indications for hip arthroplasty are not rigid but are two in number:

1. Hip pain
2. Hip deformity

If either or both are present when conservative treatment fails, then surgery should be considered.

In our series of 600 hips subjected to cup arthroplasty over a fifteen-year period, the general results showed that 50 per cent of the cases were greatly improved, 25 per cent were moderately improved and 25 per cent *failed*. Patients with rheumatoid arthritis had a higher incidence of poor results than those with osteoarthritis, and also those with complete joint ankylosis showed lesser gains in function than patients with preoperative mobile joints.

In the main, three types of arthroplasties are now performed: (*a*) cup or mold, (*b*) prosthetic replacement, (*c*) total hip replacement affords early return to function because there is no tissue healing at the joint proper. One must only wait for good wound healing, whereas in cup arthroplasty a minimum of four months is necessary for formation of suitable fibrocartilage in the acetabulum and on the femoral head. During this time, touchdown gait and crutches must be used.

It is our feeling that the cup arthroplasty has certain advantages over a metallic femoral head replacement, in that bone of the femoral head is preserved, two opposing surfaces adapt to a gliding motion, the cup is durable for at least a ten-year period, and if infection occurs the cup can be changed. The prosthesis has an advantage in that patients seem to recover function more rapidly.

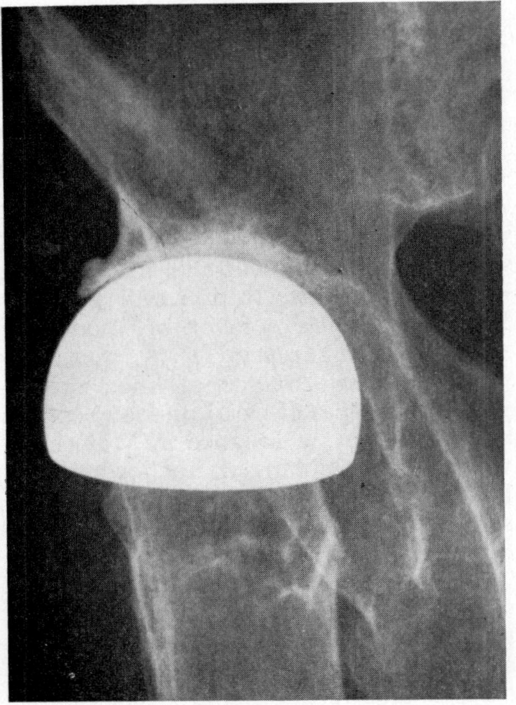

FIG. 39–12.—Roentgenogram of a successful shaft-cup arthroplasty for sepsis, following previous hip surgery. The patient had full range of painless motion and no recurrence of sepsis seven years after operation.

Arthroplasty of the Knee

As in other major joints, this operation is a challenging procedure for any reconstructive orthopedic surgeon.[34] The procedure of forming a new, painless, stable, functioning joint is an enormous one. Indeed, most patients demand that this be performed rather than arthrodesis, osteotomy, or some other form of surgery. All wish to have normally moving knee joints.

While the indications for arthroplasty are not rigid, the following factors should be considered:

1. Knees stiffened and painful due to adhesions.
2. Painful knees due to loss of hyaline cartilage.
3. Ankylosis in a flexed position.
4. Muscles that can acquire adequate strength.
5. Absence of severe osteoporosis, bone cysts or collapsed bone.

For a twelve-year period, ending about 1956, we had experience with 125 knee arthroplasties, utilizing a thin sheet of nylon as an interpositioning membrane.

While many of these patients were greatly helped, others had gradual loss of function and developed additional deformities of varus and valgus. This was attributed to the soft arthritic bone.

Therefore, metallic replacement of the upper tibial surface was instituted about 1958.[38] To date we have performed about 500 arthroplasties, implanting one of two types of plateau replicas.[39] The advantages of this type of operation are that a minimum of bone is removed at operation, thereby preserving the articular strength, and the metallic surface is a long-lasting gliding mechanism.

Other forms of metallic replacements have been used in the knee, such as the Waldius[57] or Shier[50] hinge joint, or the Aufranc[1] femoral cap replacement.

While these forms of joint reconstruction seem very formidable, good results have been attained in many cases, but in others there have been poor results because of infection, soft bone with subsequent collapse, and re-ankylosis Since the introduction of acrylic cement,[13] the total knee replacements have shown a decided improvement in overall ratings. A firm anchorage enhances the joint function and tends to prevent loosening of the prosthesis.

The arthritic knee develops a four phased deformity during the progress of the joint disease as follows:[46]

1. Flexion.
   Due to the pull of the contracted, strong hamstring muscles and opposed by the weaker quadriceps muscles, the tibia is flexed on the femur. This is aided by gravity when in the sitting position, or putting pillows behind the knees when supine to assume a comfortable position.
2. Subluxation.
   Normally the tibia glides backward on the femoral condyles when flexion takes place. The knee does not move as a simple hinge joint. The double parabolic curve of the lower end of the femur augments this glide and is stabilized in part by the posterior cruciate ligament. In long-standing cases of flexion contracture this ligament is shortened and holds the tibia in a partially dislocated position.
3. Valgus.
   This distressing component of knee deformity is caused by an intrusion of the lateral femoral condyle into the tibial plateau. It is aided by the strong pull of the tensor fascia and biceps muscle. On rare occasions there is lateral shift of the tibia on the femur in extreme cases of valgus deformity.
4. External rotation.
   The tibia rotates outwards in relationship to the femur, which is caused by arthritic deformities of the foot, tight ilio-tibial band, or tight bed clothes for long periods.

Therefore, in the correction of the knee deformity, all contributing factors must be dealt with, if adequate alignment of the leg is to be accomplished. Occasionally, multiple staging of procedures must be done to correct the several parts of knee deformity; *i.e.* in a case of moderate flexion deformity with loss of joint motion, an arthroplasty would first be done, followed in three weeks by a posterior capsulotomy to straighten the joint. Between the two scheduled operations a good trial of split Russell's traction will often decrease the flexion deformity by 50 per cent, thereby favorably modifying the soft tissue surgery.

In the performance of knee arthroplasty two types of tibial plateau replicas are available, one designed by McKeever, which has a biflanged anchoring keel, the other by MacIntosh that is "D" shaped. Both are manufactured in various sizes and thicknesses.

Each type is designed to perform a specific replacement. The McKeever prosthesis provides firm anchoring in the tibia without using acrylic cement. The chance of migration and dislocation is very slight because of the T-shaped fins, locked into the cortex of the tibial plateau. Variable thicknesses allow for correction of either knee varus or valgus by insertion of a thicker implant at the

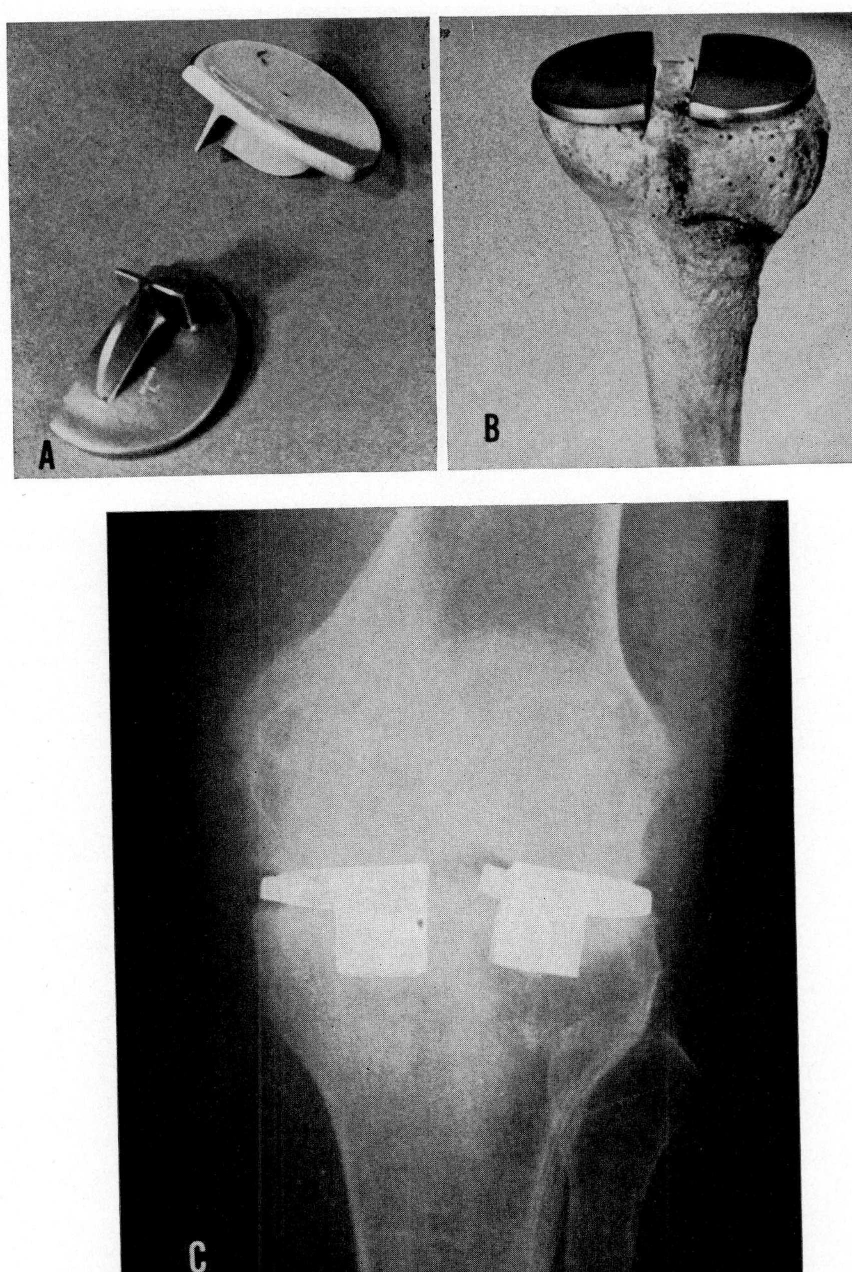

FIG. 39–13.—Arthroplasty of the knee joint. *A*, The metallic McKeever tibial plateau prosthesis is designed to be self-containing, durable and replaces the upper surface of the tibial plateau. *B*, The anatomical model illustrates the placement of the prostheses with the cruciate fin locking device within the tibia. *C*, Roentgenogram of an arthritic joint showing placement of the metallic McKeever prosthesis.

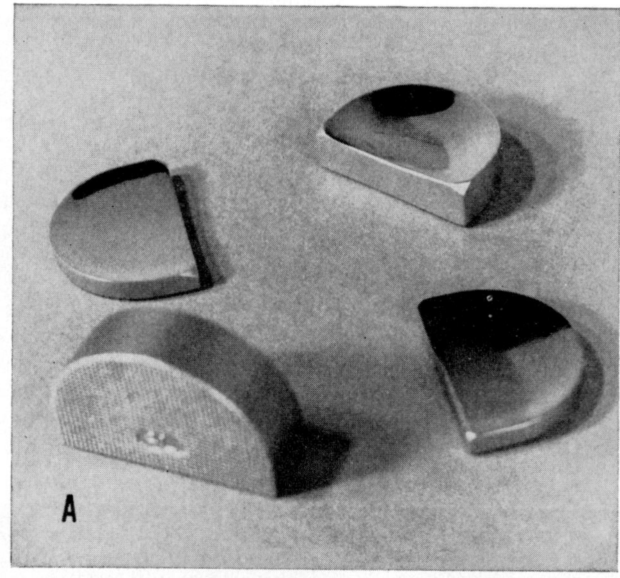

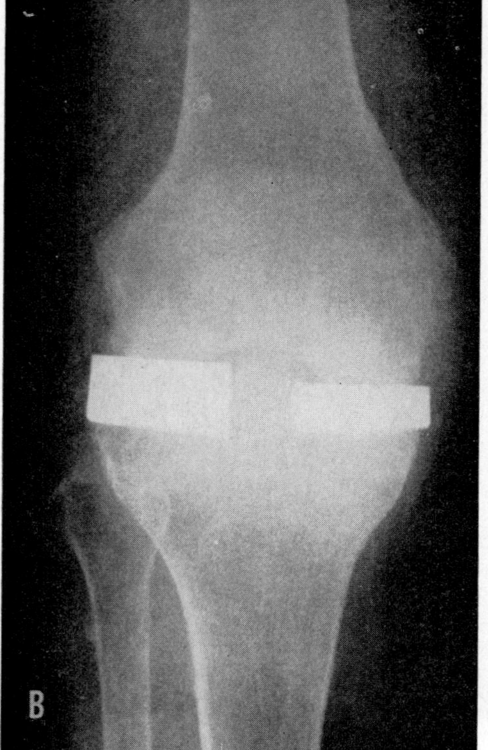

FIG. 39–14.—*A*, The "D"-shaped metallic plateau prostheses designed by MacIntosh are available in twelve sizes of variable widths and thicknesses. This replica can be used as a tibial insertion to correct varus or valgus deformities of the knees while providing a gliding joint surface. *B*, Roentgenogram of the "D"-shaped prostheses inserted into an arthritic knee joint.

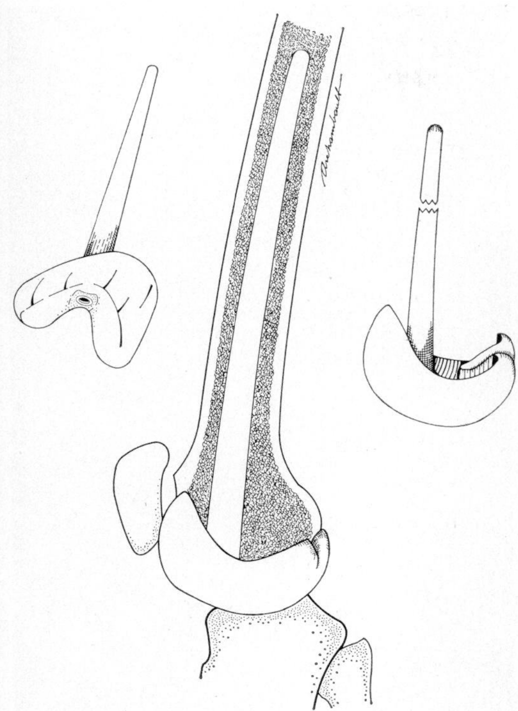

FIG. 39–15.—The femoral replacement Vitallium prosthesis of the M. G. H. design. Diagrams show the general contour in anterior and lateral views. Insertion (lateral view) shows the stem in the femoral canal and the flanges fully covering the condyles.

concave side of the deformity. The MacIntosh prosthesis has a serrated inferior surface and a highly polished articular side. The difference in the friction load of these two surfaces determines the stability. In a small group of our rheumatoid patients, migration and angular tilting of this implant have occurred.

Correction of angular deformity can also be accomplished by the variable thicknesses of the MacIntosh prosthesis.

A long-term follow-up of our first 200 cases of metallic tibial implants shows that there was a success rating of good to excellent in 63 per cent of the patients.[46] The most gratifying factor in all cases was the relief of pain.

Debridement of a Joint

This procedure is employed most often at the knee joint but can be used in all of the major joints. It is often referred to as a "house cleaning procedure." Originally popularized by Magnusson, debridement implies that all the patho-

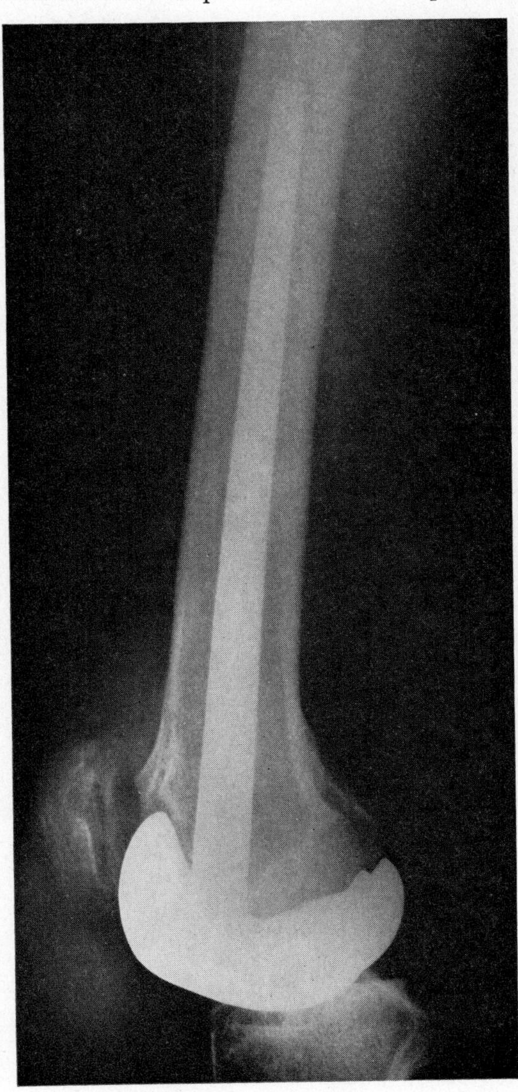

FIG. 39–16.—Roentgenogram of the knee arthroplasty, using femoral stem design of Aufranc and Jones. The Vitallium device is anchored into the medullary canal without cement and completely replaces the femoral condyles. Motion obtained is smooth, gliding, and pain free.

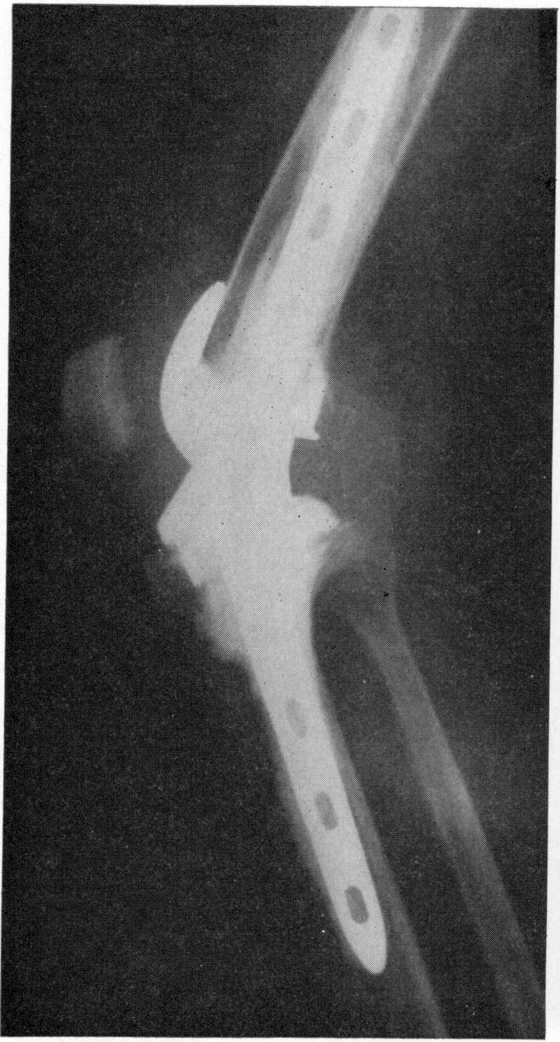

FIG. 39–17.—Roentgenogram of a Waldius Total Knee Replacement, used for a destroyed joint in rheumatoid arthritis. The femoral and tibial components have been anchored into place with acrylic cement. Rigid fixation is accomplished while a 90 degree range of motion is possible.

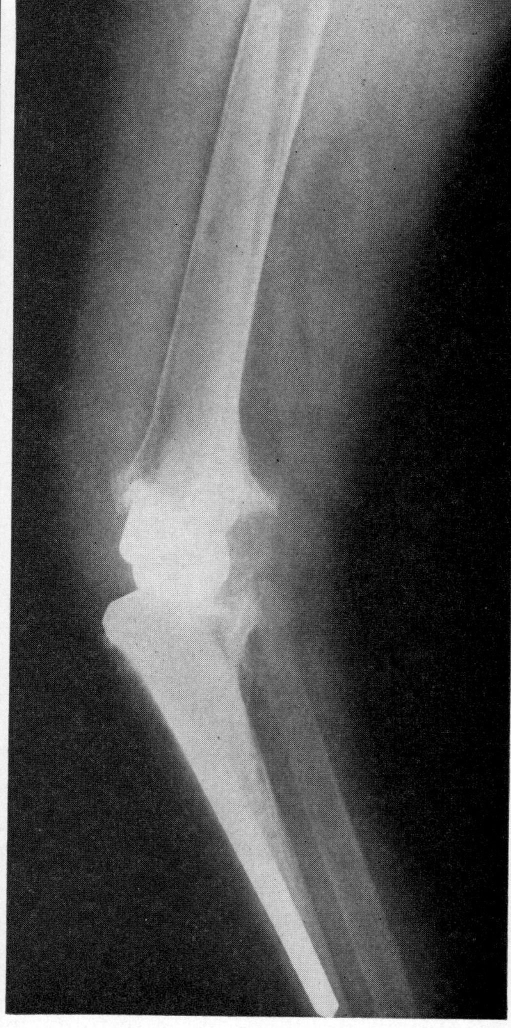

FIG. 39–18.—Roentgenogram of Shier's total knee prosthesis, showing the lateral view of the knee after insertion of the metal hinge. Fixation has been accomplished by acrylic cement, anchoring the device within the bone. Motion obtained was painless and knee was stable.

logically unacceptable material is removed. Gross adjustments are avoided and certainly hyaline cartilage must be preserved.[47] This procedure varies depending upon the pathological changes. Usually thickened synovial tissue, loose bodies, bony spurs or ridges and degenerated semilunar cartilages are removed.[54] Anything within the joint which interferes with function is removed but little if any alteration is made in the articular surfaces. It has been found that if the articular surfaces are not reshaped at the knee, and if there is much atrophy of the joint,

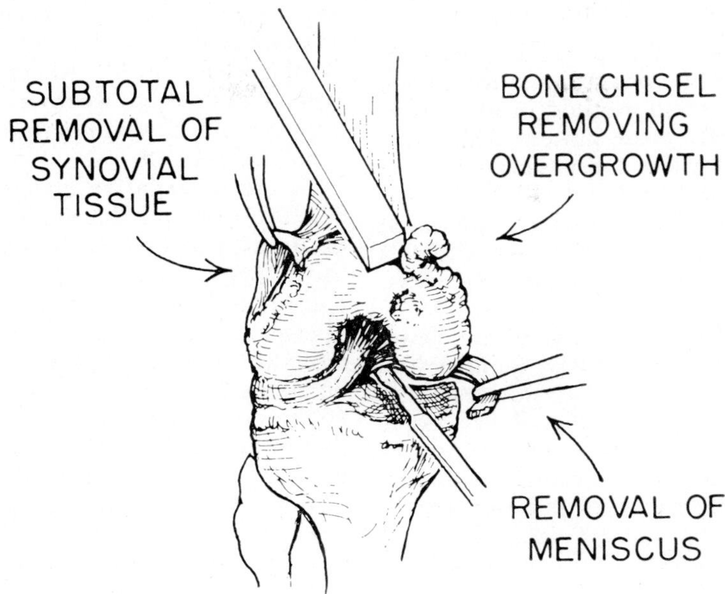

FIG. 39–19.—Debridement of a knee: This operation includes the removal of all pathological tissue which interferes with function.

collapse or telescoping of the tibial plateau does not occur. When collapse of a tibial condyle has already occurred, a metallic prosthesis can be applied to the depressed tibial plateau in combination with this procedure.

THE CORRECTION OF DEFORMITIES IN SPECIFIC JOINTS

Knees

The tendency for individuals with arthritis of the knee is to flex the knee to decrease pain and to relieve the tension and the pull of the hamstring muscles upon the posterior portion of the joint capsule. This results in shortening of the hamstring muscles and contracture of the capsule, and leads to further flexion of the knee.[38] This deformity usually is begun by allowing a pillow to be placed beneath the knee. Further contractures lead to subluxation of the knee and external rotation of the tibia on the femur.

Correction of Flexion Deformities of the Knees[28]

If flexion deformities have occurred (usually from poor treatment or from failure of the patient to adhere to treatment), conservative orthopedic management may be sufficient to restore these to a practically normal position.

A flexed knee causes shortening in the extremity, resulting in equinus of the foot and unstable weight-bearing. The latter produces abduction and external rotation of the hip to obtain a broader base on which to stand. Later, there follows a tilt of the pelvis and shoulders to the shorter side with lateral deviation of the spine (scoliosis).[41] Thus, flexion deformities of the knee may precipitate a traumatic flat foot, strain of the internal lateral ligament of the knee, knock-knee and traumatic synovitis, later followed by changes in the hip and scoliosis.

Canvas Cuff Sling Suspension

The use of the canvas cuff sling suspension may help prevent subluxation at the knee and is a good method of exercising the muscles before the patient walks.

Apparatus for this consists of: canvas—6 to 8 inches wide and 18 inches in length; heavy elastic cord (as in home exerciser sets) 2 to 3 feet long; and felt padding, the same width as the canvas, 8 inches long and ¼ inch thick.

The 8-inch ends of canvas are sewn together forming a canvas cylinder (or cuff), the elastic cord is attached to this as shown in Figure 39–20. The cord is suspended from a horizontal bar (approximately 4 feet above the mattress) running lengthwise over the bed as an overhead frame, with the canvas loop hanging from its lower end.

Use posterior molded plaster splints from the hip to the toes, removing these several times daily for hot fomentations, joint motion (if possible), and for massage to the surrounding muscles in elderly patients if the acute stage of the process has passed. Splints permit muscular relaxation often with progressive decrease in the deformity. Make new splints every two or three weeks as the condition improves until maximal improvement has been maintained.

As an alternative procedure, Buck's extension or split-Russell's traction may be used applying traction in the line of the deformity. The leg should be shaved and tincture of benzoin should be applied liberally to the skin before applying moleskin adhesive. The weights should be about 4 pounds for children and about 10 pounds for adults. The foot of the bed should be raised several inches. Traction must be supervised carefully.[43] It must be kept on constantly, usually for several weeks to secure correction. When the deformity has been overcome, the position may be maintained by a light plaster cast. In some patients, the flexion deformity is not completely overcome by serial plaster splints. In these, the remaining flexion contracture can often be corrected by gentle manipulation under

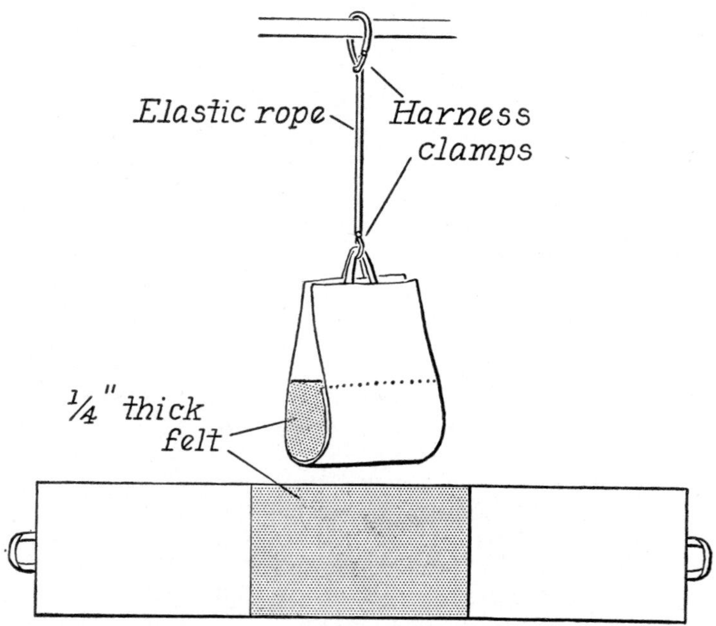

Fig. 39–20.—*Canvas cuff sling suspension* for support of the leg and for assistance in exercises in patients with arthritis of the knees.

anesthesia, followed by application of a light plaster cast to maintain the correction.

Caliper Splints

These are useful for the individual with slight flexion of the knees and in whom one wishes to avoid further flexion when the patient is up and about. The main features of these splints are as follows:

Calipers can be used to correct slight flexion deformity (less than 30°) either in bed or while the patient is ambulatory. They are used for several periods a day with the knee held as near as possible in full extension.

Forceful apparatus or wedging and turnbuckle casts have been used to correct flexion deformities. They frequently cause subluxation and fascial adhesions. They have been discarded for the most part, as better methods of correction have become available.[4]

If deformities do not respond to splints, traction, or manipulation in a reasonable period of time (three to six weeks), one may resort to surgical procedures.

Supports for the Knee

Elastic Bandages.—Strapping should be begun below the knee joint and continued upward, covering an area of about 5 inches on each side of the joint. A 4-inch ACE elastic cotton bandage is often used in milder inflammation and weakness.

A layer of 4-inch elastic bandage is wound loosely around the knee (for 4 or 5 inches above and below the patella) and then two long ovoid pieces of sponge rubber are applied, one on each side of the patella; this is followed by another layer of elastic bandage with firm traction applied at each turn. The rubber sponges are approximately 8 inches long, 2½ inches wide and ¼ inch thick. Felt strips ½ inch thick and 2 inches wide and 10 inches long can be applied in a similar fashion on either side of the patella.[32]

Elastic knee supports, with or without lacing, are often of great value in weak

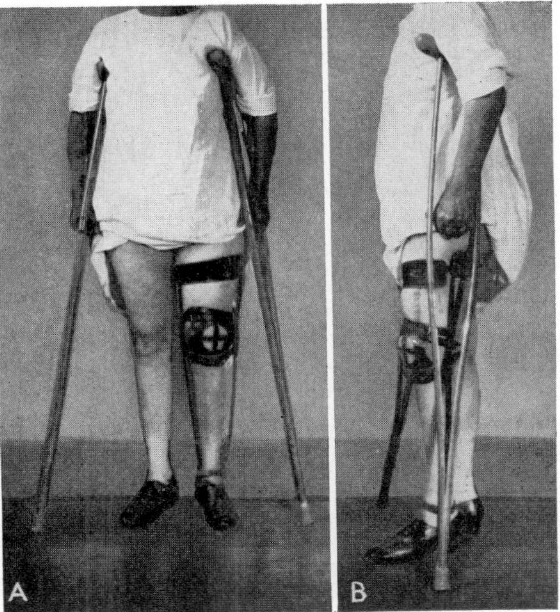

Fig. 39–21.—Caliper splint to correct flexion at the knee. This is also used to maintain full extension in walking when the muscles are weak. *A*, Anterior view. *B*, Lateral view.

Correction of Deformity at the Knee

1. The knee joint, the largest joint in the body, is often involved because it is a weight-bearing joint and is frequently subjected to sprain and other injuries.
2. Pain, swelling and fixed flexion are the first signs of impending deformity, followed soon by atrophy of muscles and ligaments about the joint, narrowing of the joint space, external rotation, subluxation of the tibia on the femur, fixation of the patella against the femoral condyles, contracture of the hamstring muscles, joint capsule and periarticular structures, and occasionally ankylosis.
3. Splint early in a bivalved cast as near full extension as possible. Begin exercises as soon as this can be done without pain. Apply heat several times a day.
4. If flexion deformities are present, these may be corrected by the application of serial casts, or by traction in the line of the deformity if casts do not bring correction. Gentle manipulation under anesthesia followed by the application of a plaster cast is advised to maintain the correction. If plaster casts are used, these should be bivalved within forty-eight hours in most instances, using the posterior half as a resting shell. The knee joint should be moved through as full a range of painless motion as possible each day.
5. If serial casts or plaster shells are used to reduce flexion contractures, these are renewed as improvement occurs.
6. When correction of deformity has been obtained, this may be maintained by exercises to strengthen the extensor muscles and by wearing a plaster cast at night. The cast and exercises may be discontinued when the muscles are strong and all inflammation has subsided.
7. If casts and manipulation fail to correct the deformity, surgery must be considered. This may require lengthening of contracted soft tissues. If there is bony ankylosis, an osteotomy or arthroplasty may be necessary.
8. Weight-bearing should not be begun until the patient can raise the lower leg and hold the leg extended horizontally over the side of the bed. If the quadriceps muscles are well developed, the patient may then attempt weight-bearing with support of the knee.
9. In patients confined to bed for long periods with arthritis of the knee, the knee must be supported more firmly when weight-bearing is begun. One may employ caliper splints or a plaster cylinder cut into an anterior and posterior half. This is held together in walking by straps or a bandage.
10. The atrophied muscles should receive daily physical and occupational therapy. After operation, exercise in a Hubbard tank is helpful. Later, resistive exercises should be given.

knees; if lacing is used, the felt pads as described above may be used on either side of the patella.

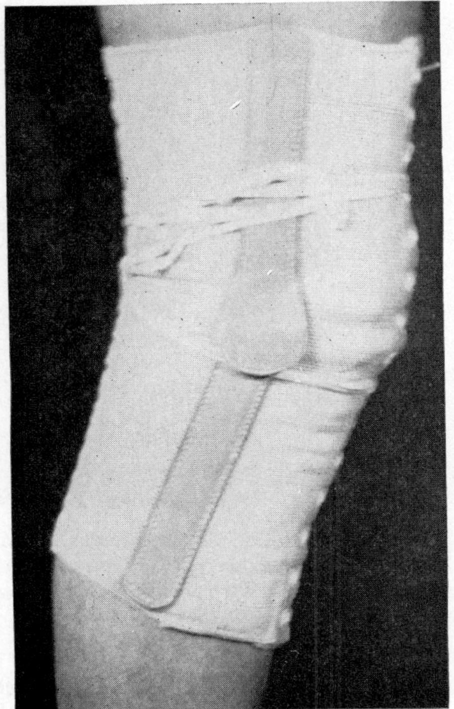

Fig. 39–22.—Elastic knee brace with lacing and side hinges used for ambulatory support in arthritis of the knee.

Elastic knee supports with hinged side joints: In place of the lateral felt pads, thin steel strips may be incorporated into the outside of the laced elastic knee support. Such steel strips may be approximately 10 to 12 inches long for adults, $\frac{3}{4}$ inch in width and made of 14- to 16-gauge steel; these are hinged so that the joint comes at the level of the knee joint. The supports may be laced up the front.

Correction of Deformity at the Hip

In arthritis of the hip, pain may be referred to the knee or to the thigh medially. The first sign of deformity in arthritis of the hip is inability to extend the leg completely at the hip due to a flexion contracture. Muscular spasm results in flexion, adduction and in some cases external rotation.

A fixed flexion and adduction deformity of the hip produces a functional and apparent shortening of the leg.

Measures of value in arthritis involving the hip joint include:

1. Elimination of weight-bearing by rest in bed; this relieves muscular spasm and pain.
2. The patient should lie on his back on a firm, non-sagging mattress most

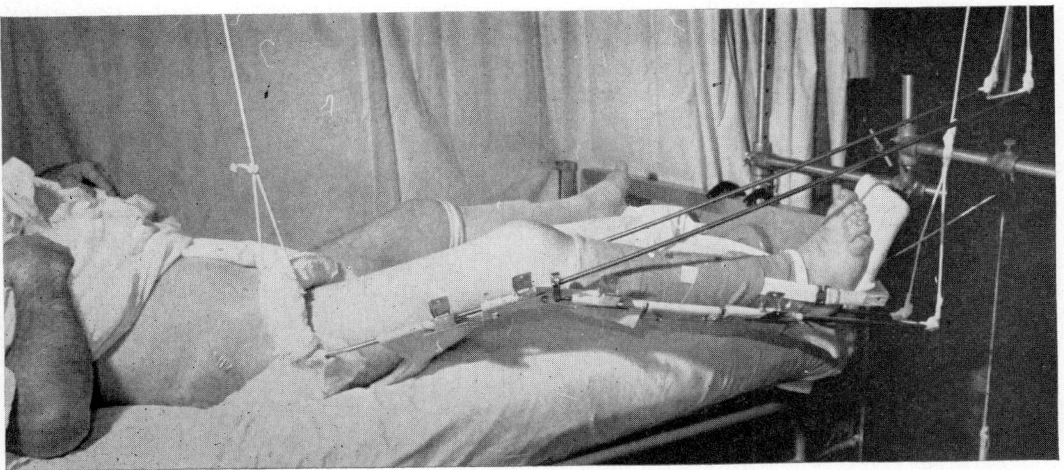

Fig. 39–23.—Balanced suspension with leg traction gives an even, gentle pull on the hip joint, relaxing muscles, correcting deformity and providing a comfortable apparatus for exercising therein.

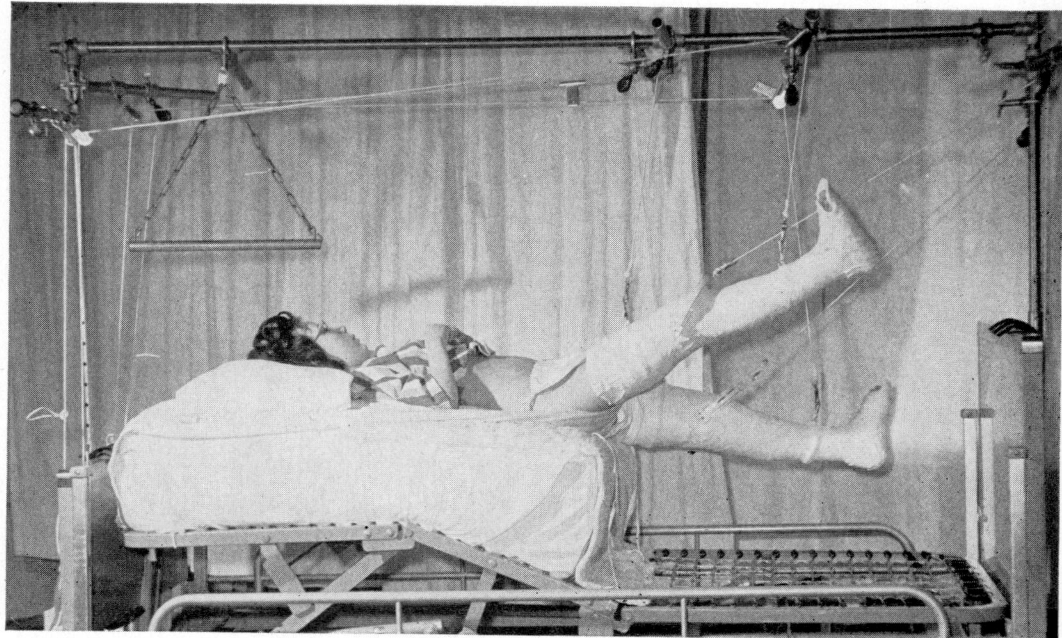

Fig. 39–24.—Schwartz balanced leg traction is useful to correct hip flexion deformities in arthritic children. Long leg solid plasters, through which skeletal traction, using K wires in the lower femurs, and attached to balanced overhead traction, completes the apparatus. By alternating flexion and extension on a split mattress, the deformities are stretched out.

of the time. Lying flat on the face also stretches a flexion deformity at the hip.

3. Maintain extension of the hip by sand bags, casts or balanced traction.
4. A long plaster spica is the most effective early method of correcting flexion, adduction and external rotation at the hip. The spica can be changed when further correction of the deformity is possible.
5. Occasionally, traction with Buck's extension or balanced suspension may be used early, or in the presence of severe pain, with the leg in adduction.
6. Intra-articular steroid injection into the hip usually relieves pain temporarily.
7. When complete extension of the hip has been obtained, continue the use of a bivalved spica and remove this daily for exercises and physical therapy.
8. The patient should not get out of bed until he can keep the thigh fully extended (*i.e.*, flex one knee with the other leg in full extension without arching the back).
9. Weight-bearing is not permitted until all muscular spasm has disappeared, and partial weight-bearing is permitted with use of crutches.
10. If necessary, use surgical procedures such as manipulation under anesthesia, followed by use of a plaster cast spica, or operative procedures such as cup arthroplasty, total hip replacement, or high femoral osteotomy can be contemplated.

Support for the Hip

This may be obtained by a figure-of-8 application of wide elastic bandage to the pelvis and thigh as a spica, with strips of ½-inch-thick felt incorporated in the bandage at the lateral side.

Correction of Deformity at the Hip

1. The first symptom may be pain referred to the anterior portion of the thigh and medial aspect of the knee.
2. Examination usually reveals muscle spasm and a flexion deformity. If improperly treated, the process will usually progress to permanent flexion deformity and marked muscular atrophy with adduction and external rotation.
3. Hip flexion may be corrected in some early cases by having the patient lie prone (on his abdomen) in bed at least thirty minutes several times per day.
4. If the flexion deformity is slight, it can sometimes be corrected by hot fomentations (twenty to thirty minutes, 3 times a day) and traction in the line of deformity, later traction in abduction.
5. Muscle tone may be preserved by supporting the lower leg in a padded canvas cuff which may be suspended by an elastic cord from an overhead frame. This permits the patient to exercise that leg almost as easily as in a Hubbard tank.
6. In acutely painful hip joints, it may be necessary to apply a unilateral or bilateral plaster spica to secure relief. It may be changed every week or ten days as an improved position is secured.
7. If a deformity is present without bony ankylosis, much of this can often be corrected by gentle manipulation under anesthesia with maintenance of the correction by plaster spica casts.
8. When the patient becomes ambulatory, a light-weight spica cut into an anterior and posterior half may be worn; this may be removed when desired for physical therapy. Crutches should be used at first.
9. If ankylosis appears inevitable, the hip should be held in full extension, about 10° of abduction and without rotation.
10. If conservative measures have failed to correct deformity, or if ankylosis has occurred in a poor position in the hip, operative release of the soft tissues, osteotomy, or an arthroplasty with the aid of a Vitallium cup, metallic endoprosthesis, or total hip replacement should be considered.

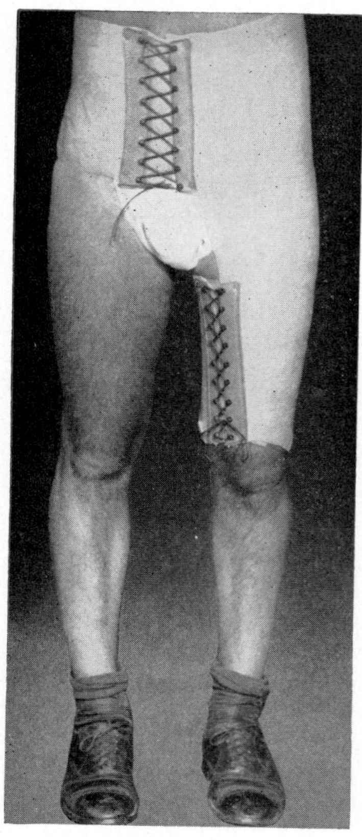

Fig. 39–25.—Unilateral plaster hip spica to provide support in arthritis of the hip joint. Lacing permits easy removal for bathing or physical therapy.

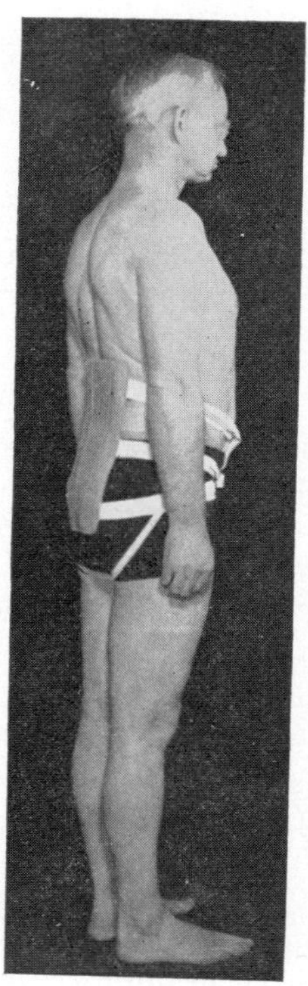

Fig. 39–26.—Support for lumbosacral spine. Anteroposterior pad, with leather reinforced posterior support, and anterior abdominal pad, used for arthritis of lumbar spine.

An ischial weight-bearing caliper can be employed but usually partial relief of weight on the hip by crutches is adequate to relieve symptoms. With less severe inflammation at the hip, a firm corset or a leather pelvic belt may be used. A short leather or plastic spica is sometimes used to relieve pain only in debilitated or aged individuals when surgery is contraindicated.

Support for the Low Back

Lumbosacral and Sacroiliac Joints.—Adhesive strapping is the simplest form of support for the low back. A firm corset may be required. This should be a back lace corset which tends to hold the low back flat and the lower abdomen in. Low back and abdominal supports and corsets are valuable only when they are fitted properly to the individual patient in an anatomic and physiologic manner.[3] A firm canvas belt may be worn. This should come firmly over the sacroiliac joints. For more severe disability a back brace may be required.[44] This should hold the low back relatively flat and the front pad should hold the lower abdomen in. The physician should determine that the spinal support is properly fitted and worn, otherwise it is of little value. With any disability in the low back, a firm bed should be used. Postural exercises should also be prescribed.

Correction of Deformities in Spondylitis

1. The rib joints are frequently involved and the chest tends to become fixed in the position of expiration. Breathing exercises to increase expansion of the chest should be given.
2. Heat should be given to the back to lessen muscular spasm and pain.
3. In ankylosing spondylitis, the patient should use a *firm, non-sagging bed* and may obtain relief by the use of *hot fomentations* to the back. Boards may be placed between a thin, hair mattress and the springs. In bedridden patients, a *posterior plaster body shell* may suffice temporarily.
4. The patient with very severe ankylosing spondylitis may require immobilization in a plaster body jacket, and later in a leather or plastic body jacket. The jacket may be removed for the use of heat and exercise. Plaster jackets are changed as further correction occurs.
5. In *arthritis of the cervical spine*, rotation and lateral tilting of the head may be prevented and corrected by a *Thomas collar*, felt collar or plaster head piece. If the patient with cervical arthritis is confined to bed, sand bags may be used to hold the head in place and *head traction* may be required if severe spasm has occurred or if severe pain is present. *Hot fomentations* are useful in relieving pain and muscle spasm.
6. The special positions mentioned under Posture will help to correct deformities.
7. Postural and breathing exercises should be continued until soreness is gone.
8. Operative correction of spinal deformity is required in seriously deformed patients.

Support for the Thoracic Spine

Adhesive strapping is the simplest form of support. If necessary, one may use a back brace with shoulder straps.

By the use of plaster jackets, spasm of the erector spinae muscles is relieved and flexion deformities of the spine may be prevented. If the patient is in bed, a plaster shell may be adequate. If a body cast is used, this should be high in front and should come to the apex of the forward bowing posteriorly. A snug fit is desirable around the abdomen; it is looser above this to encourage the patient to move the chest in breathing. It may be desirable to use a head-chin traction or a chin support while the cast is in place, if there is much forward flexion of the cervical spine.

Strapping for the Thoracic Spine.—1. The part to be strapped is shaved if necessary and is then painted with compound tincture of benzoin.

2. Adhesive tape 2 inches wide is used.

3. The strapping runs obliquely from the clavicle downward across the back to the loin.

4. The first strip begins at the base of the neck and runs downward and inward.

5. The second strip begins on the outer side and runs downward in the opposite direction.

6. At least six strips are used on each side, alternately applying the right and the left, each one overlapping the previous strip on that side. Each succeeding strip begins further laterally.

7. This will remain in position better if finally two or three strips of adhesive are placed longitudinally over this on each side of the spinal column, from above downward.

8. Powder is dusted over the adhesive strapping.

Support for the Cervical Spine

Thomas Collar.—This is easily made and consists of layers of cotton sheet wadding over thin felt or cardboard covered with gauze or stockinet. This is wrapped around the neck and fastened in position by 3 thin straps. A satisfactory support may be obtained by wrapping around the neck a piece of thick felt about 3 feet long, and 4 inches wide at one end, tapering to 2½ inches at the other. (*See* Fig. 39–39, p. 671.)

A Thomas collar may prove very useful in the patient with arthritis involving the cervical spine. If felt is not available, a piece of cardboard may be used at home. This should be approximately 4 inches wide, being curved high to fit under the ears and cut out below to fit over the trapezius muscles. It should dip down in front to fill the distance between the mandible and clavicles. The collar may be fastened in the back of the neck by a gauze tie or buckles. Semi-rigid collars are available through most surgical supply stores and are supplied in various sizes. This affords a comfortable fit for most patients. This will relieve some of the strain on the cervical spine by allowing the weight of the head to be borne in part directly upon the shoulders. If pain is severe or there is much spasm, a plaster head piece may be made and worn constantly.[27] In patients with severe spasm in the cervical muscles, it may be necessary to employ traction by means of the Sayre head sling attached by a cord, passing over a pulley at the head of the bed. Weights of about 10 pounds are used to produce traction as tolerated. When muscular spasm has been relieved by traction, a light felt or leather collar may be utilized. Exercises and physiotherapy are prescribed.

THE RHEUMATOID FOOT

The foot is involved in 90 per cent of all patients who have had rheumatoid arthritis for any period of time. Involvement of the tarsal joints is frequently observed and most arthritis of the foot is augmented by some preceding static disability.

The first disability found is most often in the metatarsophalangeal joints and in the tarsal joints, particularly the talonavicular joints. With involvement of the metatarsophalangeal joints, some subluxation and deformities of the toes occur. Involvement of the tarsal joints leads to stiffness of the longitudinal arch and to a spastic flat foot. Cavus and equinus deformities come later. During the active stage of rheumatoid arthritis one finds tenosynovitis, particularly in the extensor tendons. Rheumatoid nodules and inflamed bursae may be found also. Atrophy of the fat pads follows stiffness and ulceration and local osteomyelitis occurs where there has been a persistent excessive pressure or the existence of a necrotic rheumatoid nodule.

The following conditions are those that must be considered as commonly occurring in the rheumatoid foot:

Rigid Flat Foot

This occurs in about 50 per cent of all patients who have rheumatoid arthritis of the foot and is a most common deformity. Flat foot increases with the duration of the disease and the deformity consists of a flattening of the longitudinal arch, pronation of the forefoot, increasing heel valgus, inward rotation of the legs, and loss of demonstrable supination and pronation. Peroneal spasm is present which gives an outward rotation of the foot. The talonavicular joint is most often affected and in our series occurred in 25 per cent of patients with foot involvement. The navicular bone, being the keystone of the arch, is most vulnerable to rheumatoid arthritis resulting in peroneal spasm and flat foot. The stiffening of the flat foot is caused by inflammatory scar about the joint, by marginal osteophytes, or by fibrous ankylosis of the mid-tarsal joints. In addition, there is hyaline cartilage loss in the tarsal area that leads to excessive pain due to lack of tarsal motion. Treatment should be primarily conservative. This includes the wearing of suitable shoes, properly fitted arch supports, and inner heel wedges to overcome the pronation of the foot.[40] Probably the most important treatment for all foot disabilities is graduated foot exercises and various therapy modalities, especially the whirlpool bath. If conservative treatment fails surgery should be considered. This is particularly true if the x-rays show advanced tarsal disintegration. Manipulation of the foot under general anesthesia and the application of a retention cast with the foot inverted should be tried initially. If this fails to relieve the condition after a period of three to five weeks, then triple arthrodesis will maintain a painless alignment of the mid-foot.

Spread of the Forefoot

Widening of the metatarsal area occurs in about 40 per cent of the patients with rheumatoid arthritis. This is not always

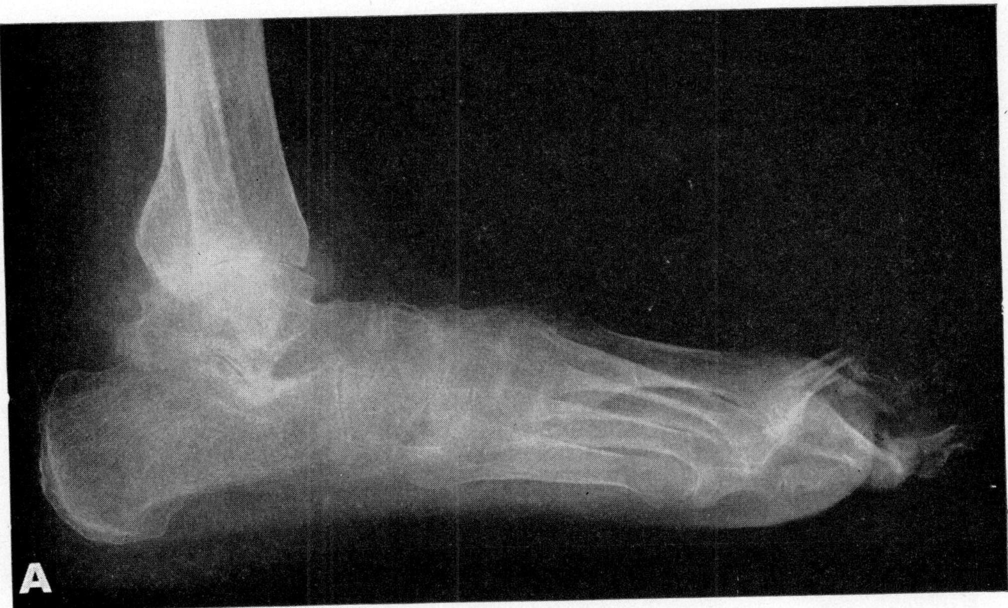

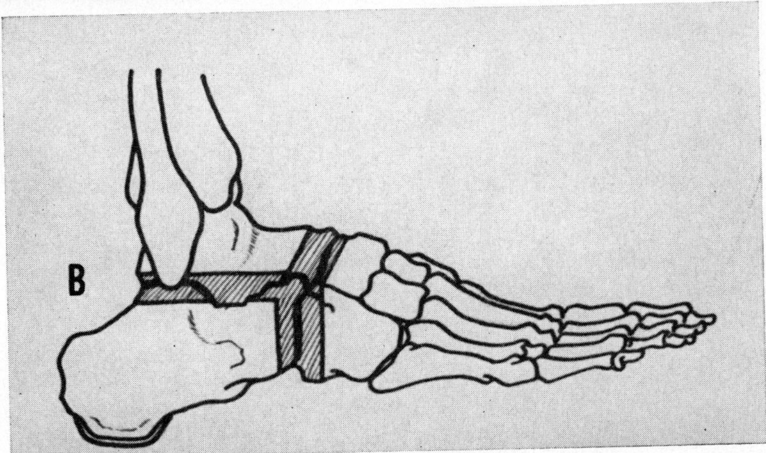

Fig. 39–27.—*A*, The roentgenogram of a rigid flat foot showing the flattening of the longitudinal arch with narrowing of the mid-tarsal joints. *B*, Diagrammatic sketch of a triple arthrodesis noted by shaded areas. This procedure maintains a painless alignment of the arthritic foot.

associated with a flat foot condition. A helpful clinical sign is that of calluses beneath the metatarsal heads. The deformity is due to overstretching of the plantar ligaments of the deep transverse arch, allowing migratory spread of the forefoot; *i.e.* the first and fifth metatarsal will spread to the greatest degree.

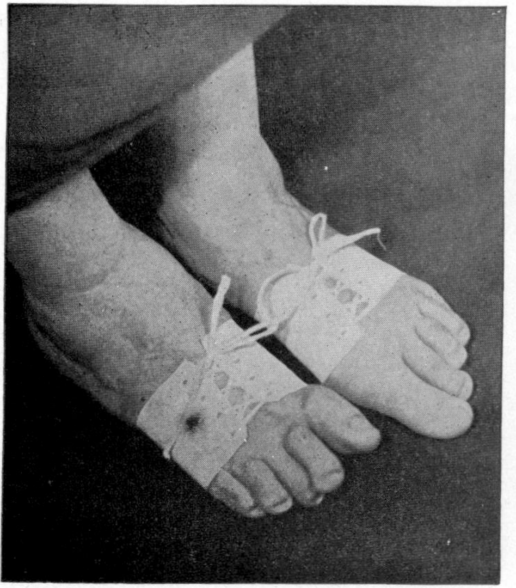

Fig. 39–28.—*Leather cuff worn about the forefoot* for spreading of the anterior arch and flexion deformity of the toes. (Kuhns, courtesy of Rheumatism.)

Treatment consists of prevention of this lateral spread by either leather metatarsal adjustable foot cuffs or by means of broad oxfords to prevent pinching of the toes and, at night, posterior resting plaster shells may be utilized. Usually, when the acute inflammatory aspect of rheumatoid arthritis subsides, the forefoot spread will decrease, but the relaxation of the lateral ligament in overstretching in most cases is usually so severe that a normal configuration of the forefoot is never attained. Synovectomy of the metacarpophalangeal joints may prevent forefoot spread.

Cavus Foot

An abnormally high longitudinal arch occurs in about 4 per cent of the cases of rheumatoid arthritis. It is usually associated with hammer-toes and painful metatarsal calluses. The patient finds that it is difficult to obtain proper shoes and one notices that the heel rolls outward. A continuous foot strain develops from muscle fatigue in an attempt to support

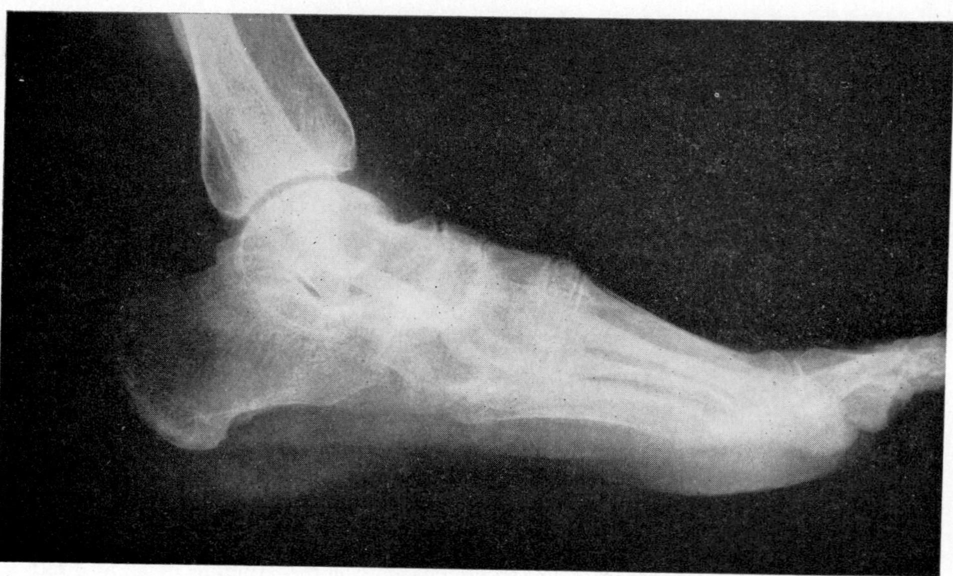

Fig. 39–29.—Roentgenogram of rheumatoid foot after talonavicular fusion. The tibial bone graft has incorporated in six months. Pain and deformity has disappeared. Compare with Figure 39–27.

the high longitudinal arch. Children may develop cavus feet, associated with a calcaneal deformity from pressure of blankets.

Conservative treatment consists of proper shoes with arch supports, physical therapy and, particularly, stretching exercises for tight heel cords and tight toe extensor tendons. If this fails, one should consider *talonavicular fusion with bone graft*. In our experience, it has been a successful operation in seventy consecutive cases. If severe cavus fixed deformity has occurred, a wedge osteotomy with the base up should be considered. If the metatarsal heads are very prominent and there

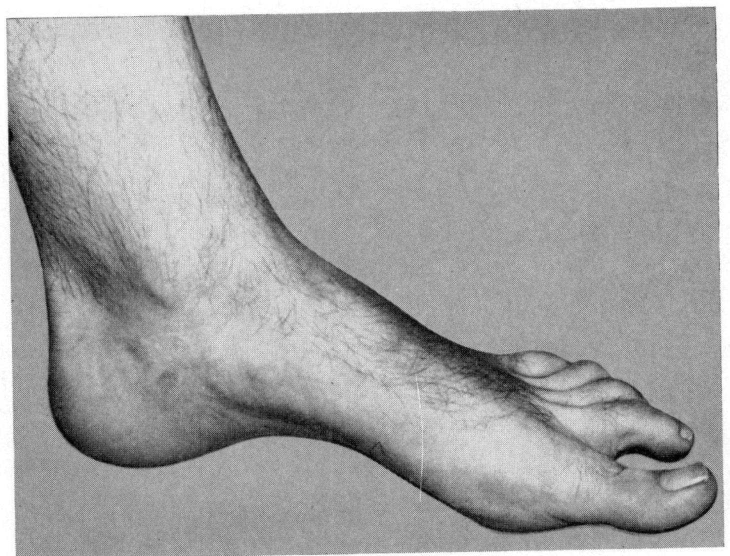

A

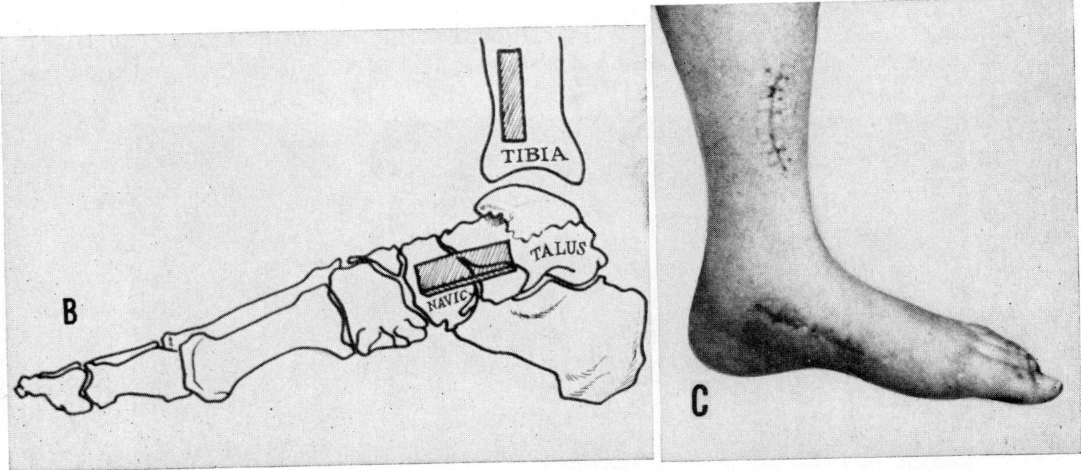

Fig. 39–30.—*A*, The cavus foot or abnormally high longitudinal arch occurs in the rheumatoid foot from over-pull of the extensor tendons. Cock-up toes and large plantar calluses occur. *B*, Drawing of the talonavicular fusion with bone graft obtained from the lower tibial cortex. This procedure stabilizes the mid-foot, preventing arthritic pain. *C*, Postoperative view of the rheumatoid foot, following talonavicular fusion with bone graft.[46]

are painful calluses on the plantar aspects of the sole a metatarsal resection of all the metatarsal heads might be considered.[19] It has given very gratifying results in a great number of cases. While some prefer a dorsal incision, it has been our experience that plantar incisions allow an excellent view of the deformity.[26] The rheumatoid bursae are readily removed, as are the protruding metatarsal heads. A wedge of plantar skin including the callouses is removed, thereby correcting the soft tissue deformities of the toes. Healing is good and partial weight-bearing with wooden-soled shoes can be started in 10 days.

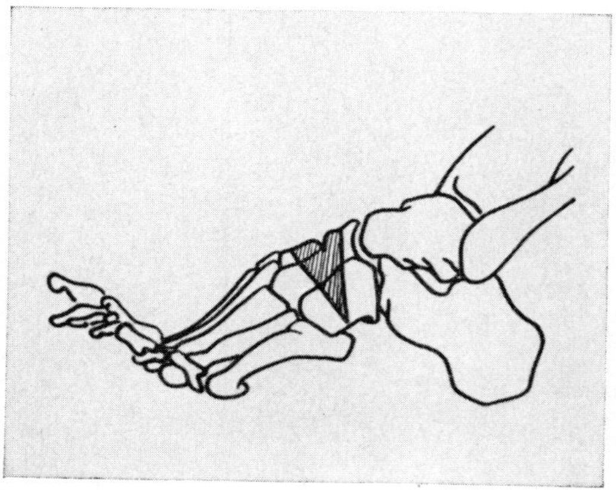

FIG. 39–31.—Wedge osteotomy of the tarsal area with the base upward corrects the severe cavus deformity in the chronic rheumatoid foot.

Hallux Valgus

This condition occurs in 23 per cent of the patients with foot involvement in rheumatoid arthritis. An angle of 20 degrees or more between the first metatarsal and the base phalanx constitutes the deformity of hallux valgus. The causes of hallux valgus are many, such as tight bedclothes, pointed shoes, or the stretching of the medial toe ligaments with erosion of the sesamoid ridge. Dislocation of the sesamoid occurs with spreading of the forefoot. There is a lateral bending of the great toe, a bursa develops containing a pseudo-cavity. Underneath, there is an exostosis of the first metatarsal head medially, and dislocation of the extensor hallucis longus tendon laterally, which becomes shortened and acts as a bow string increasing the deformity. Once the valgus deformity of the great toe begins there is very little chance of correction by conservative means. Surgical treatment for the painful, deformed toe consists of a variety of orthopedic procedures, the simplest of which is the removal of the exostosis and the overlying bursa. Exostectomy in the aged rheuma-

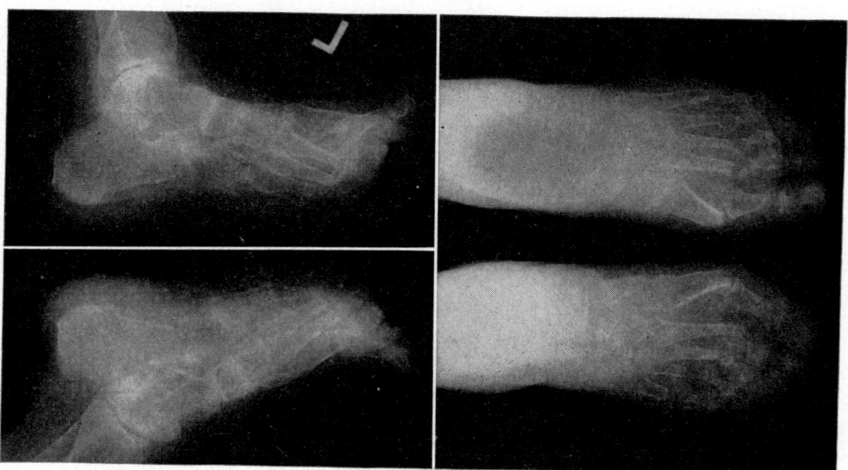

FIG. 39–32.—Arthritic foot after removal of the metatarsal heads for subluxation and deformity.

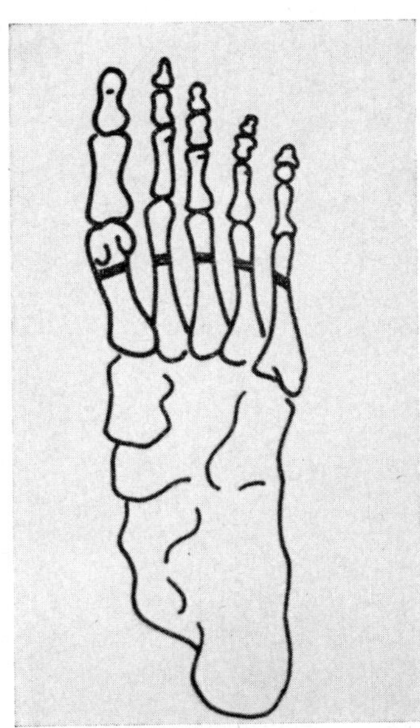

FIG. 39–33.—Metatarsal head removal (Hoffmann operation) showing the line of bone division through the metatarsal neck as a corrective procedure for markedly prominent painful metatarsal heads.

toid patient often affords gratifying relief from the painful bunion although the valgus toe is not corrected. Metatarsal head resection, resection of the base phalanx, corrective osteotomy and a re-aligning of the first metatarsal shaft, and tendon relocation procedures have been used. All have merit but must be adapted to the particular deformity. Arthrodesis of the first metatarsophalangeal joint may be considered. This operation is performed particularly in women who prefer to wear high-heeled shoes. If the fusion is attained with approximately 30 degrees dorsiflexion, an excellent result is obtained from a cosmetic standpoint, and a pain-free first metatarsal take-off segment is provided.

Cock-up Toe or Claw-toe

Cock-up deformity or claw-toe occurs in roughly 60 per cent of the patients with rheumatoid arthritis. The proximal phalanx is dorsiflexed and the distal joints are in a plantar flexed position. Cock-up toe is caused by weakness of the intrinsic muscles and contracture of the long toe extensor tendon. There is usually a dorsal dislocation of the metatarsophalangeal joints, especially in cases of long-standing disease. Cock-up toe occurs rapidly at the beginning of rheumatoid arthritis and, if the foot is involved over a ten-year period, almost every patient will have varying degrees of cock-up toe deformity.

Cock-up toe deformity becomes rigid due to contracture of the collateral ligaments.

Conservatively, one might prescribe toe-stretching exercises, manipulation of the toes, and a resting retention splint. Adhesive taping of the toes has been found to be very effective in preventing the friction callus over the dorsum of the toe and simple felt or sponge rubber pads lessen the pain due to friction with the shoe. When the deformity is severe or when there is overlapping of toes, surgery is the best treatment. Resection of the metatarsal head, resection of the phalanx, osteotomy of a phalanx, mid-shaft resection, or removal of the base phalanx all have been used. We have found that arthrodesis of the interphalangeal joint with intramedullary wire fixation, extensor tenotomy, and capsulotomy has given uniformly good results.

Bursitis

Various forms of bursitis occur in approximately 9 per cent of patients with rheumatoid arthritis, principally at the Achilles tendon attachment to the os calcis where pain and swelling in front of the tendon, pain on walking, and on dorsiflexion of the foot occurs. X-rays show a soft tissue mass beneath the tendon and erosion of the calcaneus. Spontaneous healing occurs, leaving calcaneal erosions as noted by x-ray. If protection of the bursa by an overlying adhesive pad fails then surgical removal should be considered.

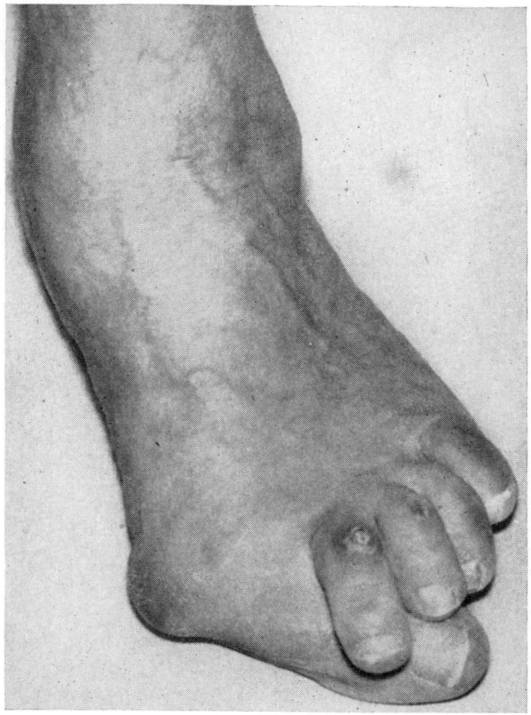

FIG. 39–34.—Hallux valgus with spread of the forefoot, cock-up toe deformity with corns and swelling of the ankle in a patient with rheumatoid arthritis.

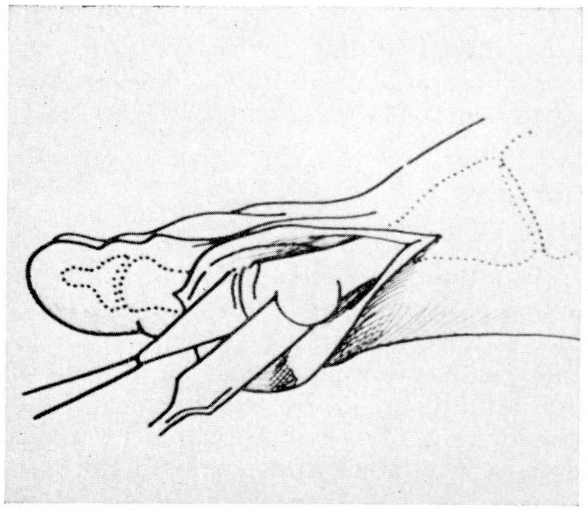

FIG. 39–35.—Simple exostectomy of the first metatarsal head relieves the painful pressure of the bunion and is often the procedure of choice in the chronic rheumatoid hallux valgus patient.

Tenosynovitis

This condition occurs in approximately 6 per cent of rheumatoid patients. The tendons most often involved are the peroneal group, tibialis anterior, and the extensor digitorum longus. Symptoms of pain, locking or swelling may occur but, in other cases, there is no deformity whatsoever. Occasionally, there is a spontaneous rupture of a posterior tibial tendon.[15]

Physical therapy, strapping, rest in a plaster boot, and occasionally the injection of corticosteroid into the tendon sheath may help. If massive swelling persists, surgical excision should be considered. Prophylactic removal of the chronic tenosynovitis may prevent tendon rupture. If this occurs, surgical repair of the ruptured tendon should be performed immediately.

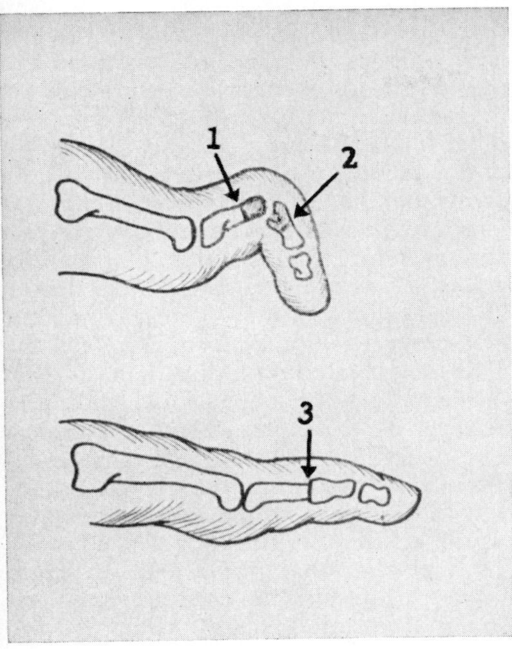

FIG. 39–36.—Surgical correction of cock-up toe deformity by partial resection (1) of the base phalanx, (2) resection of middle phalanx and (3) invagination of the cut bone ends to produce an arthrodesis.

Ankle Joint Involvement in Rheumatoid Arthritis

The ankle joint is rarely involved in rheumatoid arthritis, occurring in less than 9 per cent of patients. Ankylosis seldom occurs and if present, does not interfere seriously with walking. A common error, when there is pain and swelling in the region of the ankle joint, is that of failure to recognize involvement of the talonavicular joint.

The wearing of high shoes, a figure-8 ankle strap, and protection with a plaster walking boot may help. If serious joint damage has occurred, then arthrodesis must be considered with the ankle in equinus. This varies between men and women but usually, for the former at 95 degrees plantar flexion and for the latter approximately 100 to 105 degrees plantar flexion. Arthrodesis should not be performed if the knee is involved. We have found that a fused ankle places considerable abnormal stress on the diseased knee.

Other Deformities of the Rheumatoid Foot

Many other conditions may occur in the chronic rheumatoid foot: tight heel

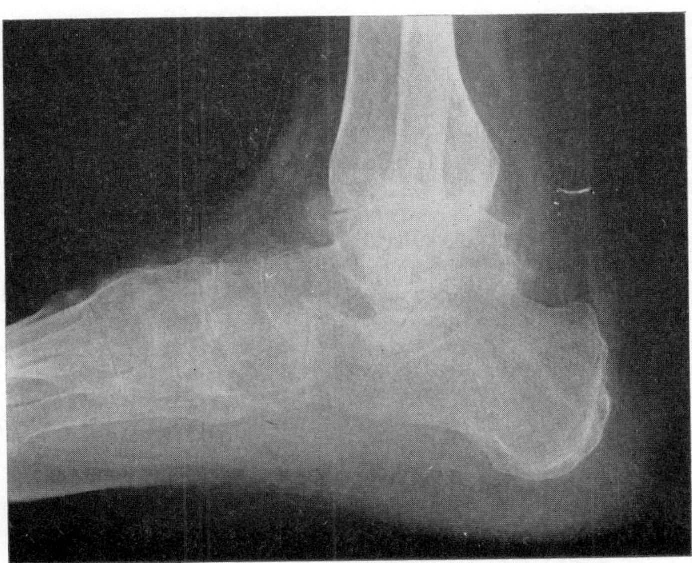

FIG. 39–37.—X-ray of a rheumatoid foot, showing narrowing of the *ankle joint*. There is soft tissue swelling about the anterior and posterior aspects of the joint.

cords may be present, particularly in children and young adults, as the result of wearing high-heeled shoes or from the pressure of bedclothes. Rheumatoid nodules occur over pressure points. A rheumatoid nodule located in the web space between the third and fourth toes often mimics the signs and symptoms of the Morton's neuroma. Surgical removal of the nodule will afford complete relief of the burning pain in this condition. Acute flexion deformities of the great toe due to elongation of the extensor hallucis longus tendon from edema and overstretching occur. This painful deformity can be corrected by fusion. Hallux rigidus or loss of motion in the first metatarsal phalangeal joint occurs. This is associated with dorsal exostosis at the metatarsophalangeal joint leading to a very painful take-off on each step. The wearing of a stout-soled shoe reinforced by a plantar metal bar placed within the leaves of the sole leather may afford relief Surgical arthrodesis with the metatarsophalangeal joint in slight extension should be considered. Base phalanx resection has afforded uniform correction of the deformity, loss of pain, and various degrees of motion. Probably, the most common soft tissue lesion in rheumatoid arthritis is an ingrown toenail.[6] If the usual conservative measures fail, the outer and inner $\frac{1}{4}$ inch of the nail

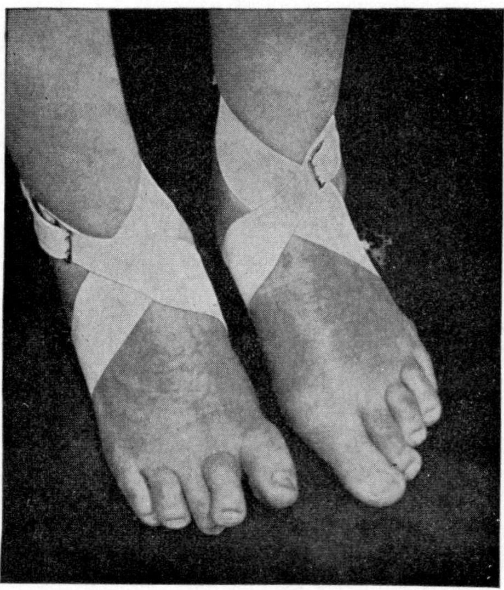

Fig. 39–38.—Ankle strap to support the mid-foot and relieve strain about the ankle. (Kuhns. courtesy of Rheumatism.)

Correction of Deformities of the Feet

1. Limited weight-bearing if the feet are painful and swollen.
2. Apply a plaster cast holding the feet in a good position for walking, at right angles to the leg with no varus or valgus. If the foot cannot be placed in this position at first, correct the deformity as much as possible and change the cast as soon as an improved position can be obtained.
3. Use heat or warm foot baths to lessen inflammation.
4. Give exercises to stretch contractures and strengthen muscles.
5. Strapping of the foot with adhesive plaster which is changed at weekly intervals will often correct spasmodic valgus.
6. When deformities are resistant, manipulation of the foot should be performed. After manipulation the foot is held in the corrected position with a plaster cast for one week. This is followed by exercises as soon as soreness subsides.
7. Ankylosis, in a faulty position for weight-bearing, can be corrected by wedge osteotomy.
8. Operations are used to correct hallux valgus, hammer toe and dislocation of the metatarsal heads. After operation or other correction of deformity, support is given to the foot until normal strength returns.
9. Crutches are often required when walking is first resumed.
10. Proper shoes are described in the chapter on Painful Feet.

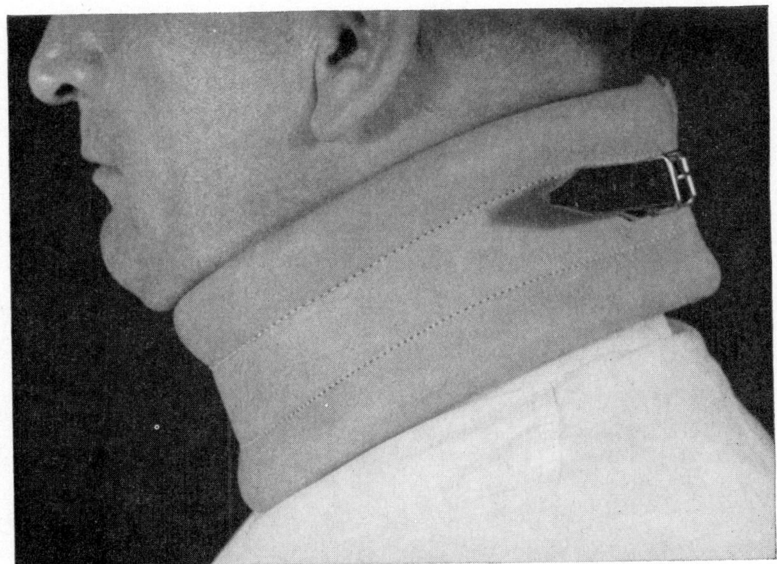

Fig. 39–39.—Leather Thomas collar used for ambulatory support in arthritis of the cervical spine.

is removed. The nail bed is curetted and portions of the nail removed to prevent a recurrence of the disability.

Arthritis of the Temporomandibular Joint

1. Limited motion occurs frequently, but ankylosis is rare.
2. Intra-articular steroid injections are useful in the acute stage.
3. Limitation of motion may be prevented by the chewing of gum after the subsidence of the acute symptoms.
4. The range of motion may be increased by cork or wooden wedges inserted between the teeth. Manipulation under anesthesia is at times helpful.
5. Arthroplasty of the temporomandibular joint may be needed in severe cases.

REHABILITATION

When deformities and disabilities of the arthritic patient have been corrected as far as possible, the physician's responsibility is not ended.[31] (*See* Chapter 36 on Rehabilitation of the Arthritic Patient.)

BIBLIOGRAPHY

1. Aufranc, O. E.: Bull. Rheum. Dis., *14*, 355, 1964.
2. Aufranc, O. E.: *Mold Arthroplasty of the Hip.* St. Louis, C. V. Mosby Co., 1962.
3. Baker, L. D.: Postgrad. Med., *13*, 428, 1954.
4. Blumberg, B.: Bull. Rheum. Dis., *6*, 93, 1955.
5. Blount, W. P.: J. Bone Joint Surg., *46A*, 1297, 1964.
6. Boylston, B. F.: Texas State J. Med., *50*, 16, 1954.
7. Broomhead, R.: Physiotherapy, *41*, 3, 1955.
8. Bunnell, S.: J. Bone Joint Surg., *37A*, 759, 1955.
9. Caruthers, F. W.: Western J. Surg., *68*, 383, 1960.
10. Charnley, J.: Physiotherapy, *49*, 180, 1963.
11. Charnley, J.: Lancet, *2*, 1129, 1961.
12. Charnley, J.: Reconstr. Surg. Traumat., *11*, 9, 1969.
13. Charnley, J.: *Acrylic Cement in Orthopedic Surgery*, Baltimore, The Williams and Wilkins Co., 1970.
14. Clayton, M. L.: Clin. Orthop., *16*, 136. 1960.
15. Clayton, M. L.: J. Bone Joint Surg., *45A*, 1517, 1963.
16. Coventry, M. B.: J.A.M.A., *191*, 487, 1965.
17. Coventry, M. B.: J. Bone Joint Surg., *47A*, 984, 990, 1965.
18. Duthrie, J. J. R.: Practitioner, *166*, 22, 1951.

19. Ferguson, A. B.: J. Bone Joint Surg., *46A*, 1159, 1964.
20. Flatt, A. L.: Geriatrics, *15*, 733, 1960.
21. Fowler, A. W.: J. Bone Joint Surg., *41B*, 507, 1959.
22. Grant, G. H.: J. Bone Joint Surg., *46*, 904, 1964.
23. Harris, N. H.: Proc. Royal Soc. Med., *58*, 879, 1965.
24. Hirsch, C.: Acta Orthop. Scand., *30*, 129, 1960.
25. Hollander, J. L.: J. Bone Joint Surg., *35A*, 983, 1953.
26. Hoffman, P.: Am. J. Surg., *9*, 441, 1911.
27. Jackson, J. P. and Waugh, W.: Proc. Royal Soc. Med., *53*, 888, 1960.
28. Jackson, J. P. and Waugh, W.: J. Bone Joint Surg., *43B*, 746, 1961.
29. Jones, W. N., Aufranc, O. E. and Kermand, W. L.: J. Bone Joint Surg., *49A*, 1022, 1967.
30. Kelly, M.: Lancet, *1*, 1158, 1954.
31. Key, J. A.: West J. Surg., *52*, 385, 1944.
32. Kuhns, J. G.: J. Amer. Geriat. Soc., *2*, 519, 1954.
33. ————: Brit. J. Phys. Med., *18*, 270, 1955.
34. ———: J. Bone Joint Surg., *46A*, 448, 1964.
35. Kuhns, J. G. and Potter, T. A.: *Current Practice in Orthopedic Surgery*, St. Louis, C. V. Mosby & Co., 1963.
36. Larmon, W. A. and Kuntz, J. F.: J. Bone Joint. Surg., *40A*, 30, 1954.
37. Lewis, G. B.: Bull. Hosp. Joint. Dis., *21*, 71, 1960.
38. McKeever, D. C.: In *Clinical Orthopedics*, DePalma, A. F. (Ed.), Philadelphia, J. B. Lippincott Co., 1960, p. 86.
39. MacIntosh, D. L.: J. Bone Joint Surg., *40A*, 1431, 1958.
40. Maslock, D. I.: Ann. Phys. Med., *10*, 236, 1970.
41. Mennell, J.: Arch. Phys. Med., *28*, 685, 1947.
42. Moore, A. T. and Bohlman, H. R.: J. Bone Joint Surg., *25*, 688, 1943.
43. Murley, A. H. G.: J. Bone Joint Surg., *42B*, 502, 1960.
44. Peabody, C. W.: J. Michigan Med. Soc., *54*, 317, 1955.
45. Pemberton, R. and Osgood, R. B.: *Medical and Orthopedic Management of Chronic Arthritis*, New York, Macmillan Co., 1934.
46. Potter, T. A.: Surg. Clinics of North America, *49*, 41, 1969.
47. Preston, R. L.: New York State J. Med., *53*, 2887, 1955.
48. Roberts, S. M. and Joplin, R. J.: New Engl. J. Med., *216*, 646, 1937.
49. Schwartzman, J. R.: J. Bone Joint Surg., *41A*, 705, 1959.
50. Shier, L. G. P.: J. Bone Joint Surg., *42B*, 31, 1960.
51. Shier, L. G. P.: J. Bone Joint Surg., *36B*, 553, Nov. 1954.
52. Smith-Peterson, M. N., Larson, C. B. and Aufranc, O. E.: J. Bone Joint Surg., *27*, 1, 1945.
53. Steindler, A.: Bull. New York Acad. Med., *36*, 97, 1960.
54. Straub, L. R.: Bull. Rheum. Dis., *12*, 265, 1962.
55. Vainio, K.: Annales Chirurgiae etc. Gynocologiac, *45*, Suppl. #1, 1956.
56. Wardle, E. H.: Surg., Gynec. & Obst., *115*, 61–64, 1962.
57. Waldius, B.: Acta Ortho. Scand., *30*, 137, 1960.
58. Wilson, P. D.: Med. Clin. North America, *21*, 1623, 1937.

Chapter 40

Correction of Arthritic Deformities of the Upper Extremity

By Adrian E. Flatt, M.D.

It is tempting to rest a painful upper limb in a sling. This support often succeeds in relieving pain and reducing the activity of the disease, but the limb frequently becomes stiff because of the immobility. Rest over a prolonged period may reduce function in many joints of the limb and may produce secondary pain from such causes as bursitis or fasciitis.[6]

Protective muscle spasm within the limb can produce deformities throughout its length: internal rotation and adduction of the shoulder, elbow flexion, limited pronation and supination of the forearm and complex deformities of the wrist and hand. Early surgical treatment of the joint primarily affected will restore function to the joint and allow regression of generalized protective muscle spasm so that the function of other joints will be maintained.[21]

Many modalities of treatment are needed in the rehabilitation of the rheumatoid patient. In recent years, surgery has been increasingly used in the treatment of various degrees of this disease in the upper limb.

There are three distinct phases of the disease in which operative treatment can be of value. It is used (1) prophylactically to prevent future destruction of joint surfaces when drug therapy has been unable to control synovitis; (2) late in the disease to salvage function from grossly involved tendons and joints, and (3) in the stage of adaptation (middle phase) of disease, surgery can be of value but is not used as commonly as in the other two phases.

Operations can restore potential range of motion and relieve pain, but it is fruitless to operate in the face of apathy, self-pity or the general aura of despair which is so frequently associated with rheumatoid disease. Surgeons share a common responsibility with physicians in other disciplines to treat the disease—and the patient—as a whole and must not confine themselves to one specific area. The rheumatoid patient is best served by a team with one person in overall charge.[9]

Of particular importance are physical and occupational therapy. The tragic wasting of muscles and stiffening of joints which often occur in these patients are sometimes so gross that rehabilitation may be impossible. Patients must be taught to become active participants in the care of their disease and they must be taught to rebuild the muscles which control and protect the joints of the limbs.

Preoperative physical therapy is of vital importance. It restores tone and strength to the limb and enables the patient to cooperate in postoperative exercises. These exercises are taught to the patient before surgery so that their purpose is fully understood before the operation is performed.

The tissue primarily affected is synovium. Only later is the articular cartilage destroyed by pannus formation and invasion of the subchondral bone. The intra-articular swelling of the synovium stretches and weakens the joint capsule and ligaments. This interference with joint integrity allows an imbalance of forces to occur over the joint and can produce grotesque deformities such as are sometimes seen in the hand.

In the past it has been said that surgery must be delayed until the disease is "burned out." This is not true. While it would clearly be foolish to operate during a generalized acute "flare" of disease, active local disease or a raised sedimentation rate is not a contra-indication to surgery.[25] Vainio has recorded a personal series of over 6500 operations in which he used similar criteria and in which he did not see any case of local flare-up or general deterioration attributable to the operation. It is becoming increasingly recognized that synovectomy of an acutely inflamed joint often leads to a marked postoperative improvement in the general state of the patient. In the upper limb almost all operations can be performed under axillary block anesthesia. It is routine for these patients to be out of bed with the arm in a sling the day after the operation.

Operations on the elbow, wrist or hand are carried out under pneumatic tourniquet applied to the arm. The combination of local axillary block and tourniquet control of bleeding produce no significant shock. Cortisone therapy is not a contra-indication to surgery and has not been observed to produce any adverse general effects on the patients or to delay local wound healing. Preoperatively, all patients on cortisone are weaned to their minimum maintenance dose, but once this dose has been established no special efforts have been made by me to load or increase this dose as a precaution against operative shock in upper limb surgery.* The usual dosage is continued throughout the operative and postoperative periods. In a personal series of over 400 consecutive upper limb operations, I have followed this routine with excellent results.

* Some surgeons, however, insist on increasing the corticosteroid dosage on the day of operation and during the period of postoperative stress. (*See* Chapter 31.) Ed.

Many patients presenting for possible surgery in the upper limb often require surgery in other areas, particularly the feet. It is sensible in planning an operative program to first perform a simple operation in the hand (such as median nerve decompression) or a simple foot operation (such as metatarsal head resection). The successful result will encourage the patient to undertake more elaborate and time-consuming operations that may also be necessary.

Many factors enter into the choice and timing of an operation. More than thirty years ago Wilson[30] listed certain questions which should be answered, so that a reasonable operative plan could be formed:

1. Is the arthritis still active?
2. Is the patient in good enough physical condition to permit extensive surgical procedures?
3. Considering the age of the patient, his physical state and the number of operations required, is the expected gain in function from operation worth the effort?
4. Should the operation be delayed for any reason for institution of other therapy?
5. Will the patient be able to cooperate in after-care with the proper morale and willingness to endure some pain?
6. Are the facilities necessary for successful treatment present in the hospital?
7. Will the patient be able to receive proper after-care on leaving the hospital?
8. Is the patient's financial status such that he can go through the entire treatment or have the resources of the community been mobilized to care for such treatment?

The ideas behind many of these questions are still valid today. Adequate financial support for the patient during the frequently prolonged postoperative period is essential. It is equally essential that the operation be performed in a hospital which can provide all the necessary facilities for good postoperative treatment.

In the final analysis, it is the patient who must request the operation. To try to "sell" a patient an operation is to do him a disservice, and it is my policy to try to introduce potential candidates for surgery to others who have had the proposed operation. A short private discussion between the two patients usually rapidly answers all potential questions and allows a decision to be made without external pressures.

Safeguards Against Shoulder Deformity

1. Use of a firm, flat bed with only one small pillow, if any, beneath the head.
2. The patient should lie with his hands clasped beneath his head several times a day for short periods of time. This position will produce abduction and external rotation of the shoulder.
3. A sling may be helpful in relieving acute pain around the shoulder, but the distal portions of the limb must be exercised several times a day. Injections of corticosteroid suspension in the shoulder joint or adjacent bursae are often helpful.
4. Various forms of external heat applications may be helpful in relieving pain and muscular spasm and are particularly valuable when they are followed by active or passive exercises which put the joint through a maximum range of painless motion.
5. After an acute attack of arthritis or periarticular capsulitis, heat, massage and active exercises are all of value in attempting to regain motion.
6. Manipulation is frequently considered but this can be undertaken only by those skilled in these procedures. The bones of the average rheumatoid patient are often so osteoporotic that the risks of fracture are too great to justify manipulation.

Shoulder

Stiffness, pain and deformity at the shoulder can be produced by local disease or be secondary to immobility produced by disease in more distal portions of the limb. A painful hand or elbow will inevitably lead to reduced activity in the limb and increase the chances of stiffness occurring in the shoulder. It is vitally important that mobility be maintained in the limb so that the risks of shoulder-hand syndrome are minimized. Exercises and proper positioning of the shoulder are important at all times but particularly important after an episode of acute disease either in the shoulder or in other portions of the limb. The common position of deformity adopted by the shoulder is adduction and internal rotation and treatment should be directed to preventing this deformity.

A very common cause of limitation of shoulder joint motion is disease of the subacromial bursa or the acromioclavicular joint. Involvement of the subacromial bursa restricts scapulothoracic motion because such movement tends to increase the tension within the bursa.[6] Local corticosteroid injections can be of help, but long-term relief is best provided by acromionectomy which will effectively decompress the joint. This operation relieves the pain of the bursitis by removing one of the two bony surfaces between which the swollen bursa was compressed. By removing the outer portion of the acromion, any accompanying acromioclavicular disease is also relieved.

The operation is usually done through a "saber-cut" skin incision over the top of the shoulder. The acromion is cleanly divided in a line extending backwards from the acromioclavicular joint. The ligaments and deltoid muscle are dissected clear of the loose piece of bone, the deltoid origin sewn back to the acromioclavicular ligament and portions of the

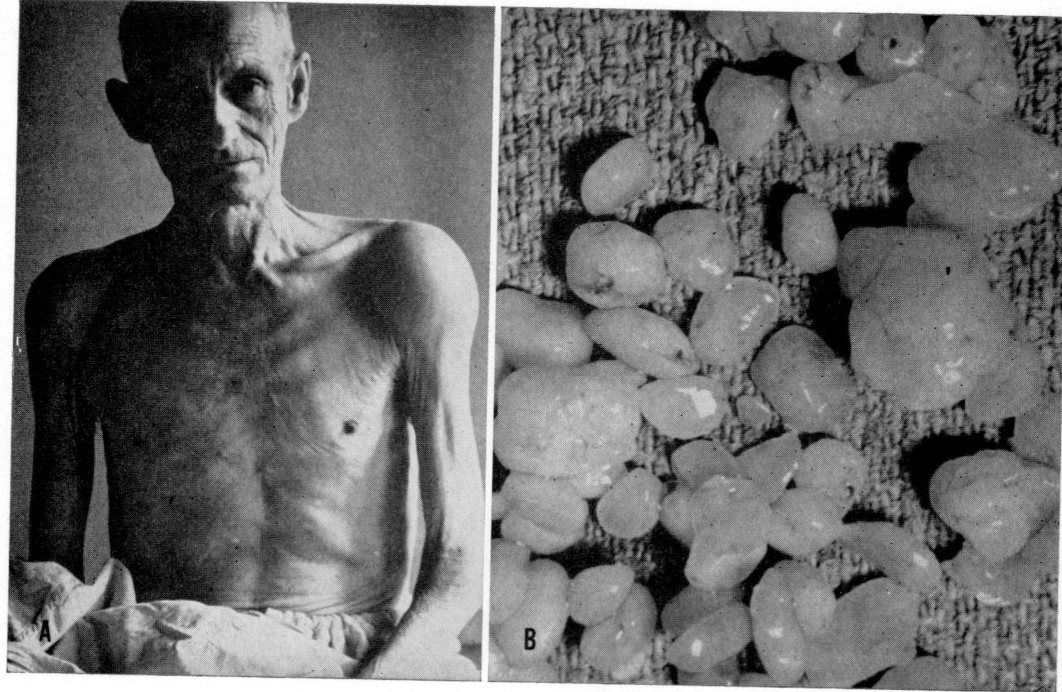

Fig. 40–1.—Rheumatoid disease of shoulder. *A*, Gross disease of the joint tissues and rice body production can greatly hinder movement of the joint. *B*, Shows some of the rice bodies removed during debridement of this patient's joint.

reflected periosteum. Postoperative immobilization is not encouraged but a sling is permissible. Pendulum exercises of the shoulder are started as soon as the operative site is comfortable, and active exercises commenced about three weeks after the operation.

Glenohumeral disease is common in varying degrees, but it is uncommon for it to produce crippling limitation of shoulder joint motion. Gross incongruity of the articular surfaces can occur and is usually associated with varying degrees of necrosis of the humeral head. It is important to relate the clinical and radiological findings; often the symptoms and limitation of motion may be far less than might be expected from the x-ray findings.

Severe disease of the joint and its surrounding bursae may produce large painful swellings which can be relieved by surgical excision. Complete synovectomy of the joint is not easy to accomplish but excision of as much diseased tissue as possible, drainage of excess fluid and removal of rice bodies often gives considerable symptomatic relief (Fig. 40–1).

Fusion of the joint is very rarely performed for rheumatoid disease. Arthroplasty of the shoulder joint is occasionally performed, particularly to relieve pain which is causing a restriction of motion. The Neer intramedullary prosthesis can be used to replace a deformed humeral head (Fig. 40–2). This prosthesis is designed to leave the muscles attached to the greater and lesser tuberosities of the humeral head.[14] The recovery period for this operation is usually about six weeks, but it can often demand a high degree of perseverance on the part of the patient to obtain the maximum range of motion and muscle strength.

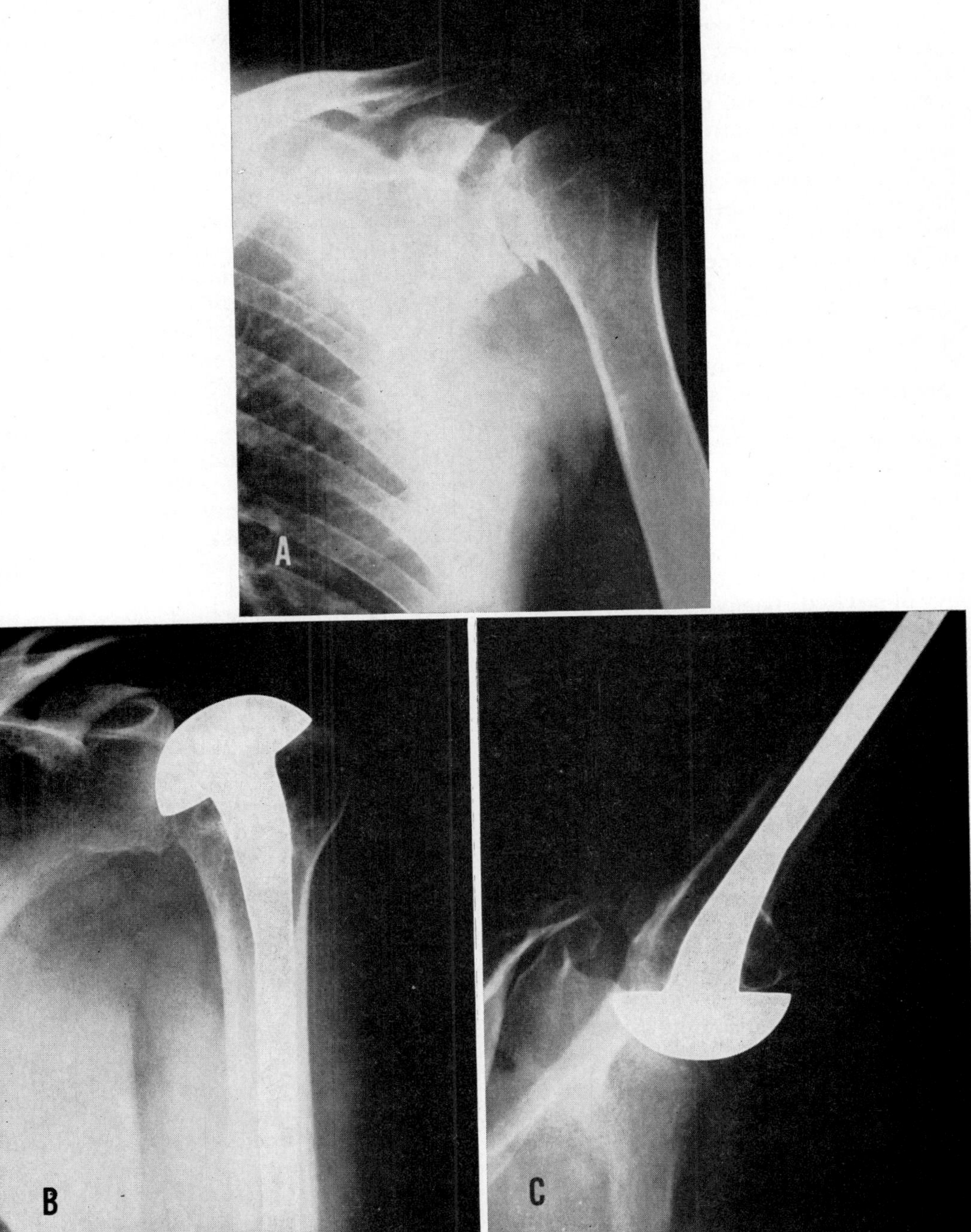

FIG. 40–2.—Prosthetic replacement of humeral head. Occasionally rheumatoid disease of the joint leads to such destruction of the humeral head that movement is almost impossible. The insertion of the Neer prosthesis can restore a satisfactory range of motion. *A*, Shoulder x-ray before surgery. *B* and *C*, at 11-year follow-up, showing extent of abduction. (Illustrations courtesy of Dr. Charles Neer.)

Elbow

The elbow joint consists of two articulations with different movements: flexion and extension and pronation and supination. The synovial cavity of the elbow is common to both articulations and deformity which occurs usually affects both joints, producing an elbow held in flexion and pronation. Surgery can frequently restore a considerable range of functional movement.

During the stage of acute synovitis the joint is rested best by molded plaster splints in about 60° of flexion. These splints are for resting and not for immobilization. The splints are removed several times a day and active motions insisted upon. There is a distinction between discomfort and pain. The patient is taught that discomfort during motion is acceptable but that pain is not. Pain is produced by too great a range of motion and is more commonly produced by ill-advised passive motion than by active contractions of the patient's muscles. Patients are taught that the elbow is not a weight-bearing joint and that to use it as such via crutches or canes will greatly aggravate the condition of the joint.

Limitation of extension is common and is not a great functional handicap. This limitation should be accepted because the elbow notoriously responds adversely to manipulation, either by a therapist or by the patient lifting buckets of sand or other similar weights. It is better to accept some limitation of extension than to provoke further reaction and subsequent further flexion by ill-considered manipulations.

When the synovial swelling within the joint has not responded to drug therapy and the pain is producing limitation of motion, synovectomy should be considered. The operation will relieve pain and perhaps increase the range of motion. It will certainly remove the considerable swellings at the side of the olecranon. Smith-Petersen has pointed out that the head of the radius is frequently involved and often shows a considerable degree of anterior dislocation.[21] The synovectomy is therefore frequently combined with excision of the radial head.

The operation is done through a lateral approach (Fig. 40–3). The muscle attachments are reflected from the lateral condyle and the epicondylar ridge. Both the anterior and posterior compartments are cleared of diseased synovium and the radial head is usually excised. Early postoperative motion is encouraged and the patients are often more comfortable in a plaster of paris gutter than in voluminous compression dressings.

Fusion of the elbow can be done, but it is rarely advisable because of the vital importance of retaining elbow motion. Rheumatoid disease affects many joints and there are therefore great risks in fusing an elbow joint. Subsequent disease may so stiffen the opposite arm that the patient would be made helpless with the two hands held away from the body. On the other hand, arthroplasty of the humero-ulnar joint is an excellent operation and yields good long-term results. The operation necessarily destroys some of the stability of the joint but this is more than compensated for by the loss of pain and increase in range of motion.

Good muscle control is essential for the success of an arthroplasty operation and this is particularly important at the elbow because it is a hinge joint in the middle of a long lever arm. Both degenerative and rheumatoid disease can be treated by this procedure. The patient in Figure 40–4 has now been followed for over sixteen years. Absorption of bone has occurred but this has not adversely affected the result. Care must be taken in the selection of patients because the joint will not necessarily be sufficiently stable to support the extra force of crutch or cane walking. The operation is usually done through a posterior incision with the humerus being approached through a slit made in the triceps muscle. Enough bone has to

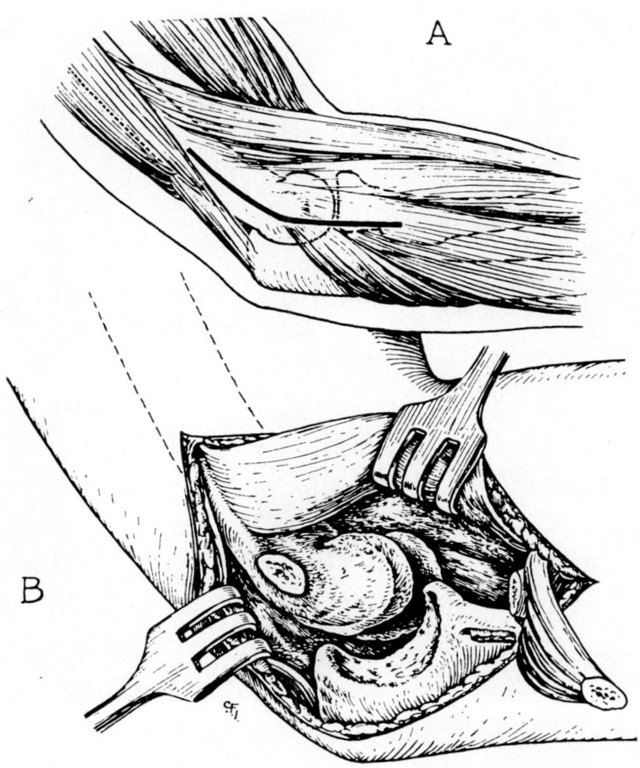

FIG. 40–3.—Synovectomy of elbow. Surgical excision of the elbow joint synovium is a useful operation which relieves pain and restores movement. It is done through a lateral approach and both anterior and posterior compartments are cleared of diseased synovium. (Campbell's *Operative Orthopedics*, courtesy of The C. V. Mosby Co.)

be removed from the lower end of the humerus and the trochlear notch of the ulna to produce a loose joint. No attempt is made to reproduce the exact bony contours and only one condyle is made on the distal end of the humerus. The head of the radius is usually excised at the junction of the head and neck.

The raw bone ends are covered by a large rectangular sheet of fascia lata cut from the thigh. The sheet is folded in half and one half is sewn around the lower end of the humerus. The other half is used to cover the raw bone of the ulna and is also tucked down between the radius and ulna.

Postoperatively the arm is immobilized in a cast at 90° of flexion and in addition is fixed in a shoulder abduction splint for the first two weeks in order to prevent rotational deformity. The skin sutures are then removed and during the next week the arm is held at rest in a gutter splint at 90° of elbow flexion. Active movement of the finger muscles arising in the forearm is encouraged throughout the postoperative period It is vital to maintain finger motion and prevent circulatory stasis in the hand.

After three weeks a sling is used in the daytime, but the gutter splint is retained at night for about two months from the time of operation. Active elbow exercises are started three weeks after the operation and must be continued for about six months. After this time, prog-

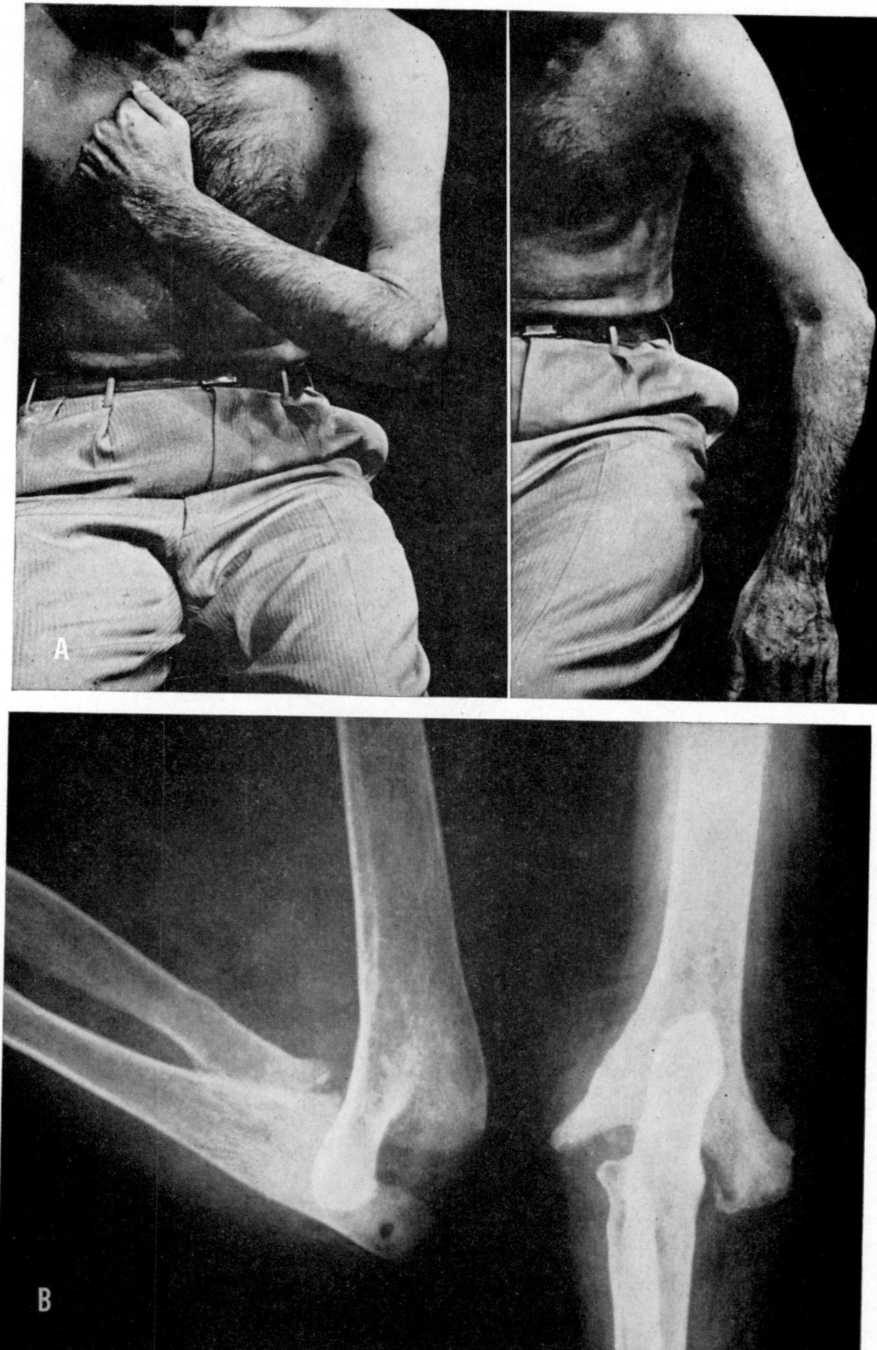

FIG. 40–4.—Elbow arthroplasty. *A,* Restoration of a considerable range of motion can be achieved by elbow arthroplasty; this patient shows his range of motion sixteen years after surgery. *B,* The roentgenogram shows that there has been a slow destruction of the lower end of the humerus but this does not interfere with function. (Courtesy of J. Amer. Phys. Therapy Assoc.)

ress both in strength and range of motion will continue at a slow rate until the maximum result is achieved, about two years after surgery.

The Wrist

The wrist is a key joint in so many functions of the hand that its impairment influences function to a far greater degree than merely limiting motion of the joint itself.[5] Two joints combine to produce wrist motion: the distal radio-ulnar joint and the radiocarpal joint.

Rheumatoid disease frequently attacks the distal radio-ulnar joint and because the joint shares a common synovial cavity with the radiocarpal joint both are frequently involved in the destructive synovitis.

The expanding synovium loosens and even destroys the ligaments supporting the radio-ulnar articulation, allowing a dorsal dislocation of the ulna to occur in relation to the distal end of the radius.[1] This dislocation not only restricts pronation and supination, but also creates a hazard for the long extrinsic extensor tendons. These tendons become tightly stretched against the radial side of the distal end of the ulna. Whenever the fingers are moved, the tendons rub against the irregular surface of the bone and attrition ruptures can, and do, occur.[27]

The operation of excision of the distal end of the ulna is therefore used to remove an actual or potential hazard to the tendons and to increase the range of pronation and supination. Care must be taken in advising this operation. It is best done when there are no signs of disease or instability of the radiocarpal joint. If extensive destruction of this joint has occurred, the distal end of the ulna may be a useful prop in stabilizing the wrist; its excision may so tip the balance that complete dislocation of the wrist can occur.

After the operation, physical therapy is directed more towards the restoration of pronation and supination rather than to wrist motion. Some discomfort can be expected at the elbow as increasing movement develops around the head of the radius. This discomfort should not be allowed to stop treatment. Stabilization of the lower end of the ulna in relation to the radius often relieves some of the discomfort that occurs during exercising.

Destruction of the radiocarpal joint from either degenerative or rheumatoid disease can often be stabilized and made relatively painless by the use of a molded leather wristlet which is held in place by lacing or velcro strapping. Cock-up splints made of plastic, metal or plaster are also useful in immobilizing the wrist and restoring some degree of function.

Fusion of the wrist is a useful operation in either degenerative or rheumatoid disease, when the pain is crippling, when the wrist has stiffened in a non-functional position or when the joint is completely unstable. The choice of the angle of fusion is of vital importance. The position usually recommended is about 30° of dorsiflexion in the so-called functional position. This position is that used by the wrist in an otherwise normal limb. The rheumatoid patient's limb is usually far from normal, and the flexion deformity of the wrist occurs because this is the functional position for many of the most vital uses of the hand. During feeding or dressing, the wrists are almost always flexed and perineal toilet is impossible with the wrists held in the so-called functional position.

In the rheumatoid patient, the wrist should be fused in a neutral position and, on occasions, in slight flexion. The operation is done through a dorsal incision over the wrist and a bone graft is needed to supply stability to the fusion. The graft is usually taken from the outer side of the ilium and laid into the dorsum of the wrist passing from the lower inch of the radius across the carpal bones to the bases of the metacarpals. The extensor tendons are replaced over the graft and the lower end of the ulna is usually excised before the skin wound is sutured (Fig. 40–5).

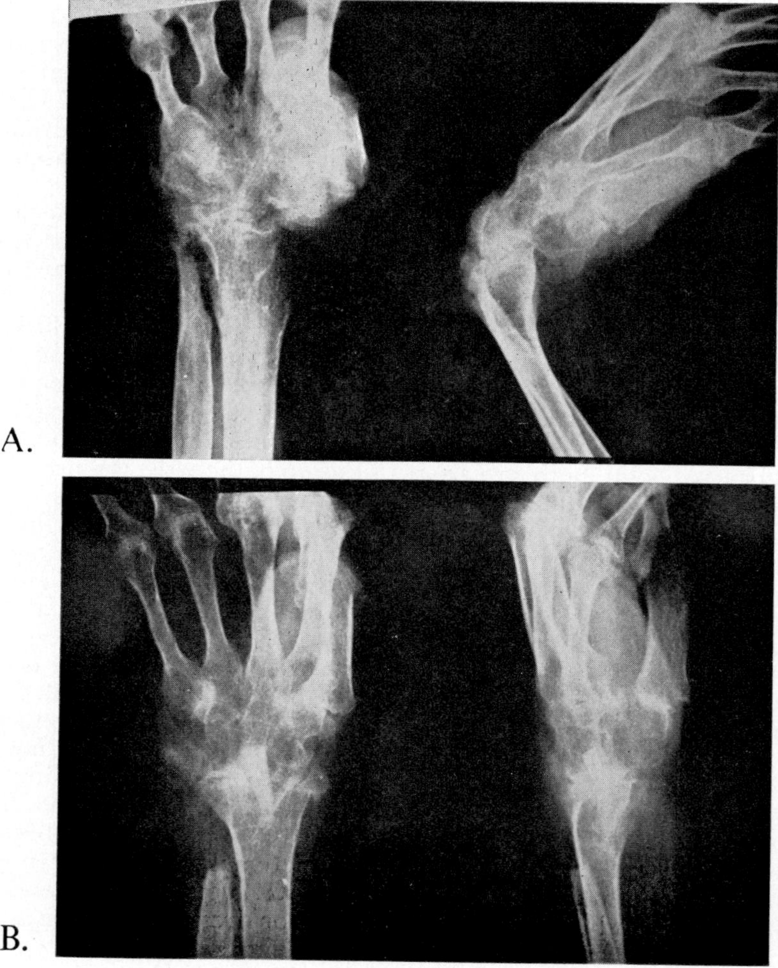

FIG. 40–5.—Wrist fusion. Stabilization of the wrist is a valuable procedure but the angle of fusion should be chosen with great care. It is not advisable to fuse the wrist in dorsiflexion because of the limitation in function imposed by such a position. *Example*—A. Preoperative malposition in palmar flexion; B. Postoperative fusion in neutral position allowing improved function of the hand.

The patient is usually in a below-elbow cast for about three months, but during this time finger movement exercises are constantly practiced. After the fusion is solid, exercises are done to improve both pronation and supination and the strength of grip. The fusion stabilizes the carpus on the radius and frequently adds power to the grip by allowing the extrinsic flexor and extensor tendons to act solely on the fingers instead of wasting their power on an unstable wrist.

The Hand

The hand is affected by three major types of arthritis and functional improvement can be obtained in each by appropriate reconstructive procedures.

The three types of arthritis to be considered are osteoarthritis, gouty arthritis and rheumatoid arthritis. Some dignify traumatic arthritis as a separate entity but from the point of view of the restoration of function it differs from degenerative arthritis only because it accelerates the inevitable normal degenerative processes.

Osteoarthritis

Osteoarthritis in the joints of the hand is usually proportional to the amount of abuse of the joints. Symptoms usually do not occur until the fifth decade and are commonly precipitated by a sprain or transmission of an unusual force through the joint. Once these symptoms have started, they are unlikely to completely disappear (Fig. 40–6). Probably the most common joint to be involved is the carpometacarpal joint of the thumb. Because the thumb carries a high proportion of the work load of the hand, it is common to find degenerative arthritic changes in the first carpometacarpal joint. In prehensile activities the thumb is one-half of the hand and arthritis at its base seriously interferes with all its functions. Conservative treatment, analgesics and splinting are all helpful but frequently the symptoms are so disabling that operation has to be considered.[9] Two operations are possible, fusion or arthroplasty. Neither operation is ideal; each has its advocates and both require several months of treatment before postoperative recovery is complete.

It is generally considered that, in the younger patient, the fusion operation is preferable because the relatively small loss of mobility of the thumb is well compensated by the painless stability achieved. The operation consists of excision of the contiguous arthritic joint surfaces, impaction of the two raw bone ends and their immobilization by a bone graft driven into both bones.[14] The graft is commonly

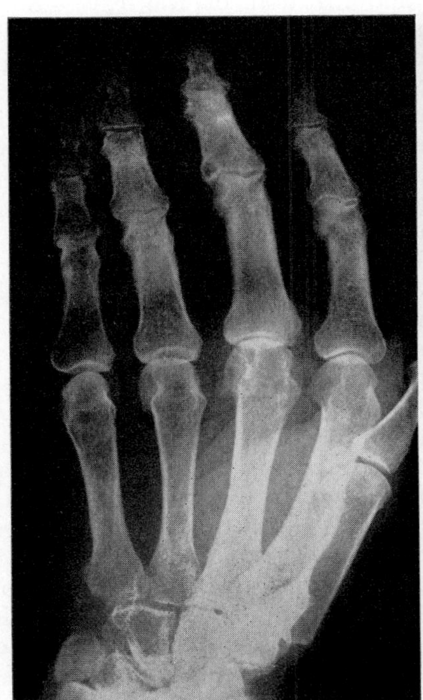
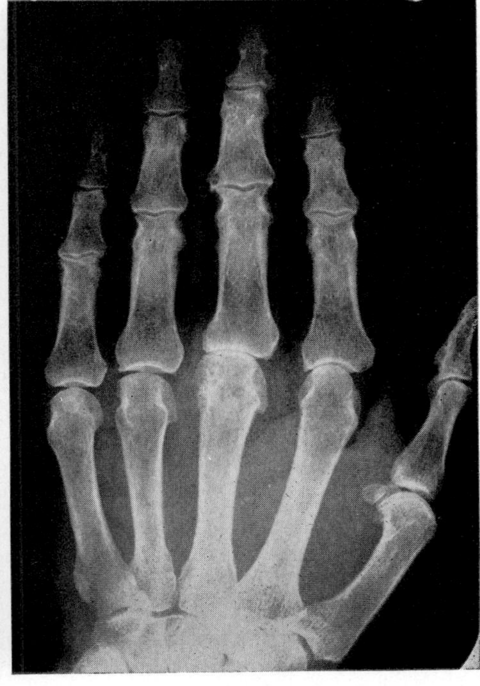

Fig. 40–6.—Degenerative arthritis of fingers. This hand of a professional wrestler shows the results of repeated traumatic insults to the digital joints.

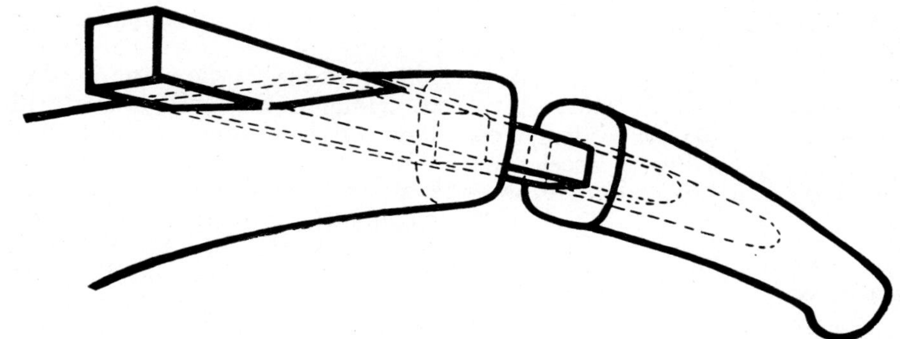

FIG. 40–7.—Digital joint fusion. The use of a squared bone peg driven across the joint insures a strong bony fusion. A proximal interphalangeal joint is illustrated. (Moberg and Hendrikson, courtesy of Acta Chir. Scand.)

taken from the tibia or occasionally the ilium. Immobilization in a cast which includes the thumb will be necessary for three to four months following the operation.

The arthroplasty operation is achieved by excision of the greater multangulum and immobilization of the thumb in an abduction cast for three to four weeks. Technically it can be very difficult to excise all of the bone and experience is needed to achieve a good result. Stability in the arthroplasty is provided by a combination of local scar and the actions of the muscles passing over the joint. In recent years I have found that the operation provides a good level of painless function and I believe it is the operation of choice for the elderly patient.

Osteoarthritis of the digital joints is common, but rarely produces deformity severe enough to result in loss of function or to require surgery. It frequently follows trauma which is usually associated with extensive soft tissue damage. The scarring produced by the soft tissue trauma is often of greater functional importance than the changes in the joint surfaces.

The usual treatment for such joints, if they are sufficiently painful to require surgery, is to fuse them in a functional position. Fusion of a single digital joint yields good function, but fusion of two of the three joints is rarely done. To achieve the best results the two fused joints should be separated by a movable joint.

Several methods of arthrodesis of digital joints are practiced, and all are based upon the principle of internal immobilization of the raw bone ends until union occurs. Immobilization can be obtained by Kirschner wire fixation or by a bone graft bridging the excised joint surface (Fig. 40–7). Union is probably achieved a little earlier by bone grafting but in either method six to eight weeks of immobilization are usually required.

Movement can be provided for these joints either by arthroplasty or prosthetic replacement. Both operations have severe drawbacks and are not commonly practiced in osteoarthritic finger joints. Arthroplasty or excision of the degenerated joint surfaces can be of use in the long and ring fingers because lateral support is supplied on the borders of the hand by the index and little fingers. Attempts to supply movement by arthroplasty in the border fingers will usually lead to gross lateral instability and severe limitation of function. Prosthetic replacement of individual finger joints has been tried and the early results were encouraging.[2] Long-term follow-up of isolated prosthetic replacement of a single digital joint has shown that bone absorption occurs around the prosthesis and that function steadily deteriorates as time goes by.

Gouty Arthritis

Both Riordan[19] and Straub[23] have reviewed gout as it affects the hand and they have shown that there is little indication for surgical intervention. Considerable symptomatic relief can be given by aspiration of tense joint effusions. There is general agreement that large tophi should be excised if they are a mechanical block to joint movement, or if there is a danger of their becoming infected. Draining sinuses and their causative tophi may need to be excised. Occasionally, bony destruction or urate deposits may be so massive that amputation of part or all of a finger may be required (Fig. 40–8). Degenerative changes of the interphalangeal joints may be so great that fusion in a functional position may be necessary. There are no published reports of attempts at prosthetic replacement in gouty finger joints.

Rheumatoid Disease of the Hand

In recent years the surgical literature has contained an increasing number of papers concerned with rheumatoid disease of the hand.[3,7,8,11,18,22,28] No thorough studies of long-term results have yet been published, but enough informa-

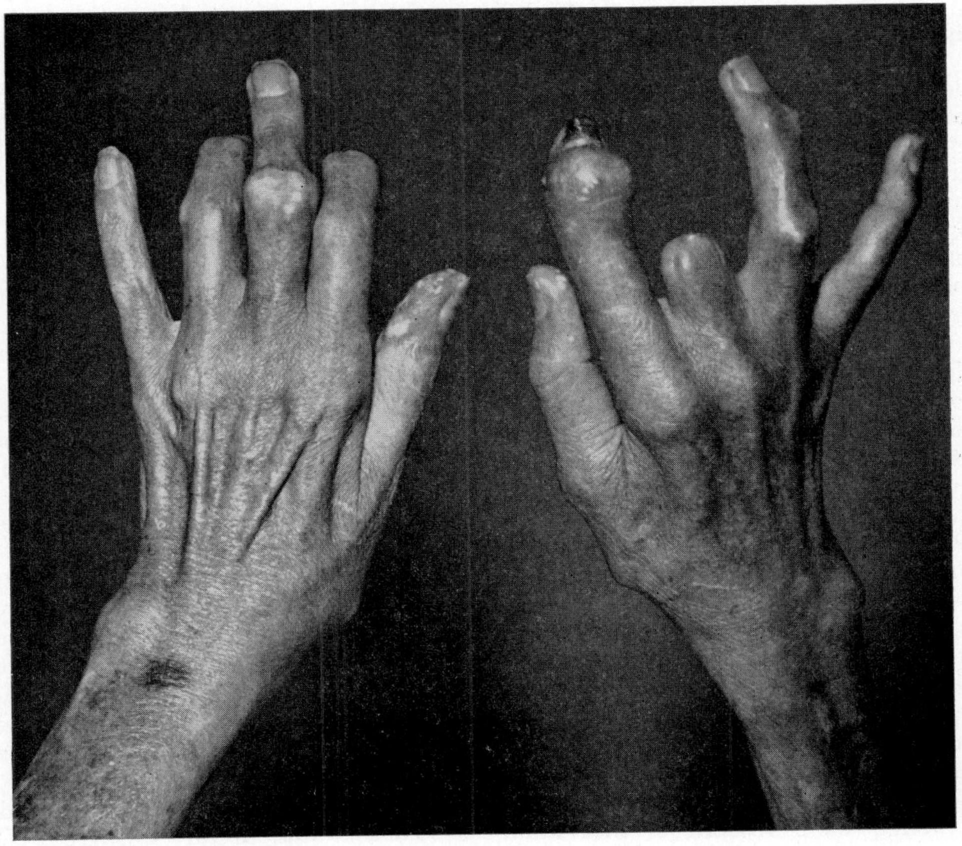

Fig. 40–8.—Gout of the hand. These hands of a 53-year-old woman illustrate the classic problems encountered in the hands of both sexes. Selective amputation has already been necessary in several digits. (Converse [Chapter 59] *Reconstructive Plastic Surgery*, courtesy of W. B. Saunders Co.)

tion is now available to establish the general principles of surgical care. The disease attacks the hand by first involving the synovium. The great majority of deformities that develop are secondary to the synovial disease and are not produced by primary involvement of the digital joint surfaces.

Splinting is of limited value in the care of rheumatoid disease of the hands. Three major types are available; passive immobilization, remedial and assistive splints.[8] Passive immobilization splints provide rest during acute disease, remedial splints can be of use in overcoming contractures and assistive splints help compensate for joint distortions and muscle weakness.

Splinting the hand effectively is an art. Much harm can be done by ill-designed or ill-fitting splints. Stiffness of the hand will inevitably occur if an ill-designed splint forces the fingers into a non-functional position or if they are held for long periods in positions which strain the joint capsules. There is a virtue in simplicity. Many ingeniously designed complex mechanisms lie neglected in closets because too great demands are made on the patient's tolerance.

The wrist is the key joint to the position of function of the hand. During an acute phase of the disease, continuous passive immobilization may be necessary. As soon as symptoms begin to subside, intermittent, properly controlled muscle-building exercises are added. Many materials are now available for making splints and none is completely superior to any other. A gutter-type flexor surface splint is made with the wrist in maximum of 20° of dorsiflexion, the fingers in their normal functional arches[8] with the palm and the thumb abducted at least 20°. Pressure is usually more evenly distributed throughout the forearm when the splint is held in place by a bandage wrap instead of individual straps.

Remedial splinting is infinitely more satisfactory than manipulation of contractures within the hand. The gradual pull of dynamic traction creates a gentle persistent force to which contracted tissue will yield; manipulation frequently produces tearing of tissues, bleeding and adhesion formation. The states which respond best to remedial splinting are adduction contracture of the thumb, flexion contracture of the digital joints, and stiffness of the interphalangeal joints. The late Dr. Sterling Bunnell pioneered the development of remedial splints for the hand, and his reversed knuckle-bender, miniature knuckle bender and the Oppenheimer attachment are all of considerable value.

Assistive and prophylactic splinting is principally used in the treatment of varying degrees of ulnar drift. Prophylactic splinting is used in an attempt to prevent a deformity increasing by counteracting the imbalance of forces producing the deformity. Assistive splints are prescribed to restore function by reinforcing the power of weakened muscle groups. It is common experience that most patients will not tolerate the indefinite use of these splints. It is probably fair to say that most hand surgeons would prefer to correct the internal dynamic imbalance by surgery rather than impose an external corrective framework on the hand. These splints are occasionally of value in the immediate postoperative period and the most satisfactory types are based upon the family of splints devised at Rancho Los Amigos Hospital in Los Angeles to aid paralytic poliomyelitis patients.

The operations available for the rheumatoid hand can be grouped into prophylactic, reparative and salvage procedures. All recent publications have stressed the value of early or prophylactic surgery. Operations early in the disease are designed to prevent the extension of disease to still unaffected areas or to prevent further destruction after limited destruction has already occurred. The operation common to all prophylactic procedures is synovectomy.

Swelling of the synovium may produce

pain from pressure symptoms, such as compression of the median nerve within the carpal canal. The swelling can obliterate the blood supply of tendons and thereby lead to rupture of either the flexor or extensor tendons. Within digital joints the swollen synovium can produce tension pain, but also it can destroy the integrity of the joints by loosening and detaching the supporting ligaments.

One of the most important results of rheumatoid synovitis of the flexor compartment is compression of the median nerve (Fig. 40–9). Unfortunately the symptoms produced by the compression are frequently dismissed as "rheumatic pains" and the condition allowed to deteriorate. Injection of hydrocortisone into the synovial sheath at the wrist is usually ineffective because the drug

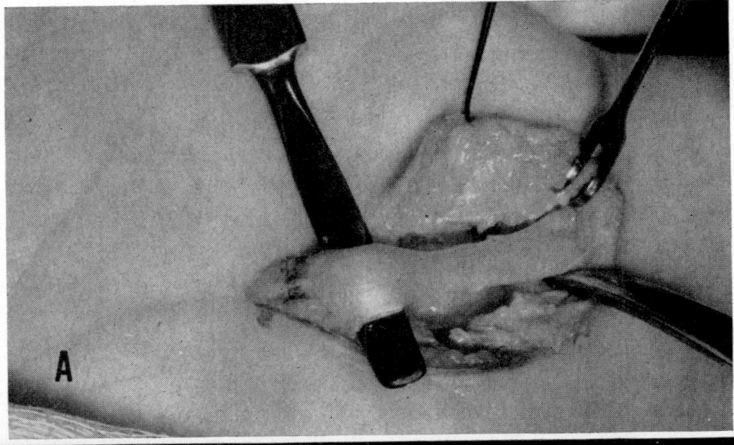

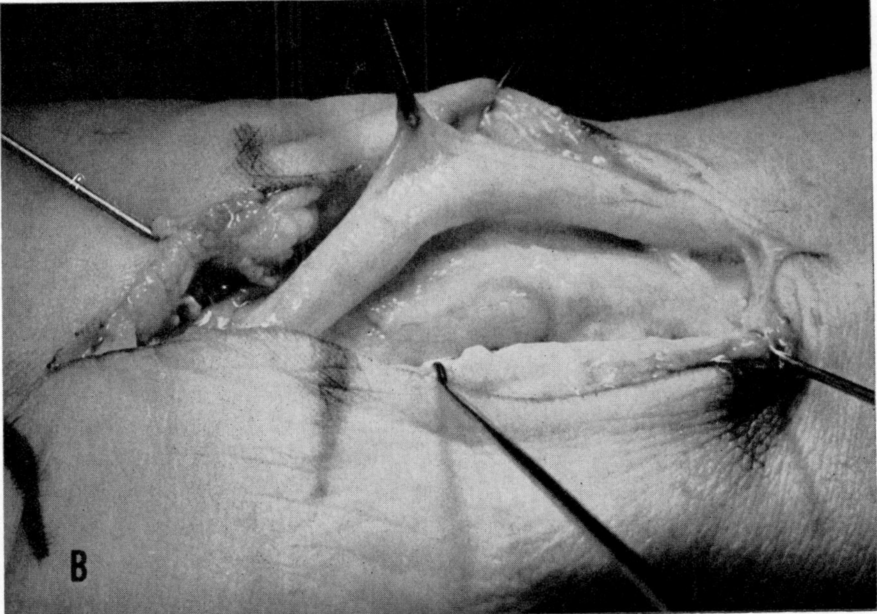

Fig. 40–9.—Median nerve decompression. Two types of involvement of the median nerve can occur. The typical hour-glass constriction produced by external pressure is seen in *A*. The more uncommon adhesive or "strangling" type of synovitis is seen in *B*. (Flatt, *Care of the Rheumatoid Hand*, courtesy of The C. V. Mosby Co.)

cannot penetrate throughout all the diseased synovium. Temporary shrinkage of the synovium may give short-term symptomatic relief but only an operation can lead to a permanent cure. Relief of median nerve compression can be achieved by incision of the transverse carpal ligament, but the operation is usually more extensive. An S-shaped longitudinal incision is made from the distal palmar crease proximally into the lower part of the forearm. All the synovium around the flexor tendons is removed even as far distally as the origin of the lumbrical muscles. This apparently drastic operation yields excellent results and can be recommended without hesitation.

A similar operation can be performed on the extensor tendons and yields equally good results if the operation is done early enough in the disease. The extensor retinaculum is peeled back and hinged on either the radial or ulnar side. After all the tendons have been cleaned of diseased synovium, the retinaculum is replaced deep to the tendons, lying between the deep surface of the tendons and the dorsum of the wrist joint. The tendons do not "bowstring" significantly during movement of the wrist, and the extra deep layer of tissue prevents subsequent involvement of the tendons by any future wrist disease. Early movement has been the treatment of choice after synovectomy of either the flexor or extensor tendons. The patient should be encouraged to begin moving the wrist and fingers forty-eight hours after the operation and a full range should be possible when the sutures are removed twelve to fourteen days after the operation.

Localized disease of the tendon may produce a trigger finger. The nodule in most trigger fingers occurs at the level of the proximal opening of the flexor tendon sheath. The surface marking of this level is the line of the distal palmar crease. In the thumb the common level is the flexor crease over the metacarpophalangeal joint. Surgical relief is frequently needed, but a preliminary trial injection of about 0.5 ml. (15 mg.) of hydrocortisone suspension intrasynovially is justified.

The operation is usually done through a small incision, under local anesthesia, in the distal palmar crease. The flexor sheath is incised longitudinally for a sufficient length to allow free travel to the tendons. Immediate use of the hand can be allowed after the operation and a Band-Aid is usually sufficient dressing.

If, in a trigger finger, a nodule cannot be felt in the palm, the flexor aspect of the proximal phalanx should be examined. Nodules occur in the profundus tendon within the finger and are usually found at the level of the decussation of the sublimis tendon. Hydrocortisone injections do not usually relieve the symptoms, and operative removal of the nodule is the best treatment. The operation is done under local anesthesia through a transverse skin incision centered over the nodule when the finger is held extended. The nodule can usually be removed by dissection with the point of a knife or by cutting off with curved or flat scissors. Caution must be used, since total clearance of all diseased tissue would usually leave a transected tendon. The postoperative care for the patient is the same as that for the more common palmar trigger finger.

Synovectomy of the digital joints is an operation which is currently enjoying immense popularity. It is designed to relieve symptoms and prevent subsequent destruction of articular surfaces. The operation is most frequently done at the metacarpophalangeal joints, often at the proximal interphalangeal joints and only rarely at the distal interphalangeal joints.

There is a profound lack of precise, long-term follow-up studies of surgical synovectomy. It is this gap in our knowledge that is responsible for the greatest controversy in the care of the rheumatoid hand. Some challenge the use of the term "prophylactic" when applied to early synovectomy, and others counter that they have yet to see a sufficient number of patients early enough to test a prophylactic procedure adequately. I have no doubt that the operation gives symptomatic relief but I believe that only in the very earliest disease is it reasonable to hope that irreversible joint changes can be prevented. (*See also* Chapter 38.) My own follow-up studies[7a] and others that are now beginning to appear in the literature[4,26] show a significant percentage of "recurrence" of rheumatoid synovitis and the higher rates are in those patients suffering from more severe disease.

The operation is done through an incision directly over the joint and the synovium is removed after the tendons on the dorsum of the joint have been retracted laterally. The technical problem is to remove all the synovium of the joint; it is particularly important to remove completely the tongue of synovium which lies between the collateral ligaments and the neck of the proximal bone of the joint. It is this tongue which is largely responsible for the detachment of the collateral ligament from the bone and for the destruction of the subchondral cortical bone.

Synovectomy of a digital joint is commonly combined with other procedures but when the operation is performed by itself the usual postoperative treatment is early active motion. Passive motion should be avoided and the patient advised to exercise to the limits of discomfort; if true pain is produced the exercise program is reduced.

Reparative Surgery

The majority of reparative operations are concerned with attempts to restore muscle balance within the hand. The common causes of muscle inbalance are tendon rupture, intrinsic muscle contracture or joint instability as in ulnar drift.

The most satisfactory treatment for

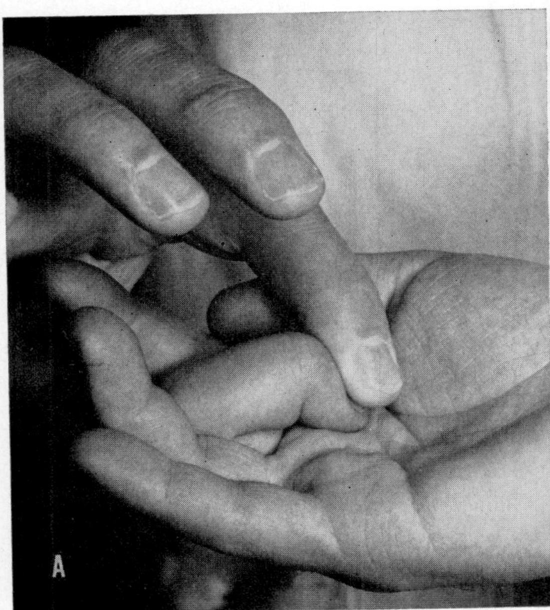

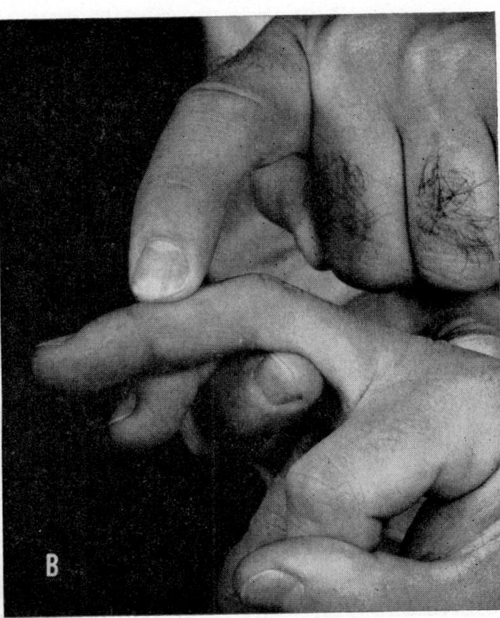

FIG. 40–10.—*A*, Intrinsic muscle tightness. To test for tightness of the intrinsic muscles to a finger it must first be passively folded into the palm to show there is no adherence of the extensor mechanism. *B*, Intrinsic tightness. The metacarpophalangeal joint is then held hyperextended and the proximal interphalangeal joint passively flexed. Resistance to flexion will demonstrate the presence of tightness within the intrinsics.

rupture of either the flexor or extensor tendons is transfer of power by suturing the distal portion to another intact tendon. Direct suture of the ruptured tendon ends is usually not possible because of destruction of a considerable length of tendon. On the flexor aspect of the wrist or hand, a sublimis tendon or a wrist flexor can be used. On the dorsum of the hand, the extensor indicis proprius, the extensor carpi radialis longus or the extensor carpi ulnaris are mostly used.

The operation is not difficult and usually produces excellent results. Postoperative therapy is essential and should start about three weeks after the operation. The early exercises are concentrated on the transferred action and its range. When a satisfactory range has been achieved strengthening exercises are added.

Swan-neck deformity of the finger is common and can be caused by a variety of conditions.[29] Probably the most common is contracture of the intrinsic muscles within the hand. The contracture is a tightness in the muscle which can be tested for by attempting to flex passively the proximal interphalangeal joint (Fig. 40–10). The excess tension can be relieved by the Littler release operation. The triangular hood is excised from either side of the finger, thereby abolishing the pull of the intrinsic muscles on the central extensor tendon (Fig. 40–11). After the operation, great care must be taken to prevent the proximal interphalangeal joints from returning to their previous hyperextended condition. Many weeks of active flexion exercises are usually needed to obtain maximum improvement. The muscles of the thumb are subject to the same disturbance, and the metacarpophalangeal joint is held in flexion, with the interphalangeal joint in hyperextension. A similar operation at the level of the metacarpophalangeal joint will produce a considerable improvement in function.

Nalebuff has pointed out that in some patients this deformity can be caused by a weakness of the extrinsic extensor muscles and is only indirectly due to overaction by the intrinsic muscles.[15] This deformity therefore needs very careful analysis before the correct operative plan can be made.

Ulnar Drift

No single factor can explain the development of this deformity. It is certainly secondary to an imbalance of power over the metacarpophalangeal joints.[20] Contributing factors are weakness of the intrinsic muscles, destruction of the collateral ligaments and the normal tendency to use the hand in an ulnar direction. Prolonged swelling of the metacarpophalangeal joints allows the extensor tendons to slip to the ulnar side of each joint.

The early stages of ulnar drift can be greatly helped by surgery if this is performed before subluxation or dislocation of the metacarpophalangeal joints has occurred. The operative plan usually includes synovectomy and tightening of the collateral ligaments of the metacarpophalangeal joints and relocation of the dislocated extensor tendons (Fig. 40–12). Transfer of the extensor indicis proprius to the radial side of the index finger may be of help but follow-up studies have shown that this tends to produce a flexion contracture of the metacarpophalangeal joint. A transfer operation which appears to be more promising is selective release of tight ulnar intrinsics and their transfer to the radial side of the next adjacent ulnar digit.[7b] By this means a deforming factor is removed and used as a corrective factor. The operation is done through a transverse dorsal incision over the metacarpophalangeal joints. The sutures are removed about two weeks after the operation and therapy begun. It is vital to re-educate these patients in the proper use of their hands and they are taught conscientiously to avoid the normal usage of the hand towards ulnar deviation. Considerable time is needed for this re-education but

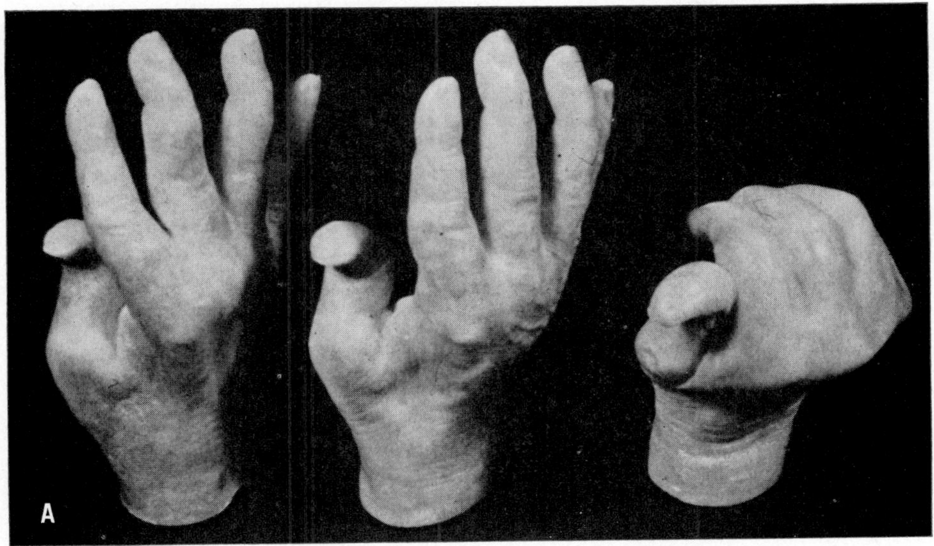

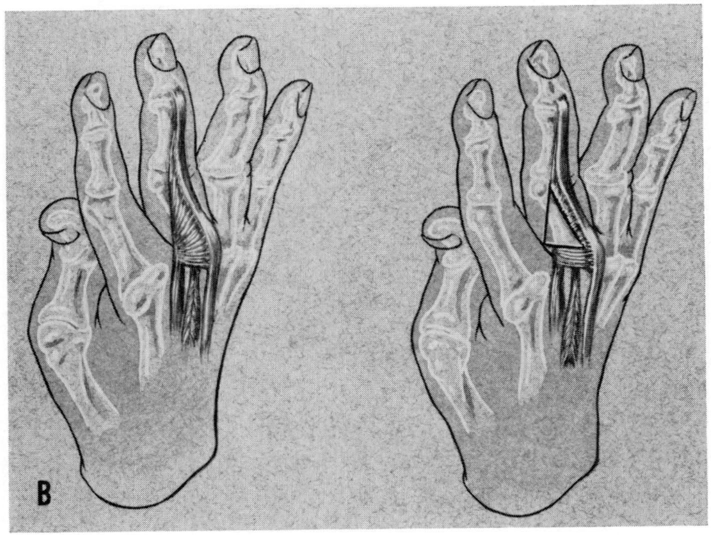

Fig. 40–11.—Intrinsic release operation. The three casts shown in *A* were taken of a patient's hand before surgery (left) two weeks after surgery (center) and two months after surgery (right). The central cast shows reversal of the "swan-neck" deformity and the cast on the right shows the flexion obtained after an intensive exercise program. The hands in *B* are traced from the above casts and show the triangular area which is excised in the Littler intrinsic release operation. (*A*, Flatt, courtesy of Rheumatism; *B*, Flatt, *Care of the Rheumatoid Hand*, courtesy of The C. V. Mosby Co.)

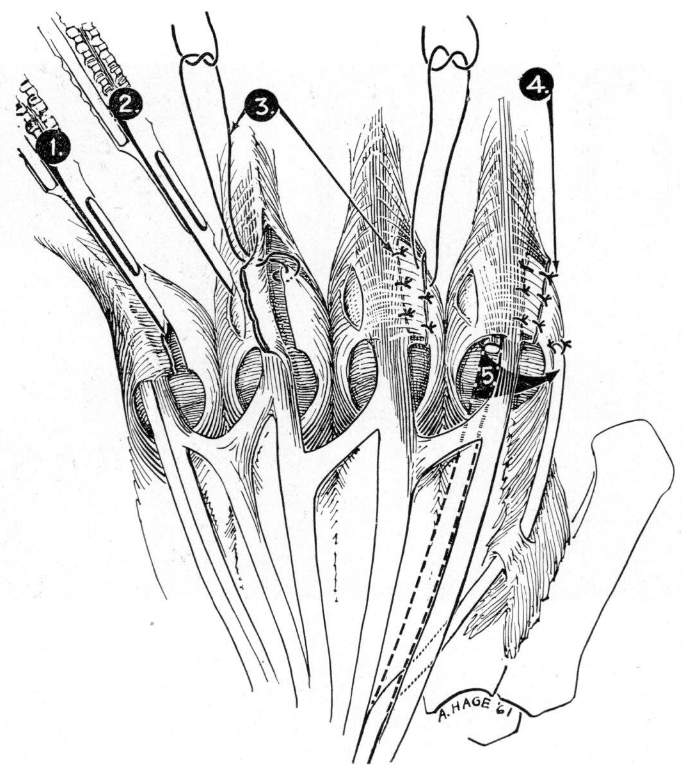

Fig. 40–12.—Early ulnar drift correction. (1) The radial side of the joint is opened and the synovium removed. (2) A relieving incision allows the extensor tendon to be centralized. (3) A double breasting of the radial tissues anchors the tendon in the normal place. (4) An imbrication rather than a "double-breasting" is usual on the index finger. (5) The extensor indicis proprius tendon may be transferred to assist the first dorsal interosseous muscle, but experience shows that this may lead to a flexion contracture of the index metacarpophalangeal joint. (Converse [Chapter 59], *Reconstructive Plastic Surgery*, courtesy of W. B. Saunders Co.)

for the surgery to be successful the therapy program must be continued for many weeks.

Salvage Procedures

The salvage operations are largely confined to attempts to restore some degree of function in grossly damaged joints. The normal integrated system of arches in the hand has been destroyed and varying procedures are used to try to restore the balance between the flexor and extensor tendons within the fingers.

Fusion of digital joints is of value in extreme cases but is not generally employed, since it may impair necessary hand function.

Movement can be maintained or restored to digital joints by either arthroplasty or prosthetic replacement. Neither operation can be done unless there is adequate and balanced muscle control of flexion and extension of the involved joint. The extrinsic flexors are frequently stronger than the extensor mechanism and the patients may need a preoperative period of strengthening exercises for the extensor muscles.

Arthroplasty operations are commonly

used at the metacarpophalangeal joint. The operation does not give a full range of movement but the combination of stability and limited motion produces a satisfactory functional result. The operation is done from the dorsum of the hand through a transverse incision over the center of the joints. There are several technical variants of the operation but all consist of excision of the roughened articular surfaces, attempts to re-attach the collateral ligaments and shortening of the extensor mechanism. The joints are usually immobilized by Kirschner wires which remain in place for about three weeks. After the wires are removed, gentle movements are begun. Progression should be slow, and some limitation of flexion accepted as a satisfactory result.

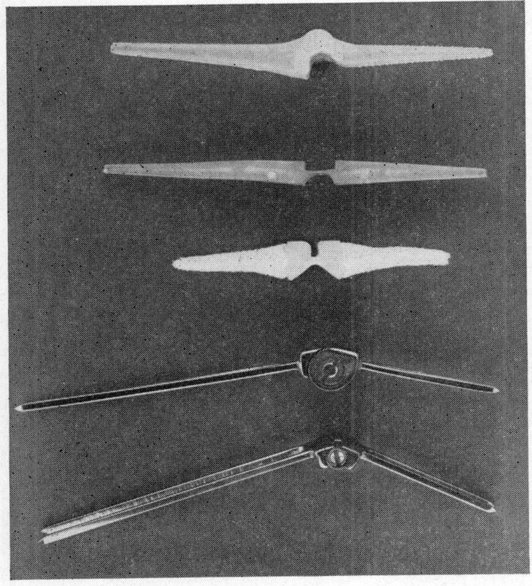

Fig. 40–13.—Prostheses. Several designs for prosthetic replacement of finger joints are currently under clinical trial. This lateral view emphasizes the different concepts of "hinge" design. The top three are "plastic" prostheses in which the top (Swanson) and third (Niebauer) are made of silicone rubber. The second (Calnan) is made of polypropylene. The bottom two metal prostheses show the difference in hinge size and axis placement between the upper, new design and the lower, old design which is no longer used.

Prosthetic replacement of rheumatoid finger joints has been tried as an experimental procedure since 1957. Theoretically, a prosthesis combines the stability of a fusion with the movement of an arthroplasty. The disadvantage of a prosthesis is that it has no lateral movement in its joint, and it is not yet known how long a prosthesis will function within human tissues.

At the 1968 meeting of the American Society for Surgery of the Hand, Swanson[24] and Niebauer each reported the early results of their trials of a prosthesis made from a carefully shaped bar of silicone. The properties of this material are such that it provides both stability and motion without the need for any form of mechanical hinge. At the 1969 workshop on Artificial Finger Joints, Reis and Calnan[17] reported the use of a polypropylene prosthesis. These three types of prostheses have significant differences of design (Fig. 40–13). I have used several prostheses of each type, and it will be most interesting to follow the long-term results of these trials. It does appear, at this time, that the elasticity of silicone may provide important biomechanical advantages over other more rigid materials.

The indications for the use of these prostheses are very limited. They have found their most satisfactory use in preexisting fusions, in fixed swan-neck deformity of the proximal interphalangeal joints, in gross dislocation or ulnar deviation of the metacarpophalangeal joints.

When a prosthesis is inserted into a proximal interphalangeal joint, two small incisions are made along either side of the joint. The joint surfaces are excised and the prosthesis inserted. The patient need only remain in the hospital for four or five days, and movement is usually started within about forty-eight hours of the operation. The maximum range of motion obtained in these joints does not approach that of a normal finger but it is often sufficient to supply some form of grasp to a hand which previously was virtually a flipper.

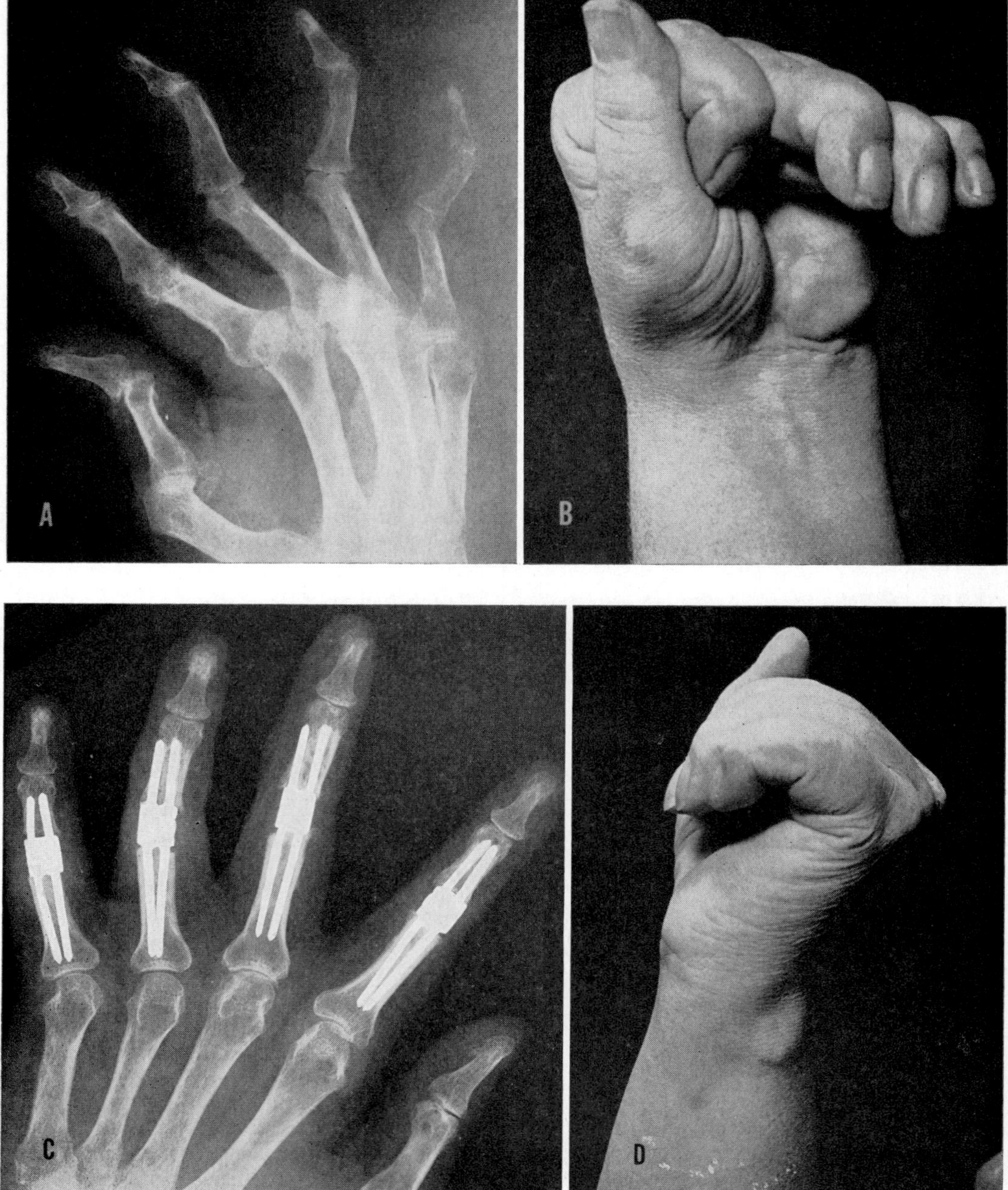

FIG. 40–14.—Middle finger joint prostheses. *A* and *B* show the pre-operative state of a hand which could not be flexed into a fist because of destruction of the proximal interphalangeal joints. *C* and *D* show prostheses in place across the hand and an acceptable, though far from normal, attempt at fist-making. (Flatt, *Care of the Rheumatoid Hand*, courtesy of The C. V. Mosby Co.)

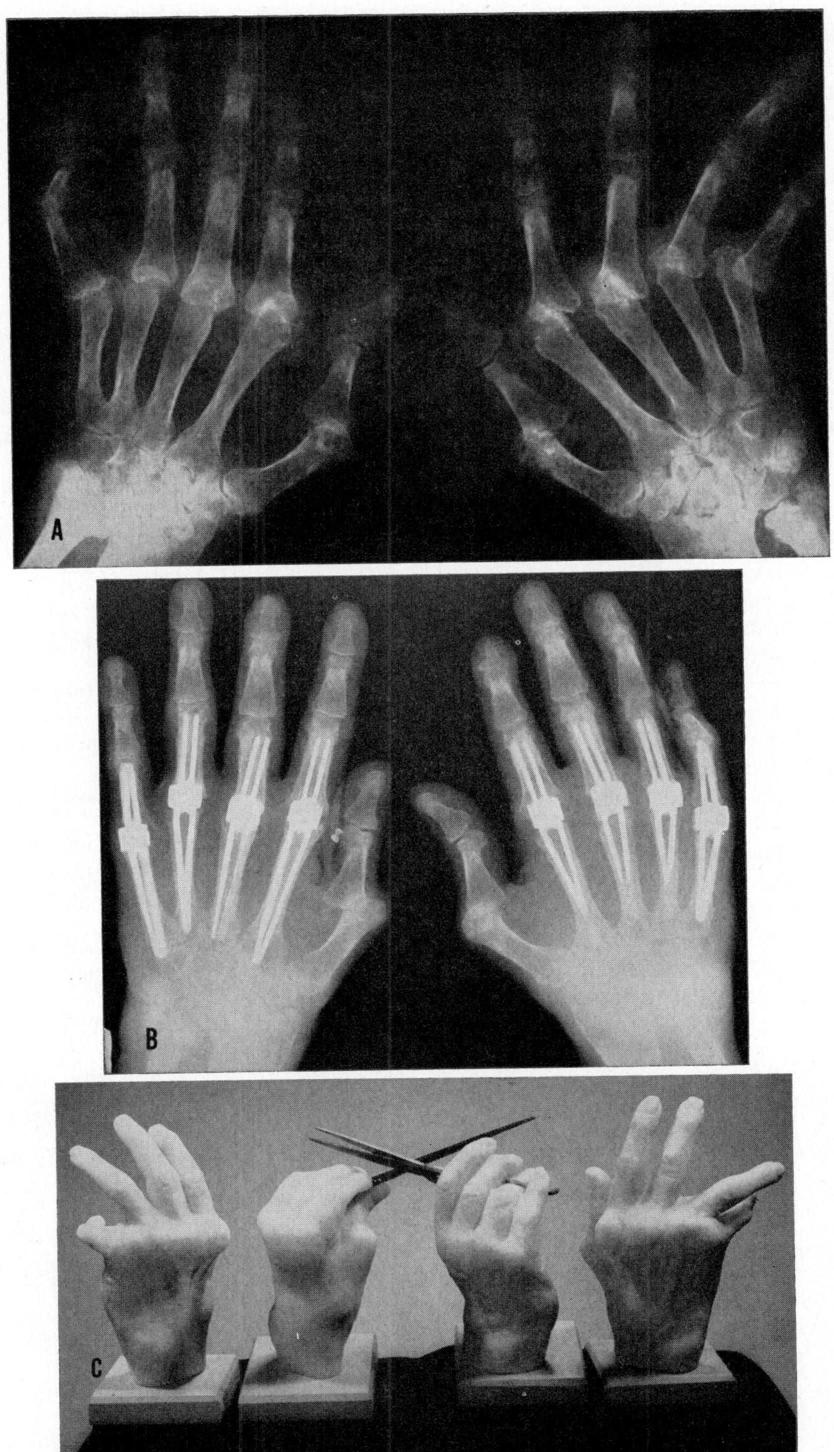

Fig. 40–15.—Proximal finger joint prosthesis. *A*, The state of a barber's hands twelve years after the onset of rheumatoid disease. *B*, Prosthetic replacement of all proximal finger joints enabled him to return to work. *C*, Shows casts of the hands made before and after the operations. The outer casts were taken before surgery and the inner ones show his hands after he had returned to work. (Flatt, ***Care of the Rheumatoid Hand***, courtesy of The C. V. Mosby Co.)

Metacarpophalangeal joint prostheses are inserted through the standard dorsal incision. Sufficient bone is excised from either side of the joint to leave room for insertion of the hinge after the bones have been placed in normal anatomical relation. The extensor tendons are often dislocated from the top of the joint and have to be held in place by appropriate suturing after the prosthesis has been inserted. Patients are usually in the hospital less than a week, but movement is not started until about two weeks after the operation in order that the tendons may heal into their proper place. The best results are obtained in patients who can devote sufficient time to a course of therapy designed to strengthen and increase the amplitude of the finger muscles. The exercises can be done as an out-patient and especial care should be given to building up the extrinsic extensor tendons.

Prosthetic replacement and other salvage procedures do not, and cannot, restore normal hand function. The greatest benefit from surgery is seen in properly selected cases of early disease. Early synovectomy must still be considered a particularly valuable procedure and its judicious use may eventually abolish the need for many currently practiced salvage procedures.

BIBLIOGRAPHY

1. Backdahl, M.: Acta Rh. Scand. Suppl. 5, 1963.
2. Brannon, E. W. and Klein, G.: J. Bone Joint Surg., *41A*, 87, 1959.
3. Brewerton, D. A.: Ann. Rheumat. Dis., *16*, 183, 1957.
4. Brown, P. W.: *In Early Synovectomy in Rheumatoid Arthritis.* Edited by Hijmans, W., Paul, W. D. & Herschel, H., Amsterdam, Excerpta Medica Fdn., 1969.
5. Bunnell, S.: *Surgery of the Hand*, 5th Ed., Philadelphia, J. B. Lippincott Co., 1970, p. 313.
6. *Campbell's Operative Orthopedics*, 5th Ed., St. Louis, C. V. Mosby Co., 1971, p. 1002.
7. Clayton, M. L.: J. Bone Joint Surg., *44A*, 1376, 1962.

7*a*. Ellison, M. R., Kelly, K. J. and Flatt, A. E.: J. Bone Joint Surg., *53A*, 1041, 1971.

7*b*. ———: J. Bone Joint Surg., *53A*, 1061, 1971.

8. Flatt, A. E.: *Care of the Rheumatoid Hand*, St. Louis, C. V. Mosby Co., Ch. 2, 1963.
9. Flatt, A. E., Larson, C. B. and Cooper, R. R.: J. Amer. Phy. Ther. Assoc., *44*, 604, 1964.
10. Flatt, A. E.: Converse, *Reconstructive Plastic Surgery*, Philadelphia, W. B. Saunders Co., Ch. 59, 1964.
11. Henderson, E. D. and Lipscomb, P. R.: J.A.M.A., *175*, 431, 1961.
12. Law, W. A.: J. Bone Joint Surg., *34B*, 215, 1952.
13. Marmor, L. and Upshaw, M. J.: J. Amer. Phy. Ther. Assoc., *44*, 729, 1964.
14. Muller, G. M.: J. Bone Joint Surg., *31B*, 540, 1949.
15. Nalebuff, E. A.: Bull. Hosp. Joint Dis., *29*, 119, 1968.
16. Neer, C. S.: J. Bone Joint Surg., *46A*, 1607, 1964.
17. Reis, N. D. and Calnan, J. S.: Ann. Rheum. Dis., *28*, 59, 1969.
18. Riordan, D. C. and Fowler, S. B.: J. Bone Joint Surg., *40A*, 1431, 1958.
19. Riordan, D. C.: Amer. J. Ortho., *2*, 256, 1960.
20. Smith, E. M., Juvinall, R. C., Bender, L. F., and Pearson, J. R.: Arth. and Rheum., *7*, 476, 1964.
21. Smith-Petersen, M. N., Aufranc, O. E. and Larson, C. B.: Arch. Surg., *46*, 764, 1943.
22. Straub, L. R.: Clin. Ortho., *15*, 127, 1959.
23. ———: J. Bone Joint Surg., *43A*, 731, 1961.
24. Swanson, A. B.: The Hand, *1*, 38, 1969.
25. Vainio, K.: Bull. Rheum. Dis., *15*, 360, 1964.
26. Vainio, K.: In *La main Rheumatoide*. Paris, Expansion Scientifique Francaise, 1969, p. 111.
27. Vaughan-Jackson, O. J.: J. Bone Joint Surg., *30B*, 528, 1948.
28. ———: J. Bone Joint Surg., *40A*, 1431, 1958.
29. ———: J. Bone Joint Surg., *44B*, 764, 1962.
30. Wilson, P. D.: Med. Clin. North America, *21*, 1623, 1937.

PART VI

Important Rheumatic Diseases Resembling Rheumatoid Arthritis

Section Editor: CURRIER McEWEN, M.D.

Chapter 41

Ankylosing Spondylitis

By Metro A. Ogryzlo, M.D.

Spondylitis, in the broad sense, means arthritis of the spine, from the Greek *spondylos*, meaning vertebra.

The vertebral bodies, the intervertebral cartilaginous discs, the posterior intervertebral (apophyseal) and costovertebral joints constitute the principal structures of the spine. The only true joints of the spine are the small posterior intervertebral (apophyseal) and the costovertebral articulations; these are diarthrodial or synovial joints. The articulations formed by the vertebral bodies and the cartilaginous discs are devoid of synovial membrane and represent synchondroses. The sacroiliac joints, although not strictly belonging to the spine, must be included in discussion because their involvement constitutes an integral part of ankylosing spondylitis.

Ankylosing spondylitis is a chronic inflammatory disease of unknown etiology, which affects principally the sacroiliac, apophyseal and costovertebral articulations along with the adjacent soft tissues. Usually the process begins in the sacroiliac joints and gradually spreads upwards to involve the synovial joints of the spine at increasingly higher levels. However, its manifestations may be considerably more extensive, with involvement of synchondroses, sites of ligamentous attachment, peripheral joints and even fibrous structures unassociated with bony attachment. Particularly characteristic are calcific and osseous changes which develop in the anulus of the intervertebral discs.

Historical Sketch

Descriptions and photographs of skeleton specimens in various museum collections give evidence that ankylosing spondylitis has existed from the earliest times. Ruffer and Reitti described the skeleton of a man who lived during the third dynasty (2980 to 2900 B.C.) whose spinal column from the fourth cervical vertebra to the coccyx, and presumably in its total length, was diseased and transformed into a solid block because of new bone formation in the longitudinal ligaments. Other ligaments were involved also, but the vertebrae and the intervertebral spaces were unaffected. A skeleton found in Nordpfalz, dated (by tomb gifts enclosed) about 400 B.C., was reported by Arnold as showing similar changes. Several skeletons of ancient Nubian bones (from a negroid tribe in eastern Africa between Egypt and Abyssinia which existed between the sixth and fourteenth centuries), studied by Professor Elliot Smith and exhibited at the Royal College of Surgeons Museum, illustrate changes. It is of academic interest that ankylosing lesions of the spine have been found in a variety of animals including horses, prehistoric crocodiles and sacred monkeys.

Probably the first acceptable description of the disease was made in 1695 by Bernard Connor,[13] who wrote: "I have lately seen in France part of a human skeleton consisting of the os ilium, the os sacrum, the five vertebrae of the loins, ten of the back, five entire ribs on the right side and three on the left;" . . . "all of these bones which naturally are separate and distinct from one another were here so straightly and intimately joined, their ligaments perfectly bony and their articulations so effaced that they really made one uniform continuous bone, so that it was as easy to break one of the vertebra in two as to disjoint or separate it from the other vertebrae, or the os sacrum from those of the os ilia," . . . "the oblique apophyses of the vertebrae were so confounded and lost that it was not possible to observe any marks of them." From the anatomical data at his disposal it is noteworthy that Connor deduced some of the outstanding clinical features associated with the malady: "From this construction of the parts, the body of this person must have been immovable, that he could neither bend nor stretch himself out, rise up, nor lie down, nor turn upon his side" . . . "and his breathing must have been short." Other early descriptions, probably of ankylosing spondylitis, were made by Wilks (1858), von Thaden (1863), Blezinger (1864), Bradhurst (1866), Virchow (1869), Harrison (1870), Flagg (1876), and Strumpell (1884).

A fairly accurate early clinical description of the disease is credited to von Bechterew. In 1893 he described what he considered to be a new neurologic disease characterized by stiffness of part or all of the spine, dorsal kyphosis, paresis of the muscles of the back, neck and extremities, atrophy of the back and shoulder girdle, diminished skin sensitivity over areas supplied by the cervical and other spinal nerves, and other symptoms of nerve root irritation including thoracic girdle pain.

In 1897, Strumpell reported a group of cases with gradually developing ankylosis of the spine and hip joints. In 1898, Marie[40] described six cases characterized by an ascending type of ankylosis in which the sacroiliac joints became ankylosed early, and the cervical spine was least and last involved. His cases showed greater involvement in the hips than in the shoulders and little or no involvement of other joints in the body. Marie probably was the first to correlate the clinical and anatomical pictures of what is now known as ankylosing spondylitis. In 1904, Fraenkel presented a rather full account of the disease and labeled it spondylitis ankylopoietica.

The pathologic features of ligamentous calcification and normal intervertebral discs were pointed out by March in 1895. Marie and Leri (1899) noted that the posterior intervertebral (apophyseal) articulations were diseased and that most of them were ankylosed in a patient who came to autopsy. Simmonds (1904) and Fraenkel (1904) emphasized the importance of the involvement of small posterior articulations and emphasized that the intervertebral spaces and the vertebral bodies were unaffected. Valentini (1899) described roentgenograms demonstrating the typical bamboo spine of ankylosing spondylitis, and Schlager (1906) first demonstrated roentgenographically ankylosis of the posterior intervertebral joints. Clear-cut descriptions of the clinical and roentgenographic features of the disease did not emerge, however, until after the development of improved roentgenologic techniques during the 1930s; significant correlation of diagnostic data can be attributed to studies by Krebs (1930), Buckley (1935), Scott (1936) and Forrestier (1939).

Synonyms and Eponyms

A myriad of synonyms and eponyms for ankylosing spondylitis have appeared in the literature.[26] These have resulted from disagreement regarding the basic nature of the disease and from descriptions based on variations of the clinical and pathologic pictures. Such varied terms as the following have been offered: Rhizomelique spondylitis (Marie), Marie-Strumpell's disease, spondylitis ossificans ligamentosa (Knaggs), von Bechterew's syndrome, rheumatoid spondylitis, adolescent or juvenile spondylitis, spondylarthritis ankylopoietica, spondylitis deformans, atrophic spondylitis, spondylitis atrophica ligamentosa and pelvospondylitis ossificans. Although the term rheumatoid spondylitis was used by the American Rheumatism Association until 1963, many authorities preferred the designation ankylosing spondylitis even prior to that time, and in 1963 the American Rheumatism Association also adopted that name.

Nature of the Disease

Ankylosing spondylitis is no longer considered to be simply an expression of rheumatoid arthritis as it affects the spine.[26,42,18] Evidence that it is an independent disease is based on the following: (1) the prominent ligamentous calcification and ossification, seen in the later stages, is not a feature of rheumatoid arthritis as it involves peripheral joints; (2) the sex ratio in spondylitis favors men while peripheral rheumatoid arthritis favors women; (3) whereas chrysotherapy may provoke remissions in some cases of peripheral rheumatoid arthritis, it seems to be ineffective in ankylosing spondylitis; (4) whereas roentgen therapy may be of value in spondylitis, it fails to alter the course of rheumatoid arthritis; (5) in contrast to the findings in rheumatoid arthritis, the incidence of positive tests for rheumatoid factor is very low in patients with spondylitis;[42] (6) although the microscopic appearance of synovial lesions is similar in rheumatoid arthritis and spondylitis, the gross pathologic features differ, as do also the cardiac lesions occurring in the two diseases. (7) Rheumatoid arthritis and ankylosing spondylitis have different inheritance patterns[17]; (8) rheumatoid nodules, one of the most characteristic features of rheumatoid arthritis, do not occur in ankylosing spondylitis; (9) the clinical and roentgenologic features of spinal involvement in rheumatoid arthritis differ from those in ankylosing spondylitis[18] and (10) bony ankylosis of joints is rare in rheumatoid arthritis but almost always occurs in ankylosing spondylitis.

Nevertheless, certain similarities do exist. Involvement of peripheral joints indistinguishable clinically, roentgenographically and pathologically from rheumatoid arthritis, occurs in about 25 per cent of patients with ankylosing spondylitis. Microscopic changes in the active phase resemble those found in rheumatoid arthritis. Both rheumatoid nodules and rheumatoid factor are absent in a significant proportion of patients with otherwise typical rheumatoid arthritis.

Incidence

Contrary to general belief, ankylosing spondylitis is a common cause of back disability, especially in young men. The most satisfactory data regarding its prevalence in the general population were compiled by West: In Bristol, England, an incidence of 1 in 2000 among the population at large was found.[56] Large series of cases have been reported, ranging from 100 to 1035.[49] In civilian series approximately one case of ankylosing spondylitis has been observed to every thirteen to nineteen cases of rheumatoid arthritis. Because the disease has a predilection for young men of military age it was a common cause of disability among military personnel during World War II. Eighteen per cent of all soldiers with chronic backache admitted to one army general hospital had the disease.[4] At a United States Army Rheumatism Center, 1084 cases of spondylitis were admitted during a period of two years. These comprised 18.1 per cent of 6000 consecutive admissions for all types of rheumatic disease, almost as many soldiers being admitted for spondylitis as for rheumatoid arthritis. At one British installation the disease made up 5.2 per cent of admissions for rheumatic complaints.[52]

Etiology

Ankylosing spondylitis usually begins between the ages of 15 and 50 years, the onset being most common between the ages of 20 and 40 years. In different series the onset of symptoms began between the ages of fifteen and nineteen years in 14 to 15 per cent, between the ages of twenty and twenty-nine years in 60 to 69 per cent and between the ages of thirty and thirty-nine years in 16 to 23 per cent.[4,46]

Ankylosing spondylitis has a striking predilection for men, the sex incidence varying from 4:1 to 8:1.[19,44]

The cause of ankylosing spondylitis is unknown. However, a number of studies support the view that hereditary factors play an important role. Occurrence of the disease in twins, brothers, father and son, mother and daughter, or other blood relatives has frequently been reported.[29] Stecher and colleagues[53] studied the families of 50 persons with spondylitis and secondary cases were detected in 7 of 297 relatives. The disease was found to be 30 times more prevalent among the relatives of spondylitic patients than among the relatives of nonspondylitic controls. The disease appeared to be inherited as a single autosomal factor with 70 per cent penetrance in men and 10 per cent penetrance in women, with susceptible individuals numbering 6 in 10,000 persons among the general population. Karten *et al.* found 4 cases of ankylosing spondylitis among 281 relatives of spondylitic patients, and by contrast found only one instance of peripheral rheumatoid arthritis.[36] De Blecourt *et al.* found the incidence of ankylosing spondylitis among the relatives of 100 spondylitic patients to be 22.6 times higher than among a similar number of controls.[17] Other studies have suggested a somewhat lower incidence.[21]

Such possible precipitating factors as trauma, physical exposure, infections of various types, psychic strain and preceding subnormal health were studied by Boland and Present.[4] In 80 per cent of cases no possible immediate precipitating or predisposing factor could be elicited, and in the remaining 20 per cent no constant factor was found. In 8 per cent the first symptoms were dated to minor back trauma.

General constitutional features, such as an increased erythrocyte sedimentation rate, low-grade fever, weight loss, hypochromic anemia and fatigue, together with pathologic evidence of inflammatory synovitis in the involved diarthrodial joints, suggest that ankylosing spondylitis may be an infectious disease. However, no specific organism has ever been identified.

The concept that ankylosing spondylitis resulted from gonococcal infection was prevalent in older publications. Marie[40] held that gonorrhea could cause this disease, while Forestier[22] further suggested that the toxic products from the genitourinary tract reached the pelvic and spinal joints by way of the lymphatics. Romanus[50] and Mason[41] also shared this view, although they presented evidence which indicated that the prostatic infection need not be gonococcal. However, gonorrhea is not uncommon in men of an age for which spondylitis has a predilection. It is more likely that the occasional appearance of gonorrhea in temporal relationship to the onset of spondylitis is coincidental. Boland and Present[4] found the incidence of gonorrheal infection to be approximately the same in patients with ankylosing spondylitis, rheumatoid arthritis and also in patients without evidence of arthritis. It is of interest in this regard that ankylosing spondylitis develops in some patients who initially exhibit urethritis, conjunctivitis, arthritis and other salient features of Reiter's syndrome. However, complement-fixing antibodies to Bedsonia antigen, such as occur in a significant proportion of patients with Reiter's syndrome, have not been found in ankylosing spondylitis.[38]

In some of the earlier reports the possibility of an etiologic relationship with tuberculous infection was considered, because of the relatively high incidence of pulmonary tuberculosis that was observed in patients with ankylosing spondylitis. It was also suggested that tuberculous infection of the genitourinary tract or sacroiliac joints might predispose to the disease. However, these views have lacked confirmation in more recent studies and it is more probable that tuberculosis may occur as a complication of the disease or an incidental phenomenon. Moreover, fibrosis of the upper lobes of the lungs with cavitation or cyst formation has been observed in these patients in the absence of demonstrable tuberculous infection.[11,33a]

Other concepts of etiology, such as metabolic, allergic and endocrine, have little foundation.

Pathology

Early knowledge of the pathologic anatomy in ankylosing spondylitis was based on necropsy examinations of the spine and studies of museum skeletons of patients with long-standing and advanced disease. Subsequently, much of the information was derived from roentgenographic observations made at various stages of the process. Even today few histopathologic studies of the diarthrodial joints of the spine, made during active phases of the disease, have been reported. Those available, however, afford sufficient data to allow certain conclusions.[16]

The most important pathologic alterations occur in the sacroiliac, posterior intervertebral (apophyseal) and costovertebral articulations. In general, the early changes are inflammatory in nature and resemble microscopically those found in peripheral joints in rheumatoid arthritis. They consist of synovitis, chondritis and juxta-articular osteitis. The first changes are in the synovial membrane and consist of an infiltration of lymphocytes and plasma cells arranged in nests around the small subsynovial blood vessels. Soon the synovial membrane actually proliferates (villous synovitis), and at the same time some degree of joint effusion occurs. It may take months or even years for the process to proceed to or beyond this point. Gradually granulation tissue grows out from the inflamed synovial membrane and invades the articular cartilage, eroding and destroying it. The joint space becomes filled with granulation tissue, and later tissue adhesions produce a fibrous synostosis. Simultaneously the juxta-articular bone undergoes changes which from radiographic evidence consist of both destruction and sclerosis. The articular surfaces appear roughened, chewed up or moth eaten; the joint space becomes irregular, being wide at one point and narrow at another. Areas of spotty and generalized osteoporosis appear in the subchondral regions. The joint capsule frequently shows parallel changes with infiltration by chronic inflammatory cells, though of less severe degree. In synchondroses such as the sacroiliac articulations, portions of the cartilage and adjacent bone are replaced by granulation tissue in which scattered nests of chronic inflammatory cells are found; concomitantly subchondral bony sclerosis develops in varying degrees. As the disease progresses the joint space becomes progressively more narrowed, and the ultimate picture is that of bony ankylosis with disappearance of all vestiges of the joint.

Calcification and ossification of the anulus of the intervertebral discs give rise to the well-known picture of a "bamboo spine." The cause of the calcification and ossification remains a subject of controversy. Mild inflammatory changes may often be observed in the outer layers of the anulus fibrosus and eventually the intervertebral disc.

Calcification, ossification and even the extension of cancellous bone through the central part of the discs may occur. In these cases the involved spine may structurally resemble a long bone. Such findings, however, represent an extreme and uncommon change. Usually the intervertebral spaces appear normal roentgenographically even in advanced cases, and the vertebral bodies usually remain uninvolved except for secondary bone atrophy. In contrast to osteoarthritis of the spine, exostoses are relatively uncommon.

The most striking early feature in ankylosing spondylitis is the involvement of the sacroiliac joints, which are usually though not always, the first joints to be affected radiologically.[5,14,46] Rarely, however, the disease may begin in the lumbar, thoracic or even in the cervical region.[51] Involvement of the peripheral joints, accompanied by swelling, tenderness and limitation of movement, may occur in as many as 35 per cent of cases at some stage of the disease. If the hips and shoulders are included with the peripheral joints, the incidence is even higher. Virtually any peripheral joint may become involved, but the order of frequency is usually the hips, shoulders, knees, metacarpophalangeal, metatarsophalangeal and proximal interphalangeal (finger or toe) joints. While involvement of the hips and shoulders usually leads to permanent damage, it is of interest to note that other joints often resolve without residual disability.[51] Equally important is the observation that the initial symptoms may appear in the peripheral joints in as many as 20 per cent of patients. The histopathological changes observed in the synovial membrane and cartilage in the peripheral joints are indistinguishable from those seen in rheumatoid arthritis.[16] In contrast to rheumatoid arthritis, involvement of synchondroses such as the manubriosternal joint and symphysis pubis is common in ankylosing spondylitis. There is often a mild osteitis with infiltration by chronic inflammatory cells and the proliferation of vascular fibrous tissue. Periosteum, cartilage and even bony trabeculae are invaded by granulation tissue leading to bony erosion and destruction of the entire joint tissues. Some sclerosis of adjacent bone accompanies the process with eventual replacement of the joint by fibrous tissue or complete ossification.[16]

Attention has recently been drawn to a form of heart disease peculiar to ankylosing spondylitis, consisting of an aortitis with aortic valve incompetence.[12,25,49] Early clinical manifestations may include tachycardia, precordial pain and A-V conduction defects with prolonged P-R interval, or sometimes an associated pericarditis. Free aortic regurgitation with left ventricular hypertrophy eventually supervenes.

Spondylitic heart disease is rather uncommon, occurring in less than 5 per cent of cases, usually in the later stages of the disease. Serologic tests for syphilis have consistently been negative, excluding syphilis as a possible cause. Pathologically, both the gross and the microscopic changes are quite different from those found in the aorta or aortic valve in syphilis, rheumatic fever, rheumatoid arthritis, relapsing polychondritis or Marfan's syndrome.[16]

The pathological changes are usually confined to the root of the aorta where it arises from the left ventricle, although they have also been observed in the descending aorta and even in the abdominal aorta. There is dilatation of the aortic valve ring at the level of the anulus fibrosus, with ballooning of the sinuses of Valsalva. The valve cusps may be thickened and shortened, with rounded margins and sometimes calcification, giving rise to incompetence and allowing the valve leaflets to sag into the cavity of the ventricle. The ascending aorta tends to be thickened and dilated, with pale, wrinkled, non-calcified intimal plaques. Microscopically there is patchy destruction of the elastic tissue of the media of the aorta, with fibrous tissue replacement and foci of chronic inflammatory cells, particularly around the vasa vasorum. The fibrosis often extends into the membranous septum to involve the A-V bundle and sometimes the mitral ring. Otherwise, the other valves have usually been normal. No Aschoff nodules or other significant lesions have been observed in the myocardium, although there may be a fibrous pericarditis.[25]

No pathological studies are available on the iritis which occurs in about 25 per cent of patients. Amyloidosis, reported in about 8 per cent of cases coming to autopsy, has shown the classical distribution of the secondary type.[16] Apical pulmonary fibrosis has been described, sometimes associated with cavitation and in the absence of evidence of pulmonary tuberculosis.[11,33a]

Clinical Picture

Mode of Onset.—Ankylosing spondylitis should be considered in any young man with complaints of low back pain. The delay in its recognition for more than three years after its onset in approximately half the cases is largely due to a lack of awareness of the disease. Early symptoms are often mislabeled as low back strain, fibrositis, herniated intervertebral disc, muscular rheumatism or psychoneurosis.[51]

The onset is insidious in about 80 per cent of cases, with the initial symptoms almost invariably being referred to the lower back. Intermittent episodes of aching pain associated with a sense of stiffness, lasting for periods of days or weeks and then subsiding, are the most frequent early complaints. Sometimes these symptoms are persistent from the onset. The aching and stiffness present qualitative characteristics of "fibrositis," that is, they are most pronounced in the morning on arising, are accentuated by physical inactivity and ameliorated by mild exercise, are made worse by weather changes, and are temporarily relieved by local heat and by acetylsalicylic acid. Although the intensity varies, the early symptoms are mild in most cases. In a few, disabling attacks often described as "lumbago" occur. Later, the aching and stiffness tend to be more persistent and to lose their typical "fibrositis" characteristics.

Less often the first symptoms consist of transient sharp pains or catches in the buttocks, hips, sacral or lumbar regions. These may be precipitated by twisting, jolting, lifting, coughing or sneezing, but at times they occur spontaneously. Eventually aching and stiffness accompany such pains. As the disease progresses the pain tends to become a constant, dull discomfort, sometimes described as a "deep ache," a "tired feeling" or a "soreness," usually aggravated by activity which entails weight-bearing or movement of the back. Commonly the discomfort is worse during the early morning hours; the patient may be awakened about three or four o'clock in the morning and lies in discomfort unless he takes a hot bath or gets up and moves around.

Pain referred down the sciatic distribution is not uncommon. This is rarely severe, is seldom accompanied by neurologic findings, and frequently is found to alternate from side to side. Occasionally thoracic girdle pains or radicular pains in the costovertebral angle, abdomen or inguinal region, simulating visceral disease, are the initial symptoms. Sometimes progressive limitation of back motion without actual discomfort is the only complaint.

General constitutional symptoms such as fatigue, weight loss, anorexia and low-grade fever may accompany the onset. Their intensity varies with the severity of the disease, but in general they are not as pronounced as in peripheral rheumatoid arthritis. Peripheral joint involvement indistinguishable from rheumatoid arthritis is observed in as many as 35 per cent of patients at some stage, while a larger proportion may have peripheral joint or muscle pain without objective changes. Peripheral joint involvement may be the initial manifestation of the disease in 20 per cent of cases.[35 51]

Symptoms and Findings.—The overall pattern of ankylosing spondylitis is fairly characteristic, but the clinical picture at the time of examination will vary, depending on a number of factors. These include (1) the severity, rate of progression and duration of the disease, (2) the extent of spinal involvement, and (3) the activity of the process at individual levels of the spine. The disease may be mild, moderate or severe. It may be localized in the sacroiliac joints, or at the other extreme all the synovial joints of the spine may be involved. One area

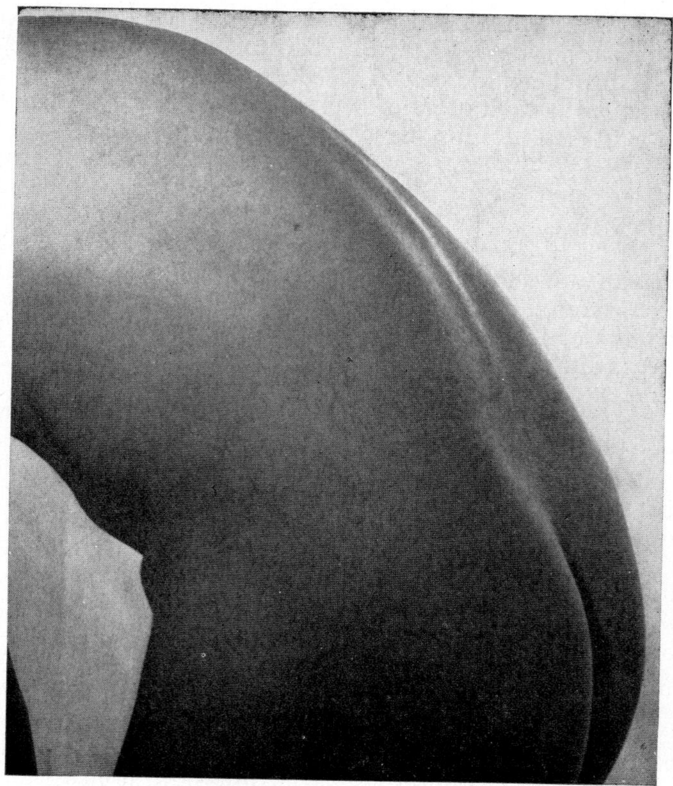

Fig. 41–1.—Contour of a normal back. When the disease is confined to the sacroiliac joints the back contour may be normal and physical signs lacking. (Boland and Present, courtesy of J.A.M.A.)

may be quiescent and silent and another area active and symptomatic.

The disease may begin at any level in the spine but most frequently it begins in the sacroiliac joints. Although the process may subside temporarily or may terminate permanently at any point, the tendency is toward gradual spread to increasingly higher levels. Thus, in most instances the sacroiliac joints are involved at the time of examination and, as a rule, the lumbar spine is affected before symptoms appear in the thoracic region. Sometimes, however, the disease may bypass one or even two segments; consequently different combinations of symptoms and findings are encountered. It would be impractical to describe all possible variations but an enumeration of the features resulting from involvement in individual segments may be useful.

Sacroiliac Involvement. — Involvement of the sacroiliac joints is usually associated with aching, stiffness and pain in the lower back, often accompanied by tenderness on percussion or deep palpation over the affected joints. Orthopedic maneuvers which produce sacroiliac joint movement tend to aggravate the pain. Once these joints have become ankylosed, the pain and tenderness may disappear. Pain referred to the lower extremities, superficially resembling sciatica, may be observed in about 50 per cent of patients at some stage. It differs from true sciatic pain in that it rarely extends below the knee and often involves both limbs or may alternate from one

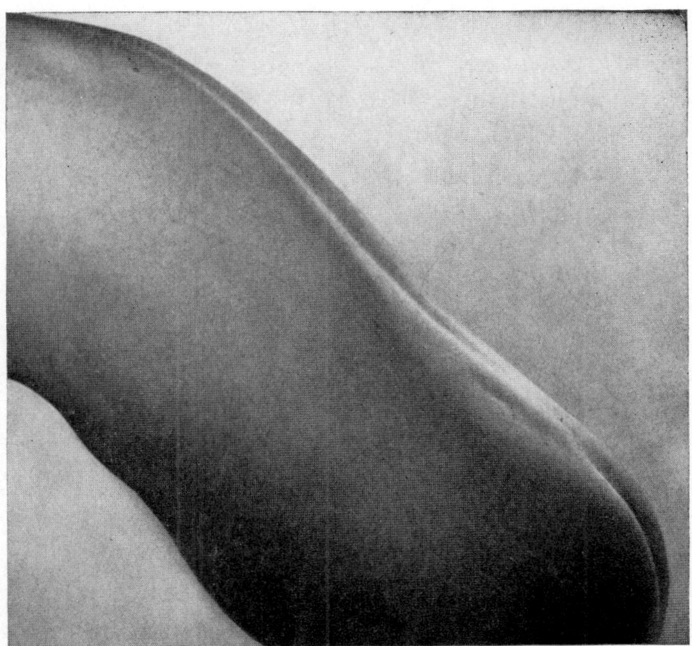

FIG. 41–2.—Ankylosing spondylitis involving the sacroiliac joints and the lumbar spine. Note the straightening of the lumbar spine and the "ironed out" appearance of the lower back.

limb to the other. Neurologic findings are characteristically absent. However, the resemblance may be so striking that occasional patients have been subjected to myelography and even laminectomy.[51]

Mild paravertebral muscle spasm with some restriction of lumbar motion is common, but when these findings are more pronounced, they usually indicate lumbar apophyseal joint involvement as well. In mild or quiescent cases without lumbar involvement, the physical signs may be minimal or entirely absent (Fig. 41–1).

Lumbar Involvement.—This segment is rarely involved alone as almost invariably the disease has extended upward from the sacroiliac joints. Pain, aching and stiffness as already noted remain the dominant symptoms; but they are not of great localizing value. Among the signs which signify involvement of the lumbar spine the following may be included: (1) limitation of motion of the lumbar spine, (2) paravertebral muscle spasm, (3) straightening of the lumbar spine, (4) tenderness to percussion and deep palpation over the lumbar spine, (5) pain on attempted forced flexion and extension of the lumbar spine, (6) muscle atrophy, especially in the lower portion of the lumbar segment, which when combined with straightening of the lumbar spine gives the lower back an "ironed out" appearance (Fig. 41–2).

Thoracic Involvement.—When the thoracic segment is affected the same localizing signs are present as are outlined for the lumbar segment, but at a higher level. In addition the following special features usually develop: (1) thoracic girdle pains, (2) chest pain on deep inspiration, (3) diminished chest expansion, (4) flattening of the anterior chest (expiratory position), and (5) thoracolumbar kyphosis (Fig. 41–3).

Cervical Involvement.—Involvement of the cervical spine often results in a

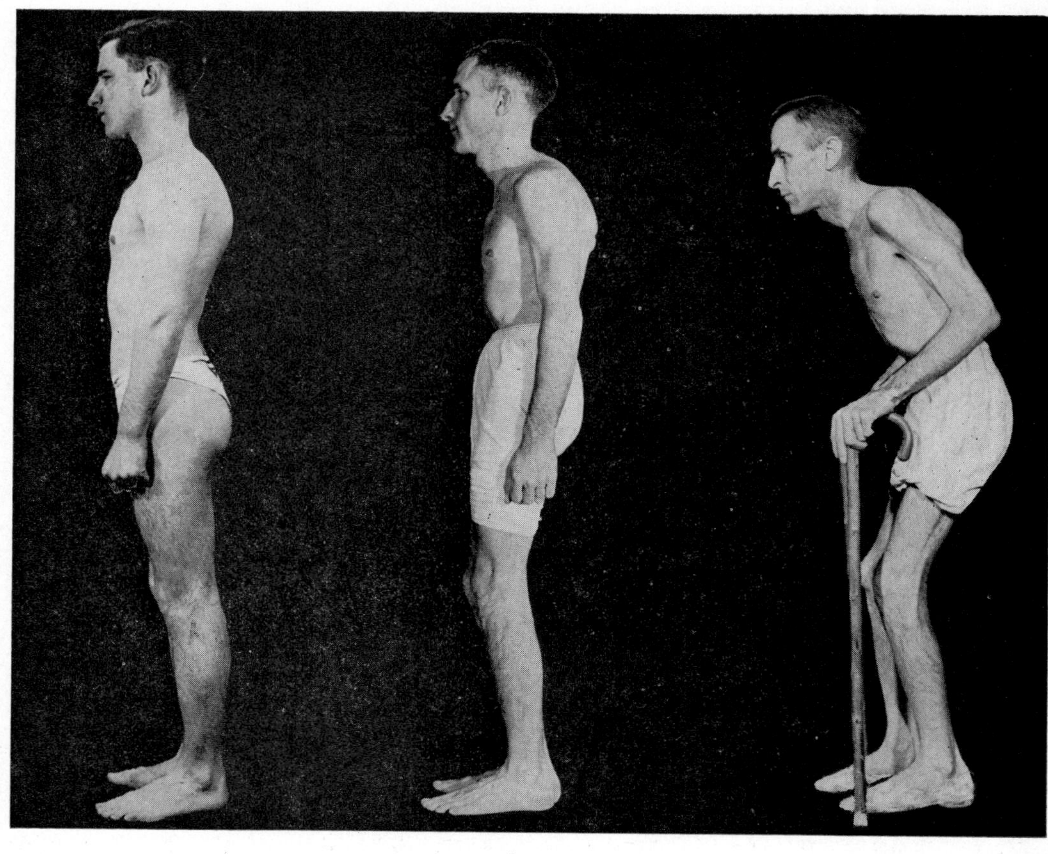

a *b* *c*

Fig. 41–3.—Ankylosing spondylitis showing progression over 20 years. Note (*a*) normal posture at age 22 years, (*b*) forward protrusion of neck and high dorsal kyphosis at age 32 years and (*c*) accentuation of deformity due to flexion contracture of hips and compensatory flexion of knees at age 42 years. (Ogryzlo and Rosen, courtesy Postgraduate Medicine.)

forward protrusion of the head and neck, superimposed conspicuously on a high dorsal kyphosis (Fig. 41–3). Movements in all directions become markedly impaired and the patient may have to pivot his whole body in order to look sideward. Usually, however, the atlanto-occipital joint does not become solidly ankylosed so that a small amount of nodding and rotary movement is preserved. Spasm of the cervical muscles may be pronounced with subsequent muscle atrophy. Cervical radicular pain may be referred up over the occiput or down the arms. The rigid cervical spine is particularly prone to injury, due to loss of its normal resilience and minor falls have been known to result in fractures, occasionally complicated by paraplegia.[33]

Peripheral Joint Involvement.—It is important to remember that the initial manifestations of the disease may appear in the peripheral joints in as many as 20 per cent of patients,[46] with pain, swelling and sometimes effusion into the joint space, indistinguishable from rheumatoid arthritis. However, as many as 35 per cent of patients exhibit peripheral joint involvement at some stage, including the knees, ankles, elbows, wrists and the small joints of the hands and feet. Often only a few joints may be so affected, in an asymmetrical manner.[51] Structural damage may also occur, leading to permanent deformity as in rheumatoid arthritis, but it is not unusual for them to undergo complete resolution without deformity. If one includes the hips and shoulders with the peripheral joints, the incidence may be as high as 64 per cent.[42b] These two joints are involved in one-third and one-half of cases respectively and sustain permanent damage in most instances.[18,42b] Some degree of flexion contracture at the hips is not uncommon in the later stages of the disease, necessitating flexion at the knees to maintain an erect posture and giving rise to a characteristic, rigid gait (Fig. 41–3.)

Other sites may also be involved. There may be pain with swelling and tenderness over the sternomanubrial, sternoclavicular or temporomandibular joints, as well as pain and tenderness over the weight-bearing surface of the heels or ischial tuberosities.

Non-articular Involvement.—Tachycardia is not uncommon, but when this is associated with evidence of *cardiac enlargement*, *pericarditis* or a *conduction defect*, one should consider the possibility of **spondylitic heart disease.**[1,12,25,38,49] The prevalence of this complication has varied from about 3 per cent of cases with a 15-year history of spondylitis, to 10 per cent after 30 years of spondylitis, occurring almost twice as frequently in patients with peripheral joint involvement. The presence of aortic insufficiency with a diastolic murmur, in the absence of causes such as syphilis or rheumatic fever, is highly suggestive of spondylitic aortitis. The lesion is progressive over a period of years, with increasing disability from dyspnea and sometimes accompanied by anginal pain. The evolution of the lesion is rather gradual with an average survival of 7 to 10 years after the onset of free regurgitation. Occasionally the aortic valve may show calcification with an element of aortic stenosis as well.

As many as 25 per cent of patients may experience one or more attacks of **iritis** during the course of their illness, when this is followed over a prolonged period.[46] It appears to be unrelated to the severity of the spondylitis, but occurs more frequently in patients with peripheral joint involvement. The iritis usually responds to corticosteroid therapy with complete resolution, although there may occasionally be some residual visual impairment and rarely complete loss of vision.

Some 8 per cent of patients may develop evidence of **amyloidosis,** usually in the later stages of the disease. It cannot be distinguished from the amyloidosis which occurs as a secondary complication of rheumatoid arthritis or other chronic inflammatory diseases. Proteinuria with evidence of hypoproteinemia and progressive renal damage are the prominent findings.

Spondylitis similar to ankylosing spondylitis occurs in association with certain **intestinal disorders,** including ulcerative colitis, regional enteritis or rarely Whipple's disease.[42a,57] Ulcerative colitis antedates or begins synchronously with the spondylitis in more than half of these cases.[42a,42b] The precise relationship between these diseases is somewhat confused because each of the intestinal disorders mentioned may also be associated with polyarthralgia or arthritis of the peripheral joints or even sacroiliac involvement as an isolated finding.

Involvement of the **cauda equina** may occur during the later stages of ankylosing spondylitis, at a time when the disease has appeared to become inactive.[7] The onset is insidious with incontinence of urine due to loss of bladder sphincter control, diminished bladder and rectal sensation, muscle wasting and pain followed by sensory loss in the sacral distribution. Bilateral involvement is the rule although this may not be symmetrical. The mechanism involved in the production of this lesion is not clear although myelography may show an enlarged lumbar sac with prominent posterior diverticula, and may indicate a pre-existing arachnoiditis with fibrosis around the dorsal roots.

Earlier reports suggested that patients with ankylosing spondylitis were more prone to develop pulmonary tuberculosis, the incidence varying from 6 to 10 per cent. This has not been the experience in more recent reviews. Studies of respiratory function indicate that respiratory disability need not be great even when the thorax is severely affected. While lung compliance may vary widely, diffusing capacity tends to be normal while residual volume and functional residual capacity may be increased. Vital capacity is not reduced until the thorax is severely restricted.[59] Recently two reports have described a form of **pulmonary fibrosis** occurring in ankylosing spondylitis affecting the upper lung fields. The lesions closely resembled tuberculosis and some progressed to cavitation, although acid-fast organisms were never demonstrated.[11,33a]

General Symptoms.—These may be minimal or absent in mild cases and many patients are able to pursue useful occupations for years without appreciable alteration in general health. In severe or moderately severe cases on the other hand, weakness or weight loss may be sufficiently pronounced to raise a suspicion of malignancy, tuberculosis or some other debilitating disease. In general, the degree of constitutional reaction parallels the height of the erythrocyte sedimentation rate, but it is seldom pronounced in the ordinary case unless peripheral joints are involved also. Fever is usually absent or it is slight, rarely exceeding 100° F.

Laboratory Findings

Few of the laboratory parameters generally used for the investigation of rheumatic patients are of value in assessing ankylosing spondylitis. The most frequent abnormality is an elevation of the erythrocyte sedimentation rate during the active phase of the disease. In most studies this has been increased (over 20 mm. in 1 hour, Westergren method) in about 70 per cent of patients.[28] It serves as a rough gauge of disease activity, but does not correlate well with fluctuations in disease activity as it does in rheumatoid arthritis. A mild secondary anemia and slight leucocytosis may be observed in about 20 per cent of cases.

Serologic test results for rheumatoid factor (sheep cell agglutination, latex fixation test, etc.) have been negative in the vast majority of patients with ankylosing spondylitis, even when the peripheral joints are involved. The occurrence of positive results has rarely exceeded 1 or 2 per cent of cases.[58] Test results for LE factor have similarly been negative. The serum proteins are usually normal, although a few patients with severe peripheral joint involvement may show some elevation of the alpha-2 and gamma globulins.[45] Slight elevation of the cerebrospinal fluid proteins has also been reported.[6,40] Complement levels in joint fluid may be increased, such as occurs in Reiter's disease.[48]

Roentgenographic Findings

The roentgen-ray findings in ankylosing spondylitis are quite characteristic.[1,24,43,47] In general they reflect those pathologic changes which occur in the sacroiliac and apophyseal articulations and in the paraspinal ligaments. So-called "squaring" of the vertebral bodies often is present in the lateral view. In this view the usual anterior concavity of the vertebral bodies is lost and the antero-superior and antero-inferior corners of the bodies appear as though eroded away. In some patients the vertebral bodies may show varying degrees of bony demineralization with so-called "ballooning" of the intervertebral discs.[18,30] In others the disc spaces may appear slightly to moderately narrowed. Ossification of the anulus fibrosus and overlying connective tissue produces the appearance of the "bamboo" spine.

Roentgenographic alterations of the

spinal synovial joints result from destruction of articular cartilage and from changes in the subchondral bone. If the pathologic process is restricted to the synovial membranes, the roentgenograms appear normal. Synovitis may exist for months or even years before cartilage or bone is modified sufficiently to be recorded on roentgenograms. Thus, the disease may be present for long periods before roentgenographic diagnosis is possible. Similarly, in patients with ascending disease there may be a lag of years between the development of physical findings and roentgenographic changes.

Sacroiliac Joint Changes.—The normal sacroiliac joints have fairly clearly defined margins (Fig. 41–4). An alteration from this normal appearance of the sacroiliac joints usually constitutes the earliest and diagnostically most helpful roentgenographic finding in ankylosing spondylitis.[18,24,43,46] Although not always symmetrical in degree at the outset, characteristically they are bilaterally involved.[42b] Rarely, unilateral involvement may be observed during the early stages of the disease[46] (Fig. 41–5).

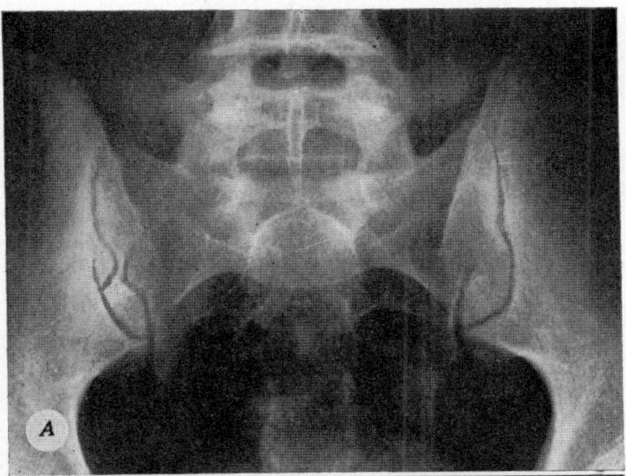

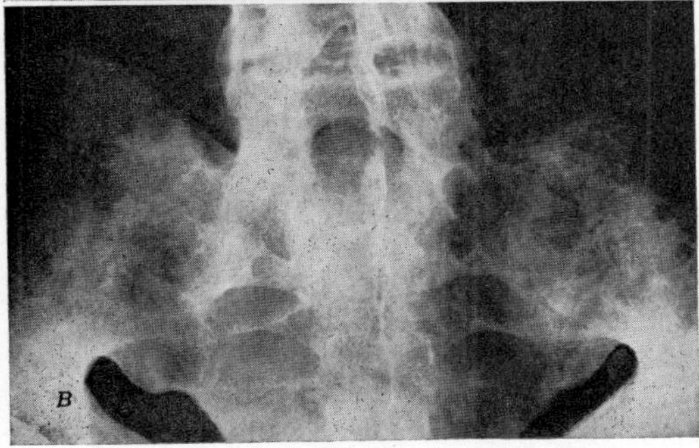

Fig. 41–4.—(*a*) Normal sacroiliac joints. Note the well-defined articular margins and clear joint spaces. (*b*) Advanced ankylosing spondylitis with obliteration of articular margins due to solid bony ankylosis.

The first changes consist of a sclerosis of the subchondral bone often with spotty rarefaction, located in the juxta-articular portion of the ilium, particularly in the lower and anterior portion of the joint. Later the juxta-articular portion of the sacrum shows similar changes. The outlines of the sacroiliac joints tend to become hazy and indistinct, with loss of definition of the articular margins. Areas of bony erosion may give a false impression of irregular widening and narrowing of the joint space. With disease progression the irregular demineralization and bony condensation cover a wider subcortical zone, and varying degrees of joint dissolution may be evident. As healing ensues, ossification takes place and bony trabeculae may be seen traversing the articular space. The joint space gradually becomes more narrowed and eventually fusion becomes complete (Fig. 41–4).

After ankylosis has occurred, the bony sclerosis slowly fades and eventually the density of the ilium and sacrum appears normal or even rarefied. In many patients the clinical severity of the spondylitis is reflected by the qualitative roentgenographic changes in the sacroiliac joints, although occasionally sacroiliac changes may be observed in the absence of significant pain. When ankylosis is complete the pain often disappears.

It should be remembered that similar sacroiliac changes may be observed in a proportion of patients with psoriasis, ulcerative colitis, regional enteritis, Whipple's disease, Reiter's disease and also in Still's disease.

Apophyseal and Costovertebral Joint Changes.—Alterations in the apophyseal and costovertebral articulations are neither as constant nor as readily demon-

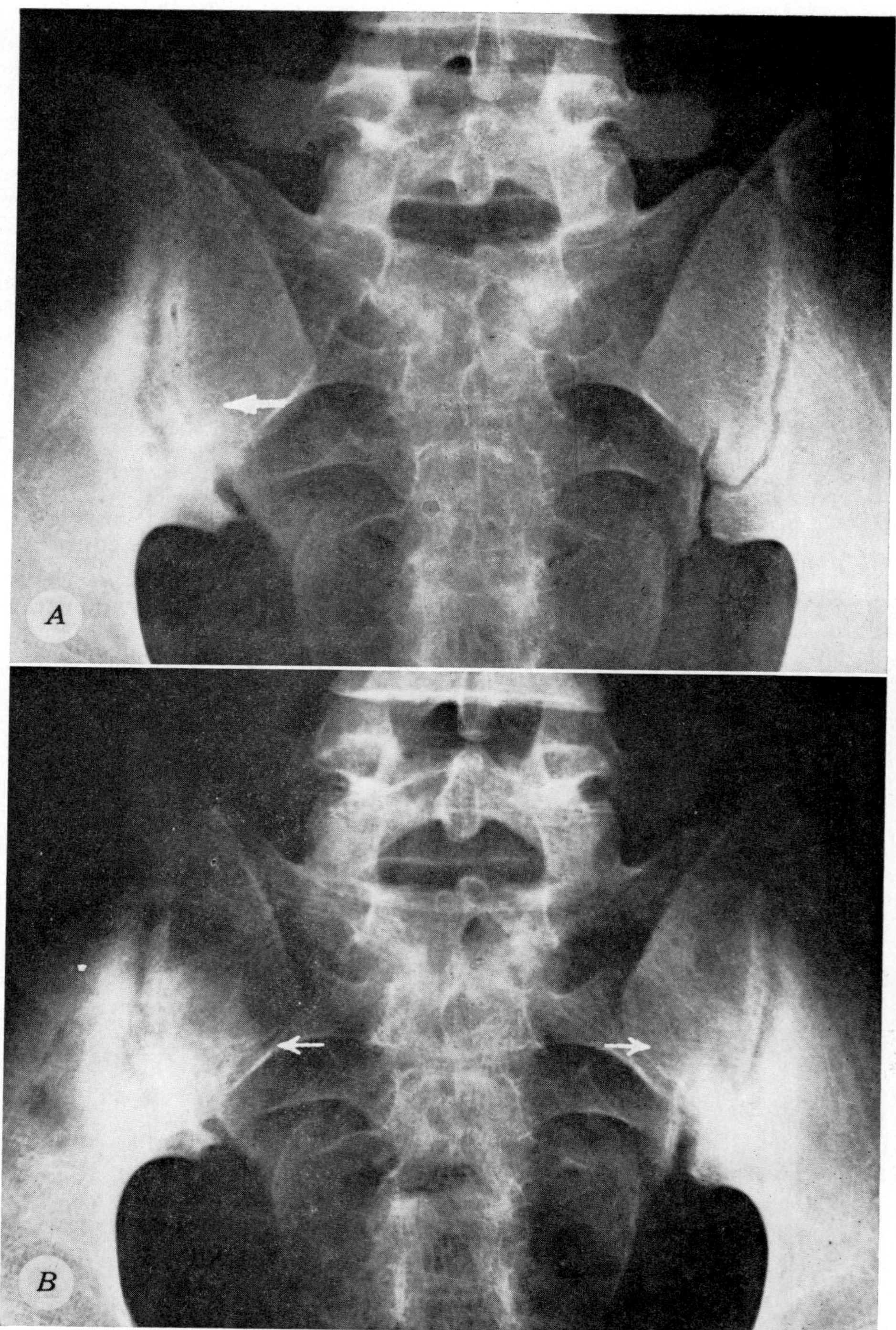

FIG. 41–5.—Ankylosing spondylitis showing (*a*) unilateral sacroiliac joint involvement after one year of symptoms, and (*b*) bilateral sacroiliac joint involvement in same patient after two years of symptoms; indicated by arrows.

Differential Diagnosis of Sacroiliac Disease

1. Ankylosing Spondylitis
2. Reiter's Disease
3. Ulcerative Colitis
4. Regional Enteritis
5. Whipple's Disease
6. Psoriasis
7. Still's Disease
8. Osteitis Condensans Ilii
9. Osteoarthritis

No. 1–7 are indistinguishable radiologically

strated as those which occur in the sacroiliac joints. Even with the use of special techniques, detailed studies may yield disappointing results. The apophyseal joint changes are best observed in the lumbar and cervical segments of the spine, but often only a few scattered joints are abnormal while intervening ones appear normal. Involved joints may become hazy and indistinct with irregular sclerosis and erosion of the articular surfaces (Fig. 41–6). As in the sacroiliac joints, the final event consists of bony fusion, although not all the joints of an involved segment may become ankylosed. Involvement of the costovertebral joints is responsible for the reduced chest expansion, usually in the expiratory position. As in rheumatoid arthritis, there may be subluxation of the odontoid process, with a wide atlanto-dental interval (more than 2.5 mm.) and sometimes erosion of the odontoid itself. The subluxation is readily demonstrated in lateral views of the neck in full flexion or with tomography.

Changes in the Paraspinal Ligaments.—Calcification and ossification of the anulus fibrosus and paravertebral ligaments usually do not develop until relatively late in the disease. The characteristic syndesmophytes which give rise to the so-called "bamboo" appearance often are considered to be due to calcification of the longitudinal ligaments. This calcification occurs first, however, in the anulus fibrosus of the intervertebral discs; and the longitudinal ligaments become involved only in advanced cases, and then only the strands adjacent to the anulus are apt to be affected. On the other hand, true calcification and ossification of the interspinous and other posterior ligaments are quite common. This often parallels the appearance of bambooing; but not infrequently, bambooing or ligamentous calcification may occur to an advanced degree with little or no roentgenologic evidence of the other. In contrast to the marginal, beak-like, heavy osteophytes of degenerative disease of the spine, the syndesmophytes of ankylosing spondylitis begin as linear, poorly defined calcifications adjacent to the margins of the vertebral bodies and

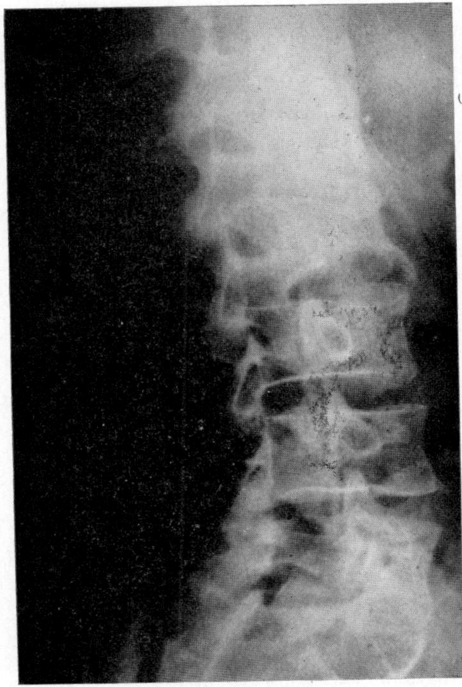

Fig. 41–6.—Involvement of the posterior intervertebral (apophyseal) joints. The articular facets of L-3 and 4 show mottled rarefaction with irregularity of the joint spaces and juxta-articular sclerosis. (Boland and Present, courtesy of J.A.M.A.)

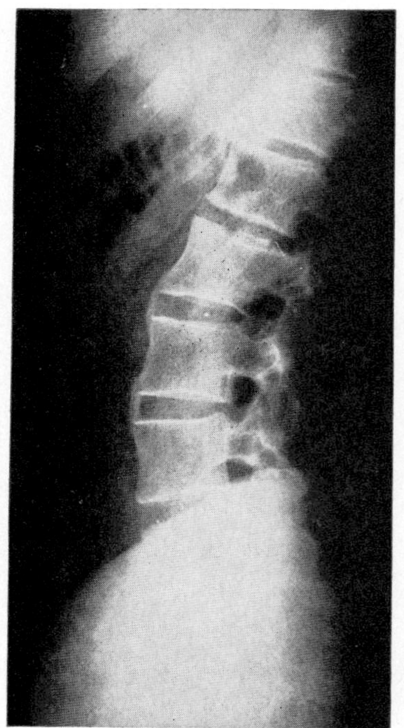

Fig. 41–7.—Calcification of anulus fibrosus.

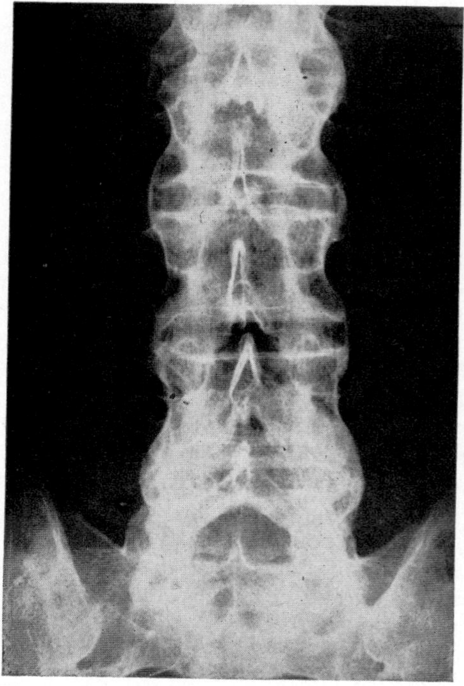

Fig. 41–8.—Typical "bamboo spine" and complete ankylosis of the sacroiliac and posterior intervertebral (apophyseal) joints.

intervertebral discs and extend vertically (Figs. 41–7, 8 and 9).

In a rare, exceptional case, bambooing and/or calcification of the spinal ligaments may be present with only minimal or early changes in the sacroiliac articu-

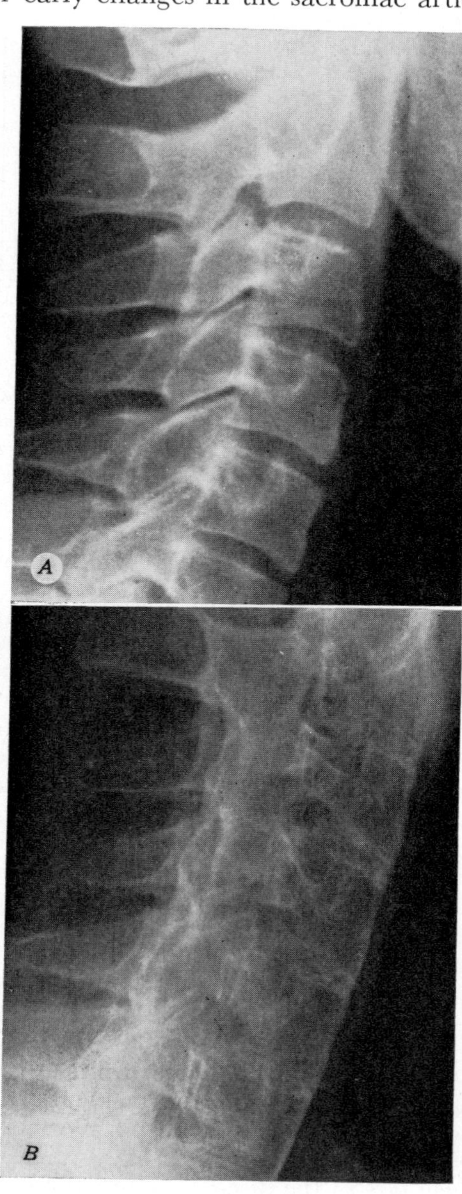

Fig. 41–9.—Cervical spine in ankylosing spondylitis showing (*A*) normal appearance after five years of disease and (*B*) complete bony fusion after seventeen years of disease. (Ogryzlo and Rosen, courtesy of Postgraduate Medicine.)

lations, but usually the latter are advanced before the paraspinal calcifications are apparent.

Spondylodiscitis.—Destructive lesions of the intervertebral discs and adjoining vertebral bodies have been described in the later stages of ankylosing spondylitis.[35,46,38a] Characteristically these are observed in the lower dorsal or upper lumbar segments of the spine, often after there has been some evidence of paraspinal ossification. Sometimes there is a history of a preceding injury leading to speculation that the lesion may be initiated by a traumatic fracture. They may also be misinterpreted as representing tuberculous or pyogenic infection or even a tumor. However, many cases have been observed in the absence of a history of injury and it appears more likely that the lesions are a feature of the spondylitic process. Moreover, they closely parallel the changes observed in the sacroiliac joints and other cartilaginous joints.

Typically the lesion appears as an erosion of the adjacent margins of two vertebral bodies with condensation of the subchondral bone (Fig. 41–10). Eventually the erosive changes become more pronounced with destruction of the disc itself and the adjacent vertebral bodies. Angulation of the spine may occur at the site, with fracture of the posterior laminae. Pain is a prominent feature in most cases but may sometimes be inconspicuous. Cord compression with paraplegia is an occasional complication. The lesion is best treated conservatively, perhaps with some temporary support to the spine.

Other Bone and Joint Changes.—Certain cartilaginous joints are also prone to develop changes strikingly similar to those usually observed in the sacroiliac joints. The sternomanubrial joint and the symphysis pubis are two such examples.[1,24,46] Early bony sclerosis, erosions and a haziness of the joint margins may later be followed by solid bony ankylosis (Fig. 41–11). Ossification of the iliolumbar, coracoclavicular and other ligaments may occur.[24] Irregular periosteal new bone formation may be evident in sites such as the ischial tuberosities or iliac crests, and bony erosions of the posterior cortex of the os calcis, greater tubercles of the humeri or greater trochanters.[1,24] The os calcis may show erosions on its weight-bearing plantar surface at the site of attachment of the plantar ligament, where it is prone to

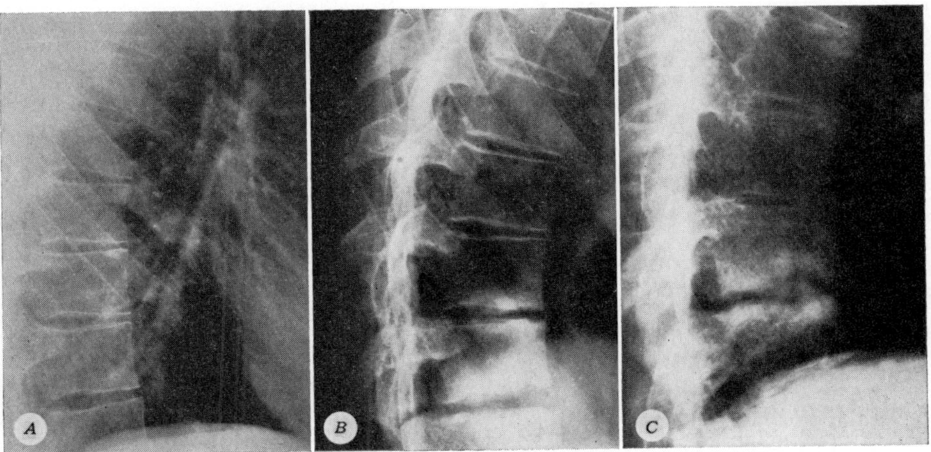

Fig. 41–10.—Spondylodiscitis. Note normal dorsal spine during early stage of disease in (*A*), erosive changes and sclerosis at margins of intervertebral disc five years later in (*B*) and further erosion with destruction of disc after another five years in (*C*). (Ogryzlo and Rosen, courtesy of Postgraduate Medicine.)

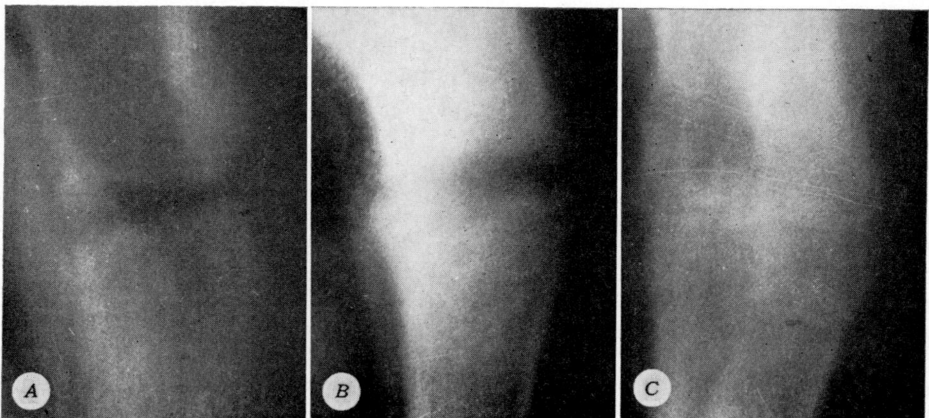

Fig. 41–11.—Sternomanubrial joint showing open joint early in the disease at (*A*), sclerosis and partial fusion after two years at (*B*) and complete bony fusion after a further eight years at (*C*). (Ogryzlo and Rosen, courtesy of Postgraduate Medicine.)

develop a bony spur. Peripheral joint changes, when they occur, resemble those in rheumatoid arthritis but are usually less severe. However, involvement of the hip joints differs in the greater tendency toward bony ankylosis.

Clinical Course

The course of ankylosing spondylitis is extremely variable and is determined to a large extent by the severity of the disease process. The concept that the disease usually progresses to complete ankylosis with eventual relief from pain has not been borne out in most studies. In contrast the degree and the extent of the ankylosis, as well as the rapidity of its development, have been totally unpredictable. Moreover, the symptoms of the disease may subside temporarily at any stage, although there is always the risk of recrudescence in later years. Occasionally the remission may be permanent without apparent evidence of further progression.

Perhaps as many as 40 per cent of cases may be characterized by insidious onset, without severe or disabling back pain, minor constitutional symptoms, little or no elevation of the erythrocyte sedimentation rate and radiological changes showing predominantly juxta-articular sacroiliac sclerosis without evidence of extensive paravertebral ossification. Such patients may run a relatively benign course with exacerbations and remissions in their symptoms, but with minimal or no apparent progression in the disease manifestations over a ten- to twenty-year period.

In the remaining patients the disease tends to be more severe, and disability due to back pain is usually of sufficient degree to cause the patient to seek medical aid early in the course of the disease. Patients with peripheral joint involvement or whose disease has begun in the peripheral joints, more often fall into this group. Progression of the disease with increasing back deformity is more rapid, the erythrocyte sedimentation rate is almost invariably elevated and the roentgenograms reveal changes which signify a higher degree of disease activity. Restriction of back motion, diminished chest expansion, lumbodorsal stoop and neck involvement may all be evident within a period of ten years or less. Nevertheless, even in this group there may be alternating periods of temporary improvement and exacerbations.

About 5 per cent of cases are characterized by an unfavorable course from the onset, rapidly progressing to severe disability and sometimes permanent invalidism within a few years. For most patients however, the disease does not interfere seriously with their ability to continue at remunerative employment or their socioeconomic status. This is especially true when a good therapeutic program is instituted early, making it possible for 80 to 90 per cent of patients to remain gainfully employed with little tendency to absenteeism. Ankylosing spondylitis does not appear to contribute to mortality with the exception of those who suffer from complications of treatment, spondylitic heart disease, amyloidosis or severe debilitating disease.

Diagnosis

The diagnosis is not difficult when the disease has progressed to a degree that there are characteristic physical and roentgenographic findings. These include such clinical features as *progressive limitation of spinal motion*, *persistent paravertebral muscle spasm*, *straightening of the lumbar spine*, *dorsolumbar kyphosis*, *restricted chest expansion*, *lumbar muscle atrophy*, *flattened anterior chest*, *protrusion of the neck*, etc. Roentgenographic alterations, such as *bilateral sacroiliitis*, *apophyseal joint changes*, *straightening of the lumbar spine*, *syndesmophytes* and *calcification of paravertebral ligaments* serve to confirm the diagnosis. Additional evidence is supplied by an *elevated erythrocyte sedimentation rate*, *general systemic symptoms or coexisting arthritis of peripheral joints*.

The spondylitic derelict with poker spine deformity can be diagnosed at a glance. Early cases, however, may offer considerable difficulty in diagnosis. This is especially true of mild cases with normal erythrocyte sedimentation rates which are observed before roentgenographic changes have developed. Certain points summarized axiomatically may be of aid in the early recognition of the disease (*see* Box Summaries).

Osteoarthritis of the spine (hypertrophic spondylitis, degenerative joint disease of the spine) is seldom difficult to differentiate from ankylosing spondylitis. Symptoms are rare before the fifth decade, the sedimentation rate is normal and constitutional symptoms are lacking. Sacroiliac joint changes are usually absent or limited to exostoses at the inferior margins. Occasionally in patients over the age of fifty, bridging or fusion across the lower portion of the sacroiliac joint may give rise to some confusion. The intervertebral spaces are often narrowed due to disc degeneration, with osteophytes or exostoses at the edges of the vertebral bodies. These tend to extend laterally from the vertebra, as "parrot-beak" bony projections. They differ substantially from the thinner, more vertical syndesmophytes of ankylosing spondylitis which

Ankylosing Spondylitis Should Be Suspected:

1. In a young man with persistent or recurring low back pain, stiffness and an elevated erythrocyte sedimentation rate.
2. In a young man with recurring sciatic pain, particularly if it alternates from side to side and is associated with stiffness or pain in the lower back.
3. In a young man with an asymmetrical or a monoarthritis of the lower limbs, or recurring iritis and history of back symptoms.
4. In the presence of thoracic girdle pains, especially if associated with aching, stiffness or restriction of spinal movement or limitation of chest expansion.
5. In the presence of roentgenographic evidence of bilateral sacroiliitis or characteristic abnormalities in the apophyseal joints and in the absence of other disease.
6. In the presence of characteristic clinical signs and symptoms, despite the absence of typical X-ray changes. Several months or years may elapse before these are demonstrable.

form in the outer layer of the anulus fibrosus. Occasionally opposing exostoses may fuse to form bony bridges between two vertebrae, frequently unilateral or asymmetrical in their distribution. In the so-called "senile ankylosing hyperostosis" of elderly patients, the osteophytes may extend as a continuous thick sheet of new bone over the anterior or lateral aspects of several vertebral bodies and disc spaces, occurring most commonly in the lower dorsal segments.[23] The lack of sacroiliac damage in roentgenograms is of great aid in differentiating this disorder from ankylosing spondylitis.

In *osteitis condensans ilii*, the dense bony sclerosis occurs only on the iliac side and does not affect the sacroiliac joint itself.[34a]

Osteochondritis juvenilis dorsi (adolescent kyphosis) must be differentiated at times.[13] In this condition the process is restricted to the dorsal and upper lumbar regions; the x-ray findings are different; and constitutional reaction is absent. Anterior wedging of the vertebral bodies occurs, and osteophytes grow out from the superior and inferior tips of the vertebra at the epiphyseal sites. At times minor spotty calcification may occur in connective tissues anterior to the spine, but in general the x-ray picture does not resemble that of ankylosing spondylitis and the *sacroiliac joints are not involved.*

Sacroiliac epiphysitis in adolescents may be confused with ankylosing spondylitis. Similar symptoms are encountered, including low back pain and stiffness, tenderness over the sacroiliac joints and sciatic pain. Roentgenograms, however, usually show widening and irregularity of the involved joint without mottling or subchondral sclerosis. *More often the process is unilateral.* In sacroiliac epiphysitis the sedimentation rate is normal and the process is self-limiting, usually subsiding with rest and conservative measures.

Since sciatic pain is not uncommon during the early stages of the disease, ankylosing spondylitis must be differentiated at times from other causes of chronic low back disability accompanied by sciatica, especially from cases of ruptured intervertebral disc. Occasionally the onset of spondylitis is dated to a back injury, and in early cases when physical or roentgenographic signs are minimal or absent differentiation may be difficult. Increases in the protein content of the cerebrospinal fluid may occur in both spondylitis and ruptured intervertebral discs; thus spinal fluid examinations are of little differentiating value. *However, the sciatica in spondylitis usually is mild, often alternates from side to side, and is unaccompanied by neurologic signs such as sensory or reflex changes.* Nevertheless the clinical picture may resemble disc protrusion so closely that myelograms have been performed on some patients and rarely even myelography.[51]

It has already been mentioned that involvement of the sacroiliac joints may also be observed in a variety of other diseases. In ulcerative colitis, regional enteritis and the rare examples of intestinal lipodystrophy, the gastrointestinal symptoms usually direct attention to the disease in question. Similarly, the typical skin lesions of psoriasis and of Reiter's

**Ankylosing Spondylitis—
Diagnostic Criteria**

1. Low back pain of over three months' duration, not relieved by rest.
2. Pain and stiffness in the thoracic region.
3. Limited chest expansion.
4. Limited motion in the lumbar spine.
5. History or evidence of iritis or its sequelae.
6. Bilateral sacroiliac disease characteristic of ankylosing spondylitis.
7. Syndesmophytes typical of the disease.

Diagnosis requires four of the five clinical criteria or No. 6 and one other criterion. Exclusions: other causes of sacroiliac disease and spondylitis.

disease, together with the predominant involvement of peripheral joints, serve to differentiate these disorders in most instances. Occasionally, however, a clear distinction between Reiter's disease and ankylosing spondylitis simply cannot be made on the basis of the clinical and radiological findings alone. Finally, considerable difficulty may sometimes be experienced in differentiating between early ankylosing spondylitis and the juvenile form of rheumatoid arthritis (Still's disease), with accompanying sacroiliac changes.

TREATMENT

There is no specific therapy for ankylosing spondylitis, but much can usually be accomplished toward ameliorating symptoms and preventing or minimizing spinal deformity—especially when appropriate measures are applied early. In instituting a program of management, two long-range objectives should be kept in mind: (1) to retard or halt progression of the disease, if possible by suppressing inflammatory activity, and (2) to prevent spinal deformity, its resultant mechanical disability, and its attendant interference with social and economic independence. An immediate objective, of course, is to relieve pain and other symptoms which contribute to the patient's suffering and incapacity.

No single therapeutic regimen is applicable to all patients with the disease. The activity of the process, its over-all severity and duration, the extent of spinal involvement and deformity, involvement of hips and shoulders and of other joints, and amount of constitutional reaction differ from patient to patient; these and other factors must influence the selection of measures for the individual patient. Obviously, the therapeutic problem is considerably different with the patient whose disease is severe and relentlessly progressive than with the patient who has mild involvement restricted to the sacroiliac articulations, or with a patient with fixed spinal deformity and only low-grade residual activity. Furthermore, the degree of inflammatory reaction varies from time to time in an individual patient; accordingly, the measures indicated during an exacerbation may be quite different from those required during periods of relative quiescence.[3]

Education of the Patient.—As in other chronic disorders, good cooperation is more likely to be achieved if the patient is familiarized with the facts relating to the disease. Instruction regarding the nature of the disorder, potential risks relating to deformity and disability, and what may be expected from following a good treatment program, is of paramount importance. Furthermore, adherence to a program of postural and other exercises in the home constitutes an essential part of a spondylitic regimen.

General Measures.—Measures designed to improve the general health of the patient are of great importance in those cases with the more severe and rapidly progressing forms of the disease. These should include adequate nutrition to maintain normal weight, correction of anemia where this is present, and adequate rest. Complete bed rest is rarely necessary except in patients with severe disease. In such circumstances, admission to a hospital or preferably to a sheltered rheumatic disease center, for the initial treatment program, has obvious advantages. Regular rest periods during the day are advocated to allay fatigue and in an attempt to overcome the tendency to develop a forward stoop.

Posture and Exercises.—Patients should be taught to stand and sit erect, as well as to sleep in the supine position on a firm mattress, using only a small pillow under the head. Physical activity which places undue strain on the back muscles or causes subsequent back discomfort should be avoided. Occupations which involve prolonged bending or stooping are potentially harmful, and a change to one which permits adherence to the principles of treatment may be necessary. Rarely external supports or braces may be helpful in maintaining good posture, but they are disliked by most patients and are not a substitute for a good postural and exercise program.

Properly regulated exercises are fundamental to good treatment, with emphasis on mobilization and strengthening of muscle groups that oppose the direction of potential deformities (extensors rather than flexors of the spine).[10] It is in respect to the exercise program that a period of indoctrination in a rheumatic disease center can play a most important role. Some means of recording changes in posture and spinal movement are desirable in order to assist in the early detection of postural deformities in subsequent years. These may include the use of a spondylometer or tape measure on the spine, marked off at 10-cm. intervals, as well as measurement of the distance from the occiput to the wall when standing erect with the back to the wall or from the fingertips to the floor while bending forward to touch the toes.

Initially patients should receive detailed instructions under the supervision of a qualified physical therapist, and instructed to continue these at home after leaving hospital. They should be taught trunk stretching exercises both in the erect and supine positions, calf and hamstring stretching exercises, exercises to correct specific postural defects and deep breathing exercises. These should be continued at least twice daily at home as preventive measures, even though postural deviations have not yet developed. Swimming in a therapeutic pool probably constitutes the best form of recreational exercise available and is to be encouraged. Otherwise patients should be permitted to lead normal active lives, avoiding only unnecessary trauma and strenuous or contact type of sports. Finally, regular re-examination or attendance at an arthritis clinic assures better adherence to the treatment program.

Relief from pain is essential to obtain maximum patient cooperation. Simple anti-inflammatory agents such as **salicylates** in divided doses of 3 to 4.5 gm. daily, may give adequate relief in many patients. Where salicylates do not suffice, other analgesics or anti-inflammatory agents may be tried as noted below. However, narcotics are rarely required and should be avoided. Where pain and muscle spasm are more severe, the application of various forms of dry heat or occasionally ice packs may do much to relax the muscles.

Prevention of Deformities.—In the majority of patients with early postural deformities, correction may be accomplished by postural exercises alone. Spinal braces are usually reserved for those cases with more severe disease and with deformities which cannot be corrected or maintained by exercise alone. Sometimes spinal braces may also be necessary when pain and muscle spasm cannot be relieved by other means. Plaster half-shells in bed may be employed when other methods fail and are sometimes helpful in controlling pain and muscle spasm.

Anti-inflammatory Agents.—**Phenylbutazone** (*see* Chapter 30) is frequently helpful in the symptomatic control of spondylitis, but because of potential toxic properties it must be employed with caution.[32 55] The drug is an effective analgesic agent and has anti-inflammatory as well as pain-relieving properties. Its use is indicated for patients not sufficiently relieved by salicylates and a good general comprehensive program. The specificity of this drug for symptomatic relief is sufficiently great to prompt review of the diagnosis in the event significant relief is not obtained. It may afford worthwhile relief even when far-advanced ankylosis is present. Patients who respond well during the first 6 months of administration usually continue to do so over long periods.

For long-term therapy total daily doses of 100 to 300 mg. should not be exceeded. Initial doses of 100 mg. 3 to 4 times daily, for approximately a week, are recommended and the dosage is then gradually reduced to maintenance levels. Because toxic reactions are usually related to dosage the minimal amount required should be utilized. The physician must be thoroughly familiar with the drug's potential toxic effects and must be ready to discontinue therapy or lower dosage if they appear. He must be particularly vigilant for such reactions as skin rash, symptoms of peptic ulcer (including bleeding), fluid retention, suppression of hematopoiesis (agranulocytosis, aplastic anemia, etc.) and hepatitis. A blood count should be accomplished routinely at least every month during continuous therapy, and nonabsorbable alkalis should be ingested with each dose of the drug. **Oxyphenbutazone,** a derivative of phenylbutazone, is also an accepted analgesic and anti-inflammatory agent for which the same precautions should be taken (*see also* Chapter 30).

Indomethacin, given in doses of 100 to 150 mg. a day may maintain symptomatic improvement comparable to that achieved with similar milligram amounts of phenylbutazone. Doses larger than 150 mg. a day may be attended by headache, mental dullness and other adverse reactions. The drug is not without danger and gastrointestinal complications, including peptic ulceration, have been reported (*see also* Chapter 30).

Corticosteroid Therapy.—The administration of synthetic corticosteroid preparations or adrenocorticotropic hormone (ACTH) is not required for the control of symptoms in most patients with ankylosing spondylitis. However, in severe and progressive disease uncontrolled by other measures, long-term steroid therapy may be justified as an alternative to prolonged invalidism. When a decision has been made to use this form of therapy, the best policy is to administer the smallest dose that will relieve pain, stiffness and muscle spasm. As a general rule, this should not exceed 10 mg. of prednisone or its equivalent daily. On the other hand, corticosteroids may be the treatment of choice for the control of severe iritis or uveitis. Whether or not long-term steroid therapy may halt the progression of spondylitic aortitis remains to be determined. The use of intra-articular injections of steroids to control severe peripheral joint arthritis is governed by the same principles as in rheumatoid arthritis (*see also* Chapter 32).

Treatment with gold salts or the chloroquines has not been found of benefit in ankylosing spondylitis. The known hazards incident to use of such drugs are not justified in this disease.

Roentgen Therapy.—It is generally agreed that x-ray therapy applied to the sacroiliac joints and other involved regions of the spine does result in symptomatic relief of pain and stiffness in about 60 per cent of patients. However with the passage of time many patients experience a return of symptoms to a degree comparable to that prior to therapy. There is no evidence that the natural course of the disease is altered in any way. In those who are helped, the improvement may last from six months to a year, although occasional patients may claim lasting benefit.[51] The usual pattern has been to administer 200 roentgen units to each of five areas on successive days; the two sacroiliac joints, lumbar, dorsal and cervical spine. This normally constitutes one course of treatment. Such courses have been repeated at intervals of several weeks or a month. Usually more than one course is administered, the average varying from two to five depending on the degree of relief obtained. Alternatively only those areas which are symptomatic may be so treated. Side effects include radiation sickness, occurring in about 75 per cent of patients, and bone marrow depression with leukopenia in about 50 per cent. Transient eosinophilia has also been observed.

In recent years roentgen therapy has fallen into disrepute, largely because of the increased risk of inducing either irreversible bone marrow aplasia or alternatively leukemia. Studies have shown that demonstrable aplasia of the bone marrow during the first six months following roentgen therapy, occurs in virtually all patients and that regeneration is incomplete for as long as fourteen years.[54] It has also been shown that such treatment induces extensive chromosomal damage in the leukocyte component of the blood, which may persist for five years or more after exposure.[9] Furthermore, it has been estimated that the risk of developing leukemia is ten times that of nonirradiated patients or of the general population.[14,15] In view of these untoward effects roentgen therapy has been abandoned by most authorities except in the rare patient who cannot be controlled by any other means.

Orthopedic Measures.—Indications for the use of corsets, braces or plaster half shells have already been discussed. Patients who have marked flexion deformity of the spine but who are otherwise well, may sometimes be greatly improved by spinal osteotomy, most often in the lumbar segment. Candidates selected for this procedure must be carefully screened, and close collaboration between the physician and surgeon is essential. Severe involvement at the hips with flexion deformity and loss of motion, can often be improved by arthroplasty. Considering the various procedures that are available, a total hip replacement usually gives the most satisfactory end result. Atlanto-axial subluxation or spinal fracture may require prolonged immobilization or possibly fusion. Painful calcaneal spurs are best treated with properly fitted sponge insoles to distribute weight or by steroid injection.

BIBLIOGRAPHY

1. Berens, D. L.: Clin. Orthoped. & Related Research, *74*, 20, 1971.
2. Boland, E. W.: Med. Clin. North America, *41*, 553, 1957.
3. ———: Arth. & Rheum., *4*, 645, 1961.
4. Boland, E. W. and Present, A. J.: J.A.M.A., *129*, 843, 1945.
5. Boland, E. W. and Shebesta, E. M.: Radiology, *47*, 551, 1946.
6. Boland, E. W., Headley, N. E., and Hench, P. S.: Ann. Rheum. Dis., *7*, 196, 1948.
7. Bowie, E. A. and Glasgow, G. L.: Brit. Med. J., *2*, 24, 1961.
8. Buckley, C. W.: Brit. Med. J., *2*, 4, 1943.
9. Bucton, K. E., Jacobs, P. A., Court-Brown, W. M. and Doll, R.: Lancet, *2*, 676, 1962.
10. Calabro, J. J. and Mody, R. E.: Bull. Rheum. Dis., *16*, 408, 1966.
11. Campbell, A. H. and MacDonald, C. B.: Brit. J. Dis. Chest, *59*, 90, 1965.
12. Clark, W. S., Kulka, J. P. and Bauer, W.: Amer. J. Med., *22*, 580, 1957.
13. Connor, B.: Phil. Trans., *19*, 21, 1695.
14. Court-Brown, W. M. and Abbatt, J. D.: Lancet, *1*, 1283, 1955.
15. Court-Brown, W. M. and Doll, R.: Brit. Med. J., *2*, 1327, 1965.
16. Cruikshank, B.: Clin. Orthoped. & Related Research, *74*, 43, 1971.
17. DeBlecourt, J. J., Polman, A. and DeBlecourt-Meindersma, T.: Ann. Rheum. Dis., *20*, 215, 1961.
18. Dilsen, N., McEwen, C., Poppel, M., Gersh, W. J., DiTata, D., and Carmel, P.: Arth. & Rheum., *5*, 341, 1962.
19. Dunham, C. L. and Kautz, F. G.: Amer. J. Med. Sci., *201*, 232, 1941.
20. Editorial: Lancet, *2*, 703, 1962.
21. Emery, A. E. H. and Lawrence, J. A.: J. Med. Genet., *4*, 239, 1967.
22. Forestier, J.: Radiology, *33*, 261, 1939.
23. Forestier, J. and Lagier, R.: Clin. Orthoped. & Related Research, *74*, 65, 1971.
24. Graham, D. C.: Can. Med. Assoc. J., *82*, 671, 1960.
25. Graham, D. C. and Smythe, H. A.: Bull. Rheum. Dis., *9*, 171, 1958.
26. Graham, W.: Arth. & Rheum., *3*, 88, 1960.
27. ———: Arth. & Rheum., *4*, 649, 1961.
28. Graham, W. and Ogryzlo, M. A.: Can. Med. Assoc. J., *57*, 16, 1947.
29. Graham, W. and Uchida, I. A.: Ann. Rheum. Dis., *16*, 334, 1957.
30. Hanson, C. A., Shagrin, J. W. and Duncan, H.: Clin. Orthoped. and Related Research, *74*, 59, 1971.
31. Hart, F. D.: Brit. Med. J., *1*, 619, 1954.
32. ———: Proc. Roy. Soc. Med., *48*, 207, 1955.
33. ———: The Lancet, *2*, 1340, 1968.

33*a*. Jessamine, A. G.: Canad. Med. Assoc. J., *98*, 25, 1968.

34. Julkunen, H.: Acta Rheum. Scand. (Supplement 4), 1962.

34*a*. Julkunen, H. and Rokkanen, P.: Acta Rheum. Scand., *15*, 224, 1969.

35. Kanefield, D. G., Mullins, B. P., Freehafer, A. A., Furey, J. G., Horenstein, S. and Chamberlin, W. B.: J. Bone and Joint Surg., *51-A*, 1369, 1969.

36. KARTEN, I., DITATA, D., MCEWEN, C. and TANNER, M.: Arth. & Rheum., *5*, 131, 1962.
37. KINSELLA, T. D., MACDONALD, F. R. and JOHNSON, L. G.: Can. Med. Assoc. J., *95*, 1, 1966.
38. KINSELLA, T. D., NORTON, W. L. and ZIFF, M.: Ann. Rheum. Dis., *27*, 241, 1968.
38*a*. LITTLE, H., UROWITZ, M. B. and ROSEN, P. S.: Arth. & Rheum., *13*, 333, 1970.
39. LUDWIG, A. O., SHORT, C. L. and BAUER, W.: New Engl. J. Med., *228*, 306, 1943.
40. MARIE, P.: Rev. de med., *18*, 285, 1898.
41. MASON, R. M., *et al.*: Brit. Med. J., *1*, 1073, 1958.
42. MCEWEN, C., ZIFF, M., CARMEL, P., DITATA, D., and TANNER, M.: Arth. & Rheum., *1*, 481, 1958.
42*a*. MCEWEN, C., LINGG, C., KIRSNER, J. B., and SPENCER, J. A.: Amer. J. Med., *33*, 923, 1962.
42*b*. MCEWEN, C., DITATA, D., LINGG, C., PORINI, A., GOOD, A., and RANKIN, T.: Arth. & Rheum., *14*, 291, 1971.
43. MIDDLEMISS, J. H.: J. Faculty of Radiologists, *7*, 155, 1956.
44. MIKKELSEN, W. M. and DUFF, I. F.: Med. Clin. North America, *45*, 1307, 1961.
45. OGRYZLO, M. A., MACLACHLAN, M., DAUPHINEE, J. A. and FLETCHER, A. A.: J. Clin. Invest., *27*, 596, 1959.
46. OGRYZLO, M. A. and ROSEN, P. S.: Postgrad. Med., *45*, 182, 1969.
47. OPPENHEIMER, A.: Amer. J. Roentgenol. & Rad. Therap., *49*, 49, 1943.
48. PEKIN, T. J., MALININ, T. I. and ZVAIFLER, N. J.: Excerpta Med., *143*, 13, 1967.
49. POLLEY, H. F.: Med. Clin. North America, *39*, 509, 1955.
50. ROMANUS, R.: Acta med. Scand. (Suppl.), *280*, 186, 1953.
51. ROSEN, P. S. and GRAHAM, D. C.: Arch. Interamer. Rheum., *5*, 158, 1962.
52. SAVAGE, O.: Brit. Med. J., *2*, 336, 1942.
53. STECHER, R. M.: Med. Clin. North America, *39*, 499, 1955.
54. STEWART, J. W. and DISCHE, S.: Lancet, *2*, 1063, 1956.
55. TOONE, E. C. and IRBY, W. R.: Ann. Intern. Med., *41*, 70, 1954.
56. WEST, H. F.: Ann. Rheum. Dis., *8*, 143, 1949.
57. WILSKE, K. R. and DECKER, J. L.: Bull. Rheum. Dis., *15*, 362, 1965.
58. ZIFF, M.: Bull. Rheum. Dis., 7 (Suppl.), 13, 1956.
59. ZORAB, P. A.: Quart. J. Med., *31*, 267, 1962.

Chapter 42

Psoriatic Arthritis

By John W. Sigler, M.D.

The association of arthritis and psoriasis was noted as early as 1822[12] but the first comprehensive clinical study of these allied conditions was recorded by Bourdillon in 1888.[9]

Various names have been applied to the combination of arthritis and psoriasis; these include psoriatic arthritis, psoriasis arthropathica, arthropathia psoriatica, and psoriasis arthritica, but the application of these terms should be restricted, as some cases merely represent psoriasis occurring coincidentally with unrelated joint disease. For example, the occurrence of psoriasis with degenerative arthritis is considered to be merely a matter of chance.

Incidence

It is now generally agreed that the association of an arthritis resembling the rheumatoid type with psoriasis is significant, and not merely the coincidence of two rather common diseases.[20,21,25] The incidence of various forms of arthritis in patients with psoriasis has been reported as low as 0.2 per cent, and as high

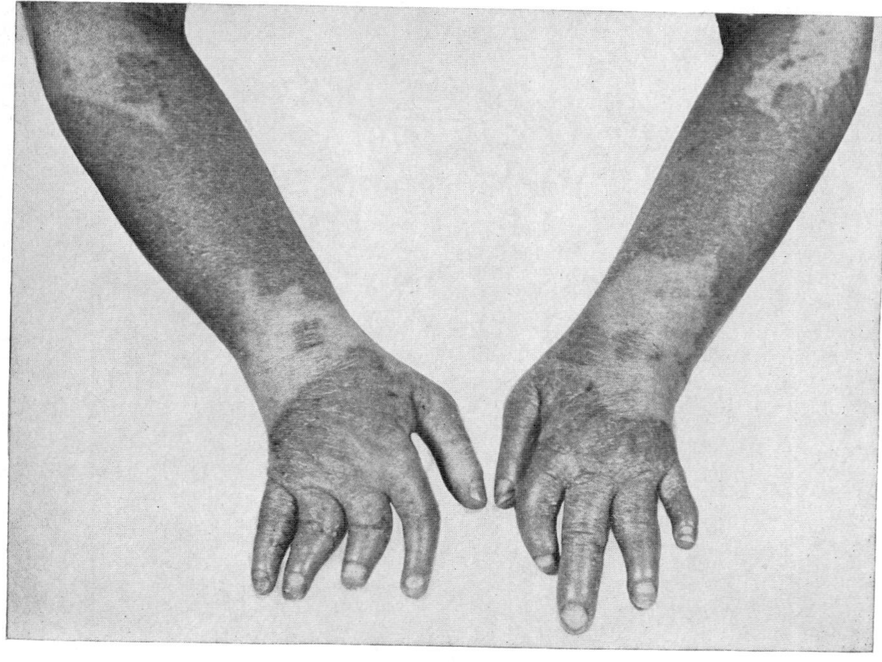

Fig. 42–1.—Psoriatic arthritis.

as 25 per cent,[2,29,34] but the extremes probably are distorted. The higher figure probably results from the inclusion of unrelated miscellaneous musculoskeletal disorders. Probably the incidence of arthritis related to psoriasis is not more than 5 to 7 per cent of patients with the cutaneous disease.

Etiology

The etiology of the arthritis and the psoriasis remains obscure but there is little doubt that they are causally related. Investigations of the families of 100 patients have suggested that heredity may play a significant role. Family histories disclosed psoriasis in 13 per cent, rheumatic disorders in 12 per cent, and both arthritis and psoriasis in 2 per cent.[35]

Pathology

In early efforts to classify various forms of arthritis[3] the fact that the histologic features of psoriatic arthritis are similar to those of rheumatoid arthritis led to the conclusion that most examples of arthritis in patients with psoriasis represented merely the coexistence of rheumatoid arthritis and psoriasis. Nevertheless the gross involvement of distal interphalangeal joints was so distinctive that it was accepted as different and truly psoriatic.[3] Bauer and his associates[3] examined minutely the finger and toe joints of a patient with only distal interphalangeal joint involvement who had died of another cause. Marked articular destruction and resorption of bone with pronounced shortening of the middle phalanges had occurred at the terminal joints. In the distal phalanges the resorptive changes were less marked but there were cup-like deformities at the proximal ends of these bones due to pronounced marginal overgrowth of bone at the sites of tendon insertions. The diffuse atrophy usually seen in rheumatoid arthritis was not present. Dense acellular fibrous tissue replaced the joint space in most of the digits. In the years since that report, advancing knowledge of the pathology of rheumatic diseases has clearly shown that, with rare exceptions, the histologic features of the various non-bacterial forms of inflammatory arthritis are very similar. Hence the earlier conclusion, based on histologic similarities, that most arthritis in patients with psoriasis is *rheumatoid* is no longer tenable.[37a]

Sherman obtained material by biopsy, or in the course of reconstructive surgery, from 33 involved joints of patients suffering from psoriatic arthritis.[33] In early lesions (two to eight weeks), the synovial membrane had the gross appearance of pale, edematous granulation tissue extending out from the joint and a few millimeters along the shaft of bone. At a somewhat later stage the synovium was thickened and injected, often eroding the articular margins, but without pannus formation. Destruction of the adjacent bone accounted for the "gnawing away" of the shaft seen in roentgenograms. In late stages the joint was completely destroyed, with articulating ends of bone represented by cancellous stubs embedded in fibrous tissue, which often surrounded the shaft of bone. Biopsies were performed on uninvolved joints in two patients with "typical psoriatic arthritis," and on normal knees in three patients with psoriasis uncomplicated by arthritis; no abnormalities were observed. The pathologic changes found in psoriatic arthritis were not considered sufficiently specific to permit histologic differentiation from rheumatoid and other similar arthritides.[33]

Clinical Features

Certain features characterize psoriatic arthritis and distinguish it from rheumatoid arthritis:[37a]

a. Any joint may be affected, but the distal interphalangeal joints of the fingers and toes are most characteristically involved and psoriatic lesions may be found in the adjacent nails. Asymmetrical joint involvement is common. The spine and sacroiliac joints may be affected.

b. Exacerbations and remissions of the joint manifestations may occur synchronously with those of the skin.

c. Articular remissions tend to be more frequent, rapid, and complete than in rheumatoid arthritis.

d. Tests for rheumatoid factor in the serum are negative.

e. Subcutaneous nodules are absent.

f. Radiologic features of joint destruction are often unlike those seen in typical rheumatoid arthritis.

The age of onset of psoriatic arthritis does not differ significantly from that of rheumatoid arthritis. Psoriatic arthritis is most often antedated by a long history of chronic psoriasis, but the onset of arthritis may coincide with or precede the appearance of the skin lesions.[2,22,26]

The joint symptoms may be acute, insidious, monarticular, or polyarticular. They may involve any peripheral joint or affect the spine, hips, or sacroiliac regions. Characteristically, the distal interphalangeal joints of the fingers and toes are very frequently affected in psoriatic arthritis (Figs. 42–2 and 3). The reported frequency of such involvement in psoriatic arthritis has varied from a quarter to half of all patients.[2,26] In a recent report[26] the frequency rose from 66% to 73% in a group of patients followed over a 10-year period; and in a group of 39 patients with psoriatic arthritis and spondylitis, the distal interphalangeal joints were involved in every one.[26]

The usual symmetry of small joint involvement in rheumatoid arthritis is often lacking in psoriatic arthritis. Constitutional symptoms of fatigue, stiffness, and fever may accompany the synovitis. Joint examination may reveal synovial thickening, effusion, erythema, increased warmth, and limitation of motion. Cervical and low back pain may precede or accompany the initial peripheral joint symptoms.

There is no definite parallelism between the severity of the cutaneous and the articular lesions, although correlations have been noted.[2] Likewise, terminal interphalangeal joint involvement and adjacent nail changes bear no constant relationship.[2,28,37] However, in patients who develop "arthritis mutilans" there is a high incidence of psoriatic changes in the adjacent nails. The changes principally seen are pitting, discoloration, thickening of the nail plate, ridging, splintering, detachment, and erosions[5] (Figs. 42–2 and 3).

In general, the activity of the disease and ultimate deformity is less in psoriatic arthritis than in rheumatoid arthritis, although some patients with psoriatic arthritis develop severe crippling deformities and ankylosis is not unusual.[2,36] It has been suggested that all patients with a seronegative inflammatory polyarthritis should be examined carefully and at frequent intervals for unrecognized psoriasis.[2]

Laboratory Features

There are no specific diagnostic tests for psoriatic arthritis. These patients may have a hypochromic type of anemia but this is much less a feature than in rheumatoid arthritis. The erythrocyte sedimentation rate usually is rapid.[2] Not infrequently the serum uric acid level is above normal, probably as a result of increased cell turnover in the psoriatic cutaneous lesions.

Numerous studies have shown that tests for rheumatoid factors in the serum are positive no more often than in normal subjects.[25,39] Recently Tapanes, Rawson and Hollander[34a] have studied the concentration of anti-immunoglobulins of both IgG and IgA type in rheumatoid and psoriatic arthritis. The levels were above those in control subjects in rheumatoid arthritis, even in patients who were seronegative by conventional tests. In contrast, the levels in psoriatic arthritic patients were *uniformly within the control range*. This suggests that the pathogenesis of articular damage in

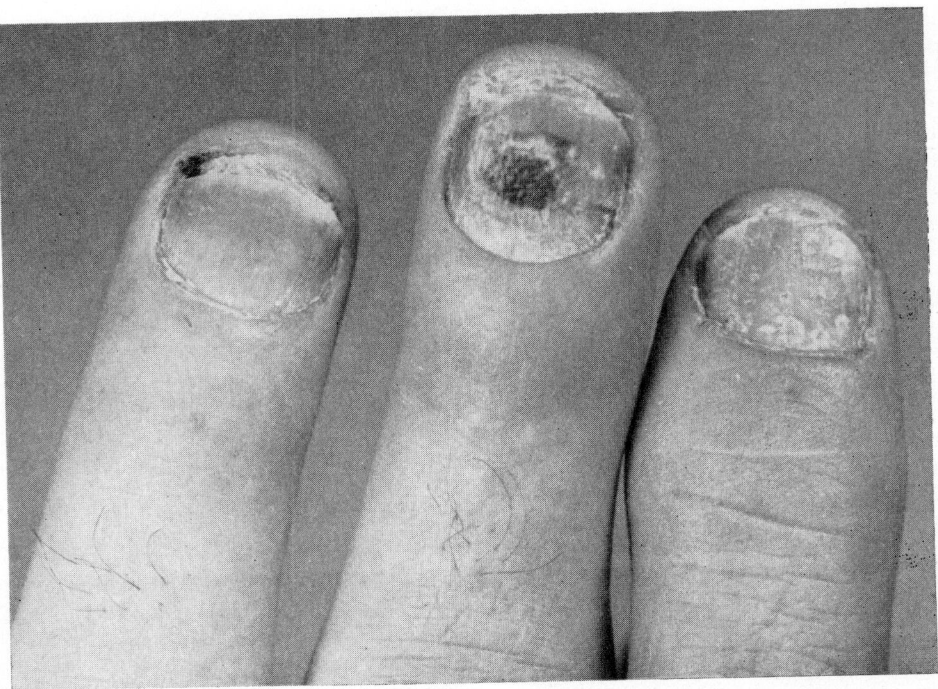

FIG. 42–2.—Psoriatic arthritis with discoloration, thickening and erosions of fingernails. Note swelling of terminal interphalangeal joint of index finger.

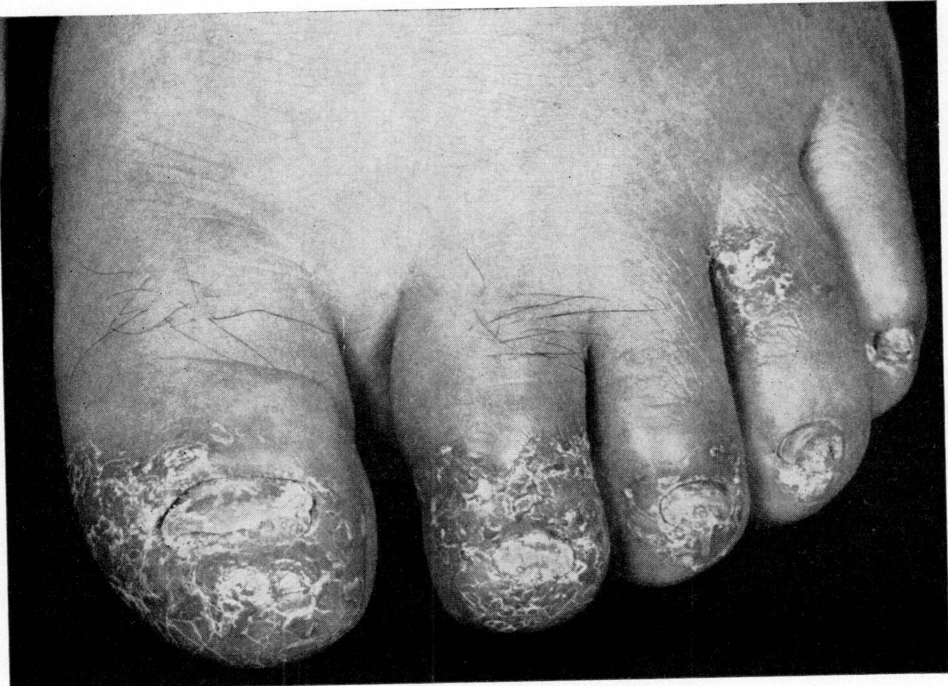

FIG. 42–3.—Foot of patient with psoriatic arthritis showing severe nail and skin changes. Note blunt, sausage-shaped digits.

psoriatic arthritis is different from that in rheumatoid arthritis.[34a]

Synovial fluid examination reveals an inflammatory exudate. The synovia is turbid, lemon yellow in color, and the mucin clot friable. The total leukocyte count ranges from 5,000 to 40,000 with neutrophils the predominant cell type. Macrophages may be seen on differential count which have ingested an intact but non-viable neutrophil. Cytoplasmic inclusions seen as spherical vacuoles are common. However, rheumatoid factor is negative as determined by the differential sheep cell agglutinating titer. Crystalline inclusions are absent although hyperuricemia is observed in some patients. If a patient with psoriasis and hyperuricemia develops an acute monarthritis suggestive of gout, the absence of urate crystals in synovial fluid or exudative leukocytes usually excludes gout and suggests psoriatic arthritis. Although synovianalysis may be helpful in the differential diagnosis from other specific arthritides such as crystal-induced, tuberculous and septic arthritis, there is no specific diagnostic feature for psoriatic arthritis.[7a]

Differential Diagnosis

The differential diagnosis from rheumatoid arthritis most frequently poses the greatest problem. The clinician may be misled by failure to recognize that psoriatic arthritis affects joints other than those of the terminal phalanges. Rheu-

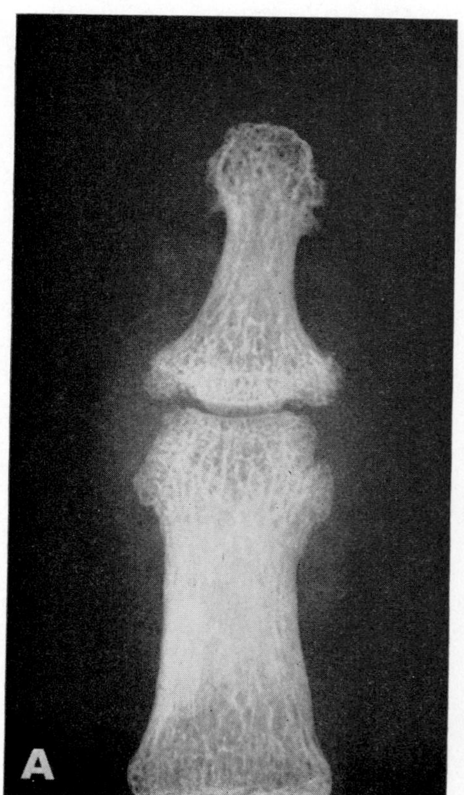

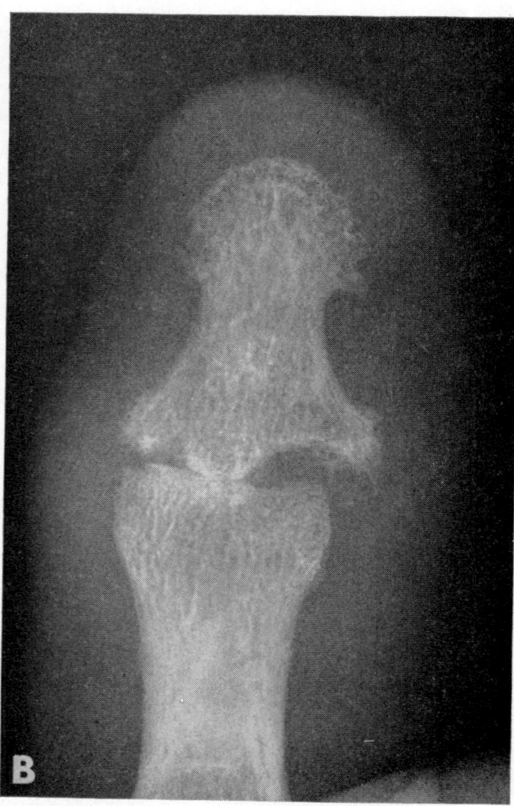

FIG. 42–4.—*A*, Psoriatic arthritis with early erosive changes of the terminal interphalangeal joint of the finger. Note destruction of joint margins and adjacent bone. *B*, Psoriatic arthritis with widening of the joint space of terminal interphalangeal joint of the thumb. (Central portion of joint space is narrowed but erosion to each side of this area gives appearance of widening of joint space.)

matoid arthritis and psoriasis may occur together but not more often than would be expected from the chance coexistence of two fairly common diseases. The presence of rheumatoid nodules excludes the diagnosis of psoriatic arthritis.[8] Other conditions which must be considered include ankylosing spondylitis, gout and Reiter's syndrome.

As with psoriatic arthritis, patients with ankylosing spondylitis are sero-negative for rheumatoid factor and do not have subcutaneous nodules. In both conditions, the sacroiliac joints are involved, and apophyseal joint changes and ligamentous ossifications may occur.[2,13,14,16,17,26,37] Although peripheral joints are often affected in ankylosing spondylitis, the distal interphalangeal

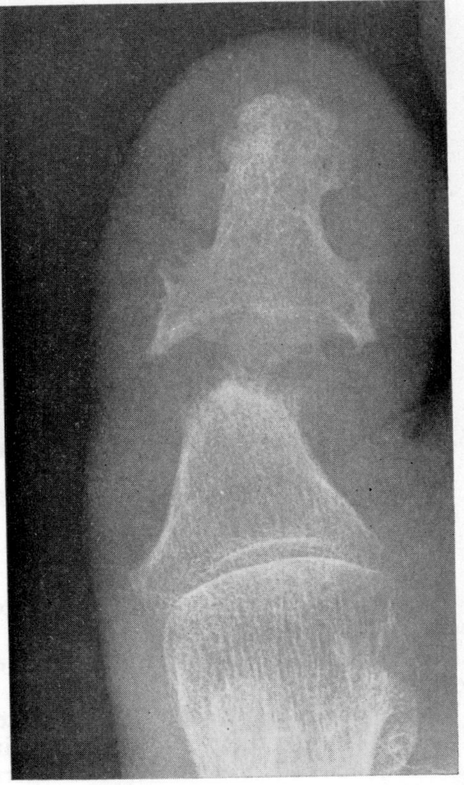

Fig. 42–5.—Psoriatic arthritis with destruction of the distal end of the proximal phalanx of the great toe. Bone spicules are seen along the margins of the distal phalanx.

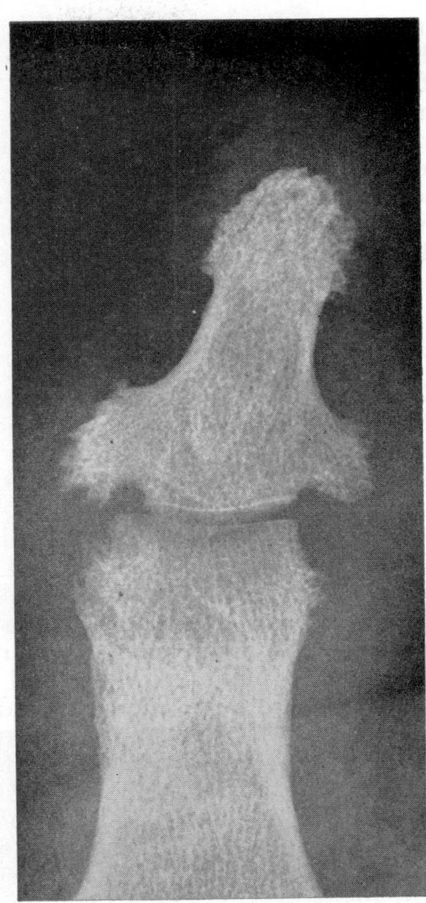

Fig. 42–6.—Psoriatic arthritis with proliferation about the base of the distal phalanx.

joints are not prominently involved. There are no skin changes and the syndesmophytes of psoriatic spondylitis often have a different appearance.[26]

The skin lesions of Reiter's syndrome and psoriasis may be indistinguishable; likewise, nail and joint changes may be similar. Non-specific urethritis and mucous membrane lesions are usually absent in psoriatic arthritis. A link between Reiter's syndrome and psoriatic arthritis has been suggested by the high incidence of ocular and sacroiliac involvement in both,[38] similarities in the spondylitis accompanying the two diseases,[26] and reported instances of apparent transfor-

ible hepatoxicity versus the seriousness of the arthritis. The treatment with methotrexate of patients with psoriatic arthritis should be reserved for unrelenting, rapidly progressing disease which has not responded to conventional management. Accordingly, in our experience, only six patients have met this criterion in the last four years and five have tolerated the drug without discernible hepatotoxicity. The one instance of intolerance was an unusual hematopoietic sensitivity. Dosage of methotrexate in the above patients consisted of 10–15 mg. of methotrexate in a single oral dose once each week. Significant improvement in subjective and objective symptoms was obtained within six weeks and sequential joint x-rays suggested that erosive changes were arrested. However, when the drug was withdrawn empirically, joint symptoms and signs recurred in two to four weeks.

Although other immunosuppressive agents hold promise for the treatment of more resistant psoriatic arthritis, their potentially serious side effects must be appreciated and their careful administration must be reserved for the clinician experienced in their use.[19a]

BIBLIOGRAPHY

1. Avila, R., Pugh, D. G., Slocumb, C. H. and Winkelmann, R. K.: Radiology, *75*, 691, 1960.

1a. Baer, R. L. and Witten, V. H.: *Yearbook of Dermatology*, Chicago, Yearbook Publishers, Inc., 1961–62, p. 9.

2. Baker, H., Golding, D. N. and Thompson, M.: Ann. Int. Med., *58*, 909, 1963.

3. Bauer, W., Bennett, G. A. and Zeller, J. W.: Trans. Assoc. Amer. Physicians, *56*, 349, 1941.

4. Baumann, R. R. and Jillson, O. F.: J. Invest. Derm., *36*, 105, 1961.

5. Beerman, H. and Pastras, T.: Amer. J. Med. Sci., *241*, 522, 1961.

5a. Berge, G., *et al.*: Brit. J. Derm., *82*, 250, 1970.

6. Black, R. L. and O'Brien, W. M.: A.I.R., *7*, 44, 1964.

7. Black, R. L., O'Brien, W. M., Van Scott, E. J., Auerbach, R., Eisen, A. Z. and Bunim, J. J.: J.A.M.A., *189*, 743, 1964.

7a. Bluhm, G. B., Riddle, J. M. and Barnhard, M. I.: Personal communication, 1970.

8. Bollet, A. J. and Turner, R. E.: Ann. N.Y. Acad. Sci., *73*, 1013, 1958.

9. Bourdillon, C.: Psoriasis et Arthropathies, These de Paris, No. 298, 1888.

10. Cecil, R. L.: Chicago Med. Soc. Bull., *51*, 747, 1949.

10a. Coe, R. O. and Bull, F. E.: J.A.M.A., *206*, 1515, 1968.

11. Cornbleet, T.: J. Invest. Derm., *26*, 435, 1956.

12. Dawson, M. H.: Med. Clin. North America, *21*, 1807, 1937.

13. Dawson, M. H. and Tyson, T. L.: Trans. Assoc. Amer. Physicians, *53*, 303, 1938.

14. Dixon, A. St. J. and Lience, E.: Ann. Rheum. Dis., *20*, 247, 1961.

15. Eisen, A. Z. and Seegmiller, J. E.: J. Clin. Invest., *40*, 1486, 1961.

16. Fletcher, E. and Rose, F. C.: Lancet, *1*, 695, 1955.

17. Forestier, J. F. J. and Rotes-Querol, J.: *Ankylosing Spondylitis*, Springfield, Charles C Thomas, 1956, p. 207.

18. Goeckerman, W. H.: Northwest Med., *24*, 229, 1925.

19. Golding, D. N., Baker, H. and Thompson, M.: Ann. Physical Med., *7*, 133, 1963.

19a. Greaves, M. W. and Dawber, R.: Brit. Med. J., *2*, 237, 1970.

20. Hench, P. S.: Ann. Int. Med., *11*, 1089, 1938.

21. Hench, P. S.: *Acute and Chronic Arthritis*, Nelson Loose-Leaf Surgery, New York, Thomas Nelson & Sons, 1935.

21a. Hench, P. S. *et al.*: Ann. Intern. Med., *15*, 1002, 1941.

22. Hollander, J. L., Brown, E. M., Jr., Jessar, R. A., Udell, L., Cooperband, S. and Smukler, N. M.: Arth. and Rheum., *2*, 513, 1959.

23. Hollander, J. L., McCarty, D. J., Jr., Astorga, G. and Castro-Murillo, E.: Ann. Int. Med., *62*, 271, 1965.

24. Kaplan, D., Plotz, C. M., Nathanson, L. and Frank, L.: Ann. Rheum. Dis., *23*, 50, 1964.

25. McEwen, C., Ziff, M., Carmel, P., Ditata, D. and Tanner, M.: Arth. and Rheum., *1*, 481, 1958.

26. McEwen, C., DiTata, D., Lingg, C., Porrini, A., Good, A. and Rankin, T.: Arth. & Rheum., *14*, 291, 1971.

27. Rawson, A. J., Abelson, N. M. and Hollander, J. L.: Ann. Int. Med., *62*, 281, 1965.

28. Reed, W. B.: Acta Dermatovener, *41*, 396, 1961.
29. Reed, W. B. and Becker, S. W.: A.M.A. Arch. Derm., *81*, 577, 1960.
30. Reed, W. B., Becker, S. W., Rohde, R. and Heiskell, C. L.: Arch. Derm. *83*, 541, 1961.
31. Sharp, J.: Brit. Med. J., *1*, 975, 1957.
32. Shelley, W. B., Harun, J. S. and Pillsbury, D. M.: J.A.M.A., *167*, 959, 1958.
33. Sherman, M. S.: J. Bone Joint Surg., *34A*, 831, 1952.
34. Sterne, E. H., Jr. and Schneider, B.: Ann. Int. Med., *38*, 512, 1953.
34*a*. Tapanes, F. J., Rawson, A. J. and Hollander, J. L.: Arth. & Rheum., *15*, 153, 1972.
35. Vilanova, X. and Pinol, J.: Rheumatism, *7*, 197, 1951.
36. Wright, V.: Ann. Rheum. Dis., *20*, 123, 1961.
37. Wright, V.: Amer. J. Med., *27*, 454, 1959.
37*a*. ———: Bull. Rheum. Dis., *21*, 627, 1971.
38. Wright, V. and Reed, W. B.: Ann. Rheum. Dis., *23*, 12, 1964.
39. Ziff, M.: J. Chron. Dis., *5*, 644, 1957.

nective tissue[16,59a,75a] origin of which is still debated. They are located usually near blood vessels and are particularly common in the posterior wall of the left

deformities of these patients are so extensive that they may by themselves explain the congestive failure and the consequent exitus, although some Aschoff

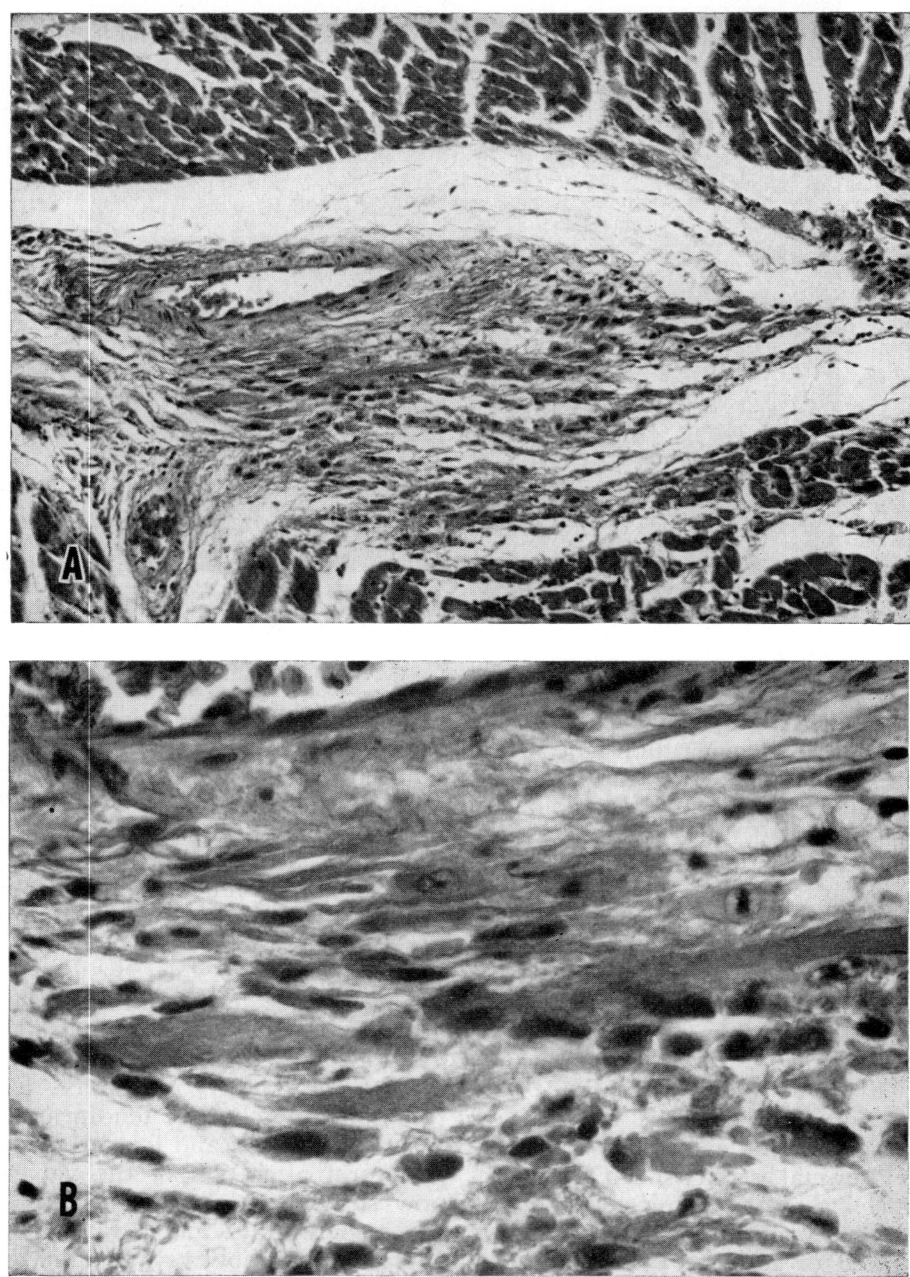

Fig. 43–2.—Aschoff body in the ventricular myocardium of a patient who had died of acute rheumatic fever. *A*, Low power; *B*, High power. (Histologic preparation obtained through the courtesy of Dr. Bradley Bigelow.)

bodies, often partly fibrotic, may still be found. The heart is regularly much enlarged because of both dilatation and hypertrophy.

In recent years biopsy specimens of atrial appendages from patients undergoing mitral commissurotomy have provided an opportunity to look at a "preview" of the histopathology of the heart, long before the patient's death and well after any acute rheumatic attack. Rather surprisingly, Aschoff bodies have been found with an incidence ranging from 16 to 67 per cent of cases in a number of different studies (reviewed in ref. 122). Whether this difference in incidence is due to the patients, to the pathologists, or to both remains uncertain. Also uncertain is the clinical correlation of these findings. The Aschoff bodies in the auricular appendage specimens are certainly not associated with clinically active disease in the conventional sense, but may be more frequent in patients with marked pre-operative worsening of heart failure.[19] Aschoff bodies may also be more frequent (not only in the auricular appendage, but in the heart as a whole) in rheumatic heart disease patients dying with clinical evidence of "rheumatic activity" than in those without it.[55a] There is a suggestion that Aschoff bodies may be made to disappear with cortisone.[82]

Arthritis[56,65,100]

The articular and periarticular structures are swollen and edematous, but there is never erosion of the joint surface or pannus formation. The exudate is turbid but never purulent. At the outset it contains mostly polymorphonuclear leukocytes; later, mononuclear cells increase. Fibrin with enmeshed exudate cells may overlay the lining mesothelial membrane, which is proliferated and damaged. The deeper synovial layers may be infiltrated with polymorphonuclear leukocytes, small round cells and multinucleated cells; the connective tissue fibers may be swollen and "fibrinoid" degeneration may be present.

Chorea[6,17,55]

The few pathologic observations available, usually on patients who had died of carditis with concomitant chorea, have revealed arteritis, cellular degeneration, and occasional emboli and infarctions. Such alterations involve areas scattered throughout the cortex, basal ganglia, substantia nigra and cerebellum. The significance of these changes is unclear because of the lack of a consistent localization and because similar findings have been reported in rheumatic fever *without* chorea.[20,67]

Subcutaneous Nodules[7,52]

Subcutaneous nodules contain much fibrinoid material in strands with clear spaces between the strands. There is much edema and relatively few cells, most of which are fibroblasts or histiocytes with an occasional lymphocyte and a rare polymorph. Vascular "islands" are present, but there is no clear demarcation in concentric zones, and there is little palisading of cells. Fibrosis is not prominent. These characteristics allow differentiation from the subcutaneous nodules of adult rheumatoid arthritis but not from those of Still's disease.[7] Essentially similar nodules may occur in an isolated fashion, without any evidence of systemic disease.[103]

Less common pathologic lesions and more details on the lesions described above are discussed in a review by Murphy.[71]

ETIOLOGY

It has long been known that rheumatic fever is often preceded by pharyngitis, with or without the exanthem of scarlet fever. From this observation of a time relation came the hypothesis that the pharyngitis *causes* rheumatic fever; and soon after scarlet fever was recognized as a streptococcal infection, the theory that rheumatic fever is a streptococcal "after-disease" was proposed.[11,95] Since a large proportion of rheumatic fever cases are not preceded by a symptomatic pharyngitis, and most streptococcal pharyngitides are not followed by rheumatic fever, it was assumed that streptococcal pharyngitis could be a cause of rheumatic fever, but a cause neither necessary nor sufficient.[117]

The development of streptococcal antibody tests has allowed the demonstration that virtually all patients with rheumatic fever, whether they have had the symptoms of pharyngitis or not, have suffered a recent streptococcal infection.[98,112] That this is not a mere time relation leading to the "post hoc, ergo propter hoc" fallacy, but an actual relation of cause and effect was strongly supported by the successful prevention of rheumatic fever recurrences by streptococcal prophylaxis, in the form of continual administration of sulfonamides to patients with previous rheumatic fever.[12] This hypothesis was further strengthened by the prevention of first attacks of rheumatic fever by adequate cure of streptococcal infections with penicillin.[119] Additional support was provided by the following observations: (1) the few attacks of rheumatic fever which do occur in the general population despite penicillin treatment of streptococcal infections can be traced to failure of the treatment to eradicate the organism from the throat,[8] and (2) the few recurrences of rheumatic fever which do occur in patients on continual antistreptococcal prophylaxis can also be traced to streptococcal infections occurring despite prophylaxis.[126]

The fact still remains, however, that only a small percentage of group A streptococcal infections are followed by rheumatic fever. Therefore, streptococcal infections are a necessary, but not a sufficient, cause of this disease. Host factors may affect the outcome, or streptococcal infections may be heterogeneous, in that only some of them are capable of causing rheumatic fever. The accessory role of a virus has often been postulated,[6a] but direct evidence for it is wanting.

Bacteriology of Streptococci as Related to Rheumatic Fever

Streptococci are spherical or oval gram-positive bacteria that tend to grow in chains. On blood agar plates streptococcal colonies may cause an area of slight hemolysis with greenish discoloration (alpha-hemolysis) or of clear and complete hemolysis (beta-hemolysis) (Fig. 43–3). They may also cause no hemolysis at all and then they are called gamma-streptococci. As a rule, only beta-hemolytic organisms are primary pathogens in man.

Streptococci can also be classified into groups by means of antisera against cellular polysaccharides. Most primary human pathogens belong to group A, some to group C ("human strains"), and very few to group G. Among the organisms isolated from streptococcal infections in man, the most common belong to group A and are beta-hemolytic, but a sizable minority are beta-hemolytic organisms of other groups, and an occasional organism belongs to group A but is non-hemolytic.[15,38b] Inspection of sur-

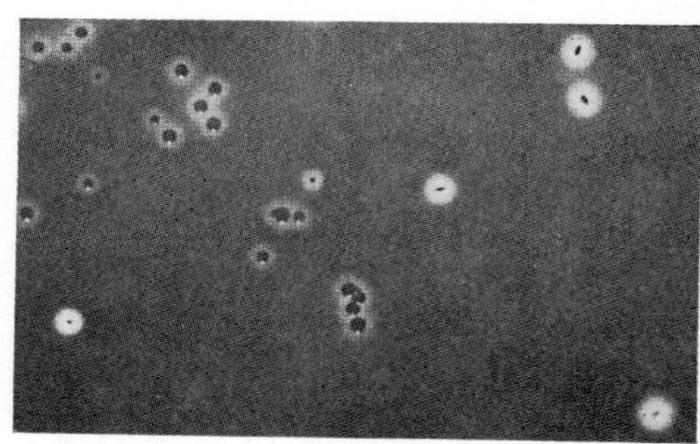

FIG. 43–3.—Pour-streak plate with beta-hemolytic streptococcal colonies on the surface and deep in the blood agar. Note the smooth, round, convex colonies, on which the light reflects itself, and the small zone of beta hemolysis surrounding them. Note also the spindle-shaped subsurface colonies surrounded by a more marked zone of beta hemolysis. (From Taranta & Moody, courtesy of Pediatric Clinics of North America.)

face growth on blood agar plates is thus not always enough to screen for group A infections. Deep growth in pour-plates may be useful in such cases because some strains which cause no hemolysis on the surface of the plate are hemolytic when imbedded in the blood agar (Fig. 43–3). Alternatively, one may incubate the plates in reduced oxygen tension.[105a]

Within group A, streptococci may be classified into over 50 types by means of antisera against the M proteins. These are antigens present on the surface of the streptococci and called M because the colonies of organisms producing them have a "matt" surface. The M proteins protect the organisms from phagocytosis, and antibodies against them overcome the protection.[59]

Hyaluronic acid is another surface

Table 43-1.—Known Extracellular Products of Group A Streptococci

	Inhibition by Antibody	*Main Characteristics*
Streptolysin O	+	Oxygen-labile (hence the name). Determination of antibody against it is the most common serologic test for streptococcal infections.
Streptolysin S	—	Extractable by serum (hence the name) but also by Tweens, nucleotides, etc. It causes the hemolysis on the surface of blood agar plates.
Hyaluronidase	+	Produced *in vitro* by most strains of type 4 and 22; *in vivo* by most strains of all types.
Streptokinase	+	Activates plasminogen, normally present in the serum, to plasmin, a proteolytic enzyme which easily digests fibrin.
Nicotinamide adenine dinucleotidase (Diphosphopyridine-nucleotidase)	+	Production more common in some serotypes and associated with leukotoxicity.
Deoxyribonuclease	+	Four antigenically distinct proteins with the same enzymatic activity. One or the other is produced by all strains.
Erythrogenic Toxin	+	Causes the rash of scarlet fever. Three antigenically distinct toxins.
Streptococcal Proteinase and Precursor	+	Production of proteinase is associated with decreased virulence, because the M protein is digested by it.
Amylase	?	
Esterase	—	
Mitogen	?	Induces "transformation" of human peripheral blood lymphocytes cultured *in vitro* into large, blast-like cells capable of mitosis.

component which protects the organisms from phagocytosis. Unlike M protein, it forms capsules around the cocci. The appearance of colonies of organisms which produce hyaluronic acid is mucoid. There are no antibodies against it, probably because it is chemically identical to the hyaluronic acid of the human body. Streptococci isolated during epidemics of streptococcal pharyngitis are often provided with both hyaluronic acid and M protein in large amounts, while those from sporadic cases of non-exudative streptococcal infections are frequently deficient in either one or both.[99] Streptococci devoid of both hyaluronic acid and M protein are unable to resist phagocytosis even in the virtual absence of all antibodies, as in the colostrum-deprived piglet.[97]

Streptococci release in their culture media many extracellular products, listed and briefly described in Table 43–1, which are usually the same in groups A, C and G. Antibodies cannot distinguish the extracellular products of group A from those of group C or G streptococci and therefore, strictly speaking, one should not make a specific diagnosis of group A streptococcal infection from an elevated titer of such streptococcal antibodies. However, "bona fide" group C and G infections are sufficiently rare for this inaccuracy to be inconsequential.

A newly described streptococcal extracellular product, the streptococcal mitogen,[104] appears to be produced exclusively by group A streptococci.[104b]

EPIDEMIOLOGY

Streptococcal infections of the skin (streptococcal impetigo or pyoderma) are not followed by rheumatic fever, although they may be followed by the other major streptococcal sequel, acute glomerulonephritis. Infections of the skin differ from those of the throat in at least three respects: 1. obviously, the site of infection; 2. the M and T type of the responsible organisms[118a]; 3. the antibody responses (which are weaker to streptolysin O and to nicotinamide adenine dinucleotidase, but not to deoxyribonuclease B, in the skin infections).[42a] Which one—if any—of these differences may account for the difference in the capacity to elicit sequels remains to be determined.

The epidemiology of rheumatic fever resembles that of group A streptococcal pharyngitis, but is not identical to it, because rheumatic fever is a sequel of these infections, but of only a small minority of them. Thus, interpersonal contagion is the rule in streptococcal pharyngitis, but is the exception in rheumatic fever. Moreover, some characteristics of the host as well as of the streptococcus influence the attack rate of rheumatic fever following streptococcal pharyngitis. Therefore, the epidemiology of streptococcal pharyngitis *per se* will be presented first, followed by a discussion of the factors affecting the rheumatic fever attack rate following streptococcal pharyngitis. Finally, information on the epidemiology of rheumatic fever and of its major sequel, rheumatic heart disease, will be reviewed.

Epidemiology of Streptococcal Pharyngitis

Group A streptococcal infections of the throat are ubiquitous and frequent, but become more frequent and more severe whenever interpersonal contacts increase. Thus, they are more common in children, who go to school, than in infants or in adults, who usually do not.[74] The exceptions to the latter statement prove the rule, because streptococcal infections are common and severe among those adults who are restricted to military camps, where 30 or 40 inductees often sleep in the same one-room barrack.[118] Moreover, streptococci appear 4 times more frequently in the throat of pre-school children and infants who have siblings who go to school, than in the throat of those who do not have such siblings.[39] This epidemiologic behavior may be explained in part by the experiments and observations that follow.

If one streaks a swab with hemolytic streptococci on the throat of a human volunteer, symptoms may appear after forty-eight hours. The organisms, which could not be recovered from the throat in the first thirty-two hours after inoculation, reappear shortly before symptoms, and persist until penicillin is administered (Fig. 43–4). If penicillin is not given, or is given in insufficient amounts in naturally occurring infections, the streptococci persist in the throat and in the nose for weeks or months, although symptoms and signs of disease disappear in a few days. The number of organisms which can be recovered from each patient decreases, so that meticulous technique and special media, such as Pike's, are often needed to demonstrate their continuing presence. They disappear from the nose earlier than from the throat.[77] These changes may reduce the infectivity of the carriers (Fig. 43–5). Moreover, the streptococci themselves change, in that they produce less and less and eventually no detectable M protein.[83] They thus become progressively more susceptible to phagocytosis even in the absence of specific antibody, and, if inoculated on the pharynx of a monkey, become unable to establish themselves there.[77] However, they are the direct descendents of the same organisms which originally caused the symptoms, because if they are "passed" through a few mice, they again start producing M protein of the same serologic type. The prolonged persistence of streptococci coincident with the loss of a virulence factor and with the development in the host of specific protective antibodies[58] is paradoxical, but not without parallel.[85]

Indirect contagion by contaminated dust and fomites does not occur,[118] although contaminated milk can cause epidemics.[62] In military barracks the rate of acquisition of streptococcal infections decreases with increasing distance from the bed of the nearest infected soldier (Fig. 43–6). It thus appears that direct interpersonal contact in the earliest stage of a streptococcal infection is essential for contagion, which probably occurs via droplets of saliva and nasal secretions, and that rapid serial transfers of the organism from throat to throat are made possible by the short incubation period.

Multiple interpersonal contacts may lead to an epidemic, not only because they increase the possibility of contagion, but also because serial transfers from pa-

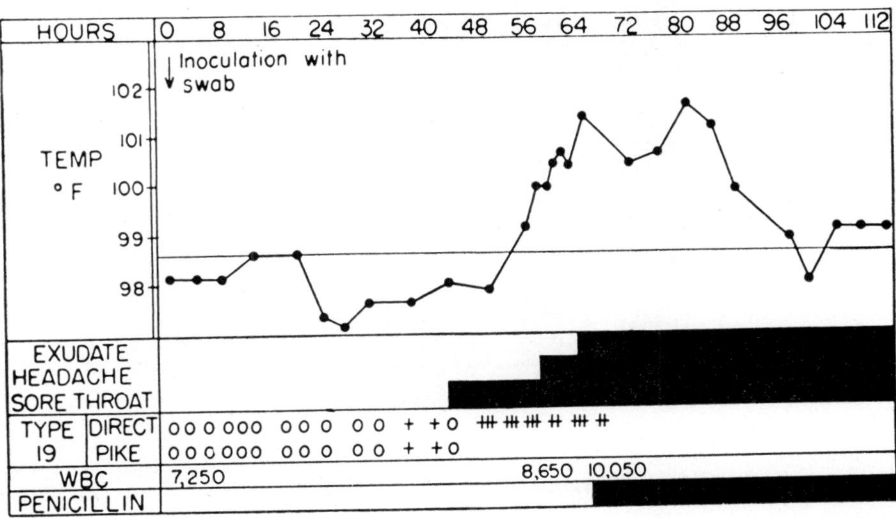

FIG. 43–4.—Time sequence of events following inoculation of group A streptococci in a human volunteer. (Rammelkamp, courtesy of Harvey Lecture Series.)

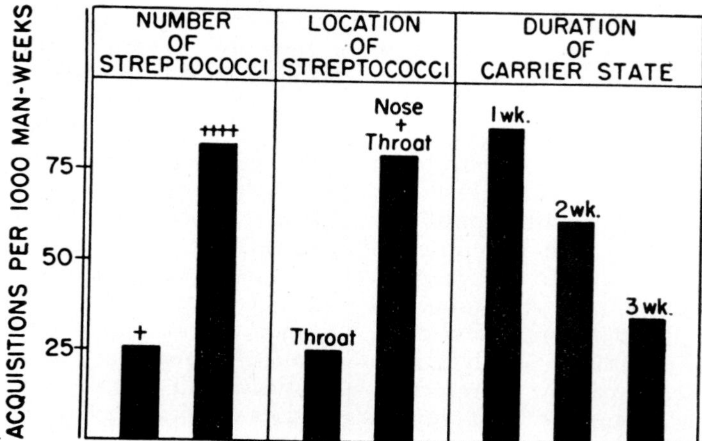

Fig. 43–5.—Characteristics of the carrier which alter the transmission, or communicability, of streptococci. Transmission was measured by the number of "acquisitions" of streptococci from the carrier by other soldiers. Transmission was greater when many streptococci rather than few streptococci were present in the throat culture of the carrier; it was greater if the streptococci were present in the nose and throat than if they were present in the throat only; and it decreased progressively with the duration of the carrier state. (Rammelkamp, courtesy of Harvey Lecture Series.)

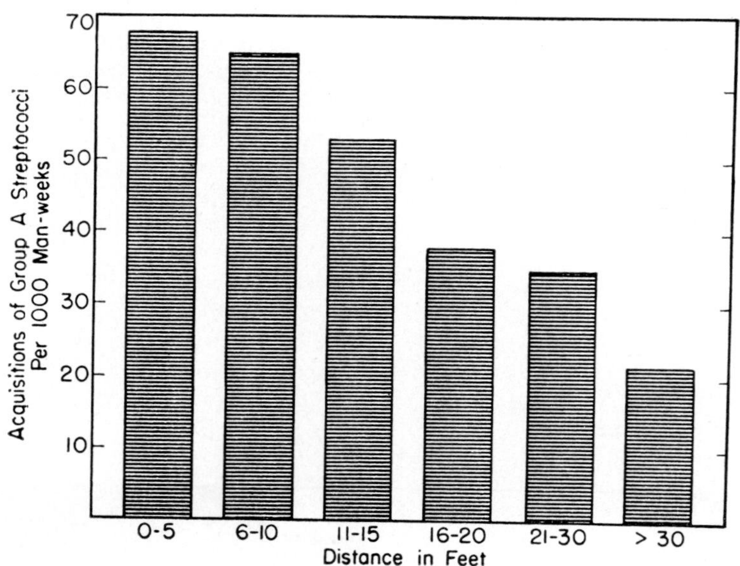

Fig. 43–6.—Acquisition rates for group A streptococci according to bed distance from the nearest carrier. (Wannamaker in McCarty, *Streptococcal Infections*, courtesy of Columbia University Press.)

tient to patient may lead to selection of those streptococcal mutants which produce most M protein and hyaluronic acid, in a manner analogous to what is artificially accomplished in the laboratory by "passage" of a strain through a series of mice. Although such increase in virulence of a streptococcal strain has never been actually documented in the successive phases of human epidemics, the information that "epidemic" strains differ from "sporadic" ones in that the former produce more M protein and hyaluronic acid than the latter is consistent with this interpretation.[99]

Recently, variation of M protein (from type 12 to a hitherto undescribed type) has been reported to occur in a streptococcal strain under conditions of natural endemic infection in man.[64a] This important observation suggests that "new" M proteins may arise whenever the streptococci need them to survive and propagate.

Age Variations.—Age influences both the incidence and the clinical manifestations of streptococcal infections. As indicated above, incidence increases from infancy to childhood; it then decreases in adolescence and reaches very low levels in adulthood.[74] The clinical picture in infants and small children is that of a subacute illness, often characterized by otitis and adenitis, while older children, adolescents and adults tend to have an acute illness more localized to the pharynx.[76]

Geographic Variations.—There is no detailed information on the frequency of streptococcal infections in various parts of the world. However, using scarlet fever, for which better and more extensive data are available (Fig. 43–7), as an indicator of streptococcal infections, it appears that these infections are frequent in both temperate zones, and become progressively rarer as one approaches the equator. A similar conclusion can be reached on the basis of the few surveys of streptococcal antibody titers done so far.[14,77] Although the major cause of this variation is likely to be the decreased tendency to congregate in warm climates, a more direct effect of the environment may also be involved.

Factors Affecting the Rheumatic Fever Attack Rate Following Streptococcal Infections

First Attacks.—Rheumatic fever follows group A streptococcal infections with an incidence of 0.3 to 3 per cent or higher, depending on the definition of both "rheumatic fever" and "streptococcal infection." Using a strict and now standard definition of rheumatic fever,[41] Rammelkamp and his associates showed that the attack rate of rheumatic fever, following *untreated*, *epidemic*, *exudative* streptococcal pharyngitis was approximately 3 per cent.[77] This rate remained constant over many years, regardless of the streptococcal type causing the disease, and irrespective of the geographic origin of the patient and of the initial ASO (antistreptolysin O) titer. The rheumatic fever attack rate increased with increasing antibody response but wide overlaps in antibody response occurred between the patients who developed rheumatic fever and those who did not.[94] In patient groups treated with antibiotics, rheumatic fever occurred only among those patients in whom the treatment failed to eradicate the streptococci.[8] Moreover, the attack rate of rheumatic fever was decreased significantly by eradication of the streptococci as long as nine days after onset of symptoms, by which time maximum antibody stimulation had already occurred.[9] These observations indicate that persistence of the organism in the host is critically important for the development of rheumatic fever.

If the definition of rheumatic fever is less strict and allows inclusion of patients with minor electrocardiographic alterations, fever or arthralgia even without clinical carditis, arthritis or chorea, the attack rate may be as high as 15 per cent.[79] These mild disturbances probably represent the low end of the spectrum of rheumatic fever severity.

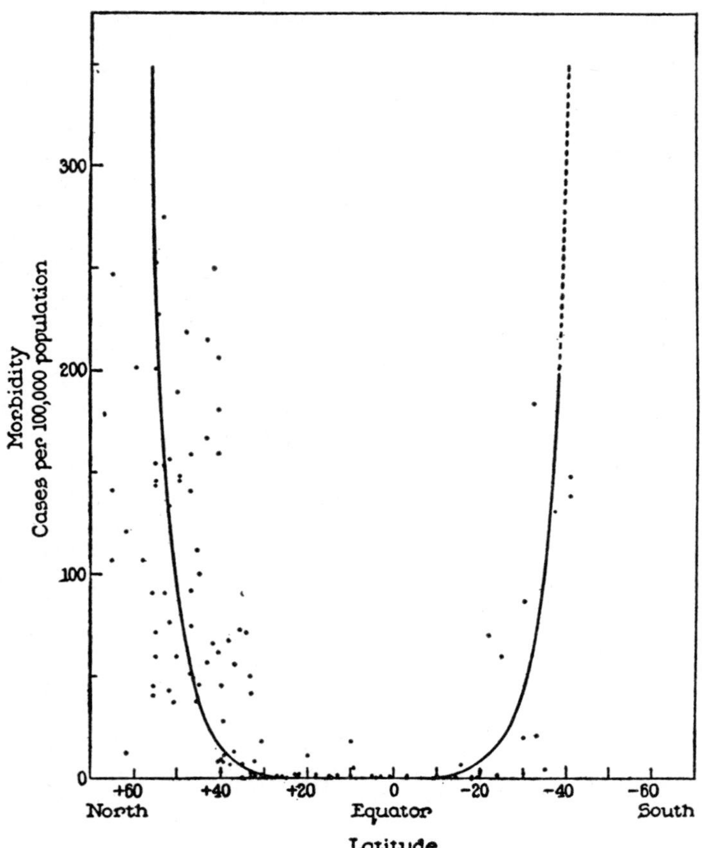

Fig. 43–7.—Relation of scarlet fever morbidity in various countries and mean latitude of the country. (Schwentker *et al.*, courtesy of Amer. J. Hygiene.)

Since they are difficult to diagnose with certainty and appear to be benign, their exclusion from the current definition of rheumatic fever seems justified on practical if not on theoretical grounds.

In recent years attention has been called to the milder forms of streptococcal parasitism and to the rarity with which they lead to rheumatic fever. Saslaw and Streitfeld showed that 45 per cent of school children in Florida harbored group A beta-hemolytic streptococci in their throat at least once during a school year.[88] This high cumulative incidence of positive cultures contrasts with the alleged rarity of rheumatic fever in that state, but it must be noted that only 4 per cent of the children studied had an ASO titer greater than 250. In a comparable group of children in San Francisco, Rantz found 35 per cent of such elevated titers.[81] It thus appears that the host-parasite relation in most of the children observed by Saslaw was more akin to commensalism (*i.e.* to "carrier state") than to parasitism, and that this type of relation does not lead to rheumatic fever.

The variety of host-parasite relations in a symptomatic pediatric group is well illustrated in a careful study by Siegel *et al.*[91] Of 2545 children with clinical pharyngitis, 47.7 per cent were found to harbor beta-hemolytic streptococci in their throats, and of these 85 per cent were group A strains. However, only 21.5 per cent of the children had typable strains (*i.e.* strains producing M protein) and only 21.7 per cent had a significant ASO rise. These latter percentages are much lower than in epidemic situations among adults.[77] Treatment was withheld in one-half of the children, and rheumatic fever occurred only twice among the 1293 untreated children. The variations of the attack rate of rheumatic fever according to the definition of the pharyngitis are illustrated in Table 43–2. It will be noted that the attack rate was very low in the whole group with symptomatic pharyngitis, and it increased progressively with increasing clinical and laboratory evidence of severity of the infection. It is noteworthy that the two cases of rheumatic fever occurred in patients who had exudative pharyngitis, significant antibody rise and convalescent carriage of the strain for more than twenty-one days. Only 81 patients of the entire untreated group met these criteria, giving an attack rate of 2.5 per cent.

It must be remembered that approximately one-third of rheumatic fever attacks follow streptococcal infections which are wholly asymptomatic,[128] and can be diagnosed only in retrospect on the basis of elevated streptococcal antibody titers. The attack rate of rheumatic fever following such asymptomatic infections is difficult to determine in the general population, but may be presumed to be lower than that after symptomatic infections on the basis of analogy with the data on recurrences (see below).

Genetic factors have been implicated in the epidemiology of rheumatic fever because siblings of patients with rheumatic fever are more likely to develop the disease than siblings of "controls." Not only genes, however, are shared by blood relatives, but also income, housing, and level of medical care, all of which may influence the frequency of untreated streptococcal infections and therefore of rheumatic fever. Moreover, families with more than one affected member are more likely to be represented in a rheumatic fever clinic or hospital population than families with only one affected member, thus biasing all studies based on hospital or clinic populations.

Comparison of concordance, *i.e.*, simi-

Table 43-2.—Attack Rates of Rheumatic Fever in Untreated Pharyngitis in Children*

Diagnostic Categories	*With or Without Exudate*		*With Exudate*	
	No.	*Per cent with Rheumatic Fever*	*No.*	*Per cent with Rheumatic Fever*
Pharyngitis	1293	0.15	310	0.65
Pharyngitis with Throat Culture Positive for Beta-hemolytic Streptococci	608	0.33	216	0.9
Pharyngitis with Throat Culture Positive for Group A Streptococci	519	0.39	186	1.0
Pharyngitis with ASO Rise	228	0.9	95	2.1
Pharyngitis with Convalescent Carriage of Streptococci for at Least 21 Days	202	0.91	81	2.5

*Based on data of Siegel *et al.*[91]

larity in being affected by the disease, between monozygotic (or "identical") and dizygotic twins of rheumatic patients may shed some light on the relative roles of genetic and environmental factors, because the genes of monozygotic twins are identical, while those of dizygotic twins are not, and the environment is common to both kinds of twins. Early case reports suggested that monozygotic twins are always concordant, which, if true, would support the argument that rheumatic fever is a "genetic" disease. A systematic study of this problem failed to confirm this impression,[50] and a more modern study of 56 twin pairs done with the advantage of more accurate diagnosis of both rheumatic fever and zygosity, has shown that the majority of monozygotic twin pairs are, like the ones illustrated in Figure 43–8, discordant for rheumatic fever, the concordance rate

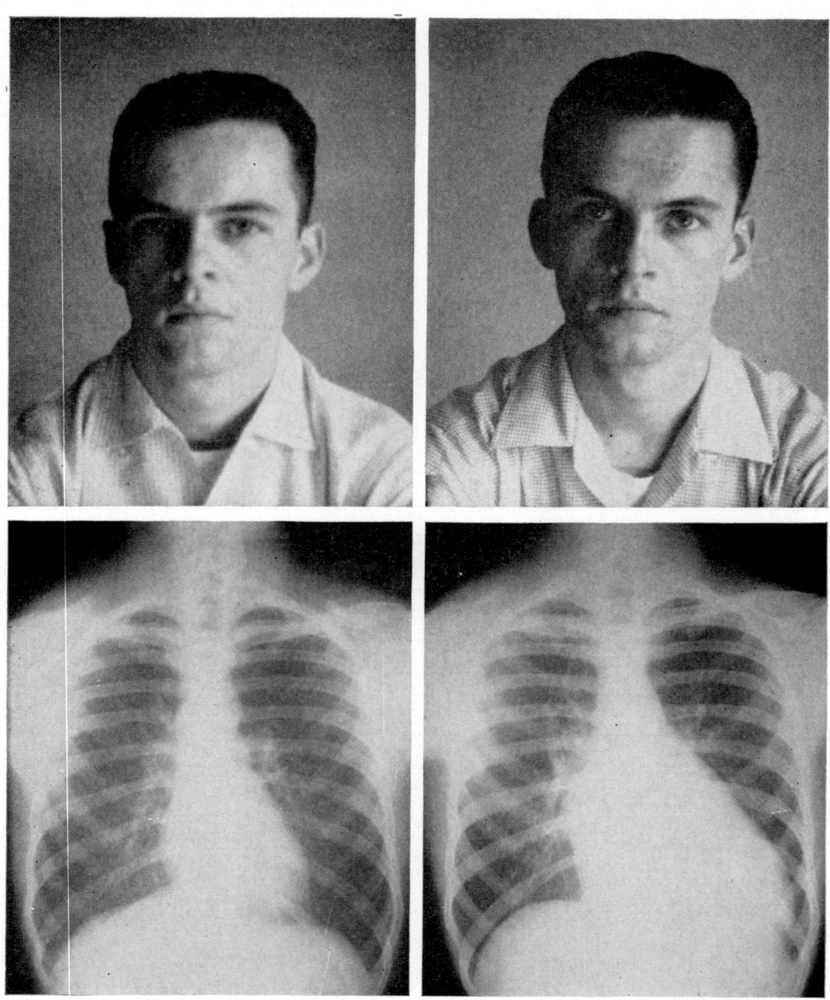

Fig. 43–8.—Monozygotic twin pair discordant for rheumatic fever. Richard, on the right, died 10 years after an attack of rheumatic fever and 9 years after subacute bacterial endocarditis, with advanced rheumatic heart disease. Robert, on the left, although sharing the same room with Richard all his life, escaped rheumatic fever and has now a normal heart. (From Taranta *et al.*, courtesy of Minerva Med.)

being only 18.7 per cent.[108] However, the concordance rate in *dizygotic* twins is even lower (2.5 per cent). This suggests that genetic predisposition may indeed play a role, though minor, comparable to that played by it in paralytic poliomyelitis[35] (see Table 43–3).

Attempts to pin down this vague trend to a specific Mendelian mode of inheritance have generally failed, with the exception of the studies of Wilson *et al.*, which suggested a recessive, autosomal gene with high penetrance,[123] but have not been confirmed.[114] Similarity of the clinical manifestations of rheumatic fever among affected siblings has recently been reported.[92a]

If the human population is indeed genetically heterogeneous in its susceptibility to rheumatic fever, what is the molecular basis of the susceptibility? Glynn *et al.*[29] have suggested that patients who develop rheumatic fever may do so because the streptococcus may bind to a component of the pharyngeal secretions and make it antigenic, with consequent production of autoantibodies. The postulated "autoantigen" is a blood group substance present in the saliva of "ABH non-secretors" and not in that of "secretors." These authors have shown a significant, but not marked, difference in percentage of non-secretors between patients with rheumatic fever (27.5 per cent) and non-rheumatic controls (21.2 per cent).[29] The significance of this difference has been both confirmed[10] and questioned[22] and further investigation is required.

Recurrent Attacks.—The attack rate of rheumatic fever following streptococcal infections is much higher in patients who have already had rheumatic fever than in those who have not. The rate is highest in the first few years after the rheumatic attack (though it may be low in the first few months after the attack in adults)[77] and declines thereafter.[105] It is not quite clear whether this decrease is due to the length of time elapsed since the last attack or to the increasing age of the patient. Nor is it clear whether the high attack rate of patients who have already had the disease is due to the preceding attack or, conversely, the preceding attack is due to a pre-existing special susceptibility to rheumatic fever. Whatever its origin, this susceptibility decreases with the passage of time, but is still present many years after the last rheumatic attack and well into adult life.[40,77,104a]

Rheumatic fever recurrences occur only among those patients who develop a streptococcal antibody response. Mere acquisition of beta-hemolytic streptococci without a rise in streptococcal antibodies

Table 43-3.—Rheumatic Fever in 56 Twin Pairs*

	Concordant Pairs	*Discordant Pairs*	*Concordance Rate (Per cent)*
16 Monozygotic Twin Pairs	3 (4†)	13 (12†)	18.7 (25†)
40 Dizygotic Pairs	1 (2†)	39 (38†)	2.5 (5†)
Paralytic Poliomyelitis in 47 Twin Pairs‡			
14 Monozygotic Twin Pairs	5	9	35.71
33 Dizygotic Twin Pairs	2	31	6.06

* Based on data of Taranta *et al.*[108]
† Taking into account pairs of questionable concordance.
‡ Based on data of Herndon and Jennings.[35]

is never followed by rheumatic fever, regardless of the presence or absence of clinical pharyngitis.[109] Clinical pharyngitis with positive throat culture and no antibody rise may be due to viral infections concomitant with the streptococcal carrier state.

One-half of the rheumatic fever recurrences (in patients on prophylaxis) follow asymptomatic streptococcal infections[109] but the recurrence rate per infection is lower in asymptomatic than in symptomatic infections. Among the latter, it increases with the severity of the symptoms.[24,92]

In those patients with antibody response, the recurrence rate per infection increases with the magnitude of the antibody rise and ranges from 15 per cent in infections characterized by the minimum significant ASO rise to 70 per cent in infections characterized by the maximum antibody rise observed. By contrast, the *pre-infection* antibody titer has no relation to the recurrence rate. It thus appears that although the recurrence rate is increased by a previous attack of rheumatic fever, it is not increased by a previous attack of streptococcal pharyngitis.[105,109] More recent, statistically controlled studies ascribe a greater role to symptoms of pharyngitis than to ASO rise as predictors of recurrences.[92]

Streptococcal infections are more likely to lead to recurrences of rheumatic fever in patients with pre-existing rheumatic heart disease than in patients with previous rheumatic fever but no heart disease. In patients with heart disease, the attack rate is higher in patients with marked cardiomegaly than in those with little or no cardiac enlargement. The attack rate per infection also increases with increasing number of preceding rheumatic attacks, and decreases with age, but these differences may not be significant and are difficult to interpret due to concomitant changes in multiple parameters. By contrast, the increase in recurrence rate with increasing heart disease appears to be definite and genuine, since it cannot be ascribed to concomitant variations in age, in the number of previous attacks, or in antibody response (Table 43–4).

Epidemiology of Rheumatic Fever and Rheumatic Heart Disease.—Rheumatic fever is not a reportable disease in most states and therefore morbidity data are scanty. The few data available must be unreliable since mortality in some instances exceeds morbidity.[63] The prevalence of rheumatic heart disease can be studied by population surveys, but the error involved in the method used for primary screening, *i.e.*, auscultation of the heart, is high,[72,102] and automatic analysis of heart sounds and murmurs is still in the experimental stage.[38a,106] Despite all these limitations, data are sufficient to substantiate the statements which follow.

Table 43-4.—Ratio of Rheumatic Recurrences to Streptococcal Infections in Patients Stratified for Pre-Existing Rheumatic Heart Disease and for ASO Rise*

ASO Rise in Number of Tube Dilutions	*Pre-existing Heart Disease*	*No Pre-existing Heart Disease*
0–1	3:24 (13%)	1:79 (1%)
2	10:38 (26%)	3:50 (6%)
3	6:16 (38%)	5:34 (15%)
4+	9:16 (56%)	9:26 (35%)

* From data of Taranta *et al.*[105]

The incidence of rheumatic fever has been decreasing for many decades. The decline started well before the introduction of sulfonamides and of penicillin and has become more obvious since. The severity of the disease may also have decreased (see next chapter). Mortality from rheumatic fever and from rheumatic heart disease has certainly decreased.[93] The decrease of rheumatic fever may well be due primarily to the improvement in the standard of living, and especially to decreased crowding in the homes since the incidence of rheumatic heart disease is directly related to the number of persons per room (Fig. 43–9).

Rheumatic fever is more common in the temperate than in the tropical and sub-tropical climates,[11] although it is not as rare in the latter as it was once thought to be.[27] In the United States, rheumatic fever is common in the Rocky Mountain and in the Northeastern areas, and rare in southern California and Florida. Figure 43–10 depicts the incidence of rheumatic heart disease in a number of localities at various latitudes. A rough parallelism with the geographic distribution of scarlet fever (Fig. 43–7) is apparent.

Rheumatic fever has a *seasonal variation* in incidence, which reaches its peak in early spring in this country. This is probably due to the progressive build-up

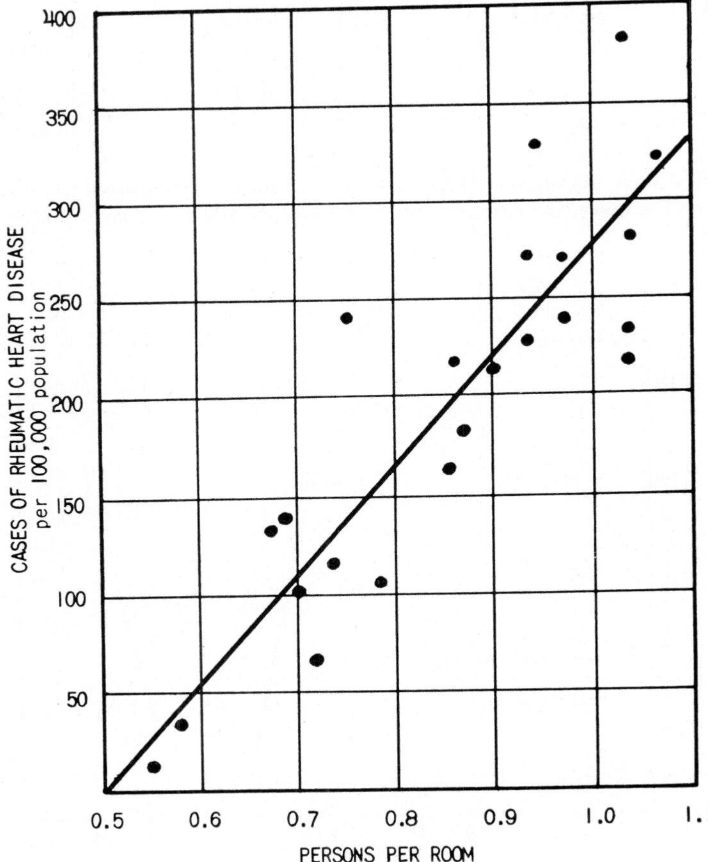

Fig. 43–9.—The relation between density of persons per room and incidence of rheumatic heart disease. (Perry and Roberts, courtesy of Brit. Med. J.)

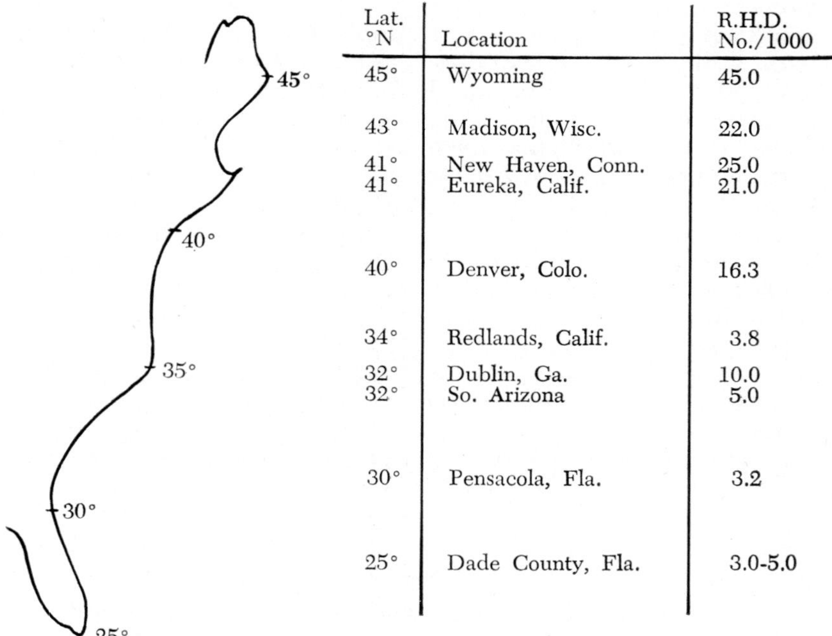

Lat. °N	Location	R.H.D. No./1000
45°	Wyoming	45.0
43°	Madison, Wisc.	22.0
41°	New Haven, Conn.	25.0
41°	Eureka, Calif.	21.0
40°	Denver, Colo.	16.3
34°	Redlands, Calif.	3.8
32°	Dublin, Ga.	10.0
32°	So. Arizona	5.0
30°	Pensacola, Fla.	3.2
25°	Dade County, Fla.	3.0-5.0

FIG. 43–10.—Prevalence of rheumatic heart disease in various localities arranged according to latitude. The line on the left represents the eastern coast of the United States. (Saslaw and Streitfeld, courtesy of A.M.A. J. Dis. Child.)

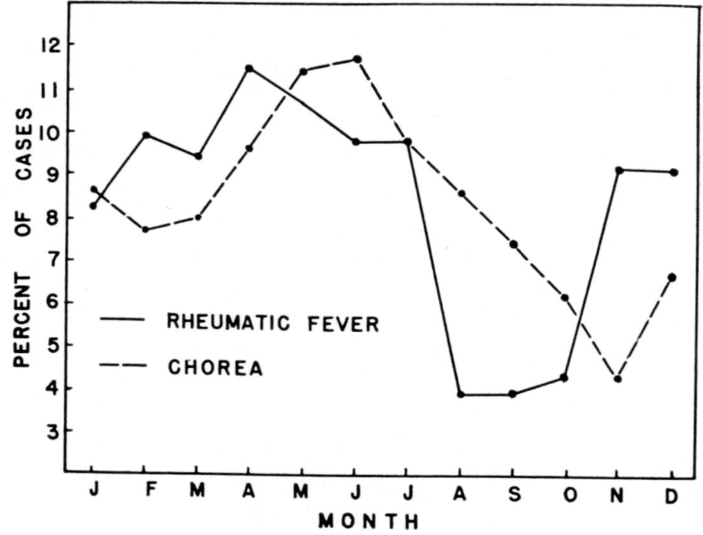

FIG. 43–11.—Seasonal incidence of chorea and of other manifestations of rheumatic fever in Chicago. (Gibson, in Brennemann's *Practice of Pediatrics*, courtesy of W. F. Prior Co.)

of streptococcal epidemics through the winter months, which reach their peak at the end of winter and are then dispersed by the decreased human aggregation which prevails with good weather. It is interesting that the peak incidence of chorea follows the peak incidence of other manifestations of rheumatic fever by an interval of two months, so that the curve of the seasonal incidence of chorea is roughly parallel to that of the other manifestations, but delayed with respect to it (Fig. 43–11). This epidemiologic peculiarity may be explained by a longer latent period between streptococcal infections and chorea as compared to the latent period between streptococcal infections and the more common rheumatic manifestations[104,107] (see next chapter, under "*Chorea*").

Age variation in the incidence of rheumatic fever is striking, and is not wholly explained by age variations in the incidence of streptococcal infections. Streptococcal infections occur in the first two years of life, but rheumatic fever does not, or, at least, is exceptional.[76,80,82a] By contrast, the other major streptococcal sequel, glomerulonephritis, occurs frequently in the first two years.[1] These discrepancies suggest that *repeated* streptococcal infections are necessary for rheumatic fever (but not for nephritis); or that the infant is inherently incapable of the tissue responses of rheumatic fever, and that he acquires this capacity later by a process of normal maturation.

Unfortunately, the data on children followed since birth with throat cultures and antibody studies[80] are not sufficiently extensive to settle this important question. Changes in the *manifestations* of the disease also occur with age (see next chapter).

A fairly large group of patients with heart disease clinically, and, as far as we know, pathologically indistinguishable from rheumatic heart disease *denies any history of rheumatic fever attacks*. It is generally assumed that all of these patients had an attack of rheumatic fever involving the heart, but without congestive failure, and sparing the joints and the brain. In such cases the physician may not be consulted because of the ill-defined nature and deceptive mildness of the disease, which may thus run its early course unrecognized. This explanation is supported by known cases of this kind which have come under the physician's observation accidentally, but the possibility that the heart disease in some of these patients might have an origin other than rheumatic fever deserves consideration.[6a]

PATHOGENESIS

Although the etiology of rheumatic fever has been elucidated, the mechanism by which group A streptococcal infections lead to rheumatic fever remains uncertain. It is not even clear whether single or multiple mechanisms are involved in the pleomorphic manifestations of the disease. From the pathologic dissimilarity among the exudative lesions of joints and pericardium, the proliferative lesions of the myocardium and the destructive and sclerosing alterations of the valve leaflets, one might infer that diverse mechanisms are at work. The effectiveness of anti-inflammatory treatment in the arthritis, but not in the endocarditis of rheumatic fever, may support this inference. The extremely long "latent period" often encountered in Sydenham's chorea seems to demand an "ad hoc" pathogenetic hypothesis. Because of the overriding importance of carditis, however, most of the efforts have centered on elucidating the mechanisms leading to it.

Rigorous definition of the pathogenesis of rheumatic fever is of interest not only in its own right, but may provide, in addition, a direction to therapeutic attempts. It may also suggest clues for the investigation of other diseases which share with rheumatic fever some clinical and pathologic features, but whose etiology is unknown.

Cogent arguments have been advanced in favor of disparate hypotheses; the most credible of them are reviewed below.

Direct Invasion by the Group A Streptococci

In most diseases of infectious etiology the causative agent is demonstrable, during at least one phase of the illness, at the site of primary tissue damage. There it exerts its action by invasion and destruction of cells and other *local* mechanisms. The possibility that the streptococcus is actually present in the lesions of rheumatic fever is intriguing. The exudate of rheumatic joints is characteristically sterile, but the sterility of the other lesions is in doubt. Three papers in 1939–1940 reported that beta-hemolytic streptococci, shown, whenever tested, to be group A, could be cultured from the heart valves affected by acute rheumatic endocarditis in 89,[30] 60[16] and 50[111] per cent of patients who had died of acute rheumatic carditis. These organisms could not be recovered from the blood or from normal valves of the same patients, but were cultured also from their myocardium, pericardial fluid, spleen, lung, mediastinal lymph nodes and brain, the latter in a case of chorea. This was clearly more than was bargained for. Collis voiced skepticism on the significance of these findings, which were, in part, his own,[16] and suggested three possible explanations for them: (1) contamination at the time of the autopsy; (2) agonal or postmortem dissemination and proliferation of streptococci; or (3) arrival of streptococci in the affected tissues well before the agonal period, and with a genuine pathogenetic role.

Repetition and extension of this work were hampered by the discovery of penicillin. Very few patients now die of rheumatic carditis without having received some form of penicillin treatment. One study, however, which was completed in the last pre-antibiotic years suggested that contamination at the time of autopsy might possibly explain the previous findings, since cultures from affected heart valves were positive for group A streptococci in 2 of 7 patients autopsied without special precautions, but were negative in the last four patients, who were autopsied with surgical aseptic techniques.[124] This is not a significant difference, however. It is intriguing that in 2 of these last 4 cases, despite the meticulous asepsis, streptococci were cultured from mediastinal lymph nodes.

Relevant to the interpretation of these old findings are the modern attempts to treat rheumatic fever with penicillin,[69] which are reviewed in the section on treatment in the next chapter. Suffice it to say at this time that these therapeutic attempts have not been clearly successful and have thus failed to strengthen the hypothesis that living group A streptococci cause rheumatic fever by direct invasion of the affected tissues.

Direct Invasion by L Forms Derived from Group A Streptococci

In the absence of "prima facie" evidence for the presence of the streptococcus in the specific lesions of rheumatic fever, interest has developed in the possible role of streptococcal L forms. These variants of the parent organism are devoid of cell wall but are capable of producing toxins.[26] They are fastidious in their growth requirements, which may explain their absence from routine cultures. Interestingly, their development is enhanced in the presence of penicillin, and therefore their demonstration, in contrast to the parent organism, would not be hampered in rheumatic fever patients treated with penicillin.

Recovery of streptococcal L forms has been reported from various organs of mice, months after intraperitoneal inoculation with group A streptococci.[57,68] Streptococcal L forms obtained *in vitro* have been reported to survive *in vivo*.[10a,88a] Moreover, transitional forms of growth which may be related to L forms of beta-hemoloytic streptococci have been reported in blood cultures of rheumatic fever patients.[42,125] Confirmation of these latter findings and extension of them to the specific lesions of rheumatic fever are eagerly awaited.

Toxic Action

Streptococci release into the surrounding media a multitude of extracellular products, many of which have attracted attention because they are enzymes, toxins or both (Table 43–1). At least twenty streptococcal extracellular products reach the human antibody-forming cells in the course of streptococcal infections, as evidenced by as many precipitin lines in immunoelectrophoresis of streptococcal filtrates developed with human gamma globulin pools.[32] In addition there may be non-antigenic products, of which one, streptolysin S, has been recognized because of its specific toxic action.[113] Still other products may be released in amounts too small to be recognized.

One or more of these soluble extracellular products could be the direct means by which streptococci, without leaving the pharynx, cause the lesions of rheumatic fever in the heart and other distant organs, as *Corynebacterium diphtheriae* causes neuritis without invading the nerves, and carditis without lodging in the heart. Interestingly, a "latent period" not unlike that of rheumatic fever is also a frequent feature of these complications of diphtheritic infections.[61] Several streptococcal products could play a role in rheumatic fever analogous to that of diphtheria toxin in diphtheritic myocarditis:

Streptolysin S is a leading candidate for such a role. Its lack of antigenicity[38,96] is compatible with the clinical information that one or more bouts of rheumatic fever do not lead to immunity. Streptolysin S can be produced by resting (non-dividing) streptococci,[3] as those lingering in the throat *after* an acute infection and during the latent period of rheumatic fever probably are. The action of streptolysin S can be inhibited by a serum lipoprotein, which has been found to be decreased in patients with rheumatic fever,[96] thereby possibly permitting an increased susceptibility to the toxic action of streptolysin S. The nature of this action in human infections is unknown, but observations *in vitro* indicate that, in addition to red blood cells, streptolysin S can disrupt lysosomes.[121] These intracellular organelles contain a number of autolytic enzymes, which, when released by disruption of their outer membrane, may provoke secondary cellular and tissue damage. Although this lysosome-disrupting ability is not unique, but shared by other hemolytic toxins,[5] streptolysin S is a more effective disruptor of lysosomes than the other streptococcal hemolysin, streptolysin O, when compared with it at equal hemolytic titer.[121]

Streptolysin S had been reported to elicit the transformation into large blast-like cells capable of mitosis, of peripheral blood lymphocytes from normal humans, or from patients with other diseases, but not from patients with rheumatic fever.[37] It has since been shown that streptolysin S is inactive in this respect, and that the mitogenic effect is due to another streptococcal extracellular product, released by most group A strains (including a streptolysin S-deficient mutant[104d]) but not by strains of other groups,[104b] and is chromatographically separable from streptolysin S.[104c] The low response of lymphocytes from rheumatic fever patients to crude streptolysin S preparations (containing the streptococcal mitogen as an impurity) has been confirmed, but similar decreases have been observed in other diseases.[18b,27b]

Streptolysin O is highly toxic to isolated organ preparations of frog and rabbit heart and to rat and rabbit heart cells in tissue culture.[4,53,110a] It is also cardiotoxic in the intact rabbit,[31] but in it hemolysis occurs and the consequent hyperpotassemia complicates the picture. Like streptolysin S, streptolysin O disrupts lysosomes *in vitro*.[121] Increased production of streptolysin O by strains recovered from rheumatic fever patients as compared to strains cultured from nonrheumatic controls has been reported[13] but not confirmed.[34]

The major objection to streptolysin O as the agent of tissue damage in rheumatic fever is that this toxin is antigenic. Although tetanus may be cited as an example of disease which is caused by an antigenic toxin, yet may leave no immunity, the comparison is untenable because of the failure of production of tetanus antitoxin in such patients,[23] which contrasts with the almost regular production of antistreptolysin O after streptococcal infections. In fact, antistreptolysin O is present, though at a low or moderate titer, in most human sera. It is, therefore, hard to explain how even first attacks of rheumatic fever may come about, and it is even harder to explain the recurrences. To obviate these objections an "ad hoc" hypothesis seems necessary:[31] that the complex of streptolysin O and its antibody is not eliminated rapidly from the circulation, as is the fate of other antigen-antibody complexes,[101] but is retained so that, due to its dissociability, a specific substrate in the heart may compete effectively for the toxin with the specific antibody. This hypothesis is ingenious, but there is no experimental evidence to support it as yet.

Streptococcal proteinase injected into rabbits provokes heart lesions which have been likened to rheumatic myocarditis.[54] Since streptococcal proteinase is antigenic,[73] the objection voiced above against streptolysin O is valid here also.

C-polysaccharide-peptide complexes of high molecular weight, but not intact streptococcal cells, tend to remain in the tissues of rabbits after injection and to induce a chronic and relapsing nodular inflammation.[18] The damage produced by these complexes is not mediated by an immune mechanism, since it starts after 3 hours only and is not affected by repeated injections; it must therefore be classified as "toxic" in a broad sense.

The long duration of this inflammatory reaction, in the absence of demonstrable living streptococci, is an attractive feature of this model because of the similarity to the prolonged inflammatory state in the absence of demonstrable living streptococci in rheumatic fever. Moreover, adaptation of this model to the mouse has led to a number of pathologic changes, including chronic inflammation of endocardium, myocardium, and pericardium. These changes followed intraperitoneal injection of a crude sterile extract of sonically disrupted group A streptococci. (The amount injected was massive, at least for a mouse: 4 ml containing 3.56 mg of rhamnose.) A similar extract of group D streptococci proved lethal to more than half the injected mice, but the survivors showed only acute, not chronic, heart damage, which was limited to the myocardium. The chronic lesions caused by the group A extract were more prominent on the left side of the heart (like those of rheumatic fever). Both the aortic and the mitral valves were affected, with diffuse inflammation and focal nodular lesions. The latter lesions resembled Aschoff bodies, though the authors reserved definitive judgement.[18a,73a]

Combined effect of soluble toxin(s) and particulate streptococcal cell component(s) was recently postulated as a variant of the toxic action theory.[28a] This variant is based on the observation that streptococcal extracellular products injected intravenously into rabbits cause areas of necrosis in the heart and liver where macrophages laden with streptococci preferentially migrate and persist. The soluble toxin involved may be one of unusually low molecular weight[27a]; the macrophages laden with streptococci may be "Trojan horses" bringing at the site of acute damage the streptococcal cellular components described in the previous section as capable of inducing chronic inflammation.

Allergic Reaction

Serum sickness resembles rheumatic fever because it affects the joints, the skin and even the heart,[60] although in a different manner (see next chapter, under *Differential Diagnosis*). A less superficial similarity is that a latent period of only slightly longer duration than that observed between the injection of serum and the development of serum sickness[118] intervenes between the streptococcal infection and the onset of rheumatic fever. The latent period in the case of serum sickness is known to be due to the time needed for antibody production; could the latent period of rheumatic fever be due to the same cause?

There are several arguments against this general formulation of the allergic hypothesis: (1) the latent period of serum sickness decreases on repeated exposure to the same antigen[115] in keeping with the immunologic tenet that the secondary antibody response is faster than the primary. The latent period of rheumatic fever, however, is not any shorter in recurrences than in first attacks;[78] (2) when the newly synthesized antibody reacts with the antigen to produce serum sickness in experimental animals, complement is fixed in the process and therefore the level of serum complement falls.[89] By contrast, in rheumatic fever the level of serum complement increases;[25] (3) serum sickness can be elicited by a number of disparate antigens but rheumatic fever follows only streptococcal infections; (4) although fibrinoid degeneration is a pathologic feature common to both serum sickness and rheumatic fever, the Aschoff body is specific to the latter only.

The allergic hypothesis may, however, be formulated in an alternate and more specific form, as follows: a specific streptococcal product is bound to the tissues involved by rheumatic fever and a subsequent immune response against it produces the tissue damage, in a manner analogous to the second phase of nephrotoxic nephritis.[51] The peculiarities of the localization of tissue damage in rheumatic fever and its etiologic and pathologic specificity could thus be explained by the specific binding of the streptococcal product, just as in the second phase of nephrotoxic nephritis the localization of damage is explained by the specific binding of the anti-kidney antibody.[51] The immune reaction against the localized streptococcal product could be of the cellular rather than the humoral type, in which case a fall of complement would not be expected. The lack of shortening of the latent period is more difficult to explain away, but one may postulate a peculiar type of immune reaction, not shortened by re-exposure, *e.g.*, because of a non-immunologic determinant of the latent period (build-up of a streptococcal product which is continuously being produced during the latent period is an acceptable alternative). Although this "specific" form of the allergic hypothesis explains more features of rheumatic fever than the "general" form, no direct data support it. Specifically, streptococcal antigens have not yet been found in the heart in rheumatic carditis. Continuation of activity in this field may be rewarding, although data on streptococcal antigens localized in the tissues will be difficult to interpret due to the immunologic cross-reactions between streptococcal and tissue antigens (see below under *Autoimmunity*).

Autoimmunity

A number of investigators over the last 35 years have shown that during the course of rheumatic fever substances appear in the serum which bind with human heart preparations *in vitro* (reviewed in ref. 43). These substances are gamma globulins with a relative specificity for heart preparations and are therefore considered antibodies. They are significantly more frequent in patients with rheumatic carditis than in patients with rheumatic fever without carditis. They are also found, though less frequently, in patients with *previous* rheumatic fever, regardless of the presence or absence of residual rheumatic heart disease (Table 43–5).

Antibodies with similar or identical specificity are found in a high percentage of patients who have recently undergone mitral commissurotomy.[36,43] Since the

Table 43-5.—Heart Antibodies in Various Conditions*

Diagnostic Categories	*No. of Subjects*	*Per cent Positive*
Acute Rheumatic Fever	171	41.5
with Carditis	71	63.4
with Doubtful Carditis	26	26.9
without Carditis	74	26.0
Rheumatic Subjects (inactive)	201	16.4
with Heart Disease	66	12.1
without Heart Disease	135	18.5
Rheumatic Subjects Post-commissurotomy	19	63.1
Miscellaneous Cardiac Diseases	39	6.3
Acute Glomerulonephritis	26	7.7
Connective Tissue Diseases	40	0
Miscellaneous Diseases	12	0
Normal Individuals	66	3.0

* From data of Hess *et al.*[36] The antibodies were demonstrated by an immunofluorescent technique; only the sera giving a staining with a subsarcolemmal or intermyofibrillar pattern are considered positive in this table. All tests were done "blindly," *i.e.*, without knowing the clinical diagnosis.

antibodies of these patients have been shown to react with the patients' own auricular tissue, biopsied during the operation, they can be properly called *auto*-antibodies. By analogy, it has been assumed that the antibodies of the other categories of patients are also auto- rather than iso-antibodies. Indirect support for auto-antibody activity *in vivo* is provided by the finding of massive deposits of gamma globulin in the myocardium of children who have died of rheumatic carditis.[45] Definitive proof of the antibody nature of these deposits, such as could be provided by their elution and subsequent specific reaction with heart muscle, is still lacking, but it appears likely that, in a fairly high percentage of rheumatic fever patients, antibodies capable of reacting with the patient's own heart circulate in the blood. What is their origin? What is their role, if any, in the pathogenesis of rheumatic fever?

Damaged tissues may elicit the formation of auto-antibodies in the very animals to which the tissues belong (as, for instance, antibodies to liver after carbon tetrachloride administration[120]) and it is perfectly plausible that such a mechanism may be at work in the case of rheumatic carditis. Antibodies to heart may occur after myocardial infarction and although their immunofluorescent staining pattern differs from that encountered in rheumatic fever[36] the mechanism of elicitation may be the same in both diseases. In the case of myocardial infarction it is hard to imagine elicitation by an antigen other than the cardiac tissue damaged by ischemia. In rheumatic fever the primary event may be damage to the heart or to the striated muscle tissue (reviewed in ref. 71) or to both, followed by release of slightly altered muscle antigens. The immunologic response to these antigens may then be a late epiphenomenon of no pathogenetic significance.

On the other hand, auto-antibodies to the heart might arise as a reaction to *foreign* antigens, which cross-react immunologically with the heart. Cross-reactions between pathogenic microorganisms and tissue antigens of certain animal species have been repeatedly demonstrated by means of antisera prepared in *other* animal species;[2,84] and the hypothesis has been advanced that such cross-reactions enhance the microorganisms' virulence by impeding the production of antibodies, due to the animal's immunologic tolerance to his own tissue antigens, and therefore to the microorganisms' antigens cross-reacting with them.[7a,84,126a]

A cross-reaction between *streptococcal* antigens and mammalian tissues was first suggested by Markowitz *et al.* because of a slight nephritogenic effect in the rat of a rabbit anti-type 12 streptococcal serum.[64] Subsequently, Kaplan demonstrated that rabbit antisera against certain group A streptococci react with human heart preparations in the immunofluorescent test[46] and that goat anti-human heart sera precipitate streptococcal extracts.[47] More importantly, he demonstrated a cross-reaction in *human sera* by means of absorption of some precipitating antibodies against streptococcal extracts with human heart preparations.[49] Not all streptococcal-precipitating antibodies were absorbed, however. The converse cross absorption of human auto-antibodies to heart with streptococcal extracts gave equivocal results,[48] which means that not all the auto-antibodies to heart can be absorbed with the streptococcal antigens (absorption of only a portion of the auto-antibodies would not be revealed by the immunofluorescent technique used for this experiment).

The streptococcal antigen involved in this cross-reaction was extracted by acid from cell wall and is closely related to the M protein, but not identical with it.[47] Cross-reacting antibodies were demonstrated in the serum of 55 per cent of 51 patients with rheumatic fever and in 60 per cent of 10 patients with glomerulonephritis, but were absent in 20 patients with rheumatoid arthritis.[49] In recent years, workers in this field have been confronted by an embarrassment of riches. Table 43–6 is a synopsis of their findings. Each one of these cross-reactions could have a role in pathogenesis (either by fooling the host's immune system, thus facilitating infection—or by breaking the host's self-tolerance, thus leading to autoimmunity). But there is no direct evidence for either role. And to view these findings in perspective, one should be mindful that cross-reactions between mammalian and bacterial antigens are plentiful[39a,126a]; perhaps the most remarkable thing about them is how com-

Table 43-6.—Cross-Reactions Between Streptococci and Human Heart

Streptococcal Antigens	*Cardiac Antigens*	*Authors (Year)*
M-like protein in cell wall of some group A strains	Myocardium	Kaplan & Meyserian (1962)[46]
Cell membranes of all group A strains	Myocardial sarcolemma?	Zabriskie & Freimer (1966)[126b]
Type 1 streptococcal cells	Myocardial intercalated discs	Lyampert *et al.* (1966a)[60a]
Four distinct antigens in acid extracts of streptococcal cells	Four distinct myocardial antigens	Lyampert *et al.* (1966b)[60b]
Group A polysaccharide	Glycoproteins of heart valves	Goldstein *et al.* (1967)[29a]
Hyaluronic acid preparations	Myocardial sarcolemma	Sandson *et al.* (1968)[85a]

monly they are found when they are deliberately looked for. Human red cells, for instance, cross-react with nearly 50% of gram-negative bacterial strains[92b] as well as with pneumococcus type XIV.[2] The latter cross-reaction has a definite, albeit iatrogenic, pathogenetic significance: patients with pneumococcus type XIV pneumonia treated with specific antiserum used to develop acute hemolytic anemia. Whether any of the other cross-reactions between acute and bacterial antigens play a pathogenetic role remains to be shown.

BIBLIOGRAPHY

1. Aldrich, C. A.: Nephritis, in *Brennemann's Practice of Pediatrics*, Vol. 3, Ch. 28, Hagerstown, Md., W. F. Prior Co., 1943.
2. Beeson, P. B. and Goebel, W. F.: J. Exp. Med., *70*, 239, 1939.
3. Bernheimer, A. W.: J. Exp. Med., *90*, 373, 1949.
4. Bernheimer, A. W. and Cantoni, G. L.: J. Exp. Med., *81*, 295, 1945.
5. Bernheimer, A. W. and Schwartz, L. L.: J. Bact., *87*, 1100, 1964.
6. Buchanan, D. N.: Amer. J. Dis. Child., *62*, 443, 1941.

6*a*. Burch, G. E., Giles, T. D. and Colcolough, H. L.: Amer. Heart J., *80*, 556, 1970.

7. Bywaters, E. G. L., Glynn, L. E., and Zeldis, A.: Ann. Rheum. Dis., *17*, 278, 1958.

7*a*. Cahill, J. F., Ide, B. C., Wiley, B. B. and Ward, J. R.: Infection & Immunity, *3*, 24, 1971.

8. Catanzaro, F. J., Rammelkamp, C. H., Jr., and Chamovitz, R.: New Engl. J. Med., *259*, 51, 1958.
9. Catanzaro, F. J., Stetson, C. A., Morris, A. J., Chamovitz, R., Rammelkamp, C. H., Jr., Stolzer, B. L. and Perry, W. D.: Amer. J. Med., *17*, 749, 1954.
10. Clarke, C. A., McConnell, R. B., and Sheppard, P. M.: Brit. Med. J., *1*, 21, 1960.

10*a*. Clasener, H. A. L., Enscring, H. L. and Hijmans, W.: J. Gen. Microbiol., *62*, 195, 1970.

11. Coburn, A. F.: *The Factor of Infection in the Rheumatic State*, Baltimore, The Williams & Wilkins Co., 1931.
12. Coburn, A. F. and Moore, L. V.: J. Clin. Invest., *18*, 147, 1939.
13. Coburn, A. F. and Pauli, R. H.: J. Clin. Invest., *14*, 755, 1935.
14. ———: J. Immunol., *29*, 515, 1935.
15. Colebrook, L., Elliott, S. D., Maxted, W. R., Morley, C. W. and Mortell, M.: Lancet, *2*, 30, 1942.
16. Collis, W. R. F.: Lancet, *2*, 817, 1939.
17. Colony, H. S. and Malamud, N.: Neurology, *6*, 672, 1956.
18. Cromartie, W. J.: Reactions of Connective Tissue to Cellular Components of Group A Streptococci, in *The Streptococcus, Rheumatic Fever and Glomerulonephritis*, J. W. Uhr, editor, Baltimore, The Williams & Wilkins Co., 1964.

18*a*. Cromartie, W. J. and Craddock, J. C.: Science, *154*, 285, 1966.

18*b*. Cuppari, G., Quagliata, F., Ieri, A. and Taranta, A.: Unpublished data.

19. Dalldorf, F. G. and Murphy, G. E.: Amer. J. Path., *37*, 507, 1960.
20. De Gortari, A., Pellon, R. and Costero, I.: Amer. Heart J., *33*, 716, 1947.
21. Dixon, F. J.: Ann. Rev. Med., *9*, 257, 1958.
22. Dublin, T. D., Bernanke, A. D., Pitt, E. L., Massell, B. F., Allen, F. H., and Amezcua, F.: Brit. Med. J., *2*, 775, 1964.
23. Eckmann, L.: *Tetanus: Prophylaxis and Therapy*, New York, Grune & Stratton, p. 89, 1963.
24. Feinstein, A. R., Wood, H. F., Spagnuolo, M., Taranta, A., Tursky, E. and Kleinberg, E.: Ann. Int. Med., *60*, Suppl. 5, 68, 1964.
25. Fischel, E. E., Frank, C. W., Boltax, A. J. and Arcasoy, M.: Arthritis Rheum., *1*, 351, 1958.
26. Freimer, E. H., Krause, R. M., and McCarty, M.: J. Exp. Med., *110*, 853, 1959.
27. Garcia-Palmieri, M. D.: Amer. Heart J., *64*, 577, 1962.

27*a*. Gazit, E., Ginsburg, I. and Harris, T. N.: Circulation, *42*, Suppl. 3, 103, 1970.

27*b*. Gery, I., Brand-Auraban, A., Benezra, D., Jacob, A. and Davies, A. M.: Clin. Exper. Immunol., *3*, 717, 1968.

28. Gibson, S.: Rheumatic Fever, in *Brennemann's Practice of Pediatrics*, Vol. II, Ch. 19, Hagerstown, Md., W. F. Prior Company, 1940.

28*a*. Ginsburg, I., Gallis, H. A., Cole, R. M. and Green, I.: Science, *166*, 1161, 1969.

29. Glynn, A. A., Glynn, L. E., and Holborow, E. J.: Brit. Med. J., *2*, 266, 1959.

29*a*. Goldstein, I., Halpern, B. and Robert, L.: Nature, *213*, 44, 1967.

30. Green, C. A.: Ann. Rheum. Dis., *1*, 86, 1939.
31. Halbert, S. P., Bircher, R., and Dahle, E.: J. Exp. Med., *113*, 759, 1961.
32. Halbert, S. P. and Keatinge, S. L.: J. Exp. Med., *113*, 1013, 1961.
33. Hall, E. M. and Anderson, L. R.: Amer. Heart J., *25*, 64, 1943.
34. Hardin, R. A., Quinn, R. W., and Avery, R. C.: J. Infect. Dis., *99*, 84, 1956.
35. Herndon, C. N. and Jennings, R. G.: Amer. J. Hum. Genet., *3*, 17, 1951.
36. Hess, E. V., Fink, C. W., Taranta, A. and Ziff, M.: J. Clin. Invest., *43*, 886, 1964.
37. Hirschhorn, K., Schreibman, R. R., Verbo, S. and Gruskin, R. H.: Proc. Nat. Acad. Sci. U.S.A., *52*, 1151, 1964.
38. Humphrey, J. H.: Brit. J. Exp. Path., *30*, 345, 1949.
38*a*. Ieri, A., Taranta, A., Spagnuolo, M. and Greenberg, M.: J.A.M.A., *202*, 703, 1967.
38*b*. James, L. and McFarland, R. B.: New Engl. J. Med., *284*, 750, 1971.
39. James, W. E. S., Badger, G. F. and Dingle, J. H.: New Engl. J. Med., *262*, 687, 1960.
39*a*. Jenkin, C. R.: Advances Immunol., *3*, 351, 1963.
40. Johnson, E. E., Stollerman, G. H., and Grossman, B. J.: J.A.M.A., *190*, 407, 1964.
41. Jones, T. D.: J.A.M.A., *126*, 481, 1944.
42. Kagan, G. J.: International (8) Congress for Microbiology, Abstracts, p. 125, 1962.
42*a*. Kaplan, E. L., Anthony, B. F., Chapman, S. S., and Wannamaker, L. W.: J. Clin. Invest., *49*, 1405, 1970.
43. Kaplan, M. H.: Amer. J. Cardiol., *24*, 459, 1969.
44. ———: Fed. Proc., *24*, 176, 1965.
45. Kaplan, M. H., Bolande, R., Rakita, L. and Blair, J.: New Engl. J. Med., *271*, 637, 1964.
46. Kaplan, M. H. and Meyeserian, M.: Lancet, *1*, 706, 1962.
47. Kaplan, M. H. and Suchy, M. L.: J. Exp. Med., *119*, 643, 1964.
48. Kaplan, M. H., Svec, K. H., Kushner, I., Arana-Sialer, J. and Suchy, M. L.: Fed. Proc., *22*, 217, 1963.
49. Kaplan, M. H. and Svec, K. H.: J. Exp. Med., *119*, 651, 1964.
50. Kaufmann, O. and Scheerer, E.: Z. Menschl. Vererb. Konstitutions, *21*, 687, 1938.
51. Kay, C. F.: Amer. J. Med. Sci., *204*, 483, 1942.
52. Keil, H.: Medicine (Balt.), *17*, 261, 1938.
53. Kellner, A., Bernheimer, A. W., Carlson, A. S., and Freeman, E. B.: J. Exp. Med., *104*, 361, 1956.
54. Kellner, A. and Robertson, T.: J. Exp. Med., *99*, 495, 1954.
55. Kernohan, J. W., Woltman, H. W. and Barnes, A. R.: Arch. Neurol. & Psychiatry, *42*, 789, 1939.
55*a*. Klibanoff, E., Frieden, J., Spagnuolo, M. and Feinstein, A. R.: J.A.M.A., *195*, 895, 1966.
56. Klinge, F.: *Der Rheumatismus*, Munich, J. F. Bergman, 1933.
57. Krause, R. M.: Presented at the A.R.A. Interim Scientific Session, 1954.
58. Kuttner, A. G. and Lenert, T. F.: J. Clin. Invest., *23*, 151, 1944.
59. Lancefield, R. C.: J. Immunol., *89*, 307, 1962.
59*a*. Lannigan, R. and Zaki, S. A.: J. Path. Bact., *93*, 449, 1967.
60. Longcope, W. T.: Medicine (Balt.), *22*, 251, 1943.
60*a*. Lyampert, I. M., Danilova, T. A., Bordyuk, N. A. and Beletskaya, L. V.: Folia Biol., *12*, 108, 1966.
60*b*. Lyampert, I. M., Vedenskaya, O. I. and Danilova, T. A.: Immunol., *11*, 313, 1966.
61. Mackenzie, I.: The Circulation in Infectious and Toxic Processes Including Acute Endocarditis, in *Oxford Medicine*, H. A. Christian, editor, Vol. III, Part I, New York, Oxford University Press, p. 322, 1949.
62. Madsen, T. and Kalbak, K.: Acta Path. Microbiol. Scand., *17*, 305, 1940.
63. Marienfeld, C. J., Robins, M., Sandidge, R. P. and Findlan, C.: Public Health Rep., *79*, 789, 1964.
64. Markowitz, A. S., Armstrong, S. H., and Kushner, D. S.: Nature (London), *187*, 1095, 1960.
64*a*. Maxted, W. R. and Valkenburg, H. A.: J. Med. Microbiol., *2*, 199, 1969.
65. McEwen, C.: J. Clin. Invest., *14*, 190, 1935.
66. Miescher, P. A., Wiedermann, G., Hirschhorn, R. and Weissmann, G.: J. Clin. Invest., *43*, 1266, 1964.
67. Mitkov, V.: World Neurol., *2*, 920, 1961.
68. Mortimer, E. A.: Proc. Soc. Exp. Biol. & Med., *119*, 159, 1965.
69. Mortimer, E. A., Vaisman, S. B., Vignau, A. I., Guasch, J. L., Schuster, A. C., Rakita, L., Krause, R. M., Roberts, R., and Rammelkamp, C. H., Jr.: New Engl. J. Med., *260*, 101, 1959.

70. Murphy, G. E.: Medicine, (Balt.), *42*, 73, 1963.
70*a*. Murphy, G. E. and Becker, C. G.: Amer. J. Path., *48*, 931, 1966.
71. Murphy, G. E.: The Histopathology of Rheumatic Fever: A Critical Review, in *Rheumatic Fever*, L. Thomas, editor, Minneapolis, University of Minnesota Press, 1952.
72. Naiman, R. A. and Barrow, J. G.: Circulation, *29*, 708, 1964.
73. Ogburn, C. A., Harris, T. N., and Harris, S.: J. Immun., *81*, 396, 1958.
73*a*. Ohanian, S. H., Schwab, J. H. and Cromartie, W. T.: J. Exper. Med., *129*, 37, 1969.
74. Paul, J. R.: *The Epidemiology of Rheumatic Fever*, New York, Amer. Heart Ass., p. 22, 1957.
75. Perry, C. B. and Roberts, J. A. F.: Brit. Med. J. (Suppl.), p. 154, Aug. 28, 1937.
75*a*. Pichaar, J. G. and Price, H. M.: Amer. J. Path., *51*, 1063, 1967.
76. Powers, G. F. and Boisvert, P. L.: J. Pediat., *25*, 481, 1944.
77. Rammelkamp, C. H., Jr.: Harvey Lectures, Series *51*, 113, 1955–56.
78. Rammelkamp, C. H., Jr. and Stolzer, B. L.: Yale J. Biol. & Med., *34*, 386, 1961.
79. Rantz, L. A., Boisvert, P. J. and Spink, W. W.: Arch. Int. Med., *79*, 401, 1947.
80. Rantz, L. A., Maroney, M. and Di Caprio, J. M.: Pediatrics, *12*, 498, 1953.
81. Rantz, L. A., Randall, E., and Rantz, H. H.: Amer. J. Med., *5*, 3, 1948.
82. Robles-Gil, J. R., Rodriguez, H. and Ibarra, J. J.: Amer. Heart J., *50*, 912, 1955.
82*a*. Rosenthal, A., Czoniczer, G. and Massell, B. F.: Pediatrics, *41*, 612, 1968.
83. Rothbard, S. and Watson, R. F.: J. Exp. Med., *87*, 521, 1948.
84. Rowley, D. and Jenkin, C. R.: Nature (London), *193*, 151, 1962.
85. Russell, W. T.: Med. Res. Counc. Spec. Rep. (London) No. 247, 1943.
85*a*. Sandson, J., Hamerman, D., Janis, R. and Rojkind, M.: Trans. Assoc. Amer. Physicians, *81*, 249, 1968.
86. Saphir, O. and Langendorf, R.: Amer. Heart J., *46*, 432, 1953.
87. Saslaw, M. S. and Streitfeld, M. M.: A.M.A. J. Dis. Child., *92*, 550, 1956.
88. ———: Dis. Chest, *35*, 175, 1959.
88*a*. Schmitt-Slomska, J., Sacquet, E. and Caravano, R.: J. Bacteriol., *93*, 451, 1967.
89. Schwab, L., Moll, F. C., Hall, T., Brean, H., Kirk, M., Hawn, C. v. Z. and Janeway, C. A.: J. Exp. Med., *91*, 505, 1950.
90. Schwentker, F. F., Janney, J. H. and Gordon, J. E.: Amer. J. Hyg., *38*, 27, 1943.
91. Siegel, A. C., Johnson, E. E. and Stollerman, G. H.: New Engl. J. Med., *265*, 559, 1961.
92. Spagnuolo, M., Pasternack, B. and Taranta, A.: New Engl. J. Med., *285*, 641, 1971.
92*a*. Spagnuolo, M. and Taranta, A.: New Engl. J. Med., *278*, 183, 1968.
92*b*. Springer, G. F., Williamson, P. and Brandes, W. C.: J. Exper. Med., *113*, 1077, 1961.
93. Stamler, J.: Amer. J. Cardiol., *10*, 319, 1962.
94. Stetson, C. A., Jr.: The Relationship of Antibody Response to Rheumatic Fever, in *Streptococcal Infections*, M. McCarty, editor, New York, Columbia University Press, p. 208, 1953.
95. Stollerman, G. H.: Int. Arch. Allergy, *12*, 287, 1958.
96. Stollerman, G. H. and Bernheimer, A. W.: J. Clin. Invest., *29*, 1147, 1950.
97. Stollerman, G. H., Ekstedt, R. D., and Cohen, I. R.: J. Immunol., *95*, 131, 1965.
98. Stollerman, G. H., Lewis, A. J., Schultz, I. and Taranta, A.: Amer. J. Med., *20*, 163, 1956.
99. Stollerman, G. H., Siegel, A. C., and Johnson, E. E.: Mod. Conc. Cardiov. Dis. *34*, 45, 1965.
100. Talalajew, W. T.: Klin. Wschr., *8*, 124, 1929.
101. Talmage, D. W., Dixon, F. J., Bukantz, S. C. and Dammin, G. J.: J. Immun., *67*, 243, 1951.
102. Taranta, A.: Changing Clinical Concepts in Rheumatic Fever, in *The Streptococcus, Rheumatic Fever and Glomerulonephritis*, J. W. Uhr, editor, Baltimore, Williams & Wilkins Co., 1964.
103. Taranta, A.: New Engl. J. Med., *266*, 13, 1962.
104. ———: New Engl. J. Med., *260*, 1204, 1959.
104*a*. Taranta, A.: Annual Review of Med., *18*, 159, 1967.
104*b*. Taranta, A. and Cuppari, G.: Circulation, (Suppl. III to vols. *41*, *42*), 104, 1970.
104*c*. Taranta, A., Cuppari, G. and Quagliata, F.: J. Exper. Med., *129*, 605, 1969.
104*d*. ———: Nature, *219*, 757, 1968.

105. Taranta, A., Kleinberg, E., Feinstein, A. R., Wood, H. F., Tursky, E. and Simpson, B. A.: Ann. Int. Med., *60*, Suppl. 5, 58, 1964.

105*a*. Taranta, A. and Moody, M. D.: In *Symposium on Laboratory Diagnosis*. Ped. Clin. North America, *18*, 125, 1971.

106. Taranta, A., Spagnuolo, M., Snyder, R., Gerbarg, D. S. and Hoffler, J. J.: Ann. N. Y. Acad. Sci., *115*, 1062, 1964.

107. Taranta, A. and Stollerman, G. H.: Amer. J. Med., *20*, 170, 1956.

108. Taranta, A., Torosdag, S., Metrakos, J., Jegier, W. and Uchida, I.: Proceedings X Int. Congress of Rheumatology, Torino, Minerva Med., p. 96, 1961.

109. Taranta, A., Wood, H. F., Feinstein, A. R., Simpson, R. and Kleinberg, E.: Ann. Int. Med., *60*, Suppl. 5, 47, 1964.

110. Thomas, L.: New Engl. J. Med., *270*, 1157, 1964.

110*a*. Thompson, A., Halbert, S. P. and Smith, U.: J. Exper. Med., *131*, 745, 1970.

111. Thomson, S. and Innes, J.: Brit. Med. J., *2*, 733, 1940.

112. Todd, E. W.: J. Path. Bact., *47*, 423, 1938.

113. Todd, E. W.: Brit. J. Exp. Path., *13*, 248, 1932.

114. Uchida, I. A.: Amer. J. Hum. Genet., *5*, 61, 1953.

115. von Pirquet, C. F. and Schick, B.: *Serum Sickness*, Baltimore, The Williams & Wilkins Co., 1951.

116. Wagner, B. M. and Tedeschi, C. G.: A.M.A. Arch. Path., *60*, 423, 1955.

117. Waksman, B. H.: Medicine (Balt.), *28*, 143, 1949.

118. Wannamaker, L. W.: The Epidemiology of Streptococcal Infections, in *Streptococcal Infections*, Maclyn McCarty, editor, New York, Columbia University Press, 1953.

118*a*. Wannamaker, L. W.: New Engl. J. Med., *282*, 23 and 78, 1970.

119. Wannamaker, L. W., Rammelkamp, C. H., Jr., Denny, F. W., Brink, W. R., Houser, H. B. and Hahn, E. O.: Amer. J. Med., *10*, 673, 1951.

120. Weir, D. M.: Lancet, *1*, 1147, 1961.

121. Weissmann, G., Keiser, H., and Bernheimer, A. W.: J. Exp. Med., *118*, 205, 1963.

122. Wilson, M. G.: *Advances in Rheumatic Fever, 1940–1961*, New York, Hoeber Medical Division, Harper & Row, p. 57, 1962.

123. Wilson, M. G., Schweitzer, M. D. and Lubschez, R.: J. Pediat., *22*, 468, 581, 1943.

124. Watson, R. F., Hirst, G. K., and Lancefield, R. C.: Arth. and Rheum., *4*, 74, 1961.

125. Wittler, R. G., Tuckett, J. D., Muccione, V. J., Gangarosa, E. J. and O'Connell, R. C.: International (8) Congress for Microbiology, Abstracts, p. 125, 1962.

126. Wood, H. F., Feinstein, A. R., Taranta, A., Epstein, J. A. and Simpson, R.: Ann. Int. Med., *60*, Suppl. 5, 31, 1964.

126*a*. Zabriskie, J. B.: Advances Immunol., *1*, 147, 1971.

126*b*. Zabriskie, J. B. and Freimer, E. H.: J. Exper. Med., *124*, 661, 1966.

127. Zabriskie, J. B., Freimer, E. H. and Seegal, B.: Fed. Proc., *23*, 343, 1964.

128. Zagala, J. G. and Feinstein, A. R.: J.A.M.A., *179*, 863, 1962.

Chapter 44

Rheumatic Fever: Clinical Aspects

By Angelo Taranta, M.D.

Rheumatic fever consists of a number of clinical manifestations, the most important of which are carditis, polyarthritis and chorea, which follow streptococcal infections and tend to occur in the same patients, simultaneously or in close succession, with a much greater frequency than would be expected from chance alone. They may occur singly, however, or in various combinations in any individual patient. The consequent heterogeneity of the population of patients who receive the diagnosis of rheumatic fever causes some difficulty in relating, and indeed in understanding, the natural history of the disease. As expounded below, it will begin with a "pre-history": streptococcal infections and latent period; it will deal with each clinical manifestation individually and collectively; and then with the recurrences, mortality and long term sequelae, *i.e.*, with information of prognostic importance. Subsequent sections will concern clinical pathology, nosology, diagnosis, treatment and prevention.

NATURAL HISTORY

The Preceding Streptococcal Infection

Although antibody studies have shown that rheumatic fever is preceded regularly by streptococcal infections (see previous chapter), a sizable percentage of patients with this disease, 13,[78] 19[154] or 33 per cent,[197] do not remember having had any illness in the preceding few weeks. A small percentage report having had a non-respiratory illness (10 per cent)[78] or an illness characterized by upper respiratory symptoms, but not by sore throat (12 per cent[78] or 21 per cent[197]). The largest single group remembers having had a sore throat (46 per cent[197] or 40.3 per cent[78]), often mild, and seldom seen by a physician.[74,200] In those patients who have consulted a physician but later develop rheumatic fever, one finds that the physician usually has failed to culture the throat;[78] and if he has prescribed antibiotics, the prescription has not conformed to the recommendation for the prevention of rheumatic fever, or the patient has failed to take the full course of oral medication. (For a fuller discussion of this problem, see below under *Prevention.*)

To what extent the high frequency of asymptomatic streptococcal infections as an antecedent of rheumatic fever is due to the forgetfulness or the inattentiveness of some patients to their own bodily symptoms is difficult to guess. However, even in a military camp, closely studied for streptococcal infections, 52 per cent of rheumatic fever attacks were preceded by streptococcal pharyngitides which were either asymptomatic or both afebrile and non-exudative.[143] Moreover, in patients with previous rheumatic fever, studied prospectively and to whom medical care was readily available, asymptomatic streptococcal infections accounted for 54[178] to 70 per cent[91] of rheumatic recurrences. In such patients forgetfulness and inattentiveness may be expected to play a lesser role; but the observations made on them cannot be extrapolated safely to the population at large because patients with previous rheumatic fever have an increased susceptibility to the disease.

Streptococcal infections of the skin are not followed by rheumatic fever, although they may be followed by acute glomerulonephritis.

The Latent Period

When streptococcal pharyngitides cause symptoms, they do so only for a few days, even in the absence of treatment. The time between the onset of symptoms of the pharyngitis and the onset of symptoms of rheumatic fever constitutes the "latent," "silent," or "lag" period of rheumatic fever.[143] According to this definition, the early or first phase of the latent period is characterized by the clinical manifestations of the streptococcal infection, while the second phase, to which the term "latent" or "silent" more literally applies, is characterized by the lack of symptoms. In patients monitored with periodic throat cultures and antibody determinations, streptococcal infections can be dated even if they are asymptomatic, in which case the latent period can be defined as extending from the onset of the asymptomatic infection to the onset of rheumatic fever.[171] In addition to the latent period of rheumatic fever as a whole, one may also consider the latent period of each individual manifestation.[171,177] However defined, this period is of crucial interest for the pathogenesis of rheumatic fever (see previous chapter), but little is known about it, in part because the low attack rate of rheumatic fever makes it necessary to recall periodically or to hospitalize a large number of patients with streptococcal infections to be able to observe, in a few, the period immediately preceding the onset of rheumatic fever.[145]

The terms "latent" or "silent" imply a lack of disease manifestations in this period, and, to be sure, overt manifestations of rheumatic fever are absent from it by definition, but whether this clinical "silence" indicates a true absence of disease process has been questioned.[145] Temperature and pulse come down to normal long before going up again at the onset of rheumatic fever, but the ESR, though declining, may remain higher in patients who go on to develop rheumatic fever than in patients who do not. Streptococci usually linger in the throat, although meticulous technique may be required to demonstrate them. ECG abnormalities such as P-R prolongation and T wave inversion may appear as early as the ninth day after the onset of the streptococcal infection and seven days before the onset of arthritis (Fig. 44–1).

The length of the apparent latent period in patients with symptomatic infections ranges from a minimum of 0 to a maximum of more than forty-five days,[143,154,197] but there are reasons to doubt the validity of both these extremes. In a carefully conducted prospective study the patients with an apparent latent period of less than six days already had elevations of the ASO titer by the time the pharyngitis became manifest, and the titers did not rise significantly thereafter. This suggests that the streptococcal infections of these patients had actually started considerably *before* they became symptomatic.[143] In patients with an apparent latent period longer than thirty-five days, reinfections with another serologic type of streptococci are quite common[143,187] and the reinfection, rather than the initial infection, may be the cause of the ensuing rheumatic fever attack. Excluding the latter patients, the average interval between onset of the symptoms of pharyngitis and onset of the symptoms of rheumatic fever was 18.6 days.[143] Additional exclusion of the patients with apparently short latent periods would increase by a few days this mean "true" latent period. Interestingly, the latent period was no shorter in patients with previous rheumatic fever than in those without.[143]

The Mode of Onset of Rheumatic Fever

The onset is typically acute when, as in the majority of cases, the presenting

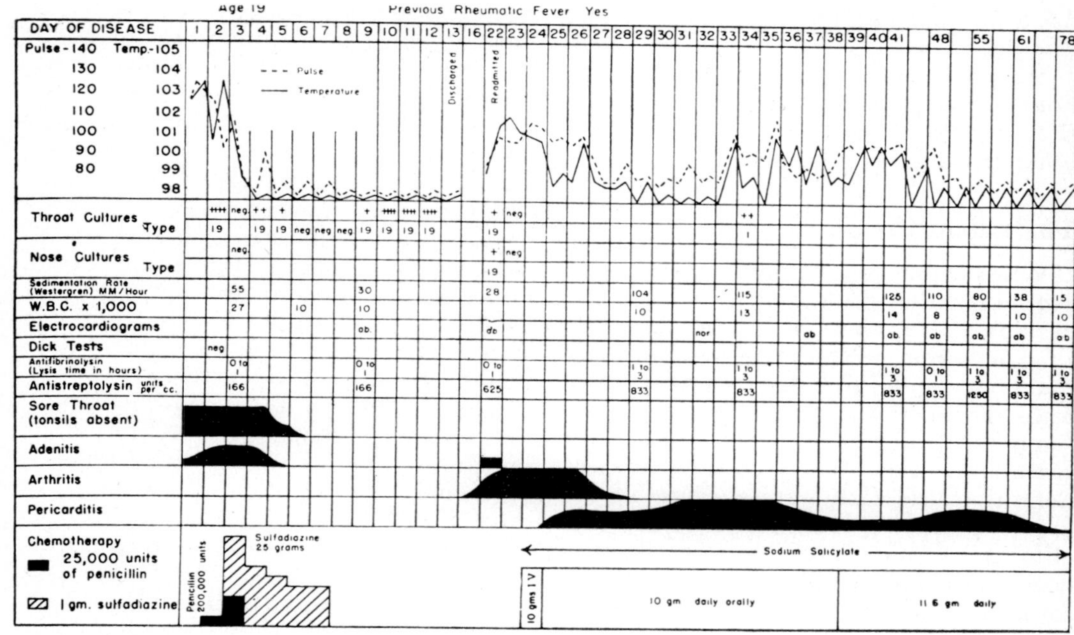

FIG. 44–1.—Clinical course of streptococcal pharyngitis followed by arthritis and pericarditis in a patient under continual observation for most of the latent period. Notice the presence of ECG alterations (sharp inversion of T waves in all leads) on the ninth day of observation, the persistence of streptococci in the throat, and the failure of sulfadiazine and of small doses of penicillin to eradicate them, and to prevent rheumatic fever. (Rantz *et al.*, courtesy Arch. Int. Med.)

manifestation is arthritis. By contrast, onset is usually gradual when heart failure due to rheumatic carditis is the presenting manifestation. The onset of chorea may appear to be acute, but is often preceded by subtle behavioral changes which are interpreted as part of chorea only in retrospect. (Subcutaneous nodules and erythema marginatum are almost never the presenting manifestations of rheumatic fever.)

The Clinical Manifestations of Rheumatic Fever

These are classified as major (polyarthritis, carditis, chorea, erythema marginatum and subcutaneous nodules) and minor (arthralgia and fever) on the basis of their diagnostic usefulness.[92,152,167] Other clinical manifestations which are less common, less characteristic or both will be dealt with later in the section. Arthritis and arthralgia will be described together under "Joint Involvement."

Joint involvement is the most common clinical manifestation of rheumatic fever. It runs the gamut from arthralgia, *i.e.*, pain in a joint (not in the muscles or other periarticular structures) *without* objective signs of inflammation and *without* limitation of movement or tenderness to touch, to arthritis, *i.e.*, joint pains *with* objective evidence of inflammation, such as swelling, redness or heat, or at least *with* tenderness to touch or limitation of motion (in the latter case the joint involvement is sometimes called "tender arthralgia").[56] The difference between arthralgia and arthritis is probably only quantitative; moreover, if arthralgia is due to rheumatic fever, it must be due to inflammation and thus, strictly speaking, to arthritis; nevertheless, the distinction between arthralgia and arthritis is important from the point

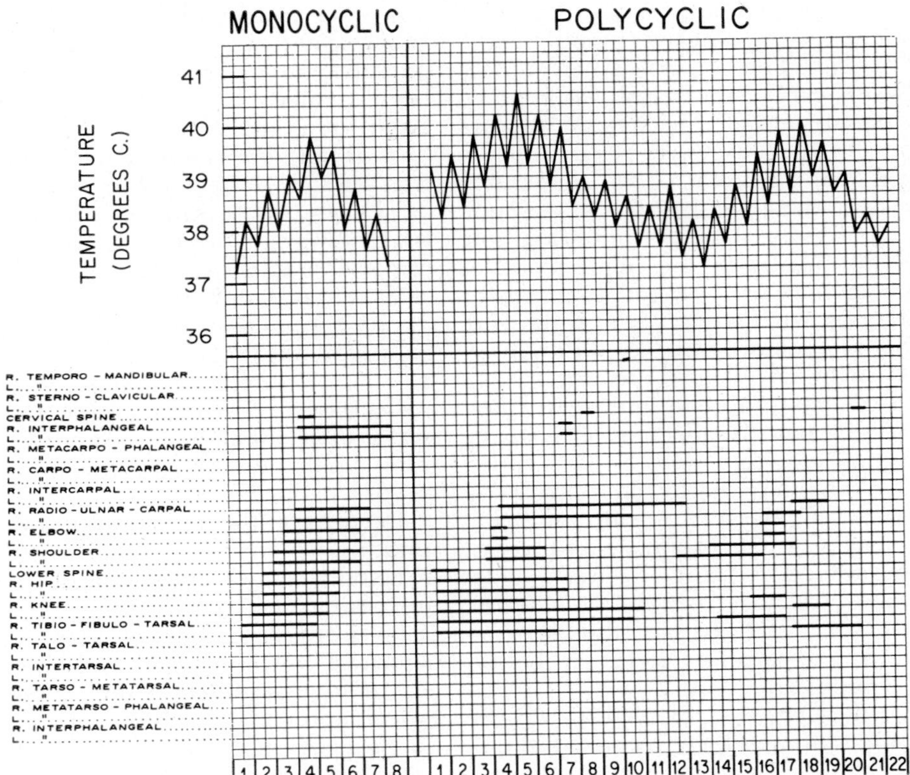

FIG. 44–2.—Clinical course of untreated rheumatic polyarthritis, with detailed notation of the involvement of individual joints in a "monocyclic" and in a "polycyclic" attack. Notice the short duration of the arthritis in each individual joint; the longer duration of the "polyarthritis," for which all joints are considered collectively; and the time overlap of the involvement of each individual joint. Redrawn from the original charts of Friedländer.[65]

of view of diagnosis because arthralgia is a less specific manifestation, and it is more difficult to be sure of its presence. Both arthralgia and arthritis usually affect more than one joint in rheumatic fever and are then called respectively *polyarthralgia* and *polyarthritis*.

In general, joint involvement becomes more common with increasing age of the patient, a trend related to the parallel decrease in incidence of carditis and chorea.[40,56,135] Arthritis occurs early in the rheumatic attack and, with the possible exception of abdominal pain (see below), it is on the average the earliest *symptomatic* manifestation of it. Rheumatic polyarthritis may be excruciatingly painful, but is always transient (for an extremely rare or questionable exception see below under *Sequelae*). The pain is usually more prominent than the objective signs of inflammation: one often sees in this disease joints which are markedly painful, tender to touch and limited in their motions because of pain, and yet have little swelling, redness or heat. Conversely, one seldom sees a definitely swollen joint with only little pain.

In the classical, untreated case, the arthritis of rheumatic fever affects several or many joints in quick succession, and each one for a short time. This characteristic behavior contributed much to the delineation of the clinical entity which we call rheumatic fever, and to its separation from other "rheumatisms" (Fig. 44–2). The arthritis often affects the lower limbs first and later may spread to the arms. The terms "migrating" or "migratory" are often used to describe the polyarthritis of rheumatic fever, but these designations are not meant to signify that the inflammation always disappears in one joint when it appears in another. Rather, the various localizations usually overlap in time, and it is the onset, more than the full course of the arthritis, which, so to speak, "migrates" from joint to joint. In most cases, each joint is affected only once, but may be affected twice or even more times. This may occur in untreated, severe cases in which two or occasionally three "cycles" of polyarthritis and fever, of generally decreasing severity, may follow and partially overlap each other (Fig. 44–2).[65,77,169] It may also occur in "rebounds" of treated cases (see below under *Treatment*).

When the disease is allowed to express itself fully, unhampered by anti-inflammatory treatment, the number of affected joints may be as high as 16, and about half the cases develop arthritis in more than 6 joints.[77] Each joint is maximally inflamed for only a few days, or a week at the most, after which the inflammation decreases, occasionally as fast as if aspirin had been administered, but usually more slowly. Milder and decreasing inflammation may linger on for another week or two before disappearing completely. Considering *all* joints, the polyarthritis may be severe for a week in two-thirds of the patients, and for two or at the most three weeks in the others, and may then persist in a mild form for another week or two.[77] X-ray examination never reveals structural abnormalities of the joint surface that were not present before rheumatic fever occurred.

Under the usual circumstances of medical practice most patients with arthritis are treated with aspirin, if not with steroids, so that arthritis subsides quickly in the joint(s) already affected and does not "migrate" to new joints. In a recent large series of rheumatic fever patients with arthritis, most of whom had been treated, involvement of only one large joint was common (25 per cent). One or both knees were affected in 76 per cent and one or both ankles in 50 per cent.

Elbows, wrists, hips, or small joints of the feet were involved in 12 to 15 per cent of patients and shoulders or small joints of the hand in 7 to 8 per cent. The lumbosacral, cervical, sternoclavicular or temporomandibular joints were affected in 2, 1, $\frac{1}{2}$ and $\frac{1}{2}$ per cent of patients respectively. Involvement of the small joints of the hands or feet and not of other joints occurred in only 1 per cent of the attacks.[56]

Carditis is the most important manifestation of rheumatic fever because it is the only one which may cause disability and death. In contrast to the seriousness of its prognosis, rheumatic carditis often causes no symptoms of its own and is most commonly diagnosed in the course of the examination of a patient with arthritis, on the basis of detection of one or more organic murmurs. It is therefore reasonable to infer that patients with carditis do not come to medical attention if (1) other symptomatic manifestations of rheumatic fever are absent, and (2) the carditis is not severe enough to cause congestive failure, and is not accompanied by prolonged fever or by the precordial pain of pericarditis. Such patients with undiagnosed carditis may later come to medical attention with the characteristic *signs* of rheumatic heart disease, but without the *history* of a rheumatic fever attack.

It should be noted that the comprehensive term "carditis" owes its wide currency to two factors: (1) the distinction of the clinical manifestations of myocarditis from those of endocarditis or valvulitis is often problematic; (2) in patients who die with severe rheumatic carditis the endocardium, the valves and the myocardium are usually all involved. The pericardium is often involved as well. The term carditis is inclusive of both endocarditis and myocarditis and, sometimes, of pericarditis also. The term pancarditis is used to emphasize the involvement of *all* three cardiac layers. In the discussion that follows, carditis will refer to the appearance of significant murmurs with or without cardiomegaly and congestive heart failure ("clinical carditis"), and no attempt will be made to disentangle myocarditis from endocarditis (or valvulitis). By contrast, pericarditis can be diagnosed clinically with some assurance, and therefore will be discussed separately.

The time when carditis appears in the course of a rheumatic attack is of interest with respect to prognosis and to the evaluation of therapy. In an unselected series of patients with rheumatic fever, murmurs indicative of carditis were already present on the physician's first examination, during the first week of the illness, in 76 per cent of all the patients who eventually received the diagnosis of carditis. Another 11 per cent became manifest in the second or third week of illness and only 14 per cent of the total number of patients with carditis appeared to develop it after the fourth week.[122] In another series, carditis seldom appeared after treatment was begun.[181] It must be noted that in some cases the late onset of carditis may be artifactual, due to delayed *detection* rather than to delayed *development* of a significant murmur.[51] ECG alterations, such as P-R prolongation and T wave inversion, may have an earlier onset, during the "latent" period (see above under *Latent Period*), but their relation to clinical carditis is practically nil (for P-R prolongation)[52,122,128] or unclear (for T wave inversion).

The most important manifestations of a clinically significant carditis are organic murmurs, enlargement of the heart and congestive heart failure, which carry a progressively worse prognosis in the order indicated. Organic murmurs are practically always present in clinically significant carditis. However, they may be difficult to hear if the heart rate is very fast, in some cases with congestive heart failure, and in the presence of pericarditis, which may mask the murmur with a rub, or, rarely, dampen it with a large effusion.

The murmurs of rheumatic carditis are essentially three, in the following order of decreasing frequency:

(1) *Apical systolic murmur* of at least grade 2 intensity, but usually grade 3 or more on a scale of 6,[104] occupying the whole of systole. The quality of this murmur is characteristically blowing; the pitch is relatively high, but not as high as that of aortic regurgitation. This murmur is heard best at the apex, radiates to the axilla, at times to the base of the heart and occasionally to the back, and is not obliterated by inspiration or by change in posture. It indicates mitral regurgitation and is difficult or impossible to distinguish from the murmur of long-standing mitral regurgitation as heard in cases of inactive rheumatic heart disease. It can and must be differentiated, however, from *physiologic* murmurs which are also called *functional* or *innocent* murmurs. These are usually faint, and then cause no diagnostic perplexity, but may be loud, especially in presence of fever and anemia (see below under *Diagnosis*).

The mitral regurgitant murmur of acute carditis may be due to dilatation of the mitral valve ring and of the surrounding and supporting cardiac muscle, even without significant valvular deformity, as some autopsy descriptions of patients dying early in the attack suggest (see under *Pathology*). However, it must be noted that in the less severe and more common cases, which do not come to autopsy, organic systolic murmurs are often found in the absence of cardiac enlargement demonstrable by X-ray.[11] In these cases valvulitis seems the most likely cause of the regurgitant murmur.

(2) *Apical mid-diastolic murmur* (*Carey Coombs murmur*) starting with the third heart sound and ending distinctly before the first heart sound. Although described first in rheumatic carditis, it is not pathognomonic of it, since it can also be found in severe anemia, thyrotoxicosis, established mitral regurgitation in inactive rheumatic

heart disease, and, in general, in instances of increased flow through the mitral valve.[188] It should be differentiated from the murmur of established, organic, or "absolute" mitral stenosis on the basis of the absence of opening snap and the lack of presystolic accentuation; the latter, however, is also lacking when mitral stenosis is complicated by atrial fibrillation. The presence of a diastolic apical thrill speaks definitely in favor of mitral stenosis. In addition, in mitral stenosis the first heart sound is typically accentuated at the apex, and the pulmonary second sound is accentuated at the base. According to the prevailing interpretation, the mid-diastolic murmur of rheumatic fever is due to "relative" stenosis of the orifice of the mitral valve in relation to the dilated ventricular chamber, plus increased flow due to fever. It is usually present for only a few days or weeks.[188]

(3) *Aortic diastolic murmur*, high-pitched decrescendo blowing, heard best along the left sternal border on the third or second and at times fourth interspace, or occasionally on the second right intercostal space parasternally. This basal diastolic murmur may be short and faint and therefore difficult to hear.[51] It is most likely due to inflammation of the aortic valves.

Other auscultatory findings in acute carditis are tachycardia, gallop, and alteration of the first heart sound. The tachycardia often persists after the temperature has returned to normal and, unlike emotional tachycardia, persists during sleep. The gallop rhythm results from a loud third heart sound (protodiastolic gallop) or, less frequently, from an accentuation of the usually inaudible fourth heart sound (presystolic gallop) in tachycardic patients. At times a "summation gallop" or quadruple rhythm may develop due to an accentuation of both the third and fourth heart sounds in conjunction with tachycardia. The first heart sound often loses its distinctive muscular quality and becomes indistinct, "impure," "mushy" or "murmurish." Decrease of intensity of the first heart sound may be due to a first degree heart block, which, delaying ventricular contraction, may allow the mitral leaflets to float back up towards the atria before they are closed by systole.[104]

Enlargement of the heart occurs only in some of the patients with organic murmurs. It may be detected clinically, or by X-ray examination, which is more reliable, especially when the enlargement is only moderate. The enlargement of the cardiac shadow is often diffuse and it may be difficult to ascertain whether it is due to a large heart or to pericardial effusion.

Congestive heart failure occurs only in patients with enlarged heart, but many patients have a large heart without failure. In children with rheumatic fever, congestive heart failure is often asymptomatic, or, at least, is discovered because of its right-sided signs before symptoms appear. Although dyspnea is the most frequent symptom, it is often absent; when present, it is seldom accompanied by rales, which occur only in the most severe cases.

A dry cough, abdominal ache, often localized to the liver, and nausea are rather frequent symptoms. Tenderness of the liver, probably due to sudden distension, occurs in the early stage of congestive failure; enlargement, often without tenderness, persists in later stages. Leg edema is less frequent, but distended neck veins are common.[50]

As detailed in the previous chapter (p. 736), congestive heart failure is the more likely due to myocarditis, the earlier heart failure occurs in the "rheumatic career" of a given patient.

Pericarditis is not, by itself, a severe manifestation because it is seldom accompanied by a large effusion, and therefore only exceptionally may cause cardiac tamponade. Pericarditis itself leaves no clinically significant sequelae. However, it tends to occur in patients with severe involvement of the myocardium, endocardium, or both,[60,122] and therefore acquires a "guilt by association." Pericarditis may cause precordial pain, but it is more frequently diagnosed on the sole basis of a pericardial friction rub. This is a noise with a characteristic superficial, scratchy, grating, crackling or leathery quality, which occurs usually both in systole and in diastole. It is most commonly heard towards the base of the heart and may change in intensity and in character depending on the pressure with which the stethoscope is applied to the chest. Unlike murmurs, pericardial friction rubs persist only a few days or weeks; therefore, they are never observed in inactive rheumatic heart disease.

On X-ray, rapid enlargement of the heart and rapid decrease of its size, especially with anti-inflammatory therapy ("accordion heart"), are characteristic of pericarditis. The enlargement is accompanied by a sudden change in shape, with obliteration of the normal contour, straightening of the left border, and increase in width of the vascular pedicle. The heart shadow may come to resemble a pear, a carafe or an onion.[11]

The *electrocardiogram* may provide confirmatory evidence for a diagnosis of pericarditis when the auscultatory findings are in doubt. The S-T segments may be elevated more than 1 mm. in the standard leads and more than 2 mm. in the precordial leads. In later stages the T waves may become flattened or inverted. Because minor degrees of S-T elevations may occur in normal children[198] some authors disregard the ECG entirely in the diagnosis of pericarditis,[56] but this seems unwarranted.

Prolongation of the P-R interval, indicative of first degree atrioventricular block, occurs during the acute attack in 28 per cent[122] to 40 per cent[128] of patients with significant murmurs and in 24[122] to 33 per cent[128] of patients without them. It does not correlate with residual rheumatic heart disease.[52] *It is not, therefore, a manifestation of clinically significant carditis*, and the suggestion has been made that it is due to heightened vagal tone.[96] However, it is much more frequent in children with rheumatic fever, irrespective of carditis, than in patients with other febrile illnesses (4 per cent) or in children with another post-streptococcal sequela, acute glomerulonephritis (5 per cent)[128] or in adults convalescent from streptococcal pharyngitis (8 per cent).[147]

Second and third degree heart block, nodal rhythm, premature contractions, and other disturbances of rhythm may occur, but they are less frequent. Flattening and inversion of T waves may also occur. The apparent incidence of all these abnormalities increases with the frequency with which electrocardiograms are taken and may reach 60 per cent for abnormalities of T waves according to one statement.[137] The Q-T interval (electrical systole) may be prolonged.[29] Although these abnormalities must originate from some kind of involvement of the conducting system and of the myocardium by the rheumatic process, they are usually benign.

It should be noted that similar changes in the ECG have been described in a number of other acute illnesses, including mumps, typhoid, typhus, rheumatoid arthritis, influenza and lobar pneumonia (reviewed in ref. 147), diseases which are almost never associated with clinically significant myocarditis. By inference, the clinical significance of these ECG changes in rheumatic fever is probably minor, although their frequency appears to be higher than in the other diseases mentioned.

Chorea (Sydenham's chorea, chorea minor, popularly "St. Vitus' dance") is the most puzzling manifestation of rheumatic fever. It is a neurologic disorder characterized by involuntary movements, muscular weakness and emotional lability. The movements are abrupt and purposeless, not rhythmic or repetitive. They disappear during sleep, but occur at rest and superimpose themselves on voluntary activity, interfering with its orderly execution. They can be stilled by willful inhibition temporarily; when the inhibition is overcome, they are likely to be more active than before. Inhibition is not effective on more than a few functional groups of muscles at a time: therefore, characteristic choreic movements can be elicited in doubtful cases by asking the patient to assume a cumulative series of postures (*e.g.*: "stretch your hands in front of you; stretch your fingers out; close your eyes; stick your tongue out;" by the time the tongue is stuck out, the fingers wriggle or the eyelids flutter).

The involuntary movements may affect

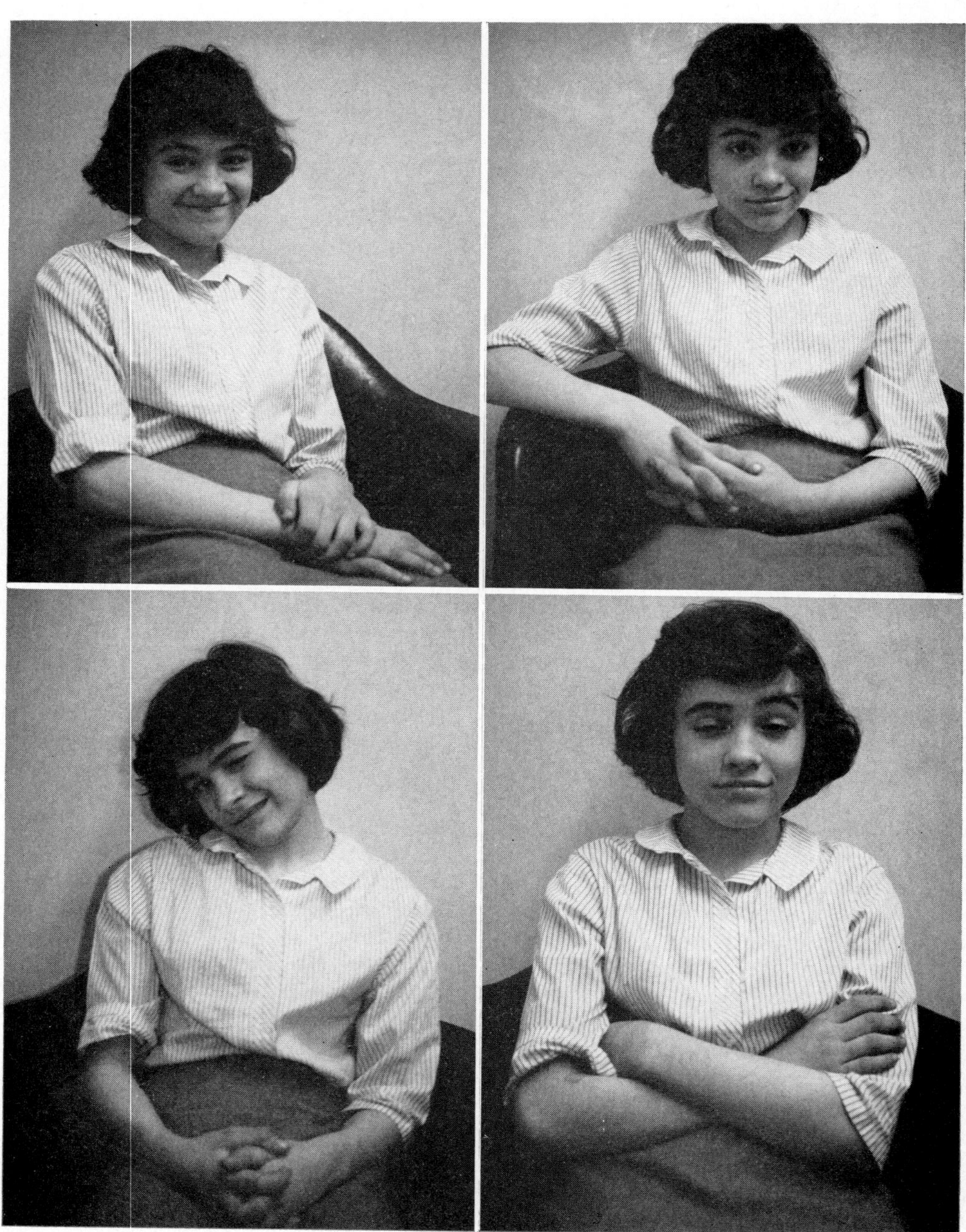

Fig. 44–3.—Grimaces in a patient with chorea.

all muscles, but the involvement of the hands and of the face is usually the most obvious. Bizarre grimaces and inappropriate grins are common (Fig. 44–3). The tongue is often affected by irregular movements of its component muscles and has been compared in such cases to a "bag of worms"; if protruded, it is often involuntarily retracted ("darting tongue"). Handwriting usually becomes clumsy or even impossible (a convenient way of following the patient's course is to ask him to write the same words on a sheet of paper each day). Speech is often halting, explosive, jerky or slurred. The movements are commonly more marked on one side; occasionally they are almost completely unilateral ("hemichorea").

The muscular weakness may be severe ("chorea mollis") but is usually moderate or slight, in which case it is expressed mostly by inability to sustain a steady muscular contraction and is best revealed by asking the patient to squeeze the examiner's hands, which results in variations of pressure, characterized by sudden releases alternated with renewed contractions ("milking sign" or "milkmaid's grip," or "relapsing grip").

The emotional lability manifests itself in outbursts of crying, restlessness, giddy, inappropriate behavior, and litigiousness. It must be noted that at least some of these symptoms may result from frustration at being unable to control one's body and to perform the activities of daily living competently, as well as from the anger at being made fun of by children, or scolded by adults. Projective tests suggest that patients with active chorea are withdrawn, unassertive and unable to handle hostility effectively.[153] In exceptional cases, the psychologic manifestations may be quite severe, and result in transient psychosis ("chorea insaniens").

The neurologic examination does not reveal sensory losses or pyramidal tract involvement. The knee-jerk may have a "hung-up" or pendular quality, *i.e.*, the leg may remain elevated longer than in normal subjects or may go up, down (not completely) and up again (Gordon's sign). There may be diffuse hypotonia. In addition, two maneuvers result in postures which are characteristic: when the arms are projected straight forward, the hands tend to assume a posture consisting of flexion of the wrist, hyperextension of the metacarpophalangeal joints, straightening of the fingers and abduction of the thumb ("spooning" or "dishing" of

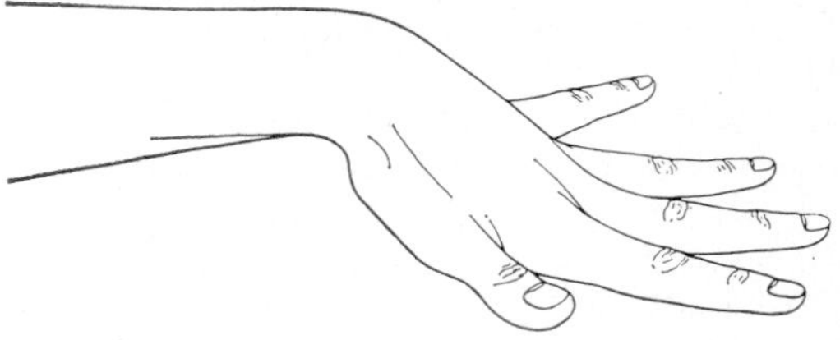

Fig. 44–4.—"Spooning" or "dishing" of the hands in a patient with chorea. Notice the flexion of the wrists, the hyperextension of the metacarpophalangeal joints, the straightening of the fingers and the abduction of the thumb.

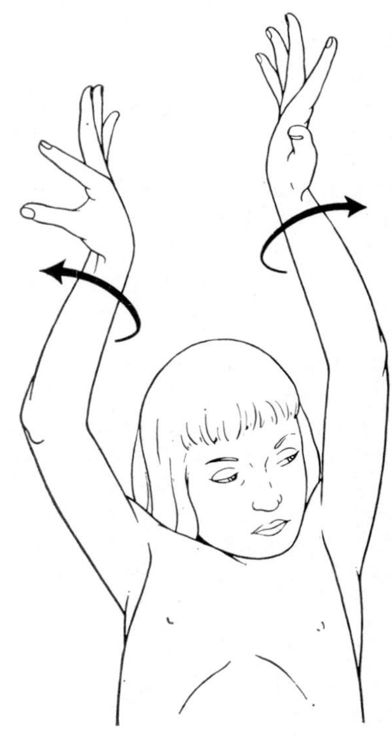

Fig. 44–5.—"Pronator sign" in a patient with chorea. When the patient raises her hands above her head she also tends to pronate her hands.

the hands) (Fig. 44–4). When the patient is asked to raise her arms above her head, she also tends to pronate one or both hands ("pronator sign") (Fig. 44–5). The electroencephalogram frequently shows abnormal slow waves.[42]

The duration of chorea in hospitalized patients ranges from 1 to 117 weeks, with a mode of 8, a median of 15 and a geometric mean of 13.7[103] but non-hospitalized cases may be milder and shorter. Unusual complications and further details may be found in a comprehensive review.[4]

Relation of Chorea to Other Rheumatic Manifestations. Chorea may appear in an isolated fashion, or in a more or less close time relation to other rheumatic manifestations. In this, it does not differ from arthritis and carditis, both of which occur frequently in an isolated manner. What makes chorea peculiar is that: (1) when it occurs alone, the CRP test result is usually negative, and the ESR is normal.[168] The test results are regularly positive in untreated cases with carditis, arthritis, or both, and have thus become the hallmark of "rheumatic activity"; their negativity in "pure" chorea may appear to be "prima facie" evidence against its rheumatic origin; (2) when chorea occurs alone, the titers of anti-streptococcal antibodies are frequently low;[177] since they are regularly elevated in patients with arthritis (but not always in patients with carditis alone),[32] their low titers have suggested the non-streptococcal etiology of this disorder; (3) when chorea occurs in patients with other manifestations of rheumatic fever, it seldom occurs at the same time as arthritis;[177] (4) patients who develop chorea as an apparently isolated manifestation, in later years have a relatively high incidence of rheumatic fever attacks with carditis[4] as well as of rheumatic heart disease.[4,13] These puzzling features may be explained in part by the following hypotheses and observations.

Chorea follows streptococcal infections after a latent period which is more variable in duration, and longer on the average, than the latent period of other rheumatic manifestations in general[177] and, in particular, of the other regularly symptomatic manifestation of rheumatic fever, rheumatic polyarthritis. Support for this hypothesis comes from recent observations of patients receiving anti-rheumatic prophylaxis. While it has long been known that "chorea sometimes alternates with acute rheumatism,"[3] the frequency of recurrences had obscured the fact that, after a single streptococcal infection, chorea does not "alternate," but rather "follows" (Fig. 44–6). In cases with an interval of one to seven months between the preceding rheumatic manifestation and the onset of chorea, intercurrent streptococcal infections were ruled out by serial determinations of streptococcal antibodies. A representative case of this sequence of events is shown in Figure 44–7.

Chorea does not, by itself, cause alterations of the ESR and of the CRP test,[168] and when these alterations coexist with it, they are due to other rheumatic manifestations or to non-rheumatic causes. Therefore, by the time chorea appears in patients with long latent periods both the acute phase reactants and the streptococcal antibody titers may have come back to normal.[13,177] This is known to occur in patients who had developed other rheumatic manifestations after their streptococcal infection, but before chorea.[13,177] (In these cases the chorea is "rheumatic" by history, but may appear non-rheumatic by laboratory examination, because it lacks the hallmark of the acute-phase reactants.) A similar sequence of events may be hypothesized in patients who have not had other symptomatic manifestations of rheumatic fever, after their streptococcal infection, and have no evidence of such manifestations on physical examination, and therefore present as "pure" or isolated chorea. Observations on three patients who developed chorea as an isolated manifestation while being closely followed in a rheumatic fever prophylaxis clinic are consistent with this hypothesis,[171]

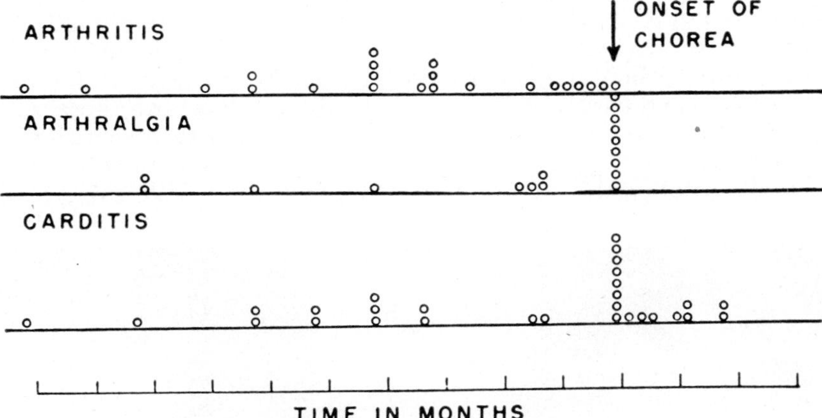

FIG. 44–6.—Time relationship of the onset of chorea to the onset of polyarthritis, polyarthralgia and carditis in the same patients. Notice that arthritis preceded chorea in all cases but one, in which their onsets coincided. Coincidence of the onset of arthralgia and of chorea was more common. In three cases of "hemichorea" the joint pains were limited to the side affected by chorea, and it is not unlikely that many of these "arthralgias" were actually due to the chorea itself, perhaps caused by the violent, involuntary movement ("painful chorea" of old). The frequent apparent coincidence of the onset of carditis and of chorea was due to the asymptomatic nature of most instances of carditis: carditis was detected *because* the patients developed chorea, and the true time of onset of carditis could not be ascertained. (Taranta and Stollerman, courtesy of Amer. J. Med.)

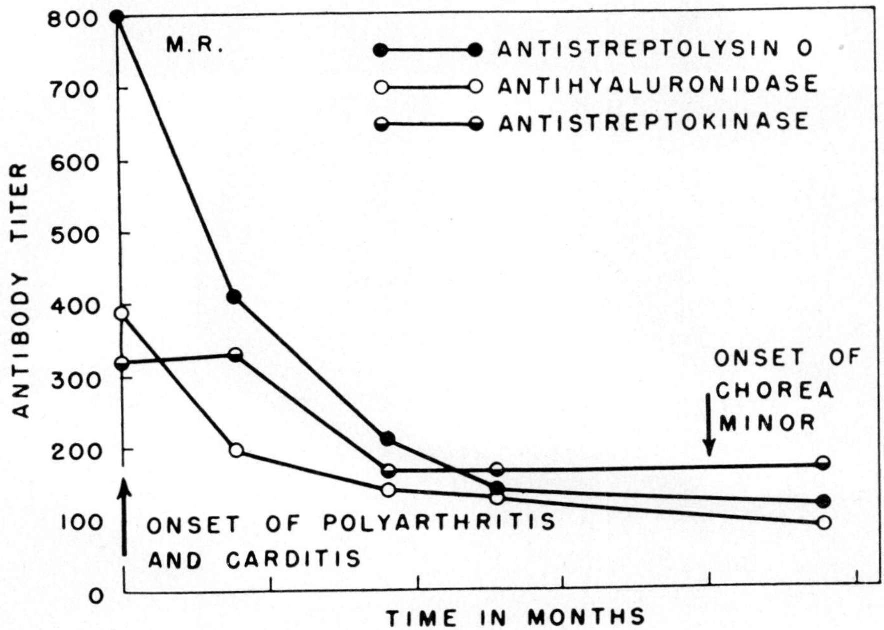

FIG. 44–7.—Chorea appearing four months after the onset of polyarthritis and carditis. Intercurrent streptococcal infections were ruled out by the falling titers of three streptococcal antibodies. (Taranta and Stollerman, courtesy of Amer. J. Med.)

and so is the observation that patients with "pure" chorea have elevated ASO titers with the same frequency as patients in the *second* month of their attack of rheumatic polyarthritis and carditis.[177]

Some of the patients presenting with "pure" chorea may have had, after the streptococcal infection, but before chorea, an asymptomatic, mild and transient carditis. This hypothesis, if correct, would explain the high incidence of chorea (66 per cent) in the first attack of rheumatic fever of those patients who have no detectable carditis in the first attack, but seem to develop carditis for the first time with the *second* attack of

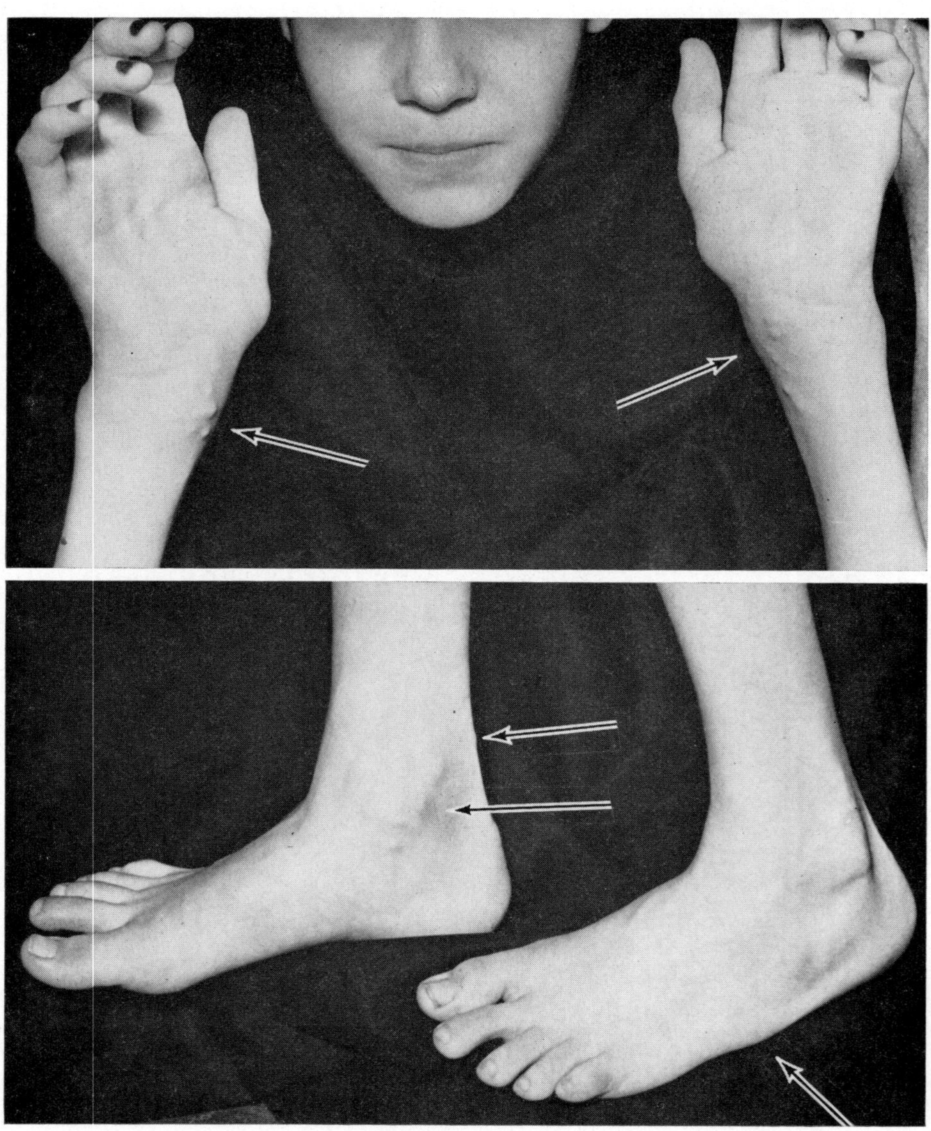

Fig. 44–8.—Subcutaneous nodules in a child with rheumatic fever (indicated by the arrows). Notice that some of them are difficult to see; often they can be more easily felt than seen. (Courtesy of Dr. Eugenie F. Doyle.)

rheumatic fever[100] (see below under *Recurrences*), as well as the relatively high and otherwise unexplained incidence of heart disease in the follow-up of patients with "pure" chorea[13] (23 per cent after 20 years).

The **subcutaneous nodules** of rheumatic fever are firm and painless. The skin overlying them is not inflamed, and almost invariably can be moved over them. The nodules are approximately round and their diameter varies from a few millimeters to 1, or less commonly, 2 cm. Occasionally they may be larger and soft. They are located over bony surfaces or prominences or in proximity to tendons (Fig. 44–8); their number varies from one to a few dozen and averages 3 or 4; when numerous, they tend to be symmetrical. Their duration is one or more weeks, and rarely exceeds a month. They thus tend to be smaller and to last for a shorter period of time than the nodules of rheumatoid arthritis. Although in both diseases the elbows are the site most frequently involved, the rheumatic nodules are more common at the point of the olecranon and the rheumatoid nodules 3 or 4 cm. distal to it.[98]

Rheumatic subcutaneous nodules tend to appear only after the first few weeks of illness and then almost only in patients with carditis.[122] Nodules are more frequently found among patients with severe than with mild carditis,[7,122] and thus are associated with a relatively poor prognosis, especially if the nodules appear in recurrent crops.[7] Occasionally, patients may have nodules without carditis, but then only in small numbers;[122] however, among patients with carditis and nodules the number of nodules is not related to the severity of heart involvement.[7]

The usual location of the nodules between the skin and hard, incompressible structures suggests that minor, repeated traumata may be involved in their formation. This hypothesis is supported by the observation that subcutaneous nodules appear over the olecranon after injection of autologous blood, followed by repeated applications of frictional pressure, in 90 per cent of patients with active rheumatic fever but in none of suitable controls.[123]

Erythema marginatum is an evanescent, non-pruritic skin rash, pink or faintly red, which affects usually the trunk, sometimes the proximal parts of the limbs, but never the face. It is composed of a variable number of individual skin lesions, starting as a solid erythema which may be slightly raised. This extends centrifugally while the skin in the center returns gradually to normal; hence the name "erythema marginatum." The outer edge of the lesion is sharp, while the inner one is diffuse (Fig. 44–9). The margin of the lesion is usually continuous, making a ring; hence the name "erythema annulare." Some authors[97] distinguish the "annulare" from the "marginatum" variety because the "marginatum" may be raised[141] while the "annulare" is purely macular,[101] but this distinction is not essential, as raised and macular lesions may occur together[97] and their course, distribution and association with other manifestations are the same. Therefore, modern authors do not differentiate between the two and speak of erythema marginatum as including the annulare, or purely macular, variety.[22,122]

The individual lesions may appear and disappear in a matter of hours, usually to return. They may change in shape and size almost as fast as smoke rings, which they resemble in shape, and in the centrifugal manner in which they expand and dissolve. The lesions may coalesce while expanding and thus acquire a circinate, gyrate or festooned pattern. A hot bath or shower may make them more evident, or even reveal them for the first time.

Erythema marginatum usually occurs in the early phase of the disease (in 11 of 14 cases it was present at the onset).[22] It often persists or recurs later, even after all other manifestations of disease have disappeared; or it may occasionally appear for the first time (or be noticed for the first time?) late in the course of the illness, or even during convalescence (1 of 14 cases[22]; unspecified proportion of cases).[56,116,164] It occurs almost only in patients with carditis,[22,56,122] but the carditis of these patients is not particularly severe.[56,122] Since subcutaneous nodules also appear almost only in patients with carditis (see above) it follows that the incidence of erythema marginatum is about doubled in the patients with subcutaneous nodules, and conversely, the incidence of nodules is about doubled in patients with erythema marginatum,[122] when compared with unselected patients with rheumatic fever.

Fever is almost regularly present at the onset of rheumatic polyarthritis; it is often present in isolated carditis, but seldom in isolated chorea. It is a remittent type of fever, without wide swings, which usually does not exceed 104° F[111] and returns to normal or near-normal in two or three weeks in most cases, even in the absence of treatment[44,77] (Fig. 44–15). Very high fevers may occur in exceptional cases and may be due to salicylate toxicity[111] or to very severe chorea which may end fatally ("hyperpyretic cerebral rheumatism" of old).[103,129]

Abdominal pain may occur in rheumatic fever as a manifestation of congestive heart failure, due to distension of the liver (see above). It may also occur in rare but important instances without heart failure and before any other manifestation has declared the rheumatic nature of the illness. In these cases the pain may be periumbilical and severe, is presumably due to mesenteric adenitis, and occasionally leads to an unnecessary appendectomy.[43,56]

Anorexia, nausea and vomiting often occur,

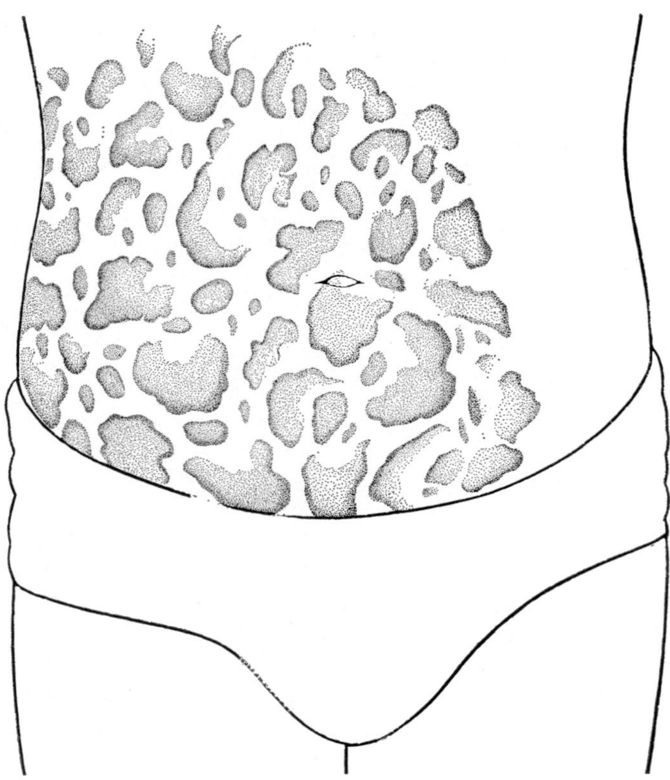

Fig. 44–9.—Erythema marginatum in a child with rheumatic fever. Most, but not all the individual lesions are outlined by closed rings. Some of the lesions have a circinate or festooned appearance.

but mostly as manifestations of congestive failure, or of salicylate toxicity. The incidence of *epistaxis* has decreased considerably from a maximum of 48 per cent in the early thirties[34] to 4 to 9 per cent in the late fifties.[56] *Fatigue* is a vague and infrequent symptom, unless heart failure is present.

Other clinical manifestations, which are seldom seen nowadays, include *erythema nodosum*, pleurisy, and "rheumatic pneumonia."[71] These were not mentioned in a large series recently reported.[122] In another recent series, erythema nodosum was seen in 0.7 per cent of patients, and pleurisy and "rheumatic pneumonia" in none.[56] It must be noted that congestive heart failure may simulate both pleurisy and pneumonia, with a pleural transudate and with pulmonary congestion, respectively. Moreover, the old-time description of rheumatic pneumonia, with patchy, shifting areas of infiltration,[148] is suspiciously similar to that of "viral" pneumonia. Therefore "rheumatic pneumonia," if indeed it exists as a clinical entity, is both rare and difficult or impossible to diagnose.

Minor Post-Streptococcal Disease: "Streptococcal Fever"

About 12 per cent of patients with streptococcal pharyngitis may show evidence of a continuing disease characterized by persistent elevation of the ESR, P-R prolongation (8 per cent) and T wave inversion (5 per cent) in the ECG, lymphadenopathy and occasionally fever, malaise or both.[145] Arthralgia may also be encountered.[58] Although these patients do not meet the standard diagnostic criteria for rheumatic fever, they probably represent "formes fruste" of it, constituting the lowest end of a continuum in the severity spectrum of the disease.

Sequence of Appearance of Manifestations

Figure 44–10 summarizes in a schematic and approximate manner the information on this subject, as detailed in the preceding pages. Most attacks of rheumatic fever present with joint symptoms, but in a small minority abdominal pain may precede them. When a physician is consulted, clinical evidence of carditis may or may not be present. If it is not already present, it usually does not appear later; if it appears, it usually does so in the first three weeks. Electrocardiographic alterations may be detected during the "latent period."

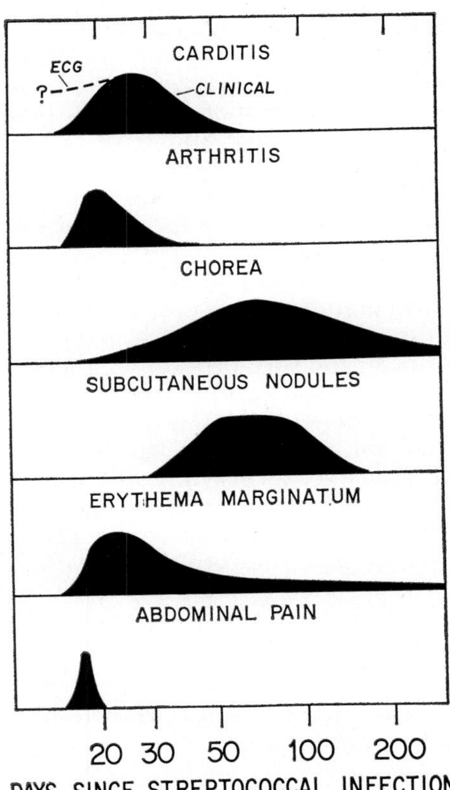

Fig. 44–10.—Approximate schema of the sequence of appearance of the various rheumatic fever manifestations. The maximum height of each curve indicates the time at which most of the cases of a given manifestation "appear," *i.e.*, become known to a medical observer. Due to the concentration of events early in the attack, time is represented on a logarithmic scale.

Patients who present with chorea may have a heart murmur and no acute phase reactants, suggesting that carditis has preceded it. Patients who present with polyarthritis may develop chorea later. Nodules are exceptional in the first three weeks of the attack and tend to appear later. Erythema marginatum is observed most frequently at the onset of a rheumatic attack, but may also appear for the first time later.

It thus seems that among the major clinical manifestations the "latent period" is shortest in arthritis, but it may be even shorter in the rare prodrome, abdominal pain; in clinical carditis the latent period may be longer, but this may be partly artifactual, due to the gradual rather than sudden onset of symptoms in isolated carditis and to delayed recognition of murmurs. The average latent period is longer in subcutaneous nodules than in erythema marginatum, in which it is usually short; and it is longest, but very variable, in chorea.

Incidence of the Clinical Manifestations of Rheumatic Fever

Variations with Age and Other Factors.— The incidence of the clinical manifestations of rheumatic fever, in patients who receive this diagnosis, varies in reported series according to the age and sex of the patients, the diagnostic criteria used, the geographic origin of the patients and the period, recent or remote, in which the reported series were collected. It also differs in recurrences as compared to first attacks. The variations with age are represented schematically and approximately in Figure 44–11.

Arthritis is the most common major manifestation of rheumatic fever; it becomes increasingly frequent with increasing age. In the few children who develop rheumatic fever between the ages of eighteen months and three years, arthritis was reported to be present only in 46 per cent of patients,[110] but in a more recent series in 80 per cent of the cases.[149a] In this age group carditis may actually be more frequent than arthritis. The incidence of arthritis in children with first attacks of rheumatic fever was 66, 70, 78, 80 and 82 per cent respectively in the age groups three to six, seven to nine, ten to eleven, twelve to thirteen and fourteen to seventeen.[56] Arthritis may also be longer and more severe in the older age groups.[26] In first attacks of rheumatic fever in adults, arthritis may be even more frequent than in the older adolescents.[49,135] Arthritis may be more common in boys (83 per cent) than in girls (67 per cent).[56] The incidence of arthritis has not varied recently. It may be less common in the tropics, but this has been debated.[67]

Clinically significant carditis is almost as frequent as arthritis, but its incidence varies with age in an opposite manner. It was present in 92 per cent[110] and 90 per cent[149a] of children with rheumatic fever under the age of three. It decreased progressively from 50 per cent in the three to six age group to 32 per cent

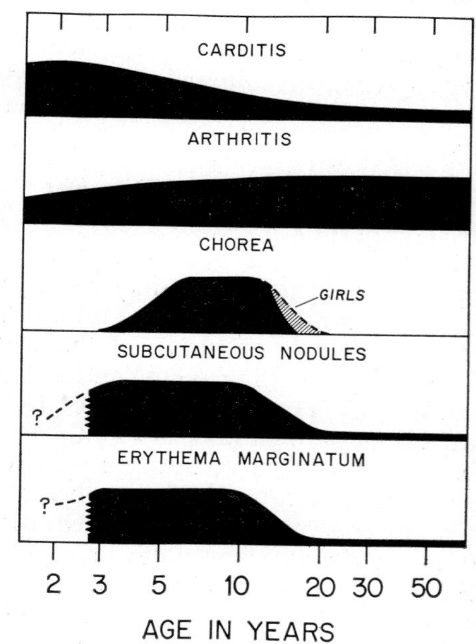

FIG. 44–11.—Schematic representation of the variations with age of the incidence of the major manifestations of rheumatic fever. The maximum height of each curve indicates the age at which a given manifestation attains its maximum incidence among patients with rheumatic fever.

in the fourteen to seventeen age group[56] in first attacks, but does not fall to zero after the age of twenty-five, as it has been suggested editorially.[64] Clinically significant carditis was present in 36 per cent of carefully studied adults with first attacks of rheumatic fever.[135] Although it is possible to argue that some of these patients had had an unrecognized previous attack of the disease, there is no evidence that this is so; moreover, one patient who developed carditis in this series actually had been examined *before* the development of rheumatic fever and found free of heart disease, and several other such cases are known to our group. Some of the decrease in incidence of carditis with age may be due to a decrease of patients presenting with isolated carditis, but even if the analysis is restricted to patients with polyarthritis, the incidence of carditis is significantly lower in adults than in children.[40]

It must be noted that carditis, quite predictably, is present in all patients with "rheumatic fever" in the series assembled by authors who make carditis, however defined, a *prerequisite* for the diagnosis of rheumatic fever (see, for instance, ref. 191). Many others define carditis to include minor electrocardiographic alterations, in the absence of murmurs or other clinical evidence of cardiac involvement (see above under *Carditis*); still others blandly assume that carditis is always present and call it "B" if loud murmurs are present, and "A" if they are not.[26] In all these cases, of course, the incidence of "carditis" is much higher than that stated in the previous paragraph. The incidence of carditis, as well as its severity, may have decreased in recent years,[12,120,125] but how much this is due to changed admission policies of hospitals and to decrease in recurrent attacks of the disease is uncertain.

Chorea is the only major manifestation which has unequivocally decreased in incidence out of proportion to the others in recent decades (from 52 per cent,[15] 43 per cent[120] and 41 per cent[125] of all the patients with rheumatic fever, to 8 per cent,[56] 15 per cent[120] and 19 per cent[125]) for reasons which are not understood. Chorea is also the manifestation which occurs in the most limited age range;* it does not occur under three years of age[1,10] is rare after puberty and does not occur in adults[4,135] with the possible exception of rare cases during pregnancy.[106] Finally, it is the only manifestation with a definite sex preference, being twice as frequent in girls as in boys;[4] after puberty this sex preference increases.[134]

Subcutaneous nodules appear to be frequent in patients in England (34 per cent,[26] 21 per cent),[181] rather common in those in Boston (10 per cent)[122] but rare in those in New York (1 per cent)[56] and in Baltimore (2 per cent).[116] Whether this is a true geographic variation, or is due to differences in the thoroughness of the physical examinations performed, is a matter for speculation.

Nodules appear to occur very seldom, or not at all,[110] in patients under the age of three; they are also quite rare in adults with rheumatic fever,[135] although they are common in adults with rheumatoid arthritis.

Erythema marginatum has been reported in 13[181] and 10[122] and as low as 4 per cent[56] of rheumatic fever attacks. It is particularly rare in adults,[135] but may occur.[93] Before the age of three "erythema" was observed, but it was not specified whether it was "marginatum."[110]

Associations Among the Various Manifestations of Rheumatic Fever

These may be positive or negative. Thus, subcutaneous nodules and erythema

* These two observations may be related. They could be explained if chorea tended to occur only after many closely spaced streptococcal infections, while other manifestations had no such requirement. If this were true, the first manifestation to disappear with a decrease in incidence of streptococcal infections, either in individuals, with increasing age, or in populations, with changes in living conditions, would be chorea. There is no direct evidence, however, to support this hypothesis.

marginatum are much more frequent in the presence than in the absence of carditis[98,101] and each one of them is about twice as frequent in the presence of the other.[122]

On the negative side, "pure" chorea is, by definition, associated with no other clinical manifestations; nevertheless, it may be associated with *subclinical* carditis, as suggested by the high incidence of delayed appearance of heart disease.[13] Carditis is much more frequent in the absence than in the presence of arthritis, but this difference arises by definition, since a patient without arthritis must have carditis (or chorea) to come to medical attention.[56] In addition, carditis is more likely to be *severe* in patients with arthralgia only, than in patients with definite arthritis, and, in general, the incidence and severity of carditis has an inverse relation to the incidence and severity of joint involvement.[56] This inverse correlation may be due, in part, to the opposite age variation of the incidence of arthritis and carditis, as noted above. It may also be influenced by factors of selection since patients with arthralgia may not be admitted to a hospital if they have no carditis; by the fact that carditis is more likely to be diagnosed if it is severe than if it is mild; and by the fact that patients with arthritis are confined to bed, which may prevent heart failure (which in turn is considered an indication of severity of carditis).

Duration of Rheumatic Fever

Duration as a whole (as opposed to the duration of each manifestation, which is considered above) varies according to the criterion used to determine it and to the clinical manifestations present. It is shortest in attacks characterized by arthritis alone; it is longer in the presence of chorea, and longest in the presence of carditis.[55,77] It is generally shorter if the end-point is the disappearance of acute clinical manifestations,[77] and longer if the end-point is the return to normal of the "acute phase reactants," although in some cases certain major clinical manifestations (chorea, and occasionally erythema marginatum and nodules) may persist or even appear for the first time after the acute phase reactants have returned to normal.

The duration of the disease is difficult to ascertain if anti-inflammatory treatment is administered (see under *Therapy*) and is best determined in series of unselected, untreated cases,[26,44,65,77,90] although the details reported are often insufficient. In a series in which the criteria for termination were mainly clinical, cases of rheumatic fever with polyarthritis in adults lasted less than forty-six days in 32 per cent of the cases, between forty-six and seventy days in another 32 per cent, and seventy to eight-six days in 36 per cent.[77] In a more recent series the average ESR fell to conventionally "normal" values by the eighth week, and reached lower and stable values by the end of twelve weeks.[44] In still another series, the ESR was normal on admission in 18 per cent of the cases; among the others, in whom the ESR was elevated, it remained so in one-third of the cases for one to three weeks, in another third for four to nine weeks and in the last third for ten or more weeks.[90] In a series of patients with first attacks of rheumatic fever receiving only little or no antirheumatic treatment, all evidence of active rheumatic fever had subsided within twelve weeks in almost 80 per cent of the cases and within fifteen weeks in almost 90 per cent.[122] In a series comprising both treated and untreated cases (not randomly selected) the duration of the disease was 109 ± 57 days.[53]

"Chronic" Rheumatic Fever

In a small proportion of cases (3 per cent or less) the active rheumatic process appears to continue for more than six months[166] or for more than two hundred and twenty-three days (= mean duration of rheumatic fever + 2 standard deviations).[176] The majority of these attacks occur in patients who have already had one or more attacks, and the incidence of such protracted attacks increases with the number of preceding attacks. It is to be noted that in some of these patients definite clinical and pathologic evidence of fresh manifestations such as arthritis, nodules, pericarditis, and endocarditis may be found peculiarly late in the attack and despite immunologically confirmed absence of intercurrent streptococcal infections.[176]

Sequelae of Rheumatic Fever

Sequelae are essentially limited to the heart, and depend on the presence and severity of carditis. In addition, patients who have had rheumatic fever tend to develop it again after streptococcal infections, with an attack rate much higher than in the general population. This increased sensitivity to the rheumatogenic effect of streptococcal infections, which may also be interpreted as a "sequela," is most marked in patients with rheumatic heart disease, but is also present in patients without it (see below, under *Recurrences*; and in previous chapter, under *Epidemiology*).

The structural and functional alterations of the heart caused by rheumatic fever and referred to collectively as "rheumatic heart disease" are described in detail in textbooks of cardiology. They will be dealt with here only briefly, and mostly in terms of their relation to the acute attacks. Among large series of patients followed in recent years from their acute attack onwards, rheumatic heart disease has not developed in those who had no clinical evidence of carditis during the acute attack (*i.e.*, in patients

Table 44-1.—Prognosis in Relation to Cardiac Status at Start of Treatment*

Cardiac Status at Start of Treatment	*No. of Cases Observed for 5 Years*	*Per Cent with No Murmur after 5 Years*	*No. of Deaths in 5 Years*
No carditis	71	96	0
Questionable carditis	32	84	0
Apical systolic murmur, grade I only‖	39	82	0
Apical systolic murmur, grades II or III only	60	68	2
Apical systolic and apical mid-diastolic murmurs	44	48	1†
Basal diastolic with or without other murmurs	45 (15)‡	53 (27)‡	1
Failure and/or pericarditis	33	30	1
Pre-existing heart disease without failure and/or pericarditis	80	30	5§
Pre-existing heart disease with failure and/or pericarditis	22	0	6

* The combined results of all three treatment groups. Modified from U.K. and U.S. Joint Report.[182]

† Death from acute nephritis and uremia.

‡ Excluding one U.K. center which had exceedingly high incidence of basal diastolic murmurs.

§ Includes 1 death from acute intestinal obstruction.

‖ Grades I, II and III are increasingly loud, but all refer to murmurs considered organic in this classification.

who at that time had no murmurs or only physiologic murmurs, irrespective of ECG alterations).[52,60,181,182,183] An exception may be noted in patients whose first attack of rheumatic fever took the form of "pure" chorea, who may develop rheumatic heart disease, usually mitral stenosis, gradually and insidiously over the years (23 per cent rheumatic heart disease after twenty years).[13] Some of these patients, according to the hypothesis advanced above (under *Chorea*) may actually have had transient carditis shortly before the onset of chorea. The evidence of heart damage, gone by the onset of chorea, may have reappeared later. A similar sequence, of carditis detectable during the acute attack, fol-

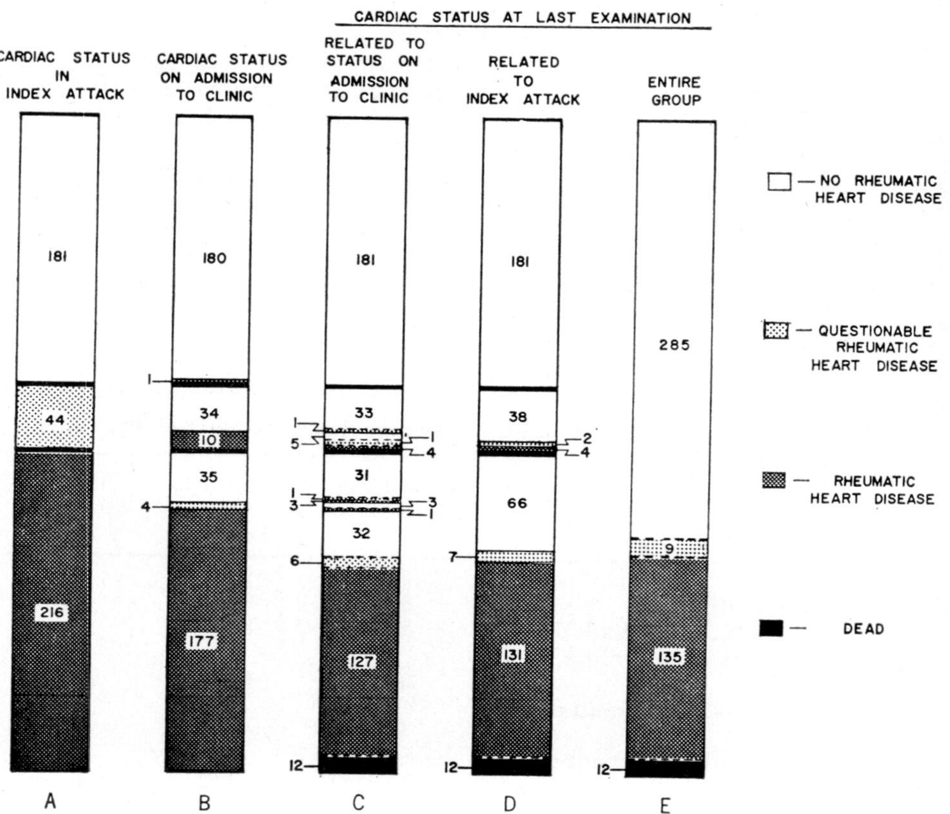

FIG. 44–12.—Cardiac status in different groups of 441 patients at three different times of observation. In each rectangle, the cardiac status is indicated by appropriate shading, and the number of patients is marked. The heavy solid horizontal lines of column A, showing division of the 441 patients into three cardiac categories during the index attack of rheumatic fever, are also maintained in the next three columns to show the course of each numbered group. In column B, which shows cardiac status on admission to the clinic, thin solid horizontal lines have been added to show the subdivisions of each previous category. Columns C, D, and E all show the cardiac status at the last follow-up examination about 8 years later. The dashed lines of column C show the outcome of the groups demarcated in column B. Column D depicts the final results in the patients shown in column A. Column E rearranges the entire final group, irrespective of previous status, with dashed, heavy horizontal lines to show the new divisions.

The results show disappearance of heart disease in many patients who previously had it, but no "insidious" development of heart disease in patients free from it during the index attack. (Feinstein *et al.*, courtesy of Ann. Int. Med.)

lowed by apparent healing and finally by reappearance of organic murmurs, actually has been observed in other patients with rheumatic fever.[60] It is interesting to remember in this connection that mitral stenosis in women is frequently preceded by a mild attack of carditis;[183] and that these patients with chorea were predominantly women and, if they had carditis before chorea, it must have been mild, since it was asymptomatic.

It must be noted that in some earlier studies the insidious development of heart disease in patients who had no carditis in their first attack of rheumatic fever was apparently a frequent occurrence.[14,15] The fact that chorea was frequent in past decades and is infrequent nowadays may explain, in part, this discrepancy between old and new studies. Other possible explanations, including observer's error, have been discussed elsewhere.[173]

Among patients with clinical evidence of carditis during the acute attack, the incidence of residual rheumatic heart disease parallels the severity of the initial carditis. Thus, in one study (Table 44–1) the incidence of residual heart disease was higher in patients who, at the time of the initial carditis, had systolic *and* mid-diastolic apical murmurs than in those who had systolic murmurs only, and among the latter it was higher in those who had loud murmurs. The incidence of residual heart disease was highest in patients who had congestive failure, pericarditis, or both during the acute attack.[182] In another study, the incidence of residual heart disease (eight years after the attack) among patients with initial carditis was maximum in patients with marked enlargement of the heart during the acute attack, and minimum in patients with organic murmurs but no cardiomegaly during the acute attack (Fig. 44–12). In both series the incidence of residual heart disease was higher after recurrences than after first attacks.

It is of interest that mitral stenosis, which after five years was present only in approximately 1.4 per cent of patients, increased to approximately 5 per cent by the end of ten years;[183] and that mitral stenosis was usually preceded by a severe attack of rheumatic carditis in males (6 of 8 cases had had failure, pericarditis, or both) but not in females (only 5 of 16 cases had had the manifestations mentioned). For unknown reasons, Indians develop mitral stenosis at a much earlier age than Westerners,[150a] up to one third of all mitral commissurotomies being performed before age 20.[32a]

Other sequelae of rheumatic fever are rare, questionable, or both. *Jaccoud's polyarthritis* or *chronic post-rheumatic fever arthritis* has been described repeatedly in the European literature and recently here[151a,201] as appearing after frequent, prolonged and severe attacks of rheumatic fever. It is characterized by ulnar deviation of the fingers and hyperextension of the proximal interphalangeal joints, without bone destruction. The deviation affects primarily the 4th and 5th digits and is at first correctable, but later becomes fixed. The joints affected cause little or no symptoms; the functional capacity is good and the erythrocyte sedimentation rate is normal. (The term "arthritis" may therefore be a misnomer for this condition which might be better described as a fibrotic residuum.) Due to its rarity and to the possible concomitance of rheumatic fever and mild rheumatoid arthritis, the existence of a specific entity of chronic post-rheumatic fever arthritis is still in doubt.

Neurologic and psychiatric disorders have been described occasionally on follow-up of patients with rheumatic fever, and especially with chorea. Some observers believe their incidence is higher than would be expected by chance alone.[4,62,189]

Recurrences of Rheumatic Fever

Recurrences are one of the most striking and common features of the disease, and set it apart from other diseases with an infectious etiology. The factors affecting the recurrence rate are discussed under *Epidemiology* in the previous chapter; the clinical manifestations and sequelae of recurrences will be dealt with here.

The same clinical manifestations present in the initial attack of rheumatic fever seem to reappear in recurrent attacks with a frequency greater than would be expected from chance alone[150] (Table 44–2). Conversely, manifestations absent in the first attack tend to be absent in recurrent attacks. This is of particular interest in the case of carditis. The studies dealing specifically with the outcome of recurrences in patients who had escaped rheumatic heart disease during a previous attack are summarized in Table 44–3. It will be seen that the incidence of carditis during the recurrent attack, as well as of residual heart disease after it, is lower than would be expected in an unselected group of rheumatic fever attacks. The study with the highest incidence of carditis during the recurrent attack[100] had a large proportion of patients who had chorea as their first attack; this, for the reasons detailed above (under *Chorea*) may have influ-

Table 44-2.—Major Clinical Manifestations of Rheumatic Fever Recurrences According to Manifestations of the First Attack*

	Manifestations of Recurrences (isolated or combined with others)		
Manifestations of First Attack (isolated or combined with others)	*Polyarthritis*	*Carditis*	*Chorea*
Polyarthritis (N = 149)	110 (74%)	51 (34%)	18 (12%)
Carditis (N = 89)	44 (49%)	62 (70%)	2 (2%)
Chorea (N = 68)	11 (16%)	10 (15%)	54 (79%)

* Data of Roth *et al.*[150]

Table 44-3.—Appearance and Persistence of Rheumatic Heart Disease with Recurrent Attacks of Rheumatic Fever in Patients Who had Escaped Rheumatic Heart Disease during a Previous Attack of Rheumatic Fever

Studies	*Patients with Rheumatic Fever Recurrences*	*Patients with Carditis During Recurrences*	*Patients with Persistent Rheumatic Heart Disease*
Retrospective:			
Boone and Levine, 1938[17]	68	?	4 (6%)
Brown and Wolff, 1940[19]	42	?	0
Feinstein and Spagnuolo, 1960[53]	71	10 (14%)	10 (14%)
Kuttner and Mayer, 1963[100]	50	13 (26%)	6 (12%)
Prospective:			
U.K. and U.S. Cooperative Study, 1964[183]	10	?	0
Feinstein *et al.* 1964[58]	11	2 (18%)	0

Table 44-4.—Incidence of Rheumatic Heart Disease According to Number of Previous Attacks of Rheumatic Fever*

Previous Attacks	*Number of Patients*	*Number of Patients with Heart Disease*
0	797	264 (33%)
1	280	170 (60%)
2	57	43 (75%)
3	31	25 (81%)
4	4	4 (100%)

* Adapted from Taranta *et al.*[176]

enced the results. It must be noted that patients with recurrent attacks tend to be older than patients with first attacks, and that rheumatic fever causes less carditis in first attacks in older patients; this may explain, in part, the benign nature of these recurrent attacks.

Although patients who escape carditis in the first attack tend to escape it again in recurrent attacks, the incidence of heart disease increases progressively with the number of previous attacks (Table 44–4).[176] This observation seems incompatible with the one expounded in the previous paragraph, but it is not. In all probability, the higher incidence of heart disease in patients with repeated attacks is due to the increased tendency of patients with heart disease to develop recurrences,[174] (see above under *Epidemiology*) more than to the acquisition of heart disease by patients initially free of it.

Mortality Caused by Rheumatic Fever

It is remarkable that of the considerable number of deaths due to rheumatic fever, only a minority occur during an acute attack, and of these only very few during the first attack of the disease. The majority of deaths occur *after* the acute attack, due to the circulatory embarrassment caused by valves which have become regurgitant, stenotic, or both.

Thus, in three large recent series the mortality during *the acute attack* of rheumatic fever, comprising both first and recurrent attacks, was 1 per cent.[56,181] *In first attacks*, it was 0.36 per cent,[56] 0.6 per cent[181] and 1.6 per cent.[122] The first percentage may have been biased because it was obtained in a convalescent home, to which rapidly fatal first attacks would not be referred. In *recurrent attacks*, the mortality was higher: 2.3 per cent[181] and 3 per cent.[56] Both in first and recurrent attacks, the mortality was nil in patients without heart involvement and occurred only in patients with congestive heart failure, giving a percentage of 3.2 among all patients with significant murmurs and of 24 in patients with failure.[122]

In the years subsequent to the acute attack the mortality used to be high,[15] due mainly to recurrent attacks, but is now only moderate. Thus, in two recent long-term follow-up studies the mortality was 2.9 per cent (calculated from the end of treatment for the acute attack to the end of the fifth year since the beginning of the attack);[182] an additional 1 per cent died between five and ten years after the attack.[183] This gives a cumulative mortality of 4 per cent from the beginning of treatment to ten years hence, which contrasts with the 20 per cent ten-year mortality which prevailed twenty years ago.[15] In another recent study, the death rate was 2.7 per cent over an eight-year period.[60] In the latter series none of the deaths was directly caused by a recurrence of rheumatic fever, but in both series deaths were more common among those who had had more than one attack.

In the older series, mortality was higher in the first than in the second decade of follow-up (20 versus 10 per cent; cumulatively 30 per cent);[15] therefore, one might expect that the low death rates observed in current series in the first decade of follow-up will become even lower in the second decade. However, much of the early mortality in the older series was due to recurrences, while this is not true now.[60] With recurrences largely controlled by prophylaxis, and mortality due mostly to deterioration of cardiac status in the absence of recurrences, the anticipated further fall of mortality in the second decade after the attack may not occur.

CLINICAL PATHOLOGY

The contributions of the laboratory to the clinical work-up of patients suspected of having rheumatic fever cluster in two main areas: (1) the diagnosis of a recent streptococcal infection and (2) the detection of an inflammatory state. The first diagnosis cannot be made by other than laboratory means since streptococcal and viral pharyngitides are hard to distinguish on clinical grounds (with the possible exception of scarlet fever, which presents a clinical picture typical enough to be diagnostic of streptococcal infection). The contributions of the laboratory in the second area are less essential, since fever and other manifestations of inflammatory disease do not necessarily need laboratory confirmation.

The diagnosis of a recent streptococcal infection is made tentatively by throat culture and definitively by antibody determinations. Throat cultures are useful in detecting a streptococcal infection if the organisms are still present at the time of the examination (see preceding chapter). However, by the time rheumatic fever appears the throat culture is often negative, especially if the patient has already been given antibiotics. If it is positive, one cannot be sure that it indicates the tail end of an infection, *i.e.* the convalescent "carrier state," rather than commensalism, *i.e.*, the non-convalescent "carrier state." Streptococcal antibody determinations are more useful because they reach their peak titer shortly after rheumatic fever appears (Fig. 44–13), and they are a more definite indication of an actual *infection*, since by definition they do not rise in the non-convalescent carrier state.

The antistreptolysin O titer (ASO) is 200 units per cc. or more in the great majority of cases of rheumatic fever; when this test is negative, one or more of the other antistreptococcal antibody tests will regularly detect an antibody response. Thus, in one series, studied within two months of the onset of rheumatic fever, a streptococcal antibody response was detected by ASO tests in 78 per cent of the cases; this percentage rose to 90 when anti-hyaluronidase was also determined and to 95 per cent when antistreptokinase determination was added[166] (Fig. 44–14). The chances of detecting a significant antibody response are greatest shortly (about two weeks) after the onset of the attack (Fig. 44–13) and decline thereafter. Lower titers may be detected in patients who present with Sydenham's chorea,[171,177] probably due to a longer latent period of this manifestation. Lower titers have also been reported in a few cases of isolated carditis[32] which may have come to medical attention relatively late in their course. Deceptively high titers may be due to non-antibody inhibitors of streptolysin O in hepatitis, biliary obstruction and nephrosis[5b,82,158,163] or to monoclonal IgG in myeloma.[108a]

The newer streptococcal antibody tests, anti-DPN-ase,[9] (anti-diphosphopyridine-nucleotidase) and anti-deoxyribonuclease B, may also be helpful. Anti-deoxyribonuclease B is particularly interesting because it appears to remain elevated longer than other streptococcal antibodies.[186] Therefore, in chorea this anti-

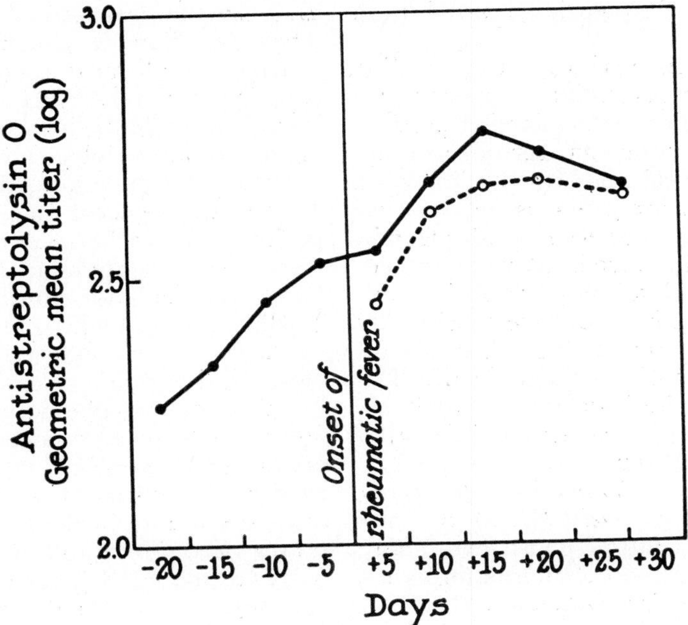

FIG. 44–13.—Mean antistreptolysin O titer in relation to the time of onset of rheumatic fever. Upper curve (solid line): 23 cases of rheumatic fever following scarlet fever. Lower curve (broken line): 45 cases of sporadic rheumatic fever. (McCarty in *Rheumatic Fever*, courtesy of University of Minnesota Press.)

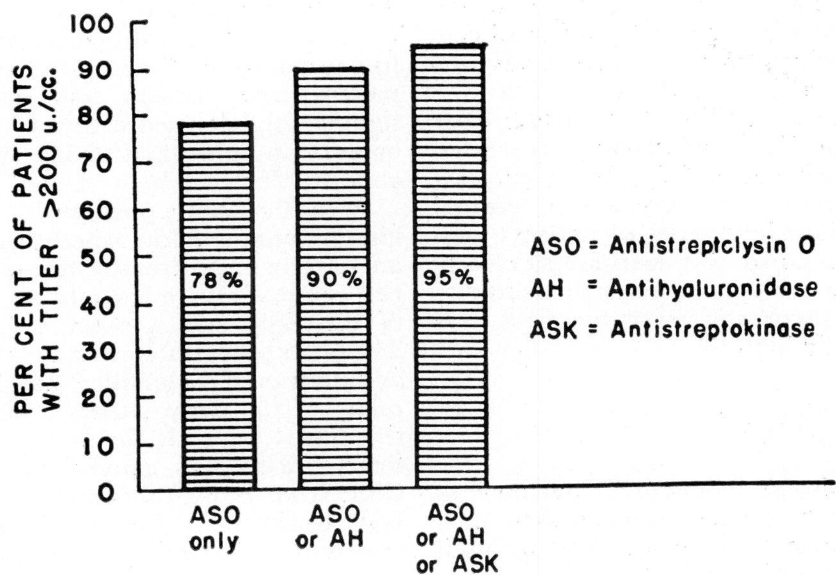

FIG. 44–14.—Streptococcal antibody titers in 88 patients studied within 2 months of onset of rheumatic fever. (Stollerman *et al.*, courtesy of Amer. J. Med.)

body is more frequently elevated than others.[5a]

In the presence of low or borderline titers, repeated determinations of streptococcal antibodies, determined if possible at the same time on serum samples obtained at weekly or biweekly intervals ("serial runs") are often useful, because in some patients a streptococcal infection may cause an increase in titer not exceeding the "normal values," but still significant. Two-tube increases are consistently reproduced in most laboratories and therefore are considered significant. Decreases in titer indicate less recent infections, which may, however, still be related to the disease at hand.

The erythrocyte sedimentation rate (ESR) and the C-reactive protein (CRP) are the laboratory procedures most commonly used for the detection of an inflammatory state. The ESR is elevated and the CRP test is positive in virtually all patients with recent untreated rheumatic fever, with the exception of those presenting with chorea only. The CRP test reverts to negative before the ESR returns to normal values.

In some patients, the ESR remains elevated for a very long time in the absence of any other evidence of disease and without any prognostic significance.[85,176]

The elevated ESR of rheumatic fever is traditionally considered to be decreased by congestive heart failure[138,140] but, if it is, is usually not decreased to normal values, since in a series of patients with episodes of congestive heart failure closely associated with other clinical manifestations of rheumatic fever the ESR was consistently high.[160]

Clinical Significance of Laboratory Tests

It should be underscored that none of the tests mentioned is *specific* for rheumatic fever. None of these tests can by itself establish the diagnosis of rheumatic fever as, for instance, a strongly positive lupus erythematosus (LE) preparation can establish the diagnosis of systemic lupus. They can, however, make the diagnosis of rheumatic fever questionable if the results are negative. Since rheumatic fever is no longer defined on clinical grounds alone, but also etiologically, as a sequel of streptococcal infections, the absence of a recent streptococcal infection is incompatible with the diagnosis of rheumatic fever (the exceptions of isolated Sydenham's chorea and, possibly, of isolated carditis, should be kept in mind).

On the other hand, the presence of an elevated titer does not carry great weight in favor of the diagnosis of rheumatic fever, because streptococcal infections are frequent, especially in children. Thus, in San Francisco 28 to 35 per cent of normal children in the five to twelve age group were shown to have an ASO titer of 250 or more.[144] The chance of having not only a positive throat culture, but also an elevated ASO titer unrelated to the disease the patient is being observed for is therefore considerable, and it varies with the local epidemiology of streptococcal infections and with the age of the patient.[146] To be on the safe side, some clinicians consider "significant" only ASO titers of 400 or more.[122] A committee of the American Heart Association has recommended taking the age of the patient into account and considering significantly elevated a titer of 250 units or more in adults and of 333 or more in children.[167]

As for the "acute phase reactants," any kind of inflammation, whether caused by an infective agent or by necrotic tissue, can cause, if severe enough, an elevation of the ESR and a positive CRP test. The latter test has unfortunately acquired an undeserved rheumatic "aura" because many of the early papers reporting on this test dealt with rheumatic fever patients. This was purely coincidental; CRP is no more "rheumatic" than the ESR or any of the other "acute phase reactants." Even the local inflammatory reactions to benzathine penicillin injections can cause elevation of the ESR and a positive CRP test.[79] The *absence* of such indicators of inflammation, however, is unusual in untreated rheumatic fever (with the exception of Sydenham's chorea) and should make one wary of the diagnosis.

A number of other changes occur in the serum proteins and mucoproteins of patients with rheumatic fever[10,72] but the tests to demonstrate these are more elaborate and the results have not yet been shown in any conclusive manner to be more specific for rheumatic fever than the ESR and the CRP test. The serum concentrations of gamma globulins, alpha-2 globulins, mucoproteins and polysaccharides are increased, and that of albumin is decreased. Among the gamma globulins, the concentration of gamma-1-A has been reported to be disproportionately high.[89] Interestingly, plasma volume appears to be increased, which may account, at least in part, for the apparent mild or moderate anemia frequently encountered in this disease.[117]

A new contribution of the laboratory to the study of patients with rheumatic fever may come from the field of *anti-heart antibodies*.[21a,95] In a "blind" study, these antibodies were present in 63 per cent of patients with carditis but in only 26 per cent of patients without carditis.[88] Their titer has been reported to be higher in patients with rheumatic fever than in patients with uncomplicated streptococcal infections.[196a] Studies of *intracellular enzymes* which leak from the damaged myocardium into the serum, so useful in the diagnosis of myocardial infarction, have been disappointing so far in rheumatic fever. An initial report pointed out the frequent elevation of serum glutamic oxaloacetic transaminase (SGOT) in patients with rheumatic fever.[133] It has since been found that the administration of aspirin frequently causes an increase in the concentration of this enzyme in the serum,[47,118] thus decreasing the potential diagnostic usefulness of this test and possibly discouraging further studies.

Abnormal urinary metabolites, 5-methoxytryptamine[80] and vanillacetic acid[33] have been reported in rheumatic fever patients, and the ability of the erythrocytes of rheumatic fever patients to deaminate 5-methoxytryptamine has been reported to be deficient.[81] These interesting findings await confirmation and interpretation.

NOSOLOGY

The main historical function of the term "rheumatic fever" has been the conceptual separation of the various manifestations that go under its name (carditis, arthritis, chorea, etc.) from those of rheumatoid arthritis, gout, and other diseases affecting the joints. The nosologic distinctions among these disease entities are now undisputed and clear-cut, although the differential diagnosis in individual instances may not be so (see below under *Diagnosis*). Since the manifestations of rheumatic fever are heterogeneous and may occur in isolated fashion, one may question the continuing usefulness of the comprehensive term "rheumatic fever."[56,64,173] As expounded below (under *Diagnosis*) the collective term "rheumatic fever" should always be qualified by specifying the clinical manifestations detected during the attack. With this proviso, the term rheumatic fever still fulfills a useful function and should be retained, because it reminds the physician that these disparate clinical manifestations not only have a common etiology but occur concomitantly or in close succession with great frequency.

Distinction of Rheumatic Fever from Other Post-Streptococcal Diseases

Although rheumatic fever is defined as a post-streptococcal sequela, it is distinct from other diseases which also follow streptococcal infections, because they very seldom occur concomitantly. Thus, glomerulonephritis was considered a different disease from rheumatic fever even before it became known that most cases follow infection with only a few "nephritogenic" strains, while rheumatic fever seems to occur after infection with any type of group A streptococci. The reason for this nosologic distinction was the rarity of the concomitance of rheumatic fever and glomerulonephritis.[6] The same reason is valid for the nosologic distinction of erythema nodosum, Schönlein-Henoch purpura and scleredema adultorum from rheumatic fever. In addition, their streptococcal etiology is not well established.[25,105,184]

Distinction of Rheumatic Fever from Its Cause and Its Sequelae

Since rheumatic fever follows pharyngitis, the latter has sometimes been considered a part of the former, but should be distinguished from it, because only a small minority of pharyngitides are followed by rheumatic fever. Although it is possible that some of the sore throats which occasionally *coincide* with the onset of rheumatic fever are a manifestation of it, rather than of a streptococcal or viral infection,[143] the evidence is inconclusive and it is safer not to include pharyngitis in the clinical picture of rheumatic fever *per se*. A distinction should also be made between rheumatic fever and its own sequelae, which are structural alterations of the heart, mainly of its valves, with little or no evidence of residual inflammation. This distinction is usually clear-cut, in which case the term "inactive rheumatic heart disease" should be applied to the sequela, but it is occasionally difficult to make.[176]

Rheumatic Fever as an Acute and as a Chronic Disease

Rheumatic fever has been defined either way. Originally, attention was attracted by the joint manifestations, which are undeniably acute and transient —hence the name "acute rheumatic fever." Later, emphasis shifted to the cardiac lesions, which are often permanent, and to the frequency of recurrences, which, before prophylaxis, was high indeed. Moreover, the relation of the recurrences to intercurrent streptococcal infections was not known, so that the recurrences were often interpreted as spontaneous exacerbations of a continuous, simmering, subclinical process. For all these reasons rheumatic fever was redefined as a chronic disease. Recently, the use of prophylaxis has curtailed recurrences. More importantly, the necessary role of streptococcal infections in initiating recurrences as well as first attacks of the disease has been recognized. Partly as a result of these developments, rheumatic fever is not generally considered a chronic disease nowadays, with the following provisos: patients who have had rheumatic fever, and especially those with residual cardiac damage, are left with a "chronic" enhanced tendency to develop rheumatic fever after a streptococcal infection; patients with rheumatic heart disease have "chronic" disabilities and permanent structural alterations (both of which may improve or worsen with time); and a small minority of patients, especially after repeated acute attacks, may go on to develop inflammatory rheumatic manifestations of a duration much greater than the usual.[176] With the exception of the latter group of patients, who may appropriately be termed "chronic," the best name for the disease is plain "rheumatic fever," without the adjective "acute" before it, because even in uncomplicated first attacks the disease lasts a month or more and the manifestations may have, especially in the case of carditis, a subacute course.

Distinctions within the Rheumatic Fever Syndrome

The manifestations of rheumatic fever are disparate. Rheumatic polyarthritis is a regularly benign disorder which leaves behind no structural alteration; when it occurs alone, some suggest calling it "post-streptococcal arthritis" rather than rheumatic fever.[39a,64] In favor of this proposal it may be noted that the term rheumatic fever, in the past, was often thought synonymous with serious cardiac crippling. This misunderstanding may still occur, and therefore the term rheumatic fever may disturb the patient unnecessarily. As detailed below, the diagnosis of rheumatic fever should be always accompanied by the diagnosis of the individual manifestations, and if this is done and the terms are explained to the patients, no unnecessary worry will be caused and the useful collective term of rheumatic fever can be retained.

DIAGNOSIS

The diagnosis of rheumatic fever, like that of any other disease, is based on a thorough and critical analysis of the history, physical examination and laboratory data. Unlike other diseases, however, rheumatic fever has no single clinical or laboratory manifestation which is sufficiently typical to "make the diagnosis." Therefore, reliance has been placed on particular *combinations* of disease manifestations.*

The diagnosis of rheumatic fever, unlike most other diagnoses, covers a wide variety of cases with manifestations which differ not only in degree, but also in kind. The diagnosis of pneumonia applies only to patients with an inflammation of the lungs. The diagnosis of rheumatic fever applies just as well to a patient with isolated carditis as to a patient with isolated polyarthritis, but the difference between the two patients is remarkable. Therefore, the diagnosis of rheumatic fever has little meaning if not supplemented by the diagnosis of the specific manifestations present. In the case of carditis, mention of the specific valvular lesion, and especially of cardiomegaly and of heart failure, if present, adds to the usefulness of the diagnosis.

The diagnostic criteria originally proposed by Jones[92] and subsequently modified[152] and revised[167] (Table 44–5) have proved valuable. They are designed to establish the diagnosis in patients during the acute stage of rheumatic fever, not the diagnosis of inactive rheumatic heart disease.

The manifestations of the disease have been classified as major and minor on the basis of their diagnostic usefulness only, not on the basis of severity. The *major* manifestations are clinical: carditis, polyarthritis, chorea, erythema marginatum and subcutaneous nodules. The *minor* criteria may be clinical: previous rheumatic fever, arthralgia and fever; or they may be laboratory manifestations: acute phase reactions (*i.e.* elevated erythrocyte sedimentation rate, positive CRP test result, or leukocytosis) and a prolonged P-R interval. In addition, in the last revision of the criteria[167] supporting evidence of preceding streptococcal infection (increased ASO or other streptococcal antibodies; positive throat culture for group A streptococcus; recent scarlet fever) fulfills a unique confirmatory role.

The presence of two major manifestations, or of one major and two minor manifestations, indicates with a high probability that the disease considered is rheumatic fever, if a preceding streptococcal infection can be demonstrated. If it cannot, the diagnosis remains dubious, except in chorea† and possibly in carditis.

* It has been pointed out that medical diagnoses are either tautologies, *i.e.*, restatements in new words of facts already known, or hypotheses, *i.e.*, interpretative assumptions susceptible to disproof.[194] The clinical diagnosis of rheumatic fever partakes of both definitions, but, although it can be confirmed by residual rheumatic heart disease clinically and by Aschoff bodies pathologically, it is not disproved by the absence of either (see under *Sequelae;* see pathologic section in ref. 176). The only "disproof" of a clinical diagnosis of rheumatic fever made according to the criteria outlined above is the appearance of features typical of another disease, which must be able to encompass the features originally thought due to rheumatic fever.[59,176] Most studies of diagnosis, however, have ignored this problem and have concentrated on a "first-level" or tautologic confirmation of diagnosis, *i.e.*, on the question whether the diagnosis made met academically approved clinical criteria.

† It should be noted that in the case of chorea other major and minor manifestations may be absent. Such cases of "pure" chorea, on the basis of the evidence discussed above (under *Chorea*) are probably post-streptococcal and rheumatic. I believe they should be diagnosed as "rheumatic fever—chorea only."

Table 44-5.—Jones Criteria (Revised) for Guidance in the Diagnosis of Rheumatic Fever*

MAJOR MANIFESTATIONS	MINOR MANIFESTATIONS
Carditis	Clinical
Polyarthritis	Fever
Chorea	Arthralgia
Erythema marginatum	Previous rheumatic fever or rheumatic heart disease
Subcutaneous nodules	
	Laboratory
	Erythrocyte sedimentation rate, C-reactive protein, Leukocytosis
	Prolonged P-R interval

PLUS

Supporting evidence of preceding streptococcal infection (increased ASO or other streptococcal antibodies; positive throat culture for Group A streptococcus; recent scarlet fever).

The presence of two major criteria, or of one major and two minor criteria, indicates a high probability of the presence of rheumatic fever if supported by evidence of a preceding streptococcal infection. The absence of the latter should make the diagnosis suspect, except in situations in which rheumatic fever is first discovered after a long latent period from the antecedent infection (*e.g.*, Sydenham's chorea or low-grade carditis).

* Courtesy of the American Heart Association.

The individual clinical manifestations have been described in detail under *Natural History*, and only diagnostically useful aspects will be reviewed here, following the Jones criteria and commenting on them on the basis of experience with errors in diagnosis.[59]

Carditis is almost always associated with one or more *significant* (*organic*) *murmurs*. In a patient without pre-existing heart disease, carditis is diagnosed essentially on the basis of a significant apical systolic murmur, an apical mid-diastolic murmur, or a basal diastolic murmur. In a patient with pre-existing heart disease, carditis may be diagnosed on the basis of the appearance of a new murmur, or of a "definite change in character" of any of the pre-existing murmurs. (The latter is hard to define exactly and its evaluation is difficult. Skepticism should be encouraged in its evaluation.)

Both over-diagnosis[182] and under-diagnosis[51] may result from faulty auscultation. The aortic diastolic murmur is notoriously easy to miss, and good training of the ear under supervision is essential to learn to detect it. Over-diagnosis is less commonly a problem (although it apparently occurred in one of the centers cooperating in a study[182]). It will be avoided by remembering that this typical high-pitched, decrescendo murmur starts at the end of the second sound and has a definite *duration*. Over-diagnosis is more commonly the result of auscultation at the apex. Physiologic third heart sounds may be mistaken for mid-diastolic murmurs. Differentiation of the two rests mainly on the perceptible *duration* of the latter. Functional systolic murmurs may be mistaken for the organic systolic murmur of mitral regurgitation, especially when their loudness is increased by fever or anemia. Most functional murmurs are heard best along the left sternal border, in the third or second interspace (Still's murmurs, innocent ejection-type murmurs); they are limited to the first two-thirds of systole and tend to have a mid-systolic accentuation. Their pitch is generally low and they lack the "blowing" or "steam-jet" quality of mitral regurgitation murmurs. Some functional murmurs have a "groaning" or "twanging-string" quality; they are often heard better along the lower left sternal margin or between it and the apex.

Other manifestations of carditis are cardiomegaly, congestive failure and pericarditis. When they are caused by rheumatic fever, murmurs are also present, so that the diagnosis does not depend on them. Exceptions should be noted when marked tachycardia interferes with auscultation, when a loud pericardial rub temporarily masks a murmur, or a pericardial effusion dampens it, and in rare cases of pericarditis without residual murmurs, as well as in exceptional cases of severe heart failure.

Over-diagnosis of enlargement of the heart is common, and may result from comparison of films taken in different phases of respiration, and from misinterpretation of the slight curvature of the barium-filled esophagus as evidence of left atrial enlargement.[56] The tachypnea of salicylate toxicity may be mistaken for the dyspnea of *cardiac failure*, but the former is not aggravated by lying down. Over-diagnosis of *pericarditis* may result from faulty ECG interpretations, since inverted T waves in the right precordial leads, normal in children and adolescents,[198] may be mistaken as evidence of pericarditis.

"*Polyarthritis*" is a term that should be restricted to cases with objective evidence of inflammation such as swelling, heat, and redness, or at least spot tenderness or limitation of motion (when only the last two are present the term "tender polyarthralgia" is sometimes used). When such evidence is lacking and joint pains are present, the term "polyarthralgia" is more appropriate. Both symptoms and signs must be localized to the joint proper to avoid confusion with myalgia, tendonitis, or bursitis. When one joint only is involved the prefix mono- should be substituted for poly-.

Chorea must be differentiated from normal hyperactivity and from "tics." The latter are stereotyped, localized, repetitive movements.

Subcutaneous nodules must be differentiated from enlarged lymph nodes (especially in rubella). *Erythema marginatum* may be confused with *cutis marmorata*, which is a fixed, reticular, bluish discoloration of the skin.

Among the minor criteria, *the history of previous rheumatic fever* or *pre-existing rheumatic heart disease* increases the index of suspicion in evaluating any manifestation. The history must be well documented, or the evidence of pre-existing heart disease clear-cut (the latter means that the patient must have been examined before, or that the cardiac lesions present are of the kind that cannot develop during an acute attack: mitral stenosis or aortic stenosis). *Fever* should be considered present only when the rectal temperature exceeds 100.4° F (38° C). In evaluating the acute phase reactants, one should be mindful that the ESR may be elevated in anemia;[193] the CRP may be a consequence of congestive heart failure *per se*;[48] and leukocytosis may be caused by steroid administration.[66]

According to the revised Jones criteria, ASO titers of at least 250 units in adults and 333 units in children over five years are considered to be increased and indicative of a recent streptococcal infection.[167] One should be aware that, depending on the general prevalence of streptococcal infections, a varying percentage of the normal population or of patients with unrelated diseases may show titers of this magnitude. As indicated above under *Clinical Pathology*, non-specific ASO elevations may occur, but seldom cause diagnostic problems.

DIFFERENTIAL DIAGNOSIS

The diagnosis of rheumatic fever is usually direct, but a significant minority of patients present differential diagnostic problems because their combination of symptoms, signs and historical data suggest at the same time rheumatic fever and one or more other diseases.[59,83] Such differential diagnoses run the gamut from the commonplace (rheumatic fever *vs.* rheumatoid arthritis) to the esoteric (rheumatic fever *vs.* berylliosis).

Rheumatoid Arthritis

This is more common in adults, and starts most commonly in middle age, while rheumatic fever is more common in children. "Morning stiffness" is a feature of rheumatoid arthritis but not of rheumatic fever. The onset is almost always sudden in the arthritis of rheumatic fever, while it is usually less so in rheumatoid arthritis. Involvement of the small joints, especially if exclusive, and symmetrical arthritis favor rheumatoid arthritis. Arthritis of the neck and of the temporomandibular joints is rare in rheumatic fever but not in rheumatoid arthritis. Given the same objective evidence of inflammation, the arthritis of rheumatic fever may be more acutely painful than that of rheumatoid arthritis.

A salmon pink, maculopapular rash is indicative of juvenile rheumatoid arthritis,[69] while erythema marginatum is indicative of rheumatic fever. In an adult with arthritis, the presence of nodules favors rheumatoid arthritis; in a child, it favors rheumatic fever.[119] However, nodules do occur in juvenile rheumatoid arthritis and are identical histologically with those of rheumatic fever.[24] (*See also* Chapter 24.)

Organic systolic murmurs or diastolic murmurs are strongly suggestive of rheumatic fever and can be diagnostic of it if one can be sure that they are of recent origin and that bacterial endocarditis is ruled out. Pericarditis may occur in either disease but is more frequently diagnosed clinically in rheumatic fever; gallop rhythm, tachycardia out of proportion to fever, and signs of congestive heart failure all point to rheumatic fever. Even in the absence of clinical carditis a prolonged P-R interval favors the diagnosis of rheumatic fever; so do electrocardiographic abnormalities in general.

A period of high fever without any localizing sign and persisting for weeks or even for more than a month may occur in juvenile rheumatoid arthritis, but not in rheumatic fever. The fever of juvenile rheumatoid arthritis tends to have wide swings; and the variations in temperature do not correlate with the ESR while they do in rheumatic fever.[111]

Acute phase reactants are more regularly altered in the arthritis of rheumatic fever than in that of early rheumatoid arthritis. Elevation of streptococcal antibody titers favors the diagnosis of rheumatic fever, especially in the adult, but one should be mindful that streptococcal infections are frequent, especially in the young (28 per cent of patients with *juvenile* rheumatoid arthritis may have elevated ASO titers).[151] More importantly, the exclusion of a recent streptococcal infection by a battery of streptococcal antibody tests virtually rules out the diagnosis of rheumatic fever in the presence of arthritis. A reliable test for rheumatoid factor is almost never positive in rheumatic fever, but will be positive in rheumatoid arthritis in direct proportion to the sensitivity of the method used.[180]

After the first few weeks of disease, the diagnosis becomes easier because of the tendency of rheumatoid arthritis to persist and of rheumatic polyarthritis to vanish. Rheumatoid nodules also tend to persist longer than rheumatic nodules and the incidence of positive results of rheumatoid factor tests increases with the passage of time in rheumatoid arthritis. Diagnostic doubts, however, will persist in some cases, especially in adults. (*See also* Chapters 24 and 25.)

Systemic Lupus Erythematosus (SLE)

This disease is uncommon in the pediatric age group, in which most first attacks of rheumatic fever occur. Onset of the disease after exposure to sunlight, during the first three months after a delivery or after the administration of a drug, suggests SLE; history of a preceding sore throat favors rheumatic fever.

A butterfly rash is typical of SLE: nephritis points strongly to this disease, while the appearance of organic murmurs suggests rheumatic fever. As usual, elevated antistreptococcal antibody titers favor the diagnosis of rheumatic fever and, more importantly, the absence of any serologic evidence of a recent streptococcal infection practically rules out this diagnosis in the presence of arthritis. A positive reaction to an LE cell test or antinuclear antibody test will be given by most patients with SLE. Serum complement is often low in this disease (even in the absence of nephritis) while it is usually elevated in rheumatic fever.

One should be mindful that chorea has been reported in association with SLE[4,27] but mostly during "active" stages of the latter disease. (*See also* Chapter 51.)

Serum Sickness

Serum sickness is accompanied by arthralgias and arthritis in a high percentage of cases, but definite articular effusion is uncommon. Historical data may provide clues (especially a history of administration of animal serum, but a serum-sickness type of reaction may also follow penicillin administration). However, when penicillin is given to treat a streptococcal pharyngitis, the history becomes thoroughly confusing. Urticarial and other pruritic rashes point to serum sickness; erythema marginatum, subcutaneous nodules, and chorea point to rheumatic fever. Although ECG abnormalities may occur in serum sickness, murmurs do not develop. The laboratory may help in ruling out a preceding streptococcal infection by means of streptococcal antibody determinations (this would virtually exclude rheumatic fever); or by demonstrating heterophile antibodies (distinguishable from those of infectious mononucleosis by differential absorption), skin sensitizing antibodies or eosinophilia (all of which would point to serum sickness). (*See also* Chapter 52.)

Subacute Bacterial Endocarditis (SBE)

Subacute bacterial endocarditis must be considered whenever a patient with rheumatic heart disease develops an unexplained fever lasting longer than a few days, and this diagnostic hypothesis must be tested with repeated blood cultures. Arthritis of one or more joints occurs frequently in children with SBE[46] and may thus mimic rheumatic fever. Lack of response of fever to aspirin is exceptional in rheumatic fever but common in SBE. The appearance of petechiae, Osler's nodes, microscopic hematuria or splenomegaly favor strongly this diagnosis, but are often late manifestations. Earlobe histiocytosis[75] and positive results of rheumatoid factor tests[190] are frequent in SBE and may be diagnostically useful.

Infectious Arthritis

This may be polyarticular. It does not respond to salicylate treatment. Purulent synovial fluid and demonstration of the causative organism by gram-staining and by culture are diagnostic. Thayer-Martin plates should be included among the culturing media whenever gonococcal arthritis is suspected. History, examination of urethral secretions and fluorescent antibody tests may be useful in the latter case.

Osteomyelitis

Osteomyelitis has occasionally been misdiagnosed as rheumatic fever. Radiology is of no help in the first week or ten days of the disease, but resistance to salicylate therapy and persistent monoarticular location are early warning signs for this diagnosis.

Rubella Arthritis

Rubella arthritis must be considered, especially in women, if arthritis is preceded by a macular skin rash and accompanied by retrocervical and suboccipital adenopathy.[94] Virus neutralization tests and streptococcal antibody tests may be useful in dubious cases. Arthritis may also follow rubella vaccination. (*See* Chapter 68.)

Sarcoidosis

Sarcoidosis in its acute, early phase can be manifested (especially in young women) by erythema nodosum and polyarthritis.[131] This combination has occasionally been misdiagnosed as rheumatic fever. Chest x-rays usually show enlarged lymph nodes in the perihilar region, and the arthritis is not very sensitive to salicylates.[107] (*See also* Chapter 70.)

Sickle-Cell Anemia

This may cause diagnostic confusion in a patient wholly or partly Negro, because of joint pains, fever and heart murmurs (not only systolic but also apical mid-diastolic). The sedimentation rate is usually elevated in rheumatic fever, but not in sickle-cell anemia. A sickle-cell preparation should be part of the laboratory work-up of such doubtful cases. The coexistence of sickle-cell disease and rheumatic fever can be particularly confusing.[5] (*See* Chapter 71.)

Gout

This rarely causes diagnostic confusion with rheumatic fever because the first attack is typically monoarticular. Serum uric acid determinations and examination of the synovial fluid by polarized light to reveal negatively birefringent crystals are most useful in questionable cases. Family history is often positive in gout. The arthritis responds to colchicine administration. (*See* Chapter 59.)

Poliomyelitis

Poliomyelitis, non- or pre-paralytic, may cause diagnostic confusion because of limb pains and fever. No true arthritis is detectable, however. Signs of meningeal irritation and pleocytosis of the cerebral spinal fluid are diagnostically useful.

Rheumatic-like Subcutaneous Nodules

These nodules constitute an entity which is probably distinct from rheumatic fever.[172] This diagnosis should be made in children who present with nodules clinically and histopathologically indistinguishable from those of rheumatic fever and rheumatoid arthritis, but with no other evidence of either.

Miscellaneous

Less common differential diagnoses have been discussed elsewhere, as follows: brucellosis;[139] cat-scratch fever;[108] meningococcemia;[39] miliary tuberculosis;[63] ascariasis;[45] juvenile hyperparathyroidism;[16] Weber-Christian panniculitis;[20] Hodgkin's disease;[136] berylliosis[161] and "irritable hip syndrome."[28]

TREATMENT

The treatment of rheumatic fever is unsatisfactory because the most important manifestation, carditis, is the most resistant to therapy. Nevertheless, a number of measures may contribute to the patient's well-being. They fall under the headings of general measures, and of anti-streptococcal, anti-inflammatory, and cardiotonic medication. Chorea presents its own therapeutic problems which will be discussed separately.

General Measures

Patients with rheumatic fever may be treated at home, if adequate family nursing is available, or in the hospital. In either case the patient should be examined daily by a physician during the first two or three weeks to ascertain whether carditis develops and to provide prompt treatment should heart failure appear. After the first two or three weeks of illness fewer new cases of carditis develop and the need for daily supervision diminishes.

Recommendations for physical activity have varied whimsically from one extreme (bed rest for months or years even in patients without carditis) to the other (ambulation within forty-eight hours even in patients with carditis).[70] The former regimen has no rational basis. Moreover, it engenders cardiac neurosis and physical wasting in the patients, and overprotectiveness in their parents. The latter regimen may well precipitate cardiac failure in patients with carditis, and has little to recommend it in a disease which is not frequently attended by thromboembolic complications. In patients treated with prednisone, a controlled study showed no greater incidence of residual cardiac damage in patients allowed full in-hospital activity soon after normalization of the ESR than in patients kept at bed rest throughout the 12 weeks of prednisone therapy.[77a] The following recommendations seem reasonable to me (Table 44–6).

All patients should be in bed for the first three weeks of illness, because carditis is present in some and may appear in others. However, strict bed rest (*i.e.* without bathroom privileges) should be limited to patients with arthritis of the lower limbs and to those with carditis and cardiomegaly. After this initial period of observation the bed rest regimen should be tailored to the manifestations of the disease.

Patients with *polyarthritis* have no joint symptoms as a rule after the first three weeks. If they have no evidence of carditis, they may be allowed out of bed, even if they are receiving aspirin. Rebounds may occur after discontinuation of therapy and may make bed rest necessary again, but in these patients the rebounds will not involve the heart.

Patients with *carditis* evidenced by *significant murmurs* but *no definite cardiac enlargement* and *no heart failure* should be kept in bed for a month. The bed rest need not be strict, however, and in the last several weeks it may be mitigated by a period of well-supervised ambulation

Table 44-6.—Suggested Schedule of Bed Rest and Physical Activity in Rheumatic Fever

No Carditis	Carditis, but *no* cardiomegaly and *no* heart failure	Carditis, *with* cardiomegaly but *no* failure	Carditis, *with* cardiomegaly *and* heart failure
Bed rest for three weeks; then gradual ambulation (even if on aspirin).	Bed rest for a month after carditis is detected; then gradual ambulation (even if on aspirin).	Strict bed rest first two weeks after detection of cardiomegaly; then modified bed rest for four weeks; then gradual ambulation (even if on treatment); modified bed rest again during the "rebound period" (first two weeks after cessation of treatment); then, gradual ambulation.	Strict bed rest as long as heart failure is present; if failure is severe, patient should be washed and fed by aides; after subsidence or control of failure, modified bed rest until a month after cessation of treatment if no rebound ensues; or until two weeks after spontaneous subsidence of rebound; then, gradual ambulation.

for a few hours a day. Patients with *carditis and cardiomegaly but no congestive failure* should be kept on bed rest for the first month and a half, mitigated by bathroom privileges for the final four weeks. Cautious ambulation within the ward or the room may be started at this time, but should be stopped again during the first two weeks after cessation of therapy because of the possibility of a rebound affecting the heart. After this "rebound" period is passed, gradual ambulation can be resumed.

Patients with *congestive heart failure* should be on strict bed rest as long as this complication lasts and, if the failure is severe, should be fed and washed by aides. After subsidence of failure or control of it by cardiotonic medication, these patients may be allowed bathroom privileges, but should otherwise be kept in bed until a month after treatment is stopped if no rebound ensues, or until two weeks after the spontaneous subsidence of a rebound. Only then should they be gradually allowed up, starting with two or three half-hour periods on a chair each day.

Pericarditis per se does not need an especially strict regimen. If failure is not present, patients with pericarditis should be handled like the patients with cardiomegaly, essentially because it is difficult to rule out enlargement of the heart in the presence of pericardial effusion. *Persistently elevated* ESR occurs in some patients in the absence of any other clinical or laboratory manifestation of activity,[85,176] and does not need special treatment.

A month after treatment has been stopped, or two weeks after spontaneous subsidence of a post-therapeutic rebound, most patients can return to their normal lives. Patients without heart disease should not be restricted in their physical activities in any way. *This should be made clear to the patients or to their parents and to school authorities, who are likely to believe that all patients with rheumatic fever are left with a "rheumatic heart" and should not exert themselves.* Patients who are left with rheumatic heart disease but no heart enlargement should be allowed normal physical activities, but should be limited in their competitive sports. Patients with heart enlargement often have diminished cardiac reserve or are in chronic overt cardiac failure. In these patients physical activities should be limited in such a way as to eliminate or minimize symptoms. Patients with normal cardiac reserve should be allowed normal activities but no competitive sports.

Antistreptococcal Treatment

It has become customary in many centers to administer an "eradicating dose" of penicillin (see section on *Prophylaxis*) to all patients with rheumatic fever as soon as the diagnosis is made, even if the throat culture is negative for group A streptococci. No controlled study has shown the efficacy of this regimen in ameliorating the course of rheumatic fever, yet this procedure is logical and innocuous enough to be recommended, at least as a protection for other patients on the ward. Patients with rheumatic fever are, by definition, convalescent from a streptococcal pharyngitis and it is known that the offending organisms may linger in the throat for months, and that they may not be detected by an occasional throat culture. An exception to this recommendation should be noted if SBE is a diagnostic possibility, in which case the administration of the streptococcal eradicating dose may mask temporarily the manifestations of SBE and thus delay the diagnosis.

Continual antistreptococcal prophylaxis should be started immediately after the "eradicating course," as detailed in the section on *Prevention*. It should be noted that some cases of apparently "chronic" rheumatic fever have been shown to be associated with inapparent intercurrent hospital infections with beta-hemolytic streptococci.[176]

The administration of courses of penicillin more intensive and longer than the usual "eradicating" ones has been advocated. This is based on the rationale that: (1) the persistence of streptococci, perhaps in the heart, may be the mechanism of tissue damage in rheumatic carditis (see section on *Pathogenesis* in the preceding chapter) and (2) these persisting streptococci may need a particularly intensive treatment for their eradication.

A clinical study was made of the effect of the administration of 48-million units of penicillin over a six-week period in children with rheumatic fever as compared with a control group which received no penicillin. There was no difference in the duration of the attack between the two groups. At follow-up one year later, the penicillin group had a somewhat lower incidence of heart disease, but this was limited to patients having "unfixed valvulitis," *i.e.*, auscultatory findings changing from significant murmurs to insignificant or to no murmurs and vice-versa during the acute attack.[129] Further studies of this therapeutic regimen have failed to confirm the original findings.[30,183a] If no better evidence is presented in their favor, there seems to be little point in administering these "larger-than-eradicating" courses in other than experimental situations.

Anti-inflammatory Treatment

Many manifestations of the disease disappear with salicylate or steroid therapy faster than without treatment, but the incidence of residual heart disease seems unaffected by treatment. Most clinicians have the impression that mortality during the acute attack is decreased by steroids, but this impression is still unsupported by a well-controlled clinical trial. Cessation of treatment is sometimes followed by reappearance of manifestations of the disease; these tend to be most frequent and severe after treatment schedules which are most effective in suppressing inflammation.

It is often stated that anti-inflammatory therapy does not shorten the duration of the disease or of "rheumatic activity." However, when the course of the disease has been compared in treated and in untreated patients, it has been shown that arthritis, fever and acute phase reactants disappear faster in the patients treated with steroids, or even only with aspirin, than in the untreated controls.[44,90] Therefore the *actual* duration of these manifestations of illness is indeed reduced by treatment. What is meant appears to be something else, namely that manifestations of illness may reappear if treatment is stopped before the time the attack would have ended spontaneously, *i.e.*, in the absence of treatment. It is this *potential* duration, dependent on discontinuation of therapy, which seems to be unaffected by treatment. Unfortunately it is impossible to be certain that the disease is "potentially" terminated as long as anti-inflammatory medication is administered. Therefore, in some studies the disease is assumed to continue during the period of suppressive medication, and it is considered ended only after spontaneous subsidence of post-therapeutic rebounds, or at the termination of therapy not followed by rebounds.[55] According to this definition, of course, medication can only prolong the disease, and, if one elected to continue medication indefinitely, the "duration" of the disease would stretch indefinitely also.

It is important to realize that this "duration" is potential, and largely assumed; it thus differs from the actual duration of illness measured by the length of time in which manifestations are present. Due to the reappearance of manifestations after cessation of therapy, the actual duration sometimes results from the summation of two periods, before and after therapy.

Claims have been made that very large doses of *salicylates* have a truly curative effect on rheumatic carditis.[35] These claims have never been substantiated, and because of the risk of mortality involved in such massive treatment[170] (see also under *Fever* above) most authors have used moderate or small doses in recent years.

In high doses sodium salicylate or aspirin causes tinnitus and hyperventilation. The latter may be mistaken for the dyspnea of heart failure, but can be distinguished from it because the patient appears to be comfortable in a horizontal position. There are some observations which suggest a possible deleterious effect of aspirin on cardiac failure,[26] which may be mediated by an increase of oxygen consumption.[1] Further studies are needed to confirm these observations.

Steroids achieve the same therapeutic results as aspirin, only faster, more completely and more dangerously. In controlled trials of aspirin versus steroids in groups of comparable patients, steroids have generally reduced arthritis, fever and ESR at a faster rate than aspirin (Figs. 44–15, 44–16 and 44–17) and the suppression of these manifestations has been more complete.[44,181] Even subcutaneous nodules, which present a productive rather than an exudative type of inflammatory reaction and are thus similar to the myocardial Aschoff bodies,

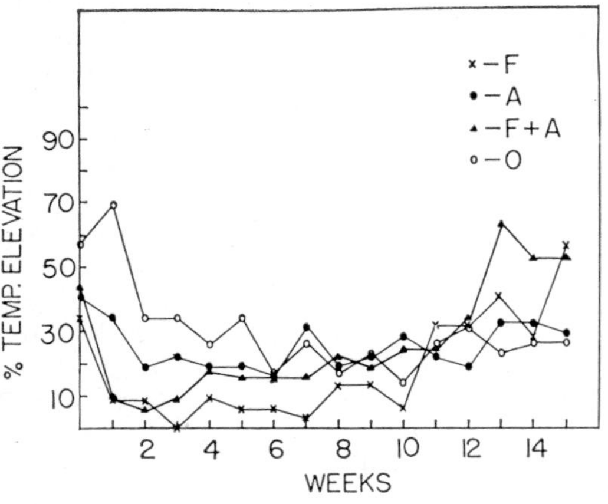

Fig. 44–15.—Percentage of patients with fever (38° C. or higher) among patients with rheumatic fever, untreated (O) and treated with aspirin (A) hydrocortisone (F) and aspirin and hydrocortisone (F + A). Hydrocortisone was given for eight weeks at full doses, then decreased stepwise for the following four weeks. Aspirin was given for nine weeks and then decreased stepwise. The observations started 9.4 (± 4.6) days after onset of the disease. The same explanations apply to the following figure. (Dorfman *et al.*, courtesy of Pediatrics.)

seem to disappear faster in patients treated with steroids than in patients given aspirin, and to appear more frequently in patients given aspirin than in those treated with steroids;[90,119,181] and there are a few observations which suggest that the Aschoff bodies themselves or at least their cellular inflammatory components may be made to disappear with steroid hormones.[149,176] Because of these observations, and also because inflammation has been traditionally considered to play a deleterious role in rheumatic fever, the expectation was widespread that suppression of inflammation by means of steroids would lessen the deleterious consequences of rheumatic fever, namely residual heart disease and mortality during the acute attack. These expectations, as detailed below, have been largely frustrated, the former more definitively than the latter.

A possible inference to be drawn from this failure is that inflammation in rheumatic fever is not deleterious but rather is indifferent or useful. It may be a reparatory reaction to a primary tissue damage which is not caused by inflammation, but instead causes it (see under *Pathogenesis* in the preceding chapter). This primary tissue damage, unlike the subsequent inflammation, may not be prevented or ameliorated by steroids. It is pertinent to recall that inflammatory changes are prominent in the histopathology of pneumococcal pneumonia, but their suppression by corticosteroids can hardly be called helpful.

The studies on the therapeutic effect of steroids in rheumatic fever can be aptly divided into "those done with enthusiasm but no controls and those with controls and no enthusiasm."[23] Only the latter kind will be reviewed here. One of the best therapeutic trials ever designed was the United Kingdom and United States Joint Study, which compared the effect of aspirin, cortisone and ACTH administered for six weeks to patients under sixteen with definite attacks of rheumatic fever. Most of the variables which could influence the outcome were carefully

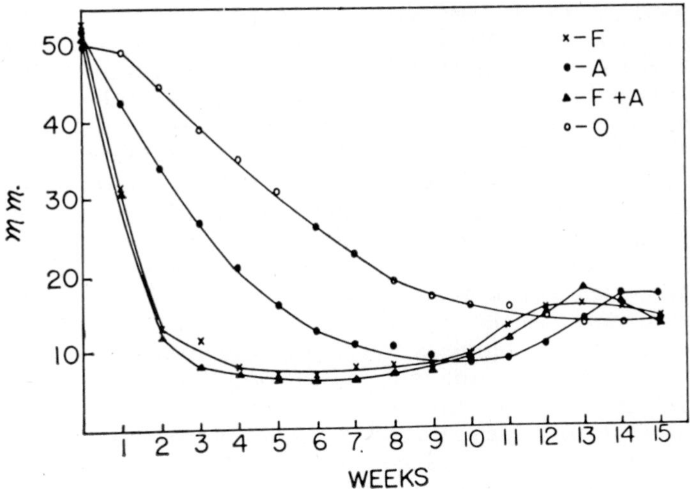

FIG. 44–16.—Average values of the ESR (Wintrobe, uncorrected) in the same groups of patients as in the preceding figure. Notice the slow but steady fall of the ESR in the untreated patients. The ESR fell more rapidly in the group treated with aspirin and even faster in the groups treated with hydrocortisone. All of the treated groups had an elevation of the average ESR after discontinuation of therapy. (Dorfman *et al.*, courtesy of Pediatrics.)

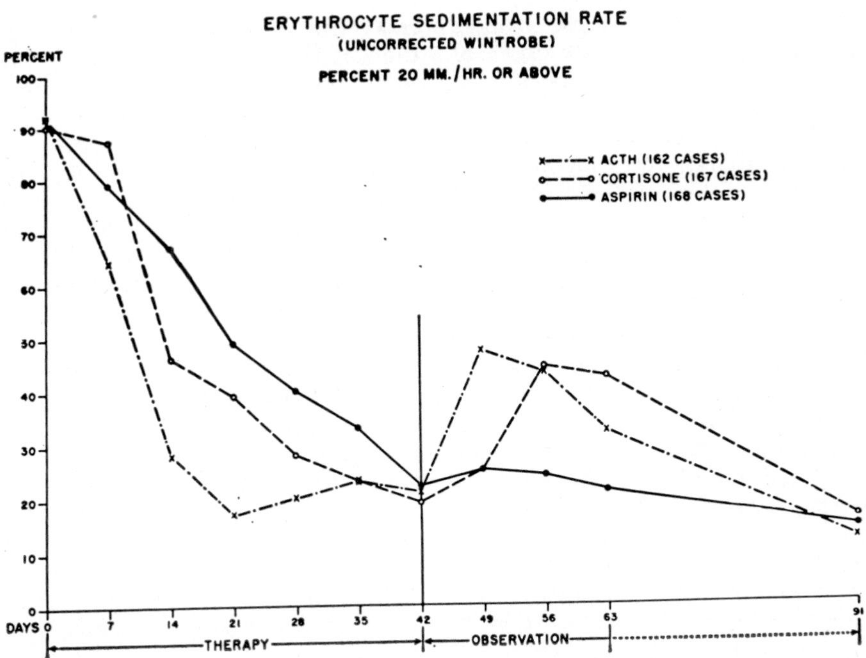

FIG. 44–17.—Per cent of patients with elevated ESR (Wintrobe, uncorrected) in patients with rheumatic fever treated with aspirin, cortisone and ACTH. The ESR "rebounded" much more frequently after the hormones than after aspirin treatment. (From the U.K. and U.S. Joint Report, courtesy of Circulation.)

taken into account (previous attacks, carditis on admission, age, pre-admission interval). The doses of hormones were moderate and amounted to totals of 1,160 U.S.P. units of ACTH and 4,050 mg. of cortisone. After the first week of treatment, fever and arthritis were controlled more completely in the hormone-treated patients, but reappeared in a higher percentage of patients after cessation of therapy than in the aspirin-treated group. More importantly, at the end of one-year,[181] five-year,[182] and ten-year[183] follow-up periods there was no significant difference in the incidence and severity of rheumatic heart disease among the three groups. Harris *et al.* treated a smaller group of patients with similar regimens of hormone therapy and compared the results obtained with those of a control group which received no medication. There was no significant difference in cardiac status between the two groups either during the acute attack[84] or five to eight years later.[66]

Following the results of these studies it was hypothesized that larger doses of hormones given for a longer period of time might be necessary for therapeutic results, and uncontrolled series seemed to support this approach.[76,115] However, a controlled study of first attacks of rheumatic fever with moderate to severe rheumatic carditis and pre-treatment intervals no longer than twenty-eight days did not confirm this hypothesis.[36] Twenty-nine patients allotted to the hormone treatment received 3 grams of prednisone over a twelve-week period. Twenty-eight patients were assigned to aspirin treatment. Four of these were shifted to prednisone because their condition was critical and it was felt that their chances of survival would be better on prednisone, but one of them died. Two of the other three had rheumatic heart disease (RHD) after one year. Of the 28 patients assigned originally to prednisone, 57 per cent had rheumatic heart disease after one year. Of those originally assigned to aspirin, one had died, as mentioned above, and 10 had RHD one year after, for a total of 39 per cent unfavorable results. One patient of the aspirin group was lost to follow-up.

In these calculations the patients transferred from aspirin to prednisone therapy are still considered part of the aspirin group; if they were not, the comparison would be even more favorable to aspirin. The only criticism one can direct to this study is that it was neither continued to include a predetermined number of patients, as in conventional therapeutic trials, nor was it continued until a predetermined level of significance was reached, as in "sequential" analysis. It may thus conceivably have been influenced by a "run of bad luck."

More favorable to the steroid therapy was a report by Dorfman *et al.*,[44] which compared hydrocortisone for twelve weeks to aspirin, to a combination of the two, and to no treatment. A smaller number of patients with residual rheumatic heart disease were found at follow-up in patients treated with hydrocortisone than in those receiving aspirin or nothing. However, the carditis in this series was peculiarly mild (only 2 of the 85 patients with carditis had congestive heart failure; only 26 had diastolic murmurs, and these were more frequent in the aspirin and in the no treatment group). These features make the report difficult to interpret with confidence.

Claims have been advanced that high-dose, short-term steroid treatment is particularly effective in preventing permanent cardiac damage.[192] Recently, the effect of prednisone, 3 mg. per pound per day for a week or two, followed by aspirin for eight weeks, has been compared to the effect of aspirin given for nine weeks.[37] One year later, heart disease was present in 56 per cent of 34 patients initially assigned to the prednisone group. Of 39 patients originally allotted to the aspirin group, 1 died and 3 were transferred to the prednisone group because their condition was critical. It was felt that their chances of survival would be enhanced by prednisone. Including the latter 3 patients as part of the aspirin group, 67 per cent of the aspirin-treated patients had residual heart disease or had died. Although this percentage was 11 per cent higher than in the group treated with prednisone, there were more patients with severe carditis initially in the aspirin group, which may well account for this minor difference.

In summary, the controlled studies of the last twelve years indicate that steroid treatment does not have a definite beneficial effect on residual heart disease. The studies are not sufficiently extensive, detailed and unanimous in their results, however, definitely to rule out the possibility of an ameliorating effect, if not on all patients with rheumatic carditis, then on some special subgroups. The one most likely to be benefited is that of patients with carditis severe enough to threaten the life of the patient during the acute attack. Such patients have usually been shifted from the aspirin to the steroid group, pointing out at the same time the conviction of the investigators that steroids are, in this respect, superior to aspirin, and the difficulty of proving the correctness of this conviction by means of a controlled clinical trial. The superiority of steroids over aspirin in respect to mortality in the acute phase is also suggested by a detailed, but retrospective and not fully controlled, clinical analysis.[38] The overall impression is that one can at least delay, and possibly avert, a lethal outcome by treating with steroids the most severe cases of rheumatic carditis.

If steroids were innocuous, one could endorse their wide use lightheartedly, but they are attended by unpleasant and occasionally deadly complications.[73] The most important of these is decreased resistance to infections, which can transform a regularly benign disease such as chickenpox into a lethal one. Osteoporosis, pathologic fractures, peptic ulcers with consequent G.I. bleeding, and psychosis are all serious complications which occur occasionally. Steroid diabetes is a rare and easily reversible condition. Striae are common and may cause permanent cosmetic damage which may be quite bothersome to women. Rarely may a nodular panniculitis develop *after* steroid therapy is discontinued.[175] All of these complications are related to the intensity and to the duration of steroid administration (*see also* Chapter 31).

I firmly believe that further therapeutic trials, with a finer subdivision of patients according to the initial clinical status, are indicated, since the results obtained in the various studies may have been influenced by clinical heterogeneity of the experimental and control groups, such as by a different percentage of patients with severe carditis (compare ref. 44 and 181). Another point that needs clarification is the natural history of the first few days of the rheumatic fever attack. It is now assumed that therapeutic decisions can be based on the presence or absence of murmurs on the first examination: it is essential to define exactly the percentage of patients who have no carditis at the onset but will develop it later. In the meantime, the following recommendations seem reasonable (Table 44–7).

Patients with mild arthritis or arthralgia and no carditis may be treated with analgesics only, such as codeine or propoxyphene as needed. Two goals will be thus accomplished: (1) The diagnosis may be made more certain by the appearance of definite arthritis in some of the initially questionable cases. This greater diagnostic certainty is useful for an informed decision on prophylaxis; (2) The duration of hospitalization or of close observation at home will be decreased, because many of the patients will get well in two or three weeks; moreover, one will not have to worry about, and deal with, post-therapeutic rebounds.

Patients with moderate or severe arthritis and no carditis, or with carditis, but without failure, will be treated with aspirin, $\frac{2}{3}$ of a grain per pound per day for the first two weeks, and then decreased to $\frac{1}{2}$ grain per pound per day for the following six weeks. In some patients, higher doses, up to $1\frac{1}{4}$ grains per

Table 44-7.—Suggested, Tentative Schedule of Anti-inflammatory Treatment in Rheumatic Fever

Arthralgia or mild arthritis; no carditis	Moderate or severe arthritis; no carditis, or carditis *with or without* cardiomegaly, but without failure	Carditis with failure; with or without joint manifestations
Analgesics only, such as codeine or propoxyphene.	Aspirin, $\frac{2}{3}$ of a grain per pound per day for two weeks; increased if necessary; $\frac{1}{2}$ grain per pound per day for the subsequent 6 weeks.	Prednisone, 40–60 mg. per day; increased if necessary; I.V. methyl prednisolone sodium succinate in fulminating cases; after 2 to 3 weeks, slow withdrawal to be completed in 3 more weeks. Aspirin to be continued for a month after discontinuation of prednisone.

pound per day, may be necessary to control arthritis. Ambulation may be started without waiting for the discontinuation of therapy. With this regimen the discomfort of arthritis is reduced, the fever with its attendant additional demands on the work of the heart is controlled, while toxic drug effects and a high incidence of rebounds are avoided.

Patients with carditis and heart failure should receive prednisone, starting with a dose of 40 to 60 mg. per day, to be increased if control of heart failure is not achieved.

In cases of extreme acuteness and severity, therapy should be started with intravenous administration of methyl prednisolone sodium succinate and may then be continued with oral medication. After two or three weeks of such therapy, prednisone may be slowly withdrawn, at which time aspirin, $\frac{2}{3}$ grain per pound per day, is started. The withdrawal of prednisone may be completed in three more weeks. Aspirin will be continued for one month after cessation of prednisone. This procedure will delay, decrease or prevent rebounds.

Cardiotonic Medication

Heart failure of patients with carditis can often be controlled with steroids alone. If these do not suffice, diuretics may be used first and then digitalis. The reason for this preference is that both acute carditis and digitalis can cause disturbances of cardiac rhythm and it may not be wise to compound these two risks unnecessarily. The therapeutic range of digitalis is reduced in rheumatic carditis, according to the older literature. Although recent data suggest that there are no more instances of digitalis toxicity in "active" than in "inactive" rheumatic heart disease, these data[160] were gathered in a convalescent home and therefore may not have had a representative share of recent rheumatic carditis. In patients with severe congestive failure, however, there may be no time to waste and it may be necessary to use the full therapeutic resources at once. In the presence of dyspnea or cyanosis, oxygen is indicated. Morphine and rotating tourniquets are indicated in pulmonary edema.

Treatment of Chorea

Chorea is likely to disturb patients and their parents because of the clumsiness of body movements, the frustration attending it, and the emotional lability or moodiness. Administration of sedatives or of tranquilizers is moderately effective. Aspirin seems to be totally ineffective. Although steroids have been reported to be successful in the treatment of chorea, the variability and unpredictability of the duration of chorea make these reports difficult to evaluate. Moreover, even if steroids were indeed effective, it would be unwise to use such potentially dangerous agents in any but the most severe cases of chorea.

Rebounds

After anti-inflammatory treatment is stopped, clinical and laboratory manifestations of the disease may reappear, usually fleetingly. These transient episodes, called rebounds or relapses, are more common after steroids than after aspirin (Fig. 44–17). Their appearance late in the course of the rheumatic attack may stretch, so to speak, its total duration over a period longer than in untreated cases (Fig. 44–16). The rebounds or relapses may be *clinical*, and then comprise those manifestations which are most influenced by treatment (fever and arthritis; less commonly carditis, as evidenced by congestive heart failure and occasionally by new murmurs). Clinical rebounds are regularly accompanied by elevation of the ESR, reappearance of a positive CRP test or both. Milder rebounds may be evidenced by *laboratory* tests only, *e.g.*, positive CRP and elevated ESR, without any clinical evidence of disease activity. These milder rebounds, often referred to as "laboratory rebounds," are more common than the clinical rebounds.[57]

Most rebounds occur in the first week after treatment has been stopped, although seldom in the first day or two. This delay may be due to the persistence of the anti-inflammatory drugs or of their effect, but rebounds may occur, with decreasing probability, over a two-month period after cessation of therapy (Fig. 44–18). The later rebounds resemble the spontaneously occurring polycyclic pattern of the disease (see under *Arthritis* above) and may be due to spontaneous fluctuations in inflammatory activity. After two months, manifestations of active disease do not reappear, unless preceded by a streptococcal infection.[166] These then constitute recurrences, rather than spontaneous relapses or rebounds.

The incidence and severity of rebounds may be decreased by using aspirin rather than steroids, by discontinuing these medications gradually rather than abruptly, and by administering aspirin during or after the discontinuation of steroids. Mild clinical rebounds and laboratory rebounds are better left untreated, but severe rebounds, especially in the presence of carditis with heart failure, may necessitate resumption of treatment.[159] Interestingly, rebounds have been provoked experimentally during convalescence of rheumatic fever by the administration of short courses of anti-inflammatory medication.[54]

PREVENTION

In contrast to the dubious effects of therapy, prevention of rheumatic fever *can be* effective. Treatment of streptococcal infections drastically reduces the attack rate of subsequent rheumatic fever, and continual antistreptococcal prophylaxis in patients who have already had the disease cuts down to minimal levels the rate of rheumatic recurrences. Unfortunately, not all streptococcal infections which can lead to rheumatic fever are symptomatic and thus amenable to treatment. Regrettably, the knowledge which has accumulated on preventive techniques is *not* generally applied. The combination of these remediable and irremediable handicaps has impeded thus far the eradication of the disease.

A national outcry[1a,47a,165a,128a] has re-

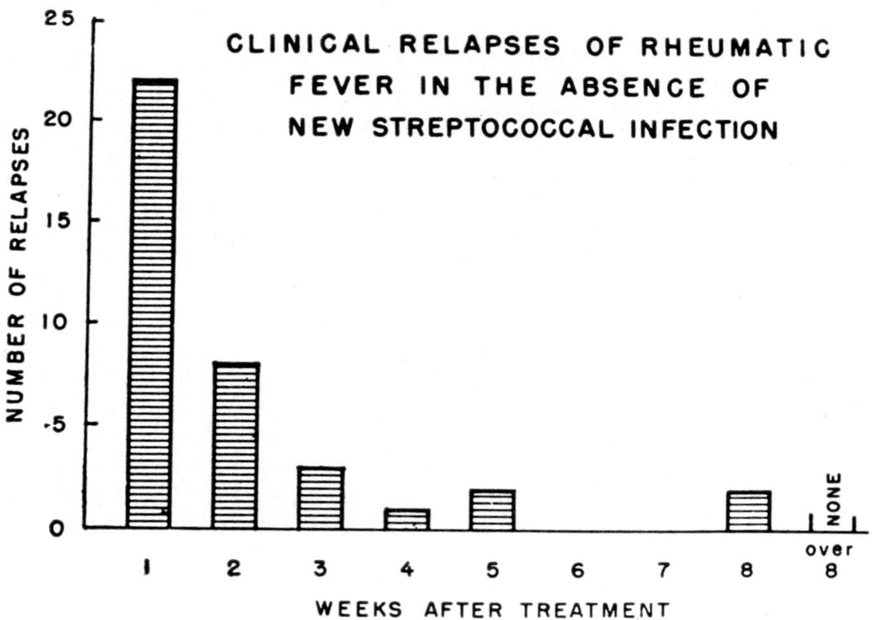

FIG. 44–18.—Time distribution of the onset of clinical relapses or "rebounds" in thirty-four patients with rheumatic fever following cessation of treatment with aspirin or cortisone. (Stollerman *et al.*, courtesy of Amer. J. Med.)

cently followed the realization that prevention of rheumatic fever in this country falls far short of optimal practice.[148a] Organizational and logistic aspects of prevention have been dealt with in detail by a government advisory commission.[148a] Rheumatic fever having been arguably defined as "an occupational disease of students,"[111a] a model program for its prevention, centered in the school, has been described.[141a] Thus, the "revolution of rising expectations" may finally catch up with us and close the gap (wide indeed in this field) between the promise of science and the delivery of medicine.

Prevention of Rheumatic Fever by Treatment of Streptococcal Infections

A number of investigators in the late forties and early fifties showed that treatment of streptococcal pharyngitis with penicillin prevents the development of rheumatic fever in children with previous rheumatic fever[121,124] and in military recruits.[41,187] Subsequent studies have shown that failure to prevent rheumatic fever correlates with failure to eradicate the streptococci from the throat.[31] Hence, regimens are recommended which, by providing effective blood levels for at least ten consecutive days, are most efficacious in eradicating the streptococci (see below).

There is every reason to believe that such regimens are equally effective in children with no previous rheumatic fever, but in them the risk of developing rheumatic fever may be slight. Rheumatic fever did not occur in several large series of children with streptococcal infections adequately treated with antibiotics,[18,113,162] but these series did not include untreated controls. In the only large controlled study available thus far,[156] rheumatic fever did not occur among 605 children with pharyngitis and positive throat culture for group A streptococci treated with 600,000 units of benzathine penicillin I.M., but occurred only in 2 patients among 608 untreated controls (see previous chapter). This report, as well as a previous one from England,[21] has pointed out the frequency of "benign" streptococcal sore throats, *i.e.*, of pharyngitides associated with the presence of beta-hemolytic streptococci in the throat, but with very low incidence of post-streptococcal sequelae.

Siegel *et al.* have emphasized that their two cases of rheumatic fever occurred in patients who had had *exudative* pharyngitis.[156] If this finding is confirmed by more extensive studies, *i.e.*, if rheumatic fever is shown to occur exclusively after exudative pharyngitis, it may provide a useful guide for treatment. One is currently confronted with an apparent paradox: studies of streptococcal pharyngitis suggest that mild, non-exudative infections may be non-rheumatogenic[21,156] but studies of rheumatic fever patients indicate that one-third of them have had streptococcal infections so mild as to escape the patient's awareness.[154,197] A reasonable explanation is that mild streptococcal infections are much more frequent than severe ones, so that despite a very low attack rate of rheumatic fever, they may cause a substantial fraction of rheumatic fever cases. Whether treatment should be restricted to exudative streptococcal pharyngitis or should be extended to the milder forms of the disease is debatable, and depends on how badly the physician wants to avoid rheumatic fever (and glomerulonephritis) and how much he fears penicillin allergy. Other factors of a psychologic and economic character, unfortunately, also influence the decision.

The risk of penicillin allergy is not very great, in terms of either death or disability. It can be, and must be, further reduced by taking an accurate history and, probably in the near future, by screening skin tests. Almost one million injections of benzathine penicillin G have been given to United States naval recruits without any known fatality, and immediate anaphylactic reactions have been extremely rare.[165] Allergic reactions, mostly of minor import, occur in about 1 per cent of cases after benzathine penicillin administration and in about 0.4 per cent after a ten-day course of orally administered penicillin. In children, the incidence of allergic reactions is even lower.[165] Unlike rheumatic fever and glomerulonephritis, penicillin reactions almost never result in chronic disease and disability. Because of these findings, I believe that a certain largesse in prescribing penicillin is justified, according to the principles detailed below. I also hope that progress in the differentiation of potentially rheumatogenic from benign streptococcal infections will soon make these recommendations obsolete.

The diagnosis of streptococcal pharyngitis is difficult to make on clinical findings alone. Of all the various clinical syndromes involving the upper respiratory tract, the pharyngitis with sudden onset, fever, headache, dysphagia, beefy red throat with exudate, and tender cervical lymph nodes is the one most frequently due to hemolytic streptococci. Even this "typical" picture, however, is not always of streptococcal origin, but may be due to adenoviruses, to Coxsackie viruses and even to influenza infections.[127,155] The diagnostic uncertainty is greater in milder, non-exudative pharyngitides. Therefore it is advisable to take a throat culture in all patients who present with pharyngitis, regardless of the presence or absence of other symptoms and signs. Administration of penicillin by mouth may be started in patients with the "typical" picture described above, in those with a scarlatinal rash, or in those who appear "toxic," and may be withheld in the others for the day or two necessary to get the result of the throat culture. Immediate treatment is advisable, however, if one wants to avoid glomerulonephritis (which has a shorter latent period than rheumatic fever[142]) whenever nephritogenic strains are prevalent in the community.

Throat cultures can be easily processed in the doctor's office or in the clinic. All one needs is a sterile cotton (or Dacron) swab, a Petri dish filled with sheep-blood-agar (available commercially in ready-made and disposable form), and a small, inexpensive incubator. Confirmation of the streptococcal nature of any beta-hemolytic colony will depend on microscopic examination of a Gram-stained smear. If beta-hemolytic streptococci are *not* recovered on culture, the oral penicillin treatment may be stopped in patients with exudative pharyngitis. If beta-hemolytic streptococci are recovered, treatment will be continued in these patients, and will be started in those who had presented with non-exudative pharyngitis.

For those physicians who are unwilling to perform these tests, diagnostic bacteriologic services, to which throat swabs can be mailed, are available in an increasing number of localities. In addition to the identification of beta-hemolytic streptococci, these services provide diagnosis of the streptococcal group of the isolated strains, which they obtain by a precipitin reaction, or by bacitracin inhibition (specific for group A) or by immunofluorescent technique. The latter allows a more rapid determination of group. Any one of these techniques for streptococcal grouping can also be carried out in the doctor's office. If a strain of beta-hemolytic streptococci isolated from a patient with pharyngitis turns out to be not of group A, one may discontinue the administration of the eradicating course of antibiotic. If facilities for grouping are not available, one is justified in treating all beta-hemolytic streptococcal infections as if they were group A, because most of them actually are. (Throat cultures and the identification of group A streptococci are discussed in detail elsewhere.[175a] A brochure describing the technique and the interpretation of throat cultures is available from the American Heart Association and its affiliates.)

Various schedules of antibiotic treatment can provide an effective blood level for ten consecutive days, and are effective in eradicating the streptococcus from the throat (Table 44–8); the choice among them depends largely on social and psychological considerations. Whenever the physician can rely on the full cooperation of the patient (or of the patient's parents), 10 days of oral administration of 200,000 to 250,000 units of penicillin 3 to 4 times a day, depending on the age of the patient, may be preferable, because the incidence of allergic reactions is less after oral than after parenteral administration,[165] and because the physician can start the treatment while bacteriologic diagnosis is pending, and can discontinue it later if the group A streptococcal nature of the illness is not confirmed. However, oral administration may be less effective than injection, largely because of uncooperativeness of the patients. In clinics and emergency rooms it has been found that adherence to the prescribed ten-day schedule of oral medication is rare indeed.[8]

Whenever the cooperativeness of the patient or of his parents is dubious (and this is by far the most frequent situation), benzathine penicillin in a single injection of 600,000 to 1,200,000 units, according to the age, is the preferred treatment. This is highly effective, irrespective of cooperativeness, but is followed frequently by local inflammatory (non-allergic) reactions which may cause discomfort and pain sometimes accompanied by fever, elevated ESR and positive CRP for a day or two.[79] Alternatively, one may prescribe oral penicillin or various combinations of oral and injectable penicillin (see Table 44–8). The symptoms of streptococcal pharyngitis, however, disappear in two or three days. The patient and his parents (and at times even his doctor) find it difficult to understand the need to treat an asymptomatic condition. Therefore, benzathine penicillin in a single injection is the optimum treatment in most instances.

Whenever a patient has a history of penicillin allergy, 125 to 250 mg. of erythromycin, 4 times a day, should be given instead. Under ideal circumstances, whatever the treatment administered, a

Table 44-8.—Recommended Treatment Schedules for Streptococcal Pharyngitis[2]

Intramuscular Penicillin	*Oral Penicillin*	*Combined Therapy*	*Other Antibiotics*
Benzathine penicillin G†			
Children—one intramuscular injection of 600,000 to 900,000 units.† (The larger dose is probably preferable for children over 10 years of age.) Adults—one intramuscular injection of 900,000 to 1,200,000 units.†	Children and adults—200,000 or 250,000 units‡ three or four times a day for *a full 10 days*. Therapy must be continued for the *entire ten days* even though the temperature returns to normal and the patient is asymptomatic.	Various combinations of oral and intra-muscular penicillin should be effective provided adequate coverage is continued for 10 days. For example, one or more injections of procaine penicillin G (600,000 units every 12 to 24 hours) might be followed by oral penicillin G in recommended doses.	Erythromycin is the drug of choice in patients who are sensitive to penicillin. Lincomycin is similarly effective, but diarrhea may be bothersome. Both drugs should be given for ten days. A few strains resistant to these antibiotics have already appeared. Tetracyclines should not be used because of the high prevalence of resistant strains.

A pamphlet covering all aspects of prevention of rheumatic fever may be obtained from local Heart Associations.

† Mixtures containing shorter acting penicillin in addition to benzathine penicillin have not been shown to be superior to benzathine pencillin alone. If such a mixture is used, it must contain benzathine penicillin in the doses noted above.

‡ Of the various oral forms available, buffered penicillin G is satisfactory and less expensive. Although higher blood levels may be achieved with alpha-phenoxymethyl penicillin (penicillin V) or alpha-phenoxyethyl penicillin (phenethicillin), especially when taken near meals, their superiority in the prevention of rheumatic fever has not been documented.

follow-up culture is advisable to ascertain the eradication of the streptococci. In some cases, failure to eradicate beta-hemolytic streptococci has been ascribed to the concomitant presence in the patient's throat of penicillinase-producing staphylococci,[157] but the evidence is inconclusive.

Also, under ideal circumstances, throat cultures should be taken from the relatives of patients with streptococcal pharyngitis. If the result of throat culture is positive, treatment should be administered even to asymptomatic contacts, because the chances are that the strain is the same in the whole family and that it is a virulent one.

Under less ideal circumstances, therapeutic decisions may have to be made without the benefit of a throat culture. This happens not uncommonly with uneducated or underprivileged patients, who demand instant treatment and will switch to another doctor or to another clinic if such treatment is not administered. The conscientious physician will make an effort to educate these patients, and, if this fails, will obtain their cooperation by administering symptomatic treatment when first consulted, and by providing antibiotic medication one or two days later, if indicated on the basis of the result of the throat culture. Still, there are situations in which the physician will treat either "now or never"—and in the latter case will not only lose his patient, but will cause the patient to miss his treatment. In such cases, which hopefully will become less common with improved health education, the physician may be aided in his therapeutic decision by the symptoms and signs most frequently associated with a streptococcal infection, and also by whatever knowledge he has of the prevalence of streptococcal or viral respiratory diseases in his community at any given time.

Prevention of Rheumatic Fever by Preventing Streptococcal Infections

Rheumatic fever can also be prevented by *preventing*, rather than treating, streptococcal infections. This can be accomplished by the continual administration of sulfonamides, or of antibiotics, in doses generally smaller than those indicated for treatment. This approach is uneconomical in the general population,

Table 44-9.—Prophylaxis and Attack Rates of Streptococcal Infections and of Rheumatic Fever Recurrences on 3 Prophylactic Regimens*

	Parenteral Benzathine Penicillin (1,200,000 u. every 4 weeks)	*Oral Penicillin (200,000 u. daily by mouth) ½ hour before breakfast*	*Oral Sulfadiazine (one gram daily by mouth)*
Number of patient-years	560	545	576
Number and *rate* of all streptococcal infections	34 (*6.1*)	113 (*20.7*)	138 (*24.0*)
Number and *rate* of all streptococcal infections, exclusive of carrier state	24 (*4.3*)	101 (*18.5*)	102 (*17.7*)
Number and *rate* of rheumatic recurrences	2 (*0.4*)	30 (*5.5*)	16 (*2.8*)

* From Wood *et al.*[195] *Rates* listed in parentheses as number per 100 patient-years.

but is used with advantage in patients who have had rheumatic fever, because they have a much higher attack rate of rheumatic fever following streptococcal infections. It is therefore desirable to protect them from *all* streptococcal infections, whether they are symptomatic (and can therefore be diagnosed and treated) or asymptomatic (and can therefore be neither diagnosed nor treated).

The most effective way of preventing recurrences of rheumatic fever is the monthly injection of 1,200,000 u. of benzathine penicillin every 4 weeks, which results in a recurrence rate as low as 0.4 per hundred patient-years in children[195] (see Table 44–9). The success of this form of prophylaxis may be due largely to its relative independence from the cooperation of the patient, or, to put it more precisely, to its immunity from hidden lack of cooperation (a patient on injectable benzathine penicillin prophylaxis either comes to the clinic and then receives his full prophylaxis, or does not come and then is dropped from the clinic; a patient on oral prophylaxis may come regularly to the clinic and yet comply only occasionally, if at all, to the instructions of taking the medication regularly[73a]). A minor drawback of this prophylactic regimen is the local reaction to the injection (see above). In highly structured clinics staffed by committed and enthusiastic workers,[68] patients who are put on this kind of prophylaxis generally stay on it. However, changes to other prophylactic regimens may become necessary in 16 per cent of the cases, as opposed to 4 per cent in patients originally put on sulfadiazine.[196] Under less favorable circumstances, patients may discontinue prophylaxis altogether because of the pain and discomfort caused by this particular type of prophylaxis. In such cases, a form of oral prophylaxis is indicated.

Although sulfonamides are ineffective in preventing rheumatic fever through *treatment* of an established streptococcal infection, they are quite effective in preventing the establishment of such infections. They are therefore valuable drugs in preventing recurrences of rheumatic fever if they are administered continually. In fact, patients receiving sulfadiazine (1 gm/day in a single dose) had a rheumatic fever recurrence rate of 2.8 per hundred patient-years; they thus fared better than those maintained on oral penicillin (200,000 units/day in a single dose one-half hour before breakfast), who had a recurrence rate of 5.5 per hundred patient-years[195] (Table 44–9). In a subsequent study, doubling the daily dose of penicillin virtually eliminated this difference, but still failed to make penicillin a better prophylactic agent than sulfadiazine.[61] Although sulfonamide-resistant streptococci have arisen during mass-prophylaxis in military installations, they have been very rare in civilian practice, at least in the United States. Patients receiving sulfonamides should have a white count and differential after two weeks of prophylaxis and also whenever a rash develops together with fever or sore throat. Sulfonamides should be discontinued if the white count is less than 4,000, or the neutrophils are less than 35 per cent. Authenticated penicillin allergy has been conspicuously absent in young patients on either form of continual prophylaxis (oral or injectable),[196] but it still may constitute a potential hazard, at least in the older age groups. One final consideration is that microorganisms in the mouth (other than group A streptococci) may become resistant to penicillin[126,132] (although this does not seem to happen in patients receiving benzathine penicillin by injection[160a]). One may conjecture that after dental procedures, or even spontaneously, these organisms may invade the blood stream and cause subacute bacterial endocarditis (SBE), which may be harder to treat because of the resistance of the organisms to penicillin. A preliminary survey has suggested that penicillin resistance may indeed be more common among the organisms isolated from SBE cases previously on penicillin than in those main-

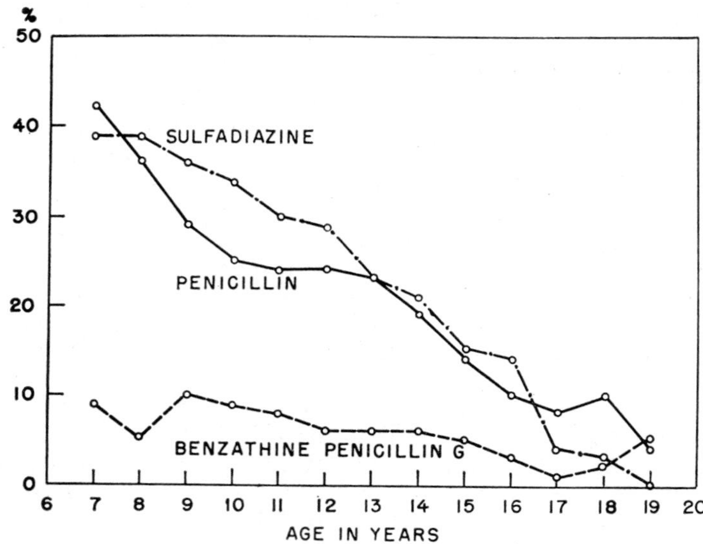

FIG. 44–19.—Rates of streptococcal infection per patient-year for each year of age by prophylaxis group (Wood *et al.*, courtesy of Ann. Int. Med.)

tained on sulfadiazine[46] but the clinical implications of all these findings remain to be evaluated. Taking all of these considerations into account, I believe that sulfadiazine is somewhat preferable to penicillin as an oral prophylactic agent. The question of how long prophylaxis should be continued in patients who have had rheumatic fever, or are discovered to have rheumatic heart disease, cannot be answered unequivocally in all cases, but one can base an informed decision on the data which follow.

Patients with rheumatic heart disease have a higher recurrence rate per streptococcal infection (30 per cent) than patients with a history of rheumatic fever but no residual heart disease (10 per cent).[174] Patients who have had carditis in the first attack are much more likely to develop carditis in a recurrent attack (69 per cent) than patients who escaped carditis in their first attack (17 per cent).[58] The incidence of streptococcal infections decreases with age[195] (Fig. 44–19), and the recurrence rate *per streptococcal infection* decreases also with increasing age and time elapsed since the last rheumatic attack.[174] It is still higher, however, in adults with previous rheumatic fever than in the general population.[91] It is up to the individual physician and to his patient to decide which course to take, weighing on one side the discomfort, expense and risk of continual prophylaxis (the latter is virtually nil), and on the other the danger of a rheumatic recurrence, which at best is a painful inconvenience and at worst causes incapacitation and death. In my eyes the balance tips in favor of prophylaxis in almost all instances, with the possible exception of adolescents and adults who have not had carditis during their first attack, an historical detail which may not always be easy to ascertain. Several clinics are now attempting to define precisely the risk involved in discontinuing prophylaxis in such patients.

The present state of prophylaxis implementation is a far cry from ideal. If one excludes the patients followed by aggressive research clinics,[68] as many as 50 per cent of patients in the lower socioeconomic groups discontinue prophylaxis after one or one and a half years.[102,185]

The situation in the higher social groups cannot be much better, if only 12 per cent of 9,044 United States college students with previous rheumatic fever are taking prophylaxis, although 51 per cent took it sometime in the past.[112] Doubtless, the percentage of patients on prophylaxis is even lower in the poorer countries, where the cost of prophylaxis is a real deterrent. Cost is no object here (or should not be) but administrative inefficiency, moral indifference, simple ignorance, or "denial of illness" may counterbalance the benefits of affluence.

Prevention of Subacute Bacterial Endocarditis

Patients with rheumatic heart disease are prone to develop subacute bacterial endocarditis spontaneously or after tooth extractions, oral surgical procedures, manipulation of periodontal tissues, removal of tonsils and adenoids, bronchoscopy and surgery or instrumentation of the genitourinary tract or the lower gastrointestinal tract.[2] Even mild dental procedures, such as cleaning and filling of teeth, have been associated occasionally with the development of endocarditis.[87] Since bacteremia has been reported after chewing of a resistant mass in patients with diseased teeth,[130] good dental care is particularly important in all patients with rheumatic heart disease.

Antibiotics should be administered to patients with rheumatic heart disease undergoing the following procedures:

1. *All dental procedures that are likely to cause bleeding*, *removal of tonsils or adenoids*, and *bronchoscopy*. These patients should receive 600,000 units of procaine penicillin and 200,000 units of crystalline penicillin intramuscularly (a commercially available mixture) 1 hour before the procedure and once daily on each of the 2 following days.

Intramuscular penicillin is preferred over oral penicillin, but if the former cannot be administered for any reason the patient should receive 0.5 gram of penicillin V (potassium phenoxymethyl penicillin) or 1,200,000 units of buffered penicillin G 1 hour before the procedure and then half this dose at 6-hour intervals for the remainder of that day and for the following 2 days. Patients allergic to penicillin or maintained on continual *oral* penicillin (whose throat and mouth may contain increased numbers of penicillin-resistant microorganisms[160a]) should receive erythromycin. The dose for adults is 500 mg. 1½ hours before the procedure, followed by 250 mg. every 6 hours for the remainder of that day and for the following 2 days. Small children should receive 20 mg. per kg. orally 1½ to 2 hours prior to the procedure and then 10 mg. per kg. every 6 hours for the remainder of that day and for the 2 following days.

2. *Surgery or instrumentation of the genitourinary tract (especially urethral manipulations), of the lower gastrointestinal tract (especially of the colon and rectum), surgery of the gallbladder*, and *obstetrical complications such as septic abortion or complicated deliveries*. (The indications for prophylaxis in uncomplicated deliveries are not firmly established.) These patients should receive streptomycin, 1 to 2 grams intramuscularly, 1 hour prior to the procedure and once daily for the 2 following days (small children should receive 20 mg. per kg. 1 hour prior to the procedure and then 10 mg. per kg. every 6 hours for the remainder of that day and for the 2 following days) plus one of the following drugs: (I) penicillin in the doses noted above, or (II) ampicillin, 25 to 50 mg. per kg. orally or intravenously 1 hour prior to the procedure, and then 25 mg. per kg. every 6 hours for the remainder of that day and for the 2 following days. Patients suspected of being allergic to penicillin should receive (III) erythromycin in the doses noted above or (IV) vancomycin, 0.5 to 1.0 gm. intravenously 1 hour prior to the procedure and then 0.5 gm. intravenously every 6 hours for the remainder of that day and for the 2 following days (small children should receive 20 mg. per kg. 1 hour prior to the

procedure and then 10 mg. per kg. every 6 hours for the remainder of that day and for the 2 following days).[2a]

BIBLIOGRAPHY

1. Alexander, W. D. and Smith, G.: Lancet, *1*, 768, 1962.

1a. Altman, L. K.: New York Times, Dec. 30, 1970.

2. American Heart Association, Rheumatic Fever Committee of the Council on Rheumatic Fever and Congenital Heart Disease. Circulation, *43*, 983, 1971.

2a. American Heart Association, Rheumatic Fever Committee and Committee on Congenital Cardiac Defects of the Council on Rheumatic Fever and Congenital Heart Disease. Circulation (in press).

3. Anonymous: *Syllabus, or Outlines of Lectures on the Practice of Medicine.* London, 1820, Cited by Osler, W.

4. Aron, A. M., Freeman, J. M. and Carter, S.: Amer. J. Med., *38*, 83, 1965.

5. Aycock, E. K. and Weston, W., Jr.: J. South Carolina Med. Assoc., *56*, 89, 1960.

5a. Ayoub, E. and Wannamaker, L. W.: Pediatrics, *38*, 946, 1966.

5b. Badin, J. and Denne, A.: Ann. Biol. Clin., *28*, 247, 1970.

6. Baehr, G. and Schifrin, A.: Libman Annu. *1*, 125, 1932.

7. Baldwin, J. S., Kerr, J. M., Kuttner, A. G., and Doyle, E. F.: J. Pediat., *56*, 465, 1960.

8. Bergman, A. B. and Werner, R. J.: New Engl. J. Med., *268*, 1334, 1963.

9. Bernhard, G. C. and Stollerman, G. H.: J. Clin. Invest., *38*, 1942, 1959.

10. Bernstein, S. H. and Allerhand, J.: Amer. J. Med. Sci., *247*, 431, 1964.

11. Besterman, E. M. M. and Thomas, G. T.: Brit. Heart J., *15*, 113, 1953.

12. Bland, E. F.: New Engl. J. Med., *262*, 597, 1960.

13. ———: Transactions of the American Clinical and Climatological Association, *73*, 209, 1961.

14. Bland, E. F. and Jones, T. D.: J.A.M.A., *113*, 1380, 1939.

15. ———: Circulation, *4*, 836, 1951.

16. Bogdonoff, M. D., Woods, A. H., White, J. E. and Engel, F. L.: Amer. J. Med., *21*, 583, 1956.

17. Boone, J. A. and Levine, S. A.: Amer. J. Med. Sci., *195*, 764, 1938.

18. Breese, B. B. and Disney, F. A.: New Engl. J. Med., *259*, 57, 1958.

19. Brown, M. G. and Wolff, L.: New Engl J. Med., *223*, 242, 1940.

20. Brudno, J. C.: New Engl. J. Med., *243*, 513 1950.

21. Brumfitt, W., O'Grady, F., and Slater J. D. H.: Lancet, *2*, 419, 1959.

21a. Burgio, G. R., Severi, F., Vaccaro, R. and Rossini, R.: Schweiz. med. Wschr., *96*, 431, 1966.

22. Burke, J. B.: Arch. Dis. Child., *30*, 359, 1955.

23. Bywaters, E. G. L.: Circulation, *14*, 1153, 1956.

24. Bywaters, E. G. L., Glynn, L. E., and Zeldis, A.: Ann. Rheum. Dis., *17*, 278, 1958.

25. Bywaters, E. G. L., Isdale, I. and Kempton, J. J.: Quart. J. Med. (New Series), *26*, 161, 1957.

26. Bywaters, E. G. L. and Thomas, G. T.: Brit. Med. J., *1*, 1628, 1961.

27. Cammarata, R. J., Rodnan, G. P. and Crittenden, J. O.: J.A.M.A., *184*, 971, 1963.

28. Caravias, D. E.: Arch. Dis. Child., *31*, 415, 1956.

29. Carmichael, D. B.: Amer. Heart J., *50*, 528, 1955.

30. Carter, M. E., Bywaters, E. G. L., and Thomas, G. T.: Brit. Med. J., *1*, 965, 1962.

31. Catanzaro, F. J., Rammelkamp, C. H., Jr., and Chamovitz, R.: New Engl. J. Med., *259*, 51, 1958.

32. Chamberlain, E. N., Hill, C. A. St., and Cope, S. R.: Brit. Heart J., *20*, 183, 1958.

32a. Cherian, G., Vytilingam, K. I., Sukumer, I. P., and Gopinath, N.: Brit. Heart J., *26*, 157, 1964.

33. Choremis, K. B., Constantsas, N., and Danelatos-Athanassiadis, K.: Clin. Chim. Acta, *8*, 814, 1963.

34. Coburn, A. F.: *The Factor of Infection in the Rheumatic State*, Baltimore, The Williams & Wilkins Co., 1931.

35. ———: Bull. Johns Hopkins Hosp., *73*, 435, 1943.

36. Combined Rheumatic Fever Study Group: New Engl. J. Med., *262*, 895, 1960.

37. ———: New Engl. J. Med., *272*, 63, 1965.

38. Czoniczer, G., Amezcua, F., Pelargonio, S. and Massell, B. F.: Circulation, *29*, 813, 1964.

39. Daniels, W. B: Arch. Int. Med., *81*, 145, 1948.

39a. Davis, E.: Lancet, *1*, 1043, 1970.

40. Deliee, E. M., Dodge, K. G. and McEwen, C.: Amer. Heart J., *26*, 681, 1943.
41. Denny, F. W., Wannamaker, L. W., Brink, W. R., Rammelkamp, C. H., Jr. and Custer, E. A.: J.A.M.A., *143*, 151, 1950.
42. Diamond, E. F. and Tentler, R.: J.A.M.A., *182*, 685, 1962.
43. Doliopoulos, T.: Rheumatism, *7*, 42, 1951.
44. Dorfman, A., Gross, J. I. and Lorincz, A. E.: Pediatrics, *27*, 692, 1961.
45. Doumer, E., Lorriaux, A., and Belbenoit, C.: Bull. Soc. Med. Hosp. Paris, *67*, 801, 1951.
46. Doyle, E. F., Spagnuolo, M., Taranta, A., Kuttner, A. G. and Markowitz, M.: J.A.M.A., *201*, 807, 1967.
47. Drivsholm, A. and Madsen, S.: Scan. J. Clin. Lab. Invest., *13*, 442, 1961.
47*a*. Editorial. J.A.M.A., *214*, 361, 1970.
48. Elster, S. K., Braunwald, E. and Wood, H. F.: Amer. Heart J., *51*, 533, 1956.
49. Engleman, E. P., Hollister, L. E. and Kole, F. O.: J.A.M.A., *155*, 1134, 1954.
50. Feinstein, A. R. and Arevalo, A. C.: Pediatrics, *33*, 661, 1964.
51. Feinstein, A. R. and Di Massa, R.: New Engl. J. Med., *260*, 1331, 1959.
52. ———: New Engl. J. Med., *260*, 1001, 1959.
53. Feinstein, A. R. and Spagnuolo, M.: New Engl. J. Med., *262*, 533, 1960.
54. ———: J. Clin. Invest., *40*, 1891, 1961.
55. ———: J.A.M.A., *175*, 1117, 1961.
56. ———: Medicine, *41*, 279, 1962.
57. Feinstein, A. R., Spagnuolo, M., and Gill, F. A.: Yale J. Biol. & Med., *33*, 259, 1961.
58. Feinstein, A. R., Spagnuolo, M., Wood, H. F., Taranta, A., Tursky, E., and Kleinberg, E.: Ann. Int. Med., *60*, Suppl. 5, 68, 1964.
59. Feinstein, A. R., Taranta, A. and Di Massa, R.: N.Y. State J. Med., *60*, 2835, 1960.
60. Feinstein, A. R., Wood, H. F., Spagnuolo, M., Taranta, A., Jonas, S., Kleinberg, E., and Tursky, E.: Ann. Int. Med., *60*, Suppl. 5, 87, 1964.
61. Feinstein, A. R., Wood, H. F., Spagnuolo, M., Taranta, A., Tursky, E., and Kleinberg, E.: J.A.M.A., *188*, 489, 1964.
62. Foster, D. B.: Arch. Neurol. & Psychiat., *47*, 254, 1942.
63. Freud, P., Weisz, A., and Brunhofer, A.: Amer. J. Dis. Child., *79*, 676, 1950.
64. Friedberg, C. K.: Circulation, *19*, 161, 1959.
65. Friedländer (initial not given): Verhandl. d. kong. f. Inn. Med., *5*, 381, 1886.
66. Friedman, S., Harris, T. N., and Caddell, J. L.: J. Pediat., *60*, 55, 1962.
67. Garcia-Palmieri, M. R.: Amer. Heart J., *64*, 577, 1962.
68. Gavrin, J. B., Tursky, E., Albam, B., and Feinstein, A. R.: Ann. Int. Med., *60*, Suppl. 5, 18, 1964.
69. Gauchat, R. D. and May, C. D.: Pediatrics, *19*, 672, 1957.
70. Gibson, M. L. and Fisher, G. R.: J. Dis. Child., *96*, 575, 1958.
71. Goldring, D., Behrer, M. R., Brown, G. and Elliott, G.: J. Pediat., *53*, 547, 1958.
72. Good, R. A.: In *Rheumatic Fever, a Symposium*, L. Thomas editor, Minneapolis, University of Minnesota Press, 1952.
73. Good, R. A., Vernier, R. L., and Smith, R. T.: Pediatrics, *19*, 95, 272, 1957.
73*a*. Gordis, L., Markowitz, M., and Lilienfeld, A.: J. Pediat., *75*, 957, 1969.
74. Goslings, W. R. O., Valkenberg, H. A., Bots, A. W., and Lorrier, J. C.: New Engl. J. Med., *268*, 687, 1963.
75. Greenberg, M. S.: Ann. Int. Med., *61*, 124, 1964.
76. Greenman, L., Weigand, F. A., and Danowski, T. S.: Ann. Rheum. Dis., *12*, 342, 1953.
77. Graef, I., Parent, S., Zitron, W. and Wyckoff, J.: Amer. J. Med. Sci., *185*, 197, 1933.
77*a*. Grossman, B. J.: Amer. J. Dis. Child., *115*, 557, 1968.
78. Grossman, B. J. and Stamler, J.: J.A.M.A., *183*, 985, 1963.
79. Haas, R. C., Taranta, A. and Wood, H. F.: New Engl. J. Med., *256*, 152, 1957.
80. Haddox, C. H., Jr., and Saslaw, M. S.: J. Clin. Invest., *42*, 435, 1963.
81. Haddox, C. H., Jr., Saslaw, M. S., Seligman, B. and Stauffer, J.: Biochim. Biophys. Acta, *81*, 184, 1964.
82. Hallen, J.: Acta Path. Microb. Scan., *57*, 301, 1963.
83. Hallidie-Smith, K. A. and Bywaters, E. G. L.: Arch. Dis. Child., *33*, 350, 1958.
84. Harris, T. N., Friedman, S., Needleman, H. L., and Saltzman, H. A.: Pediatrics, *17*, 11, 1956.
85. Harris, T. N., Friedman, S. and Tang, J.: Amer. J. Med. Sci., *234*, 259, 1957.
86. Harris, T. N. and Vandegrift, H. N.: Pediatrics, *25*, 80, 1960.
87. Harvey, P. W. and Capone, M. A.: Am. J. Cardiol., *7*, 793, 1961.
88. Hess, E. V., Fink, C. W., Taranta, A. and Ziff, M.: J. Clin. Invest., *43*, 886, 1964.

89. Hong, R. and West, C. D.: Arth. and Rheum., *7*, 128, 1964.
90. Illingworth, R. S., Lorber, J., Holt, K. S., Rendle-Short, J., Jowett, G. H., and Gibson, W. M.: Lancet, *2*, 653, 1957.
91. Johnson, E. E., Stollerman, G. H., and Grossman, B. J.: J.A.M.A., *190*, 407, 1964.
92. Jones, T. D.: J.A.M.A., *126*, 481, 1944.
93. Kamermann, J. S.: Ann. Rheum. Dis., *21*, 59, 1962.
94. Kantor, T. G. and Tanner, M.: Arth. and Rheum., *5*, 378, 1962.
95. Kaplan, M. H., Meyeserian, M. and Kushner, I.: J. Exp. Med., *113*, 17, 1961.
96. Keith, J. D.: Quart. J. Med., *7*, 29, 1938.
97. Keil, H.: Ann. Int. Med., *11*, 2223, 1938.
98. ————: Medicine, *17*, 261, 1938.
99. Kouvalainen, K., Hjelt, L. and Hallman, N.: Ann. Pediat. Fenn., *10*, 164, 1964.
100. Kuttner, A. G. and Mayer, F. E.: New Engl. J. Med., *268*, 1259, 1963.
101. Lehndorff, H. and Leiner, C.: Z. Kinderheilk, *32*, 46, 1922.
102. Lendrum, B. L. and Korbin, C.: J.A.M.A., *162*, 13, 1956.
103. Lessof, M. H. and Bywaters, E. G. L.: Brit. Med. J., *1*, 1520, 1956.
104. Levine, S. and Harvey, W. P.: *Clinical Auscultation of the Heart*, 2nd. Ed., Philadelphia, W. B. Saunders Co., 1959.
105. Lewis, I. C.: Arch. Dis. Child., *30*, 212, 1955.
106. Lewis-Johnsson, J.: Acta Paediat. (Stockholm) Suppl. *76*, 1, 1949.
107. Löfgren, S.: Acta Medica Scandinavica, *145*, 424, 1953.
108. Lyon, R.: Lancet, *2*, 555, 1956.
108*a*. Mansa, B. and Kjems, E.: Acta Path. Microbiol. Scand. (Section B), *78*, 467, 1970.
109. McCarty, M.: The Immune Response in Rheumatic Fever, in *Rheumatic Fever, a Symposium*, L. Thomas editor, Minneapolis, University of Minnesota Press, 1952.
110. McIntosch, R. and Wood, C. L.: Amer. J. Dis. Child., *49*, 835, 1935.
111. McMinn, F. J. and Bywaters, E. G. L.: Ann. Rheum. Dis., *18*, 293, 1959.
111*a*. Marienfeld, C.: Amer. J. Pub. Health, *56*, 647, 1966.
112. Marienfeld, C. J., Robins, M., Sandidge, R. P., and Findlan, C.: Public Health Reports, *79*, 789, 1964.
113. Markowitz, M.: Amer. J. Dis. Child., *105*, 12, 1963.
114. Markowitz, M., Bruton, H. D., Kuttner, A. G. and Cluff, L. E.: Pediatrics, *35*, 393, 1965.
115. Markowitz, M. and Kuttner, A. G.: Pediatrics, *16*, 325, 1955.
116. ————: *Rheumatic Fever, Diagnosis, Management and Prevention*, Philadelphia, W. B. Saunders Co., 1965.
117. Mauer, A. M.: Pediatrics, *27*, 707, 1961.
118. Manso, C., Taranta, A. and Nydick, I.: Proc. Soc. Exp. Biol. Med., *93*, 84, 1956.
119. Massell, B. F.: Med. Clin. North America, *42*, 1343, 1958.
120. Massell, B. F., Amezcua, F., and Pelargonio, S.: J.A.M.A., *188*, 287, 1964.
121. Massell, B. F., Dow, J. W., and Jones, T. D.: J.A.M.A., *138*, 1030, 1948.
122. Massell, B. F., Fyler, D. C. and Roy, S. B.: Amer. J. Cardiol., *1*, 436, 1958.
123. Massell, B. F., Mote, J. R., and Jones, T. D.: J. Clin. Invest., *16*, 125, 1937.
124. Massell, B. F., Sturgis, G. P., Knobloch, J. D., Streeper, R. B., Hall, T. N. and Norcross, P.: J.A.M.A., *146*, 1469, 1951.
125. Mayer, F. E., Doyle, E. F., Herrera, L. and Dodge Brownell, K.: Amer. J. Dis. Child., *105*, 146, 1963.
126. Michael, T. M., Michael, J. G. and Massell, B. F.: Amer. J. Med. Sci., *248*, 152, 1964.
127. Moffet, H. L., Cramblett, G. H. and Smith, A.: Pediatrics, *33*, 11, 1964.
128. Mirowski, M., Rosenstein, B. J. and Markowitz, M.: Pediatrics, *33*, 334, 1964.
128*a*. Mortimer, E. A.: Pediatrics, *47*, 1, 1971.
129. Mortimer, E. A., Jr., Vaisman, S. B., Vignau, I. A., Guasch, L. J., Schuster, C. A., Rakita, L., Karuse, R. M., Roberts, R. and Rammelkamp, C. H., Jr.: New Engl. J. Med., *260*, 101, 1959.
130. Murray, M. and Moosnick, F.: J. Lab. & Clin. Med., *26*, 801, 1941.
131. Myers, G. B., Gottlieb, B. A. M., Mattman, P. E., Eckley, G. M. and Chason, J. L.: Amer. J. Med., *12*, 161, 1952.
132. Naiman, R. A. and Barrow, J. G.: Ann. Int. Med., *58*, 768, 1963.
133. Nydick, I., Tang, J., Stollerman, G. H., Wroblewski, F. and LaDue, J. S.: Circulation, *12*, 795, 1955.
134. Osler, W.: *On Chorea and Choreiform Affections*. Philadelphia, P. Blakiston, Son & Co., 1894.
135. Pader, E. and Elster, S. K.: Amer. J. Med., *26*, 424, 1959.
136. Paquet, E. and Delage, J. M.: Canad. Med. Ass. J., *76*, 927, 1957.
137. Pardee, H. E. B.: *Clinical Aspects of the Electrocardiogram*, New York, Paul B. Hoeber, Inc., 1941.

138. Payne, W. W. and Schlesinger, B.: Arch. Dis. Child., *10*, 403, 1935.
139. Peery, T. M.: Postgrad. Med., *19*, 323, 1956.
140. Perry, C. B.: Arch. Dis. Child., *9*, 285, 1934.
141. ———: Arch. Dis. Child., *12*, 233, 1937.
141*a*. Phibbs, B., Taylor, J., and Zimmerman, R. A.: J.A.M.A., *214*, 2018, 1970.
142. Rammelkamp, C. H., Jr.: in *The Streptococcus, Rheumatic Fever and Glomerulonephritis*, J. W. Uhr editor, Baltimore, The Williams & Wilkins Co., 1964.
143. Rammelkamp, C. H., Jr. and Stolzer, B. L.: Yale J. Biol. Med., *34*, 386, 1961.
144. Rantz, L. A., di Caprio, J. M. and Randall, E.: Amer. J. Med. Sci., *224*, 194, 1952.
145. Rantz, L. A., Boisvert, P. J. and Spink, W. W.: Arch. Int. Med., *76*, 131, 1945.
146. Rantz, L. A., Randall, E. and Rantz, H. H.: Amer. J. Med., *5*, 3, 1948.
147. Rantz, L. A., Spink, W. W. and Boisvert, P. J.: Arch. Int. Med., *77*, 66, 1946.
148. Reimann, H. A.: *Pneumonia*, Springfield, Charles C Thomas, 1954.
148*a*. Rheumatic Fever and Rheumatic Heart Disease Study Group (Chmn., A. Taranta; members: J. Fiedler, C. W. Frank, B. S. Gilson, L. Gordis, C. Hufnagel, M. Markowitz and L. Wannamaker): Circulation, *41*, A–1, 1970.
149. Robles-Gil, J., Rodriguez, H., and Ibarra, J. J.: Amer. Heart J., *50*, 912, 1955.
149*a*. Rosenthal, A., Czoniczer, G. and Massell, B. F.: Pediatrics, *41*, 612, 1968.
150. Roth, I. R., Lingg, C. and Whittemore, A.: Amer. Heart J., *13*, 36, 1937.
150*a*. Roy, S. B., Bhatia, M. L., Lazaro, E. J. and Ramalinga-Swami, V.: Lancet, *1*, 1193, 1963.
151. Roy, S. B., Sturgis, G. P., and Massell, B. F.: New Engl. J. Med., *254*, 95, 1956.
151*a*. Ruderman, J. E. and Abruzzo, J. L.: Arth. & Rheum., *9*, 640, 1966.
152. Rutstein, D. D., Bauer, W., Dorfman, A., Gross, R. E., Lichty, J. A., Taussig, H. B. and Whittemore, R.: Circulation, *13*, 617, 1956.
153. Sacks, L., Feinstein, A. R. and Taranta, A.: J. Pediat., *61*, 714, 1962.
154. Saslaw, M. S. and Vieta, A. G.: J. Pediat., *64*, 552, 1964.
155. Schultz, I., Gundelfinger, B., Rosenbaum, M., Woolridge, R. and DeBerry, P.: J. Lab. Clin. Med., *55*, 497, 1960.
156. Siegel, A. C., Johnson, E. E. and Stollerman, G. H.: New Engl. J. Med., *265*, 559, 1961.
157. Simon, H. J. and Sakai, W.: Pediatrics, *31*, 463, 1963.
158. Slomska-Schmitt, J., Kozlowska, E., Baczynska, K., Torun, L. and Danielewicz, D.: Zakl. Mikrobiol. i Serol, Inst. Rheumatol., Warszawa-Rheumatologia, *2*, 133, 1964.
159. Spagnuolo, M. and Feinstein, A. R.: Yale J. Biol. Med., *33*, 279, 1961.
160. ———: Pediatrics, *33*, 653, 1964.
160*a*. Spencer, W. H., Thornsberry, C., Moody, M. D. and Wenger, N. K.: Ann. Intern. Med., *73*, 683, 1970.
161. Sprague, H. B. and Hardy, H. L.: Circulation, *10*, 129, 1954.
162. Stillerman, M. and Bernstein, S. H.: Amer. J. Dis. Child., *107*, 35, 1964.
163. Stollerman, G. H.: J. Clin. Invest., *32*, 607, 1953.
164. ———: Acta Rheumatologica, Documenta Geigy, *1*, 9, 1960.
165. ———: J.A.M.A., *189*, 145, 1964.
165*a*. Stollerman, G. H.: New Engl. J. Med., *283*, 872, 1970.
166. Stollerman, G. H., Lewis, A. J., Schultz, I. and Taranta, A.: Amer. J. Med., *20*, 163, 1956.
167. Stollerman, G. H., Markowitz, M., Taranta, A., Wannamaker, L. W., Whittemore, R.: Circulation, *32*, 664, 1965.
168. Stollerman, G. H., Glick, S., Patel, D. J., Hirschfeld, I. and Rusoff, J. H.: Amer. J. Med., *15*, 645, 1953.
169. Swift, H. F.: J.A.M.A., *92*, 2071, 1929.
170. Taran, L. M. and Jacobs, M. H.: J. Pediat., *27*, 59, 1945.
171. Taranta, A.: New Engl. J. Med., *260*, 1204, 1959.
172. ———: New Engl. J. Med., *266*, 13, 1962.
173. ———: in *The Streptococcus, Rheumatic Fever and Glomerulonephritis*, J. W. Uhr editor, Baltimore, The Williams and Wilkins Co., 1964.
174. Taranta, A., Kleinberg, E., Feinstein, A. R., Wood, H. F., Tursky, E., and Simpson, R.: Ann. Int. Med., *60*, Suppl. 5, 58, 1964.
175. Taranta, A., Mark, H., Haas, R. C., and Cooper, N. S.: Amer. J. Med., *25*, 52, 1958.
175*a*. Taranta, A., and Moody, M. D.: Pediatr. Clin. North Am., *18*, 125, 1971.
176. Taranta, A., Spagnuolo, M. and Feinstein, A. R.: Ann. Int. Med., *56*, 367, 1962.

177. Taranta, A. and Stollerman, G. H.: Amer. J. Med., *20*, 170, 1956.
178. Taranta, A., Wood, H. F., Feinstein, A. R., Simpson, R., and Kleinberg, E.: Ann. Int. Med., *60*, Suppl. 5, 47, 1964.
179. Ticktin, H. E. and Robinson, M. M.: Ann. N. Y. Acad. Sci., *104*, 1080, 1963.
180. Toumbis, A., Franklin, E. C., McEwen, C. and Kuttner, A. G.: J. Pediatrics, *62*, 463, 1963.
181. United Kingdom and United States Joint Report: Circulation, *11*, 343, 1955.
182. ————: Circulation, *22*, 503, 1960.
183. ————: Circulation, *32*, 457, 1965.
183*a*. Vaisman, S. B., Guasch, J., Vignau, A. I., Correa, E. I., Schuster, A. C., Mortimer, E. A., and Rammelkamp, C. H., Jr.: J.A.M.A., *194*, 1284, 1965.
184. Vernier, R. L., Worthen, H. G., Peterson, R., Colle, E., and Good, R. A.: Pediatrics, *27*, 181, 1961.
185. Wallace, H. M. Losty, M. A., Oliver-Smith, F., Azzaretti, L., and Rich, H.: Amer. J. Public Health, *46*, 1963, 1965.
186. Wannamaker, L. W.: in *The Streptococcus, Rheumatic Fever and Glomerulonephritis*, J. W. Uhr editor, Baltimore, The Williams & Wilkins Co., 1964.
187. Wannamaker, L. W., Rammelkamp, C. H., Jr., Denny, F. W., Brink, W. R., Houser, H. B., Hahn, E. O., and Dingle, J. H.: Amer. J. Med., *10*, 673, 1951.
188. Werbin, B. Z.: Amer. J. Cardiol., *4*, 356, 1959.
189. Wertheimer, N. M.: J. Chron. Dis., *16* 223, 1963.
190. Williams, R. C., Jr. and Kunkel, H. G. J. Clin. Inv., *41*, 666, 1962.
191. Wilson, M. G.: *Advances in Rheumatic Fever* 1940–1961, New York, Harper & Row, 1962
192. Wilson, M. G. and Lim, W. N.: New Engl J. Med., *260*, 802, 1959.
193. Wintrobe, M. M.: *Clinical Hematology* Philadelphia, Lea & Febiger, 1961.
194. Wittgenstein, L.: *The Blue Book*, New York Harper & Row, 1958.
195. Wood, H. F., Feinstein, A. R., Taranta, A. Epstein, J. A. and Simpson, R.: Ann. Intern Med., *60*, Suppl. 5, 31, 1964.
196. Wood, H. F., Simpson, R., Feinstein, A. R. Taranta, A., Tursky, E. and Stollerman G. H.: Ann. Int. Med., *60*, Suppl. 5, 6 1964.
196*a*. Zabriskie, J. B., Hsu, K. C., and Seegal, B. C.: Clin. & Exper. Immunol., *7*, 147, 1970.
197. Zagala, J. G. and Feinstein, A. R.: J.A.M.A., *179*, 863, 1962.
198. Ziegler, R. F.: *Electrocardiographic Studies in Normal Infants and Children.* Springfield, Charles C Thomas, 1951.
199. Zimdahl, W. T.: Brit. Heart J., *14*, 70, 1952.
200. Zimmerman, R. A., Siegel, A. C., and Steele, C. P.: Pediatrics, *30*, 712, 1962.
201. Zvaifler, N. J.: New Engl. J. Med., *267*, 10, 1962.

Chapter 45

Intermittent and Periodic Arthritic Syndromes

By George E. Ehrlich, M.D.

Almost all the diseases considered in this book are characterized by intermittent manifestations of some of their symptoms. However, it is the symptom, superimposed on a progressive anatomic lesion, which is intermittent, and not the underlying disease. An example would be the stiffness experienced by patients who have rheumatoid arthritis in the mornings and after rest; though the stiffness may fluctuate, one cannot pretend that this manifestation represents a fluctuation of rheumatoid arthritis. The rhythmicity of symptoms thus reflects the patterns of nature, not the natural history of the disease itself. Nor are remissions and exacerbations exceptions to the rule in most disorders, even in gout (where hyperuricemia and tophi persist between attacks, unless altered by successful treatment).

A handful of disorders, however, produce intermittent symptoms, often with disease-free intercritical periods. While some have been lumped together as periodic disease, others clearly present different pictures. The only link among these disorders seems to be their intermittency; they are relatively uncommon, their causes remain unknown, and their existence is controverted by some. With the possible exception of familial Mediterranean fever, which appears to be a heritable disease, these intermittent entities should be regarded as syndromes rather than diseases. Their definitions emphasize intermittently occurring symptom complexes, and, for their diagnosis, a certain basic number of symptoms must occur concurrently. The more that is known about a disease, the fewer symptoms must be present for its diagnosis; if the etiology is known, no symptoms need be present for accurate diagnosis as long as the causative agents are recoverable. Syndromes aspiring to separate existence must establish their credentials, and are not granted the luxury of *form fruste* existence. If *some* basic symptoms become unnecessary for the diagnosis of the syndrome, what is to prevent the diagnosis if only a single symptom is present? Is urethritis alone Reiter's syndrome? Aphthous stomatitis, Behçet's syndrome? Though some of the disorders to be discussed in this chapter may eventually turn out to be diseases, the vexing problem of diagnosis can be eased if they are regarded as syndromes, a convenient way of grouping apparently related symptoms. Intermittent hydrarthrosis is characterized by periodic monarticular swelling with little pain. Palindromic rheumatism adds signs of local inflammation to swelling, with redness, tenderness, and heat over the joint. Familial Mediterranean fever may present joint symptoms only, but they are accompanied by fever; however, there are generally other systemic features as well. In Behçet's syndrome and the Stevens-Johnson syndrome, joint manifestations are overshadowed by involvement of other areas of the body, more distressing, more severe, and more dramatic. Other syndromes often characterized by intermittency, such as Reiter's syndrome, the arthritis of ulcerative colitis, and the arthritis of sarcoidosis, are discussed elsewhere in this volume (*see also* Chapters 65, 46 and 70).

Certain feedback mechanisms seem to account for some periodic syndromes, such as cyclic neutropenia,[2] but as yet, these mechanisms have not been related to the syndromes under discussion in this chapter.

Intermittent Hydrarthrosis (Periodic Arthrosis).—This designates a pattern of recurrence of joint effusions, usually of the knees, of long-term, even life-long, duration. These recurrent attacks usually maintain a predictable periodicity. They begin at or shortly after puberty in many cases, but sometimes not until the geriatric period of life. For the diagnosis to be tenable, neither evidence of local inflammation nor systemic signs must develop. However, a similar pattern may characterize the early stages of rheumatoid arthritis[4] or of other periodic syndromes.

Ragan attributed the first report to Perrin (in 1845).[6] A scant 200 cases have been reported since then,[8] probably because there has been little new to say about this condition. Most practicing rheumatologists can recall a handful of such cases, often with the diagnosis made retrospectively. Perhaps because the condition is uncommon and benign, it has attracted little research interest.

In previous editions of this book, the comment was made that the Rheumatism Reviews took little notice of this syndrome.[7] They thus reflected a lack of attention to the syndrome in clinical reports. However, an occasional case of intermittent hydrarthrosis is included in larger series attempting to delineate certain laboratory features;[4] perhaps the largest such group, consisting of 14 cases, was reported by investigators seeking a microcrystalline etiology for rheumatic disorders.[8]

Etiology.—Nothing is known about the cause. Even feedback mechanisms fail to explain the patterned rhythmicity.[2] While most cases begin early in life, the syndrome may commence at any time. Women are vastly more susceptible to the disorder than men,* and in many, the joint manifestations parallel the menses. Although familial occurrence has been claimed,[8] other disorders may have been confused with intermittent hydrarthrosis. Because some patients have a strong allergic history, or develop giant urticaria, urticarial lesions of the joint have been suggested.[10] Unfortunately, antihistamines and other antiallergic medications have proved unsuccessful in controlling the disorder.

Symptoms.—Regular periodic recurrence of effusion of joints is the rule. Almost always, a single knee is involved. Rarely, the disease may be bilateral, and some cases involving the elbow, hip, or ankle have been reported. While the average interval between attacks is from one to two weeks, intervals of up to a month are not unusual, particularly when joint swelling accompanies the menses. The effusion is relatively painless, without local warmth, tenderness, or other signs of inflammation. Neither adjacent muscular spasm nor muscular atrophy occurs. However, because of the marked effusion, local mechanical difficulty in moving does occur. In some cases, the effusions cease about twenty years after onset, but in others, intermittent hydrarthrosis is a life-long condition. Generally, patients fail to consult physicians after the first few attacks, as they have learned by then that very little can or need be done about the swelling. While the fluid rapidly accumulates over a period of 12 to 24 hours, it absorbs more slowly, a period of two to four days being required for restitution to the premorbid state.

Laboratory Data.—Hemogram, erythrocyte sedimentation rate and other acute

* While many American authors would subscribe to this statement, Bywaters considers both sexes to be equally at risk[1] and some series actually cite a preponderance of men.[9]

phase reactants all remain normal, even during the attack. Latex fixation and other rheumatoid factor tests remain negative, LE cells are never seen, antinuclear factors are absent. Serum uric acid is generally within normal limits, though elevations resulting from doses of aspirin may lead to the erroneous presumptive diagnosis of gout. Development of abnormalities of acute phase reactants or serologic tests should cast some doubt on the validity of the diagnosis in the specific case.

Joint fluid does not contain crystals.[9] Cell counts vary from none to the low thousands (frequently polymorphonuclear leukocytes). The cells contain no characteristic inclusions. Serum and joint fluid complement levels are normal,[5] though some authors claim a decrease in C1 esterase inhibitor.[8] Synovial fluid is of normal viscosity and forms a solid clump in acetic acid. Tests for rheumatoid factor in joint fluid are likely to be positive unless the fluid is first digested with hyaluronidase.[11]

Typical Cases.—It has become customary to illustrate this condition with case histories. One patient, aged 30, had her menarche at age 13. A year later, concurrent with the onset of her menstrual period, she experienced a swollen left knee, unaccompanied by pain or other signs of inflammation. After four days, the swelling disappeared, only to recur in 27 days, upon advent of the next menstrual period. And so the pattern was set, with recurrent swelling of the left knee, unaccompanied by any signs of systemic disease or local inflammation. The numerous studies that her perplexed physicians had ordered were always unrewarding; therapy with salicylates, gold salts, and corticosteroids proved unavailing. With the benefit of hindsight, the probable correct diagnosis of intermittent hydrarthrosis was arrived at during the patient's thirtieth year. Watchful expectancy and optimism replaced drug therapy. At all times, synovial fluid removed from the joint displayed normal characteristics, and corticosteroids instilled into the joint failed to prevent the usual recurrence.

Not so fortunate was a 46-year-old man who had undergone some six years of regularly recurring effusions of the left knee at 14 day intervals. The effusion, unaccompanied by other signs of inflammation or by pain, but interfering mechanically with the extremes of range of motion, contained fluid of normal characteristics, with the exception that latex fixation test for rheumatoid factor was positive in dilutions of 1:40 to 1:1280 before digestion of the fluid with hyaluronidase, and negative thereafter. Chrysotherapy, anti-inflammatory compounds, corticosteroids, and colchicine proved unavailing. Corticosteroids were instilled after the frequent aspirations, and, ultimately, the effusion failed to subside even during the expected intercritical periods. Synovectomy ultimately was performed, the synovium displaying the features to be described below. Even synovectomy has failed to halt the recurrent effusions, which still continue.

Pathology.—Only few cases have come to surgery, providing a dearth of material for study. Villous proliferation of the synovium has been a constant feature, but the degree of round cell infiltration has varied. Some portions of removed synovial membranes have resembled changes of early rheumatoid arthritis, with lymphocytic aggregates and large numbers of plasma cells; in a previous edition, Ragan called these consistent with the first stage of rheumatoid arthritis.[7] Nevertheless, pannus has never been described, and these nonspecific synovial changes, in the presence of normal joint fluid and normal acute phase reactants and serologic tests, make a firm diagnosis of rheumatoid arthritis untenable.

Roentgenography.—The diagnosis of intermittent hydrarthrosis demands that no abnormalities more dramatic than soft tissue swelling be identified at the involved joint.

Prognosis.—In some patients, the disorder runs a finite course, whose total length is unpredictable. In others, joint swelling recurs throughout the patient's lifetime. The similarity of intermittent hydrarthrosis to an early stage of rheumatoid arthritis or related rheumatic disease makes prognostic judgment difficult even if the disorder has recurred for some time. However, the longer recurrences continue without apparent conversion to a more serious disorder, the more likely it is that crippling will be avoided.

Treatment.—No satisfactory treatment is available. Most of the standard treatments have been recommended at some time, including most of the treatments thought to be successful in aborting acute attacks or chronic progression of other rheumatic diseases. The constant possibility of spontaneous remission and the small number of total cases invalidate most claims for successful therapy. Unfortunately, as Ragan has pointed out, sustained effusions, sometimes with evidence of inflammation, may follow enthusiastic intra-articular corticosteroid instillation.[7] Observation and optimism ultimately serve the patient best.

Palindromic Rheumatism

The safest way to make the diagnosis of palindromic rheumatism is by retrospection. The term *palindromic* comes from the Greek, meaning to run back or to recur. It was to describe a type of rheumatism that recurs intermittently that the term was chosen by Hench and Rosenberg;[6,7] however, palindromes are more familiar to us as word games in which the word or sentence read forward or backward is the same, such as the name, 'Otto', or the classic, "Able was I ere I saw Elba."

Hench and Rosenberg published a detailed account of 34 cases in 1944,[7] and every investigator since then has been forced essentially to paraphrase their work. However, the definition has been made more precise, more has become known of the fate of some of the patients who seem to have this disorder, and increased employment of the diagnostic laboratory has lent further credence to speculations of etiology.

Clinical Picture.—Palindromic rheumatism is characterized by intermittently recurring attacks of painful swelling of the joints. It differs from intermittent hydrarthrosis in that there are obvious signs of inflammation at the affected joint, but resembles the latter in the absence of systemic manifestations.

Joint pain begins suddenly, somewhat resembling a gouty attack. Pain is variable, ranging from a dull ache in some patients to an intense bursting experience in others. The crescendo of pain reaches its maximum within a few hours, and then begins to decline. The duration of the attack therefore varies from a few hours to a few days, rarely more than three. The attack commonly begins late in the afternoon. Swelling consistently accompanies pain, at least in joints where it is clinically detectable, and warmth and redness may be found overlying the joint.[1] The redness is fairly characteristic, varying from a bright pink to crimson.

The diagnosis of palindromic rheumatism should not be made because of the recurrence of mere arthralgias. The cardinal signs of inflammation are required, comprising pain and tenderness, redness, heat, and particularly, swelling and dysfunction. Most authors have rejected the diagnosis when swelling has not been present. However, functional disability is usually mild and, in many patients, does not compromise their ability to work. Morning stiffness and gelling after rest rarely develop, and, when they do, are confined to the involved joint at the time of acute involvement.[7] The occurrence of generalized stiffness should direct the clinician to another diagnosis.

The pattern of joint attacks tends to be characteristic in a given patient. One or a limited number of joints is involved at a time, though symptoms may wax in new joints while waning in those affected during the previous attack. Intervals between attacks, thus, may vary from none at all to months. On the whole, the established pattern continues relatively unchanged for the duration of the illness, thus satisfying both Greek definitions of palindromic, "recurrence" and "reading the same, backward and forward." Although the original description claimed a distinct predilection for finger joints,[7] the knee is probably the most frequently involved joint, followed by wrist, dorsum of the hand, metacarpophalangeal and proximal phalangeal joints of the fingers, ankle, shoulder, elbow, temporomandibular or sternoclavicular joint, hip, small joints of the foot, and cervical vertebral articulations.[3,8,9]

Para-articular attacks also occur in about one-third of the patients. These consist of painful swellings of variable size at the heels, finger pads, distal phalanges, flexor and dorsal surfaces of the forearms, thumb pads, and Achilles tendons. Though resembling angioneurotic edema, they are tender and do not pit on pressure, and do not cause itching or burning paresthesia. When present, these lesions are said to be characteristic of palindromic rheumatism.[2,7]

Transient subcutaneous nodules are also a feature of this disorder. These nodules usually overly the tendons in the hands and fingers, though some have been described at the proximal extensor surfaces of the forearm, the most common site for rheumatoid nodules. The main differentiating feature from rheumatoid nodules at these locations is the relatively short duration the nodules are present, in almost all cases less than a week. Mattingly reported a strong family history of palindromic rheumatism and a high incidence of joint disease in mothers of his patients.[8]

Laboratory Data.—If palindromic rheumatism is to be considered as a separate entity, one should probably exclude patients with signs of systemic disease not otherwise explainable. Thus, the majority of patients who bear this diagnosis evince no abnormalities of hemogram, and at most *transient* abnormalities of acute phase reactants. Erythrocyte sedimentation rates, which are normal between attacks, may be modestly elevated during attacks (rarely above 35mm./hr., Westergren method).[8] Tests for rheumatoid factor, antinuclear factors, LE cells, and serum complement should be normal. Uric acid should likewise be normal, unless it is elevated as a result of small doses of salicylates taken to curb the pain.[9]

The findings in joint fluid are relatively unremarkable, with normal viscosity, mucin clot, cellular constituents, and proteins,[8,9] and low collagenase.[5] Only few biopsy specimens have been examined, usually obtained by needle. During the acute attack, polymorphonuclear leukocyte invasion of synovial tissues characterizes the intense inflammation. The cell population changes to round cells during subsidence, and synovial tissues are normal between attacks.[2] The subcutaneous nodules and tendon nodules are nonspecific, though some investigators claim a similarity to rheumatoid nodules.[8]

Roentgenographic Findings.—Except for soft tissue swelling at the time of attack, no specific abnormalities result from palindromic rheumatism. Those patients who develop changes consistent with rheumatoid arthritis probably suffer from rheumatoid arthritis of episodic onset.

Prognosis.—For the true syndrome of palindromic rheumatism, the prognosis in a given patient may be poor for recovery but good as far as crippling is concerned. In many patients the series of attacks will cease as abruptly as they began, with causes for their cessation as mysterious as those for their initiation. A follow-up of 140 patients with palindromic rheumatism seen at the Mayo Clinic for at least five years[10] revealed that more than half (73) suffered continued attacks. Eleven, or less than 10 per cent, experienced complete remissions during the interval of observation, while more than a third (50) eventuated into rheumatoid arthritis, with gout, systemic lupus erythematosus, and other diagnoses accounting for the remainder. The distribution of patients reflects the hazards of this diagnosis, as an appreciable number of patients who seem to have palindromic rheumatism actually have an episodic onset of rheumatoid arthritis, for which the prognosis is obviously not as favorable. Some patients will develop a related rheumatic syndrome or even malignant diseases, such as multiple myeloma,[11] though it is doubtful that the episodic arthritis of such long duration can be regarded as heralding malignant tumors.

In occasional cases, palindromic rheumatism seems to be a response to an irritant or an allergen.[4] Whether such cases are perhaps examples of urticarial joint lesions remains unsettled. Ultimately, therefore, discussions of prognosis hinge upon the validity of the concept of palindromic rheumatism as a separate entity. The safest course to take appears to be to make the diagnosis only after extended period of observation.

Treatment.—Acute attacks may well end before treatment for them can become effective. Anti-inflammatory drugs, anti-allergic medications, and colchicine have all been tried and generally found wanting. Claims for one drug or another have been made in individual cases, but the variability of this disorder makes such claims suspect. Vacations and administration of gold salts[8,9] have so far seemed to promote the most benefit, but the effectiveness of the latter, at least, raises some doubts as to the validity of diagnosis in the given patients (who might have been experiencing early but episodic rheumatoid arthritis). As in most cases of acute arthritis, corticosteroids instilled into the joint may promote a more rapid return to normal, but their use is seldom justified in a disorder in which return to normal after a relatively brief attack is the rule. Because of the expected repetitive attacks, administration of narcotics for relief is fraught with danger and should be avoided.*

ARTHRITIS OF FAMILIAL MEDITERRANEAN FEVER

Familial Mediterranean fever is a genetic disorder, apparently inherited as an autosomal recessive with complete penetrance.[14] Though it occurs primarily in people originating in the greater Mediterranean area, chiefly Sephardi and Iraqui Jews,[18] Levantine Arabs,[33] Turks,[28] and Armenians[34] (accounting for the name), it has been described in other groups and individuals as isolated cases as well.[6,32] Many instances were undoubtedly included in series reported as periodic diseases,[4,19,33,40] benign or

* Editor's note—continuous prophylaxis with indomethacin 25 mg. b.i d. or t.i.d. or phenylbutazone 100 mg. b.i.d. or t.i.d. has prevented or greatly ameliorated acute attacks in 8 straight cases.

THE PATTERN OF FAMILIAL MEDITERRANEAN FEVER

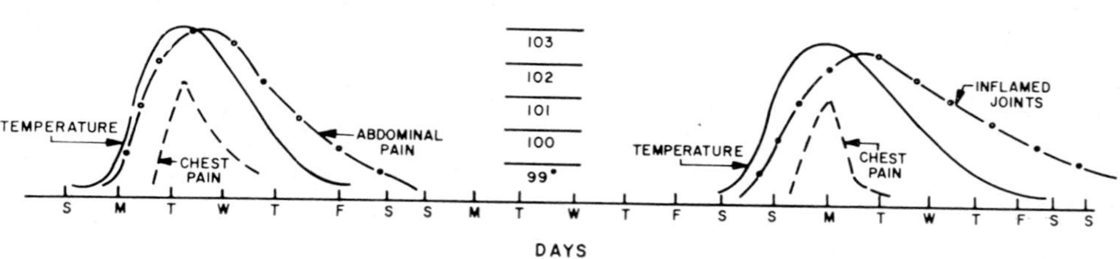

FIG. 45–1.—Typical clinical pattern of attacks of familial Mediterranean fever.

familial paroxysmal peritonitis,[38,39] or recurrent polyserositis.[29,30] The characteristic symptoms include intermittent fever and pain in the abdomen, chest, or joints. Amyloidosis (which is genetically determined) occurs in at least 40 per cent of Sephardi Jews who have the disorder; in some, it may be the sole phenotypic expression of the disease (phenotype 2).[1,12] Amyloidosis develops only rarely when the disease occurs in patients *other* than Sephardi Jews[8] or Turks.[20,28]

Clinical Picture.—Familial Mediterranean fever first appears in childhood or adolescence, and recurs intermittently throughout life. No true sex predilection has as yet been determined, though more men than women seem to be affected.[42] The family history may reveal siblings or other close relatives who have the disease. Often there is a history of consanguineous marriage among the forebears.[42]

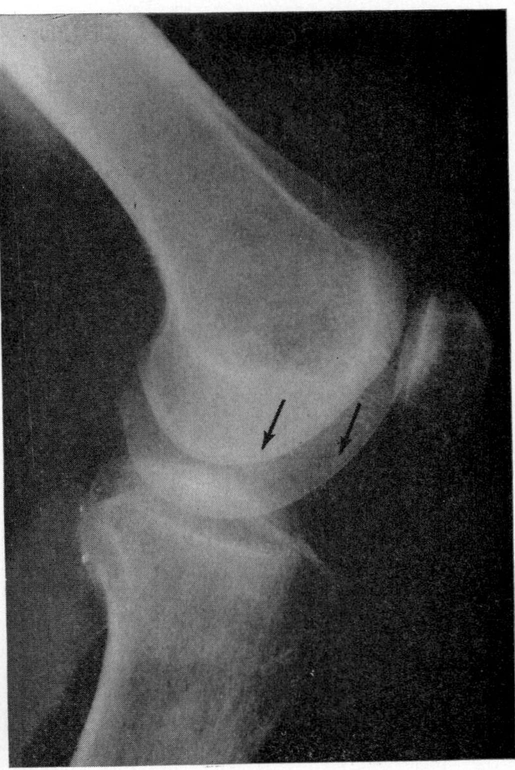

FIG. 45–3.—Roentgenogram of knee. In this adult who no longer has symptoms of joint disease, the double-contoured "eggshell" line is present despite the recovery from osteoporosis.

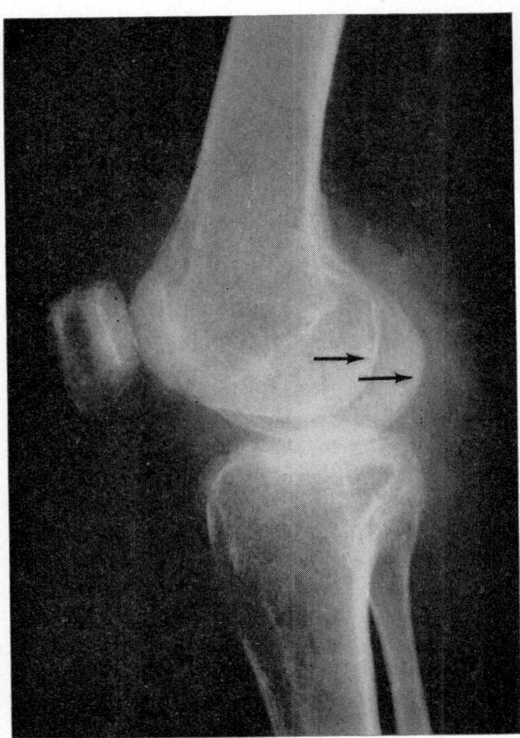

FIG. 45–2.—Roentgenogram of knee. The femoral condyles are large. Soft tissue swelling and osteoporosis are readily apparent. A double-contoured "eggshell" line outlines the femoral condyles.

Fever probably accompanies every attack but does not give rise to shaking chills or other constitutional symptoms, and usually lasts but a few hours. Temperature elevations vary from persistent low grade to spikes up to 103.1° F. (39.5° C.).[42]

The abdominal crises resemble acute peritonitis, last from twelve to twenty-four hours, and rarely for three or four days.[42] Serous fluid in the abdominal cavity is the only abnormal finding on laparotomy. Occasionally, abdominal pain simulates pelvic inflammatory disease.[5] Acute chest pain commonly involves only one hemithorax with referral

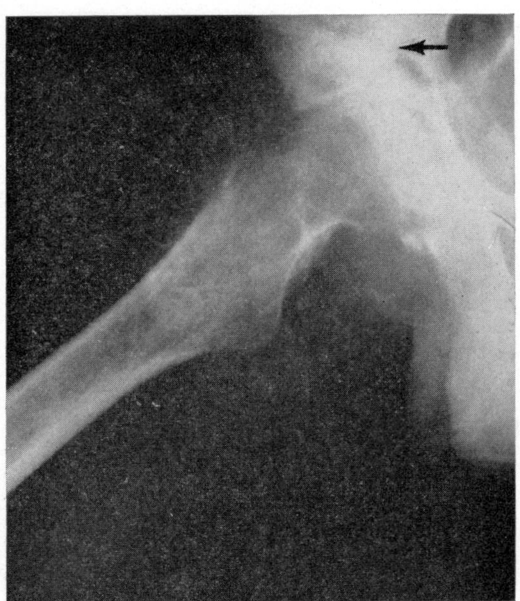

FIG. 45–4.—Roentgenogram of hip (frog lateral). Marked degenerative changes include pseudocysts, periosteal proliferation and osteoporosis of the femur, and narrowing of the joint space, marginal spurs, and a triangular iliac density at the acetabulum.

to the corresponding shoulder. It is also of short duration, and is usually accompanied by minimal evanescent pleural effusion[42] or pericarditis.[31] Many patients experience recurrent attacks of intense tenderness and redness around the ankle. This erysipelas-like erythema is probably not related to underlying joint disease. Intestinal obstruction of serious proportion,[26,36] varying types of renal disease,[9] and cyclic emotional states[6,39] are sometimes considered part of the disease. Amyloidosis characteristically produces nephrotic syndrome progressing to early death in renal failure.[3,8,17,22]

The musculoskeletal attacks may occur together with, or independently of, other manifestations in approximately 70 per cent of patients. When they occur alone, the later course or the family history confirms the diagnosis. The distribution of attacks is asymmetric, with large joints more usually involved. The affected joints, in order of decreasing frequency, are knees, ankles, hips, shoulders, feet and toes, elbows, wrists and hands, and the remaining synovial joints.[16] Isolated disease of the temporomandibular joints[21] or the sacroiliac joints[16] has been described. Arthritis is commonly monarticular. Subsequent attacks tend to adhere to the established pattern. Attacks are intermittent, not periodic, and of varying duration. They generally last longer than other manifestations of this disease. All afflicted patients experience attacks which terminate in less than a week. Not infrequently, attacks may persist for two or three weeks, and rarely, for months.[6,16]

Localized pain is the predominant, and at times, the sole symptom. The joint and periarticular area are usually exquisitely tender so that the slightest touch cannot be tolerated. At the knees, ankles, elbows, and shoulders, swelling is usually present, accompanied at times by massive effusion. However, it is usually not as pronounced as the dramatic pain would imply. Limitation of motion and severe functional impairment result. During an attack, the muscles around the joint are in spasm. However, morning stiffness in the involved or other joints does not occur. The patients do not develop gelling of joints and muscles after rest. Although the involved joints may be somewhat warm initially, the warmth does not persist as long as the pain or functional impairment. Except for the occasional erysipelas-like erythema, redness is notable by its absence. Thus, *an intermittently occurring asymmetric or monarthritis characterized primarily by pain, tenderness, and impaired joint function disproportionate to the amount of swelling and unaccompanied by warmth or redness should alert the physician to the possibility that he is dealing with the arthritis of familial Mediterranean fever*.

Joint function recovers completely between attacks. Disuse atrophy, which develops in prolonged attacks and may be marked, is also reversible. Demonstrable residua of attacks are extreme rarities. However, when the hip becomes involved by a prolonged attack, functional recovery may not be as likely. In a recent study, sixteen of eighteen affected hips developed moderate to marked anatomical and functional changes, with narrowing and sclerosis of the joint space and progressive limitation of motion. Destructive changes occasionally supervene requiring surgical intervention.[28a] Tendon contractures do not occur.[16]

During acute attacks, superficial vessels often dilate over the involved joints. This is especially true at the knee where they can be readily detected with infrared illumination.[13]

Acute tenderness and swelling of the lower thigh or upper calf may mimic arthritis at the knee. Inflammation of bursal areas may be responsible, as has infrequently been the case at the hip.[16] Various types of trauma may precipitate attacks. In different patients, overexertion, bruising, heat, cold and even paracentesis of joints have been implicated. The type of trauma is specific to the patient, but many attacks are not preceded by a recognizable precipitating event.[16]

Arthrodesis has occasionally been performed when the disease was so severe as to be mistaken for tuberculous arthritis. Surgical fusion thus prevented functional recovery, which might otherwise have been inevitable.[16]

Amyloidosis is probably the basis for the frequently encountered splenomegaly. Although many patients come from the area where infectious diseases result in enlarged spleens, patients who have familial Mediterranean fever rarely seem to develop intercurrent illnesses.[42]

Among the negative features that permit differential diagnosis are the absence of nodules, urethritis, stomatitis, balanitis, conjunctivitis, uveitis, choroiditis, and dermatitis.

Clinical Features—Arthritis of Familial Mediterranean Fever

Sex incidence—men slightly more frequently than women
Race — Armenians, Sephardi and Iraqui Jews, Levantine Arabs, Turks
Inheritance—autosomal recessive
Family history—usually present
Age of onset—childhood or adolescence
Prodromes—none
Onset—Acute, with fever and abdominal, chest or joint pain
Frequency of joint involvement—knee, ankle, hip, shoulder, elbow, or other synovial joints
Duration of attacks—four days to a year
Periodicity—intermittent
Prominent symptoms — exquisite tenderness, pain on motion and functional impairment
Other symptoms—swelling, minimal warmth, no redness, asymmetric involvement
Muscular atrophy—after prolonged attack
Skin changes—erysipelas-like erythema at ankle
Functional recovery—complete
Response to therapy—none proved

Laboratory Data.—Most of the laboratory findings in familial Mediterranean fever are nonspecific. Erythrocyte sedimentation rate and fibrinogen level are elevated or at upper reaches of normal between attacks and soar precipitously with the onset of attacks. Within days they return to previous levels.[11] Anemia may be related to a malabsorption syndrome that has sometimes been demonstrated. Leukocytosis or leukopenia, the latter in the presence of splenomegaly, is an inconsistent feature. Urinary abnormalities appear only if there is amyloidosis, and consist primarily of massive proteinuria. Serum albumin is often decreased. Gamma globulins may be normal or increased but elevations of the alpha 2, alpha 2m and beta 2m globulins, haptoglobin, and lipoproteins are common.[10] The electrophoretic pattern is similar to that seen in amyloidosis even when this latter feature is not demonstrable. Latex fixation tests for rheumatoid factor are negative, or only transiently positive in low dilutions (1:160 or less).[6,16] Other serologic tests and L.E. preparations are negative. Uric acid and etiocholanolone levels[2] are not elevated. Whole serum complement and C1 esterase inhibitor may be deficient.[35]

Early in the attacks, the joint fluid contains many polymorphonuclear leukocytes, but these are later replaced by lymphocytes. Viscosity is poor, but the mucin clot is fairly adequate. Protein and sugar are unaltered, and cultures are negative.[6,16] Foamy cells have also been described.[42]

Roentgenography.—The bone age is generally younger than the chronological age, leading to the paradoxic finding of degenerative changes while the epiphyses are still patent. When the arthritis is prolonged, coarse trabecular metaphyseal osteoporosis forms pseudocysts. Protracted involvement of the knee leads to enlargement of the femoral condyles. All these findings are nonspecific features of long-term immobilization during bone growth, such as occurs in poliomyelitis.[37]

During the acute phases, soft tissue enlargement can be seen. With chronicity, the joint space narrows and proliferative marginal bony changes develop. This is particularly true at hips and knees and is partly reversible. The changes may represent periosteal reaction to marginal destruction. True cysts are encountered only rarely. A triangular condensation of the ilium above the acetabulum characterizes chronic hip involvement.[16]

In osteoporosis of the femur, the femoral condyles appear as thin eggshell lines separated from the trabecular pattern by a narrow radiolucent zone. With the arthritis of familial Mediterranean fever this eggshell line may be found on both sides of the radiolucent zone.[16] Though it has been described in only a few patients, it may be a specific finding. The line tends to remain even when other roentgenographic changes disappear.

Though there is no clinical evidence of ankylosing spondylitis, some sacroiliac joints are widened and others sclerosed.[13] Rarely, patchy calcified bridges can be seen in the lower spine.[7] Osteitis condensans ilii is frequently present.[20] In fact, various sacroiliac abnormalities tend to be found in a disproportionate number of cases, so that familial Mediterranean fever should always be included in the differential diagnosis of radiologic abnormalities of the sacroiliac joints.[15] However, the changes may reflect more the character of the population at risk than results of the disease. The occurrence of sacroiliac changes in populations where tropical diseases are prevalent[27] makes the significance of this finding questionable.

Pathologic Anatomy.—The changes seen in biopsies from inflamed joints are nonspecific. Irregular aggregates of round cells surround small blood vessels, but true perivascular cuffing does not occur. There is increased vascularity, and stromal fibroblasts[16] and polymorphonuclear leukocytes[21] are present in increased number. Lytic lesions of bone are filled with fibrous tissue. Post-mortem examina-

Laboratory Features—Arthritis of Familial Mediterranean Fever

Blood count—variable
Urinalysis—variable
Latex fixation—negative
L.E. preparation—negative
Uric acid—normal
Fibrinogen—elevated, spiking during attack
ESR—elevated, spiking during attack
Etiocholanolone—not elevated
Roentgenograms—degenerative changes, retarded bone age, osteoporosis, "eggshell line," sacroiliac changes
Biopsy — non-specific inflammatory changes, perireticulin amyloidosis

tions of joints that had been involved but had recovered reveals no abnormalities.[16]

The amyloidosis encountered in familial Mediterranean fever, though primary, is distributed as if it were of the secondary variety.[14] The amyloid is deposited in the perireticulin areas of blood vessels, and is especially concentrated in spleen and kidney.[8,11] It has occasionally been demonstrated around blood vessels in or near inflamed joints.[16]

Treatment.—No therapy has yet proved either curative or consistently palliative. Temporary partial relief of joint pains may be achieved by the combined use of analgesic preparations and moist, hot applications. Corticosteroids are singularly ineffective, both by systemic and by intra-articular administration. In fact, unresponsiveness to corticosteroids may be used as a differential diagnostic criterion.[16] Administration of other anti-inflammatory agents has never yielded reproducible amelioration of symptoms and signs. Colchicine[22] and the gamut of immunosuppressive drugs[23] have been subjects of favorable reports, but the series are small, and other investigators have yet to confirm these results. Fat-free diets,[24,25] recommended at one time, have been found wanting.[41] Physical therapy and exercises can, however, speed functional recovery after an attack. In view of the recurrent nature of this disorder, narcotics must be assiduously avoided. Since there is complete functional recovery from arthritis, operative interference with joints is not indicated. However, appendectomy should perhaps be done early since acute appendicitis cannot readily be distinguished from the abdominal manifestations of this disease.

Prognosis.—Functional recovery from individual attacks and asymptomatic remissions are the rule, except when the hip joint is involved during a protracted attack. Those with the greatest experience with this disease believe that the vast majority of patients in whom the occurrence is familial will succumb to amyloidosis at a relatively young age.[17] In ethnic groups other than those commonly affected, prognosis seems far more favorable.

BEHÇET'S SYNDROME

Behçet's syndrome is a multisystem disorder whose limits are even now being expanded. Originally described as a triple symptom complex consisting of recurrent oral and genital ulcerations and relapsing iritis,[4] the syndrome was rapidly seen to include manifestations in most other bodily systems as well. While the original cases were described in countries bordering the Mediterranean, large series have been collected in the rest of Europe and the Middle East, Japan, and lately, the United States. In part, the syndrome resembles Reiter's syndrome, but is generally differentiated from the latter because of its intermittent recurrent nature and potentially fatal outcome. Arthralgias and arthritis have lately been recognized as frequent and prominent manifestations.[22,36]

Behçet's syndrome has been recognized under this name only since 1937, though a similar case was described in 1931 by Adamantiades,[1] whose name is sometimes linked with Behçet's in the eponym. However, the disease is by no means a recent arrival. Hippocrates provided a rather accurate clinical description,[12] and the various manifestations have subsequently been grouped in reports of other observers, including biographers (for example, the great American historian Francis Parkman is believed to have been a victim of the disease[3]). The true prevalence is difficult to estimate, as many cases probably go undetected or undiagnosed, others assume the labels "Reiter's syndrome," "Stevens-Johnson syndrome," or even "periodic disease," and others go unrecognized because of the unfamiliarity of physicians with the symptom complex.

Etiology is unknown. Proponents of allergic or "autoimmune" causation, including most English investigators, prefer to include Behçet's syndrome among the connective tissue disorders.[19] Meanwhile, French and Turkish investigators have vigorously sought evidence of viral etiology. In a recent symposium held in England, the opponents of viral etiology carried the day mainly on evidence collected by Dudgeon.[9] However, various investigators have discovered inclusion bodies in cells recovered from synovial fluid of patients with Behçet's syndrome,[6,24] and others have seemingly isolated a filterable agent from various sources (blood, CSF).[33]

Clinical Picture.—The triple symptom complex of *oral* and *genital ulcers* and *iritis* is crucial to the diagnosis, though some investigators have recently been satisfied with two of the three, with at least three other accompanying systemic involvements.[22] The oral lesions resemble aphthous stomatitis and consist of recurrent ulcers, single or multiple, distributed anywhere in the mouth and pharynx.[13] The ulcers prove particularly resistant to therapy, are larger than the usual aphthous lesions, may occur in crops, and can be provoked by trauma to the mucosa. They are accompanied by scanty fungiform papillae of the tongue,[8] plaque-like lesions of the pharynx and larynx, and oral foetor. The classic ophthalmic lesion is hypopyon iritis. However, episcleritis, conjunctivitis, keratitis, iridocyclitis, retinal thrombophlebitis,[35] papilledema,[17] and optic atrophy are also frequently encountered.[35] Ulcerative lesions of the penis and scrotum are usually painful; those of the vulva and vagina are not, and are thus easily missed.[21] Skin lesions are extremely common, especially pyoderma with tiny or large pustular lesions.[27] Such lesions can be produced by any needle puncture of the skin, and even surgical tracts become infected to their full extent.[27] Lesions resembling erythema nodosum commonly accompany the syndrome. Gangrene of fingertips and toes,[25] thrombosis of superficial veins,[10] migratory thrombophlebitis, thrombosis of the inferior vena cava (especially in the very young),[10,16] inflammatory disease of any portion of the gastrointestinal tract,[29]

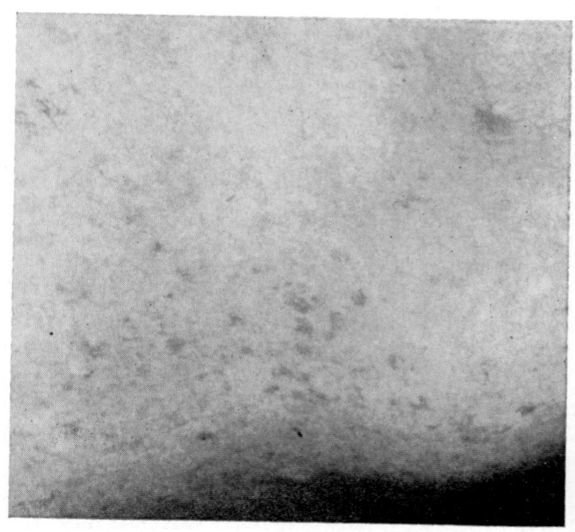

Fig. 45–7.—Cutaneous pustules in patient with pyoderma of Behçet's syndrome (Courtesy of Norman A. Cummings, M.D.).

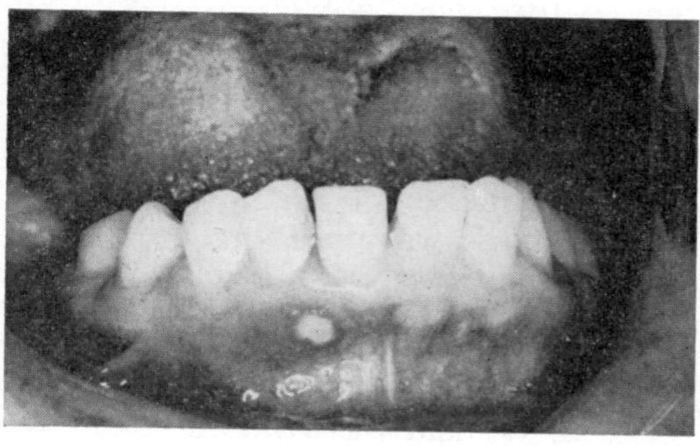

Fig. 45–5.—Aphthous ulcer on buccal surface of lower gum in a patient with Behçet's syndrome (Courtesy of Norman A. Cummings, M.D.).

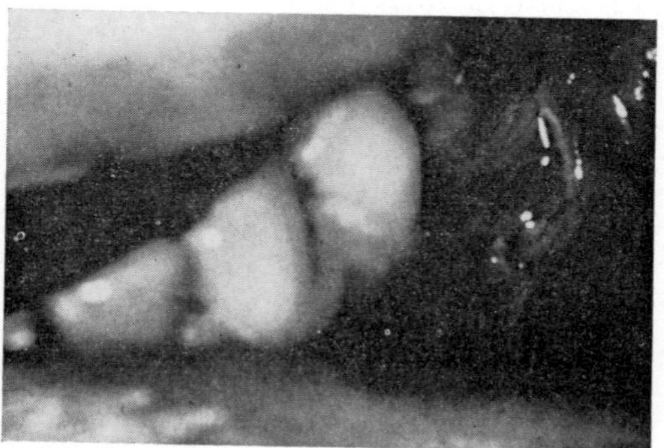

Fig. 45–6.—Deep ulcer in buccal mucous membrane in patient with Behçet's syndrome (Courtesy of Norman A. Cummings, M.D.).

and a host of nervous system disorders are part of the syndrome.[2,12] Prognosis of some of the patients is determined by nervous system involvement, including meningitis, myelitis, brain stem syndrome, and organic confusional states. As may be expected in a multisystem disorder which is both chronic and recurring, and which produces numerous genital lesions, psychiatric disorders are frequent.[11] Many authors point to the social stigma of venereal disease, with which the genital lesions may be confused, as a reason for the nonreporting of the disorder by patient or physician. Family clustering has been observed.[22]

As is true of the other intermittent and periodic syndromes, joint involvement in Behçet's syndrome tends to be monarticular or oligoarticular. While arthralgias are more frequent than true arthritis, the latter, too, occurs in most patients who have Behçet's syndrome. The knee is the joint most frequently involved, followed by ankles, wrists, elbows, and other synovial joints.[22,26,36] The manubriosternal joint[7] and the sacroiliac joints may be involved, but the small joints rarely are; fingers and toes may occasionally pain, but are not commonly swollen or deformed. Joint swelling may be so painless as to be confused with intermittent hydrarthrosis, or so painful, with gout, or, because of associated symptoms, Reiter's syndrome or rheumatoid arthritis. Onset is usually insidious and duration is extremely variable, ranging from but few weeks to several years.[22] Intervals between arthritic attacks tend to be longer than between attacks of extra-articular manifestations of Behçet's syndrome, but arthralgias of relatively brief duration occur much more frequently. During the course of arthritis, effusion is almost always present, with significant morning stiffness in the involved areas. The joints are warm, tender, and slightly reddened. Permanent changes and disability of the joints rarely develop.

Nearly all attacks are accompanied by fever and other constitutional signs. Myalgias are frequent.

There is no usual sequence of development of the various symptoms, but oral lesions tend to be first in most patients.[29] Nevertheless, joint lesions may precede the onset of other involvement or may not set in until years after the first manifestation has begun elsewhere.[22]

Laboratory Findings.—Acute phase reactants tend to be abnormal during an attack, including rapid sedimentation rate, strongly positive C-reactive protein, and elevation of alpha-2 globulins.[13] Anemia is common. A polyclonal gammopathy is characteristically found in this disorder. Unlike recurrent aphthous stomatitis, Behçet's syndrome is not associated with impairment of lymphocyte stimulation.[14] Inclusion bodies are found in mucosal cells derived from oral and vaginal mucosa,[33] and from leukocytes recovered from joint fluid.[6,24]

Results of tests for rheumatoid factor and L.E. cells are negative, and antinuclear antibodies are not present in the serum. Various antibodies against mucosa are demonstrable.[20] They rise with relapses and fall with remissions.[18,34] Cryoglobulins have been demonstrated in 20 to 25 per cent of cases investigated by Cummings.[7a]

Roentgenography.—There are no significant roentgenographic changes in the joints, even after the disease has been present for a long time. However, gastrointestinal roentgenography may show evidence of colitis or enteritis and chest films commonly show some pulmonary fibrosis.[29] Venograms may reveal blockage of large and small vessels by thrombi, including thrombosis of renal veins and the inferior vena cava, and in rare cases, of the superior vena cava.

Differential Diagnosis.—Depending upon the mode of presentation, confusion with other rheumatic syndromes is likely. Intermittent hydrarthrosis, rheumatoid arthritis, systemic lupus erythematosus, Reiter's syndrome, Stevens-Johnson syndrome, and any of the forms of arthritis associated with erythema nodosum, may be suggested by the appropriate symptom complex when joints are involved.[36]

There is no clear-cut way of differentiating Behçet's syndrome from other disorders it may resemble, and the differentiation is ultimately based on long-term observation and clinical superficialities. Enthusiasts would make of Behçet's syndrome a leading member of the connective tissue disease family; skeptics would classify most cases otherwise. Because so many of the cases are described in areas where other periodic syndromes, such as familial Mediterranean fever, are common, confusion with these is likely.[17]

Pathology.—Basic to all the ulcerative lesions of Behçet's syndrome is vasculitis.[19] The vasculitis is so reminiscent of other "autoimmune" disorders that it has fueled claims for inclusion of the disorder among the "autoimmune connective tissue" syndromes. A preparation derived from freshly epithelized skin lesions of the scrotum, called Behçetin, injected intracutaneously, produces large red edematous infiltrated reactions consisting, 36 hours after injection, of lymphocytes and polymorphonuclear leukocytes.[21] This reaction is said to be positive only during the active phase of the disease, however.[34] Mucocutaneous lesions in laboratory animals resembling those of Behçet's syndrome in humans have been produced experimentally by injections of mycobacteria and Freund's adjuvant, which more commonly produces arthritis, and can also result in dermal, genital, and ocular lesions.[30]

Behçet's Syndrome

Major Criteria:

1. Mouth (aphthous) ulcers
2. Iritis (with hypopyon)
3. Genital ulcers

Minor Criteria

4. Skin lesions*
   a. Pyoderma
   b. Nodose lesions
5. Arthritis
   a. of major joints
   b. arthralgias
6. Vascular disease
   a. Migratory superficial phlebitis
   b. Major vessel thrombosis
   c. Aneurysms
   d. Peripheral gangrene
   e. Retinal and vitreous hemorrhage, papilledema
7. Central nervous system disease
   a. Brain stem syndrome
   b. Meningomyelitis
   c. Confusional states
8. Gastrointestinal disease
   a. Malabsorption
   b. Meteorism
   c. Nonspecific bloating, pains, "dyspepsia"

* Considered a major criterion by many.

Treatment.—As yet, no effective treatment has been described, though various immunosuppressive agents, such as azathioprine[32] and cyclophosphamide,[5] hold some promise. Corticosteroids have had indifferent success.[17] Fibrinolytic compounds have found some favor.[23] Blood transfusions have seemingly induced remissions.[15,28]

On the whole, symptomatic therapy of the various expressions of the disease is moderately successful. Injections should be avoided whenever possible as needle punctures provoke purulent skin lesions. In severe cases, enucleation of the eye, amputations, major vascular surgery, and craniotomies have been performed.

Prognosis.—Though Behçet's syndrome does not necessarily compromise life expectancy, the advent of nervous system symptoms and signs is an ominous event.[7b] Behçet's syndrome ought therefore be considered as a generally benign disease subject to serious or fatal complications.

STEVENS-JOHNSON SYNDROME

In a sense, the Stevens-Johnson syndrome does not belong to the realm of rheumatology. Joint and muscle involvement consists of transient pains only, which may well be mere reflections of the severity of the disease. But because there are so many similarities or potential points of confusion between the Stevens-Johnson syndrome and Behçet's syndrome or Reiter's syndrome, it will be discussed here.

By general agreement, Stevens-Johnson syndrome is included among the oculocutaneous syndromes. Most informed clinicians regard it as a variant of erythema multiforme exudativum presenting with systemic manifestations and a potentially grave prognosis. Though there seem to be earlier reports, the description by Hebra[11] is considered the classic depiction of the cutaneous syndrome. In 1922, Stevens and Johnson elaborated the constitutional symptoms of the syndrome that now bears their name.[16]

The onset of Stevens-Johnson syndrome is heralded by high fever and extensive stomatitis. While this may superficially resemble monilial stomatitis, it rapidly develops into a series of ulcerated lesions of the oral mucous membranes, and on the conjunctiva, the nasal mucosa, and the genitalia and anus.[4] Within a few days, a bullous and erythematous skin eruption develops anywhere on the body, and erythematous plaques form on the extremities. Pneumonitis is frequently present, either as a precursor or as a concomitant.[13] To make the diagnosis, the eruption of erythema multiforme accompanied by bullae or vesicles and stomatitis is required; documented fever, balanitis, vaginitis or urethritis, and conjunctivitis also occur, though they need not all be present simultaneously in the same patient.

Widespread arthralgias and myalgias of relatively transient nature are complained of. These are rarely accompanied by actual signs of arthritis.[8]

The syndrome is particularly prevalent in the pediatric age group, though it may occur at any age; the risk of developing the syndrome is greatly reduced after the age of twenty. All reports emphasize a male preponderance.

The syndrome begins in one of three ways. It may suddenly appear in a setting of good health, without apparent exogenous factors. Secondly, there may be symptoms suggestive of an upper

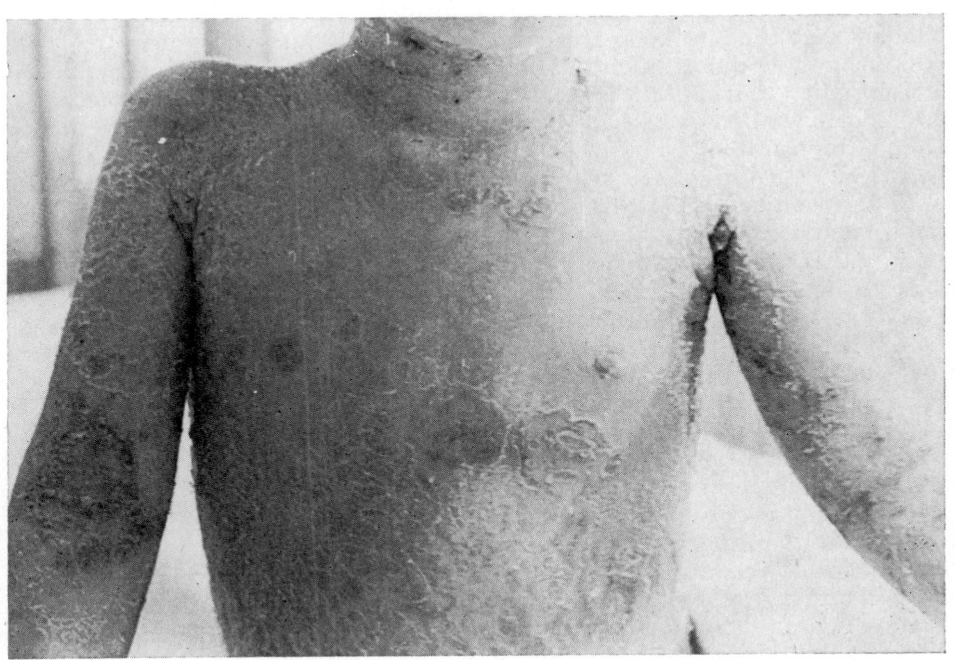

Fig. 45–8.—Bullous and crusting cutaneous eruption in a patient with Stevens-Johnson syndrome (erythema multiforme exudativum).

respiratory tract[9] or urinary tract infection,[14] for which drug therapy is initiated. While only about one-fifth of the patients present with the first pattern, half develop the syndrome after prodromata for which some treatment is afforded. In these cases, the prior illness occurs in bodily areas later to be affected by Stevens-Johnson syndrome. The third mode of presentation also follows drug treatment, but this time for disorders seemingly remote from the Stevens-Johnson syndrome. As an example, epilepsy seems unrelated to Stevens-Johnson syndrome, but the administration of anti-convulsants may directly precede the onset of the syndrome.

Laboratory and Roentgenographic Features.—There are no specific abnormalities of laboratory tests or roentgenographic examination that would support the diagnosis of Stevens-Johnson syndrome. However, in a large number of cases, mycoplasma pneumoniae are recoverable from the pharynx,[9] sputum,[6] and exudates of the bullous lesions;[13] moreover, rises of specific hemagglutination inhibition and complement fixation antibodies are recorded during the disease, with fall of these antibodies during the recovery phase.[15] Leukocyte-bound immunoglobulin is also demonstrable.[18]

Etiology.—The causes of this syndrome are still the subject of controversy.[13] Mycoplasma pneumoniae has a clear edge on other microorganisms as a provocative agent.[3,6,12] Other viruses, fungi, and bacteria have also been implicated. The majority of cases follow drug therapy, with sulfonamides clearly leading the way.[1,17] Warning labels have been affixed to certain long-acting sulfa drugs naming them as potential precursors of Stevens-Johnson syndrome,[7] but recent careful reviews of the evidence have found it wanting.[1,4] A few recorded cases followed administration of drugs in common use for treatment of rheumatic diseases, including aspirin and phenylbutazone.[1] Laxatives and sedatives, many non-prescription, are also culpable. Measles vaccination has preceded the onset.[10] In many cases, no causal relationship to a preceding event can be demonstrated.

Treatment.—When a specific microorganism seems responsible for the syndrome, appropriate antibiotic therapy, usually with tetracycline, may prove beneficial.[12] In some cases, corticosteroids are employed, with mixed success (it may be a matter of selection as some patients worsen while others improve). Other nonspecific supportive measures should be taken, of course.

Prognosis.—Though fatalities have been recorded, the outlook is not unfavorable, particularly in older patients. Infants and small children bear the greatest risk.[19]

The *periodicity* of the syndrome results from renewed provocation by the offending factor. Multiple episodes are likely when the syndrome is precipitated by a non-prescription medication, as this is beyond the physician's control unless he knows about it. Other cases recur because the patient fails to give a complete history and the offending drug is prescribed again.

As the Stevens-Johnson syndrome occurs in conjunction with ulcerative colitis[5] and disorders of the reticuloendo-

Stevens-Johnson Syndrome

Major Criteria
1. Skin lesions
   Erythema multiforme exudativum
2. Stomatitis (ulcerative)
3. Genital or anal ulcers

Minor Criteria
4. Pneumonitis—preceding or coexistent
5. History of upper respiratory or genitourinary infection treated with sulfonamides or antibiotics
6. Arthralgias
7. Conjunctivitis
8. History of ingestion of wide variety of drugs, both prescription and non-prescription.

INTERMITTENT AND PERIODIC SYNDROMES	joints	skin	eyes	buccal mucosa	genitalia	colon	cent nerv sys	fever	other
Palindromic rheumatism	√								
Intermittent hydrarthrosis	√								
Familial Mediterranean fever	√	√						√	pleura peritoneum
Behcet's syndrome	√	√	√	√	√	√	√	√	veins
Arthritis of ulcerative colitis	√	√	√	√	√	√	√	√	
Stevens-Johnson syndrome	√	√	√	√	√			√	
Reiter's syndrome	√	√	√	√	√	√	√	√	
Henoch-Schoenlein purpura	√	√				√		√	kidney

Fig. 45–9.—Summary of clinical features of the intermittent and periodic arthritic syndromes.

thelial system, including leukemias[2] (though it is usually in response to some therapeutic agent used for these various disorders), underlying diseases should always be sought.

Provocative tests with suspected drugs should never be attempted.

OTHER INTERMITTENT SYNDROMES

Many diseases exhibiting rheumatic symptoms and signs may recur after they have seemingly run their course. *Acute tropical polyarthritis*, an oligoarticular disorder affecting chiefly the large joints of adults, accompanied by fever and abnormalities of the acute phase reactants is one such disease. While the attack is usually single, and can be aborted with aspirin, recurrent attacks may develop after an indeterminate interval. Descriptions of this disease have thus far been limited to Africa, though they resemble the *epidemic polyarthritis of Northern Australia*, which is associated with Group A arbovirus infection.[1]

Thus, a number of syndromes exist with overlapping symptoms. They have been dignified with different names, but their manifestations suggest that there may well be certain basic underlying mechanisms common to all. As attention paid to esoterica often results in deeper understanding of more common problems, the periodic and intermittent syndromes may lead the way to better understanding of the mechanisms of joint inflammation and the rhythms of nature.

BIBLIOGRAPHY

General

1. Greenwood, B. M.: Quart. J. Med., *38*, 295, 1969.
2. Morley, A. and Stohlman, F.: New Engl. J. Med., *282*, 643, 1970.

Intermittent Hydrarthrosis

1. Bywaters, E. G. L. and Ansell, B.: in *Textbook of the Rheumatic Diseases*, Copeman, W. S. C., ed. 4th Ed., London, E. & S. Livingstone Ltd., pg. 525 ff., 1968.
2. Cronkite, E. P.: New Engl. J. Med., *282*, 683, 1970.
3. Denis, F., Franchimont, P., and Van Cauwenberge, H.: Rev. Med. de Liege, *24*, 604, 1969.
4. Fourteenth Rheumatism Review: Ann. Intern. Med., *56*, Supplement 1, 1962.

5. PELTIER, A. P.: J. Belge de Rhum. et de Med. Phys., *22*, 276, 1967.
6. PERRIN, E. R.: J. de med., *3*, 82, 1845.
7. RAGAN, C.: in *Arthritis*, Hollander, J. L., ed. 7th ed., Philadelphia, Lea & Febiger, pg. 755 ff., 1966.
8. REIMANN, H. A.: Geriatrics, *24*, 146, 1969.
9. SERRE, H., SIMON, L. and SANY, J.: J. Med. Montpellier, *3*(5), 37, 1968.
10. SCHLESINGER, H.: Die intermittirenden Gelenkschwellungen, Vienna, A. Holder, Nothnagel's Specielle Pathologie und Therapie, *7*, 3, 1903.
11. WEINER, A. D. and GHORMLEY, R. K.: J. Bone Jt. Surg., *38A*, 1039, 1956.

Palindromic Rheumatism

1. ANSELL, B. M. and BYWATERS, E. G. L.: Ann. Rheum. Dis., *18*, 331, 1959.
2. BYWATERS, E. G. L. and ANSELL, B. M.: in *Textbook of the Rheumatic Diseases*, Copeman, W. S. C., ed., 4th ed., London, E. and S. Livingstone Ltd., pp. 524 ff, 1968.
3. DENIS, F., FRANCHIMONT, P., and VAN CAUWENBERGE, H.: Rev. Med. de Liege, *24*, 604, 1969.
4. EPSTEIN, S.: Ann. Allergy, *27*, 343, 1969.
5. HARRIS, E. D., JR., COHEN, G. L., and KRANE, S. M.: Arth. & Rheum., *12*, 92, 1969.
6. HENCH, P. S. and ROSENBERG, E. F.: Proc. Mayo Clin., *16*, 808, 1941.
7. ————: Arch. Intern. Med., *73*, 293, 1944.
8. MATTINGLY, S.: Ann. Rheum. Dis., *25*, 307, 1966.
9. RENIER, J. C., BREGEON, C., and BESSON, J.: Rev. Rheum., *36*, 583, 1969.
10. WARD, L. E., and OKIHIRO, M. M.: Arch. Inter-Amer. Rheum., *2*, 208, 1959.
11. ZAWADZKI, Z. A. and BENEDEK, T. G.: Arth. & Rheum., *12*, 555, 1969.

Familial Mediterranean Fever

1. BLUM, A., GAFNI, J., SOHAR, E., SHIBOLET, S. and HELLER, H.: Ann. Intern. Med., *57*, 795, 1962.
2. BONDY, P. K., COHN, G. L., HERRMANN, W. and CRISPELL, K. R.: Yale J. Biol. & Med., *30*, 395, 1958.
3. CATTAN, R.: Presse med., *63*, 237, 1955.
4. CATTAN, R. and MAMOU, H.: Bull. et mem. Soc. mem. hop. Paris, *67*, 1104, 1951.
5. EHRENFELD, E. N. and POLISHUK, W. Z.: Isr. J. Med. Sci., *6*, 9, 1970.
6. EHRLICH, G. E.: Clin. Orthop., *57*, 51, 1968.
7. EISINGER, J. B., LUCCIONI, R., ACQUAVIVA, P., MOULARD, J. C., and RECORDIER, A. M.: Marseille Med., *107*, 427, 1970.
8. ELIAKIM, M.: Isr. J. Med. Sci., *6*, 2, 1970.
9. ELIAKIM, M., RACHMILEWITZ, M., ROSENMANN, E. and NIV, A.: Isr. J. Med. Sci., *6*, 228, 1970.
10. FRENSDORFF, A., SHIBOLET, S., LAMPRECHT, S. and SOHAR, E.: Clin. Chim. Acta, *10*, 106, 1964.
11. FRENSDORFF, A., SOHAR, E., and HELLER, H.: Ann. Intern. Med., *55*, 448, 1961.
12. GAFNI, J., RAVID, M., and SOHAR, E.: Isr. J. Med. Sci., *4*, 995, 1968.
13. GAFNI, J., SOHAR, E. and HELLER, H.: Communicazione al X. Congresso della Lega Internazionale contro il Reumatismo, *2*, 1031, 1961.
14. ————: Lancet, *1*, 71, 1964.
15. HART, F. D.: Lancet, *1*, 740, 1968.
16. HELLER, H., GAFNI, J., MICHAELI, D., SHAHIN, N., SOHAR, E., EHRLICH, G. E., KARTEN, I., and SOKOLOFF, L.: Arth. & Rheum., *9*, 1, 1966.
17. HELLER, H., SOHAR, E., GAFNI, J., and HELLER, J.: Arch. Intern. Med., *107*, 539, 1961.
18. HELLER, H., SOHAR, E. and SHERF, L.: Arch. Intern. Med., *102*, 50, 1958.
19. HITZIG, W. H. and FANCONI, G.: Helvet. paediat. Acta, *8*, 326, 1953.
20. HURWICH, B. J., SCHWARTZ, J. and GOLDFARB, S.: Arch. Intern. Med., *125*, 308, 1970.
21. JESSOP, J. D.: Proc. Roy. Soc. Med., *62*, 199, 1969.
22. MAMOU, H.: Sem. Hop. Paris, *31*, 388, 1955.
23. ————: Sem. Hop. Paris, *46*, 2030, 1970.
24. MELLINKOFF, S. M., SCHWABE, A. D., and LAWRENCE, J. S.: Arch. Intern. Med., *108*, 80, 1961.
25. MELLINKOFF, S. M., SNODGRASS, R. W., SCHWABE, A. D., MEAD, J. F., WEIMER, H. E., and FRANKLAND, M.: Ann. Intern. Med., *56*, 171, 1962.
26. MICHAELI, D., PRAS, M., and ROZEN, N.: Brit. M. J., *2*, 30, 1966.
27. MOHR, W.: Verh. Deutsch. Ges. Rheum., *1*, 70, 1969.
28. OZDEMIR, A. I. and SOKMEN, C.: Amer. J. Gastroent., *51*, 311, 1969.
28*a*. PRAS, M., SOHAR, E., SNEH, E., and GAFNI, J.: Presented at the VII European Rheumatology Congress, Brighton, June, 1971.
29. PRIEST, R. J. and NIXON, R. K.: Ann. Intern. Med., *51*, 1253, 1959.
30. RACHMILEWITZ, M., EHRENFELD, E. N. and ELIAKIM, M.: J.A.M.A., *171*, 2355, 1959.
31. RAVIV, U., RUBINSTEIN, A. and SCHONFELD, A. E.: Amer. J. Dis. Child., *116*, 442, 1968.

32. Reich, C. B. and Franklin, E. C.: Arch. Intern. Med., *125*, 337, 1970.
33. Reimann, H. A.: J.A.M.A., *136*, 239, 1948.
34. ———: Medicine, *30*, 219, 1951.
35. Reimann, H. A., Coppola, E. D., and Villegas, G. R.: Ann. Intern. Med., *73*, 737, 1970.
36. Schrager, G.: J. Pediat., *74*, 966, 1969.
37. Shahin, N., Sohar, E. and Delith, F.: J. Roentg. & Radiation Therap., *84*, 269, 1960.
38. Siegal, S.: Ann. Intern. Med., *23*, 1, 1945.
39. ———: Amer. J. Med., *36*, 893, 1964.
40. Siguier, F., Zara, M., Funck-Brentano, J. L. and Lagrue, G.: Sem. Hop. Paris, *29*, 3649, 1953.
41. Sohar, E., Gafni, J., Chaimow, M., Pras, M. and Heller, H.: Arch. Intern. Med., *110*, 150, 1962.
42. Sohar, E., Gafni, J., Pras, M. and Heller, H.: Amer. J. Med., *43*, 227, 1967.

Behçet's Syndrome

1. Adamantiades, B.: Ann. Oculist., *168*, 271, 1931.
2. Alema, G. and Bignami, A.: in *Behcet's Disease*, Monacelli, M. and Nazzaro, P., ed., Basel, S. Karger, 1966; p. 52 ff.
3. Atwater, E. C.: Bull. Hist. Med., *41*, 413, 1967.
4. Behçet, H.: Derm. Wschr., *105*, 1152, 1937.
5. Buckley, G. E., III, and Gills, J. P., Jr.: J. Allergy, *43*, 273, 1969.
6. Cabanel, G., Phelip, X., Renaudet, J., Gras, J. P., and Seigneurin, J. M.: Rev. Lyon Med., *18*, 657, 1969.
7. Currey, H. L. E., Elson, R. A. and Mason, R. M.: J. Bone & Joint Surg., *50B*, 836, 1968.
7*a*. Cummings, N. A.: Personal communication.
7*b*. Cummings, N. A.: Postgrad. Med., *49*, 134, 1971.
8. Davis, E. and Melzer, E.: Arch. Intern. Med., *124*, 720, 1969.
9. Dudgeon, J.: Proc. Roy. Soc. Med., *54*, 104, 1961.
10. Enoch, B. A., Castillo-Olivares, J. L., Khoo, T. C. L., Grainger, R. G. and Henry, L.: Postgrad. Med. J., *44*, 453, 1968.
11. Epstein, R. S., Cummings, N. A., Sherwood, E. B., and Bergsma, D. R.: J. Psychosom. Res., *14*, 161, 1970.
12. Fowler, T. J., Humpston, D. J., Nussey, A. M., and Small, M.: Brit. Med. J., *2*, 473, 1960.
13. Francis, T. J.: Oral Surg., *30*, 476, 1970.
14. Francis, T. J., and Oppenheim, J. J.: Clin. Exper. Immunol., *6*, 573, 1970.
15. Haim, S., and Sherf, K.: Israel J. Med. Sci., *2*, 69, 1966.
16. Jackson, B. T. and Thomas, M. L.: Brit. Med. J., *1*, 18, 1970.
17. Kalbian, V. V. and Challis, M. T.: Amer. J. Med., *49*, 823, 1970.
18. Lehner, T.: Brit. Med. J., *1*, 465, 1967.
19. ———: J. Path., *97*, 481, 1969.
20. ———: Arch. Oral Biol., *14*, 843, 1969.
21. Marchionini, A. and Müller, E.: in *Behçet's Disease*, op. cit., p. 6 ff.
22. Mason, R. M. and Barnes, C. G.: Ann. Rheum. Dis., *28*, 95, 1969.
23. Menon, I. S., Cunliffe, W. J. and Dewar, H. A.: Postgrad. Med. J., *45*, 62, 1969.
24. Mitrovic, D., Kahn, M. F., Ryckewaert, A. and deSeze, S.: Sem. Hop. Paris, *44*, 2527, 1968.
25. Mowat, A. G. and Hothersall, T. E.: Brit. Med. J., *2*, 636, 1969.
26. Nasr, F. W.: Rev. Rhum., *36*, 81, 1969.
27. Nazzaro, P.: in *Behçet's Disease*, op. cit., p. 15 ff.
28. O'Duffy, J. D., Carney, J. A., Deodhar, S.: Ann. Intern. Med., *75*, 561, 1971.
29. Oshima, Y., Shimizu, T., Yokohari, R., Matsumoto, T., Kano, K., Kagami, T., and Nagaya, H.: Ann. Rheum. Dis., *22*, 36, 1963.
30. Pearson, C. M., Waksman, B. H., and Sharp, J. T.: J. Exper. Med., *113*, 485, 1961.
31. Pekin, T. J., Malinin, T. A., and Zvaifler, N. J.: Arth. & Rheum., *9*, 531, 1966.
32. Rosselet, E., Saudan, Y., and Zenklusen, G.: Ophthalmol., *156*, 218, 1968.
33. Sezer, F. N.: Amer. J. Ophthal., *36*, 301, 1953.
34. Shimizu, T., Katsuta, Y. and Oshima, Y.: Ann. Rheum. Dis., *24*, 494, 1965.
35. Smith, R. B. W., Prior, I. A. M., and Sturman, D.: Brit. Med. J., *2*, 220, 1967.
36. Strachan, R. W. and Wigzell, F. W.: Ann. Rheum. Dis., *22*, 26, 1963.

Stevens-Johnson Syndrome

1. Bianchine, J. R., Macaraeg, P. V. J., Jr., Lasagna, L., Azarnoff, D. L., Brunk, S. F., Hvidberg, E. F. and Owen, J. A.: Amer. J. Med., *44*, 390, 1968.
2. Billiet, I. and Uyttendaele, K.: Arch. Belg. Derm. Syph., *23*, 89, 1967.
3. Blattner, R. J.: J. Pediat., *72*, 554, 1968.
4. Bukantz, S. C.: D. M., pp. 3 ff., 1969.
5. Cameron, A. J., Baron, J. H. and Priestly, B. L.: Brit. Med. J., *2*, 1174, 1966.

6. Cannell, H., Churcher, G. M. and Milton-Thompson, G. J.: Brit. J. Derm., *81*, 196, 1969.
7. Carroll, O. M., Bryan, P. A. and Robinson, R. J.: J.A.M.A., *195*, 691, 1966.
8. Coursin, D. B.: J.A.M.A., *198*, 113, 1966.
9. Fleming, P. C., Krieger, E., Turner, J. A. P., Watty, E. I., Quinn, P. A., Bannatyne, R. M.: Canad. Med. Assoc. J., *97*, 1458, 1967.
10. Galili, S.: Israel J. Med. Sci., *3*, 903, 1967.
11. Hebra, F. v.: cited in ref. 19.
12. Jones, M. C.: Thorax, *25*, 748, 1970.
13. Kalkoff, K. W.: Bull. Schweiz. Akad. Med. Wiss., *23*, 427, 1968.
14. Shaw, D. J. and Jacobs, R. P.: Johns Hopkins Med. J., *126*, 130, 1970.
15. Sieber, O. F., John, T. J., Fuginiti, V. A. and Overholt, E. C.: J.A.M.A., *200*, 185, 1967.
16. Stevens, A. M. and Johnson, F. C.: Am. J. Dis. Child., *24*, 526, 1922.
17. Taylor, G. M. L.: S. Afr. Med. J., *42*, 501, 1968.
18. Watanabe, N.: Paediat. Univ. Tokyo, *15*, 41, 1968.
19. Wilk, V. F. and Scholz, R.: Wien Med. Wschr., *118*, 663, 1968.

Chapter 46

Enteropathic Arthritis

By Richard H. Ferguson, M.D.

Attention will be directed in this chapter to the joint involvement of certain inflammatory bowel diseases and to rheumatic syndromes encountered in virus hepatitis and Laennec's cirrhosis. Arthritis associated with Reiter's syndrome, Behçet's syndrome, and lupoid hepatitis is considered in Chapters 65, 45 and 51 respectively.

ARTICULAR MANIFESTATIONS OF CHRONIC ULCERATIVE COLITIS AND REGIONAL ENTERITIS

Arthritis was emphasized by Bargen in 1929 as the major extracolonic complication of chronic ulcerative colitis.[4] In 1935 Hench provided a clear description of a pattern of peripheral joint involvement in ulcerative colitis which he regarded as distinct from rheumatoid arthritis on the basis of its clinical course.[17] Little attention was given this concept in the literature for more than two decades until the advent of tests for rheumatoid factors stimulated a general renaissance of interest in those joint diseases which resemble rheumatoid arthritis but differ serologically. Since 1958 a number of studies have almost uniformly supported the earlier suggestion that there is a type of peripheral arthritis associated with ulcerative colitis which merits classification as a separate entity. The Thesaurus sponsored by the American Rheumatism Association in 1965 applied the term "Arthritis—ulcerative colitis" for this disease[32]; others have referred to this as "colitic arthritis"[41] or "acute toxic arthritis."[14]

An inordinately high prevalence of ankylosing spondylitis in ulcerative colitis was pointed out by Steinberg and Storey in 1957[34] and has been subsequently confirmed by numerous others. The classification of spondylitis in ulcerative colitis remains unsettled. Many prefer to regard this as the coexistence of two diseases, but McEwen has suggested the term "spondylitis accompanying ulcerative colitis."[26]

Regional enteritis (Crohn's disease, granulomatous colitis, transmural colitis) exhibits many clinical, x-ray, and pathologic features which distinguish it from ulcerative colitis. However, it shares with ulcerative colitis a tendency to be complicated by an apparently identical form of peripheral arthritis and spondylitis, and by such features as erythema nodosum and uveitis. For the sake of brevity the joint manifestations accompanying these intestinal diseases will be considered together.

Peripheral Arthritis

Prevalence.—Contemporary estimates of the peripheral arthritis associated with ulcerative colitis range from 9 to 20 per cent,[7,14,41] excluding those patients with spondylitis and other rheumatic diseases. In Ansell and Wigley's series of patients with regional enteritis, 6.5 per cent had polyarthritis at the time of study and an additional 13 per cent gave a past history of one or more bouts of arthritis presumably related to the bowel disease.[3] The sex incidence of this arthritis is approximately equal in both ulcerative colitis and regional enteritis. The usual age of onset is most commonly between 25 and 45, but it may range from childhood to old age.

Course.—A bout of arthritis accompanying ulcerative colitis or regional enteritis commences rather abruptly and reaches the zenith of intensity within the first day or so in 84 per cent.[26] There is a strong tendency toward an oligoarticular pattern of involvement with the number of individual joints affected in an episode usually being less than eight. In McEwen's series 85 per cent of bouts were limited to three joints or less,[26] and 20 of 31 patients reported by Wright had a monarticular onset in the initial attack.[41] There is often a migratory pattern of involvement. There may be a severe inflammatory reaction with erythema, warmth, splinting, swelling, and marked tenderness. In other instances localized or migratory arthralgia with meager or no objective findings may characterize the attack.

The small distal joints in both arms and legs are much less commonly affected than in rheumatoid arthritis, and knees and ankles are the most commonly involved joints.[41] Joints in the lower extremities are more frequently involved than the uppers.[41] An earlier suggestion that toe interphalangeal joint synovitis was a valuable diagnostic clue in ulcerative colitis[7] has not received support in later studies.[26,41]

Duration of an individual attack was less than one month in one-half and less than two months in three-quarters of the episodes studied by McEwen.[26] Only 10 per cent of the bouts persisted longer than one year and these often continued to exhibit partial remissions and flares paralleling the colitis.[26]

Although some individuals experience one or two attacks per year, in most the recurrences tend to be rather infrequent. There was an average of 1.4 attacks in the first year after the onset of arthritis accompanying ulcerative colitis, an average of 2 attacks in patients followed 5 years, 2.3 attacks in those followed 10 years, and 2.5 attacks in those followed 15 years.[26]

Relation to Bowel Disease.—An arthritic flare shortly after an exacerbation of colitis has been recognized as a characteristic but inconstant phenomenon since Hench's description in 1935.[17] Recent authors have recognized some parallel pattern in the course of the bowel and joint reactions in 60 to 74 per cent of patients.[26,41] Even those patients whose arthritis antedates recognized onset of colitis frequently have synchronous exacerbations and remissions later. Only 7 to 11 per cent of patients were observed to experience arthritis prior to bowel symptoms.[7,26] In one series, one-quarter developed arthritis within six months following onset of colitis, but another one-quarter did not experience joint symptoms until after more than ten years of colitis.[41]

Associated Features.—Arthritis has been noted to occur four times as frequently in patients with chronic continuous or intermittent colitis as in those with acute fulminating disease or proctitis alone.[41] Some correlation has been found between the incidence of arthritis and the extent of bowel involvement in women, but this trend has not been seen in men.[41] Patients with *pseudopolyps* or *perianal disease* are two to three times as apt to have arthritis as those without these complications.[41] *Erythema nodosum* is found in approximately 5 per cent of all colitis patients[20] but occurs in 21 to 26 per cent of those with ulcerative colitis having peripheral joint manifestations.[7,14,26,41] *Pyoderma gangrenosum*, on the other hand, has no correlation with the occurrence of arthritis.[26] Patients with ulcerative colitis having recurrent *oral ulceration* are 4.5 times as apt to have arthritis and those with *uveitis* have a threefold increase in peripheral joint disease.[26,41] Uveitis, erythema nodosum, aphthous stomatitis, and peripheral arthritis often flare concurrently with exacerbations of colitis.[26]

Laboratory Studies.—The histologic appearance of the synovial membrane may be indistinguishable from that of rheumatoid arthritis. Synovial fluid analysis has revealed cell counts ranging from 4,000 to 42,400 with 75 to 98 per cent polymorphs. Protein content may be low, but the relative viscosity is at times higher than would be expected.[7] Blood leukocyte counts and sedimentation rate determinations are usually high and hemoglobin values often reduced, probably reflecting the severity of the bowel disease more than the articular reaction. Total complement in synovial fluid has been normal in isolated instances.[16,18] Test results for rheumatoid factors are reported to be positive in about the frequency anticipated for a normal population,[7,25,41] and the L.E. cell preparation is only rarely positive.

Radiologic Manifestations. — X-ray changes are usually nonspecific and minor. Soft tissue swelling and juxta-articular osteoporosis may appear. Small bony erosions are seen at times, but these tend to heal. Periosteitis may be seen in mild degree in cases with more persistent inflammation; this tends to resolve or meld in with the bone.[7]

Differential Diagnosis.—Diagnostic problems may arise particularly in those instances where bowel disease is inapparent or mild. The migratory polyarthritis may result in confusion with rheumatic fever. Monarticular involvement of a knee or ankle can suggest gout. Reiter's syndrome with a diarrheal onset must often be included in the differential considerations. Ankylosing spondylitis with peripheral joint manifestations must always be kept in mind in cases of ulcerative colitis or regional enteritis, since sacroiliac or spinal manifestations may not be evident for several years after the initial peripheral joint flares. Whipple's disease may need to be excluded by appropriate studies.

Rheumatoid arthritis is occasionally impossible to exclude in those instances where chronicity and some deformity ensue and particularly where there is lack of correlation in the course of the joint and bowel disease. Positive test results for rheumatoid factors settle the issue in many instances, but even the passage of time may not eliminate uncertainty as to the most appropriate classification in those that remain seronegative. In three extensive series of colitis patients the prevalence of the peripheral arthritis of ulcerative colitis was thought to be from eight to twenty-five times that of coexisting rheumatoid arthritis[7,26,41]; however, Fernandez-Herlihy concluded that there were 18 with rheumatoid arthritis and 49 with arthritis of ulcerative colitis in a large retrospective study of 550 patients.[14] Most observers currently believe that the prevalence of rheumatoid arthritis in ulcerative colitis and regional enteritis is no different from that in the population generally.

Prognosis.—The prognosis in most instances is quite good with regard to articular function even after repeated attacks. Perhaps one-fourth of the patients sustain residual limitation or contractures which are usually trivial or minor.[26]

Therapy.—Treatment should be directed primarily at the underlying bowel disease. Joint symptoms can usually be managed adequately with a conservative regimen of rest, salicylates, and simple measures of physical therapy. Intra-articular steroid administration is a useful maneuver at times, but *systemic steroid therapy is rarely*, if ever, *indicated for the joint disease alone.* If steroid therapy is required for control of colitis, the arthritis as a rule is rapidly suppressed. The use of *indomethacin is contraindicated in the presence of inflammatory bowel disease.*

Arthritis accompanying ulcerative colitis or regional enteritis should almost *never be the primary indication for surgery,* although resection of diseased bowel is likely to prevent recurrent joint attacks. In Wright's experience colectomy almost invariably resulted in a prolonged remission.[41] However, others have not had results this favorable.[7,14,25] At times recurrent or residual bowel inflammation has been associated with renewed or initial attacks of arthritis. In Fernandez-Herlihy's series, ten of eleven patients classified as rheumatoid arthritis failed to have improvement in joint disease after colectomy.[14] Four of ten in another study who were regarded as having the arthritis of ulcerative colitis continued to have arthritis after total colectomy; of these four, one had progressed to a "chronic deforming" arthritis preoperatively.[25]

Spondylitis

Prevalence.—Over the last 15 years, a number of studies have demonstrated a prevalence of spondylitis resembling ankylosing spondylitis in patients with ulcerative colitis ranging from 2.6 to 6.4 per cent.[1,14,31,42,44] Similarly, five of 92 patients with regional enteritis were found to have spondylitis.[3] In the general population the prevalence of ankylosing spondylitis has been estimated to be .05 per cent.[36] Hence, the rate at which spondylitis is encountered in ulcerative colitis and regional enteritis may be 50 to 100 times that expected.

Course.—The clinical picture of spondylitis seen with colitis or regional enteritis seems indistinguishable from that occurring without accompanying bowel disease so far as age of onset, radiologic features, course, and response to therapy are concerned. A slightly increased frequency of associated hip, shoulder, and knee involvement has been observed in the spondylitis with colitis; other peripheral joints are affected to approximately the same degree as in ankylosing spondylitis.[26]

Relationship to Bowel Disease.—Spondylitis often antedates the appearance of ulcerative colitis or regional enteritis. This sequence has been observed in 27 per cent of the patients reported in five recent series.[14,26,31,42,44] Furthermore, there is little correlation between the manifestations of the bowel disease and the spinal symptomatology. In one study, there appeared to be a tendency for parallel flares and remissions of both processes to occur in 25 per cent,[26] but others have concluded that there is no significant relationship.[14,31,42] Colectomy and other surgical measures have not favorably influenced the course of spondylitis as a rule even when the bowel disease has been controlled.[14]

Sex Ratio.—The usual ratio of men to women with ankylosing spondylitis is thought to be in the neighborhood of 9:1.[30] However, male predominance seems much less striking in spondylitis associated with ulcerative colitis. A total of 55 men and 22 women has been recorded as having both processes in five large series,[14,26,31,42,44] giving a sex ratio of only 2.5:1.

Some British prospective studies have reported sacroilitis by x-ray in about 18 per cent of each sex with ulcerative colitis and regional enteritis.[3,40,42] Only one-third of such patients had enough clinical evidence at the time of study to warrant a diagnosis of spondylitis and these patients were predominantly male.[3,42]

Therapy.—The treatment and prognosis of spondylitis accompanying ulcerative colitis and regional enteritis are identical with those of ankylosing spondylitis, and as mentioned earlier, the spinal and bowel processes seem to run independent courses in spite of their remarkable tendency to coexist.

Etiologic Considerations

While there has been some confusion in the past regarding colonic involvement in these two diseases, there has been growing acceptance of certain criteria which serve to distinguish the two entities. In ulcerative colitis rectal involvement is almost constant with variable degrees of proximal spread in continuity to the remainder of the colon and on occasions the terminal ileum. The pathology is characteristically limited to the mucosa, which is universally inflamed, friable, and frequently contains crypt abscesses. Toxic megacolon, massive hemorrhage, or spontaneous bowel perforation may complicate fulminating exacerbations, while shortening of the involved colon with loss of haustral markings, pseudopolyposis, and carcinoma tend to be encountered later.[13] Regional enteritis may involve either the small or large bowel or both in what is usually a segmental discontinuous pattern. Transmural inflammation featuring granulomas, fissuring, discrete ulceration, serositis, and mesenteric lymphadenitis is commonly found. Strictures, fistulas, and inflammatory masses are frequent complications, but carcinoma is not.[13]

While the two diseases seem to be distinctive entities on the basis of pathology and course, they do share certain immunologic abnormalities in addition to some apparently identical extracolonic clinical manifestations. Circulating colonic antibodies are found in both in similar incidence and titer; such antibodies are not constantly present in either condition and are also found in lesser frequency in lupus erythematosus and other diseases associated with autoimmune phenomena.[11] In addition lymphocytes from patients with chronic ulcerative colitis or regional enteritis have been found to have cytotoxic effects in vitro on colonic epithelial cells. This property can be induced in normal lymphocytes by incubation for four days in serum from ulcerative colitis patients or by incubation with an extract of *E. coli* 0119:B14.[33] While this phenomenon has thus far been clearly identified only in chronic ulcerative colitis and regional enteritis, it may not prove to be specific and for the present cannot be assumed to represent delayed hypersensitivity.[33]

Etiology of both diseases remains a mystery and such diverse possibilities as infection, allergy, autoimmunity, psychosomatic disturbances, nutritional deficiency, or an enzyme defect continue to merit consideration.[39] Furthermore, frequent positive Kveim reactions in patients with regional enteritis have led to speculation about its interrelationship with sarcoidosis.[28]

While causation of these two enteric diseases remains unknown, it is tempting to postulate a common basis for the arthritis and spondylitis which complicate them. Pathogenetic hypotheses include: (1) absorption from a damaged bowel of an endogenous or exogenous antigen which stimulates an immune reaction producing peripheral inflammation, (2) a generalized autoimmune process with a common antigen in all of the involved tissues, (3) an infectious disease with the same organism causing bowel and peripheral involvement, (4) an abnormal bowel mucosa allowing an enteric pathogen to reach the synovial membrane and other sites, (5) the production of non-immunologic toxins in the diseased bowel wall causing synovitis.[38,26] None of these theories adequately accounts for the prior onset of spondylitis and its lack of correlation with the course of inflammatory bowel disease.

WHIPPLE'S DISEASE

In 1907 Whipple reported a patient "characterized by gradual loss of weight and strength, stools consisting chiefly of neutral fat and fatty acids, indefinite abdominal signs, and a peculiar multiple arthritis."[37] Since then, at least 125 patients have been recorded with a male predominance of 9:1.[24] In addition to the findings in Whipple's patient, such features as fever, a tendency to hypotension, hyperpigmentation of the exposed areas, peripheral lymphadenopathy, and pleural reactions have been noted frequently. The presence of periodic acid-Schiff (PAS) staining granules in macrophages in the intestinal mucosa and lymph nodes was observed in 1949[5] and this greatly facilitated the recognition of the disease subsequently. In recent years electron microscopy has demonstrated the constant presence of rod-shaped organisms infiltrating the lamina propria of the intestinal mucosa. This organism was originally described by Whipple using light microscopy in his remarkable case study. The PAS staining granules are believed to represent incompletely digested components of the bacteria. While it has not been possible as yet to transmit disease to experimental animals or to culture these rod-shaped structures, their disappearance with antibiotic therapy coincident with clinical recovery constitutes impressive evidence for a causal relationship.

Peripheral joint manifestations somewhat similar to those described in ulcerative colitis and regional enteritis have been a prominent feature in 65 to 90 per cent of the reported cases of Whipple's disease.[19,24] In about one-half of the patients joint complaints antedated the development of diarrhea, and in one-third articular signs or symptoms appeared five years or more before bowel manifestations.[19,24] In one instance, arthritis persisted for 35 years before other features of Whipple's disease appeared.[8] Onset of illness most commonly occurs between 30 and 50 with a range from 11 to 64.[19] Parallel exacerbations of arthritis and diarrhea have not impressed most observers in this disease; indeed, arthritis often regresses as bowel symptoms develop.

Arthritis is usually episodic, of abrupt onset, and tends to have a migratory pattern. Involvement lasts from hours to days in a given joint, and is frequently interspersed with long remissions. Only 3 per cent of those with arthritis have been reported to develop chronic or residual clinical signs, while 10 per cent have been found to have some nonspecific roentgenologic changes.[19] Involvement has usually been bilateral, but occasionally unilateral or monarticular disease occurs. The knees, ankles, fingers, hips, wrists, and elbows have been noted to be involved in descending order of frequency.[19]

In a review of reports of 95 patients with Whipple's disease, two were recorded as having bilateral sacroiliac fusion and another had unilateral fusion.[19] Eighteen of the 95 were reported to have had low back pain in conjunction with peripheral joint complaints. Although a few of these patients had physical findings suggestive of spondylitis, there has been no well-documented report as yet of typical ankylosing spondylitis in Whipple's disease.

Results of tests for rheumatoid factors have been uniformly negative. Synovial biopsies have shown features of mild inflammation[8] and periodic acid-Schiff positive macrophages have been reported in an isolated instance in synovium.[43] Studies of synovial fluid have been unremarkable aside from a higher proportion of mononuclear cells than in most inflammatory fluids. Typical rheumatoid nodules, hand deformities, and erosive bone changes have not been reported.

Diagnosis of this condition is dependent on the demonstration of PAS positive inclusion bodies in macrophages of small intestinal mucosa, mesenteric nodes, or, less constantly, in more peripheral tissues. Peroral jejunal biopsy currently is the most appropriate diagnostic approach since the disease is thought to be consistently present and most severe in the mucosa of the upper small intestine.

Prolonged treatment with antibiotics, most commonly penicillin and streptomycin for ten days followed by tetracycline 1 gram daily for one year, has been found to result in an almost uniformly favorable response. Arthralgias usually clear in five to thirty days along with other manifestations of the disease.[24] It is not yet known what effects such treatment may have on patients with spinal symptoms or findings.

The prolonged duration of articular symptoms prior to bowel manifestations is difficult to reconcile with our current knowledge of the disease. One possibility might be that prolonged occult intestinal disease exists and in some way produces arthritis. Alternatively, this may prove to be a systemic infection which in many instances affects joints only for many years.

ARTHRITIS ASSOCIATED WITH VIRAL HEPATITIS

For many years there have been reports of arthritis or arthralgia occurring in the prodromal period of occasional patients with viral hepatitis. Recent studies tend to confirm some earlier suggestions that articular manifestations are found chiefly in serum hepatitis[2,21] but may also occur in infectious hepatitis.[13a]

Serologic investigations of the Australia antigen are consistent with the interpretation that it is either the virus of serum hepatitis or an antigen which has a specific association with that virus. Krugman and others have clearly demonstrated one strain of infectious hepatitis (MS-1) in human experiments which does not result in the development of Australia antigen;[6,22,23] others have reported the appearance of a specific antibody in spontaneous epidemics of infectious hepatitis unassociated with Australia antigen.[10] Thus present data would suggest that there are at least two viruses which produce hepatitis, both of which may be transmitted either orally or parenterally.[23]

In several serum hepatitis epidemics following mass inoculations during and after World War II the incidence of arthralgia during the prodromal pre-icteric phase was 25 to 38 per cent.[12,15,27] Occurrence of joint manifestations in patients regarded as having infectious hepatitis during this same era ranged up to 11 per cent,[9,15,35] but recent virus studies now cast doubt on the validity of the classification of hepatitis in the earlier literature. There is generally a symmetric polyarticular pattern most commonly involving hands, wrists, elbows, knees, and ankles. Swelling, tenderness, limited motion, or redness have not been prominent, and in some series no objective changes have been recognized.[12,15,27] Rest pain, motion pain, and stiffness after inactivity have been the usual features. A rash which is often pruritic and urticarial has been frequently associated with the arthralgia. The articular syndrome may last from a few days to more than a month and tends to clear as jaundice develops.[13a]

Seven patients with hepatitis who had arthralgias or arthritis associated with fever or urticarial rash in the pre-icteric phase were found to have circulating Australia antigen together with significant depletion of total serum complement and one or more of the early complement components. It was postulated that circulating immune complexes, presumably the Australia antigen and homologous antibody, had activated the complement system and resulted in a serum sickness syndrome.[2] A normal serum complement was observed in one patient with arthritis followed by infectious hepatitis in whom Australia antigen was not present.[13a]

ARTHRITIS AND LAENNEC'S CIRRHOSIS

A mild inflammatory polyarthritis has been described during the recovery phase of some patients with Laennec's cirrhosis. Twelve of thirteen such patients in one report were female alcoholics in hepatic decompensation. Rheumatic complaints generally first appeared with substantial improvement in liver function. The clinical picture was compatible with mild sero-negative rheumatoid arthritis. Shoulders, elbows, and knees were the most prominently involved joints. Pain, swelling, tenderness, morning stiffness, and limitation of motion were characteristic. Synovial fluid showed mild and nonspecific inflammatory changes. On x-ray there was some juxta-articular demineralization and an apparent tendency toward calcification of the rotator cuff in the shoulders and the triceps attachment at the olecranon. Osseous erosions, loss of joint space, and residual deformities of significance did not develop. Studies for L.E. cells, rheumatoid factor, antinuclear antibody, and gamma globulin levels revealed no essential differences between cirrhotic patients with arthritis and those without arthritis. There was a tendency for remission or marked improvement to occur within one year. The pathogenesis of this disorder remains obscure. Conceivably, it may represent the emergence of rheumatoid arthritis which had been previously suppressed by the well-known anti-rheumatic effect of hepato-cellular damage.[29] (*See also* Chapter 16, p. 276.)

BIBLIOGRAPHY

1. Acheson, E. D.: Quart. J. Med., *29*, 489, 1960.
2. Alpert, E., Coston, R. L., and Schur, P. H.: Arth. & Rheum., *13*, 303, 1970, (Abstract).
3. Ansell, B. M. and Wigley, R. A. D.: Ann. Rheum. Dis., *23*, 64, 1964.
4. Bargen, J. A.: Ann. Intern. Med., *3*, 335, 1929.
5. Black-Schaffer, B.: Proc. Soc. Exp. Biol. Med., *72*, 225, 1949.
6. Boggs, J. D., Melnick, J. L., Conrad, M. E., and Felsher, B. F.: J.A.M.A., *214*, 1041, 1970.
7. Bywaters, E. G. L. and Ansell, B. M.: Ann. Rheum. Dis., *17*, 169, 1958.
8. Caughey, D. E. and Bywaters, E. G. L.: Ann. Rheum. Dis., *22*, 327, 1963.
9. Conrad, M. E., Schwartz, F. D., and Young, A. A.: Amer. J. Med., *37*, 789, 1964.
10. DelPrete, S., Costantino, D., Doglia, M., Graziina, A., Ajdukiewicz, A., Dudley, F. J., Fox, R. A., and Sherlock, S.: Lancet, *2*, 579, 1970.
11. Deodhar, S. D., Michener, W. M., and Farmer, R. G.: Amer. J. Clin. Path., *51*, 591, 1969.
12. Dull, H. B.: J.A.M.A., *176*, 413, 1961.
13. Farmer, R. G., Hawk, W. A., and Turnbull, R. B., Jr.: Amer. J. Dig. Dis., *13*, 501, 1968.

13*a*. Fernandez, R., and McCarty, D. J.: Ann. Intern. Med., *74*, 207, 1971.

14. Fernandez-Herlihy, L.: New Engl. J. Med., *261*, 259, 1959.
15. Hawley, W. L., McFarlan, A. M., and Steigman, A. J.: Lancet, *1*, 818, 1944.
16. Hedberg, H.: Acta Med. Scand. (Suppl. 479), *1*, 137, 1967.
17. Hench, P. S.: Nelson's *Loose-Leaf Surgery*, New York, Thomas Nelson and Sons, pp. 104, 1935.
18. Hunder, G. G.: Personal communication.
19. Kelly, J. J. and Weisiger, B. B.: Arth. & Rheum., *6*, 615, 1963.
20. Kirsner, J. B., Sklar, M., and Palmer, W. L.: Amer. J. Med., *22*, 264, 1957.
21. Krugman, S.: Personal communication.
22. Krugman, S., Giles, J. P., and Hammond, J.: J.A.M.A., *200*, 365, 1967.
23. Krugman, S., and Giles, J. P.: J.A.M.A., *212*, 1019, 1970.
24. Maizel, H., Ruffin, J. M., and Dobbins, W. O.: Medicine, *49*, 175, 1970.
25. McEwen, C., Lingg, C., Kirsner, J. B., and Spencer, J. A.: Amer. J. Med., *22*, 923, 1962.
26. McEwen, C.: Clin. Orthop., *57*, 9, 1968.
27. Mirick, G. S. and Shank, R. E.: Trans. of Amer. Clin. & Climatological Assoc., *71*, 176, 1959.
28. Mitchell, D. N., *et al.*: Lancet, *2*, 496, 1970.
29. Pachas, W. N. and Pinals, R. S.: Arth. & Rheum., *10*, 343, 1967.
30. Polley, H. F.: Med. Clin. N. A., *39*, 509, 1955.
31. Rotstein, J., Entel, I., and Zeviner, B.: Ann. Rheum. Dis., *22*, 194, 1963.
32. Ruhl, M. J. and Sokoloff, L.: Arth. & Rheum., *9*, 97, 1965.
33. Shorter, R. G., Huizenga, K. A., ReMine, S. G., and Spencer, R. J.: Gastroenterology, *58*, 843, 1970.
34. Steinberg, V. L. and Storey, G.: Brit. Med. J., *2*, 1157, 1957.
35. Swift, W. E., Gardner, H. T., Moore, D. S., Streitfield, F. H., and Havens, W. P.: Amer. J. Med., *8*, 614, 1950.
36. West, H. F.: Ann. Rheum. Dis., *8*, 143, 1949.
37. Whipple, G. H.: Bull. Johns Hopkins Hospital, *18*, 382, 1907.
38. Wilske, K. R. and Decker, J. L.: Bull. Rheum. Dis., *15*, 362, 1965.
39. Wright, R.: Gastroenterology, *58*, 875, 1970.
40. Wright, R., Lumsden, K., Luntz, M. H., Sevel, D., and Truelove, S. C.: Quart. J. Med., *34*, 229, 1965.
41. Wright, V. and Watkinson, G.: Brit. Med. J., *2*, 670, 1965.
42. ———: Brit. Med. J., *2*, 675, 1965.
43. Zollinger, cited by Rutishauser, E., and Boner, F.: Schweiz. med. Wschr., *89*, 397, 1959.
44. Zvaifler, N. J. and Martel, W.: Arth. & Rheum., *3*, 76, 1960.

Chapter 47

Sjögren's Syndrome and Connective Tissue Disease with Other Immunologic Disorders

By Norman Talal, M.D.

SJÖGREN'S SYNDROME

Definition.—Sjögren's syndrome is a chronic inflammatory disease characterized by diminished lacrimal and salivary gland secretion (the sicca complex) resulting in keratoconjunctivitis sicca (KCS) and xerostomia. The glandular insufficiency is secondary to lymphocytic and plasma cell infiltration. Half of the patients have rheumatoid arthritis and a few have another connective tissue disease. This disorder belongs in the category of autoimmune diseases.

History.—A number of patients with various combinations of dry mouth, dry eyes and chronic arthritis were described by European clinicians between the years 1882 and 1925. In 1892, Mikulicz[15] reported a man with bilateral parotid and lacrimal gland enlargement associated with massive round cell infiltration. In 1925, Gougerot[6] described three patients with salivary and mucous gland atrophy and insufficiency progressing to dryness. Two years later Houwer[10] emphasized the association of filamentary keratitis (the major ocular manifestation of the syndrome) with chronic arthritis. In 1933, Henrik Sjögren[24] reported detailed clinical and histologic findings in 19 women with xerostomia and keratoconjunctivitis sicca, of whom 13 had chronic arthritis. In 1953, Morgan and Castleman[16] concluded that Sjögren's syndrome and Mikulicz's disease were the same entity.

Etiology.—Recognition of the inherent relationship of the sicca complex to rheumatoid arthritis and appreciation of the multiple autoantibodies present in patients' serum have classified Sjögren's syndrome among the connective tissue and autoimmune diseases.

A current concept of pathogenesis for these disorders implicates immunologic and viral factors.[29] A probable genetic predisposition may also contribute. According to this concept, susceptible individuals have an abnormal immune system which renders them likely to react immunologically against viral or viral-altered host antigens. For example, antigenic alteration of salivary gland antigens could lead to sensitization, lymphocytic infiltration and the production of antitissue antibodies. The role of immune mechanisms, such as delayed hypersensitivity, and the exact relationship of chronic viral infection are not known. It is noteworthy that the New Zealand Black and hybrid mice who are genetically predisposed to the spontaneous development of Coomb's-positive hemolytic anemia, L.E. cells and lupus glomerulonephritis also develop salivary gland lymphocytic infiltrates similar to those seen in Sjögren's syndrome.[12]

Pathology

The classic lesion is a lymphocytic and plasma cell infiltrate of salivary, lacrimal and other exocrine glands in the respiratory tract, gastrointestinal tract, and vagina. Both major (parotid, submaxillary) and minor (gingival, palatine) salivary glands are involved.[3,30] The term "benign lymphoepithelial lesion" has been applied to describe the characteristic histologic appearance in the salivary glands.[5] These lesions may be present without xerostomia and other features of Sjögren's syndrome.[4] The earliest infiltrates may be scattered around small intralobular ducts. The histologic picture is varied and includes acinar atrophy generally in proportion to the extent of lymphoid infiltration, occasional germinal center formation, and proliferative or metaplastic changes in the duct lining cells. The proliferation may progress to form the characteristic epimyoepithelial islets (Figure 47–1) which are seen in about 40 per cent of parotid biopsy specimens.[1,34] In some patients, adipose replacement may be more prominent than lymphoid infiltration. Typically, the lobular architecture is preserved; some lobules may be spared while others are virtually destroyed.

When mucosal glands in the trachea and bronchi are involved, benign-appearing lymphoid infiltrates are again a prominent feature. More extensive lymphoid infiltrates may involve the lung, kidney or skeletal muscle, resulting in functional abnormalities of these organs.

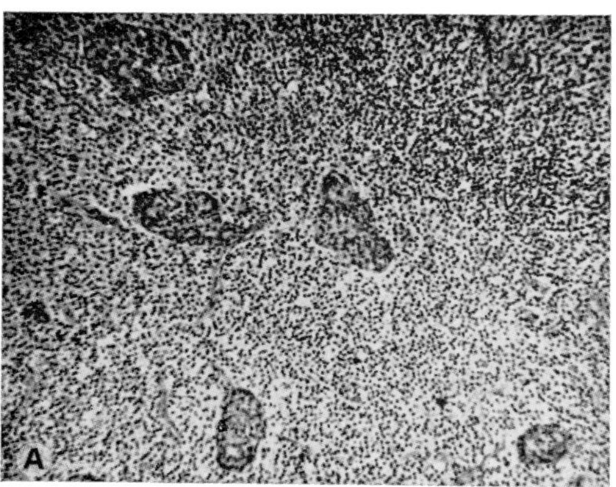

FIG. 47–1.—Extensive lymphoid proliferation and formation of epimyoepithelial islets in the parotid gland of a patient with Sjögren's syndrome. (Courtesy of Medicine, reference 1).

In some patients the lymphoid infiltrates in salivary glands, lymph nodes or parenchymal organs will be more pleomorphic, more primitive or more invasive, and they will raise the possibility of malignancy. Lymph node architecture can be destroyed and frank reticulum cell sarcoma may be diagnosed if such abnormal cells predominate.[31] It may be impossible to decide between a benign or malignant process, in which case the term "pseudolymphoma" has been employed.[32]

Clinical Features

More than 90 per cent of patients are females with a mean age of 50 years. The disease occurs in all races and in children. The two most common presentations are: (1) the insidious and slowly progressive development of the sicca complex in a patient with chronic rheumatoid arthritis, and (2) the more rapid development of a severe oral and ocular dryness, often accompanied by episodic parotitis, in an otherwise well patient.

About 50 per cent of patients with KCS have additional features of Sjögren's syndrome.[27] The most common ocular complaint is a foreign body sensation, described as "gritty" or "sandy." Other symptoms include burning, accumulation of thick ropy strands at the inner canthus (particularly upon awakening), decreased tearing, redness, photosensitivity, eye fatigue, itching, and a "filmy" sensation that interferes with vision.[8]

Patients will complain of *eye discomfort*, difficulty reading or watching television. Inability to cry is not a common complaint. Lacrimal gland enlargement occurs infrequently. Ocular complications include corneal ulceration, vascularization or opacification, followed rarely by perforation.

The distressing *symptoms of salivary insufficiency* include: difficulty with chewing, swallowing, and phonation; adherence of food to buccal surfaces; fissures and ulcers of the tongue, buccal membranes, and lips (particularly at the corners of the mouth); frequent ingestion of liquids (especially at meal times); and rampant dental caries. Patients are unable to swallow a dry cracker or toast without ingesting fluids, and will express displeasure at the suggestion. They may carry bottles of water or other lubricants in their purse, and may awake at night for sips of water. The dentist may notice that fillings are loosening.

Dryness may also involve the *nose*, the *posterior pharynx*, the *larynx*, and the *tracheobronchial tree*, and may lead to epistaxis, hoarseness, recurrent otitis media, bronchitis, or pneumonia.

Half of the patients have *parotid gland enlargement* (Figure 47–2). This is often recurrent and symmetrical, and can be accompanied by fever, tenderness, or erythema. Superimposed infection is rare. Rapid fluctuations in gland size are not unusual. A particularly hard or nodular gland may suggest a neoplasm.

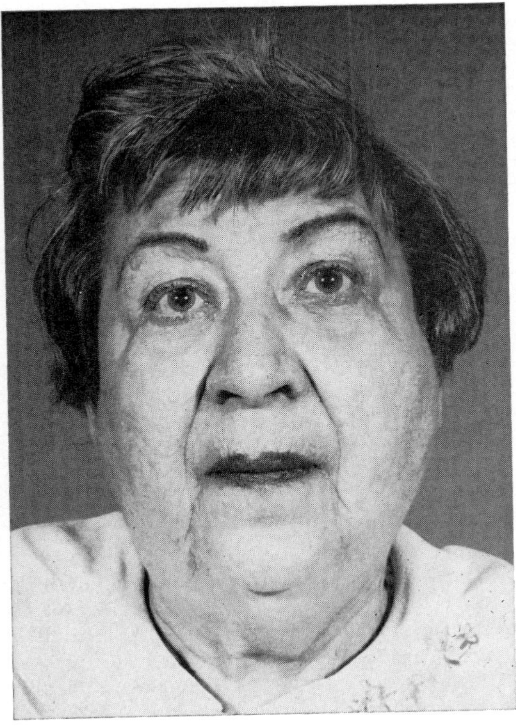

Fig. 47–2.—Bilateral parotid gland enlargement in a patient with severe xerostomia and Sjögren's syndrome.

The *arthritis of Sjögren's syndrome* resembles classical rheumatoid arthritis in its clinical, pathologic, and roentgenographic features. KCS develops in about 10 to 15 per cent of patients with rheumatoid arthritis.[9,26] Arthralgias and morning stiffness not progressing to joint deformity may occur in patients with the sicca complex. Fluctuations in the course of the arthritis are not accompanied by parallel alterations in the sicca symptoms. Splenomegaly and leukopenia suggestive of Felty's syndrome, and vasculitis with leg ulcers and peripheral neuropathy may appear even in the absence of rheumatoid arthritis. *Raynaud's phenomenon* occurs in 20 per cent of patients.

Skin or *vaginal dryness* and allergic drug eruptions occur frequently. Episodic lower extremity purpura, sometimes preceded by itching or other prodromata, may be the presenting complaint. Glomerulonephritis develops rarely and resembles lupus nephritis histologically. Overt or latent *abnormalities of the renal tubules* (diabetes insipidus, renal tubular acidosis, Fanconi syndrome) occur with greater frequency.[17,22,33]

Severe *proximal muscle weakness* and rarely tenderness may be early symptoms, leading to a diagnosis of polymyositis.[1,23] Weakness may also be associated with electrolyte imbalance, nephrocalcinosis and the clinical findings of renal tubular acidosis.[22,23] Peripheral or cranial neuropathy may cause symptoms of dysesthesia or paresthesia. Facial pain and numbness can accompany trigeminal neuropathy[11] and contribute to the oral discomfort caused by the dryness.

Although *chronic thyroiditis* of the Hashimoto type is present in 5 per cent of patients, clinical hypothyroidism is rare. Biliary cirrhosis and chronic active hepatitis, gastric achlorhydria, acute pancreatitis[2] and adult celiac disease[18] have been reported in Sjögren's syndrome. Cervical or other lymph node enlargement may be the first indication of malignant lymphoma or pseudolymphoma (Figure 47–3).

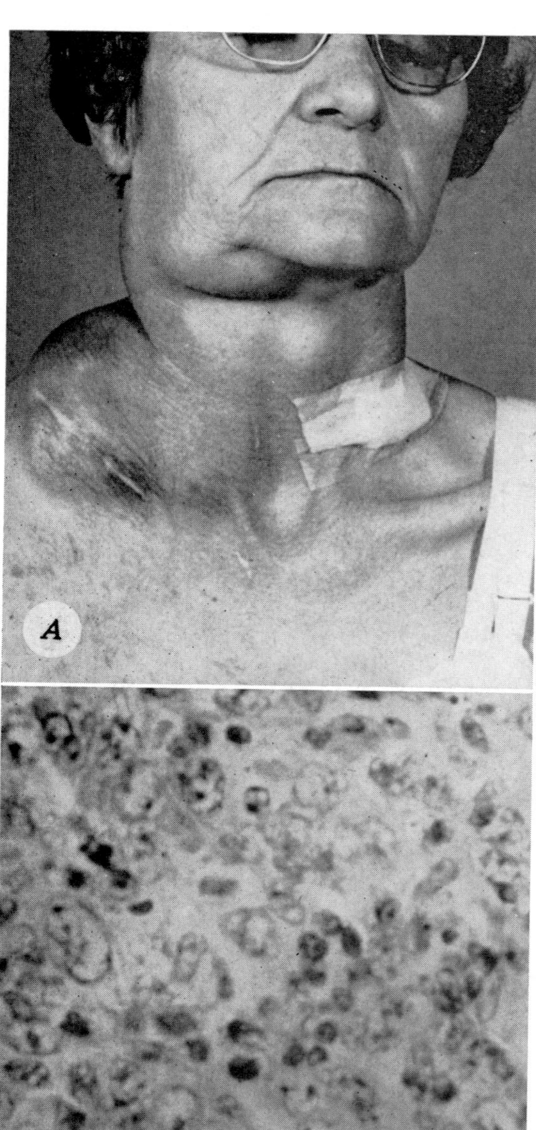

FIG. 47–3.—Several hard matted lymph nodes are present in the neck and submandibular region in this patient with Sjögren's syndrome of twenty years' duration. She had suffered from intermittent cervical lymphadenopathy for the last 6 years, with a histologic diagnosis of pseudolymphoma made on four occasions. On biopsy now, many abnormal reticulum cells with large nuclei and prominent nucleoli were found. The diagnosis was reticulum cell sarcoma. (Courtesy of The Pediatric Clinics of North America.)

Physical Findings

The extreme picture of an elderly woman with joint deformities, reddened eyes and parotid enlargement should immediately suggest the diagnosis. However, in many instances the findings are less obvious. The parotid glands may have any consistency, but are usually firm and non-tender. Severe bilateral parotid swelling may give rise to the so-called "chipmunk facies."

Gross inspection of the eyes may reveal nothing abnormal, a mucous thread, or conjunctival congestion. Lacrimal enlargement may not be apparent even when these glands are involved. The Schirmer test, in which a strip of Whatman No. 41 filter paper is folded and placed in the lower conjunctival sac, is a simple but crude measure of tear formation.[20] After 5 minutes the moistened portion normally measures 15 mm. or more. Most patients with Sjögren's syndrome moisten less than 5 mm. More reliable diagnostic signs are obtained using rose bengal dye and biomicroscopy. Normally, no stain is visible a few minutes after dye instillation. Grossly visible or microscopic staining of the bulbar conjunctiva or cornea indicates the presence of small superficial erosions. Biomicroscopy may reveal increased amounts of corneal debris and attached filaments of corneal epithelium (filamentary keratitis).[8]

The tongue and mucous membranes are characteristially dry, red, and "parchment-like." The lips may be dry and cracked. The tongue depressor will adhere to oral surfaces and the normal pool

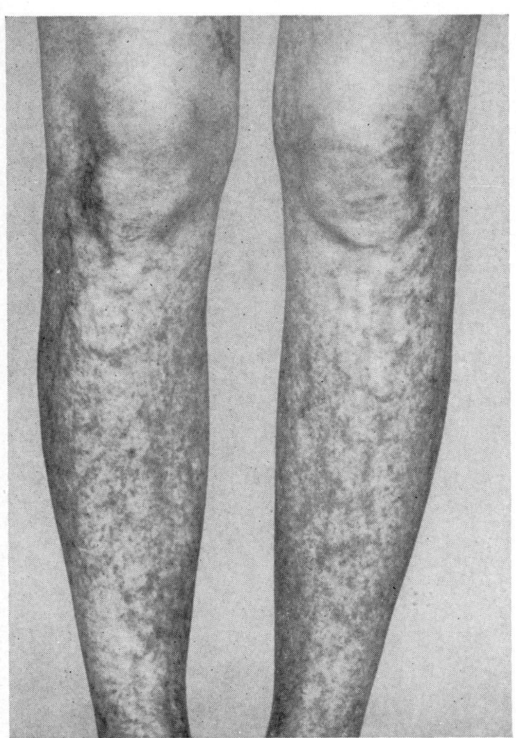

FIG. 47–4.—Characteristic appearance of the legs of a patient with Sjögren's syndrome and intermittent, dependent, non-thrombocytopenic purpura.

of saliva in the sublingual vestibule, visible when the tongue is elevated, is not present. A residual brownish pigmentation over the shins suggests past episodes of purpura (Figure 47–4). Cervical or other lymph node enlargement may be the first indication of malignant lymphoma or pseudolymphoma. Splenomegaly occurs in 25 per cent of patients.[32]

Laboratory Findings

Parotid salivary flow rates can be measured by means of Lashley cups placed over the orifices of the parotid ducts and secured by suction. Flow is stimulated by placing lemon juice on the tongue. Parotid secretion varies greatly depending upon age, sex and other factors, but should be about 1.0 ml./5 min./gland. Flow rates are markedly reduced or unobtainable in Sjögren's syndrome.

Two techniques can be employed for visualization of the salivary glands. Secretory sialography[1] is performed by introducing a radiopaque contrast medium through a small polyethylene catheter inserted into the parotid duct orifice. Following injection of 0.5 to 1.0 ml. of material, the catheter is plugged and radiographs made (injection phase). The catheter is then removed and emptying encouraged by stimulation with lemon juice. After 5 minutes, films are again taken (secretory phase). A normal sialogram shows fine arborization of parotid ductules with relatively little retention of contrast medium. In Sjögren's syndrome, there is gross distortion of the normal pattern with marked retention. The sialectasis may appear punctate, globular or cavitary (Figure 47–5).

The second method, developed more recently, depends upon the uptake, concentration and excretion of the radionuclide ^{99m}Tc-pertechnetate by the salivary glands. Twenty patients were studied by sequential salivary scintigraphy in which the gland image is recorded visually on a gamma scintillation camera over a 60- 80-minute period. Sixteen of them showed decreased function.[19] The scintigraphic findings paralleled the degree of xerostomia, salivary flow rate determinations, and results of secretory sialography (Figure 47–6).

Involvement of minor salivary glands in the lower lip has made it possible to perform lower lip biopsies and obtain histologic confirmation of the diagnosis in large numbers of patients.[3] This procedure is performed under local anesthesia with the patient seated in a dental chair. The specimen can be obtained either by punch biopsy or with a scalpel. Patients will generally experience discomfort for 24 to 48 hours; occasional patients will complain of more persistent localized numbness. The extensive degree of lymphoid infiltration is diagnostic of Sjögren's syndrome in about 75 per

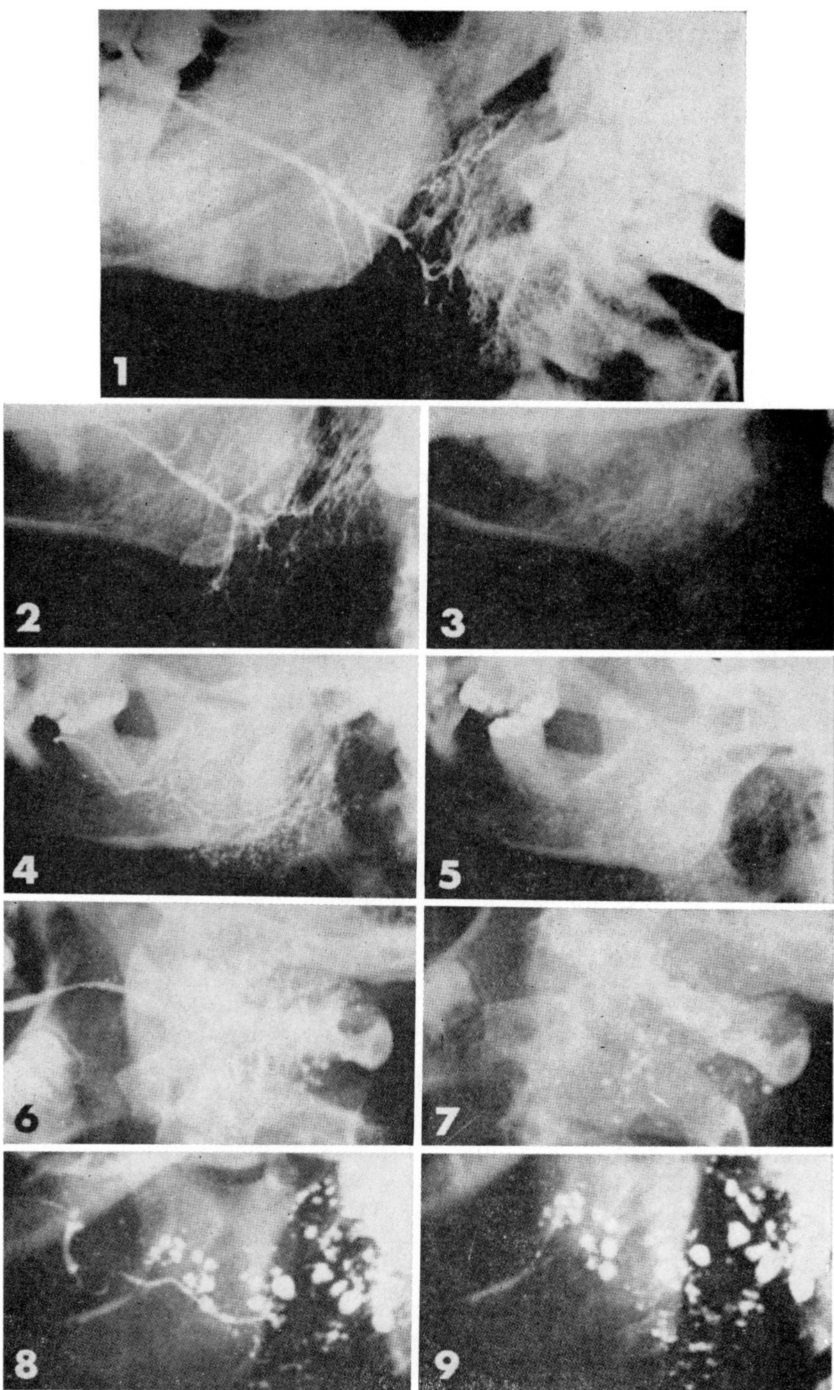

FIG. 47–5.—Appearance of secretory sialography in normal individuals and patients with Sjögren's syndrome. (1)—Injection phase, normal pattern. (2)—Injection phase, punctate sialectasis. (3)—Secretory phase, punctate sialectasis. (4)—Injection phase, punctate sialectasis with intermediate duct involvement. (5)—Secretory phase, punctate sialectasis with intermediate duct involvement. (6)—Injection phase, globular sialectasis. (7)—Secretory phase, globular sialectasis. (8)—Injection phase, cavitary and destructive sialectasis. (9)—Secretory phase, cavitary and destructive sialectasis. (Courtesy of Medicine).

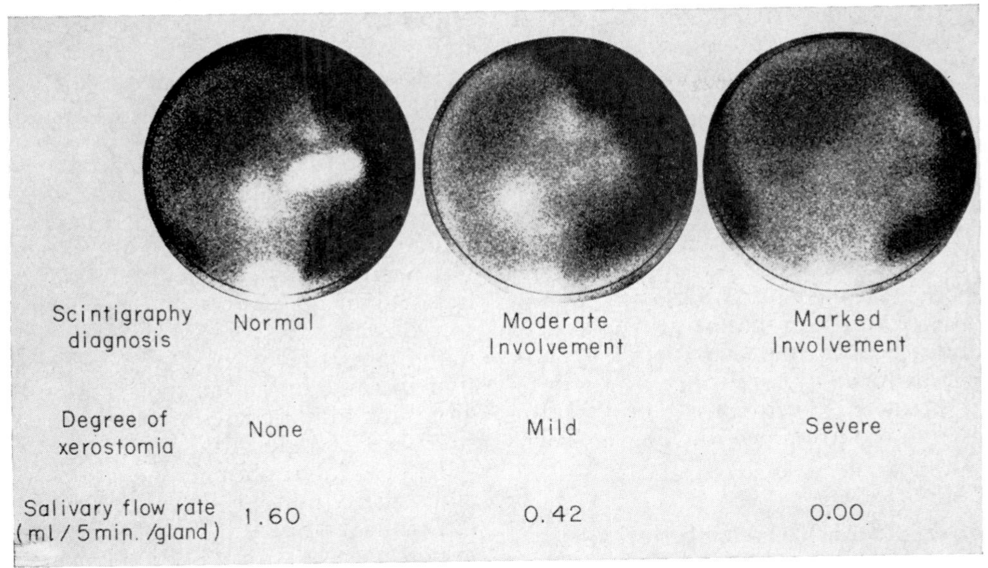

FIG. 47–6.—Comparative studies of salivary function in Sjögren's syndrome illustrating the results achieved with scintigraphy employing ^{99m}Tc-pertechnetate.

cent of patients. The infiltrating cells synthesize large amounts of immunoglobulin and macroglobulin.[30] Although the diagnosis can be made on clinical criteria alone in many instances, the complete evaluation of a patient should include a lip biopsy.

A mild normocytic, normochromic anemia occurs in about 25 per cent of patients, leukopenia in 30 per cent, eosinophilia (above 6 per cent eosinophils) in 25 per cent, and an elevated erythrocyte sedimentation rate (greater than 30 mm. per hour by the Westergren method) in over 90 per cent.

Half of the patients have hypergammaglobulinemia. This is a diffuse elevation of all immunoglobulin classes, and is most marked in patients who lack rheumatoid arthritis but have polymyopathy, purpura, or renal tubular acidosis. Cryoglobulinemia (often of the 19S-7S type) is seen in patients with glomerulonephritis or pseudolymphoma. Waldenström's macroglobulinemia, but not myeloma, occurs. Some patients with reticulum cell sarcoma have hypogammaglobulinemia. A mild hypoalbuminemia is common.

Rheumatoid factor is detected in over 90 per cent of sera when pooled human F II gamma globulin is used as antigen, and in 75 per cent when rabbit gamma globulin is employed. Thus, many patients who lack rheumatoid arthritis have rheumatoid factor. Rheumatoid factor may disappear, or diminish markedly in titer, when reticulum cell sarcoma develops.[31]

The L.E. cell phenomenon is present in 20 per cent of patients who also have rheumatoid arthritis, but rarely in others with Sjögren's syndrome. It is not found in association with nephritis or renal tubular disorders.

Antinuclear factors, giving a homogeneous or speckled pattern of immunofluorescence, are present in about 70 per cent of patients.[1] Antibodies to native DNA are occasionally present in low titer. Several precipitating or complement-fixing antibodies reacting with poorly characterized nuclear or cytoplasmic antigens occur most commonly in patients who lack rheumatoid arthritis. An antibody specific for salivary duct epithelium has been observed by indirect immunofluorescence in 50 per cent of patients.[7,14] Thyroglobulin antibodies, detected by hemagglutination, are present in about 35 per cent.

An impaired lymphocyte transformation response to phytohemmagglutinin and streptolysin-O and a diminished capacity to developed delayed hypersensitivity to dinitrochlorobenzene occur in about 50 per cent of patients.[13] This defect is most apparent when rheumatoid arthritis, lymphoma, or pseudolymphoma is present with Sjögren's syndrome.

Lymphoma and Macroglobulinemia

As already indicated, lymphoid infiltration is a prominent feature of Sjögren's syndrome. In some patients, lymphoproliferation is not benignly confined to glandular tissue but becomes more generalized to involve regional lymph nodes or distant sites such as nodes, lung, kidney, spleen, bone marrow, muscle, or liver. When such "extraglandular" lymphoproliferation occurs, diagnosis is often difficult, and clinically and histologically the disease may simulate frankly malignant lymphoproliferative disorders such as Waldenström's macroglobulinemia, reticulum cell sarcoma, or other lymphomas.[32] Since the subsequent clinical course is frequently that of the lymphoma, ending fatally, the early recognition of extraglandular lymphoproliferation in SS and prompt institution of appropriate therapy are important.

In the vast majority of patients, significant lymphoproliferation remains confined to salivary and lacrimal tissue, resulting in a chronic benign course of stable or progressive xerostomia and xerophthalmia. In some, however, after even fifteen years or more of benign disease, there appears evidence of extension of lymphoproliferation to extraglandular sites.

The extraglandular lymphoid infiltrates are of two general types. They may be highly pleomorphic and include small and large lymphocytes, plasma cells, and large reticulum cells. In a lymph node the cells may distort the normal architecture and extend beyond the capsule, making the diagnosis between a benign and malignant lesion very difficult. The term "pseudolymphoma" has been applied when the lesions show tumor-like aggregates of lymphoid cells but do not meet histologic criteria for malignancy (Figure 47–7). PAS-positive intranuclear inclusions and macroglobulins may be present, as in Waldenström's macroglobulinemia.[32]

In pseudolymphoma, the site of extraglandular lymphoproliferation determines the clinical presentation. There may be hyperplasia of lymph nodes near salivary glands, and striking regional lymphadenopathy may be the predominant clinical feature. On the other hand, lymphoid infiltration may be selectively excessive in a distant organ such as kidney or lung. The involved organs may become functionally impaired, giving rise to renal abnormalities or pulmonary insufficiency. Renal tubular acidosis may arise through such a mechanism.[33]

Features that should alert the clinician to the possibility of extraglandular lymphoproliferation in a patient with Sjögren's syndrome are regional or generalized lymphadenopathy, hepatosplenomegaly, pulmonary infiltrates, renal insufficiency, purpura, leukopenia, hypergammaglobulinemia, or elevated serum macroglobulin.[32] Vasculitis may be associated but arthritis is rare in such patients. The entity of pseudolymphoma cannot be clearly defined but occupies the middle portion of the spectrum of lymphoproliferation, merging with benign disease (e.g., with hypergammaglobulinemic purpura) on the one end, and with frankly malignant disease such as Waldenström's macroglobulinemia or reticulum cell sarcoma on the other.

The other type of extraglandular lymphoid infiltrate is histologically malignant, enabling the specific diagnosis of a

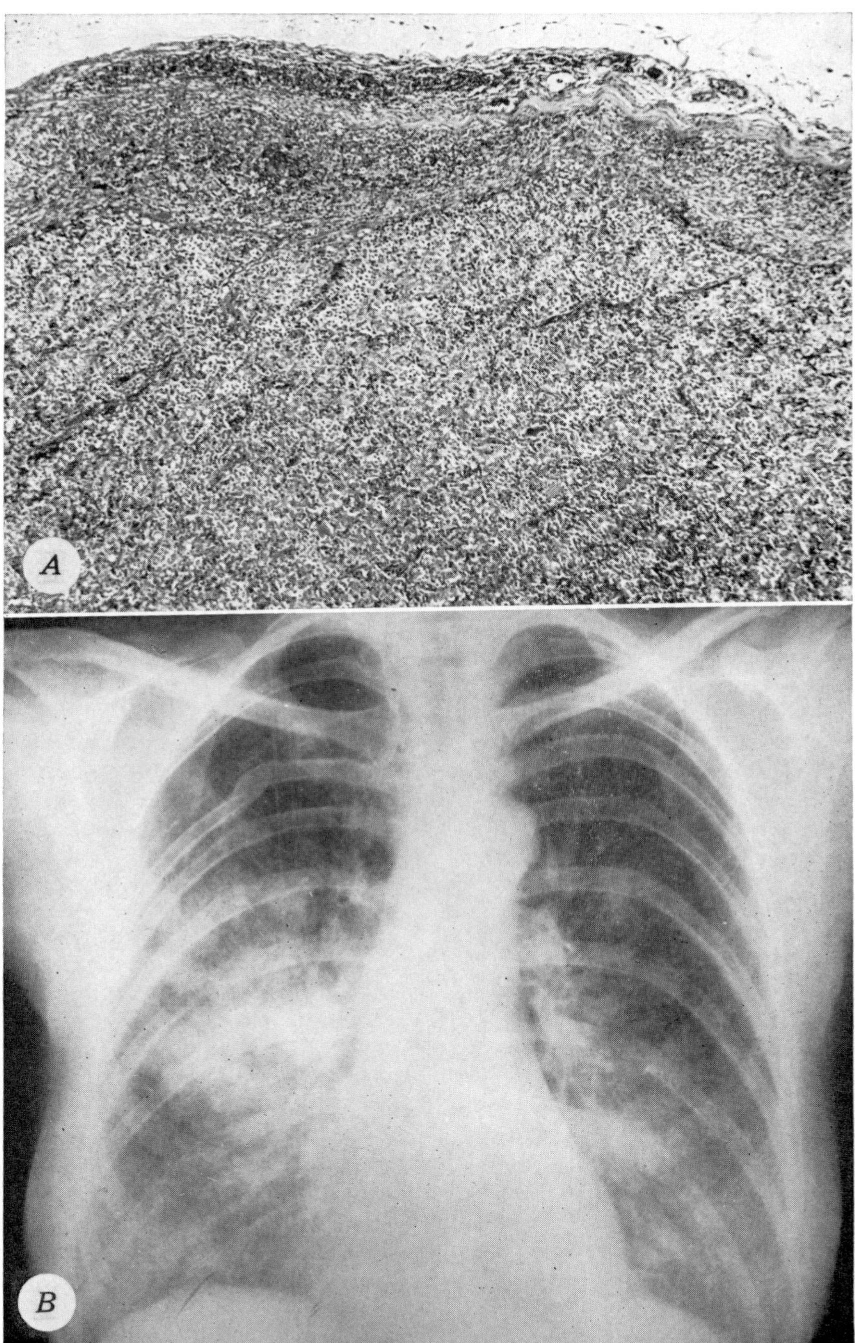

Fig. 47–7.—Pseudolymphoma can distort the normal lymph node architecture with penetration of cells through the capsule, or may appear as pulmonary infiltrates on chest x-ray (Courtesy of American Journal of Medicine).

lymphoproliferative neoplasm. These lesions may also appear after several years of apparently benign disease, may or may not be preceded by pseudolymphoma, and are often highly resistant to therapy. The most common malignant lymphoproliferation is a highly undifferentiated reticulum cell sarcoma or unclassifiable primitive or stem cell lymphoma.[31]

A low IgM level may herald the presence or development of malignant lymphoproliferation and is a poor prognostic sign. A fall in serum IgM is often accompanied by a reduction in the rheumatoid factor titer and may precede the onset of generalized hypogammaglobulinemia.

To date, there have been 40 cases reported of generalized or malignant lymphoproliferative disease associated with Sjögren's syndrome or with benign lymphoepithelial lesions of the parotid gland. These include 10 with pseudolymphoma, 13 with reticulum cell sarcoma or stem cell lymphoma, 7 with Waldenström's macroglobulinemia and 10 with miscellaneous lymphomas.

Diagnosis

Sjögren's syndrome can be considered both as an entity unto itself and as a constellation of findings that can occur in any one of the other connective tissue diseases. The diagnosis should be suspected in any patient with rheumatoid arthritis and can be made when any two of the three major clinical features (keratoconjunctivitis sicca, xerostomia, rheumatoid arthritis) are present. Another connective tissue disease (*e.g.* scleroderma,[21] systemic lupus erythematosus,[25] polymyositis[23]) may substitute for rheumatoid arthritis in this definition. Generally, the arthritis precedes or appears concurrent with the sicca complex.

Many patients will present with symptoms of oral and ocular dryness but without an underlying connective tissue disease. Such patients would appear to have Sjögren's syndrome as a primary disease entity. If arthritis does not develop within the first twelve months of the sicca complex, the chances are only 10 per cent that it will appear later.

As with many diseases, the history is the important first step in making the diagnosis of Sjögren's syndrome. Many patients, on casual questioning, will reply that their mouths feel dry. A more significant response is the fact that they require frequent fluids during the course of the day, or that they awake at night because of oral dryness. The dramatic negative response to the thought of ingesting a dry cracker is a helpful clue. Attempt to have patients describe their ocular complaints. Often they will use the expression "gritty" or "sandy" to characterize the discomfort of xerophthalmia.

Objective evidence of salivary or lacrimal gland insufficiency should be sought in any patient giving a suggestive history. This includes a careful ophthalmologic examination with biomicroscopy, measurement of salivary flow, secretory sialography and salivary gland scintigraphy. If the diagnosis is supported by any of these studies, a lower lip salivary gland biopsy should be performed for histologic confirmation.

The varied clinical presentation and multisystem nature of Sjögren's syndrome may make the diagnosis obscure. As indicated in Table 47–1, the disease may present in several different ways. A unilateral or asymmetric glandular enlargement may suggest a possible tumor. Twenty to 30 per cent of patients with hyperglobulinemic purpura will have other features of Sjögren's syndrome.[28] The initial symptoms may be related to a renal tubular disorder (*e.g.* renal gravel or calculi) or suggest a severe degenerative or inflammatory muscle disease. Peripheral neuropathy may be a prominent feature, and trigeminal involvement can cause facial discomfort. Rarely, the disease may present as a chronic active hepatitis or biliary cirrhosis. Pulmonary disease may be related to dryness and infection or to lymphoid infil-

Table 47-1.—Clinical Presentation of Sjögren's Syndrome

1. Sicca complex—dry eyes and dry mouth
2. Rheumatoid arthritis—or other connective tissue disease
3. Parotid tumor
4. Purpura—non-thrombocytopenic; hyperglobulinemic
5. Renal tubular acidosis—or other tubular disorder
6. Polymyopathy
7. Neuropathy—trigeminal
8. Chronic liver disease
9. Chronic pulmonary disease
10. Lymphoma—local or generalized
11. Immunoglobulin disorder—cryoglobulinemia; macroglobulinemia

tration of the lung. Presentation as a malignant lymphoma or immunoglobulin disorder is not unusual.

Treatment

Most often, Sjögren's syndrome is a benign disease that is not limiting of life. Consequently, conservative management is the best guide to therapy.

The sicca complex is treated with fluid replacement supplied as often as necessary. There are several readily available ophthalmic preparations (Tearisol; Liquifilm; 0.5% methyl cellulose) that will adequately replace the deficient tears. In severe situations, patients will instill these as often as every half to one hour. If corneal ulceration is present, eye patching and boric acid ointment may be necessary.

It is more difficult to compensate for the salivary insufficiency. The frequent ingestion of fluids, particularly with meals, is often the best solution. Patients should see their dentists every four months and pay scrupulous attention to proper oral hygiene. The careful use of a water pick after eating may reduce the incidence of caries.

Proper humidification of the home environment is helpful in reducing respiratory infections and other complications of the sicca complex. Patients should be encouraged to live with their disability. They require sympathetic understanding from those who have never personally experienced the unpleasant discomfort of the sicca symptoms.

The management of rheumatoid arthritis or other associated disorders is in no way altered by the presence of Sjögren's syndrome. There are no controlled studies evaluating the efficacy of corticosteroids or immunosuppressive drugs in the treatment of the sicca complex. In view of the benign nature of this problem, and the potential hazards of these agents, such therapy does not seem justified at this time.

On the other hand, corticosteroids or immunosuppressive drugs seem indicated in the treatment of pseudolymphoma, particularly when there is renal or pulmonary involvement. Cyclophosphamide at a dosage of 75 to 100 mg. daily has diminished extraglandular lymphoid infiltrates and restored salivary gland function in selected patients treated at the National Institutes of Health.

Frank malignant lymphoma should be treated with intensive chemotherapy, surgery, and/or radiotherapy as indicated by the location and extent of disease. These are highly malignant and often fatal lesions which require rapid and skilled intervention. One of the earliest patients reported with unequivocal reticulum cell sarcoma of the inguinal nodes is living and well ten years after treatment with radical surgery and radiotherapy.[31]

CONNECTIVE TISSUE DISEASE WITH OTHER IMMUNOLOGIC DISORDERS

Hypogammaglobulinemia and Connective Tissue Disease

The functions of the immune system can be divided between those dependent upon the secretion of antibody by plasma cells and those dependent upon an intact thymus and specifically sensitized lymphocytes. These two functional categories are termed humoral and cellular immunity respectively, and one or both may become deranged as a consequence of disease.

A deficiency of humoral immunity results in a failure to produce specific antibody, a severe depression of serum gamma globulin concentration, and the absence of germinal center formation in lymph nodes and spleen. In recent years, immunologists have discovered five immunologically and structurally distinct classes of gamma globulin (called IgG, IgM, IgA, IgD and IgE). All immunoglobulin classes may be depressed simultaneously in any one patient, or selective deficiencies may be present with normal or elevated levels of the remaining classes. The term "disgammaglobulinemia" has been applied to describe the latter condition. If the absolute level of gamma globulin is abnormally low, as is generally the case, the diagnosis of hypogammaglobulinemia can be made. The term agammaglobulinemia is less accurate, since a total deficiency of all immunoglobulin classes is rarely found.

Hypogammaglobulinemia may be congenital or acquired. There are several varieties of the congenital disease which are distinguished one from the other by such factors as sex-linkage, normal or abnormal cellular immune and thymic function, and the classes of immunoglobulin involved. The congenital disease is generally manifest in childhood. The acquired disorder occurs in both sexes and at any age of life. Both congenital and acquired hypogammaglobulinemia may be accompanied by an enhanced susceptibility to bacterial and other infections, watery diarrhea and malabsorption producing a sprue-like syndrome, a chronic arthritis indistinguishable from rheumatoid arthritis, or other connective tissue or lymphoproliferative diseases.

Clinical Features

Good and Rotstein found joint involvement consistent with rheumatoid arthritis in five of 27 pediatric and adult patients with hypogammaglobulinemia.[12,13] An additional 3 patients had probable rheumatoid arthritis, and another had possible systemic lupus erythematosus, for an overall 33 per cent incidence of connective tissue disease associated with depressed serum immunoglobulins. Others[8,15] have noted the association of hypogammaglobulinemia with chronic arthritis, scleroderma,[29] systemic lupus erythematosus and dermatomyositis.[17]

Three of Good and Rotstein's patients with arthritis developed characteristic subcutaneous nodules in the elbow region which histologically resembled rheumatoid nodules. These patients were 7, 33 and 44 years old respectively. A four-year-old boy with subcutaneous nodules, polyarthritis and severe hypogammaglobulinemia has been described recently.[4]

Many characteristic features of rheumatoid arthritis, such as morning stiffness and symmetrical joint swelling, are present in these patients. X-rays show demineralization of the bones and narrowing of the joint spaces but erosions and extensive joint destruction have not been reported.

Synovial biopsies show chronic inflammatory changes but typical plasma cells are not found. Likewise, plasma cells are absent from the bone marrow and lymph nodes.[4]

There was a high incidence of rheumatoid arthritis in relatives of two patients with arthritis and hypogammaglobulinemia.[12] Relatives of another patient showed elevations of gamma globulin.[4]

Laboratory Findings

The characteristic finding is a markedly depressed concentration of gamma globulin reported on routine paper electrophoresis of the serum. Every patient should then be studied by immunoelectrophoresis and should have quantitative immunoglobulin determinations for each immunoglobulin class. This can be performed in any general clinical laboratory with the use of commercially available immunoglobulin plates supplied with reference standards.

A depression of the three major immunoglobulin classes (IgG, IgM, IgA) will be found most often, although selective depressions with other classes being normal or even elevated can occur. Rheumatoid factor is absent from the serum.

Although immunoglobulins are classically reduced or absent in the serum, they are present in the synovial fluid, in mononuclear cells present in synovial biopsy specimens, and in inclusion granules contained in leukocytes.[4,23] Moreover, the total hemolytic complement and B_1C globulin concentration of synovial fluid are low, suggesting that immunoglobulin synthesis and immune complex formation may be occurring locally in the synovium in these patients.

Some patients have a selective IgA deficiency associated with autoimmune disease or with serologic abnormalities suggestive of autoimmunity. In these individuals, serum IgA may be undetectable whereas the other four immunoglobulins are present in normal concentration. In one study, 8 of fifteen patients had antibody to IgA itself, 3 had rheumatoid factor, several had antithyroid antibodies and 9 had antibodies to raw milk.[2] The clinical presentations associated with selective IgA deficiency include rheumatoid arthritis,[16] systemic lupus erythematosus,[3,8,15] Sjögren's syndrome,[9,15] and thyroiditis. Cellular immunity is generally normal in this condition.

Treatment

Patients with hypogammaglobulinemia should be treated with injections of gamma globulin at regular intervals. One patient, receiving 4 cc. of gamma globulin intramuscularly every 3 weeks, showed a marked regression of arthritis and clearing of subcutaneous nodules over a 16-month period.[4]

Etiology

Two major facts emerge from study of these patients who represent true experiments of nature. First, serum rheumatoid factor is not required for the development of rheumatoid arthritis. Second, the immunologic events occurring locally in the synovium and joint space in these patients may be very similar to those in more typical rheumatoid arthritis despite the hypogammaglobulinemia and impaired ability to produce specific antibody.

The pathogenesis of the autoimmune and connective tissue diseases probably depends upon genetic, immunologic and viral factors. The immunologic deficiency present in these patients predisposes them to pyogenic respiratory tract infections and to unexplained diarrhea and malabsorption, as well as to autoimmunity. It is possible that their altered immune status renders them more susceptible to pathologic events induced by unusual pathogens such as latent viruses. The peculiar susceptibility related to selective IgA deficiency supports this concept. IgA, the major secretory immunoglobulin, may play an important host defense role in the respiratory and gastrointestinal tract. Deficiency of IgA in these critical areas may permit the entry and establishment of foreign invaders which induce antigenic alterations and contribute to the development of autoimmunity.

Hyperglobulinemic Purpura

Clinical Features

This condition affects women predominantly and is characterized by hypergammaglobulinemia and episodes of lower extremity purpura. It was described orginally by Waldenström,[31] and is not to be confused with another entity,

Waldenström's macroglobulinemia. Patients often have no other associated illness, although myeloma,[24,25] arthritis and Sjögren's syndrome may develop.[27] Prodromata such as burning or itching of the legs may precede by several hours and announce the onset of another episode of purpura. A chronic brownish pigmentation of the skin often appears as the residue of these attacks.

Laboratory Findings

The erythrocyte sedimentation rate and gamma globulin concentration are elevated. Rheumatoid factor and antinuclear factor are frequently present in the serum.

Recent studies indicate that antigamma globulins of the IgG type are a regular feature of this disease and result in immune complexes with sedimentation properties intermediate between 7S and 19S immunoglobulins.[7] These "intermediate complexes" are formed by interactions of the IgG anti-IgG with itself and with other normal IgG molecules. The resulting pattern on serum paper electrophoresis is generally polydispersed (*i.e.* polyclonal) but may at times appear monoclonal. Indeed, 11 of 16 of these proteins when studied structurally showed evidence of restricted heterogeneity such as occurs in true myeloma proteins.[7]

Etiology

This disorder seems to occupy a middleground between autoimmune and lymphoproliferative diseases. It is distinguished immunologically from rheumatoid arthritis by the presence of IgG rather than IgM rheumatoid factor (*i.e.* anti-IgG antibody). The homogeneity of this unusual antibody suggests that the immunogen contains a limited number of antigenic determinants, or else that there may be a highly restricted host immune response.

The relationship of the hypergammaglobulinemia to the purpura is not understood. It is likely that the circulating IgG immune complexes become deposited in small blood vessels, giving rise to vascular injury and extravasation of blood.

Cryoglobulinemia

Cryoglobulins are immunoglobulins which have the physicochemical characteristic of precipitation in the cold followed by resolution upon warming. Cryoglobulins are often monoclonal or homogeneous proteins (usually IgG or IgM) produced by proliferating cells in multiple myeloma or Waldenström's macroglobulinemia. However, cryoprecipitability may also occur as a consequence of immunoglobulin interaction, *e.g.* between IgM and IgG proteins.[19] Such cryoglobulins are immune complexes and are often associated with features suggestive of a connective tissue disease.[21] Small amounts of cryoglobulins containing IgG and complement also occur in systemic lupus erythematosus.[14]

Clinical Features

Cryoglobulins of either monoclonal or immune complex ("mixed") nature may produce Raynaud's phenomenon, numbness, urticaria, vascular occlusions, tissue infarction and digital ulcerations.

Mixed cryoglobulins may also be associated with a symptom complex occurring predominantly in women that includes arthralgias, purpura (especially involving the lower extremities), weakness, vasculitis and diffuse glomerulonephritis.[21] Rheumatoid factor is present and Sjögren's syndrome or thyroiditis may occur.

Meltzer and Franklin[21] studied 12 patients whose cryoglobulins contained rheumatoid factors, a figure representing almost half of their series of 29 subjects with cryoglobulinemia. They emphasized the rapid onset of diffuse glomerulonephritis progressing swiftly to fatal acute renal failure in three patients. A low serum complement was present in seven patients tested. Immunoglobulins and complement can be demonstrated by fluorescence microscopy in the glomerular lesions,[11,21,28] suggesting that the nephritis is due to immune complex deposits.

Laboratory Findings

The outstanding laboratory finding which makes the diagnosis is the cryoglobulin in the serum. It may require up to 24 hours in the cold to precipitate the cryoglobulin from serum. Anywhere from 20 to 60 per cent of the mixed cryoprecipitate is IgM. It requires the presence of IgG to precipitate, and behaves like an antibody to IgG. Cryoprecipitation occurs without the presence of complement although complement may be associated with the complex and serum complement levels are generally depressed. The IgM is a fairly typical rheumatoid factor. The binding is to the Fc portion of IgG. The IgM may be a monoclonal (Waldenström-type) paraprotein.[32] Mixed IgA-IgG cryoglobulinemia has also been reported.[30]

In one patient with mixed cryoglobulinemia, Sjögren's syndrome and pulmonary lymphoid infiltrates, there was an associated hypogammaglobulinemia and increased susceptibility to bacterial infection.[32] The IgM was monoclonal and reacted specifically with IgG subclasses 1, 2 and 4 but not with subclass 3. Serum concentrations of IgG 1, 2 and 4 were 10 per cent of normal. These three subclasses also showed reduced synthesis and shortened survival, whereas IgG 3 had a normal synthetic rate and survival. The hypogammaglobulinemia was due in part to a rapid elimination of IgG through its interaction with the IgG-reactive monoclonal IgM.

Three patients with hyperviscosity due to an IgM-IgG interaction have been reported.[18,21] All had rheumatoid arthritis. Another patient with polyarthritis, polymyositis and the hyperviscosity syndrome had 13S aggregates which were composed of IgG.[1]

Treatment

The treatment of mixed cryoglobulinemia has recently been reviewed.[20] Corticosteroids, immunosuppressive drugs, penicillamine and splenectomy have been employed with limited success.

Etiology

The "mixed cryoglobulins" probably represent a special example of an immune complex phenomenon which has highly unusual physicochemical properties both *in vitro* and *in vivo*. The cold precipitability *in vitro* makes it possible to identify, isolate and characterize the invidual components of the complex. The *in vivo* properties of the complex probably contribute in a major way to the findings of vascular insufficiency. The purpuric lesions may be caused by cryoprecipitation in the small skin capillaries which achieve a temperature range (30° C.) at which these aggregates are known to precipitate. The complexes may also induce glomerulonephritis and be responsible for hypogammaglobulinemia with increased susceptibility to infection.

These cryoglobulins serve to illustrate in a very impressive way the dramatic pathologic consequences that ensue upon immune complex formation and deposition. They shed no light on the mechanism leading to their production, although their ready availability in serum may contribute to further investigation aimed at this question. If viral or tissue antigens are involved in the initial stages of their production, then the specificity of antibodies in the cryocomplex may conceivably be directed against such antigens.

Connective Tissue Disease and Malignant Lymphoma

There are now enough published reports of this association of two rare conditions to suggest that a mere coincidental relationship may not be the best explanation. The association of Sjögren's syndrome and lymphoproliferation is covered earlier in this chapter.

Nine patients with coexisting systemic lupus erythematosus and malignant lymphoma have been reported.[6,22,26] Four patients had Hodgkin's disease, two had lymphosarcoma, one each had mixed cell lymphoma, reticulum cell sarcoma and chronic lymphocytic leukemia. All but two died of the malignancy. Two of them had hypogammaglobulinemia. One patient had hematoxylin bodies, onion skin lesions in the spleen, and hypogammaglobulinemia with an increase in IgM. The IgM showed cryoprecipitability, was an anti-nuclear factor and contained only λ light chains.[26]

The association of rheumatoid arthritis and monoclonal gammopathies is noteworthy. In one series of 16 patients with arthritis, 6 had multiple myeloma, 8 had an asymptomatic monoclonal immunoglobulin "spike" on serum protein electrophoresis, and one each had Waldenström's macroglobulinemia or heavy chain disease.[33] These patients had rheumatoid factor and their arthritis antedated by as much as 26 years the development of the paraprotein. Such patients should be distinguished from cases of multiple myeloma or Waldenström's macroglobulinemia in which amyloid deposition or the bony lesions themselves can mimic rheumatoid arthritis.[5,10]

The connective tissue disease may predispose to the subsequent development of lymphoid or plasma cell malignancy. This might arise as a consequence of chronic viral infection or prolonged antigenic stimulation, perhaps coupled with impaired cellular immunity and immunologic surveillance.

BIBLIOGRAPHY

Sjögren's Syndrome

1. Bloch, K. J., Buchanan, W. W., Wohl, M. J. and Bunim, J. J.: Medicine, *44*, 187, 1965.
2. Cardell, B. S. and Gurling, K. J.: J. Path. and Bact., *68*, 137, 1954.
3. Chisholm, D. M. and Mason, D. K.: J. Clin. Path., *21*, 656, 1968.
4. Cruickshank, A. H.: J. Clin. Path., *18*, 391, 1965.
5. Godwin, J. T.: Cancer, *5*, 1089, 1952.
6. Gougerot, H.: Bull. Med. (Paris), *40*, 360, 1926.
7. Halberg, P., Bertram, U., Soborg, M. and Nerup, J.: Acta Med. Scand., *178*, 291, 1965.
8. Henderson, J. W.: Am. J. Ophth., *33*, 197, 1950.
9. Holm, S.: Acta Ophth., *33*, 1, 1949.
10. Houwer, A. W. M.: Ophthal. Soc. U. K., *47*, 88, 1927.
11. Kaltreider, H. B. and Talal, N.: Ann. Intern. Med., *70*, 751, 1969.
12. Kessler, H. S.: Amer. J. Path., *52*, 671, 1968.
13. Leventhal, B. G., Waldorf, D. S. and Talal, N.: J. Clin. Invest., *46*, 1338, 1967.
14. MacSween, R. N. M., Goudie, R. B., Anderson, J. R., Armstrong, E., Murray, M. A., Mason, D. A., Jasani, M. K., Boyle, J. A., Buchanan, W. W. and Williamson, J.: Ann. Rheum. Dis., *26*, 402, 1967.
15. Mikulicz, J.: Medical Classics, *2*, 165, 1937.
16. Morgan, W. S. and Castleman, B.: Amer. J. Path., *29*, 471, 1953.
17. Morris, R. C. and Fudenberg, H. H.: Medicine, *46*, 57, 1967.
18. Pittman, F. E. and Holub, D. A.: Gastroenterol., *48*, 869, 1965.
19. Schall, G. L., Anderson, L. G., Wolf, R. O., Herdt, J. R., Tarpley, T. M., Cummings, N. A., Zeiger, L. S. and Talal, N.: J.A.M.A., *216*, 2109, 1971.
20. Schirmer, O.: Arch. Ophth., *56*, 197, 1903.
21. Shearn, M. A.: Ann. Intern. Med., *52*, 1352, 1960.
22. Shearn, M. A. and Tu, W. H.: Ann. Rheum. Dis., *27*, 27, 1968.
23. Silberberg, D. H. and Drachman, D. A.: Arch. Neurol. and Psychiat., *6*, 428, 1962.
24. Sjögren, H.: Acta Ophthal. (Kbh), *11*, 1, 1933.
25. Steinberg, A. D. and Talal, N.: Ann. Intern. Med., *74*, 55, 1971.
26. Stenstam, T.: Acta Med. Scandinav., *127*, 130, 1947.
27. Stoltze, C. A., Hanlon, D. G., Pease, G. L. and Henderson, J. W.: Arch. Intern. Med., *106*, 513, 1960.
28. Strauss, W. G.: New Engl. J. Med., *260*, 857, 1959.
29. Talal, N.: Arth. & Rheum., *13*, 887, 1970.
30. Talal, N., Asofsky, R., and Lightbody, P.: J. Clin. Invest., *49*, 49, 1970.

31. Talal, N. and Bunim, J. J.: Amer. J. Med., *36*, 529, 1964.
32. Talal, N., Sokoloff, L. and Barth, W. F.: Amer. J. Med., *43*, 50, 1967.
33. Talal, N., Zisman, E. and Schur, P. H.: Arth. & Rheum., *11*, 774, 1968.
34. Vanselow, N. A., Dodson, V. N., Angell, D. C. and Duff, I. F.: Ann. Intern. Med., *58*, 124, 1963.

Connective Tissue Diseases Associated with Other Immunologic Disorders

1. Abruzzo, J. L., Heimer, R., Giuliano, V. and Martinez, J.: Amer. J. Med., *49*, 258, 1970.
2. Ammann, A. J. and Hong, R.: Clin. Exper. Immunol., *7*, 833, 1970.
3. Bachmann, R., Laurell, C. B., and Svenonius, E.: Scand. J. Clin. and Lab. Invest., *17*, 46, 1965.
4. Barnett, E. V., Winkelstein, A. and Weinberger, H. J.: Amer. J. Med., *48*, 40, 1970.
5. Calabro, J. J.: Arth. & Rheum., *10*, 553, 1967.
6. Cammarata, R. J., Rodnan, G. P. and Jensen, W. N.: Arch. Intern. Med., *111*, 330, 1963.
7. Capra, J. D., Winchester, R. J. and Kunkel, H. G.: Medicine, *50*, 125, 1971.
8. Cassidy, J. T., Burt, A., Petty, R. and Sullivan, D.: New Engl. J. Med., *280*, 275, 1968.
9. Claman, H. N., Merrill, D. A., Peakman, D. and Robinson, A.: J. Lab. Clin. Med., *75*, 307, 1970.
10. Goldberg, A., Brodsky, I. and McCarty, D.: Amer. J. Med., *37*, 653, 1964.
11. Golde, D. and Epstein, W.: Ann. Intern. Med., *69*, 1221, 1968.
12. Good, R. A. and Rotstein, J.: Bull. Rheum. Dis., *10*, 203, 1960.
13. Good, R. A., Rotstein, J. and Mazzitello, W. F.: J. Lab. Clin. Med., *49*, 343, 1957.
14. Hanauer, L. B. and Christian, C. L.: J. Clin. Invest., *46*, 400, 1967.
15. Hobbs, J. R.: Lancet, *1*, 110, 1968.
16. Huntley, C. C., Thorpe, D. P., Lyerly, A. D. and Kelsey, W. M.: Amer. J. Dis. Child., *113*, 411, 1967.
17. Janeway, C. A., Gitlin, D., Craig, J. M. and Grice, D. S.: Trans. Amer. Assoc. Phys., *69*, 93, 1956.
18. Jasin, H. E., LoSpalluto, J. and Ziff, M.: Arth. & Rheum., *12*, 304, 1969.
19. LoSpalluto, J., Dorward, B., Miller, W., Jr. and Ziff, M.: Amer. J. Med., *32*, 142, 1962.
20. Mathison, D. A., Condemi, J. J., Leddy, J. P., Callerame, M. L., Panner, B. J. and Vaughan, J. H.: Ann. Intern. Med., *74*, 383, 1971.
21. Meltzer, M. and Franklin, E. C.: Amer. J. Med., *40*, 837, 1966.
22. Miller, D. G.: Ann. Intern. Med., *66*, 507, 1967.
23. Rawson, A. J., Hollander, J. L., Abelson, N. M., Reginato, A. and Torralba, T.: Arth. & Rheum., *9*, 534, 1966 (abstract).
24. Rogers, W. R. and Welch, J. D.: Arch. Intern. Med., *100*, 478, 1957.
25. Savin, R. C.: Arch. Derm., *92*, 679, 1965.
26. Smith, C. K., Cassidy, J. T. and Bole, G. G.: Amer. J. Med., *48*, 113, 1970.
27. Strauss, W. G.: New Engl. J. Med., *260*, 857, 1959.
28. Talal, N., Zisman, E. and Schur, P. H.: Arth. & Rheum., *11*, 774, 1968.
29. Van Gelder, D. W.: South. Med. J., *50*, 43, 1957.
30. Wager, W., Mustakallio, K. K. and Rasanen, J. A.: Amer. J. Med., *44*, 179, 1968.
31. Waldenström, J.: Nord. Med., *20*, 2288, 1943.
32. Waldmann, T. A., Johnson, J. S., and Talal, N.: J. Clin. Invest., *50*, 951, 1971.
33. Zawadzki, Z. A. and Benedek, T. G.: Arth. & Rheum., *12*, 555, 1969.

Chapter 48

Relapsing Polychondritis

By Carl M. Pearson, M.D.

Relapsing polychondritis is a fairly rare human disorder whose manifestations are often widespread and are clinically and pathologically impressive, or even dramatic. The essential features are inflammation with progressive loss of structural integrity of some cartilaginous tissues, and involvement of organs of special senses such as the eye, the middle and inner ears and the vestibular apparatus. More recently aortic insufficiency has been described in some cases.

The condition was considered to be a medical oddity until about 1960.[1] Prior to that time the medical literature contained only ten single case reports.[8] Since the general recognition of this condition within the last ten years, at least an additional 64 cases have been described.[2,4,6]

Many of the earlier authors did not realize that similar instances had been described before and each invented his own descriptive terms for the condition. Thus relapsing polychondritis was previously known as "systemic chondromalacia," "panchondritis," "chronic atrophic polychondritis," and by other titles. "Relapsing polychondritis"[8] seems to describe best the undulating clinical course that this syndrome follows, although admittedly it does not take into account the frequent affliction of some non-cartilaginous structures.

CLINICAL FEATURES

The earliest identifiable report of relapsing polychondritis was published in 1923 by the German, Jaksch Wartenhorst.[5] His patient, a 32-year-old brewer, first became ill with arthritic swellings and pain in several finger joints and then in the wrists, left hand, right knee and the toes of the right foot. There was also a febrile response. One and a half months later, burning pain developed in both external ears, which slowly swelled and within the next three months receded and shrank, leaving a flabby deformity of both auricles. Two or three months later, without pain, the mid-segment of the nose slowly collapsed leaving a saddle-nose deformity. At that time there was nearly complete stenosis of both auditory canals and some diminution of hearing, even when the canals were held open. There was also associated dizziness and tinnitus. Somewhat later crepitation developed in both knees and in the spine.

On the basis of Jaksch Wartenhorst's original clinical description[5] and speculations and upon a review of the entire literature as summarized by Pearson *et al.*,[8] Dolan *et al.*,[2] and Kaye and Sones,[6] it is now possible to construct a reasonably clear composite picture of relapsing polychondritis. This picture is, however, barely more complete than that noted in the 1920's.

The disease occurs equally in both sexes and is most common in the middle decades of life. It has also been reported in children, young adults and in the elderly. It is often fatal. Dolan *et al.*[2] calculated that the life span of eleven patients who died was 7.1 years from the time of appearance of the symptoms. The spectrum of survival ranged widely

Table 48-1.—Incidence of Various Clinical Features in Relapsing Polychondritis*

Manifestation	*No. affected/No. reported*	*Frequency, %*
Ear cartilage involvement	45/51	88
Nasal cartilage involvement	40/49	82
Fever	21/26	81
Arthropathy	40/51	78
Laryngotracheal involvement	33/47	70
Episcleritis or conjunctivitis	29/48	60
Defective hearing	21/44	48
Costochondral cartilage involvement	21/45	47
Iritis	11/41	27
Labyrinthine vertigo†	—	25
Aortic valve lesion with insufficiency‡	10/74	14

* Modified from Dolan et al.[2]
† Rough approximation of incidence. These organ systems were not always clearly described.
‡ From Pearson et al.,[9] Hughes et al.,[4] and others

from 10 months to over 20 years. The causes of death were usually respiratory failure due to airway stenosis (or collapse) and complicating pulmonary infection and cardiovascular failure due to intractable aortic insufficiency.[4,9] Table 48–1 summarizes many of the clinical manifestations and their incidence.

Involvement of isolated or multiple cartilages predominates, often with an initial febrile response and involvement of one or several structures of the eye. Onset is usually acute in the first and subsequent attacks, unless the latter are modified by corticosteroid therapy. Classically, the pinnas, or cartilaginous portions of the ears, swell and become purplish-red and exquisitely tender, so that it is impossible to press them on the pillow. The soft earlobes are always spared. The external auditory canals, especially the meatus, also swell and may close almost completely; hearing is thereby reduced markedly. Sometimes the cartilaginous portion of the bridge of the nose may be similarly involved in the first or later episodes. Often the episclerae are inflamed. A labyrinthine type of vertigo may develop. Joint inflammation or simple arthralgias may occur during these attacks.

An attack may last from a few days to many weeks, and may, if left untreated, progress in a subacute or smoldering fashion to involve more and more cartilaginous structures and special sense organs. As the inflammatory phase subsides the external ear may shrink, at which time it is then realized that the cartilage has been thinned or has lost its structural integrity altogether, so that the pinna droops forward from lack of support (Figure 48–1). This may occur during the first episode or not until after several or many attacks. Similarly, the cartilaginous nasal septum may disappear (Figure 48–2), leaving a step-shaped or saddle nose which is also characteristic for this condition.

The two most serious and life-threatening, or even fatal, complications of relapsing polychondritis are: (a) an involvement of the cartilaginous structures of the respiratory tract, and (b) progressive aortic insufficiency. In the mildest forms of the disease the respiratory tract involvement consists of hoarseness, slight cough and minimal tenderness of the

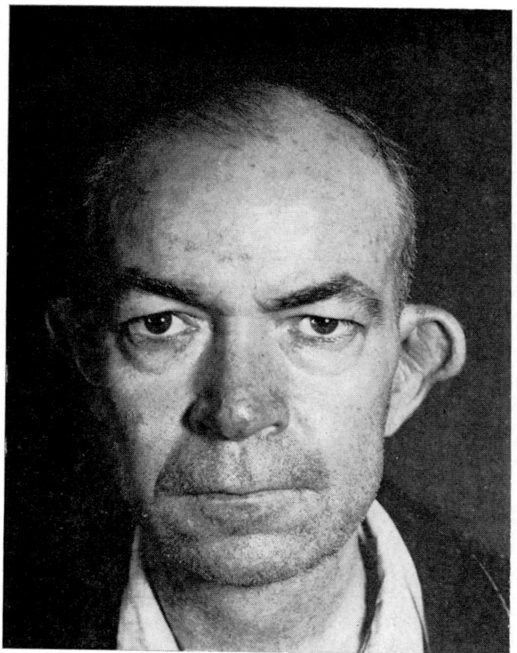

Fig. 48–1.—Classical drooping of the left external ear in a man who has had recurrent episodes of polychondritis of that ear.

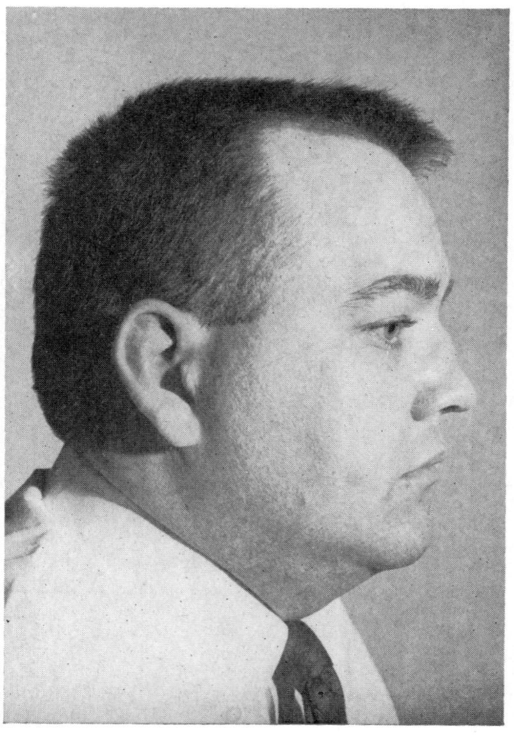

Fig. 48–2.—Characteristic saddle-nose deformity which developed painlessly three months earlier.

larynx and trachea. In more severe and complicating cartilaginous involvement there may be extensive inflammation and edema of the laryngeal and epiglottal cartilages, necessitating emergency tracheostomy. A similar process may also involve the tracheal and bronchial rings so that diffuse narrowing of the airways may ensue. This latter, of course, presents a great hazard to the patient since asphyxia and/or superimposed respiratory infection may occur in these situations. Moreover, in such circumstances tracheostomy may not prove to be adequate to maintain proper pulmonary aeration. If the patient survives one or more chondrolytic attacks on the air passages, the cartilages may be left with some loss of structural support in the involved regions. The trachea and bronchi may then become diffusely or focally narrowed because of varying degrees of stenosis, or the cartilages may lose all or nearly all of their architectural support. They then appear at autopsy as floppy collapsible tubes. In such patients intubation is useless because of the collapse throughout even the smallest bronchi. Two of the cases that we originally described[8] met this fate and were reviewed subsequently in anatomical detail by Verity *et al.*[13] As if such serious involvement of the respiratory apparatus is not enough, further embarrassment to breathing may on occasion be caused by tenderness and swelling of one or several costosternal cartilages which may, in rare instances, even go on to partial or complete dissolution, leaving a flail anterior chest plate.

The other serious complication, namely aortic regurgitation, has been recognized only more recently, since the first report of this complication by Yamazaki and his associates in 1966.[15] Two of the patients that we have seen at the UCLA School of Medicine have suffered this complication. These were reported in 1967.[9] To date the total number of reported patients with aortic insufficiency numbers 10 out of 74 cases of relapsing polychondritis so far described.[4] The aortic regurgitation is not due to a valvulitis of the aortic valve, but rather it results from progressive dilatation of the aortic ring and frequently also of the ascending aorta. Several patients have had successful prosthetic valves operatively inserted.

The eye lesions are not serious, although they occur quite commonly. They include episcleritis and conjunctivitis and, less commonly, iritis. Usually they smolder at a low rate or resolve as an attack subsides. Rarely have serious sequelae resulted, but cataracts, severe keratitis, and even blindness have been described in isolated instances.

Likewise, the arthropathy is quite variable and usually consists of subacute swelling and pain in one or several large joints of the extremities. The articulations of the spine, either of the true apophyseal cartilages or of the intervertebral discs, are rarely involved. Serious peripheral joint damage has not been a common occurrence. However, it may resemble low grade rheumatoid arthritis or secondary osteophytosis with some limitation of joint mobility.

Dolan and his associates[2] also mention hematopoietic, hepatic and renal involvement in some patients. However, these systemic complications are, in our experience, relatively minor and they may even represent secondary phenomena.

The most curious clinical feature is the selectivity that the chondrolytic process seems to achieve. Not only are some cartilages and cartilaginous structures spared while others are extensively involved, but there exists in a few patients a remarkable unilaterality so that only one ear or one eye may be affected, even after multiple attacks.

LABORATORY OBSERVATIONS

As may be anticipated, aside from specific biopsy findings, the laboratory features are quite nonspecific.[2] The most common findings are noted during the active disease process and these consist of an increased sedimentation rate, some degree of anemia, occasional low titer positively for rheumatoid factor, and moderate serum protein alterations which are also nonspecific. The latter include a decrease in serum albumin and increases in alpha and gamma globulins.

Roentgenographic findings, aside from tracheal stenosis, are of little consequence or diagnostic significance in the usual case. Occasionally, after multiple inflammatory attacks the external ears may show calcific deposits. This finding is, however, not specific for relapsing polychondritis and may result from other

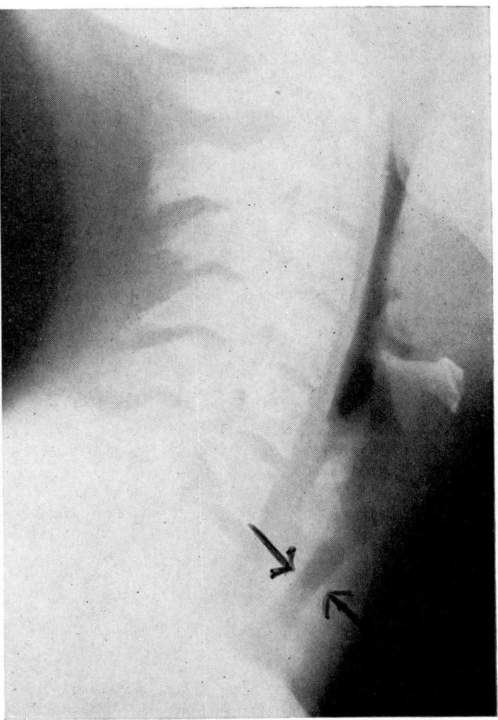

FIG. 48–3.—Significant stenosis of the tracheal airway as demonstrated by air tomography in a 50-year-old woman with classical relapsing polychondritis.

inflammatory lesions affecting the external ears. The joints may show moderate destructive changes, often spotty and asymmetric, but sometimes quite suggestive of rheumatoid arthritis. The most startling finding is narrowing of the major air passages, especially diffuse closure of focal stenosis of the trachea. This may be most clearly visualized by tracheal tomography[3] (Figure 48–3). In the presence of aortic insufficiency, cardiomegaly is, of course, commonly found.

PATHOLOGY

The histopathology of relapsing polychondritis has been examined by several workers, but most extensively by Verity, Larson, and Madden[13] in two of our cases. Acidophilic or pinkish coloration of the cartilage matrix (in contrast to the usual basophilic or bluish hue) by routine hematoxylin and eosin staining is seen. Dissolution or lysis of cartilage seems to occur from its margins inward (Figure 48–4), in addition to the loss of basophilia of the cartilage matrix. Focal or diffuse infiltration by lymphocytes and plasma cells occurs in the perichondrial tissues (Figure 48–5). Invasion by active fibroblastic granulation tissue into cartilage leads to degeneration and fibrillation as well as partial sequestration of the cartilage matrix (Figure 48–4). Evidence of thrombosis or necrotizing angiitis is lacking. Tubercle bacilli, spirochetes and fungi have never been demonstrated by special stains. The elastic tissue fibers in the submucosal elastic laminae of the blood vessels appeared to be normal in the peripheral vessels. Examination of the ocular globe in one case revealed a minimal increase in fragmentation of the elastic tissue at the scleroconjunctival angle. Mast cells, plasma cells and lymphocytes were scattered about the episcleral vessels.

Examination of the cardiac and aortic structures has shown the aortic valve leaflets to be normal, whereas the ascending aorta, especially the aortic ring, in each case has been stretched or dilated with histochemically a loss of basophilia along with degeneration, necrosis and fibrosis. The primary pathology in the aortic ring and ascending aorta was in the media, with a loss of elastic tissue, a decrease in basophilia and collagenous replacement. In addition, associated focal acute and chronic inflammation occurred in these areas as well as in the adventitial blood vessels and those of the vasa vasorum.

Histochemical studies[13] confirmed these findings and revealed a loss of metametachromasia in the residual cartilage matrix with some preservation of metachromasia in the cytoplasm and in the immediate perilacunar zones around chondrocytes. In the aorta there was a moderate loss in neutral or acidic polysaccharides by either the toluidine blue, azure A (pH 2.0) or by PAS-alcian blue methods. Hale's method for sulfated mucopolysaccharides showed marked depletion in these components in the abnormal aortas and aortic rings.

ETIOLOGIC SPECULATIONS

The etiology of relapsing polychondritis is, up until the present time, unclear. The condition is sufficiently rare to make diagnosis difficult in most instances and speculations concerning etiology have been summarized in various recent publications.[2,6,8,13] In general the loss of acid mucopolysaccharides and many of the other changes which may be secondary could be caused by release of lysosomal enzymes, especially proteases, either from chondrocytes or from some more remote sites. Many lysosomal labilizers or releasers are known and these include bacterial endotoxins,[14] pyrogenic steroids, streptolysins O and S, bile salts, progesterone, digitonin, and many others. Presumably many immunological or "autoimmune" reactions could also induce release of lysosomal enzymes following cell damage.

The interesting observation by Thomas[10] and McCluskey[7] that intra-

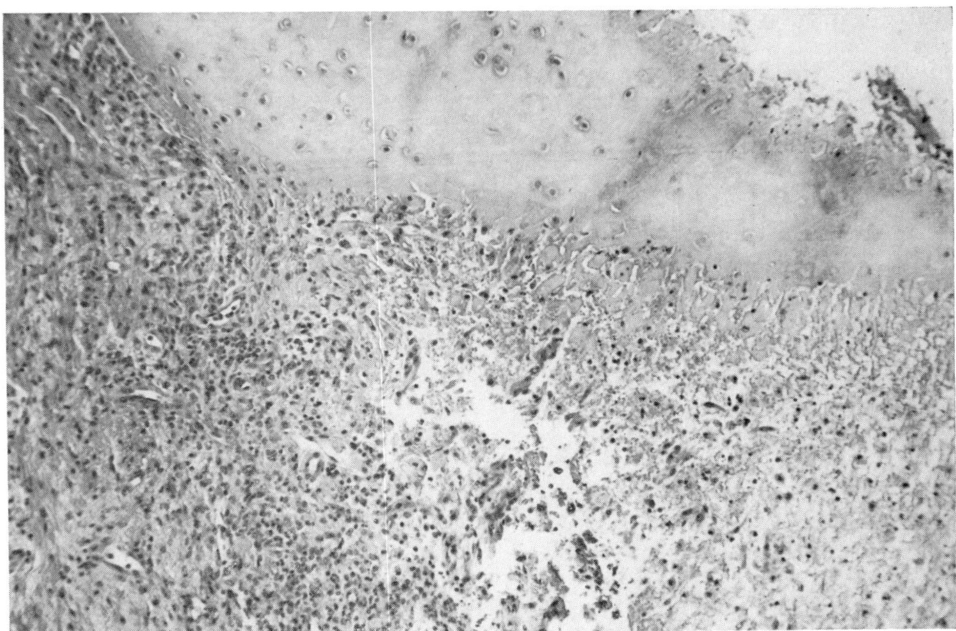

FIG. 48–4.—Extensive loss of ear cartilage basophilia, aggressive destruction and sequestration of segments of cartilage by invading fibroblastic tissue and some inflammatory response. These features are characteristic of the cartilaginous histopathology in relapsing polychondritis.

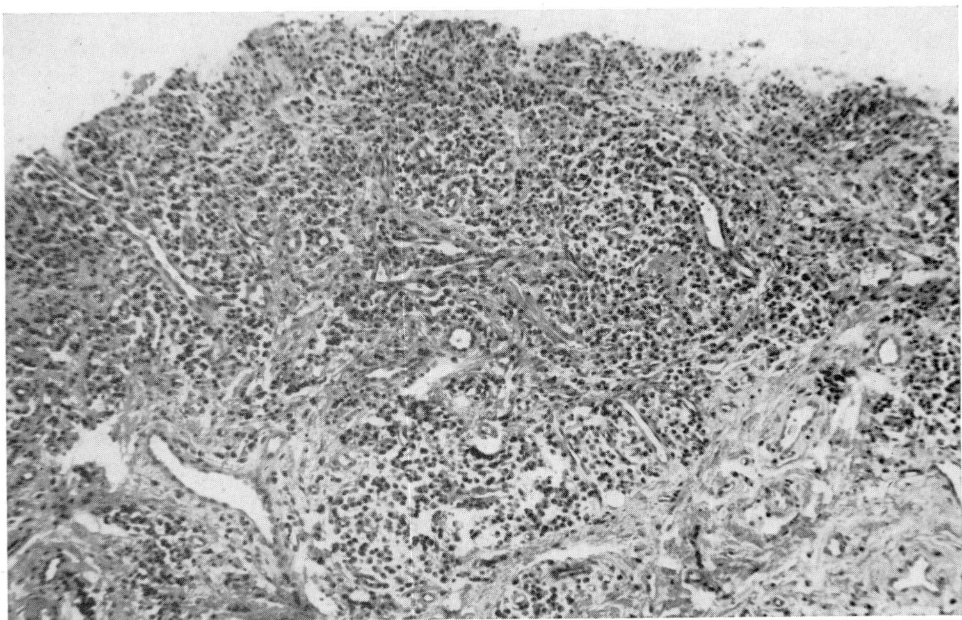

FIG. 48–5.—Marked inflammatory infiltrate, composed of lymphocytes and plasma cells in the perichondrial tissues in relapsing polychondritis. Note also connective tissue proliferation and increase in vascular channels.

venously administered crude papain, a proteolytic enzyme, induces dissolution of the ear cartilages of rabbits within four hours may be pertinent since in this model there is also a rapid loss of cartilage metachromasia and appearance of acidic mucopolysaccharides in the urine. Further, Tsaltas[11] showed that chondroitin sulfate was lost from the cartilage matrix by dissociation from its protein component in cartilage.

In a more recent observation Tsaltas[12] has also noted, again in rabbits, that from three to six weeks after a single intravenous injection of crude papain, changes occur in the ascending aorta and arch. These consist of focal plaque lesions due to alterations of connective tissue of the media which go on to metaplasia into cartilage and even into fully developed bone. Aside from a description of PAS-positive material about the margins of the lesions, no other histochemical results are reported and no mention is made of the aortic insufficiency or aneurysm in these animals.

Tsaltas[12] reasoned that the basis for these lesions may be the release, by papain, of large amounts of sulfated mucopolysaccharides which may in turn become deposited in various organs and especially in the aortic wall. One could suppose that a similar mechanism may be operative in relapsing polychondritis, but here either an endogenous proteolytic enzyme is present or a protease released from lysosomes may be responsible for the chondrolysis.

It also seems plausible that the *in situ* release of lysosomal enzymes from chondrocytes in cartilage and in the aortic wall could be responsible for such lesions, possibly through immunological mechanisms. Moreover, lysosomal membrane labilizing factors such as intermittent systemic endotoxin release may, in some instances, be responsible for the recurrent attacks.

The aortic insufficiency that occurs in relapsing polychondritis has a number of challenging similarities with the aortic regurgitation that occurs in ankylosing spondylitis, Reiter's syndrome and certain other rheumatic diseases (Table 48–2).

Table 48-2.—Aortic Insufficiency

Valvulitis	Rheumatic fever Rheumatoid arthritis Ankylosing spondylitis* Endocarditis Reiter's syndrome* Behçet's syndrome*
Congenital	Bicuspid aortic valve, etc.
Dilatation of valve ring	Marfan's syndrome Syphilis Relapsing polychondritis Secondary to dissecting aneurysm Idiopathic

* Also dilatation of valve ring

THERAPY

Aside from prosthetic valve replacement for aortic insufficiency, therapy has consisted primarily of supportive measures and the use of corticosteroids, especially prednisone. In a number of instances an acute inflammatory attack on affected cartilages may be moderated or brought under complete control with the use of prednisone, 20 to 60 mg. a day in divided dosages. As the attack quiets down the dosage may then be reduced to a low maintenance level of 10 to 15 mg. daily. Experience has shown that often the anti-inflammatory and protective effects of the corticosteroids gradually diminish over months or years so that the maintenance dosage will gradually have to be raised in order to prevent further severe attacks. In three of our cases it was necessary to eventually maintain levels of 30 mg. of prednisone daily in order to provide a tolerable degree of suppression of inflammation of cartilages and of episcleritis. Corticosteroids seem to have no obvious effect on inhibiting the development of the aortic lesions.

Theoretically some of the immunosuppressive agents such as azathioprine or cyclophosphamide might be of value in the early management of some cases, especially if one could eventually implicate an autoimmune mechanism. However antibodies against cartilage matrix or aortic wall tissues have not been demonstrated so far, therefore such therapy should probably be reserved at the present time either for purely research studies or in the occasional corticosteroid-refractory patient.

BIBLIOGRAPHY

1. Bean, W. B., Drevets, C. C. and Chapman, J. S.: Medicine, *37*, 353, 1958.
2. Dolan, D. L., Lemmon, G. B. and Titelbaum, S. L.: Amer. J. Med., *41*, 285, 1966.
3. Horns, J. W. and O'Loughlin, B. J.: Amer. J. Roentgen., *87*, 844, 1962.
4. Hughes, R. A. C., Curry, H. and Lessof, M. H.: Proc. Roy. Soc. Med., *64*, 664, 1971.
5 Jaksch Wartenhorst, R.: Wein. Arch. Intern. Med., *6*, 93, 1923.
6. Kaye, R. L. and Sones, D. A.: Ann. Intern. Med., *60*, 653, 1964.
7. McCluskey, R. T. and Thomas, L.: J. Exper. Med., *108*, 371, 1956.
8. Pearson, C. M., Kline, H. M. and Newcomer, V. D.: New Engl. J. Med., *263*, 51, 1960.
9. Pearson, C. M., Kroening, R., Verity, M. A. and Getzen, J. H.: Trans. Assoc. Amer. Phys., *80*, 71, 1967.
10. Thomas, L.: J. Exper. Med., *104*, 245, 1956.
11. Tsaltas, T. T.: J. Exper. Med., *108*, 507, 1958.
12. ———: Nature, *106*, 1006, 1962.
13. Verity, M. A., Larson, W. M. and Madden, S. C.: Amer. J. Path., *42*, 251, 1963.
14. Weissmann, G. and Thomas, L.: J. Exper. Med., *116*, 433, 1962.
15. Yamazaki, N., Yawata, H., Hannya, H. and Kimura, E.: Jap. Heart J., *7*, 188, 1966.

Chapter 49

Non-Articular Rheumatism and the Fibrositis Syndrome

By Hugh A. Smythe, M.D.

Better definition of the field of non-articular rheumatism has been hampered by:

(1) difficulties in establishing precise diagnosis,
(2) ill-defined diagnostic categories,
(3) archaic terminology,
(4) neglect by academic medicine.

These factors have permitted the persistence of patterns of uncritical clinical analysis and quaint nomenclature which would be intolerable were they not traditional.

Patients commonly present with musculoskeletal pain and tenderness not due to disease in the regional joints. Often these symptoms are due to obvious disease in other local structures, and can then be more precisely described as a bursitis, a muscle tear with hematoma, a panniculitis, etc. But often the origin of the complaints is not immediately obvious, with soreness, stiffness, and, especially, local tenderness, in a tissue which objectively seems normal. These tender points have been called "fibrositic," and the chronic presence of many such areas is the "fibrositis syndrome."

History

The name fibrositis was introduced by Sir William Gowers[8] in 1904 in an article on lumbago, in which he used the term to denote a symptom complex due to hypothetical inflammatory changes in the fibrous structure of the lumbar muscles. Stockman[26,27] was the first to relate a specific pathology to the fibrositic nodule, describing an infiltration of mononuclear cells and patchy fibrosis in one muscle biopsy specimen. He concluded that the essential change was "a condition of chronic inflammation of the white fibrous tissue." Histological studies by other investigators usually failed to reveal such lesions and the occasional presence of such minor "abnormalities" in control material[5,6,25] has lead to an almost unanimous rejection of this explanation of the pathology. At present the term "fibrositis" continues to be used in the absence of a better and widely accepted alternative, recognized as an inexact and temporary designation for a common clinical syndrome of uncertain pathogenesis.

Classification

The syndrome can be classified as (1) *primary*—without demonstrable cause or underlying systemic disease, and (2) *secondary*—to other rheumatic diseases, bone diseases, infections or other chronic illness.

The use of the term "psychogenic rheumatism" as a synonym for fibrositis has drawn attention to an important contributing factor (discussed later), but has not served the patients well. Most patients and many doctors have understood this term to imply that the pain is imaginary or hysterical in origin, which is very rarely the case. The fibrositis syndrome lacks the bizarre features of symbolic psychogenic regional pain. The symptoms are similar from patient to patient, and the tender points predictable and relatively constant in location. The term "tension rheumatism" more accurately describes the psychogenic mechanism involved, but fails to account for the pain and tenderness found over bony prominences and other non-muscular areas.

PRIMARY FIBROSITIS

Clinical Picture

The syndrome is characterized by *pain and stiffness* felt in a widespread distribution through deep tissues such as muscles, tendon insertions and bony prominences, aggravated by fatigue, tension, immobility or chilling, and eased by heat, massage, activity or a holiday. Although the pain may be diffuse, there is a tendency for concentration, and points of excessive *local tenderness* may be found, the majority at precisely predictable symmetrical sites. These include the midpoint of the upper border of the trapezius muscle, the origin of the spinati above and below the medial end of the scapular spine, the rhomboids, the regions immediately medial and lateral to the posterosuperior spines, and the upper outer buttock. In the limbs the areas in front of the lateral and medial epicondyle, and the fat pads medial to the knee are often acutely tender. Most of these areas are regions of high tissue density, and are slightly tender in normal individuals. To describe these local areas of tenderness the term "trigger point" is often used and is especially apt when pressure on these areas induces a characteristic sudden dramatic writhing leap, called the "jump sign."[13] Palpation commonly induces a marked erythema of overlying skin, and this dermographia may vary with the severity of complaints. There may be cutaneous as well as deep hyperalgesia. Temporary relief with ethyl chloride spray may be dramatic.[11,13] Some observers claim to distinguish fibrositic nodules, *i.e.* pea-sized to plum-sized tender indurations. Hench said that these were "only accessible to the finger of faith";[10] usually they represent areas of muscle spasm, fatty lumps, or normal variations in muscle density. When chronic "nervous tension" is a major pathogenetic factor, active movements such as abduction of the arms are often carried out slowly and jerkily, with facial grimacing and obvious spasmotic overactivity of antagonists as well as prime movers. Voluntary range is frequently limited, but full passive movement may be obtained with gentle persistence. Grip testing reveals a variable end point, approached slowly and irregularly. Symptoms are variable, and shift in location of their maximum severity, but rarely disappear completely. A marked weather effect is often described with increased pain and stiffness with chilling, or before storms. The patients complain of chronic fatigue, and nearly all sleep badly, with marked morning stiffness. The syndrome tends to begin in middle life, and the excellent preservation of musculature and generally youthful appearance in later years are in striking contrast to the patient's accounts of chronic misery. Blood studies, including cell counts, erythrocyte sedimentation rate, serum proteins, and serum enzyme levels are usually normal.

Criteria for Diagnosis

The following criteria have been found useful in clinical studies.

I. *Obligatory Criteria* (all must be present)
   1. Subjective aching of more than 3 months' duration
   2. Subjective stiffness of more than 3 months' duration
   3. Local point tenderness
   4. Point tenderness in 2 other sites
   5. Normal ESR, SGOT, rheumatoid factor test, ANF, muscle enzymes and sacroiliac films

II. *Minor Criteria*

1. Chronic fatigue
2. Emotional distress
3. Poor sleep
4. Morning stiffness

Prognosis.—Objective evaluation continues to indicate excellent general health, and muscle bulk and range of passive joint movement remain normal. Temporary alleviation of discomfort can be obtained with a variety of programs, but loss of all symptoms is extremely unusual. Interruption of employment can be a disaster. Very few of these patients ever return to full productive capacity if failing performance due to pain and exhaustion causes them to be fired or to resign. The meager effects of the most intensive multidisciplinary efforts at rehabilitation of these apparently fit patients are in striking contrast to the relative ease with which major functional improvement can be effected in most patients with rheumatoid arthritis.

Prevalence

Non-articular rheumatism is probably more common as a source of disability than rheumatoid arthritis and peripheral joint osteoarthritis combined, although the evidence is fragmentary and of varying reliability. Formal studies of the prevalence of various rheumatic diseases have generally avoided discussion of this problem, but provide data from which some inferences may be drawn. Of the adults screened in the U.S. Public Health Survey, 22 per cent of men and 32 per cent of women reported morning stiffness, and 13 per cent joint pain and tenderness.[24] Symptoms of arthritis or rheumatism, joint swelling or morning stiffness were described by 39 per cent of patients free of rheumatoid arthritis in each of 2 surveys in Pittsburgh and Jerusalem.[2,1] Scant information is available on the contribution of osteoarthrosis or other common degenerative problems to these symptoms. In a survey of joint disease in New Haven, Connecticut, 21 per cent of the individuals surveyed described symptoms of arthritis or rheumatism, 30 per cent complained of morning stiffness, and 19 per cent of night pain. The symptoms were about half as common in those with little evidence of osteoarthrosis in films of the hand, and much more common when extensive evidence of osteoarthrosis was present.[23] In the Tecumseh study, one-third of those surveyed reported pain or aching, and about 15 per cent described joint swelling, morning stiffness, and previous arthritis or rheumatism, with much higher frequencies in older age groups. "Definite" rheumatoid arthritis was evident in less than 1 per cent of men, and 2.5 per cent of women, and osteoarthritis in 2.2 per cent of men, and 5 per cent of women. These data suggest that the majority of patients with these symptoms do not have rheumatoid arthritis or obvious degenerative joint disease.[21] British figures provide some direct evidence of the contribution of "non-articular rheumatism" to disability. Rheumatic complaints accounted for 10.9 per cent of absences from work due to incapacity, and 10.5 per cent of days lost. Non-articular rheumatism accounted for nearly one-half of these illnesses, and for one-fourth of the days lost, ranking well ahead of any other form of arthritis, and about equal to back complaints.[30]

Pathogenesis

Three factors seem to interact to produce the syndrome:

1. Local factors
2. Reflex phenomena associated with chronic pain of deep origin
3. Psychogenic factors

The contribution of each factor may vary greatly from patient to patient. This variation and the differing sensitivites of the examining physicians, plus real difficulties in diagnosis, may explain most of the diagnostic variations. It is hypothesized that local factors determine the sites of involvement, and that the extended duration and severity of the disability are due to the interaction of a chronic tension state with the reflex phenomena that accompany deep pain.

Deep Pain

The brain is capable of localizing superficial stimuli with great accuracy, but has no mechanism for precisely identifying the site of origin of pain arising in deep structures. Exact knowledge of the position in space of such structures as the hand are essential to its function, and a mental image of the hand can be summoned at any time. Thus a "body image" of the superficial parts of the body exists,[17] and is based on specialized cerebral cortical representation. However no such image is formed of deeply lying structures. No matter how hard one concentrates, one cannot tell in which direction the appendix is pointing, guess the level in which the pancreas lies, nor detail (without anatomical training) the anatomy of the discs and apophyseal joints. No part of the brain is detailed to keep an exclusive running account of events in these structures, and they do not lie within the "body image." Pain of deep origin *must* be referred; *i.e.* misinterpreted as arising in other areas within the body image. Lewis and Kellgren[14,15,18] showed that pain following stimulation of immediate subcutaneous fascia may be localized with reasonable accuracy. However following stimulation of deeper ligaments, fasciae and muscles, pain localization was grossly inaccurate, with spread of pain sensation to other tissues broadly sharing the same nerve supply, deep enough to share the quality of deep pain, but superficial enough to be included in the body image.

Persistent pain of any origin gives rise to reflex changes, protective in nature. These include muscle spasm, inhibition of voluntary movement, increased blood flow, and cutaneous or deep hyperalgesia. Since neural localization may be wildly inaccurate when pain is of deep origin, these reflex effects may be found in areas far removed from the original site of pathologic change. Not only may the interspinous ligament be tender in patients with a herniated disc, but also the buttock, hamstrings, and calf. The patient with pain referred to the arm will often have a weak grip in the absence of any other evidence of nerve root involvement. Hyperalgesia is probably more important as a cause of deep tenderness than is muscle spasm, as the muscles are often electromyographically silent,[7,13,11] and the tenderness is not restricted to muscle bellies. Much more extreme tension without pain is seen in patients with pyramidal tract disease or parkinsonism. The intensity of referred pain and tenderness is rarely uniform throughout its segment of distribution,[12,28] but tends to be exaggerated at sites that are normally tender, such as the midpoint of the upper trapezius, coracoid process, costochondral junctions, and the crowded muscular attachments to scapula, epicondyles, and pelvis. It is no accident then that "trigger points" are characteristically located at these sites in patients with the fibrositis syndrome.

Deep pain may at first be referred because of simple misinterpretation, but later the referred pain is reinforced and prolonged by reflex hyperalgesic mechanisms, dependent in part on impulses arising from the tissue of reference. If pain reference is due to simple misinterpretation, local anesthesia of the area of reference will give no relief. If reflex deep hyperalgesia is present, local anesthesia will result in abolition or marked diminution of pain. The pain associated with reflex hyperalgesia may be aggravated by many factors, of which cold is the best studied.[16] The effects of local anesthesia and ethyl chloride spray are puzzling and inconstant.[11]

This has been a sketchy review of the phenomena associated with referred pain, staying away from areas of continuing uncertainty and controversy. But, from a consideration of the few points covered, certain corollaries become evident:

1. The localization of pain to a deep structure does *not necessarily* estab-

lish the presence of histopathology in that site.

2. The presence of local tenderness in a deep tissue does *not necessarily* establish the presence of histopathology in that site.
3. The relief of local pain and tenderness following procaine injection does *not necessarily* establish the presence of histopathology in that site, but may be evidence of a state of referred deep hyperalgesia.
4. Stiffness or resistance to stretching of a hyperalgesic muscle is *not necessarily* evidence of local histopathology, either in the muscle or the adjacent joint.
5. Referred deep hyperalgesia *may* persist for a time after the initiating stimulus has subsided, and be aggravated by cold, and probably by other factors, such as tension.
6. The area of pain reference may be altered by previous pain experience. Thus when two or more painful conditions coexist (*e.g.* angina pectoris and cervical disc disease) they may be impossible to distinguish on the basis of the site and quality of the pain.

Sites of Origin of Referred Pain.—The considerations listed above may make identification of the primary site of pathology extremely difficult. Most fibrositic pains are in the wide areas of reference of the lower cervical and lower lumbar spine, and it is perhaps likely, though not easily proved, that a state of reflex hyperalgesia exists in these segments because of mechanical stresses in deeply situated, but pain sensitive, structures associated with the discs and apophyseal joints. Clinically, deep tenderness can usually be demonstrated in the lower cervical interspinous ligaments, and forced lateral flexion or rotation, combined with mild compression of the neck, is commonly painful. In their studies of the distribution of referred pain, Kellgren and Lewis noted that painful stimulation of deeply lying tissue in the trunk gave rise to a wide distribution of pain, often extending well into the limbs; however pain arising in the deep tissue of the extremity tended to be referred only to tissue within the limb. Thus pain in the limb may well come from the spine, but pain in the spine is less likely to be referred from the limb. However, some proximal spread of pain may occur, particularly if spinal degenerative change coexists with a painful peripheral lesion. It is common to have an exacerbation of cervical symptoms in association with an acute supraspinatus tendinitis. (Conversely, subacromial pain when lowering the abducted arm is common in cervical disc disease.) Diagnosis is further confused by the frequent change in character of referred symptoms in the distal portion of the extremity, from aching pains in the proximal portion to a feeling described as numbness, heaviness, or a deadness in the hand or foot. This description suggests impaired neural function, but is common in angina, and has been described in association with radiating pain following the injection of hypertonic saline solution into interspinous ligaments.[18]

The referred pain hypothesis should be summarized at this point. It is suggested that the usual explanation for the diffuse aching, the stiffness and the trigger points of the fibrositic syndrome is to be found in a state of deep reflex hyperalgesia. The difficulties inherent in accurate diagnosis leave the source of the initial painful stimuli often in doubt, but one's attention must be drawn to those sites where pathology steadily accumulates (*i.e.* the spine and major joints) rather than to sites where pathology is rarely found (the muscles and fibrous tissues).

Psychological Aspects.—Four kinds of psychological mechanisms may be important in the pathogenesis of the fibrositis syndrome.[9] The first is a chronic tension state, the significance of which will be discussed further. The second is an exaggeration of suffering, a low tolerance to pain because of a perfectionistic attitude toward the function of the body or because of a fear of underlying serious disease. The third mechanism resembles hysteria but does not necessarily require the presence of other features of severe psychoneurosis. Pain may become identified with and symbolize psychological injury, or the fact of illness itself may be useful to the patient, for example, in helping form stronger bonds within a disintegrating family. The peripheral component of such pain may be trivial, but often pain originating in damaged tissues may be "used" and rendered bizarre and distorted by the emotional illness. The fourth possibility is conscious malingering. This is probably rare, because most patients can successfully conceal from themselves the relations between the persistence of symptoms and the secondary gain.

All these mechanisms are clinically important, but the "simple" chronic tension state must be examined in more detail. Other psychiatric disturbances may be present or absent, but evidence of a chronic tension state will be found in a high proportion of patients with the fibrositis syndrome. The increase in muscle tone which is the key somatic component of this state reinforces the muscle "spasm" occurring as a reflex response to pain, and this interaction may perpetuate a state of reflex deep hyperalgesia, through a pain-spasm-pain cycle. The development of a tension state in response to an acute psychological challenge is recognized to be a normal event, the body reacting with responses appropriate for a physical effort. Thus the concentration of an athlete before a sporting event enhances his motor responses and the anxiety of a student before examination is similarly associated with muscle tension and familiar visceral and vasomotor responses. These are not abnormal responses, and even if the changes are inappropriate to the event, they are so closely allied with the state of heightened concentration that is necessary for optimum performance that they cannot easily be lessened without affecting performance. In the acute tension state, the challenge that requires a special effort is an unusual event, and the relation between symptoms and challenge is readily apparent. However, if the problems of each day require a concentrated effort for solution, then a tension state may become chronic, and the clear relation between the symptom and the challenge may be blurred. The term "chronic tension state" no longer seems appropriate, and is now described as "anxiety." The presence of symptoms of a chronic tension state has often been used as an indication of psychological inadequacy; they may be considered more appropriately as an index of effort. Whether the effort is adequate or unsuccessful is another question, which must be assessed independently.

Sleep Disturbance in Primary Fibrositis

Chronic exhaustion with inability to obtain deep sleep is almost invariably described by patients with the fibrositis syndrome. Electroencephalograms in 4 such patients showed very abnormal electrophysiological sleep patterns with absent stage 4, and very little stage 3 sleep. REM sleep was normal, and there was no evidence of increased EMG activity in tender muscles. The use of diazepam to restore deep sleep decreased morning tenderness as tested by a dolorimeter. Preliminary studies in normal controls indicate that experimental deprivation of stages 3 and 4 sleep can strikingly increase morning dolorimeter scores.[22] The data suggest that deprivation of deep sleep increases sensitivity to pain, apart from the simple coincidence of tenderness and sleeplessness in tense individuals. These observations may be of importance both pathogenetically and therapeutically.

Other Etiologic Considerations: Local Lesions.—Not all investigators are satisfied that "fibrositis" does not exist as a pathological entity, and a very few detailed, carefully controlled studies of the pathology of this condition have been published. Miehlke and co-workers[19,20] compared histological and biochemical findings in the muscle of several groups of patients with muscle pain and stiffness. The "control" groups consisted of anxious, tense patients with diffuse and variable muscle aching, but no "trigger points" or palpable nodules. Biopsy specimen was taken from the upper mid-portion of the trapezius muscle. The other groups consisted of patients with constantly located "trigger points" or tender indurations, and biopsy specimens were taken from the most tender spot. Several differences were observed. The most common change was a mild dusting of fatty droplets through the muscle fibers, detected with fat stains. When a definite induration had been evident clinically, there was often an increase in interstitial connective tissue nuclei. Occasionally clumps of lymphocytes and plasma cells were seen, but never granulocytes. The muscle fibers did not show necrosis or loss of striation, although some variation in size and staining was apparent in the nodular lesions. There was a slight reduction in the enzyme content of the muscles from the focal lesions as compared with the controls. This group also reported the presence of an agglutinating antibody against muscle antigen in some of these patients, but no control experience was reported. It seems possible that the histological differences were due to the varying site of origin of the biopsy specimens. "Indurations" are more likely to be found close to origin or insertions of muscles, *i.e.* at musculofibrous junctions. The "control" material was taken from the mid-portion of the trapezius muscle, and a difference in connective tissue density and organization would be expected. The occasional presence of lymphoid cells was in accord with the control experience of others. A later report from this group was confused by the inclusion of patients with rheumatoid arthritis or other serious disease.[20]

Nodular areas within muscle have been found in many people who do not suffer the symptoms of fibrositis. In 500 soldiers examined by Copeman and Pugh[4] non-tender nodules were found with equal frequency in those with and those without symptoms, but local tenderness was present in only 3 per cent of those who did not give a history of pain and stiffness, and in 30 per cent of those who did.

Another focal lesion which may be responsible for fibrositic symptoms is the fat hernia described by Copeman.[3] These lesions consist of knuckles of fat protruding through defects in deep fascia. However, they do not seem commonly to be a source of pain, and must very rarely be responsible for all the widespread aching of a well-developed fibrositis syndrome.

Trauma and Occupation.—Trauma in the form of a single incident or repeated strain may be a common cause of fibrositis, although adequate statistics regarding this point are not available. The discomfort following major trauma is usually of relatively short duration, but theoretically discomfort may be prolonged by a soft tissue lesion which results in mechanical instability of a pain-sensitive structure, by a tension state, or by consideration of secondary gain. The interrelations of these factors may be very difficult to evaluate, but have considerable medicolegal significance. Fibrositis in specific areas supposedly subject to excess strain has been described associated with certain occupations, such as cervical fibrositis in taxi drivers, and back and gluteal fibrositis in bus drivers. Complaints in these areas have a high incidence in the population in general, and these claims are rarely supported by properly gathered evidence.

Exposure.—Exposure to cold, wet, drafts and sudden changes in weather may precipitate or aggravate symptoms, by mechanisms not fully understood. Kellgren[16] studied the effect of cooling on pain, and noted that "when deep hyperalgesia is present, even slow cooling of the affected part causes severe and prolonged pain, and the analgesia which normally accompanies cooling develops imperfectly unless the tissues are cooled to low temperature (10° C.)." This phenomenon must at least contribute to the weather effect noted by so many patients (*see also* Chapter 15).

Diagnosis

The first decision to be made by the clinician may be one of the most difficult: is the pain arising from joints or is it referred to regions close to joints? Often a preliminary examination of the area under discussion will simplify the task of history-taking. In peripheral joints (elbows, knees, and more distal articulations) the pain and tenderness are usually localized with sufficient accuracy that pain and tenderness restricted to the joint region are readily recognized, but rheumatoid patients may also describe pain between joints and may be seen in a remission, so that in the absence of objective findings a difficult diagnostic problem remains. Pain from more central joints presents greater problems because it is always referred. One cannot feel pain between the femoral head and the acetabulum because one is aware of no such structure, and hip pain is referred to the groin, greater trochanter, or anterior thigh. Thus pain on movement or weight-bearing, and limitation of movement are very important diagnostic points, which can only be assessed confidently if the patient is relaxed and relieved of the worst of his pain. If the pain is restricted to one region and tenderness sharply localized, the problem of diagnosis and treatment

Fibrositis Syndrome: Diagnostic Check

PART ONE: ARE SYMPTOMS CONSISTENT WITH "FIBROSITIS SYNDROME"?

If single site or segment is involved: Recheck history; maintain diagnosis if multiple sites were involved in past six months, otherwise diagnose nature of local disease.

If pain is localized to peripheral joints: Recheck history and findings; *continue* diagnosis if pain spreads beyond confines of joints and objective findings, otherwise diagnose nature of joint disease.

If muscle weakness or numbness is present: Check objective findings. If subjective limitation only, continue diagnosis. Otherwise diagnose neurological or muscular disease.

PART TWO: IS THERE SERIOUS UNDERLYING DISEASE?

Medical (Diagnose on total evidence):
- (*a*) Rheumatic disease group
- (*b*) Bone disease
- (*c*) Neurologic disease; especially parkinsonism
- (*d*) Myopathy
- (*e*) Chronic systemic infections
- (*f*) Endocrinopathy, especially myxedema

Psychiatric: (Suspect because of bizarre features; diagnose by extended history, and, if necessary, psychologic testing.)
- (*a*) Depression
- (*b*) Chronic mild schizophrenia
- (*c*) Psychopathic personality (including malingering)
- (*d*) Hysteria
- (*e*) Other chronic psychoneuroses

PART THREE: HAS THERE BEEN RECENT SOCIAL, OCCUPATIONAL OR EMOTIONAL CHALLENGE? (Answer nearly always: yes.)

If major, acquire details, further appropriate help may be necessary.
If minor, use in explanation of tension factor.

is somewhat simpler. However, further inquiry often reveals a shifting pattern of symptoms over a period of years, so that the present local episode may be merely one event in a more complex series. If the patient presents with widespread aches, stiffness, and tenderness, localized at characteristic sites, and close examination reveals no evidence of associated joint disease, no gross mucle weakness or atrophy, and no neurological findings, then one may temporarily apply the label "fibrositis syndrome."

The next challenge is to recognize associated disease. The pathogenetic role of associated degenerative change in the cervical and lumbar spine is controversial. Mild tenderness on forced movement or deep palpation of the interspinous ligaments is common in any population, but if symptoms and signs are prominent in these areas, appropriate local therapy is indicated. Any of the inflammatory rheumatic diseases may be associated with this syndrome, and the most easily missed will be ankylosing spondylitis. Some of these patients may retain close to normal rib and lumbar movement, but the syndrome can be suspected because of characteristic night pain, marked morning stiffness, or pain around the lower ribs. Radiological examination may support the diagnosis by revealing sacroiliac damage. One must be alert for a history of recent decline in strength, weight or performance, and laboratory findings of anemia and increased sedimentation rate as markers of occult but serious generalized disease.

The clinician must also evaluate the thought processes of his patient with care. A tension state is usually obvious, manifested by a furrowed brow, restless movements, cold wet hands, dripping axillae, sleeplessness, fatigue, headache, or dyspepsia. However, one must often remove the stigma of inadequacy from the tension before it can be freely discussed, and the idea that "tension is an index of effort" is a useful lever. Once the patient is talking freely, inadequacies or bizarre features usually become apparent. Depression is perhaps the most difficult alteration of emotional state to spot, and a history of sleeplessness in the early hours of the morning is of great value. Should psychopathology be identified, the diagnostic problem becomes much more difficult, because it may be extremely difficult to detect serious organic pathology in a patient with inappropriate reactions and bizarre distortions of memory.

PSYCHOGENIC REGIONAL PAIN

Not uncommonly patients with widespread non-articular pain will describe their symptoms in a manner which must be clearly differentiated from the usual fibrositic pattern. The discomfort is no longer described simply as "aching," "stiffness" and "soreness," but acquires dramatic and bizarre qualities, using emotionally loaded metaphors, for example: "The pains burn through my left breast and out my back." The pain is not segmental, but may spread diffusely across multiple anatomical boundaries. The usual aggravation and relief patterns often disappear, and the pain becomes unvarying. In such patients the pain has acquired a symbolic meaning, and the problem of treatment a new dimension. (*See also* Chapter 13.)

The presence of strong central coloring of the symptom complex establishes the presence of a psychological disturbance, but may be associated with a wide variety of personality structures. The symbolic use of pain may be symptomatic of schizophrenia, depression, various psychoneuroses, psychopathic personality, and even of organic psychoses. The name "psychogenic regional pain" has been proposed for this large clinical group,[29] reserving the term "hysteria" for the small number of patients showing all the psychopathologic features of the classical hysteria syndrome. The diagnosis of psychopathology does not by any means rule out the presence of organic disease, but greatly magnifies the difficulties in assessment and therapy.

SECONDARY FIBROSITIS

Discomfort similar to that of primary fibrositis is, of course, common as an accompaniment of a wide variety of other disorders. These range from such well-known but pathologically ill-defined complaints as those following unaccustomed exercise or associated with influenza, to diseases like rheumatoid arthritis in which histologic lesions can be demonstrated in muscles and connective tissues. The diagnosis in these instances is made clear by recognition of the primary disorder. The pain of polymyalgia rheumatica can easily be mistaken for fibrositis when the patient is first seen, but the special features, and particularly the rapid erythrocyte sedimentation rate, should soon point to the correct diagnosis (*see also* Chapter 50).

TREATMENT OF FIBROSITIS

The patient with the fibrositis syndrome comes to the doctor feeling threatened, by his illness and by his associated problems. He is therefore on the defensive, and will react negatively to any message he interprets as a further threat. The task of explanation may challenge all the physician's skill, training and imagination. It is relatively easy to prescribe an analgesic regimen, but it can be extremely difficult to give the patient an adequate account of the origins of his symptoms, and in particular to deal with the relationship between pain and tension. Patients expect doctors to use euphemisms, and will examine words carefully for unfavorable underlying meanings. Thus the suggestion that symptoms are of emotional origin, or the use of the word anxiety, may be translated by the patient into an accusation of inadequacy or willful malingering. The physician is further handicapped by the complexities of the explanation he must give. The account can be confusing or unconvincing. The physician must therefore assess the needs and understanding of the patient with great care. The intelligent, curious and imaginative patient may need a thorough, general discussion of the nature of referred pain and the origin of tension before his own problems and program are discussed. A simple and extroverted patient may need

Management of Fibrositis

1. *Reassure:* No crippling or serious disease.
2. *Explain Origin of Pain,* in greater or lesser detail depending on needs of patient.
   (*a*) Referred pain as a necessary mistake in localization ("No matter how hard you concentrate, you cannot feel your 6th cervical vertebra").
   (*b*) Reflex muscle spasm and muscle tension as source of pain.
   (*c*) Pain-spasm-pain cycle extending symptoms after initiating stresses eased.
   (*d*) Tension as part of normal response to challenge, inevitable with concentration, an index of effort.
3. *Analgesic and Antispasmodic Therapy.*
   (*a*) Salicylates or other analgesics to break pain-spasm-pain cycle.
   (*b*) Heat, massage, exercise to relieve spasm.
   (*c*) Treatment of painful primary foci, *e.g.* cervical traction.
   (*d*) Sedatives, relaxants, injections, surgery and placebos.
4. *Reorientation of Life Pattern.*
   (*a*) Challenges accepted give life meaning; accept within limitations recognizing necessary cost in effort and tension.
   (*b*) Break tension with rest, diversion, exercise and escape.

reassurance and a positive program (of almost any kind), and would be badly served by a dreary academic discussion. The patient who is terribly threatened and no longer able to cope may need hospitalization and a period of sympathetic protection before recovering sufficient strength of will to reconstruct his habits and attitudes. Attention should be paid to specific areas of local pain. Pain about the neck and shoulders may subside after a period of cervical traction or the use of a collar, and pain referred from the lower back may respond to a period of bed rest. Injection of procaine into persistently tender points may abolish the local symptom, as may chilling of the overlying skin with ethyl chloride.

These maneuvers help solve a short-term problem. However, the ultimate goal of therapy must be to establish a way of life which permits meaningful, useful activity despite some cost in tension. A varied diet of rest, diversion, exercise and escape can enable the patient to "get out from under" when the pressures are too great, and the remaining symptoms can be accepted as fatigue that is the reward of dedicated effort.

BIBLIOGRAPHY

1. Adler, E. and Abramson, J. H.: Israel J. of Med. Sci., *4*, 210, 1968.
2. Cobb, S., Warren, J. E., Merchant, W. K., and Thompson, D. J.: J. Chron. Dis., *5*, 636, 1957.
3. Copeman, W. S. C. and Ackerman, W. L.: Quart. J. Med., *13*, 37, 1944.
4. Copeman, W. S. C. and Pugh, L. G. C.: Lancet, 2, 553, 1945.
5. Cruickshank, B.: J. Path. & Bact., *54*, 21, 1952.
6. Davison, S., Spiera, H. and Plotz, C. M.: Arth. & Rheum., *9*, 18, 1966.
7. Elliot, F. A.: Lancet, *1*, 47, 1944.
8. Gowers, W. R.: Brit. Med. J., *1*, 117, 1904.
9. Halliday, J. L.: Proc. Roy. Soc. Med., *31*, 167, 1938.
10. Hench, P. S.: Ann. Intern. Med., *10*, 880, 1936.
11. Hockady, J. M. and Whitty, C. W. M.: Brain, *90*, 19, 1967.
12. Inman, V. T., and Saunders, J. B. de C. M.: J. Nerv. Ment. Dis., *99*, 660, 1944.
13. Kraft, G. H., Johnson, E. W., and LaBan, M. M.: Arch. Phys. Med. & Rehab., *49*, 155, 1968.
14. Kellgren, J. H.: Clin. Sci., *3*, 174, 1938.
15. Kellgren, J. H.: Clin. Sci., *4*, 35, 1939.
16. Kellgren, J. H., McGowan, A. M., and Hughes, E. S. R.: Clin. Sci., *7*, 13, 1948.
17. Kellgren, J. H.: Lancet, *1*, 943, 1949.
18. Lewis, T. and Kellgren, J. H.: Clin. Sci., *4*, 47, 1939.
19. Miehlke, K., Schulze, G. and Eger, W.: Ztschr. f. Rheumaforsch., *49*, 310, 1960.
20. Miehlke, K.: Bull. Rheum. Dis., *12*, 276, 1962.
21. Mikkelsen, W. M., Dodge, H. J., Duff, I. F., and Kato, H.: J. Chron. Dis., *20*, 351, 1967.
22. Moldofsky, H., Smythe, H. A., and Sauks, J.: Unpublished data.
23. O'Brien, W. M., Clemett, A. P., and Acheson, R. M.: Excerpta Medica Found., 398, 1968.
24. P. H. S. Publication No. 1000, Series 11, Number 17, U.S. Government Printing Office, Washington, D. C., 1966.
25. Sokoloff, L., Wilens, S. L., Bunim, J. J., and McEwen, C.: Amer. J. Med. Sci., *214*, 33, 1950.
26. Stockman, R.: *Rheumatism and Arthritis*, Edinburgh, E. & S. Livingstone, 1920.
27. Stockman, R.: Ann. Rheum. Dis., *2*, 77, 1940.
28. Travell, J., and Bigelow, N. H.: Fed. Proc., *5*, 106, 1946.
29. Walters, A.: Brain, *84*, 1, 1961.
30. Wood, P. H. N.: Brit. Med. Bull., *27*, 82, 1971.

Chapter 50

Polymyalgia Rheumatica

By Louis A. Healey, M.D.

Despite its name which suggests a wastebasket for musculoskeletal aches, polymyalgia rheumatica can be defined as a specific clinical entity. It is a syndrome of older patients, characterized by pain and stiffness of proximal muscles, persisting for at least a month, without weakness or atrophy, accompanied by a rapid sedimentation rate and dramatically relieved by steroid treatment.[7,14]

History

In 1957, Barber[2] introduced the term "polymyalgia rheumatica" for a group of patients with muscular pain and elevated sedimentation rate who did not have arthritis. This same illness had previously been reported under various names, including senile arthritis, myalgic syndrome of the aged, anarthritic rheumatoid disease, periarthrosis humeroscapularis, and pseudopolyarthrite rhizomelique dating back to 1888 when Bruce, in Scotland, described five elderly patients with muscular pain which he called senile rheumatic gout. The very rapid erythrocyte sedimentation rate suggested this might be a specific clinical entity, and, in 1956, Paulley pointed out its similarity to the prodromal symptoms of temporal arteritis.[13] This was confirmed by Alestig and Barr in 1963, when they found giant cell arteritis on biopsy of asymptomatic temporal arteries in patients with polymyalgia rheumatica.[1] Despite frequent reports from England, France, and Scandinavia, this syndrome received little attention in the United States. First report of a single case appeared in 1963[10] and the first series of patients were reported in 1966[4] and 1967.[15] This is the first edition of this book to include polymyalgia rheumatica as a separate chapter, attesting to recent recognition of its importance.

Clinical Picture

Although its exact incidence is unknown, polymyalgia rheumatica is not rare. It has been estimated to be as frequent as gout and it is the experience of several rheumatologists that an average of one new patient with the disease is seen each month. All patients have been

Table 50-1.—Definition of Polymyalgia Rheumatica

1. Pain in proximal muscles, not joints, persistent for a month or longer. Morning stiffness is marked; no muscle atrophy or weakness.
2. Patients at least 55 years of age; usually older.
3. Erythrocyte sedimentation rate greater than 50 mm. in one hour; often 100 mm. or more.
4. Relief of symptoms within four days by as little as 10 mg. of prednisone daily.

Exclusions: Intrinsic muscle disease
Rheumatoid arthritis
Multiple myeloma or other neoplasm
Systemic lupus erythematosus

older than 50 years of age and most older than 65. It is seen more often in women than men and seems to be more common in Caucasians. Patients complain of severe pain in neck, back, shoulders, upper arms and thighs. Often the onset may be abrupt; patients go to bed feeling well and awaken as uncomfortable as if they had chopped a cord of wood. Weakness is not prominent but pain on motion makes rising from a chair or climbing stairs difficult. Morning stiffness is marked and some patients need help from their spouse to get out of bed. Chewing may produce pain in the jaw. Nonspecific symptoms include fever, anorexia, weight loss, lassitude, apathy and depression. Weight loss may be extreme. Some patients' symptoms are confined to the region of the pectoral *or* the pelvic girdle; most, however, have both girdles involved. Joint tenderness does occur and effusions of the knees have been seen.

In view of the severity of complaints it is surprising that physical examination is entirely normal. Specifically, patients show no rash, nodules, arteritis, synovitis, muscle weakness or atrophy. X-rays are equally unrevealing. Confirmation of the diagnosis is found in one laboratory test, the erythrocyte sedimentation rate. This is always elevated, often greatly so and may exceed 100 mm./hr. (Westergren method). Hematocrit is often decreased and may be as low as 29 per cent. This anemia is due to a block in utilization of iron.

Fibrinogen levels are high and protein electrophoresis is normal except for an elevation of alpha II globulin fraction. Both of these correlate with the rapid sedimentation rate as indicators of inflammation. Rheumatoid factor and antinuclear antibodies are not present. Muscle enzyme levels in serum and electromyograms are normal, reflecting normal muscle tissue found at biopsy.

Differential Diagnosis

Since the constellation of findings in polymyalgia is not specific, it must be differentiated from a number of other conditions. The pain and stiffness persist for at least a month in contrast to the myalgia of "flu syndrome" and other viral illnesses. Apathy, depression and lack of physical findings suggest that complaints might represent a depressive reaction in elderly patients, but the rapid sedimentation rate indicates something more. The sedimentation rate also indicates it is not osteoarthritis. Polymyalgia rheumatica is most often confused with rheumatoid athritis, particularly soon after onset when it may be difficult to tell the two apart. Distinction relies on physical examination which demonstrates synovitis in wrists, hands and knees; weak grip and limited wrist motions are usually present in the patient with early rheumatoid arthritis. Rheumatoid factor, if present, is also helpful.

Table 50-2.—Conditions to Be Distinguished from Polymyalgia Rheumatica

1. Viral myalgia. Duration is less than a month.
2. Rheumatoid arthritis. Examination detects synovitis of joint; rheumatoid factor is often present.
3. Polymyositis. Muscle enzyme levels are elevated in serum; muscle biopsy and electromyogram are abnormal.
4. Multiple myeloma. Gamma globulin spike on protein electrophoresis; plasma cells in bone marrow.
5. Osteoarthritis. Erythrocyte sedimentation rate is usually normal.
6. Fibrositis. Normal sedimentation rate.
7. Depression and psychogenic symptoms. Normal sedimentation rate.
8. Occult infection. Appropriate x-rays and cultures needed.
9. Occult malignancy. Appropriate x-rays are needed. May require brief trial of steroid therapy.

Muscle pain and stiffness of polymyalgia may seem like the weakness of polymyositis. The two are separated by elevated muscle enzyme levels and abnormal electromyogram and muscle biopsy, diagnostic of polymyositis. The very high sedimentation rate itself raises the possibility of multiple myeloma, infection or malignancy which are excluded by appropriate investigations. A brief trial of steroid treatment may save an elderly patient from an expensive and uncomfortable search for occult malignancy.

Treatment

The cliché "dramatic response" truly describes the effect of steroids on the symptoms of polymyalgia. This response is so invariable that if it is not seen within a week, the diagnosis should be questioned. Some[15] prefer to start treatment with 40 mg. of prednisone a day, decreasing the dose 5 mg. a week while others[14] prefer to begin with only 10 mg. a day. Although once thought to be a brief self-limited condition, it is now recognized that most patients will require treatment for at least two years or more. Despite the risks of steroids in older patients, the maintenance dose which averages 7.5 mg. a day is safe and well tolerated. This must be continued until it is apparent that symptoms and rapid sedimentation rate do not return upon its discontinuance. Aspirin and other anti-inflammatory drugs have not proved to constitute effective treatment.

Etiology

The cause of polymyalgia rheumatica is not known. No infectious agent or toxin has been found. Despite the pain, muscles appear normal on histologic examination. Tests such as rheumatoid factor, antinuclear antibodies and increased immunoglobulins, often associated with "autoimmune diseases," are lacking. Several attempts to demonstrate a serum antibody to a constituent of muscle or artery have been unsuccessful. Patients with polymyalgia have been followed for at least five years and have not developed other neoplastic or rheumatic disease which might account for the syndrome. Of great interest has been the possible relationship between polymyalgia rheumatica and giant cell arteritis.

GIANT CELL ARTERITIS

In 1932, Horton[9] described temporal arteritis in two elderly patients who had severe headache and high sedimentation rates. As he predicted, "this is a focal localization of an unknown systemic disease." It is now well recognized that giant cell arteritis may involve medium and large-sized arteries throughout the body, of which the temporal artery is only the most superficial and accessible. The recognized complication of blindness, for example, is due to occlusion of the ophthalmic artery. Autopsy studies have shown that the aorta and most of the larger arteries may be involved, but, in contrast to polyarteritis (periarteritis nodosa), smaller arterioles are spared. Missen's dissections show that the vertebral, internal carotid and coronary arteries may become occluded, resulting in fatal cerebral or myocardial infarction.[11] Pulmonary and renal arterioles are spared and these organs do not show clinical

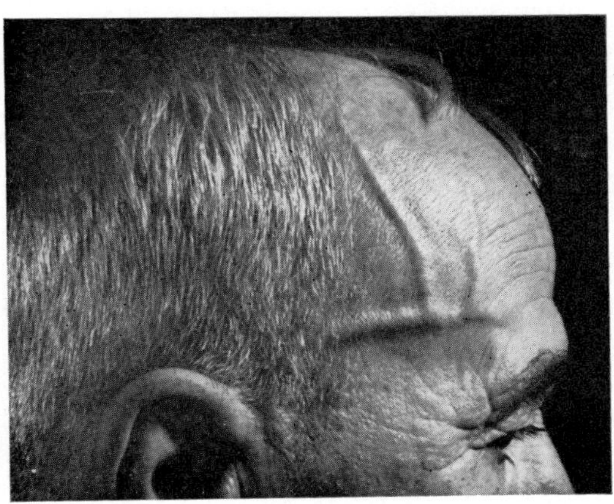

Fig. 50–1.—Temporal arteritis. The swollen temporal artery is tender, painful and pulsates.

involvement. Giant cell arteritis has produced such diverse symptoms as jaw pain, tongue pain, intermittent claudication, peripheral nerve dysfunction, and various manifestations of cerebrovascular insufficiency.[7] Anemia, due to inability to utilize iron and responsive to steroid treatment, has been described as a primary manifestation of giant cell arteritis.[8]

Table 50-3.—Manifestations of Giant Cell Arteritis

Common	Polymyalgia rheumatica Headache Blindness Anemia Fever
Less common	Claudication Jaw pain, tongue pain Cerebral, such as aphasia, vertigo, depression, psychosis, stupor, coma, "stroke" Peripheral neuropathy, such as diplopia, parasthesias, brachial paralysis
Rare	Myocardial infarction Scalp necrosis Tongue gangrene

Pathology

The earliest change is a ribbon-like, patchy infiltrate composed of fibrinoid necrosis, necrotic smooth muscle cells, lymphocytes and small mononuclear cells located on either side of the internal elastic lamina. Later, intimal thickening, fibroblasts, small round cells, epithelioid cells and foreign body giant cells are found (Fig. 50–2). The elastic lamina shows patches of destruction. In the late stage, the lumen may be fibrotic and obliterated. Electron microscopy has

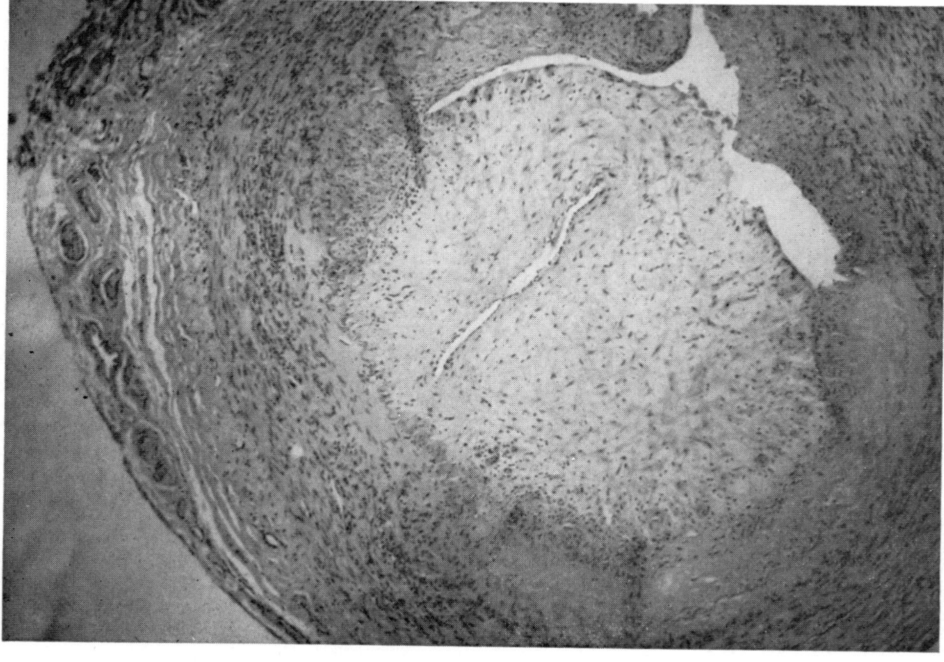

Fig. 50–2.—Giant cell arteritis. Cross section of temporal artery showing inflammatory infiltrate, giant cells, fragmentation of elastic lamina and intimal thickening; the lumen is almost occluded by thrombus.

shown that most of the cells involved are histiocytes or macrophages but has thus far not shed any further light on the cause. It is important to note that these pathological changes are random and focal and interspersed with areas of normal artery.[7]

Relationship to Polymyalgia Rheumatica

Polymyalgia is often a manifestation of giant cell arteritis. There are documented examples of both conditions occurring in the same patient, either concurrently or at different times.[6,12,15] As previously mentioned, Alestig and Barr[1] showed that arteritis may be found in an asymptomatic temporal artery of a patient with giant cell arteritis. This finding has been confirmed by others.[6,12,15] Bevan[3] found that the histologic appearance was the same, whether the temporal artery was symptomatic or not. Some feel that polymyalgia is always a manifestation of giant cell arteritis and ascribe a normal biopsy specimen to chance sampling of an uninvolved section of artery in which inflammation is distributed in patches.[6,12,15] Others, however, prefer to regard the cause of this syndrome as unknown in those patients who lack a positive biopsy specimen.[7,14] Patients with polymyalgia have been reported who later suffered a loss of vision.[5] Unfortunately, the small maintenance dose of prednisone is *not* reliable protection against blindness. At present, all patients with polymyalgia rheumatica have to be considered at some risk, however small, of developing this complication. The most prudent course is to instruct patients to increase the steroid dose and contact the physician if persistent temporal headache appears.

At present, polymyalgia rheumatica is a descriptive syndrome. It is in the early phase of definition and more will be learned as time goes on. Criteria for diagnosis given here, leaning heavily on exclusions, serve to describe a specific group of patients. These criteria will certainly be altered in light of future investigation and experience.

Acknowledgment.—The assistance of Kenneth R. Wilske, M. D., in the preparation of this chapter is gratefully acknowledged.

BIBLIOGRAPHY

1. Alestig, K. and Barr, J.: Lancet, *1*, 1228, 1963.
2. Barber, H. S.: Ann. Rheum. Dis., *16*, 230, 1957.
3. Bevan, A. T., Dunnill, M. S. and Harrison, M. J. G.: Ann. Rheum. Dis., *27*, 271, 1968.
4. Davison, S., Spiera, H. and Plotz, C. M.: Arth. & Rheum., *9*, 18, 1966.
5. Fessel, W. J. and Pearson, C. M.: New Engl. J. Med., *276*, 1403, 1967.
6. Hamrin, B., Jonsson, N. and Landberg, T.: Lancet, *1*, 397, 1964.
7. Healey, L. A., Parker, F. and Wilske, K. R.: Arth. & Rheum., *14*, 138, 1971.
8. Healey, L. A., and Wilske, K. R.: Arth. & Rheum., *14*, 27, 1971.
9. Horton, B. T., Magath, T. B. and Brown, G. E.: Proc. Mayo Clin., *7*, 700, 1932.
10. Levey, G. S., Carey, J. P. and Calabro, J. J.: Arth. & Rheum., *6*, 75, 1963.
11. Missen, G. A. K.: Brit. Med. J., *1*, 419, 1966.
12. Olhagen, B.: Acta Rheum. Scand., *9*, 157, 1963.
13. Paulley, J. W.: Lancet, *2*, 946, 1956.
14. Plotz, C. M. and Spiera, H.: Bull. Rheum. Dis., *20*, 578, 1969.
15. Wilske, K. R. and Healey, L. A.: Ann. Intern. Med., *66*, 77, 1967.

PART VII

The Diffuse Connective Tissue Diseases

Section Editor: LAWRENCE E. SHULMAN, M.D.

Chapter 51

Systemic Lupus Erythematosus

By Lawrence E. Shulman, M.D., and A. McGehee Harvey, M.D.

Systemic lupus erythematosus (SLE), formerly called "disseminated lupus erythematosus," is a connective tissue disorder with varied clinical manifestations. Although the disease may be fulminating, it usually runs a chronic undulating course characterized by variable periods of activity interspersed with remissions. One or more of a multitude of serum protein abnormalities may develop, among them being the factor (or factors) responsible for the formation of the L.E. cell (*see also* Chapter 10). Among the characteristic pathologic lesions seen in this syndrome are: fibrinoid degeneration in the connective tissue; the altered nuclear material represented by "hematoxylin bodies," verrucous endocarditis and focal glomerulonephritis. There may be, however, a striking disparity between the extent and severity of the clinical manifestations and the morphological findings. The relationship between SLE and rheumatoid arthritis (RA) is interesting and unsettled.

Attention was first called to the systemic form of the disease by Kaposi[86] in 1872. Prior to that time, lupus erythematosus had been considered to be a chronic, but relatively harmless, disorder of the skin. Osler,[118] in 1895, in his description of the erythema group of diseases, outlined virtually all of the varied clinical manifestations that may be seen in SLE, and it seems reasonable to assume that among his patients were some with this disease. He pointed out that skin lesions were not invariably present. His excellent clinical description is as follows: "by exudative erythema is understood a disease of unknown etiology with polymorphic skin lesions—hyperemia, edema, and hemorrhage—arthritis occasionally, and a variable number of visceral manifestations, of which the most important are gastro-intestinal crises, endocarditis, pericarditis, acute nephritis and hemorrhage from the mucosal surfaces. Recurrence is a special feature of this disease and attacks may come on month after month or even throughout a long period of years. Variability in the skin lesions is the rule . . . The attacks may not be characterized by skin manifestations; the visceral symptoms may be present, and to the outward view the patient may have no indications whatever of erythema exudativum . . . Five of the cases had swelling about and pain in the joints . . ."

Specific pathologic lesions were not recognized until 1924 when Libman and Sacks[103] described the verrucous endocardial changes. In 1932 Gross[64] discovered the presence of "hematoxylin bodies" in the cardiac lesions, and these bodies have since been found in other organs as well. The first collection of cases for clinical and pathological review was made in 1935 by Baehr, Klemperer and Schifrin[9] who noted that all but one of their 23 cases were in females. The impression was subsequently gained that this was an acute, highly lethal disorder. The discovery of the lupus erythematosus (L.E.) cell by Hargraves, Richmond and Morton[69] in 1948 was shortly followed by the demonstration that adrenocortical steroid therapy could alleviate promptly, and at times dramatically, the active manifestations of the disease. As a result of these important advances, interest in SLE increased and many more cases were recognized. Since that time several comprehensive reviews of this syndrome have appeared. Such clinical studies have led to an appreciation that SLE is characteristically a chronic disease punctuated by episodes of acute illness and not uniformly fatal as originally thought. Simultaneously, investigations by Holman,[78] Kunkel[94] and many others into the nature of the L.E. cell and the hematoxylin bodies in the tissues using immunological and histochemical techniques have produced evidence that these are the result of alterations in the immune mechanism with the formation of multiple antinuclear antibodies. Moreover, patients with SLE possess a striking ability to produce a multitude of various autoantibodies. Many of these participate in tissue injury in SLE. It has now been shown conclusively that circulating immune complexes of DNA and anti-native DNA antibodies are responsible for the renal lesions in most patients with SLE. The mechanisms by which these patients manufacture large amounts of autoantibody, and the factors responsible for antigen release remain to be elucidated. There is interesting recent evidence in support of genetic and viral influences (*see also* Chapter 10).

INCIDENCE

SLE is predominantly a disease of women in the childbearing age group (Fig. 51–1). In the several large series reported, 70 to 91 per cent of cases were in females. It begins usually in the third or fourth decade, but may start as early as two years of age, or as late as ninety-seven years. Female predominance is also a feature of SLE in children and the elderly. No geographical predisposition or immunity has been noted except in African populations where SLE seems rare. Clearly, its incidence is higher than estimated previously. Since the advent of the L.E. cell test, it is not uncommon for a general hospital to admit 10 to 30 new patients annually. There is, however, no convincing evidence that the disease is increasing. An epidemiological study of SLE in New York City revealed no increase in incidence from

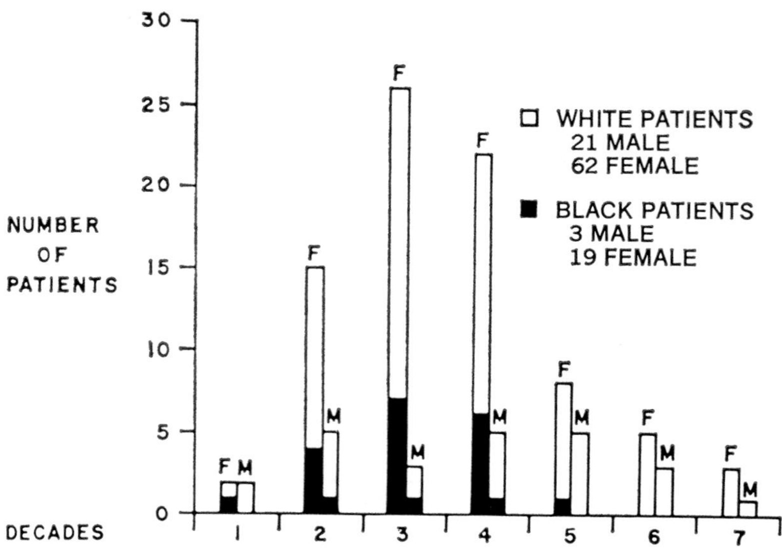

Fig. 51–1.—Age at onset and incidence by sex and race in 105 cases of systemic lupus erythematosus. (Shulman and Harvey, courtesy of Disease-A-Month.[140])

1951 through 1959. Of interest is that there were higher frequencies in non-white, than in white, populations.[143]

ETIOLOGY

A variety of precipitating factors may be associated with the onset of the disease or its exacerbations. Exposure to sunlight or ultraviolet rays not only may produce a violent cutaneous reaction, but may be followed by the development of acute SLE. Patients may relate the onset of the disease to a local infection, such as a sore throat or a pneumonia. There may be a story of a reaction to one or more drugs, or to the administration of a foreign protein such as tetanus antitoxin. The administration of gold, sulfonamides, penicillin or other antibiotics may precede the onset or an exacerbation of the process. Many patients state that they have been under emotional tension for a period before the first symptoms appeared. There is no clear evidence that any of these factors plays a primary role in pathogenesis. However, there is good evidence that many of them may exacerbate or precipitate a fulminating phase with fatal outcome.[7]

The concept that SLE is an immunopathic, perhaps autoimmune, disorder[78] is based upon the multitude of protein abnormalities described, and, in particular, the antinuclear factors, of which the L.E. cell-promoting factor is one (*see* Chapter 10 for a comprehensive discussion of L.E. and antinuclear factors). Suggestive also that an autoimmune mechanism may be operative are: (1) the drug-induced form of SLE (p. 909); (2) "lupoid hepatitis" (p. 908); (3) the demonstration of complement-fixing reactions between normal tissue antigens and immunoglobulin autoantibodies from patients with SLE; and (4) the demonstration that both gamma globulin and serum complement become fixed to the renal[52] and other lesions of SLE. There is considerable variability in the development of the different protein factors among the cases. A close correlation has been reported between the level of serum complement and the state of clinical activity of the disease.[163] The L.E. cell factor is an IgG immunoglobulin which crosses the placental membrane and may be demonstrated in the infants of mothers with SLE. These infants, however, are not ill, and do not display any of the clinical manifestations of the disease. Additional evidence of autoimmunity in SLE is the delayed cutaneous reaction after the intradermal injection of autologous leukocytes,[53] the specificity of which, however, has been questioned.

Genetic influences are suggested in different ways. There are numerous reports of the occurrence of SLE in two or more family members, including identical twins[19,71] and in more than one generation;[71] also in families with hypergammaglobulinemia[99] or agammaglobulinemia.[57] The results of controlled family studies, however, are conflicting: some reported higher frequencies of connective tissue diseases and/or serologic abnormalities among relatives than controls;[99,143] another did not.[6] There is a recent report of identical twins discordant for SLE.[24] Some have proposed that SLE is an autoimmune disease regulated by inheritance factors and somatic mutation. Such would seem to be the situation in the experimental model of SLE in New Zealand mice (*vide infra*).

Recently several investigators have described myxovirus-like inclusions in capillary endothelial cells of kidney, skin and muscle of patients with SLE.[65,116] The inclusions are not specific for SLE. To date, viruses have not been culturable from such lesions. Immunologic studies have failed to demonstrate specific myxovirus antigens in active SLE lesions or serum antibodies to endothelial inclusions. However, patients with SLE have been shown to have significantly elevated antibody titers to several viruses (measles, parainfluenza, EB virus). One group has correlated the antibody titers with serum globulin levels, and suggested that the viral antibodies are, too, non-specific, being the consequence of generalized immunologic hyperreactivity.[123]

The reason for the high incidence of SLE in young adult and middle-aged women is not clear. Exacerbations of SLE have been reported to occur frequently during the first trimester of pregnancy and shortly after delivery.

A potentially highly significant advance in our understanding of SLE is that certain inbred strains of New Zealand mice have been reported with both an autoimmune hemolytic anemia and a disorder which closely simulates SLE having both glomerular lesions and L.E. cells.[74] Viruses may play an important role in this experimental model.[110] Antinuclear factors have also been shown to occur spontaneously in certain other inbred strains of mice developed in the United States.[53] There is evidence to suggest that environmental factors may play a role in their pathogenesis.[139] Dogs with a disease resembling SLE and with L.E. cells have also been reported.[102]

PATHOLOGY

It should be emphasized, before describing the pathology of SLE, that even in the patient dying in the acute fulminating stage, only a few histological lesions may be found at postmortem examinations, even after the most meticulous search. This is, however, not the rule.

The changes in the connective tissue include a variety of lesions, some nonspecific and others which are relatively characteristic. The fibrinoid change which may be widely distributed in the connective tissue ground substances has been described in a variety of other disease states. It may be found in the walls of blood vessels as well as in the connective tissue elsewhere and is often accompanied by a cellular infiltration. According to Klemperer,[91] fibrinoid in SLE contains deoxyribonucleic acid (DNA) and thereby differs from the fibrinoid found in other conditions. He believed that it represents a substance deposited in normal connective tissue ground substance while other investigators, such as Altschuler and Angevine,[4] conceived of it as a local alteration of the acid mucopolysaccharides of the ground substance.

Among the more specific and characteristic pathologic changes in SLE are: (1) the verrucous endocarditis of Libman and Sacks; (2) segmental thickening of the basement membrane of the glomerular tuft of the kidney ("wire-loop" lesion); (3) periarterial concentric fibrosis of the spleen ("onion-skin" lesion); and (4) "hematoxylin bodies." Of these, only "hematoxylin bodies" are pathognomonic for SLE. Although first described in the heart, "hematoxylin bodies" are found in other areas including kidney, lung, lymph nodes, spleen, serous and synovial membranes. Klemperer *et al.*[92] recognized these bodies in 41 of 45 cases they studied. In hematoxylin-eosin preparations they are homogeneous purple globules, the size of cell nuclei, and may form large aggregates. The prevailing basic similarity between the hematoxylin body and the inclusion body of the L.E. cell, and the identity of the two substances has been established conclusively by the histochemical studies of Godman and his associates.[59] They showed that in the transformation from normal nucleoprotein to hematoxylin or L.E. cell bodies, there was no loss of DNA and thus DNA was not depolymerized, as previous experiments had seemed to indicate. They found the protein content of the L.E. body to be greater than that of normal nuclei; and since less histone (the basic protein which combines with DNA to form nucleoprotein) than normal could be detected, they concluded that histone was displaced from, and a new protein added to, nucleoprotein. Other observations have demonstrated that this added protein is gamma globulin, probably closely related to or identical with that responsible for L.E. cell formation.

Although biopsy specimens of skin, muscles and lymph nodes are obtained frequently for diagnostic purposes and alterations compatible with SLE may be found, it is unusual for specimens to reveal pathognomonic changes. In a study of the histopathology of 119 skin samples McCreight and Montgomery[104] concluded that they could not differentiate the chronic discoid type from the systemic variety, and found no single specific pathological lesion. However, a combination of hyperkeratosis, keratotic plugging of hair follicles, degeneration of the basal cell layer, edema of the cutis, dilatation of superficial capillaries, a cellular infiltrate mainly lymphocytic, and a lack of obliterative or proliferative change in the deeper blood vessels would suggest this diagnosis. Palmar lesion specimens stained for alkaline phosphatase activity have revealed interesting, consistent capillary abnormalities.[145] Immunofluorescent examination of skin biopsy samples has demonstrated the presence of immunoglobulins and complement in the epidermal-dermal junction[161] in 90 per cent of SLE lesions and in 60 per cent of skin uninvolved in SLE.[165] These observations emphasize the generalized nature of SLE. The procedure may be useful in diagnosis. In discoid lupus, immunoglobulins are demonstrable in 58 per cent of involved areas, but not in uninvolved sites.[165]

According to Cruickshank,[35] the lymph nodes in SLE at biopsy show primarily disease in the sinuses with necrosis and cellular proliferation, the follicles being spared. This picture contrasts sharply with the follicular hyperplasia seen in rheumatoid arthritis. Nevertheless, these changes in the nodes of SLE are entirely nonspecific, similar ones being encountered in other diseases of varying etiology. At times, they are so striking that on the basis of the biopsy the patient with SLE is thought to have a primary lymphatic disease. Virtually all investigators are agreed that muscle biopsies are of little or no diagnostic value, except in the rare patient with an associated polymyositis.

Renal biopsy may be helpful not only for diagnosis, but also in following the course of the renal involvement. The abnormalities seen may range from a focal glomerulitis to a diffuse glomerulonephritis.[115] Electron microscopy of the renal lesions has revealed electron-dense deposits which consist of immunoglobulins, complement and fibrin-related components;[33] their location is either subepithelial or subendothelial. They are not specific for SLE.

Cruickshank[36] has described the histopathology of the joint and tendon sheath lesions in 10 autopsied cases of SLE. In synovial tissue the most striking change was the presence of a thick layer of eosinophilic, fibrin-like material on or under the surface merging with the adjacent synovium and often containing pyknotic nuclei. The synovial cells were often diminished in number so that this material lay directly on the subsynovial tissue. Hematoxylin bodies were found with regularity among the synovial cells. Inflammatory change was not prominent and vascular lesions were seldom seen. Damage to articular cartilage was noted in 5 of 6 finger joints, and in 3 there was marginal erosion with granulation tissue where the cartilage had disappeared. Fibrin-like material was found on or beneath the surface of 6 tendon sheaths examined and the inflammatory reaction was more marked than in the joints. The exudate usually contained lymphocytes and plasma cells.

The author states that these pathological features, while nonspecific, when present in combination are diagnostic of SLE. It is of interest that the destruction of cartilage is usually at the articular margins which probably accounts for the infrequent occurrence of gross joint disorganization.

Occasionally, however, the loss of articular cartilage is extensive and the clinical joint disease is then indistinguishable from classical rheumatoid arthritis. Moreover, subsequent studies by needle biopsy have shown more synovial lining cell proliferation, inflammation and vascular lesions.[96] Hematoxylin bodies were infrequent. The synovial histopathology was, therefore, considered to be nonspecific, resembling closely that of rheumatoid arthritis. Endothelial cytoplasmic tubular (virus-like) inclusions were seen by electron microscopy in the synovial venules of two of four patients with SLE.

Hyperplasia of thymic epithelial cells in SLE has been described.[81] The changes differ from that of infection, but resemble those found in other autoimmune diseases.

CLINICAL FEATURES

The clinical picture of SLE at onset is highly variable. In some cases only a single organ system may be involved, suggesting that the patient has a localized, rather than a generalized, process; in others, several systems may be implicated. Most frequently affected singly are the joints and the skin, but the disease may begin as a disorder of any of the organ systems.[7] Table 51–1 lists the initial manifestations of SLE in order of frequency. One sees that, in addition to involvement of particular organ systems, in many instances constitutional symptoms and signs—fever, fatigability, generalized weakness and weight loss—provide the first evidence of illness. Moreover, even when specific organs are involved at the start, the history may be so ill-defined that it is difficult to determine when the disease has actually begun. For example, the patient may report that she "has always been sensitive to the sun," or "my joints have ached off and on for years."

Table 51-1.—Initial Manifestations in Systemic Lupus Erythematosus in Order of Frequency

1. Acute polyarthritis	9. Nephritis
2. Fever	10. Pneumonitis
3. Erythematous eruption	11. Raynaud's phenomenon
4. Fatigability, malaise, weakness	12. Generalized lymph node enlargement
5. Arthralgias	13. Bruising, bleeding
6. Weight loss, anorexia	14. Paresthesias
7. Pleurisy	15. Pericarditis
8. False positive serologic test for syphilis	16. Diplopia or ptosis

There is also no characteristic pattern of the disease as it unfolds. Often it appears to be a puzzling combination of clinical events involving many systems and having little continuity. The recurrent cutaneous and articular episodes are helpful in indicating the correct diagnosis.

The *joints* are involved in approximately 90 per cent of patients at some time during the course of the disease.[7,71] Arthritis with or without other manifestations is present during the first episode of illness in two-thirds of the cases. Most characteristic is the development of polyarthralgia with little or no evidence of inflammation. The pain is typically more intense than one might expect from the objective changes. Symmetrical polyarthritis, resembling that of rheumatic fever or of early rheumatoid arthritis, is frequently observed. Commonly involved are the proximal interphalangeal and metacarpophalangeal joints of the hands, the wrists, elbows, shoulders, knees, and ankles. Morning stiffness is a frequent complaint.[96] Erosive deforming arthritis is rare. Mild deformities may develop, including correctable subluxations with ulnar deviation or "swan neck" deformities. Contracture or ankylosis is unusual. Tenosynovitis, usually localized, may be the dominant rheumatic feature. Occasionally, subcutaneous nodules are observed, which may closely simulate those of rheumatoid arthritis.[67]

Generalized or juxta-articular atrophy of muscles may be present, and rarely there is widespread muscle tenderness and weakness suggesting the presence of a primary muscle disorder such as polymyositis.

Aseptic bone necrosis, usually of the femoral heads, but also of the humeral heads and other sites, is a feature of SLE;[44] steroid therapy may play a role in its pathogenesis. Surgical therapy may be needed.

Cutaneous lesions, usually erythematous in character, develop at some stage in most cases of SLE. The eruption most frequently appears on the face, neck, V-area of the chest, back and the extremities, and tends to be symmetrical. It may be fleeting or chronic. The classical "butterfly" distribution of the dermal involvement of the face (Fig. 51–2) occurs in less than half the cases. It must be differentiated from acne rosacea or seborrheic dermatitis. Less common but very characteristic are the erythematous lesions of the fingertips, around the nails, and scattered over the palms. Other cutaneous changes which may be seen include purpura, urticaria or angioneurotic edema, bullae, hyperpigmentation, vitiligo and thickening of the skin mimicking scleroderma. Alopecia often develops and may be diffuse or focal. Disorderly, broken hairs about the forehead (Fig. 51–2) have suggested the name "lupus-hair."[7] There may be a history of exposure to the sun prior to the development of the dermatitis. It is important to distinguish early cutaneous lupus from polymorphic light eruption. Patients with SLE who are photosensitive are reactive only to wavelengths shorter than 3200 Å.[46]

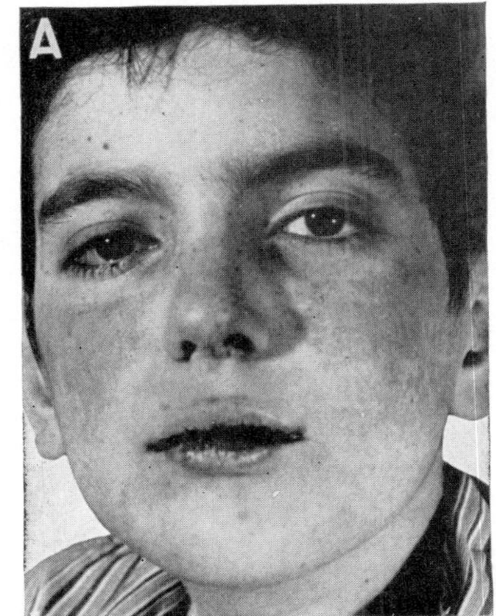

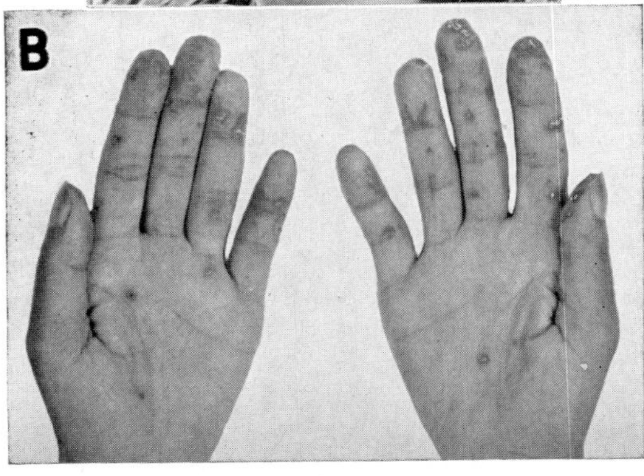

Fig. 51–2.—*A*, Characteristic "butterfly" distribution of facial eruption. *B*, Lesions of the fingers, especially at the tips. (Shulman and Harvey, courtesy of Disease-A-Month.[140])

The typical lesion in the chronic discoid form consists of red plaques with scaling and follicular plugging. Healing develops in the center and, as it spreads outward, the skin becomes atrophic and scarred. Discoid lupus is usually confined to the face, neck, ears, and scalp, but there is a generalized, "chronic disseminated" form. Although in most cases of chronic discoid lupus the systemic form of the disease does not appear, there are numerous cases on record in which the patient, after many years of uncomplicated dermal disease, developed widespread systemic manifestations with the appearance of L.E. cells. On the other hand, in a systematic study of 51 patients with discoid lupus followed for five years, none developed SLE.[107] In another study of 120 patients, antinuclear antibody was found in 42, but L.E. cells in only 2 patients. Other abnormalities were also observed, but it was concluded that the risk of patients with discoid lupus developing SLE was less than 5 per cent.[13]

Oral "vasculitic" lesions or shallow ulcerations are often seen in patients with active SLE. Similar lesions are seen in nasal or pharyngeal mucosa.

Dyspnea and chest pain are common complaints which may be associated with pleural disease, pneumonitis or carditis with heart failure. Half the cases have *pleurisy* often accompanied by a small effusion. An atelectasizing pneumonitis (Fig. 51–3), often termed "anaphylactic" and resembling "virus pneumonia," develops at one or both lung bases in 20 per cent of cases. Scattered rales may be heard, but dullness and abnormal breath sounds are unusual. It should be noted that bacterial infections of the lungs are common during the course of SLE and may be confused with "lupus pneumonitis." When roentgenograms of the chest reveal a combination of bilateral pleural disease, plate-like atelectases at the lung bases, and cardiomegaly, SLE should be suspected. Moreover, there may be pulmonary dysfunction, even in the absence of pulmonary symptoms, signs or roentgenographic abnormalities.[80] The abnormalities include a low vital capacity suggestive of restricted ventilation, reduced lung compliance and a reduced diffusing capacity. Exercise tolerance may be poor.

Some type of *cardiac* involvement develops in the majority of cases. Pericarditis is the most common, being manifested by precordial pain, friction rub or slight enlargement of the cardiac silhouette. An effusion of sufficient magnitude to impair function is rare but patients with SLE may present with acute pericardial tamponade. Myocarditis is also common, but only occasionally is it sufficiently severe to result in heart failure. Cardiac arrhythmias are infrequent, and usually preterminal. There may be an apical systolic murmur, which is difficult to interpret when fever and anemia are present. The correlation between such a murmur and Libman-Sacks lesions at autopsy is not good. Functional aberrations due to SLE valvular disease are uncommon. Aortic insufficiency from thinning of valve cusps and perforated leaflets without verrucous endocarditis is a newly recognized feature of SLE.[16] *Raynaud's phenomenon* has been recorded in as high as one-fourth of patients by some observers.[40] It is often severe, and may be associated with

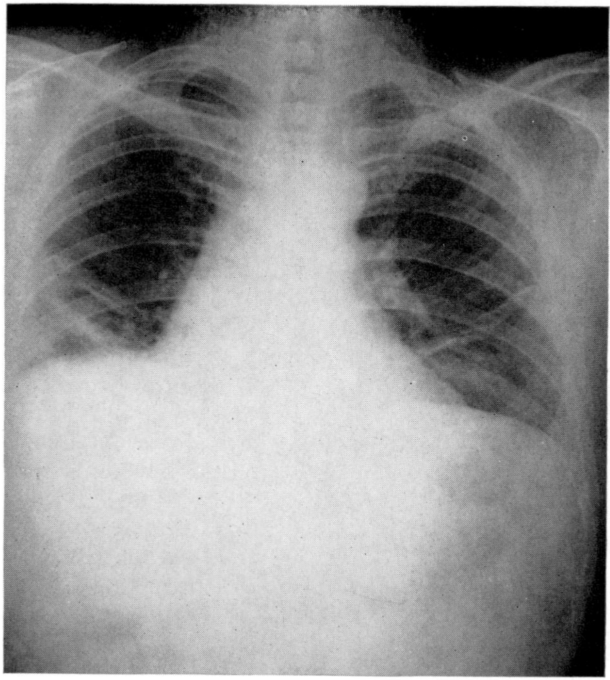

Fig. 51–3.—Roentgenogram of the chest of a patient with SLE in full inspiration. Note the elevation of the diaphragm and the plate-like atelectases.

esophageal disease as in scleroderma.[153] *Hypertension* is usually absent until moderately advanced renal disease has developed.[22] There may be gangrene of the fingers or toes, presumably from arteritis.[43]

The most serious and critical feature of SLE is its *renal* component. Kidney involvement is found in 75 per cent of the autopsied cases and is the most frequent cause of death. The nephritis has a variable clinical pattern, however, and does not *per se* indicate a poor prognosis. Serial needle biopsies have been utilized to document the progress of the renal lesions.[115] The earliest abnormality is a focal glomerulitis. There follows an increase in the thickness of the basement membrane, with deposition of fibrinoid. Adhesions develop between the glomerular tufts and Bowman's capsule, simulating subacute glomerulonephritis. The tubules degenerate and, terminally, the picture is that of a subacute or chronic glomerulonephritis. From needle biopsies, glomerular lesions may be divided into three groups; (1) focal glomerulitis, (2) membranous glomerulonephritis, and (3) proliferative glomerulonephritis. The first two signify a favorable prognosis.[128]

The renal disease may progress rapidly or develop slowly. In the earlier stages it may simulate pyelonephritis with numerous white cells in the urinary sediment. Microscopic hematuria may be the first sign of kidney involvement.[7] Subsequently, various other elements appear and the patient slowly develops renal incompetence. Many cases develop a protein-losing kidney disorder with the classical nephrotic syndrome. During the early active phase of lupus nephritis, the urinary protein may contain up to 50 per cent of gamma globulin.[154] Care must be taken not to overlook a urinary tract infection which may be mistaken for active SLE nephritis. Renal vein thrombosis has been reported to complicate lupus nephritis and contribute to the proteinuria.[68] A latent renal tubular acidosis was reported in 12 patients with SLE.[164]

The common *gastrointestinal* symptoms are anorexia, nausea, vomiting and abdominal pain. When these are severe, an acute surgical condition may be suspected. The causes of abdominal pain include peritonitis (perihepatitis, perisplenitis) or other lesions in the alimentary tract, as well as pancreatitis. Dysphagia occurs in association with impaired esophageal peristalsis or ulcerative esophagitis secondary to the arterial lesions of SLE. Extensive involvement of the intestine may produce the picture of paralytic ileus or bloody diarrhea with abdominal pain. Gross melena is unusual. Roentgenographic studies of the alimentary tract may reveal: esophageal dilatation, impaired peristalsis, or ulceration; narrowing of the gastric antrum; segmental dilatation of the duodenum, jejunum or ileum; or evidence of colitis.

Although hepatomegaly is recorded in one-third of cases, it is often transient and the result of chronic passive congestion. No histologic abnormalities characteristic of SLE are found either with *liver* biopsy or at autopsy. Fatty infiltration and/or fibrosis may be seen. Jaundice is rare. The problem of "lupoid hepatitis" will be discussed separately.

Over half of the cases demonstrate regional or generalized lymph node enlargement. In many instances the lymphadenopathy is so impressive that the patient is thought to have a primary disease of the reticulo-endothelial system or a blood dyscrasia. Enlargement of the spleen is no longer considered to be a cardinal feature of SLE, surveys indicating slight or moderate splenomegaly in only 15 to 20 per cent of cases.[71]

Nervous system abnormalities are being recognized with increasing frequency and consist mostly of mental disturbances, seizures, and cranial nerve signs.[84] The different psychological reactions include anxiety, hyperirritability, confusion, hallucinations and paranoia. Psychoses have been reported in as many as 50 per cent of cases and are usually associated with exacerbations of SLE.[151] Psychoses of SLE are not correlated with preexisting emotional disturbances.[117] Convulsions may antedate other manifestations of SLE by years.[132] More commonly, they appear during periods of active SLE, and may be accompanied by signs of meningitis and such spinal fluid abnormalities as increased protein or pleocytosis. Seizures of the grand-mal type are frequent terminally, either with or without uremia. Other neurological findings include: ptosis, diplopia, chorea, hemiparesis and motor aphasia. Four cases of transverse myelitis have been recently reported.[120] *Peripheral neuritis* due to nutrient involvement is less common, up to 8 per cent.[84] There may be albuminocytologic dissociation simulating infectious polyneuronitis. The neuropathologic findings are chiefly occlusive lesions of arterioles and capillaries, resembling those of thrombotic thrombocytopenic purpura, and unlike the vasculitis of polyarteritis.[84] The vascular changes in cerebral cortex and brain stem result in microinfarcts which correlate well with the clinical signs. Neurologic abnormalities may occur early in SLE and be mild and transient.

Cytoid bodies (Fig. 51–4), fluffy white exudates in the nerve fiber layer of the retina, may be of diagnostic importance.[108] However, funduscopically they are indistinguishable from the exudates of hypertensive or diabetic retinopathy. Thirteen of 24 patients with SLE had symptoms referable to the cornea and 21 of the 24 had fluorescein staining of cornea.[147]

In patients with SLE there seems to be an unusually high incidence of abortions, stillbirths and premature births.[58] As one might expect, there may be deterioration of renal function during pregnancy in SLE.

LABORATORY FINDINGS

Virtually every patient with SLE has one or more hematologic abnormalities during the course of the disease. In a few patients a blood disorder is the presenting or dominant feature. About 80 per cent of cases have a mild to moderate,

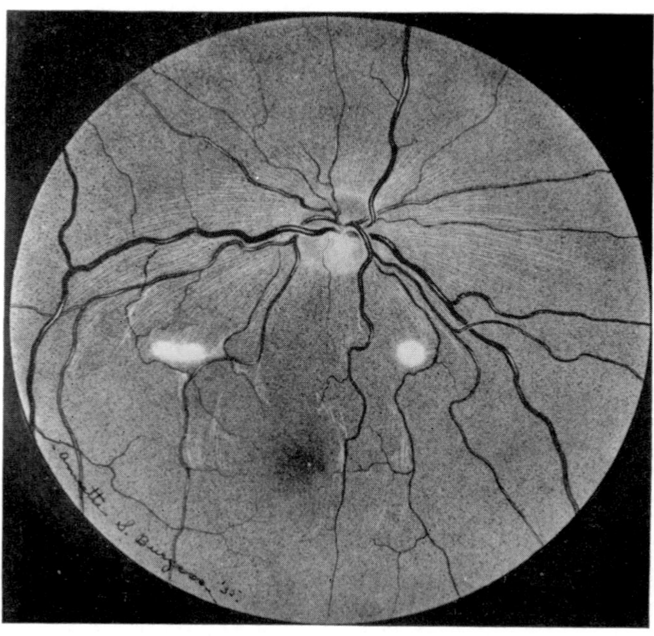

Fig. 51–4.—Typical cytoid bodies in the retina of a patient with SLE.

normocytic, normochromic anemia, which is the result of retarded erythropoiesis. Anemia may become severe with superimposed renal failure or infection. About 5 per cent of the cases have an acute hemolytic anemia of the autoimmune type with hyperbilirubinemia, reticulocytosis, a positive Coombs' reaction and splenomegaly.[71] Splenectomy is usually of little value, but the hemolytic activity can be suppressed by adrenal corticosteroid therapy. Anemia may also result from gastrointestinal hemorrhage or thrombocytopenic purpura.

The frequent development of purpura is usually the consequence of the vascular lesions of SLE, uremia, or corticosteroid therapy. In the occasional case thrombocytopenic purpura may be the first or outstanding feature of SLE. It is frequently mistaken for "idiopathic" thrombocytopenic purpura.[48] In contrast to the experience with hemolytic anemia, splenectomy is corrective in most instances. Adrenal corticosteroids are useful before and during splenectomy to suppress the bleeding. Platelet antibody is found in most (88 per cent) patients, although only a few (6 per cent) have thrombocytopenia.[87] Rarely, purpura is the result of a circulating anticoagulant.

Usually the white cell count is slightly reduced or in the low normal range. Neutropenia *per se* is uncommon; the reduction in white cells involves all forms. Extreme leukopenia, below 2000 per cubic millimeter, is rare. A deficit in white cells may interfere with the L.E. cell test; under such circumstances, one combines the patient's serum with the buffy coat from a normal individual. Leukocytosis usually indicates a complicating infection or an effect of adrenal corticosteroids. These hematologic abnormalities can be transmitted neonatally. Seip[136] reported hemolytic anemia, leukopenia, and thrombocytopenia in both a mother with SLE and her newborn infant.

A multitude of plasma protein abnormalities has been observed, many of which may not have any qualitative or quantitative correlation with the degree of clinical activity of the disease. Certain of these abnormalities, such as the false positive serologic test for syphilis, may antedate the onset of clinical disease by years.[70] In half the cases the serum globulin concentration is elevated; in many, over 4.0 gm. per cent. The serum albumin is frequently reduced, especially in those with nephritis. Plasma fibrinogen levels are increased. The erythrocyte sedimentation rate is almost uniformly elevated, and it may remain high during clinical remissions.

By electrophoretic analysis, some of the globulin elevation is found to be in the alpha-2 fraction, which contains much carbohydrate; high serum levels of both hexosamine[20] and mucoprotein[63] have been recorded. Most of the gamma globulins in SLE belong to the IgG class of immunoglobulins. Moreover, although various autoantibodies may be found in all three immunoglobulin classes, in SLE the greatest elevations are found in the IgG component.

Other evidences of plasma protein dysfunction include autoagglutination of red cells, a circulating anticoagulant,[34] positive Coombs' reaction, cryoglobulins[30] and lowered serum complement activity. The chronic, biologic false positive serologic test reaction for syphilis occurs in 10 to 20 per cent of patients with SLE.[71] Conversely, SLE was found in 14 of 192 false positive reactors, an incidence of 7 per cent.[70] False positive reactions to the fluorescent treponemal antibody (FTA) test with an atypical "beading" pattern have been recently reported in 10 per cent of patients with SLE.[95]

The most significant protein abnormalities are those concerned with the formation of L.E. cells and other antinuclear factors (*see* Chapter 10 for full discussion). It deserves emphasis that not all patients demonstrate this abnormality. The physician should not consider a positive L.E. cell test result as an absolute criterion for the diagnosis of SLE.[152] Although L.E. cells may no longer be found or may be greatly reduced in number in clinical remissions, there are exceptions. This test is not a dependable index of the degree of activity of the disease nor a reliable prognostic guide. L.E. cells may also be found in the Wright's stained sediment of synovial, pleural, or pericardial fluid.[77] Antinuclear antibodies comprise a group of gamma globulins with an affinity for nuclear material; most are IgG immunoglobulins although some are IgA and IgM. They are found in the sera of almost all patients with SLE. They are not specific for SLE, but a negative result makes the diagnosis of SLE unlikely. Anticytoplasmic factors may also be found in the sera of patients with SLE;[38] and results of tests for "rheumatoid factor" are positive in an appreciable number of patients (*see* section on "Diagnosis"). Many centers now use the antinuclear antibody test for screening purposes; and perform L.E. cell tests only in those with positive antinuclear antibody reactions. However, since there are patients with positive L.E. cells and negative antinuclear antibody reactions, it seems prudent to use both tests in diagnosis.

Antibodies reacting with native DNA are detectable in the sera of some patients with active SLE and nephritis.[162] Moreover, free native DNA is found in the sera of a few of such patients. The important concept thus arose that DNA antigen-antibody complexes were important in the pathogenesis of the renal lesions of SLE. It was later shown that there was a good correlation between clinical evidence of active SLE, especially lupus nephritis, and the presence of anti-DNA antibodies;[131,134] and that antinuclear antibodies reacting with DNA were concentrated in and could be eluted from the glomeruli of SLE patients.[94] Similar complexes are deposited in splenic vessels,[157] dermal arterioles,[161] and the choroid plexus.[8]

Reduced serum complement usually indicates active SLE, especially with respect to its nephritis.[163] There is frequently an inverse relationship between serum complement levels, on the one hand, and serum anti-nucleoprotein activity or antinative-DNA antibody levels[134] on the other. Decreased serum complement levels have also been associated with cold-insoluble immune complexes (cryoproteins) which are demonstrable in one-third of patients with SLE.[148]

Precipitating antibodies to synthetic double-stranded RNA were found in the sera of 16 of 89 patients with SLE.[133] Most of the reactive sera also contained antibody to ribosomes and/or DNA. Since mammalian RNA is probably single stranded it is likely that these antibodies to double-stranded RNA in lupus sera are probably directed against foreign antigen(s).

Cytoplasmic antibodies are found in 40 per cent of unselected SLE sera.[31] The cytoplasmic antigen used may be derived from a number of human tissues. Also, human leukocyte lysosomal antigen and antibodies thereto have been discovered in lupus sera;[14] this system may be the consequence of prior inflammation.

Cytotoxic antibodies directed against lymphocytes have been found in 74 per cent of lupus sera.[113] The antibody is an IgG immunoglobulin and is dependent on complement. It is suggested that a component of lymphocyte membrane becomes in some way antigenic; the antibodies lyse the lymphocytes discharging intracellular contents which in turn may be an important source of DNA for anti-DNA antibody formation. These lymphocytotoxic antibodies in SLE are correlated with leukopenia, lowered serum complement levels, and active SLE, but not with nephritis. Furthermore, Stastny and Ziff have shown that lymphocytes from patients with active SLE undergo lysis when exposed to rabbit (but not to human) complement.[149]

Some patients with SLE have a delayed "hypersensitivity" reaction to intradermal injection of a suspension or homogenate of autologous leukocytes.[53]

However, this reactivity is not specific for SLE. This, along with the plethora of circulating autoantibodies and hypergammaglobulinemia, has led to the concept that a generalized immunologic hyperreactivity is an important feature of SLE. However, numerous studies have shown that, for the most part, patients with SLE have normal antibody responses to several exogenous antigens;[17] and resemble normal individuals in numerous tests of delayed hypersensitivity.[17] In fact, SLE patients have a curious hyporeactivity to tuberculin, and to immunization with certain bacterial antigens. The latter has been attributed to a reduced productivity of macroglobulin (IgM) antibody, and may explain, at least in part, the lowered resistance to infection in SLE.

The synovial fluid white blood cell count is usually low, less than 3000/mm.^{3}, with a predominance of mononuclear cells.[96] Viscosity is usually normal. The synovial fluid complement may be reduced even though the serum complement level is normal.

Pleural effusions usually have the characteristics of an exudate, the protein concentration usually being greater than 3 gm./100 ml. The glucose concentrations in pleural fluid are usually not low in SLE, in contrast to the low concentrations found in rheumatoid pleural effusions; this measurement may, therefore, be helpful in differential diagnosis.

DIAGNOSIS

Diagnosis is no problem when the patient presents the classical clinical picture of SLE with multisystem involvement, several of the characteristic laboratory abnormalities, including the L.E. globulin, and compatible histopathologic changes in biopsy. Frequently, however, the course of the disease is a chronic one which unfolds episodically over many years. At any given point, whether at the onset or later, a single manifestation may dominate the illness, such as arthritis, nephritis, or hemolytic anemia, making diagnosis more difficult.

In these cases in which a single feature, such as, for example, pleuritis, dermatitis, or thrombocytopenic purpura, dominates the clinical expression of the disease, careful study of the history may reveal that the patient has had a series of illnesses in the recent past, some of which had not been adequately explained. As an example, a patient presenting with a symmetrical migratory polyarthralgia, resembling early rheumatoid arthritis, also had had undue photosensitivity for years, a bout of pleurisy one year earlier, and two months previously an unexplained febrile illness. When one manifestation of SLE such as thrombocytopenic purpura or the nephrotic syndrome is severe, other accompanying symptoms which furnish the necessary clue to the correct diagnosis, such as polyarthralgia, are easily overlooked. It is the combination of signs, symptoms and laboratory findings which directs one's attention to this diagnosis rather than any single characteristic development.

Although SLE manifests itself in so many different and often bizarre ways, certain developments are encountered with such frequency that they call this diagnosis to mind early in the patient's evaluation. These include: unexplained fever with leukopenia, "idiopathic myocarditis," unexplained nephritis, "aseptic meningitis," or a chronic false positive reaction for syphilis. These situations are only a sample of the indications for performing the test for L.E. cells or antinuclear antibodies. A more complete listing is presented in Table 51–2. If the result is negative in patients in whom the diagnosis seems likely, repeat studies should be carried out at appropriate intervals. The diagnosis can at times be confirmed by appropriate biopsy specimens. A committee of the American Rheumatism Association is currently constructing and testing diagnostic criteria (or more properly, criteria for classification) for SLE.[31a]

The differentiation of SLE from other

Table 51-2.—Clinical Features Which Should Lead the Physician to Suspect Systemic Lupus Erythematosus

1. Fever of unknown origin	8. "Bacterial endocarditis"
2. Unexplained or bizarre skin lesions	9. Nephrotic syndrome
3. Migratory polyarthritis suggesting rheumatic fever or rheumatoid arthritis	10. Thrombocytopenic purpura
4. Pleurisy	11. Acute hemolytic anemia
5. Pneumonia unresponsive to antibiotics	12. Idiopathic epilepsy
6. Raynaud's syndrome	13. Aseptic meningitis
7. Idiopathic myocarditis	14. Latent syphilis
	15. Drug reaction

diseases primarily involving connective tissue may be difficult. Rheumatic fever is distinguished on the basis of: an antecedent streptococcal sore throat followed by a proper incubation period; leukocytosis; and an elevated antistreptolysin-O titer. However, patients with SLE do have streptococcal infections and under certain circumstances, leukocytosis. Moreover, the arthritis of SLE may resemble the synovitis of rheumatic fever and the response to salicylates may be dramatic.

The distinction between SLE and other "connective tissue diseases" such as polyarteritis, progressive systemic sclerosis and dermatomyositis is further complicated by the apparent overlap among these disorders both clinically and pathologically. In certain patients considered to have SLE both during life and at necropsy, necrotizing arteritic lesions typical of polyarteritis may be found; scleroderma-like changes may be seen in the skin; or the muscle may reveal both the inflammatory and degenerative changes of dermatomyositis. Conversely, in each of these other "connective tissue disorders," cases demonstrating L.E. cells have been reported. There seems to be a relationship between Sjögren's syndrome and SLE,[72,76] but this has not been fully delineated.

SLE and Thrombotic Thrombocytopenic Purpura.—There also may be a relationship between SLE and thrombotic thrombocytopenic purpura (TTP).[101] This is a rare, febrile, multisystem disease affecting principally young adult females, the major features of which are thrombocytopenic purpura, hemolytic anemia and changing neurological signs. The presence of bizarre red blood cells ("schizocytes") facilitates diagnosis. The white count is usually elevated. The lesions involve arterioles, capillaries and venules, and consist of subendothelial hyaline, eosinophilic deposits and thromboses. They are most prominent in the heart, kidneys and brain. Inflammatory cells are not seen. SLE is frequently diagnosed ante mortem and cases have been recorded in which lesions typical of both SLE and TTP were found at post-mortem examination. Among the reported findings in TTP are: nonbacterial verrucous endocarditis, false-positive serologic reactions for syphilis and L.E. cells.[160] There are, however, important pathologic differences, and, for the present, the two disorders should be considered to be separate and distinct from each other.

SLE and Rheumatoid Arthritis.—An analysis of the relationship between SLE and RA presents certain difficulties. Although there are typical and easily recognizable clinical forms of both SLE and RA, neither disease can be defined clinically with precision. At the present time universally acceptable standards for the diagnosis of early and mild cases of either disorder are lacking. In each disease the cause is unknown. There are serologic overlaps between SLE, RA and other autoimmune disorders.[76] The

Table 51-3.—Features of Systemic Lupus Erythematosus Which Aid in Distinguishing it From Other Connective Tissue Disorders

1. 85 per cent of cases occur in females, usually young adults.
2. Characteristic facial butterfly rash and periungual erythema.
3. Serositis (pleuritis, pericarditis, peritonitis, arthritis) especially in combination.
4. Disc-like atelectases at one or both lung bases.
5. Nephritis, especially the nephrotic syndrome.
6. Retinal exudates ("cytoid bodies") in the absence of hypertension and diabetes.
7. Severe anemia, especially if hemolytic.
8. Thrombocytopenic purpura.
9. Leukopenia.
10. Chronic biologic false positive serologic reactions for syphilis in 10 to 20 per cent of cases.
11. L.E. cells and antinuclear antibodies in most, but not all, cases.

various extra-articular lesions of RA are now more fully appreciated, and the term "rheumatoid disease" has gained wider usage. Articular involvement is common in SLE and is often indistinguishable from that of RA.

In a review of the literature,[169] 28 of 83 cases of SLE had a positive reaction for rheumatoid factor. If whole serum was used, rheumatoid factor was demonstrable in 32 of 64 cases of SLE whereas with a cold-precipitable fraction of serum a positive reaction was found in only 1 of 30.[156] Kellgren and Ball,[88] in reporting rheumatoid factor in 17 of 41 clinically diagnosed cases of SLE, commented: "Among those in which the sheep cell test was positive, articular and/or peripheral vascular lesions were prominent, whereas in patients without these lesions, the test was usually negative."

Among various reported series of patients with RA, the L.E. cell test result has been positive in from 0 to 27 per cent. Opinions vary as to whether any clinical differences exist between patients with RA with a positive L.E. cell reaction and those without. Friedman *et al.*[54] found L.E. cells in 25 of 91 cases of RA and in a detailed analysis of numerous features could find no differences between the two groups including the incidence of gold or adrenal steroid administration.

Sigler *et al.*[144] found L.E. cells in 11 of 45 patients with RA followed over a two-year period. Nine of the eleven showed only a few cells on repeated preparations and did not develop any features of SLE during the period of observation. The other two consistently demonstrated greater numbers of L.E. cells and developed the clinical picture of SLE. Six of Sigler's 11 cases had subcutaneous nodules. Kievits and his associates,[90] in analyzing a larger series, reported L.E. cells or "rosettes" in 17 per cent and interpreted them as false positive L.E. test results in patients with rheumatoid arthritis. There was, however, a greater incidence of pneumonitis, splenomegaly, abnormal urinary sediment and false positive serologic test results for syphilis in those cases with L.E. cells. On the other hand, there were no significant differences between the two groups with respect to fever, rash, arthritis or proteinuria. In addition, when these cases were reinvestigated five years later,[62] the differences between the two groups were less pronounced, in some no longer statistically significant, and the mortality rate was the same in both groups. The authors concluded that they found no convincing arguments that rheumatoid arthritis with L.E. cells "should be regarded as a mono- or oligosymptomatic form of systemic lupus erythematosus." In still another study,[61] comparing three groups of patients with rheumatoid arthritis (1) with L.E. cells, (2) with a negative reaction to L.E. cell test, and (3) without a test having been performed, no differences were found except that in the group with L.E. cells the mean leukocyte count was lower and the mean serum globulin concentration was higher than in the other two groups.

In another similar study, all 18 rheumatoid patients with L.E. cells had multisystem disease with involvement of 3 to 8 organ systems in addition to arthritis.[127] Their two groups were comparable in regard to type and degree of articular involvement. Of the 20 with negative L.E. tests, 10 had arthritis alone and 7 had only one other system involved. Bateman, Malins and Meynell[11] noted L.E. cells in 28, or 16 per cent, of 176 patients diagnosed as having R.A. Evidence of systemic disease, usually transient, was recorded in 15 of 28 cases, and they concluded that these were cases of SLE with rheumatoid manifestations. Two of the 28 patients died, and in the one autopsied, no lesions characteristic of SLE were noted. The patients of Willkens and Decker[168] with rheumatoid arthritis and antinuclear antibodies (including L.E. cells) also had impressive extra-articular involvement; much of this, however, could be ascribed to the lesions of rheumatoid disease.

The appearance of rheumatoid factor in "rheumatoids" with L.E. cell globulin seems to be at least as frequent as in the general population of patients with RA; and according to one study, the titers in the former are unusually high. When the cold-precipitable fraction of serum was used, the results of rheumatoid factor tests tend to remain positive, behaving more like rheumatoid than SLE serum.

From these various reports the general impression is gained that: (1) a weakly positive L.E. cell test reaction may be found in some patients with RA uncomplicated by extra-articular disease; (2) on the whole, patients with RA who exhibit the L.E. cell phenomenon do not seem to have or develop the type of multisystem disease that is characteristic of SLE; and (3) rheumatoid factor seems to be just as prevalent in the patient with RA and L.E. globulin as in the rheumatoid population as a whole.

Periarticular subcutaneous nodules histologically indistinguishable from those of RA have been found in patients with lupus nephritis.[67] The latex fixation test result was negative in some of these patients. These interesting observations suggest that subcutaneous nodules may not be entirely pathognomonic for RA and/or that the two diseases are interrelated.

"LUPOID HEPATITIS"

Another provocative finding is the demonstration of L.E. cells in certain patients with liver disease. This was first described in 1955 in 2 patients with chronic active viral hepatitis.[85] One year later, 2 additional cases with chronic hepatitis and L.E. cells were reported.[73] Both groups considered the L.E. cells to be "false positive." Mackay, Taft and Cowling[105] found L.E. cells in 6 patients with active liver disease who simultaneously or subsequently developed a multisystem disorder of connective tissue manifested by fever, rash, arthritis and involvement of serous membranes. To characterize these cases they coined the term "lupoid hepatitis." They considered the hepatic disease to be the primary event and believed that these cases provided evidence that SLE is an autoimmune disorder, the antigen in these instances being some undefined substance associated with the hepatitis. Bearn *et al.*[12] observed that among 26 young women with chronic liver disease and hypergammaglobulinemia a few had clinical manifestations suggestive of SLE, and 1 of 10 had L.E. cells. Bartholomew and associates[10] analyzed retrospectively the medical records of 7 women with chronic liver disease and L.E. cells. All had symptoms or signs consistent with SLE for varying periods of time before the evidence of hepatic involvement appeared. Six had periodic fever, 4 sensitivity to sunlight and 4 pleurisy. All 7 had joint involvement with objective evidence of arthritis in 5, and arthralgia in 2. Four of these patients subsequently died, seemingly of liver disease; at autopsy none had characteristic lesions of SLE. Moreover, two patients with chronic active hepatitis who died of lupus nephritis have been reported.[15]

The significance of the L.E. cell in these cases of so-called "lupoid hepatitis" is obscure. According to one study, the clinical course of patients with chronic active hepatitis was the same, irrespective of the presence or absence of L.E. cells.[167] The possibilities to be considered are: (1) that the hepatic disease is a specific manifestation of SLE; (2) that it is an infectious hepatitis occurring coincidentally in a patient with SLE; (3) that it is a viral hepatitis modified in its course by the hepatic process, becomes antigenic and the L.E. cell phenomenon represents an autoimmune response. However, in contrast to acute viral hepatitis, hepatitis-associated (Australia) antigen (HAA) is not found in patients with chronic active (or aggressive) hepatitis either with or without L.E. cells.[25] In classical SLE histologic evidence of hepatitis is unusual. More information is needed before final conclusions on this subject can be drawn. The prognosis of lupoid hepatitis is poor: death usually results from hepatic incompetence. Most authors now think that this disorder is distinct from SLE, and question the designation, "lupoid hepatitis." These patients also have antibodies to smooth muscle and bile canaliculi. Serum antibodies, however, are probably not important in the pathogenesis of the chronic hepatitis, since neither bound immunoglobulin nor complement could be detected in the liver of these patients.[158]

THE DRUG-INDUCED LUPUS-LIKE SYNDROME

In 1954 several groups of investigators[45,122] reported the development of reactions simulating early RA or SLE in 7 to 10 per cent of patients receiving hydralazine (Apresoline) for hypertension. These reactions appeared after several months of treatment at doses of 400 mg. or more daily. The initial symptoms were feverishness, chilly sensations and "rheumatic" aches, which disappeared if the hydralazine was discontinued. If continued, additional features suggestive of SLE developed including: (1) photosensitivity and erythematous eruptions; (2) arthritis; (3) pleural and pericardial effusions; (4) lymphadenopathy and splenomegaly; (5) anemia and leukopenia; (6) an elevated sedimentation rate; (7) increase in the serum alpha and gamma globulin concentrations; (8) a transient false positive serologic test result for syphilis; and, in some cases, (9) L.E. cells.

Atypical for SLE were the rarity of renal abnormalities and reversibility after the hydralazine was stopped. If the drug was then reinstituted at a lower dose, 200 mg. or less daily, there was either no reaction or merely the early "rheumatic syndrome." The relation of this reaction to drug dosage and duration of treatment suggests a direct "toxic" effect, and not one of hypersensitivity. In spite of two initially encouraging reports,[21,32] numerous investigators have been unable to produce this syndrome or lesions of SLE in experimental animals by long-term administration of hydralazine (*see also* p. 184).

Of interest is the clinical evidence that affected individuals are predisposed to this syndrome, *i.e.* have a "lupus diathesis."[2,141] In a study of 50 cases, the authors concluded that hydralazine-induced SLE is indistinguishable from SLE. Moreover, there was evidence of a lupus diathesis in the past histories in 74 per cent of the 50 patients, as compared to only 13 per cent in 100 hypertensive controls; and in several patients, clinical or laboratory manifestations of SLE persisted or reappeared after the hydralazine was discontinued. However, in some of these patients, the hypertension for which the hydralazine had been given may have been caused by "idiopathic" SLE.

Similar lupus-like reactions, usually with LE cells, have been reported after the prolonged administration of other drugs including various anticonvulsants (dilantin and other hydantoin compounds, trimethadione),[82,141] isoniazid,[171] methyldopa,[137] propylthiouracil[5] and procainamide.[97] Although, after the offending drug has been discontinued, some of the manifestations may persist, most usually disappear. Also, the prognosis of "drug-induced SLE" is generally much better than for SLE as a whole.[82]

There are several reports of the induction of an SLE-like syndrome after weeks or months of antituberculosis chemotherapy. From epidemiologic data, the frequency of these reactions is low.[142] However, Cannat and Seligmann[26a] have reported that antinuclear antibody was found in 14 per cent of patients receiving isoniazid for one year or longer as compared to 4 per cent in controls. Rothfield and her associates found an even higher incidence of 26 per cent during antituberculous therapy and 4 per cent prior to therapy.[129] The incidence and titers were both higher in those on longer therapy.

It is now clear that procainamide is the most frequent and potent inciter of drug-induced SLE,[18,50] occurring in up to 30 per cent of patients receiving this drug. The syndrome may appear as early as 2 weeks or as long as 6 years after the drug has been instituted; but usually begins after 6 to 18 months of treatment. The most frequent clinical manifestations are arthritis, pleuritis, pneumonitis, pericarditis and hepatosplenomegaly; and mild anemia and leukopenia. There is no renal involvement. It occurs almost as frequently in men as in women, and uncommonly in nonwhite patients.

All patients develop antinuclear antibodies and/or L.E. cells. The antinuclear antibodies are found in all 3 immunoglobulin classes IgG, IgA and IgM. In prospective studies antinuclear antibodies appear in 50 to 74 per cent of those taking the drug: only a minority of these develop clinical symptoms. In contrast to SLE serum complement is never reduced. This and the absence of nephritis are both readily explained by the interesting report that circulating antibodies to native (double-stranded) DNA, found in 60 per cent of patients with SLE, were not detected in any of 14 patients with procainamide-induced SLE.[93] This procainamide form of drug-induced lupus, therefore, differs significantly from SLE and would not appear to depend on a lupus diathesis.

TREATMENT

It is difficult to evaluate the efficacy of a therapeutic agent in SLE because of the variation in the organ systems which may be involved and the tendency for spontaneous improvement to occur. Assessment must rely on careful evaluation of the various clinical and laboratory findings, since there is no specific and reliable index of actvity of SLE. The number of L.E. cells may diminish with improvement, but there is not always a satisfactory correlation. Thus far, quantitation of antinuclear antibodies have also failed to provide a satisfactory means of evaluating the level of activity of the disease process. The level of serum complement activity seems to be a useful indicator of the activity of the nephritis of SLE.[163]

Before reviewing the value of individual therapeutic agents, it is well to recall that there are certain general measures which may be useful in the management of the patient with SLE. Sponging with water or alcohol may lower a hazardously high fever. One should be on the alert for complicating infection so that proper antibiotic therapy may be instituted. A careful history of any previous allergic reaction to the selected antibiotic should be sought, since patients with SLE may have a high incidence of drug hypersensitivity. The routine prophylactic use of antibiotics in SLE, even in patients receiving adrenal corticosteroids, is not recommended. The development of cardiac insufficiency is an indication for limitation of activity, digitalization, sodium restriction and diuretics if necessary. Severe anemia may require blood transfusions. Although it has been rare in our experience, some observers report that transfusion reactions are fairly frequent and severe in SLE patients.

The patient's activity should be limited during periods of acute illness, but in more chronic periods activity to tolerance should be allowed. The patient should be advised to avoid exposure to the sun if there is a history of photosensitivity, since severe systemic as well as dermal manifestations may develop or increase after such exposure. At the first interview the physician can prevent much anxiety on the part of the patient by presenting an optimistic outlook, while at the same time outlining the variability of the course of the disease and the need for close medical supervision.

The most widely used agents in the treatment of SLE are salicylates, antimalarials, corticosteroids, and immunosuppressive agents.

Salicylates induce prompt defervescence in many patients and alleviate joint symptoms in some.[71,126] They may be helpful in the acutely ill patient, and their administration may reduce the maintenance dose of corticoids required by the chronically ill.

Antimalarials.—In 1951 Page[119] first described the favorable effects of *atabrine* in 17 patients with chronic discoid lupus erythematosus and in one with SLE. These observations have been confirmed repeatedly by many workers for the chronic discoid form, complete inactivation or major improvement occurring in 50 to 75 per cent of cases. After discontinuing therapy, however, the recurrence rate is high. *Chloroquine* or *hydroxychloroquine* has almost completely replaced atabrine, since they do not cause the skin to become yellow. The initial dose of chloroquine, 500 to 750 mg. daily, is given briefly until the maximum response is produced; it is then reduced to 250 mg. or less daily and maintained.

The evidence for the efficacy of chloroquine in the systemic disease is less substantial. Dubois[41] in a study of 14 patients found that: all 4 with the "chronic systemic" form (no L.E. cells) improved; 3 or 5 with "subacute systemic" disease benefited greatly; but there was improvement in only 3 of 10 patients with "classical acute" SLE. It was concluded that the less active the SLE, the better the result. Ziff and associates[170] felt that during the administration of an antimalarial there was significant reduction of the required maintenance dose of corticoid in their patients with SLE. Soffer[146] noted that, while the eruption subsided within several days after chloroquine was begun, the severe manifestations of SLE did not improve. Various side reactions to antimalarials have been reported including a lichenoid or exfoliative dermatitis; gastrointestinal disturbances; neuromyopathy; dizziness, psychosis or convulsions; corneal opacities due to pigment deposits; and, infrequently but seriously, bone marrow depression or retinopathy with loss of vision. Among these, the retinal toxicity is the most worrisome; according to one report, it occurs frequently in SLE.[75] Many now recommend low dosage and a maximum duration of one year. The analogue, hydroxychloroquine, has not proven to be much less toxic (*see also* Chapter 30).

Corticosteroids.—The introduction of corticotropin and cortisone in 1950 provided the first significant advance in the management of patients with SLE. These agents have continued to demonstrate their effectiveness and predictability in suppressing most of the clinical manifestations of active SLE. However, although the inflammatory reaction may be dramatically suppressed, the basic disease process is not fundamentally altered by adrenal corticosteroid therapy. In some cases the response to treatment is insufficient. In others, particularly after prolonged therapy, the dose has to be reduced because of serious side effects.

Since there is no reliable measure of disease activity, the decision as to when to institute treatment with adrenal corticosteroids may be a difficult one. In the absence of appreciable constitutional manifestations or evidence of active disease in vital organ systems, such as the kidneys, heart or central nervous system, corticoid therapy is usually both unnecessary and inadvisable.

The principles in regard to selection of corticoid, indications for altering the dose, and the recognition, prevention and management of side reactions, as described for rheumatoid arthritis (*see* Chapter 31), apply to the corticosteroid treatment of SLE as well, with the following important exceptions. Both the initial and maintenance dosages may have to be considerably higher in the patient with SLE. For example, in the critically ill individual, the effective initial dose of prednisone may be 60 mg. daily or higher. However, in the seriously, but not critically, ill patient, it is our practice to start at a moderate dose, *e.g.* 20 or 30 mg. of prednisone daily. If after a few days there is no response, this dose is increased in a stepwise manner until improvement occurs. After maximal benefit has been achieved, the daily dose is gradually reduced. Judgment as to the rapidity at which this is done is based on the general clinical condition of the patient with particular attention to the functional status of the vital organs involved. It is to be emphasized that one does not "treat" an elevated sedimentation rate, an elevated serum globulin concentration, or a persistently positive reaction to L.E. cell test. In some cases it may be possible over weeks or months to stop corticosteroid therapy altogether without recurrence of disease activity. In others in whom it is necessary to maintain therapy for longer periods further attempts should be made at frequent intervals to lower the daily dose or discontinue treatment.

Since the doses of corticosteroid required for control of SLE are often higher than in RA, side reactions develop more frequently. It is difficult at times to decide which is the greater risk to the patient, some degree of activity of the SLE on the one hand or the potential hormonal side reactions (such as peptic ulcer or osteoporotic fractures) on the other. When some new event develops in the patient with SLE under treatment with corticoids, it is often difficult to decide whether this represents a side reaction to the hormone, an expression of active SLE or some intercurrent process. Examples would be the appearance of abdominal pain due either to a corticosteroid-induced peptic ulcer or to SLE peritonitis; pleurisy with effusion from either tuberculosis or SLE; or an acute psychosis from either corticosteroid therapy or disease activity. Such decisions obviously have great practical importance. If the difficulty is the result of excessive corticoid, then treatment should be stopped or the dose decreased; if indicative of enhanced SLE activity, the hormonal dose should be raised; while if unrelated to either, a totally different plan of management may be required. Such decisions must be based on the careful evaluation of all the available clinical and laboratory evidence.

Alternate-day corticosteroid therapy on high dosage (100 to 120 mg prednisone every other day for 6 to 8 months), designed to minimize or prevent corticosteroid toxicity, has been reported to be effective according to histologic and functional parameters in a small group of patients with lupus nephritis.[1] In many patients on such a regimen, however, we have observed signs of activity of SLE on the days when prednisone is not given.

Opinions as to the effectiveness of corticoids and the optimal regimen in the treatment of the nephritis of SLE have been modified as experience has accumulated. The initial evidence suggested that corticosteroid therapy was neither harmful nor beneficial. Then Pollak and his associates[124] reported, on the basis of survival and the study of serial renal biopsy specimens, that significant improvement may result from large doses of prednisone (45 to 60 mg. daily) given for weeks or months, in contrast to results with lower dosage regimens. Contrariwise, the findings of Rothfield *et al.*[130] indicated that patients with SLE and nephritis responded favorably to the generally low doses required to treat the extrarenal manifestations of the disease. In the individual patient it seems advisable to use both renal and extrarenal parameters, as well as immunologic data.

Immunosuppressive Agents.—Many patients with SLE, especially those with nephritis, require large doses of corticosteroids for long periods, and develop serious toxicity. Thus, as the evidence accumulated convincingly that the renal, and perhaps other, manifestations of SLE were caused by immunopathologic mechanisms, increasing numbers of reports appeared of therapeutic trials in SLE with various *immunosuppressive agents*, used in the treatment of neoplastic disorders and transplantation. Although the first favorable report appeared more than a decade ago,[37] the efficacy of these agents in SLE remains unclarified (*see also* Chapter 33). These agents include both alkylating compounds and antimetabolites; mechlorethamine (nitrogen mustard), azathioprine (Imuran), and cyclophosphamide (Cytoxan) have been reported most frequently. It is important to appreciate that these compounds have cytotoxic, immunosuppressive, and also anti-inflammatory properties. In the vast majority, they have been given together with corticosteroids. A summary of the literature of cytotoxic agents in lupus nephritis from 1963 to 1970 indicates that 10 per cent entered into remission (clinical features controlled, proteinuria absent), 40 per cent improved, and 50 per cent were unchanged or worse, or died.[26] The results with each of the three agents listed above were similar. Whether this experience is superior to that with steroids alone cannot be determined. It is likely that in most of the reported cases the severity of SLE was above average. There have been only a few controlled therapeutic trials. In one, comparing 18 patients on steroids with 19 patients on azathioprine and "necessary" corticosteroids, azathioprine seemed to prolong survival, delay the occurrence or progression of nephritis, and be corticosteroid-sparing.[159] A double-blind trial (with corticosteroids) of cyclophosphamide in 11 patients revealed improvement in over half on the drug compared to none on placebo.[150] However, in another trial in 14 patients with SLE, cyclophosphamide given alone was significantly less useful than prednisone; in fact, the former afforded no benefit whatsoever.[55] Clearly, more data are needed.

The toxic effects of these immunosuppressive agents are numerous. Many of them mimic the signs of active SLE. They include bone marrow depression, gastrointestinal toxicity, hepatic damage, pulmonary infiltrates, alopecia, cystitis, amenorrhea and fetal abnormalities. The last of these are especially pertinent to the young female population with SLE. Also, on these agents patients become more susceptible to numerous types of common and unusual bacterial, fungal and viral infections. Moreover, there is a long-term threat of developing neoplastic disease, particularly lymphoma, which has appeared in persons treated with cytotoxic agents, and to which patients with SLE may be unusually susceptible.

In the experimental mouse (NZB/NZW) model of SLE the data on these agents are, in general, also somewhat encouraging but conflicting. Pretreatment with cyclophosphamide can prevent or reduce the severity of the nephritis in NZB/NZW mice.[28] The established disease is improved somewhat by such treatment. However, this was accomplished with high doses (8 mg./kg./day); lower doses (1 mg./kg./day) similar to those used in man failed to prevent the disease.[166] In another study, azathioprine (5 mg./kg./day) alone was less effective than prednisone alone or both drugs in preventing lupus nephritis in NZB/NZW mice, although all 3 regimens were equally immunosuppressive.[66]

At present, therefore, such immunosuppressive therapy probably has some role in the treatment of SLE, but in view of the very significant toxicity, it should be reserved for corticosteroid-resistant or corticosteroid-toxic patients; and further therapeutic investigations are needed.

Thymectomy in 3 SLE patients produced neither clinical improvement nor change in the immunologic status of the patients.[112]

PROGNOSIS

The many difficulties that arise in attempting to derive meaningful prognostic figures in a chronic disease such as SLE have been described.[111] In this study, which employed the "life-table" techniques used by insurance companies, the death rate after diagnosis was found to be rapid during the first three months and then to be constant at 10 per cent per year thereafter. The date of diagnosis was selected as the reference point because the onset of SLE is frequently so vague. It must be emphasized that these prognostic figures are average values. Since this earlier study, the prognosis in SLE has improved steadily, so that by 1966 Leonhardt reported survival after diagnosis to be 70 per cent after 5 years and 51 per cent after 10 years.[100] In the individual patient no prediction can be made because the natural course of the disease is so varied. The average prognosis in the patient without kidney disease is better than for SLE as a whole.[47,89] Renal disease is the most common cause of death. Central nervous system involvement is next.[47] The prognosis in children under 14 years of age is generally less favorable than in adults,[109] but not as grim as previously described. Bacterial infection and nephritis are the leading causes of death in children.[109] To what extent corticoid therapy has modified the prognosis of SLE is uncertain, although it appears to have been beneficial.

BIBLIOGRAPHY

1. Ackerman, G. L.: Ann. Intern. Med., *72*, 511, 1970.
2. Alarcon-Segovia, D., Walkim, K., Worthington, J., and Ward, L. E.: Medicine, *46*, 1, 1967.
3. Allison, J. H. and Beetley, F. R.: Lancet, *1*, 288, 1957.
4. Altschuler, C. H. and Angevine, D. M.: Amer. J. Path., *25*, 1061, 1949.
5. Amrhein, J. A., Kenny, F. M., and Ross, D.: J. Pediat., *76*, 54, 1970.
6. Ansell, B. M., and Lawrence, J. S.: Arth. & Rheum., *6*, 260, 1963.
7. Armas-Cruz, R., Harnecker, J., Ducach, G., Jalil, J., and Gonzalez, F.: Amer. J. Med., *25*, 409, 1958.
8. Atkins, C., Kondon, J., Quismorio, F. P., and Friou, G. J.: Arth. & Rheum., *14*, 148, 1971.
9. Baehr, G., Klemperer, P., and Schifrin, A.: Trans. Assoc. Amer. Physicians, *50*, 139, 1935.
10. Bartholomew, L. G., Hagedorn, A. B., Cain, J. C., and Baggenstoss, A. H.: New Engl. J. Med., *259*, 947, 1958.
11. Bateman, M., Malins, J. M., and Meynell, M. J.: Ann. Rheum. Dis., *17*, 114, 1958.
12. Bearn, A. G., Kunkel, H. G., and Slater, R. J.: Amer. J. Med., *21*, 3, 1956.
13. Beck, J. S. and Rowell, N. R.: Quart. J. Med., *35*, 119, 1966.
14. Bell, D. A., Leddy, J. P., and Vaughan, J. H.: Arth. & Rheum., *14*, 369, 1971.
15. Benner, E. J., Gourley, R. T., Cooper, R. J., Jr., and Benson, J. A., Jr.: Ann. Intern. Med., *68*, 405, 1968.
16. Bernhard, G. C., Lange, R. L., and Hensley, G. T.: Ann. Intern. Med., *71*, 81, 1969.
17. Block, S. R., Gibbs, C. B., Stevens, M. B., and Shulman, L. E.: Ann. Rheum. Dis., *27*, 311, 1968.
18. Blomgren, S. E., Condemi, J. J., Bignall, M. C., and Vaughan, J. H.: New Engl. J. Med., *281*, 64, 1969.
19. Blumenfeld, H. B., Kaplan, S. B., Mills, D. M., and Clark, G. M.: J.A.M.A., *185*, 667, 1963.
20. Boas, N. and Soffer, L.: J. Clin. Endocrinol., *11*, 39, 1951.
21. Braverman, I. M. and Lerner, A. B.: J. Invest. Derm., *39*, 317, 1962.
22. Brigden, W., Bywaters, E. G. L., Lessof, M. H., and Ross, I. P.: Brit. Heart J., *22*, 1, 1960.
23. Brunjes, S., Zike, K., and Julian, R.: Amer. J. Med., *30*, 529, 1961.
24. Brunner, C. M., Horwitz, D. A., and Davis, J. S., IV: Arth. & Rheum., *14*, 373, 1971.

25. Bulkley, B. H., Heizer, W. D., Goldfinger, S. E., Isselbacher, K. J., and Shulman, N. R.: Lancet, *2*, 323, 1970.
26. Cameron, J. S., Boulton-Jones, M., Robinson, R., and Ogg, C.: Lancet, *2*, 846, 1970.
26*a*. Cannat, A., and Seligmann, M.: Clin. Exp. Immun., *3*, 99, 1968.
27. Carr, D. T., Lillington, G. A., and Mayne, J. G.: Mayo Clin. Proc., *45*, 409, 1970.
28. Casey, T.: Blood, *32*, 436, 1968.
29. Christian, C. L.: New Engl. J. Med., *280*, 878, 1969.
30. Christian, C. L., Hatfield, W. B., and Chase, P. H.: J. Clin. Invest., *42*, 823, 1963.
31. Clark, G., Reichlin, M., and Tomasi, T. B., Jr.: J. Immunol., *102*, 117, 1969.
31*a*. Cohen, A. S., *et al.*: Bull. Rheumat. Dis., *21*, 743, 1971.
32. Comens, P.: J. Lab. Clin. Med., *47*, 444, 1956.
33. Comerford, F. R., and Cohen, A. S.: Medicine, *46*, 425, 1967.
34. Conley, C. L. and Hartmann, R. C.: J. Clin. Invest., *31*, 621, 1952.
35. Cruickshank, B.: Scottish Med. J., *3*, 110, 1958.
36. ————: Ann. Rheum. Dis., *18*, 111, 1959.
37. Damashek, W. and Schwartz, R.: Trans. Assoc. Amer. Physicians, *78*, 113, 1960.
38. Deicher, H. R., Holman, H. R., and Kunkel, H. G.: Arth. & Rheum., *3*, 1, 1960.
39. Drinkard, J. P. *et al.*: Medicine, *49*, 411, 1970.
40. Dubois, E. L.: Ann. Intern. Med., *38*, 1265, 1953.
41. Dubois, E. L.: Ann. Intern. Med., *45*, 163, 1956.
41*a*. Dubois, E. L.: *Lupus Erythematosus*, New York, McGraw-Hill, 1966, p. 479.
42. Dubois, E. L.: Medicine, *48*, 217, 1969.
43. Dubois, E. L. and Arterberry, J. D.: J.A.M.A., *181*, 366, 1962.
44. Dubois, E. L. and Cozen, E. L.: J.A.M.A., *174*, 966, 1960.
45. Dustan, H. P., Taylor, R. D., Corcoran, A. C., and Page, I. H.: J.A.M.A., *154*, 23, 1954.
46. Epstein, J. H., Tuffanelli, D. L., and Dubois, E. L.: Arch. Derm., *91*, 483, 1965.
47. Estes, D. and Christian, C. L.: Medicine, *50*, 85, 1971.
48. Eversole, S. L.: Bull. Johns Hopkins Hosp., *96*, 210, 1955.
49. Evans, A. S., Niederman, J. C., and Rothfield, N. F.: Arth. & Rheum., *14*, 160, 1971.
50. Fakhro, A. M., Ritchie, R. F., and Lown, B.: Amer. J. Cardiol., *20*, 367, 1967.
51. Farquhar, M. D., Vernier, R. L., and Good, R. A.: J. Exper. Med., *106*, 649, 1957.
52. Freedman, P. and Markowitz, A. S.: J. Clin. Invest., *41*, 328, 1962.
53. Friedman, E. A., Bardawil, W. A., Merrill, J. P., and Chim, C. H.: New Engl. J. Med., *262*, 486, 1960.
54. Friedman, I. A., Sickley, J. F., Poske, R. M., Black, A., Bronsky, D., Hartz, W. H., Jr., Feldhake, C., Reeder, P. S., and Katz, E. M.: Ann. Intern. Med., *46*, 113, 1957.
55. Fries, J. F., Sharp, G. G., McDevitt, H. O., and Holman, H. R.: Arth. & Rheum., *13*, 316, 1970.
56. Friou, G. J. and Teague, P. L.: Science, *143*, 1333, 1964.
57. Fudenberg, H., German, J. L., III, and Kunkel, H. G.: Arth. & Rheum., *5*, 565, 1962.
58. Garsenstein, M., Pollak, V. E., and Kark, R. M.: New Engl. J. Med., *267*, 165, 1962.
59. Godman, G. C.: J. Mt. Sinai Hosp., *26*, 241, 1959.
60. Gold, W. M., and Jennings, D. B.: Am. Rev. Resp. Dis., *93*, 556, 1966.
61. Goldfine, L. J., Stevens, M. B., Masi, A. T., and Shulman, L. E.: Ann. Rheum. Dis., *24*, 153, 1965.
62. Goslings, J., Kievets, J. H., Hazevoet, H. M., Hijmans, W., and Cats, A.: In *Proc. Xth Congress Internat. League against Rheumatism*, *1*, 328, 1961.
63. Greenspan, E.: Adv. Intern. Med., *7*, 116, 1956.
64. Gross, L.: In *Contributions to the Medical Sciences in Honor of Dr. Emanuel Libman by his Pupils, Friends and Colleagues*, New York, The International Press, 1932, Vol. 2, p. 527.
65. Gyorkey, F.: New Engl. J. Med., *280*, 333, 1969.
66. Hahn, B. H.: Arth. & Rheum., *14*, 387, 1971.
67. Hahn, B. H., Yardley, J. H., and Stevens, M. B.: Ann. Intern. Med., *72*, 49, 1970.
68. Hamilton, C. R., and Tumulty, P. A.: J.A.M.A., *206*, 2315, 1968.
69. Hargraves, M. M., Richmond, H., and Morton, R.: Proc. Staff Meet., Mayo Clinic, *23*, 25, 1948.
70. Harvey, A. M.: J.A.M.A., *182*, 513, 1962.
71. Harvey, A. M., Shulman, L. E., Tumulty, P. A., Conley, C. L., and Schoenrich, E. H.: Medicine, *33*, 291, 1954.

72. Heaton, J. M.: Brit. Med. J., *1*, 466, 1959.
73. Heller, P., Zimmerman, H. J., Rosengvaig, S., and Singer, K.: New Engl. J. Med., *254*, 1160, 1956.
74. Helyer, B. J. and Howie, J. B.: Nature, *197*, 119, 1963.
75. Henkind, P. and Rothfield, N. F.: New Engl. J. Med., *269*, 433, 1963.
76. Hijmans, W., Doniach, D., Roitt, I. M., and Holborow, E. J.: Brit. Med. J., *2*, 909, 1961.
77. Hollander, J. L.: Personal communication.
78. Holman, H. R.: Amer. J. Med., *27*, 525, 1959.
79. Howie, J. B., and Helyer, B. J.: Advances Immunol., *9*, 215, 1968.
80. Huang, C. T., Hennigar, G. R., and Lyons, H. A.: New Engl. J. Med., *272*, 288, 1965.
81. Hutchins, G. M., and Harvey, A. M.: Bull. Johns Hopkins Hosp., *115*, 355, 1964.
82. Jacobs, J. C.: Pediatrics, *32*, 257, 1963.
83. Jessar, R. A., Lamont-Havers, R. W., and Ragan, C.: Ann. Intern. Med., *38*, 717, 1953.
84. Johnson, R. T., and Richardson, E. P.: Medicine, *47*, 337, 1968.
85. Joske, R. A. and King, W. E.: Lancet, *2*, 477, 1955.
86. Kaposi, M. K.: Arch. f. Dermat. u. Syph., *4*, 36, 1872.
87. Karpatkin, S., and Siskind, G. W.: Blood, *33*, 795, 1969.
88. Kellgren, J. H. and Ball, J.: Brit. Med. J., *1*, 523, 1959.
89. Kellum, R. E. and Haserick, J. R.: Arch. Intern. Med., *113*, 200, 1964.
90. Kievits, J. H., Goslings, J., Schuit, H. R., and Hijmans, W.: Ann. Rheum. Dis., *15*, 211, 1956.
91. Klemperer, P.: Pathology of Systemic Lupus Erythematosus, in *Progress in Fundamental Medicine*, J. A. A. McManus, Ed., Philadelphia, Lea & Febiger, 1952.
92. Klemperer, P., Gueft, B., Lee, S. L., Leuchtenberger, C., and Pollister, A. W.: Arch. Path., *49*, 503, 1950.
93. Koffler, D., Carr, R. I., Agnello, T., *et al.*: Science, *166*, 1648, 1969.
94. Koffler, D., and Kunkel, H. G.: Amer. J. Med., *45*, 165, 1968.
95. Kraus, S. J., Haserick, J. R., and Lantz, M. A.: New Engl. J. Med., *282*, 1287, 1970.
96. Labowitz, R., and Schumacher, H. R., Jr.: Ann. Intern. Med., *74*, 911, 1971.
97. Ladd, A. T.: New Engl. J. Med., *267*, 1357, 1962.
98. Lamont-Havers, R. W., ed.: Arth. & Rheum., *6*, 401, 1963.
99. Leonhardt, T.: Acta Med. Scand., Suppl. 416, 1964.
100. Leonhardt, T.: Acta Med. Scand., Suppl. 445, 1966.
101. Levine, S. and Shearn, M. A.: Arch. Intern. Med., *113*, 826, 1964.
102. Lewis, R. M., Schwartz, R., and Henry, W. B., Jr.: Blood, *25*, 143, 1965.
103. Libman, E., and Sacks, B.: Arch. Intern. Med., *33*, 701, 1924.
104. McCreight, W. G. and Montgomery, H.: Arch. Dermat. & Syph., *61*, 1, 1950.
105. Mackay, I. R., Taft, L. E., and Cowling, D. C.: Lancet, *2*, 1323, 1956.
106. Maher, J. F., and Schreiner, G. E.: Arch. Intern. Med., *125*, 293, 1970.
107. Marten, R. H. and Blackburn, E. K.: Arch. Derm., *83*, 430, 1961.
108. Maumenee, A. E.: Amer. J. Ophth., *23*, 971, 1940.
109. Meislin, A. G., and Rothfield, N.: Pediatrics, *41*, 37, 1968.
110. Mellors, R. C., Aoki, T., and Huebner, R.: J. Exp. Med., *129*, 1045, 1969.
111. Merrell, M. and Shulman, L. E.: J. Chronic Dis., *3*, 12, 1955.
112. Milne, J. A., Anderson, J. R., and MacSween, R. N.: Brit. Med. J., *1*, 461, 1967.
113. Mittal, K. K., Rossen, R. D., Sharp, J. T., Lidsky, M. D., and Butler, W. T.: Nature, *225*, 1225, 1970.
114. Molina, J., Dubois, C. L., Bilitch, M., Bland, S. L., and Friou, G. J.: Arth. & Rheum., *12*, 608, 1969.
115. Muehrcke, R. C., Kark, R. M., Pirani, C. L., and Pollak, V. E.: Medicine, *36*, 1, 1957.
116. Norton, W. L.: J. Lab. Clin. Med., *74*, 369, 1969.
117. O'Connor, J. F., and Musher, D. M.: Arch. Neurol., *14*, 157, 1966.
118. Osler, W.: Amer. J. Med. Sci., *110*, 629, 1895.
119. Page, F.: Lancet, *2*, 755, 1951.
120. Penn, A. S., and Rowan, A. J.: Arch. Neurol., *18*, 337, 1968.
121. Percy, J., and Smyth, C.: J.A.M.A., *208*, 485, 1969.
122. Perry, H. M., Jr. and Schroeder, H. A.: J.A.M.A., *154*, 670, 1954.
123. Phillips, P. E., and Christian, C. L.: Arth. & Rheum., *14*, 180, 1971.
124. Pollak, V. E., Pirani, C. L., and Kark, R. M.: J. Lab. Clin. Med., *57*, 495, 1961.

125. Reiner, M.: Proc. Soc. Exper. Biol. Med., *74*, 529, 1950.
126. Ropes, M. W.: Medicine, *43*, 387, 1964.
127. Ross, S. W. and Clardy, E. K.: South. Med. J., *49*, 553, 1956.
128. Rothfield, N. F., Baldwin, D. S., Lowenstein, J., Gallo, G., and McCluskey, R. T.: Arth. & Rheum., *12*, 293, 1969.
129. Rothfield, N. F., Bierer, W. F., and Garfield, J. W.: Arth. & Rheum., *14*, 182, 1971.
130. Rothfield, N. F., McCluskey, R. T., and Baldwin, D. S.: New Engl. J. Med., *269*, 537, 1963.
131. Rothfield, N. F., and Stollar, B. D.: J. Clin. Invest., *46*, 1785, 1967.
132. Russell, P. W., Haserick, J. R., and Zucker, D. M.: Arch. Intern. Med., *88*, 78, 1951.
133. Schur, P. H., and Monroe, M.: Proc. Nat. Acad. Sci., *63*, 1108, 1969.
134. Schur, P. H., and Sandson, J.: New Engl. J. Med., *278*, 533, 1968.
135. Schwartz, S. and Cooper, N.: Arch. Intern. Med., *108*, 400, 1961.
136. Seip, M.: Arch. Dis. Child., *35*, 364, 1960.
137. Sherman, J. D., Love, D. E., and Harrington, J. F.: Arch. Intern. Med., *120*, 321, 1967.
138. Shulman, L. E.: J. Chronic Dis., *16*, 489, 1963.
139. Shulman, L. E., Gumpel, J. M., D'Angelo, W. A., Souhami, R. L., Stevens, M. B., Townes, A. S., and Masi, A. T.: Arth. & Rheum., *7*, 753, 1964.
140. Shulman, L. E. and Harvey, A. M.: Systemic Lupus Erythematosus, in *Disease-A-Month*, Chicago, The Yearbook Publishers, Inc., (May), 1956.
141. Shulman, L. E. and Harvey, A. M.: in *Proc. Xth Congress International League Against Rheumatism*, *2*, 595, 1961.
142. Siegel, M., Lee, S. L., and Peress, N.: Arth. & Rheum., *10*, 407, 1967.
143. Siegel, M., Lee, S. L., Widelock, D., Gwon, N. V., and Kravitz, H.: New Engl. J. Med., *273*, 893, 1965.
144. Sigler, J. W., Monto, R. W., Ensign, D. C., Wilson, G. M., Jr., Rebuck, J. W., and Lovett, J. D.: Arth. & Rheum., *1*, 115, 1958.
145. Smith, E. W. and Kurban, A.: Bull. Johns Hopkins Hosp., *110*, 202, 1962.
146. Soffer, L. J.: J. Mt. Sinai Hosp., *26*, 292, 1959.
147. Spaeth, G. L.: New Engl. J. Med., *276*, 1168, 1967.
148. Stastny, P., and Ziff, M.: New Engl. J. Med., *280*, 1376, 1969.
149. ————: Arth. & Rheum., *14*, 414, 1971.
150. Steinberg, A. D., Kaltreider, H. B., Staples, P. J., Goetzl, E. J., Talal, N., and Decker, J. L.: Arth. & Rheum., *13*, 351, 1970.
151. Stern, M. and Robbins, E. S.: Arch. Neurol., *3*, 334, 1960.
152. Stevens, M. B., Abbey, H., and Shulman, L. E.: Arth. & Rheum., *7*, 472, 1965.
153. Stevens, M. B., Hookman, P., Siegel, C. I., Esterly, J. R., Shulman, L. E. and Hendrix T. R.: New Engl. J. Med., *270*, 1218, 1964.
154. Stevens, M. B. and Knowles, B.: New Engl. J. Med., *267*, 1159, 1962.
155. Sturgill, B. C., and Preble, M. R.: Arth. & Rheum., *10*, 538, 1967.
156. Svartz, N. and Schlossman, K.: Ann. Rheum. Dis., *16*, 73, 1957.
157. Svec, K. H., and Allen, S. T.: Science, *170*, 550, 1970.
158. Svec, K. H., Blair, J. D., and Kaplan, M. J.: J. Clin. Invest., *46*, 558, 1967.
159. Sztienbok, M., Chase, P. H., and Kaplan, D. A.: Arth. & Rheum., *12*, 337, 1969.
160. Talbott, J. H. and Ferrandis, R. M.: *Collagen Diseases*, New York, Grune & Stratton, 1956.
161. Tan, E. M. and Kunkel, H. G.: Arth. & Rheum., *9*, 37, 1966.
162. Tan, E. M., Schur, P. H., Carr, R. I. and Kunkel, H. G.: J. Clin. Invest., *45*, 1732, 1966.
163. Townes, A. S., Stewart, C. R., Jr., and Osler, A. G.: Bull. Johns Hopkins Hosp., *112*, 202, 1963.
164. Tu, W. H., and Shearn, M. A.: Ann. Intern. Med., *67*, 100, 1967.
165. Tuffanelli, D. L., and Fukuyama, K.: Arch. Derm., *99*, 652, 1969.
166. Walker, S. L., and Bole, G. G., Jr.: Arth. & Rheum., *14*, 189, 1971.
167. Willcox, R. G. and Isselbacher, K. J.: Amer. J. Med., *30*, 185, 1961.
168. Willkens, R. F. and Decker, J. L.: Arth. & Rheum., *6*, 720, 1963.
169. Ziff, M.: J. Chronic Dis., *5*, 644, 1957.
170. Ziff, M., Esserman, P., and McEwen, C.: Arth. & Rheum., *1*, 332, 1958.
171. Zingale, S. B., Minzer, L., Rosenberg, B., and Lee, S. L.: Arch. Intern. Med., *112*, 63, 1963.

Chapter 52

Polyarteritis and Other Arteritic Syndromes

By Lawrence E. Shulman, M.D., and A. McGehee Harvey, M.D.

Polyarteritis is characterized pathologically by inflammation and fibrinoid necrosis of medium-sized or small arteries and clinically by a variable multisystem disorder, the manifestations of which depend on the location of the histological lesions. It is of importance to rheumatologists because of the prominence of muscle and joint complaints and the possible relationships, as yet unclarified, between this disorder and the vascular lesions of rheumatoid arthritis, systemic lupus erythematosus, rheumatic fever, and possible adrenocortical steroid therapy.

The etiology of polyarteritis is not entirely understood. The evidence suggests that, as in rheumatoid arthritis, there may be several variants of polyarteritis and some of these will be described briefly at the end of this section. The relationships between each of the variants and the parent disease, if there is one homogeneous entity, remain to be elucidated. Clearly, some of the variants are separate and distinct entities.

Nomenclature

The term "periarteritis nodosa" was first introduced in 1866 by Kussmaul and Maier[65] to describe a systemic disease characterized by nodules along the course of medium-sized arteries, palpable under the skin and visible in various viscera at postmortem examination. Many observers have abandoned the designation "nodosa" since nodular lesions are found in only a few cases. "Polyarteritis," or "panarteritis," is replacing "periarteritis" since the process involves the entire thickness of the arterial wall. "Arteritis" is considered by some to be restrictive, since the veins may also be affected. As a result, some investigators use "necrotizing angiitis" as a generic term to include all vascular lesions showing inflammation and necrosis, and then subdivide the angiitides into various types, one of which is the disease of Kussmaul and Maier.

Karsner[59] has pointed out that arteries most commonly become involved as a result of extension from neighboring foci of inflammation or by deposition of microorganisms in their walls. Inflammation of arteries may also occur in the course of certain infectious diseases. These forms of arteritis in which the cause is known are designated as "secondary arteritis." Those in which the etiology is obscure are termed "primary arteritis." Polyarteritis falls into this latter category.

Incidence

The incidence of polyarteritis is difficult to estimate since no specific diagnostic test is available. The use of muscle biopsy has limitations since only one-third have positive results in patients later proven to have polyarteritis at autopsy.[75,78] Furthermore, there may be mild cases which heal completely, in which the diagnosis is not suspected and no biopsy material is studied.

From the scanty epidemiologic data and experiences in large hospitals, the incidence of polyarteritis would seem to be appreciably lower than that of systemic lupus erythematosus. Some investigators believe that polyarteritis has become more common as more potentially sensitizing drugs and other agents have been introduced. For example, all but 3 of the 320 cases reported from the Armed Forces Institute of Pathology occurred after 1939.[78]

Males predominate, the sex ratio being 3:1. It is largely a disease of young adults and the middle-aged. Although the peak age incidence at onset lies between twenty and fifty years, the range varies from one month of age to seventy-eight years. Twenty-four cases in infants under one year of age and one case of neonatal transmission have been reported.[11]

Pathology

In the classical syndrome the lesions involve mainly arteries of medium and small caliber with necrosis, fibrinoid change and infiltration with leukocytes. It has been thought that this process begins in the media and later extends to the intima and adventitia. Frequently there is disruption of the internal elastic lamina. The leukocytic infiltration is present both in and around the wall of the vessel. In the early stages it consists largely of polymorphonuclear neutrophils and, in many cases, eosinophils. Eosinophils need not be present in order to make this diagnosis. Mononuclear cells (lymphocytes, monocytes and plasma cells) then appear, and later there is healing and fibrosis. Giant cells are usually absent.

The following changes may be seen in varying combinations during periods of disease activity and repair: (1) healing; (2) excessive fibrosis, which may be sufficiently extensive to form gross nodules; (3) intimal proliferation leading to thrombosis and arterial occlusion with infarction; (4) weakening and aneurysmal dilatation of the arterial wall which may rupture; or (5) arterial dissection. Typically, only one or more segments of a vessel are affected. The process may involve the entire circumference of the vessel or only part of it. Characteristically both fresh and healing lesions may be found together in the individual case.

No single set of vessels is involved uniformly and thus no single clinical finding is invariably present. Virtually any organ in the body may be involved, but most frequently affected are the kidneys and the heart. Lesions are also common in the lungs, liver, spleen, gastrointestinal tract, adrenals, testes, brain and peripheral nerves.

In hypersensitivity angiitis, which Zeek[125] separates from classical polyarteritis, only the smallest arteries and veins participate. The cellular reaction is intense and abounds with eosinophils. In the individual case the lesions are all of the same age. McCombs[72] calls such cases "systemic allergic vasculitis" and reports a more favorable prognosis in his series of 72 cases.

Etiology

For decades the favorite hypothesis has been that polyarteritis is a disease of hypersensitivity. Indeed, the experimental and fragmentary clinical evidence on which this concept rests stimulated the idea that other connective tissue disorders might have an "allergic" background. Gruber[43] in 1925 was the first to suggest that polyarteritis was a general response to hypersensitivity. In 1937 Clark and Kaplan[23] reported necrotizing arteritis in the heart and testes of 2 patients dying of serum sickness. Rich[93] in 1942 described polyarteritic lesions in the viscera and muscles of 7 patients with serum sickness or allergic reactions to sulfonamides. In the following year Rich and Gregory[95] produced lesions resembling human polyarteritis in rabbits by repeated injections of horse serum. These observations were confirmed in 1946 by Hopps and Wissler,[50] who noted glomerulonephritis as well, and by Hawn and Janeway[46] in 1947 with bovine serum in rabbits. It is of interest that the bovine albumin fraction produced arteritic lesions almost exclusively, whereas the gamma globulin fraction resulted in mainly glomerular and, to a lesser degree, heart lesions. Germuth and his associates[35] demonstrated that the arteritis induced by these protein fractions appeared at the same time as the union between antigen and antibody, and that bovine albumin could produce marked glomerular, as well as arterial lesions.

From studies with fluorescein-labeled rabbit antihuman fibrin, Gitlin and his associates[37] suggested that fibrinoid material is actually fibrin. Other investigations using immunofluorescent methods have revealed that arteritic lesions may contain gamma globulin,[32,77] albumin,[84] and complement.[66] Mellors and Ortega[77] thought that the gamma globulin might be antibody to vascular antigen. Paronetto and Strauss,[84] however, presented evidence that made this unlikely. They could not show precipitation of soluble human artery antigen by serum from a patient with polyarteritis, and the patient's serum, labeled with fluorescein, failed to localize in his arteritic or normal vessels. Subsequently, Paronetto[83] has found some patients with polyarteritis in whose arteries he was able to identify gamma globulin, fibrinogen and complement. These observations support the concept that the vascular damage in polyarteritis is caused by circulating immune (antigen-antibody) complexes, as demonstrated in experimental serum sickness in rabbits in detail by Dixon.[26] Recently, a cytotoxic serum factor has been found in the serum of nine patients with polyarteritis, and interestingly, in the serum of some of their asymptomatic relatives.[124] It is an IgG immunoglobulin active against human leukocytes and human kidney cells in culture.

In addition to the sulfonamides, there have been descriptions of polyarteritis associated with allergic reactions to various other drugs; namely, iodides, thiouracil and related compounds, arsenicals, bismuth, dilantin, penicillin, and thiazides. The apparent increase in the incidence of polyarteritis is used by some as an argument that the disease is caused by drug allergy.[78] Recently, necrotizing angiitis indistinguishable from polyarteritis was described in 14 young drug abusers.[22] Many drugs had been taken, but methamphetamine seemed to be the common denominator.

However, as Rich[94] emphasized, the "basic identity of lesions is not a proof of identity of etiology," and "while it is now established that periarteritis nodosa can result from anaphylactic reactions, both in experimental animals and in man, we are not at liberty to conclude that necrotizing vascular lesions can be caused only by hypersensitivity." In a majority of cases there is no history of a reaction to a drug or foreign protein or a record that a sensitizing drug was administered before the onset of the disease. The history of polyarteritis following the administration of a drug does not in itself prove that the drug caused the disease. In the reported cases it is often difficult to exclude the possibility that the original symptoms leading to drug administration may have been those of polyarteritis.

Zeek[125] believed that the vascular lesions found in hypersensitivity reactions, whether in man or in the experimental animal, are not identical with those of polyarteritis nodosa. They divided the necrotizing angiitides into five distinct types: (1) periarteritis nodosa, (2) hypersensitivity angiitis, (3) rheumatic arteritis, (4) allergic granulomatous angiitis of Churg and Strauss[21] and (5) temporal or cranial arteritis. Many observers have been unable to fit all of their own cases neatly into one or another of these categories. It has been particularly difficult to distinguish clearly "hypersensitivity angiitis" from "periarteritis nodosa."[98]

Over the years various infectious agents have been implicated as etiological factors, but the evidence in support of any one of them has not been substantial.

Glaser, Dammin and Wood[38] described a higher incidence (29 per cent) of necrotizing arteritis in the coronary arteries of rats given repeated intrapulmonary injections of hemolytic streptococci than in their controls. They reported only the cardiac findings. Rose and Spencer[98] after a detailed analysis of their 104 cases believed that an abnormal immune response to bacterial infection may be a likely cause in many patients. They separated out 32 cases with lung involvement and found that a respiratory illness (bronchitic, pneumonic or asthmatic) had antedated other manifestations of polyarteritis in two-thirds of them by at least one year, and that in those who had taken sulfonamides the drug had been given for the respiratory disease. A beta-hemolytic streptococcus was detected in 5 of 22 patients, and 12 per cent had a history of or a definite clinical episode of rheumatic fever. The patients with lung involvement, in contrast to those without, had an impressive blood and tissue eosinophilia; and granulomatous arteritis and necrotizing lesions not clearly related to arteries were common. Three additional cases of apparent streptococcal etiology have been described.[30] We have observed a patient with four exacerbations of polyarteritis following streptococcal infections. Many viral illnesses in man, such as influenza, may evoke a vasculitis, but not a necrotizing arteritis. Recently, Gocke *et al.*[40] reported finding Australia (SH) antigen in the sera of four patients with polyarteritis, and in the arteritic lesions of one of them. They also reported evidence to suggest the presence of circulating immune complexes with Australia antigen. However, Prince and Trepo[88] found the correlation between SH immune complexes and polyarteritis in 15 patients to be poor. Moreover, polyarteritis is an important feature of Aleutian mink disease, which is an interesting immunopathic disorder of viral etiology.

The spontaneous occurrence of arteritis has been recorded in several animal species, including cats,[70] elderly Sprague-Dawley rats,[123] and an outbred strain (PN) of New Zealand mice.[119] Arteritis has also been induced in other animal models by various means, such as administering carcinogens or creating experimental hypertension.

According to Zeek and her co-workers,[62] the periarteritis nodosa of Kussmaul and Maier[65] is the result of severe hypertension, and not of hypersensitivity. This opinion is based on the observation that necrotizing and inflammatory lesions may be produced in the rat by hypertension induced by wrapping the remaining kidney in silk after unilateral nephrectomy. Such polyarteritic-like lesions seem to be confined to the hypertensive rat; lesions similarly produced by hypertension in the dog or the rabbit reveal necrosis of arteries, but no inflammation. After careful analysis of their clinical material Rose and Spencer[98] conclude that hypertension is the result, and not the precursor, of renal polyarteritis or glomerulitis, occurring only in those with healing or healed lesions.

It seems reasonable to conclude that there may be several syndromes associated with arterial necrosis and inflammation, and that more basic knowledge concerning etiology and pathogenesis is needed.

Clinical Features

The presenting symptoms and clinical findings are so protean, depending as they do on the extent and severity of the vascular lesions, that no standard description is possible. The disease may begin abruptly or evolve gradually. The clinical problem at the initial visit may be that of: (1) a fever of unknown origin with loss of weight; (2) a primary disease of the kidneys, often thought to be glomerulonephritis; (3) unexplained hypertension; (4) abdominal manifestations which may simulate a condition requiring emergency surgery; (5) bronchial asthma or focal pulmonary infiltrates suggesting infection; (6) myocardial infarction or coronary insufficiency; (7) muscular aching, tenderness and wasting with or without objective signs; or (8) peripheral neuritis.

Fever occurs at some stage in the majority of the cases. There is no characteristic febrile pattern. The patients complain frequently of chilly sensations, but shaking chills are uncommon. Usually the pulse rate parallels the temperature, but there may be a relative tachycardia if cardiac disease is present.

Three-fourths of patients have *renal* involvement. In one series of 300 cases 60 per cent had proteinuria and 40 per cent hematuria.[122] Among the frequent complaints are back pain, nocturia, dysuria, gross hematuria or oliguria. Pathologically, one may find renal arteritis, glomerulonephritis, or both in varying combinations. Renal biopsy may facilitate diagnosis. Renal vein thrombosis has been reported. *Hypertension* is recorded in approximately 60 per cent of cases. There are conflicting opinions about the relationship of hypertension to the renal lesions in polyarteritis. According to Rose and Spencer,[98] elevation of the blood pressure is preceded by renal involvement as evidenced by proteinuria or hematuria. In another series,[91] of 20 patients with hypertension 3 had no evidence of nephritis; and of 24 with nephritis, only 17 had hypertension. In a study of their cases, Knowles, Zeek and Blankenhorn[62] found that hypertension antedated the onset of polyarteritis nodosa and concluded that it may be a causal factor. From the practical viewpoint the diagnosis of polyarteritis should be considered in all cases of severe or rapidly advancing hypertension, especially when accompanied by fever, leukocytosis or other systemic features. Patients with polyarteritis may develop acute oliguric renal failure early in the course of the disease.[67]

Abdominal pain is a frequent complaint, appearing in 65 per cent of cases. The pain which may be severe is commonly periumbilical or in the right upper quadrant. It may be accompanied by anorexia, nausea, vomiting or diarrhea, often with bloody stools. Acute appendicitis, intestinal obstruction, a bleeding ulcer or malignancy, or a perforated viscus may be mistakenly diagnosed leading to surgical intervention. The abdominal symptoms result from involvement within the viscera as well as the gastrointestinal tract. There is frequently mesenteric arteritis with thrombosis and infarction of bowel. When smaller vessels are involved, the result is mucosal ulceration with hemorrhage or perforation. The clinical picture may thus superficially resemble that of ulcerative colitis or peritonitis.

Widespread lesions may be present in the *liver* and gallbladder leading to the development of symptoms similar to those produced in a variety of diseases involving the biliary system. Jaundice may be present. Approximately half of the cases of massive hepatic infarction have been due to polyarteritis. Liver biopsies may be falsely negative, because of the sampling problem. Hepatic angiography may reveal small aneurysms and help in diagnosis. Involvement of the gallbladder may lead to its rupture. Pancreatitis with or without diabetes mellitus has also been reported.

Pleural vasculitis may produce pain accompanied by a hemorrhagic effusion. In the *lungs*, where the vascular bed is complex and lesions may be found in both the bronchial and *pulmonary* arterial tree, the resulting clinical manifestations may assume various forms. Thrombosis of a pulmonary artery may occur leading to infarction with cavitation, with or without hemoptysis, resembling tuberculosis or pyogenic lung abscess. When multiple lesions develop, numerous discrete opacities may be seen on x-ray suggesting metastatic disease. "Anaphylactic pneumonitis" has been reported in those cases which follow drug reactions. Hypertrophic pulmonary osteoarthropathy may be associated with the lung involvement.

In 1939 Rackemann and Greene[89] reported the syndrome of asthma, peripheral neuropathy and eosinophilia in 8 cases; polyarteritis was found in 7. In a review of 300 cases of polyarteritis Wilson and Alexander[122] found that 18 per cent had asthma. Eosinophilia was present in 94 per cent of cases with asthma but in only 6 per cent without asthma. The eosinophilia varied from 11 to 84 per cent, averaging over 50 per cent of the total white count. The diagnosis in these patients was thought to be bronchial asthma with subsequent development of polyarteritis. In 1951, Churg and Strauss[21] reported granulomas in the tissues of 13 of 14 patients with asthma, fever, eosinophilia and polyarteritis. They believed these cases to be different from ordinary polyarteritis, and coined the term "allergic granulomatous angiitis." They further suggested that Loeffler's syndrome might be a milder form of the same process, although patients with this syndrome have died from generalized polyarteritis.

The most frequent changes seen in the *heart* are in the myocardium, although endocardial and pericardial lesions have been described. Arteritis of a medium-sized coronary vessel may lead to myocardial infarction which is similar both clinically and electrocardiographically to that seen in coronary artery sclerosis. In 66 autopsied cases of polyarteritis, 41 had myocardial infarction, which was usually silent.[49] Commonly, however, in both polyarteritis and hypersensitivity angiitis, involvement of small vessels produces multiple areas of necrosis. This change may lead to cardiac enlargement with circulatory insufficiency, and precordial discomfort is a frequent complaint. Death occurs as a result of circulatory failure secondary to coronary arteritis or hypertension, or pericardial tamponade from rupture of a coronary aneurysm.

Arteritic involvement of the central and/or peripheral nervous system occurs in 79 per cent of cases.[29] Arteritis of the *central nervous system* may be responsible for a number of manifestations including various behavioral disturbances, headache, convulsions, hemiplegia, aphasia, cerebellar signs and subarachnoid hemorrhage. Such events may occur early in the course of polyarteritis and not merely as pre-terminal events. Ocular manifestations include episcleritis, choroiditis and retinal arteritis in polyarteritis (*i.e.* in patients without evidence of giant-cell arteritis).

One-half of the cases have a *peripheral neuritis* which is frequently bilateral, and tends to be asymmetrical. The upper as well as the lower extremities may be involved but the dysfunction is usually more prominent in the legs. The cardinal findings are paresthesias, burning pain, nerve tenderness, and motor weakness.

Polyarteritis of *muscle* may express itself as aching and tenderness which are in some cases accentuated by activity and relieved by rest. Extensive atrophy may develop. More commonly, intravascular lesions may be found without any accompanying clinical manifestations. Three patients presenting with leg pain have been recently reported to have an unusually benign course.[41]

The *articular* manifestations of polyarteritis have not been fully studied. Arthralgia, coincident with muscle soreness, is a common complaint, especially early in the course of the disease. McCall and Pennock[71] found joint pain or muscle pain in all of 12 cases, but joint swelling (without redness) was present in only 2. Thirty of Lowman's[69] 43 cases had muscle and joint symptoms but again only 4 had joint swelling which was monarticular in 3. The arthralgia was usually migratory. Rose noted a polyarthritis, resembling rheumatoid arthritis, in 8 of 104 cases of polyarteritis nodosa.[5] In 7 of the 8, the arthritis antedated other manifestations of the disease. In a later communication[97] he described arthritis in 18 (27 per cent) of 66 patients without lung involvement. In 6, it was acute and transient, simulating rheumatic fever; in 8 it resembled chronic rheumatoid arthritis.

In a few cases studied by biopsy there has been a nonspecific synovitis associated with vascular lesions typical of polyarteritis.

Dermal lesions are described in 25 per

patients with rheumatoid arthritis have an increased susceptibility to "arteritis of the polyarteritis-nodosa type." No visceral granulomas were seen. There was no history of allergy. Only 2 of the 5 patients had received adrenal steroids, and 1 of the 2 for only seven days before death.

In 1957 Bywaters[16] described ischemic changes leading to ulceration and/or gangrene in the hands of 6 patients with rheumatoid arthritis, and in a seventh case, gangrene of all four extremities as well as vascular changes in the viscera at postmortem examination. Although the lesions showed largely intimal proliferation, their distribution was similar to that of polyarteritis. None of these patients had had adrenal steroids. Ischemia was noted in 3 other steroid-treated patients. A peripheral neuropathy in 10 rheumatoid patients, only 4 of whom had been given steroids, was reported by Hart *et al.*[45]

According to some observers, however, the incidence of severe disseminated vasculitis in rheumatoid arthritics has increased since the extensive use of corticosteroids in their management. Kemper, Baggenstoss and Slocumb[61] found generalized lesions similar to those of classical polyarteritis in 4 of 14 patients at autopsy who had been treated with cortisone. In contrast, of 38 autopsied patients who had never received steroids none showed such extensive changes, although 3 had a milder acute vasculitis confined to one organ, and 5 had perivascular concentric fibrosis interpreted as a lesion of rheumatic fever. The difference between the diffuse arteritis in the two groups was thought to be significant and the conclusion was drawn that "in certain susceptible patients with rheumatoid arthritis, the administration of cortisone may precipitate the development of diffuse necrotizing arteritis." Black and his associates[10] reported the development of polyarteritis in 4 of 39 patients with rheumatoid arthritis treated with prednisone, demonstrated in two instances by muscle biopsy and at autopsy in the others.

A peripheral neuritis in 6 steroid-treated patients with rheumatoid disease was described by Irby, Adams and Toone.[54] Five of the 6 were men, and the youngest was forty-seven years of age. All had long-standing arthritis. Histological evidence indicated that an arteritis of nutrient vessels was responsible for the neuropathy. Johnson and associates[58] added 3 fatal cases of steroid-treated rheumatoid arthritis with disseminated panarteritis at autopsy. The first manifestation of arteritis in all 3 was a febrile polyneuropathy, followed by multiple organ involvement and gangrenous skin changes. They also reported the appearance of peripheral neuritis in 14 of 138 other patients with rheumatoid arthritis given corticoids. Of interest is that 11 of the 14 had subcutaneous nodules, 13 had a postive reaction to Rose test and L.E. cells were not found in the 13 tested. A purpuric eruption, mainly over the distal parts of the extremities, preceded the neuritis in 10 of the 14 cases.

Epstein and Engleman[28] described 9 cases of typical rheumatoid arthritis, all with deformities and subcutaneous nodules, in 8 of whom a neuropathy appeared during prednisone therapy, with moderate to severe vascular occlusions in 7. All of these patients had a high content of rheumatoid factor in the serum, but 20 per cent of another series without this neurovascular syndrome also had high titers. They speculated that the arterial occlusions might have been caused by intravascular deposition of rheumatoid factor, but noted that in Franklin's[31] cases with particularly high titers the dominant extra-articular features were splenomegaly, anemia and leukopenia. L.E. cells were found in 3 of the 9 patients, and also in 1 of 3 fatal cases of Johnson *et al.*[58] In the comprehensive review of 293 cases of rheumatoid arthritis by Short, Bauer and Reynolds[105] neither dermal gangrene nor neuropathy is specifically mentioned although 34.8 per cent of cases had paresthesias, 20.8 per cent cyanosis, and 11.3 per cent "vascular spasm."

The problem was summarized by Sokoloff and Bunim,[108] as follows: "The occurrence of inflammatory vascular lesions in rheumatoid arthritis is becoming more commonly recognized. The lesions present a wide spectrum of changes varying in their histologic character, location, and frequency in different patients. In a proportion of cases, they cannot be distinguished from polyarteritis nodosa. The increasing frequency with which the changes are seen currently, offers cause for concern that in many instances they may possibly result from the deleterious effect of steroid therapy. Nevertheless, such changes unquestionably have occurred in patients who had never been treated with these compounds and there is, at present, no substantial basis to estimate the magnitude of the postulated increased risk of their occurrence as a result of such therapy. As in many other circumstances, the enhanced interest in the subject must increase the frequency and diligence with which the lesions are sought, found, and reported." These authors also hold the opinion that "polyarteritis nodosa in rheumatoid arthritis may be interpreted as an exaggerated form of rheumatoid arthritis rather than as an independent or incidental finding." This was also the opinion of Schmidt and co-workers,[101] as a result of a comprehensive study of many cases. The role, if any, of corticosteroids has not been clarified.

Course and Prognosis

The prognosis in patients with polyarteritis, who have clinically evident multisystem disease, is poor with death the usual outcome after weeks or months of illness. Only 20 of 152 patients reviewed by Boyd[13] lived longer than one year. Fifty-one of Rose's[97] 54 cases of classical polyarteritis (without lung involvement), not treated with cortisone or corticotropin, died; one-third within three months, two-thirds within six months. Renal lesions were responsible for death in 65 per cent. Uremia was the immediate cause in those succumbing early, while hypertension was responsible for the later deaths. Most of the remaining cases died of either coronary or gastrointestinal arteritis. Frohnert and Sheps[33] found that the presence or absence of pulmonary involvement did not influence the course or prognosis of polyarteritis.

Rose pointed out that these and other figures are weighted heavily by cases in which the diagnosis was first made at postmortem examination. A better estimate of prognosis may be obtained from an analysis of cases diagnosed during life by biopsy material and not having received adrenal steroid therapy. In one such study[97] of 16 cases collected before the introduction of steroid therapy 11 died, 10 within a year. Two continued to have active disease after eight and eleven and one-half years of illness. The remaining 3 cases had a remission; one developed transient hematuria lasting three months; the other two with only skin and joint involvement improved after five and seven years, respectively. In a more recent report from the Mayo Clinic, of 20 patients with polyarteritis not receiving steroids, the five-year survival after diagnosis was 13 per cent.[33]

There are numerous case reports in the literature of survival for several years, even a decade or longer. Complete recovery from hypersensitivity angiitis has also been recorded. Cases of polyarteritis associated with rheumatoid arthritis, in general, have longer survivals than those with polyarteritis as a whole. In contrast, hypertension and renal involvement with polyarteritis are, as one might expect, unfavorable prognostic features.[33]

Treatment

There are a variety of general measures which may be helpful in the management of the patient with polyarteritis. These include analgesics for pain, transfusions for blood loss, digitalization and sodium restriction for heart failure, and antihypertensive drugs. In view of the possible role of hypersensitivity, a careful search for potentially offending antigens should be made, and every effort exerted to eliminate them.

The initial enthusiasm which followed the first reports of treatment with adrenocortical steroids has been dampened by subsequent experience. Relief from many of the symptoms and signs of illness may be observed promptly after initiating treatment with corticoids or corticotropin. This clinical improvement has been confirmed histologically. In serial biopsy specimens one may see resolution of the arterial inflammation within a few weeks. There have been several reports of an increased incidence of infarction, chiefly in the kidneys, heart and alimentary tract, during adrenal steroid therapy. However, infarction is a feature of the untreated disease and its supposedly greater incidence during steroid therapy is not based on data from well-controlled studies. Large doses are often required to control the active manifestations of polyarteritis and the side reactions may be troublesome.

Adequate data are not available to determine whether or not life is prolonged by steroid therapy. In one study[76] the survival rate at the end of one year in a series of 17 treated cases was compared with the rate in a retrospective control series of 19 untreated cases. At the end of one year after diagnosis by biopsy 14 (82 per cent) of the 17 cortisone-treated cases were alive, whereas only 7 (37 per cent) of the 19 untreated cases survived. However, at the time of biopsy, hypertension, an unfavorable prognostic factor, was significantly more common in the controls (42 per cent) than in the steroid-treated group (6 per cent). In 1958 Shick[104] reported that 21 of 30 treated patients were in clinical remission one to five years after the initial course of steroids. However, there were no controls and "in most there is evidence of residual vascular damage." In a more recent report from the Mayo Clinic, the five-year survival rate for 110 patients receiving steroids was 48 per cent.[33]

VARIANTS OF POLYARTERITIS

In discussing polyarteritis one must consider the entire gamut of conditions in which inflammation and/or necrosis of arteries is encountered. During the past several years numerous syndromes have come to be recognized which in certain respects resemble polyarteritis nodosa, but have distinguishing features such as: (1) the nature of the population affected; (2) the mode of onset; (3) the organ systems involved; (4) the frequency of eosinophilia; (5) the clinical course; (6) the distribution of the vascular lesions; (7) the size of the vessels involved; (8) the presence of extravascular pathology; or (9) one or more histopathological details with respect to the arteritis itself.

A list of such possible variants is presented in Table 52–1. In a broad sense all of these disorders can be classified as "angiitis," "vasculitis" or "arteritis." The reason for considering them here as variants is that all are characterized by some degree of necrosis and/or inflammation of blood vessels, and from careful

Table 52-1.—Possible Variants of Polyarteritis

1. Hypersensitivity angiitis
2. Allergic granulomatous arteritis
3. Rheumatic arteritis
4. Polyarteritis with lung involvement
5. Wegener's granulomatosis
6. Rheumatoid vasculitis
7. Corticosteroid-induced arteritis
8. Giant cell arteritis (cranial arteritis)
9. Aortic arch arteritis
10. Arteritis of serum sickness
11. Anaphylactoid purpura
12. Cryoglobulinemia
13. Erythema nodosum
14. Arteritis following resection of coarctation
15. Arterial lesions of hypertension
16. The isolated arteritic lesion
17. Secondary arteritis—*e.g.* influenza

analysis of these syndromes, clues as to the etiology and pathogenesis of widespread inflammatory disease of the vascular system may be developed.

Several of these variants have been mentioned already. Others will be reviewed here.

WEGENER'S GRANULOMATOSIS

The pathological features of this syndrome are: (1) necrotizing granulomatous lesions in the upper air passages or in the lower respiratory tract, or both; (2) generalized focal necrotizing vasculitis, involving both arteries and veins, almost always in the lungs and more or less widely disseminated in other sites; (3) glomerulitis or glomerulonephritis.[39]

Clinical Features

It usually affects young or middle-aged adults of either sex. In two-thirds of the cases the disease begins as a sinusitis or rhinitis; in the other third, it presents as a persistent pneumonitis. Other manifestations including fever, rash, arthralgia, muscle symptoms, peripheral neuropathy and nephritis occur concomitantly or follow the respiratory disease. The course is variable with death the usual outcome after five weeks to four years, the average duration being five months.[118] The cause of death is respiratory failure, uremia, or cardiac insufficiency. Most patients (97 per cent) are anemic. Leukocytosis (68 per cent) and eosinophilia (46 per cent) are common. The majority (83 per cent) develop renal failure, but only 24 per cent have hypertension. Chest x-rays reveal multiple round lesions bilaterally in over half the cases; a bronchopneumonic picture is found in another one-fourth.

Diagnosis

It seems possible that some of the cases referred to by Rose and Spencer[98] as "polyarteritis with lung involvement" and by Churg and Strauss[21] as "allergic granulomatous angiitis" had this syndrome. Immunofluorescent studies by Paronetto[83] revealed gamma globulin and complement in the vessels of one case of the Churg and Strauss syndrome, but not in the vessels of one case of Wegener's granulomatosis; no such deposits were found in the granulomas in both disorders. All lesions contained fibrinogen.

A more limited form of Wegener's granulomatosis was described by Carrington and Liebow[18] in 16 patients: 9 had only pulmonary lesions, and 7 had also extrapulmonary lesions, but nephritis was absent. Four additional cases of this limited form have been reported;[19] in them, the efficacy of prednisone therapy was uncertain.

Certain cases of Loeffler's syndrome may represent a milder and reversible form of Wegener's disease. The relationship to midline granuloma is not clear, but Spear and Walker[109] have reported histopathological differences. However, in a few instances of the disease called "midline granuloma" polyarteritis has been reported.[120] Relationships to Goodpasture's syndrome have been described,[57] but are not convincing.

Treatment

Antibiotics are often needed to combat secondary infections in the upper and lower respiratory tracts. In Wegener's granulomatosis corticosteroids are even less effective than in polyarteritis. However, there have been numerous reports of benefit from several immunosuppressive agents, including chlorambucil,[74] mechlorethamine,[48] azathioprine,[12,82] methotrexate,[17] and cyclophosphamide.[86] Long-term, and at times maintenance, therapy is usually required.

CRANIAL ARTERITIS
(Giant Cell Arteritis)

A more benign and distinct variant of polyarteritis is cranial arteritis, first described by Jonathan Hutchinson[53] in 1890 and defined as a syndrome by

Horton[51] in 1934. It is better known as "temporal arteritis," but this name is not sufficiently inclusive. It has also been recently referred to as "giant cell arteritis"; this is probably the best designation. Characteristically one or more branches of the carotid artery are involved in individuals of either sex, who are usually over fifty-five years of age. Three-fourths of the patients are women.

Pathology

Microscopically, it is a panarteritis. There is diffuse fibrotic thickening of the intima with narrowing of the lumen and often thrombosis. The internal elastic lamina may be disrupted. Maximal inflammatory change is found in the media where one sees focal necroses and granulomas containing numerous giant cells. In some patients with normal findings on routine histopathologic examination, electron microscopy revealed degeneration of smooth muscle cells in the media.[92]

Involvement of the temporal arteries is most frequent. However, disease of the retinal vessels is common and the process may affect others including the carotid, subclavian, coronary, renal, mesenteric and pulmonary, as well as those of the extremities. Involvement of extra-cranial arteries is usually discovered at autopsy, not being associated as a rule with detectable clinical manifestations. The lone exception to this is polymyalgia rheumatica with which cranial arteritis seems to be intimately associated. (*See* Chapter 50.)

Clinical Features

Cranial arteritis begins with headache and a variety of other manifestations such as fever, malaise, weight loss, weakness, muscle and joint pains, mild anemia and leukocytosis. The headache is often severe and boring in character. It is usually bilateral but more intense on one side. The temporal arteries become prominent, tortuous, red and tender and then nodular. Pain may also be felt in neighboring structures such as the scalp, face, jaws, neck and eyes.

Thirty to 50 per cent of patients may complain of ocular pain, photophobia, diplopia or loss of vision. Examination may reveal weakness of the ocular muscles and in the severe cases the fundi may show signs of occlusive central retinal arteritis. Listening for vascular bruits, especially over the eyeballs, is another diagnostic aid. Intracerebral arteries of large, medium and small caliber may be involved resulting in such manifestations as confusion, convulsions, hemiparesis or coma. The cerebrospinal fluid protein concentration may be elevated.

One-fourth to one-half of patients with polymyalgia rheumatica have giant cell arteritis, confirmed by temporal artery biopsy.[14,52] In many of these patients the temporal arteries are normal on examination, and there may be no cranial symptoms.[8]

Laboratory Findings

Temporal artery biopsy is the most important laboratory procedure. Temporal arteriography provides an additional useful diagnostic tool per se, and may assist in selecting the optimal site for biopsy.[36] The typical arteriogram shows many long, dilated and stenotic segments in arterial branches. The erythrocyte sedimentation rate is usually greatly elevated in almost all patients, and provides a useful index in regulating the dosage of corticosteroids. Serum alpha-2-globulin and fibrinogen levels are both raised; but gamma globulins are normal and test results for rheumatoid factor, L.E. cells and antinuclear antibody are negative.[2,121]

Treatment

Cranial arteritis is a self-limited but protracted illness, most patients recovering after two months to five years of illness. However, during this period of active disease the risk of blindness is 30 per cent.[9] Steroid therapy can prevent blindness, but can not promote recovery of vision, once impaired. With steroid therapy in moderate doses, the headache and other features usually disappear promptly.

Because cranial arteritis is a disease almost exclusively of the elderly, its pathogenesis may be an unusual reaction to some degenerative process arising in the intima of the proximal arteries.

AORTIC ARCH ARTERITIS

This syndrome has also been referred to as "aortic arch syndrome," "pulseless disease," "Takayasu's disease," "young female arteritis," or "branchial arteritis." The first description by Takayasu in 1909 was based on the combination of unusual ophthalmoscopic findings and absent radial pulses. Thereafter, additional Japanese cases were reported and, until the 1950's, the disease was thought to be peculiar to that country.[63] During recent years, however, numerous cases have been described in the European and American literature from a large number of countries all over the world. The majority have been females from nine to forty-five years of age. The recent literature emphasizes systemic manifestations[110] and immunologic abnormalities.[4]

Pathology

The elastic arteries originating from the aortic arch and the thoracic aorta are involved by a segmental panarteritis. The adventitia and media are infiltrated with lymphocytes and plasma cells.[1] Necrosis is most pronounced in the media. Thrombosis is frequent. There may be secondary arteriosclerosis with calcification of the aorta and its branches.[20]

Clinical Features

The pulses are absent in the neck, head and upper extremities. There is evidence of collateral circulation about the shoulders and elsewhere. Usually, the blood pressure is unobtainable in the arms and elevated in the legs. Typically, a high-pitched basilar murmur, systolic or continuous, is audible. A minority of cases have angina pectoris. Heart failure is common terminally. The hands are cool, symptoms of claudication develop in the upper extremities, and wasting may be noted in the upper half of the body. The face appears drawn and atrophic. Other manifestations include loss of teeth and hair, ulcers on the lips and the tip of the nose, and perforation of the nasal septum. Headache, syncope, mental confusion, reduced visual acuity and convulsions may result from reduced cerebral blood flow. Funduscopic examination may reveal a "crown-like" collection of dilated vessels about the optic discs, thought to represent arteriovenous anastomoses. Many of the symptoms, particularly reduction in visual acuity, are accentuated by physical activity.

Features of Polyarteritis Which Aid in Distinguishing It from Other Connective Tissue Disorders

1. Approximately 70 per cent of cases occur in men.
2. Bronchial asthma is a common feature.
3. Painful peripheral neuritis with foot drop and/or wrist drop.
4. A high incidence of severe abdominal pain with bloody diarrhea.
5. Hypochromic, microcytic anemia due to blood loss.
6. Leukocytosis in 80 per cent; with increases in polymorphonuclears, eosinophils or both.
7. Eosinophilia is frequently associated with bronchial asthma or other varieties of pulmonary involvement.
8. Biopsy material shows typical inflammation and necrosis of small arteries.

Also reported are fever, weight loss, anemia, leukocytosis, elevated sedimentation rate and a high serum gamma globulin concentration. One must differentiate this form of arteritis from various congenital abnormalities of the aorta and its branches, aortic aneurysm, syphilitic aortitis, chronic dissection of the aorta, ball-valve thrombus of the left atrium, and atrial tumor. It is separable from classical polyarteritis by its high incidence in young females, the size of the arteries involved and the distribution of the lesions.

Pathogenesis, Prognosis and Treatment

Serum immunoglobulin levels (IgG, IgA, and IgM) are all raised.[4] Antibodies against aorta have been found in two studies by Japanese[55,79] but not in three other studies.[4,47,110] This interesting difference deserves further exploration. Reports differ too with respect to the presence or absence of rheumatoid factor, antinuclear antibodies and L.E. cells. Roberts *et al.*[96] described an unusual patient with aortic arch arteritis, monoclonal gammopathy, and endocardial disease with septicemia.

The cause is unknown, although the preponderance in females suggests some endocrine abnormality. The prognosis is poor, most cases dying from cerebral or cardiac insufficiency. A favorable response to corticosteroids has been reported;[47] they may be most useful in the early systemic phase of the disease. Selected lesions such as renal artery stenosis may be corrected by arterial surgery.

SERUM SICKNESS

As originally described, serum sickness is an adverse reaction caused by the administration of heterologous serum, especially horse serum, into man. It was a very common disorder a generation ago when diphtheria and tetanus antitoxin and pneumococcal antisera were widely used. The classical description of serum sickness was published in 1905 by Von Pirquet and Schick.[115] It is a delayed systemic reaction, to be differentiated from the immediate type of anaphylactic reaction, which occurs in previously sensitized individuals.

Pathogenesis

Serum sickness is a disease caused by antigen-antibody interaction. Its pathogenesis has been well delineated by investigations of experimental models by Rich, Germuth, Dixon and others. At a critical time soluble antigen-antibody complexes are formed which cause vascular lesions by mobilizing the phagocytic and complement systems. The kinetics of these reactions have been summarized in detail by Dixon.[26] Similar mechanisms are involved in delayed allergic reactions to certain drugs, such as penicillin, and in the pathogenesis of systemic lupus erythematosus and polyarteritis. In serum sickness the data suggest a primary role for the IgG-precipitating type of antibody, and also reaginic antibodies, in inducing urticaria.

Clinical Features

The symptoms of primary serum sickness begin one to two weeks after the injection of serum. They may appear earlier, one to three days, in those who have been previously sensitized (accelerated serum sickness). The illness usually lasts four to ten days, but may persist for three weeks or longer. It consists of fever, urticaria, lymphadenopathy, myalgia, and arthralgia or arthritis. Erythema may occur at the injection site. Other cutaneous manifestations include diffuse or macular erythema, and purpura.

Joint involvement usually occurs in the more severe cases of serum sickness. It may be the outstanding feature of the illness, and the last to disappear. It usually involves large and medium-sized joints, although any joint may be affected. The arthritis is often migratory, and thus resembles that of rheumatic fever. Synovial fluid leukocytes may be as high as 20,000 per mm.[3]; usually polymorphonuclear leukocytes predominate.

Other manifestations in severely affected patients include vasculitis, glomerulonephritis, and neuritis. The vasculitis may involve many organs. Special features of the neuritis of serum sickness are involvement of the brachial plexus and the Guillain-Barré syndrome.

Laboratory abnormalities, that may be found, are mild leukocytosis, eosinophilia, increased sedimentation rate, proteinuria and hematuria, and reduced serum complement.

Treatment

As the disease is self-limited, most patients are well managed by epinephrine, antihistamines, soothing lotions and analgesics. For persistent symptoms and more serious and severe manifestations, such as glomerulonephritis or neuritis, corticosteroids are highly effective. The risks are minimal, since the duration of treatment is brief.

ANAPHYLACTOID PURPURA

(Henoch-Schönlein Purpura, Purpura Rheumatica, Allergic Purpura, Acute Vascular Purpura)

In its fully-developed state, this syndrome consists of: (1) non-thrombocytopenic purpura, (2) arthralgia or mild arthritis, (3) abdominal pain and gastrointestinal hemorrhage, and (4) renal disease. It occurs mostly in children, more frequently boys, and in young adults. Schönlein described the articular component in 1837, and Horton, the gastrointestinal and renal involvement in 1874. The distinction between Schönlein purpura and Henoch's purpura is artificial, since most patients are affected in both systems.

Etiology and Pathogenesis

The basic pathologic lesion is a widespread diffuse angiitis, involving arterioles and capillaries, of all affected organs, including the synovium.[81] There is a perivascular infiltrate with polymorphonuclear leukocytes (and at times eosinophils), extravasation of erythrocytes, endothelial cell swelling, and leukocyte-platelet thrombi.[113]

Although most patients with anaphylactoid purpura give a history of antecedent respiratory tract disease, the evidence of streptococcal infection from bacterial cultures and antistreptolysin-O titers is not impressive. Hypersensitivity to various foods and drugs has also been implicated,[1] but here too the evidence is at best presumptive.

The mechanisms by which these possibly etiologic agents produce the angiitis have not been elucidated. Vernier *et al.*[113] postulated that antigen-antibody complexes induce endothelial cell damage which leads to edema, hemorrhage and thrombosis. Little supporting data utilizing sophisticated immunologic techniques are available.

Clinical Features

The disease begins abruptly with varying combinations of rash, arthralgia and abdominal pain. The initial cutaneous manifestations consist of erythematous macules or urticarial papules distributed symmetrically over the extensor surfaces of the lower, and to a lesser degree, the upper extremities. They then darken, enlarge and coalesce, and gradually fade in approximately three weeks. One or more recurrences are common.

Two-thirds of the cases develop joint pain, usually after the onset of purpura. The joints may be tender and swollen, but other signs of inflammation are usually absent.[34] Most frequently affected are the knees and ankles, and occasionally the wrists and fingers. The arthritic symptoms subside after a few days leaving no residual deformity. Joint x-rays reveal only soft tissue swelling.[3]

The abdominal symptoms of crampy pain and melena also follow the onset of purpura. They may simulate an acute surgical abdomen. Children under five years of age may develop intussusception.

Renal involvement, with the urinary findings of acute glomerulonephritis, may end in fatal renal failure.[6] Proteinuria is found only in patients with hematuria.[3] The histopathology is that of focal or diffuse glomerulonephritis.

After the initial attack which lasts from one to five weeks, 40 per cent of patients have recurrences which consist mostly of purpura.[3] Articular recurrences are unusual. The prognosis is very good if renal and abdominal manifestations are mild.

Treatment

Only supportive treatment, *e.g.* transfusions, may be required. Salicylate therapy usually does not relieve the joint pain.[34] The role of corticosteroid therapy is not clear. Many of the acute manifestations respond promptly, but whether or not corticosteroids can favorably influence the renal disease is uncertain.

ERYTHEMA NODOSUM

Erythema nodosum is a relatively uncommon inflammatory disease consisting primarily of painful subcutaneous nodules of the legs. It occurs as an idiopathic disorder or a cutaneous feature of several diverse systemic diseases. It is associated with fever, malaise, and, in most cases, articular manifestations.

Pathogenesis

It is generally considered to be a poorly understood form of hypersensitivity to a variety of agents. Over thirty conditions have been associated with erythema nodosum. The most common, depending largely on the geographic location of the group studied, are: tuberculosis, sarcoidosis, coccidioidomycosis, and streptococcal infections. It is an infrequent complication of ulcerative colitis or regional enteritis. Five per cent are drug-induced; sulfonamides are the principal offenders.[100]

In two-thirds of the cases, however, no coexisting disease is found after thorough search.[100] The illness runs a benign, self-limited course usually subsiding in a few weeks or months.

Clinical Picture

Females are affected more often than males. Although the incidence is greatest in young women, the syndrome has been reported in a wide range of ages. In typical cases, there are constitutional symptoms at the onset with fever which may rise to 105° F.[56] The characteristic skin eruption occurs early in the course of the disease and consists of nodules in and under the skin which appear in crops at intervals of several days (Fig. 52–1). They are raised, definitely tender and seldom more than 2 inches in diameter. Their color varies from rose-pink to plum, and the overlying skin is often so shiny and tense that suppuration appears likely, although it almost never occurs. As the lesions subside there is an ecchymotic, residual discoloration, and most completely heal without scar. In most cases, the lesions are confined to the legs below the knees, although in severe cases both upper and lower extremities may be involved.

Joint manifestations occur in 60 to 75 per cent of cases.[56,112] They usually precede the nodules, but may come on concomitantly, or shortly thereafter. Joint pains may be severe, and there may be synovial effusion. Knees and ankles are most commonly involved, and then, wrists, fingers, shoulders, elbows and hips in order of frequency.[112] In ulcerative colitis[73] and sarcoidosis[44] arthritis is more common in those with erythema nodosum. Although joint manifestations usually disappear in a few weeks, articular symptoms have been known to last for as long as twelve months.[112]

Laboratory Findings

The erythrocyte sedimentation rate is usually very high. Serologic and skin tests are helpful in identifying specific

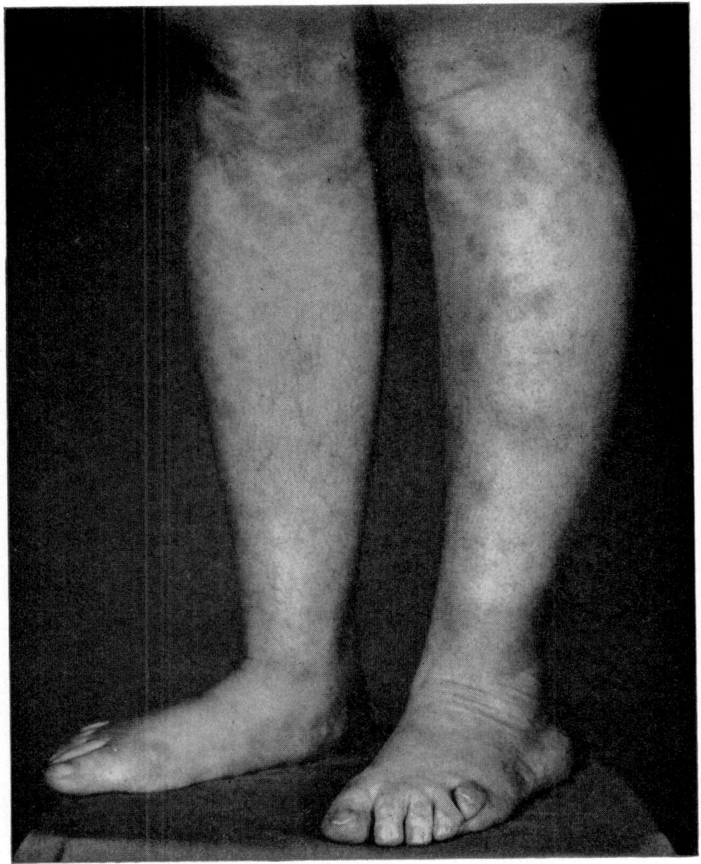

FIG. 52–1.—Patient is a thirty-two-year-old woman with two- to three-week history of morning stiffness and polyarthralgia. The skin lesions are typical of erythema nodosum. (See description in text.)

disease states associated with erythema nodosum. Some patients have hypergammaglobulinemia and positive sensitized sheep cell tests in low titer.[112] In contrast to nodular vasculitis, immunofluorescent study of erythema nodosum lesions failed to reveal deposits of IgG, IgM, complement or fibrinogen.[27] On chest x-ray hilar adenopathy (Fig. 52–2) may be found in the idiopathic and specific (*e.g.* sarcoidosis) forms of erythema nodosum.

Treatment

Elevation of the legs and analgesics may alleviate the symptoms of erythema nodosum. Corticosteroids are highly beneficial, but should be reserved for severe cases only, because of the benign, self-limited nature of the disease and the threat of fostering an undetected infection. Intravenous colchicine was promptly effective in one patient with idiopathic erythema nodosum but not in three with sarcoidosis.[116]

MISCELLANEOUS

Rheumatic Arteritis

Several workers have postulated a possible relation between rheumatic fever and polyarteritis. Aschoff bodies have been described in hearts of patients with

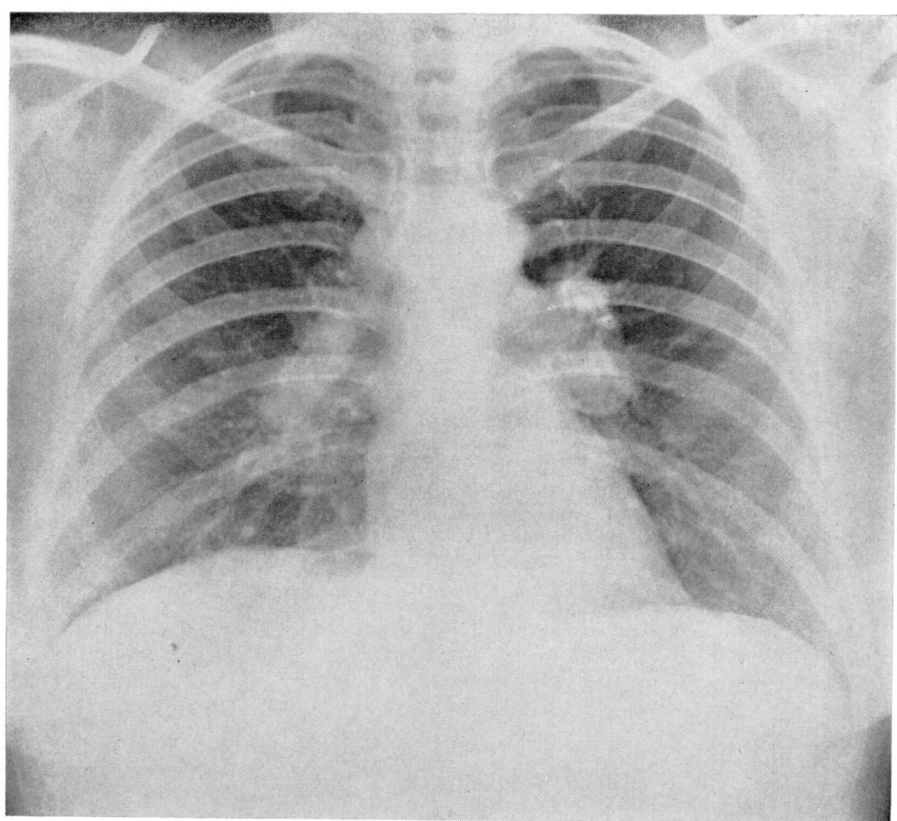

Fig. 52–2.—Chest x-ray of patient shown in Figure 52–1, demonstrating hilar adenopathy sometimes seen in erythema nodosum.

polyarteritis. Conversely, Von Glahn and Pappenheimer[114] reported an arteritis in 10 of 47 autopsies of patients with rheumatic fever. They differentiated these arteritic lesions from classical polyarteritis by an absence of thrombosis, involvement of only small arteries, and a paucity of eosinophils and plasma cells. Moreover, the lesions were sparse. According to Zeek[125] rheumatic arteritis is found in cases of fulminating rheumatic fever. Occasionally, it may involve the veins as well. It is usually confined to the heart and lungs, but rarely may be widespread. It simulates hypersensitivity angiitis, but is differentiated by the presence of Aschoff bodies. Healing results in nonspecific scarring.

Rose and Spencer[98] speculated that the association between the two disorders is that they "share a common relation to streptococcal infection, or that some patients may in addition be particularly prone to both diseases." It is possible that the vascular involvement in rheumatic fever is explained by the fact that the vessels are in the vicinity of and participate in the basic inflammatory reaction in the connective tissue. As rheumatic fever has become less common and fulminant, rheumatic arteritis has become rare.

Arterial Lesions of Hypertension

In the presence of rapidly advancing hypertension one may see arteriolosclerosis or arteriolonecrosis. In the arteriolonecrotic lesion there is a pink-staining alteration, which has the appearance of fibrinoid, and pyknotic cells of endothelial and smooth muscle cell origin. Inflammatory cells are only occasionally noted, and such hypertensive changes are rarely confused with polyarteritis.

Lesions are also frequently seen in the small muscular arteries, particularly those of the kidney, in patients dying with hypertension. Most commonly, there is an endarteritis obliterans, with endothelial cell proliferation and intimal scarring. Less frequently the scarring may extend into the media, inflammatory cells may be present and these lesions may resemble those seen in polyarteritis. Distinguishing features from polyarteritis are: (1) absence of adventitial involvement; (2) alterations in the entire circumference of the vessel wall (which may not be the case in polyarteritis); (3) edema, but little necrosis; and (4) absence of eosinophils.

Arteritis Following Resection of Coarctation of the Aorta

Seven cases have been recently reported of an arteritis with thrombosis of small mesenteric arteries occurring three to five days after surgical correction of aortic coarctation.[107] In one case symptoms did not begin until three months postoperatively. Some observers believe that these arterial changes may result from the sudden increase in pulse pressure while others consider them to be a special form of polyarteritis.

BIBLIOGRAPHY

1. Ackroyd, J. F.: Amer. J. Med., *14*, 605, 1953.
2. Alestig, K., and Barr, J.: Lancet, *1*, 1228, 1963.
3. Allen, D. M., Diamond, L. K., and Howell, D. A.: Amer. J. Dis. Child., *99*, 147, 1960.
4. Asherson, R. A., Asherson, G. L., and Schrire, V.: Brit. Med. J., *2*, 589, 1968.
5. Ball, J.: Ann. Rheum. Dis., *13*, 277, 1954.
6. Ballard, H. S., Eisinger, R. P., and Gallo, G.: Amer. J. Med., *49*, 328, 1970.
7. Bennett, G. A., Zeller, J. W., and Bauer, W.: Arch. Path., *30*, 70, 1940.
8. Bevan, A. T., Dunnill, M. S., and Harrison, M. J. G.: Ann. Rheum. Dis., *27*, 271, 1968.
9. Birkhead, N. C., Wagener, H. P., and Shick, R. M.: J.A.M.A., *163*, 821, 1957.
10. Black, R. L., Yielding, K. L., and Bunim, J. J.: J. Chronic Dis., *5*, 751, 1957.
11. Boren, R. J., and Everett, M. A.: Arch. Derm., *92*, 568, 1965.
12. Bouronola, B. A., Smith, E. J., and Cuppage, F. E.: Amer. J. Med., *42*, 314, 1967.
13. Boyd, L. J.: Bull. N.Y. Med. Coll., *1*, 219, 1938.
14. Bruk, M. S.: Ann. Rheum. Dis., *26*, 103, 1967.
15. Butler, K. R. and Palmer, J.: Canad. M.A.J., *72*, 686, 1955.
16. Bywaters, E. G. L.: Ann. Rheum. Dis., *16*, 84, 1957.
17. Capizzi, R. L., and Bertino, J. R.: Ann. Intern. Med., *74*, 74, 1971.
18. Carrington, C. B., and Liebow, A. A.: Amer. J. Med., *41*, 497, 1966.
19. Cassan, S. M., Coles, D. T., and Harrison, E. G., Jr.: Amer. J. Med., *49*, 366, 1970.
20. Cheitlin, M. D., and Carter, P. B.: Arch. Intern. Med., *116*, 283, 1965.
21. Churg, J. and Strauss, L.: Amer. J. Path., *27*, 277, 1951.
22. Citron, B. P., *et al.*: New Engl. J. Med., *283*, 1003, 1970.
23. Clark, E., and Kaplan, B. I.: Arch. Path., *24*, 458, 1937.
24. Cunliffe, W. J.: Lancet, *1*, 1226, 1968.
25. Dahl, E. V., Baggenstoss, A. H., and DeWeerd, J. H.: Amer. J. Med., *28*, 222, 1960.
26. Dixon, F. J.: In "*Immunological Diseases*" (2nd Ed.), M. Samter *et al.* (Eds.), Boston, Little, Brown & Co., 1971, Ch. 14.
27. Epstein, W. L.: in *Immunological Diseases*, 2nd Ed., Samter, M. *et al.*, Ed., Little, Brown & Co., Boston, 1971.
28. Epstein, W. V. and Engleman, E. P.: Arth. & Rheum., *2*, 250, 1959.
29. Ford, R. G., and Sickert, R. G.: Neurology, *15*, 114, 1965.
30. Fordham, C. C., III, Epstein, F. H., Huffines, W. D., and Harrington, J. T.: Ann. Intern. Med., *61*, 89, 1964.
31. Franklin, E. C., Kunkel, H. G., and Ward, J. R.: Arth. & Rheum., *1*, 400, 1958.
32. Freedman, P., Peters, J. H., and Kark, R. M.: Arch. Intern. Med., *105*, 524, 1960.

33. Frohnert, P. P., and Sheps, S. G.: Amer. J. Med., *43*, 8, 1967.
34. Gairdner, D.: Quart. J. Med., *17*, 95, 1948.
35. Germuth, F. G., Jr., Flanagan, C., and Montenegro, M. R.: Bull. Johns Hopkins Hosp., *101*, 149, 1957.
36. Gillanders, L. A., Strachan, R. W., and Blair, D. W.: Ann. Rheum. Dis., *28*, 267, 1969.
37. Gitlin, D., Craig, J. M., and Janeway, C. A.: Amer. J. Path., *33*, 55, 1957.
38. Glaser, R. J., Dammin, G. J., and Wood, W. B., Jr.: Arch. Path., *52*, 253, 1951.
39. Godman, G. C. and Churg, J.: Arch. Path., *58*, 533, 1954.
40. Gocke, D. J., Hsu, K., Morgan, G., Bombardier, S., Lockshin. M., and Christian, C. L.: J. Clin. Invest., *29*, 35, 1970.
41. Golding, D. N.: Brit. Med. J., *1*, 277, 1970.
42. Gresham, G. A. and Phear, D. N.: Amer. J. Med., *23*, 671, 1957.
43. Gruber, G. B.: Virchow's Arch. Path. Anat., *258*, 441, 1925.
44. Gumpel, J. M., Johns, C. J., and Shulman, L. E.: Ann. Rheum. Dis., *26*, 194, 1967.
45. Hart, F. D., Golding, J. R., and Mackenzie, D. H.: Ann. Rheum. Dis., *16*, 471, 1957.
46. Hawn, C. V. Z., and Janeway, C. A.: J. Exper. Med., *85*, 571, 1947.
47. Hirsch, M. S., Aikat, B. K., and Basu, A. K.: Bull. Johns Hopkins Hosp., *115*, 329, 1964.
48. Hollander, D., and Manning, R. T.: Ann. Intern. Med., *67*, 393, 1967.
49. Holsinger, D. R., Osmundson, P. J., and Edwards, J. E.: Circulation, *25*, 610, 1962.
50. Hopps, H. C. and Wissler, R. W.: J. Lab. Clin. Med., *31*, 939, 1946.
51. Horton, B. T., Magath, T. B., and Brown, G. E.: Arch. Intern. Med., *53*, 400, 1934.
52. Hunder, G. G., Disney, T. F., and Ward, L. E.: Mayo Clin. Proc., *44*, 849, 1969.
53. Hutchinson, J.: Arch. Surg. (London), *1*, 323, 1890.
54. Irby, R., Adams, R. A., and Toone, E. C.: Arth. & Rheum., *1*, 44, 1958.
55. Ito, I.: Jap. Circ. J., *30*, 75, 1966.
56. James, D. G.: Brit. Med. J., *1*, 853, 1961.
57. Johnson, J. R. and McGovern, V. J.: Austral. Ann. Med., *11*, 250, 1962.
58. Johnson, R. L., Smyth, C. J., Holt, G. W., Lubshenco, A., and Valentin, E.: Arch. & Rheum., *2*, 224, 1959.
59. Karsner, H. T.: *Acute Inflammation of Arteries*, Springfield, Charles C Thomas, 1947.
60. Kellgren, J. H. and Ball, J.: Brit. Med. J., *1*, 523, 1959.
61. Kemper, J. W., Baggenstoss, A. H., and Slocumb, C. H.: Ann. Intern. Med., *46*, 831, 1957.
62. Knowles, H. C., Zeek, P. M., and Blankenhorn, M. A.: Arch. Intern. Med., *92*, 789, 1953.
63. Koszewski, B. J.: Angiology, *9*, 180, 1958.
64. Krupp, M. A.: Arch. Intern. Med., *71*, 54, 1943.
65. Kussmaul, A. and Maier, R.: Deutsches Arch. Klin. Med., *1*, 484, 1866.
66. Lachmann, P. J., Muller-Eberhard, H. J., Kunkel, H. G., and Paronetto, F.: J. Exp. Med., *115*, 63, 1962.
67. Ladefoged, J., Nielsen, B., Raaschou, F., and Sorensen, A. W. S.: Amer. J. Med., *46*, 827, 1969.
68. Lofgren, S.: Scand. J. Resp. Dis., *48*, 348, 1967.
69. Lowman, E. W.: Ann. Rheum. Dis., *11*, 146, 1942.
70. Lucke, V. M.: Vet. Rec., *82*, 622, 1968.
71. McCall, M. and Pennock, J. W.: Ann. Intern. Med., *21*, 628, 1944.
72. McCombs, R. P.: J.A.M.A., *194*, 157, 1965.
73. McEwen, C.: Clin. Orthoped., *57*, 9, 1968.
74. McIlvanie, S. K.: J.A.M.A., *197*, 90, 1966.
75. Maxeiner, S. R., McDonald, J. R., and Kirklin, J. W.: Surg. Clin. North America, *32*, 1225, 1952.
76. Medical Research Council: Brit. Med. J., *1*, 1399, 1960.
77. Mellors, R. C., and Ortega, L. G.: Amer. J. Path., *32*, 455, 1956.
78. Mowrey, F. H. and Lundberg, E. A.: Ann. Intern. Med., *40*, 1145, 1954.
79. Nakao, K., *et al.*: Circulation, *35*, 1141, 1967.
80. Nasu, T.: Angiology, *14*, 225, 1963.
81. Norkin, S., and Wiener, J.: Amer. J. Clin. Path., *33*, 55, 1960.
82. Norton, W. L., Suki, W., and Strunk, S.: Arch. Intern. Med., *121*, 554, 1968,
83. Paronetto, F.: In *Textbook of Immunopathology*, P. Miescher and H. J. Miller-Eberhard (Eds), New York, Grune and Stratton, 1969, Ch. 59.
84. Paronetto, F. and Strauss, L.: Ann. Intern. Med., *56*, 289, 1962.
85. Paulley, J. W. and Hughes, J. P.: Brit. Med. J., *2*, 1562, 1960.
86. Pearson, C. M., and Novack, S. N.: Arth. & Rheum., *14*, 408, 1971.
87. Plaut, A.: Amer. J. Path., *27*, 247, 1951.
88. Prince, A. M., and Trepo, C.: Lancet, *1*, 1309, 1971.

89. RACKEMANN, F. M. and GREENE, J. E.: Tr. Assoc. Amer. Physicians, *54*, 112, 1939.
90. RAGAN, C.: J. Chronic Dis., *5*, 688, 1957.
91. RALSTON, D. E. and KVALE, W. F.: Proc. Staff Meet., Mayo Clin., *24*, 18, 1949.
92. REINECKE, R. D., and KNWABARA, T.: Arch. Ophthal., *82*, 446, 1969.
93. RICH, A. R.: Bull. Johns Hopkins Hospital, *71*, 123, 1942.
94. ———: Harvey Lectures, *42*, 106, 1946–7.
95. RICH, A. R. and GREGORY, J. E.: Bull. Johns Hopkins Hosp., *72*, 65, 1943.
96. ROBERTS, W. C., MCGREGOR, R. R., DEBLANC, H. J., JR., BEISU, A. D., and WOLFF, S. M.: Amer. J. Med., *46*, 313, 1969.
97. ROSE, G. A.: Brit. Med. J., *2*, 1148, 1957.
98. ROSE, G. A. and SPENCER, H.: Quart J. Med., *26*, 43, 1957.
99. ROSS, R. W.: Quart. J. Med., *28*, 471, 1959.
100. SAMS, W. M., and WINKELMANN, R. K.: Southern Med. J., *61*, 676, 1968.
101. SCHMIDT, F. R., COOPER, N. S., ZIFF, M., and MCEWEN, C.: Amer. J. Med., *30*, 56, 1961.
102. SCHREINER, G. E.: Ann. Intern. Med., *42*, 826, 1955.
103. SCOTT, J. T., HOURIHANE, D. O., DOYLE, F. H., STEINER, R. E., LAWS, J. W., DIXON, A. S., and BYWATERS, E. C. G.: Ann. Rheum. Dis., *20*, 224, 1961.
104. SHICK, R. M.: Med. Clin. North America, *42*, 959, 1958.
105. SHORT, C. L., BAUER, W., and REYNOLDS, W. E.: *Rheumatoid Arthritis*, Cambridge, Harvard University Press, 1957.
106. SINCLAIR, R. J. G. and CRUICKSHANK, B.: Quart. J. Med., *25*, 313, 1956.
107. SINGLETON, A. O., JR., MCGINNIS, L. S., and EASON, H. R.: Surgery, *45*, 665, 1959.
108. SOKOLOFF, L. and BUNIM, J. J.: J. Chronic Dis., *5*, 668, 1957.
109. SPEAR, G. S. and WALKER, W. G., JR.: Bull. Johns Hopkins Hosp., *99*, 313, 1956.
110. STRACHAN, R. W., WIGSELL, F. W., and ANDERSON, J. R.: Amer. J. Med., *40*, 560, 1966.
111. TALBOTT, J. H. and FERRANDIS, R. M.: *Collagen Diseases*, New York, Grune & Stratton, 1956.
112. TRUELOVE, L. H.: Ann. Rheum. Dis., *19*, 174, 1960.
113. VERNIER, R. L., WORTHEN, H. G., PETERSON, R. D., COLLE, E., and GOOD, R. A.: Pediatrics, *27*, 181, 1961.
114. VON GLAHN, W. C., and PAPPENHEIMER, A. M.: Amer. J. Path., *2*, 235, 1926.
115. VON PIRQUET, C. F., and SCHICK, B.: *Die Serum Krankheit*, Leipzig, Wier, 1905.
116. WALLACE, S. L., BERNSTEN, D., and DIAMOND, H.: J.A.M.A., *199*, 525, 1967.
117. WALLACE, S. L., LATTES, R., and RAGAN, C.: Amer. J. Med., *25*, 600, 1958.
118. WALTON, E. W.: Brit. Med. J., *2*, 265, 1958.
119. WIGLEY, R. D., and COUCHMAN, K. G.: Nature, *211*, 319, 1966.
120. WILLIAMS, H. L.: Ann. Otolaryngol., *58*, 1014, 1949.
121. WILSKE, K. R., and HEALEY, L. A.: Ann. Intern. Med., *66*, 77, 1967.
122. WILSON, K. S. and ALEXANDER, H. L.: J. Lab. Clin. Med., *30*, 195, 1945.
123. YANG, Y. H.: Lab. Invest., *14*, 81, 1965.
124. YUST, I., SCHWARTZ, J., and DREYFUSS, F.: Amer. J. Med., *48*, 472, 1970.
125. ZEEK, P. M.: New Engl. J. Med., *248*, 764, 1953.

Chapter 53

Polymyositis and Dermatomyositis

By Carl M. Pearson, M.D.

Polymyositis and dermatomyositis are diffuse inflammatory and degenerative disorders of striated muscle, which cause symmetrical weakness and, to a lesser degree, atrophy of muscle. They are perplexing diseases of unknown cause which occur in all age groups, but predominate in mid-adult life and are more common in women. They are usually grouped with the collagen or connective tissue diseases and such a classification is permissible since some overlapping clinical and laboratory features commonly occur, especially with rheumatoid arthritis or scleroderma, and less frequently with systemic lupus erythematosus or polyarteritis. In addition, a link seems to exist between certain cases of myositis and visceral malignancy.

CLASSIFICATION

Any classification of polymyositis and dermatomyositis will probably be inaccurate and incomplete because it is probable that under this category are included a number of different but moderately similar disorders which have as their principal features muscular weakness, sometimes associated skin lesions, and variable degrees of inflammatory reaction in muscle. This variability in clinical and pathological features relative to classification has been handled differently by various authors.[7,22,56,45] No classification has so far proved to be wholly satisfactory.

The chief merit of the classification to be suggested below seems to be that it provides a guide for prognosis and especially to segregate those forms of disease which will respond favorably, or otherwise, to therapy, especially corticosteroids. With this aim in mind, the following groupings of cases are offered (Table 53–1). Certain features such as Raynaud's phenomenon, subacute arthritis or mild scleroderma may occur in any of the types.

Table 53-1.—Classification of Polymyositis

Type	*Name*
I	Typical polymyositis
II	Typical dermatomyositis
III	Typical dermatomyositis (occasionally polymyositis) with malignancy
IV	Childhood dermatomyositis
V	Acute myolysis
VI	Polymyositis in conjunction with Sjögren's syndrome

GENERAL DISCUSSION

Polymyositis and dermatomyositis encompass a group of disorders in which muscular weakness is the principal clinical feature. Pathologically inflammatory and degenerative changes are found in the muscles in these conditions. Rarely, if ever, can the diagnosis be made in the absence of demonstrable decline in strength, although elevation of serum enzymes and histological alterations alone may be present in the earliest phase of the disease before clinical weakness has developed.

About one-half of all cases of polymyositis are linked either with one of the collagen or connective tissue disorders, or with a malignant tumor. The remainder develop as isolated primary myopathies or occur in conjunction with skin manifestations (dermatomyositis).

Although the first recorded case of polymyositis was described by Wagner as long ago as 1863[54] this condition has received comparatively little attention until recently. The more dramatic and clinically apparent subgroup dermatomyositis, first outlined by Unverricht,[53] has held the spotlight for more than half a century as the predominant inflammatory myopathy.

It is only within the past decade that we have realized that most of the myositides do not show dermal lesions at all, or at best these often occur in unusual forms. The reasons for the delay in appreciation of the disease spectrum of polymyositis have been several: (a) infrequent use of muscle biopsy as a diagnostic procedure until recent years. The histopathology thus viewed has assisted in the separation of several types of primary myopathy of adult life, especially chronic polymyositis, from the forms of muscular dystrophy which have their onset in adulthood; (b) realization came slowly that myositis may have a very insidious onset and that muscular pain and tenderness are often non-existent; (c) cases of polymyositis without skin changes were once thought to be rare, but actually have been shown to comprise about one-half of the total cases.

Within the past two decades a number of excellent reviews on the topic of polymyositis and its variants have appeared and the reader is referred to these for more details of specific features about individual cases and series.[3,4,22,32,39,42,44,56]

INCIDENCE

Polymyositis and dermatomyositis may occur at virtually any age. Documented cases have been described before 2 years of age or as late as the eighth decade. Generally, however, the largest proportion arises in the fifth and sixth decades (Table 52–2).

Table 53-2.—Age and Onset in 432 Cases of Polymyositis*

Age Range (years)	*Number of Cases*	*Total (per cent)*
0–15	69	16
16–30	56	15
31–45	108	24
46–60	157	36
61–	42	9

* From Barwick and Walton (1963).

Women are affected twice as commonly as men. In a composite of 414 cases from several series,[40] 279 (67 per cent) were female and 137 (33 per cent) male.

The general frequency of polymyositis is difficult to assess so that only estimates of its incidence are possible. It is not very rare, as shown by combined reports of about 800 cases which have accumulated in the literature in a span of 12 years, although most of these were reviews of clinic and hospital series built up over previous years. Rose and Walton[45] saw 89 new cases during a 12-year span between 1954 and 1965, from an estimated regional population of 3.3 million persons. They calculated, based upon a 1961 census of the United Kingdom of 52.6 million persons, that 150 to 200 new cases occur per year in that population, an estimated incidence of 1 case per 280,000 per year. In our own clinical service with 600 teaching beds, we routinely see about ten to fifteen new cases per year. A personal series of 145 cases has thus been accumulated within the past 12 years. For comparison, about 90 new cases of rheumatoid arthritis are seen in our clinics and hospital each year, as are 30 cases of lupus erythematosus, 16 of scleroderma, 3 of polyarteritis, 4 of endogenous Cushing's disease, and 30 of gout.

Of the primary myopathies which affect the proximal muscle groups of the pelvis, shoulder girdle and limbs, polymyositis is about as common as muscular dystrophy in adult life, whereas in childhood it is much less common.[56]

PRELIMINARY SYMPTOMS

Polymyositis and dermatomyositis may start in one of several ways and there is no stereotyped manner of onset. Based upon an analysis of many of my own cases and those drawn from Walton and Adams[56] series a total of 100 in all, Table 53–3 defines the first observable symptoms in the cases of this group.

The initial diagnosis of myositis is uncommonly made in the early stages. Reasons for this include: (a) general unfamiliarity with the condition; (b) variability in the mode of onset, as outlined in Table 53–3; (c) insidious onset of weakness in many cases simulating muscular dystrophy; (d) the initial symptom is nonmuscular in more than one-third of the cases.

In Table 53–4 are tabulated the initial diagnoses in 95 cases, again from Walton and Adams' series[56] and from some of my own.

Table 53-3.—The First Symptom in 100 Cases

	Number
Muscular weakness	
Legs	44
Arms	8
Dysphagia	2
Skin rash	24
Joint or muscular pains	15
Other feature*	7

* Includes fever, chills, general fatigue, sore throat, Raynaud's phenomenon, etc.

Table 53-4.—Initial Clinical Diagnosis in 95 Cases*

	No. of Times Diagnosed†	
Neuromuscular		
Progressive muscular dystrophy	26	
Polymyositis and dermatomyositis	19	
Myasthenia gravis	12	
Polyneuritis	10	78
Poliomyelitis	3	
Progressive muscular atrophy	5	
Paralytic myoglobinuria	2	
Tumor of muscle	1	
Rheumatic		
Rheumatoid arthritis	12	
Systemic lupus erythematosus	10	
"Acute rheumatism"	2	27
"Collagen disease"	2	
Fibrositis	1	
Dermatological		
Scleroderma	7	
Seborrheic dermatitis	4	
Exfoliative dermatitis	2	18
Other dermatoses	5	
Other Conditions		
Streptococcal pharyngitis	2	3
Addison's disease	1	

* From Walton and Adams[56] and Pearson.[40]

† Multiple diagnosis in some cases.

PRECIPITATING FACTORS

Although a wide variety of factors have been incriminated as inciting agents in individual cases, the fact remains that in the great majority of instances no initiating cause is evident. Some cases have been preceded by a febrile illness,[23] an exanthem[46] or benign infection or trauma.[7] Photosensitization is common in dermatomyositis and exposure to sunlight may initiate an eruption on the face, arms and upper trunk which can be the first clinical evidence of that disease.[48,57,24] Moreover, some cases have developed after, or have been intensified by, sulfonamide[48,57] or penicillin therapy. Prior infection or intensification by drugs suggests a hypersensitivity mechanism. However, one should keep in mind the greater likelihood that the disease was already present in a subclinical form and that it was merely brought to the point of clinical recognition by one of the aforementioned factors.

Malignancy occurs in a far greater proportion of cases than would be expected by pure chance[21] and commonly there is evidence for its existence months or years prior to the onset of muscular weakness. Among the 145 cases of polymyositis with which we have dealt personally, 22 have had a malignant tumor. Evidence of tumor existed before development of myositis in 8 of them, although it was not diagnosed until later in some. Whether tumor can actually be called a "precipitating factor" is a debatable point. More likely, in those cases where it coexists, it plays a complex etiological role.

Table 53-5.—Percentage of Clinical Signs and Symptoms in 200 Cases of Polymyositis*

Musculature	*Per cent*
Weakness:	
Proximal muscles	
Lower extremities	95
Upper extremities	76
Distal muscles	27
Neck flexors	62
Dysphagia	47
Facial muscles	6
Extraocular muscles	2
Pain or tenderness	48
Contractures	27
Atrophy	50
Skin	
"Typical" dermatomyositis	44
"Atypical" features	20
Other	
Raynaud's phenomenon	30
Arthritic or rheumatic features	24
Intestinal disorders	8
Pulmonary disorders	4

* From Walton and Adams,[56] Eaton,[22] Barwick and Walton[4] and personal series.

CLINICAL CHARACTERISTICS

Not only is the early clinical picture of polymyositis variable in type and form, but also in tempo or rate of onset and progression of symptoms, whether muscular, dermal, articular or other. Moreover, in some chronic cases the clinical course is one of "spontaneous" exacerbations and remissions. This variability from one case to another usually persists throughout the disease and makes it nearly impossible to give a unified clinical portrait of the disease. The extremes are seen in (*a*) acute polymyositis, with or without an edematous skin rash, severe constitutional symptoms and rapid loss of strength, and (*b*) the gradual appearance of weakness in the pelvic girdle musculature over a 5- to 7-year period with no other features, except perhaps for Raynaud's phenomenon or slight evidence of scleroderma of the hands and arms.

Some of these variables will be dealt with below under classification. What follows is a general picture of myositis as it affects the various systems. In Table 53–5 is shown the overall incidence of symptoms in 200 cases collected from several sources.

MUSCULAR MANIFESTATIONS

Muscular weakness is present in *all* cases of polymyositis and in its absence the clinical diagnosis cannot be made with assurance. In subacute or chronic cases the weakness comes on slowly, first affects the lower limbs and closely resembles muscular dystrophy. Hence difficulty in arising from the floor or getting out of a bathtub is often mentioned in retrospect, as initial evidence of weakness. Likewise it may become impossible to climb up on a high bus step. Soon difficulty is experienced when arising from a low lounge chair and then from a higher chair. Stairs can be ascended only with the assistance of a hand-rail and the gait becomes clumsy and waddling. There is a tendency to fall after which it is impossible to arise without assistance.

At some point, usually after the appearance of pelvic girdle weakness, loss of strength in the shoulder girdle becomes clinically manifest. Hence two or three books cannot be placed on a high shelf unless two hands are used and combing the hair or keeping the arms elevated for more than a few moments is impossible. Later the arms cannot be abducted to the horizontal, even against gravity alone. Weakness of the anterior neck muscles is shown by an inability to raise the head from the pillow while in bed but the patient is rarely aware of this feature until it is called to his attention. Involvement of the posterior pharyngeal muscles gives a picture of partial bulbar palsy with dysphagia and dysphonia. The latter is usually manifest as a nasal voice.

In severe or advanced cases the weakness may be extreme and the patient is bedridden, or at best confined to a wheelchair. In such cases progressive involvement of the respiratory muscles may prove fatal. Such cases are, in our experience, extreme rarities unless a very acute myolytic process exists from the start, or a coexistent malignancy makes the muscular disease refractory to corticosteroid therapy.

In a few cases muscular pain, tenderness and induration are present in the early stages and are accompanied by the erythematous rash of dermatomyositis. Pain is most often manifest about the shoulders, upper back and in the upper arms and forearms. It is usually less obvious in the thighs and elsewhere.

Contractures or shortening of muscles rarely occurs early. They are features of advanced or long-standing disease. They involve the biceps brachii, producing contractures at the elbows; the wrist flexors, preventing full extension of the wrists without flexion of the fingers; and the hamstrings, producing shortening. Atrophy of muscles is also a late event and is usually mild or moderate in extent; this is another point of differentiation from advanced dystrophy, in which atrophy is often extensive. Calcinosis of the muscles may result from a severe bout of acute myositis and occurs most often in children. Occasionally, ulcerations over the bony prominences or elsewhere may extrude calcium.

DERMAL FEATURES

The typical rash of dermatomyositis occurs in about 40 per cent of the patients. In addition, another one-quarter of the patients will show a variety of dermal atrophy (poikiloderma) to transient erythema or a scaling eruption resembling 'eczema.'

It is not at all uncommon in any type of polymyositis to find, in conjunction with active muscle disease, dusky red patches which are slightly elevated and smooth or slightly scaly on the elbows, on the knuckles, over the knees and on the medial malleoli at the ankles. Sometimes there are linear hyperemic streaks on the backs of the hands and fingers with accentuation over the extensor surface of the joints. In conjunction, there is also hyperemia about the base of the fingernails, along the sides of the nails and on the ends of the fingers (Fig. 53–1). These areas become shiny, red, somewhat atrophic and the skin is constantly flaking or peeling.

Emphasis has been placed upon these features since they are commonly overlooked. When recognized they may provide the needed clinical clue in an otherwise puzzling case. During the active phases of the myositis the plaques may become tender and elevated and occasionally they ulcerate and drain. In

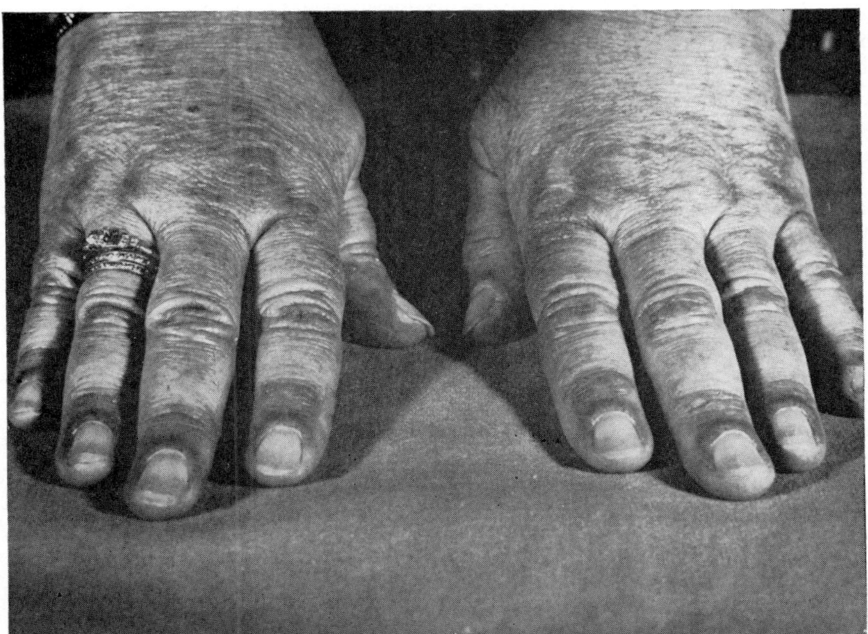

FIG. 53–1.—Diffuse erythema about the base of all the nails in a classical case of dermatomyositis. Also shown moderately well are erythema and scaling of the knuckles with extension up the forearms.

quiescent periods, usually with corticosteroid suppression, they become smaller but remain as whitened atrophic patches. On several occasions a recoloration of these areas, in association with an increase in tenderness, has heralded a reactivation of the myositic process.

The "typical" rash of dermatomyositis consists of a dusky erythematous eruption on the face, especially in the "butterfly" distribution, in the periorbital regions, occasionally on the forehead, and also on the neck, shoulders, front and back of the upper chest and proximal or distal portions of the arms (Fig. 53–2). The erythema may be mottled or diffuse and intensely red or cyanotic. On the upper eyelids a peculiar dusky lilac suffusion can be seen, sometimes as the most prominent feature of an otherwise faint erythema of the face. This has been called the heliotrope rash and is quite pathognomonic for dermatomyositis. In conjunction with facial erythema scaly rash can be found on the extensor surfaces of the forearms along with erythematous plaques on the elbows, knuckles and elsewhere as described above.

In very acute cases the erythema of the shoulders, arms and neck may be accompanied by intradermal and subcutaneous edema. In association with underlying edema and extreme tenderness of the muscles, these dermal changes contribute to the characteristic clinical picture of acute dermatomyositis. Other less common dermal features include, in addition to moderate sclerodermatous thickening of the hands and arms, diffuse or focal hyperpigmentation or vitiligo, telangiectasia of the face, anterior chest and shoulders, and some loss of scalp hair.

The comment was made above that in the absence of muscular weakness the diagnosis of polymyositis cannot be made. However, I have for some time observed five women who show the completely typical erythematous and heliotrope eruption as described above in association with erythematous plaques on the elbows and elsewhere. In none of them can I find evidence of muscle disease, nor any other disorder. One woman has been observed repeatedly for 8 years. Hence it may be possible to dissociate the dermal from the muscular component in these very rare instances, whereas in many other cases the myositic process may occur without any dermal feature. In six other persons (4 women and 2 men) the rash is florid whereas weakness and EMG changes are very slight in degree. This variant could be called amyopathic dermatomyositis.

RAYNAUD'S PHENOMENON

As in the other collagen or connective tissue diseases, to which polymyositis has some relation, Raynaud's phenomenon occurs with considerable frequency. In a large series it is found in about one-third of all patients with polymyositis. It is usually not of severe degree, and never, in my experience, does it proceed to necrosis or permanent and serious change. The bluish cyanosis or total blanching of one or several fingers occurs as a result of local or general cooling. Emotional stress may likewise incite an attack. Most persons with polymyositis who exhibit Raynaud's phenomenon are also the ones who have mild features of scleroderma or acrosclerosis.

RHEUMATIC MANIFESTATIONS

Mild or transitory arthritis or rheumatic symptoms occur in from about

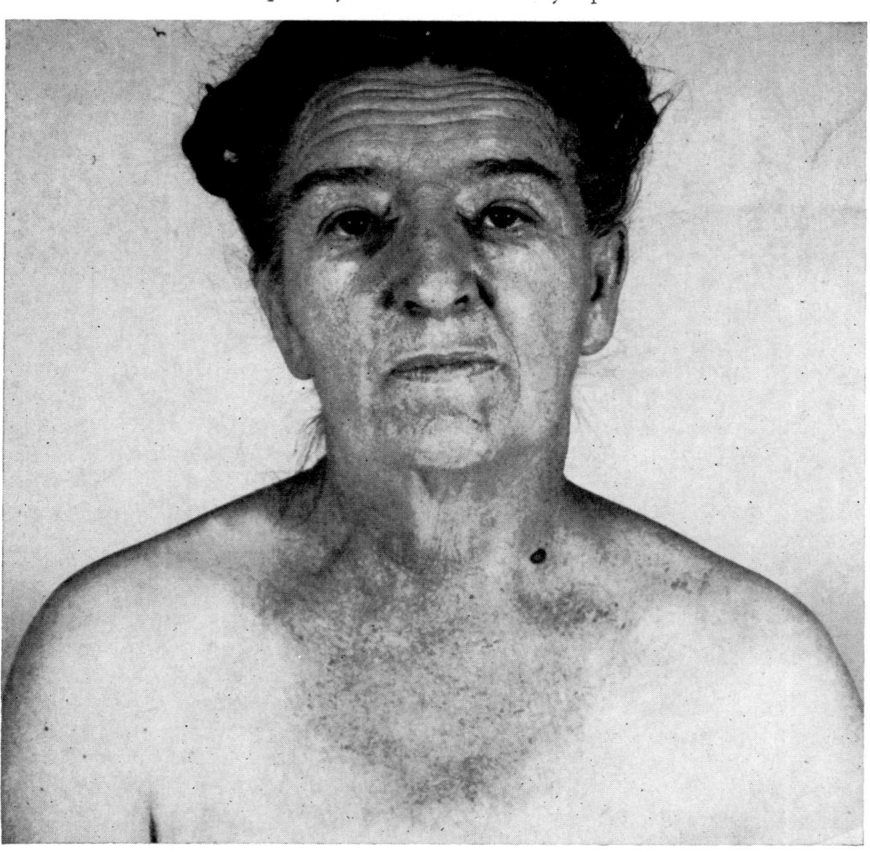

FIG. 53–2.—Classical dermatomyositis with diffuse erythema of the face, neck and V of the upper anterior chest as shown. There was also diffuse erythema and cyanosis of the upper eyelids and some periorbital edema.

one-third (Table 53–5) to one-half of all cases.[38] The clinical disease may be heralded by acute arthralgias or arthritis with effusions especially in wrists, knees and finger joints. In this phase the disease is identical with early rheumatoid arthritis. In a few cases articular symptoms have been present for one or many years before muscle weakness appears,[41] or rarely, they may develop after the myositic process is in evidence. All articular and rheumatic symptoms have responded promptly to corticosteroid therapy and no residual articular deformities have been seen except in a few patients who have had fairly typical, perhaps coexistent, rheumatoid arthritis for 3 or more years prior to the appearance of proximal muscle weakness and evidence of myositis on muscle biopsy.

Myopathic weakness typical of that seen in chronic polymyositis has been observed in two of the present cases, and has been described in detail in several others,[50] in conjunction with Sjögren's syndrome. The latter diagnosis is usually based upon the triad of keratoconjunctivitis sicca, xerostomia (with or without enlargement of the salivary glands) and rheumatoid arthritis. Recently, however, many other organs and systems have been found to be involved and multiple "autoantibodies" may occur.[5,10] In one of our cases arthritis was present and in another it was not. Both had severe proximal weakness and massive inflammatory infiltrates within the muscle. Bunim[10] has observed myopathic weakness in 4 out of 40 cases of Sjögren's syndrome and these were described in detail by Silberberg and Drachman.[50]

OTHER CLINICAL FEATURES

Pure neurological symptoms do not occur, and deep tendon reflexes are normal or depressed in accordance with the associated muscular weakness though less so than in muscular dystrophy. Visceral manifestations of polymyositis are rare but have been described as affecting almost every organ. A transitory pneumonitis has been reported. Involvement of the cardiac muscle is said to occur,[56] causing non-specific T-wave changes in the electrocardiogram and interstitial fibrosis pathologically. It rarely causes clinical symptoms but very occasionally pericarditis is observed. Renal involvement is likewise a rarity but it has been reported,[56] as have various ocular and nervous system defects.

Two components, namely weakness of the pharyngeal musculature and hypotonicity of the esophagus, may contribute to the dysphagia in patients with polymyositis. The pharyngeal weakness is demonstrated radiographically by a pooling of barium in the valleculae and pyriform sinuses and is the major cause of dysphagia. In about 30 per cent of cases a hypomotility or atonicity of the esophagus is found.[19] It is identical to that observed in scleroderma. Often, but not invariably, these persons also have mild cutaneous evidence of scleroderma or acrosclerosis.

In three of our patients with advanced weakness due to polymyositis and very mild sclerodermatous skin changes, marked evidence of disease of the small intestine also existed. Severe hypomotility was the most obvious clinical disorder, with accompanying abdominal bloating, constipation and other signs. Radiographically, loss of haustrations and other classic features were seen, and a moderate malabsorption syndrome, as manifested by low serum carotene, was present in each case. The disease of the small bowel was identical to that seen in advanced systemic scleroderma (progressive systemic sclerosis), yet the dermal evidence of this condition was minimal and the myositic weakness was advanced.

ASSOCIATION WITH MALIGNANT DISEASE

An unequivocal association has been established between malignancy and polymyositis or dermatomyositis in a sizable proportion of cases. Nearly all such combined disease has been noted in adults, usually beyond the age of 40 years. Cases accumulated from several sources in the literature[21,49,58] indicate that this relationship has been noted more than 150 times. The overall incidence of tumor, when all cases of myositis are included, is nearly 20 per cent, or five times more common than would be expected on the basis of pure chance in a matched population of comparable age.[21] However, when dermatomyositis develops in a man over the age of 40 there is more than a 50 per cent chance that he will eventually demonstrate a tumor,[2] and if the myositis appears after the age of 50 cancer will be found in 71 per cent of men and 24 per cent of women.[49] Even more impressive is the comment by Shy[49] that among men over 50 who developed myositis and were followed for 3 or more years all nine had associated neoplasia.

The myositis is usually associated with skin lesions which are typical of dermatomyositis. Proximal muscular weakness is the rule and dysphagia is common. It may develop in conjunction with a recognized tumor or more commonly precedes its detection by 2 or more years. Twenty-two of our 145 patients had a neoplasm, and three of these were not found until autopsy, even though a diligent search had been made for them during life.

From the reports that have been submitted so far certain points can be made concerning the interrelationship of myositis and malignancy. They include: (*a*) from among all cases of myositis, about 15 to 20 per cent will harbor a malignant neoplasm; (*b*) with one or two rare exceptions, all of these cases have occurred in adults in the "tumor-bearing age" over 40; (*c*) almost without exception the muscular disorder takes the form of a florid dermatomyositis which is easily recognized. In a few persons the skin changes are only minor; (*d*) in almost all cases the neoplasm is a carcinoma, although occasionally leukemia or even a thymoma has been present; (*e*) muscular weakness is characteristically proximal in distribution and dysphagia may be a particularly prominent complication; (*f*) dermatomyositis may be overt and the neoplasm symptomatically minor or unrecognized even up to the time of death; and (*g*) therapeutic response to corticosteroids is generally poor in contrast to that noted in Types I and II of polymyositis.

The growth is usually a carcinoma, which may originate in the lung, prostate, female genitalia (ovary or uterus), breast, or large intestine. However, less common sites, such as stomach, gallbladder, parotid gland, tonsil and others, have been the source of a primary tumor. Even lymphoma or Hodgkin's disease has occurred in a very few cases, but the association here is too infrequent to be, so far, more than suggestive. Of particular interest are several recent reports of the association of myositis with either a benign or a maligant thymoma, in at least one of whom a classical picture of myasthenia gravis appeared after thymectomy, at which time the clinical and histopathological evidences of myositis had completely resolved.[30]

The simultaneous occurrence of these two pathological conditions in such a high incidence strongly suggests a causal interrelationship, the nature of which is as yet unclear. Despite the fact that tumor exists in these cases, death almost always occurs from the progressive and relentless muscular weakness with eventual fatal involvement of the respiratory and pharyngeal musculature. Corticosteroids are less effective in treating this type of disease than in practically any other form.

Involvement of the central or peripheral nervous system, separately or in conjunction with muscular weakness and wasting, has commanded increased attention within the past several years.[9,14] Myopathy, including myasthenia gravis, comprises about 20 per cent of these cases, most of which are associated with carcinoma of the lung.

SPECIFIC CLINICAL FEATURES OF THE VARIOUS TYPES OF POLYMYOSITIS AND DERMATOMYOSITIS

Typical Polymyositis (Type I)

This is the most common variety, comprising about 35 per cent of cases which will be seen in any large series. It occurs almost exclusively in women in a ratio of 3:1 and especially in the third to the fifth decades. The clinical onset is insidious with gradual appearance of weakness in muscles of the pelvic girdle and the thighs. Difficulty may first be experienced climbing stairs or in arising from a low chair or from the floor. Later, it may become difficult to raise the arms above the head or even to the horizontal. Dysphagia and dysphonia appear, due to weakness of the laryngeal and the posterior pharyngeal muscles. A number of patients may have a more mild and protracted course with spontaneous partial remissions and exacerbations Many show no dermal manifestations. On the other hand, a few demonstrate an "atypical" skin rash, especially moderately erythematous atrophic eruptions on the knuckles and elbows, or mild evidence of scleroderma or Raynaud's phenomenon. A moderate arthritis and arthralgia, sometimes with joint effusions and positive laboratory tests for rheumatoid factor, may accompany this form of the disease.

Typical Dermatomyositis (Type II)

This type of myositis comprises about 25 per cent of all cases and its usual clinical course is commonly either an acute or subacute muscular weakness, chiefly proximal in distribution, as the main feature. The typical skin rash is a diffuse erythematous, sometimes edematous, eruption on the face, about the eyes, on the anterior and posterior neck and the shoulders, the arms and the upper chest (Fig. 53–2). A characteristic feature in some patients is peri-orbital edema with a dusky lilac coloration on the upper lids which has been called the "heliotrope eruption." Also a scaly erythematous and often atrophic rash may occur on the extensor surfaces of the knuckles (Fig. 53–1), elbows, knees and the medial malleoli. The skin rash may frequently precede or accompany the development of muscular weakness. Systemic features such as malaise, leukocytosis and muscular symptoms of pain, tenderness and induration are common in this form of the disease. Subacute joint symptoms occur quite commonly at the onset of this disease. In persons over 40 years of age who have a skin rash of dermatomyositis and symmetrical proximal muscle weakness, a detailed search should be made for the presence of a visceral malignancy.

Typical Dermatomyositis with Malignancy (Type III)

Almost all of these cases arise in the years after the age of 40 and, hence, occur in the "tumor-bearing age."[2,21] In contrast to the other two forms, Type III occurs somewhat more commonly in men. In some cases the malignancy is evident before or concurrent with the onset of skin rash and muscular weakness. In the majority, however, the insidious onset of proximal muscle weakness and dysphagia may antedate for as much as two or three years the detection of malignancy.[49,58] A skin rash characteristic of dermatomyositis occurs in almost all of these cases and provides a valuable initial clue to the possible presence of malignancy, especially in men over 40 years of age. The sites of origin of malignancy, in order of their frequency, are the lungs, female pelvic organs, prostate, female breast, stomach, esophagus, colon and other rare sites such as the gallbladder, parotid, thymus, and the thyroid gland.[58]

It is of interest that although a tumor is present in these cases, the direct effects of the tumor are rarely serious. Rather, the indirect effects on the striated musculature, and to a lesser degree on the skin, are the most serious of the clinical features. Thus, the weakness is progressive, symmetrical, and predominantly proximal and often includes dysphagia and respiratory muscle weakness. Death is almost invariably from progressive muscular enfeeblement which includes severe dysphagia, malnutrition and aspiration or respiratory failure with superimposed pulmonary infection. It is worth making the point that complete surgical resection of a malignancy has occasionally been followed by total remission of the myopathy.[58]

Childhood Dermatomyositis (Type IV)

This form is frequently a serious and often crippling disorder of childhood. The traditional skin rash of dermatomyositis occurs in the majority of the children and is often associated with a classical erythematous, atrophic, scaly eruption on the extensor surfaces of the joints especially on the knuckles, elbows and knees. In a very rare case the dermal lesions are absent or are grossly atypical. The disease may occur in any age during childhood but it more commonly begins between the ages of 4 and 10. Proximal muscular weakness is more prominent than loss of strength in the distal muscles. Pain and stiffness are moderate. Sensory abnormalities do not occur. The evolution of the disease in childhood is quite variable. In some children, the weakness is rapidly progressive over weeks or months so that severe involvement of chewing, deglutition, phonation and respiration occurs and the child soon is totally incapacitated.[46] In others, the disorder is characterized by exacerbations and remissions in the muscular symptoms, although the skin manifestations may persist relatively unchanged. A few children have a very mild but persistent course with minimal slowly increasing weakness over a number of years. In many there is a tendency to the development of contractures and severe atrophy, especially of the arms and legs. These characteristics must be diligently guarded against by appropriate use of physical therapy and other measures. In late or in advanced disease subcutaneous calcifications (calcinosis universalis, Fig. 53–3) and brawny thickening of the skin are common features.[13]

Another unique manifestation in childhood dermatomyositis is abdominal pain. This may occur early in the disease as was the case in 6 of 40 children studied by Banker and Victor.[3] It was associated with hematemesis and melena and these complications commonly led to death. At autopsy multiple ulcerations and perforations of the gastrointestinal tract were found in these cases, some of which had never been treated with corticosteroids. Pathologically the

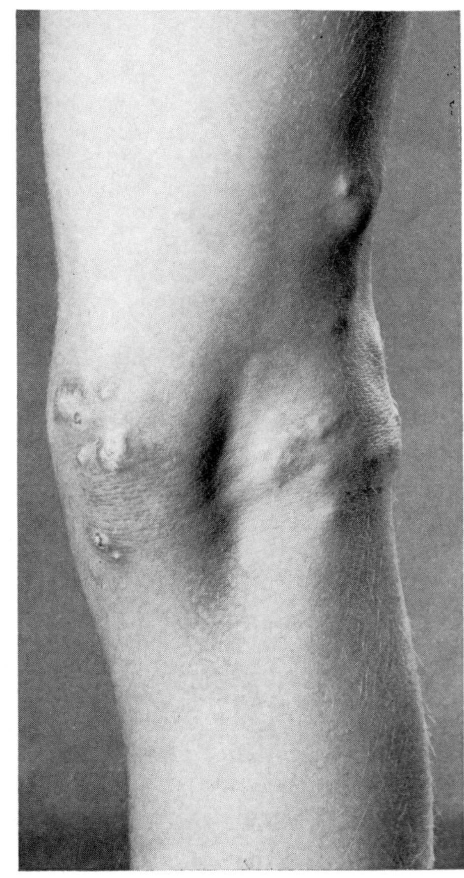

Fig. 53–3.—Calcinosis in a 12-year-old boy who suffered from dermatomyositis of 3 years' duration. The popliteal area shows multiple calcified nodules presenting beneath and in the skin and elsewhere.

factor responsible for the gastrointestinal involvement was a severe vasculitis, sometimes with vascular thrombosis. Similar ischemic changes were noted in striated muscles in children in contrast to the relative infrequency of such lesions in the adult.

Acute Myolysis (Type V)

This form is an acute and frequently fatal disease which is fortunately rare, comprising about 3 per cent of all cases. It is an episodic disease which is difficult to separate completely from idiopathic paroxysmal myoglobinuria. It may be differentiated from the latter, perhaps somewhat artificially, by the fact that acute myolysis develops suddenly and sporadically, often separated by an interval of several years, and there is no family history of similar disorder.[40,42] No known inciting lesion has been discovered, although in some cases an infectious disease such as measles or virus infection seems to precede development of the acute symptoms. Most cases occur in the first or second decades of life.

The attacks are characterized by a rapid onset of generalized muscular weakness involving the proximal as well as the distal musculature, in addition to the bulbar and sometimes the facial musculature. Severe muscle pain and edema are common features. Mechanical support of respiration is often necessary. Serum enzymes are all very high and myoglobinuria is usually grossly evident. It is possible that acute myolysis is a metabolic and not an inflammatory disease since only minimal inflammatory infiltrations are usually found.

Polymyositis in Sjögren's Syndrome (Type VI)

Classically, Sjögren's syndrome includes hypofunction of the lacrimal glands, hypertrophy of the salivary glands with diminished salivary secretions and typical or atypical rheumatoid arthritis. Various other organ system features and overlaps with other collagen or connective tissue diseases have also been noted and circulating "antibodies" have been frequently described.[10]

Occasionally muscular involvement occurs in Sjögren's syndrome and when it does a slowly progressive weakness chiefly involves the proximal muscles of the limbs and girdles.[49] Dysphagia is also a prominent symptom, and a skin rash is not characteristic. This type also is rare, making up only about 5 per cent of all cases of polymyositis. Also, the incidence of muscular weakness in cases of Sjögren's syndrome is low, having been reported to be approximately 10 per cent in 40 cases which were described by Bunim.[10]

LABORATORY FINDINGS

Results of most of the routine laboratory tests are normal, with the exception of an elevation of the sedimentation rate and an alteration of other acute phase reactants.[18] In acute cases a neutrophilic leukocytosis may occur but anemia is rare unless severe debility or an accompanying neoplasm coexist. LE cells were not found in any of our patients, even where the facial rash resembles that found in lupus, and they have been found infrequently in cases reported in the literature. Abnormal urinary findings are likewise a rarity.

The serum and urine levels of creatine and creatinine are frequently abnormal, but these abnormalities are not specific for myositis.[13] Production and excretion of these substances are influenced by many extramuscular conditions as well as by the total muscle mass. Hence the level of these substances in body fluids cannot be uniformly relied upon to lend any degree of assistance in differential diagnosis.

An abnormality of serum proteins occurs in more than one-half of these cases. The changes, although nonspecific, are helpful in the overall evaluation of the case. They include particularly an elevation of the α_2- and β-globulins. Likewise results of tests for circulating rheumatoid factor, such as the latex fixation or sensitized sheep cell procedures, are positive in about 50 per cent of cases.[38]

Of greatest diagnostic and prognostic help, although again not pathognomonic, are elevation in the serum levels of various enzymes. In acute polymyositis, nearly every enzyme which normally resides within skeletal muscle fibers is liberated from diseased muscle and appears in the serum. In our laboratory we find that transaminases (glutamic or pyruvic), creatine phosphokinase (CPK) or aldolase are sensitive indicators.[42,44] Lactic dehydrogenase and malic dehydrogenase are also elevated, but somewhat less predictably.

The actual state of the myositic activity can be predicted with a reasonable degree of certainty by serial measurements of one or several enzymes levels. In active disease the levels are high, and they often return promptly toward normal as the myopathic process responds to corticosteroid therapy. Their decline usually precedes by 3 to 4 weeks any significant improvement in strength. Likewise, relapses have been foretold by recurrent serum enzyme rises as long as 6 weeks in advance of recurrent clinical weakness as corticosteroid therapy was being reduced. In advanced cases of chronic polymyositis, in which much muscle has been replaced by connective tissue or in which progression is very slow, the serum enzyme levels are normal or the aldolase and CPK values are only slightly raised. Elevation of serum enzymes occurs in some forms of muscular dystrophy but these do not respond to any form of therapy. The enzymes are not usually elevated in cases of neuropathic muscular wasting.

ELECTRICAL ABNORMALITIES

Electrical Stimulation

In polymyositis the contraction which follows the application of either a faradic or a galvanic stimulus occurs promptly, but its amplitude is diminished in proportion to the amount of atrophy of the muscle. A reaction of degeneration is not found, which indicates that there is no significant involvement of motor nerves in this condition. In support of this view Lambert, Sayre and Eaton[31] have shown that nerve conduction time in the ulnar nerve is normal in polymyositis, but it is invariably prolonged in polyneuritis and usually in progressive muscular atrophy.

Electromyography

The details of the electromyographic alterations in polymyositis, and their value in diagnosis, have been recognized only relatively recently. A triad of findings, although not absolutely specific, is characteristic of polymyositis. These include (*a*) spontaneous fibrillation and positive or saw-tooth potentials which are indistinguishable from those found in denervation and occur at complete rest or after mild mechanical irritation, (*b*) complex polyphasic or short-duration potentials which appear on voluntary contraction and are greatly reduced in amplitude when compared with normal motor unit potentials and (*c*) salvos of repetitive potentials or "pseudomyotonic" chains of oscillations of high frequency which are evoked by mechanical stimulation of the muscle or movement of the electrode. The latter are distinguished from the "dive bomber" sound of true myotonia by their lesser intensity and by the fact they cease abruptly.

In the large majority of my cases, and this has been the experience of others, the triad is complete. However, in a few only one or two of its components can be shown. Hence in two cases, both chronic in course, only denervation potentials could be found despite histological evidence of unequivocal myositis. In each of these cases the volitional activity was only questionably diminished. The precise explanation for the presence of "denervation" potentials in this disease is not clear. A neuronitis does not seem to be present, unless this affects the terminal nerve twigs in addition to the muscle fibers. The "pseudomyotonic" response can be explained on the basis of an abnormal irritability of the muscle fibers, whereas the volitional polyphasic potentials of decreased amplitude are the result of a patchy loss of muscle fibers from independent motor units.

In addition to the diagnostic assistance that one can derive from electromyography in polymyositis we have used this procedure to indicate the most favorable site for muscle biopsy. Hence, in a moderately weakened, or even in a strong muscle, if electrical abnormalities are plentiful, a biopsy specimen from such a muscle, or preferably, its partner on the opposite side, will almost invariably show pathological changes.

PATHOLOGY

The site for muscle biopsy should be carefully selected in accordance with electrical abnormalities as mentioned just above. The site should also be selected by clinically choosing a muscle which is neither profoundly weakened and atrophic nor of normal strength. Readily accessible muscles such as the gastrocnemius are usually to be avoided. They rarely show classical pathologic features. Preferably, a proximal muscle is chosen for sampling, such as the quadriceps femoris, or the deltoid. When such criteria are followed, myopathological changes will be found in nearly every case in the first biopsy specimen. However, it should be remembered that in some cases focal cellular infiltration has resulted from the insertion of a needle for electromyography a few days before. Hence it is the best practice to electromyographically sample the muscles of the upper and lower extremities on one side of the body and obtain a biopsy specimen from the opposite side so as to avoid the chance sampling of an area of previous needle insertion.

The term "polymyositis" suggests that inflammatory infiltrates are to be found in many muscles, yet it is a notable fact that infiltrates are not uncommonly absent in some clinically typical cases although changes are usually present. Several authors have commented upon this point.[22,56] In many respects the pathological features are remarkably variable from one case to another. The alterations that are found in muscle are, in order of their frequency, as follows:

1. focal or extensive primary degeneration of muscle fibers sometimes with vacuolation of individual fibers (Fig. 53–4);
2. basophilia of some fibers with prominent and central positioning of nuclei, both features of which are evidences of attempts at regeneration;
3. necrosis of parts or entire groups of muscle fibers, sometimes with phagocytosis of their contents;
4. infiltrates of chronic inflammatory cells usually near or surrounding blood vessels (Fig. 53–5) or between the individual muscle fibers (Fig. 53–4). These cells are predominantly small lymphocytes and sometimes plasma cells;
5. interstitial fibrosis which varies in degree and extent especially with the duration of the disease and to some extent with the type of disease. Interstitial fibrosis is much more likely to occur if (*a*) there has been massive acute necrosis of muscle fibers early, (*b*) if therapy was not initiated early, or (*c*) if there is a significant element of scleroderma in conjunction with the myositic process;
6. variation in cross-sectional diameter of fibers. Variation in diameter indicates partial regeneration of the total volume of muscle fibers in this evolving process.

The degenerative and regenerative features of muscle in polymyositis and dermatomyositis have been described in considerable detail in a number of reviews.[1,56] In both children and to a greater extent in adults, the clinical and pathological features of proximal muscu-

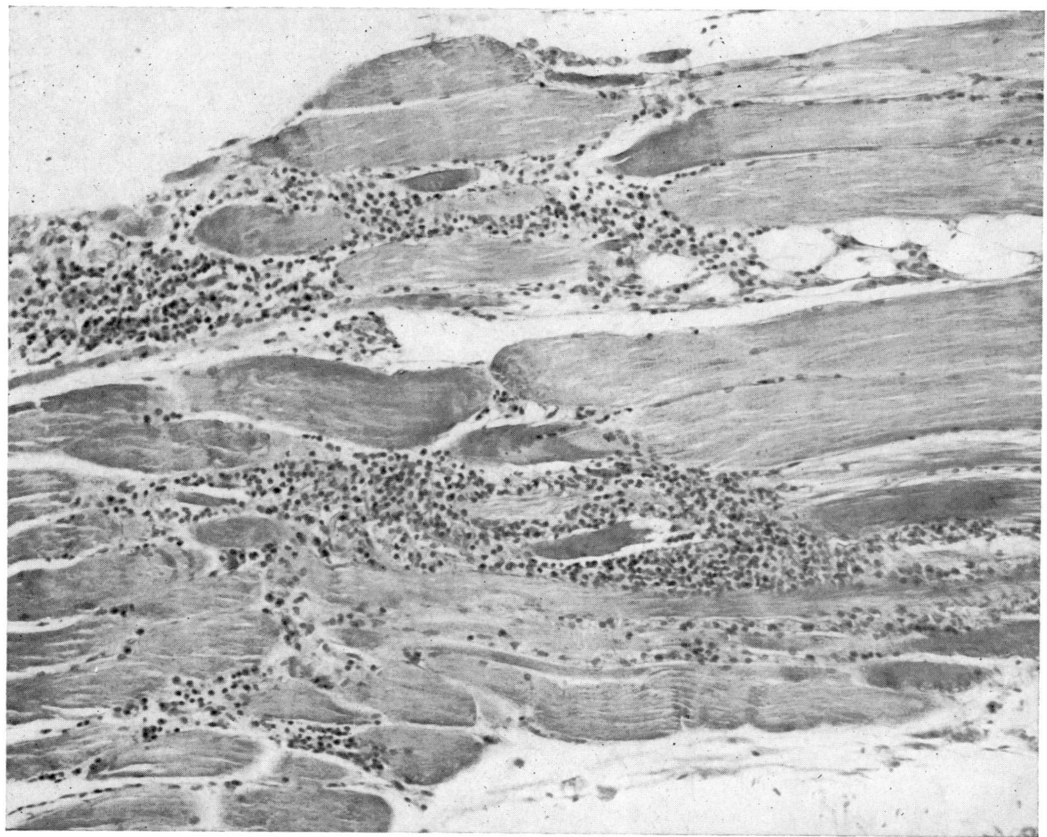

Fig. 53–4.—Classical muscle biopsy specimen from a patient with polymyositis (Type I). There are diffuse inflammatory infiltrates comprised primarily of lymphocytes, a few plasma cells as well as other nonspecific monocytes. Some muscle fibers are in the process of being damaged.

lar weakness make it difficult to differentiate between polymyositis and muscular dystrophy.[20]

In type IV, childhood dermatomyositis, some different pathological features have been outlined, especially in the review by Banker and Victor.[3] These authors gave a detailed account based upon extensive clinical and postmortem studies of eight children with this disease. They reviewed this series and compared it with the muscle biopsy material from many other children that survived their illness. The characteristic features were proximal weakness, skin changes, low grade fever, dysphagia, as well as contractures and widespread subcutaneous calcinosis (Fig. 53–3). The children that died usually died of abdominal complications including abdominal pain and melena. Pathologically there was widespread gastrointestinal ulceration and major pathologic abnormalities were found in relation to the blood vessels of the connective tissues of the skin, gastrointestinal tract, muscles, fat and small nerves. There was significant arteritis with necrosis and thrombosis as well as phlebitis. Such severe evidence of angiitis is rarely found in polymyositis or dermatomyositis in adults.

The electron microscopic features of polymyositis have recently been described in three reports in which a total

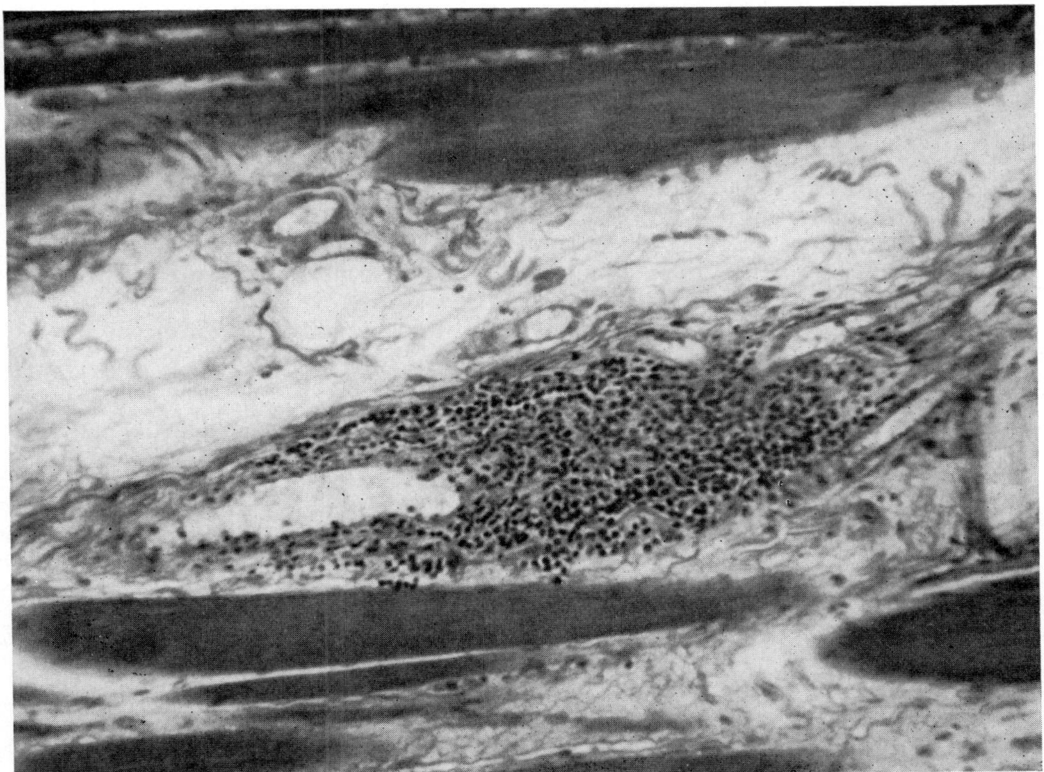

Fig. 53–5.—Classical perivascular (perivenular) infiltrate in muscle biopsy specimen in polymyositis. Other minor or moderate alterations of muscle fibers are seen on the margins of the photograph.

of about 20 cases are examined.[35,44,47] It is not surprising to learn that a wide range of variable changes are noted in muscle fibers in polymyositis when viewed under the electron microscope. In addition, some semi-distinct changes are also found in the small intermuscular blood vessels. The most prominent muscle fiber change consists of focal degeneration of myofibrils (leading in some cases to "targetoid" structures), formation of "cytoplasmic bodies," shredding of myofilaments and hyaline degeneration. Also noted were the formation of autophagic vacuoles and increase in the lipid globules and lipofuscin granules in some muscle fibers. The changes in the intramuscular blood vessels primarily affected capillaries and small arterioles. These consisted of an increase in thickness of the endothelium as well as homogeneous thickening of the basement membrane of capillaries, sometimes up to seven times their normal thickness. Fairly recently[37a] endothelial inclusions have been noted in the small capillaries in cases of dermatomyositis as well as in some patients with systemic lupus erythematosus and scleroderma.

In one recently described case[12] clusters of filamentous tubules resembling myxovirus strands were seen with the electron microscope in both sarcolemmal nuclei and cytoplasm. None of the other authors described above reported the presence of such structures in their cases, but it is possible that these filaments were only present in minor numbers and they could have been overlooked or mistaken for fragmented myofibrils.

PROGNOSIS

Rose and Walton[44] compared 51 cases in their Groups I and II (which include nearly all patients in our major categories except for those with malignancy) with 38 patients described by O'Leary and Waisman in 1940.[37] The latter group was, of course, not treated with corticosteroids whereas the majority of Rose and Walton's patients had been so treated. Although the two groups were not strictly comparable in regard to age, length of follow-up period and certain other features, it was noted that 58 per cent of those treated with corticosteroids had virtually recovered whereas only 10 per cent of O'Leary and Waisman's series had improved to a similar degree. Moreover, only 14 per cent of Rose and Walton's patients had died whereas 50 per cent of O'Leary and Waisman's 38 patients had succumbed by the time of the study.

It is generally concluded that the prognosis is much better in the young age groups and the mortality rate is, in general, directly proportional to the age of onset of the disease process.[32,44] In one series 80 per cent survived for between 1 and 4 years if their disease onset was below age 20, 62.3 per cent survived in the age group of 21 to 40 and only 33.3 per cent were still alive after a comparable period of time if the onset of their disease was age 41 or over. In Rose and Walton's series[44] the mortality rate in their entire group of patients was 30 per cent. However, after the exclusion of patients with carcinoma it was only 16 per cent, and the majority of these patients were treated with corticosteroids. After the age of 51 years the incidence of malignant disease becomes the most important factor that determines the mortality rate. A carcinoma was found in only 2 of 48 patients under 51 years in Rose and Walton's series[44] but malignant disease was present in 12 of 41 patients over the age of 51 years so that 29 per cent of the deaths in this age group were due to carcinoma. The mortality rate in their series from all causes over the age of 51 years was 42 per cent.

SPECULATIONS ABOUT ETIOLOGY

The causes of polymyositis and dermatomyositis are not known. Due to the frequent finding of inflammatory infiltrates in muscle, a multitude of infective agents has been suspected but none has been proved. Physical agents such as sunlight exposure or contact with metals or drugs have also been implicated in individual cases.[56] Most likely these contacts were coincidental in these isolated cases since no single thread of continuity of this type can be found in any sizable series.

The simultaneous occurrence of neoplasm and dermatomyositis is of great interest from an etiologic viewpoint. An interrelationship between the two disorders is inescapable. The explanation for such an association could include: (*a*) by-products of the tumor exert a direct effect upon the metabolism of the muscle fibers, thereby inducing fiber necrosis, clinical weakness, and so on; (*b*) one or more basic defects in the individual's "resistance" allow for the simultaneous emergence of myositis and a tumor; or both could be products of a single pathogenetic agent; (*c*) the development of myositis causes or predisposes to the formation of a neoplasm, especially after 40 years of age; or (*d*) the presence of a neoplasm in the body induces the myositis through immunological or hypersensitivity mechanisms. In the latter case the myositis would be the result of an autoimmune reaction perhaps directed against a common or similar antigen in the muscle and in the tumor. Currently, this hypothesis seems to be the most likely one, although proof for its existence has not as yet been obtained. The fact that polymyositis is frequently associated with features of other "collagen" diseases[25] which may likewise be due to autoimmunity, and that other specific tissue responses such as cerebellar degeneration[8] and peripheral neuropathy[17,27] may occur in conjunction with a remote carcinoma, all suggest some type of common denominator, of which hypersensitivity seems to be the most likely at present.

Some possible support for this idea comes from the studies by Grace and Dao[26] who demonstrated a skin-sensitizing antibody to tumor extract in a patient with carcinoma of the breast. A similar observation was made in another single patient by Curtis, Heckaman and Wheeler[15] who showed a similar skin-sensitizing antibody in a tumor extract from a patient with dermatomyositis and metastatic carcinoma of the lung which had originally arisen in the sigmoid colon.

In a further search for the presence of circulating antibody or antibodies and other immune-reacting proteins, Caspary, Gubbay and Stern[11] examined the serum of 25 of Walton's patients with polymyositis as well as certain other myopathies and neuromyopathies for the presence of antibody against myosin, for antinuclear factor and for immunoconglutinin. The results of these studies are shown in Table 53–6.

From these rather interesting and rather surprisingly inconclusive negative results one can see that although antimyosin antibody and certain other reactants are found quite commonly in polymyositis, similar findings are also observed in dystrophy and neurogenic muscular atrophy. Antinuclear factors were found slightly more frequently in polymyositis. The strikingly high incidence of antimyosin antibody in controls, using the tanned-red cell method, is completely unexplained unless one concedes an extreme degree of sensitivity to the test method and some inhibitory agent or factor in the circulation of patients with various muscular and neuromuscular diseases. In another report[52] similar essentially negative results were found for circulating antibodies against muscle extracts and nuclei.

As can be told from the foregoing, the etiology of polymyositis in any of its forms continues to remain a mystery although there is no doubt that many cases appear to be related in some fashion to the collagen-vascular diseases or to malignancy which would suggest the operation of some type of hypersensitivity of autoimmune response. In one experimental study which seemed to approach this problem fairly directly[16] guinea pigs were given injections of heterologous (rabbit) muscle mixed with Freund's adjuvant. It was reported that these animals developed a generalized myositis which was quite similar to

Table 53-6.—Antibody Studies in Muscular Diseases*

	Antimyosin antibody		*Immunoconglutinin*		*Antinuclear factor*	
Group	*No. tested*	*No. positive*	*No. tested*	*No. positive*	*No. tested*	*No. positive*
Polymyositis	25	12	25	20	23	9
Muscular dystrophies	27	12	27	16	23	3
Neurogenic muscular atrophy	24	13	24	20	24	7
Controls	76	36	54	30	41	0

* from Caspary et al.[11]

polymyositis and this was borne out by some illustrated photographs. Only a very small proportion of animals which received adjuvant alone developed minor evidences of myositis. When the guinea pigs were skin-tested with heterologous or homologous muscle many were said to show delayed-type responses. Even autoclaving of the muscle suspension used for the injection did not appear to diminish its antigenicity. The author concludes that the myositis so produced can be included among the "experimental auto-allergies."

In other provocative studies[28,29] 40 well-differentiated tissue cultures of newborn rat skeletal muscle were each treated with 4 million viable lymph node cells from rats which had been given 3 injections of homogenized rabbit skeletal muscle plus adjuvant. Thirty-eight of these tissue cultures were completely destroyed or inactivated from within 2 to 6 days; whereas 7 of 40 similar cultures were destroyed when lymph node cells from untreated rats were added, and 6 of 40 cultures were destroyed following the addition of cells from rats that had been given adjuvant only. Necrotic muscle lesions were observed in all 10 rats that had been sensitized to muscle and in lesser numbers that had been given adjuvant alone. The author interprets the findings as evidence that a cell (the lymphocyte) in certain circumstances may cause muscle fiber necrosis. Moreover, the fundamental lesion of human polymyositis may be due to the effects of "sensitized" lymphocytes on muscle because of the development of an autoimmune reaction.

Mention has already been made of the recent reports by Chou[12] and by Norton and associates[37a] of the presence of intranuclear and intracytoplasmic aggregates of filamentous tubular structures or particulate bodies in the endothelium of capillaries in muscle in polymyositis. The possible roles of viruses or other similar agents in the induction or perpetuation of some cases of polymyositis or dermatomyositis deserve a great deal of additional study and the final decision concerning virus etiology of some cases of this type has yet to be decided upon.

TREATMENT

Over the years a great many agents have been tried in the treatment of polymyositis, without significant benefit. With the advent first of ACTH and then of the various corticosteroids, it seems quite definite that the natural course of the disease has been altered and that satisfactory suppression is possible in most cases. Based on our experience, we believe that every patient with acute polymyositis should receive corticosteroids. The initial dosage in adults should be from 50 to 60 mg. of prednisone in three or four divided daily doses. In some children and in adults with coexistent malignancy or Sjögren's syndrome, the response will be poor or only temporarily good. In almost all other patients it will be quite gratifying.

Within the past several years a number of papers have described the patterns of polymyositis and the response of these various forms to treatment.[4,36,41,44]

Serial analysis of serum enzyme levels provides one with the best early prognostic tools. If the enzyme levels tend to return toward normal, even though clinical weakness is still severe or increasing, I have been encouraged to predict that reversal of the ominous trend and recovery of strength will soon occur, and this has happened in almost all cases. The prednisone dosage is then very slowly reduced, and the serum enzyme levels are monitored serially during the reduction. Rapid lowering of the dosage or attempts to discontinue therapy have almost invariably been met with recurrent elevations of serum enzyme levels and the reappearance of clinical weakness several weeks later. Maintenance therapy with 7.5 to 20 mg. of prednisone daily (average 12.5 mg.) has been adequate to control the myositis but this dosage level has been reached only about six months after a cautious stepwise reduction from the initial large dosage. In only a very few of the cases in my series have I found it possible to discontinue therapy completely after it has proved to be successful. On the other hand, in ten instances in eight cases a clinical and/or chemical relapse has occurred once the prednisone was omitted or lowered beyond a critical point. Each of these patients has responded again to an increase in prednisone dosage, although some further residual weakness persisted after each relapse.

All patients receiving high-dosage prednisone therapy are given frequent antacids and potassium supplements, and these are continued until a low maintenance dosage of prednisone is achieved or even longer if necessary. Among 60 patients treated in this manner over fairly long periods there has been only one complication, namely, severe sepsis. Bed rest, of course, is imperative during the acute or subacute stages of the disease, and hot applications may lessen the muscular soreness. We have not been impressed with the necessity for a specific program of physical therapy or exercise, except when contractures seem to be developing. As strength returns, cautious exercise, taking care to avoid overstretching, may be used to hasten the recovery.

In general, we have observed three fairly predictable responses to corticosteroid therapy in adults with polymyositis:

1. A fairly prompt decline in serum enzyme levels and return of strength in persons with *acute* or *subacute* polymyositis or dermatomyositis of Types I and II in whom treatment is begun within two months after the appearance of clinical weakness.

2. A modest but definite improvement in muscular power in persons with *chronic* myositis of Types I and II of several months' or years' duration. Serum enzyme levels, which are only moderately elevated, slowly revert towards normal. Strength is not fully regained, but improvement over the pretreatment status averages 50 to 70 per cent. Moreover, improvement is maintained and the fluctuating but progressive decline is reversed.

3. An initial modest decline in serum enzyme levels and some improvement in strength in patients with polymyositis and coexistent malignancy (Type III) and/or in Sjögren's syndrome (Type VI). These benefits are soon reversed, within 3 to 6 months, when slowly progressive weakness and elevation of enzyme levels reappear while the patient is receiving a constant amount of corticosteroid. Increasing the quantity of prednisone has only a transitory effect or none at all, and the disease progresses with the development of severe dysphagia, dyspnea and diminished respiratory excursion, leading soon to death from anoxia or complicating infection.

4. Unpredictable but usually ineffective response to corticosteroids is the myositis of early age as exemplified in Types IV and V.

IMMUNOSUPPRESSIVE THERAPY

It has become increasingly apparent that there are a number of cases of any type of polymyositis or dermatomyositis that predictably may not respond to corticosteroids, even in full doses over a long period of time. Based upon these observations, plus the fact that some cases of polymyositis may represent examples of altered immune response or an autoimmune response, Malaviya and associates[33] described the beneficial effects of intermittent high-dose intravenous methotrexate in four patients with dermatomyositis, three of whom have recently proved to be refractory to corticosteroids. Based upon this report Sokoloff, Goldberg and Pearson[51] recently reported an extension of these studies in which seven patients with corticosteroid-resistant polymyositis were treated similarly with intravenous methotrexate. The initial dosage of methotrexate was 25 mg. intravenously given once per week with an average level of 35 to 40 mg. per week. Five of seven patients improved significantly as demonstrated by (1) improvement in muscle strength and in skin lesions; (2) return of at least three of the four serum enzymes to normal or near-normal levels; and (3) ability to taper prednisone without causing deterioration in the first two features. Toxicity attributable to methotrexate was not important and careful monitoring of liver function parameters was always undertaken.

In an extension of these studies I have now treated 15 corticosteroid-refractory patients with intravenous methotrexate by the methods outlined by Sokoloff. Ten have shown an excellent or moderate response and all have been maintained on low dose prednisone (average 10 to 15 mg. daily). Five have not responded at all but three of these have far advanced disease, presumably intramuscular fibrosis, and had progressed to such an extent that improvement could hardly have taken place in any case. Two patients who proved to be failures on both methotrexate, intermittently, and corticosteroids appeared to respond moderately well to the use of intravenous and then oral cyclophosphamide over a several-week or several-month period of time. The dosages of cyclophosphamide have not been fully worked out as yet. Two patients treated by me were given cyclophosphamide intravenously, 5 to 7 mg./kg./day for 2 to 3 days until leukopenia was induced, then several days later oral cyclophosphamide was administered, starting with a dosage of 150 to 200 mg. daily with careful monitoring for leukopenia, forcing fluids to avoid hemorrhagic cystitis. Despite these precautions a number of annoying or potentially serious side effects developed, as expected. Nevertheless, improvement in these two patients was quite gratifying with considerable return of strength and lowering of serum enzymes, as well as improvement or complete disappearance of dysphagia.

It is quite clear that selective treatment of polymyositis and dermatomyositis must eventually depend upon a fuller understanding of the etiology or etiologies of these conditions. It is entirely possible that eventually treatment must be selective so that some patients may respond to corticosteroids, others may require immunosuppressive agents, and yet others may eventually require therapy with anti-viral agents, if and when such factors are found to be responsible for the muscle degeneration in certain selected cases.

BIBLIOGRAPHY

1. Adams, R. D., Denny-Brown, D. and Pearson, C. M.: *Diseases of Muscle; a Study of Pathology*, 2nd ed., New York, Hoeber, 1962.
2. Arundell, F. D., Wilkinson, R. D., and Haserick, J. R.: Arch. Derm. Syph., *82*, 772, 1960.
3. Banker, B. Q. and Victor, M.: Medicine, *45*, 261, 1966.
4. Barwick, D. D. and Walton, J. N.: Amer. J. Med., *35*, 646, 1963.
5. Bloch, K. J., Buchanan, W. W., Wohl, M. J. and Bunim, J. J.: Medicine, *44*, 187, 1965.
6. van Bogaert, L. and Radermecker, M. A.: Acta Neurol. Belg., *1*, 1952.
7. van Bogaert, L., Radermecker, M. A., Lowenthal, A. and Ketelaer, C. J.: Acta Neurol. Belg., *11*, 869, 1955.
8. Brain, W. R., Daniel, P. M., and Greenfield, J. G.: J. Neurol. Neurosurg. Psychiat., *14*, 59, 1951.
9. Brain, L., and Norris, F. H.: *The Remote Effects of Cancer on the Nervous System*, New York and London, Grune and Stratton, 1965.
10. Bunim, J. J.: Ann. Rheum. Dis., *20*, 1, 1961.
11. Caspary, E. A., Gubbay, S. S. and Stern, G. M.: Lancet, *2*, 941, 1964.
12. Chou, S. M.: Science, *158*, 1453, 1967.
13. Christianson, H. B., O'Leary, P. A. and Power, M. H.: J. Invest. Derm., *27*, 431, 1956.
14. Croft, D. B. and Wilkinson, M.: Brain, *88*, 427, 1965.
15. Curtis, A. C., Heckaman, J. G. and Wheeler, A. H.: J.A.M.A., *178*, 571, 1961.
16. Dawkins, R. L.: J. Path. Bact., *90*, 619, 1965.
17. Denny-Brown, D.: J. Neurol. Psychiat., *11*, 73, 1948.
18. Diessner, G. F., Howard, F. M., Winkelmann, R. K., Lambert, E. H. and Mulder, D. W.: Arch. Intern. Med., *117*, 757, 1966.

19. Donoghue, F. D., Winkelmann, R. K. and Moersch, J. H.: Ann. Otol., *69*, 1139, 1960.
20. Dowben, R. M., Vawter, G. F., Brandfonbrenner, A., Sniderman, S. P. and Kaegey, R. D.: Arch. Intern. Med., *115*, 584, 1965.
21. Dowling, G. B.: Brit. J. Dermat., *67*, 275, 1955.
22. Eaton, L. M.: Neurology, *4*, 245, 1954.
23. Ford, F. R.: *Diseases of the Nervous System in Infancy, Childhood and Adolescence*, 3rd ed. Springfield, Charles C Thomas, 1952.
24. Garcin, R., Lapresle, J., Gruner, J. and Scherrer, J.: Rev. Neurol., *92*, 465, 1955.
25. Glaser, G. H.: Int. J. Neurol., *1*, 319, 1960.
26. Grace, J. T. and Dao, T. L.: Cancer, *12*, 648, 1959.
27. Henson, R. A., Russell, D. and Wilkinson, J.: Brain, *77*, 82, 1954.
28. Kakulas, B. A.: Nature, *210*, 1115, 1966.
29. ————: J. Path. Bact., *91*, 495, 1966.
30. Klein, J. J., Gottleib, A. J., Mones, R. J., Appel, S. H. and Osserman, K. E.: Arch. Intern. Med., *113*, 142, 1964.
31. Lambert, E. H., Sayre, G. P. and Eaton, L. M.: Trans. Amer. Neurol. Assoc., *79*, 64, 1954.
32. Logan, R. G., Bandera, J. M., Mikkelsen, W. M. and Duff, I. F.: Arch. Intern. Med., *65*, 996, 1966.
33. Malaviya, H. N., Mauy, A. and Schwartz, R. S.: Lancet, *2*, 485, 1968.
34. Maxeiner, S. R., McDonald, J. R. and Kirlin, J. W.: Surg. Clin. North America, *32*, 1225, 1952.
35. Mintz, G., Gonzalez-Angulo, A. and Fraga, A.: Amer. J. Med., *44*, 216, 1968.
36. Mulder, D. W., Winkelmann, R. K., Lambert, E. H., Diessner, G. R. and Howard, F. M.: Ann. Intern. Med., *58*, 969, 1963.
37. O'Leary, P. A. and Waisman, J.: Arch. Derm. Syph., *41*, 1001, 1940.
37*a*. Norton, W. L., Valayos, E. and Robison, L.: Ann. Rheum. Dis., *29*, 67, 1970.
38. Pearson, C. M.: Arth. & Rheum., *2*, 127, 1959.
39. Pearson, C. M., and Rose, A. S.: Res. Publ., Assoc. Nerv. Ment. Dis., *38*, 422, 1961.
40. Pearson, C. M.: Postgrad. Med., *31*, 450, 1962.
41. Pearson, C. M.: Ann. Intern. Med., *59*, 827, 1963.
42. Pearson, C. M.: Ann. Rev. Med., *17*, 63, 1966.
43. Pitkeathly, D. A. and Coomes, E. N.: Ann. Rheum. Dis., *25*, 127, 1966.
44. Rose, A. L. and Walton, J. N.: Brain, *89*, 747, 1966.
45. Rose, A. L., Walton, J. N. and Pearce, G. W.: J. Neurol. Sci., *5*, 457, 1967.
46. Selander, P.: Acta Med. Scand., Suppl. 246, 187, 1950.
47. Shafiq, S. A., Milhorat, A. T. and Gorycki, M. A.: J. Path. Bact., *94*, 139, 1967.
48. Sheard, C.: Arch. Intern. Med., *88*, 640, 1951.
49. Shy, G. M.: World Neurol., *3*, 149, 1962.
50. Silberberg, D. H. and Drachman, D. A.: Arch. Neurol., *6*, 428, 1962.
51. Sokoloff, M., Goldberg, L. S. and Pearson, C. M.: Lancet, *1*, 14, 1971.
52. Stern, G. M., Rose, A. L. and Jacobs, K.: J. Neurol. Sci., *5*, 181, 1967.
53. Unverricht, H.: Z. Klin. Med., *12*, 533, 1887.
54. Wagner, E.: Arch. Heilk, *4*, 288, 1863.
55. Wallace, S. L., Lattes, R. and Ragan, C.: Amer. J. Med., *25*, 600, 1958.
56. Walton, J. N. and Adams, R. D.: Polymyositis, Edinburgh, Livingstone, 1958.
57. Wedgewood, R. J. P., Cook, C. and Cohen, J.: Pediatrics, *12*, 477, 1953.
58. Williams, R. C.: Ann. Intern. Med., *50*, 1174, 1959.

Chapter 54

Progressive Systemic Sclerosis (Scleroderma)

By Gerald P. Rodnan, M.D.

Progressive systemic sclerosis (PSS) is a generalized disorder of connective tissue characterized by inflammatory, fibrotic and degenerative changes, often accompanied by prominent vascular lesions in the skin (scleroderma), synovium and certain internal organs, notably the esophagus, intestinal tract, heart, lung, and kidney.[9,21,74,120,162,190,203,254,290,291,312,365] Although the disease often appears to remain confined to the integument for many years and is not incompatible with long life, in many cases there is steadily and at times rapidly progressive visceral involvement, which may cause death as a result of cardiac failure, hypertensive renal disease, pulmonary complications, or intestinal malabsorption and cachexia.

The etiology and fundamental nature of PSS are presently obscure. During recent years however, the demonstration of serologic abnormalities in a high percentage of patients,[288,366] together with other findings, has given rise to the suspicion that aberrant immunity may play an important role in the pathogenesis of this disorder.

Historical Note.—Descriptions of skin conditions *compatible* with scleroderma have been found in the writings of the ancients,[291] but the first convincing account is generally credited to Carlo Curzio, a physician of Naples, in 1753.[73] (There is reason to suspect, however, that the young woman described by Curzio may have had scleredema rather than scleroderma [*see below*].) Curzio's case is cited under the designation *ichthyosis cornea* in the pioneer dermatologic texts of Willan (1808) and of his students Bateman and Alibert, the latter commenting that

> "Rien n'est plus bizarre, mais aussi rien n'est plus intéressant que la dégénération cornée du système dermoïde. Elle sera toujours pour les médicins un grand suject d'étude et de méditation . . ."[2]

The disease was rediscovered by Grisolle[127] and by Forget in 1847,[106] and designated *sclérodermie* by Gintrac.[118] Despite the fact that scleroderma was then widely recognized and that many patients were known to have serious visceral disturbances,[80,208,395] the systemic nature of the disease was not clearly appreciated until well into this century.[221,291] Gradually increasing awareness that scleroderma is the external manifestation of a more generalized disorder was crystallized in 1945, when Goetz[120] proposed that the disease be renamed progressive systemic sclerosis.

CLINICAL FEATURES

Epidemiology

Progressive systemic sclerosis has been described in people of all races and appears to be global in distribution.[9,353] Women are affected approximately two to three times as often as men. Initial symptoms usually appear in the third to fifth decade of life, but there are many patients who first become ill after age 50. The disease is relatively uncommon in childhood.[165,175]

In an analysis of cases diagnosed in the hospitals of Shelby County, Tennessee, during the period 1963–1968, and meeting specified criteria, the average annual incidence of PSS was found to be 4.5 cases per million population.[229] No significant racial differences were observed in the incidence, which increased with age, reaching a peak in the oldest age group (65 + years). A considerably higher incidence rate, 12 cases per million population per year, was noted during the period 1951–1967 in the residential population of Rochester, Minnesota.[194]

Occupational Factors

PSS has been noted to occur with unusual frequency among goldminers, coalminers, and other workers in occupations in which there is heavy exposure to silica dust.[91,292] The disease appears to be twice as common in coalminers as in non-miners, and it has been suggested that silicosis may serve as a predisposing factor.

Initial Symptoms

In most cases, the initial complaint is either Raynaud's phenomenon or insidious edema of the distal portions of the extremities or gradual thickening of the skin of the hands and fingers.[96,287] Approximately one-third of patients first have articular symptoms, most often pain and stiffness of the fingers and knees and in some cases frank polyarthritis not unlike rheumatoid arthritis.[297] In still others the onset of PSS is marked by severe muscle weakness which may be indistinguishable from polymyositis.[231] In a small proportion of cases the presenting symptoms are referable to neither the skin nor musculoskeletal structures, but to visceral involvement (PSS *sine* scleroderma).[293] In this respect one may encounter patients who have dysphagia or a disturbance in intestinal motility, or both, long before the development of cutaneous changes.

Clinical and Pathophysiologic Findings in Systemic Sclerosis

(*a*) *Skin.*—Three stages are recognized in the evolution of scleroderma, viz. edematous, indurative and atrophic. In the early or edematous phase, there is a painless, pitting edema of the hands and fingers which may also involve the forearms and the legs and feet as well as the face. The tightly swollen fingers have been compared to sausages in their appearance. The edema may last for several weeks to months and is gradually replaced by thickening and tightening of the skin, which loses its normal pliability. In all but a few instances these indurative changes first affect the fingers (sclerodactyly), dorsum of the hands, and the face. In rare instances there may be bullous lesions in the involved skin,[116] or nodules consisting of dense collagenous connective tissue.[40,330]

The induration of the skin, which is symmetrical in distribution, may remain confined to the distal portions of the upper extremity, constituting a limited form of scleroderma to which the term *acrosclerosis* has been applied. Since it may be difficult to detect thickening of the skin by palpation alone, however, estimates of the relative frequency of limited versus more generalized forms of scleroderma which do not include biopsy specimens or some other objective measurement (*see below*) must be interpreted with caution. In our experience the majority of patients with PSS have had scleroderma which spread in varying degree to the forearms, arms, upper anterior chest, abdomen and back. Although the legs and feet and to a lesser extent the thighs may be involved, the sparing of these parts in many patients with scleroderma of the upper extremity is notable. As the scleroderma progresses the skin becomes taut and shiny and may be tightly tethered to the subcutaneous structures. Contraction and hardening of the tissues lead to a loss of normal skin folds and the development of a characteristic pinched or immobile, mask-like facies (Figure 54–1). The lips become thin

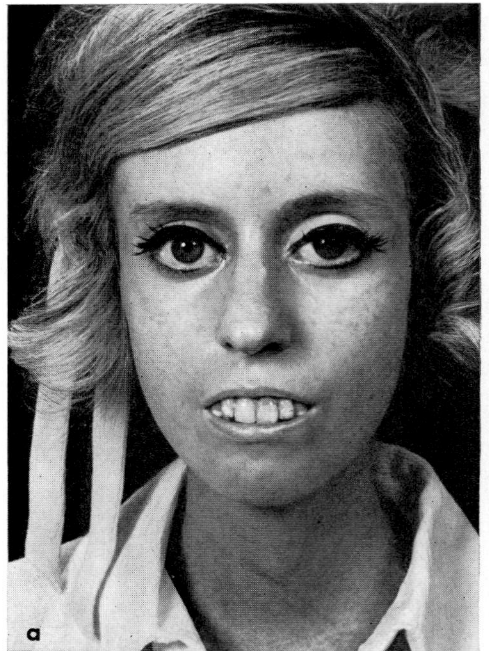

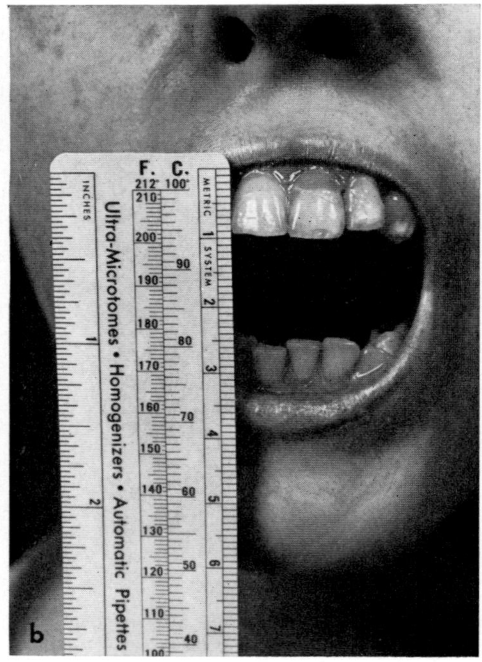

FIG. 54–1.—(*a*) Facies of young woman with PSS. Note loss of normal skin folds, retraction of lips, and numerous telangectases on cheeks. (*b*) Same patient, with her mouth open as widely as possible, illustrating reduction in oral aperture. The distance between the lips, 3.3 cm., is considerably less than normal for young women (normal = 5.8 ± .4 cm.).

and tightly pursed, and there is narrowing of the oral aperture ("tabaksbeutelmund," tobacco pouch mouth).[380] Microstomia interferes with eating and with dental care.

These skin changes are accompanied and in some instances preceded by a generalized melanotic hyperpigmentation which may become as intense as that encountered in Addison's disease, but without mucous membrane involvement. There is often spotty or patchy vitiligo in the darkened areas. Telangectases, consisting of dilated capillary loops and venules of the subpapillary venous plexus, appear on the fingers, nailfolds, face, lips, tongue, and forearms.[33,375] The patients are often plagued by ulcerations and infections of the fingertips, the dorsum of the proximal interphalangeal joints, and other bony eminences, including the lower portion of the legs where large ulcers may occur[146,365] which are extremely refractory to treatment. (Healing of the skin is otherwise normal in PSS and ordinarily there is no difficulty in the repair of surgical wounds.) Women are particularly liable to develop subcutaneous calcifications (*calcinosis circumscripta*), which occur chiefly in the palmar and lateral aspects of the terminal phalanges of the fingers (Figure 54–2) and about the metacarpophalangeal joint of the thumb and the wrist[108,182] (Figure 54–3). These vary in size from tiny punctate deposits to large conglomerate masses. The latter, which are found over the knees, elbows, and forearms, as well as other bony eminences and pressure surfaces, may be complicated by ulceration of the overlying skin and the intermittent extrusion of calcareous matter. The association between subcutaneous calcinosis and scleroderma has long been known as the *Thibierge-Weissenbach syndrome*.[355]

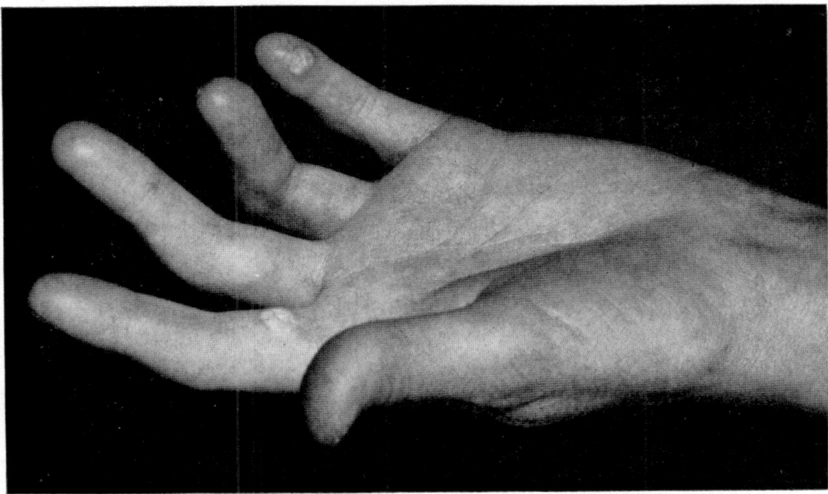

Fig. 54–2.—Hand of an adolescent white girl sufferıng from mild progressive systemic sclerosis of about 5 year's duration. Note the circumscribed lesions of calcinosis in the skin of the volar surface of the proximal portion of the second and distal portion of the fifth digits.

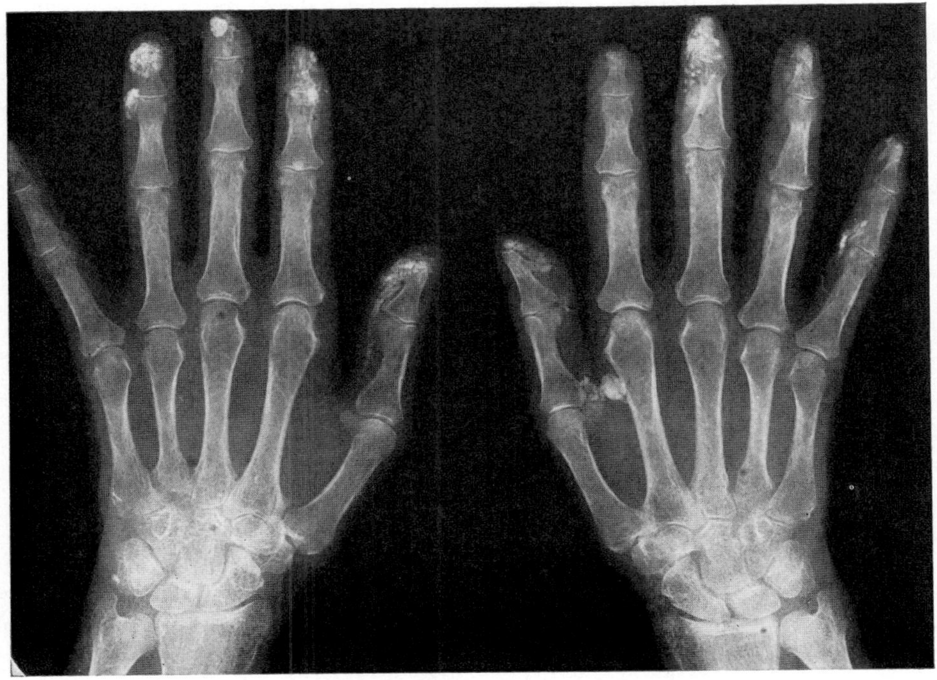

Fig. 54–3.—Roentgenogram of the hands of a woman with PSS illustrating extensive subcutaneous calcinosis in the fingers and about the metacarpophalangeal joint of the right thumb.

Skin biopsy specimens obtained from patients during the active indurative phase of scleroderma disclose a striking increase of compact collagen fibers in the reticular dermis and such other classic histopathologic changes as thinning of the epidermis with loss of rete pegs, atrophy of dermal appendages, and hyalinization and fibrosis of arterioles[88,101,252,371] (Figure 54–4). Increased melanin is found in the basal layer of the epidermis.[252] The weight and thickness of skin cores obtained during this stage of the disease are significantly increased and provide an accurate means of assessing the degree and progression of scleroderma.[295] Electron microscopic examination of sclerodermatous skin reveals numerous collagen fibers of narrow diameter and immature banding pattern and the presence of many double-stranded beaded filaments, identical to those encountered in embryonic skin, and believed to be an early form of extracellular collagen.[143,190,191,311] The process of fibrosis may extend into the trabeculae of the subcutis, but in most instances there is remarkably little or no involvement of this layer. In cases considered clinically to represent mild or "early" scleroderma, there may be only slight homogenization of the collagen bundles and confirmation of the diagnosis by means of skin biopsy specimen often proves difficult.

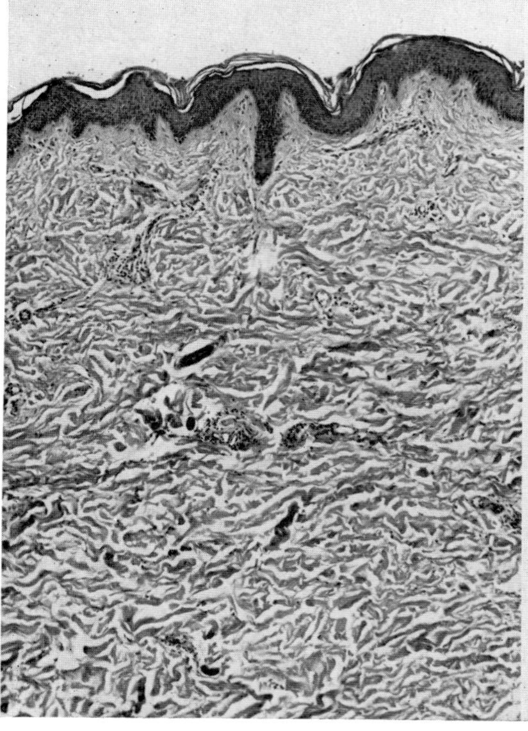

Fig. 54–4.—Photomicrograph of skin from the forearm of a woman with PSS. There is thinning of the epidermis and an increase in dermal collagen fibers which are arranged in bundles parallel to the skin surface. Note sparsity of blood vessels and absence of dermal appendages.

Later in the course of the disease, usually after a period of several years, the skin tends to soften and revert to normal thickness, or to atrophy.[24]

(*b*) *Raynaud's Phenomenon.*—Paroxysmal vasospasm of the fingers occurs in approximately 90 per cent of patients with PSS[9,287,365] and was well documented by Raynaud himself.[274,291] Less often the toes, and rarely the tip of the nose, the earlobes, and tongue are affected in this reaction. In the majority of cases the onset of this reaction is contemporaneous with the development of skin changes and/or rheumatic complaints, or precedes these by a few months to a year. On occasion, however, Raynaud's phenomenon may antedate other evidence of PSS by an interval of three years or more.[79,162,287] Typically the patient reports episodes of sudden pallor and/or cyanosis of the distal two-thirds of the fingers or of the entire digits, which become cold and numb. These attacks are initiated by exposure to environmental cold, as well as by emotional upsets. The cyclical color changes and accompanying tingling and burning sensations usually last for 10 to 15 minutes after re-warming, which elicits reactive hyperemia. Small areas of ischemic necrosis or ulceration of the fingertip are common in PSS and in some cases there may be gangrene of portions of the terminal phalanges of the fingers or toes. On rare occasions there is thrombosis of one or more of the major vessels in the extremities.[18]

Patients with Raynaud's phenomenon with or without scleroderma have an abnormally low digital pad temperature in the basal state[110,144] and a smaller capillary blood flow in their fingers in both warm and cool environments than do normal subjects.[61,62,204] These findings, together with the inability to rewarm the fingers after exposure to cold, have been interpreted as evidence of a persistent structural defect in the blood vessels. This conclusion is supported by angiographic studies which disclose narrowing and obstruction in the digital arteries of patients with PSS and Raynaud's phenomenon[31,41,108,199,341] (Figure 54–5), and the abnormal appearance and paucity of capillary loops in the nailfold.[33,162,277] The role, if any, of these vascular disturbances in the pathogenesis of PSS is unclear. Since blood flow has been found to be normal in the skin and subcutaneous tissue of the clinically involved forearm[61] it would appear that the development of skin changes is not primarily dependent upon a decrease in nutritional capillary blood flow.

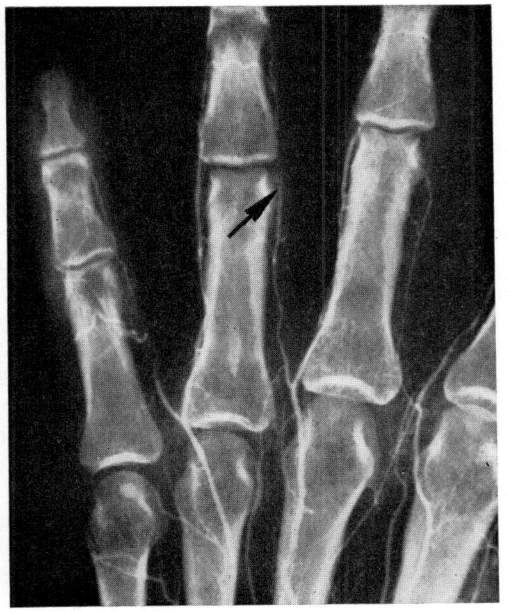

Fig. 54–5.—Brachial arteriogram of man with PSS and Raynaud's phenomenon, illustrating narrowing and irregularity of the lumina of the digital arteries with several points of apparently total obstruction.

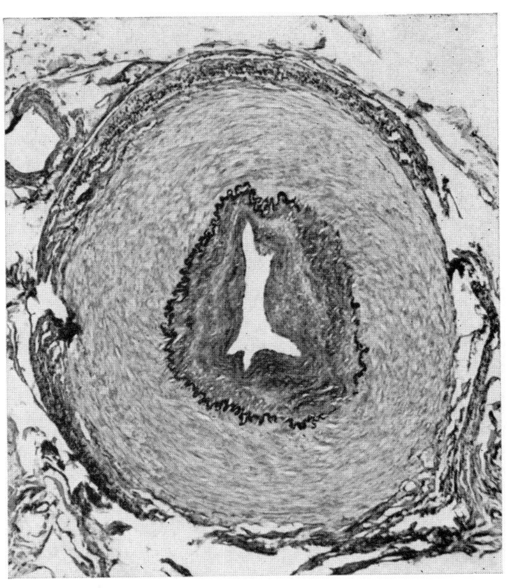

Fig. 54–6.—Photomicrograph of digital artery of man with PSS and Raynaud's phenomenon who died of malignant hypertension and renal failure. There is eccentric hyperplasia of the intima, reduplication and fraying of the internal elastic lamina, and marked thickening of the media (Verhoeff stain).

Histologic examination of digital arteries of patients with PSS obtained at necropsy has revealed abnormalities consisting of subintimal proliferation of young connective tissue, subendothelial fibrin deposits, and thickening of the basement membrane, together with reduplication and fraying of the internal elastic lamina[171,209,221] (Figure 54–6). When severe these changes lead to considerable narrowing or occlusion of the lumen. Studies of resting venous plasma catecholamine concentrations and of the urinary catecholamine excretion patterns of patients with PSS and Raynaud's phenomenon have failed to support the hypothesis that norepinephrine and/or epinephrine are neurohumors of excess in this particular form of Raynaud's phenomenon.[188,317]

Attention has been drawn to the tetrad of calcinosis, Raynaud's phenomenon, sclerodactyly, and telangectasia (*CRST syndrome*), and it has been suggested that this combination of features is associated with a benign form of PSS and more favorable prognosis.[47,147,393] (Many such cases have been and continue to be described under the designation of *Thibierge-Weissenbach syndrome*.) The telangectases found in these patients are similar in appearance and distribution to those of hereditary hemorrhagic telangectasia, and in some instances there has been serious bleeding from lesions in the gastrointestinal tract or bladder.[149,336,393] It should be noted, however, that calcinosis and telangectasia are not confined to patients with more limited scleroderma, but are often encountered in those with widespread involvement of the skin (*see above*). Although it is clear that individuals with CRST syndrome do develop typical visceral involvement[47,309,323] there are many indeed in whom the disease remains relatively confined for very long periods of time.[230]

(*c*) *Bones and Joints*.—Polyarthralgia and joint stiffness affecting chiefly the fingers, wrists, knees, and ankles are frequent complaints early in the course of PSS and are often the first manifestation of the disease.[203,254,286,287,297,312,318,346,365] There may be morning stiffness similar to that present in rheumatoid arthritis. At this stage the patients usually report little more than mild swelling of the parts, but in some cases there is appreciable tenderness, redness, and warmth. Later in the course of the disease, there is increasing stiffness of the joints and many patients become aware of creaking noises in their knees and fingers, as well as over certain tendinous areas, notably the distal portions of the legs and forearms.[286,297,334]

In the beginning one commonly finds diffuse swelling of the fingers (*see above*) and it may be difficult to ascertain to what degree limitation in motion of the interphalangeal joints is based on articular disease, as opposed to changes in the skin and para-articular connective tissues. In the case of the larger peripheral joints, however, there may be signs of frank inflammation, including synovial effusion[297,318] The synovia in such cases is turbid and contains large numbers of neutrophilic leukocytes, the cytoplasm of which contains numerous inclusions.[57,297] These particles have been found to consist of fibrin and/or fibrin breakdown products as well as immunoglobulins (IgG and IgM).[297]

Those patients who have noted creaking in their knees, as well as many who are unaware of any unusual joint noise, have a peculiar type of coarse, leathery crepitus which may be felt by placing the hand over the patella during flexion of the leg.[286] (This sign was first noted by Westphal in 1876.[382]) Similar rubs are also encountered over the tendons of the tibialis anterior and peroneal muscles and the extensor and flexor tendons immediately proximal to the wrist, as well as over the olecranon, subscapular, and other large bursae. (The occurrence of tendon rubs in PSS appears to have been discovered by Harley in 1877.[134]) These rubs have been traced to fibrinous deposits on the surfaces of the tendon sheaths and overlying fascia.[334] There may be thickening of tendons and tendon sheaths, often marked by distention of the extensor sheath on the dorsum of the hand and/or the development of median nerve compression (carpal tunnel syndrome) as a result of swelling of the flexor tendons. We have encountered several patients with striking painless enlargement of their Achilles tendons.

Many patients develop flexion contractures of the fingers, which are caused, at least in part, by a limitation in the excursion of the extensor mechanisms as a result of the attenuation of the central bands, volarward slippage of the lateral bands, and scarring of the thin layer of areolar tissue which normally separates the extensor tendons and underlying capsules and the bone.[212] These contractures, which also occur commonly in the wrists and elbows, may form within a period as short as a few months. Occasionally, patients with PSS develop hoarseness as a result of cricoarytenoid joint disease.[128]

The most common abnormality found in the bones and joints on roentgenographic examination is absorption of the tufts of the terminal phalanges of the fingers (and much less often the toes), which is frequently accompanied by atrophy of the soft tissue and subcutaneous calcinosis (*see above*).[108,121,182,286,396] The erosion of bone, which has been found in as many as 80 per cent of cases,[182] first occurs on the palmar aspect of the fingertip. Although usually limited to the tuft, this absorption may ultimately lead to complete dissolution of the terminal phalanx. In a few cases there is loss of bony substance of the middle phalanges as well (Figure 54–7), and rarely there is atrophy of the distal portions of the radius and ulna, or the acromioclavicular joint.[182] Alterations in the joints are generally confined to thickening of the periarticular soft tissues and juxta-articular osteoporosis. In most cases there is little if any loss of articular cartilage and little tendency toward subchondral bone destruction. Recently, however, we have observed two women with PSS and avascular necrosis of a femoral head ascribed to intrinsic vascular disease (*see below*).[383] Thickening of the periodontal membrane (a collagenous structure) may lead to loss of lamina dura and loosening of the teeth.[25,115,344]

Examination of the synovium of those patients with arthritis reveals an inflammatory reaction marked by hyperemia and by infiltrates of lymphocytes and plasma cells, gathered in focal aggregates or scattered diffusely throughout the tissue.[286,297] The appearance of the synovium is not unlike that of early mild rheumatoid arthritis. In those patients with joint rubs the surface of the synovium is found to be covered by a thick coat of fibrin (Figure 54–8*a*). Later in the evolution of the disease there is intense fibrosis of the synovium.[57,70,286] In some cases this affects only the more superficial portions leading to a loss of normal villous folds; in others the entire synovium is replaced by a dense, homogeneous, connective tissue which encompasses and obliterates the vascular structure (Figure 54–8*b*).

(*d*) *Skeletal Muscle.*—Although the weakness and wasting of skeletal muscle found in PSS are to a large extent the result of disuse and poor nutrition, there are many patients who exhibit clinical and biochemical evidence of a primary myopathy. Like polymyositis, this usually

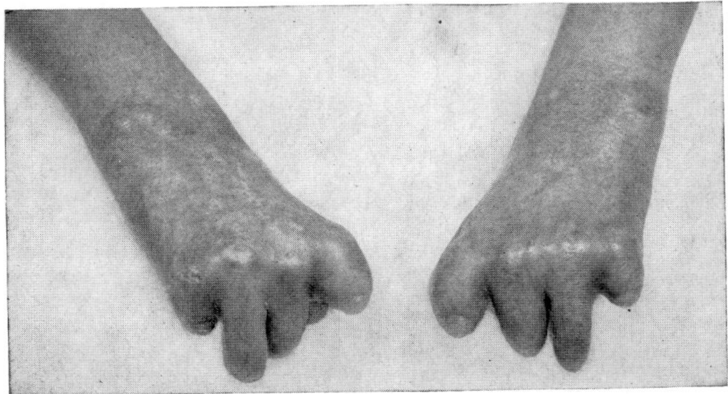

FIG. 54–7.—Hands of a sixty-two-year-old white woman showing extreme degree of digital absorption from scleroderma. The distal phalanges have disappeared but the nails on several digits have remained almost intact. The disease began with Raynaud's phenomenon thirty-five years previously and progressed to this state with little pain and no ulceration.

affects the proximal musculature.[231] The muscle disease in PSS tends to be more subdued and less incapacitating, although in some instances the degree of atrophy may be severe with differentiation from polymyositis proving difficult or impossible ("*sclerodermatomyositis*").[83,210,366] In general, serum glutamic oxalo-acetic transaminase (SGOT) and creatine phosphokinase (CPK) levels are normal, but in many cases there is an increase of serum aldolase activity and in urinary

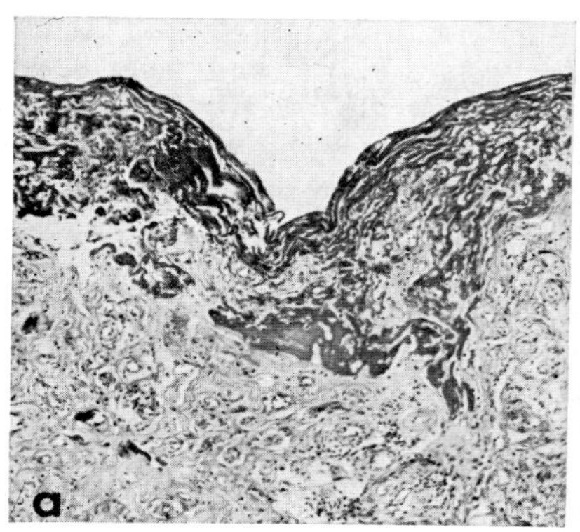
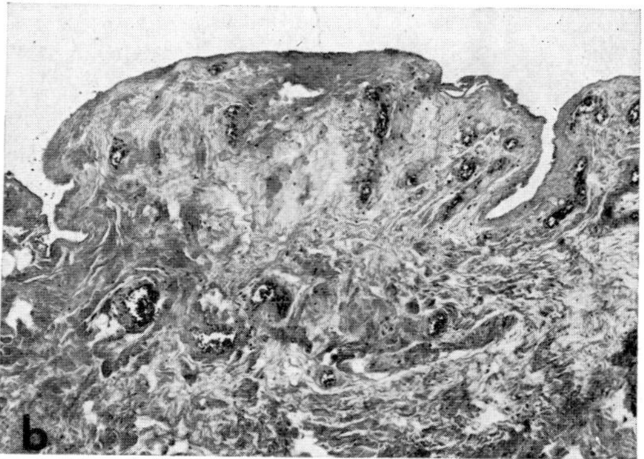

Fig. 54–8.—(*a*) Photomicrograph of synovium (suprapatellar bursa) of a man with PSS who had a loud joint friction rub, illustrating fibrosis of the subsynovialis and thick layer of fibrin on the lining surface. (*b*) Photomicrograph of synovium (suprapatellar bursa) of another man with PSS, illustrating dense fibrosis of entire subsynovialis (From Rodnan,[286] courtesy Annals of Internal Medicine).

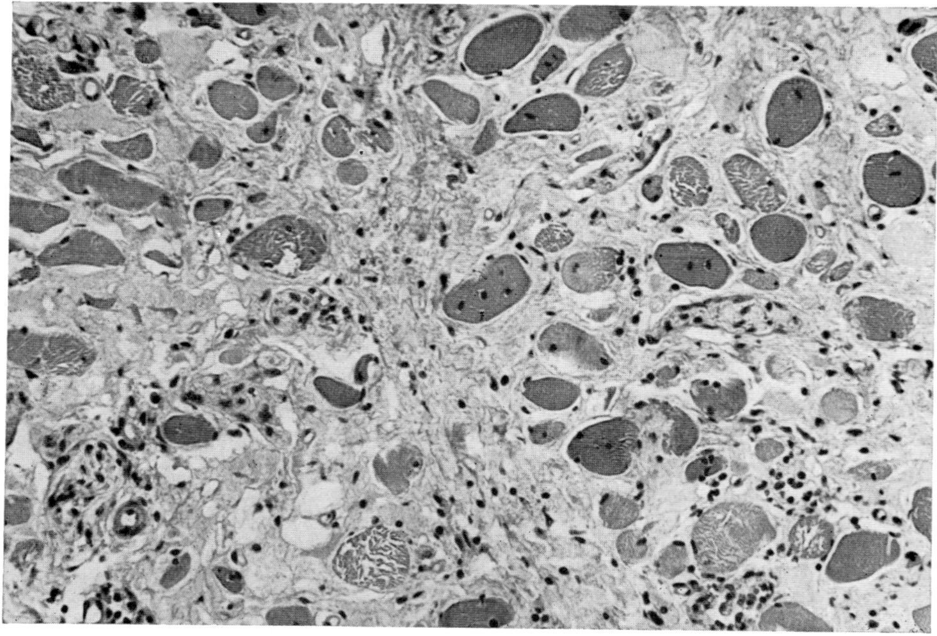

Fig. 54–9.—Photomicrograph of deltoid muscle from a woman with PSS, illustrating severe degree of atrophy of muscle fibers and extensive perimysial and epimysial fibrosis (from Medsger *et al.*,[231] courtesy Arthritis and Rheumatism).

creatine excretion which correlates well with the degree of muscle weakness.[231] Electromyographic abnormalities have been described consisting chiefly of a decrease in the amplitude and average duration of potential and an increase in the percentage of polyphasism.[262] The pathologic changes, which include atrophy and necrosis of muscle fibers, perivascular infiltrates of lymphocytes and plasma cells, and perimysial and epimysial fibrosis, are similar to those encountered in polymyositis[231,268] (Figure 54–9). The muscles most frequently affected are the deltoid, pectoral, and forearm groups, but the tongue, diaphragm, and anterior tibial musculature may also be involved.[231] In one study, electron microscopic examination of skeletal muscle revealed a diminished number of capillaries, endothelial swelling of the remaining vessels, and reduplication and thickening of the capillary basement membrane;[249] and others have failed to find any significant change in mean capillary diameter or width of the basement membrane.[357]

(*e*) *Esophagus*.—Esophageal dysfunction develops in upwards of 90 per cent of patients with PSS and constitutes the most common manifestation of internal involvement in this disorder.[7,28,315,365] In a number of cases a disturbance in swallowing occurs long before evidence of cutaneous disease, giving rise to a form of PSS *sine* scleroderma.[293] At first there may be only mild retrosternal burning pain or unusual fullness after completion of a meal. Later there is difficulty in the swallowing of solids, which tend to remain in the lower esophagus and require copious draughts of liquid in order to pass. Patients often reduce food intake and may lose large amounts of weight. Despite the frequency of peptic esophagitis,[20] esophageal hemorrhage is surprisingly unusual.[19]

Roentgenographic abnormalities are found in over three-fourths of patients, including many who are free from esophageal symptoms.[108,182] Cinefluoroscopic examination reveals a diminution to total absence of peristaltic activity in the esophagus and, later, dilatation (less often narrowing) of the lower one-half or two-thirds of the organ[7] (Figure 54–10). Gastroesophageal reflux occurs, and in many cases there is a small hiatal hernia of the sliding variety.[117] With progression of this disease the cardia tends to become widely patent; in some cases, however, peptic esophagitis is complicated by narrowing or stricture of the lower end of the esophagus. It is important to note that disturbances in esophageal peristalsis and emptying may not be apparent in the erect position, due to the effects of gravity and that these patients should be examined in recumbency.[182] Manometric measurements confirm the incoordination and loss of contractile power affecting both primary and secondary waves, which may progress to complete,

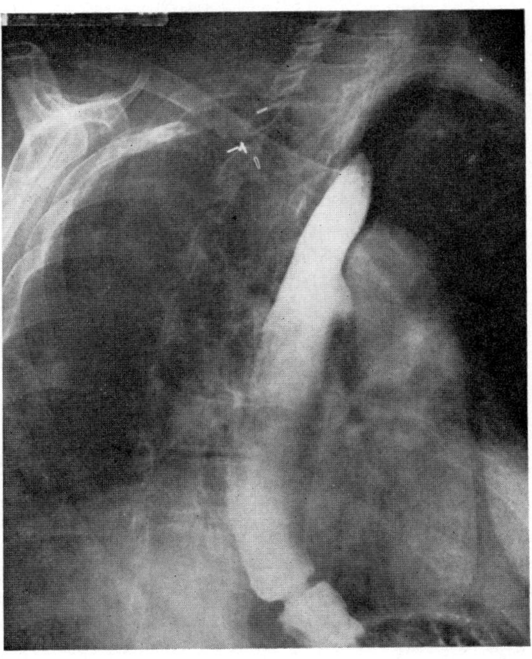

FIG. 54–10.—Roentgenogram of the esophagus of a woman with PSS, who had been troubled by increasingly severe dysphagia. There is generalized dilatation. Cinefluoroscopic examination revealed an absence of peristaltic activity. Note incidental presence of lower esophageal contraction ring and small hiatal hernia.

irreversible paralysis, and reveal a reduction in the tone of the gastroesophageal sphincter which permits the reflux of gastric juice.[7,117,359] No significant improvement in esophageal motor function follows the administration of methacholine.[315] Gastric atony and dilatation may occur, but involvement of the stomach is remarkably uncommon when compared to other portions of the alimentary tract.[156,261,365] Gastric acid secretion is unimpaired in PSS.[20]

Histologic changes are most marked in the lower two-thirds of the esophagus.[156,268] There may be thinning of the mucosa, which is often ulcerated. Increased amounts of collagen are present in the lamina propria and submucosa and there is a variable degree of atrophy of the muscularis, which may be almost totally replaced by scar tissue (Figure 54–11). The walls of small arteries and arterioles are thickened and often surrounded by periadventitial deposits of collagen. Cellular infiltrates have been noted in the submucosa and also surround and infiltrate the myenteric plexuses of Auerbach, which may be conspicuously lacking in ganglion cells,[120] but usually do not appear to be abnormal.[7,359]

(*f*) *Lungs*.—The lungs are involved in the great majority of patients with PSS,

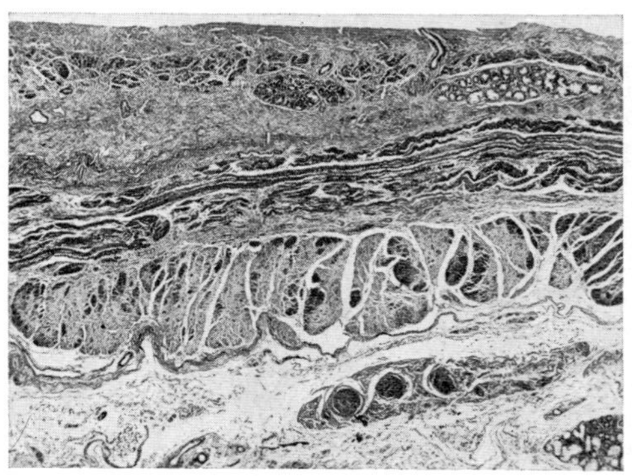

FIG. 54–11.—Photomicrograph of esophagus of man with PSS. The mucosa is missing as a result of postmortem autolysis. Note compact fibrosis of the submucosa and severe atrophy of muscularis which has been largely replaced by collagenous connective tissue (trichrome stain).

and interstitial and pulmonary fibrosis have been found in 74 to 90 per cent of cases at postmortem examination.[74,268] The most prominent symptom of this fibrosis is exertional dyspnea.[77,379] Occasionally there is a chronic cough, which is ordinarily non-productive unless there be supervening infection, and there may be one or more bouts of pleuritic chest pain. Many patients remain quite asymptomatic, however, despite evidence of severe fibrosis, presumably because of a restriction in physical activity. There may be tachypnea and basilar rales, and strikingly intense friction rubs have been noted in those individuals with pleurisy, but more often than not examination of the lungs proves unremarkable. Pneumothorax is rare.[87] In most cases the roentgenogram of the chest discloses a reticular pattern of linear, nodular, and lineonodular densities which are most pronounced in the lower two-thirds of the lung fields and which in some cases assume the appearance of diffuse mottling or honeycombing, indicative of cystic lesions.[121,182]

The most common and usually the earliest physiologic abnormality is an impairment in gas exchange.[1,49,77,158,160,283,313,379,388] Low diffusing capacities have been found in the absence of any significant alteration in ventilation or any roentgenographic evidence of fibrosis. Electron microscopic examination of the lung of a patient with a diminution in pulmonary gas exchange disclosed marked thickening of the basement membrane of alveolar lining cells and the endothelium of small blood vessels.[388] In many cases there is a restrictive ventilatory defect indicated by a reduction in vital capacity (chiefly inspiratory capacity) and decreased lung compliance,[283,313] which has been attributed to peribronchial and interstitial fibrosis. Later there is evidence of obstructive disease marked by a reduction in maximal breathing capacity and an increase in residual volume. Gross effort intolerance may develop which in some cases appears to be related to ventilation/

perfusion imbalance.[32,119] Despite these disturbances, however, the impairment of pulmonary function is rarely of sufficient severity to dominate the clinical picture or to cause death, unless there is cardiac failure or complicating infection.

The predominant histologic changes consist of diffuse alveolar, interstitial and peribronchial fibrosis.[74,379] In many cases the alveolar walls are simply thickened; in others degeneration and rupture of septa lead to the formation of cystlike cavities and small areas of bullous emphysema.[46,64,253] There may be extensive sclerosis of the small pulmonary arteries, particularly in subjects with pulmonary hypertension and cor pulmonale[74,241,360,379] (*see below*). In the early lesions the intima of small muscular arteries is swollen and contains material rich in acid mucopolysaccharides. Later one finds dense fibrosis of the intima with reduplication and fraying of the internal elastic membrane, hypertrophy of the fibromuscular tunic of pulmonary arterioles and perivascular fibrosis. With the exception of this latter change the severity of these vascular abnormalities (which usually spare pulmonary veins and bronchial vessels) may bear little relation to the degree of pulmonary interstitial fibrosis.[241,312,360] Pleural fibrosis is found in many more cases than would be suspected from the relative infrequency of pleurisy and/or pleural effusion.[74,379] Alveolar or bronchiolar cell carcinoma has been reported in at least fifteen patients with PSS.[3,46,64,399] These individuals had severe pulmonary fibrosis, either of the diffuse or of the compact cystic (honeycomb lung) variety, and the neoplasms appear to have arisen in areas of intense bronchiolar epithelial proliferation which accompanies this fibrosis. Aside from this, the association of PSS with malignant tumors is not particularly common.[42,152,220]

(*g*) *Heart.*—The nature and severity of cardiac disease depend on the degree of underlying myocardial fibrosis and on the extent to which concurrent pulmonary hypertension places an added burden on the circulation.[67,314] Many patients whose hearts are otherwise normal have an accentuation of the pulmonic second sound or a presystolic gallop rhythm, or both.[287,314] Cardiac catheterization has disclosed a high frequency of pulmonary hypertension even in patients with little or no evidence of fibrosis of the lung.[313,360] The rise in pulmonary arterial pressure is usually a modest one, but on occasion there is an elevation to the degree seen in primary pulmonary hypertension. Indeed, the latter is frequently marked by the coexistence of Raynaud's phenomenon and of arthritis, which has given rise to speculation that some cases may represent limited forms of PSS or a related connective tissue disorder.[378,394] Many patients with PSS develop cor pulmonale[241,313,314] which may progress slowly or may give rise to lethal right ventricular failure within a period of months. Extensive and severe pulmonary vascular lesions play a major role in those cases marked by a rapidly ingravescent course, while cor pulmonale of more protracted duration tends to be the result of pulmonary fibrosis which gradually obliterates more and more of the vascular bed of the lesser circulation.

There may be left ventricular or biventricular insufficiency, which tends to be very chronic; in our experience this has proven more frequent than cor pulmonale. A number of patients have chest pain not unlike angina due to coronary artery disease.[255] Cardiac arrhythmias (including complete heart block[10,206,275]) and other electrocardiographic abnormalities are commonplace, as would be expected in the case of a myocardiopathy.[77,92,206,255,389] Pericarditis and pericardial effusion, leading on occasion to cardiac tamponade, have been appreciated with increasing frequency.[14,74,233,243,255,314,348] There is a report of aortic valvulitis with perforation of an aortic cusp attributed to PSS,[305] but the prevalence of valvular lesions is no greater than that found in age-matched controls[74] and in most cases with clinically significant valvular dysfunction, it is difficult to exclude coincidental rheumatic heart disease. At autopsy there may be extensive degeneration of myocardial fibers with replacement by irregular patches of fibrosis prominent in, but not limited to, perivascular areas.[74,120,255,268,314] In addition, there may be focal infiltrates of round cells and thickening of smaller coronary vessels. The major coronary arteries are usually normal and myocardial infarction is most unusual. Study of the conduction system of two patients with complete heart block revealed replacement of the bundle branches by fibrous tissue.[206,275]

(*h*) *Intestinal Tract.*—In a small percentage of patients with PSS (including some with minimal or undetectable skin changes[3,261,293]), the illness is dominated by intestinal complaints, consisting of severe bloating, abdominal cramps, vomiting, episodic diarrhea, and constipation.[3,17,59,60,125,155,172,223,242,261,278,303,316,326,342] A number of these individuals show evidence of malabsorption (affecting water and electrolytes[265] as well as fat) which may result in extreme wasting. The hypomotility of the small intestine found in these cases is believed to favor the overgrowth of intestinal microorganisms which consume large amounts of vitamin B_{12} and interfere with normal fat absorption, presumably as a result of their deconjugation of bile salts, leading to impaired micelle formation.[28,82,172,193,232,316] (In one reported case, steatorrhea was attributed to pancreatic fibrosis.[222]) Dramatic improvement has been observed following the administration of tetracycline or other broad-spectrum antibiotics, with diminution in abdominal distention and diarrhea, increased appetite, decrease in steatorrhea, and substantial weight gain.[3,59,172,223,232,261,316]

There may be a pronounced disturbance in intestinal motility, as judged by radiographic study (even in asymptomatic patients), with prolonged retention of barium meal in the second and third portions of the duodenum, which are

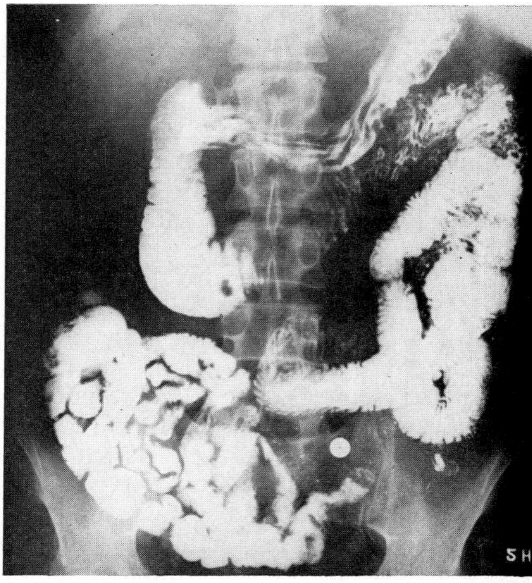

Fig. 54–12.—Roentgenogram of upper portion of gastrointestinal tract of a man with PSS (CRST syndrome) obtained 2 hours after taking barium meal. Note retention of food in stomach and in duodenum, which is widely dilated ("loop sign").

often atonic and widely dilated ("loop sign")[108,120,145] (Figure 54–12). In the remainder of the small intestine one may find irregular flocculation, localized areas of dilatation, and hypersegmentation.[28,108,121,182,278] The mucosal pattern of the distended jejunum is marked by prominent transverse folds.[261] Similar "barring" may also be found in the ileum. The atony of the bowel may be so severe as to result in an ileus with symptoms simulating mechanical obstruction,[28,125,261] and there is a report of a case in which the greatly dilated small intestine underwent volvulus.[3]

Patchy atrophy of the muscularis of the large intestine leads to the development of wide-mouthed diverticula, which usually occur along the anti-mesenteric border of the transverse and descending colon (Figures 54–13 and 54–14). In time these sacculations may disappear to be replaced by generalized colonic dilatation.[108,120,121,156,182,254,261] These sacculations may also occur in the jejunum and ileum[28] and are almost entirely unique

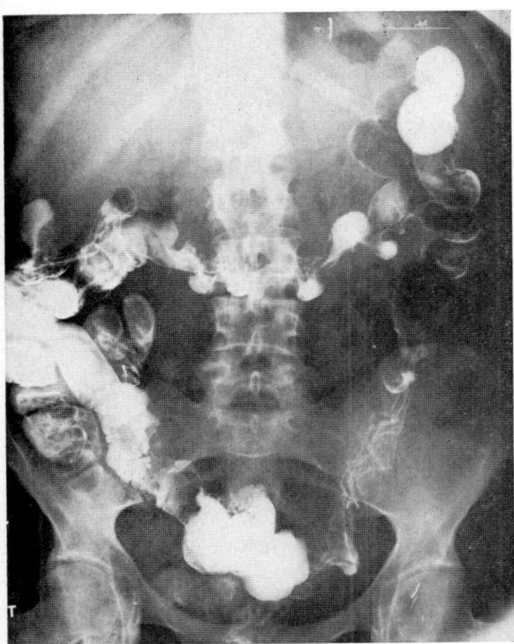

FIG. 54–13.—Roentgenogram of large intestine of a woman with PSS, illustrating numerous large-mouthed diverticula in transverse and descending colon.

to PSS, having been described to date in only one other condition, a single patient with amyloidosis.[182] Ordinarily these sacculations cause no difficulty; rarely, however, they may perforate or become impacted with fecal matter, producing obstruction.[66,156,242]

There are several reports of pneumatosis intestinalis in PSS.[48,159,232,236] This takes the form of numerous radiolucent cysts or linear streaks of gas within the wall which may dissect almost the entire length of the small intestine. (Figure 54–15*a*). Rupture of subserosal cysts leads to (benign) pneumoperitoneum. When accompanied by symptoms of partial small bowel obstruction the clinical picture may be highly suggestive of perforated viscus. The air which is present in the wall of the intestine apparently enters from the lumen through small defects in the mucosa and muscularis mucosae. (Figure 54–15*b*).

With the addition of serosal fibrosis, the chief pathologic changes in the intestinal tract are similar to those noted in the esophagus, *i.e.* fibrous thickening

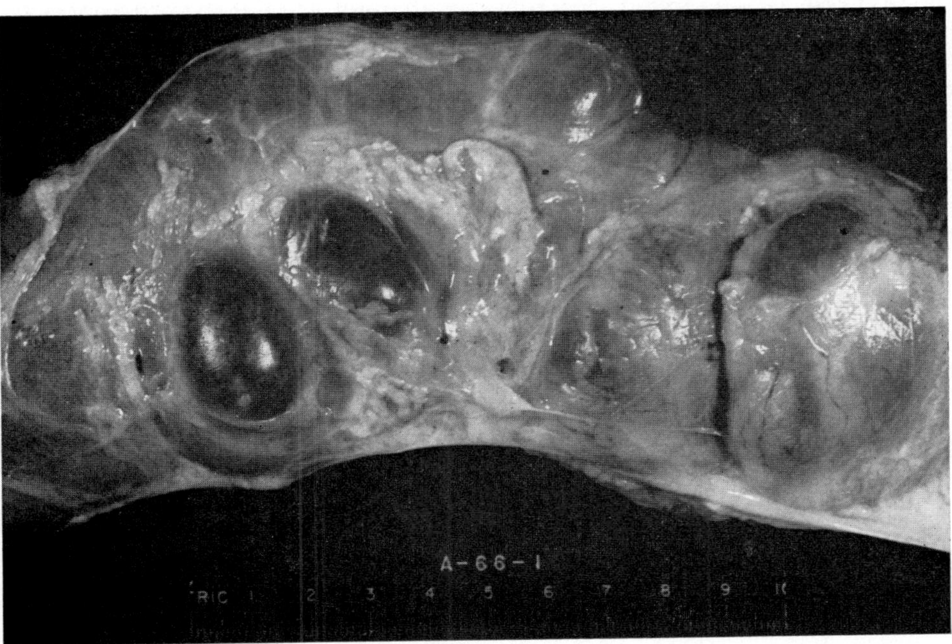

FIG. 54–14.—Gross appearance of portion of transverse colon, the roentgenogram of which is shown in preceding illustration. Note large, thin-walled sacculations.

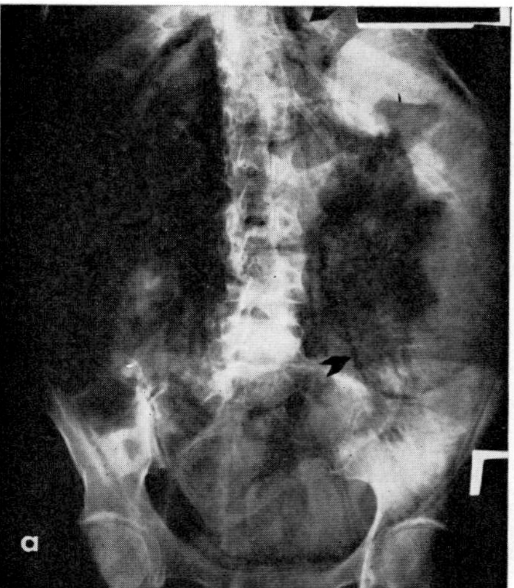

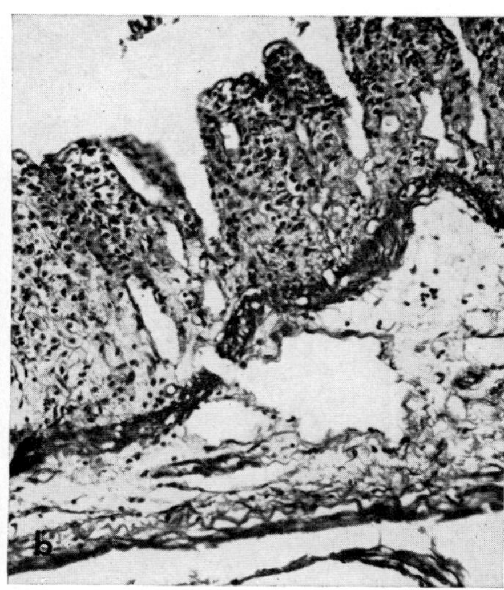

FIG. 54–15.—Pneumatosis intestinalis. (*a*) Roentgenogram of abdomen of woman with PSS, illustrating accumulation of gas in the wall of the greatly dilated small intestine. (*b*) Photomicrograph of ileum of this patient, demonstrating point of entry of air into the submucosa.

of the submucosa and atrophy of the smooth muscle, which is replaced by collagen.[3,48,74,125,156] Extensive infiltration of the lamina propria by lymphocytes and plasma cells is often found.[125,156,172,316,326] Large lipid droplets have been noted at the base of the epithelial cells, resembling those encountered in intestinal lymphangectasia;[125] this finding together with the occasional description of dilated lacteals suggests the existence of an impairment in lymph flow in some cases.[125,242] The intrinsic ganglion cells and their processes have been found to be normal in number and appearance.[3] Severe vasculitis, affecting chiefly small arteries and arterioles, has been observed[3,156] and on rare occasions there has been occlusion of larger mesenteric vessels, with infarction of portions of the ileum and colon.[86] Peroral biopsy specimens of the duodenum have revealed the presence of increased amounts of collagen surrounding and infiltrating Brunner's glands.[304,316,326] Biopsy specimens of the jejunum usually show no abnormality,[28,59,227,310] but may disclose mild villous atrophy.[326]

(*i*) *Kidney.*—Renal disease is recognized to be an important component of PSS and a major cause of death in this disorder.[230,287] Typically this involvement is manifested in the form of highly malignant arterial hypertension which is associated with the early development of rapidly progressive and irreversible renal insufficiency.[207,299,300,319,320] Most patients with this disturbance have had scleroderma for four years or less. The development of hypertension is often heralded by difficulty in vision as a result of severe retinopathy which is characterized by cotton-wool spots containing cytoid bodies, sero-fibrinous exudates, capillary hemorrhages, and papilledema.[5,216] In several days or weeks there is evidence of renal disease, indicated by proteinuria, rapidly increasing azotemia, and terminally by oliguria (at times anuria) and uremia. Extremely high plasma renin levels have been noted in two men with PSS and malignant hypertension.[331] On occasion the blood pressure may remain within normal limits,[74] but severe hypertension is the rule. These patients have succumbed to renal or cardiac failure or to cerebral hemorrhage despite treatment with a wide variety of antihypertensive medications. In a number of cases the onset of hypertension has been linked with the administration of ACTH or a corticosteroid.[300,352] There have been many instances, however, in which the patients had received none of these agents (including a few which antedate the corticosteroid era)[74,300] and the question of the role of corticosteroids in the provocation or precipitation of renal disease in these patients remains to be resolved.

The kidneys of the patients who die of renal disease usually contain a number of small infarcts. The lesions found on microscopic examination tend to be focal in distribution and consist of intimal hyperplasia of inter- and intralobular and smaller arteries marked by the deposition of a material rich in acid mucopolysaccharides, and fibrinoid necrosis of small arteries, afferent arterioles, and glomerular tufts[100,300,319,320] (Figure 54–16). These changes appear to be indistinguishable from those encountered in nonsclerodermatous malignant nephrosclerosis,[100,259] and in both conditions large amounts of fibrin have been detected in the fibrinoid material present in the walls of small vessels.[98] (It should be noted, however, that intimal hyperplasia of intralobular arteries and fibrinoid necrosis of afferent arterioles have been noted in the absence of hypertension.[74]) It is difficult to be certain of the significance of the presence of gammaglobulin and/or complement components in the glomerular lesions and necrotic areas of the renal vessels of patients with PSS and severe hypertension,[109,320] since similar findings have been reported in malignant nephrosclerosis of diverse etiology.[36,260] The possibility remains that immune complexes may be involved in the pathogenesis of the renal vascular changes. Additional immunohistologic studies prior to the development of arterial hypertension may prove helpful in this regard.

Endothelial cytoplasmic inclusions, morphologically resembling the nucleocapsid of certain paramyxoviruses and similar to those recently described in systemic lupus erythematosus[130,247] and polymyositis,[248] have been found in the kidney of at least two patients with PSS.[56,247] (These particles have also been

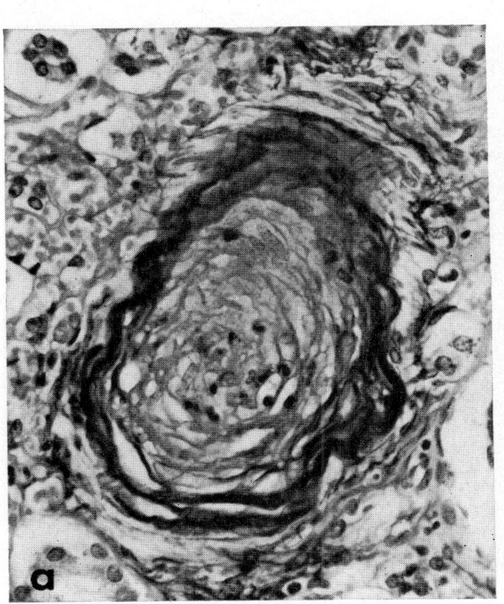

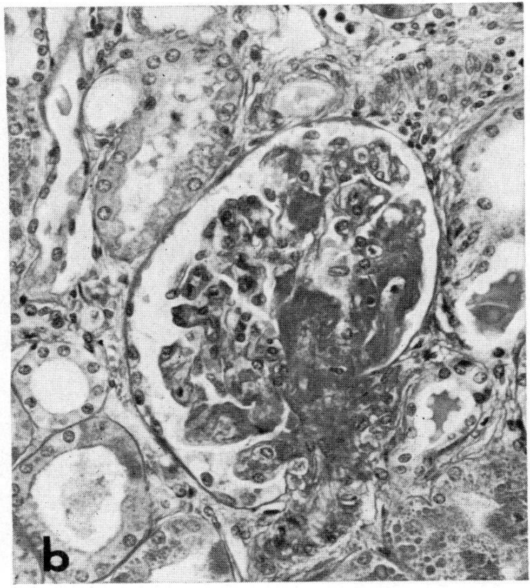

FIG. 54–16.—Photomicrograph of kidneys of two women with PSS, who died of malignant arterial hypertension and renal insufficiency. (*a*) Intimal hyperplasia of interlobular artery leading to occlusion of lumen. Note reduplication and fraying of internal elastic lamina (orcein stain). (*b*) Fibrinoid necrosis of glomerular capillaries.

seen in the skin of one patient with PSS.[129])

Angiographic examination during life and postmortem injection studies have revealed a striking constriction of the interlobular arteries and afferent arterioles and a sharp decrease in glomerular filling[299,372] (Figure 54–17). This disturbance in the renal circulation may be likened to Raynaud's phenomenon in the digital circulation (*see above*). It should be noted, however, that similar abnormalities have been observed in the kidneys of patients with nonsclerodermatous arterial hypertension.[148,228] Certain of the pathologic changes in the renal arteries are quite similar to those encountered in the distal vessels.[171]

The pathogenesis of the renal circulatory abnormalities in PSS remains unclear. In one investigation of normotensive patients with this disease, effective renal plasma flow was reduced in a majority of cases, while the glomerular filtration rate was normal in all but a few.[373] These findings were considered to be indicative of efferent arteriolar constriction. Patients with PSS who are normotensive display a hyperreactivity to angiotensin and normal cold pressor responses, which suggest the existence of an intrinsic arteriolar abnormality.[298] In some, but not all, cases with frank renal involvement we have found evidence of increased intravascular coagulation and the possibility that this mechanism[349] may play a role in the aggravation of the renal damage is worthy of additional study.

(*j*) *Liver*.—Primary disease of the liver is most unusual in PSS, and in several of the cases which have been described it is difficult to be certain of any causal connection.[11,43] There have been recent accounts, however, of the occurrence of primary biliary cirrhosis in a number of women with the CRST syndrome[43,69,239,279] (*see above*). These patients have

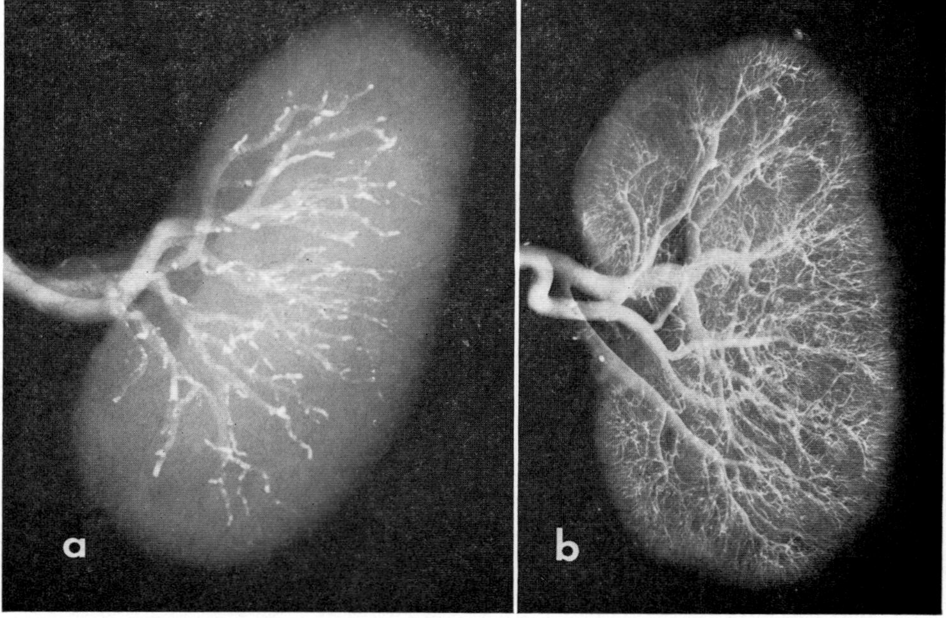

Fig. 54–17.—Roentgenograms of kidneys, injected post mortem, of two patients with PSS. (*a*) Kidney of woman who developed malignant arterial hypertension and died one month later of renal insufficiency. There is irregular narrowing of the interlobular vessels, only a few of which fill normally. (*b*) Kidney of man who died of cardiac failure and had no evidence of renal disease. There is normal filling of the interlobular arteries and cortical vessels.

had jaundice, pruritus, and hepatomegaly, with a marked elevation of serum alkaline phosphatase activity and anti-mitochondrial antibodies.[279] In addition there are isolated reports of occlusion of the extrahepatic ducts secondary to arteritis[384] and of spontaneous rupture of the liver in a woman with PSS and arterial hypertension[225] (*see above*). Pancreatic involvement in PSS appears to be a rarity.[222]

(*k*) *Hematologic Findings.*—Early in PSS the blood count is normal and the bone marrow unremarkable save for focal plasmacytosis and occasional aggregates of lymphocytes.[365,381] Later, there may be anemia associated with visceral involvement and its complications (renal failure, intestinal malabsorption, and rarely esophageal bleeding). In those patients with impaired absorption of vitamin B_{12} and of iron, the marrow may be mildly to markedly hypoplastic, but is not fibrotic. A few instances of autoimmune hemolytic anemia have been reported.[52,302] Microangiopathic hemolytic anemia has occurred in patients with renal disease. Eosinophilia (as high as 2400 or more eosinophils per mm.^{3}) occurs on rare occasions,[203,254] but ordinarily the differential white blood cell count is normal. Recently a patient with PSS and autoimmune thrombocytopenia has been reported.[161a]

(*l*) *Nervous System.*—The nervous system is rarely involved in PSS. In general the neurologic abnormalities which do occur are either purely coincidental or represent secondary manifestations of renal or cardiopulmonary involvement.[122] Exceptional patients have had mononeuropathy or polyneuropathy which has been attributed to thickening of the connective tissue sheaths of the nerve, deposition of mucoid material around the nerve fibers, and changes in the arteriae nervorum.[183,281] The occurrence of trigeminal sensory neuropathy has been described[16,351] as well as an apparently unique case of cerebral infarction resulting from arteritis localized to a single internal carotid artery.[202]

COURSE OF THE DISEASE

The natural course of PSS is extremely variable. In many cases there is steadily progressive sclerosis of the hands and fingers leading to crippling flexion contractures; in others there is spontaneous improvement in the skin which may return to a near normal condition. Most if not all patients eventually show evidence of visceral involvement which can often be detected by appropriate testing (pulmonary function studies, esophageal pressure measurements, etc.) long before the appearance of symptoms. It is difficult to judge prognosis with respect to both disability and death early in the course of the illness. In particular esophageal, intestinal, renal and other internal changes may appear in the face of minimal or apparently stable scleroderma and may or may not progress in concert with the skin.[117,293]

Survivorship

Decreased survivorship has been noted in patients who are 45 years or older at the time of diagnosis, and in men compared to women.[230] Negroes fare less well than do whites, particularly early in the course of disease.[220,230] In general the outlook is significantly poorer when there is clinical evidence of involvement of the kidney, heart, or lung at the time that PSS is first recognized, and is particularly grave in those patients who develop renal disease with malignant hypertension; as a rule these latter die within a few weeks to months.[96,230,287] The worsened prognosis in patients with rapidly progressive and more widespread scleroderma is related to the high frequency of associated changes of vital organs. Individuals with the CRST syndrome (*see above*), who have less severe visceral dysfunction tend to have a particularly favorable course.[230] In these and other cases, the disease may be only very slowly progressive and not necessarily threatening to life. In two studies employing the life-table method of analysis and based on roughly comparable populations of hospital-diagnosed cases of PSS, the cumulative survival rate after 5 years was 34 per cent and 48 per cent and after 7 years 27 per cent and 35 per cent.[230,312]

PSS and Pregnancy

We, like others,[167,237] have found that pregnancy exerts no consistent effect on the course of PSS. The disease, in turn, ordinarily does not interfere with pregnancy and parturition, although there have been a number of cases in which the development of eclampsia (in some instances superimposed upon or associated with the renal changes of PSS) was responsible for the loss of mother and child.[97,343] Others, with experience based upon a different patient population, have concluded that the pregnancy in PSS is attended by a high rate of premature deliveries, stillbirths, and abortions.[337]

METABOLISM OF CONNECTIVE TISSUE IN PSS

The fibrosis of the skin and internal organs in PSS appears to be the result of overproduction of collagen, the turnover of which is normally very limited in the adult animal.[245] This view is supported by both morphologic observations and biochemical studies. Electron microscopic examination has disclosed alterations in the dermal fibroblasts and collagen fiber population which are indicative of active fibrillogenesis (*see above*).[142,143,190,191,192,311] Measurement of the weight and hydroxyproline content of skin cores of uniform surface diameter obtained early in the course of PSS has confirmed clinical and histologic evidence of an hypertrophy of the dermis, and has shown that there is a concomitant and proportional increase in the collagen content of the thickened skin.[102,295]

Increased levels of protocollagen proline hydroxylase activity have been reported in the skin of patients with scleroderma.[180,368] In one study, greater than normal enzyme activity was found in both obviously affected as well as apparently normal skin from the same patients, the values being twice as great, however, in the abnormal skin.[180] This enzyme is responsible for the conversion of peptide-bound proline to hydroxyproline in protocollagen, the precursor of collagen, and measurements of its activity in embryonic tissues and healing wounds have been found to correlate well with the rate of collagen synthesis.[240] Additional evidence indicative of an increase in collagen synthesis in scleroderma has come from studies in which skin biopsy specimens were incubated in a medium containing radioactive proline and new collagen formation estimated from the specific radioactivity of proline in collagen[179] or from the accumulation of radioactive hydroxyproline in nondialyzable protein.[196] Judging from the rapid insolubilization of this newly synthesized radioactive hydroxyproline (collagen), there appears to be no abnormality in the maturation process whereby collagen is continuously converted into less and less soluble forms as a result of intra- and intermolecular cross-linking.[369] (Examination of the solubility of the collagen in skin biopsy specimens from patients with PSS has yielded conflicting results, some authors reporting normal or slightly decreased amounts of acetic acid- or citrate-soluble material,[137,141] others describing the extraction of increased amounts of soluble collagen.[196,370])

Collagenase has been extracted from human granulocytic leukocytes and has been detected in cultures of both skin and synovium, including the synovium of a patient with PSS.[89,114,136,200] The importance of this enzyme in the normal metabolism of collagen, as well as the question of its function, if any, in the origin and evolution of scleroderma, remains to be determined.

There is no evidence of any qualitative abnormality of the collagen in PSS, save for an increase in bound hexosamine which may be related in some way to the homogeneous appearance of this collagen.[104,311] The amino acid composition of the insoluble collagen fraction is closely similar to that of normal dermal collagen[102] and its shrinkage temperature and contractile properties are comparable to those of mature collagen.[273] Although the elimination of urinary hydroxyproline in patients with PSS maintained on a low hydroxyproline diet has generally been found to lie within normal limits,[220,340] we have noted an increased excretion (>50 mg. per 24 hours) in 19 of 69 patients, with values as high as 116 mg. per 24 hours[289,296] (Figure 54–18). Those with excessive urinary hydroxyproline have been individuals with diffuse and rapidly progressive scleroderma, many of whom were also found to have elevated levels of plasma hydroxyproline-containing collagen-like protein (hyproprotein).[205,289,296] In a number of instances urinary hydroxyproline excretion and plasma hyproprotein levels have returned to normal after the sclerodermatous process has appeared to become stable.

The reports dealing with serum mucopolysaccharide and mucoprotein levels, and with urinary mucopolysaccharide excretion in PSS are conflicting, some authors citing elevations and others normal values.[103,133,154,251,258,356,391] These discrepancies may be due in part to methodological difficulties but can also be explained by differences in the patients studied with respect to duration, severity, and rate of progression of disease. In the early stage of scleroderma there is histologic evidence of an increase in acid mucopolysaccharides in the dermis,[30] and it appears likely that water-binding by these substances accounts for the edema

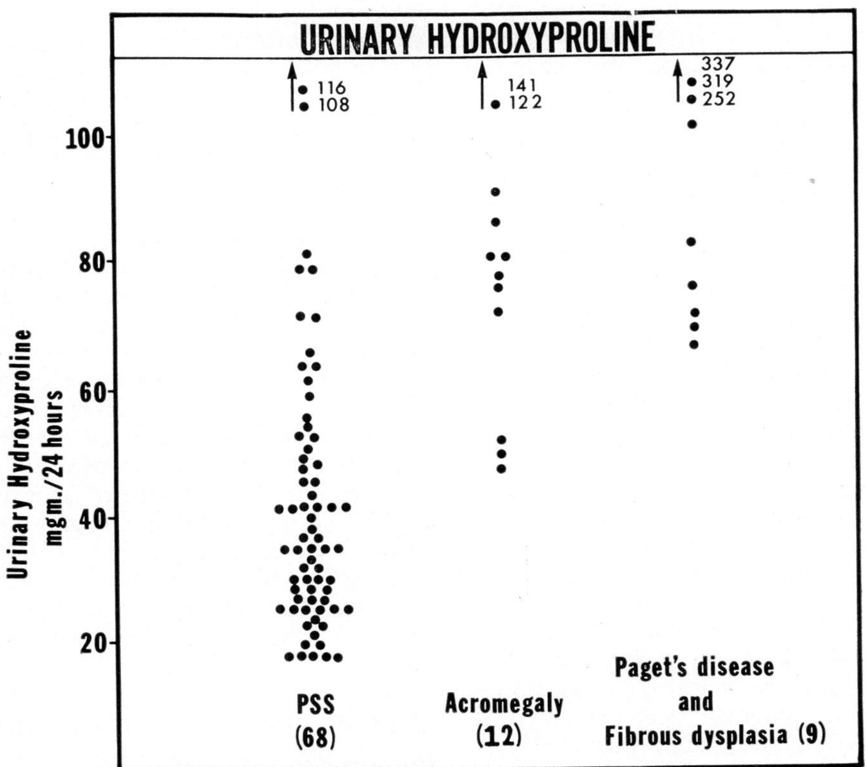

FIG. 54–18.—Urinary hydroxyproline excretion in patients with PSS, acromegaly, and Paget's disease (osteitis deformans), all of whom were maintained on a low hydroxyproline diet during collections.

which is among the first manifestations of the disease. An abnormally high intake of radioactivity in the skin of patients given an intravenous injection of $Na_2{}^{35}SO_4$ has been interpreted as indicating an increase in the rate of local synthesis of sulfated mucopolysaccharides.[78] Later in the course of scleroderma, however, there is a notable diminution or absence of such material in the skin.[101]

The factors which regulate the normal turnover of collagen are only poorly understood and the cause of the overgrowth of connective tissue in PSS remains a mystery. Based on the occurrence of a peculiar localized scleroderma-like fibrosis of the skin in a few patients with the malignant carcinoid syndrome[4, 140,398] it has been suggested that the answer may lie in a derangement of serotonin metabolism.[397] Also intriguing in this regard is the development of an inflammatory fibrosis involving the retroperitoneal tissues, thorax, and heart in patients treated with the antiserotonin agent methysergide[123] and the report of a case in which retroperitoneal fibrosis was associated with Raynaud's phenomenon and pulmonary fibrosis.[271] There is, however, little or no evidence of an underlying disturbance in serotonin metabolism in PSS, and urinary excretion of 5-hydroxyindoleacetic acid is normal.[361] It has been reported that patients with PSS (and also, in at least one case, unaffected relatives) have an abnormality in tryptophan metabolism, characterized by excretion of excessive amounts of kynurenine and other intermediary metabolites, suggestive of a deficiency in kynurenine hydroxylase.[269] This is a nonspecific finding, similar deviations having been observed in rheumatoid arthritis and various other disorders.[266] It is of interest, however, that the development of scleroderma of the trunk and extremities has recently been reported in children with phenylketonuria.[84,163,189] In this disorder, the absence of the enzyme phenylalanine hydroxylase leads to the accumulation of phenylalanine and abnormal intermediary metabolites which interfere with the normal utilization of tryptophan, leading to excessive urinary excretion of indolic compounds and decreased levels of plasma hydroxytryptamine (serotonin) and urinary 5-hydroxyindoleacetic acid. The changes in the skin and subcutaneous tissues, which have appeared at the age of 6 to 10 months, are unlike those of PSS in the sequence of their development and there has been no evidence of esophageal dysfunction or other visceral involvement. Improvement was noted when these patients were placed on low phenylalanine diet. Studies of nine other children with scleroderma, from 3 to 14 years of age, revealed normal urinary levels of both phenylalanine and o-hydroxyphenylacetic acid.[189]

Autografts of clinically normal skin transferred to the involved forearm have been reported to become progressively sclerodermatous, while forearm skin placed in the abdominal site remained thickened.[111] In contrast, the lesions of localized scleroderma (morphea) proved reversible after transplantation into normal areas.[139] The importance of extracutaneous factors in determining the localization and severity of the skin changes in PSS is further suggested by a case in which a finger that had been reattached following accidental amputation many years prior to the development of scleroderma remained unaffected while Raynaud's phenomenon and the resorption of terminal phalangeal bone took place in the remaining digits.[321] We have recently encountered a man with PSS in whom digital vasospasm and skin changes were disproportionately mild in an arm in which there was severe motor weakness (but normal sensation) as the result of childhood injury of the brachial plexus.[294]

ETIOLOGY AND PATHOGENESIS

Immunologic Abnormalities

Progressive systemic sclerosis was originally linked with rheumatoid arthritis, systemic lupus erythematosus (SLE) and certain other rheumatic diseases because these conditions have a number of clinical features in common and because they are all characterized anatomically by generalized alterations of (or in) the connective tissue, or as it was called at first, the collagen-vascular system.[186,187] Morphologic similarities in the vascular changes to the lesions of experimental and human serum sickness, polyarteritis, and drug hypersensitivity[280] led to the hypothesis that an immunologic abnormality might be a common denominator in the pathogenesis of these "collagen diseases." This concept has been strengthened in recent years by evidence drawn from a number of different lines of investigation.

(*a*) *Morphologic Changes.*—Although the most obvious change in advanced PSS is widespread hyperplasia of collagenous connective tissue, in many cases there are impressive inflammatory and vascular lesions. These are detected with particular frequency early during the course of the disease, before there has been dense overgrowth of collagen in the tissues. The most conspicuous sites of inflammation are the synovium, muscle, and gastrointestinal tract (*see above*) but collections of lymphocytes and plasma cells have also been detected in the skin and other locations.[125,156,288] Vascular lesions were first emphasized by Matsui[221] and have been described in a number of organs, including the lung, heart, gastrointestinal tract, and kidneys, as well as in the digital arteries.[250] As discussed previously the significance of the immunoglobulin and complement components found in the renal vessels of patients with PSS and malignant hypertension[109,320] is unclear, and as yet there is no convincing evidence that antigen-antibody complexes are involved in the production of the vascular lesions of PSS. The changes which take place in the vessel walls closely resemble those which occur in extravascular connective tissue, and there is a conspicuous absence of polymorphonuclear leukocytes or other cellular infiltrate. Furthermore, in contrast to discoid and systemic lupus erythematosus wherein the presence of immunoglobulins (IgG, IgA, and IgM) and complement at the dermal-epidermal junction can be demonstrated in high percentage of cases, the skin of patients with PSS has generally failed to show such deposits.[54,174,176]

Hyperplasia of the thymus with germinal follicle formation and abnormal Hassall's corpuscles has been described in a young man with PSS who died of cardiac failure.[22] The question of thymic changes requires additional study.

(*b*) *Serum Proteins.*—Hypergammaglobulinemia has been found in a quarter to a half of patients with PSS.[9,58,288,306,347] Although this is usually only moderate in degree (1.4 to 2.0 g./100 ml.) values over 4.5 g./100 ml. have been observed. In most instances the increase is chiefly in IgG; less often the levels of IgA and IgM are elevated.[306] In one study of urinary immunoglobulin excretion no free light chains were found in fourteen patients with PSS,[68] while in another report two patients with the disease were noted to have increased urinary IgG, accompanied in one by large amounts of a monoclonal kappa-type light chain.[211] There was a polyclonal hypergammaglobulinemia in this case and no evidence of myeloma.

(*c*) *Serologic Abnormalities.*—Between a quarter to a third of patients with PSS have positive tests for rheumatoid factor.[9,58,226,288,306] In most cases the serum titers have been 1:320 or less. Positive reactions tend to occur more frequently in those patients with pronounced joint disease, but this correlation is not strong. There have been numerous reports of positive LE cell reactions and of biological false positive serologic tests for syphilis.[50,58,85,287,288,308,366] A number of these individuals have had evidence of SLE and of Sjögren's syndrome.[85,366]

Antinuclear antibodies have been found in the sera of 40 to 90 per cent of patients with PSS.[12,37,94,99,170,226,284,306,327] In most cases the titers are relatively low, as compared to those present in SLE, although in some cases the titer has been 1:1024 or greater.[306] Most commonly the pattern of nuclear immunofluorescence is that of fine or large speckles[38,226,306] (Figure 54–19). Occasionally the nuclear staining is diffuse (homogeneous) or thready[39] in appearance. The antinuclear factors have been found to be present chiefly in the IgG and IgM classes of immunoglobulin, but also involve IgA and IgD.[284,306] Nucleolar immunofluorescence has been observed in 10 per cent to as high as 54 per cent of cases and is found more often in PSS than in the other connective tissue diseases.[12,13,37,99,170,284,285,327] These antibodies which are frequently confined to IgG immunoglobulins[285] are particularly common in those patients in whom PSS is associated with Sjögren's syndrome. Antibodies to DNA, to ribosomes, and to double-stranded DNA, which are detected with great frequency in SLE, have been notably unusual or absent in patients with PSS.[161,325,327] There appears to be little if any correlation between the presence or titer of antinuclear antibody and the clinical severity or duration of PSS,[12,226,306] although there is some disagreement in this matter.[37] We like others[15,38] have noted antinuclear factors in many patients with so-called primary Raynaud's disease. A variety of patterns (homogeneous, speckled, and nucleolar) has been seen in this group.

(*d*) *Serum Complement.*—Some diminution in whole hemolytic complement has been noted in an occasional patient with PSS, but in general the levels have been found to be normal,[358,386] including those in individuals with fulminating renal involvement.[324] We have examined 90 serums from 69 patients with PSS, including many in the early stages of disease, and have found values of less than 32 units/ml. in only 5 instances.

(*e*) *Cellular Immunity.*—There is no evidence of any deficit in cell-mediated immune defense mechanisms in PSS. The patients are not unduly susceptible to viral, fungal or other systemic infection.

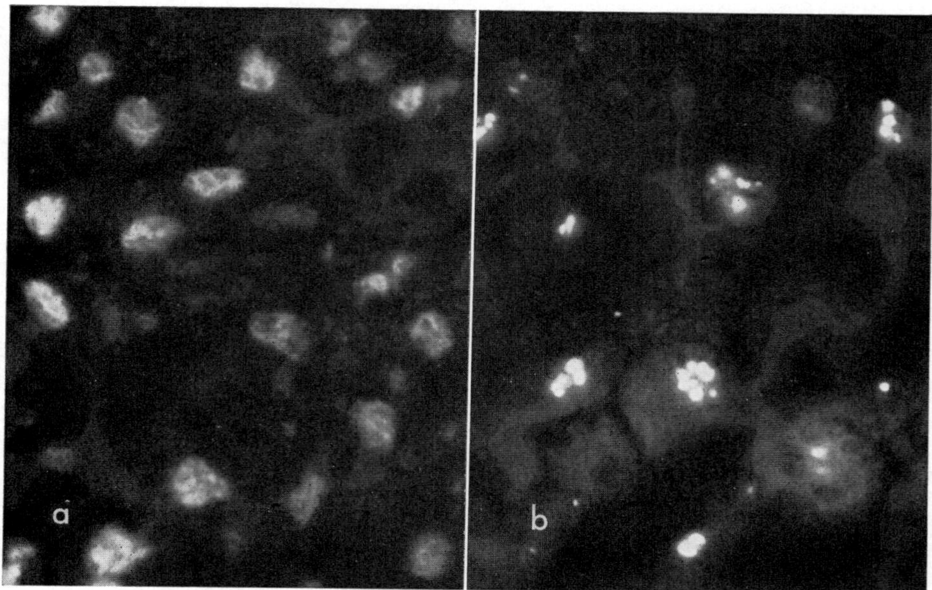

Fig. 54–19.—Patterns of nuclear immunofluorescence produced by sera of patients with PSS incubated with mouse liver slices and followed by application of fluorescein-isothiocyanate labeled rabbit antihuman immunoglobulin (IgG). (*a*) Fine speckles in reticular network. (*b*) Large discrete speckles. (From Rothfield and Rodnan,[306]courtesy of Arthritis and Rheumatism).

Cutaneous delayed hypersensitivity is intact and the proliferative response of their lymphocytes exposed to phytohemagglutinin is similar to that observed in normal subjects.[392] The intriguing possibility that aberrant cellular immunity may play an important role in the pathogenesis of this disorder remains to be investigated.

Some patients with PSS exhibit a delayed reaction after the intradermal injection of leukocytes or calf thymus DNA.[95,362] It is not clear whether this is related to an immunologic reaction.

(f) Miscellaneous Observations.—Unlike certain other connective tissue diseases PSS does not predispose to the development of overt amyloidosis. Pericollagenous amyloid deposits have been detected by means of polarization microscopy in the skin and in the internal organs, however.[153] There are two cases on record in which there was an apparently fortuitous association between primary amyloidosis and PSS.[213,312] The thickening of the skin produced by infiltration of amyloid may closely simulate the changes of scleroderma. The significance of the pleomorphic acid-fast bacteria which have been found in the skin of patients with PSS and morphea (localized scleroderma), both in tissue sections and on culture is unknown.[45]

Association of PSS with Other Connective Tissue Disorders ("Overlap Syndrome")

There are a number of patients with scleroderma and other evidence of PSS who also present certain clinical and serologic features highly suggestive of SLE, including fever, discoid rash, pleurisy, pleural effusion, pericarditis, splenomegaly, lymphadenopathy, convulsions, anemia, leukopenia, marked hypergammaglobulinemia, and positive LE cell reaction.[21,50,54,74,85,254,308,332,366] In our experience, this blend (labeled "*lupoderma*") is usually encountered in young women. These patients have been found to have extremely high titers of a hemagglutinating antibody which reacts with an extractable nuclear antigen and is associated with a speckled pattern of antinuclear immunofluorescence.[332] Comment has already been made on the similarity between the early articular disease of PSS and rheumatoid arthritis[297] and the skeletal muscle involvement which may be clinically and pathologically indistinguishable from polymyositis ("*sclerodermatomyositis*").[83,210,231,366] In our experience the number of individuals in whom there is evidence of an "overlap syndrome" has been relatively small, amounting to approximately 10 per cent of our patients with PSS. Like rheumatoid arthritis and SLE, PSS has been associated in a number of instances with Sjögren's syndrome, less often with Hashimoto's thyroiditis, and rarely with hypogammaglobulinemia.[26,288,333,366]

Familial Occurrence of PSS

Familial PSS is a rarity.[25,220,222,254,288,323] A family has been described in which the four daughters of a woman with typical PSS and Sjögren's syndrome developed Raynaud's phenomenon and variably convincing evidence of scleroderma.[44] Close relatives of patients with PSS are uncommonly affected by other connective tissue diseases, and in one instance the identical twin of a woman with scleroderma and discoid lupus erythematosus developed SLE.[85] The number of such occurrences is too few to support the notion of an heritable predisposition to these disorders, and suggests the possibility of either chance association or common exposure to some environmental agent. In this latter regard it has been found that the first degree relatives of patients with PSS occasionally have unexplained hypergammaglobulinemia and that in approximately 10 per cent of these individuals there is a low titer of serum antinuclear antibodies.[306]

Chromosomal Abnormalities

Cytogenetic studies of peripheral blood lymphocytes of patients with PSS have revealed a marked increase in simple (chromatid) and compound (chromosomal) aberrations which are inconsistent in pattern and suggestive of nonspecific breakage with resultant deletions and translocations.[157,257] Since there is no evidence of a familial (genetic) predisposition to chromosome breakage and since neither chemical nor physical factors (specifically x-radiation) appear to be wholly responsible, it has been suggested that these abnormalities may be the result of acquired damage by virus(es) or some other biologic agent.

Experimental Models of PSS

No naturally occurring disorder which mimics PSS has been identified to date in lower animals. Of interest, however, are the changes in rats which develop homologous disease after the injection of lymphoid cells from an unrelated strain of donor animals.[345] In the chronic dermatosis of homologous disease there is a great increase in dermal collagen and atrophy of the epidermis and skin appendages, with a very mild or barely discernible inflammatory reaction. The resemblance to scleroderma is apparent. Collagenous thickening of the skin has also been noted in autografts undergoing chronic rejection. Whether or not the skin changes in homologous disease (or PSS) involve a specific anti-collagen antibody remains to be determined. It is now clear that both pure and enzyme-treated collagen are capable of provoking antibodies and that the major immunogenic sites in native tropocollagen are the telopeptides present on both α1- and α2-chains.[75,234]

CLASSIFICATION OF PSS AND DIFFERENTIAL DIAGNOSIS OF SCLERODERMA

When there is diffuse induration of the skin and Raynaud's phenomenon combined with typical articular and visceral features the diagnosis of PSS is readily apparent and is confirmed by the finding of the roentgenographic, histologic and serologic abnormalities which have been discussed above. The situation may be far less obvious during the early phases of the disease, when cutaneous changes are not fully developed. Cases in which there is a minimum or absence of scleroderma (PSS *sine* scleroderma) and those in which PSS overlaps with other connective tissue disorders present special difficulties. Many of the former remain undiagnosed until the characteristic sclerosis and vascular lesions of internal organs are revealed at autopsy. There are, on the other hand, a number of diseases which may be confused with PSS, usually because of a similarity in the cutaneous manifestations.

The term scleroderma has traditionally been applied not only to the cutaneous changes of PSS but to a heterogeneous group of conditions in which there is more circumscribed or patchy sclerosis of the skin (Table 54–1).[53,55,71] The hardening, tightening and inelasticity of the

Table 54-1.—Classification of Scleroderma

A. Progressive systemic sclerosis
   1. Diffuse (acrosclerosis) or generalized scleroderma
   2. Thibierge-Weissenbach or CRST syndrome, with limited changes in the skin (sclerodactyly)
   3. "Overlap" syndromes ("lupoderma," "sclerodermatomyositis")

B. Localized scleroderma
   1. Morphea
      a. Guttate morphea
      b. Plaque
      c. Generalized morphea
   2. Linear scleroderma
      a. Linear scleroderma of the extremity
      b. Linear scleroderma *en coup de sabre*, with or without facial hemiatrophy

integument may be indistinguishable from that observed in PSS, but certain pathologic as well as clinical differences exist between these conditions and PSS. In our experience, like that of others, there has been little or no convincing evidence of internal involvement in the localized forms of scleroderma or of overlap between these conditions and PSS.[53,268]

Localized Scleroderma

Although the etiology of localized scleroderma is presently obscure, in many cases the skin changes appear soon after trauma and originate at the site of injury.[51,53,55,151] A familial incidence has been observed.[35,55] There are a few cases of probably chance association between localized scleroderma and SLE or other systemic connective tissue disease.[364]

(*a*) *Morphea.*—This variety of localized scleroderma begins with areas of violaceous or erythematous discoloration of the skin which take the form of discrete drop-like patches (guttate morphea) or plaques. As the lesions evolve they become sclerotic and waxy or ivory colored and may increase to a diameter of many centimeters. The surface is smooth and hairless and ceases to sweat. During this active phase of the disease the lesions are surrounded by a violaceous border of inflammation. After a period of several months to years there is spontaneous softening of the skin, which becomes atrophic and hyperpigmented or depigmented. Localized morphea may occur at any age and affect any site. The disease is confined entirely to the skin and subcutis, and is ordinarily of little consequence unless there is involvement of the face (sometimes with hemiatrophy[364]) or extensive dissemination of the lesions (generalized morphea) which may affect large portions of the trunk and extremities and cause much despair. The major histologic changes during the stage of thickening of the skin consist of new collagen deposition in the dermis and septa of the subcutaneous tissue and variably heavy perivascular infiltrations of lymphocytes, plasma cells and histiocytes.[53] The inflammatory reaction at the border of the lesions is much more marked than that usually encountered in PSS. There is inflammation, and later fibrosis and atrophy of underlying striated muscle;[190] in contrast to PSS, there appears to be little or no abnormality in the muscle capillaries.[235] Children with morphea are reported to have antibodies to both native and heat-denatured deoxyribonucleic acid while none were found in children with PSS.[132]

(*b*) *Linear Scleroderma.*—In this variety of localized scleroderma, which usually develops during childhood,[71] a linear streak of sclerosis develops in the upper or lower extremity, or in the frontoparietal area of the head ("en coup de sabre"). Less commonly, the trunk is affected. The band may run the entire length of the arm or leg. Occasionally there may be multiple lesions.[35] Induration extends into the deeper tissues, including muscle, and fibrosis and fixation of para-articular structures may result in contractures which seriously interfere with motion of the joint (usually fingers, elbows, or knees) and require surgical correction. There have been several instances in which linear scleroderma has coexisted in the same extremity with melorheostosis, a peculiar type of linear fibrotic hyperostosis of bone.[238] There is considerable overlap between morphea and linear scleroderma and typical lesions of each often exist contemporaneously in the same patient.[55,252,364]

Conditions with Scleroderma-Like Changes in the Skin ("Pseudoscleroderma")

There are a number of conditions in which there are skin changes that may resemble those encountered in PSS ("pseudoscleroderma") (Table 54–2). Ordinarily there is little difficulty in differentiation because most of these maladies lack the visceral components of PSS

Table 54-2.—Diseases in Which There Are Skin Changes That May Resemble Scleroderma ("Pseudo-scleroderma")

A. Edematous
  1. Scleredema (scleredema adultorum of Buschke) (A. Buschke, 1900)
  2. Scleromyxedema (papular mucinosis)

B. Indurative
  1. Carcinoid syndrome
  2. Phenylketonuria
  3. Porphyria cutanea tarda
  4. Congenital porphyria
  5. Primary amyloidosis
  6. Acromegaly

C. Atrophic
  1. Werner's syndrome (O. Werner, 1904)
  2. Progeria
  3. Rothmund's syndrome (Rothmund-Thomson syndrome) (A. Rothmund, Jr., 1868; M. S. Thomson, 1923)
  4. Acrodermatitis chronica atrophicans
  5. Lichen sclerosus et atrophicus

and/or display characteristic diagnostic features of their own.

Scleredema is characterized by firm, painless, symmetrical edematous induration of the skin of face, scalp, neck, trunk, and proximal portions of the extremities.[29,72,105,124] The hands and feet may be affected, but this is uncommon. The changes in the skin, which frequently appear in the wake of a streptococcal infection, tend to resolve spontaneously after a period of 6 to 12 months, but may persist for many years.[72,105,124] There may be hydrarthrosis, pleural and pericardial effusions, widespread involvement of muscle including the heart, and macroglossia. (It is possible that the historic patient described by Curzio had scleredema, rather than scleroderma.[73]) Since children constitute a relatively high proportion of the cases, the older term scleredema adultorum is a misnomer.[124] Histochemical studies have revealed swollen collagen bundles and the accumulation of mucopolysaccharide (probably hyaluronic acid) in the dermis, subcutis, and skeletal muscle.[29,105,124]

Scleromyxedema (lichen myxedematosus, papular mucinosis) is a rare disorder in which there is a widespread lichenoid eruption of soft pale red or yellowish papules accompanied by diffuse thickening of the skin, including the face and hands.[264] Dense deposits of acid mucopolysaccharide are found in upper portion of the dermis. Abnormal serum immunoglobulins (M-components) have been detected in several cases suggesting a relationship of this condition to myelomatosis.[65,165a,224,264]

Scleroderma-like induration of the skin and pigmentary changes occur in *porphyria cutanea tarda* usually, but not always, in sun-exposed areas. In distinction from the latter, however, bullae are rare in PSS[116] and uroporphyrin excretion is normal.[276]

Infiltration of the dermis occurs in many cases of *primary amyloidosis*. This may take the form of firm, discrete, hemispherical brown or yellow papules, but when the deposition of amyloid is diffuse and involves the fingers, hands and face, the edema and hardening of the skin are easily mistaken for scleroderma. In two such instances in our experience the correct diagnosis was suggested by the development of macroglossia.

There may be considerable thickening of the skin and subcutaneous tissues in *acromegaly*, as a result of connective tissue hyperplasia.[181] The cutaneous sclerosis which develops in some cases of the *carcinoid syndrome* and *phenylketonuria* has been described above.

The principal manifestations of *Werner's syndrome* consist of a symmetrical retardation of growth with absence of adolescent growth spurt, premature graying of hair and baldness, atrophy and hyperkeratosis of skin, juvenile cataracts, chronic ulcerations over pressure points in the feet, and, in about half of the cases, mild diabetes mellitus.[90,282] Other features of this rare hereditofamilial disorder include atrophy of subcutaneous fat and muscle, vascular calcification, hypogonadism, severe arterio- and atherosclerosis, and an increased frequency of neoplasms (particularly sarcomas and meningiomas). Evidence of an autosomal recessive mode of inheritance has been presented. The nature of the disturbance in the development and metabolism of connective tissue which appears to constitute the primary defect in Werner's syndrome is unknown.

In *progeria*, the corium and subcutis have been reported as being either thickened or atrophic[217,377] and the thermal shrinkage and solubility of skin collagen in two children with this rare autosomal recessive syndrome of dwarfism and premature senility have been found to resemble those of aged rather than normally growing connective tissue.[377] *Rothmund's syndrome*, like Werner's syndrome, is a heritable (recessive) disorder in which atrophy of the skin (poikiloderma), beginning in infancy, is associated with juvenile cataracts. Additional features include alopecia, short stature, small hands, congenital bone anomalies, hypogonadism, and a variety of other ectodermal and mesodermal defects.[354]

In *acrodermatitis chronica atrophicans*, there is an initial phase of edema and dense infiltration of the dermis by lymphocytes and histiocytes, following which the skin becomes markedly atrophic.[138] This condition, which appears to be largely restricted to adults of Northern and Central Europe, usually affects the feet and legs, less often the forearms and hands, and uncommonly the face and trunk. In some cases involvement of the joint capsules and other para-articular tissues in the inflammatory process results in limitation of motion of the hands and feet and of the shoulders.

Lichen sclerosus et atrophicus is an uncommon disorder of unknown etiology, occurring chiefly in women, in which small depigmented areas on the skin may be associated with atrophy of the vulva and perianal skin.[151] The term "*white-spot disease*" is sometimes used to describe the maculopapular lesions on the trunk and limbs, and some authors consider these to be examples of generalized guttate morphea. The histologic changes in the dermis are distinctive, and consist of a band of edematous hyalinized collagen immediately beneath the epidermis and a deeper layer of lymphocytic infiltration.

A peculiar variety of *acro-osteolysis* has been recognized in a small percentage of workmen who clean reactor-vessels containing the polymerizing agent vinyl chloride (CH_2CHCl).[81,387] These individuals develop soreness and tenderness of the fingertips, Raynaud's phenomenon on exposure to cold, nodular thickening of the skin of the dorsum of the hands and forearms, clubbing, and synovial thickening of the proximal interphalangeal joints. Roentgenograms reveal varying degrees of osteolysis of the distal phalanges of one or more or all of the fingers, as well as erosive and sclerotic changes in the sacroiliac joints.

TREATMENT

The management of the patient with PSS consists of supportive measures designed to compensate for the damage wrought to the skin, joints, and internal organs, and the use of agents which may inhibit the underlying pathological process(es) that gives rise to progressive fibrosis of the connective tissue.

The evaluation of the effectiveness of treatment has proven difficult because of the slowly progressive nature of PSS, the tendency in many cases to spontaneous improvement or remission, the potent influence of psychophysiologic factors on many of the symptoms, and the limitations in objective criteria for ascertaining improvement (or deterioration) in both the cutaneous and visceral aspects of the disease. It is questionable whether any improvement can be expected in those manifestations which are the result of severe far-advanced fibrosis of the tissue. All too often success has been judged solely on the basis of a diminution in subjective complaints and poorly documented "softening" of the skin. No single drug or combination of drugs has been proved to be of value in adequately controlled studies or is generally accepted as useful. There is an impressively long list of vitamins, hormones, pharmaceuticals, and surgical procedures which have been employed in PSS nearly all of which have been abandoned after varying periods of at first enthusiastic and later more critical trial.[93,263,390]

Although *ACTH* and the *anti-inflammatory corticosteroids* have been shown to cause atrophy of dermal collagen bundles and depletion of mucopolysaccharides[218,335] and may temporarily control cutaneous and articular manifestations in early cases,[400] their influence on visceral disease has proved disappointing. In view of the many problems involved in their administration and the possible special hazard to the kidney, we have restricted their use to those patients who have disabling myositis or who are critically ill with an "overlap" syndrome. These latter have responded very favorably to treatment with corticosteroids, showing a reduction in the swelling or tightening of the skin, relief of fever and myositis and improvement in many other manifestations of disease.[332]

The demonstration of a diminution of subcutaneous calcinosis following treatment with *sodium versenate* (disodium-ethylenediaminetetraacetate) led to widespread use of this agent in PSS, but there is little or no evidence of significant or sustained improvement in patients so treated.[112,244] *Potassium para-aminobenzoate* has been employed with reported success in both systemic sclerosis as well as localized scleroderma,[397] but there has been no confirmation of these claims.[9,159,376] The mechanism of action of the drug, which is administered over prolonged periods, is obscure and it seems to exert little if any influence on the visceral disease. In the recommended dosages potassium para-aminobenzoate is often nauseating and occasionally produces drug fever and rash. Severe hypoglycemia has occurred in patients who have continued to take the drug during periods of inadequate food intake. There are conflicting reports concerning the value of the antifibrinolytic agent *epsilon-amino caproic acid*[131,307] and *dimethyl sulfoxide*.[322,363] On the whole the evidence of therapeutic benefit is unconvincing.

Attention has been focused on the possible usefulness of *D-penicillamine* (D-3-mercapto-valine), a drug known to interfere with the intermolecular cross-linking of collagen.[246] The prolonged administration of D-penicillamine leads to a striking increase in soluble dermal collagen[137] and eventual thinning of the skin (originally observed in patients with Wilson's disease). Penicillamine appears to have several effects upon collagen metabolism. It has been reported that pharmacological doses selectively inhibit the collagen biosynthesis of embryonic organ cultures by binding ferrous ions required for the enzymatic hydroxylation of proline in protocollagen.[367,369] It blocks aldehyde groups required for the formation of new insoluble (mature) collagen.[246,267,369] Penicillamine may also accelerate the turnover of preexisting insoluble collagen, presumably by cleaving intermolecular bonds, which stabilize the fibrous structure,[246] although the evidence for this is controversial,[185] and it has been noted there is no increase in urinary hydroxyproline excretion during treatment with this substance. Despite these several theoretically desirable actions, there is, however, still insufficient evidence on which to judge the therapeutic worth of D-penicillamine. According to preliminary reports there has been little or no significant benefit (despite evidence of an improvement in skin elasticity)[27] after treatment for periods of many months and pulmonary function has generally remained unchanged.[27,113,338,390] Furthermore, many patients experience toxic reactions, including pyrexia, rash, nausea, and anorexia, hypogeusia (reversed by oral administration of copper), leukopenia, nephrotic syndrome and a lupus-like syndrome.[113,135,164,177,272] Pyridoxine is given to offset the increased excretion of this vitamin during treatment. Clearly D-penicillamine must be administered with extreme caution.

In an experimental study of the lathyrogenic agent *beta-aminoproprionitrile*, one patient with PSS developed a reversible periosteal reaction, and untoward effects were observed in four other patients taking a dose which produced only slight changes in skin collagen solubility and no apparent therapeutic benefit.[178] Efforts to reduce new collagen synthesis by use of a diet lacking in ascorbic acid (an essential cofactor in the enzymatic hydroxylation of proline in protocollagen) resulted in no discernible improvement in skin tension or pulmonary diffusing capacity.[201]

Thoracic sympathectomy in patients with PSS may be followed by an improvement (often only transitory) in the symptoms of digital vasospasm[9,23,169,268] but appears to have no significant or sustained effect on the course of the cutaneous changes or visceral sclerosis. There are many patients with so-called primary Raynaud's disease who have developed typical PSS (or some other connective tissue disease) years after sympathectomy[8,23,169]

The possible therapeutic role of *immunosuppressive agents* clearly requires additional study.[76,166,215] Since these drugs and nearly all the other "specifics" which remain in vogue carry a high risk of toxicity, it would seem appropriate to restrict their use to patients in whom there is evidence of progressive and disabling disease.

Supporting Measures

Careful discussion with the patient and family concerning the nature of PSS is the first step in supportive management. Nearly all patients have Raynaud's phenomenon and to the extent that it is precipitated by low temperatures, this may be prevented by dressing warmly and avoiding undue exposure to cold. Many patients feel more comfortable in a warm climate but those with diffuse scleroderma tend to sunburn easily and may be predisposed to heat stroke.[34] Tobacco should be avoided. Vasodilating drugs have proved disappointing in the past, but there are a number of recent reports that regular oral or occasional intra-arterial administration of *reserpine* is followed by a significant increase in peripheral blood flow during cold exposure, healing of digital ulcerations, and remarkably long-lasting relief from Raynaud's phenomenon.[62,188,301,385] Similar benefits have been claimed for *methyldopa* (taken orally)[374] and for the intravenous infusion of low molecular weight *dextran*. The latter is said to increase digital capillary flow and relieve ischemic pain of patients with PSS by reducing the viscosity of the blood;[150,151] others have been unimpressed with this treatment and have reported the course of the underlying disease to be unaffected.[184,197]

Special creams, soaps, and bath oils should be used to relieve the excessive dryness of the skin, and household detergents should be avoided. If ulcerations of the fingertips become infected, healing may be assisted by use of bacteriocidal antibiotic ointment, preceded by removal of purulent exudate and soaking with hyaluronidase to facilitate penetration of medication. The pain in these fingers is lessened by repeated application of jelly containing 2 per cent lidocaine. Articular complaints usually respond to salicylates or indomethacin and the cautious use of moist heat and other forms of physical therapy.

Patients who have difficulty in swallowing learn to masticate carefully and to avoid foods such as tough meat and dry bread that are likely to cause dysphagia. Tincture of belladonna and methacholine have been recommended, but are usually of little value.[156,315] The development of esophageal stricture may require periodic dilatation; peptic esophagitis and esophageal hiatal hernia call for appropriate measures.

The occurrence of pneumonia or other respiratory tract infection in patients with pulmonary fibrosis requires prompt treatment and vigorous efforts to maintain ventilation. Those who develop cardiac failure often respond poorly to digitalis and easily become intoxicated, so that greater reliance is placed on diuretics and the dietary restriction of sodium.

The improvement in steatorrhea and other signs of intestinal malabsorption which follows the administration of tetracycline and other broad-spectrum antibiotics has been previously mentioned.[3,59,172,223,232,316] The usefulness of medium chain triglycerides in these cases is an unsettled question.[126]

Table 54-3.—Diseases in Which There May Be Calcification of the Soft Tissues in the Extremities

I. Metastatic calcification
   A. Hypercalcemic conditions
      1. Primary hyperparathyroidism
      2. Hypervitaminosis D
      3. Milk-alkali syndrome
      4. Metastatic and other neoplasm of bone
      5. Sarcoidosis
   B. Hyperphosphatemic conditions
      1. Chronic renal failure with secondary hyperparathyroidism
      2. Hypoparathyroidism
      3. Pseudohypoparathyroidism
      4. Tumoral calcinosis (lipocalcinosis granulomatosis)

II. Dystrophic calcification (calcinosis)
   A. Connective tissue diseases
      1. Progressive systemic sclerosis, including Thibierge-Weissenbach or CRST syndrome (*calcinosis circumscripta*)
      2. Polymyositis/dermatomyositis (*calcinosis universalis*)
      3. Ehlers-Danlos syndrome
      4. Pseudoxanthoma elasticum
   B. Metabolic disorders
      1. Chondrocalcinosis articularis (pseudogout)
      2. Gout
      3. Diabetes mellitus
      4. Alkaptonuria (ochronosis)
      5. Porphyria cutanea tarda
      6. Pseudopseudohypoparathyroidism
      7. Werner's syndrome
      8. Progeria
      9. Myositis (or fibrodysplasia) ossificans progressiva
   C. Vascular diseases
      1. Medial sclerosis of arteries (Mönckeberg's sclerosis)
      2. Venous calcifications
   D. Parasitic infestations
   E. Other
      1. Neuropathic arthropathy
      2. Calcific tendonitis

CALCINOSIS

Calcinosis or pathologic calcification of the soft tissues occurs in a wide variety of systemic disorders (Table 54–3).[6,31a,63,117a,198,350a,382a] Only a few of these conditions will be dealt with here since most are considered in detail in other chapters (*see also* Chapters 60 and 62). This ectopic calcification has generally been separated into that which is basically a complication of long-continued hypercalcemia and/or hyperphosphatemia (metastatic calcification) and that which is the result of some local abnormality in the affected tissues (dystrophic calcification).

Metastatic Calcification

Calcareous deposits occur commonly in hypercalcemic states and are found in the kidney (nephrocalcinosis), stomach, lung, brain, and eyes (band keratopathy) as well as in the skin, subcutaneous and periarticular tissues and arterial walls.[198] Calcification of the articular cartilage (chondrocalcinosis), menisci and joint capsules is a well-recognized feature of hyperparathyroidism[41a,145a] and there are a number of individuals in whom an attack of calcium pyrophosphate crystal-induced synovitis (pseudogout) represents the first clinical manifestation of this disease. Accordingly the possibility of parathyroid adenoma should be carefully considered in all patients with this arthropathy (*see also* Chapter 60).

A similar pattern of soft tissue calcification (with the exception of ocular involvement) is also found in hyperphosphatemic-normocalcemic secondary hyperparathyroidism, although renal calculus formation is much less frequent than in the case of hypercalcemic states. Acute episodes of articular and periarticular inflammation, which appear to be related to the local deposition of hydroxyapatite (and, at times, monosodium urate), have been described in patients receiving periodic hemodialysis for chronic renal failure.[237a] It has been suggested that this may be related to the removal of pyrophosphate, which appears to act as a physiologic inhibitor of calcification.[311a] Treatment with aluminum hydroxide gel has resulted in a significant reduction of serum phosphorus levels and clinical relief[237a] and in the disappearance of cutaneous calcinosis.[89a] In hypoparathyroidism, pseudohypoparathyroidism, and pseudopseudohypoparathyroidism, calcification may occur in the brain, particularly in the basal ganglia, as well as in the subcutaneous tissues (*see also* Chapter 62).

Dystrophic Calcification

Many restrict the use of the term calcinosis to those cases in which the deposition of calcium salts in the soft tissues occurs in the absence of any generalized disturbance in calcium or phosphorus metabolism.

(*a*) *Calcinosis Circumscripta and Calcinosis Universalis.*—In the past efforts were made to separate calcinosis into two chief categories, *calcinosis circumscripta* and *calcinosis universalis*, a divison based largely upon the extent and location of the calcific deposits. These terms are purely descriptive, however, and carry only limited diagnostic significance. In *calcinosis circumscripta* the calcareous deposits were described as occurring chiefly in young women, being generally confined to the extremities, and being particularly frequent in the terminal phalanges, around joints and near other bony eminences. In *calcinosis universalis*, which occurred predominantly in children and young adults, there was widespread encasing calcification of the skin, subcutaneous, and periarticular tissues, as well as involvement of the deeper structures, including tendons and tendon sheaths and muscles, forming irregularly shaped plaques and nodules; this was often associated with severe joint contractures and ankylosis. Much confusion resulted from an underlying assumption that this calcification represented a primary disease process.[350,382a] It is now quite

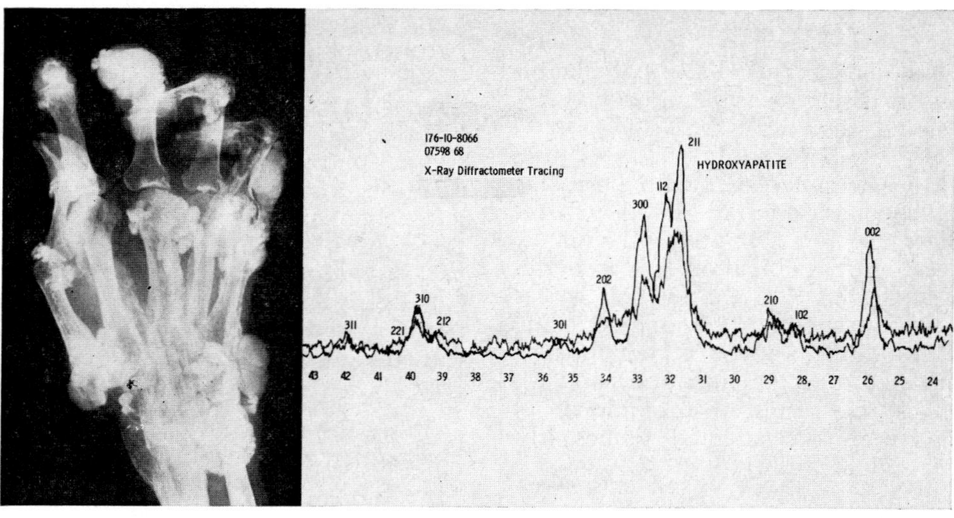

Fig. 54–20.—Calcinosis. (*Left*) Roentgenogram of hand of woman with polymyositis illustrating extensive calcinosis of subcutaneous tissues and tendon sheaths. (*Right*) X-ray diffractometer tracing of sample of calcareous matter removed from fluctuant nodule on hand, indicating identity with hydroxyapatite. (Prepared by Dr. Martin Sax.)

clear that most of the cases labeled as *calcinosis circumscripta* were in reality instances of progressive systemic sclerosis (scleroderma).[6,63,382a] These were often patients with mild and/or restricted skin changes, who would now be recognized as having the CRST or Thibierge-Weissenbach syndrome (*see above*). It is equally apparent that many cases of *calcinosis universalis* represented a late stage in the course of polymyositis (dermatomyositis (*see also* Chapter 53). The development of such diffuse calcinosis has become less common since the introduction and widespread use of corticosteroids in the treatment of polymyositis, although one still encounters patients who develop striking calcification of tendons and tendon sheaths (Figure 54–20 *left*). We have seen several older women who had large fluctuant nodules involving the tendon sheaths in the hands; aspiration of these masses yielded a creamy white substance with the consistency of toothpaste. Chemical analysis and x-ray diffraction studies of this material and of other calcinotic deposits in patients with scleroderma and dermatomyositis have demonstrated these to consist chiefly of hydroxyapatite (Figure 54–20 *right*).[6,69a,256] On microscopic examination the precipitates of calcium in the skin appear as large pleomorphic crystals, many in the shape of needles and large plates.[256]

Normal concentrations of serum calcium, phosphorus and alkaline phosphatase activity are the rule in patients who have progressive systemic sclerosis and dermatomyositis with or without apparent calcinosis. A number of these individuals have been found to be in positive calcium balance on low or normal calcium diets while others have been observed to be in negative balance.[6,69b,350,382a] In recent studies of patients with calcinosis cutis there has been evidence of hyperabsorption of calcium as well as of increased retention.[7a,219] Paradoxically, the rate of disappearance of radiolabeled calcium from an intradermal injection site was found to be faster in two patients with calcinosis cutis than in control subjects.[219] The bone resorption rate increased and the urinary excretion of calcium fell in a normal manner while the net calcium accretion rate (which includes extraosseous calcium deposition) remained constant when a woman with scleroderma and *calcinosis universalis* (not described in detail) was placed on a calcium-restricted diet.[173]

The basis for the deposition of calcium salts in the dermis of patients with progressive systemic sclerosis is unclear. A number of different forms of cutaneous, subcuticular, periarticular, and visceral calcification have been produced experimentally in the rat by the phenomenon of calciphylaxis and it has been suggested that the production of such lesions may serve as a model for the study of the underlying pathogenesis of human calcinosis.[328] In this process topical treatment with a variety of "challengers" (including metallic salts) during a critical period after "sensitization" by a systemic "calcifying factor" (*e.g.* vitamin-D compounds, parathyroid hormone) leads to local calcification, followed by inflammation and fibrosis. In the related phenomenon of "calcergy," soft tissue calcification occurs wherever "direct calcifiers" or "calcergens" (chiefly various metallic salts) come into contact with connective tissue without the need for any pre-treatment by systemic calcifying compounds.[329] The local injection of minute amounts of histamine or serotonin can elicit certain mast cell-dependent forms of this type of experimental calcinosis in which the "calcergen" is administered intravenously. The initial precipitation of calcium salts in the case of calciphylactic cutaneous calcinosis in the rat takes place in areas rich in mucopolysaccharides or, in some instances, collagen fibers, which appear to act as a matrix for this calcification.[168] However, in view of recent evidence supporting the concept that polysaccharides may "shield" reactive sites on collagen fibrils and block mineral nucleation[157a] it is tempting to consider the possibility that the calcinosis which occurs in scleroderma may be related to the diminution of mucopolysaccharides in the affected skin during later stages in the disease.

Numerous drugs and hormones as well as a host of nonspecific measures have been employed without success in the treatment of *calcinosis circumscripta* and *calcinosis universalis.* Although there have been a number of patients with scleroderma in whom cutaneous deposits disappeared for a time following the intravenous administration of large amounts of sodium versenate (disodiumethylenediaminetetraacetate)[388a] the difficulties attendant upon oft repeated infusions make such treatment impractical. It has recently been shown that certain diphosphonates (which contain the P-C-P bond) inhibit the crystallization of calcium phosphate and are capable of preventing various types of experimental pathologic calcification.[107] These are relatively non-toxic compounds which are effective when given orally and it is possible that they may prove of value in the treatment of calcinosis in man. (In this regard, see the recent report of R. L. Cram *et al.*: New Engl. J. Med. *285*, 1012, 1971.)

(*b*) *Tumoral Calcinosis.*—This rare entity, which has also been called *lipocalcinosis granulomatosis*, is characterized by the rapid development of large, multilobulated calcific masses in the subcutaneous tissue and muscle overlying the hips, shoulders, and elbows in otherwise healthy young subjects.[195,339] Smaller tumors occur adjacent to the spine, wrists, feet, lower ribs, sacrum, and ischium. These deposits, which may increase in size to a diameter of 20 cm. or larger over a period of months to years, are firm and non-tender. Usually there is little or no limitation of movement at the joints(s) unless these masses become very large or are complicated by the development of fistulous tracts from secondary infection or attempts at surgical drainage. Curiously, a number of patients have angioid streaks of the retina. There is a notable lack of visceral calcifications. On sectioning, the masses are found to be composed of multilocular cysts enclosing pockets of milky fluid or pasty microcrystalline calcareous matter. The tissue lining the walls of these cysts contains mononuclear cells which are rich in alkaline phosphatase and are believed to be responsible for the local accumulation of calcium phosphate, as well as foreign body giant cells. These mononuclear and polynuclear cells are structurally and apparently functionally similar to osteoblasts and osteoclasts, respectively.[195] Analyses of the contents of the masses have revealed pure calcium carbonate, pure calcium phosphate, or a mixture of the two salts. The majority of patients with tumoral calcinosis have normal levels of serum calcium but an increase in serum phosphorus has been noted in several cases.[195] Serum alkaline phosphatase activity is normal. There is evidence of rapid exchange of calcium between the serum and the masses and an increased intestinal absorption of dietary calcium, with no defect in the turnover of skeletal calcium.[195] Approximately half the patients with tumoral calcinosis reported to date have had affected siblings. This observation, together with the occurrence of hyperphosphatemia, has led to the suggestion that this disorder may represent a heritable disturbance in the metabolism of phosphorus.[195] Treatment at present consists mainly of early surgical excision of the calcareous masses, which rarely recur at the same site. New deposits may appear in time around other joints, but as a rule the prognosis is good although in some instances secondary infection of the deposits has led to the development of multiple discharging sinuses, profound cachexia, and amyloidosis. Although included in the category of metastatic calcification because of the frequent elevation in serum phosphorus levels and occasional elevation in serum calcium values, tumoral calcinosis is separable from other forms of metastatic calcification by the absence of visceral involvement.

(*c*) *Myositis* (*or Fibrodysplasia*) *Ossificans Progressiva.*—In this uncommon disorder there is widespread ectopic calcification and ossification in fascia, aponeuroses, and other fibrous structures related to muscle.[214] The initial symptoms of the disease usually appear in early childhood, and may or may not be preceded by local trauma. The disease progresses rapidly to a point at which there may be involvement of the entire musculoskeletal system. There are a number of associated congenital anomalies of the digits, including microdactyly or total absence of the thumbs and great toes. The initial manifestation usually consists of a localized area of swelling, redness and warmth in the neck or paravertebral area, often associated with extreme pain. After several days the signs of inflammation subside, leaving an area of residual doughy firmness which gradually ossifies over the course of the following weeks. The replacement of the tendon and muscle by bone leads to characteristic contracture deformities. Once ossification occurs there is little further change. Recurring bouts of inflammation and ossification result in progressive damage of much of the striated musculature. Death usually results from respiratory failure and/or pulmonary infection due to involvement of the muscles of the thorax or from inanition as a result of involvement of the muscles of mastication. The disease occurs in families, has been observed in homozygotic twins, and appears to be transmitted as an autosomal dominant trait with irregular penetrance. It has recently been suggested that the changes which take place in the soft tissues in myositis ossificans progressiva may result from an abnormal collagen or, alternatively, the deficiency of an inhibitor material (? mucopolysaccharide) which normally prevents the crystallization and accretion of calcium salts on collagen fibers at sites other than bone.[214] There is no evidence of any fundamental aberration in calcium metabolism *per se* in this disorder. Treatment with various drugs, including disodiumethylenediaminetetraacetate, appears to have had little effect on the course of the disease, although the use of corticosteroids may relieve the acute symptoms of inflammation.[214]

BIBLIOGRAPHY

1. Adhikari, P. K., Bianchi, F. A., Boushy, S. F., Sakamoto, A. and Lewis, B. M.: Amer. Rev. Resp. Dis., *86*, 823, 1962.
2. Alibert, J. L.: *Précis Théorique et Pratique sur les Maladies de la Peau*, Vol. 2. Paris, Caille & Ravier, 1818, pp. 168–170.
3. Alpert, L. I. and Pichel Warner, R. R.: Amer. J. Med., *45*, 468, 1968.
4. Asboe-Hansen, G.: Acta Dermatovener (Stockholm), *39*, 270, 1959.
5. Ashton, N., Coomes, E. N., Garner, A. and Oliver, D. O.: J. Path. Bact., *96*, 259, 1968.
6. Atkinson, F. R. B. and Weber, F. P.: Brit. J. Derm. Syph., *50*, 267, 1938.
7. Atkinson, M. and Summerling, M. D.: Gut, *7*, 402, 1966.
7*a*. Avioli, L. V., McDonald, J. E., Singer, R. A., and Henneman, P. H.: J. Clin. Invest., *44*, 128, 1965.
8. Baddeley, R. M.: Brit. J. Surg., *52*, 426, 1965.
9. Barnett, A. J. and Coventry, D. A.: Med. J. Austral., *1*, 992 & 1040, 1969.
10. Barr, I. M., Abramov, A., Dreyfuss, F., Yahini, J. H. and Neufeld, H. N.: Israel J. Med. Sci., *6*, 373, 1970.
11. Bartholomew, L. G., Cain, J. C., Winkelmann, R. K. and Baggenstoss, A. H.: Amer. J. Dig. Dis., *9*, 43, 1964.
12. Beck, J. S., Anderson, J. R., Gray, K. G. and Rowell, N. R.: Lancet, *2*, 1188, 1963.
13. Beck, J. S., Anderson, J. R., McElhinney, A. J. and Rowell, N. R.: Lancet, *2*, 575, 1962.
14. Bedford, D. E.: Brit. Heart J., *26*, 499, 1964.
15. Beetham, W. P., Jr. and Breslin, D. J.: Arth. & Rheum., *11*, 466, 1968 (abstract).
16. Beighton, P., Gumpel, J. M. and Cornes, N. G. M.: Ann. Rheum. Dis., *27*, 367, 1968.
17. Bendixen, G., Jarnum, S., Ottesen, O., Schmidt, H. and Thomsen, K.: Dermatologica (Basel), *137*, 26, 1968.
18. Bergan, J. J., Conn, J., Jr. and Trippel, O. H.: Ann. Surg., *173*, 301, 1971.
19. Berliner, S. D. and Burson, L. C.: Amer. J. Gastroent., *46*, 477, 1966.
20. Bettarello, A., Brito, T. and Zaterka, S.: Amer. J. Dig. Dis., *12*, 804, 1967.
21. Bianchi, F. A., Bistue, A. R., Wendt, V. E., Puro, H. E. and Keech, M. K.: J. Chron. Dis., *19*, 953, 1966.
22. Biggart, J. D. and Nevin, N. C.: J. Path. Bact., *93*, 334, 1967.
23. Birnstingl, M.: Proc. Roy. Soc. Med., *61*, 790, 1968.
24. Black, M. M., Bottoms, E. and Shuster, S.: Brit. J. Derm., *83*, 552, 1970.
25. Blanchard, R. E. and Speed, E. M.: Periodontics, *3*, 77, 1965.
26. Bloch, K. J., Buchanan, W. W., Wohl, M. J. and Bunim, J. J.: Medicine, *44*, 187, 1965.
27. Bluestone, R., Grahame, R., Holloway, V. and Holt, P. J. L.: Ann. Rheum. Dis., *29*, 153, 1970.
28. Bluestone, R., MacMahon, M. and Dawson, J. M.: Gut, *10*, 185, 1969.
29. Bradford, W. D., Cook, C. D., Vawter, G. F. and Berenberg, W.: J. Pediat., *68*, 391, 1966.
30. Braun-Falco, O.: Derm. Wschr., *136*, 1085, 1957.
31. Bron, K. and Rodnan, G. P.: Unpublished observations.
31*a*. Brooks, W. D. W.: Quart. J. Med., *3*, 293, 1934.
32. Brundin, A.: Scand. J. Resp. Dis., *51*, 160, 1970.
33. Buchanan, I. S. and Humpston, D. J.: Lancet, *1*, 845, 1968.
34. Buchwald, I. and Davis, P. J.: J.A.M.A., *201*, 270, 1967.
35. Burge, K. M., Perry, H. O. and Stickler, G. B.: Arch. Derm. (Chicago), *99*, 681, 1969.
36. Burkholder, P. M.: Immunology and Immunohistopathology of Renal Disease. In *Structural Basis of Renal Disease*, E. L. Becker, Ed., New York, Hoeber Medical Division, Harper & Row, 1968, pp. 197–237.
37. Burnham, T. K., Fine, G. and Neblett, T. R.: Ann. Intern. Med., *65*, 9, 1966.
38. Burnham, T. K., Neblett, T. R. and Fine, G.: Amer. J. Clin. Path., *50*, 683, 1968.
39. Burnham, T. K., Neblett, T. R., Fine, G. and Bank, P.: Arch. Derm. (Chicago), *99*, 611, 1969.
40. Butler, J. and Laymon, C. W.: Arch. Derm. Syph. (Chicago), *35*, 919, 1937.
41. Bywaters, E. G. L. and Scott, J. T.: Systemic Diseases of Connective Tissue. In *Progress in Clinical Rheumatology*, A. St. J. Dixon, Ed. Boston, Little, Brown, 1965, p. 114.
41*a*. Bywaters, E. G. L., Dixon, A. St. J. and Scott, J. T.: Ann Rheum. Dis. *22*, 171, 1963.
42. Calabro, J. J.: Arth. & Rheum., *10*, 553, 1967.

43. Calvert, R. J., Barling, B., Sopher, M. and Feiwel, M.: Brit. Med. J., *1*, 22, 1958.
44. Camus, J.-P., Emerit, I., Reinert, P., Guillien, P., Crouzet, J. and Fourot, J.: Ann. Méd. Int., *121*, 149, 1970.
45. Cantwell, A. R. and Kelso, D. W.: Arch. Derm. (Chicago), *104*, 21, 1971.
46. Caplan, H.: Thorax, *14*, 89, 1959.
47. Carr, R. D., Heisel, E. B. and Stevenson, T. D.: Arch. Derm. (Chicago), *92*, 519, 1965.
48. Case records of the Massachusetts General Hospital. Case 22–1968: New Engl. J. Med., *278*, 1218, 1968.
49. Cattarall, M. and Rowell, N. R.: Thorax, *18*, 10, 1963.
50. Cayla, J., Saporta, L., Delbarre, F. and Coste, F.: Bull. Soc. Méd. Hôp. Paris, *118*, 681, 1967.
51. Chamberlain, J. L., III and Bard, J. W.: South Med. J., *61*, 206, 1968.
52. Chaves, F. C., Rodrigo, F. G., Franco, M. L. and Esteves, J.: Brit. J. Derm., *82*, 298, 1970.
53. Chazen, E. M., Cook, C. D. and Cohen, J.: J. Pediat. *60*, 385, 1962.
54. Chorzelski, T. and Jablonska, S.: Acta Dermatovener (Stockholm), *50*, 81, 1970.
55. Christianson, H. B., Dorsey, C. S., O'Leary, P. A. and Kierland, R. R.: Arch. Derm. (Chicago), *74*, 629, 1956.
56. Churg, J.: Electron Microscopic Aspects of Renal Pathology. In *Structural Basis of Renal Disease*, E. L. Becker, Ed. New York, Hoeber Medical Division, Harper & Row, 1968, pp. 132–196.
57. Clark, J. A., Winkelmann, R. K., McDuffie, F. C. and Ward, L. E.: Mayo Clin. Proc., *46*, 97, 1971.
58. Clark, J. A., Winkelmann, R. K. and Ward, L. E.: Mayo Clin. Proc., *46*, 104, 1971.
59. Cliff, I. S., Herber, R. and Demis, D. J.: J. Invest. Derm., *47*, 475, 1966.
60. Clinicopathologic Conference. A patient with steatorrhea and Raynaud's phenomenon: Mayo Clin. Proc., *40*, 714, 1965.
61. Coffman, J. D.: J. Lab. Clin. Med., *76*, 480, 1970.
62. Coffman, J. D. and Cohen, A. S.: New Engl. J. Med., *285*, 259, 1971.
63. Cole, W. R.: Guy's Hosp. Rep., *102*, 56, 1953.
64. Collins, D. H., Darke, C. S. and Dodge, O. G.: J. Path. Bact., *76*, 531, 1958.
65. Colomb, D. and Creyssel, R.: Ann. Derm. Syph. (Paris), *92*, 499, 1965.
66. Compton, R.: Amer. J. Surg., *118*, 602, 1969.
67. Conner, P. K. and Bashour, F. A.: Amer. Heart J., *61*, 494, 1961.
68. Cooper, A. and Bluestone, R.: Ann. Rheum. Dis., *27*, 537, 1968.
69. Copeman, P. W. M. and Medd, W. E.: Brit. Med. J., *3*, 353, 1967.

69*a*. Cornbleet, T., Reed, C. I. and Reed, B. P.: J. Invest. Derm., *13*, 171, 1949.

69*b*. Cornbleet, T. and Struck, H. C.: Arch. Derm. Syph. (Chicago), *35*, 188, 1937.

70. Coste, F., Delbarre, F., Guiraudon, C., Saporta, L. and Bontoux, D.: Rev. Rhum., *35*, 416, 1968.
71. Curtis, A. C. and Jansen, T. G.: Arch. Derm. (Chicago), *78*, 749, 1958.
72. Curtis, A. C. and Shulak, B. M.: Arch. Derm. (Chicago), *92*, 526, 1965.
73. Curzio, C.: *Discussioni Anatomio-Pratiche di un raro e stravagante morbo cutaneo in una giovane Donna felicemante curato in questo grande Ospedale degl'Incurabili.* Napoli, G. diSimone, 1753.
74. D'Angelo, W. A., Fries, J. F., Masi, A. T. and Shulman, L. E.: Amer. J. Med., *46*, 428, 1969.
75. Davison, P. F., Levine, L., Drake, M. P., Rubin, A. and Bump, S.: J. Exper. Med., *126*, 331, 1967.
76. Demis, D. J., Brown, C. S. and Crosby, W. H.: Amer. J. Med., *37*, 195, 1964.
77. DeMuth, G. R., Furstenberg, N. A., Dabich, L. and Zarafonetis, C. J. D.: Amer. J. Med. Sci., *255*, 94, 1968.
78. Denko, C. W. and Stoughton, R. B.: Arth. & Rheum., *1*, 77, 1958.
79. DeTakats, G. and Fowler, E. F.: J.A.M.A., *179*, 1, 1962.
80. Dinkler, M.: Deutsch. Arch. Klin. Med., *48*, 514, 1891.
81. Dodson, V. N., Dinman, B. D., Whitehouse, W. M., Nasr, A. N. M. and Magnuson, H. J.: Arch. Environ. Health, *22*, 83, 1971.
82. Donaldson, R. M., Jr.: Ann. Intern. Med., *64*, 948, 1966.
83. Dowling, G. B.: Brit. J. Derm., *52*, 242, 1940.
84. Drummond, K. N., Michael, A. F. and Good, R. A.: Canad. M.A.J., *94*, 834, 1966.
85. DuBois, E. L., Chandor, S., Friou, G. J. and Bischel, M.: Medicine, *50*, 199, 1971.
86. Edwards, D. A. W. and Lennard-Jones, J. E.: Proc. Roy. Soc. Med., *53*, 877, 1960.
87. Edwards, W. G., Jr. and Dines, D. E.: Dis. Chest, *49*, 96, 1966.

88. Ehrmann, S. and Brunauer, St. R.: Sclerodermie. In *Handbuch Der Haut- Und Geschlechtskrankheiten*, J. Jadasohn, Ed. Vol. 8 (Part 2). Berlin, J. Springer, 1931.
89. Eisen, A. Z., Jeffrey, J. J. and Gross, J.: Biochim. Biophys. Acta, *151*, 637, 1968.
89*a*. Eisenberg, E. and Batholow, P. V.: New Engl. J. Med., *268*, 1216, 1963.
90. Epstein, C. J., Martin, G. M., Schultz, A. L. and Motulsky, A. G.: Medicine, *45*, 177, 1966.
91. Erasmus, L. D.: S. Afr. J. Lab. Clin. Med., *3*, 209, 1957.
92. Escudero, J. and McDevitt, E.: Amer. Heart J., *56*, 846, 1958.
93. Evans, J. A., Rubitsky, H. J. and Perry, A. W.: J.A.M.A., *151*, 891, 1953.
94. Faber, V. and Elling, P.: Acta Med. Scand., *177*, 309, 1965.
95. Fardal, R. W. and Winkelmann, R. K.: Arch. Derm. (Chicago), *91*, 503, 1965.
96. Farmer, R. G., Gifford, R. W., Jr. and Hines, E. A., Jr.: Circulation, *21*, 1088, 1960.
97. Fear, R. E.: Obstet. Gynec., *31*, 69, 1968.
98. Fennell, R. H., Jr., Reddy, C. R. R. M. and Vazquez, J. J.: Arch. Path. (Chicago), *72*, 209, 1961.
99. Fennell, R. H., Jr., Rodnan, G. P. and Vazquez, J. J.: Lab. Invest., *11*, 24, 1962.
100. Fisher, E. R. and Rodnan, G. P.: Arch. Path. (Chicago), *65*, 29, 1958.
101. ———: Arth. & Rheum., *3*, 536, 1960.
102. Fleischmajer, R.: Arch. Derm. (Chicago), *89*, 437, 1964.
103. ———: Arch. Derm. (Chicago), *89*, 749, 1964.
104. Fleischmajer, R. and Krol, S.: Proc. Soc. Exp. Biol. Med., *126*, 252, 1967.
105. Fleischmajer, R. and Lara, J. V.: Arch. Derm. (Chicago), *92*, 643, 1965.
106. Forget, C.-P.: Gaz. Méd. Strasbourg, *7*, 200, 1847.
107. Francis, M. D., Russell, R. G. G. and Fleisch, H.: Science, *165*, 1264, 1969.
108. Fraser, G. M.: Brit. J. Derm., *78*, 1, 1966.
109. Freedman, P., Peters, J. H. and Kark, R. M.: Arch. Intern. Med. (Chicago), *105*, 524, 1960.
110. Fries, J. F.: Arch. Intern. Med. (Chicago), *123*, 22, 1969.
111. Fries, J. F., Hoopes, J. E. and Shulman, L. E.: Arth. & Rheum., *14*, 571, 1971.
112. Fuleihan, F. J. D., Kurban, A. K., Abboud, R. T., Beidas-Jubran, N. and Farah, F. S.: Brit. J. Derm., *80*, 184, 1968.
113. Fulghum, D. D. and Katz, R.: Arch. Derm. (Chicago), *98*, 51, 1968.
114. Fullmer, H. M., Lazarus, G. S., Gibson, W. A., Stam, A. C. and Link, C.: Lancet, *1*, 1007, 1966.
115. Fullmer, H. M. and Witte, W. E.: Arch. Path. (Chicago), *73*, 184, 1962.
116. Garb, J. and Sims, C. F.: Dermatologica (Basel), *119*, 341, 1959.
117. Garrett, J. M., Winkelmann, R. K., Schlegel, J. F. and Code, C. F.: Mayo Clin. Proc., *46*, 92, 1971.
117*a*. Gayler, B. W. and Brogdon, B. G.: Amer. J. Med. Sci., *249*, 590, 1965.
118. Gintrac, E.: Rev. Méd. Chir. (Paris), *2*, 263, 1847.
119. Godfrey, S., Bluestone, R. and Higgs, B. E.: Thorax, *24*, 427, 1969.
120. Goetz, R. H.: Clin. Proc. (Cape Town), *4*, 337, 1945.
121. Gondos, B.: Amer. J. Roentgen., *84*, 235, 1960.
122. Gordon, R. M. and Silverstein, A.: Arch. Neurol. (Chicago), *22*, 126, 1970.
123. Graham, J. R.: Amer. J. Med. Sci., *254*, 1, 1967.
124. Greenberg, L. M., Geppert, C., Worthen, H. G. and Good, R. A.: Pediatrics, *32*, 1044, 1963.
125. Greenberger, N. J., Dobbins, W. O., III, Ruppert, R. D. and Jesseph, J. E.: Amer. J. Med., *45*:301, 1968.
126. Greenberger, N. J., Ruppert, R. D. and Tzagournis, M.: Ann. Intern. Med., *66*, 727, 1967.
127. Grisolle, M.: Gaz. Hôp. Civ. Milit. (Paris), *9*, 209, 1847.
128. Grossman, A., Martin, J. R. and Root, H. S.: Laryngoscope, *71*, 530, 1961.
129. Györkey, F., Min, K-W., and Györkey, P.: Arth. & Rheum., *12*, 300, 1969 (abstract).
130. Haas, J. E. and Yunis, E. J.: Exp. Molec. Path., *12*, 257, 1970.
131. Hall, A. P. and Scott, J. T.: Ann. Rheum. Dis., *25*, 175, 1966.
132. Hanson, V., Drexler, E. and Kornreich, H.: Arth. & Rheum., *13*, 798, 1970.
133. Hardy, K. H., Rosevear, J. W., Sams, W. M., Jr. and Winkelmann, R. K.: Mayo Clin Proc., *46*, 119, 1971.
134. Harley, J.: Med.-Chirurg. Trans. (London), *60*, 131, 1877.
135. Harpey, J. P., Caille, B., Moulias, R. and Goust, J. M.: Lancet, *1*, 292, 1971 (correspondence).
136. Harris, E. D., Jr., Cohen, G. L. and Krane, S. M.: Arth. & Rheum., *12*, 92, 1969.

137. Harris, E. D., Jr. and Sjoerdsma, A.: Lancet, *2*, 996, 1966.
138. Hauser, W.: Hautarzt, *6*, 77, 1955.
139. Haxthausen, H.: Acta Dermatovener (Stockholm), *27*, 352, 1947.
140. Hay, D. R.: New Zeal. Med. J., *63*, 90, 1964.
141. Hayes, R. L. and Rodnan, G. P.: Arth. & Rheum., *11*, 487, 1968 (abstract).
142. Hayes, R. L. and Rodnan, G. P.: Anat. Rec., *163*, 197, 1969 (abstract).
143. Hayes, R. L. and Rodnan, G. P.: Amer. J. Path., *63*, 433, 1971.
144. Heerma, van Voss, S. F. C.: Bibl. Radiol., *5*, 143, 1969.
145. Heinz, E. R., Steinberg, A. J. and Sackner, M. A.: Ann. Intern. Med., *59*, 822, 1963.
145*a*. Hellström, J. and Ivemark, B. I.: Acta Chir. Scand., suppl., 294, 1962.
146. Herman, B. E., Fischl, R., Frankel, A. and Herman, P.: J.A.M.A., *182*, 578, 1962.
147. Hodkinson, H. M.: J. Amer. Geriat. Soc., *19*, 224, 1971.
148. Hollenberg, N. K., Epstein, M., Basch, R. I. and Merrill, J. P.: Amer. J. Med., *47*, 845, 1969.
149. Holt, J. M. and Wright, R.: Brit. Med. J., *3*, 537, 1967.
150. Holti, G.: Brit. J. Derm., *77*, 560, 1965.
151. Holti, G.: Practitioner, *204*, 644, 1970.
152. Holzmann, H. and Frisch, W.: Aerztl. Forsh., *24*, 129, 1970.
153. Holzmann, H., Korting, G. W. and Missmahl, H. P.: Klin. Wschr., *47*, 390, 1969.
154. Holzmann, H., Korting, G. W. and Morsches, B.: Arch. Klin. Exp. Derm., *231*, 156, 1968.
155. Horswell, R. R., Hargrove, M. D., Peete, W. P. and Ruffin, J. M.: Gastroenterology, *40*, 580, 1961.
156. Hoskins, L. C., Norris, H. T., Gottlieb, L. S. and Zamcheck, N.: Amer. J. Med., *33*, 459, 1962.
157. Housset, E., Emerit, I., Baulon, A. and deGrouchy, J.: C. R. Acad. Sci. Paris, *269*, 431, 1969.
157*a*. Howell, D. S., Pita, J. C., Marquez, J. F. and Gatter, R. A.: J. Clin. Invest., *48*, 630, 1969.
158. Huang, C. T. and Lyons, H. A.: Amer. Rev. Resp. Dis., *93*, 865, 1966.
159. Hughes, D. T. D., Gordon, K. C. D., Swann, J. C. and Bolt, G. L.: Gut, *7*, 553, 1966.
160. Hughes, D. T. D. and Lee, F. I.: Thorax, *18*, 16, 1963.
161. Hughes, G. R. V., Cohen, S. A. and Christian, C. L.: Ann. Rheum. Dis., *30*, 259, 1971.
161*a*. Ivey, K. J., Hwang, Y.-F. and Sheets, R. F.: Amer. J. Med., *51*, 815, 1971.
162. Jablonska, S.: *Scleroderma and Pseudoscleroderma* (transl. by W. Z. Kulerski). Warsaw, Poland. Panstwowy Zaklad Wydawnictw Lekarskich (PZWL-Polish Medical Publishers), 1965.
163. Jablonska, S., Stachow, A. and Suffczynska, M.: Arch. Derm. (Chicago), *95*, 443, 1967.
164. Jaffe, I. A., Treser, G., Suzuki, Y. and Ehrenreich, T.: Ann. Intern. Med., *69*, 549, 1968.
165. Jaffe, M. O. and Winkelmann, R. K.: Arch. Derm. (Chicago), *83*, 402, 1961.
165*a*. James, K., Fudenberg, H., Epstein, W. L. and Shuster, J.: Clin. Exp. Immunol., *2*, 153, 1967.
166. Jansen, G. T., Barraza, D. F., Ballard, J. L., Honeycutt, W. M. and Dillaha, C. J.: Arch. Derm. (Chicago), *97*, 690, 1968.
167. Johnson, T. R., Banner, E. A. and Winkelmann, R. K.: Obstet. Gynec., *23*, 467, 1964.
168. Johnson, W. C., Forbes, P. D., Graham, J. H. and Gray, H. R.: J. Invest. Derm., *43*, 453, 1964.
169. Johnston, E. N. M., Summerly, R. and Birnstingl, M.: Brit. Med. J., *1*, 962, 1965.
170. Jordon, R. E., Deheer, D., Schroeter, A. and Winkelmann, R. K.: Mayo Clin. Proc., *46*, 111, 1971.
171. Justh, G. O. and Rodnan, G. P.: Arth. & Rheum., *14*, 168, 1971 (abstract).
172. Kahn, I. J., Jeffries, G. H. and Sleisenger, M. H.: New Engl. J. Med., *274*, 1339, 1966.
173. Kales, A. N. and Phang, J. M.: J. Clin. Endocrin. Metab., *31*, 204, 1970.
174. Kalsbeek, G. L. and Cormane, R. H.: Dermatologica (Basel), *135*, 205, 1967.
175. Kass, H., Hanson, V. and Patrick, J.: J. Pediat., *68*, 243, 1966.
176. Kay, D. M. and Tuffanelli, D. L.: Ann. Intern. Med., *71*, 753, 1969.
177. Keiser, H. R., Henkin, R. I., Bartter, F. C. and Sjoerdsma, A.: J.A.M.A., *203*, 381, 1968.
178. Keiser, H. R. and Sjoerdsma, A.: Clin. Pharmacol. Ther., *8*, 593, 1967.
179. Keiser, H. R. and Sjoerdsma, A.: Clin. Chim. Acta, *23*, 341, 1969.
180. Keiser, H. R., Stein H. D. and Sjoerdsma, A.: Arch. Derm. (Chicago), *104*, 57, 1971.

181. Kellgren, J. H., Ball, J. and Tutton, G. K.: Quart. J. Med., *21*, 405, 1952.
182. Kemp Harper, R. A. and Jackson, D. C.: Brit. J. Radiol., *38*, 825, 1965.
183. Kibler, R. F. and Rose, C. F.: Brit. Med. J., *1*, 1781, 1960.
184. Kirk, J. A. and Dixon, A. St. J.: Ann. Rheum. Dis., *28*, 49, 1969.
185. Klein, L. and Nowacek, C. J.: Biochim. Biophys. Acta, *194*, 504, 1969.
186. Klemperer, P.: Amer. J. Path., *26*, 505, 1950.
187. Klemperer, P., Pollack, A. D. and Baehr, G.: J.A.M.A., *119*, 331, 1942.
188. Kontos, H. A. and Wasserman, A. J.: Circulation, *39*, 259, 1969.
189. Kornreich, H. K., Shaw, K. N. F., Koch, R. and Hanson, V.: J. Pediat., *73*, 571, 1968.
190. Korting, G. W. and Holzmann, H.: *Die Sclerodermie und ihr Nahestehende Bindegewebsprobleme*. Stuttgart, Thieme, 1967.
191. Korting, G. W., Holzmann, H. and Forssmann, W. G.: Arch. Klin. Exp. Derm., *223*, 105, 1965.
192. Korting, G., Holzmann, H. and Kühn, K.: Arch. Klin. Exper. Derm., *209*, 66, 1959.
193. Krone, C. L., Theodor, E., Sleisenger, M. H. and Jeffries, G. H.: Medicine, *47*, 89, 1968.
194. Kurland, L. T., Hauser, W. A., Ferguson, R. H. and Holley, K. E.: Mayo Clin. Proc., *44*, 649, 1969.
195. Lafferty, F. W., Reynolds, E. S. and Pearson, O. H.: Amer. J. Med., *38*, 105, 1965.
196. Laitinen, O., Uitto, J., Hannuksela, M. and Mustakallio, K. K.: Ann. Clin. Res., *1*, 64, 1969.
197. Lane, P.: Brit. Med. J., *4*, 657, 1970.
198. Lathan, S. R., Block, R. A. and McLean, R. L.: Amer. J. Med., *44*, 1000, 1968.
199. Laws, J. W.: Brachial Arteriography in the Connective Tissue Disorders. In *Progress in Clinical Rheumatology*. A. St. J. Dixon, Ed. Boston, Little, Brown, 1965, p. 246.
200. Lazarus, G. S., Daniels, J. R., Brown, R. S., Bladen, H. A. and Fullmer, H. M.: J. Clin. Invest., *47*, 2622, 1968.
201. Lazarus, R. J., Kaplan, D. A., Diamond, H. S. and Emmanuel, G.: J.A.M.A., *213*, 2261, 1970.
202. Lee, J. E. and Haynes, J. M.: Neurology, *17*, 18, 1967.
203. Leinwand, I., Duryee, A. W. and Richter, M. N.: Ann. Intern. Med., *41*, 1003, 1954.
204. LeRoy, E. C., Downey, J. A. and Cannon, P. J.: J. Clin. Invest., *50*, 930, 1971.
205. LeRoy, E. C. and Sjoerdsma, A.: J. Clin. Invest., *44*, 914, 1965.
206. Lev, M., Landowne, M., Matchar, J. C. and Wagner, J. A.: Amer. Heart J., *72*, 13, 1966.
207. Levine, R. J. and Boshell, B. R.: Ann. Intern. Med., *52*, 517, 1960.
208. Lewin, G. and Heller, J.: *Die Sclerodermie*. Berlin, A. Hirschwald, 1895.
209. Lewis, T.: Clin. Sci., *3*, 287, 1937–38.
210. Lewis, T.: Brit. J. Derm. Syph., *52*, 233, 1940.
211. Lindström, F. D.: Ann. Clin. Res., *3*, 39, 1971.
212. Lipscomb, P. R., Simons, G. W. and Winkelmann, R. K.: J. Bone & Joint Surg., *51A*, 1112, 1969.
213. Lowe, W. C.: Milit. Med., *134*, 1430, 1969.
214. Lutwak, L.: Amer. J. Med., *37*, 269, 1964.
215. Mackenzie, A. H.: Arth. & Rheum., *13*, 334, 1970 (abstract).
216. MacLean, H. and Guthrie, W.: Trans. Ophthal. Soc. UK, *89*, 209, 1970.
217. Makous, N., Friedman, S., Yakovac, W. and Maris, E. P.: Amer. Heart J., *64*, 334, 1962.
218. Mancini, R. E., Stringa, S. G. and Canepa, L.: J. Invest. Derm., *34*, 393, 1960.
219. Marks, J.: Brit. J. Derm., *82*, 1, 1970.
220. Masi, A. T. and D'Angelo, W. A.: Ann. Intern. Med., *66*, 870, 1967.
221. Matsui, S.: Mitt. Med. Fak. Tokyo, *31*, 55, 1924.
222. McAndrew, G. M. and Barnes, E. G.: Ann. Phys. Med., *8*, 128, 1965.
223. McBrien, D. J. and Lockhart Mummery, H. E.: Brit. Med. J., *2*, 1653, 1962.
224. McCarthy, J. T., Osserman, E., Lombardo, P. C., and Takatsuki, K.: Arch. Derm. (Chicago), *89*, 446, 1964.
225. McCoy, D. G.: J. Irish Med. Assoc., *60*, 474, 1967.
226. McGiven, A. R., deBoer, W. G. R. M., Barnett, A. J. and Coventry, D. A.: Med. J. Austral., *2*, 533, 1968.
227. McPherson, J. R.: Dis. Colon Rectum, *8*, 425, 1965.
228. Meaney, T. F., Dodson, A. E., Poutasse, E. F. and McCormack, L. J.: Cleveland Clinic Quart., *25*, 21, 1958.
229. Medsger, T. A., Jr. and Masi, A. T.: Ann. Intern. Med., *74*, 714, 1971.
230. Medsger, T. A., Jr., Masi, A. T., Rodnan, G. P., Benedek, T. G. and Robinson, H.: Ann. Intern. Med., *75*, 369, 1971.

231. Medsger, T. A., Jr., Rodnan, G. P., Moosy, J. and Vester, J. W.: Arth. & Rheum., *11*, 554, 1968.
232. Meihoff, W. E., Hirschfield, J. S. and Kern, F., Jr.: J.A.M.A., *204*, 854, 1968.
233. Meltzer, J. I.: Amer. J. Med., *20*, 638, 1956.
234. Michaeli, D., Martin, G. R., Kettman, J., Benjamini, E., Leung, D. Y. K. and Blatt, B. A.: Science, *166*, 1522, 1969.
235. Michalowski, R.: Brit. J. Derm., *82*, 137, 1970.
236. Miercort, R. D. and Merrill, F. G.: Radiology, *92*, 359, 1969.
237. Morin, P., Kahn, F. and Waterhouse, C.: Gynec. Obstet. (Paris), *69*, 355, 1970.
237*a*. Moskowitz, R. W., Vertes, V., Schwartz, A., Marshall, G., and Friedman, B.: Amer. J. Med., *47*, 450, 1969.
238. Muller, S. A. and Henderson, E. D.: Arch. Derm. (Chicago), *88*, 142, 1963.
239. Murray-Lyon, I. M., Thompson, R. P. H., Ansell, I. D. and Williams, R.: Brit. Med. J., *3*, 258, 1970.
240. Mussini, E., Hutton, J. J. and Udenfriend, S.: Science, *157*, 927, 1968.
241. Naeye, R. L.: Dis. Chest, *44*, 374, 1963.
242. Nash, A. G. and Fountain, R.: Brit. J. Surg., *55*, 667, 1968.
243. Nasser, W. K., Mishkin, M. E., Rosenbaum, D. and Genovese, P. D.: Amer. J. Cardiol., *22*, 538, 1968.
244. Neldner, K. H., Winkelmann, R. K. and Perry, H. O.: Arch. Derm. (Chicago), *86*, 305, 1962.
245. Neuberger, A.: Ann. Rheum. Dis., *19*, 1, 1960.
246. Nimni, M.: J. Biol. Chem., *243*, 1457, 1968.
247. Norton, W. L.: J. Lab. Clin. Med., *74*, 369, 1969.
248. Norton, W. L.: Ann. Rheum. Dis., *29*, 67, 1970.
249. Norton, W. L., Hurd, E. R., Lewis, D. C. and Ziff, M.: J. Lab. Clin. Med., *71*, 919, 1968.
250. Norton, W. L. and Nardo, J. M.: Ann. Intern. Med., *73*, 317, 1970.
251. Øhlenschlaeger, K. and Friman, C.: Scand. J. Clin. Lab. Invest., *21*, 364, 1968.
252. O'Leary, P. A., Montgomery, H. and Ragsdale, W. E., Jr.: Arch. Derm. (Chicago), *75*, 78, 1957.
253. Opie, L. H.: Dis. Chest, *28*, 665, 1955.
254. Orabona, M. L. and Albano, O.: Acta Med. Scand., *160*:Suppl. 333, 1957.
255. Oram, S. and Stokes, W.: Brit. Heart J., *23*, 243, 1961.
256. Paegle, R. D.: Arch. Path. (Chicago), *82*, 474, 1966.
257. Pan, S., Rodnan, G. P. and Wald, N.: Arth. & Rheum., *14*, 407, 1971 (abstract).
258. Panja, R. K., Sengupta, K. P. and Aikat, B. K.: J. Clin. Path., *17*, 658, 1964.
259. Pardo, V., Fisher, E. R., Perez-Stable, E., and Rodnan, G. P.: Lab. Invest., *15*, 1434, 1966.
260. Paronetto, F.: Amer. J. Path., *46*, 901, 1965.
261. Peachey, R. D. G., Creamer, B. and Pierce, J. W.: Gut, *10*, 285, 1969.
262. Pende, G. and DeCarlo, M.: Arch. Maragliano, *18*, 577, 1962.
263. Perry, H. O.: Arch. Derm. (Chicago), *83*, 300, 1961.
264. Perry, H. O., Montgomery, H. and Stickney, J. M.: Ann. Intern. Med., *53*, 955, 1960.
265. Phillips, S. F. and Schmid, W. C.: Gut, *10*, 990, 1969.
266. Pinals, R. S.: Arth. & Rheum., *7*, 662, 1964.
267. Pinnell, S. R., Martin, G. R. and Miller, E. J.: Science, *161*, 475, 1968.
268. Piper, W. N. and Helwig, E. B.: Arch. Derm. (Chicago), *72*, 535, 1955.
269. Price, J. M., Yess, N., Brown, R. R. and Johnson, S. A. M.: Arch. Derm. (Chicago), *95*, 462, 1967.
270. Prockop, D. J. and Kivirikko, K. I.: Ann. Intern. Med., *66*, 1243, 1967.
271. Que, G. S. and Mandema, E.: Amer. J. Med., *36*, 320, 1964.
272. Rasmussen, K.: Acta Med. Scand., *189*, 367, 1971.
273. Rasmussen, D. M., Wakim, K. G. and Winkelmann, R. K.: J. Invest. Derm., *43*, 349, 1964.
274. Raynaud, M.: Gangrène Symétrique des Extrémités, in *Nouveau Dictionnaire de Médecine et de Chirurgie Pratiques.* Vol. 15, Paris, J. B. Baillière et Fils, 1872, p. 636.
275. Raynaud, R., Benatre, A., Brochier, M., Morand, P. and Raynaud, P.: Sem. Hôp. Paris, *44*, 489, 1968.
276. Redeker, A. G. and Bronow, R. S.: Arch. Derm. (Chicago), *85*, 705, 1962.
277. Redisch, W., Messina, E. J., Hughes, G. and McEwen, C.: Ann. Rheum. Dis., *29*, 244, 1970.
278. Reinhardt, J. F. and Barry, W. F., Jr.: Amer. J. Roentgen., *88*, 687, 1962.
279. Reynolds, T. B., Denison, E. K., Frankl, H. D., Lieberman, F. L. and Peters, R. L.: Amer. J. Med., *50*, 302, 1971.

280. Rich, A. R.: Harvey Lect., *42*, 106, 1946–47.
281. Richter, R. B.: J. Neuropath. Exp. Neurol., *13*, 168, 1954.
282. Riley, T. R., Wieland, R. G., Markis, J. and Hamwi, G. J.: Ann. Intern. Med., *63*, 285, 1965.
283. Ritchie, B.: Thorax, *19*, 28, 1964.
284. Ritchie, R. F.: Arth. & Rheum., *10*, 544, 1967.
285. Ritchie, R. F.: New Engl. J. Med., *282*, 1174, 1970.
286. Rodnan, G. P.: Ann. Intern. Med., *56*, 422, 1962.
287. Rodnan, G. P.: Bull. Rheum. Dis., *13*, 301, 1963.
288. Rodnan, G. P.: J. Chron. Dis., *16*, 929, 1963.
289. Rodnan, G. P.: Proceedings of the World Health Organization Conference on Scleroderma, 1969 (in press).
290. Rodnan, G. P.: Progressive Systemic Sclerosis (Scleroderma). In *Immunological Diseases*, M. Samter, Ed. 2nd edition. Boston, Little, Brown, 1971, pp. 1052–1072.
291. Rodnan, G. P. and Benedek, T. G.: Ann. Intern. Med., *57*, 305, 1962.
292. Rodnan, G. P., Benedek, T. G., Medsger, T. A., Jr. and Cammarata, R. J.: Ann. Intern. Med., *66*, 323, 1967.
293. Rodnan, G. P. and Fennell, R. H., Jr.: J.A.M.A., *180*, 665, 1962.
294. Rodnan, G. P. and Fraser, D.: Unpublished observations.
295. Rodnan, G. P., Lipinski, E. and Luksick, J.: Arth. & Rheum., *11*, 114, 1968 (abstract).
296. Rodnan, G. P. and Luksick, J.: Arch. & Rheum., *12*, 693, 1969 (abstract).
297. Rodnan, G. P. and Medsger, T. A., Jr.: Clin. Orthop., *57*, 81, 1968.
298. Rodnan, G. P., Shapiro, A. P. and Krifcher, E.: Ann. Intern. Med., *60*, 737, 1964 (abstract).
299. Rodnan, G. P., Shapiro, A. P., Moutsos, S. E. and Bron, K. M.: Arth. & Rheum., *8*, 464, 1965 (abstract).
300. Rodnan, G. P., Schreiner, G. E. and Black, R. L.: Amer. J. Med., *23*, 445, 1957.
301. Romeo, S. G., Whalen, R. E. and Tindall, J. P.: Arch. Intern. Med. (Chicago), *125*, 825, 1970.
302. Rosenthal, D. S. and Sack, B.: J.A.M.A., *216*, 2011, 1971.
303. Rosenthal, F. D.: Gastroenterology, *32*, 332, 1957.
304. Rosson, R. S. and Yesner, R.: New Engl. J. Med., *272*, 391, 1965.
305. Roth, L. M. and Kissane, J. M.: Amer. J. Clin. Path., *41*, 287, 1964.
306. Rothfield, N. F. and Rodnan, G. P.: Arth. & Rheum., *11*, 607, 1968.
307. Rotstein, J., Reiss, F., Lauriello, A. and Bourel, M.: Arth. & Rheum., *8*, 465, 1965 (abstract).
308. Rowell, N. R.: Ann. Rheum. Dis., *21*, 70, 1962.
309. Rowell, N. R.: Brit. Med. J., *1*, 514, 1968 (correspondence).
310. Rubin, C. E. and Dobbins, W. O., III: Gastroenterology, *49*, 676, 1965.
311. Rupec, M. and Braun-Falco, O.: Arch. Klin. Exp. Derm., *218*, 543, 1964.
311*a*. Russell, R. G. G., Bisaz, S., and Fleisch, H.: Arch. Intern. Med. (Chicago), *124*, 571, 1969.
312. Sackner, M. A.: *Scleroderma*, New York, Grune & Stratton, 1966.
313. Sackner, M. A., Akgun, N., Kimbel, P. and Lewis, D. H.: Ann. Intern. Med., *60*, 611, 1964.
314. Sackner, M. A., Heinz, E. R. and Steinberg, A. J.: Amer. J. Cardiol., *17*, 542, 1966.
315. Saladin, T. A., French, A. B., Zarafonetis, C. J. D. and Pollard, H. M.: Amer. J. Dig. Dis., *11*, 522, 1966.
316. Salen, G., Goldstein, F. and Wirts, C. W.: Ann. Intern. Med., *64*, 834, 1966.
317. Sapira, J. D., Rodnan, G. P., Scheib, E. T., Klaniecki, T. and Rizk, M.: Amer. J. Med. (in press).
318. Saporta, L., Guiraudon, C., Delbarre, F., and Coste, F.: Bull. Soc. Méd. Hôp. Paris, *118*, 669, 1967.
319. Saporta, L., Guiraudon, C., Massias, P., Cayla, J., Delbarre, F. and Coste, F.: Bull. Soc. Méd. Hôp. Paris, *118*, 1361, 1967.
320. Schäfer, H. E. and Schäfer, A.: Arch. Klin. Med., *214*, 187, 1968.
321. Scharer, L. and Smith, D. W.: Arch. & Rheum., *12*, 51, 1969.
322. Scherbel, A. L., McCormack, L. J. and Poppo, M. J.: Cleveland Clin. Quart., *32*, 47, 1965.
323. Schimke, R. N., Kirkpatrick, C. H. and Delp, M. H.: Arch. Intern. Med. (Chicago), *119*, 365, 1967.
324. Schur, P. H. and Rodnan, G. P.: Unpublished observations, 1971.
325. Schur, P. H., Stollar, B. D., Steinberg, A. D. and Talal, N.: Arch. & Rheum., *14*, 342, 1971.
326. Scudamore, H. H., Green, P. A., Hoffman, H. N., Rosevar, J. W. and Tauxe, W. N.: Amer. J. Gastroent., *49*, 193, 1968.

327. Seligmann, M., Cannat, A. and Hamard, M.: Ann. N.Y. Acad. Sci., *124*, 816, 1965.
328. Selye, H.: J. Invest. Derm., *39*, 259, 1962.
329. Selye, H. and Tuchweber, B.: Quart. J. Exper. Physiol., *50*, 196, 1965.
330. Seville, R. H.: Proc. Roy. Soc. Med., *44*, 573, 1951.
331. Shapiro, A. P. and Rodnan, G. P.: Unpublished observations, 1969.
332. Sharp, G. C., Irvin, W. S., LaRoque, R. L., Velez, C., Daly, V., Kaiser, A. D. and Holman, H. R.: J. Clin. Invest., *50*, 350, 1971.
333. Shearn, M. A.: Ann. Intern. Med., *52*, 1352, 1960.
334. Shulman, L., Kurban, A. K. and Harvey, A. M.: Trans. Assoc. Amer. Physicians, *74*, 378, 1961.
335. Shuster, S., Raffle, E. J. and Bottoms, E.: Lancet, *1*, 525, 1967.
336. Simpson, H. and O'Duffy, J.: Brit. Med. J., *3*, 536, 1967.
337. Slate, W. G. and Graham, A. R.: Amer. J. Obstet. Gynec., *101*, 335, 1968.
338. Smiley, J. D., Johnson, R. L., Jr. and Ziff, M.: Arth. & Rheum., *10*, 313, 1967 (abstract).
339. Smit, G. G. and Schmaman, A.: J. Bone & Joint Surg., *49B*, 698, 1967.
340. Smith, Q. T., Rukavina, J. G. and Haaland, E. M.: Acta Derm.-Venereol. (Stockholm), *45*, 44, 1965.
341. Soila, P.: Acta Rheum. Scand., *10*, 189, 1964.
342. Sonneveldt, H. A., van Leeuwen, P. and Blom, P. S.: Acta Med. Scand., *171*, 391, 1962.
343. Sood, S. V. and Kohler, H. G.: J. Obstet. Gynec. Brit. Commw., *77*, 1109, 1970.
344. Stafne, E. C.: Oral Surg., *6*, 483, 1953.
345. Stastny, P., Stembridge, V. A. and Ziff, M.: J. Exp. Med., *118*, 635, 1963.
346. Šťáva, Z.: Dermatologica (Basel), *117*, 135, 1958.
347. Šťáva, Z.: Dermatologica (Basel), *117*, 147, 1958.
348. Steinberg, I. and Rothbard, S.: Radiology, *83*, 292, 1964.
349. Stiehm, E. R. and Trygstad, C. W.: Amer. J. Med., *46*, 774, 1969.
350. Sunderman, F. W., Jr. and Sunderman, F. W.: Amer. J. Med. Sci., *234*, 287, 1957.
350*a*. Swannell, A. J., Underwood, F. A. and Dixon, A. St. J.: Ann. Rheum. Dis., *29*, 380, 1970.
351. Tait, B. and Ashworth, B.: Ann. Rheum. Dis., *29*, 339, 1970 (abstract). (*See* Ashworth, B. and Tait, G. B. W.: Neurology, *21*, 609, 1971.)
352. Tange, J. D.: Austral. Ann. Med., *8*, 27, 1959.
353. Tay, C. H. and Khoo, O. T.: Austral. Ann. Med., *19*, 145, 1970.
354. Taylor, W. B.: Arch. Derm. (Chicago), *75*, 236, 1957.
355. Thibierge, G. and Weissenbach, R.-J.: (a) Bull. Mém. Soc. Méd. Hôp. Paris, *30*, 10, 1910; (b) Ann. Derm. Syph. (Paris), *2*, 129, 1911.
356. Thompson, G. R. and Castor, C. W.: J. Lab. Clin. Med., *68*, 617, 1966.
357. Thompson, J. M., Bluestone, R., Bywaters, E. G. L., Dorling, J. and Johnson, M.: Ann. Rheum. Dis., *28*, 281, 1969.
358. Townes, A. S.: Johns Hopkins Med. J., *120*, 337, 1967.
359. Treacy, W. L., Baggenstoss, A. H., Slocumb, C. H. and Code, C. F.: Ann. Intern. Med., *59*, 351, 1963.
360. Trell, E. and Lindström, C.: Ann. Rheum. Dis., *30*, 390, 1971.
361. Tuffanelli, D. L.: J. Invest. Derm., *41*, 139, 1963.
362. Tuffanelli, D. L.: J. Invest. Derm., *42*, 179, 1964.
363. Tuffanelli, D. L.: Arch. Derm. (Chicago), *93*, 724, 1966.
364. Tuffanelli, D. L., Marmelzat, W. L. and Dorsey, C. S.: Dermatologica (Basel), *132*, 51, 1966.
365. Tuffanelli, D. L. and Winkelmann, R. K.: Arch. Derm. (Chicago), *84*, 359, 1961.
366. Tuffanelli, D. L. and Winkelmann, R. K.: Amer. J. Med. Sci., *243*, 133, 1962.
367. Uitto, J.: Biochim. Biophys. Acta, *194*, 498, 1969.
368. Uitto, J., Hannuksela, M. and Rasmussen, O. G.: Ann. Clin. Res., *2*, 235, 1970.
369. Uitto, J., Helin, P., Rasmussen, O. and Lorenzen, I.: Ann. Clin. Res., *2*, 228, 1970.
370. Uitto, J., Øhlenschläger, K. and Lorenzen, I. B.: Clin. Chim. Acta, *31*, 13, 1971.
371. Unna, P. G.: *The Histopathology of the Diseases of the Skin.* Transl. by N. Walker, Edinburgh, W. F. Clay; New York, Macmillan and Co., 1896, pp. 1100–1113.
372. Urai, L., Munkacsi, I. and Szinay, G.: Brit. Med. J., *1*, 713, 1961.
373. Urai, L., Nagy, Z., Szinay, G. and Wiltner, W.: Brit. Med. J., *2*, 1264, 1958.
374. Varadi, D. P. and Lawrence, A. M.: Arch. Intern. Med. (Chicago), *124*, 13, 1969.
375. Verel, D.: Lancet, *2*, 914, 1956.

376. Vickers, H. R.: Practitioner, *199*, 198, 1967.

377. Villee, D. B., Nichols, G. and Talbot, N. B.: Pediatrics, *43*, 207, 1969.

378. Walcott, G., Burchell, H. B. and Brown, A. L.: Amer. J. Med., *49*, 70, 1970.

379. Weaver, A. L., Divertie, M. B. and Titus, J. L.: Dis. Chest, *54*, 490, 1968.

380. Weidner, F. and Braun-Falco, O.: Hautarzt, *19*, 345, 1968.

381. Westerman, M. P., Martinez, R. C., Medsger, T. A., Jr., Totten, R. S. and Rodnan, G. P.: Arch. Intern. Med. (Chicago), *122*, 39, 1968.

382, Westphal, C. F. O.: Charite-Annalen (Berlin), *3*, 341, 1876.

382*a*. Wheeler, C. E., Curtis, A. C., Grekin, R. H. and Zheutlin, B.: Ann. Intern. Med., *36*, 1050, 1952.

383. Wilde, A. H., Mankin, H. J. and Rodnan, G. P.: Arth. & Rheum., *13*, 445, 1970.

384. Wildenthal, K., Schenker, S., Smiley, J. D. and Ford, K. L.: Arch. Intern. Med. (Chicago), *121*, 365, 1968.

385. Willerson, J. T., Thompson. R. H., Hookman, P., Herdt, J. and Decker, J. L.: Ann. Intern. Med., *72*, 17, 1970.

386. Williams, R. C. and Law, D. H.: J. Lab. Clin. Med., *52*, 273, 1958.

387. Wilson, R. H., McCormick, W. E., Tatum, C. F. and Creech, J. L.: J.A.M.A., *201*, 577, 1967.

388. Wilson, R. J., Rodnan, G. P. and Robin, E. D.: Amer. J. Med., *36*, 361, 1964.

388*a*. Winder, P. R. and Curtis, A. C.: Arch. Derm. (Chicago), *82*, 732, 1960.

389. Windesheim, J. H. and Parkin, T. W.: Circulation, *17*, 874, 1958.

390. Winkelmann, R. K., Kierland, R. R., Perry, H. O., Muller, S. A. and Sams, W. M., Jr.: Mayo Clin. Proc., *46*, 128, 1971.

391. Winkelmann, R. K. and McGuckin, W. F.: Acta Dermatovener (Stockholm), *45*, 212, 1965.

392. Winkelstein, A., Rodnan, G. P. and Heilman, J. D.: Ann. Rheum. Dis., *31*, 126, 1972.

393. Winterbauer, R. H.: Bull. Johns Hopkins Hosp., *114*, 361, 1964.

394. Winters, W. L., Joseph, R. R. and Learner, N.: Arch. Intern. Med. (Chicago), *114*, 821, 1964.

395. Wolters, M.: Arch. Derm. Syph., *24*, 695 & 943, 1892.

396. Yune, H. Y., Vix, V. A. and Klatte, E. C.: J.A.M.A., *215*, 1113, 1971.

397. Zarafonetis, C. J. D.: Amer. J. Med. Sci., *248*, 550, 1964.

398. Zarafonetis, C. J. D., Lorber, S. H. and Hanson, S. M.: Amer. J. Med. Sci., *236*, 1, 1958.

399. Zatuchni, J., Campbell, W. N. and Zarafonetis, C. J. D.: Cancer, *6*, 1147, 1953.

400. Zion, M. M., Goldberg, B. and Suzman, M. M.: Quart. J. Med., *24*, 215, 1955.

PART VIII

Osteoarthritis

Section Editor: Ephraim P. Engleman, M.D.

Chapter 55

The Pathology and Pathogenesis of Osteoarthritis

By Leon Sokoloff, M.D.

INTRODUCTION

Despite the almost ubiquitous occurrence of osteoarthritis in the adult population, many parameters of its pathogenesis—some quite elementary—have not been established. Although the name *osteoarthritis* is a misnomer insofar as it implies an inherently inflammatory process, it has enjoyed many decades of common use in the English speaking world and will probably continue to do so because it has greater consumer appeal than the more accurate term *degenerative joint disease*. *Arthrosis* or *osteoarthrosis*, as frequently employed in continental Europe, might offer certain advantages were it to gain general acceptance here.

Osteoarthritis is a non-inflammatory disorder of movable joints characterized by deterioration and abrasion of articular cartilage, and also by formation of new bone at the joint surfaces. Two rather different views of the relationship between the bone and joint changes have been argued over the years.

EARLY CHANGES IN ARTICULAR CARTILAGE

The anatomic features of osteoarthritis are complex and sometimes subtle. Even in the simplest lesions, it is virtually impossible to isolate a single abnormality that is not accompanied by others. For this reason, the precise sequence of histologic events in the disorder can be reconstructed with only limited confidence. The earliest changes observed microscopically in the cartilage have been described quite differently by various investigators. Among those reported have been the following:

Focal Chondromucoid Softening.—In their valuable study of the knee joint, Bennett and co-workers[12] concluded that the initial abnormality was a focal swelling of cartilage matrix associated with inincreased affinity for hematoxylin. This mucoid transformation took place close to the surface of the cartilage. Cellular changes also were present in relation to this alteration: chondrocytes adjacent and superficial to the softened matrix were more numerous, and those within it were less numerous than normal.

Focal Loss of Metachromasia.—Loss of metachromatic material, presumed to be chondroitin sulfate, from all but the deepest portion of the radial zone of the articular cartilage has been proposed as the morphologic counterpart of chondromalacia that is followed by osteoarthritis.[64] The diminution of metachromasia corresponds to a loss rather than increase of affinity for hematoxylin, as proposed in the preceding view.

Proliferation of Chondrocytes.—Clusters of small chondrocytes are a common occurrence at the margin of minute fissures in the surface of the cartilage. Many pathologists have regarded these as having proliferated in response to the dehiscence of the tissue—either as an abortive "repair" phenomenon or as a consequence of the increased access of synovial fluid.[32] Nevertheless, disorderly hypertrophy and hyperplasia of articular chondrocytes in aging mice have been an integral part of the concept of Silberberg and Silberberg[132] that growth of joint tissue is an essential element of degenerative joint disease.

Diminution of Chondrocytes.—Although the unit number of chondrocytes is lower in adult than in young joint cartilage,[160] Meachim and Collins have presented evidence that there is no further alteration of the cell count in aging of articular cartilage, once adulthood is achieved, unless osteoarthritis is present.[94] Submicroscopic evidence of chondrocyte death has been found in all layers of joint cartilage of old rabbits;[9] these may appear as whorled myelin bodies, which represent residual mitochondrial phospholipid deposits.

Fatty Degeneration.—Fine fat deposits in the interterritorial matrix have been described as an early degenerative change in cartilage; these may become larger and form coarse droplets at the capsule of the chondrocytes.[116] Fat does not, however, characteristically accumulate in the cytoplasm of degenerated chondrocytes.[25]

Alteration of Collagen Fibrils.—Although exceptional coarseness has been observed as an occasional abnormality of the collagen fibrils adjacent to senescent chondrocytes of aged articular cartilage in several species,[133] normal-sized fibers[18, 27] have been described more frequently. A progressive radial reorientation of fibrils that normally have a random disposition in juveniles was noted in the head of the human femur both by electron microscopic as well as x-ray diffraction methods.[88] This rearrangement antedated development of osteoarthritis. Amprino and others have also noted increased perpendicular arrangement of collagen fibers with the light microscope.[3] *Amianthoid* (asbestos-like) degeneration of the matrix[4] is, however, a late and inconstant manifestation of the disorder. In one study, collagen fibers that had a normal electron microscopic appearance were observed, nevertheless, to dissolve with exceptional speed in acid solution.[28] In the absence of other explanation, this finding may simply reflect the depletion of ground substance rather than intrinsic alteration of the collagen.

Surface Irregularities.—Submicroscopic undulations and fissures, less than 2 microns (.002 mm.) deep, have been observed in the surface of old articular cartilage of rabbits by electron microscopy.[9]

Weichselbaum's Lacunar Resorption.—Focal dissolution of matrix by chondroclastic cells in the cartilage lacunae was at one time regarded as a characteristic feature of osteoarthritis (Fig. 51–4*C*), a view no longer generally accepted.[12]

GROSS CHANGES IN ARTICULAR CARTILAGE

Localized areas of softening of the cartilage are associated with a fine, velvety disruption of the surface. In these areas, there is a dehiscence of the cartilage along the planes of the collagen fibrils of the matrix. When the disruption is confined to the tangential layer at the surface, the process has frequently been referred to as *flaking*; when the process has extended deeper to the radial layer, it has been described as *fibrillation* (Fig. 55–1). Abrasion of the fibrillated cartilage takes place with progressive denudation of the underlying bony cortex (Fig. 55–2). In most joints, the sites of predilection for these changes have traditionally been described as ones subjected to weight-bearing or shearing stresses. Trueta and co-workers,[61] however, have stated that in the case of the hip, the earliest erosion occurs, not at the weight-bearing surface, but medial to the latter. In the knee joint, the central portions of the facets of the patella are the site most prone to erosion. Although not a weight-bearing surface, the patella is subject to enormous loads due to leverage when the knee is flexed in the squatting position.

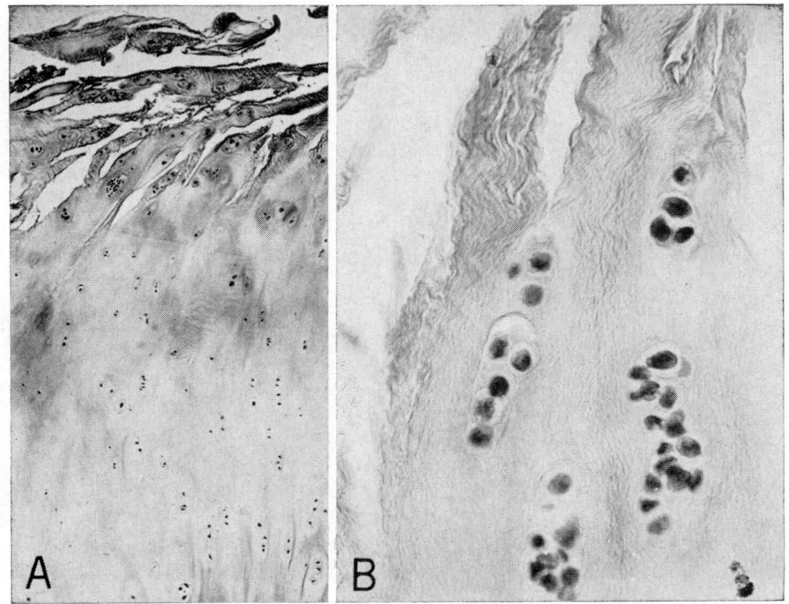

FIG. 55-1.—Fibrillation of articular cartilage. *A*, The most superficial dehiscences are oriented parallel to the surface, and then arch downward in a more vertical direction. These correspond to the fibrous planes of the cartilage. (Hematoxylin and eosin, × 40.) *B*, Higher magnification (× 240) of fibrillated edge. The collagen fibrils at the surface have been "unmasked" from the hyaline matrix and appear frayed. Clusters of chondrocytes have proliferated to form so-called "brood capsules."

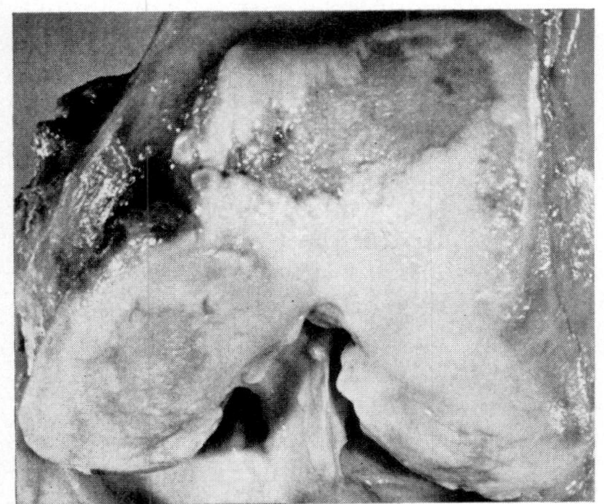

FIG. 55-2.—Degenerative joint disease, knee. Large areas of erosion of articular cartilage are present on the patellar facet and condyles of the femur. These occupy principally the central portions of the joint surfaces and spare the marginal regions.

CHANGES IN THE BONE

New bone formation takes place in two separate locations in relation to the joint surface; in exophytic growths at the margins of the articular cartilage or in the marrow immediately subjacent to the cartilage (Fig. 55-3).

The *marginal osteophytes* generally have one of two patterns of growth. One of these is as a protruberance into the joint space; the other develops within capsular and ligamentous attachments to the joint margins. In each circumstance, the direction of the osteophyte is governed by the lines of mechanical force exerted on the area of growth and generally corresponds to the contour of the joint surface from which the osteophyte protrudes. The osteophyte consists in large part of bone that merges imperceptibly with the other cortical and cancellous tissue of the subchondral bone. It is frequently capped by a layer of hyaline

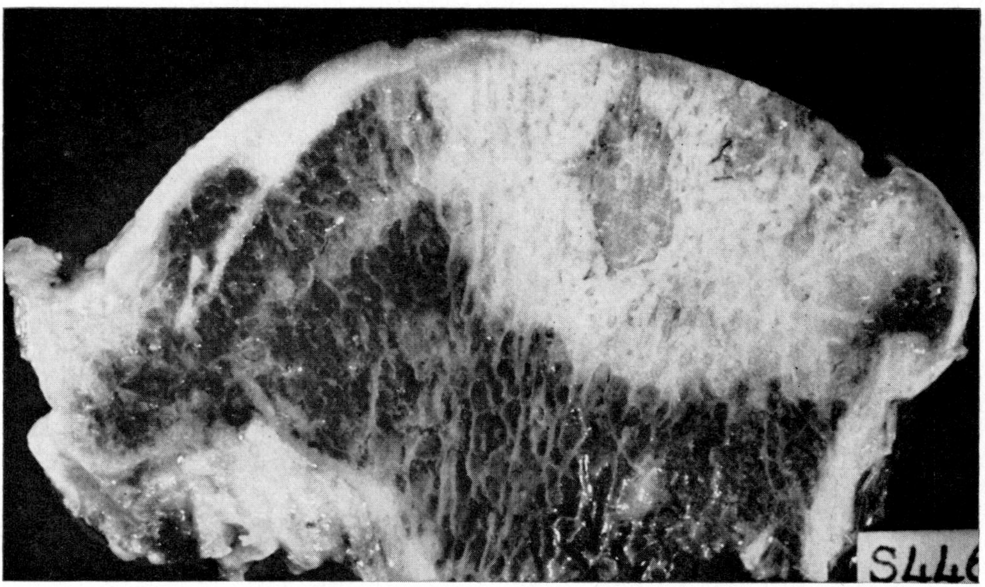

FIG. 55–3.—Advanced osteoarthritis, head of femur. The contours have been greatly deformed both by abrasion of articular cartilage from most of the surface, and also by formation of large marginal osteophytes. The spur at the left has grown not only to the side but also superiorly into the original joint cartilage. Subchondral pseudocysts approach the articular surface through slender crevices. The pallor of the eburnated tissue beneath the eroded surface reflects the condensation of bony trabeculae and avascular fibrous tissue in contrast to the darker, vascular hematopoietic marrow.

and fibrocartilage that becomes continuous with the adjacent synovial lining.

The proliferation of bone in the subchondral tissue is most marked in areas that have been denuded of their cartilaginous covering by osteoarthritic erosion. In these regions, the articulating surface consists of bone that has been rubbed smooth. The glistening appearance of this polished, sclerotic surface suggests ivory; hence the name *eburnation* for this process. In addition to this alteration, two other variants of new bone formation are also seen in relation to the articular cartilage.

"Cystic" areas of rarefaction of the bone may develop immediately beneath the joint surface (Fig. 55–3). Within these areas, the marrow undergoes mucoid or fibrous degeneration, trabeculae disappear and the entire area is encircled by a rim of reactive new bone and compact fibrous tissue (Fig. 55–4*D*). In early lesions of this sort, compact fibrinous exudate may appear in the degenerating marrow. Vascular injection studies by Trueta and co-workers[61] have demonstrated these pseudocystic areas to be deficient in blood vessels, while excessive new vessel formation develops at the periphery. Most often the apex of these areas presents directly at the eburnated surface of the joint. In some instances, however, these cysts are apparent roentgenographically before narrowing of the joint space, evidence of cartilage destruction, is demonstrable. At times, such "cysts" are located at the attachments of ligaments to the joint surfaces, *i.e.*, where the cortex is perforated by nutrient vessels. These findings are consistent with an hypothesis proposed[84] and modified as follows:[111] that there is an intrusion of pressure, if not of synovial fluid, from the articular space through a defect in the articular cortex into the subchondlar

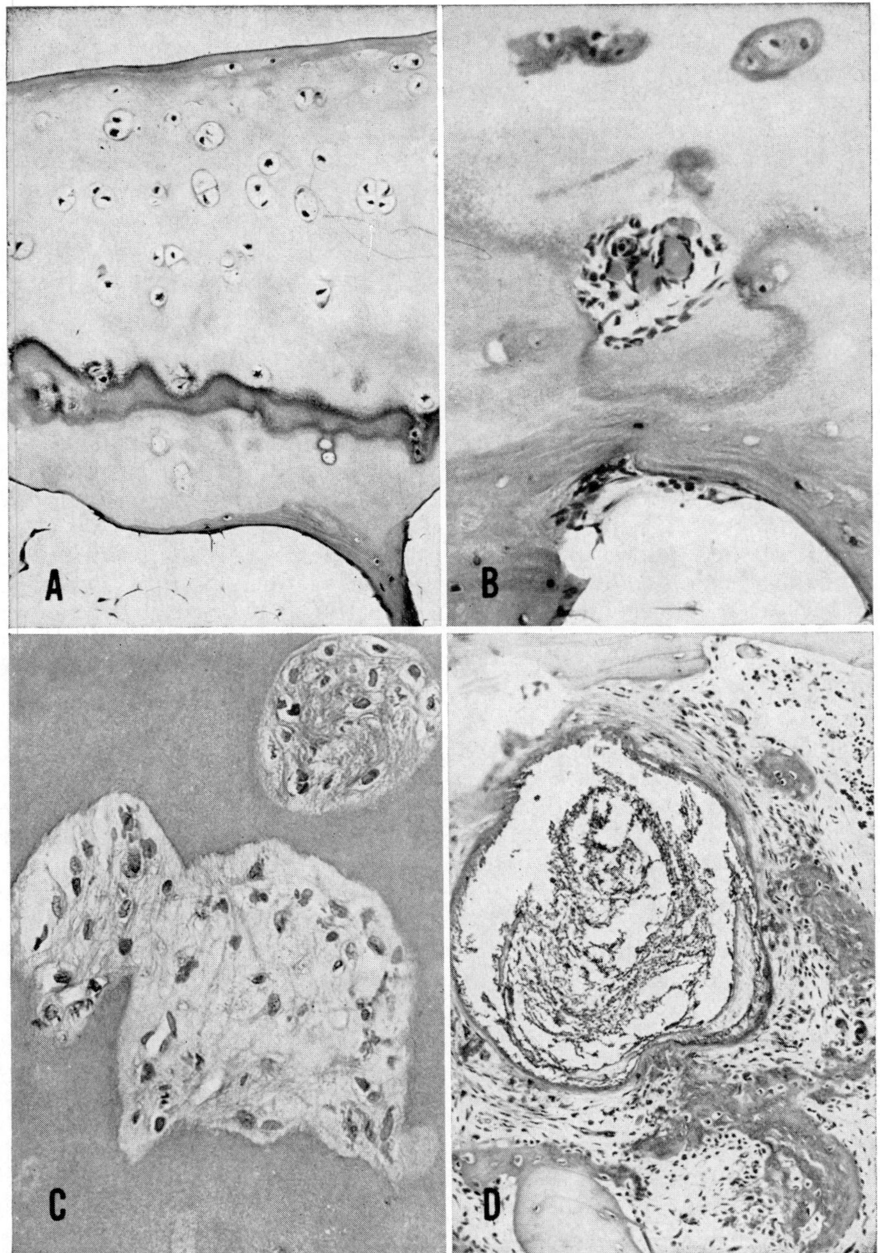

Fig. 55–4.—Miscellaneous remodeling and degenerative changes. All sections stained with hematoxylin and eosin. *A*, Reduplication of calcification "tidemark" (× 95). *B*, Vascularization of base of articular cartilage. The dark stained material in the capsules of the chondrocytes is calcific (× 183). *C*, Weichselbaum's lacunar resorption. Small, geographic areas of hyaline cartilage are replaced by loose-textured, cellular fibrous tissue (× 210). *D*, Early subchondral "cystic" degeneration. A small true cyst, filled with mucoid material, has a fibrous border. New bone formation is seen in the adjacent marrow (× 90).

bone marrow. The increased pressure is dissipated radially into the adjacent bone marrow, compressing the blood vessels in marrow and thereby leading to the retrogressive changes observed. Parenthetically it may be noted that the so-called punched-out lesions observed roentgenographically in gout and the bone cysts in hemophilic arthropathy correspond pathologically to these cysts in osteoarthritis, with the exception that the specific exudates of each of these arthropathies also lie within the degenerated marrow space.

The other type of new bone formation in this location is a focal ossific metaplasia of the base of the articular cartilage. This should be regarded as part of a general *remodeling* of the joint contour through which bone is added to a portion of the articular cortex, while other areas in the joint surface may display focal resorption of the bone.[53,73] The relationship between these changes in the bone and those in the cartilage has been interpreted in quite different ways; the theoretical implications with respect to the pathogenesis of osteoarthritis are quite important and will be discussed below.

The junction between the articular cartilage and the subchondral plate of bone is actually occupied by a zone of calcification of cartilage. During the years of skeletal growth, the epiphysis and the articular cartilage participate in the enlargement of the bone. Expansion of the epiphysis during this period is accomplished by endochondral ossification of calcified cartilage in this region. The interface between the calcified and non-calcified hyaline articular cartilage is demarcated in usual histologic preparations by a thin, wavy hematoxyphil line (sometimes called the *tidemark*) (Fig. 55–4*A*). It is a common finding in older joints to find not one, but a number of discontinuous parallel lines of this sort in this region. Their presence is clear evidence of progression of calcification of the basal portion of the articular cartilage. This probably should be interpreted much as the new bone formation in the base of the cartilage—as part of a subtle remodeling process.[58] The possibility that this process of basilar calcification may lead to an apparent thinning of articular cartilage ("senile atrophy") has received no support in one recent study.[134]

SYNOVIAL AND CAPSULAR TISSUES

The synovial tissue itself is apparently the least affected portion of the joint in osteoarthritis. A progressive increase in the amount of fibrous tissue separating the synovial capillaries from the joint space has recently been described as an age-correlated finding.[125] The suggestion that this might constitute an impediment to formation of synovia and so contribute to osteoarthritis, must be regarded as speculative. Hyaline sclerosis of minute vessels was, at one time, invoked as a cause of vascular insufficiency leading to articular degeneration. It is now recognized as a common focal finding in joints, even of young individuals, and not directly related to osteoarthritis.[45] Fibrosis of the synovial surface and even mild cartilaginous metaplasia and fibrillation are occasionally seen in the synovial surface of the patellar tendon in association with advanced osteoarthritis of the knee (Fig. 55–5). Nevertheless, inflammatory changes in the synovium are not characteristic of osteoarthritis. In the hip, fibrosis has been associated with synovial hypertrophy, and it has been a common experience in *malum coxae senilis* or severe osteoarthritis of the hip to observe a severe, chronic inflammatory infiltrate as well. This inflammatory reaction has been the source of considerable nosologic and diagnostic difficulty in malum coxae senilis; at times the disorder is indistinguishable histologically from isolated rheumatoid arthritis of the hip. Similarly, hypertrophic villous synovitis also is present in association with advanced degenerative joint disease in horses—and this too has caused confusion with rheumatoid arthritis.[60] The reason for this inflammation is uncertain, but it has been suggested that a foreign body reaction to cartilaginous and other detritus into the synovial tissue may be a mechanism.[68,89] Minute tears in the capsular tissues appear as slender fibrous or vascular seams disrupt-

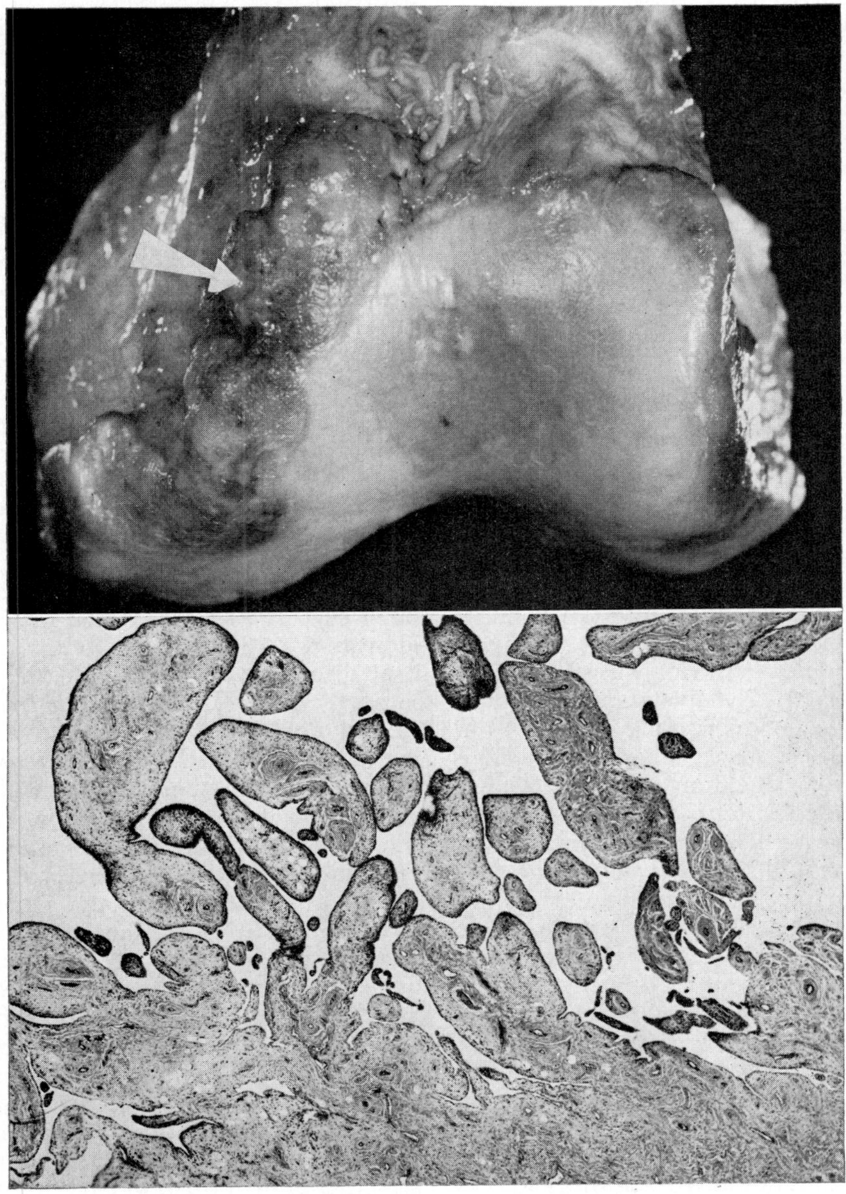

Fig. 55–5.—Synovial hypertrophy in severe osteoarthritis. The patient was a 63-year-old man whose left knee had been enlarged for 23 years following an automobile accident. There is a massive osteophyte (arrow) at the medial border of the articular surface. The adjacent synovial tissue has undergone prominent papillary thickening. Histologically, the villous processes are seen made up of compact fibrous tissue that is not infiltrated by inflammatory cells (hematoxylin and eosin, × 16).

ing the principal axis of the collagen bundles.

COMPARATIVE PATHOLOGY

Osteoarthritis, unlike rheumatoid arthritis, occurs widely in the vertebrate kingdom, regardless of the position of the species in the taxonomic scale. Osteophytic lesions, sometimes leading to ankylosis of the joints, were a relatively common finding in certain types of giant dinosaurs a hundred million years ago. The disorder has been observed in large and small mammals; in animals that swim (cetaceans) rather than bear their weight on their extremities, and also, to a mild degree in birds. It is of considerable economic importance in livestock commerce, the horse-racing industry and veterinary practice.

In small laboratory animals, it has been possible to study, under controlled conditions, a number of pathogenetic concepts of the nature of degenerative joint disease. In mice, the importance of genetic factors has been established.[145] The inheritance appeared to be polygenic and the overall behavior was of recessive type. There was no evidence of major sex linkage. Surprisingly, obesity did not appear to be a major deleterious factor in the development of the lesions. Male mice consistently develop more severe osteoarthritis than do females. Although it would seem entirely reasonable that the endogenous hormones should account for this, there is no unanimity as to the result of experimental administration of them on the production of the lesions, nor convincing evidence as to the mechanisms involved.

The genetic character of the disorder is also manifested by variable species susceptibilities and resistance to the development of osteoarthritis. Rats, for example, are generally resistant, whereas another rodent, Mastomys, develops severe generalized degenerative joint disease by the time it is two years old. Genetic contributions also are evidenced by the recently reported inheritability of osteoarthritis in certain breeds of cattle[138] and of swine.[129] The fundamental pathogenetic problem these present is whether the genetic factors involved are local articular ones related to the configuration and mechanical forces exerted on the joint (as in the common dysplastic hips of German shepherd dogs) or are more generalized, metabolic properties of the articular tissues.

DEGENERATIVE DISEASE OF THE SPINAL COLUMN

Degenerative changes in the spine affect two discrete intervertebral articular systems: the diarthrodial (apophyseal) joints, and the synchondroses (intervertebral discs). Most English-speaking rheumatologists have accepted the formulation of Collins[32] that the degenerative processes in the two structures should be differentiated. Accordingly, *spinal osteoarthritis* would describe the changes in the apophyseal joints, while *spinal osteophytosis* or *spondylosis deformans* would properly be identified with degenerative intervertebral disc disease. Although one cannot seriously quarrel with this distinction, it should not necessarily lead to a fundamental pathological dichotomy between the processes in these two sets of joints. Indeed, it is a common experience, in the cervical region, to find the lesions associated with each other, albeit on neighboring rather than the same vertebrae.[54] Aside from the fact that the degenerative changes take place in the nucleus pulposus, rather than in articular cartilage, the sequence of pathological events in the two sets of joints are remarkably similar. The nucleus pulposus becomes fissured and deformed; and fibrillary disintegration of the hyaline cartilage plates, through which it is attached to the vertebral bodies, cannot be distinguished histologically from the changes in diarthrodial osteoarthritis. Eburnation of the subchondral bony plate develops in like manner. The marginal osteophytes arise under the mechanical stimulus of horizontal pulsion of the anulus fibrosus and its periosteal attachments arising from collapse and spreading out of the nucleus pulposus.[32] Others have additionally implicated traction forces of spinal muscles on the tendinous insertions in this region. In any event, these mechanisms are not qualitatively different from those in the more movable joints.

Although the marginal osteophytes develop most often on the anterolateral aspects of the vertebral bodies, it has become increasingly recognized in recent years that posterior osteophytic protrusions also occur, and may embarrass the spinal cord and its roots. In the cervical region, antecedent spondylosis has constituted a principal neurosurgical hazard of injuries among older patients.[102] Osteophytes in the Luschka (uncovertebral, neurocentral) joints have been shown by anatomic and angiographic means to compromise the neighboring vertebral arteries. The narrowing of the lumens is most marked during rotation of the head. This provides the basis for the *posterior cervical sympathetic* or *Barré-Liéou syndrome*.[69,131]

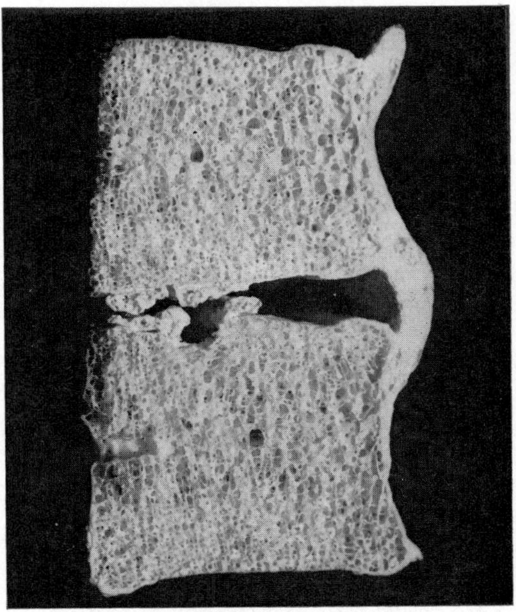

Fig. 55–6.—Hyperostotic ankylosing spondylosis, thoracic vertebrae from a 72-year-old man. Unlike the Marie-Strümpell lesion illustrated in Figure 20–9, there are marked degenerative changes in the intervertebral disc: the space between the vertebral bodies is narrowed, and the articular lamella is irregular as a result both of focal resorption and of protrusion of new bone into the disc. The cortex on the anterolateral surface of the vertebra (right) is blended with the bony bridge.

Characteristically, degenerative joint disease does not lead to ankylosis. There is, however, a form of senescent joint disease in which ossific transformation of the anterior longitudinal ligaments takes place. This is associated with degenerative changes in the intervertebral discs (Fig. 55–6) and marginal osteophytosis, and probably represents a severe form of spondylosis. The cortex of the vertebral body in the vicinity of the ligamentous ossification has a variable degree of destruction. The condition is known by a variety of names (*spondylorrheostosis, senile ankylosing vertebral hyperostosis of Forestier and Rotés-Querol, and hyperostotic spondylosis*). It is not clear whether it is identical with so-called *physiological vertebral ligamentous ossification*.[139] Hyperostotic spondylosis occurs frequently in species other than man and has been confused with Marie-Strümpell disease in them.[147] *Baastrup's syndrome* is an osteoarthritic-like change in the distal portions of "kissing" dorsal spinous processes. It is usually associated with severe spondylosis and is of roentgenologic interest primarily.

These several patterns of senescent spinal disease occur in species other than man. The direction of displacement of the nucleus pulposus differs in quadrupeds from that of man. In dogs, for example, displacement often occurs dorsally and, particularly in chondrodysplastic breeds, leads to spinal cord paralysis. In man, the upright posture leads more characteristically to displacement toward the vertebral bodies. The common development of subchondral nodules of cartilaginous and fibrous tissue beneath the subchondral plate of the vertebral bodies—the *Schmorl nodes*—is usually attributed to the displacement of nucleus pulposus into the vertebral body.[130] These islands are usually surrounded by a shell of bone and, except for their greater content of cartilage, are quite reminiscent of the subchondral "cysts" already noted in osteoarthritic peripheral joints. Rats and mice, forced to assume an upright posture through amputation of the forelimbs in infancy, ultimately acquire severe degenerative disc disease in the lumbosacral region.[165]

Degeneration of intervertebral discs that takes place normally with aging and apparently is exaggerated in instances of herniation is characterized microscopically by a depletion of metachromatic ground substance from the matrix and partial fibrous transformation of the nucleus pulposus.[153] An electron microscopic study of herniated nucleus pulposus tissue revealed the collagen fibers to be disorderly and attenuated; the cross-striations were often indistinct and the periods shortened.[35] Although swelling of the nucleus has sometimes been invoked to account for acute herniation,[29] there is reasonably consistent evidence that the water content and also the swelling pressure of the disc are reduced rather than increased in the disorder.[22,62,98] The herniation depends ultimately upon the development of tears in the anulus fibrosus.[65]

SPECIAL FORMS OF OSTEOARTHRITIS

Heberden's Nodes

Despite their great frequency, little systematic information is available on the morbid anatomy of these common marginal osteophytes that form at the base of the distal finger phalanges. In advanced cases, the lesions cannot be distinguished from osteoarthritis in other locations (Fig. 55–7). A number of specimens have, however, been clearly demonstrated to have quite a different appearance[31] that is of considerable theoretical interest. In these specimens, the articular cartilage, rather than displaying degenerative fibrillation and erosion, has actually been hypertrophic.

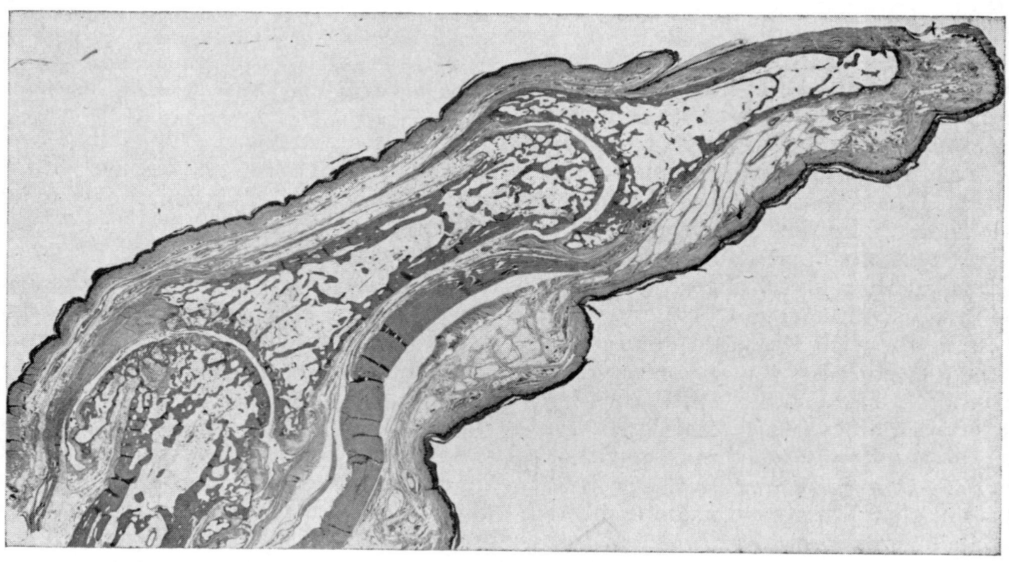

FIG. 55–7.—Heberden's node. The articular cartilage has completely disappeared from the surfaces of the distal interphalangeal joint. Bony osteophytes, directed toward the base of the finger, are present on the dorsal and palmar aspects of both articulating surfaces. Advanced osteoarthritic changes also are present in the proximal interphalangeal joint, forming a so-called Bouchard node. (Hematoxylin and eosin, × 20.)

Ossific transformation of the insertion of the tendons into joint capsule and periosteum accounted for the exophytosis. A decision as to whether these two forms correspond, as has been suggested,[32] to two clinically different types of Heberden node—the traumatic, acquired and the genetically governed type—must be kept in abeyance until further clinicopathologic information is available. In other instances, mucoid transformation of the peri-articular fibroadipose tissue, associated with proliferation of myxoid fibroblasts and cyst formation, has been seen. The fluid from cysts has been identified as hyaluronic acid.[71] This is not a unique anatomic feature of Heberden nodes. Indistinguishable changes are present at times in other osteoarthritic joints in other species; the process has certain morphologic similarities to ganglion formation or cystic degeneration of the semilunar cartilages.

Generalized Hypertrophic Osteoarthritis

Kellgren and co-workers at Manchester, England, have described a pattern of osteoarthritis that differs from other types of degenerative joint disease in its pathogenesis, so far as can be determined roentgenographically.[77] This disorder is characterized clinically by involvement of multiple joints, in addition to the formation of Heberden nodes; by affecting primarily women at the onset of menopause; and by having more conspicuous inflammatory manifestations. Radiologic examination of the joints suggested that the primary events were not erosion of the articular cartilage, but proliferation of bone into the base of the cartilage and also exophytic growth at the margins of the joint. So far as the anatomic findings are concerned, only limited information is available; postmortem examinations years after the onset of the lesions have indicated that the changes are not distinguishable from ordinary osteoarthritis. This disorder is not well recognized in the United States.

Malum Coxae Senilis

It is well known that a variety of structural abnormalities of the hip joint in childhood—congenital dysplasia, Legg-Perthes disease, slipped capital epiphysis and congenital coxa vara—leads to premature osteoarthritic degeneration. In other cases, however, none of the precursors has been clinically overt. Roentgenographic analysis of the contour of the hip joint has suggested to some investigators[164] that low-grade dysplasia has actually been the basis for most if not all these cases. The validity of this retrospective view may be questionable because subluxation has been documented roentgenographically to develop as a late manifestation of the joint deformity.[113] Reference has already been made to the synovitis that may be present.

Osteoarthritis Associated with Miscellaneous Heritable Articular Disease

Precocious osteoarthritis develops with great frequency in *multiple epiphyseal dysplasia*, a rare disease in which there is a defect of epiphyseal growth and maturation of variable portions of the axial and appendicular skeleton.[101] Allison and Blumberg have observed osteoarthritis also to develop in a rare form of heritable osteochondrosis[2] of the digits. The *nail-patella syndrome* (*hereditary osteo-onychodysplasia*, *Turner-Kieser syndrome*, *iliac horn syndrome*) also is complicated frequently by osteoarthritis. Mention has already been made of osteoarthritis complicating *congenital dysplasia of the hip*. The hereditary component of this disorder has been argued several ways.[26] In dogs, there seems to be evidence for a significant heritable contribution to the disorder, insofar as certain breeds (German shepherds) commonly develop it, while others (American greyhounds) never do.[120] The shepherd dogs also are prone to another articular dysplasia, affecting the elbows; this, too, is subject to osteoarthritic complication.

Chondromalacia Patellae

This term is used rather loosely as indicating a distinctive post-traumatic softening of the articular cartilage of the patella in young persons.[64] From a perusal of the anatomical reports on the subject, it is apparent that most authors are describing lesions indistinguishable from early osteoarthritis. One occasionally observes, as an incidental lesion at necropsy on young adults, a swollen, markedly softened articular cartilage with high water content in patellas that have no histologic evidence of osteoarthritic change. The possibility that there may exist a true type of chondromalacia, as distinguished from osteoarthritic degeneration, deserves further study.

Kaschin-Beck Disease

This interesting condition has been recognized in Eastern Siberia and Manchuria for more than a century, but only recently has come to the attention of American rheumatologists. It is a disorder of growing children but also affects other species. The disease is characterized by defective growth and maturation of the epiphyses, and leads, despite the youth of the patient, to articular changes indistinguishable from osteoarthritis.[108] The lesion apparently has a nutritional basis. One school of contemporary thought is that it derives from contamination of grain by a fungus; another[30] attributes it to defective mineral content of grain grown in the areas in which the condition is endemic.

Arthropathy in Caisson Disease

Severe, chronic degenerative joint disease is a fairly common occupational disease among sandhogs. It apparently is a late sequela of bone infarcts, although a history of "bends" frequently cannot be elicited. As in other types of bone infarcts, the epiphyseal ends of the bones are principally involved. The articular cartilage, deriving nutrition from the synovial fluid, does not undergo cell death as the subchondral bone does. Nevertheless, weakening of the bony support of the joint apparently ultimately leads to mechanical infractions of the joint surface, and the sequence of osteoarthritis ensues.[75]

Gout

The articular lesions of gout are related to the deposition of monosodium urate salts in or about the joint tissues. The form that these lesions take varies with the amount, location and duration of these deposits. Aside from massive disorganization of the articular structures by tophaceous deposits, the commonest lesion is osteoarthritis. Urate crystals are deposited not only on and in the surface of the articular cartilage, but also in the subchondral cysts, where they constitute the so-called punched-out lesions. In the areas of crystal deposition in the cartilage, chondrocytes characteristically are necrotic, and the matrix exceptionally oxyphilic.

Ochronotic Arthropathy

The articular and spinal lesions associated with alcaptonuria have many similarities to those of degenerative joint disease. The hyaline articular cartilage and the nucleus pulposus become discolored by the ochronotic pigment, and their material properties are grossly and markedly altered thereby. They are remarkably brittle despite the fact that the water content does not decrease.[96] Necrosis of chondrocytes is more conspicuous than in degenerative joint disease. Splitting off of fragments of the brittle cartilage is much more evident in ochronotic than non-ochronotic osteoarthritis. With these exceptions, the processes are very similar. Although "calcification" of the nucleus pulposus is frequently described in ochronosis, it is probable that what is seen is actually an ossific replacement of degenerated, pigmented tissue, rather than calcium deposition in the disc. Furthermore, the radiologically recognized, so-called loose bodies in the peripheral joints, actually represent a reactive polypoid, secondary osteochondromatous response of the synovial tissue to the articular detritus.

Charcot Joints

Neurogenic arthropathies may be regarded basically as examples of severe osteoarthritis, in which the destructive and hypertrophic elements are exaggerated by trauma associated with loss of articular proprioception. A sometimes postulated primary or important contributory role of neurovascular reflex atrophy of bone has received no support from experimental studies.[46]

Hemophilic Arthropathy

The joint disease that complicates the hemophilias also may be regarded as a variant of osteoarthritis. Erosion of articular cartilage is characteristic and differs, in some areas only, from other types of degenerative joint disease. In these places, the superficial portion of the cartilage is replaced by a fibrous tissue in which considerable hemosiderin is deposited. This pigment has not been recognized in intact hyaline cartilage. The pathogenesis of the condition is not fully understood, although it obviously is related to the articular hemorrhage. It has variously been proposed that toxic derivatives of the blood may develop, or that a deleterious trophic effect on the articular tissues arises from the compression by the extravasated blood and loss of motion. The subchondral cysts are filled with blood, but otherwise are analogous to those of degenerative joint disease.

CHEMICAL CHANGES IN OSTEOARTHRITIS

Any consideration of the composition of articular cartilage in relation to osteoarthritis must take into account two postulates that, when neglected in the past, have led to erroneous conclusions. The first is that the changes in articular cartilage must be studied in articular rather than other types of cartilage because there are significant biological differences between various types of cartilage in this regard. The second is that changes associated with osteoarthritis must be distinguished from those simply related to age in this cartilage.

The vascularity,[110] amianthoid degeneration,[4] pigmentation[158] and marked dehydration that occur in adult costal cartilage are not characteristic of old articular cartilage. Although costal cartilage of human adults has approximately 20 per cent less water by weight than that of children, the difference in the patellar cartilage is only about 2 per cent or less.[87,97]

Unlike the findings in osteoarthritic cartilage, intact articular cartilage from elderly persons has no reduction of hexosamine sulfate[5,93] or chondromucoprotein content.[17] This must be contrasted to a repeatedly documented reduction of hexosamine in costal cartilage[76] of older patients. A considerable increase in the keratosulfate content of costal cartilage occurs during the years of growth, and a decrease in the proportion of chondroitin sulfate to this polysaccharide (C/K ratio) has also been observed in aging nucleus pulposus[37,59,91] and certain other connective tissues. Although there have been several reports of analogous alteration of the C/K ratio in aging articular cartilage[13,56,82,83] the reservation that osteoarthritic lesions of some degree were also present in the tissues studied must be noted. There is no reason to believe, however, that future studies may not disclose, as preliminary reports suggest,[123] chemical changes in aged cartilage that are not associated with osteoarthritis.

The reduction in the chondroitin sulfate content of osteoarthritic cartilage is not accompanied by a corresponding diminution of the matrix protein according to one recent chemical study.[17] In another report on the diminution in metachromasia of osteoarthritic cartilage, in which ultraviolet microscopy rather than chemical analysis was employed, the findings were interpreted to indicate a depletion of the protein as well as the chondroitin sulfate of the interterritorial portions of the matrix.[49] The ability of the articular chondrocytes to fix sulfate, as demonstrated *in vitro* by autoradiography with $S^{35}O_4$, does not decrease with age. In osteoarthritis, the proliferating chondrocytes display increased rather than defective utilization of sulfate.[94] The fixation of sulfate by chondrocytes is ordinarily presumptive evidence of production of chondroitin sulfate. The reduction of chondroitin sulfate content at the same time that this material may be undergoing excessive production in osteoarthritic cartilage would thus be anomalous. It may, in this context, be significant that the free sulfate content of synovial fluid is somewhat elevated in osteoarthritis.[30]

Aside from the increase in the keratosulfate to chondroitin sulfate ratio already noted in aging and degenerating nucleus pulposus, a loss of water content[115] and of total polysaccharide relative to collagen,[38] and also of the viscosity of the protein-polysaccharide complex,[91] has also been reported. The type of chondroitin sulfate also changes with aging, from the 4 to a predominantly 6 form.[20] There is some evidence that the keratosulfate of old nucleus pulposus is metabolically inert.[37]

REPAIR OF ARTICULAR CARTILAGE AND POTENTIAL REVERSIBILITY OF OSTEOARTHRITIS

The persistent erosion of articular cartilage in osteoarthritis has long aroused interest in the limited ability of this tissue to grow. By all parameters studied, the metabolic activity of hyaline cartilage is very low.[160] In general, experimentally induced gaps in articular cartilage, so long as they do not penetrate into the subchondral, vascular marrow, show little tendency to be filled in with new cartilage.[24,25] These observations provide the basis for the generally held view that it is the inability of articular cartilage to repair itself that is responsible for irreversible development of osteoarthritis.

There are a number of reasons for re-examining the unqualified validity of this concept. Freezing injuries, which kill the cells but avoid thermal contraction of the collagen, show that necrosis of articular chondrocytes does not in itself suffice to cause the lesions.[136] Although the rate of repair of articular cartilage is low, it may not be, over a length of time, negligible. Recent surgical experience offers two sorts of evidence, relevant to a potential reversibility of osteoarthritis:

1. Following arthroplasties of the hip in which devitalized tissue is removed, a new articular surface, composed admittedly of imperfect hyaline articular cartilage, may form beneath the prosthesis.[157] The metallic device in this circumstance presumably has served to protect the reparative granulation tissue, destined to form the articular cartilage, from mechanical abrasion.

2. Wedge osteotomies and other procedures designed to relieve mechanical stresses on osteoarthritic hips[81,109,112] have frequently yielded impressive roentgenologic evidence of regression of the arthritic lesions. The implications of these observations with respect to the pathogenesis of osteoarthritis are that the disorder may develop not so much because the articular cartilage is incapable of repairing itself, but because there may be a disparity between factors requiring proliferation of cartilage and the limited ability of the cartilage to respond. This carries with it a certain optimism for ultimate development of methods for retarding if not reversing development of osteoarthritis.

LOCAL EXPERIMENTAL INDUCTION OF OSTEOARTHRITIS

Numerous efforts to establish mechanisms that may be involved in the pathogenesis of degenerative joint disease have been made through induction of osteoarthritis by different local manipulations. These include:

1. *Surgical Discontinuity in the Articular Surface.*—Although the literature is not wholly consistent on the subject, minute defects in the articular cartilage[11,24,25] generally have not resulted in osteoarthritis. On the other hand, larger defects, that caused deformation of the joint contour, did.[77]

2. *Physical or Chemical Injury to Articular Cartilage.*—Thermal and traumatic insults to the cartilage, as induced by local cautery or hammering, also have caused osteoarthritis.[50,159] Necrosis of chondrocytes and associated degenerative changes have also been induced by topical application of caustic agents. Synovitis, induced by intra-articular instillation of acids or other irritants[21,28] or infectious materials,[50] also has been accompanied by certain osteoarthritic changes. Of course, these same agents may also have acted on the cartilage as well as the synovium. Articular chondrocytes, which formerly were considered incapable of undergoing mitotic division in mature animals, are now known to grow readily and to synthesize sulfated mucopolysaccharides and collagen when cultured *in vitro.*[57,147]

3. *Subluxations and Luxations.* — Protracted displacements of the patella[11] and of the hip[114] have resulted in early remodeling and later degenerative changes in the articular tissues.

4. *Prolonged Compression.*—When the articular cartilages have been maintained tightly compressed to each other for even a few days, death of chondrocytes has been followed by development of osteoarthritis.[34,126,154] Under these circumstances, the compression is presumed to have hindered the normal percolation of interstitial fluid upon which the nutrition of the chondrocytes depends.

5. *Foreign Body Abrasion.*—Degenerative changes in the superficial layer of articular cartilage resulted from the intra-articular instillation of carborundum.[152] These particles, like talc[92] or cartilage fragments,[68,89] also evoked a foreign body reaction in the synovium and articular capsule. In the vicinity of the attachments of the latter to the articular surface, exostoses developed.

6. *Restriction of Joint Motion.*—There exists a sizable and somewhat inconsistent literature on the effects of immobilization on animal joints. Aside from atrophy and focal fibrous transformation of the superficial portions of the cartilage, a degree of fibrosis of the soft tissues with focal adhesions to the joint surfaces also has been described. In addition, however, degenerative changes in articular cartilage and subchondral bone, having certain resemblances to osteoarthritis, have also been reported.[47] The preponderant evidence indicates that these changes also required abnormal pressures or frictional forces for their development in addition to the restriction of motion.

7. *Chondrolytic Enzymes.*—Intra-articular injection of crude papain into young rabbits resulted in degenerative changes of articular cartilage associated with a low-grade synovitis.[103] In view of the fact that other chemical irritants may cause analogous changes, the lack of adequate controls, such as inactivated papain, makes it difficult to assess the extent to which the proteolytic effect of the enzyme on the matrix was responsible *per se* for the lesions observed.

It thus appears that a variety of procedures that embarrass the viability of articular chondrocytes and the integrity of the collagenous framework can lead to the sequence of osteoarthritic change. The procedures involving abnormal mechanical stresses on the articular cartilage, compression and dislocation, also evoke structural remodeling of the joint contours.

PATHOGENESIS OF OSTEOARTHRITIS

With this background, we can attempt to formulate some concepts of the nature of osteoarthritis.

Primary versus Secondary Osteoarthritis

It is well recognized that osteoarthritis may supervene on other types of preexisting damage to joints, inflammatory or non-inflammatory. Several special examples of these have already been noted. Such instances are classified as secondary in contradistinction to those forms in which no traumatic or other predisposing articular etiology can be assigned. In such instances, intrinsic degeneration of the articular tissue is presumed to underlie the development of the disease. This is primary osteoarthritis or degenerative joint disease. In practice, it is difficult in most instances to distinguish on anatomical grounds between the two types of osteoarthritis.

Does Osteoarthritis Begin Primarily in the Bone or in the Cartilage?

It has already been pointed out that most English-speaking authorities have concluded that the earliest evidences of osteoarthritis are to be found in the articular cartilage.[12,32,61,85] Marginal osteophyte formation, as well as the several subchondral changes already noted, is regarded as a secondary remodeling of the bone. Presumably they would develop consequent to a loss of substance of the articular cartilage and transmission of the mechanical forces, attending joint function, to other, more labile articular tissues. A rather different view has long been entertained on the European continent. Emphasis has often been placed on a primary alteration in the bone.[53] This hypothesis has been given new currency in recent years by L. C. Johnson and co-workers.[73] They have suggested that growth does not completely cease at the articular ends of the bones in the adult; furthermore, remodeling of the joints takes place, under the aegis of functional demand, independently of degeneration of the articular cartilage.[99] According to this formulation, it is only when the rate of remodeling exceeds that of orderly cartilage repair that osteoarthritis develops.

These different hypotheses are of considerable importance, both for theoretical and therapeutic reasons. If Johnson's concept is correct, the view that degenerative joint disease depends on intrinsic deterioration of cartilage must be re-evaluated. It has already been pointed out that there is considerable difficulty histologically in determining what the precise initial degenerative changes are in the cartilage. It also is true that it is difficult in many instances to ascertain, on histologic grounds, what the initial events in remodeling may be. In many joints, such as the knee, the formation of marginal osteophytes usually develops in proportion to the osteoarthritic changes in the cartilage. Nevertheless, one is frequently impressed with the disparity in the changes in the cartilage and joint. Sometimes, extensive erosion of articular cartilage and eburnation may occur without any marginal osteophyte formation. At other times, one is impressed with a great degree of marginal osteophytosis that may exist in association with little cartilage erosion.

In the lack of more definitive methods for resolving these divergent concepts, it seems useful to attempt to reconcile them: both are likely true and intimately related to each other. This formulation neither denies the possible role of metabolic factors in favoring deterioration of the cartilage, nor the significance of mechanical factors in inducing or treating osteoarthritis. The relative importance of the cartilage degeneration vis-à-vis the bone remodeling may, of course, vary in different joints and in different types of osteoarthritis.

Systemic Contributions to Osteoarthritis

In general, the most outstanding feature about the occurrence of degenerative joint disease is its relationship to age. Senescence, as an etiological factor, can mean two quite different things. It may simply represent the accretion of a series of cumulative insults to the articular tissues, or, more biologically, time-dependent molecular alterations that take place in the cartilage independent of acquired lesions. In the case of the articular cartilage, for example, a long-protracted, low-grade thermal degradation of the collagen or interaction of the collagen with metabolites, *e.g.*, certain aldehydes, might represent such a biologic aging of cartilage.[95] Dehydration of cartilage, as has been proposed in the case of spondylosis deformans, does not occur as a progressive phenomenon of aging in the articular cartilage.[87,97] Chemical alterations presumably would change the material properties of the cartilage upon which its functional integrity depends.

Aside from senescence, there are sufficient differences in the occurrence of osteoarthritis in various individuals to have aroused considerable speculation about other systemic contributory factors. Such factors might be metabolic. Ochronotic arthropathy is a rare but striking prototype of such an etiological type. We may conceive of other metabolic patterns of degenerative joint disease whose nature has not been fathomed because the metabolites involved are colorless. Endocrine factors have been suggested at times. The arthropathy complicating acromegaly has been suggested as an extreme example of somatotropin harming articular cartilage. There is little convincing evidence that thyroidal dysfunction plays a role in the human degenerative joint disease. Aside from favoring neurogenic arthropathy, diabetes mellitus has been suggested as predisposing to the development of degenerative joint disease.[161] Although it seems fairly well established that gonadal hormones contribute to osteoarthritis in mice, there is little evidence that menopausal changes affect the development of osteoarthritic lesions in women.

Genetic factors that contribute greatly to osteoarthritis in other species may operate either through certain systemic, metabolic instrumentalities, or, as in the case of the dysplasias, simply have a local effect on the joint disease. In man, one investigation has yielded evidence for genetic factors being involved in the development of Heberden nodes. The data were interpreted as indicating that a single gene was involved; its behavior in females appeared to be dominant, while in males it was recessive.[149] This type of inheritance is quite different from that described above in mice. In another study in man, degenerative joint disease of other peripheral and spinal joints also gave evidence of being influenced genetically, but the genetic influences were recessive and polygenic.[78] Several remarkable familial occurrences of chondromalacia patellae have also suggested heritable factors.[124,156]

Obesity, as a contributory factor to osteoarthritis, has been generally accepted without question because it would seem self-evident that it poses a mechanical burden on the joints undergoing abrasion. Several recent studies have dealt with this and they suggest that this is a more complicated problem than previously recognized. In mice, it has already been pointed out, obesity *per se* does not appear to have an important harmful effect on osteoarthritis.[145] Obesity was found not to contribute to formation of Heberden's nodes, osteoarthritis of the hip[36,127] or knee[100] in man.[149] Other epidemiologic studies[78] have, however, confirmed the impression that osteoarthritis and spondylosis are more common in obese than in non-obese individuals. Nevertheless, the joints so affected were not necessarily weight-bearing ones, and the role of obesity in harming them was, as a result, obscure.

In addition to congenital dysplasia of the hip, a variety of postural abnormalities of joints that are presumably associated with laxness of the ligamentous structures, also predispose to osteoarthritis. These include recurrent luxations of the patella and shoulder, genu recurvatum and knock-knees. Such laxness has been described as a feature of several systemic disorders, including Ehlers-Danlos and Marfan's syndromes. Howorth has observed that general relaxation of the ligaments occurs commonly in children growing up in New York City, but not in youngsters in many less privileged parts of the world.[67] Whether this reflects different genetic substrates or an untoward acquired consequence of urban life remains to be determined.

The "Unmasking" of Collagen

One feature common to osteoarthritic alteration of joint cartilage, to degeneration of the intervertebral discs and to senescent change in costal cartilage is a diminution of the chondroitin sulfate content relative to the collagen in the matrix. These chemical changes correspond to the histologic depletion of metachromatic ground substance and more conspicuous fibrillar elements as revealed either by silver staining methods[3] or examination under polarized light.[90] The "unmasking" of the collagen fibrils has also been demonstrated at a more minute level in electron micrographs of the degenerating nucleus pulposus.[153] *A priori* one would anticipate that this would greatly alter the material properties of the cartilage with respect to wear and tear: the matrix protein-polysaccharide ordinarily dissipates applied stresses hydrostatically.[107] In the absence of such protection, the unmasked collagen fibrils could be subjected to excessive flexural and torsional forces that might lead them to rupture.

The mechanism of depletion of the chondroitin sulfate in osteoarthritic cartilage has not been established. It has already been pointed out that although loss of chondroitin sulfate is a time-correlated event in costal cartilage, this apparently is not so in joint tissue, or at least is much less so. The proposal that this may reflect a mechanical leaching out of the chondromucoprotein as a result of excessive percolation of interstitial fluid associated with vascularization of the base of the cartilage[49] is not in complete accord with the chemical studies that it is the chondroitin sulfate and not the protein-chondroitin sulfate that is reduced in osteoarthritic cartilage.[17] Parenthetically, the vascularization should be regarded as a component of the basilar remodeling already described (Fig. 55–4*B*).

An interesting alternative hypothesis has been proposed: that there may be a local enzymatic lysis of the chondroitin sulfate by a hyaluronidase normally present in synovial fluid.[16] Hyaluronidase of testicular origin is known to reduce the metachromasia of articular cartilage.[128] Evidence has recently been presented that the affinity of osteoarthritic articular cartilage for immunofluorescent stains for protein-polysaccharides is altered from normal in a manner similar to that induced by hyaluronidase.[6] The findings were interpreted as evidence that the polysaccharides are depolymerized in these areas of orthochromatic, osteoarthritic cartilage matrix degeneration. Another chondrolytic system that may play a role in osteoarthritis has also been described recently:[48] an enzyme that exists within articular cartilage and can split the chondroitin sulfate from the protein-polysaccharide complex. The enzyme might be a cathepsin of the articular chondrocytes.[1] These chondrolytic enzymes of articular origin are to be distinguished from hematogenous ones (plasmin and leukoproteases) that gain access to synovial fluid in inflammatory processes.

Role of Mechanical Factors

Although there are some data to support a popular view that a normal turnover of articular cartilage takes place through abrasion of its surface layers,[43] it has already been noted that electron microscopic studies have not disclosed a progressive death of cells proceeding toward the tangential layer.[39] Firmer evidence for mechanical abrasion of the cartilage in osteoarthritis is provided by the anatomic findings in the joint surface and the demonstration of chards of cartilage in the synovial fluid.[66] Nevertheless, information concerning the mechanics involved is sparse.

In vitro studies of animal joints moved in the absence of synovial fluid demonstrated rapid frictional destruction of the articular cartilage.[74] Experimental instillation of testicular hyaluronidase into rabbit joints also led to *in vitro* scoring of the joint surface.[7] Although the latter experiments suggested that depolymerization of synovial mucin accounted for the friction, the possibility that the hyaluronidase may also have acted on the cartilage could not be excluded. Recently developed concepts of lubrication[104,105] make untenable widely accepted views[8,14,40,163] that the viscosity of synovial fluid is important in maintaining the low friction of joint surfaces.[117]

The state of the synovial fluid in degenerative joint disease has not been universally agreed upon. There has been some difficulty in evaluating the synovia in this condition because control values from truly normal fluid are not readily come by. Furthermore, in cases of osteoarthritis from which synovial fluid can be recovered, secondary inflammatory changes in the synovial tissue may complicate the findings. According to Ropes and Bauer,[122] the volume, hyaluronic acid content and relative viscosity of synovial fluid are not decreased in osteoarthritis, and, indeed, are sometimes increased over normal. Several recent studies have, however, yielded evidence for diminished polymerization of synovial mucin in osteoarthritis, as measured by the intrinsic[15,81,148,151] and dynamic viscosities,[14,72] as well as a reduction of the hyaluronic acid content.[15] In any event, for the reasons indicated in the preceding paragraph, none of these constitutes satisfactory evidence of defective lubrication as a factor in the pathogenesis of degenerative joint disease.

The stresses taking place in diarthrodial joints have never been measured directly, although rough estimates have been made through analyses of the forces between the feet and the ground, and also from the rate and magnitude of the excursion of the center of gravity of the body during walking.[41] Pauwels and his students have applied a computation of moments from roentgenograms to demonstrate the abnormal distribution and excessive forces on the hip in the development of coxarthrosis.[112] Analogous measurements have also been made in osteoarthritis of the knee.[137] Direct studies on the distribution of stress in the intervertebral discs have been made *in vivo* and *in vitro*.[107] The nucleus pulposus served, through its hydrostatic properties, to distribute the loads uniformly on the surrounding tissues. This purpose was effectively served even in the presence of moderate degenerative changes in the disc; only in severe disease was the hydrostatic function of the disc found to be decreased.

The elastic properties and strength of the articular cartilage are important factors governing its resistance to wear.[135] The elasticity is determined largely by the water-binding capacity of the matrix.[45,79,142] Neither the water content[87] nor the elasticity, measured either as stiffness or recovery from a standard deformation,[143] is altered in aging so long as fibrillation is absent.

The stiffness of the underlying bone has also been considered at times in relation to the development of osteoarthritis, and provided the theoretical basis for dietary manipulation of calcium and vitamin D often prescribed in the management of the disease. Although osteoporosis is characteristically present in the age groups in which degenerative joint disease is likely to occur, a direct association between these two common senescent processes in the skeletal apparatus has not been generally recognized. Nevertheless, Trueta regards osteoporosis as a neglected and prime etiologic factor in idiopathic osteoarthritis of the hip.[155] There is considerable veterinary evidence purporting to show that a variety of metabolic states in which mineralized bone is insufficient may adversely affect the articular cartilage.[141] The arthropathy that complicates hyperparathyroid osteitis fibrosa may in part reflect a lack of mechanical support from the subchondral, articular lamella;[23] this interpretation is made difficult by the presence of additional joint lesions: infractions of the surface and metastatic calcification of the cartilage. By contrast, osteopetrosis has also been cited by one observer as favoring premature osteoarthritic degeneration. It was proposed that the excessive stiffness of the bone might interfere with the normal nutritive movement of fluid in the cartilage during joint function.[55] Articular changes have not been present in the experience of other investigators.[63] Although osteoarthritis is seen in some patients with Paget's disease, Snapper is of the opinion that it is related to the age rather than the bone disease of the patient.[140] A more specific association of degeneration of articular cartilage with the osteitis deformans in the underlying bone has been reported as a rare finding in this disorder.[52]

CONCLUDING REMARKS

As in other fields of rheumatic disease, recent years have witnessed progress in our understanding of the pathogenesis of osteoarthritis. This progress has largely taken the form of inquiry in an area of disease formerly regarded as offering neither promise for comprehension by the pathologist nor hope for the patient. Apparently divergent biomechanical and biochemical concepts of the nature of the lesions seem to reaffirm an interdependence between the wear-and-tear process and the metabolic state of the articular tissues. Although it would be premature to emphasize the ultimate significance of these researches, the pathological findings should not be interpreted as proof that degenerative joint disease is an inevitable concomitant of aging, or that there is no biological potential for a degree of reversibility of the lesions.

BIBLIOGRAPHY

1. ALI, S. Y.: Biochem. J., *93*, 611, 1964.
2. ALLISON, A. C. and BLUMBERG, B. S.: J. Bone Joint Surg. (Brit.), *40B*, 538, 1958.
3. AMPRINO, R.: Z. Zellforsch. mikr. Anat., *28*, 734, 1938.
4. AMPRINO, R. and BAIRATI, A.: Z. Zellforsch. mikr. Anat., *20*, 143, 1933.
5. ANDERSON, G. E., LUDEWIEG, J., HARPER, H. A. and ENGLEMAN, E. P.: J. Bone Joint Surg., *46A*, 1176, 1964.
6. BARLAND, P., JANIS, R., and SANDSON, J.: Ann. Rheum. Dis., *25*, 156, 1966.
7. BARNETT, C. H.: J. Bone Joint Surg. (Brit.), *35B*, 567, 1956.
8. BARNETT, C. H. and COBBOLD, A. F.: J. Bone Joint Surg. (Brit.) *44B*, 662, 1962.
9. BARNETT, C. H., COCHRANE, W. and PALFREY, A. J.: Ann. Rheumat. Dis., *22*, 389, 1963.
10. BENNETT, G. A. and BAUER, W.: J. Bone Joint Surg., *19*, 667, 1937.
11. BENNETT, G. A., BAUER, W. and MADDOCK, S. J.: Amer. J. Path., *8*, 499, 1932.
12. BENNETT, G. A., WAINE, H. and BAUER, W.: *Changes in the Knee Joint at Various Ages.* New York, Commonwealth Fund, 1942.
13. BERTOLIN, A.: Rev. Franc. Études Clin. Biol., *6*, 173, 1961.
14. BLOCH, B. and DINTENFASS, L.: Australia New Zealand J. Surg., *33*, 108, 1963.
15. BOLLET, A. J.: J. Lab. Clin. Med., *48*, 721, 1956.
16. BOLLET, A. J., BONNER, W. M. and NANCE, J. L.: J. Biol. Chem., *238*, 3522, 1963.
17. BOLLET, A. J., HANDY, J. R. and STURGILL, B. C.: J. Clin. Invest., *42*, 853, 1963.
18. BONI, M. and MONTELEONE, M.: Ortop. e Traum. (Roma), *25*, 279, 1957.
19. BRAIN, W. R. and WILKINSON, M.: *Cervical Spondylosis and Other Disorders of the Cervical Spine.* Philadelphia, W. B. Saunders, 1967.
20. BUDDECKE, E. and SZIEGOLEIT, M.: Hoppe-Seyler's Z. Physiol. Chem., *337*, 66, 1964.
21. BURCKHARDT, H.: Arch. klin. Chir., *132*, 706, 1924.
22. BUSH, H. D., HORTON, W. G., SMARE, D. L. and NAYLOR, A.: Brit. Med. J., *2*, 81, 1956.
23. BYWATERS, E. G. L., DIXON, A. ST. J. and SCOTT, J. T.: Ann. Rheumat. Dis., *22*, 171, 1963.
24. CALANDRUCCIO, R. A. and GILMER, W. S., JR.: J. Bone Joint Surg., *44A*, 431, 1962.
25. CARLSON, H.: Acta Orthop. Scand. Suppl., *28*, 1957.
26. CARTER, C. O. and WILKINSON, J. A.: Clin. Orthop., *33*, 119, 1964.

27. Cecchi, E. and Bisogno, E. M.: Z. Rheumaforsch., *16*, 12, 1957.
28. Cecchi, E., Bisogno, E. M. and Rocca-Rossetti, S.: Z. Rheumaforsch., *17*, 197, 1958.
29. Charnley, J.: Lancet, *1*, 124, 1952.
30. Chepurov, K. P., Cherkasova, A. V., Makulov, N., Ostrovskii, I. I. and Martuinyuk, D. F.: *Urovskaia Bolezn.* Blagoveschensk: Amur Book Publishing House, 1955.
31. Chrisman, O. D., Bechtol, C. O., Coelho, R. R. and Brennan, R.: J. Bone Joint Surg., *40A*, 457, 1958.
32. Collins, D. H.: *The Pathology of Articular and Spinal Diseases.* London, E. Arnold, 1949.
33. Coventry, M. B., Ghormley, R. K. and Kernohan, J. W.: J. Bone Joint Surg., *27*, 460, 1945.
34. Crelin, E. S. and Southwick, W. O.: Anat. Rec., *149*, 113, 1964.
35. Dahmen, G.: Z. Rheumaforsch., *22*, 192, 1963.
36. Danielsson, L.: Acta Orthop. Scand., Suppl. *66*, 1964.
37. Davidson, E. A. and Small, W.: Biochim. Biophys. Acta, *69*, 445, 1963.
38. Davidson, E. A. and Woodhall, B.: J. Biol. Chem., *234*, 2951, 1959.
39. Davies, D. V., Barnett, C. H., Cochrane, W. and Palfrey, A. J.: Ann. Rheumat. Dis., *21*, 11, 1962.
40. Dintenfass, L.: J. Bone Joint Surg., *45A*, 1241, 1963.
41. Drillis, R.: Ann. N.Y. Acad. Sci., *74*, 86, 1958.
42. Eggers, G. W. N., Evans, E. B., Blumel, J., Nowlin, D. G. and Butler, J. K.: J. Bone Joint Surg., *45A*, 669, 1963.
43. Ekholm, R. and Norbäck, B.: Acta Orthop. Scand., *21*, 81, 1951.
44. Elmore, S. M., Malmgren, R. A. and Sokoloff, L.: J. Bone Joint Surg., *45A*, 318, 1963.
45. Elmore, S. M., Sokoloff, L., Norris, G. and Carmeci, P.: J. Appl. Physiol., *18*, 393, 1963.
46. Eloesser, L.: Ann. Surg., *66*, 201, 1917.
47. Evans, E. B., Eggers, G. W. N., Butler, J. K. and Blumel, J.: J. Bone Joint Surg., *42A*, 737, 1960.
48. Fessel, J. M. and Chrisman, O. D.: Arth. & Rheum., *7*, 398, 1964.
49. Fischer-Wasels, J. and Meyer-Arendt, J.: Frankfurt. Z. Path., *64*, 252, 1953.
50. Fisher, A. G. T.: Brit. J. Surg., *10*, 52, 1922.
51. Fletcher, E., Jacobs, J. H. and Markham, R. L.: Clin. Sci., *14*, 653, 1955.
52. Freund, E.: Virchows Arch., *274*, 1, 1929.
53. ———: Arch. Surg., *39*, 596, 1939.
54. Friedenberg, Z. B., Edeiken, J., Spencer, H. N. and Tolentino, S. C.: J. Bone Joint Surg., *41A*, 61, 1959.
55. Frost, H.: Henry Ford Hosp. Med. Bull., *8*, 415, 1960.
56. Greiling, H., Herbertz, T., and Stuhlsatz, H. W.: Hoppe-Seyler's Z. physiol. Chem., *336*, 149, 1964.
57 Green, W. T., Jr.: Clin. Orthop., *75*, 248, 1971.
58. Green, W. T., Jr., Martin, G. N., Eanes, E. D. and Sokoloff, L.: Arch. Path., *90*, 151, 1970.
59. Hallén, A.: Acta Chem. Scand., *16*, 705, 1962.
60. Hare, T.: Vet. Rec., *7*, 411, 1927.
61. Harrison, M. H. M., Schajowicz, F. and Trueta, J.: J. Bone Joint Surg. (Brit.), *35B*, 598, 1953.
62. Hendry, N. G. C.: J. Bone Joint Surg. (Brit.), *40B*, 132, 1958.
63. Hinkel, C. L. and Beiler, D. D.: Amer. J. Roentgenol., *74*, 46, 1955.
64. Hirsch, C.: Acta Chir. Scand. Suppl., *84*, 1944.
65. Hirsch, C. and Schajowicz, F.: Acta Orthop. Scand., *22*, 184, 1953.
66. Hollander, J. L., Jessar, R. A. and McCarty, D. J.: Bull. Rheum. Dis., *12*, 263, 1961.
67. Howorth, M. B.: Clin. Orthop., *30*, 133, 1963.
68. Hultén, O. and Gellerstedt, N.: Acta Chir. Scand., *84*, 1, 1940.
69. Hutchinson, E. C. and Yates, P. O.: Brain, *79*, 319, 1956.
70. Ingelmark, B. E.: Acta Anat. Suppl., *36*, 12, 1959.
71. Jackson, D. S. and Kellgren, J. H.: Ann. Rheumat. Dis., *16*, 238, 1957.
72. Jebens, E. H. and Monk-Jones, M. E.: J. Bone Joint Surg. (Brit.), *41B*, 388, 1959.
73. Johnson, L. C.: Lab. Invest., *8*, 1223, 1959.
74. Jones, E. S.: Lancet, *1*, 1426, 1934.
75. Kahlstrom, S. C., Curton, C. C. and Phemister, D. B.: Surg. Gyn. Obst., *68*, 129, 1939.
76. Kaplan, D. and Meyer, K.: Nature (London), *183*, 1267, 1957.
77. Kellgren, J. H.: Bull. Rheum. Dis., *4*, 63, 1954.
78. Kellgren, J. H., Lawrence, J. S. and Bier, F.: Ann. Rheumat. Dis., *22*, 237, 1963.

79. KEMPSON, G. E., MUIR, H., SWANSON, S. A. V. and FREEMAN, M. A. P.: Biochim. Biophys. Acta, *215*, 70, 1970.
80. KEY, J. A.: J. Bone Joint Surg., *11*, 705, 1929.
81. KNODT, H.: J. Bone Joint Surg., *46A*, 1326, 1964.
82. KUHN, R. and LEPPELMANN, J.: Liebig's Ann. Chem., *607*, 202, 1957.
83. ———: Liebig's Ann. Chem., *611*, 254, 1958.
84. LANDELLS, J. W.: J. Bone Joint Surg. (Brit.), *40B*, 123, 1958.
85. LEWIN, T.: Acta Orthop. Scand. Suppl., *73*, 1964.
86. LINN, F. C. and RADIN, E. L.: Arth. & Rheum., *11*, 674, 1968.
87. LINN, F. C. and SOKOLOFF, L.: Arth. & Rheum., *8*, 481, 1965.
88. LITTLE, K., PIMM, L. H. and TRUETA, J.: J. Bone Joint Surg. (Brit.), *40B*, 123, 1958.
89. LLOYD-ROBERTS, G. C.: J. Bone Joint Surg. (Brit.), *35B*, 627, 1953.
90. LUGIATO, P.: J. Bone Joint Surg., *30A*, 895, 1948.
91. LYONS, H., JONES, E., QUINN, F. E. and SPRUNT, D. H.: Proc. Soc. Exp. Biol. Med., *115*, 610, 1964.
92. MARTINI, D.: Clin. y Lab., *35*, 241, 1950.
93. MATTHEWS, B. F.: Brit. Med. J., *2*, 660, 1953.
94. MEACHIM, G. and COLLINS, D. H.: Ann. Rheumat. Dis., *21*, 45, 1962.
95. MILCH, R. A.: Gerontologia (Basel), *7*, 129, 1963.
96. MILCH, R. A. and ROBINSON, R. A.: J. Chron. Dis., *12*, 409, 1960.
97. MILES, J. S. and EICHELBERGER, L.: J. Amer. Geriatrics Soc., *12*, 1, 1964.
98. MITCHELL, P. E. G., HENDRY, N. G. C. and BILLEWICS, W. Z.: J. Bone Joint Surg. (Brit.), *43B*, 141, 1961.
99. MOFFETT, B. C., JR., JOHNSON, L. C., MCCABE, J. B. and ASKEW, H. C.: Amer. J. Anat., *115*, 119, 1964.
100. MOHING, M.: *Die Arthrose deformans des Kniegelenkes*. New York, Springer-Verlag, 1966.
101. MOLDAWER, M., HANOLIN, J. and BAUER, W.: In: H. T. Blumenthal (ed.) *Medical and Clinical Aspects of Aging*. New York, Columbia University Press, 1962, p. 226.
102. MUNRO, D.: New Engl. J. Med., *262*, 839 1960.
103. MURRAY, D. G.: Arth. & Rheum., *7*, 211, 1964.
104. MCCUTCHEN, C. W.: Wear, *5*, 1, 1962.
105. MCCUTCHEN, C. W.: Fed. Proc., *25*, 1061, 1966.
106. MCELLIGOTT, T. F. and COLLINS, D. H.: Ann. Rheumat. Dis., *19*, 31, 1960.
107. NACHEMSON, A.: Bull. Hosp. Joint Dis., *23*, 130, 1962.
108. NESTEROV, A. I.: Arth. & Rheum., *7*, 29 1964.
109. NISSIN, K. I.: Proc. Roy. Soc. Med., *56*, 1061, 1963.
110. NOVÁK, V.: Cesk. Morfol., *9*, 227, 1961.
111. ONDROUCH, A. S.: J. Bone Joint Surg. (Brit.), *45B*, 755, 1963.
112. PAUWELS, F.: Verhandl. Deutsch. orthopäd. Ges., 48th Congress, Berlin, 1960, p. 332.
113. PEARSON, J. R. and RIDDELL, D. M.: Ann. Rheumat. Dis., *21*, 31, 1962.
114. POLACCO, E.: Arch. Ital. Chir., *21*, 85, 1928.
115. PÜSCHEL, J.: Beitr. path. Anat. allg. Path. *84*, 123, 1930.
116. PUTSCHAR, W. G. L.: In: F. Buchner, E. Letterer and F. Roulet (eds.) *Handbuch der allgemeinen Pathologie Vol. 7, Part 2*. Berlin, Springer, 1960, p. 444.
117. RADIN, E. L., SWANN, D. A. and WEISSER, P. A.: Nature, *228*, 377, 1970.
118. RAMSEY, R. H. and KEY, J. A.: J. Bone Joint Surg., *37A*, 354, 1955.
119. RHANEY, K. and LAMB, D. W.: J. Bone Joint Surg. (Brit.), *37B*, 663, 1955.
120. RISER, W. H.: J. Sm. Animal Pract., *4*, 421, 1963.
121. ROBINS, R. H. C. and PIGGOT, J.: J. Bone Joint Surg. (Brit.), *42B*, 480, 1960.
122. ROPES, M. W. and BAUER, W.: *Synovial Fluid Changes in Joint Disease*. Cambridge, Massachusetts, Harvard University Press, 1953.
123. ROSENBERG, L., JOHNSON, B. and SCHUBERT, M.: J. Clin. Invest., *44*, 1647, 1965.
124. RUBACKY, G. E.: J. Bone Joint Surg., *45A*, 1685, 1963.
125. RUCKES, J. and SCHUCKMANN, F.: Frankf. Z. Path., *72*, 243, 1962.
126. SALTER, R. B. and FIELD, P.: J. Bone Joint Surg., *42A*, 31, 1960.
127. SAVILLE, P. D.: Arth. & Rheum., *11*, 635, 1968.
128. SCHAJOWICZ, F. and CABRINI, R. L.: J. Histochem., *3*, 122, 1955.
129. SCHILLING, E.: Z. Tierzücht. Züchtungsbiol., *78*, 293, 1963.
130. SCHMORL, G. and JUNGHANNS, H.: *The Human Spine in Health and Disease*. New York, Grune & Stratton, 1950.

131. Sheehan, S., Bauer, R. B. and Meyer, J. S.: Neurology, *10*, 968, 1960.
132. Silberberg, M. and Silberberg, R.: In: G. H. Bourne (ed.) *Structural Aspects of Ageing*. New York, Hafner, 1961, p. 85.
133. Silberberg, R., Silberberg, M., Vogel, A. and Wettstein, W.: Amer. J. Anat., *109*, 251, 1961.
134. Simon, W. H.: Arth. & Rheum., *14*, 493, 1971.
135. ———: J. Biomechanics, *4*, 379, 1971.
136. Simon, W. H. and Green, W. T., Jr.: Amer. J. Path., *64*, 145, 1971.
137. Simonet, J., Maquet, P. and de Marchin, P.: Rev. Rhum., *30*, 777, 1963.
138. Sittman, K. and Kendrick, J. W.: Genetica, *35*, 132, 1964.
139. Smith, C. F., Pugh, D. G. and Polley, H. F.: Amer. J. Roentgenol., *74*, 1049, 1955.
140. Snapper, I.: *Bone Diseases in Medical Practice*. New York, Grune & Stratton, 1957, p. 114.
141. Sokoloff, L.: Adv. Vet. Sci., *6*, 193, 1960.
142. ———: Science, *141*, 1055, 1963.
143.. ———: Fed. Proc., *25*, 1089, 1966.
144. ———: *The Biology of Degenerative Joint Disease*. Chicago, University of Chicago Press, 1969.
145. Sokoloff, L., Crittenden, L. B., Yamamoto, R. S. and Jay, G. E., Jr.: Arth. & Rheum., *5*, 531, 1962.
146. Sokoloff, L., Malemud, C. J. and Green, W. T., Jr.: Arth. & Rheum., *13*, 118, 1970.
147. Sokoloff, L., Snell, K. C. and Stewart, H. L.: Clin. Orthop., *61*, 285, 1968.
148. Stafford, C. T., Niedermeier, W., Holley, H. L. and Pigman, W.: Ann. Rheumat. Dis., *23*, 152, 1964.
149. Stecher, R. M.: Ann. Rheumat. Dis., *14*, 1, 1955.
150. Stockwell, R. A. and Barnett, C. H.: Nature (London), *201*, 835, 1964.
151. Sundblad, L.: Acta Orthop. Scand., *20*, 105, 1950.
152. Sutro, C. J.: J. Hosp. Joint Dis., *23*, 20, 1962.
153. Sylvén, B., Paulson, S., Hirsch, C. and Shellman, O.: J. Bone Joint Surg., *33A*, 333, 1951.
154. Trias, A.: J. Bone Joint Surg. (Brit.), *43B*, 376, 1961.
155. Trueta, J.: Clin. Orthop., *31*, 7, 1964.
156. Twidle, R. S.: Practitioner, *191*, 657, 1963.
157. Urist, M. R.: Clin. Orthop., *12*, 209, 1958.
158. van der Korst, J. K., Sokoloff, L. and Miller, E. J.: Arch. Path., *86*, 40, 1968.
159. von Manteuffel: Deutsch. Z. Chir., *124*, 321, 1913.
160. Wagoner, G., Rosenthal, O. and Bowie, M. A.: Amer. J. Med. Sci., *201*, 489, 1941.
161. Waine, H., Nevinny, D., Rosenthal, J. and Joffe, I. B.: Tufts Folia Med., *7*, 13, 1961.
162. Weiss, K.: Klin. Med. (Wien), *15*, 299, 1960.
163. White, R. K.: J. Bone Joint Surg., *45A*, 1084, 1963.
164. Wiberg, G.: Acta Chir. Scand. Suppl., *58*, 155, 1939.
165. Yamada, K.: Clin. Orthop., *25*, 20, 1962.

Chapter 56

Clinical and Laboratory Findings in Osteoarthritis

By Roland W. Moskowitz, M.D.

Osteoarthritis is a slowly evolving articular disease characterized by the gradual development of joint pain, stiffness and limitation of motion. The terms *degenerative joint disease* and *osteoarthrosis* have been suggested as being more accurately descriptive in nomenclature, since degeneration of cartilage represents the prominent pathologic change. Experimental[9] and clinical[40] studies have demonstrated, however, that mild to moderate synovitis may be an associated finding. Although it is true that osteoarthritis is generally a benign disease, degenerative changes may at times be severe and cause serious disability. Newer concepts of pathogenesis which appear to indicate that it is not an inevitable disease of aging may provide the framework for further studies directed toward the development of specific modes of prevention and treatment.

In the present chapter, osteoarthritis will be discussed according to its classification into two major forms, primary (idiopathic) and secondary osteoarthritis.

PRIMARY OSTEOARTHRITIS

In the primary form of the disease no definitive etiology has been proved, although a number of systemic and local factors has been implicated in pathogenesis (see Chapter 55). Degenerative changes in most patients are usually localized to one or a few joints. In some patients, however, diffuse polyarticular involvement may be seen.

Natural History

The compilation of data regarding the natural history of primary osteoarthritis has been complicated by the use of different case-finding techniques (clinical, radiologic and/or pathologic) in many of the studies reported. In addition, studies based on different joints cannot be readily compared even though similar case-finding methods have been utilized. Variations due to interobserver error may be significant[4] despite use of essentially identical protocols for study. Nevertheless, a number of studies is available which allows a reasonable attempt at delineation of the natural course of the disease.

Incidence

Autopsy studies show that degenerative changes in joints begin to appear around the second decade of life.[31] By 40, 90 per cent of all persons will have such changes in their weight-bearing joints, even though clinical symptoms are not present.[31] Roentgenographically, manifestations of the disease are not uncommon as early as the third decade of life with a progressive increase in involvement with age. In a survey of the prevalence of osteoarthritis in adults in the United States based on x rays of the hands and feet, 40.5 million or 37 of each 100 adult civilians living outside institutions had osteoarthritis in some degree.[41] The rate steadily increased from 4 per 100 among persons 18 to 24 years of age to 85 per 100 at age 75 to 79 years. Twenty-three per cent of those persons having osteoarthritis had moderate or severe disease. Under age 45, nearly all cases were mild. In studies of an adult English population based on a roentgenographic survey of a larger number of joints,[29] osteoarthritis was noted overall in approximately 52 per cent of patients studied. When minimal disease was excluded, prevalence of osteoarthritis was approximately 20 per cent. Osteoarthritis was almost universal in older age groups as evidenced by the finding that in the age range 55 to 64 years, 85 per cent of persons studied had osteoarthritis to some degree in one joint or other.

Sex and Race

In the United States survey reported by Roberts and Burch,[41] men and women were equally affected by osteoarthritis when all ages were considered. The pattern of involvement between sexes differed at various ages, however. Under age 45, prevalence among men was greater; over 55 years of age prevalence was greater in women. Moderate and severe grades of osteoarthritis were seen to a greater extent in women. In studies carried out in Great Britain on population samples from age 15 years,[24] the number of joints involved and severity by x ray were similar in men and women to age 54; thereafter, the disease was more severe and more generalized in women. The pattern of joint involvement was also similar in men and women under 55. After this age, distal interphalangeal, proximal interphalangeal, and first carpometacarpal joints of the hands were more frequently affected in women; hips were more commonly affected in men. The sex difference in patterns of joint involvement suggested that, although the same basic etiologic mechanisms may be involved in osteoarthritis in both sexes, the pattern in men may be markedly affected by trauma, occupational stress and mechanical factors.[22] Clinical symptoms appear to be somewhat more common in women.[7]

Osteoarthritis was noted to occur with approximately equal frequency in both black and white races,[6] although the pattern of joint involvement differed. Osteoarthritis of the knees was more frequent in blacks; osteoarthritis of distal interphalangeal joints of the hands and the first metatarsophalangeal joint was less frequent. Degenerative joint disease was seen in higher prevalence in the American Indian than in the general population.[41]

Climate

On the basis of geographic studies in Northern Europe and America, it has been suggested that changes of osteoarthritis are less frequent farther north.[6] In support of these observations are the findings that the prevalence of osteoarthritis may be lower in Alaskan Eskimos,[5] and less prevalent in Finland than in the Netherlands.[30] Studies comparing populations in Jamaica and Great Britain,[6] however, revealed an equal frequency in the two climates. Factors such as race, culture and environment complicate comparisons of climatic effects on disease prevalence. Clinical symptoms may be less in a warmer climate, related perhaps to higher temperatures, greater amount of sunshine and lighter-weight clothes.

Obesity

Obesity appears to affect the pattern of disease[23] with an increased frequency of involvement of weight-bearing joints. In males, obesity appears to be associated also with increased involvement of distal interphalangeal joints of the hands.[23]

Symptoms and Signs

The symptoms of osteoarthritis are local in character and related to involved joints. Involvement of a number of joints may suggest a systemic form of arthritis, since in these cases symptoms may be widespread. Frequently there may be little or no correlation between joint symptomatology and the extent or degree of pathologic or radiologic change. This disparity in the relationship between symptoms and structural disease changes was noted in the autopsy study alluded to earlier[31] wherein, by age 40, 90 per cent of all persons had degenerative changes in weight-bearing joints, even if clinical symptoms were absent. Cobb, Merchant and Rubin[10] reported that there was no association between morning stiffness and x-ray evidence of osteoarthritis and only about 30 per cent of persons with radiologic evidence of degenerative joint disease complained of pain at the relevant sites. Despite the fact that most patients with osteoarthritis will not have associated pain, studies by Lawrence, Brenner and Bier[29] showed that, except for lumbar apophyseal joints, the presence of osteoarthritis on x ray carried a definite predisposition for related symptoms to develop. This predisposition, seen most strikingly in the first metatarsophalangeal joint, appeared related to the severity of change on x ray. These studies are in concurrence with clinical observations that individuals with marked degenerative changes may have few or no clinical complaints.

The *cardinal symptom of degenerative joint disease is pain*, which at first occurs on use and is relieved by rest. The pain is usually aching in character and poorly localized. As the disease progresses, pain may occur with minimal motion or at rest. In advanced cases pain may awaken the patient during sleep due to loss of normal joint splinting which limits painful motion during the waking hours. The pain is usually of multifactorial origin and may result from elevation of the periosteum following marginal bony proliferation, pressure on exposed subchondral bone, trabecular microfractures, and pinching or abrasion of synovial villi. Additional contributing factors include synovitis, if present, and inflammation of the articular capsule. Spasm of muscles around the joint or pressure on contiguous nerves may be more painful than the primary pain of articular origin. Frequently, as with other types of joint disease, the pain is intensified just before changes in weather. *Stiffness on awakening in the morning* and after inactivity during the day is a common complaint. Such stiffness, however, is *relatively short* in duration and rarely persists for more than fifteen minutes. Studies[50] utilizing a specially designed arthrograph to measure stiffness of the knee joint in osteoarthritis revealed an increase in elastic stiffness. The findings suggested that the stiffness observed was due to a change in periarticular structures rather than to changes in the synovial fluid. Limitation of motion develops as the disease progresses, due to joint surface incongruity, muscle spasm and contracture, capsular contracture, and mechanical block due to osteophytes or loose bodies. In weight-bearing joints, abrupt giving way may occur. Objectively, joints may show localized tenderness, especially if synovitis is present. Pain on passive motion may be a prominent finding even though local tenderness may be absent. Crepitus, a feeling of crackling or grating as the joint is moved, may result from cartilage loss and joint surface irregularity. Enlargement of the joint may occur due to synovial reaction, increase in synovial fluid or proliferative changes in cartilage or bone. In the latter case, the joint will have a hard bony consistency to palpation. Late stages of the disease are associated with gross deformity and subluxation due to cartilage loss, collapse of subchondral bone and cysts, and gross bony overgrowth. Although the symptoms and signs noted are common to osteoarthritis in various locations, the clinical picture and course vary somewhat with the specific joint involved.

One of the most common manifestations of primary degenerative joint disease is the *Heberden's node*[18] (Figs. 56–1 and 56–2). This is a cartilaginous and

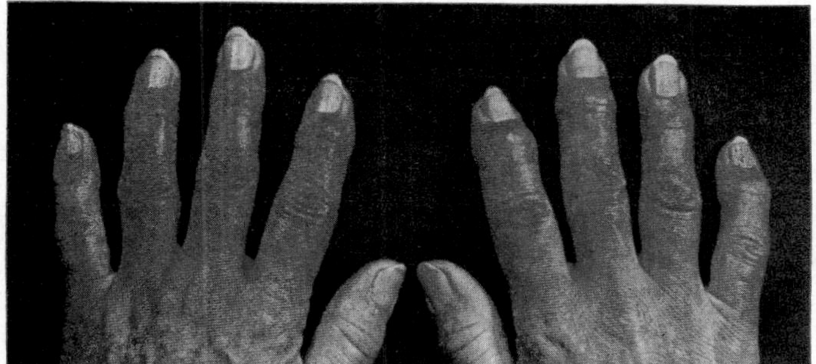

Fig. 56-1.—Typical Heberden's nodes, the signpost of osteoarthritis. Note their characteristic position at the distal interphalangeal joints. Proximal interphalangeal joints may be involved later.

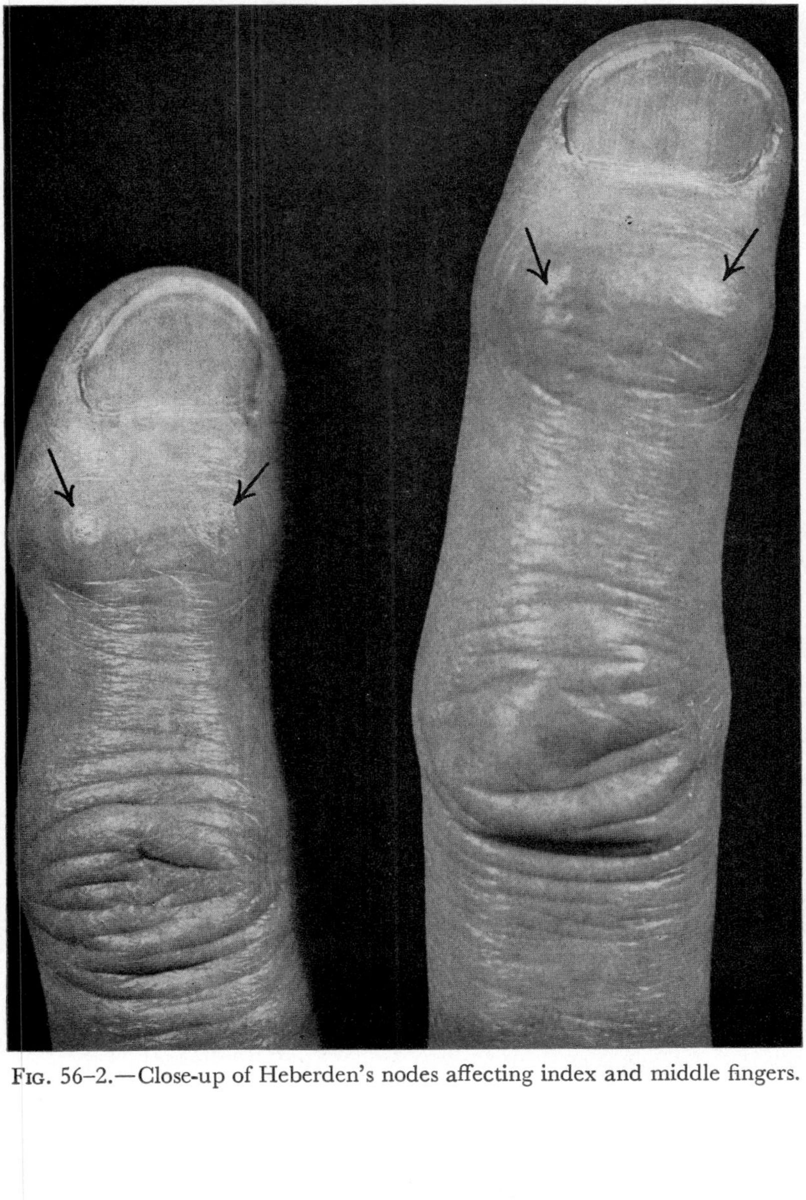

Fig. 56-2.—Close-up of Heberden's nodes affecting index and middle fingers.

bony enlargement of the distal interphalangeal joint of the finger, often associated with flexion and lateral or medial deviation of the distal phalanx. Similar nodes may be seen in the proximal interphalangeal joints and are often called *Bouchard's nodes* (Figs. 56–3*A* and *B*). Heberden's nodes may be single but usually are multiple. Although they begin most often after age 45, they are

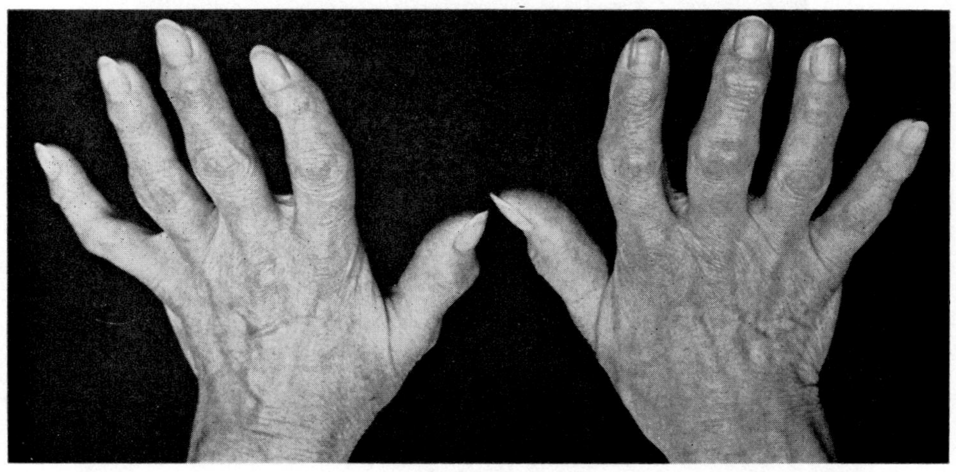

A

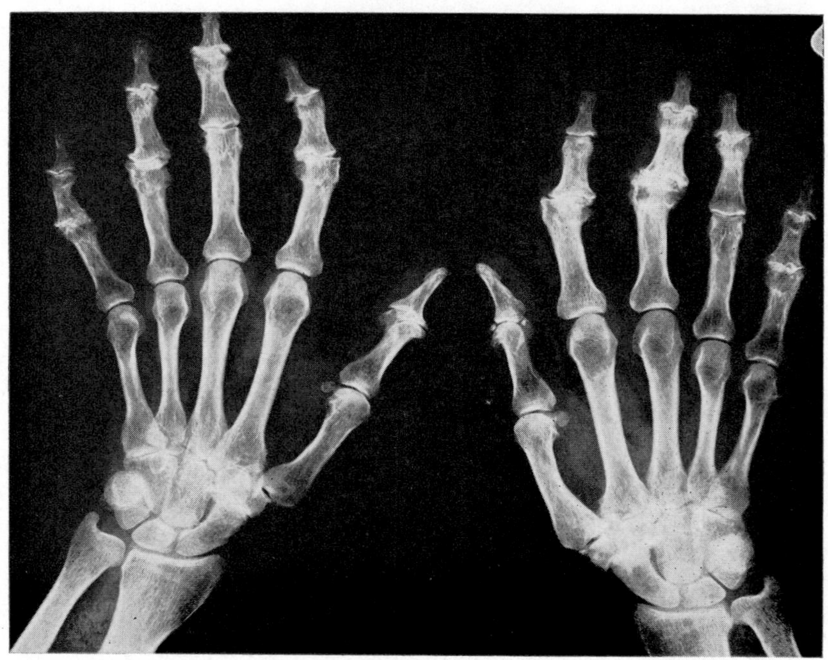

B

FIG. 56–3.—A. Primary osteoarthritis of the hands with marked proximal interphalangeal joint involvement (Bouchard's nodes) as well as distal interphalangeal joint involvement (Heberden's nodes). *B*. X-ray appearance of same hands.

not uncommon earlier. Women are affected much more frequently than men (approximately 10 to 1).[45] Stecher[44] found that heredity plays a large part in their origin, particularly in the female side of the family (mother, daughter, sister). He found that it was twice as common in mothers and three times as common in sisters of affected women as the normal expectance in the general population. It was his impression that the genetic mechanism involves a single autosomal gene, sex-influenced, dominant in females and recessive in males.[46] Penetrance is complete by the age of 70 (all who have this gene have developed disease). Although, as noted, idiopathic Heberden's nodes appear to have a genetic origin, the exact mode of transmission remains open to question since several genetic patterns fit the data presently available.[37]

Clinically, *Heberden's nodes* may develop gradually with little or no pain and progress essentially unnoticed for months or years. In other cases they appear rather rapidly with redness, swelling, tenderness and aching, particularly after use. Individuals afflicted by them may complain of paresthesias and clumsiness on use. A number of distal interphalangeal joints may be involved almost simultaneously in some patients; in others, one or two joints may be involved for a long period of time before other joints develop similar changes. The swelling may be soft and fluctuant or may be quite hard. At times the original swelling is complicated by the appearance of small, *gelatinous cysts*. These appear generally on the dorsal aspects of the distal interphalangeal joint or just proximal to it. They often are attached to tendon sheaths and resemble ganglia; they may recede spontaneously or persist indefinitely. At times they precede the appearance of the Heberden's node itself. As stated above, the proximal interphalangeal joints of the fingers may also be involved, usually after several distal joints are affected. Metacarpophalangeal joint involvement may occur but is rare.

In addition to osteoarthritis involving the interphalangeal joints of the hands, degenerative changes involving the *first carpometacarpal joint* may be symptomatically distressing. Middle-aged women are mainly involved and interference with daily household tasks is common. Pain and tenderness are noted on the dorsum or radial aspect of the hand and symptoms may suggest a stenosing tenosynovitis. There is often a tender prominence at the base of the first metacarpal bone and the joint in this area may have a "squared" appearance. Motion is often limited and painful. Typical changes of osteoarthritis are noted on x ray.

One of the most common sites of primary osteoarthritis, both clinically and radiographically, is the *first metatarsophalangeal joint* of the foot. Onset is usually insidious with gradual progression of swelling and associated pain. Symptoms may be aggravated by the wearing of tight shoes. An acute increase in swelling and pain may result from inflammation of the bursa at the medial aspect of the joint. The involved joint itself is irregular in contour and bony irregularity may be palpable. Foot symptoms may also result from osteoarthritis of the *subtalar* and other *tarsal joints*. Pain of subtalar origin is aggravated by inversion and eversion motions of the foot and symptoms may make walking difficult.

Degenerative arthritis of the *acromioclavicular joint* is frequently overlooked as a cause of shoulder area pain and disability. Symptoms are usually not well localized to the joint and shoulder motion is nearly full, though painful. Crepitus may be prominent. X-ray changes of degeneration are often minimal. Osteoarthritis of the *manubriosternal joint* is rare but may result in chest pain and tenderness. Degenerative joint disease occurs in the *temporomandibular joint* but it tends to be relatively asymptomatic.[32] Symptoms of crepitus, stiffness and pain are more likely to be due to disturbances in joint dynamics rather than to structural degenerative changes.

The *knee joints* are frequently affected by primary degenerative joint disease (Fig. 56–4*A* and *B*). Symptoms consist of pain on motion, relieved considerably by rest; stiffness, particularly after sitting or rising in the morning; and a "crunching" sensation on motion. Objectively, the joint may show very little. At times, there is localized tenderness over various aspects of the joint and pain on passive motion. Irregular hard enlargement due to cartilage and bone proliferation may be observed and felt. Mild synovitis and joint effusion may add to the swelling. A sensation of *crepitus* or crunching can often be palpated when the examiner's hand is held over the patella while the knee is flexed. Joint limitation on active or passive motion may be seen. *Muscle atrophy* about the knee may be seen, especially if disuse has been prominent. Disproportionate degenerative changes localized to the medial or lateral aspects of the knee may lead to secondary genu varus or valgus with joint instability and subluxation. Instability is further aggravated by laxity of collateral ligaments. Closely related to osteoarthritis of the knee is the syndrome of *chondromalacia patellae.*[27] Typically seen in young adults it may be a precursor to the development of patellar osteoarthritis. Articular cartilage of the patella undergoes fibrillation, softening and erosion. Later, erosions and cysts of subchondral bone are seen; eventually, sclerosis of bone and osteophyte formation develop. The syndrome is often associated with repeated trauma as in recurrent lateral subluxation of the patella. X-ray changes may be minimal or absent. Pain is present about the patella and is aggravated by activity. Symptoms may resolve with conservative therapy including heat, exercise and cylinder cast application. In some patients, however, the disease progresses and shaving of patellar hyaline cartilage, patelloplasty or patellectomy may be required.

Osteoarthritis of the hip (malum coxae senilis; morbus coxae senilis) may be extremely disabling (Fig. 56–5). Symptoms due to primary degenerative hip disease usually appear in older individ-

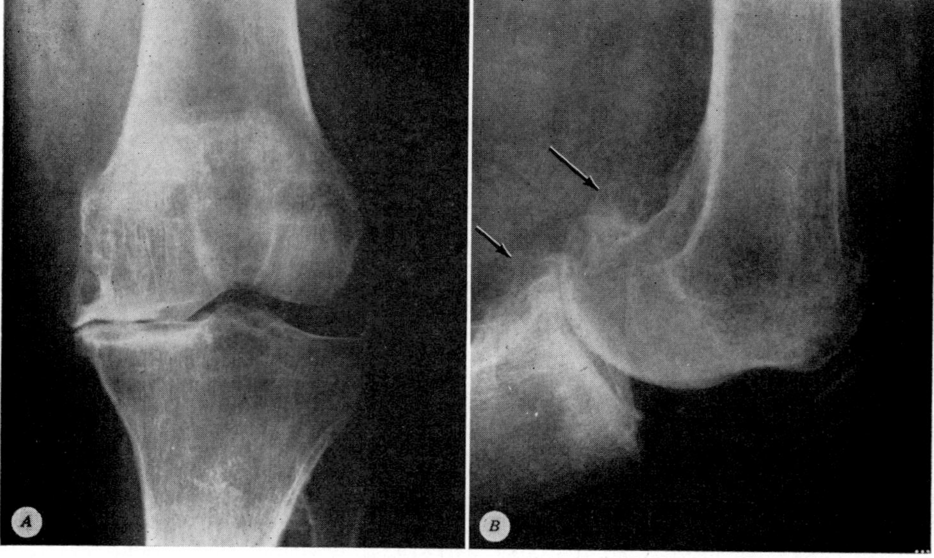

Fig. 56–4.—*A*. Osteoarthritis of the knee. Medial joint space narrowing is prominent and is associated with subchondral bony sclerosis (eburnation) and osteophyte formation. *B*. Lateral view of same knee: Large osteophytes can be seen at the posterior aspects of the femur and tibia (arrows).

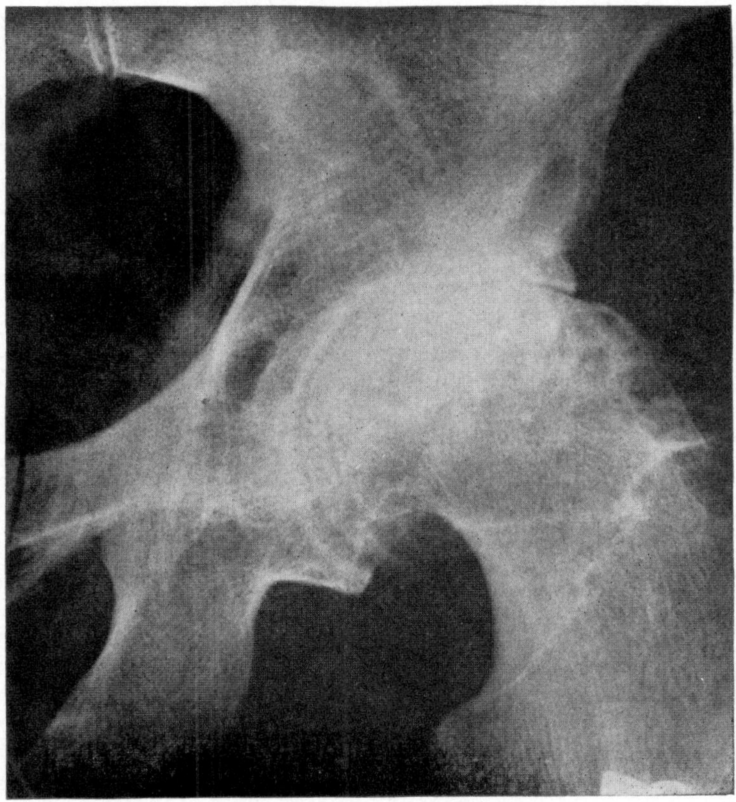

FIG. 56–5.—Osteoarthritis of the hip. Note almost complete loss of articular cartilage, flattening of the femoral head and small cystic areas in the head and neck of the femur. Subchondral bone is sclerotic.

uals; however, it is probable that degenerative changes begin at an earlier age. It occurs more frequently in men than in women and may be unilateral or bilateral. In a study of the natural history of hip osteoarthritis, Evarts[15] noted that over a period of eight years, 20 per cent of patients with unilateral hip degeneration developed bilateral disease. The main symptoms of degenerative joint disease of the hip are an insidious onset of *pain* followed by a *limp*. Pain is aggravated by motion and relieved by rest. It is important to note that pain in the region of the hip may not originate there; conversely, pain arising in the hip may present elsewhere. True hip pain is usually felt on the outer side or front of the joint, in the groin or along the inner aspect of the thigh. It may be referred to the buttocks or sciatic region and is not uncommonly referred along branches of the obturator nerve down the front of the thigh to the knee. Occasionally, most of the pain is in the knee and is so severe that its true origin is overlooked. The degree of pain varies widely and does not always correlate with the amount of cartilage and bone changes. Stiffness is common and more marked following a period of inactivity. Severe backache may result from the compensatory lordosis which follows flexion contracture. Physical examination reveals varying degrees of limitation of motion. The leg is often held in external rotation with the hip flexed and adducted. Functional shortening of the extremity may occur.

The gait is frequently awkward and shuffling. Sitting is difficult, as is rising from this position due to limitation of motion.

Degenerative joint disease of the spine is common (Fig. 56–6) and may result from degenerative changes in the intervertebral fibrocartilaginous disks, vertebral bodies or posterior apophyseal articulations. Disk narrowing may be associated with secondary subluxation of the posterior apophyseal joints. Lipping or spur formation (osteophytosis, exostosis) on the vertebral bodies is a prominent finding (Fig. 56–7). Anterior spurs are the most prevalent but are seldom related to clinical symptoms. Degenerative changes consisting of joint space narrowing, bony sclerosis and spur formation are seen in apophyseal joints. Some authors[20] make a distinction between degenerative changes involving the disks and vertebral bodies, for which they use the term *spondylosis*, and *osteoarthritis* of the *apophyseal joints*. Since these changes frequently occur together, the terms are usually used synonymously.

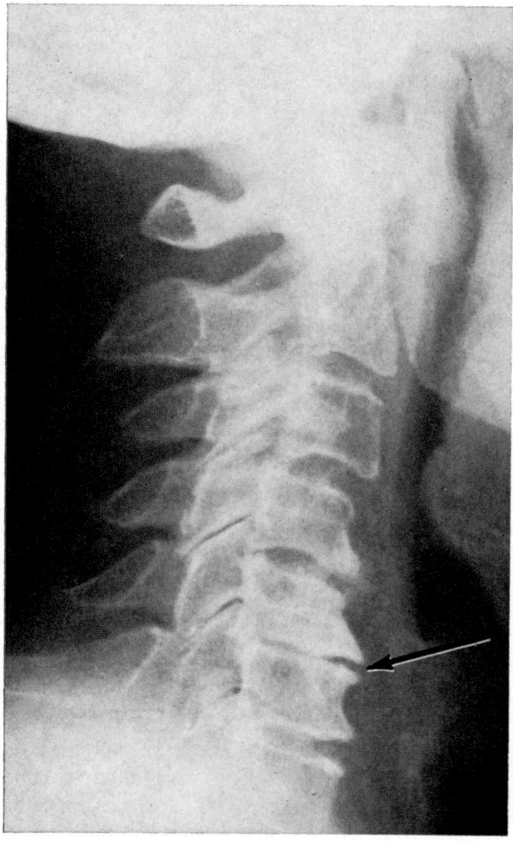

FIG. 56–6.—Osteoarthritic changes in the lower cervical spine. Spur formation is prominent. Note the marked narrowing of the intervertebral disk between C-5 and C-6 vertebrae (arrow).

Degenerative changes of all types are seen most frequently in the areas of the lordotic and kyphotic apices, C-5, T-8 and L 3-4 and correlate in general with the areas of maximal spine motion. In some older individuals, however, osteophytes may extend along the entire length of the spine with prominent involvement of the thoracic region (Fig. 56–8). At times, these exostoses may be striking in degree and coalescence with fusion may occur. Forestier[16] has suggested the name "ankylosing vertebral hyperostosis of the aged" for these severe cases which may be associated with moderate to severe spinal limitations. Pain is not pronounced. The changes may at times simulate those of ankylosing spondylitis but the two can usually be differentiated on the basis of clinical and radiologic features.

Symptoms of spinal osteoarthritis include localized *pain* and *stiffness*, and *radicular pain*. Local pain has been assumed to be due to reactions occurring in certain soft tissues including paraspinal ligaments, joint capsules and periosteum. Such reactions would help to explain spontaneous remissions and exacerbations of symptoms in the presence of persistent or progressive cartilage degeneration and spur formation. Spasm of paraspinal muscles is common and may be a major factor in causing the pain. Radicular pain may be due to compression of nerve roots or may represent pain referred along dermatomes related to the primary localized area of disease.

Neurologic involvement resulting from *nerve root compression* is common. Compression may result from impingement on the root by large spurs which com-

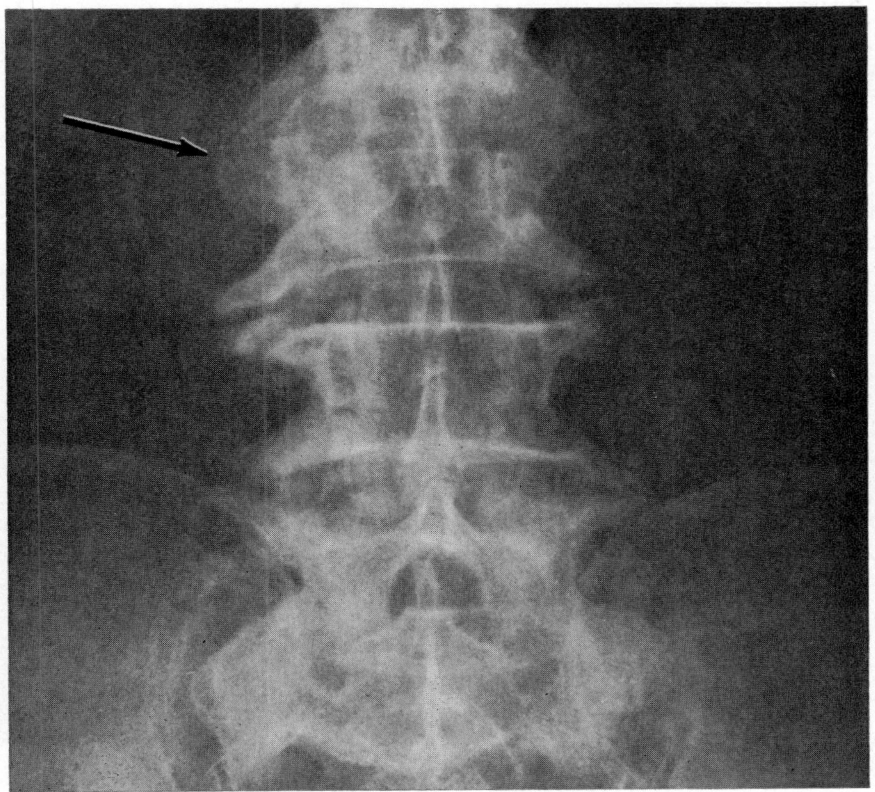

FIG. 56–7.—Osteoarthritis of the lumbar spine. Note the marked osteophyte formation with bridging of spurs between L-2 and L-3 on the right (arrow).

promise the foraminal space (Fig 56–9) or by lateral prolapse of a degenerated disk. In addition, nerve root compression may occur when foraminal narrowing results from apophyseal joint subluxation. Pressure on nerve roots may result in radicular pain, paresthesias, and reflex and motor changes in the distribution of the compressed root. Neurologic complications of this type are seen most frequently in the cervical region because of the relatively small size of the spinal canal and intervertebral foramina in this area. Involvement of similar nature is seen in other areas of the spine, however. Root compression in the dorsal spine may result in radicular pain radiating around the chest wall in a girdle distribution and may simulate symptoms caused by other disorders in this area. Involvement of nerve roots in the lumbosacral area is associated with low back pain and neurologic signs and symptoms in a sciatic distribution.

Further neurologic symptoms may be associated with cervical osteoarthritis if large posterior spurs or protruded disks compress the spinal cord. In these cases upper motor neuron and other long tract signs may be observed. Compression of the anterior spinal artery may produce a *central cord syndrome*. The blood supply to the brain may be compromised if large spurs *compress the vertebral arteries* as these vessels course upward through foramina to the brain. Transient neurologic symptoms such as vertigo and visual disturbances may result. Spinal cord lesions

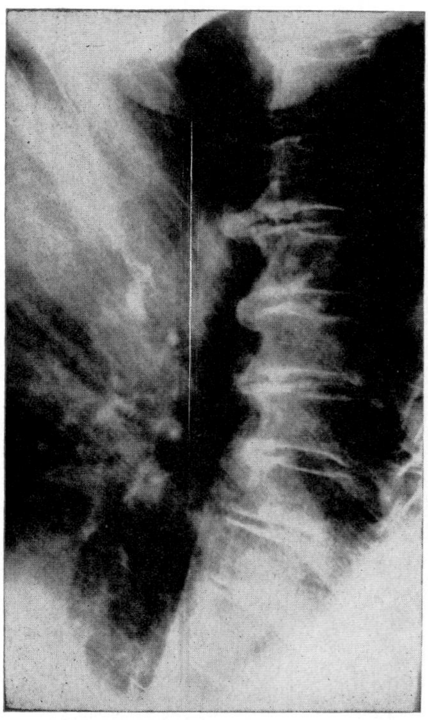

FIG. 56–8.—Osteoarthritis of the thoracic spine. Note the pronounced exostoses at the anterior vertebral margins and the narrowed intervertebral disk spaces.

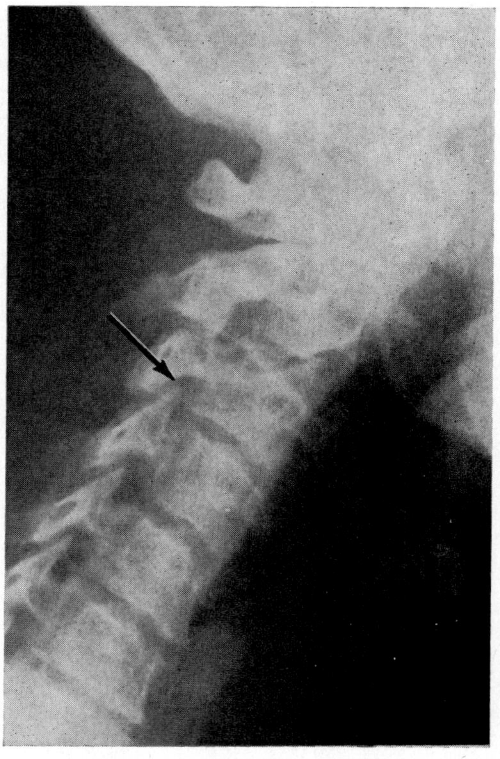

FIG. 56–9.—Osteoarthritis of cervical spine, oblique radiologic view. The foraminal space between cervical vertebrae 3 and 4 (arrow) is severely compromised by marked posterior spur formation.

as a result of osteoarthritis of the dorsal spine may occur but are rare. Cord compression is not seen with lumbosacral lesions since the spinal cord ends in the region of L-1. *Cauda equina syndrome* with sphincter dysfunction may, however, be produced.

It is to be stressed that *x-ray evidence of degenerative disease in the spine may be extensive but yet bear little relationship to the patient's symptoms. On the other hand, severe symptomatology may develop with relatively minor spur formation if the spur is located in a critical area.*

Roentgenographic changes of marginal lipping, sclerosis of articular margins and narrowing have been found in sacroiliac joints with increasing age, but it is unlikely that these changes lead to symptoms.

Laboratory Findings

There are no specific diagnostic laboratory abnormalities. The erythrocyte sedimentation rate is normal in most cases. Results of routine blood counts, urinalyses and blood chemical determinations are normal. When synovial effusions are present, study of *synovial fluid* exhibits minimal abnormalities with slight increase in cells. *Viscosity* is *good* and the *mucin clot* formed after addition of glacial acetic acid is *normal* in appearance. Synovial fluid fibrils which were thought to represent desquamated articular cartilage and to be characteristic of osteoarthritis have been described.[19] Subsequent studies[26] have shown, however, that such fibrils may be found in most synovial fluids

Symptoms and Signs of Osteoarthritis

Usually an elderly patient with few joints involved.

Joints most frequently involved: distal interphalangeal joints of the fingers, first carpometacarpal joint, hips, knees, first metatarsophalangeal joint, lower lumbar and cervical vertebrae.

Almost never involves first metacarpophalangeal joints, wrists, elbows or shoulders, except after trauma.

Usually little or no joint effusion.

Symptoms uncommon before 40 years of age, except when due to secondary causes.

Onset insidious in most cases.

Practically no systemic manifestations.

Main symptoms: Early, pain on motion; later, pain at rest. Pain aggravated by prolonged activity, relieved by rest. Localized stiffness, of short duration, relieved by "limbering-up" exercise. Associated muscle spasm common and may be painful. Limitation of motion as disease progresses.

True bony ankylosis rare.

Main signs: May be localized tenderness. Crepitus and crackling as joint is moved. Joint enlargement usually mild and with a firm consistency due to proliferation of bone and cartilage. Synovitis less common. Gross deformity late.

from patients representing a whole spectrum of rheumatic diseases. Some of these fibrillar structures are collagen fibers, not related to any particular disease entity. Although the specific origin of these collagen fibrils remains unknown, they may result from sloughing of superficial layers of cartilage in osteoarthritis or from articular cartilage erosion in inflammatory arthritis. *Fragments of cartilage,* occasionally even containing typical lacunae with chondrocytes, are frequently found in the synovial fluid.[19] (*See also* Chapter 6.)

Thermography, a method of constructing photographic images of surface temperature, was evaluated as a possible tool for the diagnosis and quantification of rheumatic disease.[17] In rheumatoid arthritis a definite picture of heat emission was noted which correlated with the degree of joint inflammation. The thermographic pattern of degenerative joint disease, on the other hand, nearly resembled that of a normal subject. Heat emission from involved osteoarthritic joints was less than that from rheumatoid arthritis, in keeping with the milder inflammatory character of the former. An exception may be seen in "erosive (inflammatory) osteoarthritis," to be described later. Here the involved joints may be prominently highlighted by this technique. Thermography may have potential in the differential diagnosis of osteoarthritis from other rheumatic disorders. Similarly, radioactive isotope studies may be helpful in differential diagnosis. Scintillation scans of joints in patients with various rheumatic disorders following the intravenous injection of radioiodinated human serum albumin[48] demonstrated distinct radioactivity over the joints in rheumatoid arthritis, systemic lupus erythematosus and gout but not in osteoarthritis. The radioactive uptake correlated with the severity of inflammation. Removal of fluid from the inflamed joint did not significantly alter the amount of radio-

Laboratory Tests and Radiologic Findings in Osteoarthritis

Erythrocyte sedimentation rate and routine blood counts normal.

Tests for rheumatoid factor negative.

Normal serum calcium, phosphorus, alkaline phosphatase and serum protein electrophoresis.

Synovial fluid: Good viscosity with normal mucin clot. May be slight increase in cells. Cartilage debris usually present.

Thermographic pattern of heat emission usually normal.

Main roentgen findings: Narrowing of the joint space (due to destruction and loss of articular cartilage); subchondral bony sclerosis (eburnation) due to new bone formation; marginal osteophyte formation due to proliferation of cartilage and bone; bone cysts; gross deformity with subluxation and loose bodies in advanced cases.

activity present and the main localization of isotope appeared to be in the synovial lining in addition to the peri-articular area and vascular bed. Uptake was insignificant in osteoarthritis. Other workers[3] utilized strontium 85 in studies of osteoarthritis based on previous findings which demonstrated that degenerative joint disease is associated with an increased rate of bone tissue turnover. Results of studies on the knee showed that, in general, ^{85}Sr-uptake was higher than normal in those areas of osteoarthritis where bony sclerosis was a prominent x-ray feature. These findings may indicate increased mineral turnover in these areas or may merely reflect the increased bone density in these regions. Although these techniques represent additional parameters by which arthropathy can be measured, their role in the diagnosis of osteoarthritis remains to be determined.

Roentgenographic Appearance

The roentgenographic appearance of osteoarthritis may be normal if the pathologic changes leading to clinical symptoms are sufficiently mild. Many gradations of abnormality may be noted as the disease progresses. *Joint space narrowing* occurs due to degeneration and disappearance of articular cartilage. *Subchondral bony sclerosis* (*eburnation*) may be noted as new bone is laid down in subarticular areas, causing the bone in this region to become more radiopaque. *Marginal osteophyte formation* takes place as a result of proliferation of cartilage and bone. *Cysts*, varying in size from several millimeters to several centimeters, may be seen as translucent areas in periarticular bone. Gross *deformity* with *subluxation* and the appearance of *loose bodies* may be seen in advanced cases.

Although *osteophytes* are usually regarded as a manifestation of osteoarthritis, the use of this feature alone in diagnosis has been questioned. Findings in long-term studies of the hip and knee[12] suggest that the presence of osteophytes does not imply later development of other radiographically demonstrable structural changes characteristic of osteoarthritis. The authors of these studies suggest that degenerative joint disease of peripheral joints should be based on x-ray findings of structural abnormalities in cartilage (degeneration with decreased joint space) or in subchondral bone (cysts and eburnation) or both. In a study of 19 patients with osteophytes of the patella followed over a seventeen-year period,[13] only one developed other structural changes and decreased range of motion. If osteophytes were present on the femoral condyles or tibial plateaus, however, 34 of 87 patients developed further structural changes. It was concluded that osteophytes in the femorotibial joint were more likely to be associated with other structural changes than were patellar osteophytes; however, even in the former, many patients may go along without development of additional structural abnormalities.

Several explanations have been advanced to explain the origin of the cyst-like cavities noted. It has been suggested that *cysts* arise from a failure in the remodeling process, in which osteoclastic outstrips osteoblastic activity in certain areas. It has also been suggested that cysts are the result of pressure transmitted from the joint surface to subarticular bone through cracks in the subchondral plate (trabecular microfractures). Cyst contents may include fluid, nonspecific detritus or a primitive mesenchymal tissue which undergoes fibrosis.

Ankylosis in osteoarthritis is uncommon. A form of ankylosis may be seen in the spine when marginal osteophyte formation is extensive and leads to coalescence of spurs.

Radiologic examination of the spine in osteoarthritis reveals osteophytic spurs (exostoses) at the margins of the vertebral bodies. Most commonly they are located on the anterior and anterolateral borders of the vertebral bodies and are best visualized on lateral roentgenograms. The amount of bony overgrowth varies considerably. Posterior spurs arising from the posterior margins of the vertebral bodies and/or from the margins of the articular facets are less common but of greater clinical importance due to their proximity to neural structures. Narrowing of intervertebral joint spaces is seen as a result of disk degeneration. As with exostoses, narrowing is most frequent and usually most marked in the lower cervical and lower lumbar regions. Sclerosis of adjacent bone is common, and sometimes there is wedging of the anterior borders of the vertebral bodies. Apophyseal joints may show joint space narrowing, sclerosis and associated spur formation. Osteoporosis is not a component of degenerative change. Many of the radiologic abnormalities noted above may be visualized on routine PA and lateral views. *Oblique views of the cervical and lumbar spine should be routinely performed, if degenerative changes involving intervertebral foramina and apophyseal joints are to be accurately delineated.* Myelography with radiopaque dyes may be of help when symptoms are severe and surgery is contemplated.

Roentgenographic study of *Heberden's nodes* reveals joint space narrowing, bony sclerosis and cyst formation. In addition, spur formation is prominent and appears to develop at the attachments of the flexor and extensor tendons to the distal phalanx. Spur formation is best seen radiologically on routine PA views. In some cases, however, spurs may be directed anteroposteriorly rather than mediolaterally. In these situations lateral views with the fingers in a spread position may be necessary to demonstrate changes present. Although the nodes may feel quite hard, some cases reveal only minimal spur formation on x ray. Most of this enlargement is apparently of soft tissue and cartilage origin. Although, as previously noted, degenerative joint disease of metacarpophalangeal joints is uncommon, hook-like osteophytes were noted on the radial side of the head of the metacarpals in 7 of 100 patients with osteoarthritis of the hands.[49] These changes, seen primarily in patients over 65 years of age, may result from tension on capsular ligaments caused by contraction of interosseous muscles at the radial side of the metacarpal head. These hook-like osteophytes, proliferative in nature, are to be differentiated from osseous hooks which develop as a result of erosion on the radial side of the metacarpal head in chronic post-rheumatic fever arthritis (*Jaccoud's arthritis*).[21] In the latter disease, ulnar deviation and volar subluxation of proximal phalanges may be seen as associated findings.

PA *roentgenographic views of the pelvis* should be obtained routinely when *osteoarthritis of the hip* is suspected. This view is especially informative in that both hips, sacroiliac joints, symphysis pubis and the pelvic bones are visualized. Special views of the hips, including lateral views and laminagrams, may be of value when pathologic changes are suspected but are not seen by routine techniques. Advanced degenerative disease may demonstrate striking abnormalities such as *protrusio acetabuli* (*arthrokatadysis*), a condition in which the floor of the acetabulum is displaced medially by the head of the femur so that it bulges into the pelvis.*

Although *degenerative changes of the knee* are usually readily seen with routine PA and lateral x-ray views, special views are often diagnostically helpful. Tunnel views taken with the knee in flexion serve to expose the intercondylar notch so that loose bodies, intra-articular spurs and changes in the tibial spines may be better identified. Skyline views taken from above allow more detailed study of the patellofemoral articulation. X rays taken in a weight-bearing standing position will allow maximal demonstration of genu varus or valgus which may result secondary to medial or lateral joint space narrowing.

Peripheral joints elsewhere affected by osteoarthritis will show characteristic radiologic changes when appropriate routine techniques are utilized.

One must be extremely careful in relating roentgenographic findings to clinical symptoms. A normal x ray does not exclude very early degenerative change as a cause of symptoms. Conversely, osteoarthritic changes seen on roentgenographic examination, even when severe, may not bear any relationship to the clinical symptoms observed. All too often, radiologic changes are used to explain any and all symptoms occurring in the area studied, when in reality the osteoarthritic changes observed are contributing little or nothing to the complaints given by the patient. X rays of the opposite side may be helpful in evaluating the clinical significance of osteoarthritic changes seen.

* This condition has also been called "Otto's pelvis." (Ed.)

Variant Forms of Primary Osteoarthritis

The clinical, radiologic and/or pathologic findings in certain patients with primary degenerative joint disease have been described as being sufficiently different from those usually seen to warrant consideration of these cases as distinct symptom complexes.[11,14,25,40] One group of cases, characterized by diffuse polyarticular involvement, has been termed "primary generalized osteoarthritis."[25] The other group, characterized by inflammatory synovitis of interphalangeal joints of the hands in association with juxta-articular bone erosions, has been termed "erosive (inflammatory) osteoarthritis."[11,14,40]

Primary Generalized Osteoarthritis

This generalized form of osteoarthritis, as described by Kellgren and Moore,[25] was seen predominantly in middle-aged women. Distal and proximal interphalangeal joints of the hands and first carpometacarpal joints were sites of predilection and often affected in succession. Involvement of distal interphalangeal joints was similar to that seen in the usual Heberden's node. Other peripheral joints including knees, hips and metatarsophalangeal joints were not uncommonly affected, as were joints of the spine. Chronic articular symptoms were frequently preceded by an acute inflammatory phase. The erythrocyte sedimentation rate was normal or slightly elevated; test results for rheumatoid factor were negative. Although the overall pattern of radiologic changes was similar to that usually seen in localized osteoarthritis, certain differences were noted. Articular facets, neural arches, and spinous processes of the vertebral column were often enormously enlarged and led to a radiologic picture characterized as "kissing spines." Examination of knee roentgenograms revealed marked narrowing of joint spaces with rounded "molten wax" osteophytes and the absence of the more usual sharply pointed osteophytes. Radiologic changes overall in advanced cases were striking and greatly in excess of the clinical findings. Joint function was often only mildly affected despite severe anatomic changes. Subsequent studies have suggested that patients with generalized osteoarthritis may be divided into at least two groups on the basis of clinical findings and hereditary patterns.[24] In the first group, in whom clinical findings of generalized osteoarthritis were as described above, symptoms were somewhat more severe and the hereditary trait was associated with Heberden's nodes. The second group, on the other hand, represents an inherited form of multiple osteoarthritis with a pattern of joint involvement which differed somewhat from that occurring in association with Heberden's nodes. This latter form was sometimes associated with an overlapping inflammatory polyarthritis which was predominantly negative for rheumatoid factor.

Erosive (Inflammatory) Osteoarthritis

Crain,[11] in 1961, described 23 patients who had a localized form of osteoarthritis involving the distal and proximal interphalangeal joints of the hands. The arthritis was characterized by degenerative changes with intermittent inflammatory episodes leading eventually to deformities and ankylosis. X-ray changes gradually became marked with narrowing of joint spaces, osteophyte formation, destruction of epiphyseal bone and subluxation of digits. Degenerative changes were also frequently noted in cervical spine apophyseal joints. His patients were predominantly women of middle age. Disease occurrence tended to be hereditary and familial. Erythrocyte sedimentation rate and rheumatoid factor test results were characteristically normal.

Peter, Pearson and Marmor,[40] in a later report, described a series of 6 women with joint findings similar to those described by Crain. Interphalangeal arthritis of the hands was characterized by painful inflammatory episodes which, although similar in many respects to idiopathic Heberden's nodes, differed from them in certain clinical and radiologic aspects. Onset of symptoms was seen in middle-aged or postmenopausal women; no cases were seen, however, in whom early menopause had been artificially induced. Symptoms usually began in the distal interphalangeal joints, followed by proximal interphalangeal joint involvement. Acute flares often recurred for many years, but patients were relatively asymptomatic after 10 years. Mucous cysts over the involved joints were common. The acute inflammation and synovial swelling were often sufficiently severe to suggest the diagnosis of rheumatoid arthritis. Bony ankylosis, rare in classic osteoarthritis, was seen. Radiologic changes included cartilage loss, osteophyte formation and subchondral sclerosis. In addition, juxta-articular bone erosions were prominent. There were no roentgenographic changes of primary generalized osteoarthritis. Study of synovium revealed an intense proliferative synovitis, often indistinguishable from rheumatoid arthritis. The erythrocyte sedimentation rate was usually normal or only slightly elevated and the result of latex-fixation study for rheumatoid factor was characteristically negative. Peter and co-workers[40] suggested that this syndrome represented a unique disease distinct from both rheumatoid arthritis and classic osteoarthritis. They suggested the name "erosive osteoarthritis" because of the prominent cartilage destruction and bony erosions.

Ehrlich[14] recently reported a similar inflammatory osteoarthritis in the interphalangeal joints of the hands in 170 patients. Mean age of onset was 50.5 years.

Earlier onset was seen in patients with exceptionally strong family histories, or after panhysterectomy. Although distal interphalangeal joints were involved more frequently than any other joints of the hands, proximal interphalangeal joints were involved in approximately half the cases. Roentgenographically, some erosive changes were demonstrated in almost all patients. Degenerative changes were noted in metacarpophalangeal joints, knees and cervical spine.

Although the findings described in the above reports on primary generalized osteoarthritis and erosive (inflammatory) osteoarthritis support the existence of variant forms of primary osteoarthritis, the validity of classifying these forms as distinct symptom complexes or entities remains open to question. Osteoarthritis may affect one or a number of joints in any given patient, so that generalized involvement may merely reflect one end of the clinical spectrum of disease severity. Acute inflammation may occur in early osteoarthritis,[40] whether localized or generalized, and its use as a differentiating characteristic is not definitive. In addition, it is difficult to rule out the coexistence of mild seronegative rheumatoid arthritis and diffuse degenerative changes in some of the patients with so-called primary generalized osteoarthritis. This could well account for the inflammatory nature of some of the cases described.

Similarly, classic osteoarthritis of the interphalangeal joints of the hands is frequently inflammatory in nature, particularly when onset is acute. McEwen[33] has suggested that erosive osteoarthritis may be merely a severe form of the same process that underlies Heberden's nodes and the proximal interphalangeal changes which often accompany them. The increased frequency of bony ankylosis seen in comparison to the usual forms of osteoarthritis of the hands may be the result of the prominent inflammatory reaction. He noted that it might be of value, nevertheless, to use the term "erosive osteoarthritis" to stress the severely erosive cases.

Although the question of the existence of variant forms of osteoarthritis is still open for discussion, attempts at classification appear worthwhile. They stimulate further study of the nature of osteoarthritis and direct attention to the necessity for critical analysis of cases for accurate differential diagnosis.

Prognosis

The outlook in patients with primary osteoarthritis is extremely variable. Involvement of distal interphalangeal joints of the hands, for example, may be associated with a moderate amount of pain but usually leads to little limitation of essential function unless fine finger motion is occupationally required. Involvement of weight-bearing joints, on the other hand, may lead to marked disability as the disease progresses. Similarly, osteoarthritis of the cervical spine may not only give rise to distressing symptoms but may lead to severe objective neurologic deficits and disability.

Studies of disease progression in specific joints suggest that not all patients with osteoarthritis inevitably deteriorate. In a review of 125 patients with osteoarthritis of the hip,[43] one-third of those available for followup showed no measurable deterioration. Disease progression was more likely if cysts were present. In a second study of osteoarthritis of the hip,[39] the average time from onset of pain to almost complete loss of motion in 400 patients reviewed was eight years, with a range of 18 months to 23 years. Active treatment may retard disease progression and is of further value in protecting contralateral joints which may be exposed to increased stress. Patients should be reassured that the outlook in general is favorable and disability uncommon, in contrast to the threat of crippling seen with rheumatoid arthritis. When indicated, however, they should be apprised that involvement of certain joints may be associated with moderate to severe pain, stiffness, and limitation of motion localized to that particular area.

In this regard, osteoarthritis is not always a benign disease.

Differential Diagnosis

The accurate differentiation of primary osteoarthritis from other disorders of the musculoskeletal system depends upon a careful correlation of clinical, laboratory and roentgenographic findings. It is apparent that osteoarthritis may be readily confused clinically with other forms of articular disease since pain, stiffness and limitation of motion are common features. Differential diagnosis is further complicated by the fact that x-ray evidence of osteoarthritis is common and frequently bears no relationship to the musculoskeletal symptoms observed.

Rheumatoid arthritis can usually be differentiated on the basis of its more inflammatory nature and the characteristic pattern of joints involved. When rheumatoid arthritis presents as monarticular disease of the knee or hip, however, differentiation from osteoarthritis may be difficult without prolonged followup. An increase in the erythrocyte sedimentation rate and a positive test result for rheumatoid factor are of value when present since they are not characteristic of degenerative joint disease. Synovial fluid analysis is of important differential value (*see* Chapter 6). Rheumatoid arthritis may be particularly difficult to differentiate from the so-called erosive form of osteoarthritis in which the interphalangeal joints of the hands may have an inflammatory component of such degree as to make the findings both clinically and pathologically suggestive of rheumatoid disease. The pattern of joint involvement is of diagnostic value since erosive osteoarthritis is limited mainly to distal and proximal interphalangeal joints of the hands; rheumatoid arthritis usually attacks metacarpophalangeal and proximal interphalangeal joints as well as peripheral joints elsewhere. Some patients with Heberden's nodes or erosive osteoarthritis may later develop rheumatoid arthritis, and a careful clinical history is necessary to identify the presence of a mixed arthritis. Mixed disease may also be present when rheumatoid arthritis leads to secondary degenerative change.

Rheumatic syndromes characterized by involvement of distal interphalangeal joints of the hands, such as psoriatic arthritis, Reiter's syndrome and the arthritis of chronic ulcerative colitis, may be confused with osteoarthritis of the Heberden's type. Associated clinical findings of the underlying disease in these cases usually suffice to clarify the diagnosis. Pseudogout syndrome (chondrocalcinosis articularis) may simulate osteoarthritis when low-grade arthralgias result from deposition of calcium pyrophosphate dihydrate crystals in articular cartilage. Symptoms related to early manifestations of localized joint disorders such as aseptic necrosis, pigmented villonodular synovitis, and chronic infectious arthritis may be mistakenly attributed to degenerative changes seen as coincidental findings on x ray. Neurologic symptoms secondary to spinal osteoarthritis must be differentiated from those seen as a result of other neurologic disorders. This is particularly true of osteoarthritis of the cervical spine where symptoms may simulate those seen in multiple sclerosis, syringomyelia, amyotrophic lateral sclerosis, progressive spinal atrophy and spinal cord tumors.

SECONDARY OSTEOARTHRITIS

The term "secondary osteoarthritis" describes those cases which appear to occur in response to some clearly recognizable underlying local or systemic factor. Some of these factors are noted in Table 56–1. A diagnosis of secondary degenerative arthritis should be particularly considered when osteoarthritis develops at an early age in life.

Secondary to Acute Trauma

Degenerative joint disease may follow acute injury. The usual history is one of trauma followed by redness, soft tissue swelling and pain over the involved joint. After several months, the acute inflammatory changes subside and are replaced by a hard painless enlargement. The deformity is localized to the injured joint. The anatomic changes which develop are similar to those seen in the primary form of the disease. Injury of this nature which involves the distal interphalangeal joints of the hands may lead to development of traumatic Heberden's nodes.[45] Acute trauma to any of the interphalangeal joints of the hands may lead to the commonly seen "baseball finger" (Fig. 56–10).

Secondary to Chronic Trauma

An increased prevalence of osteoarthritis has been noted in association with chronic trauma related to certain occupations. For example, there appears to be an increased frequency of osteoarthritis of the spine and knees in coal miners,[23] the shoulders in bus drivers,[28] and the shoulders, elbows and hands in pneumatic tool workers.[28] Although exposure of a joint to subtle chronic trauma (microtrauma) has been suggested as an etiologic factor in the development of primary osteoarthritis, the relationship between trauma and joint changes in the above cases seems more clear-cut and supports their classification as secondary forms of the disease.

Secondary to Other Joint Disorders

Local: Secondary localized osteoarthritis may follow local joint disorders of other cause, such as old fractures, aseptic necrosis, or acute or chronic infection. Early onset of osteoarthritis in the knee

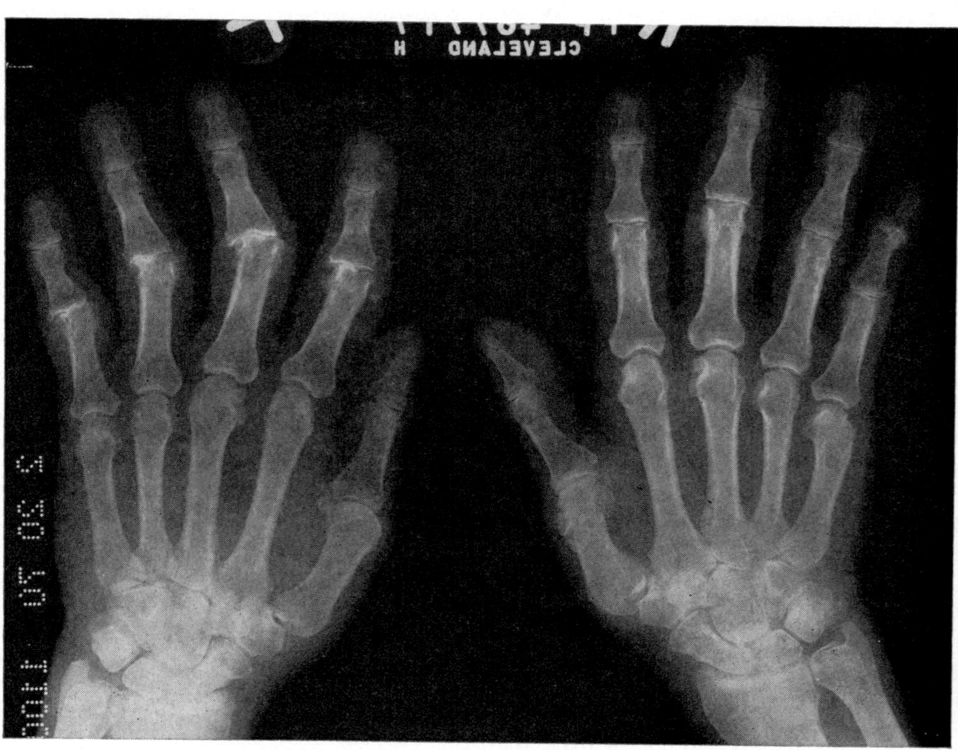

Fig. 56–10.—Secondary osteoarthritis of the 2nd, 3rd, 4th and 5th proximal interphalangeal joints of the left hand ("baseball fingers") in a patient who suffered recurrent episodes of acute trauma during a career as a semi-professional baseball player.

may be the result of torn menisci, patellar dislocation, strain resulting from obesity, or poor mechanics due to inverted feet, genu varus or genu valgus. Localized osteoarthritis of the hip may follow childhood disorders such as congenital dysplasia of the hip, slipped capital epiphysis and Legg-Perthe's disease. Osteoarthritis of the mid or hind foot may result in patients with congenital calcaneonavicular and talocalcaneal coalition.

Diffuse: Diffuse secondary degenerative changes may supervene in patients suffering from rheumatoid arthritis or in patients with bleeding dyscrasias in whom repeated hemarthroses may occur.

Secondary to Neuropathic Disorders

Severe degenerative joint disease occurs in association with neuropathic disorders, as first described by Charcot.[8] Loss of proprioceptive or pain sensation or both results in relaxation of normal joint protective mechanisms and leads to joint instability and an exaggerated response to normal daily stresses. Although first described in patients with tabes dorsalis, similar lesions may be seen in other diseases associated with neuropathy including diabetes mellitus, syringomyelia, meningomyelocele and peripheral nerve section. The distribution of affected joints depends on the area of neurologic abnormality. The degenerative changes which develop are similar qualitatively to those seen in ordinary osteoarthritis but often differ in degree, with exuberant overgrowth of bone and cartilage presenting a characteristic radiologic picture. Frequently clinical symptoms are minimal and disproportionate to the extensive pathologic changes observed.

Secondary to Overuse of Intra-articular Adrenal Corticosteroid Therapy

Development of localized osteoarthritis has been ascribed to the repeated use of intra-articular injections of adrenal corticosteroids.[1,35,47] It has been suggested that in these cases pain relief allows overuse of already damaged joints, thereby promoting degenerative change. Recent studies which have demonstrated a direct deleterious effect of corticosteroids on cartilage[36,42] suggest a second mechanism for development of the degenerative changes described.

Secondary to Metabolic Disorders

Alkaptonuria (*ochronosis*): Generalized osteoarthritis may be associated with metabolic diseases, such as alkaptonuria.[38] The latter, an inherited metabolic disease associated with an absence of homogentisic acid oxidase, is characterized by excretion of homogentisic acid in the urine and a binding of homogentisic acid to connective tissue components. Tissue

Table 56-1.—Local and Systemic Disease States which May Be Associated with Development of Secondary Osteoarthritis.

A. Trauma
   1. Acute
   2. Chronic

B. Other joint disorders
   1. Local
      a. Old fracture
      b. Aseptic necrosis
      c. Acute or chronic infection
   2. Diffuse
      a. Rheumatoid arthritis
      b. Hemarthroses associated with blood dyscrasias

C. Neuropathic disorders
   1. Tabes dorsalis
   2. Neuropathy of diabetes mellitus
   3. Syringomyelia
   4. Meningomyelocele
   5. Peripheral nerve section

D. Overuse of intra-articular adrenal corticosteroid therapy

E. Metabolic disorders
   1. Alkaptonuria (ochronosis)
   2. Gout

F. Chondrocalcinosis

deposition of brown-black pigment (ochronosis) occurs and is seen primarily in cartilage, skin and sclera. Degenerative joint disease of the spine is frequently seen; calcification of numerous intervertebral discs is a characteristic finding. Arthritis of peripheral joints such as hips, knees, and shoulders is seen less frequently and develops later. It has been suggested that the binding of homogentisic acid to collagen structures is related to the later clinical development of ochronotic arthritis.[34] (*See also* Chapter 61.)

Secondary to Chondrocalcinosis

Atkins and his associates[2] recently reported the presence of a characteristic generalized osteoarthritis in patients with idiopathic chondrocalcinosis. Large joints of the lower limbs and intervertebral joints of the lumbar spine were particularly affected. Since both chondrocalcinosis and osteoarthritis increase in incidence with advancing age, their association may be coincidental. On the other hand, the two may be causally related if calcification of cartilage predisposes it to a secondary degenerative change or if primary degenerative change predisposes cartilage to calcification (*see also* Chapter 60).

Symptoms and signs, laboratory findings and roentgenographic abnormalities related to secondary osteoarthritis are generally similar in nature to those seen in the primary form of the disease. Additional findings related to associated underlying disease states will also be present. Management of patients with osteoarthritis is similar to that outlined for patients with the primary form of the disease.

BIBLIOGRAPHY

1. Alarcon-Segovia, D. and Ward, L. E.: Arth. & Rheum., *9*, 443, 1966.
2. Atkins, C. J., McIvor, J., Smith, P. M., Hamilton, E. and Williams, R.: Quart. J. Med., *39*, 71, 1970.
3. Bauer, G. C. and Smith, E. M.: J. Nucl. Med., *10*, 109, 1969.
4. Bland, J. H., Soule, A. B., Van Buskirk, F. W., Brown, E. and Clayton, R. V.: Amer. J. Roentgen., *105*, 853, 1969.
5. Blumberg, B. S., Bloch, K. J., Black, R. L., and Dotter, L.: Arth. & Rheum., *4*, 325, 1961.
6. Bremner, J. M., Lawrence, J. S. and Miall, W. E.: Ann. Rheum. Dis., *27*, 326, 1968.
7. Bunim, J. J.: South, M. J., *52*, 1571, 1959.
8. Charcot, J. M.: Arch. de Physiol. Norm. et Path., *1*, 161 and 379, 1968.
9. Chrisman, O. D., Fessel, J. M., and Southwick, W. O.: Yale J. Biol. and Med., *37*, 409, 1965.
10. Cobb, S., Merchant, W. R., and Rubin, T.: J. Chronic Dis., *5*, 197, 1957.
11. Crain, D. C.: J.A.M.A., *175*, 1049, 1961.
12. Danielsson, L. G. and Hernborg, J.: Clin. Orthop., *69*, 224, 1970.
13. ————: Clin. Orthop., *69*, 302, 1970.
14. Ehrlich, G.: Presented at the Seventh European Rheumatism Congress, Brighton, England, June 1971.
15. Evarts, C. M.: Geriatrics, *24*, 112, 1969.
16. Forestier, J., Jacqueline, F., and Rotes-Querol, J.: *Ankylosing Spondylitis*, Springfield, Charles C Thomas, 1956.
17. Haberman, J. D., Ehrlich, G. E., and Levinson, C.: Arch. Phys. Med., *49*, 187, 1968.
18. Heberden, W.: *Commentaries on the History and Cure of Diseases*, 2nd Edition, London, T. Payne, p. 148, 1803.
19. Hollander, J. L.: Arth. & Rheum., *3*, 564, 1960.
20. Hussar, A. E. and Guller, E. J.: Amer. J. Med. Sci., *232*, 518, 1956.
21. Jaccoud, F. S.: *Lecons de Clinique medical faites a l'Hopital de la Charite*, 2nd Ed., Paris 1869.
22. Kellgren, J. H.: Brit. Med. J., *2*, 1, 1961.
23. Kellgren, J. H. and Lawrence, J. S.: Ann. Rheum. Dis., *17*, 388, 1958.
24. Kellgren, J. H., Lawrence, J. S., and Bier, F.: Ann. Rheum. Dis., *22*, 237, 1963.
25. Kellgren, J. H. and Moore, R.: Brit. Med. J., *1*, 181, 1952.
26. Kitridou, R., McCarty, D. J., Prockop, D. J. and Hummeler, K.: Arth. & Rheum., *12*, 580, 1969.
27. Lam, S. J.: Postgrad. Med., *43*, 173, 1968.
28. Lawrence, J. S.: Amer. J. Epidem., *90*, 381, 1969.
29. Lawrence, J. S., Bremner, J. M. and Bier, F.: Ann. Rheum. Dis., *25*, 1, 1966.

30. Lawrence, J. S., deGraff, R., and Laine, V. A. I.: In, *Epidemiology of Chronic Rheumatism*, J. H. Kellgren, ed., Oxford, Blackwell, 1963, Vol. 1, p. 98.
31. Lowman, E. W.: J.A.M.A., *157*, 487, 1955.
32. Mayne, J. G. and Hatch, G. S.: J. Amer. Dent. Assoc., *79*, 125, 1969.
33. McEwen, C.: Arth. & Rheum., *11*, 734, 1968.
34. Milch, R. A., Arth. & Rheum., *8*, 1002, 1965.
35. Miller, W. J. and Restifo, R. A.: Radiology, *86*, 653, 1966.
36. Moskowitz, R. W., Davis, W., Sammarco, J., Mast, W., and Chase, S. W.: Arth. & Rheum., *13*, 236, 1970.
37. Moskowitz, R. W., Klein, L., and Mast, W. A.: Bull. Rheum. Dis., *17*, 459, 1967.
38. O Brien, W. M., La Du, B. N. and Bunim, J. J.: Amer. J. Med., *34*, 813, 1963.
39. Pearson, J. R. and Reddill, D. M.: Ann. Rheum. Dis., *21*, 31, 1962.
40. Peter, J. B., Pearson, C. M. and Marmor, L.: Arth. & Rheum., *9*, 365, 1966.
41. Roberts, J. and Burch, T. A.: U.S. Public Health Serv. Publ. No. 1,000, Series 11, No. 15.
42. Salter, R. B., Gross, A. and Hall, J. H.: Canad. Med. Assoc. J., *97*, 374, 1967.
43. Seifert, M. H., Whiteside, C. G., and Savage, O.: Ann. Rheum. Dis., *28*, 325, 1969.
44. Stecher, R. M.: Amer. J. Med. Sci., *201*, 801, 1941.
45. Stecher, R. M. and Hauser, H.: Amer. J. Roentgen., *59*, 326, 1948.
46. Stecher, R. M., Hersh, A. H. and Hauser, H.: Amer. J. Human Genetics, *5*, 46, 1953.
47. Steinberg, C. L., Duthie, R. B. and Piva, A. E.: J.A.M.A., *181*, 851, 1962.
48. Strasser, N. F. and Thrift, C. B.: J. Amer. Geriat. Soc., *16*, 539, 1968.
49. Swezey, R. L., Peter, J. B. and Evans, P. L.: Arth. & Rheum., *12*, 405, 1969.
50. Wright, V., Goddard, R., Dawson, D. and Longfield, M. D.: Ann. Rheum. Dis., *29*, 339, 1970.

Chapter 57

Treatment of Osteoarthritis

By Roland W. Moskowitz, M.D.

Treatment of osteoarthritis is at present symptomatic rather than specific. Nevertheless, much can be done in most cases to relieve discomfort and, in some cases, to prevent or retard disease progression. Successful therapy, as in other forms of arthritis, requires that the patient understands the nature of the disease and the goals of management. Reassurance that the disease is generally benign may allow the patient to tolerate mild symptoms more readily so that overtreatment can be avoided. In many cases, such reassurance may be all the therapy the patient requires. On the other hand, as noted in the preceding chapter, involvement of certain joints such as the hip, knee and cervical spine may be associated with severe pain and major disability. Failure to recognize that in these cases the disease is not truly benign may result in a passive response with respect to management on the part of both the physician and patient with subsequent failure to provide measures directed toward symptomatic relief and retardation of disease progression. It is advisable to outline and explain an individual program to each patient, with proper stress that drugs constitute only one part of the program. Intelligent application of modalities of therapy presently available can lead to gratifying results.

GENERAL CONSIDERATIONS

Rest

Adequate rest of involved joints is a significant factor in treatment since excessive joint use may aggravate symptoms and accelerate degenerative changes. A joint with degenerative changes cannot endure the stresses and strains tolerated by healthy joints and normal activity may represent joint overuse in these patients. It is advisable that persons with osteoarthritis "live within their joints" if symptoms are to be diminished and disease acceleration retarded.

The amount and type of rest vary with joints involved and the severity of the disease. Few patients require complete bed rest. When weight-bearing joints are involved (knees, hips, lumbar spine), rest in bed or on a couch for at least forty-five to sixty minutes in the early afternoon or evening may be helpful. In a wage-earner, a period of rest should be arranged at noon if possible. As a rule, patients can do more, with less damage to their joints, by dividing rest periods during the day, than by trying to work throughout the day. Weight-bearing joints can be further protected during daily activity by the appropriate use of appliances such as canes, crutches or a walker since forces applied to each lower extremity when walking are increased several-fold over those at rest. When one knee or hip is involved and a single cane or crutch used, the appliance should be used in the hand opposite the involved joint when feasible. Advanced disease or bilateral joint involvement may require bilateral canes or crutches or a walker with adequate instruction in the type of gait best suited to protect affected joints. When non-weight-bearing joints are involved, resting the parts by prohibiting excess motion is sufficient.

Many individuals suffering from degenerative joint disease are obsessed with the idea that their joints will become stiff unless they exercise them continuously. It is important to stress that while a balanced therapeutic program of joint or muscle exercise is important, excessive activity may result in additional trauma or damage.

Correction of Factors Causing Excessive Strain

All factors which tend to cause excessive stress and strain on a joint should be corrected if possible. Optimally, correction of these factors should be carried out prior to the onset of degenerative changes in the hope that degeneration may be prevented. Once disease is present, correction of them assumes even greater importance.

Some experimental[44] and clinical[38] studies have suggested that obesity per se is not a factor in the induction or aggravation of degenerative joint disease; other studies[25,26] have demonstrated an increased frequency of degenerative joint disease in obese persons, particularly in weight-bearing joints. Despite these conflicting reports, weight reduction would appear prudent since present concepts of pathogenesis suggest that degenerative joint disease is initiated by increased or abnormally directed pressures on joint cartilage. Weight reduction would appear to be especially appropriate in patients with malalignment of weight-bearing joints since increased forces may be particularly deleterious when abnormally directed. Weight loss in patients with degenerative joint disease may be especially difficult since physical activity is limited. Nevertheless, strong persistent efforts toward this result should be made when indicated.

Poor body mechanics may induce or aggravate degenerative changes. Inverted feet, for example, may place extra strain upon the medial aspect of the knee. Proper foot support in the form of a lateral shoe lift shifts forces to the lateral aspect of the knee and allows a more normal force distribution. Genu varus and valgus may place severe stress on the medial and lateral knee compartments respectively. Surgical realignment can be beneficial. Faulty posture may result in extra strain on the low back and should be corrected. Chronic strain related to certain occupations may be minimized by use of proper work habits. Continuous standing, as before a machine at work or behind a store counter, is conducive to increased pain, and frequent use of a stool or chair can bring relief. When degenerative changes are severe and disabling, routine therapeutic measures may not be effective and a change in occupation may have to be considered.

Diet

Experimental studies[39] have demonstrated an increased frequency of osteoarthritis in male mice ingesting a diet enriched with lard, a saturated fat. Substitution of part of the lard by linoleic acid, an unsaturated fatty acid, resulted in a statistically significant lowering of the incidence of osteoarthritis. To my knowledge, no clinical investigations have yet been carried out in man to test the significance of these observations. There is no clinical evidence at this time that diet may play a specific role in this disease except in relation to obesity per se. Many patients exhibit concern that arthritis is due to either "too much calcium in the joints" or "too little calcium in the bones" and will undertake dietary measures incorporating decreased or increased calcium respectively. Correction of these misconceptions is usually readily accepted by the patient.

PHYSICAL THERAPY

Physical therapy measures are of value in symptomatic relief of pain and stiffness, in maintenance of joint range of motion, in recovery of range of motion already lost and in strengthening muscles to preserve joint function. Although not a cure for the disease, a properly instituted daily program of physical therapy represents an important component of the treatment program and can be instrumental in limiting disability which might otherwise occur.

Heat is effective in relieving pain and muscle spasm and allows a more effective follow-up exercise program. Heat may be applied in many forms such as baking, infrared, hot packs, electric pads, diathermy and ultrasound (*see* Chapter 34). Moist heat appears at times to be more beneficial than dry but the latter is also efficacious and may be preferred if more convenient. Although diathermy and ultrasound at times may be recommended, especially in deep-seated areas, these measures in general do not seem to offer much more than do simple and less expensive forms of heat. Painful Heberden's nodes usually are aided by hot plain water soaks, paraffin wax applications or contrast baths. In patients with a more generalized osteoarthritis, warm tub baths may be beneficial. It should be noted that in an occasional patient heat may aggravate rather than help pain. In all patients in whom the use of heat is indicated, the simplest measures are more likely to be utilized on a regular home basis.

Massage following the use of heat can be helpful for its sedative effect and for relief of muscle spasm. This therapeutic modality is of significantly less importance, however, than heat and exercise. Programmed exercises should be directed toward joint range of motion and strengthening of involved muscles. Isometric rather than isotonic exercises are generally preferred for building muscle power since joint stress is minimized. Generally exercises should be performed in two or three sessions daily, beginning with a small number of repetitions at each session and progressing to ten to fifteen repetitions at a time. Excessive exercise may aggravate pain. Discomfort persisting for more than one or two hours following exercise indicates that it has been too great and therefore should be reduced in amount. Active exercises are preferable to passive ones.

As with other chronic diseases, the patient himself, and not just articular symptoms, should be treated. Psychotherapeutic support is of great importance since emotional upset may aggravate symptoms by increasing muscle tension. A stoic person may abuse damaged joints by ignoring pain, whereas the oversensitive patient may be afraid to take enough exercise.

DRUG THERAPY

Many patients with osteoarthritis can be effectively managed for long periods of time without the help of drugs. In other patients the judicious use of analgesic and anti-inflammatory drugs can be of considerable symptomatic benefit. It is important to stress that drug therapy, when utilized, constitutes only one part of disease management and should be combined with a good general program. The basic program encompassing the general measures outlined earlier may decrease or obviate the need for drug therapy; on the other hand, the addition of drugs for relief of pain and stiffness may allow a more effective physical therapy program to be carried out.

At the present time there is no drug which has been proven consistently successful in preventing or reversing the pathologic changes of osteoarthritis. For this reason, therapeutic measures involve primarily the use of analgesic and anti-inflammatory drugs for symptomatic relief. Findings obtained in newer investigative studies of disease pathogenesis raise the hope that specific measures designed to affect the basic pathologic process will be forthcoming.

Analgesic Drugs

Acetylsalicylic acid (*aspirin*) is both analgesic and anti-inflammatory. It represents the cornerstone of drug therapy in osteoarthritis in the same fashion as does its use in rheumatoid arthritis. When used properly it is an effective agent and is associated with fewer and less severe toxic reactions than other more potent agents whose side effects limit their safe long-term use. It is essential that the patient understands that sufficient aspirin must be taken to obtain adequate therapeutic levels. Doses of 640 mg. four times a day are given initially and therapeutic effects observed. The dose is then gradually increased if adequate relief has not been obtained. Older persons may be more likely to develop aspirin toxicity and increases from the initial dosage schedule should be made with caution. If tinnitus or hearing impairment occur, aspirin should be withheld until toxic symptoms clear, at which time it can be resumed at lower dose levels. Administration of aspirin with meals and with food at bedtime will diminish gastrointestinal side reactions. Patients with gastric intolerance to plain aspirin may find it well tolerated when taken with oral antacids such as magnesium-aluminum hydroxide. Salicylate preparations designed to produce less gastrointestinal distress may be tried if such symptoms persist. Preparations of value include enteric-coated aspirin, aspirin-antacid mixtures, salicyl-salicylic acid, magnesium salicylate and choline salicylate (*see also* Chapter 28).

Other analgesic medications can be added to the baseline aspirin program if increased pain relief is required, or may be substituted if aspirin allergy or intolerance makes continued aspirin administration impractical. *Acetophenetidin* (phenacetin) has been utilized for these purposes and may be given in doses of 300 mg. four times daily. Long-term administration is not advised, however, since interstitial nephritis may develop as a complication of its use. *Acetaminophen* has analgesic value and may be similarly administered. Renal complications of significance have not been described. *Propoxyphene hydrochloride* (Darvon), 65 mg., and *ethoheptazine citrate* (Zactane), 75 mg., are comparable in analgesic effectiveness and may be given 3 or 4 times daily on a regular or demand basis. Combination preparations of these latter two drugs with aspirin may be utilized but have the disadvantage of requiring a simultaneous increase or decrease in both the basic drug and aspirin when the dosage is varied. Propoxyphene side reactions include sedation, light-headedness and gastrointestinal upset. Drug dependency may develop. Nausea, dizziness and drowsiness may be seen with ethoheptazine citrate. *Pentazocine* (Talwin) is available in oral form. In my experience it has been of benefit only in selected cases. Doses of 50 mg. three to four times daily are utilized. Side reactions which include nausea, flushing of the skin and light-headedness are frequent and often preclude its continued use. Narcotic preparations such as codeine and its derivatives are practically never required; if used, they should be administered only on a short-term basis. Local application of liniments such as methyl salicylate or chloroform as counter-irritants may provide hyperemia and temporary relief of pain.

The analgesic agents mentioned above may be helpful in controlling pain but must be used cautiously since abuse of diseased joints with subsequent deterioration may result when pain is masked.

Anti-inflammatory Agents

Anti-inflammatory agents appear to be of help in many patients with osteoarthritis. Their effectiveness may be related to synovial inflammation seen at times as a component of the basic pathologic reaction. In addition, several of the anti-inflammatory agents used have analgesic properties as well. *Indomethacin* (Indocin), an indole-3-acetic acid derivative, has been extensively tried in osteoarthritis[17,18,43,46] as well as in other rheumatic diseases (*see also* Chapter 30). Although it has been described as being especially helpful in osteoarthritis of the hip,[49] relief of pain, stiffness and limitation in other joints has similarly been noted. Beneficial effects equal to those seen with phenylbutazone have been described.[17,51] In a recent controlled study in patients with osteoarthritis of the hip and knee, Harth and Bondy[18] demonstrated that indomethacin, 50 mg., and acetylsalicylic acid, 1.3 gm., had a similar effect when administered three times daily. All patients were hospitalized, making it difficult to ascertain the true role of drugs in the improvement observed. Smyth,[43] in a recent review, concluded that the relative value of this drug in comparison to older and better known treatments of osteoarthritis is not well established at present. Nevertheless, this agent appears worthy of trial if other measures fail. It should be used with caution, if at all, in patients allergic to aspirin, particularly in those with asthma, as cross-sensitivity between these 2 drugs has been demonstrated.[35] A total daily dose of 75 to 150 mg. may be administered in divided amounts and must be given with food to minimize gastrointestinal side reactions. It is my experience that, in general, doses over 100 mg. daily are associated with a high frequency of side reactions with minimal therapeutic gain. Prominent side reactions include, in addition to gastrointestinal upset, gastrointestinal bleeding, severe postoccipital headache, light-headedness and psychic phenomena such as vague feelings of separation. It has been suggested that side effects are diminished if low doses are initially used and gradual increases made as needed.

Phenylbutazone (Butazolidin) and its derivative, *oxyphenbutazone* (Tandearil), have been recommended by various investigators[10,28,29] for treatment of osteoarthritis. Although oxyphenbutazone has been reported to be less toxic than the parent drug, the two drugs may be considered essentially similar with respect to therapeutic effects, dosage schedules and side reactions. While symptomatic improvement may be achieved in a significant number of patients, most authors feel that the clinical benefit to be expected in this generally benign disease is not commensurate with the dangers of drug toxicity. They do not influence the course of the disease. Dosage varies but in general should be kept minimal in amount and duration in order to avoid serious side reactions. When either drug is administered for acute exacerbations, 300 to 400 mg. a day for several days followed by a gradually decreasing daily dose over a period of 7 to 10 days may be efficacious. If administered over a prolonged period, doses of 100 to 200 mg. daily are associated with least side reactions. Regardless of dosage schedule, however, side reactions may be serious and include bone marrow depression, upper gastrointestinal bleeding, fluid retention and skin rash. If given on a regular basis, the total blood leukocyte count, differential white blood cell count and platelet count should be performed every other week for approximately 6 weeks and then monthly as long as the drugs are given. A history of peptic ulcer disease should generally contraindicate their use and they should be used with caution in patients with congestive heart failure. Depression of prothrombin activity by coumarin-type anticoagulants may be accentuated. Some are of the opinion that the pendulum of skepticism regarding the toxic effect of these drugs has swung too far toward ultraconservatism in their use and has deprived many patients of a useful and important antirheumatic drug.[42] Others do not use them unless debilitation is great and salicylates or indomethacin has not helped (*see also* Chapter 30).

Systemic *adrenocortical* or *adrenocorticotropic hormone therapy* has been tried in patients with osteoarthritis with somewhat equivocal results.[8,13] It was anticipated that the anti-inflammatory properties of these drugs might result in temporary alleviation of pain. The equivocal results of such therapy, however, the possible side effects associated with their long-term administration and the relatively benign nature of most forms of osteoarthritis contraindicate their general use in this disease (*see also* Chapter 31).

In contradistinction to the recommendation that oral or parenteral *adrenocorticoids* be avoided in treatment of osteoarthritis, it has been suggested that *intra-articular administration* of these medications can be of benefit and without serious hazard when used appropriately.[21,22,23,24] Hollander, Brown and Jessar[24] reported successful relief of symptoms in peripheral joints when a suspension of hydrocortisone acetate was injected directly into the joint space. Repeated injections were carried out on 231 cases for two years with complete or nearly complete relief of symptoms in 87 per cent of cases.[21] Periods of symptomatic relief after each injection varied from 3 days to several months. Therapy was least efficacious in patients with disease of the hip. In a later review of his experience, Hollander[22] stated that his group had followed nearly 1,000 patients with osteoarthritic knees who had received such injections on an "as needed" basis over a period of nine years. Nearly 60 per cent no longer required injection, not having enough pain to require additional injections. About 20 per cent were either not benefited sufficiently or were lost in follow-up studies. Although similar findings have been reported by other investigators,[50,52] many of the studies have been uncontrolled. It is important to note in this regard that intra-articular injections of suspending vehicle,[50] isotonic sodium chloride[47] or 1 per cent procaine,[47] have been shown to provide similar relief for variable periods of time in a number of patients (*see also* Chapter 32).

Various preparations of steroids, such as hydrocortisone, hydrocortisone tertiary butylacetate, triamcinolone, 6-methyl prednisolone and dexamethasone, have been used. In all cases, however, improvement has been only temporary, varying from a few days to a few months. The mechanism of pain relief with intra-articular steroids is not certain but may be related to their anti-inflammatory role since, as noted previously, synovitis may be a concomitant of the pathologic picture in osteoarthritis. While such treatment may be effective in relieving pain, one must bear in mind that the masking of such pain may result in serious overuse of affected joints with subsequent disease acceleration and joint instability.[2,32,45] Direct *deleterious effects of these drugs on cartilage*, as demonstrated in recent experimental studies,[33,36] *may add further to joint deterioration.* Other adverse effects include post-injection inflammatory flares induced in response to the injected steroid crystals[31] and joint infection. For the above reasons, intra-articular steroid therapy is not without hazard and some writers require strong justification for its use. It must be concluded that, while intra-articular steroid injection may be beneficial, this form of temporary relief must be used only as an adjunct to the previously mentioned time-honored measures. Injections should be relatively infrequent and patients must be cautioned against excessive use of injected joints. Steroid injection into pericapsular tissues alone may provide significant symptomatic relief while avoiding the hazards associated with direct intra-articular administration. A full discussion of specific techniques for intra-articular injection is given in Chapter 32.

The following anti-inflammatory agents have been studied elsewhere in treatment of osteoarthritis but their use remains *investigative* in the United States. *Ibuprofen* (2,4′-isobutylphenylproprionic acid), 0.6 gm. daily, was compared to placebo in a double-blind crossover study.[4] In the nineteen patients treated there was a slight but not significant preference by patients for the drug. No significant objective improvement was noted. Side effects, which included gastrointestinal reactions, rash, headache, and nocturia, were similar with drug and placebo. The drug was given for only a short period of time and longer term trials were suggested. *Flufenamic acid*, an anthranilic acid derivative, was similar in efficacy to phenylbutazone.[7,14] Side reactions included gastrointestinal upset, headaches, dizziness and ankle swelling.

Other Drugs and Measures

Roentgen therapy has been recommended by some workers[27] but is not utilized any longer by most experienced rheumatologists. Relief of symptoms is inconstant and the basic disease is unaltered. It appears to be of little proven value in the management of osteoarthritis. Recent reports suggesting that leukemia occurs more frequently in individuals who have received roentgen therapy should make one further hesitant to use this treatment for a generally benign condition.

The use of *estrogenic substances*, particularly in the treatment of Heberden's nodes, has been advocated by some, deplored by others. Their use was suggested by the observation that some forms of osteoarthritis appear to begin most commonly at the time of or slightly after the onset of menopause. No definitive clinical evidence in support of its value is presently available and their role remains speculative.

Mefenamic acid, another anthranilic acid derivative, was shown to be of symptomatic benefit in the treatment of osteoarthritis when a dose of 1500 mg. per day was compared to indomethacin, 75 mg. per day. Toxic reactions associated with prolonged administration may be severe, however, and it would appear to have little, if any role, in the treatment of osteoarthritis.

Muscle relaxants may be of value in decreasing pain and limitation of motion related to muscle spasm. *Chlorphenesin carbamate* (Maolate) has both muscle-relaxing and analgesic properties. Clinical response to this agent in a dose of 400 mg. four times daily was similar to that of placebo in a double-blind crossover study,[48] however, and it does not appear to be of specific value in osteoarthritis. Its effectiveness, if any, is further limited by side reactions such as upper gastrointestinal symptoms, diarrhea, and vague feelings of confusion which limit it to short-term administration.

Helal and Karadi[19] injected *silicone oil* intra-articularly in an effort to improve function of "dry joints." Functional and symptomatic improvement including pain relief, loss of crepitus and increased range of motion was noted following its use. Control studies were not performed. Protection of cartilage by this agent was postulated. Although encapsulated tumors (siliconomas) were seen in animals receiving subcutaneous injections of this material and embolism was associated with its experimental injection into blood vessels, no clinical complications were noted with use in humans. Corbett and co-workers[11] compared the intra-articular effects of silicone oil and hydrocortisone acetate. Improved range of motion was noted to an equal degree with both agents. Once again, placebo studies were not carried out. Although interesting in concept, the use of silicone oil is strictly investigative at this time.

Certain therapeutic agents, such as desiccated thyroid and vitamins of all types, are of no proven benefit in the treatment of osteoarthritis and their use, not always innocuous, should be discouraged.

Investigative Agents Directed Toward Disease Prevention, Retardation or Reversal

As described above, the present-day therapy of osteoarthritis centers about agents and measures directed toward symptomatic relief. The development of therapeutic agents capable of affecting the basic disease process would be aided by a more accurate delineation of pathogenic mechanisms. Newer studies support the view that osteoarthritis is not an inevitable concomitant of aging, but, rather, develops by way of definable biomechanical and biochemical mechanisms.[6,34] Injury to cartilage and alteration in joint surfaces by abnormal stresses appear to be key factors in disease initiation. Damage to chondrocytes as a result of these stresses may result in release of proteolytic lysosomal enzymes (cathepsins) of chondrocyte origin, which further alter cartilage matrix near the surface. Increased degradation of matrix polysaccharide by synovial fluid hyaluronidase, which cannot ordinarily penetrate cartilage, is promoted since it can now enter cartilage and act near cells with a more favorable pH environment. Degradation is followed by attempts at repair by means of increased synthesis of chondroitin sulfate and chondrocyte proliferation. Failure of reparative responses to keep pace with degradation may result in a decreased concentration of matrix polysaccharide, leading to a loss of elasticity and alteration of joint lubrication. Cell necrosis and cartilage erosion might be expected in areas where forces become excessive with breakdown exceeding repair, leading finally to the sequence of pathologic abnormalities seen in degenerative joint disease.

The above hypothesis suggests avenues of approach whereby therapeutic measures affecting the disease process itself might be developed. Redirecting or removing abnormal joint forces by appropriate surgical procedures would ameliorate the stress component which initiates the process. Therapeutic agents which prevent release of lysosomal enzymes or which directly antagonize their effects would be of value in decreasing the degradative response. *Antimalarial drugs*, which stabilize lysosomal membranes, and *epsilonaminocaproic acid*, an effective anticathepsin, are being investigated experimentally in animals in this regard. *Sodium salicylate* has been shown to decrease protein polysaccharide breakdown by chondrocyte cathepsins[41] acting either by a direct anticatheptic mechanism or by reacting with protein polysaccharide so that it is less susceptible to catheptic effects.[15] Investigative studies in rabbits whose cartilage was damaged by a scarification technique have demonstrated a healing of cartilage lesions in salicylate-treated animals, not seen in controls.[41] Recent studies in our laboratory have failed to show any effect of sodium salicylate on experimentally induced osteoarthritis in rabbits, nor did it affect in vitro degradation of protein polysaccharide by chondrocyte enzymes.

An alternative therapeutic approach lies in the use of agents which would stimulate cartilage repair so that the reparative process would maintain pace with or exceed degradative changes. Experimental studies suggest that *Rumalon*, an extract derived from calf costal cartilage or cartilage plus bone marrow, might have this potential. This agent, administered to growing male mice from the age of 1 to 6 months, stimulated hypertrophy of epiphyseal chondrocytes.[40] In vitro studies by Astaldi, Stroselli and Rinaldi[3] demonstrated that cartilage extract protects growing cartilage cells against their dedifferentiation into primitive connective tissue cells. Addition of Rumalon to fibroblast tissue cultures has been shown to result in an increase in duration and amount of polysaccharide synthesis.[5] Studies by Bollet[5] have shown an increased in vitro incorporation of ^{35}S into cartilage when Rumalon is present. This effect in rats was limited to younger animals. Similar studies with human knee cartilage revealed increased incorporation of ^{35}S into cartilage chondroitin sulfate obtained from either normal or osteoarthritic sites and no age limitation on effect was noted. In addition to its effect on ^{35}S incorporation into chondroitin sulfate, Rumalon was shown to increase incorporation of ^{3}H-uridine into RNA in cartilage fragments.

Based on the above experimental findings, a number of clinical studies with this agent have been carried out. In a double-blind study performed on 75 treatment and 75 control patients with osteoarthritis of the hip,[12] *Rumalon* in a dose of 2 ml. given intramuscularly was compared to control injections using 1:10,000 dilutions of the same agent. After 24 weeks there was no difference between therapy and control groups in respect to hip pain and range of motion. After 48 weeks, however, Rumalon-treated patients appeared to be significantly better with respect to pain on rest and pain on motion. Improvement was confined to patients with lesser x-ray changes of osteoarthritis. Radiologic studies at 0, 24, and 48 weeks revealed no differences in the rate of deterioration between treatment and control groups. The effects of Rumalon were compared to placebo in 107 patients with osteoarthritis of the knee over a six-month period.[16] A striking clinical response to placebo alone was noted after 3 months, and no decisive differences between treatment and control groups were noted after 6 months. The trend of x-ray changes after 6 months, however, favored Rumalon. Five per cent of Rumalon-treated patients showed radiologic evidence of deterioration at 6 months; 25% of the control group deteriorated. Adler, Wolf and Taustein[1] compared the effects of Rumalon in a dose of 1 ml. given 3 times a week intramuscularly with placebo given by a similar route in 106 patients with bilateral knee osteoarthritis. Sixty-four per cent of Rumalon-treated patients showed favorable results; 29 per cent of placebo patients improved. Evaluation of results was based on relief of pain at rest and motion and on objective changes in swelling, crepitation and joint range of motion. No side reactions of note were seen except for one patient who developed urticaria. The effect of *Rumalon* on osteoarthritis of the knees following *intra-articular injection* has also been studied.[37] One ml. of extract was administered every second or fourth day for a period of one to four months. Each patient received a total of 8 to 17 injections. Each injection was followed by a severe local reaction, sometimes associated with shivering, fever and malaise. Systemic reactions could be lessened by using a lower dose with concomitant administration of phenylbutazone for a 24-hour period. In twenty patients so studied, four had relief of pain and improved mobility, five had slight improvement and eleven showed no improvement. Radiologic appearances were unaltered.

Further well-controlled clinical studies will be necessary before the role of Rumalon, if any, in the treatment of osteoarthritis can be identified. Although a crude product, it appears to be clinically safe for trials in human studies. Experimental and clinical studies will be aided if the active principle responsible for its effect can be isolated. Evaluation of subjective and objective improvement in this disease is difficult. Radiologic evidence of cartilage regeneration as indicated by widening of the joint space would be strong evidence of its therapeutic efficacy in clinical tests. It has been suggested that drug trials be performed on patients with mild to moderate disease since it is likely that effects would be less dramatic in advanced cases. Similarly, the duration of drug study should bear a relationship to the natural history of the disease. Prolonged studies may provide most accurate assessment of its degree of effectiveness. Use of experimental models of osteoarthritis would facilitate its overall evaluation. The drug at present remains investigative and of unproven clinical value. The results noted in basic experimental studies, however, support its continued clinical evaluation.

SURGERY

Orthopedic surgical procedures may be of value in the management of patients with osteoarthritis. Disease progression may be retarded by correction of malalignment which produces abnormal joint stresses, as, for example, in correction of genu varus or valgus by angulation tibial or femoral osteotomy. This type of procedure may not only slow down disease progression, but may in addition provide gratifying pain relief by bringing healthier articular cartilages into apposition. Removal of free bits of cartilage or bone (joint mice) is of benefit in prevention of rapid and extensive degenerative changes which might otherwise be promoted by their presence. Relief of pain and joint locking are additional benefits associated with their removal. Debridement of large osteophytes may be helpful in lessening joint deterioration and improving function. Joint arthroplasty, resection procedures and partial or total prosthetic replacements have been designed to relieve pain and improve joint range of motion. Joint fusion, indicated at times for pain relief in severe disease, is of value although range of motion is sacrificed. Specific surgical procedures available for treatment of various joints affected with osteoarthritis are presented in the following section which outlines treatment of specific lesions of degenerative joint disease. Patients should be fully advised as to end results, value and limitation of surgery. Details regarding surgical techniques, complications and results to be expected are to be found in Chapters 39 and 40.

TREATMENT OF SPECIFIC LESIONS OF DEGENERATIVE JOINT DISEASE

Degenerative Joint Disease of the Hands

Once present, Heberden's nodes remain due to irreversible changes in the hyaline articular cartilage and subchondral bone. Patients with these nodes should be reassured that they do not have crippling arthritis; they should be supported in accepting their appearance and be reassured that the nodes will eventually become painless. When pain is present, physical therapy in the form of hot soaks, paraffin baths or contrast baths usually will give relief. Trauma which may aggravate the process should be avoided. Local steroid injections into or around the joint may be of temporary benefit; injection into large painful mucinous cysts may be particularly efficacious. A recent report described relief of pain, paresthesias, throbbing and morning stiffness when nylon or nylon-spandex gloves were worn.[14a] The latter material seemed more effective. This simple measure appears to deserve further trial. Osteoarthritis of the first carpometacarpal joint may be similarly benefited by the judicious use of intra-articular steroids. When pain is severe, surgery may be indicated. Joint arthroplasty allows retention of grip motion but grip strength is compromised. Arthrodesis, on the other hand, provides good strength but with limitation of motion.

Degenerative Disease of Acromioclavicular and Temporomandibular Joints

Acromioclavicular joint symptoms frequently respond to previously outlined measures, including the use of aspirin, indomethacin, phenylbutazone, heat or local steroid injections. When severe, symptoms can usually be relieved by surgical excision of the outer end of the clavicle. Temporomandibular joint symptoms due to osteoarthritis are uncommon.[30] Specific therapy is usually unnecessary. When indicated, however, local use of heat plus the use of mild analgesic and anti-inflammatory medications are usually effective. In some instances, intra-articular injection of steroids may be helpful. Dental malocclusion may lead to functional derangements which accelerate degeneration, and should be corrected if present. Symptoms resulting from temporomandibular joint dysfunction rather than structural changes should be carefully differentiated.

Degenerative Joint Disease of the Spine

Treatment of symptoms resulting from disease of the cervical spine should include rest, heat, gentle range of motion exercises and the correction or control of factors causing additional strain, such as occupational stress. Severe symptoms, especially those related to radicular compression, may be benefited by partial neck immobilization in mild flexion with a cervical collar. A soft cervical collar may suffice in mild cases; a more firm plastic collar is of value in advanced disease. When symptoms are acute, the collar is worn during the night and as much as possible during the day; gradual decrease in use may follow as symptoms subside. Cervical traction in mild flexion, in a sitting or reclining position, is helpful in relieving muscle spasm and nerve root compression, but should be avoided when symptoms of cord compression or vascular occlusion are present. Home traction units are readily available and can be used several times daily. Cervical spine x rays to rule out other causes of neck pain, such as metastatic neoplasms, are essential prior to institution of this form of treatment. In patients unresponsive to the use of medications and conservative measures, surgical attempts at relief should be considered, especially if neurologic complications are evident. Laminectomy is usually indicated if myelopathy is present. Fusion alone may be of benefit when root symptoms and signs only are present. Use of an anterior approach for fusion appears to be a safe procedure in experienced hands and allows early mobilization with only collar support. Pain relief may be surprisingly rapid and further neurologic loss usually avoided. Patients with symptoms due to degenerative changes in the lumbar spine may benefit from the use of a lumbodorsal corset or brace with abdominal support. A firm mattress, pelvic traction, and judiciously applied heat and massage are beneficial in most instances. Exercises to strengthen anterior abdominal muscles should be instituted when acute symptoms are absent. Surgical procedures such as laminectomy, discectomy and fusion may be considered when symptoms are severe but are only rarely to be recommended in older patients.

Hip Joint Disease

Conservative measures include rest from weight bearing, heat, systematically applied strengthening and range of motion exercises, and the use of analgesic and anti-inflammatory drugs. In patients with a movable hip, extension traction applied to the lower limb with the patient recumbent on a firm mattress is often effective in relieving pain and correcting the flexion and adduction deformity. If not well tolerated, traction in the line of deformity may be initially required. Lying prone for periods of 30 minutes two or three times daily may be of similar benefit in correcting flexion deformity. Ambulatory patients with severe disease should use crutches, canes or a walker, but several periods of recumbency each day should be insisted upon. Strain in moving between sitting and standing positions may be reduced by such simple measures as the use of cushions to raise the seat level of chairs or by elevated toilet seats.

Most forms of heat will aid in alleviating pain and muscle spasm. Intra-articular injections of steroids are sometimes helpful when pain is severe and persistent. In advanced cases with severe symptoms, surgical measures may be of benefit. Femoral osteotomy may provide significant relief of pain. Vitallium cup arthroplasty may relieve pain and improve range of motion. The need for a long rehabilitation period and maximal patient cooperation in this surgical procedure frequently contraindicates its use in older patients. Femoral head replacement by various prosthetic devices can be utilized if the acetabular component of the joint is only minimally involved. Arthrodesis provides complete pain relief but sacrifices joint motion. Fusion should not in general be carried out if there is significant disease in the opposite hip, low back or ipsilateral knee. Muscle release procedures may provide pain relief by reducing pressure on the joint. Resection of the head of the femur (Girdlestone procedure) provides pain relief; joint instability which follows, however, usually requires continued use of canes or crutches. This latter procedure may be of particular benefit in older patients in whom more extensive surgery is of prohibitive risk. Total hip replacement is now being performed in many centers. It provides pain relief in a high percentage of cases and restoration of motion approaches that of the normal hip. This procedure is particularly suited to the treatment of osteoarthritis in the aged. It will probably replace those surgical procedures that require optimal patient cooperation and a prolonged period of rehabilitation. Denervation procedures for pain relief have been of apparent value,[20] but are no longer frequently used in most centers.

Degenerative Joint Disease of the Knees

The general procedures outlined earlier usually suffice to give effective relief in osteoarthritis of the knee. Excess stresses applied to more severely involved parts of the knee may be redistributed by use of appropriate shoe lifts. A lateral lift will transfer forces to the lateral knee compartment and diminish stress on the medial aspect of the knee; a medial lift will redirect forces so as to protect lateral knee surfaces. Elastic knee supports or knee cages provide increased stability and are of benefit in some patients. Range of motion exercises help maintain or regain motion. Quadriceps-setting exercises maintain muscle tone; progressive resistive exercises build muscle strength necessary to optimal joint mechanics. Exercise should be carried out for at least ten repetitions twice daily. As in other forms of advanced osteoarthritis, surgery may be of therapeutic benefit. Joint debridement including removal of large osteophytes, torn menisci and free bits of cartilage or bone may relieve pain, promote better range of motion and retard degenerative change. Osteotomy, most commonly performed on the tibia, may serve to relieve pain and disability by redirecting stresses to that area of the joint with least degenerative change. Partial prosthetic knee replacement procedures are presently available, and total knee replacement is being used with increasing frequency. (*See* Chapter 39.)

Degenerative Joint Disease of the Feet

Subtalar osteoarthritis, either primary or secondary in origin, may be resistant

Treatment of Osteoarthritis

Adequate daily periods of rest of involved joints.

Avoidance of trauma to or abnormal use of affected areas.

Correction of factors causing excessive strain.

Reduction in weight, if obese, and weight-bearing joints are involved.

Physical therapy: heat, massage and exercise (properly administered).

Orthopedic appliances: crutches, canes or walker to relieve stress of weight bearing; corset or brace supports to the back; use of cervical collar; elastic bandages or reinforced cages for the knee.

When necessary, relief of pain by analgesic and anti-inflammatory drugs, such as aspirin, propoxyphene (Darvon), ethoheptazine citrate (Zactane), indomethacin or phenylbutazone.

Systemic adrenal corticosteroids to be avoided.

Intra-articular corticosteroids as an adjunct measure, to be used infrequently, if pain is severe and persistent in spite of above measures.

Orthopedic operative procedures to relieve pain, regain motion and correct stressful deformity in progressively deteriorating joints.

to the usual conservative measures. Canes or crutches are helpful in the reduction of pain and disease progression associated with weight bearing. Triple arthrodesis may give gratifying results in advanced cases. Inflammation and swelling of the bursa medial to the first metatarsophalangeal joint may be effectively relieved by aspiration and local steroid injection. Symptoms related directly to involvement of the latter joint can be relieved by various surgical procedures which correct deformities as well.

MEDICAL-LEGAL ASPECTS OF DEGENERATIVE JOINT DISEASE

Not infrequently, legal action is undertaken following acute joint trauma when symptoms appear to be induced for the first time or when prior joint symptoms appear to be aggravated. Although trauma has been postulated to be a major factor in disease initiation, its relationship to post-trauma symptoms is often difficult to determine. Degenerative structural changes following shortly after trauma are unlikely to be the result of that particular injury and probably represent prior idiopathic disease. Comparison review of joint x rays which might have been taken for past symptoms is helpful in deciding the question. Support for disease aggravation by trauma is strengthened when osteoarthritic changes previously shown to be stable or only slowly progressive undergo rapid deterioration. Although findings derived from long-term studies of the natural course of osteoarthritis would seem to be of value in making judgments in these cases, the clinical course in any one patient is often capricious and difficult to prognosticate. For this reason the relationship of trauma to disease changes in a given patient often remains speculative.

BIBLIOGRAPHY

1. Adler, E., Wolf, E. and Taustein, I.: Acta Rheum. Scand., *16*, 6, 1970.
2. Alarcon-Segovia, D. and Ward, L. E.: Arth. & Rheum., *9*, 443, 1966.
3. Astaldi, G., Stroselli, E. and Rinaldi, C.: Medicina Experimentalis, *2*, 349, 1960.
4. Boardman, P. L., Nuki, G. and Hart, F. D.: Ann. Rheum. Dis., *26*, 560, 1967.
5. Bollet, A. J.: Arth. & Rheum., *11*, 663, 1968.
6. ———: Arth. & Rheum., *12*, 152, 1969.
7. Brocks, B. E.: Ann. Phys. Med., *9*, 114, 1967.
8. Brown, C. Y., Jessar, R. A. and Hollander, J. L.: J.A.M.A., *147*, 551, 1951.
9. Buchmann, E.: Ann. Phys. Med., *9*, 119, 1967.
10. Compere, E. L.: J. Amer. Geriat. Soc., *2*, 673, 1954.
11. Corbett, M., Seifert, M. H., Hacking, C. and Webb, S.: Brit. Med. J., *1*, 24, 1970.
12. Dixon, A. S., Kersley, G. D., Mercer, R., Thompson, M., Mason, R. M., Barnes, C., and Wenley, G.: Ann. Rheum. Dis., *29*, 193, 1970.
13. Dowdell, W. F., Solomon, W. M., Stecher, R. M., and Wolpaw, R.: Ann. Rheum. Dis., *11*, 168, 1952.
14. Frenger, W.: Therapiewoche, *19*, 1772, 1969.

14*a*. Ehrlich, G. and DiPiero, A. M.: Arch. Phys. Med. & Rehab., *52*, 479, 1971.

15. George, R. C. and Chrisman, O. D.: Clin. Orthop., *57*, 259, 1968.
16. Hamilton, E. B. D.: Ann. Rheum. Dis., *27*, 193, 1970.
17. Hart, F. D. and Boardman, P. L.: Brit. Med. J., *2*, 1281, 1965.
18. Harth, M. and Bondy, D. C.: Canad. Med. Assoc. J., *101*, 311, 1969.
19. Helal, B. and Karadi, B. S.: Ann. Phys. Med., *9*, 334, 1968.
20. Herfort, R. A.: Arth. & Rheum., *7*, 314, 1964.
21. Hollander, J. L.: J. Bone Joint Surg., *35-A*, 983, 1953.
22. ———: Arth. & Rheum., *3*, 564, 1960.
23. ———: Maryland State Med. J., *19*, 62, 1970.
24. Hollander, J. L., Brown, E. M., Jessar, R. A. and Brown, C. Y.: J.A.M.A., *147*, 1629, 1951.
25. Kellgren, J. H.: Brit. Med. J., *2*, 1, 1961.
26. Kellgren, J. H. and Lawrence, J. S.: Ann. Rheum. Dis., *17*, 388, 1958.
27. Kuhns, J. G. and Morrison, S. L.: New Engl. J. Med., *235*, 399, 1946.
28. Kuzell, W. C., Schaffarzick, R. W., Brown, B. and Mankle, E. A.: J.A.M.A., *149*, 729, 1952.
29. Leitch, O. W.: Australian and New Zealand J. Surg., *24*, 310, 1955.

30. Mayne, J. G. and Hatch, G. S.: J. Amer. Dent. Assoc., *79*, 125, 1969.
31. McCarty, D. J. and Hogan, J. M.: Arth. & Rheum., *7*, 359, 1964.
32. Miller, W. T. and Restifo, R. A.: Radiology, *86*, 653, 1966.
33. Moskowitz, R. W., Davis, W., Sammarco, J., Mast, W. and Chase, S. W.: Arth. & Rheum., *13*, 236, 1970.
34. Moskowitz, R. W., Klein, L. and Mast, W. A.: Bull. Rheum. Dis., *17*, 459, 1967.
35. Pinals, R.: N. Engl. J. Med., *276*, 512, 1967.
36. Salter, R. B., Gross, A. and Hall, J. H.: Canad. Med. Assoc. J., *97*, 374, 1967.
37. Santamaria, A. and Barcelo, P.: Rev. Esp. Reum., *13*, 53, 1969.
38. Seifert, M. H., Whiteside, C. G., and Savage, O.: Ann. Rheum. Dis., *28*, 325, 1969.
39. Silberberg, M., Silberberg, R. and Orcutt, B.: Gerontologia, *11*, 179, 1965.
40. Silberberg, M., Silberberg, R. and Rüttner, J.: Exper. Med. Surg., *21*, 241, 1963.
41. Simmons, D. P. and Chrisman, O. D.: Arth. & Rheum., *8*, 960, 1965.
42. Smyth, C. J., *et al.*: Fourteenth Rheum. Rev., Ann. Intern. Med., Suppl. 1, *56*, 45, 1962.
43. Smyth, C. J.: Ann. Intern. Med., *72*, 430, 1970.
44. Sokoloff, L., Mickelsen, O., Silverstein, E., Jay, G. E. and Yamamoto, R. S.: Amer. J. Physiol., *198*, 765, 1960.
45. Steinberg, C. L., Duthie, R. B. and Piva, A. E.: J.A.M.A., *181*, 851, 1962.
46. Thompson, M. and Percy, J. S.: Brit. Med. J., *1*, 80, 1966.
47. Traut, E. F.: J.A.M.A., *150*, 785, 1952.
48. Waltham-Weeks, C. D.: Ann. Phys. Med., *9*, 197, 1968.
49. Wanka, J., and Dixon, A. St. J.: Ann. Rheum. Dis., *23*, 288, 1964.
50. Wright, V., Chandler, G. N., Morison, R. A. H. and Hartfall, S. J.: Ann. Rheum. Dis., *19*, 257, 1960.
51. Zachariae, E.: Nord. Med., *75*, 384, 1966.
52. Zuckner, J., Machek, O. and Ahern, A. M.: Ann. Rheum. Dis., *15*, 258, 1956.

PART IX

Metabolic Bone and Joint Diseases

Section Editor: Charley J. Smyth, M.D.

Chapter 58

The Etiology and Pathogenesis of Gout

By James B. Wyngaarden, M.D.

Definition

Gout is a metabolic disease manifested by (1) an increase in the serum urate concentration, (2) recurrent attacks of a characteristic type of acute arthritis, (3) deposits of sodium urate monohydrate (tophi), which occur chiefly in and around the joints of the extremities and may lead to joint destruction and severe crippling, (4) renal disease involving glomerular, tubular and interstitial tissues and blood vessels, and in which hypertension is common, and (5) urolithiasis.

Many gouty patients do not develop visible urate deposits, but few gouty subjects escape without some renal damage. This may be mild, only slowly progressive, and without noticeable effect upon life expectancy. Severely afflicted patients may manifest all of the features enumerated above, and in some patients renal disease or cardiovascular accidents may lead to premature death.[371]

History

Ancient Greek and Roman physicians possessed an intimate knowledge of gout. As early as the fifth century B.C., Hippocrates described gout as podagra, cheiagra or gonagra, depending on whether the big toe, wrist or knee was involved. Tophi were first described by Galen (A.D. 131 to 200).[236] The term gout, introduced in the 13th century, is derived from the Latin *gutta*, a drop, and reflects an early belief that a *noxa*, a poison, falling drop by drop into the joint was responsible for the disease.

Colchicine was known to Byzantine physicians in the fifth century under the name "hermodactyl" (finger of Hermes). A drug probably identical with colchicine was described in Ebers Papyrus (1500 B.C.). Colchicum autumnale (or meadow saffron) was introduced into Europe in 1763 by Baron Anton von Storch, physician to Empress Maria Theresa.[351] Benjamin Franklin is reported to have introduced colchicine into this country.[292] The term "colchicum" probably originates from an ancient district in Asia Minor called Colchis.

The modern clinical history of gout began with Thomas Sydenham, whose unsurpassed description of the disease, authoritatively drawn from thirty-four years of personal affliction, clearly differentiated gout from other articular disorders.[336,337] The chemical history of gout began a century after Sydenham, when, in 1776, Scheele[290] discovered uric acid as a constituent of a kidney stone. Shortly thereafter Wallaston (1797)[361] and Pearson (1798)[245] demonstrated urate in the tophi of patients with gout. Fifty years later, A. B. Garrod performed his historic experiments in which he demonstrated first by the *murexide test*[99] and later by his famous "*thread*" *test* (1854)[100] an increased amount of uric acid in the blood of gouty subjects. Through the centuries, gout has enjoyed a royal patronage, and victims of gout have been favored subjects of caricature, novels and biography. Among the illuminating articles on the history of gout are those by Rodnan,[275] Hartung[127] and Bywaters.[46]

Classification

Gout may be *primary or secondary.* In primary gout, of which there are several biochemically distinct forms, the hyperuricemia is a consequence of an inborn error of metabolism. Secondary gout is an acquired disease, in which acute and possibly chronic tophaceous gouty arthritis develop as complications of hyperuricemia caused by another disorder. It is now thought that both the acute gouty attack and chronic gouty arthritis are related to formation of crystals of sodium urate monohydrate, and that crystallization of urate may occur from the supersaturated body fluids of any hyperuricemic subject, regardless of the mechanism or disease association of the hyperuricemia. A classification of types of primary and secondary gout is given in Table 58–1.

Primary gout is commonly divided into the following stages:

Asymptomatic Hyperuricemia

There is normally a rise in serum urate concentration at puberty, greater in the

Table 58-1.—Classification of Hyperuricemia and Gout

Type	*Metabolic Disturbance*	*Inheritance*
Primary		
Idiopathic		
Normal excretion (75–80% of primary gout)	Overproduction of uric acid and/or underexcretion of uric acid (Specific defects undefined)	Polygenic Autosomal dominant forms?
Overexcretion (20–25% of primary gout)	Overproduction of uric acid (Specific defects undefined)	
Associated with specific enzyme defects		
Glucose 6-phosphatase: deficiency or absence	Overproduction plus underexcretion of uric acid; glycogen storage disease, Type I (von Gierke)	Autosomal recessive
Hypoxanthine-guanine phosphoribosyltransferase: deficiency, partial or "virtually complete" (Lesch-Nyhan syndrome)	Overproduction of uric acid	Sex-linked
Glutamine-PP-ribose-P amidotransferase: feedback resistance	Overproduction of uric acid	Unknown
Glutathione reductase variant: increased activity	Overproduction of uric acid suspected, but undetermined	Autosomal dominant
Secondary		
Associated with increased nucleic acid turnover	Overproduction of uric acid	
Associated with decreased renal excretion of uric acid	Reduced renal functional mass, inhibited tubular secretion of uric acid, enhanced tubular reabsorption of uric acid	

male than female.[359,360] This rise may be exaggerated and reach levels beyond the range of normal.[315] Many subjects may be hyperuricemic throughout the remainder of their lifetimes, without incurring any recognized deleterious effects. Only about one-third of hyperuricemic subjects develops articular gout, and the average age of onset is about forty-five years. Renal calculi composed wholly or partially of uric acid may occur in the prearticular stage or in hyperuricemic subjects who never develop gout; their significance is often overlooked. Rarely, tophi may antedate the development of articular gout. Very rarely, renal injury may occur from hyperuricemia in otherwise asymptomatic persons.

Acute Gouty Arthritis

The first attack of acute arthritis usually occurs suddenly. About one-half of initial attacks involves the great toe; other common sites of involvement are the instep, ankle, heel, knee, and wrist, or the olecranon or subdeltoid bursae. The untreated attack may last a few days to a few weeks. Recovery is generally complete.

Interval Phase of Gout

Acute attacks of gouty arthritis or bursitis are apt to recur. Initially the asymptomatic intervals may be of months' or even years' duration. Characteristically, the attacks recur with increasing frequency and severity. Later attacks are often polyarticular, longer, and perhaps febrile. Roentgenographic changes may develop, and the attacks may abate more gradually than before, but the joints recover complete symptomless function.

Chronic Gouty Arthritis

Less than one-half of gouty subjects who experience recurrent acute attacks develops chronic gouty arthritis.[17] The duration of time from the initial attack to the beginning of chronic symptoms or visible tophaceous involvement is highly variable, ranging in one large series from three to forty-two years, with an average of 11.7 years.[134] Chronic gouty arthritis may develop as a residue of an acute attack, or it may develop insidiously in a previously uninvolved joint. Acute attacks may be superimposed on the chronically affected joint; late in the chronic phase they may disappear altogether. Chronic gouty arthritis is generally polyarticular. The destructive arthritis may be totally disabling, although the tophi are relatively painless. They may ulcerate and drain chalky material. Severe tophaceous gout is almost always associated with marked hyperuricemia and limited renal excretion of uric acid.

Secondary gout may evolve through these same stages. The acute attacks are indistinguishable from those of primary gout. In secondary gout associated with hematopoietic diseases, the interval phases tend to be shorter than in primary gout, and tophaceous disease and chronic gouty arthritis occur earlier and are often more severe.

HEREDITY

Gout

The familial nature of gout has been recognized since antiquity. Galen ascribed gout to "debauchery, intemperance and an hereditary trait." English observers have reported a familial incidence of gout of 38 to 80 per cent in their cases.[57] In series reported from the United States the familial incidence has generally been from 6 to 22 per cent,[234] but the true familial incidence may be higher as reflected in the figures of 75 per cent,[339] obtained after persistent and diligent questioning. Among hyperuricemic relatives of gouty subjects the incidence of gout averaged 20 per cent in 5 series reviewed by Smyth.[312]

Serum Urate Concentrations

Impressive evidence for heredity in the determination of hyperuricemia has come from studies of serum urate values in families of gouty patients and in populations, particularly those of certain relatively isolated ethnic groups.

The first recorded observation of asymptomatic hyperuricemia in a man whose family had gout was by Folin and Lyman in 1913.[88] In 1937 Jacobson found hyperuricemia in a son of each of two men with gout, and a brother of a third.[154] The first extensive study was by Talbott[338] who reported in 1940 that 25 per cent of 136 asymptomatic blood relatives of 27 gouty persons had hyperuricemia. Smyth, Cotterman and Freyberg[313] in the United States, and Hauge and Harvald[129] in Denmark found similar incidences (24 and 27 per cent) in groups of 87 and 261 relatives respectively. In other studies, incidences from 11 per cent[329] to as high as 72 per cent have been recorded.[357]

Patterns of Transmission of Hyperuricemia

The studies of Smyth *et al.*[313] and Stecher *et al.*[329] led to the suggestion that hyperuricemia in families of gouty subjects was determined by a single autosomal dominant gene, which had a much lower penetrance in women than in men. A major factor leading to this interpretation was the apparent bimodality of the frequency histogram, a feature much less in evidence when the families of Smyth *et al.*[313] were restudied by Neel and associates[235] 18 years later. Hauge and Harvald[129] confirmed the influence of heredity in the determination of hyperuricemia, but concluded that their data were not compatible with a single gene difference, and that several, perhaps many, genes were involved.

Subsequent population studies have supported both genetic patterns. A study of 2,000 Blackfeet and Pima Indians showed strong hereditary determinants of serum urate levels, which appeared to be polygenic. Transmission patterns suggested that some of the genes were autosomal dominants, others possibly sex-linked dominants.[240] The studies of Mikkelsen *et al.*[222] in 6,000 residents of Tecumseh, Michigan, and of Hall *et al.*[123] in 5,000 residents of Framingham, Massachusetts, also favored multifactorial inheritance. The frequency histograms showed skewness toward high values without evidence of bimodality.

In contrast, the population studies of Lawrence[189] in England, of Cobb and associates[56] in Pittsburgh executives and medical students, of Decker *et al.*[60] in Filipino males living in northwest North America, and of Burch *et al.*[42] in the Chamorros and Carolinians of the Mariana Islands, all showed bimodal distributions of serum urate values. Accordingly, these studies appear to support the single dominant gene hypothesis.

An alternative view of these data is that the serum concentration is controlled by multiple genes, but that in any selected group one genetic factor may predominate. The probability of selecting out a single genetic factor increases when the basis of selection is racial, when the group is an isolate, or when the study concerns several generations of families in which gout occurs, as in the studies of Smyth[313] and Stecher.[329] Evidence for polygenic control will be more prominent when the population is heterogeneous, or when only siblings of gouty subjects are studied, as in the investigations of Hauge and Harvald.[129]

These genetic concepts imply that there may be multiple metabolic aberrations responsible for hyperuricemia, but that a single type of defect is apt to characterize a given hyperuricemic family.[295]

Good evidence for this point of view is now available within the types of hyperuricemia associated with specific enzyme or protein abnormalities. Hypoxanthine-guanine phosphoribosyltransferase deficiency is a sex-linked condition.[172] Glucose 6-phosphatase deficiency is an autosomal recessive trait[176] and so is the partial deficiency of the urate binding α_{1-2} globulin found in certain gouty families.[2] The glutathione reductase variant associated with hyperuricemia and gout in certain Negro groups is inherited as an autosomal trait manifested in both single and double gene dosage.[197] No doubt additional specific subtypes of gout remain to be recognized within and separated from the larger category of idiopathic primary gout.

Definition of Hyperuricemia

The limit of solubility of sodium urate in solutions having the sodium content of extracellular fluid is about 6.4 mg. per 100 ml.[247] An additional 0.3 or 0.4 mg. per 100 ml. may be bound to plasma proteins at 37° C,[181] so that saturation of plasma may be reached at approximately 6.8 mg. per 100 ml.

The traditional definition of hyperuricemia is based upon the statistical range of values, mean + 2 std. dev., with a given analytical method in a normal population. With modern colorimetric[79, 329] and enzymatic spectrophotometric[129, 222] methods, the upper limits of normal, thus defined, are 6.9 to 7.5 mg. per 100 ml. in adult males and 5.7 to 6.6 in adult premenopausal females. Autoanalyzer[59] (colorimetric) methods give values about 0.4 mg. per 100 ml. higher than enzymatic methods. The values in males averaged 19 per cent higher than in females in 11 studies.[369] The sex difference is in part attributable to a slightly greater renal clearance of uric acid in the premenopausal female.[359,360] In prepubertal children, mean values are 3.6 mg. per 100 ml.[125] In postmenopausal women, mean values approach[129,222] or equal[315] those in men.

The physicochemical definition of hyperuricemia is preferable to the statistical definition for a number of reasons, some theoretical, others pragmatic: (1) The distributions of plasma urate values are not symmetrical about the mean, but show skewness toward the right, so that the majority of values outside the 2 s.d. range are high ones. (2) Some frequency histograms show bimodality. (3) Serum urate values are positively correlated with body weight, surface area, ponderal index, social class, academic achievement, leadership qualities, aptitude test scores, hemoglobin and plasma protein values—"the associates of plenty."[1] (4) In a number of populations, mean values are significantly higher[42,60,265] or lower[259] than in the United States. (5) In one typical study 94 per cent of 177 analyses in 21 gouty subjects exceeded 7 mg. per 100 ml.,[104,154,343] and in 3 laboratories 98 per cent of 1190 determinations of serum urate in 234 gouty subjects were above 6.0 mg. per 100 ml.[154]

ACUTE GOUTY ARTHRITIS

Prevalence and Incidence

The prevalence of gout varies widely in different parts of the world. A figure of 0.3 per cent in Europe was recorded by Lawrence.[189] In the United States it has been estimated to be some 275 per 100,000 (0.27 per cent).[367] In the Heart Disease Epidemiology Study conducted in Framingham, Massachusetts, a prevalence of gouty arthritis of 0.2 per cent was found in a population of 5,127 subjects (2,283 men and 2,844 women) aged 30 to 59 years (mean age 44). Fourteen years later the prevalence had increased to 1.5 per cent of this population (mean age 58), 2.8 per cent in men, 0.4 per cent in women.[123] Prevalence appears to be even higher among Filipino males in Northwestern North America,[60] and very much higher among the Chamorros and the Carolinians in the Mariana Islands[42] and in the Maori of New Zealand.[265] In the last group the mean serum urate value is 7.06 mg. per 100 ml. in males and the prevalence of gout is 10 per cent![190,264] The relationship of prevalence to the serum urate level is shown in Table 58–2, which summarizes the situation in the Framingham population admitted at mean age 44 and followed for 14 years.

During World Wars I and II acute gouty arthritis was uncommon in Europe. When protein again became plentiful, the prevalence returned to prewar levels.[34,397] In Japan, where protein intake per capita has doubled since World War II, gout is becoming increasingly prevalent. These and other observations underscore the importance of dietary and environmental influences in determining whether the genetic factor or factors are expressed in subjects at risk.

Primary gout is preeminently a disease of the adult male. Since the time of Hippocrates it has been known that gout is uncommon in women. In large series, only 3 to 7 per cent of the cases of primary gout are found in women, and these are chiefly in the postmenopausal group.[16,114,144] In limited series, higher percentages of women are occasionally noted.[64,346] These series may include cases of secondary gout complicating hypertension, renal disease, or the use of diuretics.

The usual form of primary gout is uncommon before the third decade, and its peak incidence in various series is in the thirties,[351] forties,[346] or fifties.[126] In general, the higher the serum urate level, the earlier the onset of gouty arthritis.[123] In the population study in Framingham, Massachusetts, the cumulative incidence of gouty arthritis in men appeared to be approaching a plateau at mean age 58 years. This occurred in spite of the fact that only one-third of the men with urate levels of 8 mg. per 100 ml. or more had experienced an attack of gout.[123] The age factor may explain the low fraction of 21 patients with gout among 5,400 cases of arthritis (0.4 per cent) in one United States Army Arthritis Center during World War II,[144a] compared with the usual frequency of 4 or 5 per cent of gouty patients among all arthritic patients in civilian clinic populations in this country.[233,314]

Mechanism of the Acute Attack

Garrod[101] proposed in 1876 that the acute gouty paroxysm was triggered by precipitation of sodium urate crystals in the joint or neighboring tissues. In 1899, Freudweiler[94] reproduced acute gouty attacks by the injection of microcrystals of sodium urate, and also of other crystals such as those of hypoxanthine, or xanthine.[95] The subcutaneous injection of urate crystals was followed by the evolution of a histologically characteristic tophus.[142]

These observations were lost sight of, and when the measurement of serum and urinary uric acid revealed no characteristic changes during the acute attack and infusions of urate solutions[25,87] or injections of them near, or even into, the joints of gouty subjects evoked no inflammatory response,[111] the concept of a direct role of urate in the pathogenesis of the acute attack fell into disfavor. Theories of a primary vascular disturbance,[228] metabolic abnormalities, endocrine imbalance,[133,274] or allergy to food or bacterial products[348a] were then proposed.

A study of joint fluid by McCarty and Hollander[201] led to a renewed interest in crystals of sodium urate in gouty effusions,[273] and particularly in the diagnostic value of large numbers of negatively birefringent crystals within synovial fluid leukocytes during the acute attack as demonstrated with the use of polarized light[200] (Fig. 58–1). With the use of a first-order red compensator, the urate crystal may be recognized by its yellow color when oriented in parallel with the axis of the compensator and its blue color when oriented perpendicularly to it.[254] Intracellular urate crystals are virtually constant in acute gouty arthritis[302,400] and are a more reliable diagnostic criterion than the presence of crystals in the synovial membrane, which are only inconsistently observed in tissue obtained by needle biopsy.[316,395]

Following the recognition of crystals in gouty effusions (a confirmation of the *gutta-noxa* theory!), Faires and McCarty[83] and Seegmiller and associates[210,299] rediscovered the capacity of microcrystals of sodium urate to evoke an inflammatory response in the skin, subcutaneous tissues,

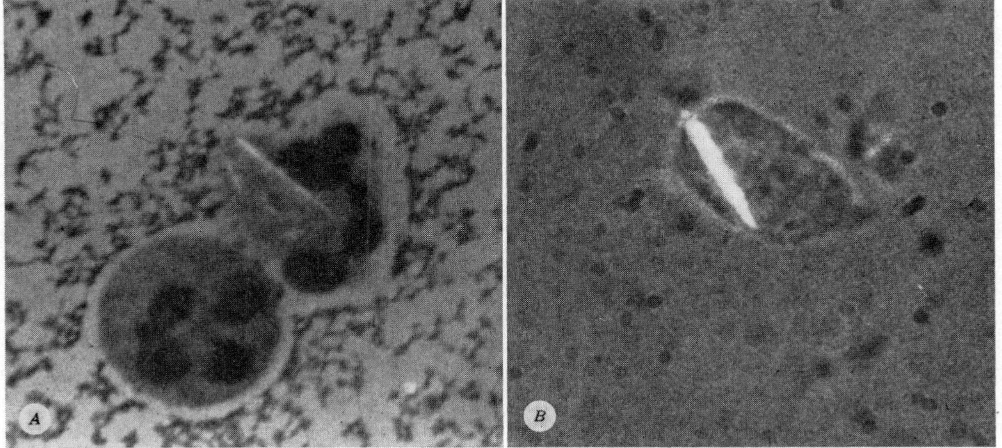

FIG. 58–1.—Crystals of sodium urate monohydrate in leukocytes of synovial fluid in acute gouty arthritis, as seen under polarized light. (Courtesy of Dr. Daniel J. McCarty, Jr.)

and joints of animals and man. In man, both normouricemic and gouty, the inflammatory response strikingly resembles the acute gouty attack. It may be successfully treated with[300] or prevented by[211] colchicine. The response is not limited to crystals of sodium urate but may also be evoked by calcium oxalate,[83] sodium orotate,[316] and certain steroids.[83]

The mechanism by which crystals induce inflammation is complex and imperfectly understood. It has been suggested that ingested crystals cause *mechanical damage* to cells by the release of intracellular substances, *e.g.*, lysosomal enzymes, into the synovial tissues and fluid, leading to the characteristic findings of inflammation.[267,356] It has also been proposed that urate crystals initiate *chemical reactions* in the synovial fluid resulting in the development of inflammatory mediators. Kellermeyer[164] proposes that the negatively charged urate crystals activate the Hageman factor, which in turn initiates a series of reactions resulting in the development of permeability-enhancing activity, perhaps PF/dil (permeability factor/diluted serum), kallikrein, or kinins. These factors can induce vasodilatation, increased vascular permeability, and leukocyte emigration through the vessel wall. It is further proposed that urate crystals may activate still another series of reactions in the synovium resulting in the activation of chemotactic factors from complement components, which then direct the movement of leukocytes to the urate crystals. Release of lysosomal proteolytic and hydrolytic enzymes from the accumulated leukocytes may enhance and prolong the inflammatory process. Thus acute gouty arthritis can be viewed as the end result of several reaction sequences, each responsible for a phase of the inflammatory process.

This hypothesis is supported by considerable data:[164] (1) the Hageman factor is activated in vitro by urate crystals;[165] (2) the Hageman factor is present in normal synovial fluid;[166] (3) permeability-enhancing factors are found in normal human synovial fluid exposed to urate crystals in vitro;[167] (4) the permeability-enhancing factors are not activated in normal human synovial fluid if the Hageman factor is inactivated by a specific antibody; (5) kinins are present in synovial fluid exudates from individuals with acute gout;[218] and (6) the chicken, which lacks the Hageman factor, does not develop an acute inflammatory response following the intra-articular injection of monosodium urate crystals.[164]

In dogs, the inflammatory response to sodium urate shows an absolute requirement for leukocytes. The response is markedly suppressed in dogs rendered leukopenic with vinblastin[252] or with antipolymorphonuclear leukocyte serum,[53] unless the leukocyte count is restored by cross circulation from a normal donor dog[252] or time for recovery is allowed.[53] Following the intra-articular injection of microcrystalline urate into a canine joint the pressure increases, and the pH of the synovial fluid falls slightly as a consequence of a rise in the concentration of lactic acid, produced by the metabolic activity of the leukocytes. The maximal pH drop is only 0.5 unit however,[148] probably inconsequential in terms of its effect upon urate solubility.[326] The ingested crystals are either destroyed by the verdoperoxidase of the leukocytes[151] or released if the leukocyte ruptures and then reingested by other leukocytes.[200] The concentration of kinin-like peptides in synovial fluid may rise as much as fiftyfold during crystal-induced attacks in man, as it does during spontaneous attacks of gout and in other inflammatory states such as rheumatoid arthritis,[218] but bradykinin is not thought to be the mediator of inflammation.[253] Complement is depleted in human serum by urate crystals,[231] and chemotactic activity develops.[248,250] A formulation of the role of the urate crystal in acute gout is presented in Figure 58–2.

The effect of colchicine upon the leukocyte and the possible relation of this action to its specific anti-inflammatory effect in gout are reviewed below.

CHRONIC GOUTY ARTHRITIS

Prior to the advent of uricosuric agents 50 to 60 per cent of gouty patients devel-

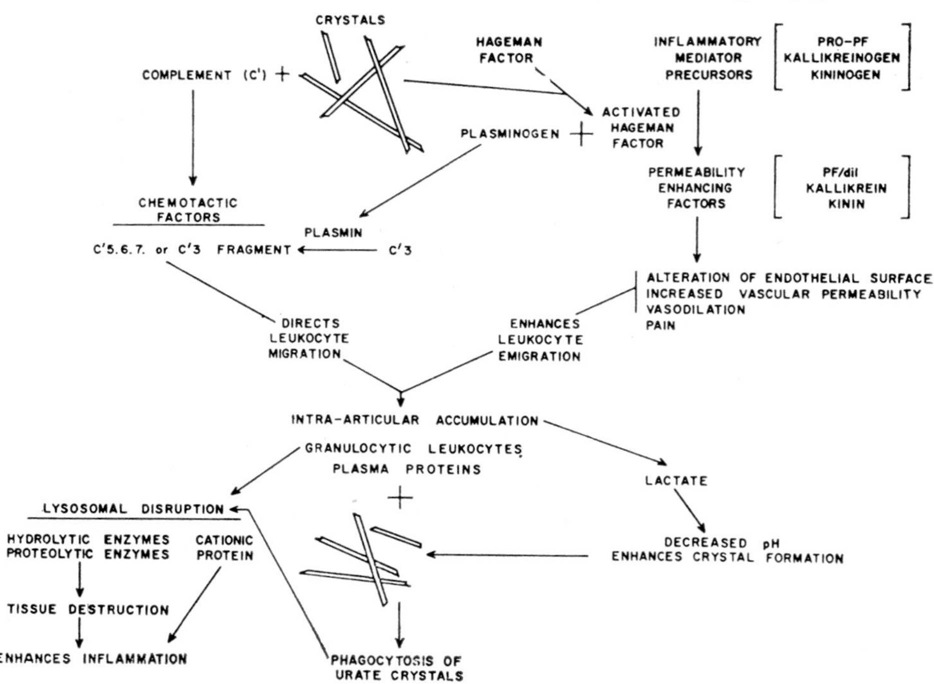

FIG. 58–2.—Hypothesis of the roles of urate crystals in the pathogenesis of acute gouty inflammatory reaction. Crystal surfaces are postulated to activate Hageman factor; ingestion of crystals by leukocytes is postulated to lead to lysosomal disruption. (From R. W. Kellermeyer[164] with permission of Arthritis and Rheumatism.)

oped visible tophi, permanent joint changes, or chronicity of symptoms.[17] In more recent series the incidence of tophi has ranged from 13 to 25 per cent.[15,340] Development of tophi is correlated with height of the serum uric acid concentration, severity of renal involvement, and duration of the disease,[112] occurring primarily in subjects who have had gout for six to ten years or more.[134,342]

Pathology

In gout, urates tend to deposit in cartilage, epiphyseal bone, periarticular structures, and kidneys. The deposits produce local necrosis and (unless the tissue is avascular) an ensuing foreign body reaction with proliferation of fibrous tissue. The characteristic tophaceous nodule consists of the multicentric deposit of urate crystals and intercrystalline matrix together with the inflammatory reaction and foreign body granuloma it has evoked. The crystals, which have been shown by x-ray crystallography to be monosodium urate monohydrate,[32,150] are acicular and arranged radially in small clusters. Granular and amorphous deposits have also been described. Calcific material deposited in the matrix may render the tophus radiopaque, and rarely this process may reach the proportions of heterotopic ossification.[193] Protein, lipid and polysaccharide components are also found in the tophus.[316]

Tophi commonly occur in the helix or antihelix of the ear, the olecranon and patellar bursae, and tendons. Less commonly, they occur in skin of fingertips, palms or soles, the tarsal plates of the eyelids, nasal cartilages, or the cornea or sclerotic coats of the eye. Rarely they occur in the corpus cavernosum and prepuce of the penis, the aorta, myocardium, aortic or mitral valves, the tongue, epiglottis, vocal cords and arytenoid cartilages. Tophi have been the cause of nerve compressions and the carpal tunnel syndrome[353] and paraplegia.[183]

The joint may develop cartilaginous degeneration, synovial proliferation, destruction of subchondral bone, proliferation of marginal bone, often synovial

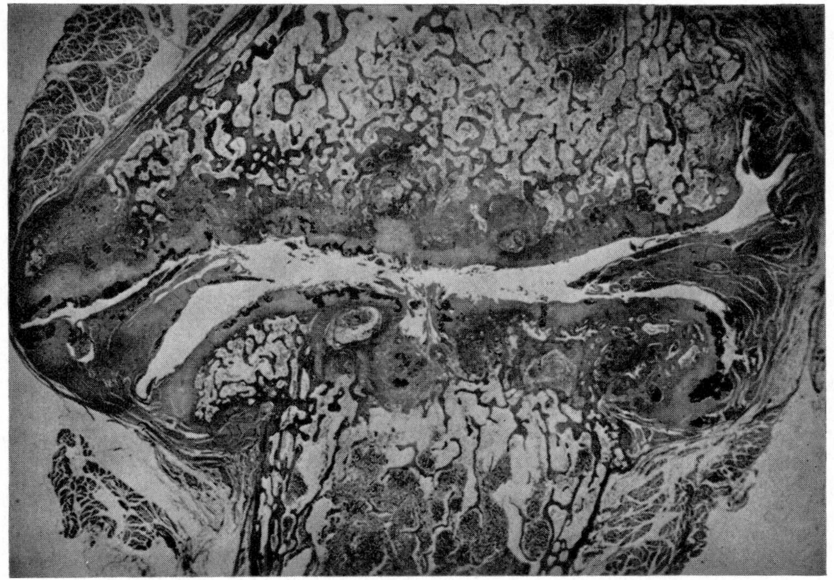

Fig. 58–3.—Chronic gouty arthritis. Urate crystals in the synovial membrane, articular cartilages, and subchondral bone appear black. Erosion of cartilage, advanced osteoarthritic changes, and marginal osteophyte formation are seen. (Sokoloff and Gleason, courtesy of Am. J. Clin. Path.)

pannus, and sometimes fibrous or bony ankylosis.[198] No joint is exempt, although those of the lower extremity are most commonly involved. Spinal joints do not escape urate deposition, but acute gouty spondylitis almost never occurs. Tophaceous involvement of the sacroiliac joint[212] and aseptic necrosis of the hip[203] are well documented but uncommon complications of gout. In vertebral bodies, urate deposits are found in marrow spaces adjacent to intervertebral discs, as well as in disc tissue itself. The punched-out lesions of bones commonly seen in roentgenograms of gouty patients represent marrow tophus deposits, which in most instances communicate with the urate crust on the articular surface through erosions and defects in articular cartilage (Fig. 58–3).

The tissues in which urates tend to deposit are relatively avascular.[127] Sokoloff[316] has pointed out that several sites of urate deposition in gout—articular and other cartilages, synovial tissues, interstitial tissue of the renal pyramid, and sclerae and heart valves—are rich in ground substance containing acid mucopolysaccharide. Cartilage has an affinity for absorbing urates in vitro,[39] and the tarsal bones of swine will cause the precipitation of needles such as are seen in gout when suspended in saturated solutions of urate.[273] Katz and Schubert[163] have identified substances from bovine nasal cartilage, which are protein polysaccharides composed of protein and chondroitin sulfate and which augment urate solubility. Unbound chondroitin sulfate or trypsin-digested material fails to exhibit this property. It is suggested that when, as a result of normal or accelerated connective tissue turnover, protein polysaccharides are destroyed, urate crystals may precipitate from the saturated tissue fluids. This concept may be integrated with the role of lysosomes in joint disease.[267,356] Lysosomes contain acid proteases capable of breaking down the protein polysaccharides of cartilage matrix. One may now envision a link between hyperuricemia, recurrent acute attacks, and chronic tophaceous gout. Injury may result in damage to the lysosomes, release of cathepsins, degradation of cartilage matrix, and, in the case of hyperuricemic individuals, perturbation of the equilibrium between solubilized and soluble urate, with the resultant crystal formation leading to the triggering of acute attacks, deposition in tophi, or both.

The Kidney in Gout

Renal disease is the most frequent complication of gout apart from arthritis.[14,345,365] Ordinarily the process is only slowly progressive and does not materially reduce life expectancy.[344,348] The incidence of proteinuria varies from 20 to 40 per cent. It may be intermittent or persistent; only rarely is the quantity heavy. Hypertension is approximately as common as albuminuria. Uusally it is benign.[345]

The only distinctive histological feature of the gouty kidney is the presence of urate crystals and surrounding giant cell reaction. These may be associated with pyelonephritic or vascular changes or both.[316] In a review of 191 gouty patients on whom clinical information and postmortem renal tissue permitted adequate evaluation, Talbott and Terplan[345] found only three that revealed neither urate crystals, nor pyelonephritic or vascular changes. In all others these features were present in variable proportions and severity. There was a strong correlation between clinical severity of gout and the severity of the histologic lesions in the kidney, both in the case of predominantly pyelonephritic changes and of predominantly vascular changes. The pyelonephritic changes included arterial and arteriolar sclerosis, and in eleven instances the changes were those of malignant renal hypertension. A total of thirty patients revealed well-developed vascular changes and pyelonephritis with extensive structural alterations from urate deposits.

A few notable exceptions in correlation between severity of clinical symptoms and severity of renal disease were also found. Some patients with severe tophaceous gout showed only minimal clinical evidence of renal insufficiency; conversely, some patients with severe renal disease had suffered only minimal articular distress. In the latter type of patient renal disease may be the cause of premature death. The extreme degree of this phenomenon may be represented by a few reports of "Gout Nephrosis" occurring without clinical evidence of gout. In four patients purported to represent this syndrome[38,71,347] no uric acid analyses had been performed during life. The concept of hyperuricemic nephropathy has been applied by Duncan and Dixon[70] to an English family in which eight members had hyperuricemia and six showed evidence of renal disease, in spite of the presence of articular gout in only two of the family.

The traditional view has been that the renal lesions stem from deposition of urates in collecting tubules with resultant obstruction, atrophy of the more proximal tubules and secondary necrosis and fibrosis.[38,224] The associated interstitial inflammatory process has been attributed to complicating pyelonephritis.[38,86] More recent studies have shown that the earliest structural abnormality in the kidney is tubular damage associated with interstitial reaction.[106] There is a distinctive glomerulosclerosis, with uniform fibrillar thickening of glomerular capillary basement membranes, different from that of nephrosclerosis, or diabetic glomerulosclerosis. Henle loops show early atrophy and dilatation, occasionally associated with brown pigment degeneration of epithelium. The interstitial reaction is maximal in the region near the changes in the Henle loops. In kidneys without tophi this reaction tends to spare the medulla and juxtamedullary cortex. The changes of chronic pyelonephritis may therefore not be of infectious origin.[105] The vessels, both arteries and arterioles, show increased basophilia and degenerative changes which are out of proportion to the parenchymal changes.

Renal failure is the eventual cause of death in from 22 to 25 per cent of gouty subjects.[216,345] The majority of gouty patients die of cardiac or cerebral vascular disease.[268] In the epidemiological study in Framingham, Massachusetts, the incidence of coronary artery disease was twice as high in gouty subjects as in the male population with normal serum urate values but was not increased in hyperuricemic subjects without clinical gout.[122] In Tecumseh, Michigan, the serum urate levels of patients with coronary disease were not significantly different from the mean of the population.[229]

PATHOGENESIS OF HYPERURICEMIA IN PRIMARY GOUT

Potential Mechanisms

In theory, hyperuricemia could result from increased absorption of precursor purines, or decreased excretion, decreased destruction, or increased production of uric acid, or from some combination of these factors. A purine-free diet results in an average reduction of serum urate level of 1 to 1.2 mg. per 100 ml. in gouty subjects[111,297] but does not correct hyperuricemia. Feeding of 4 gm. of yeast RNA per day for four days results in comparable elevations of serum urate levels in nongouty[239,297] and gouty subjects.[382] It is clear that hyperuricemia cannot be attributed to abnormal absorption of precursor purines.

Such uricolysis as occurs in man[378] can be accounted for almost entirely by action of intestinal flora upon uric acid entering the gastrointestinal tract in gastric, biliary, pancreatic and intestinal secretions which may amount to 200 or 300 mg. per day.[318] There is no evidence that extrarenal disposal of uric acid is diminished in gout, but on the contrary, it may be increased in all hyperuricemic subjects,[258,318] and may constitute the chief route of disposal of urate in gouty patients with reduced renal excretion of uric acid.[319] There is no reason to invoke impairment of uricolysis as a cause of hyperuricemia in gout.

There is considerable evidence that both increased production of uric acid and reduced renal excretion of uric acid play important roles in the pathogenesis of hyperuricemia in primary gout. These topics will be considered in some detail.

Production of Uric Acid in Primary Gout

Chemical Balance.—The rate of purine synthesis may theoretically be assessed by measurement of the difference between purine excretion and intake in the dynamic steady state. Because urinary excretion of uric acid represents a variable fraction of total purine excretion only gross estimates of purine production are achieved by urinary measurements. Purine intake may be reduced as low as 3 mg. of purine-N per day by dietary restriction. The average urinary uric acid value then becomes a minimal estimate of purine production. Values in normal adult males range from 278 to 558 mg. per day (mean 418 ± 70 mg.)[112] or from 264 to 588 mg. per day (mean 426 ± 81 mg.).[298]

The distribution of urinary uric acid values in males with primary gout extends from values of 150 mg. per day or less to values of 1,500 mg. per day or more. Low values are found in patients with overt renal damage. From 21 to 28 per cent of subjects with primary gout consistently excrete quantities of urate exceeding the mean +2 s.d.[112,298] Such patients have arbitrarily been classified as *overexcreters* of uric acid. The theoretical possibility that an increased urinary excretion is secondary to a decreased extrarenal disposal of urate has been excluded by normal urinary recoveries of injected labeled uric acid in the majority of overexcreter patients.[298] Therefore, sustained overexcretion of uric acid is evidence for excessive synthesis of purines *de novo*. However, a normal urinary excretion of uric acid does not exclude overproduction of uric acid in gouty subjects, for in the hyperuricemic subject with reduced renal urate excretion, the disposal of urate by extrarenal processes may be much increased, occasionally accounting for over 80 per cent of the urate turnover.[298]

Turnover of Uric Acid.—The isotope dilution technique for measurement of the miscible pool of uric acid and the rate of its turnover was introduced by Benedict *et al.* in 1949.[21] A quantity of isotopic uric acid is injected intravenously and isotope concentration of uric acid isolated from urine is determined during succeeding days. From these data the size of the "miscible pool" of uric acid and the rate of its turnover may be calculated.

In about 25 normal males the rapidly miscible pool of uric acid averaged 1,200 mg. (range 866 to 1,587 mg.) and its turnover averaged 695 mg. per day (range 513 to 1,108 mg. per day).[294,298,369] In gouty subjects the miscible pool is generally enlarged to 2,000 to 4,000 mg. in patients without tophi[21,27,318] and may reach 18,000 to 31,000 mg. in patients with severe tophaceous gout.[20] Even so, the value of the miscible pool may represent only a small fraction of the total urate in the body, for only the peripheral layers of tophi are readily exchangeable with urate in solution in body fluids.[20] In one patient the amount of uric acid in the tophaceous compartment participating in a slow exchange with soluble uric acid was estimated by Sorensen[319] to be some 300 times the size of the rapidly miscible pool.

Because of the possibility of exchange of labeled urate of the miscible pool with unlabeled urate of the solid phase, the rate of change of isotope concentration of the soluble phase may not be a dependable measure of the synthesis of new urate in subjects with tophaceous gout. Even so, the derived value for turnover of urate often agrees very well with another calculation of rate of synthesis,[172,298] viz.,

$$\frac{\text{Basal urinary uric acid, mg per day}}{\text{Urinary recovery of injected isotopic uric acid, fraction of administered dose}}$$

In gouty patients whose miscible pool is within, or just above, the normal range it is sometimes possible to calculate that all the urate measured in the miscible pool is in solution. In two patients meeting these criteria, Sorensen[318] found excessive turnover of uric acid. However, in five patients also meeting these criteria, Seegmiller *et al.*[298] found a normal turnover of uric acid, and these five patients also showed normal incorporations of isotopic glycine into uric acid.

Incorporation of Labeled Precursors into Uric Acid

The rate of generation of uric acid has also been studied by measurement of the rate of incorporation of isotopically labeled precursors into urinary uric acid. The purine ring is synthesized in the body from various low molecular weight precursors, which are identified in Figure 58–4. When glycine-^{15}N or -^{14}C is fed to normal man, the isotopic enrichment of urinary uric acid reaches a maximum on the second or third day and thereafter declines.[22,363] In the gouty patient the pattern of incorporation is often abnormal.[22,23,298,363] Particularly in the overexcreters the peak enrichment values are higher and occur earlier, and are followed by a more rapid decline.[302,368,373] These differences signify an accelerated rate of synthesis of uric acid.

The results of published studies conducted under standardized conditions are presented in Figure 58–5, where the data are expressed in terms of cumulative incorporation into urinary uric acid in seven days. The results show marked overincorporation of precursor glycine into urinary uric acid in all overexcreter subjects, as well as significant overincorporation in more than one-half of the normal excreter group of patients with idiopathic gout.

Several of the gouty subjects with apparently normal incorporation values had extensive tophaceous deposits and impaired renal function. Theoretically, these factors could completely mask overincorporation by lowering the isotope values in urinary uric acid. Seegmiller and co-workers[298] have corrected for the fraction of intravenously injected uric acid (labeled with a different isotope) which was not recovered in the urine during the experiment. Two of 5 gouty subjects whose uncorrected glycine-^{14}C incorporation values were normal now

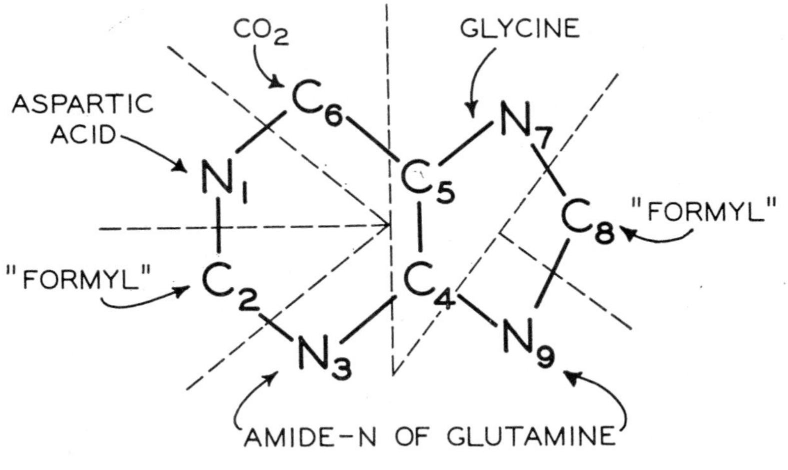

Fig. 58–4.—Origins of the atoms of the purine ring.

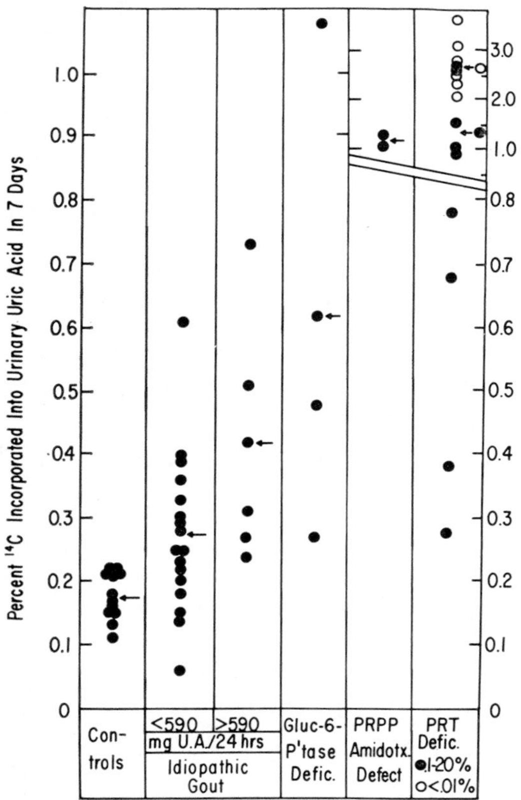

FIG. 58–5.—Summary of incorporations of glycine-1-^{14}C and glycine U-^{14}C into urinary uric acid. Values represent data from published studies[22,23,171,172,176,182,298,364,369] in which glycine was administered to subjects on purine-restricted diets.

showed excessive incorporation, but in the other 3 subjects the values were still normal. Taken altogether, the glycine incorporation studies suggest that subjects with primary idiopathic gout show a spectrum of rates of production of uric acid ranging from values within the normal range[364] to values increased four- or five-fold.

Control of Purine Synthesis in Gout

Biochemical studies have indicated that the rate of operation of the first specific reaction of purine ribonucleotide biosynthesis may control the rate of synthesis of the entire sequence.[368,370] This is the reaction in which L-glutamine and α-phosphoribosyl-1-pyrophosphate interact to form β-phosphoribosyl-1-amine, a compound which has no other utility than to be converted to inosinic acid through a series of reactions in which additional atoms of the eventual purine ring are successively added. The reactions concerned in the interconversions of purine ribonucleotides and the production of uric acid are shown in Figure 58–6. Inosinic acid may be converted to adenylic and guanylic acids, which serve as precursors of nucleotide cofactors or nucleic acids. Nucleic acids are eventually degraded by way of adenylic and guanylic acids to hypoxanthine and xanthine, the direct precursors of uric acid. Alternatively, synthesis of inosine monophosphate (IMP) in excess of needs for nucleic acids may result in its immediate degradation to inosine, hypoxanthine, xanthine and uric acid. Isotope data cited above suggest a possible accentuation of this "shunt" pathway in gouty subjects, especially the overproducers of uric acid.

The factors which control the rate of synthesis of phosphoribosylamine may be grouped in three categories:[369,370] (1) concentrations of substrates (glutamine and PP-ribose-P), (2) amount or intrinsic activity of the enzyme catalyzing production of phosphoribosylamine (glutamine phosphoribosylpyrophosphate amidotransferase), and (3) concentrations of feedback inhibitors of this enzyme.

The Role of L-Glutamine in Gout

Amino Acids and Urinary Ammonia Production in Gout.—Plasma glutamine values are normal in gout, and range from 7 to 10 mg. per 100 ml., or 0.5 to 0.7 μmoles per ml.[159,304,380] Concentration values of total amino acids in plasma, exclusive of proline and aspartic acid, are about 2.7 μmoles per ml. in both nongouty[241,380] and gouty subjects.[159,241,350] One report of hyperaminoacidemia in gout (2.6 μmoles per ml.) is probably attributable to low values in the control groups (2.02 μmoles

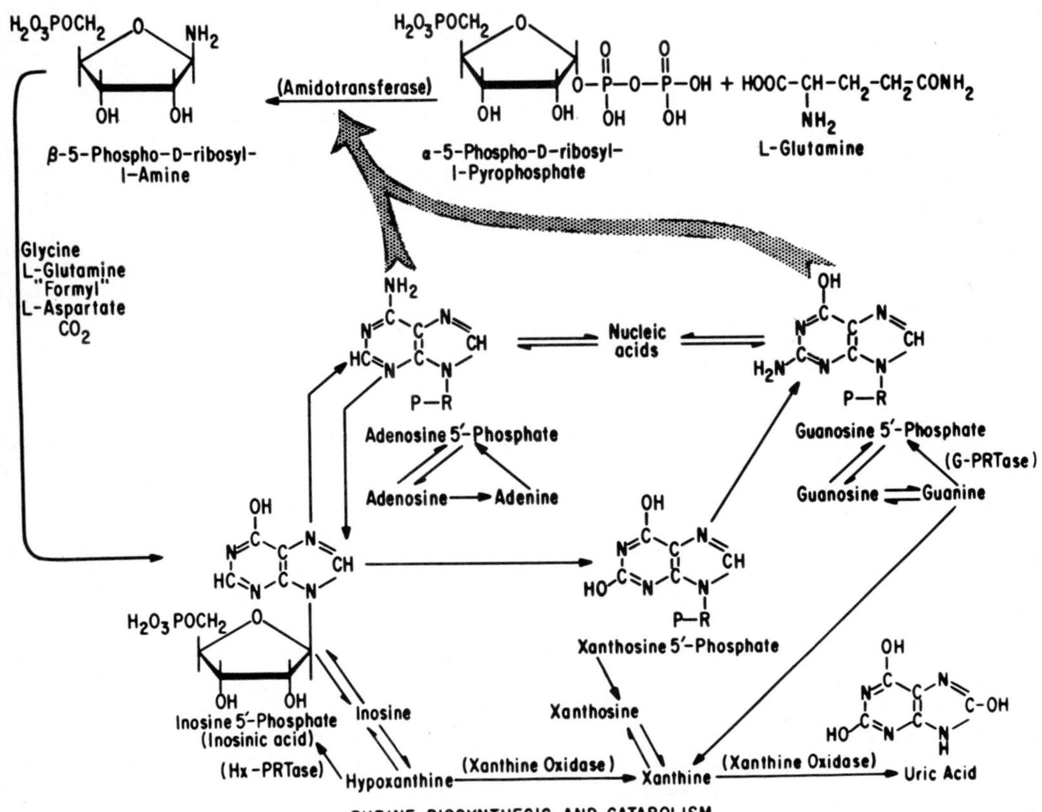

Fig. 58–6.—Purine biosynthesis and catabolism. The first reaction of the pathway is under inhibitory control of adenosine and guanosine 5′-phosphates. Key enzymes are indicated in parentheses.

per ml.) which included a large number of hospitalized subjects recovering from acute infectious illnesses.[159] Reported elevations of individual plasma amino acid values in gout largely disappear when protein intakes are standardized in the two groups.[380] An exception is glutamic acid which remains higher than in controls[141,380] even after casein loading of both groups.[241]

Renal clearances of several amino acids are less in gouty subjects than in controls.[160,380] Deficits of some degree persisted for glutamine, serine, and threonine even after protein restriction. By far the most conspicuous deficit found in the gouty subjects was in the urinary excretion and clearance of glutamine. Following glutamine loading, plasma glutamine levels rose and fell indistinguishably in gouty and control subjects, but the differences in glutamine excretion and clearance persisted.[380]

When glycine-^{15}N was administered to gouty normal and overexcreter subjects, the first-day and cumulative ammonium-^{15}N values were less than found in control subjects with equivalently acid urines. The deficit was attributed to a decrease in the quantity of ammonia produced in the gouty subjects.[117]

Gutman and Yü have suggested that the increased tubular reabsorption of glutamine, and reduced urinary excretion of ammonia in primary gout (overexcreters and normoexcreters alike) are related in some way (*see* below).

Hypothesis of Abnormal Glutamine Metabolism in Primary Gout.—When ^{15}N glycine is given to man, ^{15}N is chiefly incorporated into N–7 of the purine ring. However, nitrogen derived from glycine is also incorporated into the N–1 of purines via aspartic acid and into N-3 and N-9 by way of the amide-N of glutamine (Fig. 58–4). Chemical dissection of the urate molecule by Gutman and Yü[115,119] disclosed an increase in the percentage of ^{15}N in N-(3 + 9) in gouty subjects, relative to values observed in their control subjects. The preferential increase of labeling of N-(3 + 9) and the reduced excretion of ammonia suggested to Gutman and Yü[115] that there was a deviation of the amide nitrogen of glutamine from ammonia production into purine synthesis *de novo* in gout. A block of glutaminase I was proposed.[116] This hypothesis has been disproved by the finding of normal activities of phosphate-activated glutaminase (glutaminase I), pyruvate-activated glutaminase (glutaminase II), and nonactivated glutaminase in renal biopsy tissue from four gouty subjects by Pollak and Mattenheimer.[257] More recently, an increase in the ratio (^{15}N in N-3 + N-9)/(^{15}N in uric acid) has also been found in gouty overproducers with PRT deficiency[296,328] in whom a second specific defect leading to purine overproduction is very improbable. This finding suggests that the shift of percentage enrichment toward N-(3 + 9) in overproducers is a consequence of the complex kinetics of enrichment of precursor pools, following the administration of ^{15}N-glycine, and not specifically related to a defect of glutamine metabolism.[328]

Nevertheless the availability of glutamine may exert a significant influence on the rate of purine biosynthesis. Normal human fibroblasts grown in a glutamine-free medium for 1 or 2 days show a roughly linear increase in purine synthesis with increasing glutamine concentrations, the maximal stimulation being five- to tenfold.[266] The stimulation of purine biosynthesis *de novo* by a high-protein diet in both normal and gouty man[26] may operate by providing additional glutamine. The intracellular concentrations of glutamine are not known, but those of plasma are close to the Michaelis constant for PP-ribose-P amidotransferase.[141,279,374] Thus glutamine concentrations in liver are probably well below saturation values for this enzyme, and changes in concentration would be very likely to influence the rate of purine biosynthesis.

The Role of Phosphoribosylpyrophosphate in Gout

Concentration values of PP-ribose-P are normal in the erythrocytes and fibroblasts of gouty subjects and are not correlated with plasma or urinary uric acid values.[90,109] An exception is found in patients who are deficient in PRT activity in whom there is a gross underutilization of PP-ribose-P in purine salvage with resultant accumulation of PP-ribose-P. The maximal rates of synthesis of PP-ribose-P are not increased in PRT-deficient cells.

Hershko *et al.*[139] and Sperling *et al.*[327] have reported that erythrocytes from patients with idiopathic gout and excessive purine production exhibit an increased capacity for the synthesis of nucleotides from preformed purines as well as an increased rate of PP-ribose-P formation. The turnover of PP-ribose-P is increased in gouty overexcreter subjects.[158] Other workers[276] have not found differences in rate of PP-ribose-P formation in gouty subjects, and clarification of these important observations is awaited.

PP-ribose-P is synthesized from ribose-5-phosphate and ATP. Methylene blue will raise the intracellular concentration of PP-ribose-P in Ehrlich ascites cells in vitro,[136] in human fibroblasts in tissue culture,[109] and in human erythrocytes in vitro,[169] presumably by accelerating the regeneration of NADP in the oxidative pathway of glucose metabolism and thereby stimulating the rate of production of ribose-5-phosphate. Purine biosynthesis *de novo* is enhanced. PP-ribose-P synthesis is also stimulated in vitro by glucose, fructose, and mannose. Ingestion of fructose[109,136] or galactose, or rapid infusions of fructose,[89,246,334] mannose, or glucose,[309] lead to hyperuricemia and increased uric aciduria in man and animal. It is likely that the hexose-induced acceleration of purine biosynthesis operates at least in part by providing surplus substrate for the synthesis of PP-ribose-P. Intracellular PP-ribose-P concentrations may be reduced by stimulating PP-ribose-P consumption with allopurinol,[91] orotic acid,[170] adenine,[109] or 2,6-diaminopurine.[109] Such measures reduce the rate of purine biosynthesis *de novo*, except in PRT-deficient cells which have a surfeit of PP-ribose-P.

Normal levels of PP-ribose-P range from 1 to 5 $\times$ $10^{-6}M$ in erythrocytes; and perhaps as high as 1.3 $\times$ $10^{-5}M$ in fibroblasts in tissue culture.[90] These values are below the Michaelis constants for the PP-ribose-P-amidotransferases of avian liver,[279,374] and mammalian adenocarcinoma cells,[141] which range from 6 $\times$ 10^{-5} to 4.7 $\times$ $10^{-4}M$. Thus it is entirely reasonable to expect that measures which alter intracellular concentrations of PP-ribose-P would affect the rate of purine biosynthesis.

Glutamine-PP-Ribose-P-Amidotransferase in Gout

There are at present no data on the activity of this enzyme in gouty subjects, for current techniques do not permit the direct assay of amidotransferase activity in accessible tissue in man. No activity of this enzyme is detectable in erythrocytes. The recognition of two patients with possibly a mutant amidotransferase exhibiting reduced control features is mentioned below.

The Role of Inhibitor Ribonucleotides in Gout

The amidotransferase catalyzing the initial reaction of purine biosynthesis has special inhibitor sites that are sensitive to levels of adenylic and guanylic acids.

Disturbances of control of purine biosynthesis could result from alterations of the concentrations of active feedback inhibitors at the surface of glutamine-PP-ribose-P-amidotransferase.[52,278] In normally growing or neoplastic cells, presumably it is the removal of nucleotides into nucleic acids, or into other products, which reduces the inhibitory constraints upon the amidotransferase and allows synthesis of purines *de novo* to proceed. An abnormally rapid degradation of nucleotides might have the same effect. There are a few clues that the latter mechanism may operate in specific hyperuricemic patients. In one overproducer gouty subject studied by Seegmiller *et al*. the rate constant for the turnover of labeled adenine was twice that of two other gouty subjects and two controls.[301] In addition, fibroblasts cultured from a patient with familial gout associated with normal uric acid production showed a twentyfold increase in the rate of deamination of adenylic acid to inosinic acid,[137] which was thought possibly to correlate with an abnormally rapid rate of breakdown of azathioprine to uric acid in this patient *in vivo*.[175] Fructose-induced hyperuricemia is associated with reduction of concentration of adenyl nucleotides of liver.[205] Relaxed feedback control of the amidotransferase may account for part of the acceleration of purine synthesis *de novo* induced by fructose.

EXCRETION OF URIC ACID IN IDIOPATHIC PRIMARY GOUT

Renal Mechanisms of Uric Acid Excretion in Normal Man

The current view is that all but a small fraction of urate in plasma is freely filterable at the glomerulus, that nearly all filtered urate is reabsorbed in the tubule, and that the major fraction of excreted urate enters the tubule by a secretory process.[113,332]

Tubular secretion of uric acid, once thought to be restricted to birds and certain reptiles, has now been demonstrated in the rabbit,[261] guinea pig,[226] dog,[179,187,384] Cebus monkey,[85] and man,[120,256,262] but not the rat.[184] The first indication of this process in man was found by Praetorius and Kirk[262] in a young male with hypouricemia (plasma urate values of 0.2 to 0.6 mg. per 100 ml.), who showed urate clearances 28 to 46 per cent above simultaneous inulin clearances. These findings were explained by postulating an absence of tubular reabsorption of filtered urate and the presence of substantial tubular secretion of urate. Supporting arguments came from the analysis of the biphasic response of urate excretion to uricosuric agents by Gutman *et al.*[113,120] At low doses, salicylates,[387] phenylbutazone and sulfinpyrazone,[44,386] and probenecid[311] caused a reduction in the C_{urate}/C_{inulin} ratio; at higher doses all of these agents increased this ratio and were uricosuric.[44,214,311,386,387] These results have been explained by postulating an inhibition of urate secretion at low drug concentrations, and in addition an inhibition of tubular reabsorption at higher drug concentrations.[387] Finally, confirmatory data on tubular secretion were obtained from urate clearance values in normal man as much as 23 per cent greater than the glomerular filtration rate under experimental conditions.[120] Attempts to localize the site of urate secretion within the nephron in man have suggested that this process occurs in the proximal tubule.[256]

Evaluation of the relative roles of filtration, reabsorption, and tubular secretion depends upon the use of a technique that allows specific analysis of each component of the bidirectional transport system for urate.[121,332] Pyrazinamide is a potent inhibitor of uric acid excretion which has little or no effect on glomerular filtration rate.[383] In man, large doses of pyrazinamide or pyrazinoic acid will reduce uric acid excretion almost to the vanishing point.[121,332] On the basis of animal studies, the drug is presumed to inhibit the tubular secretion of urate.[383] Uric acid which appears in urine in subjects given full doses of pyrazinamide is presumed to represent filtered urate that has escaped reabsorption.

In the normal kidney, the excreted quantity ranges from 1.2 to 1.6 per cent of filtered urate. This value is constant over a wide range of plasma urate values.[121,332] It represents a *maximal* figure. The normal value could be lower, perhaps even zero. Apparent excretion of a small fraction of filtered urate could represent (1) incomplete inhibition of tubular secretion of urate by pyrazinamide; or (2) complete inhibition of secretion plus some inhibition of urate reabsorption. The latter effect of pyrazinamide has been demonstrated in the rat.[184] Conclusions based on the use of the pyrazinamide test, described below, should be considered tentative at present.

In spite of the constancy of the fraction of filtered urate that is reabsorbed in the normal renal tubule, the ratio C_{urate}/C_{inulin} increases as plasma urate levels are raised.[188,237–239,297,382] The near completeness of reabsorption of filtered urate suggests that the increase in clearance ratio results from increased tubular secretion of urate. A plot of the rate of uric acid excretion at various plasma levels shows that the increase in rate is more than proportional to the increment in plasma urate concentration and that there is a sharp augmentation of the rate of excretion in normal man at plasma urate concentrations of 9 or 10 mg. per 100 ml.[368] A study of this phenomenon with the use of pyrazinamide suppression confirms that the augmented excretion of uric acid at high plasma levels is attributable entirely to the increased tubular secretion of urate.

Reduced Nephron Population.—In the chronically diseased kidney, urate secretion is markedly reduced in association with a striking increase in the fractional excretion of filtered urate. When renal disease is severe, as much as 45 per cent of filtered urate may escape reabsorption and be excreted. Thus, although substrate-regulated tubular secretion is the principal homeostatic mechanism for urate excretion in normal and moderately diseased kidneys, glomerular filtration assumes this role in far-advanced renal disease.[333]

Renal Mechanisms of Uric Acid Excretion in Gout

It is also assumed that virtually all urate in the plasma of gouty man is freely filterable at the glomerulus. The binding of urate by plasma proteins,[3–5] still a controversial subject, would account for only about 4 per cent of plasma urate at 37° C., and a deficiency of a urate binding α_1-α_2-globulin in gout, as reported by Alvsaker[2,5] would result in more nearly complete filtration.

The C_{urate}/C_{inulin} ratio tends to be lower in gouty subjects than in normal controls at any specified serum urate level.[112,147,188,230,237,239,287] This ratio increases in gouty subjects as the plasma urate level is raised, as it does in normal controls, but higher plasma urate values are required in gouty subjects to achieve a given clearance ratio.[237,368]

When the data of these studies are plotted as rates of uric acid excretion at various serum urate levels, it appears that the curve of excretion rates has the same form in gouty subjects as in nongouty controls, and that the *capacity* of the excretory mechanism for uric acid is not reduced in gout (Fig. 58–7). However, the excretion curve is shifted so that gouty subjects require serum values 2 or 3 mg. per 100 ml. higher than controls in order to achieve equivalent uric acid excretion rates. The sharp augmentation of rate of urate excretion occurs at approximately 13 mg. per 100 ml. rather than at 9 or 10 mg. per 100 ml. as in normal man.

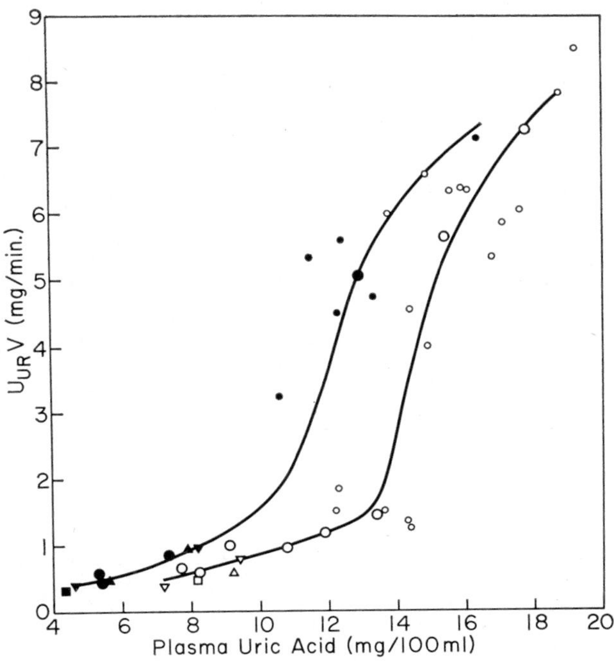

Fig. 58–7.—Rate of uric acid excretion at various plasma urate levels in nongouty and gouty subjects. Large symbols represent mean values; small symbols represent individual data of a few mean values, selected to illustrate the degree of scatter within groups. Studies were conducted under basal conditions, after RNA feeding and after infusions of lithium urate. (△, ▲[239]; ▽, ▼[297]; ○, ●[382]; □, ■[187].) (Wyngaarden,[368] *Advances in Metabolic Disorders*, courtesy of Academic Press.)

The data plotted in Figure 58–7 are from control and gouty subjects with normal functional renal mass, *i.e.*, all subjects have a glomerular filtration rate of 100 ml. per minute or greater. The displacement of the curve in gouty subjects is not a consequence of sustained hyperuricemia, for in leukemic subjects the rates of uric acid excretion are generally normal or increased in relation to the titration curve in nongouty subjects.[238,271]

Application of the pyrazinamide suppression test to the study of uric acid excretion in gouty subjects shows that a normal fraction of filtered urate escapes reabsorption in both normal producers and overproducers both at basal and increased filtered urate loads.[121,272] The augmented excretion of uric acid at high plasma urate levels is attributable to the increased tubular secretion of urate in the gouty subjects, as it is in normal man.[272] In most gouty normal producers, there was a blunted augmentation of urate secretion in the range of plasma urate values from 7 to 13 mg. per 100 ml. in comparison with controls, as one would predict from an inspection of Figure 58–7. However, in many gouty overproducers the pattern of response of urate secretion to elevated plasma urate values was not distinguishable from the normal response.

Rieselbach and associates[272] have postulated diminished renal urate secretion *per nephron* as a basis for hyperuricemia in some patients with primary gout without demonstrable overproduction of uric acid. Although this study appears to be consistent with the hypothesis that one can separate gout into two large subtypes, primary metabolic gout and primary renal gout, the data on tubular secretory response to elevated plasma urate concentrations in this study show considerable overlap of individual values, including one overproducer wholly without and one normal producer wholly within the normal range of secretory response. These observations, together with others showing low C_{urate}/C_{inulin} ratios in relation to plasma urate concentrations in certain overproducers,[112,298] suggest that it may not be appropriate to separate patients with idiopathic primary gout so sharply into two groups on the basis of mean responses. Some gouty subjects appear to be simultaneous overproducers and underexcreters.[366] However, overproducers in the specific subgroup with partial or complete PRT deficiency have no demonstrable impairment of renal handling of urate apart from the effects of renal disease and reduced functional mass.[172,297]

The explanation of the shift of the velocity-substrate curve of the tubular secretion of uric acid toward higher plasma urate values in a large fraction of patients with gout is unknown. It does not appear that this finding can be attributed to hemodynamic changes. Tubular blood flow may be reduced in gout but not enough to explain these findings.[112] There is an active transport system for uric acid in erythrocytes,[185] but little is known about the mechanism of the transfer of urate from renal cells into the tubular lumen.

REFLECTIONS ON THE METABOLIC DEFECTS OF IDIOPATHIC GOUT

The data on turnover of the uric acid pool and of glycine incorporation into urinary urate show that the majority of subjects with idiopathic gout overproduce uric acid by the *de novo* pathway. Many also underexcrete uric acid and show a reduced rate of tubular secretion of urate per nephron. At the extremes of the spectrum, pure examples of each pathogenetic type may exist, but many gouty subjects simultaneously show both excessive production and reduced secretion. In addition, patients with primary gout tend as a group to be overweight, and to have elevated serum β-lipoprotein cholesterol and serum triglyceride values.[13] In population studies and perhaps in groups of gouty patients, hyperuricemia and alcohol intake are positively correlated.[82,204,289] In one obese gouty subject Emmerson[78] found that evidence of hyperuricemia, hyperuricaciduria, increased turnover of the urate pool, increased incorporation of glycine into uric acid, and a low ratio of urate clearance to creatinine clearance all disappeared following loss of 45 pounds of weight over a two-year period. This interesting study further emphasizes the complex nature of the metabolic defects in patients with idiopathic gout, the simultaneous presence of overproduction and underexcretion in many, and the uncovering of the defects leading to hyperuricemia by dietary excesses in some. Clinical observations and population studies have long implicated both non-genetic (dietary) and genetic factors in hyperuricemia and gout. Substrate surfeit of phosphoribosylpyrophosphate and glutamine may be important in the pathogenesis of idiopathic primary gout. Present evidence implicates a surplus of PP-ribose-P somewhat more persuasively than of glutamine. The defective metabolic controls in primary gout which allow the putative overproduction of substrates for purine biosynthesis are not yet identified, but instructive examples are found among the sub-types of gout associated with well-established or tentatively identified enzyme or protein abnormalities, which will now be discussed.

GOUT ASSOCIATED WITH SPECIFIC ENZYMATIC DEFECTS

Glucose 6-Phosphatase Deficiency and Gout

Over forty cases of glycogen storage disease Type I (glucose 6-phosphatase deficiency) and gout have been recorded.[296] In addition, in some cases of "primary juvenile gout," the clinical history and physical findings are suggestive of underlying glycogen storage disease. Patients with glycogen storage disease have hyperuricemia from infancy, and may develop gouty arthritis by the end of the first decade of life, sometimes of disabling severity.[155,157,349]

Chronic tophaceous gout and gouty nephropathy may be responsible for a major portion of the morbidity in these patients as they become adults.

Hyperuricemia is rather marked, often in the range of 10 to 16 mg. per 100 ml. of plasma.[149,176] Two and perhaps three distinct pathophysiologic mechanisms contribute to the hyperuricemia. They are: reduced excretion of uric acid; increased production of uric acid *de novo*; and perhaps increased binding of urate in plasma by lipoproteins which are present in increased amounts.

Patients with glucose 6-phosphatase deficiency are unable to produce free glucose from phosphorylated carbohydrates. Recurrent hypoglycemia acts as a stimulus both to glycogenolysis and gluconeogenesis. One consequence is hyperlactacidemia.[149,156] Blood lactate levels may be 50 mg. per 100 ml. or more (normal 5 to 18 mg. per 100 ml.). Recurrent hypoglycemia also results in ketonemia.[149] Both lactate and β-hydroxybutyrate are thought to suppress tubular urate secretion.[306,391] Renal clearances of uric acid are low in Type I glycogen storage disease.[149] Nevertheless, uric acid excretion values are high when expressed in terms of body weight.[176] By tracer methods, both the turnover of the urate pool[176] and glycine-1-^{14}C incorporation into urinary urate may be excessive.[155,176] Accelerated biosynthesis *de novo* has provisionally been attributed to the overproduction of phosphoribosylpyrophosphate.[176] The intracellular surfeit of carbohydrate intermediates that cannot be released as free glucose may lead to an excessive production of phosphorylated ribose compounds, including PP-ribose-P. The active operation of the oxidative pathway of glucose 6-phosphate catabolism has been demonstrated in liver in this disease.[149]

Hypoxanthine-guanine Phosphoribosyltransferase Deficiency in Gout

One of the major advances in the study of the mechanisms of hyperuricemia was the discovery by Seegmiller and associates of a deficiency of hypoxanthine-guanine phosphoribosyltransferase (PRT) in certain patients with flamboyant overproduction of uric acid.[172,173,303]

There are two different purine phosphoribosyltransferases which are widely distributed in human tissue, and particularly active in brain, liver and erythrocytes.[135,146] Hypoxanthine-guanine phosphoribosyltransferase catalyzes the reaction of both hypoxanthine and guanine with PP-ribose-P, in the formation of inosinic and guanylic acids respectively.[135] Adenine PRT catalyzes the conversion of adenine to adenylic acid in a similar reaction (Fig. 58–5).[146] These phosphoribosyltransferase reactions operate as "salvage pathways" in minimizing the loss of purine bases from the metabolically active pools of body constituents.

Complete or virtually complete deficiency of hypoxanthine-guanine phosphoribosyltransferase activity is associated with the Lesch-Nyhan syndrome,[303] a disorder characterized by choreoathetoses, spasticity, mental retardation, and a bizarre compulsive self-mutilation. There is prodigious overproduction and overexcretion of uric acid, and renal stones and secondary renal damage are common. In a few patients, a severe gouty arthritis has occurred. All the patients are males, and the disorder is X-linked.

A high-grade, but partial, deficiency of the same enzyme has been found in a portion of adult patients with marked overproduction of uric acid.[172,173] The incidence of this enzyme defect in the gouty population is not yet known, but it is probably quite low. Six affected individuals, three of them in one family, were found among 110 gouty patients admitted for special study at the Clinical Center of the National Institutes of Health over a 14-year period. A total of 18 patients were described in a general review of the topic written in September, 1968.[172] Included in this group were several patients who had been reported earlier as examples of juvenile gout associated with marked hyperexcretion of uric acid or with neurological abnormalities.[257,319] Sperling *et al.*[325] found only one subject with a partial deficiency of PRT activity among 52 adult male gouty overproducers of urate. About 25 cases had been published throughout the world by the end of 1970.

Presenting symptoms in patients with partial PRT deficiency may be typical acute gouty arthritis, renal stones, crystalluria, or neurological dysfunction.[81] Gouty arthritis usually presents in the second or third decade. Three-quarters of known patients have formed renal stones; half of these occurred before age 10. In 20 per cent of patients there have been neurological manifestations, including mental retardation, mild spastic quadriplegia, dysarthria, cerebellar ataxia, and seizure. These suggest that there may be a relationship to the debilitating disease found in patients with complete PRT deficiency. Neurological findings have occurred in patients with 0.5 per cent or less of normal PRT activity in erythrocyte lysates.[80,81,321] As little as 1 per cent of normal enzyme activity in hemolysates is associated with no discernible neurological involvement.[182] A few patients have had a mild macrocytic anemia.[172]

Gouty subjects with PRT deficiency tend to have serum urate values above 10 mg. per 100 ml. Urinary uric acid excretion is elevated unless renal failure is present, often being well above 1,000 mg. per day. Turnover studies with labeled uric acid have disclosed enlarged urate pools and increased urate turnovers in all patients studied.[172] Glycine-1-^{14}C incorporation into urinary uric acid is excessive, particularly after correction for extrarenal disposal. Values in five patients ranged from 0.88 to 3.94 per cent of administered glycine in seven days. These values are somewhat less than may be found in patients with complete PRT deficiency (4.3 to 6.1 per cent) but very much greater than in normal subjects (0.1 to 0.3 per cent).

PRT Assays.—The clue to the discovery of PRT deficiency in the Lesch-Nyhan

Table 58-2.—Specific Activity of Phosphoribosyltransferases in Erythrocytes in Hyperuricemic Subjects

Subject	*Number*	*PRT Activity*		
		Hypoxanthine	*Guanine*	*Adenine*
		nmoles/mg protein/hr (mean ± s.d.)		
Normal Controls	32	103 ± 18	103 ± 21	31.1 ± 6.0
Gout				
Normal uric acid production	6	99 ± 13	106 ± 10	31.2 ± 6.9
Excessive uric acid production				
Normal PRT activity	10	103 ± 18	104 ± 22	30.4 ± 5.3
Partial deficiency	24	0.03–12.2	0.009–17.3	26–74
Lesch-Nyhan Syndrome	9	0.01	0.004	39–94

Sources: Kelley *et al.*,[172] except that data of Kogut *et al.*,[182] Emmerson and Wyngaarden,[81] and Sperling *et al.*,[325] on patients with partial PTR deficiency, have been added, with corrections for differences in control values. Activity with hypoxanthine and guanine was reduced in parallel in patients with partial PRT deficiency, except in the L. family of Kelley *et al.* in which activity with hypoxanthine as substrate was twentyfold greater than with guanine.

syndrome[303] was the unresponsiveness of purine biosynthesis and uric acid levels to administered azathioprine in children with this disorder.[320] Suppression of purine biosynthesis by azathioprine requires prior conversion of this compound, or one of its metabolites, to a ribonucleotide form,[35] in a reaction catalyzed by PRT.[202] Extension of the study of PRT activity to acute gouty subjects disclosed a partial deficiency in a limited number of overexcreters.[173]

Activity values in dialyzed hemolysates have ranged from 0.01 to 17 per cent of normal, with guanine as substrate (lowest activity detectable = 0.004 per cent of normal) (Table 58–2). The amount of activity with either hypoxanthine or guanine as substrate varied greatly from one family to another, but was about the same among members of the same family. Further evidence of heterogeneity among the mutant enzymes was obtained in studies of heat stability and electrophoretic migration of the protein. In one family, the mutant enzyme was less stable than normal; in another, it was more stable; and in a third, it exhibited normal thermolability.[172] Leukocytes and fibroblasts of patients with partial PRT deficiency also show low activity values, indicating that this deficiency is not confined to a single cell line.

A-PRT Activity.—An increase in the activity of the closely related enzyme, adenine phosphoribosyltransferase (A-PRT) has been a consistent observation in hemolysates of patients with complete PRT deficiency,[172] and was also observed in about one-half of patients with partial deficiency[172,325] (*see* Table 58–2). The elevated activity values have been attributed to stabilization of the enzyme by the very high concentrations of phosphoribosylpyrophosphate in the erythrocytes of PRT-deficient subjects.[107]

Purine Metabolism in Heterozygotes

All mothers of PRT-deficient patients are obligate heterozygotes, except in the case of new mutations. In most instances heterozygotes have been clinically normal, without hyperuricemia or hyperuricaciduria.[172,182,325] However, three of nine heterozygotes studied by Kelley *et al.*[172] and two of three by Emmerson and Wyngaarden[80] were hyperuricemic. Only one of nine heterozygotes of the first series and one of three of the second showed reduced PRT activity values in erythrocytes, intermediate between those of hemizygotes and normal controls. Increased urinary uric acid, enlarged urate pools, increased urate turnover, and enhanced glycine incorporation into urinary urate have been reported in several obligate heterozygotes.[80]

The fibroblasts of heterozygotes are mosaic, consisting of some cells having normal activity and some having no activity.[277] The proportion of normal cells varies from 60 to virtually 100 per cent depending on the degree of cell contact in cultures. Demonstration of PRT-deficient cells may be enhanced by the use of selective growth conditions, in which an antimetabolite is employed to kill PRT-competent cells.[220] The two cell populations have also been separated by cloning techniques.[221]

Relationship of PRT Deficiency to Accelerated Purine Biosynthesis

Accelerated purine biosynthesis *de novo* in PRT deficiency is thought to reflect an alteration of the activity of glutamine-phosphoribosylpyrophosphate amidotransferase, resulting from greatly elevated concentrative values of one of its two substrates, PP-ribose-P. Abnormally elevated values of PP-ribose-P have been found in both fibroblasts and erythrocytes from patients with complete or partial PRT deficiency.[109,276] Presumably these elevations reflect a reduced consumption of PP-ribose-P in the deficient PRT reaction. These values are sufficiently high so that modest reductions induced by orotic acid or adenine, through consumption of PP-ribose-P in other phosphoribosyltransferase reactions, do not suppress purine biosynthesis *de novo* in vitro.[170]

OTHER PROTEIN ABNORMALITIES DESCRIBED IN GOUT

Glutathione Reductase Variants and Gout

Long[196,197] has observed a highly significant association of hyperuricemia and gout with a mutant glutathione reductase, which moves faster than the normal enzyme on electrophoresis. Twenty-three of twenty-eight Negro patients with gout were found to have the glutathione reductase variant. The fast variant is 28 per cent more active than the normal enzyme.[197] Elevated activity of erythrocyte glutathione reductase has also been observed in a group of Caucasians with untreated primary gout.[196] The suggestion was made that increased activity of glutathione reductase results in an increased rate of operation of the hexose monophosphate shunt, and of synthesis of ribose-5-phosphate and PP-ribose-P. This putative mechanism is somewhat similar to that envisioned in glycogen storage disease Type I in which there is a postulated diversion of hexose phosphate toward pentose-phosphate synthesis because of glucose 6-phosphatase deficiency.[149]

Role of Abnormal Properties of Glutamine-PP-Ribose-P-Amidotransferase in Two Gouty Patients

Henderson and associates[137] found that purine biosynthesis *de novo* in fibroblasts cultured from two patients with extraordinary overexcretion and overproduction of uric acid and normal PRT activity appeared to be abnormally resistant to feedback inhibition by both 6-amino and 6-hydroxypurine compounds. These results suggested the presence of a mutation which had altered the regulatory properties of glutamine-PP-ribose-P-amidotransferase.

The situation in these two patients is unclear, however. PP-ribose-P levels were somewhat above normal in fibroblasts,[137] a result unanticipated on the basis of altered feedback properties of the enzyme. Furthermore, ^{14}C-glycine incorporation into urinary urate was normally inhibited in response to administered adenine[301] or azathioprine.[175] Also allopurinol inhibited total purine production in both subjects.[172] The question of altered responsiveness to feedback inhibitors will need to be resolved by kinetic or inhibitor-binding studies of partially purified enzyme, the technical requirements of which have not yet been solved in human tissue.

Xanthine Oxidase Activity in Gout

Carcassi *et al.*[51] have reported elevated values of xanthine oxidase activity in liver biopsy specimens obtained from eight overexcreter gouty subjects. Mean values were fourfold greater than in controls. It is not known whether the increase in xanthine oxidase activity is primary or secondary to another metabolic lesion. PRT activity was not assayed in these subjects, nor have assays been published from patients with secondary hyperuricemia, *e.g.*, associated with polycythemia vera. Xanthine oxidase is known to be an inducible enzyme in animals.[280] However, even if the elevated values are a secondary effect, increased xanthine oxidase activity would be expected to augment the conversion of hypoxanthine and xanthine to uric acid, and to reduce reconversion of hypoxanthine and xanthine to ribonucleotides in the PRT reaction, at least in liver. It is possible that this shift in the balance of competition for hypoxanthine results in a reduction of intracellular nucleotide levels, with the relaxation of end product inhibition of glutamine-PP-ribose-P-amidotransferase.

Deficiency of a Urate-binding Plasma Globulin in Gout

Alvsaker[2,4,5] has described a reduced capacity of plasma from seven gouty patients to bind urate, which he has attributed to a specific reduction in a plasma component which migrates as an α_1-α_2-globulin. This deficiency appeared to be inherited in an autosomal manner and the patients exhibiting reduced levels were heterozygous for this defect.[2] Using equilibrium dialysis, Klinenberg and Kippen[181] described reduced binding of urate in plasma proteins in three patients with severe tophaceous gout, although plasma from seventeen other gouty subjects including three with tophi exhibited a normal urate-binding capacity. The relevance of these observations to the pathogenesis of gouty arthritis and the deposition of tophi remains to be established.

SECONDARY HYPERURICEMIA AND GOUT

Acquired hyperuricemia is common, and the potential for development of gout exists in all hyperuricemic subjects. Secondary hyperuricemia is caused by either the increased turnover of nucleic acid purines or the impaired renal excretion of uric acid. Thus in secondary gout, as in primary gout, hyperuricemia appears to have a dual pathogenesis.

Hematologic Disorders

Hyperuricemia and secondary gout occur in lymphoproliferative and myeloproliferative disorders,[110,140,340,379] multiple myeloma,[37] secondary polycythemia,[317,393] certain hemoglobinopathies, thalassemia, and pernicious anemia. All of these conditions are associated with chronically increased marrow activity.[341]

In one large series of patients with leukemia, myeloid metaplasia, polycythemia vera, and multiple myeloma, hyperuricemia was noted in 66 per cent of 113 male patients and 69 per cent of 73 female patients. Only 10 patients had a history of gouty arthritis[199] and 6 of them were found among the 22 patients with myeloid metaplasia. In other series, gouty arthritis has occurred in 2 to 14 per cent (mean 6 per cent) of patients with polycythemia vera. Curiously, 84 per cent of these gouty patients have been males, although the basic disease is almost as common in females as in males.

Gutman and Yü[114] found a mean urinary uric acid excretion value of 634 mg. per 24 hour in 27 cases of secondary gout complicating hematologic disorders, as compared to a mean value of 497 mg. per 24 hour in their control group. The fractional urate clearance, $C_{uric\ acid}/GFR$, is generally normal or increased.[238,271] The miscible pool of uric acid and its turnover are increased in patients with myelogenous leukemia or polycythemia vera.[27] The incorporation of glycine-^{15}N,[186,394] glycine-1-^{14}C, and 5-aminoimidazole-4-carboxamide-4-^{14}C[362,377] into urinary purine bases and uric acid has revealed striking labeling of the bases during the first day followed by secondary maxima in bases and uric acid between 7 and 12 days. Cumulative incorporation of isotope into uric acid is approximately normal during the first few days but greatly exceeds the normal after 1 to 2 weeks.[377] These data indicate an exaggerated turnover of nucleic acid purines as the cause of hyperuricemia in these subjects.

Gouty arthritis may also complicate sickle cell disease,[10,102] hemoglobin SC disease, β-thalassemia, and other chronic hemolytic anemias.[213,242]

Drug-induced Hyperuricemia and Gout

The list of drugs which lead to hyperuricemia includes the potent diuretics, alcohol, pyrazinamide, and salicylates in low doses. Drug-induced gout has become increasingly important since the advent of the potent thiazide diuretics.[6,232]

Diuretics.—In a study of hyperuricemic men admitted to a Veterans Administration hospital, diuretics were considered the causative factor in 20 per cent.[244] Of the new cases of gout in Framingham, Massachusetts, 50 per cent have developed in subjects taking thiazides or ethacrynic acid. Hyperuricemia has been noted in up to 75 per cent of patients treated with diuretics.[65]

There are several mechanisms by which potent diuretic agents may produce hyperuricemia.[373] The work of Steele and Oppenheimer[330,331] and of Suki *et al.*[335] suggests that a prerequisite is sufficient salt and water loss to produce volume contraction. Following the administration of thiazides or of ethacrynic acid, tubular reabsorption of filtered urate is increased. In addition, inhibition of tubular secretion of urate seems likely. Neither effect appears to represent a direct action of the diuretic agent upon tubular transport of urate, for urate excretion values remain near control values when volume depletion is prevented by replacement of urinary salt and water losses with intravenous saline. Thus, secondary extrarenal influences upon the kidney may be responsible for the hyperuricemia. Volume contraction leads to a generalized increase in solute reabsorption, perhaps mediated by changes in oncotic pressure.[50,330] In addition, furosemide induces hyperlactacidemia sufficient to suppress tubular secretion of urate.

Role of Ethanol.—In his classic treatise on gout published in 1863, A. B. Garrod[98] wrote: "There is no truth in medicine better established than the fact that the use of fermented liquors is the most powerful of all the predisposing causes of gout; nay, so powerful, that it may be a question whether gout would ever have been known to mankind had such beverages not been indulged in."

The association of the acute gouty paroxysm with overindulgence in drink has at long last acquired a physiologic explanation. Hyperuricemia is common in inebriated subjects,[194] and infusions of ethanol result in hyperuricemia.[195] As ethanol is metabolized by alcohol dehydrogenase, NAD is reduced, and this may account in part for the excessive conversion of pyruvate to lactate. The levels of hyperlactacidemia achieved[195] are adequate to suppress the renal excretion of uric acid and to induce hyperuricemia,[391] thus increasing the probability of crystal formation.

More recently, MacLachlan and Rodnan[204] have observed that the combination of ethanol ingestion and fasting may be additive or synergistic with respect to the effects of each of these factors on uric acid metabolism. Epidemiologic studies have reported a correlation between serum urate levels and habitual alcohol intake.[82,289] The daily ingestion of alcohol in significant but tolerated amounts, *e.g.*, 100 ml. per 24 hours, may be associated with hyperuricemia and *increased* urinary excretion of uric acid, both of which may return toward or to normal during protracted periods (days) of abstinence and normal diet. These cycles are not explained by reduced urinary clearance of uric acid. An effect upon purine synthesis has been postulated.[61]

Hypertension

In untreated hypertensive patients without discernible renal disease the incidence of hyperuricemia ranges from 22 to 27 per cent.[33,49] When therapy and renal disease are not excluded, the incidence increases to 47 to 67 per cent.[68,152,180] Hyperuricemia is equally common in essential and renovascular hypertension.[49] Values of 59 to 67 per cent were recorded in patients in whom the disease was severe enough to warrant sympathectomy[180] or adrenalectomy.[152] Gout was observed in 11 of 105 adrenalectomized patients. The overall incidence of gout in hypertension has been variably reported as 2 to 12 per cent.[33,49]

In most hypertensive patients, hyperuricemia appears to be related to the reduced renal excretion of uric acid, attributed to a lower $C_{uric\ acid}$/GFR ratio than in nonhyperuricemic hypertensives.[310] The suggestion has been made that tubular dysfunction may be a consequence of vascular disease, tissue hypoxia, and local lactic acid excess, but attempts to relate hyperuricemia to hyperlactacidemia have been controversial.[49,152]

Chronic Renal Insufficiency

Hyperuricemia is common in renal insufficiency, but in spite of very high serum urate concentrations in some patients, gouty arthritis occurs only rarely. In a study of 496 patients with chronic renal insufficiency, Sarre[288] found 6 with gout, in 4 of whom the disease appeared to be primary. Examples have also been reported by others.[270,319] The paucity of gouty arthritis in these patients has been attributed to (1) a shortened life span; and (2) a decreased ability to respond to an inflammatory stimulus.[40]

Recurrent attacks of acute arthritis may occur in patients with chronic renal failure treated with periodic hemodialysis. The clinical features of the acute inflammatory episodes, their response to colchicine, and the tendency for their frequency to vary directly with the plasma urate level have led to the diagnosis of acute gouty arthritis.[48] However, examination of the synovial fluid frequently reveals the presence of calcium phosphate crystals rather than monosodium urate crystals. Similarly the crystals in muscle have also been identified as calcium phosphate not urate.[225]

Lead Gout

The association of gout with chronic lead poisoning led many years ago to the concept of "saturnine gout," in which gout was regarded as a complication of the nephritis of plumbism. This type of gout exists in Queensland, Australia,[76] and in France[269] where patients were exposed to leaded paint in childhood. When compared to primary gout, this group of patients has a higher incidence of renal disease prior to the first episode of arthritis, females are more frequently affected, the arthritis is milder, the mean age of onset is younger, there is a lower incidence of renal calculi, hyperlipoproteinemia is absent and a family history of gout is unlikely.[77] In the United States, saturnine gout is most often related to the habitual consumption of "moonshine" alcohol with an appreciable lead content. In a recent study at a southern Veterans Administration hospital, 37 of 43 cases of gout were found to be associated with chronic lead intoxication.[9,11]

Starvation

Total caloric restriction results in extreme degrees of hyperuricemia[58,69,191] attributable in part to a reduced renal clearance of uric acid and in part to the overproduction of uric acid. The retention of uric acid is correlated best with ketosis and with the serum concentration of β-hydroxybutyrate.[103,130,306] Refeeding of carbohydrate results in correction of ketosis, temporarily excessive excretion of uric acid, and reduction in serum urate levels.

Attacks of gouty arthritis may occur during periods of starvation,[281] but are unusual except in patients with a prior history of gout.[204]

Hyperparathyroidism

There is a high incidence of hyperuricemia in hyperparathyroidism.[47,223,293] Scott *et al.*[293] noted hyperuricemia in 11 of 12 patients, in 5 of whom they obtained a history consistent with gout. Synovial fluid examination is essential to the diagnosis of gout in these patients and must disclose urate rather than calcium pyrophosphate crystals, for pseudogout may also occur in this setting.

Psoriasis and Sarcoidosis

Hyperuricemia occurs in 30 to 50 per cent of patients with psoriasis[72] and in a like percentage of patients with sarcoid.[41,162,396] Urinary uric acid in hyperuricemic patients with psoriasis given glycine-1-^{14}C shows peak enrichment values intermediate in time between those of primary gout and those of secondary gout due to myeloproliferative disease. This has been interpreted as indicating increased nucleotide and nucleic acid turnover in the psoriatic lesions as probable pathogenetic factors in the hyperuricemia.[72] The association of sarcoidosis, psoriasis, and gout has been reported and regarded as a syndrome by some,[162] as chance concurrence by others,[54,396] or possibly as sarcoid arthritis in a hyperuricemic subject with psoriasis but without true gout.[41]

UROLITHIASIS IN GOUT

The incidence of renal calculi in various American or European series of gout is 5 to 33 per cent;[7,340] it is 75 per cent in Israel.[7] In the experience of Yü and Gutman,[389] the incidence was 22 per cent in 1,258 patients with primary gout and 42 per cent in 59 patients with secondary gout, or at least 1,000 times that of the general population. In 40 per cent of the cases of primary gout, lithiasis antedated acute arthritis, occasionally by more than 20 years. Uric acid nephrolithiasis may be associated with hyperuricemia without acute arthritis. About one-third of such patients gives a family history of gout. Over 80 per cent of calculi in gouty subjects are composed of uric acid.[389] Occasionally they may be mixed, or have only a central nidus of uric acid,[263] or contain only calcium oxalate or phosphate.[389]

Factors which predispose toward uric acid nephrolithiasis in gout include undue acidity of the urine, increased urinary excretion of uric acid, increased urinary concentration, and perhaps qualitative or quantitative abnormalities of urinary constituents which affect the solubility of uric acid.[7]

Gouty patients have a tendency toward unusually acid urine both in fasting morning specimens and throughout the day[62,67,305,358,389] and a substandard rise of urinary pH in response to oral alkali. There is no correlation between urine pH and urinary uric acid excretion.[389] In the three-fourths of gouty subjects whose urinary uric acid values fall within the normal range, the high incidence of renal stones is probably related to low urinary pH. This, in turn, is a reflection of a low NH_4^+/titratable acidity ratio, attributed by some to a subnormal ammonium excretion at a given acid load or pH[116,117,138,255,358] and by others to high values of titratable acidity.[18,62,93,219] The deficit of ammonium excretion, when present, has been assigned to the effects of occult or measurable renal damage,[219,243] aging,[324] or high purine intake[243] by some authors, but is regarded as an intrinsic defect in the production of ammonia, presumably from glutamine, by Gutman and Yü.[115,117,118] The pK_{a1} and pK_{a2} of uric acid are 5.75 and 10.3, respectively. At urinary pH values of 4.5 to 5 the predominant form should be uric acid, not sodium urate and this has been established by x-ray crystallographic studies.[150,263] The solubility of uric acid is only one-seventeenth that of sodium urate in water at 37° C. The prevalence of renal stones rises with increasing plasma urate levels in the general population and approximates 50 per cent when serum urate levels exceed 12 mg. per 100 ml. in patients with gout.[389] The influence of hyperuricemia is probably chiefly significant as it affects urinary uric acid excretion. The prevalence of urolithiasis increases from 11 per cent in patients with excretion values under 300 mg. per day to 50 per cent in patients with values over 1,100 mg. per day.[389]

Uric Acid Nephrolithiasis in Nonhyperuricemic Subjects

Only about 20 per cent of patients without clinical gout who form uric acid stones are hyperuricemic.[340] In *idiopathic* uric acid nephrolithiasis, by definition occurring in patients with normal plasma and urinary uric acid values, a consistent finding, as in gouty and in otherwise asymptomatic hyperuricemic subjects, is a tendency toward a low urine pH. The risk of uric acid stones is also increased in patients with ileostomies[24,55,66] who exhibit increased renal conservation of sodium, a decreased urinary Na/K ratio, increased urinary acid excretion, and low urinary pH values.[55]

Uric acid stones may at times be dissolved with protracted fluid and alkali therapy[8] but allopurinol is the treatment of choice.

MECHANISM OF ACTION OF DRUGS IN GOUT

Colchicine

The response of acute gouty arthritis to colchicine has long been considered specific, but this time-honored axiom has been questioned in reports of responses of acutely inflamed joints of serum sickness,[227] experimental arthritis,[145] sarcoid arthrits,[161] rheumatoid arthritis,[399] and the inflammation associated with hydroxyapatite calcific tendinitis. Some of the disagreement results from the varying criteria for an adequate colchicine effect.[228] Using rigid criteria, Wallace *et al.*[352] noted a typical response to oral colchicine in 75 per cent of 58 patients with gout, and in only 4 of 37 patients with a variety of other articular disorders.

The favored hypothesis of the action of colchicine is that it interferes with the metabolic activity of phagocytizing leukocytes. Following its intravenous infusion colchicine rapidly enters cells[192] where it is bound in a noncovalent complex to a subunit protein of microtubules.[31,206,307,355] The microtubules of human polymorphonuclear leukocytes are no longer visible in the presence of colchicine.[31] These observations led Malawista to suggest that colchicine may interfere with leukocyte locomotion, a process which requires rapid, reversible sol-gel transformations within the cell.[31,206,307,355] Colchicine inhibits a variety of leukocyte functions including adhesiveness,[207] amoeboid motility,[208] mobilization,[97] chemotaxis,[251] random motility under the influence of urate,[249] degranulation of lysosomes,[209,267] and metabolism during phagocytosis.[267,354] In addition, colchicine blocks kinin release from plasma under the influence of leukocytes.[217] The most potent inhibitory effects of colchicine are on the motility of leukocytes[249] and the development of chemotactic activity after phagocytosis of urate crystals.[251] Nevertheless it remains to be proved that the effects of colchicine in the treatment of acute gout are related to these actions upon the leukocyte.[151,300] This drug does not alter serum concentrations or renal excretion of uric acid,[340] nor does it have any significant effect upon the miscible pool of uric acid or the rate of its turnover.[20,45]

Uricosuric Drugs

This category of compounds includes salicylates,[387] cinchophen, probenecid,[311] phenylbutazone[392] and its derivatives, sulfinpyrazone and *p*-nitrophenylbutazone,[350] zoxazolamine,[43] dicumarol,[124] ethyl biscoumacetate,[323] phenylindandione,[323] acetoheximide,[381] glycine,[390] azauridine,[84] orotic acid,[171] benziodarone,[63,286,398] chlorprothixene,[132] and certain radiographic agents.[260] At the present time probenecid and sulfinpyrazone are most widely employed in this country; benziodarone and zoxazolamine are used in Europe as well.

All of these compounds increase the excretion of uric acid without causing a significant change in the glomerular filtration rate. A number have been shown to have a paradoxical effect upon uric acid excretion, consisting of an inhibition of excretion at low doses (presumably from inhibition of tubular secretion of urate) and an enhancement at high doses. The uricosuric effect of most agents studied has been attributed to inhibition of tubular reabsorption of filtered urate. Recently it has been suggested that certain drugs may be uricosuric because they enhance tubular secretion of urate. This may be the mechanism by which glycine,[390] benziodarone,[286] and x-ray contrast agents[260] increase uric acid excretion. The effect of these drugs is blocked by prior administration of pyrazinamide, whereas pyrazinamide does not block the uricosuric effect of probenecid in man.

Striking reductions of the miscible pool of uric acid have been demonstrated after the administration of adequate doses of salicylates,[20] probenecid,[28,311] phenylbutazone,[392] and cortisone.[27] These are probably accounted for entirely by the increment in urate excretion.

The uricosuric actions of probenecid, sulfinpyrazone, and zoxazolamine are suppressed by salicylates in man, in part because of a countermanding of the inhibition of tubular reabsorption of uric acid produced by uricosuric drugs. The mechanism is complex, however, and also involves effects upon the tubular secretion of uric acid by salicylates and competition between salicylates and sulfinpyrazone for binding sites on transporting plasma proteins and perhaps elsewhere.[385] Probenecid, phenylbutazone, and salicylates are reported to reduce urate binding to protein.[29] Sulfinpyrazone may have a similar though less striking effect.[30] Such an action could at best account for only a fraction of their uricosuric effects.

Xanthine Oxidase Inhibitors.—Many inhibitors of xanthine oxidase are known, various purine analogues,[153,308,369] symmetrical triazines,[96] allopurinol [4-hydroxypyrazolo-(3,4-d)pyrimidine], and oxipurinol [2,4-dihydroxypyrozolo-(3,4-d)-pyrimidine]. Only allopurinol and oxipurinol are employed therapeutically in man.

Allopurinol is an analogue of hypoxanthine in which the positions of N-7 and C-8 are reversed (Fig. 58–8). Allopurinol is metabolized to oxipurinol by xanthine oxidase.[73] The Michaelis constant of allopurinol is some 15- to 200-fold lower than that of xanthine, whereas that of oxipurinol is comparable to that of xanthine.[73] Both allopurinol and oxipurinol produce pseudoirreversible inactivation of xanthine oxidase: Inactivation occurs when allopurinol and the enzyme are incubated in the absence of substrate, but enzyme activity can be restored by prolonged dialysis. Oxipurinol has no effect on the enzyme alone, but inactivates it in the presence of xanthine.[215,284]

Allopurinol has a very short biological half-life of only 2 to 3 hours.[74] Three to ten per cent of an administered dose is excreted with a clearance rate approximately equal to the GFR.[74] The majority of allopurinol (45 to 65 per cent) is rapidly oxidized to oxipurinol in vivo, with a smaller portion being converted to allopurinol 1-N-ribonucleoside[184a] and probably allopurinol 1-N-ribonucleotide[91] (Fig. 58–8). Most of the oxipurinol formed is excreted unchanged by the kidney with a relatively long half-life (28 hr.),[74] and perhaps also to 1-N-ribonucleoside and ribonucleotide derivatives[75] (Fig. 58–9). It has been suggested that oxipurinol rather than allopurinol is primarily responsible for xanthine oxidase inhibition in vivo.[73] A direct comparison of the two drugs administered orally indicated that allopurinol was the more effective perhaps because of its better absorption from the gastrointestinal tract.[52]

The administration of allopurinol to subjects with normal renal function is followed by a prompt decrease in the serum and urinary uric acid values occurring within 24 to 48 hrs., reaching a maximum in 4 days to 2 weeks and remaining relatively constant over prolonged periods of time.[282,283,375,376] With the inhibition of urate production by allopurinol, increased amounts of the precursors, hypoxanthine and xanthine, appear in the urine, usually within 4 to 6 hours[74] (Fig. 58–9). Only trivial changes occur in the excretion of other urinary purine bases.[178] The combined increase in hypoxanthine and xanthine, though striking, usually falls far short of balancing the decrement in uric acid. Withdrawal of allopurinol results in a return to pretreatment serum urate levels within a few days and the exceptional, more prolonged effects are clearly associated with the delayed excretion of oxipurinol.[284]

When allopurinol is given, serum oxypurine levels rise only slightly, reaching 0.5 to 1.0 mg. per 100 ml.[285] or, rarely, 2.0 mg. per 100 ml[388] because of the high renal clearance of oxypurines. The oxy-

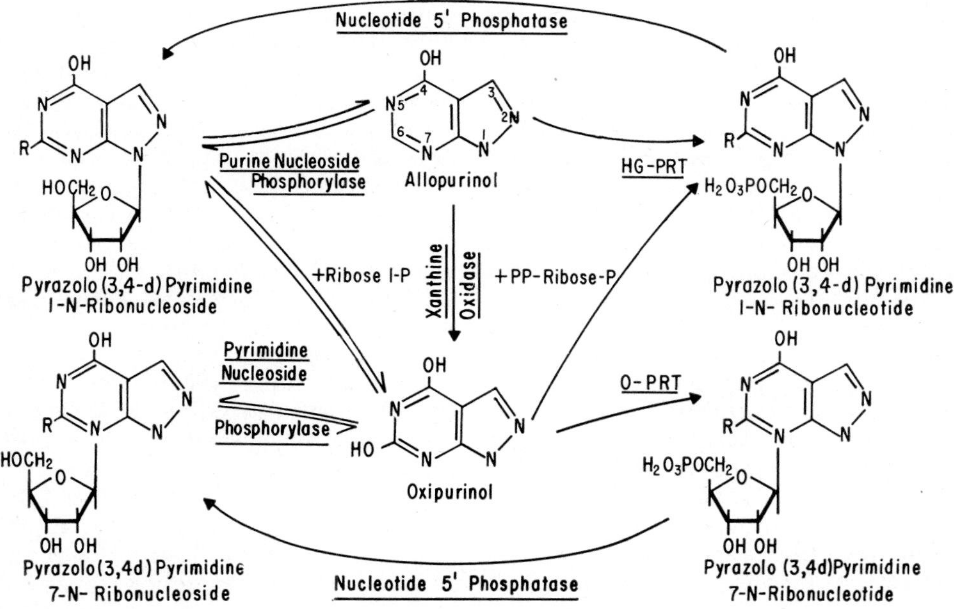

Fig. 58–8.—Reactions of allopurinol and of its oxidation product oxipurinol. Enzymes are underlined. R = H-(allopurinol) or HO-(oxipurinol).

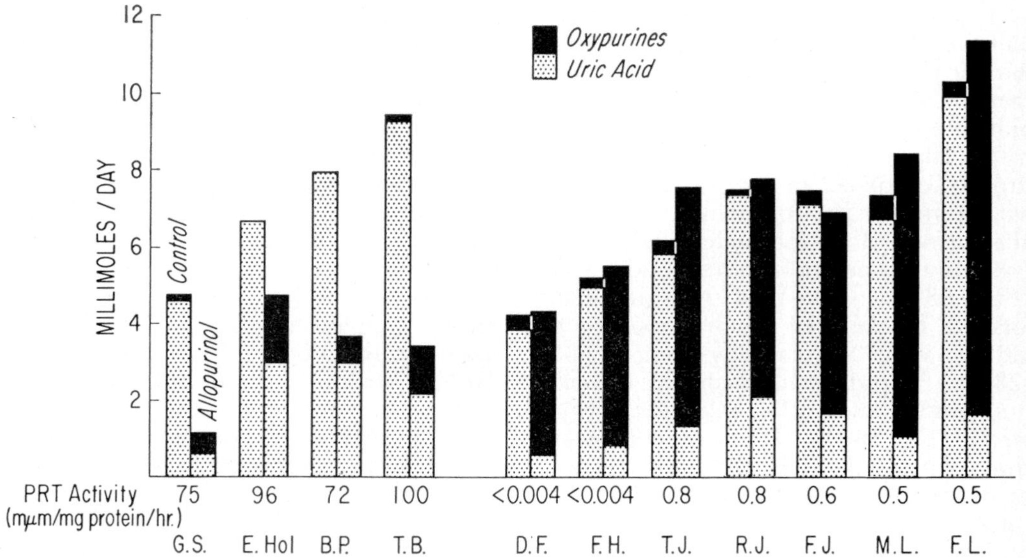

Fig. 58–9.—Effects of allopurinol on total purine excretion in patients who produce excessive quantities of uric acid. Comparison in patients with normal, virtually completely deficient, and partially deficient hypoxanthine-guanine phosphoribosyltransferase (PRT) activity. The height of each bar represents total purine excretion, oxypurines plus uric acid. (Reprinted from Kelley *et al.*[172] with permission of Ann. Intern. Med.)

purine levels achieved are well below the solubility limits of hypoxanthine or xanthine in serum.

More than one-half of the urinary oxypurine increase observed with allopurinol therapy consists of xanthine, a compound sparingly soluble in acid and neutral urine. The levels attained with full doses of allopurinol equal those which in xanthinuria subjects (who lack xanthine oxidase activity as an inborn error of metabolism) have caused the formation of urinary calculi composed of xanthine. Thus far, the development of xanthine crystalluria or lithiasis, as a complication of allopurinol therapy, has not been observed in any patient given the drug for treatment of gout or uric acid stones. Three instances of xanthine stone formation, induced by allopurinol therapy, have been reported in other circumstances. Two occurred in children with the Lesch-Nyhan syndrome[108,322] and the third in an adult patient with lymphosarcoma.[12] All three excreted approximately 1,500 mg. uric acid per day. One child, who received 9 mg. allopurinol per kg., excreted as much as 800 mg. xanthine per day while on therapy.[322,372] It appears that allopurinol should be given cautiously and in minimal doses to patients with extraordinarily great uric acid excretion values, particularly those with an inability to reutilize hypoxanthine and xanthine because of PRT deficiency.[372]

Effect of Allopurinol on Purine Synthesis De Novo.—In most patients, the replacement of urinary uric acid by oxypurines is less than stoichiometric.[143,282,285] The deficit ranges from 10 to 60 per cent and is roughly proportional to the pretreatment level of uric acid excretion.[143] The deficit may amount to several hundred milligrams of purines per day[285,388] (Fig. 58–9). In addition, the reduction in total purine excretion is associated with a decreased incorporation of isotopic glycine into urinary uric acid. These effects of allopurinol require the presence of hypoxanthine-guanine phosphoribosyltransferase[172,174] and may be due to a combination of factors, including an increased conversion of hypoxanthine to IMP,[282] the inhibitory action of purine ribonucleotides derived from IMP, or of allopurinol ribonucleotide, upon glutamine-PP-ribose-P-amidotransferase,[52,202] and to the depletion of PP-ribose-P which is an essential substrate for this enzyme.[91]

The administration of allopurinol leads to a substantial reduction of erythrocyte PP-ribose-P content within 3 to 5 hours.[91] This effect is due to the consumption of PP-ribose-P resulting from the conversion of allopurinol to its ribonucleotide. It is probably not attributable to the increased reutilization of hypoxanthine and xanthine, since erythrocytes do not contain xanthine oxidase activity. PP-ribose-P levels do not fall after oxipurinol administration.[91]

Effect of Allopurinol on Pyrimidine Synthesis De Novo.—The administration of allopurinol or oxipurinol in man is accompanied by a significant increase in the excretion of orotidine and orotic acid.[92,168,178] Studies *in vivo* and in cell culture demonstrate that this effect results from the inhibition of orotidylic decarboxylase which catalyzes a step in the conversion of orotic acid to uridine-5′-monophosphate (UMP). Allopurinol 1-N-ribonucleotide and xanthine ribonucleotide, which can be formed by action of HG-PRT, and oxipurinol-7-ribonucleotide, which can be formed by action of orotate phosphoribosyltransferase (O-PRT),[128] are potent inhibitors of orotidylic decarboxylase.[168]

Effects of Allopurinol in Patients Deficient in Hypoxanthine-guanine Phosphoribosyltransferase Activity.—Allopurinol exerts its predicted effect upon xanthine oxidase in PRT-deficient subjects. Uric acid levels in blood and urine are reduced and urinary oxypurines are increased. However, in contrast to results in other subjects, there is a stoichiometric replacement of urinary uric acid by hypoxanthine and xanthine in PRT-deficient subjects[172,174,321] (Fig. 58–9). Similarly, no reduction of total purine excretion occurs in response to azathioprine.[175] These anomalous responses are attributed to the PRT deficiency itself, as inhibition of purine synthesis *de novo* requires prior conversion of these analogue bases or of oxypurines to ribonucleotide form.[35,36,202] No reduction of intracellular PP-ribose-P content occurs on incubation of PRT-deficient erythrocytes with allopurinol.[91]

In spite of the PRT deficiency, allopurinol does result in orotidinuria in children with the Lesch-Nyhan syndrome.[19] Furthermore, in PRT-deficient fibroblasts studied *in vitro*, high concentrations of both allopurinol and oxipurinol inhibit an early step of purine synthesis *de novo*, probably glutamine-PP-ribose-P-amidotransferase.[177] These effects probably involve the formation of oxipurinol 7-N-ribonucleotide in the reaction catalyzed by O-PRT.

BIBLIOGRAPHY

1. Acheson, R. M., Chan, Y. K.: J. Chron. Dis., *21*, 543, 1969.
2. Alvsaker, J. O.: J. Clin. Invest., *47*, 1254, 1968.
3. ———: Scand. J. Clin. Lab. Invest., *17*, 467, 1965.
4. ———: Scand. J. Clin. Lab. Invest., *17*, 476, 1965.
5. ———: Scand. J. Clin. Lab. Invest., *18*, 227, 1966.
6. Aronoff, A.: New Engl. J. Med., *262*, 767, 1960.
7. Atsmon, A., de Vries, A., and Frank, M.: *Uric Acid Lithiasis*, Elsevier, Amsterdam, 1963.
8. Atsmon, A., de Vries, A., Lazebnik, J., and Salinger, H.: Amer. J. Med., *27*, 167, 1959.
9. Ball, G. V., Morgan, J. M.: Southern Med. J., *61*, 21, 1968.
10. Ball, G. V., and Sorensen, L. B.: Arth. & Rheum., *13*, 846, 1970.
11. ———: New Engl. J. Med., *280*, 1199, 1969.
12. Band, P. R., Silverberg, D. S., Henderson, J. F., Ulan, R. A., Wensel, R. H., Banerjee, T. K., and Little, A. S.: New Engl. J. Med., *283*, 354, 1970.
13. Barlow, K. A.: Metabolism, *17*, 289, 1968.
14. Barlow, K. A., and Beilin, L. J.: Quart. J. Med., *37*, 79, 1968.

15. Bartels, E. C.: Postgrad. Med., *15*, 254, 1954.
16. ———: Surg. Clin. North America, *38*, 847, 1957.
17. Bartels, E. C., and Matossian, G. S.: Arth. & Rheum., *2*, 193, 1959.
18. Barzel, U. S., Sperling, O., Frank, M., and de Vries, A.: J. Urol., *92*, 1, 1964.
19. Beardmore, T. D., Fox, I. H., and Kelley, W. N.: Lancet, *2*, 830, 1970.
20. Benedict, J. D., Forsham, P. H., Roche, M., Soloway, S., and Stetten, DeW., Jr.: J. Clin. Invest., *29*, 1104, 1950.
21. Benedict, J. D., Forsham, P. H., and Stetten, DeW., Jr.: J. Biol. Chem., *181*, 183, 1949.
22. Benedict, J. D., Roche, M., Yü, T. F., Bien, E. J., Gutman, A. B., and Stetten, DeW., Jr.: Metabolism, *1*, 3, 1952.
23. Benedict, J. D., Yü, T. F., Bien, E. J., Gutman, A. B., and Stetten, DeW., Jr.: J. Clin. Invest., *32*, 775, 1953.
24. Bennett, R. C., and Jepson, R. P.: Austral. and New Zealand J. Surg., *36*, 153, 1966.
25. Berliner, R. W., Hilton, J. G., Yü, T. F., and Kennedy, T. J., Jr.: J. Clin. Invest., *219*, 396, 1950.
26. Bien, E. J., Yü, T. F., Benedict, J. D., Gutman, A. B., and Stetten, D., Jr.: J. Clin. Invest., *32*, 778, 1953.
27. Bishop, C., Garner, W., and Talbott, J. H.: J. Clin. Invest., *30*, 879, 1951.
28. Bishop, C., Rand, R., and Talbott, J. H.: J. Clin. Invest., *30*, 889, 1951.
29. Bluestone, R., Kippen, I., and Klinenberg, J. R.: Brit. Med. J., *4*, 590, 1969.
30. Bluestone, R., Kippen, I., Klinenberg, J. R., and Whitehouse, M. W.: J. Lab. Clin. Med., *76*, 85–91, 1970.
31. Borisy, G. G., and Taylor, E. W.: J. Cell Biol., *34*, 525, 1967.
32. Brandenberger, E., De Quervain, F., and Schinz, H. R.: Helvet. med. acta, *118*, 195, 1947.
33. Breckenridge, A.: Lancet, *1*, 15, 1966.
34. Brochner-Mortensen, K.: *Epidemiology of Chronic Rheumatism*, Philadelphia, Davis, vol. 1, P. 140, 1963.
35. Brockman, R. W.: *Exploitable Molecular Mechanisms and Neoplasia*, Baltimore, Williams & Wilkins Co., 1969, pp. 435–464.
36. Brockman, R. W., and Chumley, S.: Biochim. Biophys. Acta, *95*, 365, 1965.
37. Bronsky, D., and Bernstein, A.: Ann. Intern. Med., *41*, 820, 1954.
38. Brown, J., and Mallory, G. K.: New Engl. J. Med., *243*, 325, 1950.
39. Brugsch, T., and Citron, J.: Ztschr. exper. Path. u. Therap., *5*, 401, 1908.
40. Buchanan, W. W., Klinenberg, J. R., and Seegmiller, J. E.: Arth. & Rheum., *8*, 361, 1965.
41. Bunin, J. J., Kimberg, D. V., Thomas, L. B., Van Scott, E. J., and Klatskin, G.: Ann. Intern. Med., *57*, 1018, 1962.
42. Burch, T. A., O Brien, W. M., Need, R., and Kurland, L. T.: Ann. Rheum. Dis., *25*, 144, 1966.
43. Burns, J. J., Yü, T. F., Berger, L., and Gutman, A. B.: Amer. J. Med., *25*, 401, 1958.
44. Burns, J. J., Yü, T. F., Ritterband, A., Perel, J. M., Gutman, A. B., and Brodie, B. B.: J. Pharmacol. Exper. Therap., *119*, 418, 1957.
45. Buzard, J., Bishop, C., and Talbott, J. H.: J. Biol. Chem., *196*, 179, 1952.
46. Bywaters, E. G. L.: Ann. Rheum. Dis., *21*, 325, 1962.
47. Bywaters, E. G. L., Dixon, A. St. J., and Scott, J. T.: Ann. Rheum. Dis., *22*, 171, 1963.
48. Caner, J. E. Z., and Decker, J. L.: Amer. J. Med., *36*, 571, 1964.
49. Cannon, P. J., Stason, W. B., Demartini, F. E., Sommers, S. C., and Laragh, J. H.: New Engl. J. Med., *275*, 457, 1966.
50. Cannon, P. J., Svahn, D. S., and Demartini, F. E.: Circulation, *41*, 97, 1970.
51. Carcassi, A., Marcolongo, R., Jr., Marinello, E., Riario-Sforza, G., and Boggiano, C.: Arth. & Rheum., *12*, 17–20, 1969.
52. Caskey, C. T., Ashton, D. M., and Wyngaarden, J. B.: J. Biol. Chem., *239*, 2570, 1964.
53. Chang, Y.-H., and Gralla, E. J.: Arth. & Rheum., *11*, 145, 1968.
54. Chetrick, A.: J.A.M.A., *186*, 950, 1963.
55. Clarke, A. M., and McKenzie, R. G.: Lancet, *2*, 395, 1969.
56. Cobb, S.: *The Epidemiology of Chronic Rheumatism*, Philadelphia, Davis, vol. 1, p. 182, 1963.
57. Cohen, H.: *Textbook of the Rheumatic Diseases*, ed. W. S. C. Copeman, Edinburgh, Livingstone, 1955, p. 361.
58. Cristotori, F. C., and Duncan, G. G.: Metabolism, *13*, 303, 1964.
59. Crowley, L. V. and Alton, F. I.: Amer. J. Clin.. Path., *49*, 285, 1968.
60. Decker, J. L., Lane, J. J., Jr., and Reynolds, W. E.: Arth. & Rheum., *5*, 144, 1962.

61. Delbarre, F., Auscher, C., Brouilhet, H., and de Géry, A.: La Semaine des Hopitaux, *43*, 659, 1967.
62. Delbarre, F., Auscher, C. and DuLac, Y.: Rein foie, *6*, 53, 1964.
63. Delbarre, F., Auscher, C., Olivier, J. L., and Rose, A.: La Semaine des Hopitaux, *43*, 1127, 1967.
64. Delbarre, F., Braun, S., and Saint-Georges-Chaumet, F.: La Semaine des Hopitaux, *43*, 623, 1967.
65. Demartini, F. E., Wheaton, E. A., Healey, L. A., and Laragh, J. H.: Amer. J. Med., *32*, 572, 1962.
66. Deren, J. J., Porush, J. G., Levitt, M. F., and Khilnani, M. T.: Ann. Intern. Med., *56*, 843, 1962.
67. de Vries, A., Frank, M., and Atsmon, A.: Amer. J. Med., *33*, 880, 1962.
68. Dollery, C. T., Duncan, H., and Schumer, B.: Brit. Med. J., *2*, 832, 1960.
69. Drenick, E. J., Swenseid, M. E., Blahd, W. H., and Tuttle, S. G.: J.A.M.A., *187*, 100, 1964.
70. Duncan, H., and Dixon, A. St. J.: Quart. J. Med., *29*, 127, 1960.
71. Ebstein, W.: *Die Natur und Behandlung der Gicht*, Wiesbaden, Bergmann, 1906.
72. Eisen, A. Z., and Seegmiller, J. E.: J. Clin. Invest., *40*, 1486, 1961.
73. Elion, G. B.: Ann. Rheum. Dis., *25*, 608, 1966.
74. Elion, G. B., Kovensky, A., Hitchings, G. H., Metz, E., and Rundles, R. W.: Biochem. Pharmacol., *15*, 863, 1966.
75. Elion, G. B., Yü, T. F., Gutman, A. B., and Hitchings, G. H.: Amer. J. Med., *45*, 69, 1968.
76. Emmerson, B. T.: Australasian Ann. Med., *12*, 310, 1963.
77. ————: Ann. Rheum. Dis., *25*, 622, 1966.
78. ————: Arth. & Rheum., *11*, 623, 1968.
79. Emmerson, B. T., and Sandilands, P.: Australasian Ann. Med., *12*, 46, 1963.
80. Emmerson, B. T., and Wyngaarden, J. B.: Science, *166*, 1533, 1969.
81. ————: In preparation.
82. Evans, J. G., Prior, I. A. M., and Harvey, H. P. B.: Ann. Rheum. Dis., *27*, 319, 1968.
83. Faires, J. S., and McCarty, D. J., Jr.: Arth. & Rheum., *5*, 295, 1962.
84. Fallon, H. J., Frei, E., III, Block, J., and Seegmiller, J. E.: J. Clin. Invest., *40*, 1906, 1961.
85. Fanelli, G. M., Jr., Bohn, D., and Stafford, S.: Amer. J. Physiol., *218*, 627, 1970.
86. Fineberg, S. K., and Altschul, A.: Ann. Intern. Med., *44*, 1182, 1956.
87. Folin, O., Berglund, H., and Derick, C.: J. Biol. Chem., *60*, 361, 1924.
88. Folin, O., and Lyman, H.: J. Pharmacol., *4*, 539, 1913.
89. Forster, H., Meyer, E., and Ziege, M.: Klin. Wschr., *48*, 14, 1970.
90. Fox, I. and Kelley, W. N.: Ann. Intern. Med., *74*, 424, 1971.
91. Fox, I. H., Wyngaarden, J. B., and Kelley, W. N.: New Engl. J. Med., *383*, 1177, 1970.
92. Fox, R. M., Royse-Smith, D. and O'Sullivan, W. J.: Science, *168*, 861, 1970.
93. Frank, M., de Vries, A., Atsmon, A., and Kochwa, S.: Israel Med. J., *12*, 299, 1960.
94. Freudweiler, M.: Deutsch. Arch. klin. Med., *63*, 266, 1899.
95. ————: Deutsch. Arch. klin. Med., *69*, 155, 1901.
96. Fridovich, I.: Biochemistry, *4*, 1098, 1965.
97. Fruhman, G. J.: Proc. Soc. Exper. Biol. Med., *104*, 284, 1960.
98. Garrod, A. B.: *The Nature and Treatment of Gout and Rheumatic Gout*, London, Walton and Maberly, 1863, p. 251.
99. ————: Tr. M.-Chir. Soc. Edinburgh, *31*, 83, 1848.
100. ————: Tr. M.-Chir. Soc. Edinburgh, *37*, 49, 1854.
101. ————: *A Treatise on Gout and Somatic Gout* (*Rheumatoid Arthritis*), 3d ed., London, Longmans, 1876.
102. Gold, M. S., Williams, J. C., Spivack, M., and Guann, V.: J.A.M.A., *206*, 1572, 1968.
103. Goldfinger, S., Klinenberg, J. R., and Seegmiller, J. E.: New Engl. J. Med., *272*, 351, 1965.
104. Goldthwait, J. C., Butler, C. F., and Stillman, J. S.: New Engl. J. Med., *259*, 1095, 1958.
105. Gonick, H. C., Rubini, M. E., Gleason, I. O., and Sommers, S. C.: Ann. Intern. Med., *62*, 667, 1965.
106. Greenbaum, D., Ross, J. H., and Steinberg, V. L.: Brit. Med. J., *1*, 1502, 1961.
107. Greene, M. L., Boyles, J. R., Seegmiller, J E.: Science, *167*, 887, 1970.
108. Greene, M. L., Fujimoto, W. Y., and Seegmiller, J. E.: New Engl. J. Med., *280*, 426, 1969.
109. Greene, M. L., and Seegmiller, J. E.: J. Clin. Invest., *48*, 32a, 1969.
110. Gutman, A. B.: Ann. Intern. Med., *39*, 1062, 1953.
111. Gutman, A. B., and Yü, T.-F.: Advances Intern. Med., *5*, 27, 1952.

112. ———: Amer. J. Med., *23*, 600, 1957.
113. ———: Tr. Assoc. Amer. Physicians, *74*, 353, 1961.
114. ———: Ann. Intern. Med., *56*, 675, 1962.
115. ———: Amer. J. Med., *35*, 820, 1963.
116. ———: Tr. Assoc. Amer. Physicians, *76*, 141, 1963.
117. ———: J. Clin. Invest., *44*, 1474, 1965.
118. ———: Amer. J. Med., *45*, 756, 1968.
119. Gutman, A. B., Yü, T.-F., Adler, M., and Javitt, N. B.: J. Clin. Invest., *41*, 623, 1962.
120. Gutman, A. B., Yü, T.-F., and Berger, L.: J. Clin. Invest., *38*, 1778, 1959.
121. Gutman, A., Yü, T.-F., and Berger, L.: Amer. J. Med., *47*, 575, 1969.
122. Hall, A. P.: Arth. & Rheum., *8*, 846, 1965.
123. Hall, A. P., Barry, P. E., Dawber, T. R., and McNamara, M.: Amer. J. Med., *42*, 27, 1967.
124. Hansen, O. E., and Holten, C.: Lancet, *1*, 1047, 1958.
125. Harkness, R. A., and Nicol, A. D.: Arch. Dis. Childhood, *44*, 773, 1969.
126. Harth, M., and Robinson, C. E. G.: Mil. Serv. J. Canada, *18*, 671, 1962.
127. Hartung, E. F.: Metabolism, *6*, 196, 1957.
128. Hatfield, D., and Wyngaarden, J. B.: J. Biol. Chem., *239*, 2580, 1964.
129. Hauge, M., and Harvald, B.: Acta med. scandinav., *152*, 247, 1955.
130. Healey, L. A.: Arth. & Rheum., *7*, 313, 1964.
131. Healey, L. A., and Hall, A. P.: Bull. Rheum. Dis., *20*, 600, 1970.
132. Healey, L. A., Harrison, M., and Decker, J. L.: New Engl. J. Med., *272*, 526, 1965.
133. Hellman, L.: Science, *109*, 280, 1949.
134. Hench, P. S.: J. Lab. Clin. Med., *220*, 48, 1936.
135. Henderson, J. F., Brox, L. W., Kelley, W. N., Rosenbloom, F. M., and Seegmiller, J. E.: J. Biol. Chem., *243*, 2514, 1968.
136. Henderson, J. F. and Khoo, K. Y.: J. Biol. Chem., *240*, 2349, 1965.
137. Henderson, J. F., Rosenbloom, F. M., Kelley, W. N., and Seegmiller, J. E.: J. Clin. Invest., *47*, 1511, 1968.
138. Henneman, P. H., Wallach, S., and Dempsey, E. F.: J. Clin. Invest., *41*, 537, 1962.
139. Hershko, A., Hershko, C. and Mager, J.: Israel Med. J., *4*, 939, 1968.
140. Hickling, R. A.: Lancet, *1*, 57, 1953.
141. Hill, D. L., and Bennett, L. L., Jr.: Biochemistry, *8*, 122, 1969.
142. His, W. J.: Deutsch. Arch. klin. Med., *67*, 81, 1900.
143. Hitchings, G. H.: Ann. Rheum. Dis., *25*, 601, 1966.
144. Hoffman, W. S.: Med. Clin. North America, *43*, 595, 1959.
144*a*. Hollander, J. L.: In *Arthritis and Allied Conditions*, 8th ed., Philadelphia, Lea & Febiger, 1972, p. 10.
145. Hoppe, D.: Deutsch. Gesundheitsw., *12*, 896, 1957.
146. Hori, M., and Henderson, J. F.: J. Biol. Chem., *251*, 3404, 1966.
147. Houpt, J. B., and Ogryzlo, M. A.: Arth. & Rheum., *7*, 316, 1964.
148. Howell, D. S.: Arth. & Rheum., *8*, 736, 1965.
149. Howell, R. R., Ashton, D. M., and Wyngaarden, J. B.: Pediatrics, *29*, 553, 1962.
150. Howell, R. R., Eanes, E. D., and Seegmiller, J. E.: Arth. & Rheum., *6*, 97, 1963.
151. Howell, R. R., and Seegmiller, J. E.: Arth. & Rheum., *5*, 303, 1962.
152. Itskovitz, H. D., and Sellers, A. M.: New Engl. J. Med., *268*, 1105, 1963.
153. Iwata, H., Yamamoto, I., and Muraki, K.: Biochem. Pharmacol., *15*, 955, 1969.
154. Jacobson, B. M.: Ann. Intern. Med., *11*, 1277, 1937.
155. Jakovcic, S. and Sorensen, L. B.: Arth. & Rheum., *10*, 129, 1967.
156. Jeandet, J., and Lestradet, H.: Rev. franç. etude clin. et biol., *6*, 71, 1961.
157. Jeune, M., Charrat, A., and Bertrand, J.: Arch. franç. pediat., *14*, 897, 1957.
158. Jones, O. W., Jr., Ashton, D. M., and Wyngaarden, J. B.: J. Clin. Invest., *41*, 1805, 1962.
159. Kaplan, D., Bernstein, D., Wallace, S. L., and Halberstam, D.: Ann. Intern. Med., *62*, 658, 1965.
160. Kaplan, D., Diamond, H., Wallace, S. L., and Halberstam, D.: Ann. Rheum. Dis., *28*, 180, 1969.
161. Kaplan, H.: New Engl. J. Med., *268*, 761, 1963.
162. Kaplan, H., and Klatskin, G.: Yale J. Biol. Med., *32*, 335, 1960.
163. Katz, W. A., and Schubert, M.: J. Clin. Invest., *49*, 1783, 1970.
164. Kellermeyer, R. W.: Arth. & Rheum., *11*, 452, 1968.
165. Kellermeyer, R. W., and Breckenridge, R. T.: J. Lab. Clin. Med., *65*, 307, 1965.
166. ———: J. Lab. Clin. Med., *67*, 455, 1966.
167. Kellermeyer, R. W.: J. Lab. Clin. Med., *70*, 372, 1967.
168. Kelley, W. N. and Beardmore, T. D.: Science, *169*, 388, 1970.

169. Kelley, W. N., Fox, I. H., and Wyngaarden, J. B.: Clin. Res., *18*, 457, 1970.
170. Kelley, W. N., Fox, I. H. and Wyngaarden, J. B.: Biochim. Biophys. Acta, *215*, 512, 1970.
171. Kelley, W. N., Greene, M. L., Fox, I. H., Rosenbloom, F. M., Levy, R. I., and Seegmiller, J. E.: Metabolism, *19*, 1025, 1970.
172. Kelley, W. N., Greene, M. L., Rosenbloom, F. M., Henderson, J. F., and Seegmiller, J. E.: Ann. Intern. Med., *70*, 155, 1969.
173. Kelley, W. N., Rosenbloom, F. M., Henderson, J. F., and Seegmiller, J. E.: Proc. Nat. Acad. Sci., *57*, 1735, 1967.
174. Kelley, W. N., Rosenbloom, F. M., Miller, J., and Seegmiller, J. E.: New Engl. J. Med., *278*, 287, 1968.
175. Kelley, W. N., Rosenbloom, F. M., and Seegmiller, J. E.: J. Clin. Invest., *46*, 1518, 1967.
176. Kelley, W. N., Rosenbloom, F. M., Seegmiller, J. E., and Howell, R. R.: J. Pediat., *72*, 488, 1968.
177. Kelley, W. N., and Wyngaarden, J. B.: J. Clin. Invest., *49*, 602, 1970.
178. ————: Clin. Chem., *16*, 707, 1970.
179. Kessler, R. H., Hierholzer, K., and Gurd, R. S.: Amer. J. Physiol., *197*, 601, 1959.
180. Kinsey, D.: Arth. & Rheum., *6*, 778, 1963.
181. Klinenberg, J. R., and Kippen, I.: J. Lab. Clin. Med., *75*, 503, 1970.
182. Kogut, M. D., Donnell, G. N., Nyhan, W. L., and Sweetman, L.: Amer. J. Med., *48*, 148, 1970.
183. Koshoff, Y. D., Morris, L. E., and Lubic, L. G.: J.A.M.A., *152*, 37, 1953.
184. Kramp, R. A., Lassiter, W. E., and Gottschalk, C. W.: J. Clin. Invest., *50*, 35, 1971.
184*a*. Krenitsky, T. A., Elion, G. B., Strelitz, R. A., and Hitchings, G. H.: J. Biol. Chem., *242*, 2675, 1967.
185. Lassen, U. K.: Biochem. biophys. acta, *53*, 557, 1961.
186. Laster, L., and Muller, A. F.: Amer. J. Med., *15*, 857, 1953.
187. Lathem, W., and Rodnan, G. P.: J. Clin. Invest., *41*, 1955, 1962.
188. Lathem, W., Davis, B. B., and Rodnan, G. P.: Amer. J. Physiol., *199*, 9, 1960.
189. Lawrence, J. S.: Proc. Roy. Soc. Med., *53*, 522, 1960.
190. Lennane, G. A. Q., Rose, B. S., and Isdale, I. C.: Ann. Rheum. Dis., *19*, 120, 1960.
191. Lennox, W. G.: J.A.M.A., *82*, 602, 1924.
192. Levine, M.: Ann. N.Y. Acad. Sci., *51*, 1406, 1951.
193. Lichtenstein, L., Scott, H. W., and Levin, M. H.: Amer. J. Path., *32*, 871, 1956.
194. Lieber, C. S., and Davidson, C. S.: Amer. J. Med., *33*, 319, 1962.
195. Lieber, C. S., Jones, D. P., Losowsky, M. S., and Davidson, C. S.: J. Clin. Invest., *41*, 1863, 1962.
196. Long, W. K.: Science, *138*, 991, 1962.
197. ————: Science, *155*, 712, 1967.
198. Ludwig, A. P., Bennett, G. A., and Bauer, W.: Ann. Intern. Med., *11*, 1248, 1938.
199. Lynch, E. C.: Arch. Intern. Med., *109*, 639, 1962.
200. McCarty, D. J., Jr.: Arth. & Rheum., *4*, 425, 1961.
201. McCarty, D. J., Jr., and Hollander, J. L.: Ann. Intern. Med., *54*, 452, 1961.
202. McCollister, R. J., Gilbert, W. R., Jr., Ashton, D. M., and Wyngaarden, J. B.: J. Biol. Chem., *239*, 1560, 1964.
203. McCollum, D. E., Mathews, R. S., and O Neil, M. T.: South. Med. J., *63*, 241, 1970.
204. MacLachlan, M. J., and Rodnan, G. P.: Amer. J. Med., *42*, 38, 1967.
205. Mäenpââ, P. H., Raivio, K. O., Kekomäki, M. P.: Science, *161*, 1253, 1968.
206. Malawista, S. E.: Arth. & Rheum., *11*, 191, 1968.
207. ————: Arth. & Rheum., *7*, 325, 1964.
208. ————: Arth. & Rheum., *8*, 752, 1965.
209. Malawista, S. E., and Bodel, P. T.: J. Clin. Invest., *46*, 786, 1967.
210. Malawista, S. E., Howell, R. R., and Seegmiller, J. E.: Arth. & Rheum., *5*, 307, 1962.
211. Malawista, S. E., and Seegmiller, J. E.: Ann. Intern. Med., *62*, 648, 1965.
212. Malawista, S. E., Seegmiller, J. E., Hathaway, E., and Sokoloff, L.: J.A.M.A., *194*, 954, 1965.
213. March, H. W., Schlyen, S. M., and Schwartz, S. E.: Amer. J. Med., *13*, 46, 1952.
214. Marson, F. G. W.: Quart. J. Med., *22*, 331, 1953.
215. Massey, V., Komai, H., Palmer, G., and Elion, G.: J. Biol. Chem., *245*, 2837, 1970.
216. Mayne, J. G.: Ann. Rheum. Dis., *15*, 61, 1965.
217. Melmon, K. L., and Cline, M. J.: Biochem. Pharmacol., *17*, 271, 1968.
218. Melmon, K., Webster, M. E., Goldfinger, S. E., and Seegmiller, J. E.: Arth. & Rheum., *10*, 13, 1967.

219. Metcalfe-Gibson, A., McCallum, F. M., Morrison, R. B. I., and Wrong, O.: Clin. Sci., *28*, 325, 1965.
220. Migeon, B. R.: Biochem. Genet., *4*, 377, 1970.
221. Migeon, B. R., Der Kaloustian, V. M., Nyhan, W. L., Young, W. J., and Childs, B.: Science, *160*, 425, 1968.
222. Mikkelsen, W. M., Dodge, H. J., and Valkenburg, H.: Amer. J. Med., *39*, 242, 1965.
223. Mintz, D. H., Canary, J. J., Carreon, G., and Kyle, L. H.: New Engl. J. Med., *265*, 112, 1961.
224. Modern, F. W. S., and Meister, L.: Med. Clin. North America, *36*, 941, 1952.
225. Moskowitz, R. W., Vertes, V., Schwartz, A., Marshall, G., and Friedman, B.: Amer. J. Med., *47*, 450, 1969.
226. Mudge, G. H., McAlary, B., and Berndt, W. O.: Amer. J. Physiol., *214*, 875, 1968.
227. Mugler, A.: Ann. méd., *51*, 495, 1950.
228. ————: Congrès international de la goutte et de la lithiasis urique, p. 283, Evian, 1964.
229. Myers, A., Epstein, F. H., Dodge, H. J., and Mikkelsen, W. M.: Amer. J. Med., *45*, 520, 1968.
230. Mugler, A., Pernet, A., and Friedrich, S.: *Contemporary Rheumatology*, ed. J. Goslings and H. Van Swaay, Amsterdam, Elsevier, 1956, p. 574.
231. Naff, G. B., and Byers, P. H.: J. Clin. Invest., *46*, 1099, 1967.
232. Naimark, A., and Fyles, T. W.: Canad. Med. Assoc. J., *83*, 819, 1960.
233. Nathan, L. A., Kubota, C. K., and Turnbull, G. C.: J. Lab. Clin. Med., *42*, 927, 1953.
234. Neel, J. V.: Medicine, *26*, 115, 1947.
235. Neel, J. V., Rakie, M. T., Davidson, R. I., Valkenburg, J. A., and Mikkelsen, W. M.: Amer. J. Hum. Genet., *17*, 14, 1965.
236. Neuwirth, E.: Arch. Intern. Med., *72*, 377, 1943.
237. Nugent, C. A., MacDiarmid, W. D., and Tyler, F. H.: Arch. Intern. Med., *113*, 165, 1964.
238. ————: Arch. Intern. Med., *109*, 54, 1962.
239. Nugent, C. A., and Tyler, F. H.: J. Clin. Invest., *38*, 1890, 1959.
240. O Brien, W. M., Burch, T. A., and Bunim, J. J.: Ann. Rheum. Dis., *25*, 117, 1966.
241. Pagliara, A. S., and Goodman, A. D.: New Engl. J. Med., *281*, 767, 1969.
242. Paik, C. H., Alavi, I., Dunea, G., and Weiner, L.: J.A.M.A., *213*, 296, 1970.
243. Pak Roy, R. K.: Australasian Ann. Med., *14*, 35, 1965.
244. Paulus, H. E., Coutts, A., Calabro, J. J., and Klinenberg, J. R.: J.A.M.A., *211*, 277, 1970.
245. Pearson, G.: Phil. Tr. London, *88*, 15, 1798.
246. Perheentupa, J., and Raivio, K.: Lancet, *2*, 528, 1967.
247. Peters, J. P., and Van Slyke, K. K.: *Quantitative Clinical Chemistry*, 2d ed., Baltimore, Williams & Wilkins, 1946, vol. 1, p. 937.
248. Phelps, P.: Arth. & Rheum., *12*, 197, 1969.
249. ————: Arth. & Rheum., *12*, 189, 1969.
250. ————: J. Lab. Clin. Med., *76*, 622, 1970.
251. ————: Arth. & Rheum., *13*, 1, 1970.
252. Phelps, P., and McCarty, D. J., Jr.: J. Exper. Med., *124*, 115, 1966.
253. Phelps, P., Prokop, D. J., and McCarty, D. J.: J. Lab. Clin. Med., *68*, 433, 1966.
254. Phelps, P., Steele, A. D., and McCarty, D. J., Jr.: J.A.M.A., *203*, 508, 1968.
255. Plante, G. E., Durivage, J., and Lemieux, G.: Metabolism, *17*, 377, 1968.
256. Podevin, R., Ardaillou, R., Paillard, F., Fontanelle, J., and Richet, G.: Nephron, *5*, 134, 1968.
257. Pollak, V. E., and Mattenheimer, H.: J. Lab. Clin. Med., *66*, 564, 1965.
258. Pollycove, M., Tolbert, B. M., Lawrence, J. H., and Harman, D.: Clin. Res. Proc., *5*, 38, 1957.
259. Popert, A. I., and Hewitt, J. V.: Ann. Rheum. Dis., *20*, 154, 1962.
260. Postlethwaite, A. E., and Kelley, W. N.: Ann. Intern. Med., *74*, 845, 1971.
261. Poulsen, H., and Praetorius, E.: Acta pharmacol. et toxicol., *10*, 371, 1954.
262. Praetorius, E., and Kirk, J. E.: J. Lab. Clin. Med., *35*, 865, 1950.
263. Prien, E. L., and Prien, E. L., Jr.: Amer. J. Med., *45*, 654, 1968.
264. Prior, I. A. M., and Rose, B. S.: New Zealand Med. J., *65*, 295, 1966.
265. Prior, I. A. M., Rose, B. S., Harvey, H. P. B., and Davidson, F.: Lancet, *1*, 333, 1966.
266. Raivio, K. O., and Seegmiller, J. E.: Clin. Res., *19*, 161, 1971.
267. Rajan, K. T.: Nature, *210*, 959, 1966.
268. Rakic, M. T., Valkenburg, H. A., Davidson, R. T., Engels, J. P., Mikkelsen, W. M., Neel, J. V., and Duff, I. F.: Amer. J. Med., *37*, 862, 1964.

269. Richet, G., Albahary, C., Ardaillou, R., Sultan, C., and Morel-Maroger, A.: Rev. franç, études clin. et biol., *9*, 188, 1964.
270. Richet, G., Ardaillou, R., De Montera, H., Slama, R., and Bougault, Th.: J. urol. et nephrol., *67*, 1, 1961.
271. Rieselbach, R. E., Bentzel, C. J., Cotlove, E., Frei, E., III, and Freireich, E. J.: Amer. J. Med., *37*, 872, 1964.
272. Rieselbach, R. E., Sorensen, L. B., Shelp, W. D., and Steele, T. H.: Ann. Intern. Med., *73*, 359, 1970.
273. Roberts, W.: Brit. Med. J., *2*, 61, 1892.
274. Robinson, W. D., Conn, J. W., Block, W. D., and Louis, L. H.: J. Lab. Clin. Med., *33*, 1473, 1948.
275. Rodnan, G. P.: Arth. & Rheum., *4*, 27, 1961.
276. Rosenbloom, F. M., Henderson, J. F., Caldwell, I. C., Kelley, W. N., and Seegmiller, J. E.: J. Biol. Chem., *243*, 1166, 1968.
277. Rosenbloom, F. M., Kelley, W. N., Henderson, J. F., and Seegmiller, J. E.: Lancet, *2*, 305, 1967.
278. Rowe, P. B., Coleman, M. C., and Wyngaarden, J. B.: Biochemistry, *9*, 1498, 1970.
279. Rowe, P. B., and Wyngaarden, J. B.: J. Biol. Chem., *243*, 6373, 1968.
280. ———: J. Biol. Chem., *241*, 5571, 1966.
281. Runcie, J., and Thomson, T. J.: Postgrad. Med. J., *45*, 251, 1969.
282. Rundles, R. W., Metz, E. N., and Silberman, H. R.: Ann. Intern. Med., *64*, 229, 1966.
283. Rundles, R. W., Silberman, H. R., Hitchings, G. H., and Elion, G. B.: Ann. Intern. Med., *60*, 717, 1964.
284. Rundles, R. W., Wyngaarden, J. B., Hitchings, G. H., and Elion, G. B.: Ann. Rev. Pharmacol., *9*, 345, 1969.
285. Rundles, R. W., Wyngaarden, J. B., Hitchings, G. H., Elion, G. B., and Silberman, H. R.: Tr. Assoc. Amer. Phys., *76*, 126, 1963.
286. Ryckewaert, A., Kuntz, D., Henrard, J.-C., Puel, M., and de Seze, S.: Presse Med., *77*, 1157, 1969.
287. Sala, G., Ballabio, C. B., Amira, A., Ratti, G., and Cirla, E.: *Contemporary Rheumatology*, ed. J. Goslings and H. Van Swaay, Amsterdam, Elsevier, 1956, p. 581.
288. Sarre, H.: *Congrès international de la goutte et de la lithiase urique*, Evian, 1964.
289. Saker, B. M., Tofler, O. B., Burvill, M. J., and Reilly, K. A.: Med. J. Austral., *1*, 1213, 1967.
290. Scheele, K. W.: *Opuscula*, *2*, 73, 1776.
291. Schirmeister, J., Man, N. K., and Hallauer, W.: *Progress in Nephrology*, ed. G. Peters and F. Roch-Ramel, Berlin-Heidelberg-New York, Springer-Verlag, 1969, p. 59.
292. Schnitker, M. A., and Richter, A. B.: Amer. J. Med. Sc., *192*, 241, 1936.
293. Scott, J. T., Dixon, A. St. J., and Bywaters, E. G. L.: Brit. Med. J., *5390*, 1070, 1964.
294. Scott, J. T., Holloway, V. P., Glass, H. I., and Arnot, R. N.: Ann. Rheum. Dis., *28*, 366, 1969.
295. Scott, J. T., and Pollard, A. C.: Ann. Rheum. Dis., *29*, 397, 1970.
296. Seegmiller, J. E.: In *Duncan's Diseases of Metabolism*, ed. P. K. Bondy, Philadelphia, W. B. Saunders & Co., 1969, p. 516.
297. Seegmiller, J. E., Grayzel, A. I., Howell, R. R., and Plato, C.: J. Clin. Invest., *41*, 1094, 1962.
298. Seegmiller, J. E., Grayzel, A. I., Laster, L., and Liddle, L.: J. Clin. Invest., *40*, 1304, 1961.
299. Seegmiller, J. E., and Howell, R. R.: Arth. & Rheum., *5*, 616, 1962.
300. Seegmiller, J. E., Howell, R. R., and Malawista, S. E.: J. Clin. Invest., *41*, 1399, 1962.
301. Seegmiller, J. E., Klinenberg, J. R., Miller, J., and Watts, R. W. E.: J. Clin. Invest., *47*, 1193, 1968.
302. Seegmiller, J. E., Laster, L., and Howell, R. R.: New Engl. J. Med., *268*, 712, 1963.
303. Seegmiller, J. E., Rosenbloom, F. M., and Kelley, W. N.: Science, *155*, 1682, 1967.
304. Segal, S., and Wyngaarden, J. B.: Proc. Soc. Exper. Biol. Med., *88*, 342, 1955.
305. Sérane, J., and Lederer, J.: Presse Méd., *63*, 335, 1955.
306. Shapiro, J. R., Klinenberg, J. R., Peck, W., Goldfinger, S. E., and Seegmiller, J. E.: Arth. & Rheum., *7*, 343, 1964.
307. Shelanski, M. L., and Taylor, E. W.: J. Cell. Biol., *34*, 549, 1967.
308. Silberman, H. R., and Wyngaarden, J. B.: Biochem. et biophys. acta, *47*, 178, 1961.
309. Simkin, P. A.: Arth. & Rheum., *12*, 332, 1969.
310. Simon, N. M., Smucker, J. E., O Connor, J., Jr., and Del Greco, F.: Circulation, *39*, 121, 1969.
311. Sirota, J. H., Yü, T.-F., and Gutman, A. B.: J. Clin. Invest., *31*, 692, 1952.
312. Smyth, C. J.: Metabolism, *6*, 218, 1957.
313. Smyth, C. J., Cotterman, C. W., and Freyberg, R. H.: J. Clin. Invest., *27*, 749, 1948.

314. Smyth, C. J., and Huffman, E. R.: Rocky Mountain Med. J., *52*, 513, 1955.
315. Smyth, C. J., Stecher, R. M., and Wolfson, W. Q.: Science, *108*, 514, 1948.
316. Sokoloff, L.: Metabolism, *6*, 230, 1957.
317. Sommerville, J.: Brit. Heart J., *23*, 31, 1961.
318. Sorensen, L. B.: Metabolism, *8*, 687, 1959.
319. ———: Arch. Intern. Med., *109*, 379, 1962.
320. ———: Proc. Nat. Acad. Sci., *55*, 571, 1966.
321. Sorensen, L. B., Kawahara, F., Chow, D., Benke, P. J., and Coben, L.: Arth. & Rheum., *13*, 835, 1970.
322. Sorensen, L., and Seegmiller, J. E.: Fed. Proc., *27*, 1097, 1968.
323. Sougin-Mibashin, R., and Horwitz, M.: Lancet, *1*, 1191, 1955.
324. Sperling, O., Frank, M., and De Vries, A.: Fev. Franc. etud. Clin. et Biol., *11*, 401, 1966.
325. Sperling, O., Frank, M., Ophir, R., Liberman, U. A., Adam, A., and De Vries, A.: Rev. Europ. Etudes Clin. Biol., *15*, 942, 1970.
326. Sperling, O., Kedem, O., and De Vries, A.: Rev. Franc etud. Clin. et Biol., *11*, 40, 1966.
327. Sperling, O., Ophir, R., and De Vries, A.: Rev. Europ. Etudes Clin. Biol., *16*, 147, 1971.
328. Sperling, O., and Wyngaarden, J. B.: In preparation.
329. Stecher, R. M., Hersh, A. H., and Solomon, W. M.: Ann. Intern. Med., *31*, 595, 1949.
330. Steele, T. H.: J. Lab. Clin. Med., *74*, 288, 1969.
331. Steele, T. H., and Oppenheimer, S.: Amer. J. Med., *47*, 564, 1969.
332. Steele, T. H., and Rieselbach, R. E.: Amer. J. Med., *43*, 876, 1967.
333. ———: Amer. J. Med., *43*, 868, 1967.
334. Stirpe, F., Corte, E. D., Bonetti, E., Abbondanza, A., Abbati, A., and de Stefano, F.: Lancet, *2*, 1310, 1970.
335. Suki, W. N., Hull, A. R., Rector, F. C., Jr., and Seldin, D. W.: J. Clin. Invest., *46*, 1121, 1967.
336. Sydenham, T.: *Tractatus de podagra et hydrope*, London, G. Kettilby, 1683.
337. Sydenham, T.: *The Works of Thomas Sydenham*, trans. R. G. Latham, London, Sydenham Society, 1850, vol. II, p. 214.
338. Talbott, J. H.: J. Clin. Invest., *27*, 749, 1940.
339. ———: J. Chron. Dis., *1*, 338, 1955.
340. ———: *Gout*, New York, Grune & Stratton, 1957.
341. ———: Medicine, *38*, 173, 1959.
342. ———: *Gout*, 2d ed., New York, Grune & Stratton, 1964.
343. Talbott, J. H., and Coombs, F. S.: J.A.M.A., *110*, 1977, 1938.
344. Talbott, J. H., and Lilienfeld, A.: Geriatrics, *14*, 409, 1959.
345. Talbott, J. H., and Terplan, K. L.: Medicine, *39*, 405, 1960.
346. Turner, R. E., Frank, M. J., Van Ausdal, D., and Bollet, A. J.: Arch. Intern. Med., *106*, 400, 1960.
347. Umber, F.: *Ernahrung und Stoffwechselkrankheiten*, Corban und Schwarzenberg, Vienna, 1914.
348. Ungerleider, H. E.: Ann. Intern. Med., *41*, 124, 1954.
348*a*. Villa, L., Robecchi, A., and Ballabio, C. B.: Ann. Rheum. Dis., *17*, 9, 1958.
349. Von Hogningen-Huene, C. B. G.: Arch. Intern. Med., *118*, 471, 1966.
350. Von Rechenberg, H. K.: *Phenylbutazone*, p. 48, London, Arnold, 1962.
351. von Storch, A.: An essay on the use and effects of the root of the *Colchicum autumnale*, or meadow saffron, trans. from the Latin, T. Becket and P. A. de Honet, 1764.
352. Wallace, S. L., Bernstein, D., and Diamond, H.: J.A.M.A., *199*, 525, 1967.
353. Ward, L. E., Bickel, W. H., and Corbin, K. B.: J.A.M.A., *167*, 844, 1958.
354. Wechsler, R., Wallace, S. L., Gerber, D., and Scherrer, J.: Arth. & Rheum., *8*, 1104, 1965.
355. Weisemberg, R. C., Borisy, G. G., and Taylor, E. W.: Biochemistry, *7*, 4466, 1968.
356. Weissmann, G.: Arth. & Rheum., *9*, 834, 1966.
357. Wilson, D., Collins, D. H., and Marson, R. M.: Proc. Roy. Soc. Med., *44*, 285, 1951.
358. Woeber, K. A., Ricca, L., and Hills, A. G.: Clin. Res., *10*, 45, 1962.
359. Wolfson, W. Q., Hunt, H. D., Levine, R., Guterman, H. S., Cohn, C., Rosenberg, E. F., Huddlestun, B., and Kadota, K.: J. Clin. Endocrinol., *9*, 749, 1949.
360. Wolfson, W. Q., Krevshy, D., Levine, R., Kadota, K., and Cohn, C.: J. Clin. Endocrinol., *9*, 666, 1949.
361. Wollaston, W. H.: Phil. Tr. London, *87*, 386, 1797.
362. Wyngaarden, J. B.: Metabolism, *6*, 244, 1957.
363. ———: J. Clin. Invest., *36*, 1508, 1957.
364. ———: Metabolism, 7, 374, 1958.
365. ———: Arth. & Rheum., *1*, 191, 1958.

366. ———: Arth. & Rheum., *3*, 414, 1960.
367. ———: *Metabolic Basis of Inherited Disease*, 1st ed., ed. J. B. Stanbury, J. B. Wyngaarden, and D. S. Fredrickson, New York, McGraw-Hill, 1960, p. 679.
368. ———: Advances Metab. Dis., *2*, 2, 1965.
369. ———: *Metabolic Basis of Inherited Disease*, ed. J. S. Stanbury, J. B. Wyngaarden, and D. S. Fredrickson, 2nd ed., New York, McGraw-Hill, 1966.
370. ———: Trans. Amer. Clin. Climatol. Assn., *81*, 161, 1969.
371. ———: *Principles of Internal Medicine*, ed. T. R. Harrison, R. D. Adams, I. L. Bennett, W. H. Resnik, G. W. Thorn and M. M. Wintrobe, 6th ed., New York, McGraw-Hill, p. 597, 1970.
372. ———: New Engl. J. Med., *283*, 371, 1970.
373. ———: New Engl. J. Med., *283*, 1170, 1970.
374. Wyngaarden, J. B., and Ashton, D. M.: J. Biol. Chem., *234*, 1492, 1959.
375. Wyngaarden, J. B., Rundles, R. W., and Metz, E. N.: Ann. Intern. Med., *62*, 842, 1965.
376. Wyngaarden, J. B., Rundles, R. W., Silberman, H. R., and Hunter, S.: Arth. & Rheum., *6*, 306, 1963.
377. Wyngaarden, J. B., Seegmiller, J. E., Laster, L., and Blair, A. E.: Metabolism, *8*, 455, 1959.
378. Wyngaarden, J. B., and Stetten, D., Jr.: J. Biol. Chem., *203*, 9, 1953.
379. Yü, T.-F.: Arth. & Rheum., *8*, 765, 1965.
380. Yü, T.-F., Adler, M., Bobrow, E., and Gutman, A. B.: J. Clin. Invest., *48*, 885, 1969.
381. Yü, T.-F., Berger, L., and Gutman, A.: Metabolism, *17*, 309, 1968.
382. Yü, T. F., Berger, L., and Gutman, A. B.: Amer. J. Med., *33*, 829, 1962.
383. ———: Proc. Soc. Exper. Biol. Med., *107*, 905, 1961.
384. Yü, T.-F., Berger, L., Kupfer, S., and Gutman, A. B.: Amer. J. Physiol., *199*, 1199, 1960.
385. Yü, T.-F., Dayton, P. G., and Gutman, A. B.: J. Clin. Invest., *42*, 1330, 1963.
386. Yü, T.-F., and Gutman, A. B.: Proc. Soc. Exper. Biol. Med., *90*, 542, 1955.
387. ———: J. Clin. Invest., *38*, 1293, 1959.
388. ———: Amer. J. Med., *37*, 885, 1964.
389. ———: Ann. Intern. Med., *67*, 1133, 1967.
390. Yü, T.-F., Kaung, C., and Gutman, A. B.: Amer. J. Med., *49*, 352, 1970.
391. Yü, T.-F., Sirota, J. H., Berger, L., Halpern, M., and Gutman, A. B.: Proc. Soc. Exper. Biol. Med., *96*, 809, 1957.
392. Yü, T.-F., Sirota, J. H., and Gutman, A. B.: J. Clin. Invest., *32*, 1121, 1953.
393. Yü, T.-F., Wasserman, L. R., Benedict, J. D., Bien, E. J., Gutman, A. B., and Stetten, D., Jr.: Amer. J. Med., *15*, 845, 1953.
394. Yü, T.-F., Weissmann, B., Sharney, L., Kupfer, S., and Gutman, A. B.: Amer. J. Med., *21*, 901, 1956.
395. Zeveley, H. A., French, A. J., Mikkelsen, W. M., and Duff, I. F.: Amer. J. Med., *20*, 510, 1956.
396. Zimmer, J. G., and Demis, D. J.: Ann. Intern. Med., *64*, 786, 1966.
397. Zollner, N.: Klin. Ergbn. inn. Med. Kinderh., *14*, 321, 1960.
398. Zollner, N., Stern, G., Gröbner, W., and Dofel, W.: Klin. Wschr., *46*, 1318, 1968.
399. Zuckner, J.: Arth. & Rheum., *5*, 329, 1962.
400. Zvaifler, N. J., and Pekin, T. J.: Arch. Intern. Med., *111*, 99, 1963.

Chapter 59

Diagnosis and Treatment of Gout

By Charley J. Smyth, M.D.

Definition

Gout is a disorder of uric acid metabolism manifested by hyperuricemia, recurrent attacks of acute arthritis, deposits of sodium urate in joints, subcutaneous and kidney tissues.

TYPES AND CLINICAL COURSE

Primary Gout

The term *primary gout* is used to designate cases in which the cause for hyperuricemia is an inborn error of metabolism in which there are multiple factors influencing the hereditary trait. It occurs predominantly (90 to 95%) in postpubertal men with the peak age of onset in the fifth decade and less often (5 to 10%) in postmenopausal women. Primary gout usually progresses gradually over many years but in severe cases crippling, chronic gouty arthritis and/or nephropathy may occur within only a few years. The clinical course may be divided into three stages (Fig. 59–1).

Stage I (Asymptomatic Hyperuricemia).—In hereditary gout the serum urate rises to normal or above the range of normal at puberty and will be slightly higher in males than in females. The incidence of asymptomatic hyperuricemia among

CLINICAL COURSE OF CLASSICAL GOUT

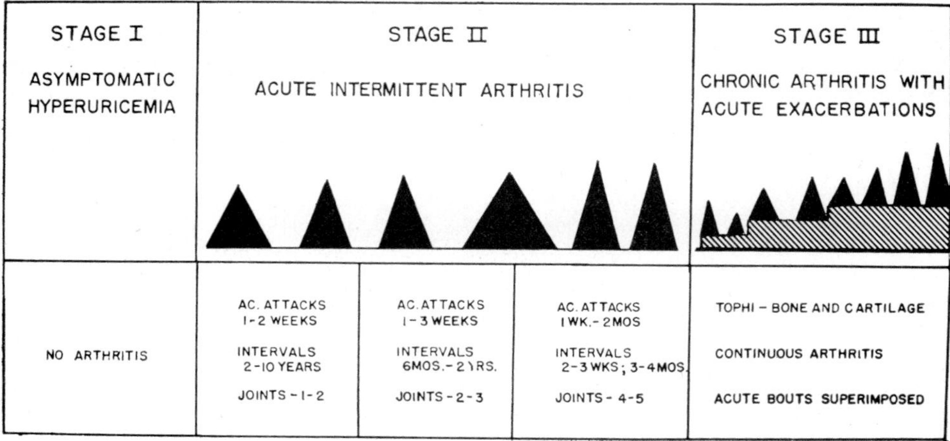

Fig. 59–1.—Basic pattern of clinical gout showing schematically the stages and the events of the usual course of this disease.

blood relatives of gouty persons ranges from 20[109] to 24 per cent.[129] It is estimated that approximately one-third of the subjects with hyperuricemia develops gouty arthritis. The remainder have elevated values throughout their lifetime without any evidence of deleterious effects.

Stage II (Acute Intermittent Gouty Arthritis).—The first clinical evidence of gout is usually the occurrence of acute arthritis in one or two joints lasting for a few days to a few weeks. This is followed by a period of complete freedom from joint symptoms and then recurrence of episodes of acute joint inflammation. The asymptomatic periods vary from months to years but during these pain-free intervals the high serum urate level persists. As time passes the duration of each individual gouty episode increases to several weeks and the number of joints affected increases.

Stage III (Chronic Gouty Arthritis or Tophaceous Gout).—The development of chronic arthritis with superimposed bouts of acute synovitis or bursitis and the presence of visible urate deposits in joints, bursae, or subcutaneous tissues mark the onset of this tophaceous phase. The duration between the first attack to the onset of continuous joint symptoms is variable, ranging in one series from 3 to 42 years with an average of 11.7 years.[38] Uric acid calculi, nephrosclerosis with deposits of urates in the kidney (gouty nephropathy), may lead to renal failure.

Secondary Gout

In secondary gout the hyperuricemia is a complication of another disease. This type is associated chiefly with blood dyscrasias (*e.g.*, polycythemia, chronic mylogenous leukemia, myeloid metaplasia), the reduced renal urate elimination from certain drugs (*e.g.*, all thiazides, diuretics, pyrazinamide), intrinsic renal disease (*e.g.*, chronic nephritis or lead nephropathy), or to conditions causing hyperlactacidemia (glycogen storage disease, preeclampsia, diabetic ketoacidosis and severe bouts of alcoholism or starvation). In contrast to primary gout, the age and sex incidence of the secondary type is that of the underlying disease. The level of serum urate in secondary gout tends to be higher than in primary gout with the concentration frequently ranging between 12 to 14 mg per cent.

Overproduction vs. Underexcretion

On the basis of the turnover rate of uric acid, gouty patients may be classified as either overproducers or underexcreters of urate. In the former, when on a low purine diet, hyperuricema is associated with a daily urinary excretion of 600 mg. of uric acid or higher.[110] One mechanism by which patients with primary gout may "overproduce" uric acid is the lack of the enzyme hypoxanthine-guanine phospho-ribosyl-transferase (HG-PRTase)[56] (*see also* Chapter 58). The lack of this enzyme results in a greatly increased urate production and may cause gout in children with the rare Lesch-Nyhan syndrome.[69] A partial lack of HG-PRTase has been found in gouty subjects, some of whom had minor neurological abnormalities.[54]

CLINICAL MANIFESTATIONS

Stage I—Asymptomatic Hyperuricemia

Inherited Disorders of Purine Metabolism.—In families in which gout occurs, the serum urate concentration rises to normal or above at puberty and will be slightly higher in males than females. The first extensive investigation of the incidence of asymptomatic hyperuricemia among blood relatives of gouty persons was by Talbott,[139] who reported that 25 per cent of 136 relatives of 27 patients with gout had elevated serum uric acid values. In a similar study, Smyth *et al.*[129] reported an incidence of hyperuricemia of 24 per cent among the relatives of gouty patients. An 18-year follow-up study of these same families revealed that 10 per cent of 291 relatives had asymptomatic hyperuricemia and 6.5 per cent had gout.[109] Hauge and Harvald[36] compared the serum urate values in the siblings of gouty patients with those of a control group and found values significantly higher in the former. These and other studies have established the fact that relatives of patients with gout have an increased incidence of hyperuricemia and gout and suggest that the serum uric acid level is controlled by multiple genes.[98,120]

The excretion of uric acid in first-degree relatives of patients with gout has shown a rough but significant graded correlation between the level of urate clearance in gouty probands and the mean clearance of their relatives.[120] It seems, therefore, that the concept of multifactorial influences applying to the level of uric acid in the blood may be extended to the handling of urate by the kidney.

The presence of hyperuricemia is also a consistent finding in the familial syndrome described by Lesch and Nyhan in which there is a deficiency of the enzyme HG-PRTase. The clinical course of the condition may also be complicated by uric acid urolithiasis[43] and less frequently by acute gouty arthritis. The use of the urinary uric acid to creatinine ratio as a screening test for inherited disorders of purine metabolism has been suggested.[53] Rosenberg *et al.* reported that, of a 22 member kindred of a previously undescribed syndrome, five had hyperuricemia, renal insufficiency, ataxia and deafness.[113] Serum urate levels were elevated in other members of the family who did not have renal insufficiency. Red cell HG-PRTase levels were normal. On the evidence recently reported, it seems clear that many factors regulate uric acid metabolism and that genetic influences make a major contribution in many patients.[90,98,147]

Other Causes of Hyperuricemia

As a result of population surveys, periodic health examinations and multiphasic laboratory screening programs, many individuals with hyperuricemia are being identified who give no history of gout, and are without any clinical evidence of gouty arthritis or other diseases known to be associated with this laboratory abnormality.[89,123] In such cases it is necessary to verify by several determinations that a consistent hyperuricemia

Table 59-1.—Causes of Hyperuricemia

Drugs	*Renal Disease*
Salicylates, 2 to 3 gm./day	*Lead Poisoning*
Diuretics—Chlorothiazide	*Cardiovascular Disease*
Hydrochlorothiazide	Hypertension
Ethacrynic Acid	Myocardial Infarction
Bendroflumethiazide	*Hereditary Disorders*
Pyrazinamide, Pyrazinoic Acid	Down's Syndrome (Mongolism)
Hematologic Disorders	Glycogen Storage Disease (Type I)
Leukemia	Primary Gout
Polycythemia vera	Lesch-Nyhan Syndrome
Hemolytic anemia	*Endocrine Disorders*
Sickle-cell anemia	Hyper- and Hypoparathyroidism
Pernicious anemia	Myxedema
Thalassemia	Obesity
Myeloid metaplasia	Idiopathic hypercalciuria
Non-tropical sprue	*Skin Diseases*
Waldenström's hyperproteinemia	Psoriasis

exists and then initiate appropriate studies to determine the cause. This search for a possible cause may require considerable time and effort because the number of conditions that have been shown to be associated with an increased serum urate level has increased rapidly in recent years. A partial list is shown in Table 59–1. The most commonly reported non-gouty causes are azotemia (20%), acidosis (20%), and diuretics (20%).[102] A large number of other poorly understood factors including race, obesity, intelligence and "drive" is known to be associated with hyperuricemia.

Regardless of cause, the presence of hyperuricemia leads to an increased risk of gouty arthritis, tophi and renal stones. The magnitude of the risk rises with the degree of hyperuricemia.[33,123] In the Framingham study, a group of middle-aged men were observed for an average of ten years.[33] One out of every six with a serum urate level between 7 and 8 mg% developed clinical gout; it developed in less than 1 per cent of those with serum urate levels below 6 mg%. Stones were also common in subjects with hyperuricemia, being found in 12.7 per cent of men with 7 mg% and in 40 per cent of those with levels over 9 mg%.

Stage II—Acute Intermittent Arthritis

Initial Gouty Attacks.—Acute gouty arthritis usually begins in men over thirty years of age. The attack is usually of sudden onset, frequently at night, lasts from three to eleven or more days and the symptoms then disappear completely with restoration of normal joint function. Although the attacks may begin in the early hours of the morning, the symptoms are usually first detected when the individual puts his foot on the floor after awakening.

The dramatic suddenness of the onset of an attack of gout is striking. The affected joint may swell markedly within a few hours and become hot, dusky red and extremely tender. The big toe joints are most often affected (podagra) and the site of maximum tenderness is on the medial side of this bunion joint where even the slightest pressure is apt to produce unbearable pain. The inflammation resembles a bacterial cellulitis and may be incised by the unwary with the intent to release pus.

Joints Involved.—The first attack of gout is usually monarticular involving most commonly the big toe, instep, heel, ankle, or knee. The big toe is affected in from 53 to 70 per cent of gouty individuals in the initial attack of the disease, and is involved sooner or later in 90 to 95 per cent of these patients. Although no joint is exempt from gout, the joints of the lower extremities are involved more frequently than the upper. The hip joint becomes involved at some time in about 2 per cent of cases.*

Diagnosis of Acute Episode

Signs and Symptoms.—An acute attack of gouty arthritis usually appears without warning or may be precipitated by minor trauma, overindulgence in food or alcohol or by a surgical procedure. The degree of pain becomes progressively more excruciating and is often described as "crushing" or "pulsating." The dramatic suddenness of the onset of acute joint pain in a middle-aged man, frequently involving the big toe joint, with complete freedom of joint symptoms and signs between attacks is almost pathognomonic of gout.

Demonstration of Crystals.—The identification of monosodium urate crystals in synovial fluid or in synovial needle biopsy material from a joint is the most positive method of diagnosing acute gouty arthritis. This involves the collection of joint fluid, using heparin as an anticoagulant (avoid oxalate), and the demonstration by compensated polarized light microscopy of needle-shaped crystals that exhibit strongly negative birefringence.[82] Polarized light microscopy with a first

* Editor's note: We have never seen gout in the temporomandibular joint. This point is helpful in the differential diagnosis of polyarthritis.

order red plate compensator imparts characteristic color changes; urate crystals turn yellow when their long axis is parallel to the direction of slow vibration of light through the compensator and blue when lying at right angles to it.[106] In contrast, the calcium pyrophosphate dihydrate crystals of pseudogout show more varied shapes and weakly positive birefringence. Synovial tissue sections show urate deposits with a radial architecture, enveloped by a granulomatous reaction, which are sufficiently characteristic to be differentiated from the crystal deposits of pseudogout.[67]

Hyperuricemia in Gout.—The demonstration of increased serum urate concentration is an essential element in the diagnosis of gout. One satisfactory definition of hyperuricemia is based upon the solubility of monosodium urate in serum which was found by Seegmiller to be 7 mg%, a figure which agrees closely with the upper limits of normal as determined from population studies. The critical level at which gout appears varies but it is rare for verified instances of untreated gout to occur with the serum urate less than 7 mg%.

Using colorimetric methods, the upper normal limits are 6.0[14,25,108] to 6.2[33] mg% in adult males and 4.9[25,33] to 5.5[108] mg% in adult females; with enzymatic uricase spectrophotometric methods the upper limits of normal values are 6.4[90] to 7.5[32,124] mg% in men and 5.4[90] to 6.6[36] mg% in women. This sex difference is an important factor in interpreting the serum urate values when considering the diagnosis of gout.

A number of drugs in common use reduces the serum urate concentration. This list includes aspirin and sodium salicylates in large doses (4.0 to 6.0 gm. daily), phenylbutazone, cortisone and its derivatives, probenecid, sulfinpyrazone, and allopurinol. Other drugs which induce a hyperuricemic state are pyrazinamide, salicylates in low dosage (less than 3.6 gm. daily) and all thiazide diuretics (Table 59–1). Thus, to obtain a valid determination of the serum urate concentration the patient should abstain from the above drugs for at least three or more days. Colchicine can be administered without altering serum urate levels.

Family History of Gout.—A positive family history of clinically overt gout varies from 6 to 18 per cent in reports from the United States.[93,112] However, Talbott observed an incidence of more than 50 per cent in families of gouty patients with two or more male members.[135]

Response to Colchicine.—An unequivocal response of an acute attack of arthritis to an adequate therapeutic trial of colchicine provides a presumptive diagnosis of gout. Although there are reports of the marked improvement with colchicine in other inflammatory diseases of joints, it remains that a dramatic response favors a diagnosis of gout. An effective therapeutic course consists of 0.5 to 0.65 mg. every hour until relief is obtained or gastrointestinal side effects occur. In a controlled study of gouty patients, Wallace *et al.*, observed that 44 of 58 patients (75%) responded to a therapeutic trial of colchicine, whereas only 3 of 62 (5%) of the patients with other types of acutely inflamed joints responded.[145]

Differential Diagnosis.—The clinical manifestations of the first attack of acute gouty arthritis may occasionally be seen in other diseases: acute rheumatic fever, gonorrheal arthritis, atypical rheumatoid arthritis, acute traumatic arthritis, cellulitis, suppurative arthritis, Reiter's syndrome, periarticular fibrositis, psoriatic arthritis, arthritis with ulcerative colitis, hemophilic arthritis, sarcoidosis, pseudogout and subdeltoid bursitis (*see also* Chapter 25). Rarely in other acute diseases of joints does the onset strike with the same suddenness or is the pain as agonizing. Palindromic rheumatism may also begin acutely (*see* Chapter 45).

The most commonly mistaken conditions are: acute rheumatic fever, gonorrheal arthritis, and atypical rheumatoid arthritis. However, the patient with acute rheumatic fever is usually young, whereas first attacks of gout occur more often after the age of forty. Migratory polyarticular involvement is much more common in rheumatic fever than in gout. In younger persons, if multiple joints are involved, fever, leukocytosis, and increased sedimentation rate may cause confusion with rheumatic fever; however, the absence of cardiac involvement, epistaxis and tachycardia favors the diagnosis of juvenile gout.

Gonorrheal arthritis occasionally exhibits recurrent attacks. In gonorrheal arthritis a genitourinary, rectal or pharyngeal involvement can often be demonstrated or obtained by history. Gonorrheal arthritis is usually polyarticular at the onset involving several large joints but usually settling in only one or two of those affected; gout in the early stages attacks only one or two joints. In gonorrheal arthritis, purulent effusions commonly occur from which cultures of gonococci may be obtained. In these cases the serum uric acid is usually normal and no urate crystals are found in the fluid (*see also* Chapter 64).

Recovery from attacks of atypical rheumatoid arthritis may be so complete and so rapid as to make one consider the possibility of gout. However, the typical patient with rheumatoid arthritis exhibits symmetrical involvement of joints, fusiform joint swellings, joint fluid findings and the insidious onset of a low-grade inflammatory reaction. The prodromal stage of rheumatoid arthritis may simulate attacks of palindromic rheumatism with intermittent episodes of sudden onset producing incapacitating arthritis in one or a few joints and acute inflammation in the adjacent soft tissues. Such attacks last only a few hours or days, are not associated with any abnormal laboratory changes and leave the affected joint area perfectly normal. The foot in gout is usually hot and dusky red in contrast to the slightly warm, clammy foot in rheumatoid arthritis. If the diagnosis is in doubt, one must study the serum urate value, search for urate crystals in synovial fluid, evaluate the results of colchicine therapy, inquire about a family history of gout, and study the course of the disease. Although the occurrence of gout and rheumatoid arthritis in the same individual has been reported, there is need for unusual caution in making both diagnoses in one person.[100]

The clinical manifestations of articular chondrocalcinosis (pseudogout) closely resemble true gout.[80,84,158] The swelling of a joint, pain on motion and heat develop quickly and reach a peak on the third or fourth day. The episodic acute inflammatory involvement subsides completely after seven to fifty days without sequelae. The knee is most often affected, followed by the ankle, wrist, elbow, hip and shoulder, in that order. Pseudogout may involve the great toe, is associated with elevated serum uric acid levels in one-third of cases and may benefit dramatically from colchicine therapy. The diagnosis is established by the demonstration of calcification of articular cartilages by roentgenographic studies and calcium pyrophosphate dihydrate crystals in the synovial fluid of affected joints[81,106] (*see* Chapter 60).

Acute joint inflammation in sarcoidosis may on occasions simulate acute gouty arthritis.[112,135] Such patients may present diagnostic difficulties because of the favorable and prompt response to oral colchicine.

DISEASES ASSOCIATED WITH GOUT

The number of reports dealing with diseases or abnormal states that are intimately or casually associated with hyperuricemia and gout has increased rapidly in recent years. It is not clear whether hypertension and atherosclerosis should be considered as complications of gout or merely incidental disorders; many observers regard them as an integral part of the disease.[29,63] The high mortality due to complication of either hypertension or atherosclerosis among 195 consecutive patients with gout led Ogryzlo to favor this view.[94] Of 23 consecutive deaths in this group of gouty subjects, he found that 52 per cent were due to myocardial infarction as opposed to 26 per cent of a control group taken from a general hospital population. An additional 9 per cent died from cerebrovascular accidents. Hypertension is common in gouty individuals and hyperuricemia is a frequent finding in nongouty, hypertensive patients with a reported incidence ranging from 27[8] to 38 per cent.[12]

Diabetes mellitus is estimated to occur in 10 per cent of patients with gout.[94,149] The role of ketone bodies in diabetic ketoacidosis[101] and from fasting in the production of hyperuricemia has been well documented.[101] Recent studies have suggested that increased blood triglycerides may be the common biochemical feature shared by patients with both diabetes and gout.

Certain disorders of hematopoiesis are commonly associated with gout. This list is long and includes polycythemia vera, secondary polycythemia, myeloid metaplasia, myeloid and lymphocytic leukemia, sickle-cell anemia, thalassemia and pernicious anemia. In these situations the hyperuricemia and articular distress are attributed to the expansion and increased turnover of the cellular elements of the bone marrow, resulting in an overproduction of uric acid.

The development of primary gout in children is rare but it occurs in association with neoplastic disease, glycogen storage disease[48,56] (Type I) and the Lesch-Nyhan syndrome.[55,69]

Hyperuricemia and an increased incidence of gouty arthritis have been recorded in a number of other disorders although the pathogenesis of the biochemical abnormality is not yet understood. Overproduction of uric acid may be a factor in the hyperuricemia in psoriasis, Reiter's syndrome, and perhaps in obesity. Decreased renal urate excretion may account for the hyperuricemia in patients with chronic nephritis and chronic hemodialysis, lead nephropathy,[1,18] hyperparathyroidism,[121] myxedema, prolonged fasting,[16] ketoacidosis and lactacidemia.

PROVOCATIVE FACTORS

A number of factors play some part in determining individual attacks of gouty arthritis and its site, but their true relation to the disease has not been determined.

Trauma.—Trauma has repeatedly been considered responsible as a provocative agent for acute attacks of gout. The first metatarsophalangeal joint is liable to trauma and chronic strain from pressure of tight shoes. Attacks may result from such minor trauma as that from long walks, incident to hunting or fishing trips, sight-seeing or golf.

Dietary Excesses.—Gouty arthritis is often provoked by dietary indiscretions associated with feast days, holidays, or weddings.

Drugs. — Medicinal provocatives include liver extracts, thiamin chloride, sulfathiazole, insulin,[39] chlorothiazide, gynergen, and adrenocorticotropin (ACTH),[37] penicillin[137] or testosterone withdrawal.[70]

Alcohol.—Some clinicians consider habitual excesses in drink the most important of all precipitating factors.

Surgical Operation.—If acute arthritis occurs during the first week after an operation, gout or pseudogout should be suspected. Linton[72] reported an incidence of 86 per cent of acute gout in gouty patients subjected to 22 surgical operations. Acute arthritis developed within the third to fifth postoperative day in 5 cases of gout reported by Ficarra and Adams.[19]

Miscellaneous Factors.—Latent gout has been activated by marked blood loss and transfusions, emotional upsets, foreign protein therapy, exposure to cold and dampness, severe purgation and x-ray therapy.

SUBSEQUENT GOUTY ATTACKS

The intervals between attacks are called *intercritical periods.* In rare instances, attacks may be eight to ten years apart with absolute disappearance of all joint phenomena between attacks. These periods become progressively shorter until acute bouts of arthritis occur several times each year, often with a certain regularity.

The recurrent attacks may or may not affect the joint initially involved. Although the first few attacks are usually afebrile, later attacks may be accompanied by a temperature of 101° to 102° F. or more and usually affect several joints.

The disease may be polyarticular (about 5 per cent of cases) with a fulminating course from the onset; this is more likely to occur in young patients, rarely involves the great toe, is accompanied by a fever which persists for weeks, and is often misdiagnosed as acute rheumatic fever.

Stage III—Chronic Gouty Arthritis or Tophaceous Gout

As the disease advances with attacks occurring at frequent intervals, the joints become stiff, enlarged, and often deformed. There is usually involvement of the joints of the hands, feet, ankles, wrists, knees, and elbows; rarely, the shoulder, the sacroiliac or the sternoclavicular joints are involved. At any time during the chronic stage acute bouts in joints and bursae are common.

Tophi (Heb.—a hardening)—Collections of sodium monourate crystals surrounded by giant cells and encircled by a granulomatous capsule are the pathognomonic lesions of gout (Fig. 59–2). They vary in size from 1 mm. to several centimeters. They are found frequently upon the helix or antihelix of the ear (Fig. 59–3). They also occur often in the olecranon and prepatellar bursae, and in the tendons of the fingers and wrists, toes, ankles, heels, and bone (Fig. 59–4). Accumulations in the carpal tunnel at the wrist may compress the median nerve and cause a carpal tunnel syndrome. Tophi have been found in the mitral valve, cardiac muscle, sacroiliac joint and vertebrae. The skin overlying large subcutaneous tophi is frequently highly vascular, thin and orange colored. Ulcers may develop in areas of pressure and the semi-solid chalky white contents having the consistency of toothpaste can be expressed.

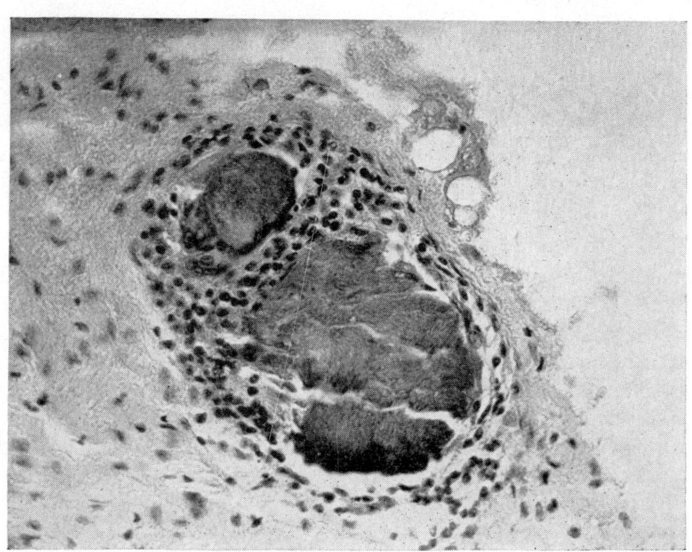

Fig. 59–2.—Gouty tophaceous deposit in synovial membrane obtained by closed needle punch biopsy. (William M. Mikkelsen, courtesy of Arch. Int. Med.)

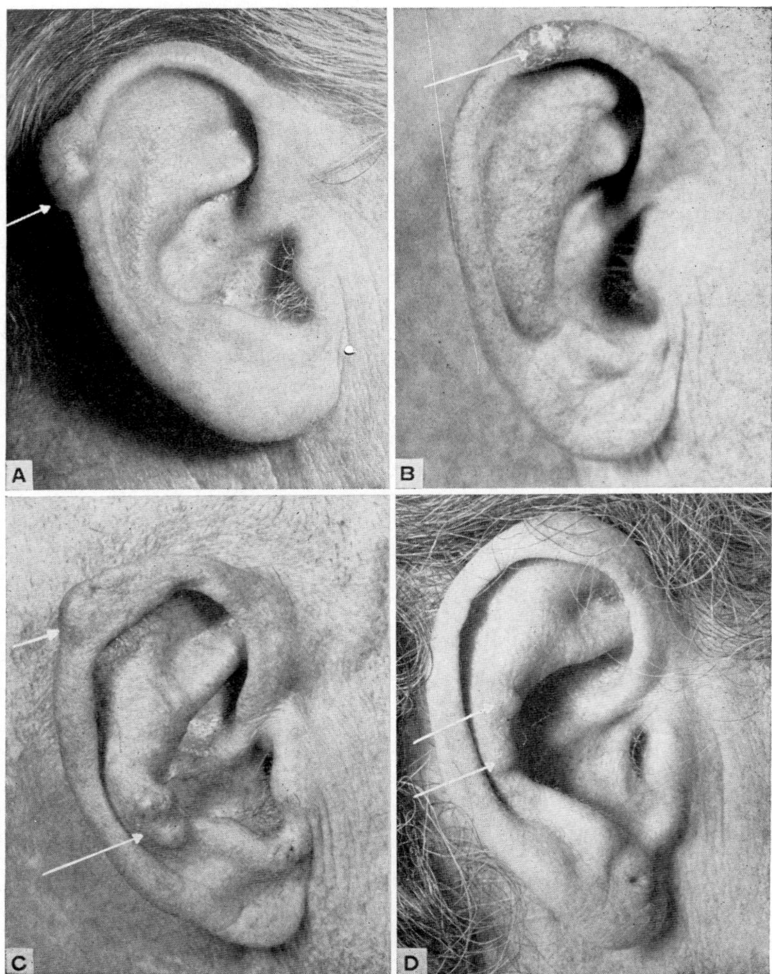

FIG. 59–3.—Tophi in ears: Large cystic tophus on the helix (*A*), ulcerated tophus (*B*), two tophi in ear, upon the helix and antihelix (*C*), subcutaneous nodules of rheumatoid arthritis, *not* gouty tophi, in a female patient (*D*).

The crystalline urate may be identified both by polarized light microscopy and by the murexide chemical test. In severe cases chronic sinus formation and secondary infection may occur.

Gouty Nephropathy and Calculi.—Subjects with tophaceous gout for several years usually show evidence of renal functional impairment. Mild proteinuria is the first evidence of this nephropathy. Later inability to concentrate and decreased clearance are demonstrated and finally marked proteinuria and nitrogen retention develop. Renal failure is the most important cause of death from gout.

The passage of uric acid stones or gravel is estimated to occur in 10 to 20 per cent of patients. During a nine-year period in one large clinic, 14 per cent of 324 gouty subjects gave a history of urinary calculi.[58] A defect in the ammonia production by the gouty kidney with the resultant persistent excess acidity is thought to be a major factor in stone formation.[156]

Schnitker and Richter[118] collected a

series of 55 cases of gout and found that 17 (31 per cent) had chronic nephritis. In the 38 gouty subjects without nephritis the kidney function was essentially normal. Brown and Mallory[10] studied five proven, autopsied cases and reported that every kidney had urate deposits in the medulla which conformed to the shape, direction and position of the collecting tubules. In most the inflammatory and foreign body reaction to the urates had destroyed the tubular structure. These cases all showed moderate to striking benign nephrosclerosis.

Ocular Changes.—Ocular inflammations associated with gout are not numerous but such cases often present a perplexing problem. They include conjunctivitis, scleritis, episcleritis, iridocyclitis, tenonitis, and rarely keratitis.[87] They are reported to improve following the reduction of blood uric acid.

Other Complications.—Thrombophlebitis is a rather unusual complication of gout and is reported in less than 1 per cent of cases.[94] Aseptic necrosis of the femoral head[45] and deposits of mixtures of hydroxyapatite and sodium urate in and about joints in chronic dialysis patients are uncommon oddities.[11]

Diagnosis of Chronic Gout

The diagnosis of chronic gouty arthritis is easy in the majority of cases. A history can almost invariably be obtained of numerous acute episodes of inflammatory joint involvement followed by complete remissions and with the attacks tending to occur with increasing frequency. This chronic stage of gout is also suggested when the bouts of synovitis do not completely subside but leave some residual, low-grade pain, stiffness and deformity. The presence of tophi and chronically enlarged, non-tender bursa over bony prominences, especially of the elbows, knee, and Achilles tendon, are additional helpful diagnostic features.

Chronic gouty arthritis may be confused with the firm and bony-hard osseous enlargements of the joints of degenerative joint disease. Also tophi overlying the fingers are sometimes mistaken for Heberden's or Bouchard's nodes. Differentiation between chronic gout and rheumatoid arthritis may present problems. Rheumatoid subcutaneous nodules and tophi both form at points of pressure and cannot be distinguished by palpation; biopsy material and histological study may be required to distinguish them. The first proven instance of the coexistence of rheumatoid arthritis and gout was reported by Owen *et al.* in 1966. It is extremely rare that these two relatively common diseases are demonstrated in the same person.[100] Patients with chondrocalcinosis (pseudogout) fre-

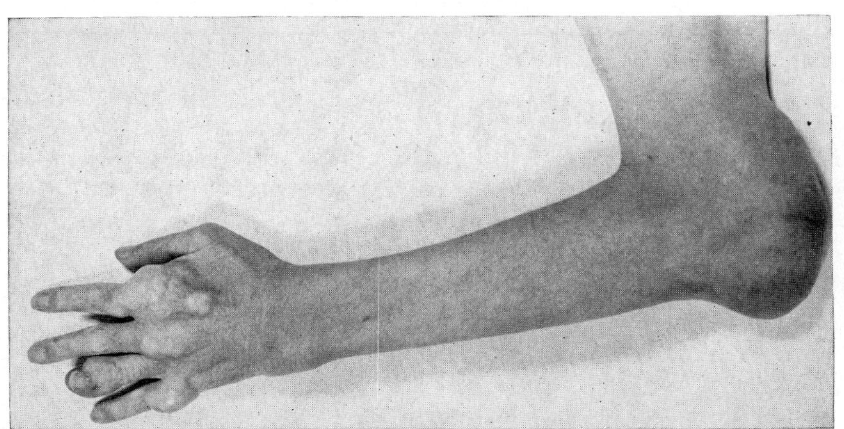

Fig. 59–4.—Chronic gouty arthritis with shortening of the fourth finger, subcutaneous urate deposits over the knuckles and extensive olecranon bursitis.

quently have progressive chronic arthritis of the larger weight-bearing joints, usually in one or both knees and less frequently one or both hips with well-defined superimposed episodic acute attacks. Not all patients with radiopaque deposits in the articular cartilages have deposits of calcium pyrophosphate crystals. Therefore, the differentiation between pseudogout and gout depends primarily on the characteristics of the crystals either in the joint fluid or within tissues obtained by articular biopsy.[80,84] Gout and pseudogout occasionally coexist.

A determination of the serum urate level is of primary importance. It is essential that the blood sample be obtained several days following a period of abstinence from drugs known to influence the concentration of serum urate.

Any chronic joint or bursal effusion should be aspirated and a drop of fluid placed on a slide and examined microscopically for the presence of urate crystals (vide supra). The same methods of crystal identification can also be used to study material from a suspected tophus.

In children with the rare Lesch-Nyhan syndrome, an assay of the erythrocytes for the enzyme HG-PRTase shows low levels.[6] A simple screening test for this enzyme deficiency is the determination of the urinary uric acid/creatinine ratio. A figure of 0.76 or over suggests a partial deficiency.[52]

Punch Biopsy

Closed biopsy with the Polley and Bickel needle[107] is a useful diagnostic procedure. It is necessary that the tissues be fixed in absolute alcohol rather than aqueous fixatives to preserve the water-soluble urates. Zeveley and associates[157] found urate deposits in 4 of 6 instances in which tissue was obtained by punch biopsy (Fig. 59–2).

The renal lesion in gout was examined by Gonick *et al.* in material from 28 biopsies and 42 autopsies.[23] His studies of the specimens showed that a distinctive glomerulosclerosis was present in 57 per cent; atrophy and dilatation and regeneration of the Henle loops were seen in 25 per cent; scars, foci of lymphocytes, macrophage and plasma cells typical of chronic pyelonephritis were found in 21 per cent. Tophus formation was rare.

Roentgen Examination

Huber in 1896 first described the specific "punched-out" areas of bone seen

Laboratory Findings

Increased serum urate—greater than 7 mg.%, almost invariably present.

Crystals of monosodium urate in synovial fluid, strongly negative bifringence with compensated polarized light.

Sedimentation rate usually normal between attacks; frequently elevated during attacks.

Roentgenograms usually negative early; of little use in diagnosis until late in disease; films of feet show changes first.

Mild or moderate leukocytosis is the rule during attacks.

Anemia is rare except in the terminal stages.

Albuminuria and decrease in renal function may occur.

Decreased HG-PRTase in erythrocytes in Lesch-Nyhan syndrome.

Urinary urate 24-hour excretion over 600 mg. on a purine-free diet indicates "overproduction."

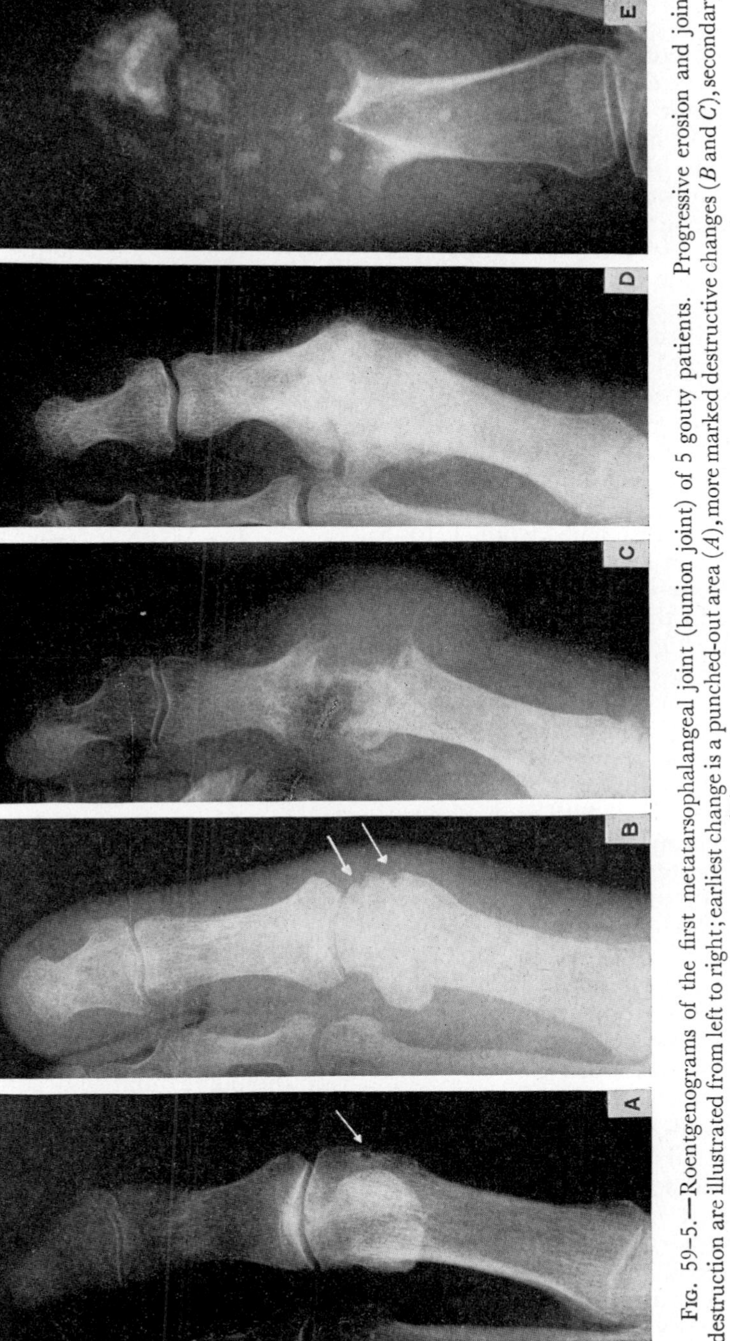

Fig. 59–5.—Roentgenograms of the first metatarsophalangeal joint (bunion joint) of 5 gouty patients. Progressive erosion and joint destruction are illustrated from left to right; earliest change is a punched-out area (*A*), more marked destructive changes (*B* and *C*), secondary hypertrophic changes (*D*), far-advanced destruction (*E*).

roentgenologically in gout.[44] These radiolucent areas represent osseous tophi containing urate crystals and, although they may be found in any bone, involvement of the lower extremities (Fig. 59–5) is more frequent than of the upper. Roentgenograms frequently indicate no changes early in the disease; bony erosions are seen in only about one-third of cases even in the later stages. The earliest roentgenologic evidence of gouty involvement of bone is a localized area of osteoporosis in the first metatarsal head and this decalcification is seen in patients with frequent prolonged, severe attacks. It is usually several years after the initial gouty attack and following repeated episodes in the same joint that the first helpful roentgen findings of gout are detected. The bony cortex becomes eroded and areas, which usually vary from 1 to 5 mm. or more in diameter, located in the subchondral bone of the base or head of the phalanges in the hand or feet can be demonstrated (Fig. 59–6). Martel has emphasized the presence of an overhanging margin of bone at the periphery of the erosion which is displaced outwardly over the tophus as though it were lifted by it gives it a shell-like configuration[79] (*see also* Chapter 7). Although characteristic, these lesions are not diagnostic of gout. They are commonly observed in rheumatoid arthritis and are also seen in other chronic diseases including degenerative joint disease, sarcoidosis, hyperparathyroidism, multiple myeloma, Hand-Schüller-Christian syndrome, syphilitic gumma, tuberculosis, yaws, metastatic neoplasms and leprosy.

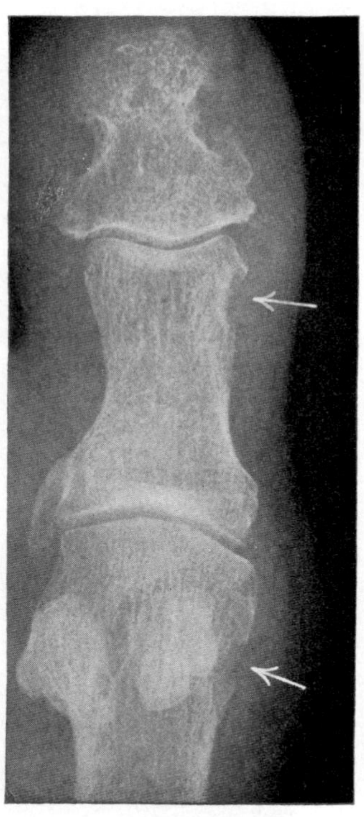

FIG. 59–6.—Punched-out areas in a sixty-two-year-old brewmaster with gout. This great toe had suffered repeated attacks of acute swelling.

Marginal bone hypertrophy or spurring is also common in joints which have been the seat of numerous attacks of gout. Localized soft tissue tumefactions, with or without calcifications, may be observed. Joints rarely involved by gout include the sacroiliac,[26] temporomandibular, sternoclavicular, spine, shoulders, or hips. Autopsy material has shown gouty erosions of the sacroiliac joints and urate deposits in the spine and jaw.

The finding of calcification of the cartilage by radiographic examination does not completely differentiate gout from pseudogout. In two studies of patients with proven gout, chondrocalcinosis was present in 5 per cent in one series[24] and in 30 per cent in another.[15] Also, certain well-defined metabolic disorders have been associated with chondrocalcinosis. These include primary hyperparathyroidism, hemochromatosis, acromegaly and diabetes mellitus. In addition, the presence of idiopathic chondrocalcinosis in 7 per cent of an elderly population casts some doubt upon the diagnostic value of this x-ray sign.[7]

TREATMENT OF GOUT

Although there is no known cure for gout, the control of the frequency and severity of acute attacks is quite satisfactory with the measures available. In contrast to other forms of arthritis, the treatment of gout is relatively effective, and, with the acute attacks properly managed, the results are frequently dramatic. With accumulating experience in the long-term use of uricosuric drugs, allopurinol and colchicine as a prophylactic agent, there is a more hopeful attitude toward the management of chronic gout. With continuous therapy chronic joint symptoms disappear, tophaceous deposits in skin, cartilage and bone can be made to shrink and with persistence can be made to disappear; acute attacks decrease in number and serum urate can be maintained at or near normal levels. There is encouraging evidence that the renal damage of gout can be prevented or, if present, can be improved and the patient maintained in a state of good renal function for many years. In advanced cases with massive urate deposits, surgical removal of tophi combined with long-term uricosuric therapy, or with allopurinol alone, may lead to marked restoration of function. This program of treatment requires a dedicated physician and a cooperative patient. If properly carried out for an indefinite period, it is one of the most satisfactory of medical experiences.

Since recent studies point to the hereditary etiology of gout, relatives of patients with active gout having hyperuricemia should live moderately and avoid obesity, fatigue, exposures to extremes of temperature, excessive trauma to joints, excessive foods high in purines, all known provocatives of acute gouty arthritis.

Acute Attack

The aim of therapy is to reduce the severity of the pain and quickly terminate the acute inflammatory process. The patient should be on restricted activity and the affected part immobilized and protected. Four drugs of proven value are available and commonly used: colchicine, phenylbutazone, indomethacin, and corticosteroids (or ACTH).

Colchicine.—If the diagnosis is in doubt, a clear-cut response to colchicine is still widely used as confirmatory evidence of gout. However, this time-honored axiom has been questioned in reports of satisfactory control of inflamed joints of patients with serum sickness,[92] sarcoid arthritis,[50] and rheumatoid arthritis.[159]

Colchicine tablets, each 0.5 and 0.65 mg., should be given, one tablet every hour or two until pain is relieved or until diarrhea, nausea or vomiting occurs. The average attack of gout requires approximately 10 tablets to suppress inflammation. Paregoric may be necessary to control the diarrhea. Once the amount of colchicine necessary to produce toxic symptoms has been established, a patient may be able in subsequent attacks to obtain a satisfactory effect by taking 1 or 2 tablets less in a course. The patient should start taking the drug at the first appearance of symptoms of a gouty attack. Delay of a few hours in the treatment after the onset of acute gouty pains may increase the severity and prolong the duration of the acute episode.[77]

The response to this drug is often dramatic. Joint pains and swelling begin to subside approximately twelve hours after the institution of therapy and in most instances pain is completely relieved in from one to two days. Over 95 per cent of acute attacks are materially benefited by a single course of colchicine. The response to colchicine is often disappointing if the drug is started several days after the onset of acute symptoms; relief is usually prompt if therapy is begun at the very onset of the attack. Should no benefit occur, a second course can be given after an interval of three days; repetition sooner might precipitate marked gastrointestinal symptoms.

Intravenous Colchicine.—Intravenous colchicine gives quick relief, is safe and is free from troublesome gastrointestinal side effects. The initial dose is 1 to 3 mg. with no more than 4 to 6 mg. in 24 hours. Care must be taken to ensure that the injection is made intravenously, as the colchicine solution is irritating outside the vein. This route is rarely necessary

Treatment of the Acute Attack of Gout

Colchicine, 0.5 mg. orally every hour until pain relieved unless toxic symptoms appear (nausea, vomiting and diarrhea); it is usually not necessary to exceed 8 to 10 doses during the first twenty-four hours. If diarrhea occurs and pain persists, colchicine may be continued (0.5 mg., 4 times a day) and the diarrhea controlled by paregoric and bismuth (4 cc. of the former every hour for 5 doses in addition to 2 gm. of bismuth subcarbonate after every liquid stool).

Intravenous colchicine in 1 to 3 mg. doses is effective and minimizes the intestinal irritation.

Phenylbutazone is as effective as colchicine and is preferred by many patients. High initial dose, 200 mg. or 400 mg. followed in two and four hours by 200 mg. on the first day. On the next two to six days, 100 mg. four times daily will usually give complete relief from an acute attack and avoid a rebound.

Indomethacin is comparable to phenylbutazone. A large initial dose (100 to 150 mg.) followed by 3 or 4 additional doses of 50 mg. each during the first day. A daily dose of 100 or 150 mg. during the next two to four days in divided doses results in the control of all signs of inflammation.

Corticotropin (ACTH) and oxyphenbutazone are also effective agents.

and inadvisable if the oral route can be used.

Phenylbutazone and Oxyphenbutazone.—The anti-inflammatory drug phenylbutazone (Butazolidin) is highly effective in terminating the acute attacks of acute gouty arthritis.[57,150] This drug has replaced colchicine and in the opinion of some[77,131] is the drug of choice in controlling acute gout. Its use is preferred largely because the gastrointestinal disturbances are avoided. It is administered orally and is rapidly and completely absorbed from the gastrointestinal tract. A large initial dose on the first day of 400 to 600 mg. is followed by intermittent administration of 100 mg. four times daily for 3 to 5 days or until the acute attack resolves. This is a reliable drug for quick (six to eight hours) control of acute joint symptoms in gout. If the patient has had joint symptoms for several days before phenylbutazone is started, it may be necessary to continue therapy for five to eight days or more to produce a resolution. The undesirable side effects include rash, nausea, bloating, vertigo, and sometimes typical ulcer symptoms. Nausea is the most frequent untoward reaction; preexisting peptic ulcers may be activated and require interruption of therapy. The reported hematopoietic toxicity following its use is rare. The clinical benefits begin within a few hours and the majority of patients experience a complete remission in forty-eight hours or less. It has been shown to be effective in patients resistant to colchicine and sometimes in patients previously treated with colchicine, the response is better to phenylbutazone.

The effects of oxyphenbutazone (Tandearil) are about the same as those of phenylbutazone with marked relief of symptoms within 24 to 48 hours. In dosages of 400 to 600 mg. daily for 4 to 7 days oxyphenbutazone will control the majority of acute attacks. In the few published reports the results and side reactions of these allied compounds are comparable and their use is preferred by most physicians to colchicine.[27]

Indomethacin.—Reports from many experienced observers indicate that this synthetic anti-inflammatory agent is quick-acting and strikingly effective in acute arthritis.[88,105,132] In comparative studies the results are comparable to those obtained with phenylbutazone.[35,104] The dosage schedule should be high for the first few days and maintained for approximately one week or until all signs of joint inflammation disappear. A large initial dose of 150 mg. followed by three or four additional doses of 100 mg. each during the first day results in prompt relief of pain and a rapid reduction in other signs of synovitis. During the next two to four days, 100 mg. in divided doses have usually given complete control of the acute episode. This or similar dosage schedules have been effective with a low frequency of side effects. Gouty patients are most tolerant of this drug and have fewer reactions than patients with chronic rheumatoid arthritis (Fig. 59–7).

ACTH and Corticosteroids.—If other measures fail, ACTH by injection or corticosteroids by mouth may be effective.[41,111] Most observers use such hormonal therapy only for patients failing to respond to other measures and it is rarely required.[133]

As a local adjunct in treatment of the acute attack of gouty arthritis, Hollander *et al.*[40,42] have injected 25 mg. of hydrocortisone acetate directly into the inflamed joint. In 17 such cases, where a gouty bunion joint, ankle, wrist or knee was so injected, there was a rapid disappearance of symptoms and signs within twelve hours in each instance.

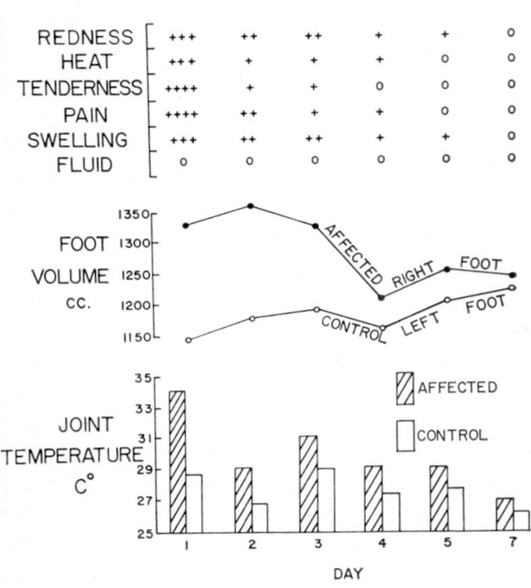

FIG. 59–7.—Clinical response in acute gouty arthritis affecting right foot treated with indomethacin for 7 days. Note reduction in inflammation foot volume and joint temperature during first 4 days of therapy. Unaffected left foot served as control of foot volume and joint temperature.

Other Measures

A large fluid intake is advisable and all alcoholic beverages should be avoided.

During the early hours of an acute gouty attack, opiates may be required to relieve severe pain; they are seldom required longer than twelve to twenty-four hours.

Premature resumption of normal activity may precipitate a flare-up. Strenuous physical therapy may provoke an exacerbation.

INTERVAL TREATMENT (STAGE II)

A plan that permits some selection and adaptability to the needs of the individual patient has been found preferable to a rigid program of strict dietary control. Such a program involves continuous urate diuretic therapy and/or allopurinol, and/or daily maintenance colchicine.

The aim of treatment in this stage of the disease is to avoid precipitating factors and to treat any acute episodes promptly. If the patient has a mild disease with no more than one attack of gout every year or two and has no evidence of renal disease and responds promptly to therapy of the acute episode, no daily drug therapy is used in the intercritical period.

Diet.—Ingested preformed purines are by no means the only source of uric acid, since uric acid is synthesized in the body (*see* Chapter 58). Complete control of urate formation by dietary regulation is therefore obviously impossible.

Since uric acid is largely derived from cell nuclei, the basic principle in the reg-

Table 59-2.—Low Purine Diet[143]

Purine Content of Foods per 100 Gm.

List A	*List B*	*List C*
(150–1000 mg.)	(50–150 mg.)	(0–15 mg.)
Sweetbreads	Meats	Vegetables
Anchovies	Fish	Fruits
Sardines	Sea Food	Milk
Liver	Beans	Cheese
Kidney	Peas	Eggs
Meat Extractives	Lentils	Cereal
	Spinach	

SPECIAL INSTRUCTIONS

1. Avoid liver, sweetbreads, brains and kidneys. A 2-oz. portion of any other meat, fish or fowl may be served twice weekly.
2. Serve cheese and eggs as meat substitute.
3. Use 1 to 2 pints of milk daily in order to meet the protein need.
4. Omit all meat extractives, broth, soups, and gravies.
5. A moderate reduction should be made in the following vegetables: beans, peas, lentils and spinach.
6. Allow fruits of all kinds—fresh, frozen, canned and dried.
7. Allow cereals of all kinds.
8. Serve sugar as desired with amount adjusted to caloric needs. Cream and butter may be restricted when a low-caloric allowance is needed or when a low-fat regimen is desired.

The approximate content of the above diet is 11 mg. of purine nitrogen or 34 mg. of uric acid.

ulation of the purine content of a diet for gout must be avoidance of those foods in which nuclei are abundant. A reasonably low purine intake is assured by omitting the foods that are included in List A, of the diet given in Table 59–2. If, in addition, moderate restrictions are placed on meats, fish, sea food, beans, peas, lentils and spinach (List B), the patient can easily obtain a balanced and palatable diet. Foods in List C may be consumed in amounts compatible with the caloric needs of the patient. The special instructions listed in the lower part of the diet schedule should be easily followed by most patients.

If the disease can be kept under good control with dietary restrictions and drug therapy, alcohol in moderation is allowed. Failure to control the frequency and duration of attacks is an indication for the complete abstinence from all alcoholic beverages.

Rarely a patient will report that a specific food or beverage will consistently induce an acute attack, apparently on the basis of an individual idiosyncrasy; avoidance of that trigger substance is clearly indicated in such cases.[27] If the patient is obese or significantly overweight, as is often the case, appropriate weight reduction should be recommended. Gutman has recently emphasized the influence of caloric restriction and weight reduction without any medications in lowering serum urate concentrations.[29] This physiological approach in the management of hyperuricemia in the obese patient with chronic gout should receive more attention.

Drugs

Colchicine.—Some experienced observers recommend colchicine in 0.5 mg. doses 1 to 3 times daily during the interval phase of gout. This practice is based upon the demonstration that maintenance colchicine has a prophylactic effect in reducing the frequency of attacks.[29,73,155] In those individuals who have less than one attack of gout per year, a few colchicine tablets may be taken at times when mild pains and aches appear in the joints.[136] Patients who recognize prodromata of an attack may abort attacks by prompt use of colchicine. In a few patients with severe gouty arthritis, 2 or 3 tablets of colchicine have been given daily for five years with no untoward effects from the prolonged ingestion of the drug. This program of prophylactic colchicine therapy, in doses of 0.5 to 2.0 mg. (1 to 4 tablets) daily, produced excellent or satisfactory results in terms of prevention of acute attacks in 94 per cent of 153 cases reported by Yü and Gutman.[155] The individual does not develop tolerance to the drug and the full course of colchicine is still just as effective in these individuals should an acute attack occur. There is increasing evidence that colchicine has a preeminent place in the prophylaxis of acute gout where there is frequent recurrence of attacks.

Urate Diuretics.—In recent years it has been clearly established that by protracted treatment with suitable uricosuric drugs, the formation of new tophi can be prevented, existing tophi made to shrink in size or disappear and the frequency of acute attacks of gouty arthritis reduced or prevented entirely. Such ideal results constitute a major therapeutic advance, but this optimistic outlook requires that the patient be willing to cooperate for long periods or perhaps for a lifetime. In chronic intermittent gouty arthritis (Stage II), urate diuretic drug therapy is used in those patients who are having frequent attacks of gout (3 to 4 attacks per year), when the disease is progressing rapidly, and in any patient with a persistently elevated serum urate level (greater than 9 mg%).[125,142]

Safe, effective, oral uricosuric drugs are probenecid (Benemid), and sulfinpyrazone (Anturane). These drugs have in common the property of increasing the urinary excretion of urates by blocking the renal tubular reabsorption of uric acid. It is the aim of long-term therapy to correct the hyperuricemia and in turn decrease the excess tissue stores of urates. This is accomplished by creating a negative urate balance with a resultant reduction of both the hyperuricemia and the enlarged miscible uric acid pool of the body. Whenever urate diuretic therapy is prescribed, it is worthwhile to take enough time to explain the objectives of therapy and to stress the necessity for complete cooperation even during the long asymptomatic periods. It is also well to point out that, during the first six months of therapy, attacks of gout are very likely to continue, but that this is no sign of failure of the program and is not an indication for stopping the drug. Time spent in such an instructional period will increase the probability of successful long-term results.

To reduce the tendency to develop renal calculi, many recommend increased fluid intake when uricosuric drugs are used. Others also advise using sodium bicarbonate in daily doses of 4 gm. or more to reduce acidity of the urine (*see also* below).

Probenecid (Benemid).—Many clinical studies[4,28,57,95] indicate that probenecid is an effective and safe uricosuric drug and of definite benefit in chronic gouty arthritis. There is general agreement that the incidence and severity of acute attacks of gout diminish with continued therapy. The amount of drug required to maintain the serum urate level at normal or near normal varies from 0.5 to 3.0 gm. per day. It is recommended that the beginning daily prophylactic dose of probenecid be 1.0 gm. taken in divided doses of 0.5 gm. each morning and evening; the maintenance dose is titrated to the serum uric acid response. Gutman[30] found the optimal daily dosage was 0.5 gm. in 10 per cent of patients, 1.0 gm. in 50 per cent, 1.5 to 2.0 gm. in 25 per cent, and 2.5 to 3.0 gm. in 15 per cent. Bartels[3] analyzed the amount of probenecid required to sustain a normal serum urate level in 95 patients with gout and found the dose ranged from 0.25 to 3.0 gm. per day, the average being 1.2 gm. per day. In some gouty patients, notably those with overt renal damage, it is impossible to lower the serum urate level below 7 mg.% even with daily doses of 2.5 to 3.0 gm.

If an acute episode of gouty arthritis occurs during uricosuric therapy, the urate diuretic should be continued during treatment with colchicine, indomethacin, or phenylbutazone. Because salicylates will block the diuretic effect of probenecid or other uricosuric drugs, aspirin or sodium salicylate should be prohibited. If an analgesic is necessary, codeine sulfate or Darvon may be tried.

Sulfinpyrazone (*Anturane*).—This drug has been shown to be a potent and safe uricosuric agent.[21,53,95,103,130,144]

In an extensive study of this drug, Yü, Burns and Gutman[153] treated 44 gouty subjects for periods up to sixteen months. A daily dose of 400 mg. was comparable to 1.5 to 2.0 mg. per day or more of probenecid. The mean initial blood uric acid level of 10.7 mg.% in this group was reduced to an average of 7.1 mg.%. The uricosuric action of sulfinpyrazone is well sustained in the recommended dose of 400 mg. per day over prolonged periods of three to twelve months.[95] The concomitant use of aspirin with this drug completely reverses the urate diuretic action. This drug is more potent as a uricosuric agent than probenecid on a weight basis and is often effective in patients refractory to other uricosuric agents.[122] These advantages are obvious and its low toxicity makes sulfinpyrazone a valuable agent for the long-term treatment of chronic gout.

Allopurinol (*Zyloprim*).—Rundles, Wyngaarden *et al.* in 1963 demonstrated that the *xanthine oxidase* blocking agent allopurinol [4-hydroxypyrazole (3, 4-d) pyrimidine] was capable of safely and effectively reducing the serum urate concentrations and producing minor increases in the urinary excretions of hypoxanthine and xanthine in patients with gout.[116] Allopurinol, by inhibiting the conversion of hypoxanthine to xanthine and xanthine to uric acid, blocks the final stages in the degradation of oxypurines to uric acid. It reduces the hazard of renal stones by reducing and spreading the total purine excretory load between uric acid, xanthine and hypoxanthine, each with its own solubility limit. Allopurinol is chiefly metabolized to form a dihydroxy compound, oxypurinol, which has a longer biological half-life than the parent drug; it inhibits xanthine oxidase and thus contributes to the suppression of uric acid formation.[17]

Dosage.—The aim of treatment is to attain a serum level of 6 to 7 mg.% and this is usually achieved by a dosage of 200 to 300 mg. per day. In some patients 400 to 600 mg. daily may be required. The dosage should be regulated to produce a satisfactory fall in the serum urate level. Like probenecid and sulfinpyrazone, allopurinol has no anti-inflammatory effects, hence, it has no place in the treatment of acute gouty arthritis (Fig. 59–8).

Clinical Use.—The clinical benefits derived from controlling the hyperuricemia in patients with chronic gout have been well established.[60,152,154,155] Most patents have progressively fewer and less severe attacks after starting treatment. However, at the beginning acute attacks may be precipitated in spite of adequate colchicine prophylaxis and the patient should be forewarned of this possibility. Progressive healing of bone lesions has been observed (Fig. 59–9) and massive tophi in bone with extensive destruction and large bursae have shown striking improvement in 6 to 8 months. Gutman and Yü treated 108 patients with uric acid nephrolithiasis in doses of 200 to

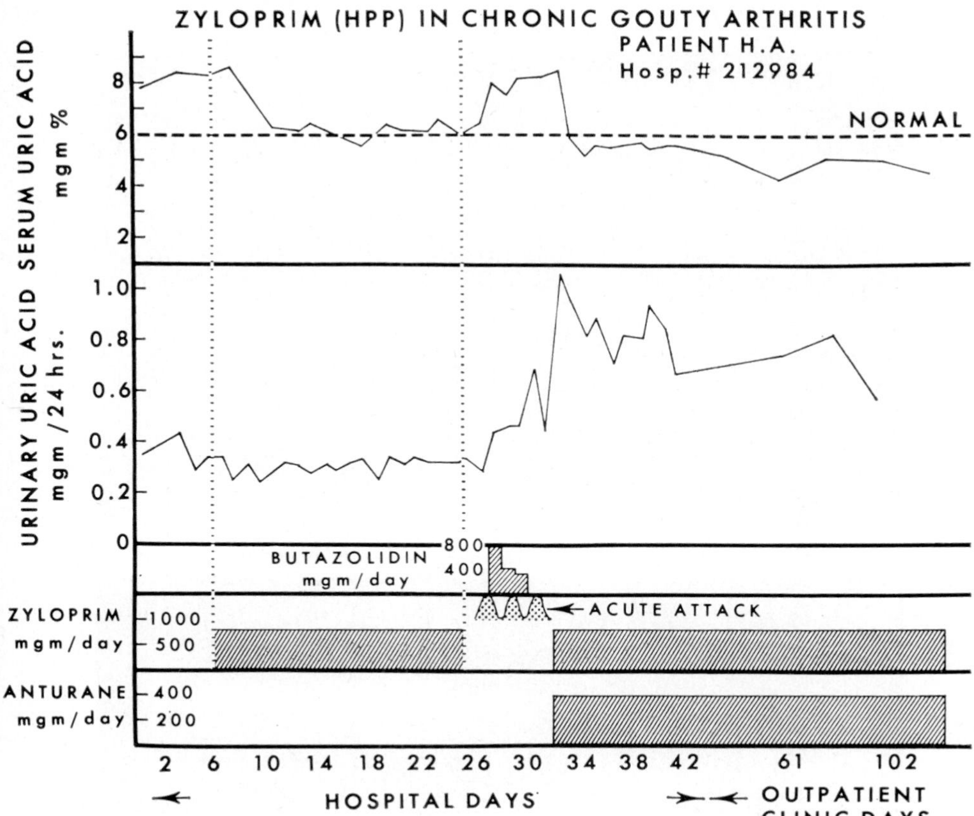

Fig. 59–8.—The prompt reduction of serum uric acid values to normal following two courses of allopurinol in this forty-two-year-old patient during study on a metabolic unit is shown above. This drug alone produced no change in the twenty-four-hour urinary excretion, but when sulfinpyrazone was added a prompt increase in the amount of urinary uric acid occurred. An acute attack of gout followed the first course of allopurinol therapy which promptly responded to phenylbutazone.

400 mg. per day and observed that the recurrence of renal calculi and the passage of sand and gravel ceased in all but 10 patients.[31]

The introduction of allopurinol marked a major advance in the treatment of chronic gouty arthritis. When this potent drug was first used there was concern about its potential for long-term toxicity. Experiences to date indicate that its continuous use for several years is well tolerated by the great majority of patients. However, there are reports of isolated instances of untoward reactions including alopecia, rashes, fever, chills, dizziness, nausea and diarrhea, bone marrow depression,[46] xanthine stones,[26] and severe hypersensitivity reactions with vasculitis and eosinophilia.[91,117,119] Recently Watts *et al.* using polarized light microscopy have demonstrated crystals of hypoxanthine, xanthine and oxypurinol in skeletal muscle biopsy specimens from gouty patients treated with allopurinol. These patients had no clinical or biochemical manifestations of muscle disease.[148]

The combined use of allopurinol plus either probenecid or sulfinpyrazone hastens the mobilization of stored urates and

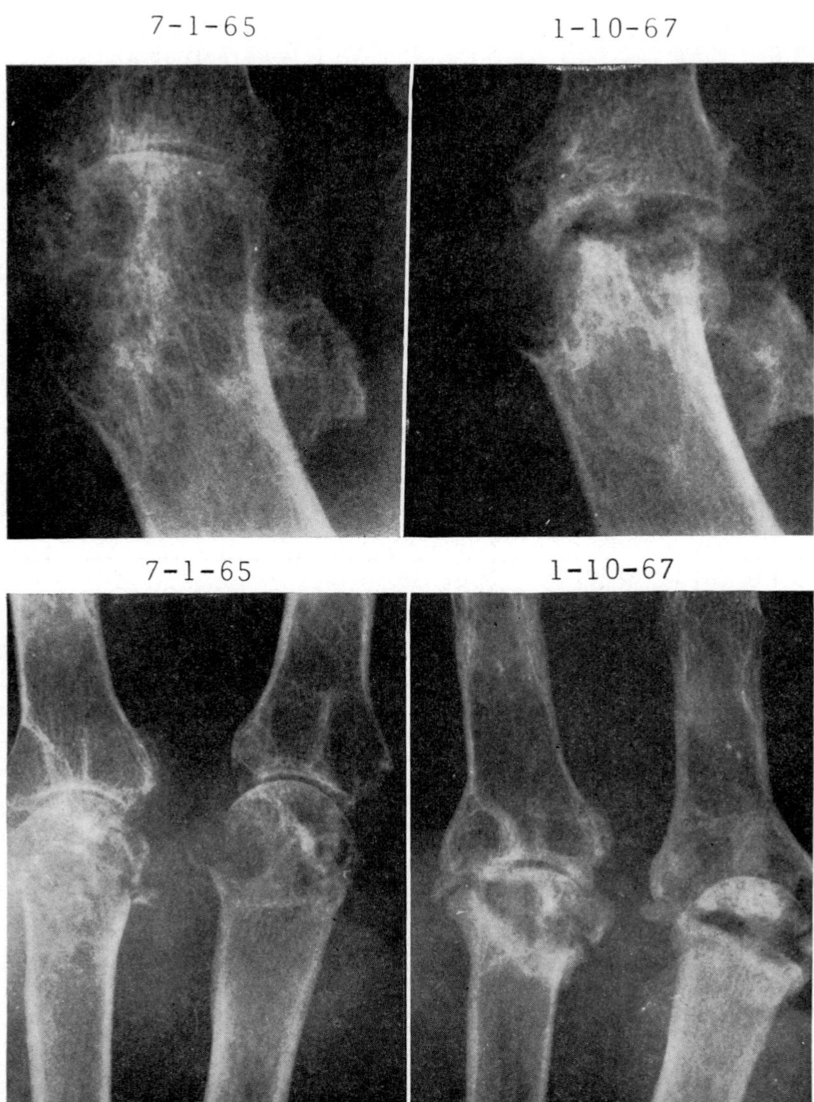

Fig. 59–9.—The roentgenograms of the left first metatarsophalangeal joint of patient K. C., showing on the left large lytic areas before therapy with allopurinol and on the right the same joint 18 months later. Note the bone resorption. The metacarpophalangeal joints of this patient show progressive destruction of bone despite treatment.

promotes more rapid disappearance of tophi (Fig. 59–10). The results obtained by increasing uric acid excretion and blocking its *de novo* biosynthesis have been uniformly excellent with a rapid resolution of extensive tophi and without the added risk of drug toxicity or urinary calculi.[22,97,128]

Indications for Allopurinol.—With the questions of the frequency of reactions to this relatively new agent still unanswered, it is the present policy to use one of the

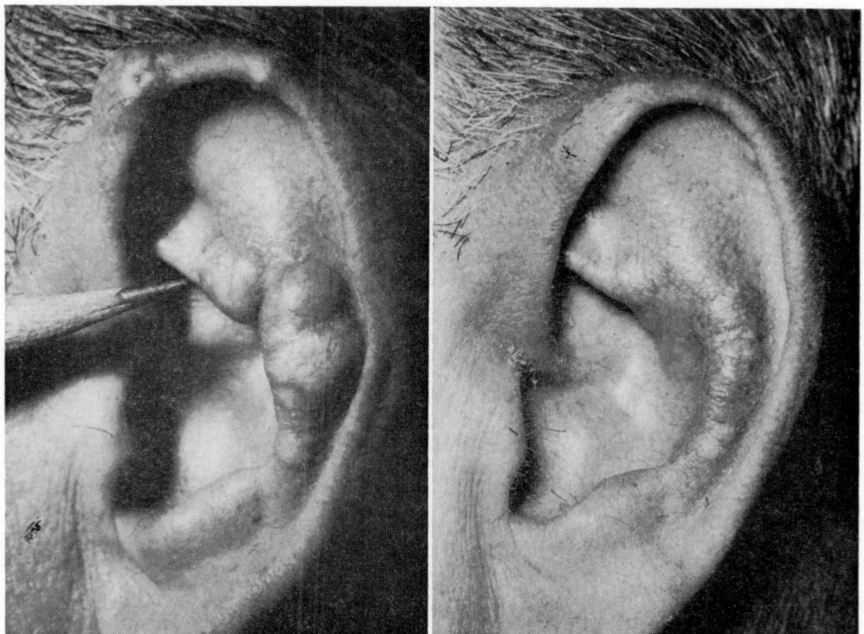

FIG. 59–10.—Left ear of patient with tophaceous gout. On left before allopurinol and probenecid therapy showing large tophaceous deposits in helix and antihelix. On right complete resolution after 10 months of therapy.

uricosuric drugs in the uncomplicated case of chronic gout and reserve allopurinol for those patients in whom probenecid and sulfinpyrazone have failed or are not tolerated, or in patients with renal failure, or who give a history of passing stones or gravel or hematuria. Allopurinol is also indicated in gouty patients who synthesize excessive amounts of uric acid, *i.e.*, with urinary uric acid excretion exceeding 700 mg. per day. It has the advantage over the uricosuric agents of being effective in the presence of renal failure.

TREATMENT OF CHRONIC GOUTY ARTHRITIS (STAGE III)

The mobilization of tophi by the protracted use of urate diuretic agents and/or allopurinol has been clearly demonstrated.[3,30,78] In patients with longstanding gout the severity and the frequency of severe attacks of gouty arthritis may be greatly reduced and the size of enlarged joints can be reduced. The drugs used in the management of the acute attacks in Stage III are the same as those used in Stage II and the manner of their administration is also the same. The response to colchicine, indomethacin, or phenylbutazone in the treatment of the acute arthritis may not be as complete nor as dramatic as in the earlier stages. Small daily doses of colchicine, 0.5 mg. twice or 3 times, are recommended by experienced observers.[138,155]

Uricosuric Drugs.—Protracted uricosuric therapy is essential in tophaceous gout. If a satisfactory result is to be obtained, the patient must adhere strictly to a program of restricted purine intake and the daily use of an effective uricosuric agent which will restore the uric acid to normal. If this is done, the formation of new tophi can be halted and established tophi made to disappear (Fig. 59–11). In a comparative long-term study of probenecid

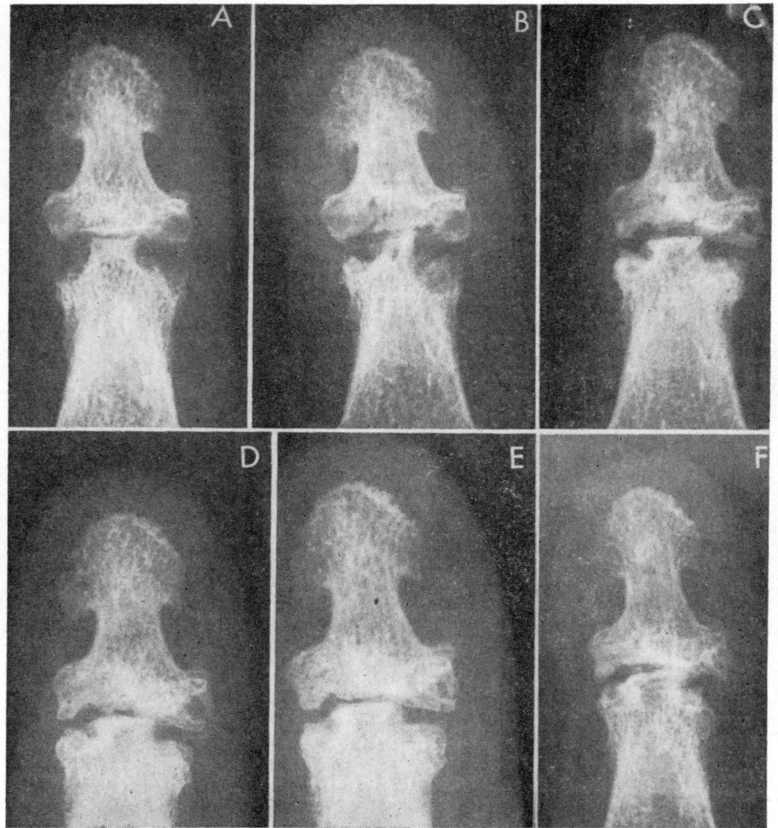

FIG. 59–11.—Roentgenograms of the same distal interphalangeal joint of the right index finger of a patient with tophaceous gout during a nine-year period of uninterrupted urate diuretic therapy. *A*, Feb. 4, 1955; *B*, Jan. 16, 1956; *C*, May 2, 1958; *D*, April 24, 1959; *E*, June 3, 1960; *F*, Feb. 21, 1968. Note the progressive regeneration of bone of the middle phalanx and the reduction in the size of the lytic area in the base of the distal phalanx.

and sulfinpyrazone in 58 patients with chronic gout, Velayos and Smyth[144] observed a more marked uricosuric effect during period of therapy with sulfinpyrazone. Seegmiller has pointed out that the greater uricosuric potency carried with it an increased potential hazard of precipitation of urate in the urinary tract, unless special attention is paid to measures for increasing the solubility of uric acid in the urine and, in preventing sudden high loads of uric acid delivered to the kidney, by careful attention to dosage.[125] The duration of uricosuric therapy depends upon the size of the mobilizable deposit of urate. When this is depleted, the dosage may be reduced or the drug withheld for periods depending on the rate of reaccumulation of the urate deposits.

Allopurinol

It has been clearly demonstrated that many patients refractory to conventional uricosuric therapy because of renal damage improve progressively with allopurinol therapy. It has also been shown that with its use the prevention of urolithiasis has been completely successful in both gouty and non-gouty subjects who formed uric acid stones. The effectiveness of allopurinol was dramatically shown by Ogryzlo *et al.* in a series of 27 consecutive stone formers with gout, who suffered a total of 63 episodes of renal colic requiring some form of surgical intervention in 14 patients during the three-year period immediately preceding therapy. In the course of 30 months of allopurinol therapy not one instance of stone formation was encountered.[97]

At present the use of allopurinol is reserved for the following circumstances: patients who have not been controlled by uricosuric drugs; patients with a history of passing stones or hematuria; and in patients with reduced renal function.

Gouty Kidney and Stones.—The appearance of proteinuria usually signals a disturbance of renal function, but this alone does not imply a serious prognosis and is not an indicator for allopurinol therapy. Because proteinuria may be observed for many years without the development of significant deterioration, such a patient should be observed and tested at intervals for concentrating ability and the clearance of creatinine or urea. The decision to start allopurinol therapy is based upon impaired renal function by these parameters. The incidence of renal injury sufficient to require prolonged therapy varies from 4 to 35 per cent with an average of 12 per cent of all patients.[2] There is agreement among observers who have studied the effect of allopurinol on the renal lesion of gout to indicate that in patients with azotemia no consistent deterioration occurs;[71,94,114,151] in some patients, renal function has shown progressive improvement.[9,126]

Since deposition of urate in the urinary tract is a potential hazard of therapy even with relatively low doses of uricosuric drugs, measures to reduce this tendency are recommended. A high fluid intake of at least 2 liters per day will increase the amount of solvent urine in which the urates are carried. Alkalinization of the urine to a pH of 7 will increase the solubility of urates in the urine. This can be readily effected by the administration of 4 gm. of sodium bicarbonate or trisodium citrate 3 to 4 times per day. For patients with hypertension or cardiac disease, in whom sodium retention must be avoided, the corresponding potassium salts may be used. Those patients who find the salts unpalatable may accept a solution composed of 100 gm. of sodium citrate, 100 gm. of potassium citrate, 70 gm. of citric acid and syrup of lemon flavoring to 1 liter administered in doses of 20 ml., 4 times per day. The availability of allopurinol has not eliminated the need for most of these measures in controlling stone formation.

Surgery in Gout.—Prior to the availability of modern drugs for the control of tophaceous deposits, the surgical removal of large and often ulcerating lesions, debridement and even amputation were occasionally necessary. Despite these remarkable advances, it may be beneficial to resect large deposits that are interfering mechanically with function (*see* Chapter 39). Tophaceous granulomatous tissue may fill the space beneath the transverse carpal ligament producing pressure of the median nerve (carpal tunnel syndrome).[99] The prompt surgical release with removal of the urate deposits will relieve pain and restore function in the affected hand (*see* Chapter 40).

PROGNOSIS

Prognosis is poorest in those whose symptoms appear early in life and best in those whose symptoms come on late in life. The severity of primary gout varies from a benign disease characterized by only a few attacks of acute arthritis to the rare but malignant course that begins at puberty and is marked by frequent recurrent episodes of crippling arthritis, the formation and passage of urate stones, a progressive loss of renal function and death from renal failure. Gout is a chronic disorder which is not cured when the acute attack has subsided. Treatment must be continued for life in order to prevent recurrence of symptoms. Faithful adherence to treatment (especially between acute attacks) will modify the course, reduce the severity and number of attacks, reduce the likelihood or prevent the occurrence of chronic gouty arthritis, and possibly postpone or avoid fatal renal and cardiovascular complications. Most patients with gout may lead a normal life by simply following a long-term plan of management, provided the disease is recognized early. Usually the life expectancy is better than the degree of renal impairment might suggest and available evidence indicates that the longevity of gouty patients is not significantly less than that of the adult male population of the United States.[140,141] The prognosis in secondary gout is usually that of the underlying disease.

BIBLIOGRAPHY

1. Ball, G. V. and Morgan, J. M.: South Med. J., *61*, 21, 1968.
2. Barlow, K. A. and Berlin, L. J.: Quart. J. Med., *37*, 79, 1968.
3. Bartels, E. C.: Ann. Intern. Med., *42*, 1, 1955.
4. Bartels, E. C. and Matossian, G. S.: Arth. & Rheum., *2*, 193, 1959.
5. Bartels, E. C.: Med. Clin. North America, *44*, 543, 1960.
6. Berman, P. H., Balis, M. E. and Dancis, J.: J. Lab. Clin. Med., *71*, 247, 1968.
7. Bocher, J., Mankin, H. J., Berk, R. N. and Rodnan, J. P.: New Engl. J. Med., *272*, 1093, 1965.
8. Breckenridge, A.: Lancet, *1*, 15, 1966.
9. Briney, W., Ogden, D., Bartholomew, B. A. and Smyth, C. J.: Unpublished data.
10. Brown, J. and Mallory, G. K.: New Engl. J. Med., *243*, 325, 1950.
11. Caner, J. E. Z. and Decker, J. L.: Amer. J. Med., *36*, 571, 1964.
12. Cannon, P. J., Stason, W. B., Demartini, F. E., Sommers, S. C. and Laragh, J. H.: New Engl. J. Med., *275*, 457, 1966.
13. Davis, J. S., Jr. and Bartfield, H.: Amer. J. Med., *16*, 218 (Feb) 1954.
14. Decker, J. L., Lane, J. J., Jr. and Reynolds, W. E.: Arth. & Rheum., *5*, 144–155 (Apr) 1962.
15. Dodds, W. J. and Steinbach, H. L.: New Engl. J. Med., *275*, 745, 1966.
16. Drenick, E. J., Swensied, M. E., Blahd, W. H., and Tuttle, S. G.: J.A.M.A., *187*, 100, 1964.
17. Elion, G. B., Yü, T. F., Gutman, A. B. and Hitchings, G. H.: Amer. J. Med., *45*, 69, 1968.
18. Emmerson, B. T.: Austral. Ann. Med., *14*, 295, 1965.
19. Ficarra, B. J. and Adams, R.: Arch. Surg., *7*, 229, 1945.
20. Gertler, M. M., Garn, S. M. and Levine, S. A.: Ann. Intern. Med., *34*, 1421, 1951.
21. Glick, E. N.: Proc. Roy. Soc. Med., *54*, 423, 1961.
22. Goldfarb, E. and Smyth, C. J.: Arth. & Rheum., *9*, 414, 1966.
23. Gonick, H. C., Rubini, M. E., Gleason, I. O. and Sommers, S. C.: Ann. Intern. Med., *62*, 667, 1965.
24. Good, A. E. and Rapp, R.: New Engl. J. Med., *277*, 286, 1967.
25. Grahame, R. and Scott, J. T.: Ann. Rheum. Dis., *29*, 461, 1970.
26. Greene, M. L., Fujimoto, W. Y. and Seegmiller, J. E.: New Engl. J. Med., *280*, 426–427, 1969.
27. Gutman, A. B.: J. Am. Geriatrics Soc., *16*, 499, 1968.
28. Gutman, A. B.: Advances Pharmacol., *4*, 91, 1966.
29. Gutman, A. B.: "*The Changing Pattern of Gout*"—(The First Richard Freyberg Lecture), New York, Hospital for Special Surgery, Nov. 12, 1970.
30. Gutman, A. B.: Lancet, *2*, 1258, 1957.
31. Gutman, A. B., Yü, T. F. and Berger, L.: Amer. J. Med., *47*, 575, 1969.
32. Gutman, A. B. and Yü, T. F.: Amer. J. Med., *45*, 756, 1968.
33. Hall, A. P., Barry, P. E., Dawber, T. R. and McNamara, P. M.: Amer. J. Med., *42*, 27, 1967.
34. Hall, A. P., Holloway, V. P. and Scott, J. T.: Ann. Rheum. Dis., *23*, 439, 1964.
35. Hart, F. D. and Boardman, P. L.: Brit. Med. J., *2*, 965, 1963.
36. Hauge, M. and Harvald, B.: Acta Med. Scand., *152*, 247, 1955.
37. Hellman, L.: Science, *109*, 280, 1949.
38. Hench, P. S.: J. Lab. & Clin. Med., *22*, 48, 1936.
39. Hench, P. S.: In *Nelson's Loose Leaf Living Surg.*, New York, Thomas Nelson & Sons. *3*, 104, 1935.
40. Hollander, J. L.: J. Bone Joint Surg., *354*, 983, 1953.
41. Hollander, J. L., Brown, E. M. and Elkinton, J. R.: Proceedings Second Clinical ACTH Conf. Philadelphia, The Blakiston Co., 1951.

42. Hollander, J. L., Brown, E. M., Jessar, R. A. and Brown, C. Y.: J.A.M.A., *147*, 1629, 1951.
43. Howard, R. S. and Walzak, M. P.: J. Urol., *98*, 639, 1968.
44. Huber: Deutsch. med Wchnschr., *22*, 182, 1896.
45. Hunder, G. G., Worthington, J. W. and Bickel, W. H.: J.A.M.A., *203*, 47, 1968.
46. Irby, R., Toone, E. and Owen, D., Jr.: Arth. & Rheum., *9*, 860, 1966.
47. Jaffe, A. and Hyman, G. A.: New Engl. J. Med., *257*, 157, 1957.
48. Jakovcic, S. and Sorensen, L. B.: Arth. & Rheum., *10*, 129, 1967.
49. Kantor, G. I.: J.A.M.A., *212*, 478, 1970.
50. Kaplan, H.: New Engl. J. Med., *263*, 778, 1960.
51. ————: New Engl. J. Med., *268*, 761, 1963.
52. Kaufman, J. M., Greene, M. L. and Seegmiller, J. E.: J. Pediat., *73*, 583, 1968.
53. Kersley, G. D., Cook, E. R. and Tovey, D. C. J.: Ann. Rheum. Dis., *17*, 326, 1958.
54. Kelley, W. N., Greene, M. L., Rosenbloom, F. M., Henderson, J. F., and Seegmiller, J. E.: Ann. Intern. Med., *70*, 155, 1969.
55. Kelley, W. N., Rosenbloom, F. M., Henderson, J. F., and Seegmiller, J. E.: Proc. Nat. Acad. Sci., *57*, 1735, 1967.
56. Kelly, W. N., Rosenbloom, F. M., and Seegmiller, J. E.: J. Pediat., *72*, 488, 1968.
57. Kidd, E. C., Boyce, K. C. and Freyberg, R. H.: Ann. Rheum. Dis., *12*, 20, 1953.
58. Kittredge, W. E. and Downs, R.: J. Urol., *67*, 841, 1952.
59. Klinenberg, J. R., Goldfinger, S., Miller, J. and Seegmiller, J. E.: Arth. & Rheum., *6*, 779, 1963.
60. Klinenberg, J. R., Goldfinger, S. E. and Seegmiller, J. E.: Ann. Intern. Med., *62*, 639, 1965.
61. Kogut, M. D., Donnell, G. N., Nyhan, W. L. and Sweetman, L.: Amer. J. Med., *48*, 148, 1970.
62. Kohn, N. N., Hughes, R. E., McCarty, J. J., Jr. and Faires, J. S.: Ann. Intern. Med., *56*, 738, 1962.
63. Kohn, P. M. and Prozan, G. B.: J.A.M.A., *170*, 1909, 1959.
64. Kuzell, W. C. and Schaffarzick, R. W.: Ann. Review Med., *2*, 367, 1951.
65. Kuzell, W. C., Schaffarzick, R. W., Brown, B. and Mankle, E. A.: J.A.M.A., *149*, 729, 1952.
66. Kuzell, W. C., Schaffarzick, R. W., Naugler, W. E., Koets, P., Mankle, E. A., Brown, B. and Champlin, B.: J. Chronic Dis., *2*, 645, 1955.
67. Kulka, J. P. and Schumacher, H. R.: Bull. Rheum. Dis., *18*, 495, 1968.
68. Lambeth, J. T.: Radiology, *95*, 413, 1970.
69. Lesch, M. and Nyhan, W. L.: Amer. J. Med., *36*, 561, 1964.
70. Leven, M. H., Fred, L. and Bassett, S. H.: Amer. J. Med., *15*, 525, 1953.
71. Levin, N. W. and Abrahams, O. L.: Ann. Rheum. Dis., *25*, 681–687, 1966.
72. Linton, R. R. and Talbott, J. H.: Ann. Surg., *117*, 161, 1943.
73. Lockie, M.: Bull. Rheum. Dis., *6*, 97, 1955.
74. Lucey, C.: Irish J. Med. Sci., *423*, 113, 1961.
75. Malawista, S. E.: Arth. & Rheum., *7*, 325, 1964.
76. ————: Arth. & Rheum., *11*, 191, 1968.
77. Mason, R. M.: Brit. Med. J., *1*, 1522, 1959.
78. Marson, F. G. W.: Brit. J. Radiol., *25*, 539, 1952.
79. Martel, W.: Radiology, *91*, 755, 1968.
80. McCarty, D. J., Jr.: Disease-a-Month, *1*, 31, 1970.
81. McCarty, D. J., Jr.: Clin. Orthop. & Rel. Res., *71*, 28, 1970.
82. McCarty, D. J., Jr. and Hollander, J. L.: Ann. Intern. Med., *54*, 452, 1961.
83. ————: Amer. J. Med. Sci., *243*, 288, 1962.
84. McCarty, D. J., Jr., Kohn, N. N. and Faires, J. S.: Ann. Intern. Med., *56*, 711, 1962.
85. McCarty, D. J., Jr. and Gatter, R. A.: Bull. Rheum. Dis., *14*, 331, 1964.
86. McCrea, L. E.: J. Urol., *73*, 29, 1955.
87. McWilliams, J. R.: Amer. J. Ophthal., *35*, 1778, 1952.
88. Michotte, L. J. and Wauters, M.: Acta Rheum. Scand., *10*, 273, 1964.
89. Mikkelsen, W. M. and Robinson, W. D.: Med. Clin. North America, *53*, 1331 (Nov) 1969.
90. Mikkelsen, W. M., Dodge, H. J. and Valkenburg, H.: Amer. J. Med., *39*, 242–251, 1965.
91. Mills, R. M., Jr.: J.A.M.A., *216*, 799, 1971.
92. Mugler, A.: Ann. Med., *5*, 51, 1950.
93. Neel, J. V.: Medicine, *26*, 115, 1947.
94. Ogryzlo, M. A.: Clinical Orthop. & Rel. Res., *71*, 46, 1970.
95. Ogryzlo, M. A. and Harrison, J.: Ann. Rheum. Dis., *16*, 425, 1957.
96. Ogryzlo, M. A., Urowitz, M., Weber, H. M. and Haupt, J. B.: Ann. Rheum. Dis. *25* (Suppl), 673, 1966.

97. Ogryzlo, M. A., Urowitz, M. B., Weber, H. M. and Haupt, J. B.: Canad. Med. Assoc. J., *95*, 1120, 1966.
98. O'Brien, W. M., Burch, T. A. and Bunin, J. J.: Arth. & Rheum., *7*, 335, 1964.
99. O'Hara, L. J. and Levin, M.: Arch. Intern. Med., *120*, 180, 1967.
100. Owen, D. S., Toone, E. and Irby, R.: J.A.M.A., *197*, 123, 1966.
101. Padova, J. and Bendersky, G.: New Engl. J. Med., *267*, 530, 1962.
102. Paulus, H. E., Coutts, A., Calabro, J. J. and Klinenberg, J. R.: J.A.M.A., *211*, 277, 1970.
103. Percellin, R. H. and Schmid, F. R.: J.A.M.A., *175*, 971, 1961.
104. Percy, J. S. and Smyth, C. J.: Unpublished data.
105. Percy, J. S., Stephenson, P. and Thompson, M.: Ann. Rheum. Dis., *23*, 226, 1964.
106. Phelps, P., Steele, A. D. and McCarty, D. J., Jr.: J.A.M.A., *203*, 508, 1968.
107. Polley, H. F. and Bickel, W. H.: Ann. Rheum. Dis., *10*, 227, 1951.
108. Primer on Rheumatic Diseases: Comm. Amer. Rheum. Assoc., J.A.M.A., *190*, 509–530, 1964.
109. Rakic, M. T., Valkenburg, H. A., Davidson, R. T., Engels, J. P., Mikkelsen, W. H., Neel, J. V., and Duff, I. F.: Amer. J. Med., *37*, 862, 1964.
110. Rieselbach, R. E., Sorensen, L. B., Shelp, W. D. and Steele, T. H.: Ann. Intern. Med., *73*, 359, 1970.
111. Robinson, W. D., Conn, J. W., Block, W. D., Louis, L. H. and Katz, J.: Ann. Rheum. Dis., *8*, 313, 1949.
112. Rosenberg, E. F.: Ann. Rheum. Dis., *2*, 273, 1941.
113. Rosenberg, A. L., Bergstrom, L., Troost, T. and Bartholomew, B. A.: New Engl. J. Med., *282*, 992, 1970.
114. Rundles, R. W.: Ann. Rheum. Dis., *25*, 694, 1966.
115. Rundles, R. W., Wyngaarden, J. B., Hitchings, G. H. and Elion, G. B.: Ann. Rev. Pharmacol., *9*, 345, 1969.
116. Rundles, R. W., Wyngaarden, J. B., Hitchings, G. H., Elion, G. B. and Silberman, H. R.: Tr. Assoc. Am. Physicians, *76*, 126, 1963.
117. Rundles, R. W., Metz, E. N. and Silberman, H. R.: Ann. Intern. Med., *64*, 229, 1966.
118. Schnitker, M. A. and Richter, A. B.: Am. J. Med. Sci., *192*, 241, 1936.
119. Scott, J. T. (ed): Ann. Rheum. Dis., *25*, (Suppl.), 599, 1966.
120. Scott, J. T., Holloway, V., Arnot, R. N. and Glass, H. I.: Ann. Rheum. Dis., *28*, 366, 1969.
121. Scott, J. T., Dixon, A. St. J., and Bywaters, E. G. L.: Brit. Med. J., *1*, 1070, 1964.
122. Seegmiller, J. E.: Bull. Rheum. Dis., *11*, 251, 1961.
123. Seegmiller, J. E.: Med. Ann. D.C., *36*, 215, 1967.
124. Seegmiller, J. E., Laster, L. and Howell, R. R.: New Engl. J. Med., *268*, 712, 764, 821, 1963.
125. Seegmiller, J. E.: Med. Clin. North America, *45*, 1259, 1961.
126. Sjoberg, K.-H.: Ann. Rheum. Dis., *25*, 688–690, 1966.
127. Smyth, C. J., *et al.*: Ann. Intern. Med., *50*, 633, 1959.
128. Smyth, C. J.: Clin. Orthop. & Rel. Res., *57*, 69, 1968.
129. Smyth, C. J., Cotterman, C. W. and Freyberg, R. H.: J. Clin. Invest., *27*, 749, 1948.
130. Smyth, C. J., Frank, L. S. and Huffman, E. R.: Arch. Interamer. Rheum., *3*, 3, 1960.
131. Smyth, C. J. and Frank, L. S.: Rheumatism, *18*, 2, 1962.
132. Smyth, C. J., Velayos, E. E. and Amoroso, C.: Acta Rheum. Scand., *9*, 306, 1963.
133. Steinberg, V. L. and Mason, R. M.: Brit. J. Clin. Pract., *16*, 173, 1962.
134. Straub, L. R., Smith, J. W. and Carpenter, G. K.: J. Bone Joint Surg., *43A*, 731, 1961.
135. Talbott, J. H.: *Gout*, 3rd Ed., New York, Grune & Stratton, 1967.
136. ————: Bull. N.Y. Acad. Med., *18*, 318, 1942.
137. ————: Veterans Adm. Tech. Bull., *10*, 90, 1953.
138. ————: Ann. Intern. Med., *42*, 1137, 1955.
139. Talbott, J. H. and Coombs, F. C.: J. Clin. Invest., *17*, 508, 1938.
140. Talbott, J. H. and Lilienfield, A.: Geriatrics, *14*, 409, 1959.
141. Talbott, J. H. and Terplan, K. L.: Medicine, *39*, 405, 1960.
142. Thompson, G. R., Duff, I. F., Robinson, W. D., Mikkelsen, W. M. and Galindez, H.: Arth. & Rheum., *5*, 384, 1962.
143. Turner, D.: *Handbook of Diet Therapy*, Chicago, Univ. Chicago Press, 1946, p. 41.
144. Velayos, E. and Smyth, C. J.: Arch. Intern. Med., *116*, 212, 1965.

145. WALLACE, S. L., BERNSTEIN, D. and DIAMOND, H.: J.A.M.A., *199*, 525, 1967.
146. WALLACE, S. L., OMOKOKA, B. and ERTEL, N. H.: Amer. J. Med., *48*, 443, 1970.
147. WATTS, R. W. E.: Proc. Roy. Soc. Med., *62*, 853, 1969.
148. WATTS, R. W. E., SCOTT, J. T., CHALMERS, R. A., BITENSKY, L. and CHAYEN, J.: Quart. J. Med., *40*, 1, 1971.
149. WHITEHOUSE, F. W. and CLEARY, W. J., JR.: J.A.M.A., *197*, 73, 1966.
150. WILSON, G. M., JR., HUFFMAN, E. R. and SMYTH, C. J.: Amer. J. Med., *21*, 232, 1956.
151. WILSON, J. O., SIMONDS, H. A. and NORTH, J. D. K.: Ann. Rheum. Dis., *26*, 136, 1967.
152. WYNGAARDEN, J. B., RUNDLES, R. W., SILBERMAN, H. R. and HUNTER, S.: Arth. & Rheum., *6*, 306, 1963.
153. YÜ, T. F., BURNS, J. J. and GUTMAN, A. B.: Arth. & Rheum., *1*, 532, 1958.
154. YÜ, T. F. and GUTMAN, A. B.: Amer. J. Med., *37*, 885, 1964.
155. ————: Ann. Intern. Med., *55*, 179, 1961.
156. ————: Ann. Intern. Med., *67*, 1133, 1967.
157. ZEVELEY, H. A., FRENCH, A. J., MIKKELSEN, W. M. and DUFF, I. F.: Amer. J. Med., *20*, 510, 1956.
158. ZITNAN, D. and SITAJ, S.: Ann. Rheum. Dis., *22*, 142, 1963.
159. ZUCKNER, J.: New Engl. J. Med., *14*, 783, 1963.

Chapter 60

Pseudogout; Articular Chondrocalcinosis

Calcium Pyrophosphate Crystal Deposition Disease

By Daniel J. McCarty, Jr., M.D.

Introduction

Microscopic examination of wet preparations of synovial fluid by compensated polarized light has provided a rapid, specific and sensitive method for identification of crystals in gout (which might be called sodium urate crystal deposition disease).[26,38] In the description of such crystals in the language of crystallographers, both monoclinic (unit cell with one obtuse and 2 right angles) and triclinic (unit cell with 3 obtuse angles) types are seen, and "twinning" or pairing of crystals is frequently observed. Specific digestion with purified uricase has established the specific chemical composition of these crystals.[26]

Application of these methods to examination of many synovial fluids led to the discovery of non-urate crystals in the joint fluid from patients with a gout-like syndrome ("pseudogout").[26,27] These biaxial crystals were identified as calcium pyrophosphate dihydrate ($Ca_2P_2O_7.2H_20$), which we hereinafter refer to as "CPPD",[20] and are illustrated in Figure 60–1*a*. Crystallographically, these exhibited monoclinic and triclinic dimorphism and frequently showed twinning. Polariscopically, they showed a *weakly positive* birefringence and inclined extinction. Some CPPD crystals are isotropic (non-refractile). Urate crystals, on the other hand, are *strongly negatively* birefringent under compensated polarized light and show axial extinction. Fluid removed from acutely inflamed joints of patients with pseudogout invariably showed phagocytosed CPPD crystals (Fig. 60–1*b*).

Both monosodium urate and calcium pyrophosphate (CPPD) crystals have been synthesized with morphologic features identical to natural crystals.[3,11] Injection of such crystals into normal human and canine joints was followed by an acute inflammatory response associated with phagocytosis by polymorphonuclear and mononuclear leukocytes. This response was completely reversible, dose related, and non-specific with regard to host species or to the chemical nature of the injected crystal. These findings confirm the older work of Riehl, His and Freudweiler[12,13,18,40] and complement the more recent findings of Seegmiller *et al.*,[45] describing an acute inflammatory response to microcrystalline sodium urate injected into the joints of gouty patients. The phrase "crystal-induced synovitis" was coined to describe the tissue reaction provoked by either type of crystal.[30]

Initially, seven arthritic patients were collected over a two-year period, using the presence of microcrystalline calcium pyrophosphate dihydrate as a common denominator (Figs. 60–2, 60–3). The interplanar spacings and relative intensities of x-ray diffraction powder patterns prepared from clinical material are compared with those of pure monoclinic and triclinic CPPD prepared by Brown *et al.*[3] in Table 60–1. After the clinical and roentgenologic findings in this group

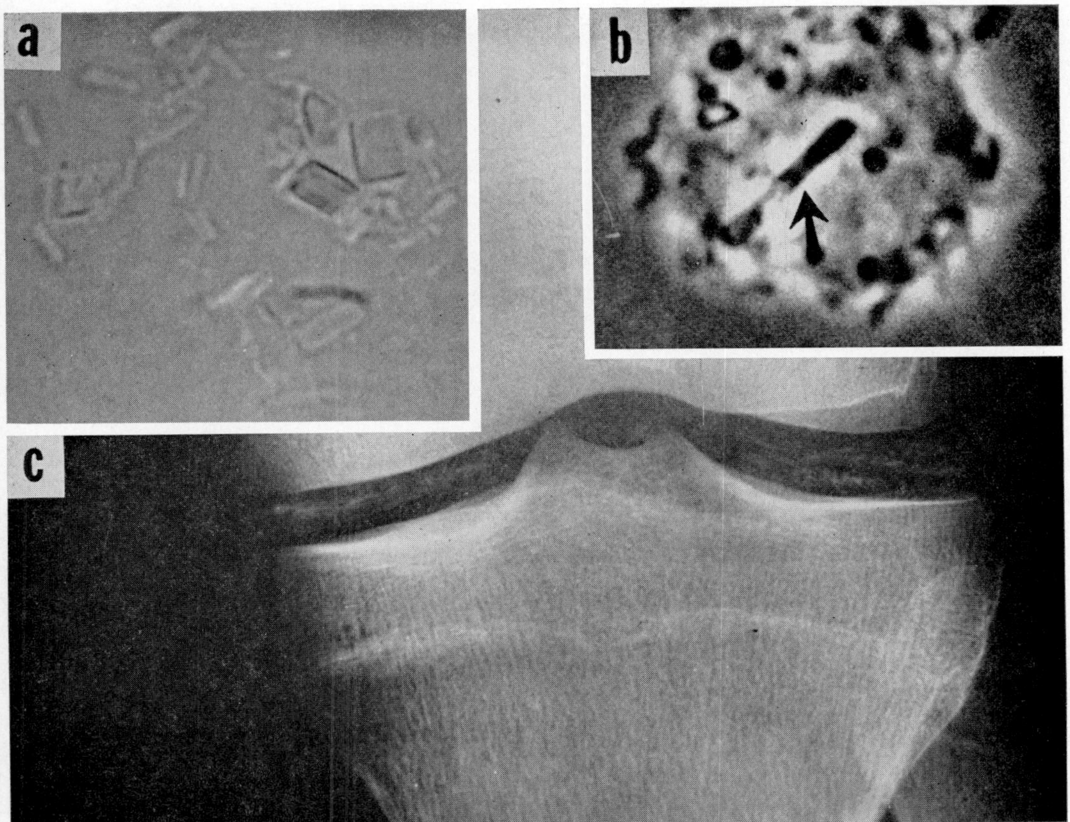

Fig. 60–1.—(*a*) Weakly birefringent monoclinic and triclinic calcium pyrophosphate dihydrate (CPPD) microcrystals in synovial fluid removed from a chronically symptomatic knee (polarized light × 1250). (*b*) Phagocytosed crystal (arrow) in a polymorphonuclear leukocyte (phase contrast × 1250). (*c*) Anteroposterior roentgenogram of the knee showing typical punctate and linear deposits of CPPD in the menisci and articular cartilage.

were analyzed, a review of the literature revealed that they were strikingly similar to the features of chondrocalcinosis polyarticularis (familiaris), as described in 1958 by the Czechoslovakian authors, Zitnan and Sitaj.[59] These workers used the highly characteristic roentgenologic appearance as the unifying diagnostic feature. They pointed out that the menisci of the knee were most commonly involved (Fig. 60–1*c*). These authors have recently reported 27 cases, 21 of which were from 5 families; moreover, 4 of the affected families were from a single village.[60] Among the cases forming the basis of our present series there are four crystallographically proved examples of familial disease.

Two types of meniscal calcification were differentiated on gross and microscopic pathologic grounds in 1927 by the Viennese surgeon Mandl.[21] A "primary" type predominated in the elderly, involved all 4 menisci with diffuse focal deposits of calcium salts, had smooth meniscal surfaces, occurred without antecedent trauma, and was frequently asymptomatic. Microscopically, punctate deposits of granular calcific material and a striking hypocellularity of the involved

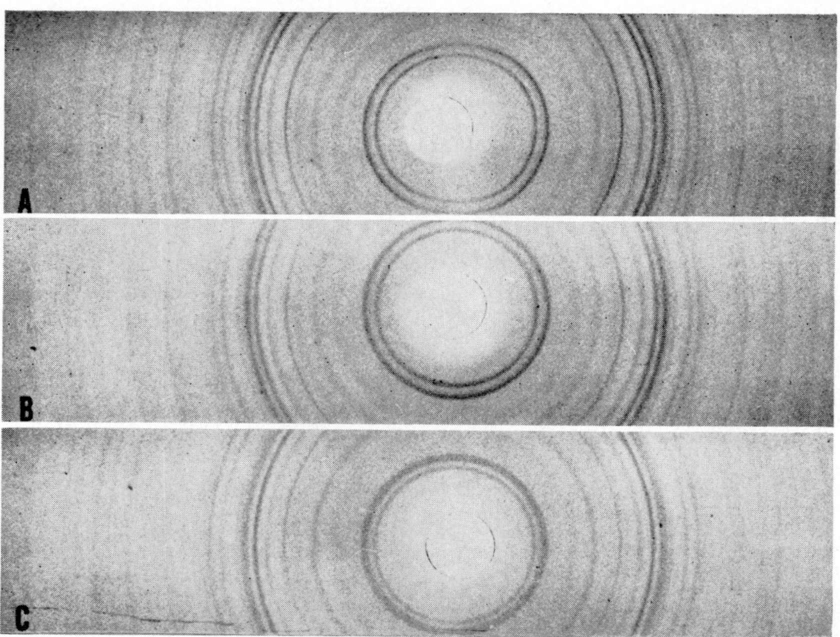

FIG. 60–2.—X-ray diffraction powder patterns of crystals harvested from fluid aspirated from the knees of 3 patients; the interplanar spacings of the crystal populations are identical. The powder pattern is known as the "fingerprint" of the crystal and is ideal for the specific identification of very small crystals such as these

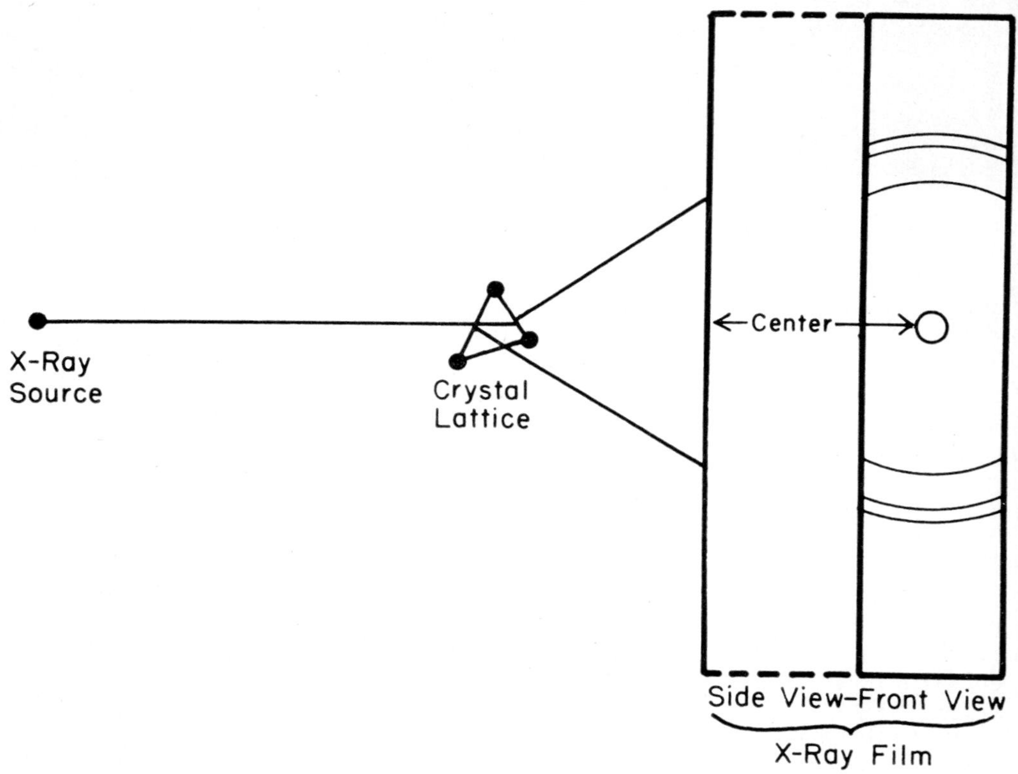

FIG. 60–3.—Diagram showing the essential features of the powder pattern technique. Low energy x rays are diffracted by sheets of atoms the arrangement of which is highly specific for a given crystal. The diffracted beams are recorded on a strip of x-ray film, located at a fixed distance from the crystals. When developed, a series of arcs are obtained. The interplanar spacings between the atomic sheets may then be calculated simply from measurements made on the arcs.

TABLE 60–1.—SUMMARY OF MAJOR INTERPLANAR SPACINGS AND RELATIVE INTENSITIES OF NATURAL CPPD (MEAN OF 78 PATTERNS*) COMPARED WITH THOSE OF SYNTHETIC CPPD.

Natural		*Synthetic*			
		Monoclinic		*Triclinic*	
d†	*i*‡	*d*	*i*	*d*	*i*
8.04	100			7.94	90
7.37	30	7.37	90		
7.01	90			6.95	90
		6.12	35		
5.50	20			5.50	20
		5.40	30		
5.25	20			5.27	20
4.61	40	4.62	100		
4.50	25			4.49	50
4.02	30			4.03	50
3.74	10	3.72	75	3.74	10
3.45	50	3.45	50	3.48	70
3.24	100	3.25	100	3.24	100
3.12	90			3.11	100
3.06	40	3.05	100	3.06	25
2.98	50			2.98	60
2.78	50	2.79	40	2.78	60
2.67	50	2.65	90	2.67	60
2.59	20	2.57	100	2.59	30
2.52	25			2.53	40
2.44	15	2.42	40		
2.40	10			2.40	35
2.34	15			2.34	25
2.30	5	2.31	40		
2.26	25			2.26	50
2.18	10	2.21	35	2.20	25
2.11	15	2.11	35	2.11	30
2.06	10			2.07	25
2.01	20	2.01	40	2.01	40
		1.91	40		
1.90	15			1.90	20
1.84	15	1.85	25	1.84	30
1.81	10			1.81	30
		1.77	30		
1.75	10	1.74	25	1.75	25
1.72	10	1.71	25	1.72	40
1.66	10			1.66	30
1.63	10			1.63	20
1.57	15	1.57	20	1.57	25

* All patterns obtained with a 114.59 mm. diameter Debye-Scherrer powder camera using nickel-filtered copper K alpha radiation (λ = 1.54050 Å).

† *d* = interplanar spacings in Angstroms.

‡ *i* = relative intensities estimated visually by assigning the value of 100 to the strongest line and comparing the other lines to this standard.

cartilage were noted. A "secondary" type, found in a younger age group, involved a localized deposit in a single meniscus in one knee; this type usually followed trauma to the joint. The cartilage surface over the deposit was roughened and the condition was always symptomatic, frequently requiring surgical intervention.

A well-studied case reported by Werwath in 1928[55] contained the first roentgenogram showing the characteristic pattern of "primary" calcification and correlated this pattern with the pathological findings at meniscectomy. Calcifiactions were found in the menisci, hyaline articular cartilage, ligaments and joint capsule; the author felt that the condition was due to a metabolic disorder and that it led to arthritis deformans (osteoarthritis). In 1929, Tobler[47] systematically examined 400 menisci from 100 necropsies of cadavers ranging in age from several days to eighty-six years. He found degenerative changes in 75 per cent and calcification in 25 per cent of menisci.

In their classic monograph on the effect of aging in the knee, Bennett, Waine and Bauer[1a] described small deposits of "granular material" in semilunar cartilages showing interstitial matrix markedly altered by degenerative changes. These deposits, observed in 2 medial menisci from cadavers in their fifth decade, were thought to represent an early stage of calcification. Marked calcifications of the "primary" type were found in the lateral meniscus of a ninety-year-old man; the medial meniscus, similarly involved, had been almost completely destroyed. Thus 3 of 63 cadavers studied showed "primary" calcification (4.1 per cent). It is important to remember that none in their series had had symptomatic arthritis during life.

Bennett *et al.*[1a] state that the menisci of the immature subject adapt to joint enlargement during the growth phase by a generative process beginning at the medial border; this observation also had been made by Tobler.[47] Semi-quantitation of articular degenerative changes, based on gross and microscopic criteria, showed an increase with age in all portions of the joints studied. The rate of increase in degeneration was accentuated markedly after age seventy in the synovial membrane, perichondral margins, and menisci as compared to the articular surfaces of the joints.

Prevalence

X-ray diffraction powder patterns were obtained from at least one tissue deposit or from crystals harvested from synovial fluid in 51 of our first 80 cases; all were CPPD. A study of over 800 menisci from 215 anatomical cadavers was undertaken, using the CPPD crystal as a "marker" (Fig. 60–4). At least 1 tiny deposit was seen in the type M roentgenogram of 22 per cent of excised menisci; most were too small to permit dissection, much less identification. Seven sets of menisci (3.3 per cent of cadavers) showed linear and punctate deposits of CPPD; 5 sets (2.3 per cent of cadavers) showed multiple punctate deposits of dicalcium phosphate dihydrate ($CaHPO_4 \cdot 2H_2O$ — DCPD) (Fig. 60–5); 3 single menisci (1.4 per cent of cadavers) showed solitary deposits of hydroxyapatite (HA). Thus there are 2 types of "primary" pathological carti-

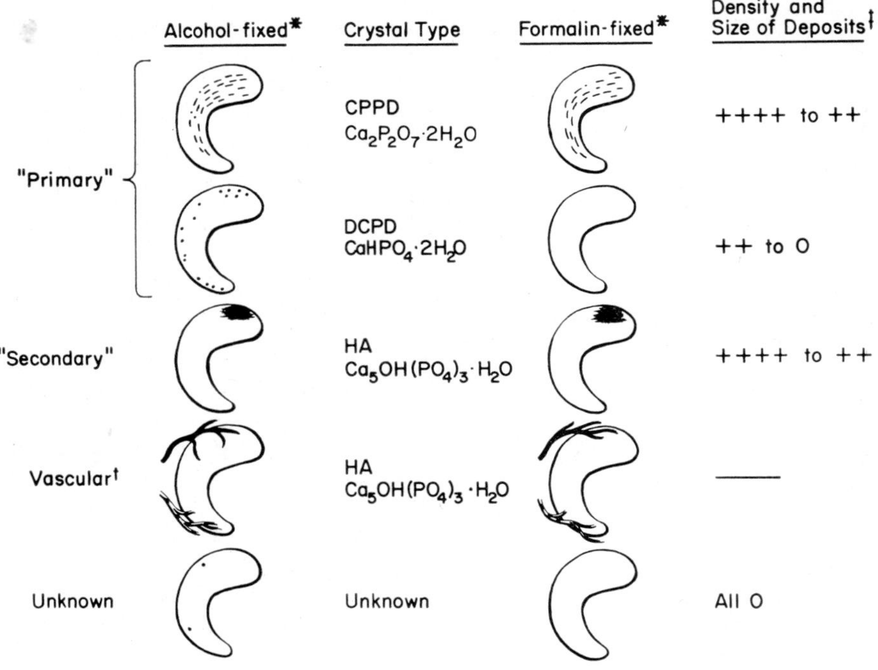

FIG. 60–4.—Summary of pathological calcifications found in over 800 menisci removed from 215 anatomical cadavers. Two types of "primary" calcification were found which, with one exception, were mutually exclusive in a given cadaver; CPPD crystal deposits were found in 3.3 per cent of cadavers, DCPD in 2.3 per cent. Both involved other cartilaginous structures in the same cadavers. Calcification of the vessels supplying the outer third of the menisci occurred frequently and usually affected all 4 menisci. Tiny radiopaque deposits, occurring in at least one meniscus in 30 per cent of cadavers, were too small to permit identification.

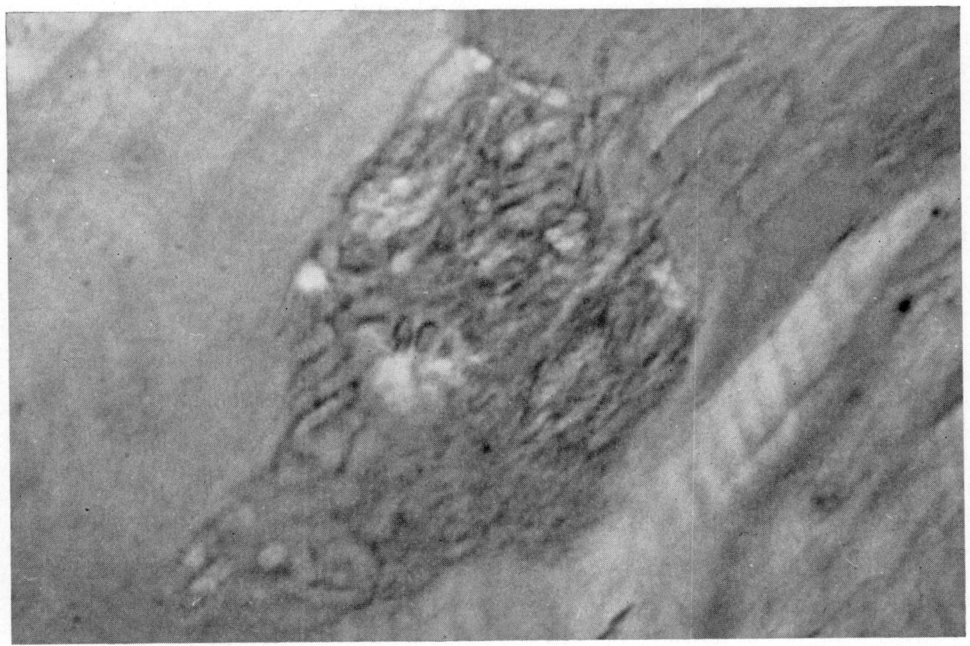

Fig. 60–5.—A focal deposit of DCPD microcrystals in fibrocartilage; these strongly birefringent crystals are relatively soluble in water and were not found in specimens fixed in aqueous formalin (unstained section by polarized light × 1250—linear magnification × 3.5 when printed).

laginous calcifications, which, with one exception, were mutually exclusive in a given cadaver. Most cadavers with "primary" meniscal deposits showed these in avascular articular structures in other joints as well. Four cadavers in this series showed sodium urate deposits in the menisci.

Although the age distribution of the cadaver population closely paralleled that of the United States population dying in 1962, no firm conclusions could be drawn with regard to prevalence because of the obviously biased nature of the sample. The figures of 3.3 per cent for CPPD and 5.6 per cent for the combination of both primary types bracket that of Bennett, Waine and Bauer (4.1 per cent).[1a]

In 1942, Weaver[54] combined 5 roentgenographic surveys of the knee joint; 52 of 12,268 films showed meniscal calcification (0.42 per cent). A recent roentgenologic survey of the knees of elderly persons by Bocher *et al.*[2] showed intra-articular calcific deposits in 7 per cent, precisely the total of significant calcification observed in the cadaver study outlined above. Although additional anatomical and roentgenologic data are needed, it is safe to conclude on the basis of the available facts that the condition is by no means uncommon pathologically. Moreover, our detection of 238 symptomatic cases in 11 years may indicate that a significant percentage of those with deposits develop arthritis.

A survey of a large number of pathologic calcifications from necropsy and surgical material using crystallographic techniques showed no calcium pyrophosphate, thus establishing the CPPD crystal as specific for pseudogout.[15]

Identification of crystals in aortic plaques, costal cartilages, and a pancreatic calcification (in one instance) obtained from CPPD patients at necropsy showed only hydroxyapatite. Thus CPPD deposits were restricted to the joints, even in pseudogout patients.

Diagnostic Criteria

A classification based on the concept of the CPPD crystal as the specific feature of the disease has been suggested;[24] cases are termed "definite," "probable" or "possible" depending on fulfillment of certain criteria. Table 60–2 contains a revised classification based on wider experience. A case is considered "definite" if CPPD crystals have been demonstrated in tissues or synovial fluid by definitive means (*e.g.* x-ray diffraction) or if crystals compatible with CPPD are demonstrated by compensated polarized light *and* typical calcifications are seen on roentgenograms. If only one of the latter criteria is found, a "probable" diagnosis is made. A clinical course compatible with symptomatic CPPD crystal deposition disease should alert the clinician to its possible presence. Many of our later cases were diagnosed on clinical grounds with subsequent confirmation by joint fluid and roentgenographic study.

Clinical Features

The features of the 2 crystal deposition diseases (gout and pseudogout) are compared in Table 60–3.

In the present series of 238 cases, 198 were "definite" and 39 were "probable" by the revised criteria. Men predominated in a 1.48/1 ratio (142/96 cases). The mean age of the present series was 72.3 years (range thirty-six to ninety-two years); the mean age at onset of symptoms of acute arthritis was fifty-seven years (range thirty to ninety years). One case (not in the series) with several affected relatives noted onset of symptoms at age twenty; at age twenty-five nearly every cartilage showed typical calcifications roentgenographically.[5]

A number of clinical studies have been published in English; these are listed in Table 60–4. All except our series showed a female predominance. The average age at time of diagnosis was lower in the Piestany and Santiago series as these included familial case stud-

TABLE 60–2.—DIAGNOSTIC CRITERIA FOR CPPD CRYSTAL DEPOSITION DISEASE (PSEUDOGOUT)

Criteria

I. Demonstration of CPPD crystals (obtained by biopsy, necropsy, or aspirated synovial fluid) by definitive means (*e.g.* characteristic "fingerprint" by x-ray diffraction powder pattern).

II. (*a*) Identification of monoclinic and triclinic crystals showing none or a weakly positive birefringence by compensated polarized light microscopy.
   (*b*) Presence of *typical* calcifications in roentgenograms.*

III. (*a*) Acute arthritis, especially of knees or other large joints with or without concomitant hyperuricemia.
   (*b*) Chronic arthritis, especially of knees and hips and if accompanied by acute exacerbations.

Categories

A. Definite—Criteria I or II (*a*) *plus* (*b*) must be fulfilled.
B. Probable—Criteria II (*a*) *or* II (*b*) must be fulfilled.
C. Possible—Criteria III (*a*) *or* (*b*) should alert the clinician to the possibility of the diagnosis.

* *i.e.* Heavy punctate and linear calcifications in fibrocartilages, articular (hyaline) cartilages, and joint capsules, especially if bilaterally symmetrical; faint and/or atypical calcifications may be due to DCPD ($CaHPO_4 \cdot 2H_2O$) deposits or to vascular calcifications. Both of these are often bilaterally symmetrical also.

Table 60–3.—Comparison of Features of the Crystal Deposition Diseases

	Sodium Urate	Calcium Pyrophosphate
Synonyms	gout	pseudogout, chondrocalcinosis
Sex (male/female)	20:1	1.4/1
Hereditary tendency	present in some cases	present in some cases
Age onset	middle decades—rare but severe in young—incidence rises with age	middle or late decades—rare but severe in young—incidence rises with age
*Prevalence**	4 of 215 cadavers	7 of 215 cadavers
Asymptomatic deposits of crystals in joints	probably occurs†	occurs frequently
Acute attacks	almost always	very common
time onset to peak intensity	abrupt (2 to 12 hours)	abrupt or gradual (2 to 72 hours)
site	small peripheral joints especially in feet—all other joints occasionally	large joints—especially knee—all other joints occasionally
precipitating factors	surgery—trauma—alcohol—exercise—dietary excesses	surgery—trauma
duration	½ day to 3 weeks	½ day to 4 weeks
colchicine	usually dramatically effective	usually ineffective
serum urate	almost always elevated	elevated in 34% cases
"*Petite*" (abortive) *attacks*	common—may outnumber classical attacks	much more common than severe attacks
Synovianalysis		
acute symptoms		
gross	inflammatory (Group II)‡	inflammatory (Group II)‡
microscopic	phagocytosed crystals	phagocytosed crystals
polariscopic	strongly negative birefringence	weakly positive birefringence or non-refractile
chronic symptoms		
gross	non-inflammatory (Group I)‡	non-inflammatory (Group I)‡
microscopic	mostly extracellular crystals	extracellular crystals found—(often—not always)
Associated diseases§	hypertension—diabetes mellitus—hyperparathyroidism—CPPD deposition disease	hypertension—diabetes mellitus—hyperparathyroidism—sodium urate deposition disease—osteoarthritis—hemachromatosis
Chronic arthritis	often present (chronic tophaceous gouty arthritis)	often present—especially in hips and knees
Gross cartilaginous deposits	almost invariable	invariable—especially in fibrocartilaginous menisci
Microscopic appearance	in superficial hyaline (articular) cartilage and often in fibrocartilaginous structures—ligaments—and joint capsules	in midzone—and with erosion—in superficial hyaline cartilage—often in ligaments and joint capsules—most marked in fibrocartilage
Roentgenograms of affected joints	may show non-specific punched-out lesion in subchondral bone	often show highly characteristic appearance (described in text)

* Refers to only comparative study available;[25] as the knee was the joint of reference, other joints containing urates could have been overlooked easily.

† Garrod[14] found sodium urate deposits in 2 of 40 first metatarsophalangeal joints from cadavers not known to have had gout during life.

‡ Group designations of Ropes and Bauer.[41]

§ No causal relationships established or implied.

TABLE 60–4.—SUMMARY OF REPORTED SERIES OF PATIENTS WITH CPPD DEPOSITION DISEASE

		Age (yrs)		*Sex*		*Associated Diseases*				
Series	*No.*	*aver.*	*range*	*M*	*F*	*hyper-uricemia*	*diabetes mellitus*	*hyper-tension*	*urate gout*	*hyperpara-thyroidism*
Cleveland[33]	24	—	46–96	7	17	6	33%	25%	2	1
Boston[46]	18	76	58–94	6	12	4	66%	33%	1	1
London[8]	35	64	32–89	14	21	10	–	–	3	2
Piestany[58]	33† (24)	53	29–84	13	20	–	–	–	‡	–
Santiago[39]	37† (19)	53.5	28–82	17	20	–	–	–	–	2

† numbers in parentheses = familial cases.
‡ 23.6% of metatarsophalangeal joints were calcified radiographically in this series.

ies and asymptomatic cases detected radiologically. The absence of diabetes, hyperparathyroidism, hypertension and urate gout in the familial cases is noteworthy.

Several patterns of arthritis have emerged and are summarized graphically in Figure 60–6. Intermittent attacks of acute arthritis (type A) constituted the most distinctive pattern and were found in 24 per cent of cases. Here, the inflammatory signs and symptoms subsided completely and the afflicted joint was normal on physical examination between attacks. These cases were frequently labeled as "gout," especially if hyperuricemia coexisted. Men were more likely to show this pattern (Fig. 60–7*a*).

There were 6 per cent of cases showing a pattern (type B) of almost continuous acute attacks, usually in a number of joints; these were often labeled "rheumatoid arthritis." Test results for rheumatoid factor were usually negative, however, and joint fluid aspirates revealed CPPD crystals.

A third pattern (type C), found in 60 per cent of cases, consisted of a progressive chronic arthritis of large joints, especially the knee and/or hip, with superimposed acute inflammatory episodes. The chronic arthritis was indistinguishable from degenerative joint disease (osteoarthritis).

A fourth pattern (type D), found in 10 per cent of cases, resembled type C but no acute episodes occurred. In both types C and D flexion contractures were fairly common; these were found in the knees most commonly, but also occurred in the fingers, wrists and elbows. Heberden's nodes were not commonly found. Often fluid could be obtained from chronically symptomatic joints but the chance of finding crystals was less than during an acute phase (Table 60–5). Trauma seemed to intensify local CPPD deposition; several cases showed marked deposition in a previously fractured joint

TABLE 60–5.—SUMMARY OF SYNOVIAL FLUID FINDINGS

	Patients	*Fluids*	*Average Leukocytes (cmm.)*	*CPPD Crystals pos.*	*neg.*	*pos.%*
Acute	126	178 (174)	21,350	172	26*	98.9
Chronic	95	252	1,800	186†	66	73.8

* Twelve "acute" fluids contained numerous phagocytosed sodium urate crystals; 4 attacks were not tabulated as "CPPD negative," as they were due to coincident gout; 8 fluids showed both CPPD and urate crystals.

† Two fluid specimens from one knee showed both sodium urate and CPPD crystals; the identity of the crystals was confirmed by x-ray diffraction. This was case #8 described in our original report.

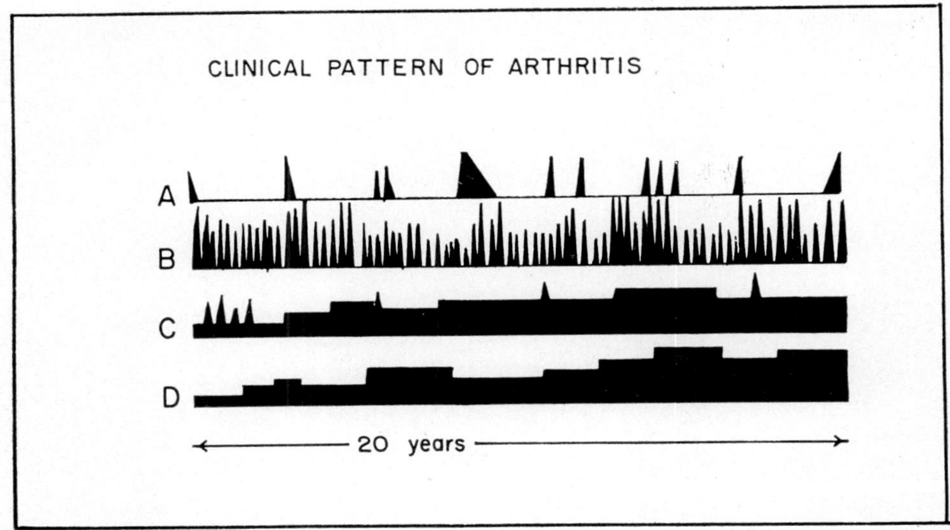

Fig. 60-6.—Diagrammatic representation of patterns of arthritis in CPPD crystal deposition disease. *Type A*—Intermittent attacks of acute arthritis constitute the most distinctive pattern; between attacks, the affected joint appears normal. *Type B*—Almost continuous acute episodes occur, usually in a number of joints. *Type C*—A progressive chronic arthritis of the larger weight-bearing joints develops (*i.e.* knee, hip and lower spine) with superimposed acute episodes. *Type D*—Chronic arthritis as in type C, but without acute exacerbations. Men predominated in type A, women in type D. Cases without clinically evident arthritis might be considered as "*type E.*"

whereas its opposite counterpart showed lighter or no deposits. Many patients stated that dampness and weather changes intensified the arthritic symptoms.

The knee was by far the most frequent site of acute arthritis, but attacks in the hip, shoulder, elbow, ankle, subastragalar, wrist, the bursa between the superficial and deep medial collateral ligaments of the knee, and calcaneocuboid joints were also observed. Fluid aspirated from these sites revealed active phagocytosis of CPPD crystals by leukocytes, supporting the diagnosis. Such fluid was obtained from an inflamed first metatarsophalangeal (bunion) joint in 8 cases. Inflammation of the smaller joints of hands and feet was observed not infrequently; acute episodes involving the lumbar or cervical spine and an extra-articular site (heel) were also noted. No fluid was obtained from these areas however; here the relationship of inflammation to crystals remains conjectural. Attacks in the temporomandibular joint were not seen.

Skinner and Cohen have reported that the mucin clot produced by acetic acid addition to joint fluid in their experience has been good or "fair-good", as opposed to other inflammatory fluids which are normally fair to poor.[46] This quantitative test for mucin was substantiated by quantitative hyaluronic acid determinations on 9 pseudogout joint fluids. Of these, 3 were in the normal range and five were in the range found in mild noninflammatory articular disease.

Stiffness, swelling, pain, local warmth and tenderness usually occurred; erythema of the overlying skin often occurred in severe attacks. In general, the acute episodes were not as severe as those of gout, although attacks more painful than the most severe gout have been observed. Typically, the signs and symptoms reached maximum intensity in twelve to thirty-six hours; they were often first noted in

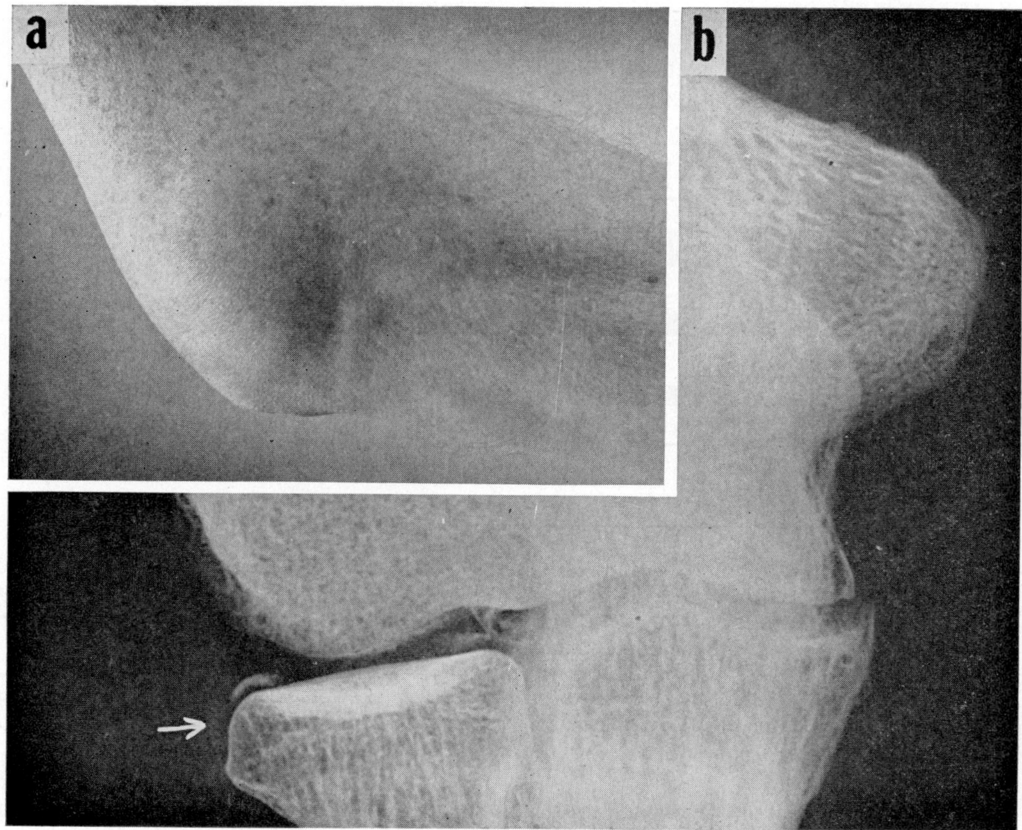

FIG. 60–7.—(*a*) Acute arthritis in the right elbow of a patient with the clinical pattern shown in Figure 60–6*A*. Severe pain, tenderness, swelling, warmth, and erythema of the overlying skin were noted; 25 ml. of inflammatory-type fluid with a leukocytic content of 65,000/c.mm. were aspirated and many phagocytosed CPPD crystals were found. (*b*) Roentgenogram of elbow showing calcific deposits in articular cartilage of humerus and of radial head; deposits, less well visualized, are also present in the articular capsule (arrow).

the morning upon attempted weight-bearing. Tossing in bed in search of a more comfortable position was described frequently. Attacks lasted from twelve hours to four weeks or longer (mean 9 days); those of longer duration may represent overlapping of acute attacks. Patients frequently experienced minor bouts of stiffness or transient aching; joint fluid, usually scant in amount, was obtained on a number of occasions during these "petite" attacks. Elevated synovial fluid leukocyte counts and active phagocytosis of CPPD crystals were found almost invariably (Table 60–4). Some patients denied ever having had an acute attack despite the synovial fluid findings. If the present concept of a dose-related inflammatory response is correct, the existence of "petite" (sub-clinical) attacks is hardly surprising. Acute attacks occurred after trauma, surgical procedures and injections of mercurial diuretics. The role of these "predisposing factors" to articular inflammation is not clear. There was a tendency for attacks to recur in joints that had been involved previously. Attacks often occurred in "clusters," one or more joints flaring closely after an isolated acute seizure. Acute attacks sometimes responded dramatically to therapeutic doses of colchicine, but the effect of this drug was less predictable than in the treatment of urate gout.

A fifth clinical pattern (type E) was exhibited by those with completely asymptomatic calcification. Two such cases were included in this series only because crystal identification was accomplished on tissue removed at necropsy. Moreover, most of the symptomatic cases showed calcific deposits on x-ray examination in joints that had never been the site of acute or chronic arthritis.

Systemic findings in an acute attack were frequently, but not invariably, present. These included low-grade fever (99 to 101° F.), leukocytosis (12 to 15,000/c.mm.) with a "left shift," elevated erythrocyte sedimentation rate and alpha 2 globulin fraction on serum protein (paper) electrophoresis.

TABLE 60–6.—CONDITIONS ASSOCIATED WITH CPPD CRYSTAL DEPOSITION DISEASE (238 cases)

	%		%
Diabetes mellitus*	40–60	Renal stone#	7.5
Hypertension*	25–40	Classic gout¶	5
Atherosclerosis†	35–50	Hemachromatosis[9,17]	none
Azotemia	34	Hyperthyroidism	3
Hyperuricemia‡	34	Inflammatory small bowel disease	2.1
Gynecomastia§	7	Paget's disease of bone	3.4
Hyperparathyroidism‖	7.2		

* Dependent on diagnostic criteria employed.
† Serum lipids, estimated in 20 cases, showed no consistent abnormality.
‡ Half of these cases had concomitant azotemia.
§ Based on 142 male cases.
‖ Parathyroid adenomas were removed in 17 cases.
¶ Urate crystals found in joint fluid.
\# Four stones were analyzed; all were calcium oxalate.

Associated Diseases

Analysis of the first 7 cases and a review of the literature at once suggested that a number of metabolic and degenerative diseases were more prevalent than might be expected by chance.[27] Although clinical studies of many additional cases have served to reinforce this notion, no proven associations may be inferred because no well-designed studies involving controls of like age and sex have been performed. Certainly no causal relationships have been established. Pragmatically, however, the clinician is well advised to keep the diseases listed in Table 60–6 in mind when confronted with a case of CPPD crystal deposition disease. Unsuspected diabetes mellitus and hyperparathyroidism have been found repeatedly when appropriate laboratory studies were performed in this group of arthritics. Conversely, when arthritis supervenes in a patient with one of these diseases, the possibility of CPPD deposition disease should be considered in the differential diagnosis. Related hyperparathyroidism has been reported frequently.[19,44a,46,51,61]

Heredity

Zitnan and Sitaj[59] originally considered the condition to be familial, but have decided in favor of an heredity factor on the basis of later work;[50] 24 of their series of 33 cases were from 5 families. In each family, only 1 parent was affected. These authors suggested 2 phenotypes: (*a*) a polyarticular form, developing at a young age with rapid and progressive involvement of many joints, (*b*) an oligoarticular form, developing at an advanced age, affecting few joints and progressing slowly or not at all. Both forms were found in each family. A female predominance (16/8) was noted in the familial cases; 10 of 32 children of an affected parent had developed calcified cartilage—3 of 18 sons and 7 of 14 daughters. Since no generation was skipped and about half of the older offspring of an affected parent developed calcifications, a dominant hereditary pattern was suggested. On the other

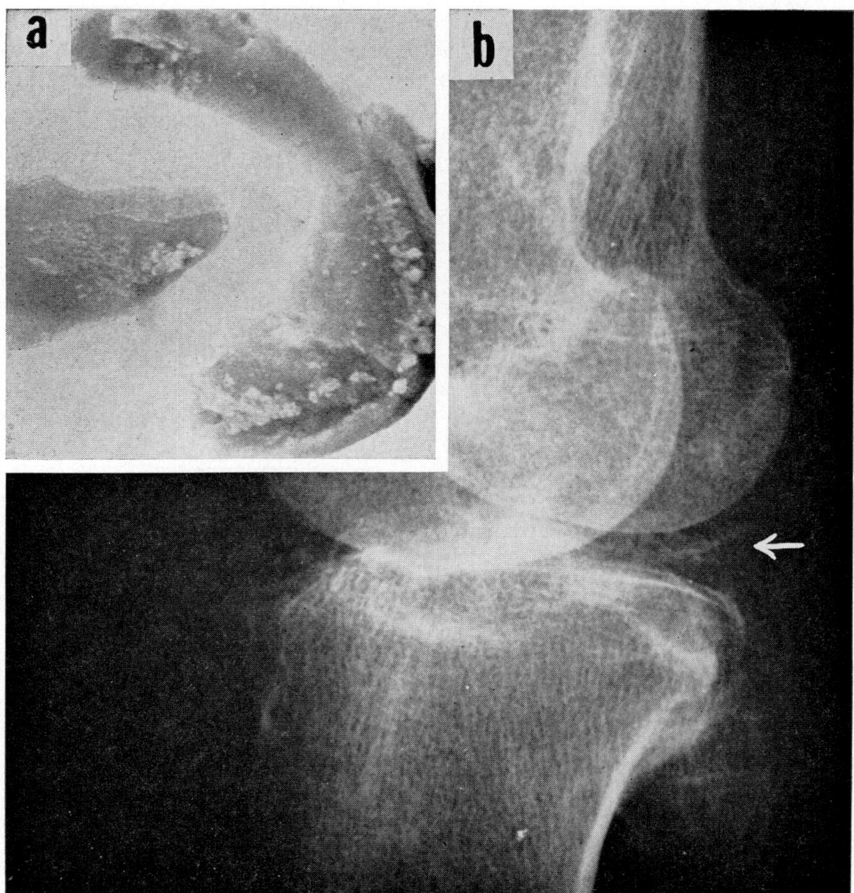

FIG. 60–8.—(*a*) Meniscus excised at necropsy showing punctate and linear aggregates of CPPD microcrystals; a wedge of articular cartilage from the tibial plateau shows similar deposits. (*b*) Lateral roentgenogram of the knee showing typical Y-shaped appearance of meniscal calcification.

hand, the localization of cases to one Slovakian village populated by Hungarians, where inbreeding was known to occur, suggested a recessive pattern. The authors could not definitely determine the mode of transmission from the data at hand.

A family study of a patient with CPPD deposition disease disclosed typical calcifications in roentgenograms of the joints of 2 siblings, while suggestive deposits were noted in a third sibling and 2 daughters.[32]

A recent genetic analysis of 6 families from the Chiloe Islands in the southern part of Chile was reported from Santiago.[39] Again the dominant pattern is evident from the data, but why is a closed population necessary to appreciate a clearly dominant trait? Since there have been no recorded instances of transmission from an affected father to a son, a sex-linked dominant trait may be postulated. It should be noted that with inbreeding, a recessive trait may appear as a dominant ("pseudodominance").

In the present series, CPPD crystals were identified in joint fluids from a father and daughter. Four other "definite" cases had asymptomatic siblings with typical calcifications on roentgenograms. Many others gave histories suggestive of CPPD crystal deposition disease in close relatives. The suspected association with heritable metabolic diseases, such as diabetes mellitus, hyperparathyroidism and hemachromatosis, supports the concept that at least some instances of CPPD disease are genetically determined.

Roentgenologic Features

Heavy CPPD crystal deposits in fibrocartilaginous structures, hyaline (articular) cartilage, ligaments and joint capsules presented a strikingly characteristic appearance that was diagnostically helpful.[24,49,57] Punctate and linear radiodensities were seen most frequently in the fibrocartilaginous menisci of the knee, and usually involved both menisci of both knees (Figs. 60–1*c* and 60–8*b*). Other fibrocartilaginous structures often calcified in this miliary fashion were the articular discs of the distal radioulnar joint (Fig. 60–9), the symphysis pubis, the glenoid and acetabular labra, and the annulus fibrosus of the intervertebral discs. The articular discs of the sternoclavicular joints were often involved, but those of the temporomandibular joint usually were spared.

Calcification of the hyaline articular

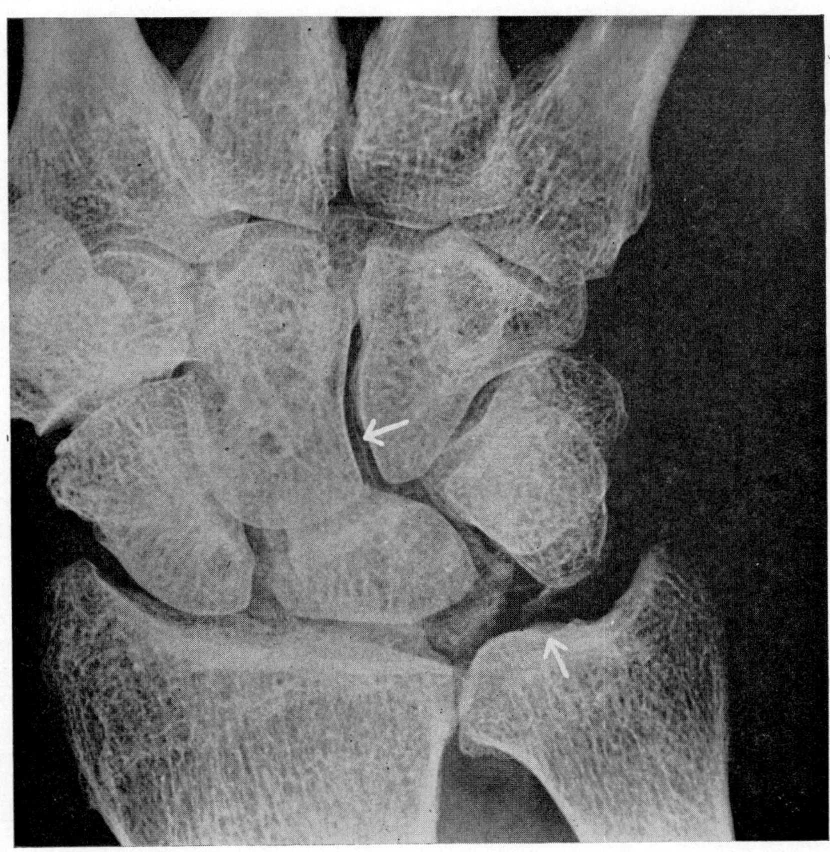

FIG. 60–9.—Anteroposterior roentgenogram of the wrist showing calcification of the fibrocartilaginous articular disc of the distal ulnar-triquetral joint and a fine line of calcification parallel to the radio-density of the underlying bone indicative of articular cartilage calcification (arrows).

cartilage was often encountered; here the deposits in the midzonal layer appeared as a radiopaque line paralleling the density of the underlying bone (Figs. 60–7*b* and 60–9). The larger joints showed these deposits most frequently although they were observed in nearly every diarthrodial joint on at least one occasion. Calcifications of articular capsules, especially of the elbow, shoulder, hip and knee were seen not infrequently; here the deposits appeared as a broader, more diffuse, faintly opaque line (Fig. 60–7*b*).

Subchondral bone cysts have been seen in many instances. These can attain a very large size. One such lesion undermined the medial tibial plateau to such an alarming degree that we elected to pack it with bone chips. Histologic examination of the walls of the lesion confirmed that it was only a bone cyst. How such lesions are related to CPPD deposition disease is unknown.

Practically, an arthritic may be screened for CPPD deposits with four suitably exposed roentgenograms: an anteroposterior (AP) view of each knee, an AP view of the pelvis, and a postero-anterior view of the wrists. If nothing diagnostic is seen on these films, it is highly unlikely that a more extensive survey will be helpful.

The deposits visualized roentgenographically were extensively studied by crystallographic techniques in 3 necropsied cases; all were CPPD.[23] The chemical composition of the crystal deposits may be inferred with confidence from *typical* roentgenograms. Caution must be exercised when the calcifications are faint or atypical however, because of the possibility of DCPD crystal deposits or vascular calcifications, both of which tend to be symmetrical.[25]

Pathology

An extensive examination of the joints was accomplished in the 3 necropsied cases and in 7 anatomical cadavers. The distribution of calcification generally paralleled that seen on x ray. Joint capsules, especially in the hip and shoulder, and the hyaline articular cartilages were often affected, but the heaviest deposits were in fibrocartilaginous structures. The menisci of the knee were involved in all (Fig. 60–8*a*). Heavy deposits were often noted in tendons and in intra-articular ligaments, such as the cruciates in the knee. Microscopically the deposits were composed of various-sized microcrystalline aggregates of CPPD (Fig. 60–10). Their diameters varied from 15 μ to 0.6 cm.; the larger ones appeared grossly as white chalky deposits. It was difficult on gross inspection to distinguish these deposits from the white chalky lesions of true gout. These were distributed diffusely in fibrocartilage, mainly in the midzonal area of articular cartilage. They appeared at the surface particularly in areas eroded by degenerative change. The smallest, and presumably the earliest, lesions seemed to be located at the lacunar margin of the chondrocytes (Fig. 60–11). The larger deposits showed a compressed fibrous stroma and were thought to arise from coalescence of smaller deposits. Although some crystals occurred in areas of degeneration, others were found in cartilage possessing normal staining properties. No categorical statement can be made at this time as to which comes first, the crystals or the degenerative changes in the cartilaginous matrix. Serial roentgenographic studies by Zitnan and Sitaj showed that the radiopaque deposits progressed in time to involve more of a given joint and to involvement of previously unaffected joints. Degenerative changes in these studies also progressed in time and clearly followed the calcification process.[58]

Synovial biopsy material obtained with the Polley-Bickel needle showed inflammatory and reparative changes consistent with the clinical state of the joint at the time of biopsy. Early in an acute attack, the edematous synovium was infiltrated with polymorphonuclear leukocytes; later, mononuclear infiltration and fibroblastic

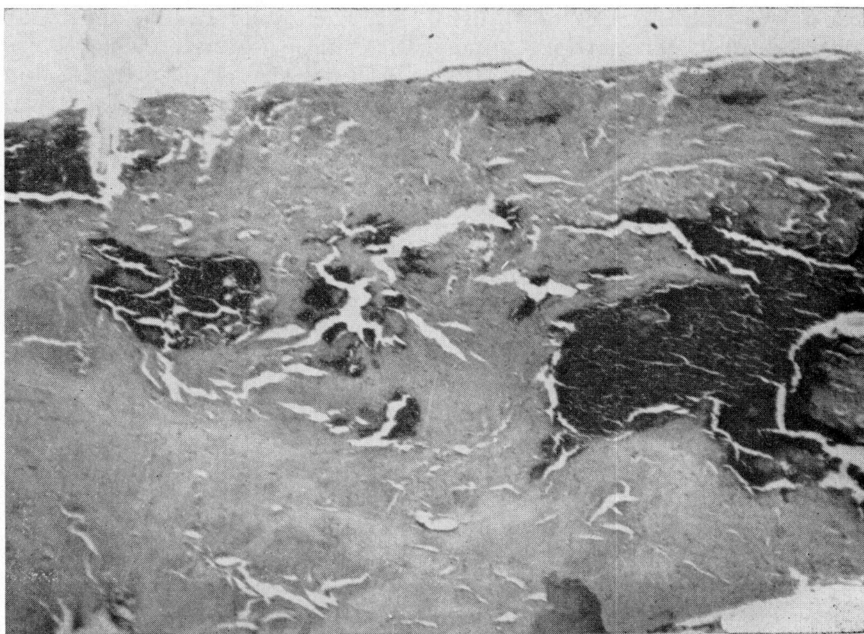

FIG. 60-10.—Photomicrograph of a section through meniscus shown in Figure 60–8(*a*); various-sized aggregates of calcified material are distributed throughout (hematoxylin and eosin × 26).

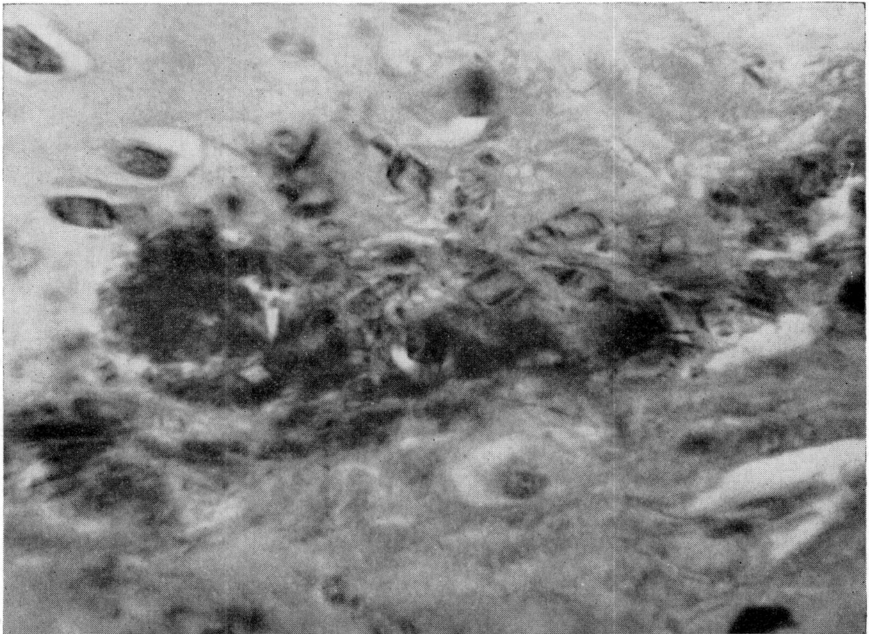

FIG. 60–11.—Photomicrograph of smallest deposits found shows them surrounding the lacunae of the chondrocytes. This process begins in the midzonal layer of articular cartilage, more diffusely in fibrocartilage. Individual crystals of CPPD are visible in this section (Alizarin red × 800; linear magnification × 3).

proliferation were seen. Crystals have been identified in the superficial synovium by polarized light. Non-specific inflammatory changes were found in chronically symptomatic joints but crystals rarely were seen.

Pathogenesis

The mechanism of calcium pyrophosphate crystal precipitation in cartilage is unknown. However, CPPD, DCPD and hydroxyapatite (HA), the 3 crystal forms identified in human cartilage, and anhydrous $CaHPO_4$, identified in the bones and joints of a gibbon[34] are all members of the 3 component system CaO-P_2O_5-H_2O. Another important compound in this system is octacalcium phosphate (OCP). These are precisely the same crystalline compounds that, used as fertilizer, are stable in soil systems.[4] A review of pertinent soil chemistry literature affords a basis for speculation because, no matter what metabolic changes in cartilaginous matrix or chondrocytes may underlie the process, the physicochemical conditions for CPPD precipitation must be satisfied. Brown and his colleagues[3] have shown (*in vitro*) that monoclinic CPPD crystals form in the presence of dilute electrolyte at pH 6 to 7 at a temperature of 45° C., conditions reasonably close to physiologic. These then convert to the more insoluble triclinic dimorph. The triclinic form has predominated in all specimens analyzed in our laboratory thus far. In fact, the interplanar spacings characteristic of the monoclinic dimorph frequently cannot be identified.

An analogy with our present ideas about sodium urate crystal deposition disease (gout)[22] may provide a unifying concept; *i.e.*, that *the crystal represents a final common pathway of a number of metabolic disturbances*. The familial prevalence noted by others[32,39,50] and proven crystallographically in 5 cases in the present series certainly suggests a specific genetic (and by implication biochemical) abnormality. The association with heredit-able metabolic and endocrine abnormalities supports this idea.

Zitnan and Sitaj have postulated a primary defect in cartilage matrix, with secondary formation of a mineral phase. We have postulated a defect in inorganic pyrophosphate (PPi) metabolism, perhaps a deficiency of an inorganic pyrophosphatase. A recent report of pseudogout in a woman with hypophosphatasia,[35] together with the suggestive evidence that PPi is a natural substrate for alkaline phosphatase,[7] suggests that deficiency of this enzyme may be causally related to CPPD deposition in joints. Inorganic pyrophosphatases hydrolyze PPi to Pi in accordance with the following equation:

$$PPi + H_2O = 2\ Pi$$

However, urinary PPi levels are elevated in hypophosphatasia but not in pseudogout.[42,43,36] Russell *et al.*[43] and McCarty *et al.*[28] have recently described elevated (4- to 8-fold) levels of PPi in synovial fluid from pseudogout patients as compared to fluids from patients with other types of arthritis (approximately 10 to 40 μg of pyrophosphate phosphorus per 100 ml.). Whether the elevated joint fluid PPi levels are merely a result of crystal dissolution or conversely, whether the CPPD crystals themselves are a result of these levels remains to be determined. If local overproduction or underdestruction of PPi occurs, it is not clear whether the defect is localization in the chondrocyte or of the synovial cell, or both.

Preliminary studies of CPPD crystal solubility showed that a level of 265 μg per 100 ml. (pyrophosphate phosphorus) was obtained in joint fluid and that 710 μg per 100 ml. was obtained in normal plasma. Protein and magnesium ions increased solubility, whereas calcium and orthophosphate ions decreased it.[28]

Russell *et al.*[43] and Yaron *et al.*[56] have recently reported decreased alkaline phosphatase activity in pseudogout joint fluid. But McCarty *et al.*[28] found no difference between pseudogout and control joint fluids against the 2 synthetic substrates P-nitrophenylphosphate and betaglycerophosphate. Studies of alkaline phosphatase isoenzymes in these same fluids showed approximately the same frequency of identification of the liver, intestine and bone enzyme as in the controls.

Decreased joint fluid levels of an enzyme transferring phosphorus from PPi to glucose (glucose phosphotransferase) in accord with the following equation

glucose + PPi = glucose 6-phosphate + Pi

have been found in both gout and pseudogout fluids as compared to other types of inflammatory arthritis. Similar levels of a potent, magnesium dependent, pyrophosphatase from erythrocytes, active at neutral pH, have been found in erythrocytes from pseudogout patients as compared to normal persons and patients with other diseases.[31] This enzyme was markedly inhibited by divalent iron, calcium, and copper leading to speculation that similar enzymes in articular tissues might be similarly inhibited in those cases of CPPD deposition associated with hyperparathyroidism, hemochromatosis and (not proven) Wilson's disease.

The pathogenesis of the acute attack

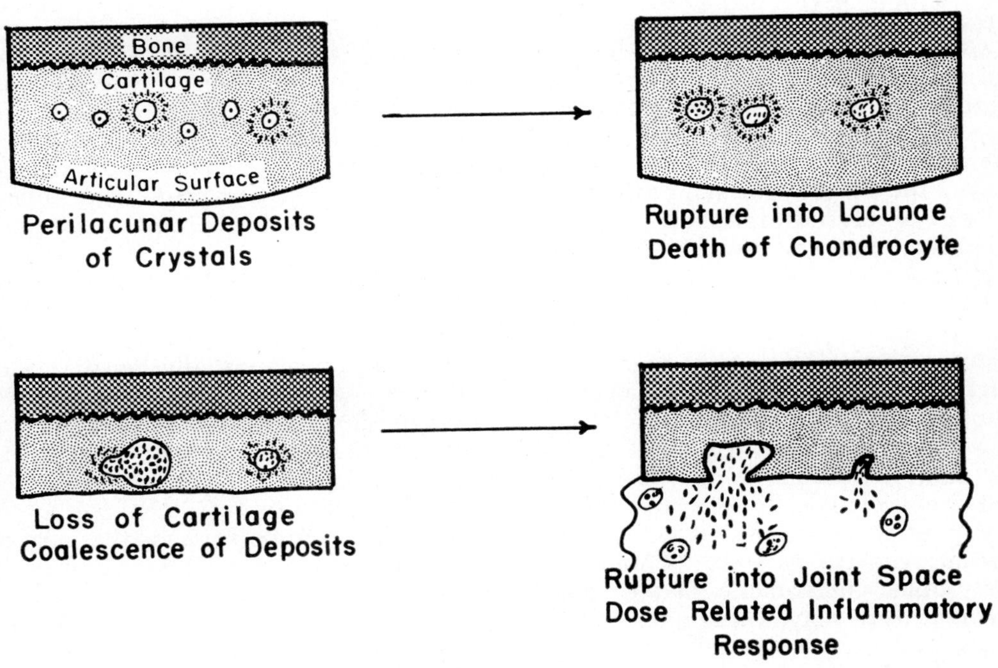

Fig. 60–12.—Hypothetical mechanism of arthritis in CPPD crystal deposition disease. The smallest, and presumably the earliest, deposits occur around the chondrocyte which subsequently dies. Replacement of cartilaginous matrix (collagen and polysaccharide) is thereby impaired, resulting in thinning of cartilage and coalescence of deposits. Rupture of a deposit into the vascular tissue (joint) space results in a dose-related inflammatory response; the rate and amount of crystal entering the joint may govern the rapidity of onset and the duration of the attack. The wide variation in severity, duration, and rapidity of onset of symptoms may be explained with this conceptual model.

may be explained by rupture of a preformed deposit into the adjacent large tissue space represented by the synovial cavity (Fig. 60–12). Crystals have been identified in virtually all fluids obtained from acutely inflamed joints in these patients. Early in an attack "rosettes" have been seen, composed of small aggregates of crystals surrounded by leukocytes. As in true gout, crystal phagocytosis is invariably present during, and for some time after, an acute attack. CPPD crystals, morphologically, chemically, and crystallographically identical to those found in joint fluid have been synthesized by the technique of Brown and his colleagues.[3] Injection of the synthetic or natural crystals into normal human and canine joints has induced an acute inflammatory response. This series of observations may be considered as analogous to fulfillment of Koch's postulates.

Conceptually, the hypothetical mechanism outlined in Figure 60–12 fits many of the clinical observations. The variation in rapidity of onset may be due to the rate of crystal release into the tissue space, the severity of symptoms to the "dose" of crystals released. The postoperative and post-traumatic attacks suggest a shared, albeit enigmatic, pathogenetic mechanism with classical gout. The progressive and often severe chronic degenerative arthritis may be related in part to the death of chondrocytes surrounded by crystal masses.

Much has been learned about the cellular and molecular events involved in inflammation induced by urate crystals.[29] Many of these events apply to CPPD crystal synovitis as well. Thus a nondialyzable, chemotactic factor, that is released from polymorphonuclear leukocytes after urate crystal phagocytosis, described by Phelps,[37] was also released after CPPD crystal ingestion. Colchicine in usual pharmacological concentrations predictably inhibited the release of this factor after urate crystal phagocytosis. But colchicine inhibition of chemotactic factor release after CPPD crystal ingestion was unpredictable.[48] Sometimes the drug worked and sometimes it did not.

Membranolytic effects of urates have been demonstrated recently against erythrocyte membranes and against polymorphonuclear leukocyte phagosomes.[52,53] This effect is believed to be mediated by hydrogen bonding between crystal surface and the membrane, as strong hydrogen-bonding compounds such as polyvinyl-pyridine-N-oxide (PVPNO) blocked the reaction. CPPD crystals appear to be much less reactive against membranes than urates and what little membranolytic effect they do exert is not blocked by hydrogen bonding agents such as PVPNO.

Weissmann and his colleagues have extended these observations.[52a] Urate, but not CPPD crystals, disrupted isolated human polymorphonuclear leukocyte (PMN) lysosomes but not isolated mitochondria, suggesting that the cholesterol content of the membranes was important for hydrogen bonding. Urates disrupted artificial membranes (liposomes) that contained androgens but not estrogens, suggesting a molecular basis for the well-known proclivity for acute gouty inflammation in men and postmenopausal women.

Sequential electron microscopic study of urate crystal phagocytosis by human PMN by Schumacher and Phelps showed that the crystals initially lay in a membranous sac (phagosome) formed by invagination of the plasma membrane during phagocytosis, but that breaks appeared in the membrane shortly thereafter.[44] The entire phagosome disappeared eventually and the enzymes that had been liberated from the lysosomes into the phagosome were released into the interior of the cell, resulting in autolysis and cell death. Andrews and Phelps[1] and Wallingford and Trend[53a] incubated urate and CPPD crystals with human PMN and measured the release of lysosomal and cytoplasmic marker enzymes. Lysosomal enzymes were released into the supernatant by both types of crystals, and lactic acid dehydrogenase (cytosol marker) was released by PMN that had phagocytosed urate after 6 hours of incubation,[53a] but not after one hour.[1] Colchicine and Indomethacin in concentrations of 10^{-6}M inhibited lysosomal release by small doses of crystals.[1]

Therapy

There is no way to halt the progressive deposition of crystals nor is there a method of removing those already deposited. Acute attacks were treated most often by thorough aspiration of the joint followed by injection of microcrystalline corticosteroid esters. Phenylbutazone, systemic corticosteroids and salicylates in large doses seem effective, but the effect of colchicine is unpredictable; some acute joints appear to respond while others do not. This may be related to the *in vitro* effect of colchicine described above. Treatment of the associated chronic arthritis is the same as that for osteoarthritis. Removal of parathyroid adenomas and careful regulation of diabetes mellitus in a number of cases did not stop the acute episodes; the long-term effectiveness of these measures in halting or reversing crystal deposition is not known.

BIBLIOGRAPHY

1. Andrews, R., and Phelps, P.: Arth. & Rheum., *14*, 368, 1971 (Abstract).

1.*a* Bennett, G. A., Waine, H., and Bauer, W.: *Changes in the Knee Joint at Various Ages*, New York Commonwealth Fund, 1942, p. 30, 39.

2. Bocher, J., Mankin, H. J., Berk, R. N. and Rodnan, G. P.: New Engl. J. Med., *272*, 1093, 1965.

3. Brown, E. H., Lehr, J. R., Smith, J. P., and Frazier, A. W.: J. Agricult. & Food Chem., *11*, 214, 1963.

4. Brown, W. E.: Soil Science, *90*, 51, 1960.

5. Bundens, W. D., Brighton, C. T. and Weitzman, G.: J. Bone & Joint Surg., *47A*, 111, 1965.

6. Bywaters, E. G. L., Dixon, A. St. J., and Scott, J. T.: Ann. Rheum. Dis., *22*, 171, 1963.

7. Cox, R. P. and Griffin, M. J.: Lancet, *2*, 1018, 1965.

8. Currey, H. L. F., Key, J. J., Mason, R. M., and Svettenham, K. V.: Ann. Rheum. Dis., *26*, 295, 1966.

9. Delbarre, F.: Presse med., *72*, 2973, 1964.

10. Eklof, G.: Nord. med., *47*, 899, 1952.

11. Faires, J. S. and McCarty, D. J.: Lancet, *2*, 682, 1962.

12. Freudweiler, M.: Deutsch. Arch. Klin. Med., *63*, 266, 1899.

13. Freudweiler, M.: Deutsch. Arch. Klin. Med., *69*, 155, 1901.

14. Garrod, A. B.: *A Treatise on Gout & Rheumatic Gout* (R.A.), London, Longmans, Green & Co. 1876.

15. Gatter, R. A. and McCarty, D. J.: Arch. Path., *84*, 346, 1967.

16. Good, A. E. and Starkweather, W. H.: Arth. & Rheum., *12*, 298, 1969. (Abstr.)

17. Hamilton, E., Williams, R., Barlow, K. A., and Smith, P. M.: Quart. J. Med., *37*, 171, 1968.

18. His, W. J., Jr.: Deutsch. Arch. Klin. Med., *65*, 156, 1900.

19. Hosking, G. E. and Clennar, G.: J. Bone & Joint Surg., *42B*, 530, 1960.

20. Kohn, N. N., Hughes, R. E., McCarty, D. J., and Faires, J. S.: Ann. Intern. Med., *56*, 738, 1962.

21. Mandl, F.: Arch. f. Klin. Chir., *146*, 149, 1927.

22. McCarty, D. J., Jr.: Arth. & Rheum., *7*, 534, 1964.

23. McCarty, D. J., Jr. and Gatter, R. A.: Arth. & Rheum., *5*, 652, 1962 (Abstr.)

24. McCarty, D. J., Jr. and Haskin, M.: Amer. J. Roent. Rad. Ther. & Nucl. Med., *90*, 1248, 1963.

25. McCarty, D. J., Jr., Hogan, J. M., Gatter, R. A. and Grossman, N.: J. Bone & Joint Surg., *48A*, 309, 1966.

26. McCarty, D. J., Jr. and Hollander, J. L.: Ann. Intern. Med., *54*, 452, 1961.

27. McCarty, D. J., Jr., Kohn, N. N., and Faires, J. S.: Ann. Intern. Med., *56*, 711, 1962.

28. McCarty, D. J., Jr., Solomon, S. D., Warnock, M. and Paloyan, E.: J. Lab. Clin. Med., *78*, 216, 1971.

29. McCarty, D. J., Jr.: Ann. Rev. Med., *21*, 357, 1970.

30. ———: Geriatrics, *18*, 467, 1963.

31. McCarty, D. J. and Pepe, P. F.: J. Lab. Clin. Med., *79*, 277, 1972.

32. Moskowitz, R. W. and Katz, D.: J.A.M.A., *188*, 867, 1964.

33. ———: Amer. J. Med., *43*, 322, 1967.

34. Murphy, R. C. and Sullivan, W. E.: Med. Radiography & Photography, *34*, 80, 1958.
35. O'Duffy, J. D.: Arth. & Rheum., *13*, 381, 1970.
36. Pflug, M., McCarty, D. J., and Kawahara, F.: Arth. & Rheum., *12*, 228, 1969.
37. Phelps, P.: Arth. & Rheum., *13*, 1, 1970.
38. Phelps, P., Steele, A. D., and McCarty, D. J.: J.A.M.A., *203*, 508, 1968.
39. Reginato, A. M., Valenzuela, F. R., Martinez, V. C., Passano, G., and Daza, S. K.: Arth. & Rheum., *13*, 197, 1970.
40. Riehl, G.: Wien. Klin. Wchsch., 761, 1897.
41. Ropes, M. W. and Bauer, W.: *Synovial Fluid Changes in Joint Disease*, Cambridge, Mass., Harvard University Press, 1953.
42. Russell, R. G. G.: Lancet, *2*, 461, 1965.
43. Russell, R. G. G., Bisaz, S., Fleisch, H., Currey, H. L. F., Rubenstein, H., Micheli, A., Boussine, I., and Fallet, G.: Lancet, *2*, 899, 1970.
44. Schumacher, H. R., and Phelps, P.: Arth. & Rheum., *14*, 513, 1971.
44*a*. Scott, J. T.: Ann. Rheum. Dis., *22*, 171, 1963.
45. Seegmiller, J. E., Howell, R. R., and Malawista, S. E.: J.A.M.A., *180*, 469, 1962.
46. Skinner, M. and Cohen, A. S.: Arch. Intern. Med., *123*, 636, 1969.
47. Tobler, T.: Schweiz. med. Wchnschr., *59*, 10, 1929.
48. Tse, R. L. and Phelps, P.: J. Lab. Clin. Med., *76*, 403, 1970.
49. Twigg, H. L., Zvaifler, N. J., and Nelson, C. W.: Radiology, *82*, 655, 1964.
50. Valsik, J., Zitnan, D., and Sitaj, S.: Ann. Rheum. Dis., *22*, 153, 1963.
51. Vix, V. A.: Radiology, *83*, 468, 1964.
52. Wallingford, W. R., and McCarty, D. J., Jr.: J. Exper. Med., *133*, 100, 1971.
52*a*. Weissmann, G. W., Rita, G., and Zurier, R. B.: J Clin. Invest., *50*, 97A, 1971 (Abstract)
53. Wallingford, W. R.: Personal communication.
53*a*. Wallingford, W. R., Trend, B.: Arth. & Rheum., *14*, 420, 1971 (Abstract).
54. Weaver, J. B.: J. Bone & Joint Surg., *24*, 873, 1942.
55. Werwath, K.: Fortschr. Gdb. Rontgenstrahlen, *37*, 169, 1928.
56. Yaron, M., Zurkowsky, P., Weiser, H. I., Yost, I., Goldschmied, A., and Hermann, I.: Ann. Intern. Med., *73*, 751, 1970.
57. Zitnan, D. and Sitaj, S.: Cesk. Rent., *14*, 27, 1960.
58. Zitnan, D. and Sitaj, S.: *Acta Rheumatologica et Balneologica Pistiniana.* Piestany, Czechoslovakia, 1966, p. 71.
59. Zitnan, D. and Sitaj, S.: Bratisl. lek. Listy., *38*, 217, 1958.
60. Zitnan, D. and Sitaj, S.: Ann. Rheum. Dis., *22*, 142, 1963.
61. Zvaifler, N. J., Reefe, W. E., and Black, R. L.: Arth. & Rheum., *5*, 237, 1962.

Chapter 61

Ochronosis, Hemochromatosis and Wilson's Disease

By H. Ralph Schumacher, Jr., M.D.

ALKAPTONURIA AND OCHRONOSIS

Definition

Alkaptonuria is an hereditary disorder characterized by the presence in the urine of homogentisic acid which, when oxidized, imparts a brownish-black color to the urine. The word "alkaptonuria," denoting an avidity for oxygen in alkaline solution, was coined by Bodeker in 1859, and is derived from fusion of an Arabic word meaning "alkali" and a Greek word καπτειν (kaptein) meaning "to suck up avidly." When the freshly passed urine is alkalinized, polymerization of homogentisic acid is accelerated and the color of the urine turns black promptly. *Ochronosis* denotes a bluish-black pigmentation of connective tissue in patients with alkaptonuria, usually apparent clinically in cartilage of ear, skin and sclera. This term was originated by Virchow in 1866 who described the microscopic appearance of this pigmentation as "ochre" (*vide infra*).

Alkaptonuria *per se* is a symptomless condition. Clinical signs and symptoms develop when pigment is deposited in cartilage and other connective tissues (ochronosis).

History

The earliest clinical observation, of a school boy who passed dark urine, was made by Scribonius in 1584. Bodeker was the first to isolate homogentisic acid from the urine of a patient with alkaptonuria (1859). Wolkow and Bauman (1891) established the chemical structure of this compound as 2,5-dihydroxyphenylacetic acid and named it homogentisic acid. A. E. Garrod[7] formulated the concept in 1902 that alkaptonuria was an "inborn error of metabolism" consisting of an inability to oxidize homogentisic acid, an intermediary metabolite of phenylalanine and tyrosine. LaDu and his collaborators[13] demonstrated for the first time (1958) the absence of the enzyme homogentisic acid oxidase in the liver of a patient with alkaptonuria and ochronotic spondylosis and peripheral arthropathy.

In 1866, Virchow published a brief report of the bizarre pigmentation in the connective tissue of a sixty-seven-year-old man who died of a ruptured aneurysm. The pigment had an ochre (dark yellow) color microscopically and Virchow designated this case as "ochronosis." However, it was not until thirty-six years later that Albrecht in 1902 and, soon thereafter, Osler in 1904 recognized the relationship between alkaptonuria and ochronosis.

Nature of the Biochemical Lesion

The metabolic pathway for the aromatic amino acid tyrosine is charted in Figure 61–1. It will be noted that nor-

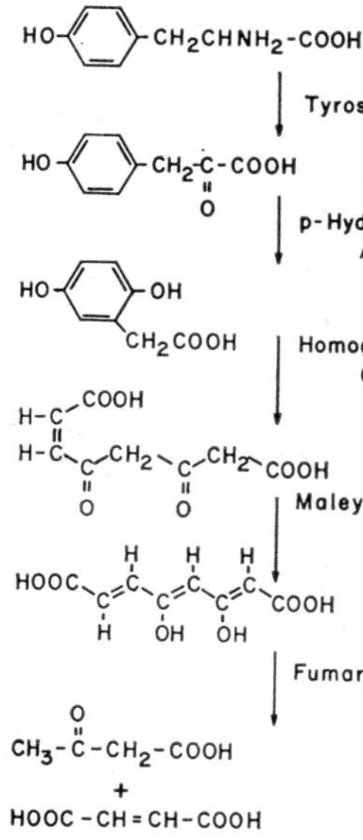

SCHEME		ENZYMES	ENZYME ACTIVITY: μMoles of substrate oxidized per hour per gram of liver — NON-ALKAPTONURIC	ALKAPTONURIC
TYROSINE	HO-C_6H_4-CH_2CHNH_2-COOH			
		Tyrosine Transaminase	36	32
p-HYDROXYPHENYL-PYRUVIC ACID	HO-C_6H_4-CH_2-C(=O)-COOH			
		p-Hydroxyphenylpyruvic Acid Oxidase	67	46
HOMOGENTISIC ACID	HO-C_6H_3(OH)-CH_2COOH			
		Homogentisic Acid Oxidase	268	<0.048
MALEYLACETO-ACETIC ACID	H-C-COOH ‖ H-C-C(=O)-CH_2-C(=O)-CH_2-COOH			
		Maleylacetoacetic Acid Isomerase†	960	780
FUMARYLACETO-ACETIC ACID	HOOC-CH=CH-C(OH)=CH-C(OH)=CH-COOH			
		Fumarylacetoacetic Acid Hydrolase	288	222
ACETOACETIC ACID AND FUMARIC ACID	CH_3-C(=O)-CH_2-COOH + HOOC-CH=CH-COOH			

Fig. 61–1.—Metabolic pathway of tyrosine; the specific enzymes that catalyze the successive reactions; and enzyme activity of liver of an alkaptonuric patient as compared to control. Note that homogentisic acid oxidase, the enzyme required to break the benzene ring of homogentisic acid, is absent in the alkaptonuric liver. (Courtesy of Ann. Intern. Med.)

mally the benzene ring of homogentisic acid is broken by the enzyme homogentisic acid oxidase and maleylaceto-acetic acid is formed. LaDu and his co-workers assayed the homogenates from samples of liver removed from a patient with ochronotic arthritis and similarly from a non-alkaptonuric patient. The sequence of enzyme steps of tyrosine oxidation were then studied with each preparation. The results revealed (Fig. 61–1) that *the pattern of enzyme activities of the alkaptonuric liver was essentially the same as the control in all respects except for homogentisic acid oxidase activity which was completely missing in the alkaptonuric patient.*

Of special interest is the demonstration that the deficiency is limited to a single enzyme system, for all the other enzymes involved in the complete metabolism of tyrosine were present in the patient's liver. Beadle and Tatum concluded from their classic studies on induced mutation in *Neurospora crassa* that the production of a single defective gene is correlated with the appearance of a metabolic block in a single biochemical reaction.[2] Alkaptonuria now furnishes an additional illustration that the principle of gene:enzyme relationship applies to man as well as mold. Of additional interest is the presence of the enzyme maleylaceto-acetic acid isomerase in the alkaptonuric liver despite the apparent absence of the substrate maleylaceto-acetic acid, which could be derived only from the metabolism of homogentisic acid which is blocked in this case. The presence of this enzyme in the absence of its substrate demonstrates that the genetic mechanism which controls the synthesis of this enzyme is not regulated by the substrate.

Genetic Factors

Alkaptonuria is felt to be transmitted by a single recessive autosomal gene. The occurrence of this disorder in successive generations of certain families is most likely the result of consanguineous marriages—homozygotes mating with heterozygotes. The present concept of the mode of transmission of alkaptonuria, originally advanced by Garrod (and challenged at times), has been substantiated by several careful family studies in which complete pedigrees were available.[12]

Laboratory Aspects of Alkaptonuria

The freshly passed urine of an alkaptonuric patient is of normal color and does not darken at once unless it is alkaline or contains less than normal concentration of vitamin C or other reducing agents. On standing, it turns brownish black as the homogentisic acid becomes oxidized. If Benedict's reagent is used in testing the urine for sugar, a yellow-orange precipitate is formed (homogentisic acid reduces the copper in Benedict's) which is usually misinterpreted as indicating glucosuria. The color of the supernatant solution in these cases is always brownish black which is diagnostic for alkaptonuria.

Using copper-reduction tablets (Clinitest) a black supernatant may also be seen with malignant melanoma and following intravenous urography with sodium diatrizoate (Hypaque) and other x-ray contrast media.[14] Specific glucose oxidase tapes (Clinistix) may not detect urine glucose in diabetics with ochronosis because of interference with the peroxidase-indicator chromagen reaction by homogentisic acid.[11,18] Spuriously increased serum and urinary uric acid determinations have been described in ochronosis with colorimetric methods. Values were normal by the uricase spectrophotometric technique.[11] Homogentisic acid in the urine may also produce false elevations in creatinine when measured by Jaffe's reaction.[21]

Diagnostic Tests for Alkaptonuria

There are several presumptive, nonspecific tests for alkaptonuria. These are color reactions based on the reducing properties of homogentisic acid. Thus in the Briggs' test[4] molybdate is reduced and a deep blue color is obtained. When a drop of urine is placed on photographic paper, a black spot indicates reduction of silver. When sodium hydroxide is added to the freshly passed urine homogentisic acid is rapidly oxidized and the urine promptly darkens in color. A specific enzymatic method for quantitative determination of homogentisic acid in urine and blood has been developed by Seegmiller *et al.*[22]

Pathology of Ochronosis

The lesions in ochronosis result from the inter- or intracellular deposition of pigment in many organs or structures. The exact chemical composition of the pigment has not yet been defined although it is believed to be a polymer derived from homogentisic acid. It has been proposed[23] that benzoquinoneacetic acid may be an intermediate compound which, when bound to connective tissue, may participate in a polymerization process leading to the final pigment formation. Homogentisic acid is concentrated preferentially by connective tissue but this is reversible until after polymerization. The typical pathological findings have been comprehensively reviewed by Lichtenstein and Kaplan.[15] Granules of highly insoluble melanin-like pigment are usually found in the skin and subcutis, cartilage of joints, intervertebral discs (annulus fibrosus as well as nucleus pulposus), tracheal cartilages, within the epithelial cells of the renal tubules and in the islets of the pancreas. Pigment granules impregnate the walls of large and medium-sized arteries and arterioles including the aorta, pulmonary, coronary and renal arteries as well as atherosclerotic plaques, fibrous patches in pericardium and myocardial infarctions. Aortic stenosis has been seen in some instances in association with deposition of ochronotic pigment.

Clinical Picture of Ochronosis

Patients with alkaptonuria who live to the fourth decade of life almost invariably develop ochronosis. The *cartilage of the ear*, especially the concha and antihelix, is frequently involved. It takes on a slate-blue discoloration, becomes irregularly thickened and inflexible. When the pinna is transilluminated the opaque pigmented areas stand out prominently. The cerumen in the external canal is often black and the periphery of the tympanic membrane grayish black. A considerable proportion of patients with long-standing ochronosis have impaired hearing. Thus, discoloration of the pinna and tympanic membrane, black cerumen and deafness may be considered the "*earmarks*" of ochronosis. Pigmentation of the *sclera* is usually localized to a small area midway between the limbus of the cornea and inner or outer canthus. The *skin* over the malar areas, nose, axilla and groin is often pigmented.

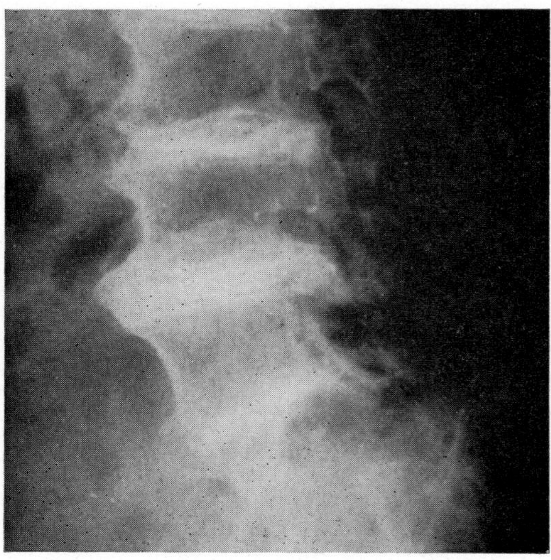

Fig. 61–2.—Roentgenogram of lumbar spine of a fifty-five-year-old man with ochronotic spondylosis. Note calcification of intervertebral discs. The osteophytes are of only moderate size.

Deposition of pigment in the intervertebral discs and articular cartilages of the large joints leads to spondylosis and peripheral arthropathy which will be discussed separately.

Loud *cardiac murmurs* (mostly systolic) have been noted in about 15 to 20 per cent of the cases of ochronosis reported in the literature.[20] Pigment deposits in the mitral and aortic valves may be associated with deformity of the leaflets or cusps and, infrequently, valvular disease.

Prostatic calculi occur in a large proportion of men with ochronosis. These are readily palpable on rectal examination. Dysuria and frequency may be present and in some cases prostatic surgery may be necessary. Calculi may be passed spontaneously or delivered surgically. They have a characteristic black color and contain ochronotic pigment and calcium phosphate salts.

Ochronotic Spondylosis

The majority of patients with ochronosis past the age of thirty develop spondylosis. Symptoms usually consist of stiffness and discomfort in the low back. They appear at an earlier age and more commonly in the male than female patient. In about 10 to 15 per cent of cases of ochronosis, onset of spondylosis occurs with herniation of a nucleus pulposus.[20] In such instances the symptoms and signs are indistinguishable from those observed in typical cases of herniated disc without alkaptonuria. The earliest site of spondylosis is in the lumbar spine; years later the dorsal and finally the cervical spine become involved. Stiffness of the low back slowly progresses to rigidity and obliteration of normal lumbar lordosis. In many cases lumbar kyphosis develops. Symptoms may be minimal despite prominent x-ray changes.

The earliest changes to appear in x rays of the spine consist of a wafer of calcification (and actual ossification) in the intervertebral disc of the lumbar spine (Fig. 61–2). Crystallographic study has shown the calcium in these discs to be hydroxyapatite.[5] Radiographic evidence of calcified intervertebral discs in adults is characteristic of ochronosis but is not diagnostic in that similar changes can also be seen in pseudogout, hemochromatosis, patients with chronic respiratory paralytic polio[8] and occasionally without detectable associated disease. There is secondary narrowing of the intervertebral spaces and relatively small osteophytes later extend from the borders of the vertebral bodies. In sharp contrast to ankylosing spondylitis, the sacroiliac joints are not fused, the interfacetal articulations retain normal radiographic appearance and annular ossification with "bamboo" pattern does not appear. The marked narrowing of multiple intervertebral spaces results in loss of several inches in the patient's linear stature. The spinal deformity and forward stoop cause the patient to stand with knees flexed and on a broad base. This posture imparts to the patient with ochronotic spondylosis a characteristic stance and gait quite similar to that of a patient with ankylosing spondylitis (Fig. 61–3).

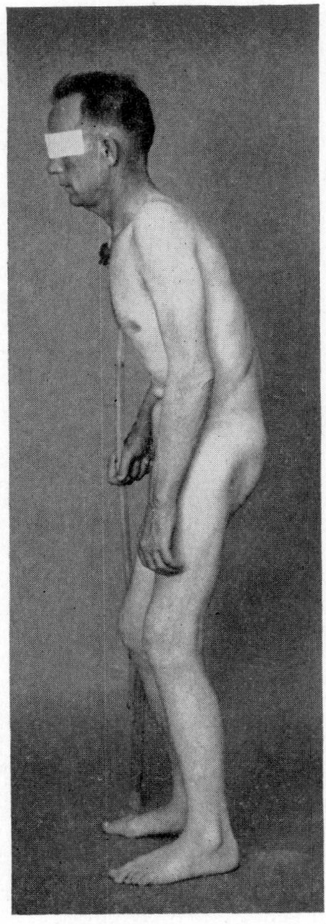

Fig. 61–3.—Typical posture and stance of a patient with ochronotic spondylosis: forward stoop, loss of lumbar lordosis, flexed hips and knees, standing on wide base. This forty-year-old man lost 6 inches in height.

Ochronotic Peripheral Arthropathy

A degenerative-type arthritis of the peripheral joints also occurs although it is less frequent and develops later than spondylosis. The joints most commonly affected are the knees, shoulders and hips, in order of descending frequency. The knees are involved in the majority of cases of peripheral arthritis. Pain, stiffness, crepitation, flexion contractures and limitation of motion are the commonest features. In the peripheral joints symptoms often antedate any visible x-ray changes. Effusion occurs in about half the cases. Synovial fluid is clear, viscous and yellow without darkening on exposure to alkali. Although homogentisic acid can be demonstrated, its concentration is much lower than in the urine. Leukocyte counts in one large series by Hüttl[10] ranged from 112 to 700 with predominantly mononuclear cells. Occasional cells have dark inclusions that appear to be phagocytized ochronotic pigment (Fig. 61–4). Synovial effusions have recently been reported to occasionally contain calcium pyrophosphate crystals[5] but without the inflammation seen in pseudogout.

Pigmentation of the articular cartilage is initially in the deeper layers with relative sparing of the surface. It is predominantly in the matrix of the tangential zone but is also seen in chondrocytes. There is necrosis of chondrocytes. The pigmented articular cartilage is brittle; minute fragments are broken off and displaced into the synovial tissue (Fig.

61–5). In this location, they sometimes evoke a foreign body reaction and new formation of bone tissue, osteochondral bodies[19] (Fig. 61–6). These bodies may be several centimeters in diameter and readily palpable in and around the knee joint. They are not tender and may be freely movable. Surgical removal may be necessary when the bodies interfere with motion.

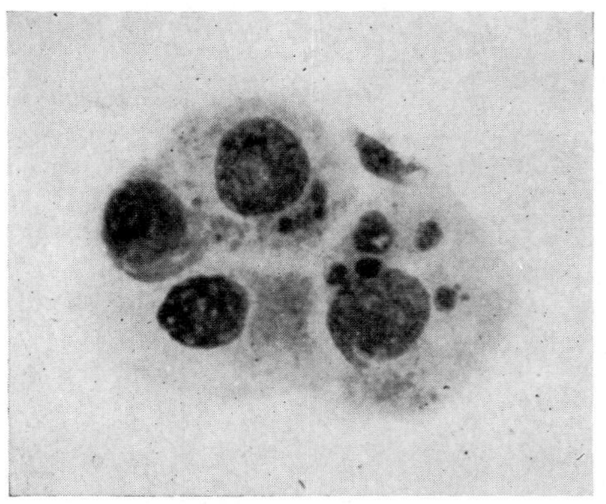

FIG. 61–4.—Synovial fluid mononuclear cells in ochronotic arthropathy. The dark cytoplasmic inclusions appear to be phagocytized pigmented debris. (Giemsa stain × 1,250). (Courtesy of S. Hüttl and Acta. Rheum. Baln. Pistiniana.)

Radiographic appearance of the peripheral joints in ochronotic arthritis is not characteristic (in contrast to that of the spine). The picture is consistent with primary osteoarthritis: narrowing of joint space, marginal osteophytes and eburnation. Ossification of the ligaments near the joints may be present. Rupture of deeply pigmented ochronotic Achilles tendons has been reported.

In contrast to rheumatoid arthritis and osteoarthritis, the small joints of hands and feet are rarely, if ever, affected in ochronosis.

Experimental and Non-Alkaptonuric Production of Ochronosis

Rats fed with 8 per cent L-tyrosine for 18 to 24 months develop pigment deposition in joint capsules and cartilages and a degenerative arthritis similar to that of spontaneous human alkaptonuria.[3] The

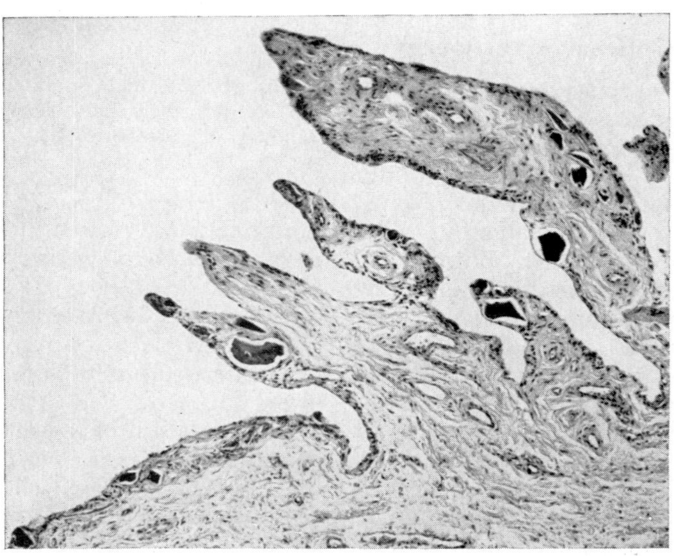

FIG. 61–5.—Synovial tissue in ochronotic arthropathy. Minute fragments of darkly pigmented cartilage lie within the superficial portion of the tissue. The sharp edges of the "chards" are quite characteristic. A foreign body cell reaction is present at the margins of a few and is accompanied by mild synovial fibrosis. (Hematoxylin and eosin × 90.)

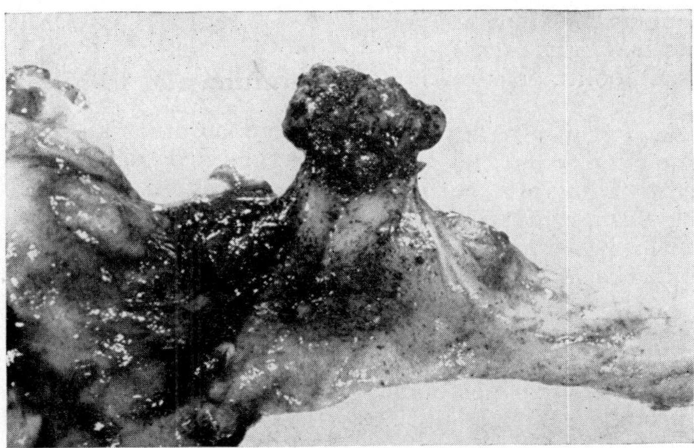

Fig. 61–6.—Synovial tissue in ochronotic arthropathy. Numerous pigmented deposits are present. A polypoid nodule has formed in the central portion as an osteochondroid reaction to the displaced cartilage fragments.

Diagnostic Features of Alkaptonuria, Ochronosis, Ochronotic Spondylosis and Peripheral Arthropathy

ALKAPTONURIA

1. Urine turns black
   a. on alkalinization
   b. on standing
   c. when tested for sugar by Benedict's reagent (in addition, yellow-orange precipitate forms)
2. Positive family history

OCHRONOSIS

1. Pigmentation of cartilage and skin
   a. pinna of ear, ear drum and cerumen
   b. sclera
   c. skin over malar area, nose, axilla, groin
2. Prostatic calculi

OCHRONOTIC SPONDYLOSIS

1. Calcification and ossification of intervertebral discs
2. Disproportionately little osteophytosis
3. Sacroiliac joints not fused and no "bamboo" spine
4. Loss of lumbar lordosis
5. Spine rigid and stooped, knees flexed, stance typical (Fig. 61–3)

OCHRONOTIC PERIPHERAL ARTHROPATHY

1. Knees, shoulders and hips most commonly affected
2. Synovial fluid contains small amounts of homogentisic acid and is non-inflammatory
3. Brittle cartilage fragments and produces pigmented "chards" in the synovium
4. Osteochondral joint bodies are fairly common
5. Small joints of hands and feet not affected

cartilage pigment is melanin-like and includes phenolic bodies as in homogentisic acid or its metabolite benzoquinone acetic acid.

Ochronosis (*i.e.*, a grossly bluish black connective tissue pigmentation) with degenerative arthritis has also been described following prolonged administration of quinacrine in the absence of alkaptonuria.[16] Application of phenol dressings has been reported to produce ochronosis with alkaptonuria and arthropathy. Cartilage pigmentation does not appear to occur in melanoma. D-Dopa may produce elevated urine homogentisic acid.[1]

Treatment

It is not yet feasible to compensate for the enzymatic deficiency of homogentisic acid oxidase. Attempts have been made to treat patients with a diet low in phenylalanine and tyrosine by Holdsworth *et al.*[9] Urinary excretion of HGA can be decreased but clinical change was minimal in patients with already advanced joint disease. The diet used is most unpalatable but was tolerated by their two patients. Initiation of this diet at early age before massive ochronosis develops has not been tried. Reduced protein intake can also decrease urine homogentisic acid but is also impractical for routine treatment. High doses of ascorbic acid, although not decreasing total urine homogentisic acid, has been reported to decrease binding to connective tissue in experimental alkaptonuria of rats.[17] Long-term use of ascorbic acid has not been studied in human ochronosis.

Symptomatic measures are of most practical value. Analgesics, braces, programs limiting joint abuse and weight reduction have all provided some help. Adrenal corticosteroids, x ray, tyrosinase, insulin, various vitamins, and phenylbutazone are among the measures tried without benefit. Corrective orthopedic procedures have been helpful in several patients.[6]

HEMOCHROMATOSIS

Definition and Clinical Picture

Hemochromatosis is a chronic disease characterized pathologically by excess iron deposition and fibrosis in many organs and tissues with ultimate functional impairment in untreated patients. Frequent clinical manifestations are hepatomegaly and cirrhosis, skin pigmentation (due mostly to increased melanin), diabetes, other endocrine dysfunction and heart failure.[7,16] Arthropathy occurs in 20 per cent or more of patients. Hemochromatosis is often idiopathic with a definite increased familial incidence. Hemochromatosis can also be a late result of alcoholic cirrhosis or occasionally of multiple transfusions, refractory anemia, and chronic excess oral iron ingestion. In all instances there is excess iron absorption. Significant overload occurs only after many years so that onset of symptoms is most common between 40 to 60 years. Hemochromatosis is less frequent in women presumably because of menstrual blood losses.

Pathology and Pathogenesis

Iron as hemosiderin can be identified histologically in all the symptomatically affected tissues as well as elsewhere. The largest iron deposits are in the liver and diagnosis is most frequently established by liver biopsy. Large amounts of hemosiderin are seen in parenchymal cells in the liver and other organs. Iron confined to reticuloendothelial tissues is termed hemosiderosis and does not produce the clinical picture seen in hemochromatosis. It should be noted that, although suspected, the iron has not been proved to be the cause of the tissue damage. Organ fibrosis, as in hemochromatosis, has not yet been produced by experimental iron overload alone. Iron may act in an additive fashion with nutritional deficiencies, alcohol or hereditary factors.

Diagnosis

The most important simple laboratory test in diagnosis is determination of serum iron and iron-binding capacity. Both are greatly elevated in hemochromatosis but can also be elevated in hemolytic anemia and other situations. Liver biopsy is needed to determine the extent of tissue iron deposition and degree of tissue damage. The plasma iron-binding proteins are usually fully saturated in this disease.

Osteopenia

Diffuse demineralization of bone can be seen but its frequency and relationship to the hemochromatosis are difficult to ascertain. A 25 to 50 per cent incidence has been estimated.[5] A diffuse osteopenia of the hands (without the periarticular demineralization as seen in rheumatoid arthritis) has been most common.[8] The mechanism for osteopenia is not known. Delbarre who studied this most extensively postulated an androgen deficiency secondary to hemochromatosis.[2] Serum calcium, phosphorus and alkaline phosphatase are normal. Biopsy specimens have shown osteoporosis rather than osteomalacia. Osteopenia can also be seen in alcoholic cirrhosis so a direct relation to the defect in iron metabolism is not established.

Degenerative Arthropathy

An arthropathy associated with hemochromatosis was first described by Schumacher in 1964[14] and since that time more than 100 cases have been reported.[3,4,6,8,10,12,18] The most frequent joint involvement is degenerative. This occurs in 20 to 50 per cent of patients with hemochromatosis.[8] Age of onset has varied from 26 to 70 but is most common in the 50's. Onset of arthropathy is usually close in time to onset of other symptoms of hemochromatosis. Joint symptoms occasionally are first noted many years later and even after completion of phlebotomy therapy.

Hands, knees, and hips are most frequently involved, although most other joints can be affected. Characteristic hand findings are a firm, only mildly tender, enlargement of metacarpophalangeal (MCP) and proximal (PIP) and distal interphalangeal (DIP) joints. The second and third MCP's are most often affected (Fig. 61–7). These joints are stiff and have limited motion but no increased warmth or erythema. Ulnar deviation is not seen. Involvement is generally symmetrical. Pain, when present, is accentuated on use. Morning stiffness is usually less than one-half hour. This arthropathy is gradually progressive. Acute inflammation has occasionally been described and whether this is always due to associated chondrocalcinosis and crystal-induced synovitis (see below) is not certain. Test results for rheumatoid factor are typically negative. Sedimentation rates are only occasionally elevated. Serum uric acid is generally normal and occasionally low.[18] Hand x rays often also show the characteristic involvement of MCP, PIP and DIP joints. There is narrowing of the joint space, cyst-like erosion, joint space irregularity, subchondral sclerosis and moderate bony proliferation (Fig. 61–8). In 30 to 60 per cent of patients with arthropathy, chondrocalcinosis is also seen. X rays of other joints show changes similar to those in the hands and are generally indistinguishable from degenerative arthritis and idiopathic chondrocalcinosis. Synovial fluid is non-inflammatory with low leukocyte counts and predominantly mononuclear cells, good viscosity and pale yellow color. Iron measurements on synovial fluid have been comparable to serum levels.[10] Occasional mononuclear cells in the synovial fluid can be shown to contain iron by Prussian blue stain.[10] Synovial tissue shows a striking deposition of iron predominantly in the synovial lining cells. On hematoxylin and eosin stains, golden brown hemosiderin granules are seen. The iron can also be stained blue by Prussian blue (Fig. 61–9). By electron microscopy the

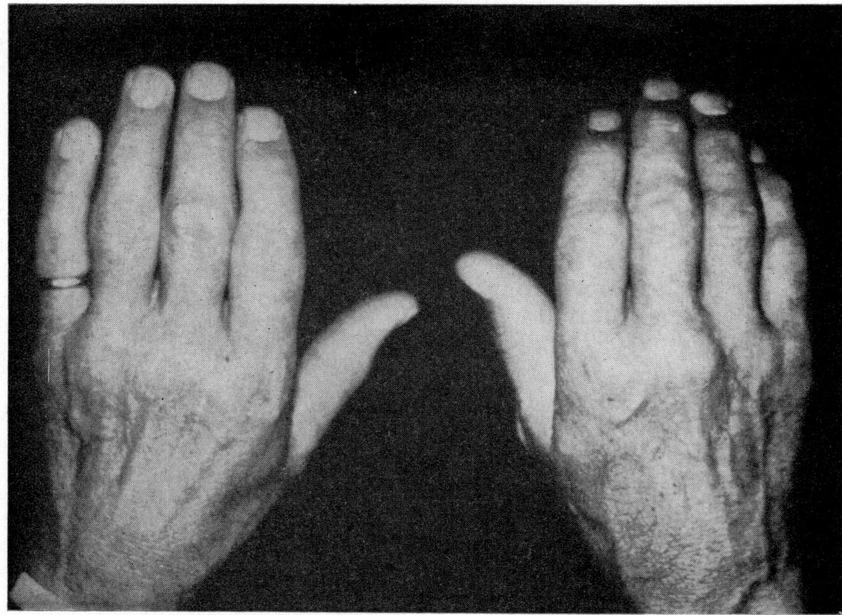

Fig. 61–7.—Photograph of hands of a 45-year-old man with hemochromatosis. Note the knobby enlargement at MCP, PIP and DIP joints. He is unable to fully extend these joints.

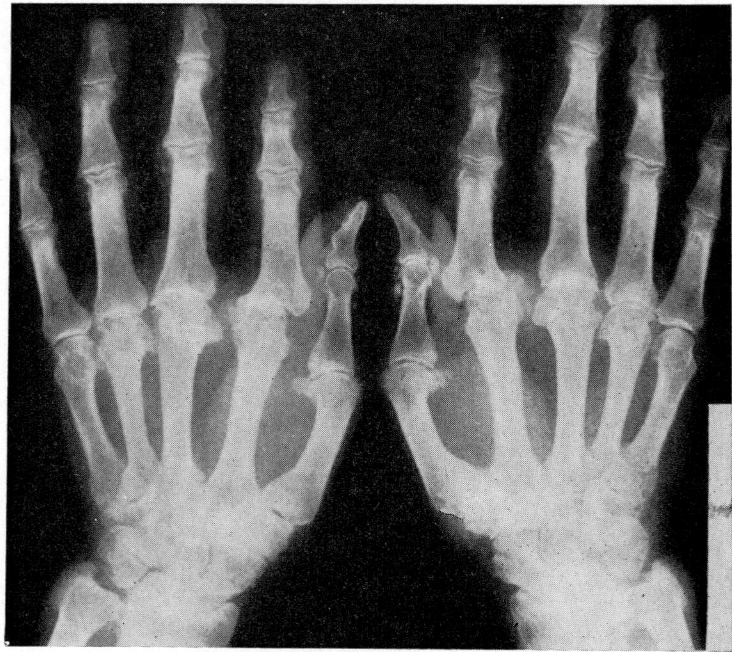

Fig. 61–8.—Hand x rays showing involvement of MCP, PIP and DIP joints with characteristic joint space narrowing, cystic subchondral lesions, joint space irregularity, subluxation, some osteophytosis, and areas of bony sclerosis. There are also multiple periarticular calcifications at the left thumb IP joint and probable chondrocalcinosis at the right ulnocarpal joint. Osteopenia is minimal in these hands.

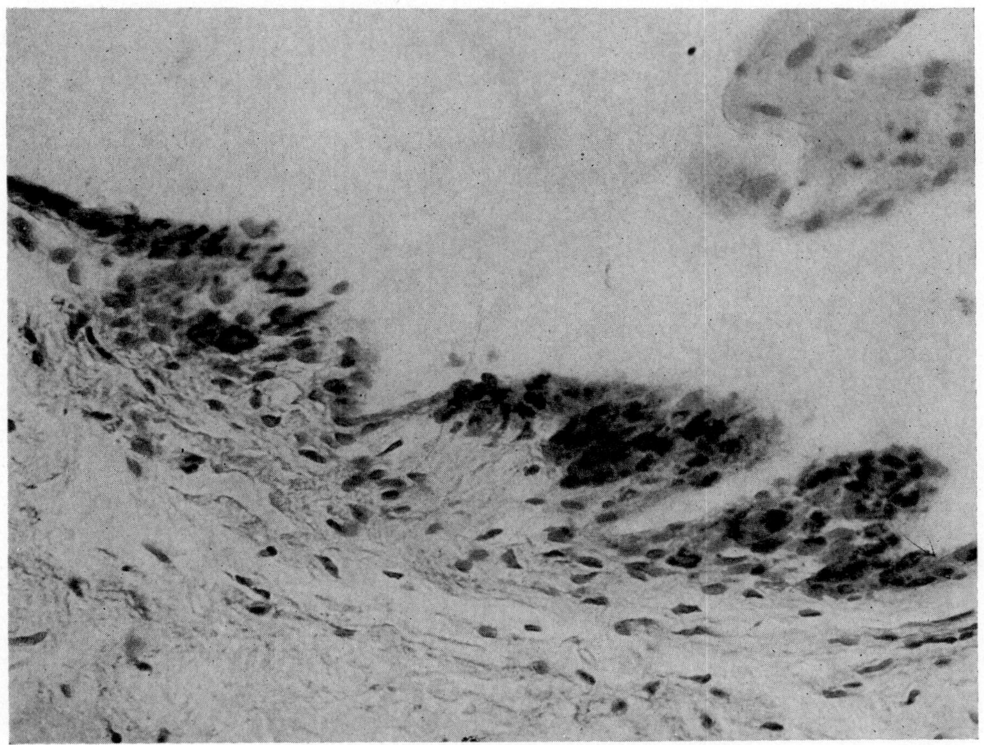

FIG. 61–9.—Synovium in hemochromatosis with dark Prussian blue-stained iron granules in the synovial lining cells. 400×.

iron is principally in the type B or synthetic type lining cells (Fig. 61–10).[15] This distribution of synovial iron differs from that in hemarthrosis, rheumatoid arthritis, and other diseases with iron presumably derived from gross or microscopic bleeding into the joint. In these conditions the iron is mostly in deeper cells and macrophages. In addition to the iron, most synovial tissue in hemochromatosis shows only mild lining cell proliferation, fibrosis, and scattered chronic inflammatory cells. Biopsies during bouts of acute inflammation have not been reported.

Chondrocalcinosis

Chondrocalcinosis occurs in up to 30 per cent of patients with hemochromatosis and, although usually associated with the degenerative arthropathy, can also be an isolated joint finding.[8] Calcification is most commonly detected in menisci and articular cartilages at the knee, but can also be seen at the wrists, fingers, elbows, shoulders, hips, ankles, toes, symphysis pubis, intervertebral discs and in the soft tissues of the heels or elsewhere. Typical acute arthritis as in pseudogout with crystals identified as calcium pyrophosphate can occur. The synovial effusion is inflammatory during such episodes. Menisci and articular cartilages can show grossly evident superficial coating with white crystals. Round intra-cartilaginous aggregates of positively birefringent crystals identical to those of pseudogout can be seen with compensated polarized light microscopy.[8,12] Iron staining of cartilage has also been seen, but this is in chondrocytes and at the line of ossification and not at the crystal deposits.[15] X-ray diffraction

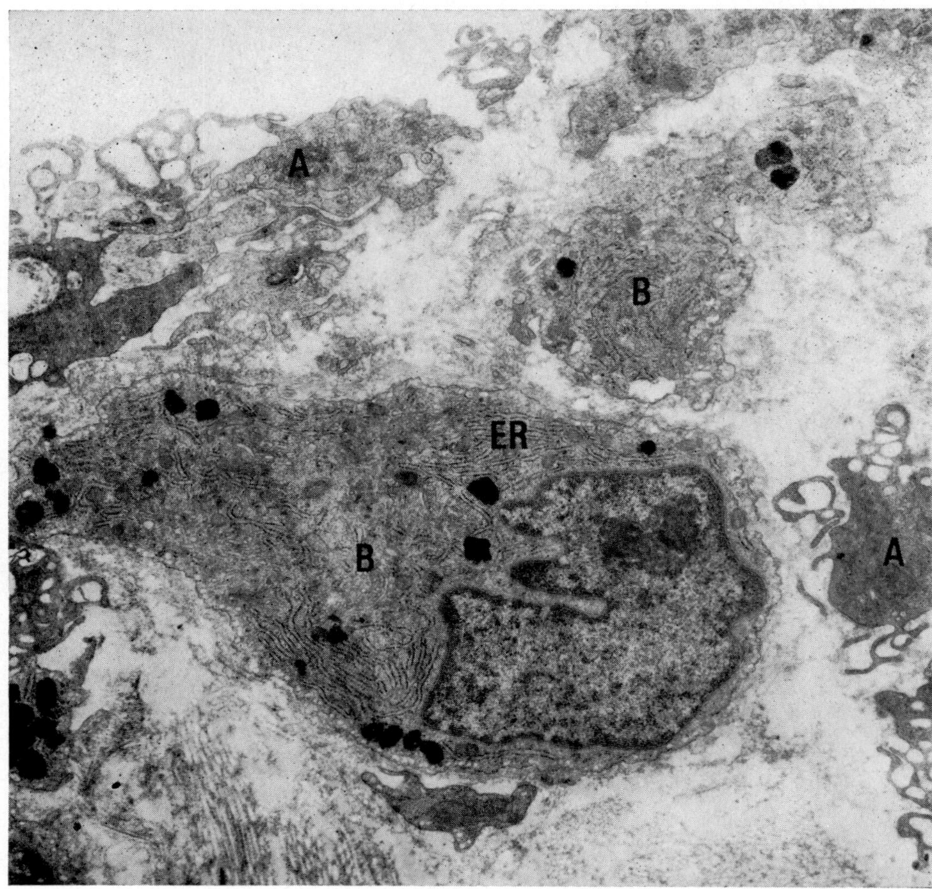

Fig. 61–10.—Electron micrograph of electron dense iron deposits in type B synovial lining cells (B) in hemochromatosis. Type B cells are primarily synthetic in function and have profuse rough endoplasmic reticulum (ER). The type A cells (A) often have prominent filopodia and vacuoles and are felt to be more active in phagocytosis. Here they contain no identifiable iron. 13,000×.

and chemical studies likewise have shown no iron at the sites of cartilage calcification.[8]

Possible Mechanisms for the Arthropathy

It is attractive to speculate that the iron directly or indirectly causes the osteoarthropathy, but this has not yet been demonstrated. The rarity of arthropathy in transfusion siderosis and Bantu siderosis suggests that factors other than the iron are required. A patient with spherocytosis has developed hemochromatosis with arthropathy and chondrocalcinosis.[6] Many patients with iron-loading anemias may not survive long enough to develop tissue damage. Kaschin-Beck disease, an endemic growth disturbance and premature generalized degenerative arthritis seen in Russia and Manchuria, has been attributed by Hiyeda to high iron content in drinking water[9], although it should be noted that Nesterov[13] recently has suggested instead that it is a result of fungal infection of grain. Hiyeda in support of this theory administered iron to vigorously exercized rabbits and felt he produced an accelerated cartilage deterioration. More recently, experimental iron loading of rabbits has been reported to produce cartilage degeneration only if started early in life suggesting that early initiation of the toxic effect of iron may be critical.[1] Iron, since localized so predominately in synthetic-type cells, might produce its joint damage by altering the protein polysaccharide or collagen produced by these cells. Ferric ion has been suggested to irreversibly oxidize ascorbic acid causing impaired hydroxylation of proline and thus deficient collagen formation.[1] Iron might produce damage by binding to connective tissue protein polysaccharides as it does *in vitro* in the Hale stain for protein polysaccharide. Some iron is in lysosomes and it could allow increased release of lysosomal enzymes.

Iron *in vitro* inhibits pyrophosphatase and might in this manner be a factor in allowing the deposition of the calcium pyrophosphate of chondrocalcinosis.[11] The primary site of joint damage is not established. The cartilage is most suspect in this degenerative process but subchondral bone involvement may also be important as could the synovial disease since cartilage is dependent on both these areas for its nutrition. No correlation has been found between the presence of advanced liver disease, generalized osteopenia, diabetes, or other endocrine disease and the arthropathy. Classical rheumatoid arthritis has been seen to coexist in several cases so that the arthropathy is not an iron-altered rheumatoid disease.

Treatment

Present therapy of hemochromatosis is directed at removal of the excess iron by phlebotomy, and this has appeared to reverse cardiac failure, improve liver function and ameliorate diabetes.[19] Improvement depends largely on the amount of existing tissue damage. Prevention certainly would be preferable so that serum iron concentrations of relatives should be checked and phlebotomy prophylaxis considered. Phlebotomy is usually started at 500 ml. per week until the development of mild iron deficiency anemia or demonstrable depletion of liver iron. Supportive treatment of the diabetes, liver disease and heart failure is pursued as needed. Phlebotomy has so far produced no beneficial effect on the arthritis, and clinical arthritis has even developed after phlebotomy therapy. Irreversible connective tissue and joint change may well have been established long before arthritis could be clinically or radiographically detected. Iron is easily demonstrable in the synovium of asymptomatic patients. Treatment of the arthritis is symptomatic with analgesics and systematic range of motion exercises being most helpful. Prosthetic hip and knee arthroplasties in advanced disease

Diagnostic Features of Hemochromatosis

1. Cirrhosis of the liver with iron deposition predominantly in parenchymal cells.
2. Iron deposition in other organs causing cardiomyopathy, diabetes or other endocrine deficiencies.
3. Increased skin pigmentation largely due to melanin.
4. Markedly elevated serum iron concentration and highly saturated iron-binding capacity.

Diagnostic Features of the Arthropathy of Hemochromatosis

1. Degenerative type arthropathy.
2. Prominent involvement of MCP's, PIP's, DIP's, hips and knees.
3. Chondrocalcinosis.
4. Iron deposition in synovial lining cells.

have been successfully performed although further breakdown after 18 months has occurred in one knee after prosthetic arthroplasty.[15]

WILSON'S DISEASE

Wilson's disease (*hepatolenticular degeneration*)[11] is an uncommon, familial disease characterized by a diagnostic ring of brown pigment at the corneal margin (the Kayser-Fleischer ring), basal ganglion degeneration and cirrhosis of the liver.[9] The condition is inherited as an autosomal recessive. Onset of symptoms may be from age 4 to 40. Neurologic symptoms are usually earliest and include tremor, rigidity, dysarthria, incoordination or personality change. Many patients also develop renal tubular disease manifested by aminoaciduria, proteinuria, glucosuria, phosphaturia, defective urine acidification or uricosuria. The latter often results in very low serum uric acid levels. Untreated disease is invariably fatal.

Characteristic disorders of copper metabolism are present. Copper concentration is increased in liver, brain and other tissues; urine copper excretion is increased; and the serum copper-binding protein, ceruloplasmin, as well as total serum copper are almost always decreased. Increased absorption of copper can be demonstrated, but whether this is a result of the diminished ceruloplasmin concentration, tissue affinity for copper, or other defect is not established. It is postulated that the copper is the cause of the tissue damage. Mobilization of copper from the body seems to produce improvement in many patients.

Osteopenia

Radiographic evidence of demineralization of bone has long been recognized as part of Wilson's disease and is described in 25 to 50 per cent of patients.[5,7] Osteopenia is seen at all ages, and usually is asymptomatic. Occasional patients have pathological fractures. Others have definite rickets[3] or osteomalacia that can be attributed to the renal tubular disease.

Arthropathy

Boudin *et al.*[1] first described articular alterations in Wilson's disease in 1957. Joint changes are rare in childhood but are seen in up to 50 per cent of adults. Most patients studied have been 20 to 40 years old. Articular involvement[2,4,5,7,8] ranges from premature osteoarthritis with marked symptoms to asymptomatic radiographic findings. Scattered subchondral bone fragmentations, cortical irregularity and sclerosis at the margin of wrist, hand, elbow, shoulder, hip and knee joints are seen (Fig. 61–11). The cartilage space is also often narrowed. Early age of onset and prominent involvement of wrists and metacarpal phalangeal joints suggest a difference from the usual osteoarthritis. Tiny periarticular cysts,[7] vertebral wedging and marginal irregularity,[8] osteochondritis dissecans and chondromalacia patellae[4] have been seen in several cases and may be related to the Wilson's disease. Periarticular calcifications are common. Many such calcifications are in ligaments, tendons and capsule insertions. Other calcifications seem to represent bone fragments or occasional chondrocalcinosis.[2,4] The nature of the calcium in these lesions has not been studied. Joint effusions are usually small. A single synovial fluid has been examined and showed clear, viscous fluid. There were 200 cells and these were mostly mononuclears. Synovial fluid copper and ceruloplasmin have not been studied.

No correlation has been found between total disease severity, spasticity and tremors, osteopenia, liver or renal disease and the arthropathy. It has been suggested that the primary defect is in the cartilage or subchondral bone but there have been no histologic or chemical studies of these tissues. Although the joint involvement in Wilson's disease is generally milder, an analogy can be made with that of hemochromatosis. In both dis-

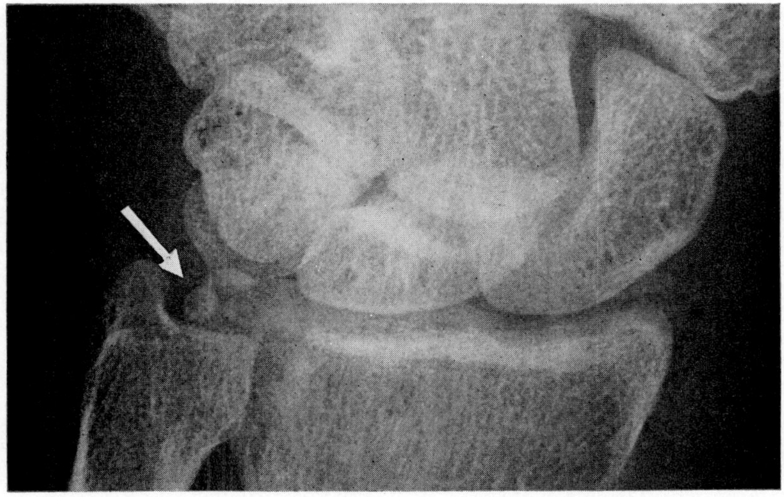

A

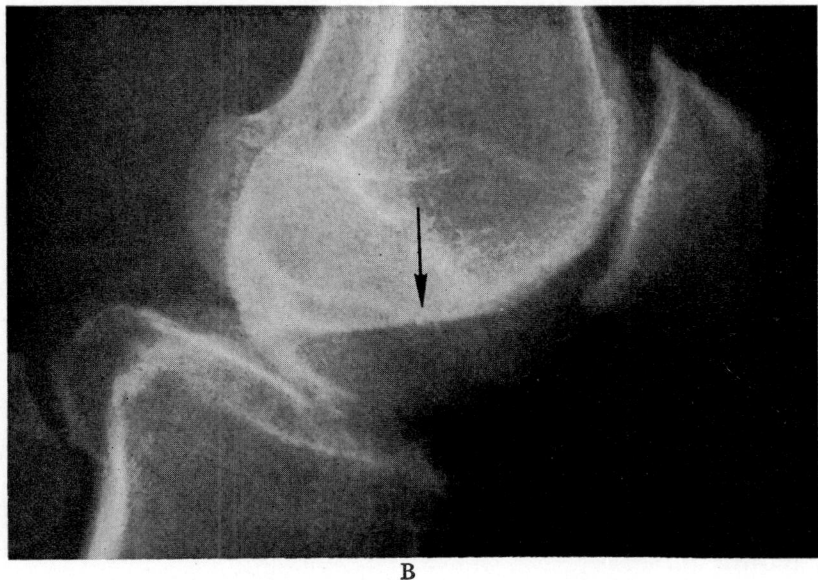

B

Fig. 61–11.—Arthropathy in a 30-year-old woman with Wilson's disease. A. Wrist. Note the bony ossicles (arrow) which have been suggested to be a result of cortical fragmentation. There is also some sclerosis at the distal radius. B. Knee. Ossicles are seen near the tibiofibular articulation. There is marked chondromalacia patellae with spurs on the posterior surface of the patella. The articular cortex of the lateral femoral condyle is slightly irregular with a suggestion of fragmentation at the arrow.

eases the metal excess is a possible mechanism for direct or indirect production of the arthropathy. Short-term experimental copper loading has not produced arthropathy. McCarty and collaborators[6] have shown *in vitro* inhibition of pyrophosphatase by cupric and ferrous ions and have suggested this as a possible mechanism for deposition of calcium pyrophosphate producing chondrocalcinosis in Wilson's disease and hemochromatosis.

Bone and Joint Changes in Wilson's Disease

1. Bone demineralization.
2. Occasionally rickets or osteomalacia attributable to renal tubular disease.
3. Premature degenerative arthritis with prominent subchondral bone fragmentation.
4. Prominent involvement of wrists, MCP's, knees and less often other joints.
5. Periarticular calcifications and bone fragments.

Treatment

Penicillamine (1 to 4 gm per day by mouth) has proved to be the most successful chelating agent for mobilizing copper from the tissue and has produced definite clinical improvement in mental and neurologic changes in many patients. Treatment is continued for life. Low copper diets and potassium sulfide may also be used to decrease copper absorption. Symptomatic disease may be preventable by early D-penicillamine treatment of asymptomatic individuals with biochemical abnormalities only.[10] Occasional patients treated with penicillamine have still developed arthropathy. Whether early and long-term treatment will decrease the bone and joint disease is not yet known.

BIBLIOGRAPHY

Alkaptonuria and Ochronosis

1. Arras, M. J.: New Engl. J. Med., *282*, 813, 1970.
2. Beadle, G. W. and Tatum, E. L.: Proc. Nat. Acad. Sci., *27*, 499, 1941.
3. Blivaiss, B. B. *et al.*: Arch. Path., *82*, 45, 1966.
4. Briggs, A. P.: J. Biol. Chem., *51*, 453, 1922.
5. Bywaters, E. G. L., Dorling, J. and Sutor, J.: Ann. Rheum. Dis., *29*, 563, 1970.
6. Detenbeck, L. C., Young, H. H., and Underdahl, L. O.: Arch. Surg., *100*, 215, 1970.
7. Garrod, A. E.: *Inborn Errors of Metabolism*, London, Oxford Univ. Press, 1909.
8. Gilmartin, D.: Clin. Radiol., *17*, 115, 1966.
9. Holdsworth, D., Barry, M. L. and Swyter, J. L.: Arth. & Rheum., *10*, 284, 1967.
10. Hüttl, S.: Acta. Rheum. Baln. Pistiniana, *5*, 1, 1970.
11. Kelley, W. M., Fox, I. H., Feldman, J. M. and Wyngaarden, J. B.: Arth. & Rheum., *12*, 673, 1969.
12. Knox, W. E.: Amer. J. Human Genetics, *10*, 95, 1958.
13. LaDu, B. N., Zannoni, V. G., Laster, L., and Seegmiller, J. E.: J. Biol. Chem., *230*, 251, 1958.
14. Lee, S. and Schoen, I.: New Engl. J. Med., *275*, 266, 1966.
15. Lichtenstein, L. and Kaplan, L.: Amer. J. Path., *30*, 99, 1954.
16. Ludwig, G. D., Toole, J. F. and Wood, J. C.: Ann. Intern. Med., *59*, 378, 1963.
17. Lustberg, T. J., Schulman, J. D., and Seegmiller, J. E.: Nature, *228*, 770, 1970.
18. Naganna, B. and Ethirajulu, G.: Brit. Med. J., *4*, 55, 1967.
19. O Brien, W. M., Banfield, W. G., and Sokoloff, L.: Arth. & Rheum., *4*, 137, 1961.
20. O Brien, W. M., LaDu, B. N., and Bunim, J. J.: Amer. J. Med., *34*, 813, 1963.
21. Sadilek, L.: Clin. Chim. Acta, *12*, 436, 1965.
22. Seegmiller, J. E., Zannoni, V. G., Laster, L. and LaDu, B. M.: J. Biol. Chem., *236*, 774, 1961.
23. Zannoni, V. G., Malawista, S. E., and LaDu, B. N.: Arth. & Rheum., *5*, 547, 1962.

Hemochromatosis

1. Brighton, C. T., Bigley, E. C. and Smolenski, B. I.: Arth. & Rheum., *13*, 849, 1970.
2. Delbarre, F.: Sem. Hop., *58*, 1, 1960.
3. ———: La Presse Med., *72*, 2973, 1964.
4. Dorfmann, H., Solnica, J., DiMenza, C., and deSeze, S.: Sem. Hop., *45*, 516, 1969.
5. Dulac, Y., DeLoux, G. and Devil, R.: Rev. Rhum., *34*, 758, 1967.
6. Dymock, I. W., Hamilton, E. B. D., Laws, J. W., and Williams, R.: Ann. Rheum. Dis., *29*, 469, 1970.
7. Finch, S. C. and Finch, C. A.: Medicine, *34*, 381, 1955.

8. Hamilton, E., Williams, R., Barlow, K. A. and Smith, P. M.: Quart. J. Med., *145*, 171, 1968.
9. Hiyeda, K.: Jap. Med. Sci., *4*, 91, 1939.
10. Kra, S. J., Hollingsworth, J. W. and Finch, S. C.: New Engl. J. Med., *272*, 1268, 1965.
11. McCarty, D. J., Pepe, P. R., Solomon, S. D. and Cobb, J.: Arth. & Rheum., *13*, 336, 1970.
12. Mitrovic, D., Mazabraud, S., Jaffres, R., Kerbrat, G., Amourous, J., Solnica, J. and deSeze, S.: Arch. Anat. Path., *14*, 264, 1966.
13. Nesterov, A. I.: Arth. & Rheum., *7*, 29, 1964.
14. Schumacher, H. R.: Arth. & Rheum., *7*, 41, 1964.
15. ———: Unpublished observations.
16. Sheldon, J. H.: *Haemochromatosis*, London, Oxford Univ. Press, 1935.
17. Sinniah, R.: Arch. Intern. Med., *124*, 455, 1969.
18. Wardle, E. N. and Patton, J. T.: Ann. Rheum. Dis., *28*, 15, 1969.
19. Whitcomb, F. F., Lummis, F. R., Mejia, J. A., and Achkar, E. J.: Lahey Clin. Fdn. Bull., *18*, 109, 1969.

Wilson's Disease

1. Boudin, G., Pepin, B., Barbizet, J., and Molinard, P.: Bull. Soc. Med. Hop. Paris, *73*, 756, 1957.
2. Boudin, G., Pepin, B. and Hubault, A.: Rev. Rhum., *31*, 594, 1964.
3. Cavallino, R. and Grossman, H.: Radiology, *90*, 493, 1968.
4. Feller, E. and Schumacher, H. R.: Arth. & Rheum. In press.
5. Finby, N. and Bearn, A. G.: Amer. J. Roentgenol., *79*, 603, 1958.
6. McCarty, D. J., Pepe, P. F., Solomon, S. D., and Cobb, J.: Arth. & Rheum., *13*, 336, 1970.
7. Mindelzun, R., Elkin, M., Scheinberg, I. H., and Sternlieb, I.: Radiology, *94*, 127, 1970.
8. Rosenoer, V. M. and Michell, R. C.: Brit. J. Radiol., *32*, 805, 1959.
9. Scheinberg, I. H. and Sternlieb, I.: Ann. Rev. Med., *16*, 119, 1965.
10. Sternlieb, I. and Scheinberg, I. H.: New Engl. J. Med., *278*, 352, 1958.
11. Wilson, S. A. K.: Brain, *34*, 395, 1912.

Chapter 62

Metabolic Bone Diseases

By David S. Howell, M.D.

Improved methods of diagnosis and discovery of previously uncharted syndromes have launched a new interest in metabolic bone diseases. Inasmuch as rheumatic symptoms are often the initial complaint and cause of chronic disablement, confusion of the diagnosis with non-articular rheumatism, fibrositis and functional back syndromes is likely. The opportunity for cure or striking palliation in certain of these diseases adds to the importance of correct diagnosis. For investigators, these maladies offer a challenge in the field of electrolyte metabolism, intermediary and hormone metabolism, as well as biophysics.

Terminology, pathologic physiology, clinical description and management of the more common disorders are reviewed briefly. References should be consulted for detailed discussion of the subject matter.[3,15,18,29,30,33,46,48,51,56,57,68]

FUNDAMENTAL PROPERTIES OF BONE

Anatomy

The two pathways of bone formation are *enchondral* and *membranous*.[46] In the first type, exemplified by epiphyseal growth in ribs and extremities, bone develops on the scaffolding of preformed cartilage (Fig. 62–1). Lengthening of the skeleton depends primarily on this first type. In the second, new bone forms *de novo* in the embryo or along the margin of cortical or trabecular bone; this type accounts for the bulk of lateral expansion in childhood as well as the remodeling processes throughout life. In both meth-

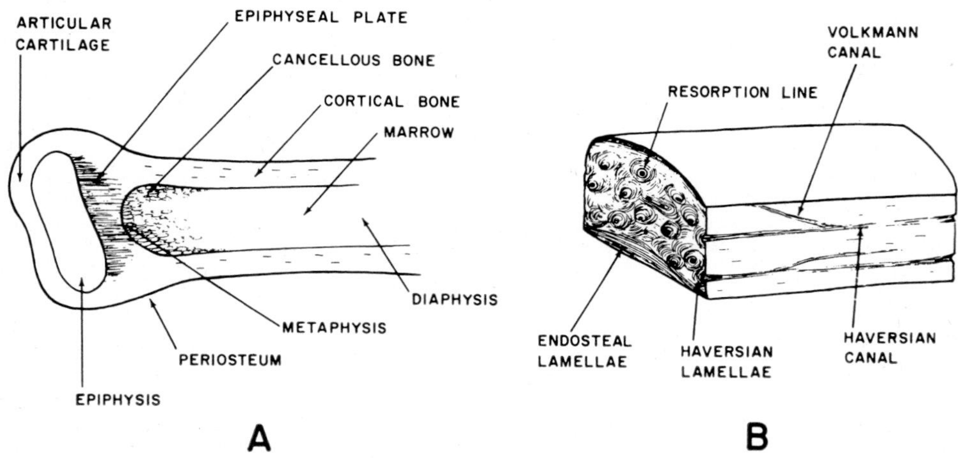

Fig. 62–1.—Diagrams of bone with regional terminology (*A*) and system of canals in osteones of compact bone (*B*).

ods of formation, there is deposition of an extracellular matrix by uninuclear lining cells (osteoblasts) with subsequent rapid deposition of minerals in the matrix. In each of the long bones, remodeling occurs within Haversian canals beneath periosteum and at endosteal surfaces. Multinuclear giant cells (osteoclasts) are important in the erosion phase of remodeling.

Cortical (compact) bone primarily consists of longitudinally oriented tubules (osteones) in the center of which traverse the Haversian canals containing blood vessels and lymph which diffuses radially to the osteocytes by canaliculi. Penetrating the surface are Volkmann canals (Fig. 62–1). In the life-long process of remodeling, as well as in childhood growth, erosion cavities are continually forming and new Haversian systems developing. These remodeling processes comprise a fascinating detailed sequence of cellular events elucidated principally in the last decade by morphometric measurements.[35] Mineral transfers by short-term exchange at open osteoid seams and by a long-term exchange process within the older or more mature portions of the skeleton.[42]

Biochemistry

The average adult, weighing 70 kg., contains a total of 1150 gm. of calcium (hereafter abbreviated Ca) confined largely to bones and teeth, in mineral phases resembling closely amorphous Ca phosphate and hydroxyapatite, $Ca_{10}(PO_4)_6(OH)_2$.[56] The remaining fraction is found primarily in extracellular fluid. Normal total Ca in adult serum is 10.0 ± 1.0 mg. per cent (5.0 ± 0.5 mEq/liter). Approximately half the Ca is bound to serum protein and most of the remainder is ionized. Ca associated with protein is not diffusible, whereas the ionized is in equilibrium with and diffused throughout body extravascular lymph spaces and cerebrospinal fluid.[45] Such fluids normally contain about 5 mg. per cent of Ca. These averages apply to the healthy state in which a serum protein of approximately 7 gm. per cent is present. Inasmuch as higher or lower values of serum protein profoundly influence the total Ca content, study of patients with bone disease should include measurement of total serum protein. Inorganic phosphorus (hereafter termed IP) in adult serum is normally 3.5 ± 0.5 mg. per cent (1.0 ± 0.3 mEq./liter) with values in children 1 to 2 mg. higher. IP is present principally as mono- and dihydrogen phosphate ions. Without parathyroid glands, Ca levels fall to 6 to 7 mg. per cent and remain approximately in that range.[51] However, in a person with intact parathyroid function, the levels of Ca and IP in the extracellular fluid are maintained in a state of supersaturation in respect to hydroxyapatite by the action of the parathyroid hormone. There is extensive evidence that parathyroid hormone mobilizes bone salt by local action and the hormone is believed to accelerate IP excretion by the kidneys, thereby preventing body accumulation of liberated IP.[51,66] Dissolution of bone salt is accelerated by systemic acidosis and depressed by alkalosis. In particular, bone phosphate is an important physiological buffer in systemic acidosis.[66]

Bone remodeling involves the following processes: (1) formation and dissolution of the osteoid matrix; (2) exchange of various ions, particularly Ca and IP, in the layer of bound water (hydration shell) and surface of hydroxyapatite microcrystals and (3) incorporation or removal of Ca atoms within the crystal lattice.[33,51] These crystals aggregate along the collagen fibrils in a periodic manner as demonstrated by electron microscopy.[19,20] Expanding mineralization probably results from seeding of specially prepared nucleation sites.[20]

In normal adult humans, studies with radioactive Ca indicate a half-life of administered ion to be *circa* two hundred and sixty days;[7] the absorbed portion of orally administered Ca immediately mixes with a miscible pool in the extracellular spaces and soft tissues. In adult man, bone accretion occurs at the rate of a few hundred mg. per day.[25,27] (*See reference 25 for detailed concepts concerning bone accretion, primary and secondary mineralization, periosteocytic deposition as well as long-term exchange.*) It has been shown that within a short period, 3 times the normal extracellular fluid content of Ca may be mobilized from bone.[24] Prolonged exposure of bone to lymph under conditions of excess resorption brings to view previously unexposed hydroxyapatite microcrystals, and, eventually, Ca loss leads to structural demineralization. Resorption of apatite and matrix follow in such close succession as to appear concomitant. In the normal individual, synthetic and catabolic processes occur simultaneously so as to remodel the newly formed bone into a specific structural arrangement which fulfills local mechanical needs.

Bone Biopsy

The iliac or tibial bone biopsy (usually with replacement of tissue by a bank graft) has become an increasingly useful diagnostic procedure as well as method for assessment of results in research studies on metabolic bone disease.[17,36,43,55] Presence of unmineralized "open" osteoid seams, ratio of linear surface in histologic sections occupied by osteogenic versus osteoclastic function,[36] number of osteocytes per unit area of compact bone, states of feathering,[17] and lacunar wall resorption are among the measurements possible at a local tissue site. Volume of new bone synthesized per unit time can be quantitated from spaced injections of tetracycline and measurement of area between fluorescent rings visualized by ultraviolet microscopy.[17] Also, two tetracyclines with different fluorescence spectra can be used to demarcate separate experimental periods.[26]

Effect of Hormones

Parathyroid hormone, identified as a polypeptide, is an important endogenous secretion (Fig. 62–2) and is believed to regulate the supersaturation of lymph with Ca and IP indirectly by its action on cells involved in mineral ion transfers. Strong evidence indicates an influence upon bone cells[48] with an additional important renal phosphaturic and intestinal absorptive effect. Parathyroid hormone produces hypercalcemia in the nephrectomized animal[62] and causes release of mineral ions from bone in organ cultures.[22] Local dissolution of cranial bone results from transplanted parathyroid tissue.[5]

Mobilization of organic matrix components along with the mineral during parathyroid hormone administration is apparent from histologic observations.[63] Also, biochemical studies of bone chip preparations incubated *in vitro* from parathyroid-treated animals recorded a striking elevation of collagenase activity in comparison to that of normal controls.[69] In other experimental preparations, increased urinary excretion of catabolic products of collagen-hydroxyproline peptides attended parathyroid hormone administration.[57]

A feedback control mechanism is believed to govern the secretion rate of parathyroid hormone mediated by the plasma concentration of ionized Ca perfusing the glands.[48] An exciting area of recent advance has been the discovery and rapid characterization of calcitonin (Thyrocalcitonin), a single-chain polypeptide hormone produced by the ultimobranchial bodies of lower life forms and produced in man by the "C" cell of the thyroid gland.[15,30] Calcitonin produces hypocalcemia and hypophosphatemia by a primary action on bone resorption. The hormone inhibits modulation of mesenchymal cells into osteoclasts and deters prompt release (Fig. 62–2) of Ca from bone via a direct action on existing bone cells. In effect, calcitonin action negates the action of parathyroid hormone. Its exact role as a regulator of Ca metabolism remains to be delineated.[9,15] Certainly, its elevated output in thyroid medullary carcinoma has not been associated with detectable bone disease.[63a]

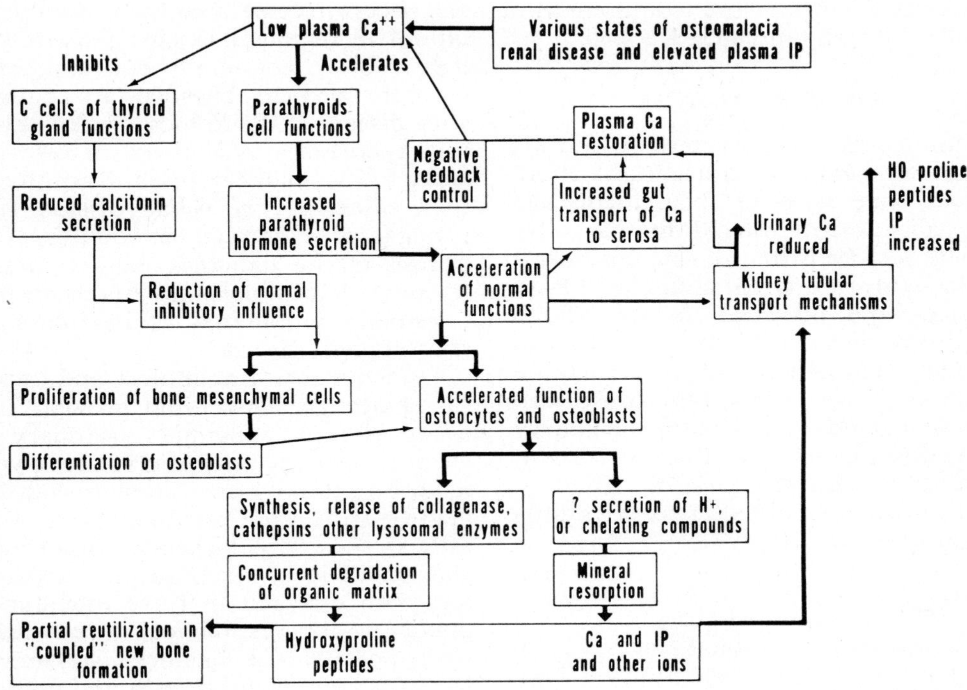

FIG. 62–2.—Diagram illustrating simplified concept of parathyroid function. Increased bone mobilization without elevated urinary phosphorus output occurs in secondary hyperparathyroidism with the negative balance from increased fecal excretion.

Vitamin D profoundly affects bone metabolism. It accelerates net absorption of Ca from the gastrointestinal tract, elevates IP excretion in the urine by decreasing renal tubular resorption and changes metabolism within osteoid cells in a manner to support bone mobilization.[3] Whether vitamin D is absolutely critical to the function of parathyroid hormone or only synergism with it exists remains controversial.[3,18]

Considerable recent progress in understanding of vitamin D metabolism has been made.[3] In man, vitamin D is partly converted to metabolites; one active metabolite (from porcine serum) is 25-hydroxycholecalciferol. Such a metabolite is believed to have a major functional role in delivery of specific vitamin D action on target organs. Derangement in fate of vitamin D and its metabolites has recently been discovered in certain disorders of calcium and bone metabolisms reviewed elsewhere in detail.[3] Thyroid hormone tends to influence skeletal remodeling as a part of a general influence on cellular metabolism without a specific regulatory action on bone. In hyperthyroidism, there is increased efflux Ca from bone secondary to accelerated bone remodeling.[37] Androgens and estrogens both have an anabolic effect on production of osteoid matrix[29] as well as decreased bone resorption. Growth hormone stimulates basal energy metabolism of osteoid cells and increases membranous bone formation as well as enchondral growth—the latter process has been adapted for the assay of this hormone. Adrenocortical oxysteroids divert amino acids from protein synthesis to glucogenesis and retard protein matrix formation. For brevity, such statements oversimplify the action of these hormones on bone and comprehensive treatises are recommended.[3,15,18,25,29,30]

OSTEOMALACIA

This disorder is characterized by widespread weakening and structural alteration of bone resulting from inadequate mineralization of osteoid matrix. The clinical picture is that of osteomalacia in adults and rickets in children. Early Romans and observers in the Middle Ages were aware of rickets, but Glisson, in 1668, provided the first scholarly description.[21] Recognition that the disease may be caused by a vitamin deficiency, the vitamin D activity of ergosterol after irradiation, and the curative effects of cod liver oil highlighted discoveries of the period from 1917 to 1922.[44,47,54]

Etiology

Classification of osteomalacia (Table 62–1) indicates the diversity of etiology. Deficiency of dietary vitamin D has become a rarity in the United States but still occurs in some undernourished populations in regions lacking adequate sunlight. More commonly encountered in modern medical practice are patients with disease of the kidney or malabsorption syndromes as a cause of osteomalacia. The malabsorption syndrome in such cases may be celiac disease, nontropical sprue, chronic pancreatitis, cystic fibrosis of the pancreas, biliary atresia, regional ileitis, intestinal lipodystrophy, intestinal lymphomas, tuberculosis or chronic liver disease.

Table 62–1.—Etiology of Osteomalacia

A. Inadequate calcium (and, rarely, phosphorus)
   1. Diet lack alone
   2. Relative dietary insufficiency during
      a. Rapid bone growth
      b. Pregnancy
      c. Hyperthyroidism
      d. Malabsorption

B. Inadequate vitamin D
   1. Absolute
      a. Dietary deficiency
      b. Malabsorption
   2. Relative
      a. Hyperthyroidism and rapid bone growth
      b. Vitamin D-resistant rickets or osteomalacia
         1. Congenital (renal tubular defects)
            a. Phosphate diabetes
            b. Fanconi-type syndromes
         2. Acquired
            a. Azotemic osteodystrophy
            b. Acquired Fanconi syndrome (*e.g.*, Wilson's disease or ingestion of degraded tetracyclines)[10]

Osteomalacia (in adults) and rickets (in children during rapid growth) may occur during azotemia secondary to chronic glomerulonephritis or pyelonephritis, usually associated to variable degrees with renal osteitis fibrosa. Vitamin D resistance hitherto considered a characteristic of the Fanconi syndrome has been detected in these much more prevalent diseases; clinical improvement with positive Ca balance, accelerated Ca absorption from the gut, and reduced renal Ca excretion has followed treatment with massive doses of vitamin D.[60]

Chronic excessive Ca loss in the urine associated with certain nonazotemic renal diseases may lead to osteomalacia. Thus, a primary tubular defect, renal tubular acidosis, results in chronic hypercalciuria, as well as natriuresis and kaliuresis.[1] Cations are lost in large amounts due to renal tubular defect in the acidification mechanism. Secondly, the Fanconi syndrome and variants which cause osteomalacia are characterized by abnormal renal loss of amino acids, phosphates and glucose. Hydrogen ion secretion fails to keep pace and the deficit is paid by a chronic loss of cations, including Ca. Vitamin D resistance is also present.[60]

Thirdly, there is a discrete phosphaturic renal tubular defect, and a fourth disorder, idiopathic hypercalciuria, appears to manifest a lowered renal threshold for Ca excretion.[1] If Ca intake is inadequate, osteomalacia may develop during the additional stress of hyperthyroidism, periods of rapid bone growth and pregnancy.

For the most part, patients with azotemia do not have hypercalciuria and their disorder of Ca metabolism results primarily from vitamin D resistance, possibly due to accelerated degradation of vitamin D metabolites.[3]

Pathophysiology

New methodologies of fundamental biochemical examinations of mineralization processes have brought forth several alternative biochemical models to explain why vitamin D lack might directly or indirectly lead to osteomalacia. For the present purposes, the bone cells in osteomalacia synthesize adequate amounts of osteoid matrix but the lymph is undersupplied with Ca and IP ions and local cellular mechanisms for mineral deposition become deranged. The same progression of clinical bone findings results regardless of the diverse etiologies just mentioned. Gradations of the syndrome in adults are conveniently described by Albright[1] as follows: (1) chemical osteomalacia manifested by reduced serum Ca and/or IP with normal serum alkaline phosphatase and no detectable bone demineralization; (2) chemical osteomalacia with high serum alkaline phosphatase and no bone disease; (3) chemical osteomalacia, elevated serum alkaline phosphatase and pseudofractures (Milkman's syndrome) described below, and (4) advanced osteomalacia, characterized by increased serum alkaline phosphatase, pseudofractures or pathologic fractures, and demineralization of bone detectable on x ray[1] (Fig. 62–3). Pseudofractures (Looser lines) probably represent small fractures at stress points which fill in with uncalcified matrix (Fig. 62–4). These pseudofractures, when bilateral in a symmetrical distribution, have been considered pathognomonic of osteomalacia. Demineralization of the spine in osteomalacia, as well as in osteoporosis and hyperparathyroidism, may produce three types of pathologic lesions observed in roentgenograms as follows: (1) "Codfish" deformities—the softened vertebrae show concave juxtaposing surfaces caused by the pressure of intervertebral discs. Their shape resembles that of codfish vertebrae. (2) Schmorl's nodes—disc material may herniate at a weak point through the surface of the vertebral body—radiologically visible as a small excrescence when calcified. (3) Compression fractures with or without wedging deformation.

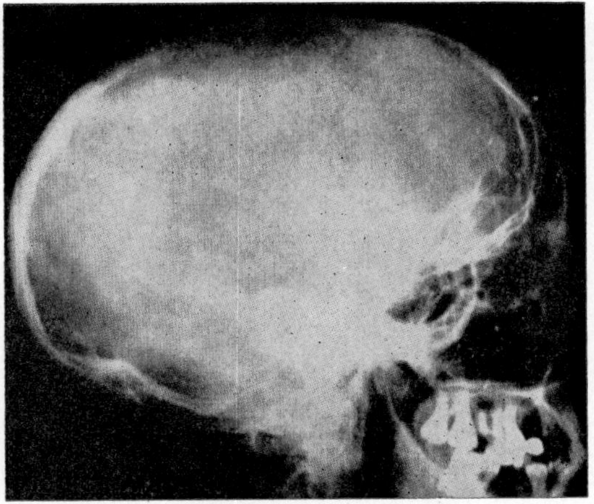

FIG. 62–3.—Osteomalacia due to renal acidosis (tubular insufficiency without glomerular insufficiency). The large decalcified area in the top of the skull resembles osteoporosis circumscripta of Paget's disease. (Stein, Stein and Beller, *Living Bone in Health and Disease*, courtesy J. B. Lippincott Co.)

Clinical Description

Initial symptoms are commonly pain and tenderness over the bones—particularly the back, hips, legs, thighs, and, less often, the ribs. Pain is usually increased by rising from a supine, sitting or kneeling position and aggravated by motion. The gait becomes awkward, hesitant and simulates a duck waddle. As a result of decreased serum ionized Ca levels there may develop increased muscle irritability, positive Chvostek's or Trousseau's signs, electrocardiographic evidence of hypocalcemia and spontaneous tetany. Radicular pain is a consequence

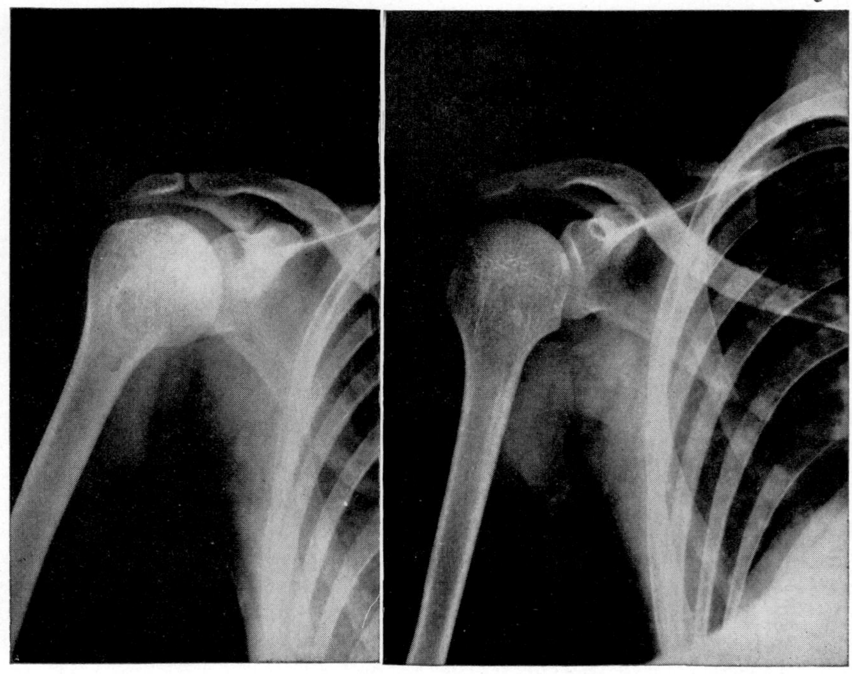

Fig. 62–4.—Osteomalacia resulting from renal acidosis (tubular without glomerular insufficiency). Note pseudofracture at the base of the acromion process. Note: before (left) and after (right) treatment with a calcifying regimen. (Stein, Stein and Beller, *Living Bone in Health and Disease,* courtesy J. B. Lippincott Co.)

of compression fractures of the vertebrae. Favorite sites of symmetrical pseudofractures are the lateral margins of the scapula, ribs, necks of the femora and rami of the pubic ischial bones (Fig. 62–4). Pathologic fractures occur, particularly of the femoral neck.

If there is a defect in gastrointestinal absorption, there will be evidence of steatorrhea, diarrhea, as well as disease-produced absorption deficiencies. Studies such as stool fat determination, triolein and oleic acid absorption and xylose tolerance tests are worthwhile to exclude a malabsorption syndrome.[13] The syndrome of renal tubular acidosis is characterized by polyuria, polydipsia, urine of low fixed specific gravity, elevated serum chloride and variable depression of sodium, potassium and bicarbonate[1] with inability to acidify the urine. These electrolytic disturbances may be accentuated for diagnostic purposes by an ammonium chloride tolerance test.[14,70] The urine of a patient on a low Ca diet should be tested also for amino acids, phosphate, glucose and Ca to exclude discrete phosphaturic as well as metabolic abnormalities of the Fanconi type. Nephrocalcinosis and nephrolithiasis frequently are present in any of the renal disorders, manifesting chronic infection or hypercalciuria except for the Fanconi syndrome.

As mentioned above, a component of vitamin D resistance should be suspected in most cases of renal azotemic osteodystrophy with evidence of osteomalacia and a cautious trial of calciferol is recommended. The dose is increased in a stepwise manner until an effect is obtained.[60]

Differential Diagnosis

Features distinguishing osteomalacia from other metabolic bone diseases are portrayed in Table 62–2. It should be noted that in primary hyperparathyroidism and osteitis fibrosa cystica generalisata, serum Ca is high rather than low. Presence of renal insufficiency with high NPN, elevated serum IP, low serum Ca, and bone cysts indicates secondary hyperparathyroidism and renal osteitis fibrosa cystica generalisata. As opposed to osteomalacia, findings of osteoporosis include normal serum Ca, IP and alkaline phosphatase; whereas the generalized bone demineralization is similar, the skull remains unaltered in osteoporosis. Paget's disease exhibits a normal serum Ca and IP, but alkaline phosphatase is elevated. In polyostotic fibrous dysplasia, bone cysts are present but Ca and IP levels remain normal; alkaline phosphatase may be moderately elevated.

Treatment

Vitamin D (calciferol), 50,000 units orally, daily, together with Ca lactate or gluconate, 5 to 10 gm. 3 times daily, should be given until the bones have healed by x-ray examination. If there is overt or incipient tetany, it is helpful to prescribe, 3 times daily after meals, Ca gluconate, 10 ml. of a 30 per cent solution, diluted in water. In vitamin D-resistant rickets, 500,000 to 1,000,000 units of vitamin D, daily, may be needed to obviate the defect. *Urinary tract lithiasis may be precipitated in secondary hyperparathyroidism by vitamin D treatment unless the dosage is cautiously regulated.* In the presence of a malabsorption syndrome, additional therapy should include vitamin B_{12}, folic acid, or crude liver extract and a low-fat, high-protein diet, together with the fat-soluble vitamins. For patients with osteomalacia due to excessive renal Ca excretion there should be cautious replacement of Ca and measures to control the acidosis. A solution containing 140 gm. citric acid, 75 gm. sodium citrate and 25 gm. potassium citrate in 1 liter of water is sometimes used. Thirty ml. of this mixture are administered orally, 5 times daily. Effect of treatment in patients with renal disease should be carefully watched until the electrolytic disturbances reach optimal control. Severity of renal disease determines prognosis in such cases. In the presence of adult phosphate diabetes administration of neutral sodium phosphate has also been recommended.[50] Management of osteomalacia, as outlined above, usually produces spectacular improvement of the bone disorder, with bone pains, tetany and pseudofractures disappearing in a short time. Serum alkaline phosphatase levels return to normal within two to six months together with x-ray evidence of bone healing.

BONE DISTURBANCE OF HYPERPARATHYROIDISM
(Osteitis Fibrosa Cystica Generalisata)

Primary and secondary hyperparathyroidism cause identical bone disease, characterized by accelerated catabolism of both hydroxyapatite and osteoid matrix with resultant cysts and giant cell tumors. Von Recklinghausen is credited with the first detailed report of this disease in 1891.[65] Thirteen years later Askanazy[2] suggested an association of the bone pathology with parathyroid adenomas, and in 1926, Mandl demonstrated the curative effect of removing a parathyroid adenoma.[40]

Etiology and Pathophysiology

Metabolic disturbances from an excess of this hormone are caused in most instances of the *primary* type by a chief cell adenoma of a single parathyroid gland, but rarely there may be multiple adenomas. *Primary* hyperplasia of all glands or carcinoma may also occur. *Secondary* hyperparathyroidism is associated with hyperplasia of multiple parathyroid glands and results from stimulation by a depressed serum ionized Ca. The underlying disease is usually chronic nephritis or chronic pyelonephritis with renal

TABLE 62–2.—METABOLIC BONE DISEASES

Disease	*Etiology*	*Histology*	*Ca*	*P*	*Alkaline Phosphatase*
Osteomalacia	Defect in supply of vitamin D and/or Ca and P. Also resistance to vitamin D.	Widened (uncalcified) osteoid seams	Normal or low	Low	Increased
Rickets	Same as osteomalacia but in children	Metaphyseal osteoid matrix increased	Normal or low	Low	Increased
Primary hyperparathyroidism	Adenoma of parathyroid or primary hyperplasia	Excessive bone destruction, cysts, giant cell tumors	High	Low	Increased
Secondary hyperparathyroidism	Kidney disease Malabsorption	Same as primary type	Normal or variably low	High—renal disease. Normal or low—malabsorption syndrome	Increased
Postmenopausal and senile osteoporosis	Unknown—(*see* text)	Decreased bone mass (*see* text)	Normal	Normal	Normal
Osteitis deformans (Paget's disease)	Unknown	Widened, patternless trabeculae; increased bone formation and destruction	Normal (may rise with immobilization)	Normal	Increased
Fibrous dysplasia	Unknown	Same as hyperparathyroidism except for areas of normal bone	Normal	Normal	Normal or moderately increased

TABLE 62–2.—METABOLIC BONE DISEASES (*Continued*)

NPN	*Other Findings*	*X-ray Findings*	*Clinical*
Normal or High (*see* text)	Usually negative balance of Ca and P	Pseudofractures, pathologic fractures, radiolucent bones	Generalized bone pain and tenderness. Localized pain at fracture sites. Signs of associated diseases, particularly of gastrointestinal tract or kidneys
Normal	Negative balance of Ca and P	Cupping of metaphyses Increased size of epiphyseal plates	Dwarfism, deformities, rachitic rosary, bowing of long bones, Harrison's groove, craniotabes; otherwise same as osteomalacia
Normal	Elevated urine output of Ca and P	Deformities, pathologic fractures, bone cysts, osteoclasts. Ground-glass texture of skull	Diffuse bone pains; localized back pain. Symptoms related to hypercalcemia, nephrolithiasis and nephrocalcinosis
Increased	High fecal, low urinary Ca, and P, but in balance	Same as in primary hyperparathyroidism	Acidosis; signs of chronic nephritis or pyelonephritis. In children—"renal rickets" and dwarfism
Normal	Hypercalciuria during immobilization	Decreased bone density, codfish deformities Schmorl's nodes, compression fractures of vertebrae	More common in women. Often asymptomatic. Back pain is localized, segmental or sciatic distribution
Normal	Nephrolithiasis nephrocalcinosis sarcomas	Coarse trabeculations enlargement, bowing, microfractures, transverse pathologic fractures	Pain at fracture sites. Immobilization leads to Ca and P loss with stone formation in kidneys
Normal	No other biochemical abnormalities detected	Often unilateral involvement. Bone cysts. Shepherd's crook deformity	Deformities and pathologic fractures. Cafe-au-lait spots and precocious menstruation indicate Albright's syndrome

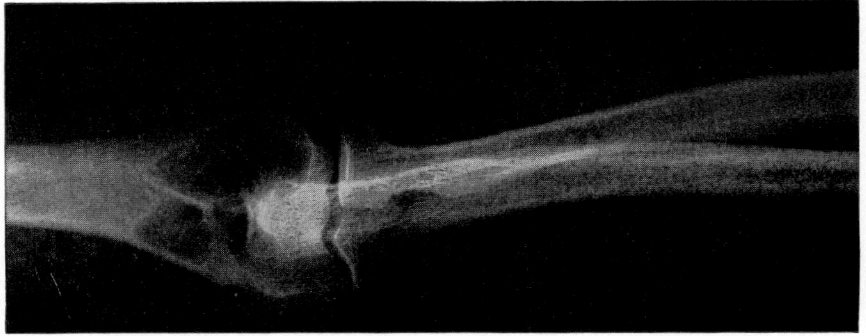

Fig. 62–5.—Primary hyperparathyroidism. Note: (1) cyst-like osteoclastoma in distal humerus, (2) medullary widening, coarsened trabeculations and thinned cortices of radius and ulna. (Stein, Stein and Beller, *Living Bone in Health and Disease*, courtesy J. B. Lippincott Co.)

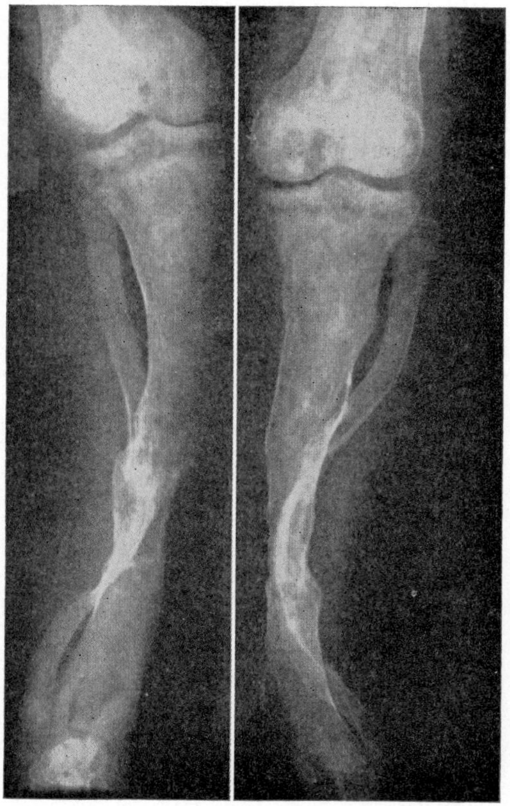

Fig. 62–6.—Renal osteitis fibrosa cystica generalisata and secondary hyperparathyroidism. General osteoclasis has resulted in the marked radiolucency and deformity with cyst formation of tibiae and fibulae. (Stein, Stein and Beller, *Living Bone in Health and Disease*, courtesy J. B. Lippincott Co.)

failure. Elevation of the serum IP (usually) and blood urea nitrogen, and moderate to severe acidosis with a low bicarbonate are found. Failure of renal excretion of IP and consequent IP retention lead to depression of plasma Ca and feedback stimulation of the parathyroids. Acquired vitamin D resistance also leads to depressed plasma Ca. Increased secretion of parathyroid hormone, thus induced, accelerates mobilization of bone Ca, increases plasma Ca and promotes hypercalciuria except in azotemic patients. Evidence of secondary hyperparathyroidism may also occur in osteomalacia with variable restoration of serum Ca to normal levels and simultaneous depression of IP. Why *hyperthyroidism* should at times be linked with this bone disturbance is unknown.

Pathologically, the bones reveal cysts and "brown tumors" which contain masses of osteoid cells (also termed osteoclastomas or osteoblastomas). They appear notably in the jaws, metacarpals, metatarsals and ends of the long bones (Figs. 62–5 and 62–6).

Clinical Description

Many patients with this disease manifest no symptoms or signs of bone disorder probably because the intake of Ca and phosphorus in the average American diet is high and keeps the influx apace with the accelerated loss. Anorexia, constipation, "indigestion," nausea, vomiting, polydipsia, polyuria, weakness, band keratopathy, psychosis, coma and evidence of nephrolithiasis or progressive renal failure may be noted. In such cases, serum alkaline phosphatase often is normal and the use of a standard low Ca diet and tests of renal phosphate reabsorption should be useful to establish the diagnosis. With a few exceptions, the cortisone suppression test of Dent has proved to be a worthwhile diagnostic measure.[12]

In patients whose dietary intake of Ca and phosphorus is average or low, rheumatic symptoms are often the primary complaint. Diffuse pains in the extremities, together with bone tenderness, are mistaken for signs of arthritis or neuritis. Back pain is frequent and often aggravated by sneezing or coughing. As bone loss exceeds bone formation, alkaline phosphatase becomes elevated possibly as a response of osteoid cells to increased stresses and strains. Compression fractures, "codfish deformity," Schmorl's nodes, kyphosis, pigeon breast deformities, bending of the long bones and bone cysts appear. Teeth may fall out due to marked softening of the jaw bones. Estimation of the severity of disease is obtained by a radiologic survey which may reveal single or multiple cysts, subperiosteal bone resorption, jagged, feathery appearance, particularly of the phalanges, mottled "ground glass" texture of the skull, metastatic calcification, nephrocalcinosis and nephrolithiasis. Rarely, giant cell tumors have been demonstrated in the mediastinum. Additional abnormalities found in this disease include slipping, tilting and fragmentation of epiphyses, particularly the femoral heads. Chronic epiphyseal involvement at the knee joint leads to genu valgum. Chondrocalcinosis and joint degeneration have been reported.[8]

Differential Diagnosis

The characteristic features of primary hyperparathyroidism are elevated serum Ca and alkaline phosphatase with depressed serum IP, whereas in osteomalacia Ca and/or IP is low and in osteoporosis Ca, IP and alkaline phosphatase usually are normal. In contrast to osteomalacia or osteoporosis, there are large bone cysts and subperiosteal bone resorption. Also, in contrast to osteoporosis, there is resorption of lamina dura and frequently skull involvement. In fibrous dysplasia of bone, lesions tend to be unilateral;[1] there is no expansion of the cortical bone by cysts, and lamina dura is normal. In addition, biopsy specimens of bone will show some areas of normal architecture on histologic section.[1] The presence of a high serum Ca and protein should suggest the possibility of metastatic malignancy, multiple myeloma or sarcoidosis. In this regard, the elevation of the prostatic fraction of acid phosphatase in carcinoma of the prostate and distinctive rapid response of hypercalcemia of sarcoidosis to cortisone administration provide useful diagnostic aids.

Treatment

Surgical removal of the parathyroid tumor is followed by rapid bone healing. Postoperatively, vigorous measures including intravenous Ca—10 to 30 ml. of 10 per cent Ca gluconate or lactate, 6 times daily—and vitamin D by mouth may be required to combat tetany. This distressing event is more severe in patients who have shown marked bone disease. *Awareness that hypomagnesemia may be the cause of tetany under these circumstances is important, particularly if response to calcium infusions is unsatisfactory.* In regard to secondary hyperparathyroidism, the most essential aspect of treatment relates to management of the underlying kidney disease, for upon its course the prognosis depends. Attempts to restore serum bicarbonate toward normal levels by the use of intravenous or oral alkalinizing agents are performed cautiously, but tetany, resulting from further depression of ionized Ca when the total level is already low, is a complication more often dreaded than encountered. Some authorities advocate a regimen which might be used on a daily basis as follows: calciferol, 50,000 units; sodium citrate, 2 to 3 gm. in 4 doses; Ca gluconate, 5 gm., for 3 doses. Although bone healing occurs on this regimen, concurrent acceleration of nephrolithiasis and nephrocalcinosis is a constant hazard. Further details of renal and electrolytic treatment are beyond the scope of this discussion.[1,60]

HYPOPARATHYROIDISM

There is (1) decrease or absence of parathyroid hormone secretion, (2) subsequent decrease of urinary phosphate excretion, and (3) rise of serum IP and fall of serum Ca. The disease is rare and most instances reported are due to inadvertent removal of parathyroid glands at thyroid surgery. Except for abnormal radio-density of bones in some instances, skeletal findings are minimal and correction of the serum manifestations is the major consideration.

In terms of differential diagnosis, pseudohypoparathyroidism is a rare disorder resembling idiopathic hypoparathyroidism with abnormally early epiphyseal union; consequent bone shortening involves usually metacarpals and metatarsals, roundness of face, shortness of stature and metaplastic islands of bone in connective tissues and skin. There are hypocalcemia and resistance to the hypercalcemic effect of daily intramuscular injections of parathyroid extract over several weeks. There are usually hyperphosphatemia, basal ganglia calcifications and history of tetany or convulsions.[41] Also, recently assays of plasma have revealed remarkable elevations of calcitonin concentrations in this disease. Pseudopseudohypoparathyroidism refers to an extremely rare disease involving a genetic defect similar to pseudohypoparathyroidism manifesting similar clinical and x-ray features but displaying no hypocalcemia or failure of tissue responsiveness to parathyroid hormone.[1]

OSTEOPOROSIS

This is by far the commonest metabolic bone disorder encountered in medical practice. In certain population samples, 1 of 4 females and 1 of 5 to 6 males over age seventy were afflicted.[64] Approximately four-fifths of patients with osteoporosis, in a recent careful study, were of the senile or postmenopausal type and the remainder were linked with a variety of diseases.[64] The term *osteoporosis* means increased porosity of bone and is employed to identify diffuse as opposed to localized bone atrophy. A characteristic feature is that the weight of whole dry bone per unit volume is reduced. Inasmuch as the "physiologic" atrophy of aging (or age-related bone loss) exhibits this as well as almost every other hallmark of osteoporosis, but to lesser degrees, it is currently almost impossible to divide the aforementioned physiologic state from osteoporosis. In this regard, recent investigations indicate that maximum bone mass is attained between age 20 and 35. This peak level of total bone mass is greater in men than in women, greater in blacks than in Caucasians, and greater in normal than in malnourished or hypogonadal subjects. Between age 35 and 75 years decrements of mineral mass occur annually with a cumulative 50 per cent loss in vertebral bodies and 20 to 30 per cent loss in several long bones. The extreme lower range of "normal" bone mass during late aging fits all the characteristics of osteoporosis. These extreme low values of mineral mass may result theoretically either from failure to attain adequate mineral mass in the third decade or from an accelerated attrition of mineral from a normal peak level of mineral mass. In addition, several factors can produce pathological accentuation of mineral loss. The diagnosis of osteoporosis becomes obvious in the presence of "bone failure" indicated by clear-cut objective changes detected radiologically (*e.g.* vertebral compression fractures, codfish deformities, etc.). Osteoporosis is readily distinguishable histologically from osteomalacia and osteitis fibrosa.

Etiology and Pathophysiology

Whether the various factors indicated in Table 62–3 are capable alone of causing osteoporosis or whether a genetically controlled predisposition is required remains unknown.[64] A very low incidence of osteoporosis in blacks, regardless of activity and diet, suggests strong genetic factors. That a chronic insufficiency of Ca intake or low net intestinal absorption effectively produces osteoporosis in animals and an influence in man has been suggested.[52] Signs of osteoporosis appear in relation to the postmenopausal state and in the presence of certain endocrine diseases wherein estrogen secretion is reduced. Lack of androgenic steroids may play a role in the osteoporosis of eunuchoid males and probably of senile patients. Cushing's syndrome and chronic iatrogenic hyperadrenocorticism share a high prevalence rate of osteoporosis, resulting from the effects on bone cells of adrenocortical oxysteroids. Also, metabolism of the bone matrix is altered with the appearance of osteoporosis in the presence of other endocrine disturbances including hyperthyroidism and acromegaly, as well as in association with malnutrition, scurvy and various chronic wasting diseases, such as rheumatoid arthritis or malignant tumors. The effects of the disease-provoking factors, above, become superimposed on the age-related bone loss to produce the observed clinical state. *Thus, postmenopausal women with rheumatoid arthritis under long-term corticosteroid treatment seem especially prone to develop osteoporosis.*[32]

Other causes of osteoporosis are prolonged immobilization, physical agents and hereditary defects. As for the first, stresses and strains normally stimulating osteoblastic activity are lacking, with the

Table 62-3.—Etiology of Osteoporosis

A. Hormonal lack*
   1. Postmenopausal, natural or induced (estrogens)
   2. Congenital ovarian agenesis (estrogens)
   3. Eunuchoidism (androgens)
   4. Senility (androgens)
   5. Diabetes mellitus (insulin)

B. Hormonal excess*
   1. Hyperthyroidism (thyroid hormone)
   2. Acromegaly (growth hormone)
   3. Cushing's syndrome or iatrogenic hyperadrenalism (adrenocortical oxysteroids)

C. Nutritional lack
   1. Inadequate diet
   2. Chronic wasting diseases, *e.g.*, malignant tumors and collagen diseases

D. Physical agents and poisons
   1. X-ray treatment—excessive
   2. Overdosage with ultrasonic waves
   3. Metal poisoning

E. Disuse (absence of stresses and strains)
   1. Paralysis
   2. Chronic wasting diseases
   3. Immobilization in casts

* The alterations of hormonal effect are undoubtedly only partly the cause of osteoporosis in these circumstances; other contributing factors are unknown.

second (*e.g.*, x-ray irradiation or ultrasound) there is injury to osteoid cells and in the last (*e.g.*, osteogenesis imperfecta) genetic factors undoubtedly are important.[61] Chronic administration of heparin was shown to cause osteoporosis,[23] and the altered environment of space flight was associated with acute calcium loss.[39]

Histologic sections of bone from patients with clinical evidence of osteoporosis in comparison to normal controls over age sixty-five have shown: (1) enlarged vascular channels and porosity with diminished number and width of trabeculae; (2) increased number of osteones less than three-fourths closed, with development of sclerotic inner margins,[36] (3) increased osteocytolysis, (4) increased number of osteocyte lacunae filled with mineral salts and (5) increased surface occupied by resorption.[17,36] Remaining bone trabeculae and compact bone show a normal or higher than normal proportion fully mineralized. In postmenopausal and senile osteoporosis, kinetic studies reveal total skeletal accretion, Ca turnover, and return of Ca from the skeleton to be increased and bone formation surfaces increased to a lesser extent. Cellular activity in some of these bone-forming sites is reduced.[25] A possible role of growth hormone lack in postmenopausal osteoporosis has been postulated[25] as well as possible increased end-organ sensitivity to parathyroid hormone, with conditioning through loss of estrogen at the menopause and decreased physical activity.[25] In the local osteoporosis adjacent to joints afflicted with rheumatoid arthritis accelerated bone turnover was found.[28]

Clinical Description

Although osteoporosis is a generalized bone disorder, it is more severe in the pelvis and spine than in the remainder of the skeleton. The commonest symptom is back pain with segmental radiation in the distribution of the affected nerve rootlets. Cord compression is uncommon. Decrease of body height, upper dorsal kyphosis and symmetrical skin folds along the base of the thoracic cage are usually found.[64] Fractures may develop either spontaneously or from minor trauma and occur more frequently than bending of the bones, observed in osteomalacia. A fracture of the femoral neck is, in many cases, the first incident to call attention to the diagnosis of osteoporosis.[6] By x ray, wedging and collapse of the vertebra, codfish deformities, Schmorl's nodes and generalized demineralization are the predominant lesions in the spine (Fig. 62–7). Newer radiologic techniques with densitometric reading systems add sensitivity and objectivity for long-term research comparisons[34] but aid little the clinician faced with an early case of osteoporosis. One investigator used the following criteria for defining

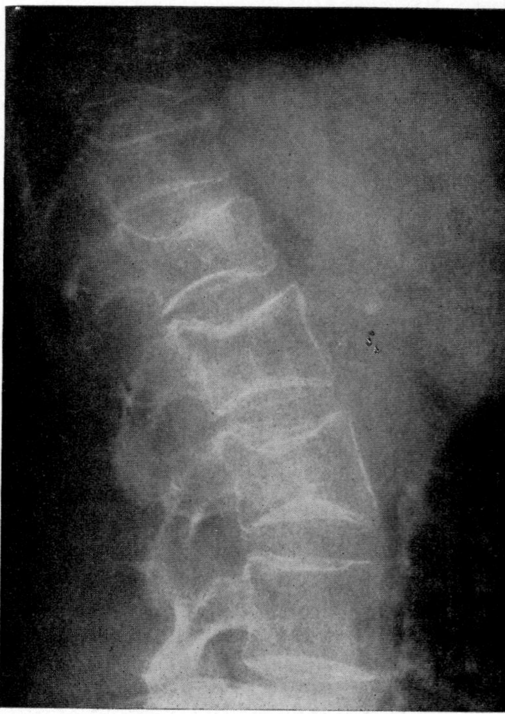

Fig. 62–7.—Roentgenogram showing advanced postmenopausal osteoporosis. Note the biconcavity of the vertebral bodies due to pressure of the intervertebral discs (so-called "codfish vertebrae") and compression fracture of the body of T 11.

the presence of osteoporosis radiologically in his studies: (1) when the ratio of the vertical height of the best centered lumbar vertebra at its narrowest point to the vertical height of the same vertebra at its anterior margin was less than 0.81 in a lateral view; (2) when the width of the cortex to total diameter at the thickest point of the femur and of the second metacarpal bone was less than 0.5 in a PA view and (3) mixed findings with both (1) and (2) indicating both peripheral and central osteoporosis.[52]

Limbs placed in casts for several weeks may develop cystic erosions (*e.g.*, tarsal bones), resembling early stages of rheumatoid arthritis (Fig. 62–8). Chronic immobilization leads to negative balance of Ca, nitrogen and phosphorus.[11] Renal stones are engendered by the hypercalciuria. In a typical patient with chronic osteoporosis, serum Ca, IP and alkaline phosphatase levels usually are within normal range; however, in rapidly developing osteoporosis, hypercalcemia may occur. Calcification of the abdominal aorta has been reported as common.[64] Serum protein concentrations will reflect the changes typical of the associated disease but in relation to the osteoporosis are either normal or slightly low. Multiple myeloma, most common in middle-aged or elderly men, often mimics osteoporosis by displaying diffuse demineralization of the ribs and spine with or without compression fractures. The classical picture of punched-out areas in the bones may be absent, and cases of several years' duration have been reported. However, there is likely to be severe bone pain and anemia. Bone marrow aspiration, serum protein electrophoresis and tests of the urine for Bence Jones protein should be performed in all doubtful cases.

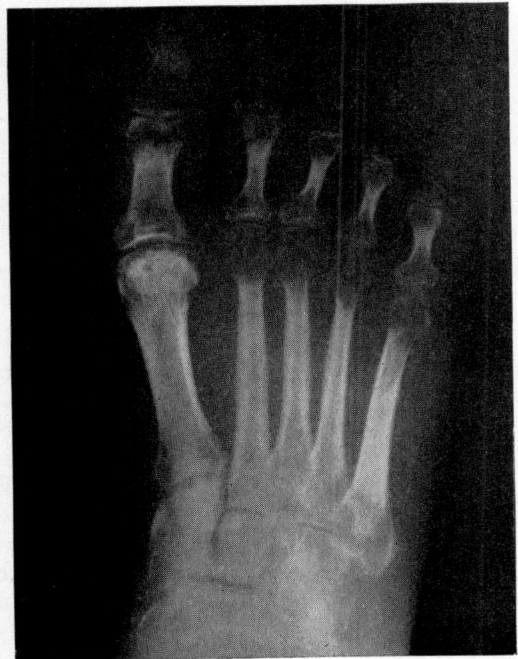

Fig. 62–8.—Osteoporosis of disuse in a sixty-year-old man. Immobilization in a cast for three months resulted in this appearance.

Treatment

The long-term goal of treatment is to arrest progression of the disease and alleviate symptoms. Except in rare instances of Cushing's syndrome, there is no satisfactory evidence that any of the treatments listed below even partially restores osteoporotic bone toward a normal state.* Also, some degree of spontaneous remission in symptoms complicates evaluation of short-term treatments, and production of a positive Ca balance alone does not prove the site of new mineral deposition, which might be extra-osseous. Nevertheless, considerable suggestive evidence of effectiveness warrants, in my own opinion, the combined use of: (1) analgesics and bracing; (2) exercises;[58,64] (3) a modestly supplemented calcium-phosphate-vitamin D intake and (4), in most cases, gonadal hormones.[25]

Specific Measures.—Pain relief often is the most immediate problem and re-

* Sodium fluoride treatment, at levels of 60 mg. per day, or calcitonin appears to influence osteoporosis favorably, but general recommendation of these treatments is withheld pending long-term evaluation.

quires proper analgesics, as well as a well-fitted Taylor-Knight brace or lumbosacral belt (*see* Chapter 82). Periods of bracing should be short to prevent muscle weakness. Intractable radicular pain may require appropriate paravertebral blocks with local anesthetics. Other aspects of management include diet, hormones and exercise. The diet should be moderate to high in protein content at a caloric level geared for weight reduction in the obese patient. Ca diphosphate, 0.5 gm. tablets sufficient to provide at least 1.6 gm. per day of Ca, along with 1,000 units of vitamin D is recommended. Maintenance of a large urine output during periods of immobilization minimizes a tendency to renal calcifications.

Androgenic and estrogenic steroids cause, under appropriate circumstances, a positive balance of nitrogen, Ca and phosphorus.[29,38] Administration is facilitated by the use of an agent such as Deladumone, containing testosterone enanthate and estradiol valerate. From a single intramuscular injection, adequate hormone levels are provided for approximately one month. Daily oral medications and shorter-acting combinations are less readily administered. Weak salt-retaining activity of estrogen causes occasional patients to develop edema, particularly if there is underlying heart disease. Oral diuretics may be used with caution in such situations. Within two weeks to a month of starting estrogen and androgen treatment for postmenopausal osteoporosis, improvement in bone pain usually occurs. This initial improvement regularly slackens within a few months. Nevertheless, long-term retardation of progression of osteoporosis occurs with postmenopausal or senile osteoporosis (arbitrarily over age sixty-five) and in patients with rheumatoid arthritis. In the light of current research results, properly administered gonadal hormones are probably warranted indefinitely in most patients.

Persistent efforts to encourage exercise are mandatory. Exercise against resistance is a stimulant to positive nitrogen and Ca balance,[58] and daily use of a stationary bicycle or swimming is recommended.[64] Patients should do specific exercises daily for strengthening back and abdominal musculature as well as for postural correction. In patients with osteoporosis, periods of immobilization for superimposed illness or fractures of the hip should be minimized. To combat osteoporosis of disuse, the postoperative period in patients with rheumatoid arthritis or other chronic inflammatory rheumatic states should include an exercise program with ambulation as soon as possible. Interestingly enough, fasting and hypoglycemia-induced levels of growth hormone which are reduced in postmenopausal women have been restored to normal or above by estrogen treatment.[16]

PAGET'S DISEASE OF BONE
(Osteitis Deformans)

Paget's disease is a chronic, widespread disturbance of the adult skeleton typified by softening, enlargement and bowing of the bones with a disarranged osseous architecture. Sir James Paget[53] described the disease in 1871 but it was frequently confused with the bone disorder of hyperparathyroidism until the latter was clarified by Mandl in 1926.[40]

Etiology and Pathophysiology

The cause of Paget's disease is unknown; information has accrued on metabolic and pathologic aspects. Histologically the trabeculae are thickened with osteoid seams developing in a disorganized, patternless manner. Both new bone formation and erosion are accelerated. There are well-demarcated areas with normal appearance—a feature which differentiates this disease from metabolic bone disturbances previously described.[1] Regions under the most stress show the greatest pathologic change. Schmorl reported (autopsy series) that bones involved in order of increasing frequency are the tibia, clavicle, left femur, pelvis, sternum, skull, right femur, spine and sacrum. Blood circulation is excessive at the site of lesions, probably due to multiple arteriovenous shunts, and as a result occasional patients develop high-output cardiac failure. Rate of Ca-45 exchange at the bone surfaces is enormously increased, as well as that of other bone-seeking radio-elements.[25] The high rate of bone turnover correlates with increased levels of plasma alkaline phosphatase, a level highest of all bone diseases per unit of bone.[49] The local acceleration of bone resorption is usually attended by concomitant accelerated bone formation, with reutilization of ions released from resorption sites. In regard to organic matrix, some of the hydroxyproline of the collagen removed at resorption sites is *not* reutilized and there is, therefore, consistently elevated urinary excretion of hydroxyproline peptides. In active Paget's disease[57] this latter parameter correlates well with bone turnover rates measured with Ca-45 and plasma alkaline phosphatase determinations. The disease may commence as an area of local destruction in the skull (osteoporosis circumscripta) preceding by years the osteoblastic changes indicative of full-blown disease.

Clinical Description

Most patients are over age forty, with men predominant, and frequently a positive family history is elicited. In a large number of patients, the disease is asymptomatic and is first discovered by the radiologist. The commonest complaint is pain, usually of a deep, aching type, often accentuated by weight-bearing. Headaches, dizziness and reduced hearing due to bony impingement on neural pathways and visual disturbances may occur. Severe increase of pain and further rise of alkaline phosphatase should suggest fracture. Incomplete fractures occur repeatedly with healing and apparently cause the deformities of bowing and elongation seen most often in the tibia and femur. With advanced disease, the skull enlarges at the calvarium; temporal arteries are engorged and tortuous; the head is held forward, chin resting on

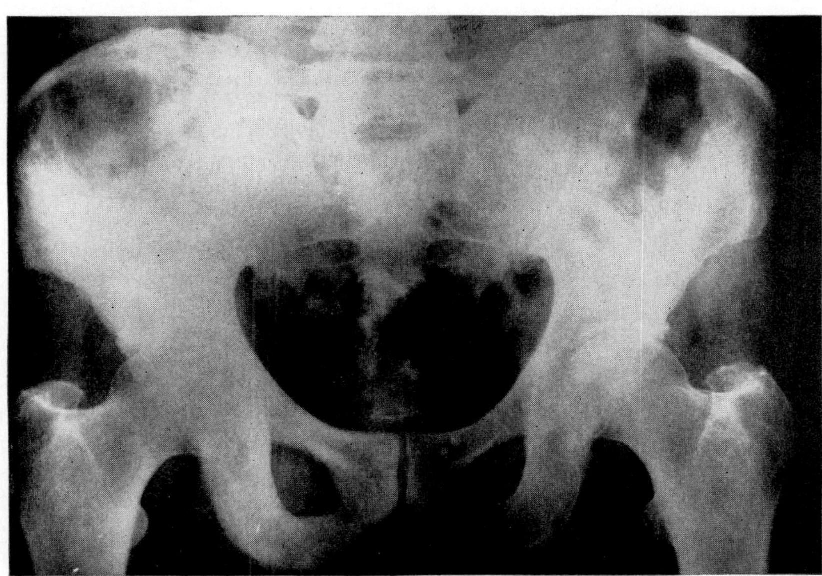

Fig. 62–9.—Paget's disease of right innominate bone. Note sclerosis, enlargement and coarsening of trabecular structure.

the sternal notch; clavicles become distorted and dorsal kyphosis develops; there is an accentuated V-shaped demarcation between chest and abdomen; the acetabulum may be thrust upward by the femoral head with tri-radiate deformity of the pelvic outlet; legs rotate outwardly, are curved and consist of massive bone; further deafness results from ossicle involvement and otosclerosis; teeth show thickening of the cementum, partial destruction of the roots and replacement of abnormal bone; and congestive heart failure may develop. Angioid streaks have been observed around the optic discs. Asymptomatic Paget's disease in one leg may lead to a painful osteoarthritis in the opposite limb. The radiologic appearance of osteitis deformans includes a mottled increase of bone density, coarse trabeculation, incomplete fractures and "tufts of cotton wool" in the skull, as well as deformities listed above (Figs. 62–9 and 62–10). Signs of arteriosclerosis appear at an earlier age than expected. The incidence of osteogenic sarcomas is increased beyond the age of forty, and may be associated with further increase of serum alkaline phosphatase.

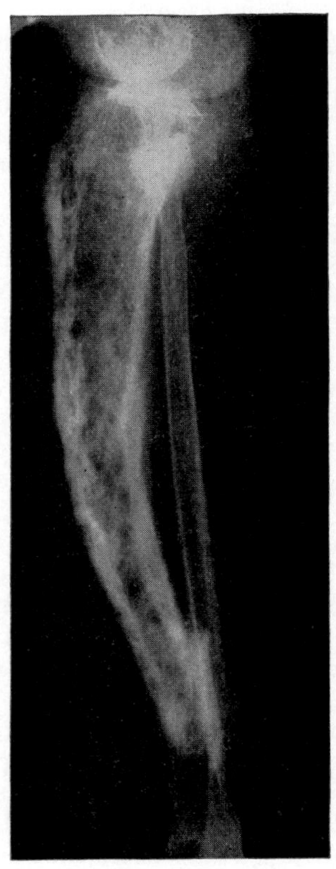

FIG. 62–10.—Paget's disease. Extensive disease of the right tibia with endosteal and periosteal proliferation with thickening and bowing of the diaphysis. There is a fracture in the lower third of the tibia and fibula.

Differential Diagnosis

The presence of normal serum Ca, IP, high alkaline phosphatase and characteristic radiologic features of Paget's disease differentiate it from the metabolic bone diseases previously discussed (Table 62–2). In the advanced stages, osteitis deformans should not be confused with any other bone disorder. Pelvic lesions may resemble those of metastatic carcinoma of the prostate, but an elevated serum *acid* phosphatase in the presence of a normal alkaline phosphatase helps label the latter condition. In fibrous dysplasia, serum alkaline phosphatase shows only moderate or no elevation, and pigmented skin lesions may be observed.

Treatment

There is no specific therapy for this disease and management is directed toward its complications. Sarcomas appear with increased frequency and should be handled early by surgery. Confinement to bed, as for treatment of fractures, reduces bone repair and leads to rapid mobilization of Ca. Hypercalcemia, hypercalciuria and renal stones result. A large fluid intake is advocated and in the presence of excessively elevated serum Ca, Fleets Phospho-soda, 4 cc. given t.i.d., is recommended. Some improvement of bone pain and reduction of disease activity have been reported from the use of acetylsalicylic acid, 3.6 to 4.8 gm. daily. Some improvement of bony symptoms and reduction of plasma alkaline phosphatase and urinary hydroxyproline have attended experimental administration of sodium fluoride, 120 mg. per day, to patients with Paget's disease.[4,59] Indomethacin, 25 mg. given t.i.d., is a helpful adjunctive measure to reduce pain, particularly with root joint involvement. When knees or other peripheral joints are affected, intra-articular corticosteroid injection produces local symptomatic relief, and may be repeated every few weeks as needed.[31]

Initial trials of *calcitonin* have appeared effective in controlling disease activity, but this agent must not be recommended yet for general usage. It has been reported that doses ranging from 6 to 200 units daily of calcitonin have been effective.[6a] Pain is often relieved, and plasma alkaline phosphatase and urinary hydroxyproline levels are apparently lowered,[23a,50a] and bone turnover is reduced.[5a]

Results of studies on patients with Paget's disease receiving *mithramycin*, a cytotoxic agent similar to actinomycin D, revealed remarkable improvement in symptoms and clinical signs of active disease concurrent with lowering of serum Ca, IP and urinary hydroxyproline excretion with a later fall of serum alkaline phosphatase. The drug is believed to act predominantly through reducing the functional activity of osteoclasts on bone resorption. The general usage of this drug is not recommended because of potential toxic effects on the liver, kidney and platelet formation in the bone marrow. Whether some exceptions to this view may be warranted in the event of severe symptomatic and rapidly advancing disease remains for further investigation.[59a,59b]

Another recent encouraging report of new agents in treatment of Paget's disease was concerned with the use of the *diphosphonates*. Disodium etidronate (EHDP) was administered in a daily oral dose of 20 mg. per kg. of body weight to 4 patients with active Paget's disease. Increased values of alkaline phosphatase in plasma and increased hydroxyproline in plasma and urine fell to half their initial values after 3 months' treatment, suggesting decrease in the excessive bone turnover.[59c] No toxic effects were reported, but it is much too early to assume that diphosphonates represent a practical advance in therapy of Paget's disease.[13a]

Although calcitonin, mithramycin and the diphosphonates are still strictly experimental drugs for treatment of Paget's disease and may not prove to be of practical value, it is indeed encouraging that, within a few years, *three* agents have been found which have a definite effect on the pathological process of the disorder.[13a]

BIBLIOGRAPHY

1. Albright, F. and Reifenstein, E. C., Jr.: *Parathyroid Glands and Bone Disease*. Baltimore, The William & Wilkins Co., 1948.
2. Askanazy, M.: Arb. A.D. Geb. D. path. Anat. Inst., zu Tubingen, *4*, 398, 1902–1904.
3. Avioli, L. V.: Chapter 11, in *The Fat Soluble Vitamins* (DeLuca, H. F. and Suttie, J. W., eds.), Madison, University of Wisconsin Press, 1970.
4. Avioli, L. and Berman, M.: J. Clin. Endocr., *28*, 700, 1968.
5. Barnicot, N. A.: J. Anat., *82*, 233, 1948.

5a. Baud, C. A., *et al.*: Schweiz. med. Wschr., *99*, 657, 1969.

6. Bauer, G.: Clin. Orthop., *17*, 219, 1960.

6a. Bijvoet, O. L. M., *et al.*: *Calcitonin 1969*. Proc. II Int. Symposium, London, 1970, p. 531.

7. Bonner, F., Harris, R. S., Maletskos, C. J., and Benda, C. A.: J. Clin. Invest., *35*, 78, 1956.
8. Bywaters, E. G. L., Dixon, A. St. J., and Scott, J. T.: Ann. Rheum. Dis., *22*, 171, 1963.
9. Care, J. D.: J. Clin. Endocr., *25*, 577, 1965.
10. Cleveland, W. W., Adams, W. C., Mann, J. B. and Nyhan, W. L.: J. Pediat., *66*, 333, 1965.
11. Deitrick, J. E., Whedon, D. G., and Shorr, E.: Amer. J. Med., *4*, 3, 1948.
12. Dent, C. E.: Brit. Med. J., *1*, 230, 1956.
13. Duffy, B. J. and Turner, D. A.: Ann. Intern. Med., *48*, 1, 1958.

13a. Editorial: Lancet, *1*, 955, 1971.

14. Elkinton, J. R., Huth, E. J., Webster, G. D., Jr., and McNance, R. A.: Amer. J. Med., *29*, 554, 1960.
15. Foster, G. V.: New Engl. J. Med., *279*, 349, 1968.

16. Frantz, A. G. and Tabkin, M. T.: J. Clin. Endocr. and Metab., *25*, 1470, 1965.
17. Frost, H. M.: J. Amer. Geriat. Soc., *9*, 1078, 1961.
18. Gaillard, P. P., Talmage, R. V., and Budy, A. M., (eds.), *The Parathyroid Glands—Ultrastructure, Secretion and Function*, Chicago, University of Chicago Press, 1965.
19. Glimcher, M. J., Hodge, A. J., and Schmitt, F. O.: Proc. Natl. Acad. Sci., *43*, 860, 1957.
20. Glimcher, M. J. and Krane, S. M.: Chapter 2, In *Treatise on Collagen* Vol. IIb (Gould, B. S. and Ramachandran, G. N., eds.), New York, Academic Press, 1968.
21. Glisson, F.: De Rachitide Sive Morbo Puerile Qui Vulgo dicitur (A treatise of rickets, being a disease common to children). Translated by Phil. Armin, London, Streator, 1668.
22. Goldhaber, P.: New Engl. J. Med., *266*, 870, 1962.
23. Griffith, G. C., Nichols, G., Jr., Asher, J. D., and Flanagan, B.: J.A.M.A., *193*, 91, 1965.
23*a*. Haddad, J. G., *et al.*: New Engl. J. Med., *283*, 549, 1970.
24. Hastings, A. B.: In *Conference on Metabolic Interrelations, Transactions of the 3rd Conference* (Reifenstein, E. C., Jr., ed.), New York, Josiah Macy Foundation, 1951, p. 38.
25. Harris, W. H. and Heaney, R. P.: New Engl. J. Med., *280*, 193, 253, and 303, 1969.
26. Harris, W. H., Haywood, E. A., Lavorgna, J., and Hamblen, D. L.: J. Bone & Joint Surg., *50A*, 1118, 1968.
27. Heaney, R. P., and Whedon, D. G.: J. Clin. Endocr. & Metab., *18*, 1246, 1958.
28. Heaney, R. P., Walch, J. J., Steffes, P., and Skillman, T. G.: Calc. Tissue Res., *2*, Suppl. 33, 1968.
29. Henneman, P. H., and Wallach, S.: Arch. Intern. Med., *100*, 715, 1957.
30. Hirsch, P. F., and Munson, P. L.: Physiol. Rev., *49*, 548, 1969.
31. Hollander, J. L.: Personal communication.
32. Howell, D. S., and Ragan, C., Jr.: Medicine, *35*, 83, 1956.
33. Howell, D. S.: J. Bone & Joint Surg., *53A*, 250, 1971.
34. Hurxthal, L. M., Dotter, W. E., Baylink, D. J., and Clerkin, E. P.: Lahey Clin. Bull., *13*, 155, 1964.
35. Johnson, L. C.: In *Henry Ford Hospital International Symposium on Bone Biodynamics* (Frost, H. M., ed.), Boston, Little, Brown, 1964, p. 543.
36. Jowsey, J.: Clin. Orthoped., *17*, 210, 1960.
37. Krane, S. M., Brownell, G. L., Stanbury, J. B., and Corrigan, H.: J. Clin. Invest., *35*, 874, 1956.
38. Lafferty, R. W., Spencer, G. E., Jr., and Pearson, O. H.: Amer. J. Med., *36*, 514, 1964.
39. Mack, P. B., Lachance, P. A., Vose, G. P., and Vogt, F. B.: Amer. J. Roentgenology, *100*, 503, 1967.
40. Mandl, F.: Arch. f. Klin. Chir., *143*, 245, 1926.
41. Mann, J. B., Alterman, S., and Hills, A. G.: Ann. Intern. Med., *56*, 315, 1962.
42. Marshall, J. H.: In *Bone as a Tissue* (Rodahl, K., Nicholson, J. T., and Brown, E. M., Jr., eds.), New York, McGraw-Hill, 1960, p. 144.
43. McClendon, J. F., Jowsey, J., Gershon-Cohen, J., and Foster, W. G.: J. Nutrition, *77*, 299, 1962.
44. McCollum, E. V., Simmonds, N., Beahm, J. E., and Shipley, P. G.: J. Biol. Chem., *53*, 293, 1922.
45. McLean, F. C.: In *The Biochemistry and Physiology of Bone* (Bourne, G. H., ed.), New York, Academic Press, Inc., 1956, p. 705.
46. McLean, F. C. and Urist, M. R.: *Bone: An Introduction to the Physiology of Skeletal Tissue*. Chicago, The University of Chicago Press, 1961.
47. Mellanby, E.: J. Physiol., *52*, 11, 1918.
48. Munson, P. L., Hirsch, P. F. and Tashjian, A. H.: Ann. Rev. Physiol., *25*, 325, 1963.
49. Nagant de Deuxchaisnes, C. and Krane, S. M.: Medicine, *43*, 233, 1964.
50. Nagant de Deuxchaisnes, C. and Krane, S. M.: Amer. J. Med., *43*, 508, 1967.
50*a*. Neer, R. M., *et al.*: J. Clin. Invest., *49*, 89a, 1970.
51. Neuman, W. F. and Neuman, M. W.: *The Chemical Dynamics of Bone Mineral*, Chicago, The University of Chicago Press, 1958.
52. Nordin, B. E. C.: In *Bone as a Tissue* (Rodahl, K., Nicholson, J. T., and Brown, E. M., Jr., eds.), New York, McGraw-Hill, 1960, p. 46.
53. Paget, J.: Med. Clin. Trans., London, *60*, 37, 1877.
54. Park, E. A. and Howland, J. J.: Bull. Johns Hopkins Hosp., *32*, 341, 1921.
55. Pirok, D. J., Ramser, J. R., Takahashi, H., Villaneuva, A. R., and Frost, H. M.: Henry Ford Hosp. Med. Bull., *14*, 760, 1969.
56. Posner, A. S.: Physiol. Rev., *49*, 760, 1969.
57. Prokop, D. J., and Kivirikko, K. I.: Ann. Intern. Med., *66*, 1243, 1967.
58. Ragan, C., Jr., and Briscoe, A. M.: J. Clin. Endocrinol., *24*, 385, 1964.

59. Rich, C., Ensick, J., and Ivanovich, P.: J. Clin. Invest., *43*, 545, 1964.
59*a*. Ryan, W. G., Schwartz, T. B. and Northrup, G.: J.A.M.A., *213*, 1153, 1970.
59*b*. Ryan, W. G., Schwartz, T. B. and Perlia, C. P.: Ann. Intern. Med., *70*, 549, 1969.
59*c*. Smith, R., Russell, R. G. G. and Bishop, M.: Lancet, *1*, 945, 1971.
60. Stanbury, S. W. and Lumb, G. A.: Medicine, *41*, 1, 1962.
61. Stein, I., Stein, R. O., and Beller, M. L.: *Living Bone in Health and Disease*, Philadelphia, J. B. Lippincott Co., 1955.
62. Stewart, G. S. and Bowen, H. F.: Endocrinology, *48*, 568, 1951.
63. Talmage, R. V. and Belanger, L. F.: *Parathyroid Hormone* and *Thyrocalcitonin* (*Calcitonin*), International Congress Series No. 159, Amsterdam, Netherlands, Excerpta Med., 1968, p. 137.
63*a*. Tashjian, A. H., Jr., Howland, B. G., Melvin, K. E. W., and Hill, C. S., Jr.: New Engl. J. Med., *283*, 890, 1970.
64. Urist, M. R., MacDonald, N. S., Moss, M. J., and Skoog, W. A.: In *Mechanisms of Hard Tissue Destruction.* (Sognnaes, R. F., ed.), Washington, D.C., American Association for the Advancement of Science, 1963, p. 385.
65. von Recklinghausen, F.: *Die Fibrose oder deformirende ostitis die osteomalacie*, in Festschrift, Berlin, Rudolph Virchow, Reimer, 1891.
66. Wachman, A., and Bernstein, D. S.: Clin. Orthop., and Rel. Res., *69*, 252, 1970.
67. Walser, M.: J. Clin. Invest., *40*, 723, 1961.
68. Whedon, G. D.: *Osteoporosis in Clinical Endocrinology II.* (Astwood, E. B., ed.), New York, Grune and Stratton, Inc., 1968, p. 349.
69. Woods, J. F. and Nichols, G., Jr.: Science, *142*, 386, 1963.
70. Wrong, O. and Davies, H. E. F.: Quart. J. Med., *28*, 259, 1959.

PART X

Arthritis Caused by or Occurring With Specific Infections

Section Editor: EPHRAIM P. ENGLEMAN, M.D.

Chapter 63

Principles of Diagnosis and Treatment of Infectious Arthritis

By Frank R. Schmid, M.D.

Infection of the joint space represents a curable disease. Specific antimicrobial agents are effective against many microorganisms that cause infectious arthritis. The joint cavity is accessible so that inflammation can be detected readily and its course monitored more easily than in any other tissue except perhaps the skin. Yet, all too frequently, eradication of the infection followed by full restoration of joint function is not accomplished.

Because poor results were obtained in the past, some earlier workers championed elaborate treatment schedules in an arbitrary and empirical manner.[11] Multiple antimicrobial agents were administered for a predetermined number of days, not only systemically but also intra-articularly, by repeated single injections or via an irrigating system through the joint. While this type of program may be successful in experienced hands, it is not required for all infections, is not easily achieved, leads to unnecessary morbidity and, in some instances, compounds the infectious synovitis by a chemical synovitis induced by high local concentrations of the instilled drug.[2,26]

In contrast, a therapeutic program based upon the principles listed in Table 63–1 can be tailored for each patient with septic arthritis. An essential element of this program is continual monitoring during treatment so that the physician can correct deficiencies before irreversible damage has developed.[55]

Table 63-1.—A Rational Therapy for Infectious Arthritis

a. Awareness of the possibility of infection.

b. Identification of the invading microorganism in synovial fluid.

c. Rapid institution of antimicrobial therapy.

d. Drainage of infected joint fluid.

e. Verification of bactericidal levels of antimicrobial agents in joint fluid.

f. Repeated assessment of the response of the joint to treatment and willingness to alter the type or dose of antibiotic or the type of drainage, if indicated.

g. Management of underlying disease which may have predisposed the patient to joint infection.

Not only is this individualized approach suitable for use with available drugs but its basic features provide guidelines that can be adapted to newer antimicrobial agents as these become available. Since infectious agents are being considered as causes for Reiter's syndrome,[20,54] systemic lupus erythematosus,[22,47] and rheumatoid arthritis,[6] knowledge gained from known infectious forms of arthritis may also prove useful for these problems in the future.

Concept of a Closed-space Infection

A rational therapeutic program requires an understanding of events that occur when a closed space is infected. Invading microorganisms usually reach the normally sterile joint cavity from the blood stream[40,60,66] but occasionally by direct penetration from neighboring structures[12,56] or from the exterior.[8] The joint cavity maintains a high level of natural protection against such intruders as overt infection is not a common accompaniment of most septicemic states. Although it may develop in normal joints, its likelihood is greater if the general resistance of the host has been impaired by prior disease[66] or after treatment with drugs that interfere with host-defense mechanisms such as corticosteroids[31,37] or immunosuppressive drugs. Sometimes previous damage by trauma or another arthritic disease[31,36] predisposes a joint to infection.

Once inside, microorganisms are more remote from the humoral and cellular defense mechanisms. Concentrations of antibody, complement and other large molecular weight substances are lower in normal synovial fluid than in plasma and most of the circulating leukocytes are excluded. But water and smaller molecules are exchanged constantly between synovial space and plasma and this flux is accentuated after the vascular synovium becomes inflamed.[51] At such times all plasma constituents have easier access to the joint space.

Small molecules such as antimicrobial agents have been demonstrated at the site of inflammation, both in the synovial fluid and in the surrounding tissue, after their administration by the systemic route.[43] Their diminished effectiveness against bacteria in a closed-spaced infection is due *not* to *sub*optimal local concentrations but rather to the fact that purulent exudates retard bacterial cell growth.[16] Dormant bacteria are able to survive in the presence of drug concentrations that otherwise would be bactericidal.

Thus, a major difference between a closed-space infection and one spread out within the tissues, such as a cellulitis, is the rate of exchange between the vascular space and the area that it supplies. This rate is slowed within the depths of the joint cavity at points removed from the interface of synovial fluid with its vasculature while it is rapid within the closely woven vascular interstitium of connective tissue elsewhere. Slowed access to and egress from the joint permits accumulation of products of inflammation. In such a miasma, pathologic conditions prevail. Fluid pressure is increased,[46] pH is lowered,[35] activated proteolytic and other enzymes abound[17,67] and bacterial metabolism is reduced.[16] It is for these reasons that the time-honored principle of drainage of pus assumes much importance and complements an effective antibiotic program.

Microorganisms Commonly Responsible for Infectious Arthritis

Successful management requires early diagnosis. This in turn is based upon a heightened sense of suspicion that a joint might be infected.

Although almost any microorganism can cause infectious arthritis, the list of

Table 63–2.—Estimate of the Incidence of Microorganisms Commonly Responsible for Acute Pyogenic Arthritis.[2,7,18,38,39,52,55,61,66]

Microorganism	*Adults (per cent)*	*Children (per cent)*
Gram-positive cocci		
Staphylococcus aureus	25	40
Diplococcus pneumoniae	10	10
Streptococcus pyogenes	10	25
Gram-negative cocci		
Neisseria gonorrhoeae	50	<1
*Hemophilus influenzae**	<1	10
Gram-negative bacilli (*E. coli*, *Salmonella* sp., *Pseudomonas*, etc.)	<5	<15

* *H. influenzae* are actually coccobacilli but are listed under "cocci" because they are frequently mistaken on smears for cocci.

common agents is quite restricted[2,7,39,52,55,61,66] (Table 63–2). In children who have a higher incidence of pyogenic arthritis than adults,[38] *Staphylococcus aureus*, beta hemolytic streptococci, pneumococci, *H. influenzae* and a variety of gram-negative bacilli are most often responsible. Gram-negative bacilli and *H. influenzae* frequently cause joint infections in the age group under 2 or 3 years.[7,39,45,52] Fink even reported cases of gonococcal arthritis in children from age 2 to 11 years, emphasizing the importance of not dismissing this possibility simply because of the patient's age.[18] In adults, gonococci, staphylococci, pneumococci and streptococci account for most cases of septic arthritis.[2,55,61,66]

The high prevalence of pyogenic invaders of the synovial cavity in part reflects the incidence of septicemia associated with these common microorganisms[2,4,10,61] but also, perhaps, an affinity of such cocci for synovial structures since these agents readily infect "normal" as well as diseased joints. The Gram-negative bacilli (other than *Hemophilus*) which are even more common causes of clinical septicemia tend to invade mainly damaged joints.

Many kinds of bacteria including *H. influenzae* in the adult,[27] *Klebsiella pneumoniae*,[64] salmonella,[63] *Vibrio fetus*,[33] *M. tetragenus*,[49] *Pseudomonas pseudomallei*,[13] *Bacteroides* sp.[1] and *Clostridium welchii*[59] can cause arthritis. An unusually high frequency of infectious arthritis caused by Gram-negative bacilli is seen in patients with malignancy.[14,65] Infection may be caused by more than one microorganism, for example, when septic arthritis of the hip follows perforation of abdominal organs.[56]

Mycobacterium sp.[32] and a variety of fungi[48,50,53,58] may cause infectious arthritis in patients of any age. These microorganisms should always be considered when examination of the synovial fluid suggests infection but routine cultures are sterile. Mycobacteria and fungi usually cause a more chronic process in contrast to the acute forms of pyogenic arthritis. However, clinical criteria can be misleading so that identification of the invading microorganism is the only reliable means of establishing the diagnosis.

Approach to the Patient with Infectious Arthritis

Recognition of Sepsis.—The classic description of pyogenic arthritis with its acute onset usually in a single but sometimes in two or more joints is recognized by most physicians.[2,3,9,39,61,65] A migratory polyarthritis may precede this phase, especially in gonococcal and meningococcal arthritis.[19,24] Most often large joints such as the knee and hip are involved but *any* articular structure including the sacroiliac and spinal joints may be affected. The infected joint is warm and painful and distended with fluid. Since bacterial entry into the joint is most often by hematogenous spread, the patient may experience high fever with chills.[31] Signs and symptoms of infection elsewhere may be present. A careful examination of the patient will reveal the lobar pneumonia that seeded the pneumococcus to the joint, the carbuncle which was the source of the staphylococcus or the history of a urethral discharge responsible for entry of the gonococcus.

Unfortunately, septic arthritis may appear under less characteristic guises. When the joint has been damaged by prior disease, the superimposed infection may be less obvious so that the physician does not easily appreciate that a new process has occurred. Patients with rheumatoid arthritis may develop infections in their joints[31] and when they do, the infected joint becomes "lost" among other painful, swollen joints. Careful questioning of the patient, however, usually demonstrates that the infected joint has become more inflamed than noted previously. Not all infected joints, however, present with extreme signs of inflammation, a difficulty that is compounded in joints remote from the skin surface such as the hip.

Differential Diagnosis.—Arthritic disorders that have an acute onset may be confused with cases of infectious arthritis. These include gout, rheumatic fever, trauma and, particularly in children, monoarticular rheumatoid arthritis. Constitutional symptoms such as high fever or chills and marked leukocytosis are uncommon in these conditions. Even when a noninfectious form of arthritis is present, the physician's orientation still must be directed toward *exclusion* of an infectious process. This requires bacteriological examination of synovial fluid. An example of infection with underlying, antecedent disease noted by me has been the development of septic arthritis in the urate crystal-laden joints of two patients with prior episodes of proven gout. Similar superimposed infections have long been recognized in patients with rheumatoid arthritis.[31]

General Studies.—A complete history and physical examination is essential. Special attention should be paid to portals of entry for infection: the upper airway passages including sinuses and the middle ear, the lungs, the skin and the rectum, urethra or pelvic areas.

Initial laboratory studies may reveal a leukocytosis with a shift to more immature leukocytes on the differential count and an elevated erythrocyte sedimentation rate. Absence of leukocytosis does not rule out pyogenic arthritis, particularly in a debilitated individual. Anemia is not likely until later unless underlying disease antedates the infectious process.

Studies to establish the type of bacterial agent responsible for the infection must be begun before chemotherapy is prescribed. At least two blood cultures for both aerobic and anaerobic organisms should be done within several hours in every patient suspected of pyogenic arthritis. A single blood culture, if positive, may be difficult to interpret because of possible contamination during collection. Two blood cultures containing the same microorganism virtually rule out contamination. Cultures should also be made of any exudate or secretion at a suspected portal of entry of infection.

Radiological Examination—Joint sepsis does not immediately damage a normal joint. Several weeks may pass before a cartilaginous or bony abnormality can be detected. Then a general rarefaction of the subchondral bone develops, followed by areas of erosion at the articular ends of the adjacent bone and narrowing of the joint space due to destruction of the articular cartilage (Fig. 63–1). When superimposed upon a diseased joint, changes due to infection may be indistinguishable from those already present.

Diagnosis of sepsis therefore may not be aided by x ray. However, films taken before treatment help assess the extent of structural damage and permit an estimate of the degree to which joint function can be restored. The contralateral joint should be included in the initial radiological examination as a control for subtle changes that might have developed on the involved side. Films should be taken sequentially to aid in monitoring the treatment program.

Joint Fluid Examination.—*Aspiration and examination of joint fluid are mandatory whenever infection is considered.* They must be done *immediately* upon suspicion of infection and must never be deferred.

The technique of arthrocentesis requires strict asepsis. The overlying skin should be scrubbed with tincture of iodine or other appropriate sterilizing agent. While equipment for the aspiration is being readied for use, a moist alcohol sponge should be kept on the skin over the site of entry.

Inadvertent introduction of a para-articular or subcutaneous infection into a sterile joint cavity represents a hazard of joint aspiration. For this reason, a careful examination of the area is required to define anatomically the exact site of infection. The needle should be introduced into the joint through uninvolved subcutaneous tissue.

The equipment tray taken to the bedside for arthrocentesis should always contain sterile tubes. A small quantity of joint fluid is inoculated into sterile tubes as well as into tubes for appropriate

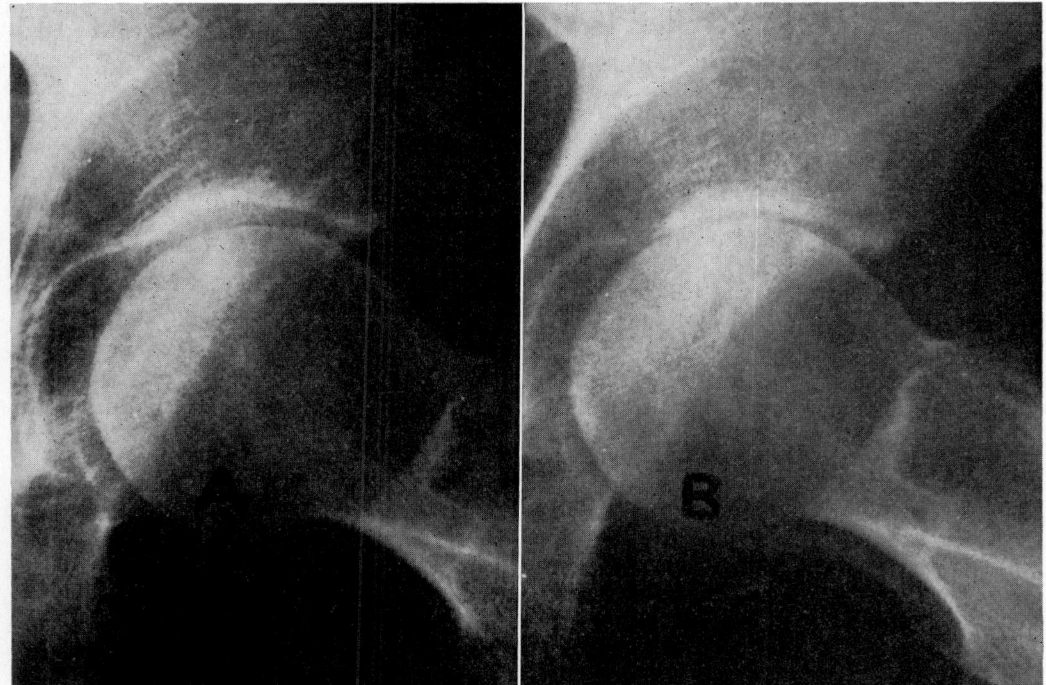

FIG. 63–1.—The hip joint of a patient with septic arthritis due to *S. aureus*. A. Radiological examination within the first week shows no abnormality. B. Film repeated 3 weeks later shows loss of cartilage and beginning bone erosion.

chemical determinations and tubes with anticoagulant (heparin or ethylene diamine tetracetate, EDTA) for cell examination. These samples should be taken at once to the laboratory *by the physician himself* rather than by an intermediary. This ensures prompt examination and inoculation of still warm fluid into appropriate bacteriologic media. For growth of fastidious microorganisms, such as the gonococcus, speed is essential. Some clinicians even recommend bedside inoculation of the fluid onto media.

Blood agar should be used routinely for culturing all synovial fluid specimens. However, *Neisseria gonorrhoeae* and *Hemophilus* sp. may not be recovered without using some form of chocolate agar. The gonococcal media described by Thayer and Martin is quite suitable for gonococcal isolation but it must be remembered that this medium contains vancomycin and colistin methanesulfonate and was designed to isolate gonococci from the mixed flora of the female genital tract.[57] Therefore, many other bacteria which might cause septic arthritis such as *Hemophilus* sp. will not grow on Thayer-Martin media. Recently, the suggestion has been made that media of higher ionic strength be utilized to facilitate the culture of gonococcal protoplasts.[28] In this report of one patient with gonococcal arthritis, standard cultures were negative but growth occurred on the special media. *Hemophilus* sp. can easily be isolated on peptic digest of blood agar which is prepared from commercially available products. Placing about 1 ml. of the synovial fluid in thioglycollate broth will allow recovery of many anaerobic and aerobic bacteria. Many microaerophilic bacteria actually grow more rapidly after primary inoculation in thioglycollate broth than on solid media. Isolation of strict anaerobes may require special anaerobic techniques. Fungal media, such as Sabouraud's, should be inoculated in most instances. However, if fungal media inadvertently are not inoculated, fungi may be recovered from the blood agar plates provided these are incubated for up to two weeks at room temperature. Drying of such blood agar plates can be retarded by sealing the plate with paraffin tape. Culture of *Mycobacterium* sp. is best done by utilizing at least two kinds of media: one, an egg-glycerol-potato medium such as A.T.S. medium and the other, a synthetic medium such as Middlebrook 7H10 agar. If a large volume of synovial fluid is available it should be concentrated by centrifugation before inoculating mycobacterial cultures. With improvements in culture media, there is no need to utilize guinea pig inoculation as a means of recovering *M. tuberculosis*. Recent studies clearly show that the guinea pig is rarely positive when mycobacterial cultures are negative.[34] Furthermore, atypical *Mycobacterium* sp., which can infect joints, are nonpathogenic for guinea pigs.

Having completed inoculation of the joint fluid into all appropriate media, smears are prepared on microscopic glass slides. These are air-dried and stained by Gram's stain, Wright's stain and appropriate stain for acid-fast organisms. Examination of these slides provides the necessary information to begin treatment.

Certain additional studies of joint fluid are regularly performed (Table 63–3). The total leukocyte count can be determined by a manual procedure or an automated cell counter provided physiologic saline solution is used as a diluent rather than the acid diluents often used for leukocyte enumeration in the blood. Acid solutions coagulate the hyaluronate of synovial fluid. The leukocytes are trapped in these clumps and the cell cell counts are falsely low. While fluids in septic arthritis often appear grossly purulent and have elevated cell counts, predominantly polymorphonuclear leukocytes, it must be remembered that high white cell counts containing many polymorphonuclear cells can appear in noninfected fluids obtained from some patients with acute gout or rheumatoid arthritis.[51] Therefore, bacteriologic stain and culture alone provide the only absolute confirmation of sepsis.

The fasting synovial fluid glucose value is usually reduced to less than half the

TABLE 63–3.—SYNOVIAL FLUID FINDINGS IN ACUTE PYOGENIC ARTHRITIS

		Inflammatory fluids	
Joint Fluid Examination	*Noninflammatory fluids*	*Noninfectious*	*Infectious*
Color	Colorless, pale yellow	Yellow	Yellow
Turbidity	Clear, slightly turbid	Turbid	Turbid, purulent
Viscosity	Not reduced	Reduced	Reduced
Mucin clot	Tight clot	Friable	Friable
Cell count (per mm^3)	200–1,000	1,000–>10,000	10,000–>100,000
Cell type	Mononuclear	PMN*	PMN*
Synovial fluid/blood glucose ratio	0.8–1.0	0.5–0.8	<0.5
Gram stain for organisms	None	None	Positive#
Culture	Negative	Negative	Positive#

* PMN = polymorphonuclear leukocyte.
# In some cases, especially with the gonococcus, no organisms may be demonstrated.

blood glucose value obtained simultaneously.[61] Reductions of similar magnitude are not usually found in inflammatory joint fluids of non-septic origin. Determinations should be made only on specimens obtained six or more hours after eating or after termination of glucose infusions to allow equilibration of glucose between blood and synovial fluid.

Transport of Antibiotics into Synovial Fluid.—The fear of many physicians that antibiotics are not transported from the blood stream into septic joints is not supported by available data.[15,25,26,38,41,43,66] To be sure, early studies of synovial fluid concentrations of penicillin showed inadequate amounts of this drug in the joint. But the dose of penicillin was small compared to the amounts currently recommended.[5,26,41] Effective synovial fluid concentrations for a number of commonly used antibiotics were documented in a study of 75 paired samples of synovial fluid and blood obtained from 29 adult patients with a presumptive diagnosis of infectious arthritis.[43] Parenteral administration of penicillin G, phenoxymethyl penicillin (penicillin V), nafcillin, cloxacillin, cephaloridine, tetracycline, erythromycin, and lincomycin in conventional doses produced bactericidal fluid concentrations within the joint (Fig. 63-2). Similar results have been reported in infants and children for ampicillin, methicillin, penicillin G and cephalothin.[38] Knowledge that antimicrobial agents may achieve effective concentrations in infected joints

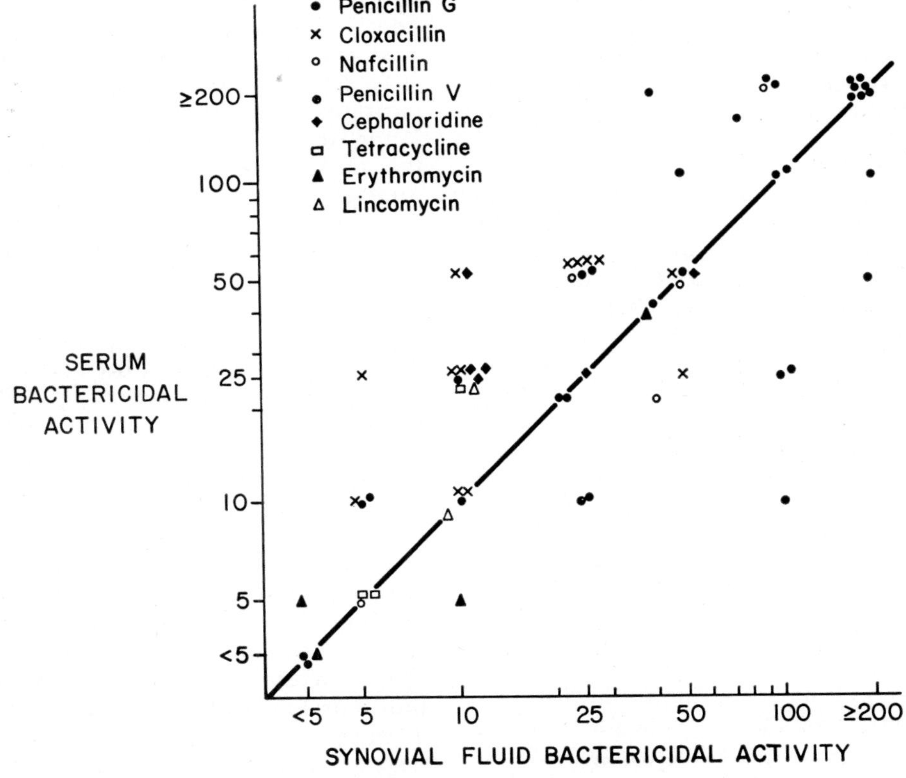

FIG. 63-2.—Comparison of the bactericidal activity of 75 paired specimens of serum and synovial fluid obtained from 29 patients during systemic antibiotic therapy. Points on the diagonal line indicate pairs with equal activity. Bactericidal activity is expressed as the reciprocal of the maximum dilution showing this activity.[43]

obviates the need for *direct* instillation of antibiotics into the joint space, thus reducing the risk of introducing a new infectious agent or producing a "chemical synovitis."[2,26] The latter complication is probably due to toxicity of excessively high local concentrations of some drugs.

Unfortunately, little information is available regarding transport of amphotericin B, polymyxins and aminoglycosides (streptomycin, kanamycin, gentamicin) into synovial fluid. These drugs are considered poorly diffusible. Therefore, until additional data are provided, it is recommended that adequate transport of these drugs be documented by *in vitro* studies of each patient in which they are used (see below). If such transport is not achieved, local instillation into the joint might be done or another antibiotic used that does enter the joint more readily.

Immediate Antibiotic Management.—Decisions regarding antibiotic management are made under three sets of circumstances: (1) initial treatment before identification of the infecting microorganism, (2) definitive treatment after the microorganism has been identified and its antimicrobial activity assayed, or (3) definitive treatment based upon a presumptive diagnosis of septic arthritis when no microorganism has been identified by either microscopy or culture.

Antibiotic treatment should begin within the first hour or two after admission to the hospital before the results of the cultures are known. Preliminary recognition of the different types of infection can be made on the basis of the initial findings noted on the Gram-stained smear of synovial fluid.

1. Septic arthritis due to Gram-positive cocci.
2. Septic arthritis due to Gram-negative cocci or coccobacilli.
3. Septic arthritis due to Gram-negative bacilli.
4. Septic arthritis suspected but no microorganism seen on the Gram-stained smear.

If no organism is detected on the smear, it is our practice to begin therapy in the adult with penicillin G given intravenously (Table 63–4). Such a procedure ensures delivery to the synovial cavity of concentrations of drug adequate for most infections caused by pneumococci, gonococci, penicillin G-susceptible staphylococci as well as a number of less common bacteria causing joint infections. Gonococcal arthritis is the most frequent example in the adult in which a negative smear occurs in the face of convincing evidence of infection.[23,29,30,44] Improvement, often within 4 to 7 days, using large amounts of penicillin G alone without anti-inflammatory drugs is often dramatic in this disease. Initial treatment in children, especially infants below 2 or 3 years of age, should be ampicillin in adequate dosage, 200 mg./kg. per day, due to the strong likelihood that *H. influenzae* might be present.

During the acute phase of the illness, antibiotics should be given parenterally. If the drug is administered intravenously the daily dose should be divided into quarters and the quarter dose added every 6 hours over a span of 30 to 60 minutes to a constantly running infusion ("piggy back" infusion). This technique is preferred to continual delivery of the drug by intravenous drip infusion since it is not surprising to find that a patient who supposedly was receiving 20,000,000 U. of penicillin G per day from the infusion flask actually received much less due to frequent interruptions caused by subcutaneous infiltration or kinking of tubing.

When a specific bacterium is seen on the Gram-stained smear, a closer approximation to definitive antibiotic therapy can be attempted. Types and doses of drugs currently recommended for several different kinds of infection are listed in Table 63–4. Infections caused by Gram-negative bacilli such as *E. coli* and *Pseudomonas* require a more aggressive approach, sometimes using two antibiotics systemically. In the case of kanamycin or polymyxin B, the possible use of intra-

Table 63-4.—Drugs Used During the Initial Treatment of Acute Pyogenic Arthritis Before Results of Culture and Anti-microbial Sensitivity of Organism Are Known*

Finding on Gram stain	*Drug*	*Dosage*	*Remarks*
Gram-positive "cocci"	Nafcillin†	25 mg./kg. q. 6 hr. I.V.	Therapy must be directed toward possible penicillin G-resistant staphylococcal infection. These drugs are also active against pneumococci and Group A streptococci.
	Cephaloridine‡	15–20 mg./kg. q. 12. hr I.M.	
	Erythromycin§	7.5 mg./kg. q. 6 hr. I.V.	
Gram-negative "cocci"	Penicillin G	50–75,000 U./kg. q. 6 hr. I.V.	In adults *Neisseria gonorrhoeae* most often will be the infectious agent and in children *Hemophilus influenzae.*
	Ampicillin‖	50 mg./kg. q. 6 hr. I.V. or I.M.	
	Tetracycline	7.5 mg./kg. q. 6 hr. I.V.	
Gram-negative bacilli	Cephaloridine	See above	Two drugs may be required in critically-ill patients with septicemia. May need to give 5 to 10 mg intra-articular doses of kanamycin or polymyxin B.
	Kanamycin	7.5 mg./kg. q. 12 hr. I.M.	
	Polymyxin B	1.25 mg./kg. q. 12 hr. I.M. or I.V.	
Smear negative	Treat as if gram-negative "cocci" were visualized.		

* Drugs listed in order of preference. Second and third choices may be used when there is allergy or inability to tolerate the first choice. The active collaboration of Dr. Richard H. Parker in these recommendations is gratefully acknowledged.

† Nafcillin is preferred over other penicillinase-resistant penicillins because of greater activity *in vitro* against both penicillinase-producing staphylococci and penicillin G-susceptible microorganisms such as pneumococci.[42]

‡ Cephalothin also provides equivalent antibacterial effect but cephaloridine is preferred because it is well tolerated intramuscularly. Cephalosporins should not be used if allergy to penicillins exists as these drugs have common antigenic determinants.

§ Lincomycin can be used as an alternative.

‖ In adults cephaloridine is preferred over ampicillin because *H. influenzae* infection is unlikely.

articular administration should be considered.

Definitive Antibiotic Management. — As soon as the exact identity of microorganism and its susceptibility to antibiotics have become known, definitive therapy can be planned according to the information provided in Table 63–5. Either the antibiotic chosen initially is continued in the same or modified dose or a more appropriate antibiotic is selected. Proof that the antibiotic being administered intravenously is actually being carried to the joint in bactericidal concentrations should be obtained by determination of antibacterial activity in paired samples of synovial fluid and serum. A simple tube-dilution technique can be performed in most clinical bacteriological laboratories utilizing either the bacterium isolated from the patient or a bacterial species with antibiotic susceptibility identical to the test microorganism.[43] The results of such a test indicate the dilution to which serum and synovial fluid can be taken and still retain bacteriostatic and bactericidal activity. A margin of *bactericidal* effect tenfold or greater than that found in undiluted synovial fluid provides sufficient antibiotic for antimicrobial action. Reliance should not be placed upon a drug program that produces only bacteriostatic activity without adequate bactericidal activity. If this occurs, the dose of antibiotic administered is increased until adequate bactericidal activity is reached or another antibiotic is substituted. An excellent correlation exists between this rather simple tube-dilution test and the more quantitative agar-diffusion technique.[43]

Parenteral antibiotic administration should be maintained until clinical signs of active synovitis and inflammatory changes in the joint fluid have begun to revert toward normal. Synovial fluid should be recultured during the initial stages of therapy to demonstrate that it has been rendered sterile. With assurance that control of the infection is being achieved, oral administration of the antibiotic may be substituted. In the earlier stages of treatment, oral therapy is unreliable because patients with sepsis have a high incidence of nausea, vomiting and other gastrointestinal disturbances.

Infections caused by staphylococci respond more slowly to treatment than those caused by the other common pyogenic microorganisms.[7] No satisfactory explanation for this is available but a change in the staphylococcal strain is not likely to be a factor. In most cases, the strain of infecting organism within the joint remains constant and is not replaced during therapy by another variety that might be drug-resistant unless such a contaminating strain is carried into the joint inadvertently during arthrocentesis. This contrasts with the greater incidence of change in bacterial flora noted during treatment of "open" infections in the respiratory or urinary tract. In addition, staphylococci do not usually show spontaneous mutation in their patterns of drug sensitivity. Thus, a strain of *S. aureus* sensitive to penicillin G at the outset will remain sensitive to this drug during treatment. The slow therapeutic response often seen with staphylococcal infection is compounded when there is inadequate removal of purulent fluid or necrotic tissue remnants from the joint.

Suggestions for antibiotic therapy provide only general guidelines for the physician. Such information quickly becomes dated as more effective drugs are discovered or changing patterns of drug resistance emerge for some strains of bacteria. For these reasons, the physician must have access to current knowledge concerning antibiotic usage. More importantly, he should establish that the program selected for each patient with septic arthritis provides effective antimicrobial control. Knowledge of drug toxicity is also essential. Renal toxicity must be considered and the dosages of antibiotic appropriately reduced if the patient has diminished renal function. Blood levels of antibiotic determined by a tube-dilution technique[43] provide this necessary information.

Drainage of Purulent Exudate.—Initially,

Table 63-5.—Preferred Treatment Schedule for Several Major Types of Septic Arthritis*

Microorganism	*Drug*	*Dosage*	*Duration*†	*Alternative Rx*
Staphylococcus aureus Penicillin G resistant	Nafcillin	25 mg./kg. q. 6 hr. I.V.	At least 2 weeks, then oral therapy for 4–6 weeks after infection is controlled	Cephaloridine Erythromycin Lincomycin
	Dicloxacillin	10–15 mg./kg. q. 6 hr. orally		
Penicillin G susceptible	Penicillin G	50–70,000 U./kg. q. 6 hr. I.V.	At least 2 weeks, then oral therapy for 4–6 weeks after infection is controlled	Cephaloridine Erythromycin Lincomycin
	Penicillin V	10–15 mg./kg. q. 6 hr.		
Diplococcus pneumoniae Group A β hemolytic streptococcus	Penicillin G	25–50,000 U./kg. q. 6 hr. I.V.	10–14 days	Cephaloridine Erythromycin Lincomycin
Neisseria gonorrhoeae	Penicillin G	50–70,000 U./kg. q. 6 hr. I.V.	10–14 days	Tetracycline Cephaloridine
Hemophilus influenzae	Ampicillin	50 mg./kg. q. 6 hr. I.M.	10–14 days	Chloramphenicol Tetracycline

* The active collaboration of Dr. Richard H. Parker in these recommendations is gratefully acknowledged.

† Duration of therapy must be individualized and related to patient's response.

drainage is accomplished by needle aspiration in almost all instances. All possible fluid is removed on a daily or if necessary on a more frequent basis. Since a small portion will always remain, some clinicians suggest washing out the joint cavity with sterile physiologic saline or Ringer's solution. In our experience this small residual has not been a problem provided aspiration is repeated whenever larger amounts of fluid reaccumulate. Needle aspiration is continued as often as necessary, observing at each time the volume and cell count and, at appropriate intervals, the fasting glucose level. In addition, certain samples serve for analysis of the bactericidal level of antibiotic in the joint.

If needle drainage does not control the accumulation of fluid or if access to the joint is difficult, as in the hip joint, open surgical drainage becomes necessary. The exact time to use surgical drainage cannot be stated with certainty but, in general, its use is considered if little or no clinical or laboratory evidence of joint improvement occurs within 4 to 7 days after the onset of therapy. In children with septic arthritis of the hip, open surgical drainage should be considered earlier or even initially because needle aspiration may not be feasible.[21,52] A catheter can be sutured to the capsule of the joint permitting irrigation with isotonic saline or other physiological solution. Antibiotics should continue to be administered parenterally and not locally.

On-going Evaluation of the Treatment Program.—At regular periods a clinical appraisal of the state of inflammation is recorded by noting changes in tenderness, heat, tissue swelling and range of motion of the joint. The frequency of joint aspirations and character of the fluid are observed. Whenever any change in the type of dose or route of administration of antibiotic is made, a tube-dilution assay of serum and synovial fluid should be performed to prove that bactericidal levels at least 10 times those required to kill the test microorganism have been achieved. When joint fluid is no longer obtainable, assay of antibiotic concentration in the blood alone provides a close approximation of drug concentration in the joint. This plan of continuous monitoring should be charted chronologically so that the results of the treatment program can be quickly and accurately assessed.

Antibiotic therapy should be continued for at least 10 to 14 days after all systemic and local signs of inflammation have subsided. In staphylococcal infections this period is extended to 4 to 6 weeks to avoid a relapse because these infections tend to respond more slowly. The patient should be observed for another few weeks after cessation of antibiotic therapy for any signs of relapse of infection.

If delay in improvement or worsening of the infection occurs during any interval in the treatment period, a review of all aspects of the program must be undertaken. The following questions should be asked:

1. Was the joint fluid rendered sterile?
2. Were bactericidal levels of antibiotic in the joint fluid achieved?
3. Did each needle aspiration remove most of the joint fluid?

Answers to these questions will dictate the appropriate change that needs to be made in either the type or dose of antibiotic administered or the method of drainage used. Consultation with the staff of the laboratory interested in infectious diseases and the orthopedic surgeon is invaluable in resolving questions that might arise.

A case history of a patient with septic arthritis illustrates the value of continual monitoring of the response to treatment (Fig. 63–3). Gram-positive cocci subsequently proven to be *S. aureus* were identified in the smear of fluid obtained from the knee. Penicillin G was administered intravenously. On the second day of treatment, more than adequate bactericidal levels of antibiotic were demonstrated against the staphylococcus recovered from the joint. However, the patient developed an intense allergic response so that penicillin was discontinued

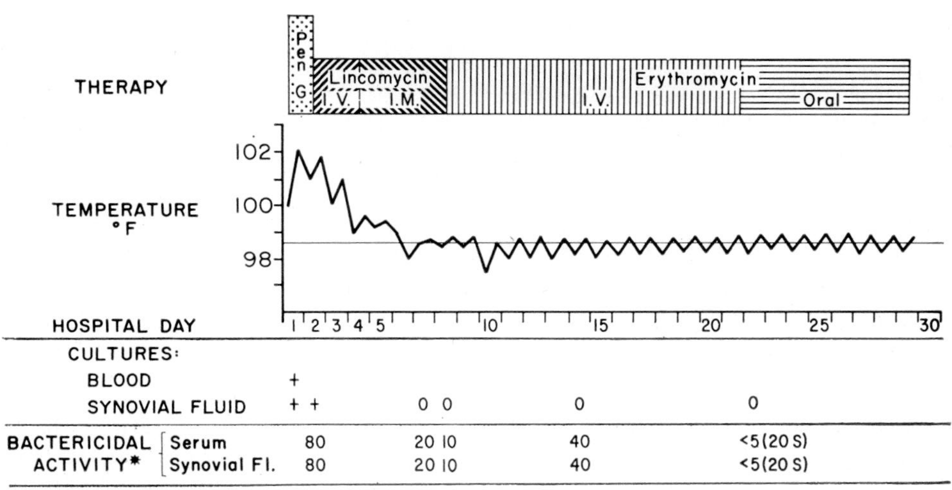

Fig. 63–3.—Response of a patient with septic arthritis to antibiotic treatment. Comparable bactericidal drug levels were achieved in the joint fluid and blood for each drug.

and lincomycin substituted. Again, suitable bactericidal drug concentrations were achieved. As improvement occurred, lesser amounts of fluid were obtained by needle aspiration from the joint. For the balance of treatment schedule, erythromycin was given. Both by the intravenous and later by the oral route, bactericidal levels of drug were noted. Following discharge from the hospital on the 29th day, oral medication was continued for another 2 weeks. Although this patient had developed septic arthritis in a joint already damaged by rheumatoid arthritis, prompt diagnosis and therapy prevented further loss of joint function.

Other Aspects of Therapy.—The affected joint must be kept at rest. During the acute phase of the process, a splint may be indicated to provide complete immobilization since this reduces pain and helps control inflammation. A posterior resting splint for the leg or arm is usually sufficient. As the process improves, attempts should be started to restore gradually range of motion and increase muscle strength. Passive exercises, followed by graded active exercises, are begun with the assistance of the physical therapist. Weight-bearing should be deferred until all signs of acute inflammation have disappeared.

In addition to specific efforts directed toward the joint infection, general principles that apply to treatment of patients with septicemia must be incorporated into the program. These include attention to the primary infection that led to the arthritis, fluid and nutritional needs of the patient and measures for control of pain.

BIBLIOGRAPHY

1. Ament, M. E. and Gaal, S. A.: Amer. J. Dis. Child., *114*, 427, 1967.
2. Argen, R. J., Wilson, C. H., Jr. and Wood, P.: Arch. Intern. Med., *117*, 661, 1966.
3. Badgley, C. E., Yglesias, L., Perham, W. S. and Snyder, C. H.: J. Bone & Joint Surg., *18*, 1047, 1936.
4. Baitch, A.: Clin. Orthop., *22*, 157, 1962.
5. Balboni, V. G., Shapiro, I. M. and Kydd, D. M.: Amer. J. Med. Sci., *210*, 588, 1945.

6. Baum, J.: Arth. & Rheum., *14*, 135, 1971.
7. Borrela, L., Goobar, J. E., Summitt, R. L. and Clark, G. M.: J. Pediat., *62*, 742, 1963.
8. Bunn, P.: Trans. Amer. Clin. & Climat. Assoc., *69*, 9, 1957.
9. Caldwell, G. A.: J.A.M.A., *98*, 37, 1932.
10. Chartier, Y., Martin, W. J. and Kelly, P. J.: Ann. Intern. Med., *50*, 1462, 1959.
11. Compere, E. L., Metzger, W. J. and Mitra, R. N.: J. Bone & Joint Surg., *49A*, 614, 1967.
12. Cutler, C. W., Jr.: Surg. Clin. North America, *18*, 549, 1938.
13. Diamond, H. S. and Pastore, R.: Arth. & Rheum., *10*, 459, 1967.
14. Douglas, G. W., Levin, R. H. and Sokoloff, L.: New Engl. J. Med., *270*, 299, 1964.
15. Drutz, D. J., Schaffner, W., Hillman, J. W. and Koenig, M. G.: J. Bone & Joint Surg., *49A*, 1415, 1967.
16. Eagle, H.: Amer. J. Med., *13*, 389, 1952.
17. Evanson, J. M., Jeffrey, J. J. and Krane, S. M.: J. Clin. Invest., *47*, 2639, 1968.
18. Fink, C. W.: J.A.M.A., *194*, 237, 1965.
19. Foley, W. B.: Proc. Roy. Soc. Med., *34*, 657, 1941.
20. Ford, D. K.: Canad. Med. Assoc. J., *99*, 900, 1958.
21. Freiberg, J. A. and Perlman, R.: J. Bone & Joint. Surg., *18*, 417, 1936.
22. Fresco, R.: Fed. Proc., *27*, 246, 1968.
23. Graber, W. J., III, Sanford, J. P. and Ziff, M.: Arth. & Rheum., *3*, 309, 1960.
24. Heberling, J. A.: J. Bone & Joint Surg., *23*, 917, 1941.
25. Heyl, J. T.: Proc. Roy. Soc. Med., *34*, 782, 1941.
26. Hirsch, H. L., Feffer, H. L., and O'Neil, C. B.: J. Lab. & Clin. Med., *31*, 535, 1946.
27. Hoaglund, F. T. and Lord, G. P.: Arch. Intern. Med., *119*, 648, 1967.
28. Holmes, K. K., Gutman, L. T., Belding, M. E. and Turck, M.: New Engl. J. Med., *284*, 318, 1971.
29. Keefer, C. S. and Spink, W. W.: J.A.M.A., *109*, 1448, 1937.
30. Keiser, H., Ruben, F. L. and Wolinsky, E.: New Engl. J. Med., *279*, 234, 1968.
31. Kellgren, J. H., Ball, J., Fairbrather, R. W. and Barnes, K. C.: Brit. Med. J., *1*, 1193, 1958.
32. Kelly, P. J. and Karlson, A. G.: Proc. Mayo Clin., *44*, 73, 1969.
33. Kilo, C., Hagemann, P. O. and Marzi, J.: Amer. J. Med., *38*, 962, 1965.
34. Klein, S. J., Craggs, E. and Konwaler, B. E.: Amer. Rev. Resp. Dis., *87*, 451, 1963.
35. McCarty, D. J., Jr., Phelps, P. and Pyenson, J.: J. Exper. Med., *124*, 99, 1966.
36. Miall, W. E.: Ann. Rheum. Dis., *14*, 150, 1955.
37. Mills, L. C., Boylston, B. F., Greene, J. A. and Moyer, J. H.: J.A.M.A., *164*, 1310, 1957.
38. Nelson, J. D.: New Engl. J. Med., *284*, 349, 1971.
39. Nelson, J. D. and Koontz, W. C.: Pediatrics, *38*, 966, 1966.
40. Oldham, J. B.: Lancet, *2*, 576, 1937.
41. Ory, E. M., Meads, M., Brown, B., Wilcox, C. and Finland, M.: J. Lab. & Clin. Med., *30*, 809, 1945.
42. Parker, R. H. and Paterson, P. Y.: J. Chron. Dis., *21*, 719, 1969.
43. Parker, R. H. and Schmid, F. R.: Arth. & Rheum., *14*, 96, 1971.
44. Partain, J. O., Cathcart, E. S. and Cohen, A. S.: Ann. Rheum. Dis., *27*, 156, 1968.
45. Peterson, J. C.: J. Pediat., *7*, 765, 1935.
46. Phemister, D. B.: Ann. Surg., *80*, 481, 1924.
47. Phillips, P. E. and Christian, C. L.: Science, *168*, 982, 1970.
48. Pollock, S. F., Morris, J. M., and Murray, W. R.: J. Bone & Joint Surg., *49A*, 1397, 1967.
49. Reimann, H. A.: J. Clin. Invest., *14*, 311, 1935.
50. Rhangos, W. C. and Chick, E. W.: South. Med. J., *57*, 664, 1964.
51. Ropes, M. W. and Bauer, W.: *Synovial Fluid Changes in Joint Disease*, Cambridge, Mass., Harvard University Press, 1953.
52. Samilson, R. L., Bersani, R. A. and Watkins, M. B.: Pediatrics, *21*, 798, 1958.
53. Sanders, L. L.: Arth. & Rheum., *10*, 91, 1967.
54. Schachter, J., Barnes, M. G., Jones, J. P., Jr., Engleman, E. P. and Meyer, K. F.: Proc. Soc. Exper. Biol. (N.Y.), *122*, 283, 1966.
55. Schmid, F. R. and Parker, R. H.. Arth. & Rheum., *12*, 529, 1969.
56. Smith, W. S. and Ward, R. M.: J.A.M.A., *195*, 1148, 1966.
57. Thayer, J. D. and Martin, J. E.: Pub. Health Rep. (Wash), *81*, 559, 1966.
58. Toone, E. C., Jr., and Kelly, J.: Amer. J. Med. Sci., *231*, 263, 1956.
59. Torg, J. S. and Lammot, T. R.: J. Bone & Joint Surg., *50A*, 1233, 1968.
60. Veal, J. R.: New Orleans Med. & Surg. J., *87*, 549, 1935.
61. Ward, J., Cohen, A. S. and Bauer, W.: Arth. & Rheum., *3*, 522, 1960.

62. Watkins, M. B., Samilson, R. C. and Winters, D. M.: J. Bone & Joint Surg., *38A*, 1313, 1956.
63. Weaver, J. B. and Sherwood, L.: J.A.M.A., *105*, 1188, 1935.
64. Weber, R. G. and Ansell, B. F., Jr.: Ann. Intern. Med., *57*, 281, 1962.
65. Willerson, J. T., Barth, W. F. and Decker, J. L.: Postgrad. Med., *45*, 127, 1969.
66. Willkens, R. F., Healey, L. A. and Decker, J. L.: Arch. Intern. Med., *106*, 354, 1960.
67. Ziff, M., Gribetz, H. J. and LoSpalluto, J.: J. Clin. Invest., *39*, 405, 1960.

Chapter 64

Gonococcal Arthritis

By John T. Sharp, M.D.

An association between arthritis and urethritis was reported as early as 1507 and repeated comments in medical writings from then until the middle of the 19th century indicate that the early recognition of this association was not forgotten.[6,10,40] In 1879 Neisser described the gonococcus and the organism was soon shown to be a common cause of urethritis. Fourteen years later, the organism was cultured from the joint fluid of a patient with acute arthritis and one year after that it was cultured from the blood of three patients with arthritis, two of whom had urethritis.[20] Following these observations, it was generally assumed that all cases of arthritis associated with urethral discharge were due to the gonococcus, although by the 1930's it was quite clear that the organism could not be cultured from the joint fluid in a majority of such cases.

In 1916 Hans Reiter[39] reported a patient with diarrhea, arthritis, conjunctivitis and non-gonococcal urethritis. Although others before him had described cases with the triad of urethritis, conjunctivitis and arthritis, the condition became known as Reiter's syndrome after Bauer and Engelman[3] reported the first case in the English literature in 1942 and referred to the previous publication of Reiter. As this syndrome became more widely recognized investigators began to look more critically at patients previously considered to have gonococcal arthritis whose joint fluid cultures were negative and some physicians raised the question of whether these cases were an incomplete form of Reiter's syndrome.

To answer this question it is first necessary to determine whether gonococcal arthritis ever occurs in the absence of positive joint fluid cultures and, if so, how frequently. In the past it has been stated repeatedly that approximately one-third of patients with gonococcal arthritis have positive joint fluid cultures but the evidence supporting the gonococcal origin in the other cases is amazingly scanty. A comprehensive review of the literature from the 1920's to the present[40] has uncovered a single case report of a patient who had simultaneously a positive blood culture and a negative joint fluid culture.[31] From personal experience I can add four more such cases. In addition discrepant results have been observed in two patients with polyarthritis. Each had one positive joint fluid culture; one patient had one additional affected joint with a negative fluid culture, and the other patient had two involved joints with negative fluid cultures. These cases establish that gonococcal infection can induce articular inflammation without infecting the synovial fluid but the frequency of this phenomenon remains undetermined.

In an attempt to determine the distribution of cases between gonococcal arthritis and Reiter's syndrome, 94 patients seen between 1962 and 1967 at the Ben Taub General Hospital and the Houston Veterans Administration Hospital with suspected arthritis of either condition were reviewed.[41] Twenty-four had gonococci isolated from joint fluid, three from blood, and one from a skin lesion characteristic of blood-borne infection. Seven patients had the Reiter's triad (Table 64–1). Among the remaining patients there were no features that established a specific diagnosis although a number had skin lesions like those found in gonococcal septicemia.[1,2,4,7,12,18,24,29,31,32] These observations are remarkably similar to data compiled by analyzing cases reported as "gonococcal arthritis" between 1931 and 1964.[40] Seven hundred ninety-one reported cases included sufficient clinical description to permit a retrospective determination of "possible Reiter's syndrome"[9,14,17,22,28,30,34,42,43,46] (Table 64–1). Twenty-six patients had conjunctivitis. Sixteen of these were stated to be catarrhal conjunctivitis in whom conjunctival cultures were negative for gonococci. In the remaining ten no comment was made about cultures. Six patients had iritis and twenty-two had keratodermia blennorrhagica. If we accept these features as more likely in Reiter's syndrome than gonococcal arthritis, then 44 of 791 or 5.6 per cent had one or more features suggesting possible Reiter's syndrome, a figure remarkably similar to that observed in the Houston population in the 1960's.

The Organism

Neisseria gonorrhoeae is a gram-negative diplococcus whose adjacent sides are slightly flattened or concave giving the organism the appearance of a pair of kidney beans. The organism does not grow well or may not grow at all on ordinary bacteriologic media but grows readily on media supplemented with serum, ascitic fluid or heated blood. Yeast and liver extracts facilitate the growth of some strains. Carbon dioxide enrichment of the atmosphere during incubation facilitates growth of many strains and is necessary for the cultivation of some. Chilling must be avoided in handling exudates and cultures. Hence it is customary to plant warmed culture media immediately after aspirating synovial fluid. The organism produces an indophenol oxidase as do other members of the genus *Neisseria* and the organism designated as *Mima polymorpha*. The gonococcus ferments glucose but not maltose. Serologic studies have identified two antigenic types of gonococci but serologic tests have not been applied to clinical material. Kellog *et al.* have identified four colony types of gonococci on morphologic grounds.[26,27] Examination of exudate from infected individuals and inoculation of human volunteers led them to associate two colony types with virulence.

The gonococcus appears to have an unusually strong affinity for synovial tissue. Among 45 reported cases of gonococcemia, 37 had arthralgia or arthritis.[40] Synovial fluid cultures were obtained on ten and were positive in eight. In contrast, in a study of pneu-

Table 64-1.—Relative Frequency of Gonococcal Arthritis and Reiter's Syndrome

	Baylor series[41]	*Literature*[40]
Gonococcal arthritis with positive cultures—synovial fluid, blood or skin lesion	28/94 (29.8%)	59/174 (33.9%)
Reiter's syndrome (complete triad)	7/94 (7.5%)	
Possible Reiter's retrospective analysis		44/791 (5.6%)
Suspected gonococcal arthritis or incomplete Reiter's	59/94 (62.8%)	

monococcal pneumonia Tilghman and Finland reported five cases of septic arthritis among 580 patients with positive blood cultures.[45]

The Disease

Epidemiology.—Gonococcal arthritis is a complication of genital tract infection in most instances. Its exact frequency is unknown. Before antibiotics were available arthritis was reported as complicating urethritis in 0.5 to 3 per cent of cases[5,10,30] but, since bacteriologic studies were not regularly performed, some of these cases may have been Reiter's syndrome.

Before effective antibiotics were available, gonococcal arthritis was considered to be more common in men than in women but in recent years proven infections have occurred more frequently in women[15,25,36,41] (Table 64–2). Some believe that the former predominance of men was due to a confusion of many cases of Reiter's syndrome with gonococcal arthritis. Others believe the current predominance of women with gonococcal arthritis is due to frequent occurrence of inapparent genital tract infections in women resulting in a lack of early, effective treatment. This concept gains support from the occasional observation of gonococcal arthritis in homosexual males who have had inapparent, untreated primary infections and the development of gonococcal arthritis in the heterosexual male who has neglected to seek treatment of an antecedent urethritis.

Table 64-2.—Fifty-one Cases of Proven Gonococcal Arthritis*

Fever	
<99.8°	5
99.8°–102.8°	39
≥103°	7
Monoarthritis	12 (23.5%)
Polyarthritis	39 (76.5%)
Skin lesions	16 (31.4%)
Male*	10 (23.3%)
Female*	33 (76.7%)
Blood cultures	Positive 7/35
Joint fluid cultures	Positive 43/47
Skin lesion cultures	Positive 1/5†
WBC—range of 4,150 to 34,200 per mm³	
<10,000	17
10,000–17,999	29
≥ 18,000	4

* Patients were seen at the Ben Taub General and the Houston Veterans Administration Hospitals. In determining sex ratio, only patients at Ben Taub General Hospital were considered.

† Numerator indicates the number of patients with positive culture, the denominator the number of patients on whom culture was performed. In addition to cultures made on skin lesions in 5 patients listed here, cultures were negative on similar lesions of 5 patients in whom a final diagnosis was not made, the blood and joint fluid cultures also being negative (see ref. 41).

Most patients with gonococcal arthritis are in the second and third decades of life but newborn infants, young children and adults in the fifth and sixth decades are occasionally affected.[33,41]

The interval from onset of genitourinary tract infection to onset of arthritis is extremely variable. In a few instances, arthritis follows the urethritis in a few days. More frequently the interval is at least one or two weeks and occasionally much longer intervals occur. Presumably some risk of arthritis remains as long as the carrier state in the genitourinary tract persists, a period reaching several years in some instances.[8,13] Among women, the interval from primary genital infection to arthritis commonly is not apparent.

The route of entry is usually the genitourinary tract but among homosexuals, entry may occur through the oral or rectal mucosa.

Clinical Manifestations

Moderate fever occurs in a majority of patients but is not always present. In a group of patients personally observed the temperature ranged from normal to 103° and averaged 101° F (Table 64–2). Shaking chills occur in a minority of patients.

Joint involvement is polyarticular in most cases (Table 64–2). In many patients onset of illness is characterized by a one- to five-day period of migratory polyarthralgia with variable signs of articular inflammation. With more prolonged episodes, the joints first involved may clear as new joints are affected, but eventually articular swelling, pain and inflammation become particularly severe and persistent at one or more sites. Persistently involved joints are usually quite severely inflamed, exhibiting marked swelling, redness and heat and exquisite pain and tenderness. After the inflammation subsides, the skin may desquamate, a phenomenon reflecting the severity of the inflammation. Effusion is usually apparent and often there is considerable periarticular swelling. The large joints are more frequently attacked, but probably any articulation may be involved. For example, the gonococcus has been cultured from fluid aspirated from finger and toe joints and a gonococcal origin has been suspected in a case of acute arthritis of the sacroiliac joint.

Several authors consider tenosynovitis to be especially characteristic of gonococcal arthritis. Tenosynovitis is relatively common in this condition but is non-specific since it is also seen in many other types of acute arthritis, both infectious and non-infectious.

A distinctive type of skin rash similar to that described by Cabot[7] occurs in about one-third of cases (Table 64–2). Skin lesions indicating a septicemic phase of the illness may precede onset or develop simultaneously with the arthritis. The earliest lesion is a small, erythematous macule, usually measuring 2 or 3 mm. in diameter which may become petechial. Some of these lesions disappear without further development. Others develop a small vesicle in their

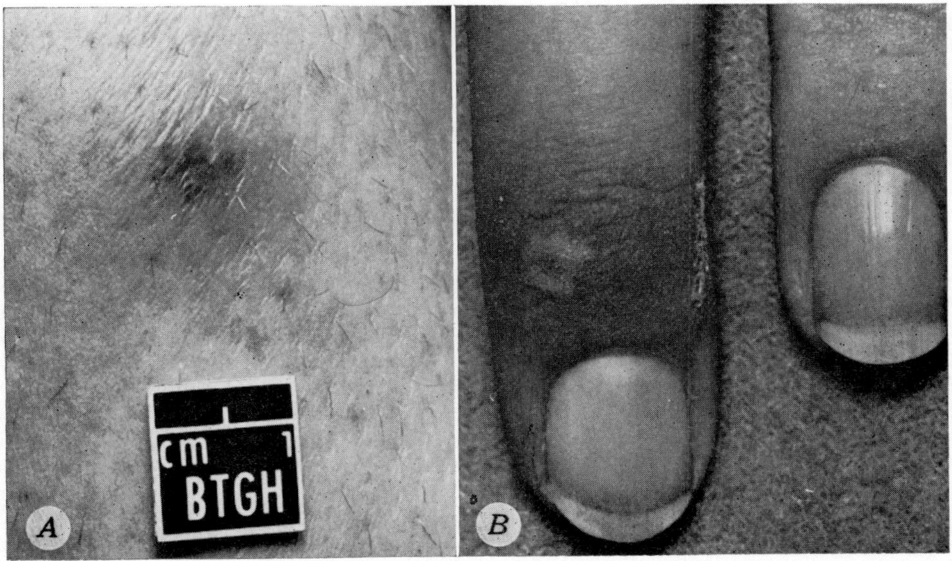

FIG. 64–1.—Skin lesions characteristic of septicemia due to *Neisseria gonorrhoeae*, *N. meningitidis*, *Streptobacillus moniliformis* and *Hemophilus influenzae*. *A*. Hemorrhagic spot 5 to 6 mm. in diameter on the upper arm. There is a gray area 1 to 2 mm. in diameter in the center indicating necrosis. *B*. Pustulovesicular lesion on finger of same patient. Necrotic center evident as dark gray area.

center. The vesicles often become pustular and a dark necrotic center tends to form in the pustule. The fully developed lesion is 3 to 8 mm. in diameter and consists from outside inward of an erythematous ring, a pustular vesicle and a dark eschar in the center (Fig. 64–1). Skin lesions in all stages of development may be present at the same time. This rash is very characteristic of gonococcemia[1,2,4,7,12,18,24,29,31,32] but is not diagnostic since identical skin lesions may be seen in septicemias due to *Neisseria meningitidis*, *Hemophilus influenzae* and *Streptobacillus moniliformis*.

Prolonged gonococcemia was occasionally seen before antibiotics were available. Many of these patients developed endocarditis[11,21,35,37,38,44,49] but this complication has been reported infrequently in recent years.

Pericarditis is an infrequent complication of gonococcal infection.[47]

Gonococcal conjunctivitis occurs in newborn infants infected during passage through the birth canal and is well recognized as frequently leading to severe impairment of vision. Catarrhal conjunctivitis was reported in the past as a frequent complication of gonococcal arthritis in the adult. In these cases, cultures of the conjunctiva were negative for gonococci. I believe that many or all of these cases were Reiter's syndrome.

Conjunctivitis has not been observed by me in 51 cases of gonococcal arthritis proven by positive synovial fluid, blood or skin cultures. Iritis previously reported as occasionally complicating gonococcal infections is also poorly authenticated and its occurrence is more likely a manifestation of Reiter's syndrome.

Pathology.—Histology of the arthritis of gonococcal infection has not been well studied. Keefer reported one patient who had a positive joint fluid culture and died of progressive sepsis.[23] The synovial membrane was thickened and injected and the surface was covered by exudate. There was loss of the superficial synovial cells. The cellular infiltrate consisted of polymorphonuclear leukocytes, lymphocytes, macrophages and plasma cells. Similar changes were seen in two synovial biopsy specimens from which gonococci were cultured, one of which is shown in Figure 64–2.

Laboratory Abnormalities.—The peripheral white blood cell count is frequently elevated but about one-third of cases personally observed had white blood counts under 10,000. Leukocytosis greater than 18,000 is occasionally seen (Table 64–2).

Among 51 proven cases of gonococcal arthritis joint fluid cultures were positive in 43. Blood cultures were positive in seven patients, four of whom had negative joint fluid cultures. Synovial fluid was not cultured in the other three. Cultures of skin lesions were positive in one patient. The joint fluid varied in gross

Fig. 64–2.—A 38-year-old man had abrupt onset of pain and swelling in terminal interphalangeal (TIP) joint left 3rd finger. One day later he developed pain and swelling in right wrist and dorsum of right hand and two days later had swelling and pain in right ankle. Ten days after onset, examination confirmed involvement of above areas. There were no skin lesions or urethral discharge. On the eleventh day of illness the left ankle became swollen and painful. Blood cultures were sterile and synovial fluid cultures from right wrist and left ankle on the 15th day of illness showed no growth. Serum uric acid, ASO titer and EKG were normal. LE cell preparations and latex fixation for anti-IgG were negative. Nineteen days after onset the left 3rd TIP and the right wrist joint remained inflamed, the other joints having cleared. Fever was present. Diagnostic biopsy was advised by the consultant on the 21st day of illness. Tissue from the wrist joint grew out *Neisseria gonorrhoeae*.

Hematoxylin and eosin stained section of biopsy specimen is shown in Figure 64–2*A* (magnification 185×) and Figure 64–2*B* (magnification 460×). The biopsy shows proliferation of new tissue including prominent neo-vascularization. Synovial lining cells are not seen on the surface of the section shown (top, right) and were infrequently present throughout the tissue. The inflammatory infiltrate consists of a mixture of cell types. Collections of polymorphonuclear leukocytes are scattered through the section, along with mononuclear cells and lymphocytes. In some areas not shown, plasma cells were prominent.

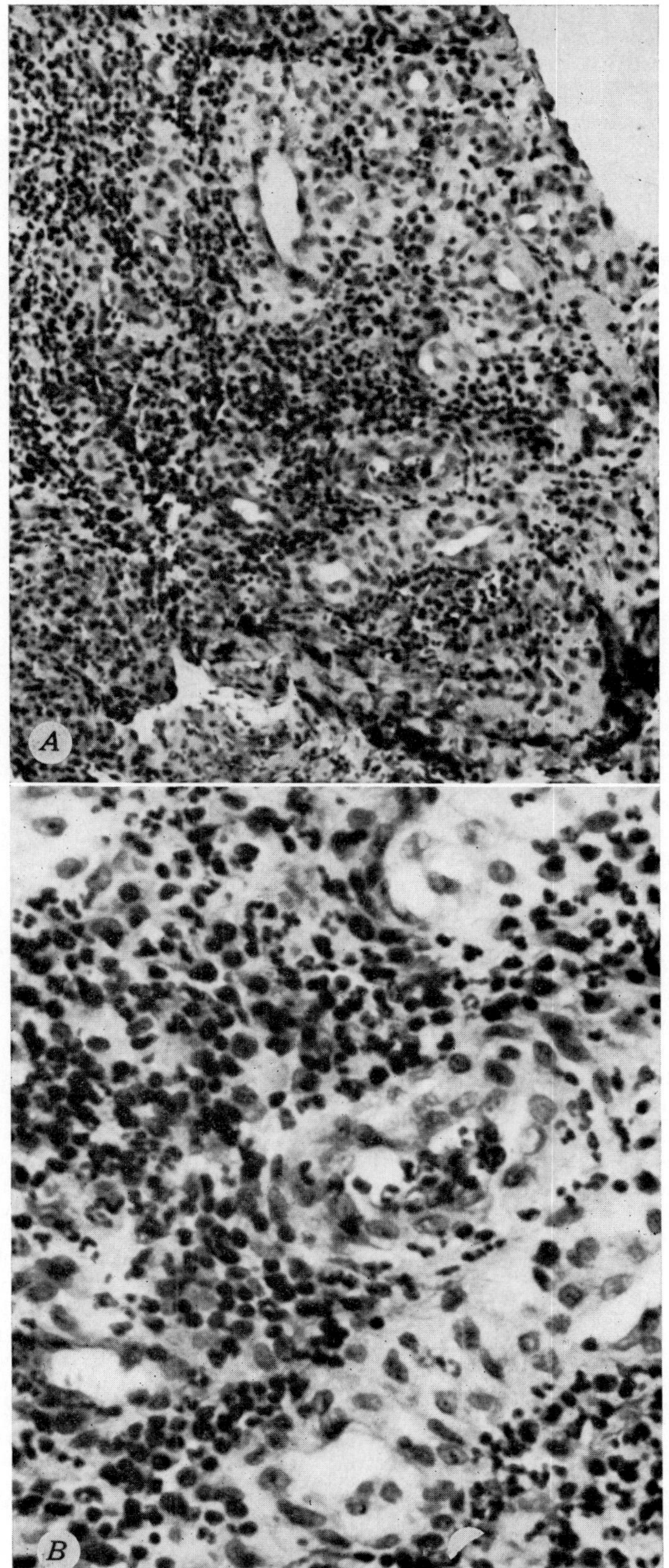

Legend on opposite page

appearance from slightly turbid to grossly purulent. Leukocyte counts ranged from 13,250 to several hundred thousand per cubic millimeter. In about one-third of cases the joint fluid sugar was less than 30 mg. per cent.

Examination of gram-stained synovial fluid fails to reveal organisms in the majority of cases of gonococcal arthritis, a not unexpected finding since the number of organisms present in the fluid is usually small. Granular material which stains with safranin is usually present in synovial fluid and is easily confused with gram-negative cocci which can lead to an erroneous diagnosis. Fortunately, unless the patient received an antibiotic before cultures were obtained, the culture will be positive in those patients who have a positive smear so that any confusion will be resolved as soon as the culture result is known.

The gonococcal complement fixation test used two and three decades ago has been discarded as having no diagnostic value. The specificity of the test was not established and positive results were thought to remain positive for prolonged periods after a genital tract infection so that the diagnostic value of the test in acute arthritis was uncertain.[16,48] Recently fluorescence techniques have been used to demonstrate gonococcal antibodies.[19] In the author's experience the test result was positive in six patients with gonococcal arthritis, three of six patients with Reiter's syndrome and 14 of 28 patients suspected of having gonococcal arthritis.[41] One-third of a group of patients attending a venereal disease clinic had positive results. In some individuals with proven gonococcal arthritis a rise in antibody titer was demonstrated during recovery and convalescence. Other serologic tests are now being studied. If a technically simple test that regularly shows a significant rise in titer during an acute infection can be developed, serologic tests for gonococcal infection will be helpful in the diagnosis of gonococcal arthritis.

X-ray changes should not be seen in

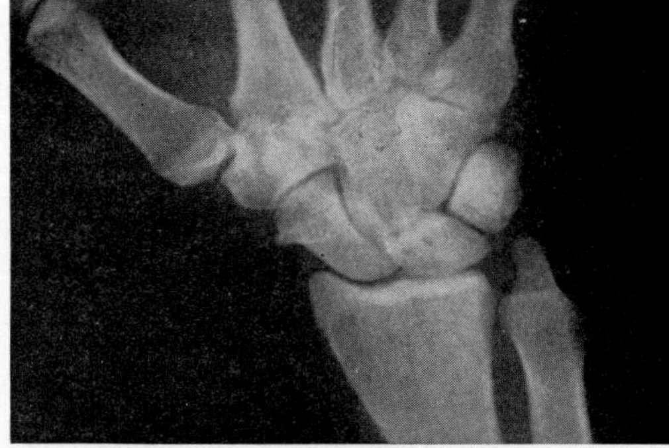

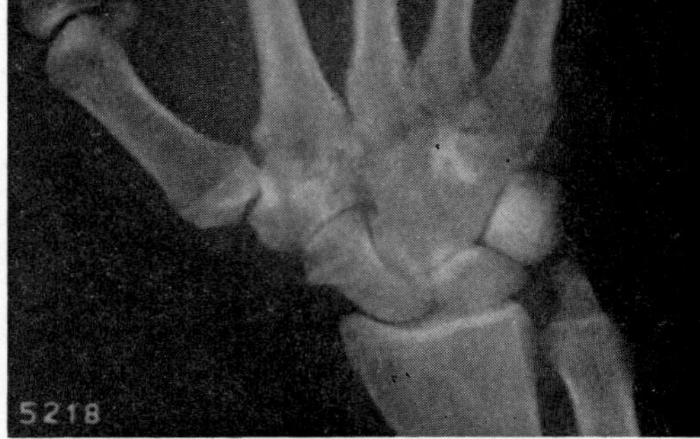

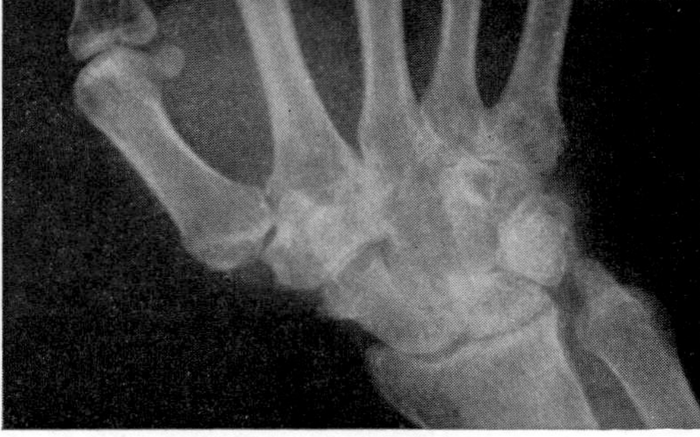

FIG. 64–3.—X rays of patient whose biopsy specimen is shown in Figure 64–2 (see legend of Figure 64–2 for history). Top film was obtained on 11th day of illness, 10 days after onset of pain and swelling in right wrist. The film is normal. The middle film was taken on the 19th day of illness. There is demineralization of carpals and metacarpals along the carpometacarpal articulations with loss of clearly defined trabecular bone markings and loss of articular cartilage in the same area. The last film was obtained 11 weeks after onset of arthritis. Remineralization has occurred. Joint space narrowing is present along the carpometacarpal row, the intercarpal articulations and the radiocarpal joints.

patients properly diagnosed and treated within the first few days of illness. Radiologic changes have been observed to develop between the tenth and fifteenth days of untreated arthritis. The earliest change is a diffuse demineralization that gives the bones a hazy or smudged appearance (Fig. 64–3). With progression, cartilage destruction becomes apparent and with advanced cases there may be extensive destruction of bone with loss of normal anatomical structure. Ankylosis can occur.

Differential Diagnosis

Differential diagnosis among male patients with evidence of genitourinary tract infection is for practical purposes confined to a consideration of Reiter's syndrome and gonococcal arthritis. If the complete Reiter's triad is present and cultures of the blood, joint fluid, and genital tract are negative, a diagnosis of Reiter's syndrome is evident. Patients who lack conjunctivitis and have the gonococcus cultured from the blood, joint fluid, or skin lesions unequivocally have gonococcal arthritis. Only a presumptive diagnosis can be made for patients whose cultures are negative and who lack the Reiter's triad. Some of these patients may have gonococcal infection of the synovial tissue without invasion of the joint fluid.[20a] Others may have an incomplete form of Reiter's syndrome. Unfortunately present methods of investigating these patients will not establish a positive diagnosis in a majority of instances.[41]

The significance of positive cultures from the genital tract has been overstressed in the past. Many authors have considered a gonococcus in the genital tract as proof of gonococcal cause of any coexisting arthritis. This has led to confusion as to what constitutes gonococcal arthritis and renders much of the older literature valueless. Positive cultures in the joint fluid or synovial tissue constitute proof of gonococcal origin and positive cultures of blood and skin lesions are acceptable evidence that the organism has spread from the portal of entry and hence is the most likely cause of concurrent articular involvement.[20a] The presence of a gonococcus in the genital tract should be considered to have about the same weight as a group A streptococcus in the pharynx in a patient with possible rheumatic fever. In both instances, the primary infection is followed by a second illness in 3 per cent or fewer instances.

In the absence of apparent genital tract infection, the differential diagnosis of the acute case of gonococcal arthritis presenting with migratory polyarthralgia or polyarthritis is much broader. The illness in some patients is indistinguishable from acute rheumatic fever and an occasional patient with systemic lupus erythematosus may present with the same symptoms and signs. At times, particularly when a single joint is involved, gout and pseudogout are serious considerations. In many patients other types of septic arthritis are the main consideration and the final diagnosis is made on the basis of bacteriologic studies.

ST- and T-wave electrocardiographic changes have been reported in gonococcal arthritis[47] but are much more likely to occur in acute rheumatic fever. Heart murmurs indicating valvular disease occur in patients with gonococcal endocarditis but this complication of gonococcemia is prevented by early treatment and significant murmurs are not present initially in gonococcal arthritis unless by coincidence.

Systemic lupus erythematosus is usually characterized by multiple system involvement and most well-developed cases have positive test reactions for antinuclear antibody. Gout and pseudogout can be diagnosed by adequate examination of synovial fluid for monosodium urate or calcium pyrophosphate crystals.

Pustulovesicular skin lesions are characteristic of infection but in addition to the gonococcus, the meningococcus, influenza bacillus or *Streptobacillus moniliformis* may be the causative organism.

Clinical Features Suggesting Gonococcal Arthritis

Patient usually febrile.

Polyarthritis often occurs early, followed by persistent synovitis in one or more joints.

Macular, hemorrhagic, vesicular or pustular skin lesions present in many patients.

Joint fluid contains from several thousand to more than 100,000 white blood cells per mm^3.

Joint fluid sugar may be reduced.

Diagnosis established by culture of blood, synovial fluid or skin lesion.

After all appropriate diagnostic studies have been done and adequate cultures have been obtained, those patients in whom a final diagnosis has not been established, but in whom gonococcal arthritis is a serious consideration, should be given an antibiotic effective against gonococci. During such a trial salicylate, indomethacin, phenylbutazone and colchicine should be withheld. Most patients improve within 72 hours after starting appropriate antibiotic treatment, but complete clearing of all signs of arthritis requires a longer period. Improvement coincident with antibiotic therapy is compatible with gonococcal origin but since acute arthritis due to many causes subsides spontaneously, such therapeutic response alone is not very strong evidence for an infectious etiology.

Treatment

Penicillin is the drug of choice and is given in divided doses that total 2.4 million or more units per day. There is little indication that the total dose given beyond an effective level influences the rapidity or completeness of recovery. However, the duration of therapy is probably important in eradicating the articular infection and the primary focus so that continuation of therapy for two weeks is recommended. In the first few days of treatment arthrocentesis is done at daily intervals if the fluid reaccumulates rapidly enough to produce a palpably tense effusion. Splinting is not required in most cases, since recovery is usually rapid. Hospitalization is usually not required beyond seven to ten days because of rapid and complete recovery of joint function. In these cases, 1.2 million units of Bicillin may be given intramuscularly at the time of discharge from hospital and 2 million units of penicillin are given by mouth daily to complete a 14 day course of treatment. Intra-articular injection of antibiotics is to be avoided since it may induce an intense inflammatory reaction making it impossible to follow the course of the infection. Since antibiotics achieve levels in the synovial fluid close to those in blood, systemic administration of antibiotics is effective and adequate therapy.

In those patients who are allergic to penicillin, 250 mg. of tetracycline are given four times daily and treatment is continued for two weeks.

Course

Some evidence of response to therapy is expected within 24 to 72 hours. In the majority of febrile cases the temperature falls to normal, the joint pain eases, and swelling and inflammation diminish. In only a few instances is response delayed beyond 72 hours. Subsidence of all signs of arthritis may occur in three to seven days and usually is complete in one or two weeks but may require longer. The rapidity of recovery depends largely on the duration and severity of illness at the time treatment is started. Patients with gonococcal arthritis tend to be irresponsible individuals and follow-up examinations have not been carried out on as many patients as desired. Three patients seen in Houston have had significant restriction of articular function at the last examination which was either at the time of hospital discharge or a return clinical visit. Two patients had permanent damage to infected wrists but treatment was delayed for 18 and 28 days due to a delay in making the correct diagnosis. A third patient, who was treated on the third day of illness, had a flexion contracture when discharged from the hospital and when seen on one follow-up visit. Further follow-up was unsuccessful. In some of our patients symptoms were present for more than seven days before hospital entry and yet permanent damage did not occur. Nevertheless, diagnostic studies should be completed with haste and treatment started as soon as appropriate cultures have been obtained to minimize the risk of residual articular damage.

The natural course of the untreated disease cannot be stated with certainty due to the inadequate diagnostic criteria adopted by most authors who studied the disease in the pre-antibiotic era. Several authors stated that the prognosis for complete recovery without residual was better for cases with negative joint fluid cultures but none of the studies reported prior to the antibiotic era separated cases into those with positive cultures and those with negative cultures. Fibrous and bony ankylosis occurred in some cases and extensive joint destruction was common. Death was infrequent but was observed occasionally. Draining fistulae did not develop.

BIBLIOGRAPHY

1. Abu-Nasser, H., Hill, N., Fred, H. L. and Yow, E. M.: Arch. Intern. Med., *112*, 731, 1963.
2. Ackerman, A. B., Miller, R. C. and Shapiro, L.: Arch. Derm. (Chicago), *91*, 227, 1965.
3. Bauer, W. and Engleman, E. P.: Trans. Assoc. Amer. Phys., *57*, 307, 1942.
4. Bruusgaard, E. and Thjotta, T.: Acta Dermatovener., *6*, 262, 1925.
5. Bunim, J. J.: Bull. U.S. Army Med. Dept., *8*, 458, 1948.
6. Burbacher, C. R. and Weiland, A. H.: J. Florida Med. Assoc., *24*, 433, 1938.
7. Cabot, R. C.: Boston Med. & Surg. J., *197*, 1140, 1927.
8. Carpenter, C. M. and Westphal, R. S.: Amer. J. Public Health, *30*, 537, 1940.
9. Coggeshall, H. C. and Bauer, W.: New Engl. J. Med., *220*, 85, 1939.
10. Culp, O. S.: J. Urol., *43*, 737, 1940.
11. Davis, D. S. and Romansky, M. J.: Amer. J. Med., *21*, 473, 1956.
12. Foster, R. C.: Ann. Intern. Med., *16*, 1018, 1942.
13. Fraser, C. K. and Dye, W. J. P.: J.A.M.A., *105*, 269, 1935.
14. Goobar, J. E. and Clark, G. M.: Arch. Interamer. Rheum., *7*, 1, 1964.
15. Graber, W. J., Sanford, J. P. and Ziff, M.: Arth. & Rheum., *3*, 309, 1960.
16. Green, F.: Canad. Med. Assoc. J., *28*, 289, 1933.
17. Hagemann, P. O., Hendin, A., Lurie, H. H. and Stein, M.: Ann. Intern. Med., *36*, 77, 1952.
18. Hazel, O. G. and Snow, W. B.: J.A.M.A., *109*, 1275, 1937.
19. Hess, E. V., Hunter, D. K., and Ziff, M.: J.A M.A., *191*, 531, 1965.
20. Hewes, H. F.: Boston Med. & Surg. J., *131*, 515, 1894.

20*a*. Holmes, K. K., Gutman, L. T., Belding, M. E. and Turck, M.: New Engl. J. Med., *284*, 318, 1971.

21. Irons, E. E.: Arch. Intern. Med., *4*, 601, 1909.
22. Keefer, C. S. and Myers, W. K.: Ann. Intern. Med., *8*, 581, 1934.
23. Keefer, C. S., Parker, F. and Myers, W. K.: Arch. Path., *18*, 199, 1934.
24. Keil, H.: Quart. J. Med. (new series), *7*, 1, 1938.
25. Keiser, H., Ruben, F., Wolinksy, E. and Kushner, I.: New Engl. J. Med., *279*, 234, 1968.
26. Kellog, D. S., Jr., Cohen, I. R., Norins, L. C., Schroeter, A. L. and Reising, G.: J. Bact., *96*, 596, 1968.
27. Kellog, D. S., Jr., Peacock, W. L., Jr., Deacon, W. E., Brown, L. and Pirkle, C. I.: J. Bact., *85*, 1274, 1963.
28. Kersley, G. D.: Proc. Roy. Soc. Med., *35*, 653, 1942.
29. Kvorning, S. A.: Danish Med. Bull., *10*, 188, 1963.
30. Lees, D.: Lancet, *1*, 640, 1931.
31. Levin, O. L. and Silvers, S. H.: New York J. Med., *37*, 1712, 1937.
32. Margolin, E. S.: Urol. & Cutan. Rev., *47*, 512, 1943.
33. MacLennon, J. M.: Brit. Med. J., *2*, 121, 1936.

34. Myers, W. K. and Gwynn, H. B.: Med. Ann. D.C., *4*, 194, 1935.
35. Newman, A. B.: Amer. Heart J., *8*, 820, 1932–33.
36. Partain, J. O., Cathcart, E. S. and Cohen, A. S.: Ann. Rheum. Dis., *27*, 156, 1968.
37. Perry, M. W.: Amer. J. Med. Sci., *179*, 599, 1930.
38. ————: Amer. J. Med. Sci., *185*, 394, 1933.
39. Reiter, H.: Deutsche med. Wchnschr., *42*, 1535, 1916.
40. Sharp, J. T.: in *Vistas in Connective Tissue Diseases*, Bennett, J. C. (ed.), Springfield, Ill., Charles C Thomas, 1968, p. 155.
41. Sharp, J. T., Lidsky, M. D. and Riley, W. A.: Arth. & Rheum., *11*, 569, 1968.
42. Spink, W. W. and Keefer, C. S.: New Engl. J. Med., *218*, 453, 1938.
43. Stecher, R. M. and Solomon, W. M.: Amer. J. Med. Sci., *192*, 497, 1936.
44. Tayer, W. S.: Amer. J. Med. Sci., *130*, 751, 1905.
45. Tilghman, R. C. and Finland, M.: Arch. Intern. Med., *59*, 602, 1937.
46. Vandervort, W. J.: Delaware Med. J., *35*, 69, 1963.
47. Vietzeke, W. M.: Arch. Intern. Med., *117*, 270, 1966.
48. Warren, C. F., Hinton, W. A., and Bauer, W.: J.A.M.A , *108*, 1241, 1937.
49. Withington, C. F.: Boston Med. & Surg. J., *151*, 99, 1904.

Chapter 65

Reiter's Syndrome

By John T. Sharp, M.D.

The development of arthritis in male patients who had recently acquired a urethral infection was observed at least as early as the 16th century. Pierre Van Forest described a patient who developed arthritis of the knee in association with urethritis in 1507[4] and Martiniere referred to arthritis as a complication of urethritis in 1664.[13] John Hunter in 1786 described a patient who had articular symptoms with several recurrences of urethral discharge.[4] Probably the first recorded association of urethritis, arthritis and conjunctivitis was by Brodie in 1818 who reported five patients suffering from this triad of clinical manifestations.[3] Almost a century later, Hans Reiter described a patient who developed non-gonococcal urethritis, conjunctivitis and arthritis following an episode of bloody diarrhea.[38] In the same year, 1916 Fiessinger and LeRoy described four cases of mild diarrhea associated with a conjunctivo-urethro-synovial syndrome.[16] In 1942 Bauer and Engleman described the first case in the American literature and noted the previous report by Reiter.[1] Since that time, the association of non-gonoccocal urethritis, arthritis and conjunctivitis generally has been referred to as Reiter's syndrome.

Some observers have proposed that the condition is a distinct disease and have suggested that patients manifesting only non-specific urethritis and arthritis suffer from the same illness. This view has gained sufficiently wide acceptance in recent years so that a majority of reports in the English language now use the term Reiter's syndrome to connote arthritis occurring as a complication of non-gonococcal urethritis. There is much logic to this view but as yet no proof for it. Extensive comparisons have not been made between patients manifesting the complete triad, and those with only urethritis and arthritis. Moreover, the identity of the two groups has not been established. Until the etiology (or etiologies) of Reiter's syndrome is discovered this question cannot be finally settled.

The main advantage to considering patients manifesting only urethritis with arthritis as having the same disease as those with the complete Reiter's triad is that a larger number of cases can be collected and studied in a short time. The main disadvantage is the greater likelihood that urethritis alone may occur coincidentally with established types of arthritis such as rheumatoid arthritis or ankylosing spondylitis, whereas those cases manifesting the complete triad appear to represent a distinct entity.

In preparing this chapter the term "Reiter's syndrome" is used to refer to those patients with the clinical triad of non-gonococcal urethritis, arthritis and conjunctivitis. It is believed that some, perhaps many, of those patients who have only arthritis and urethritis have the same illness but currently available clinical and laboratory tests cannot distinguish such cases from those due to other causes.

Epidemiology

The exact frequency of the condition is not known. During the past three decades several large series of cases have been reported indicating that Reiter's syndrome is not rare. It is believed to be more common in the military personnel and particularly in those stationed away from home. Noer stated that approximately four cases per 100,000 men per year were seen in the U. S. Navy personnel over a ten-year period.[34]

Since the cause of Reiter's syndrome is unknown, our concept of the mode of transmission is derived from circumstantial evidence. It is a remarkable fact that Reiter's syndrome apparently can be transmitted either in association with epidemic dysentery[34,36,54] or by sexual intercourse.[7,22] In most sporadic cases urethritis is the initial manifestation of illness and most of these patients give a history of an extramarital sexual relationship shortly preceding onset of the urethritis. These cases suggest that an infectious agent transmitted by sexual intercourse is the cause of Reiter's syndrome. But this does not account for all the patients with Reiter's syndrome. Several large epidemics of dysentery have been followed by outbreaks of arthritis associated with urethritis and conjunctivitis. In these patients the temporal association with the dysentery suggests a specific relationship of Reiter's syndrome to the episode of diarrhea.

Most cases of the complete triad that follow a sexual contact occur in men. The association of arthritis, conjunctivitis and cystitis in women has been proposed as the counterpart of Reiter's syndrome in the female, but there is no agreement on this point and the condition is only occasionally observed.

Among the post-dysenteric cases women frequently have been affected[36] and children occasionally have been reported as having Reiter's syndrome.[55]

Clinical Manifestations

Reiter's syndrome is defined as the association of non-bacterial urethritis, arthritis and conjunctivitis. Most patients have fever. A modest weight loss occurs in many patients and may be extensive in some. Dysentery is prominent in many patients. Skin lesions and mucous membrane involvement occur in a majority of instances. In addition to conjunctivitis ocular involvement may include keratitis, iritis, retinitis and optic neuritis. Complications in the genitourinary tract include hemorrhagic cystitis, prostatitis and hydronephrosis. Lymphadenopathy, splenomegaly and pericarditis are occasionally seen. Neurological and pulmonary involvement have been reported but their specificity is uncertain.

Articular Involvement

Articular involvement usually is the second or third feature of the illness with urethritis, diarrhea or conjunctivitis or a combination of these features preceding the synovitis. Arthritis is more frequent in the large joints but toes and fingers are commonly involved. The weight-bearing joints are affected more frequently than those of the upper extremities. Arthritis is usually polyarticular but the number of joints involved is quite variable. Involvement is usually not symmetrical. Arthritis may be mild with minimal objective signs of synovitis or severe with marked swelling, redness, heat and pain. During the early phase of illness, synovitis may develop in new articulations every few days. In many patients an initial period of polyarthritis is followed by more persistent inflammation in only a few joints for several weeks or longer. Back pain occurs in a few patients during the acute illness.

Genitourinary Tract Involvement

Urethral discharge is the characteristic feature of genitourinary tract involvement. In most patients the discharge is mucopurulent or mucoid. Dysuria may accompany the discharge but, in some instances, urethritis is nearly asymptomatic. In those patients who give a history of an extramarital sexual relationship the interval from intercourse until onset of urethritis varies from a few days to approximately a month.[7,22,52]

Prostatitis is frequently present in addition to urethritis.[52] The prostatic gland is enlarged, soft and tender, and the prostatic secretions contain large numbers of pus cells. Prostatic abscesses occasionally develop.[6]

Hemorrhagic cystitis is a frequently observed complication.[22,52] In these cases dysuria, frequency and suprapubic pain are present and examination of the urine reveals pyuria and gross or microscopic hematuria. Cystoscopic examination reveals edema, superficial ulceration and petechial hemorrhages. Reduction in bladder capacity may be marked. Colby[6] and Hall and Finegold[22] reported hydronephrosis in several cases, a complication which may result from obstruction of the ureters due to edema in the bladder wall.

Ocular Involvement

Conjunctivitis is the first manifestation of involvement of the eye in most cases. Usually the inflammation is mild and accompanied only by a slight burning sensation and some adhesiveness of the lids in the morning. In some instances the conjunctivitis is unilateral although in most cases both eyes are involved. Iritis develops in 5 to 10 per cent of patients during their first attack and has been reported to occur in from 20 to 50 per cent of patients when long-term follow-up is carried out, taking into account multiple attacks in many patients.[7,22,23,52] Zewi reported the frequent occurrence of keratitis and described optic neuritis in two cases of incomplete Reiter's triad.[55] Both of these cases were associated with diarrhea. Retinitis and macular edema have been described.[31]

Skin and Mucous Membrane Involvement

Superficial ulcers on the penis, particularly around the urethral meatus, are commonly observed. Coalescence of lesions on the glans may give rise to a circular or scalloped border which is called balanitis circinata (Fig. 65–1).

Small, painless superficial ulcers with an erythrematous base are frequently seen on the buccal mucosa and the tongue.[32] The lesions vary from a few millimeters in diameter to more than a centimeter. Patients are often unaware of their presence.

Involvement of the skin is most commonly seen on the palms of the hands and the soles of the feet but may occur

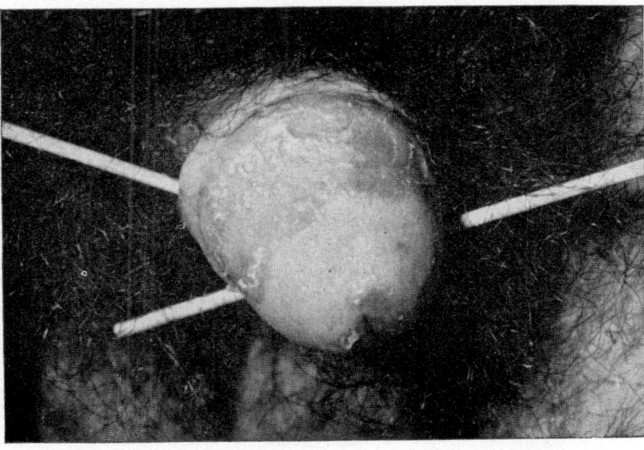

Fig. 65–1.—Circinate lesions on glans penis (balanitis circinata) in a patient with Reiter's syndrome. Note also ulceration around meatus.

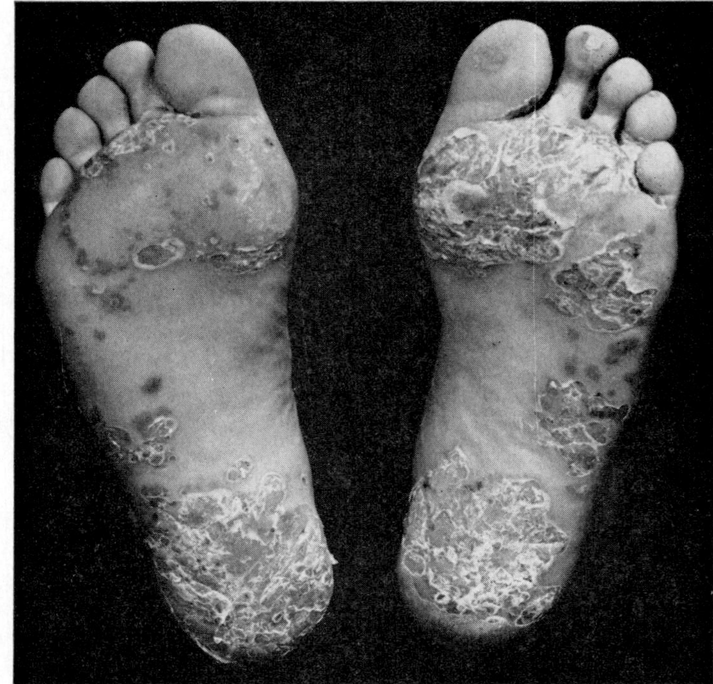

Fig. 65–2.—Keratodermia blennorrhagica of feet in a patient with Reiter's syndrome.

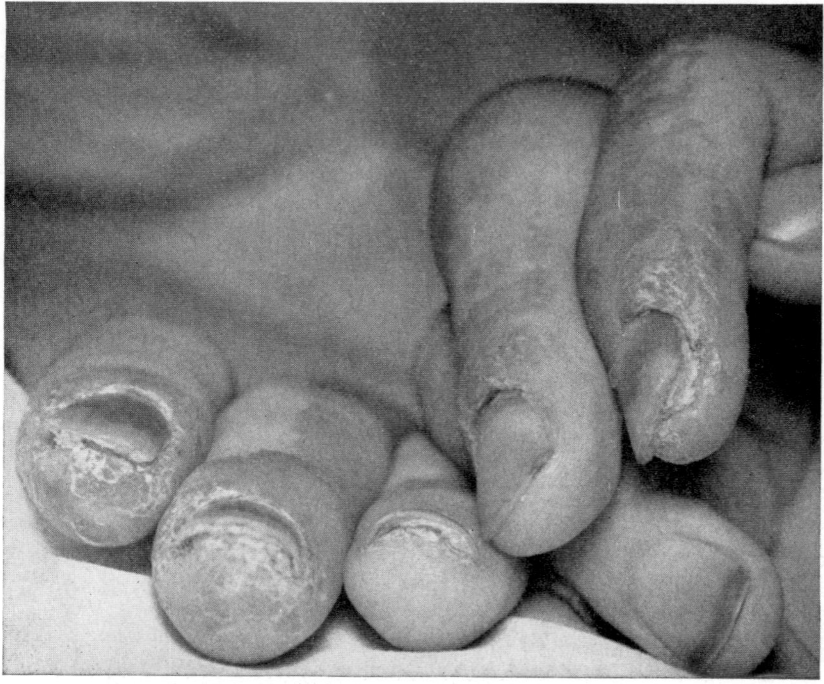

Fig. 65–3.—Keratotic lesions of fingernails in a patient with Reiter's syndrome.

anywhere on the extremities, trunk or scalp. The initial skin lesion is a small papule which rapidly develops a pustular appearance, but when opened this lesion contains only keratotic material. Individual lesions are a few millimeters in diameter but when large numbers are present they may become confluent so that a large area is covered by a thick keratotic crust (Fig. 65–2). Eventually the crust peels from the underlying skin and when it does it leaves no scar. Keratosis also occurs under the finger- and toenails and may lead to separation of the nails from the nail beds (Fig. 65–3).

These skin lesions which are referred to as keratodermia blennorrhagica usually develop several weeks after onset of other manifestations of the Reiter's syndrome. The skin lesions are self-limiting but usually last for several weeks. Lesions on the skin are less common than mucous membrane lesions and frequently occur in patients who already have lesions on the genitalia or in the oral cavity. Histologically, lesions are the same on the skin and mucous membranes but the constant moisture on the mucous membrane prevents the keratosis so that the characteristic crusts do not form.[26]

Gastrointestinal Involvement

Gastrointestinal involvement is manifested by diarrhea, which may be quite mild and brief or severe and prolonged. Occasionally the diarrhea is bloody. Diarrhea usually occurs one to three weeks before onset of the other manifestations of the illness but may follow other features of the syndrome.

Epidemic dysentery has been associated with Reiter's syndrome in several instances. The most widely studied epidemic, due to infection with *Shigella flexneri*, was estimated to have involved 150,000 people.[36] Features of Reiter's syndrome were observed in 334 patients, 233 of whom had the complete triad. Epidemiologic studies have been too few to determine whether post-dysenteric arthritis is associated with specific Shigellae strains.

Cardiovascular Involvement

Pericarditis occurs infrequently in the acute stage of Reiter's syndrome. Electrocardiographic abnormalities including prolongation of the PR interval and ST- and T-wave changes may be seen but cardiomegaly and congestive failure have not been observed in the initial attacks.[12,22,36,51,52]

Valvular heart disease has been reported as an infrequent sequela (see below).

Neurologic Involvement

Peripheral neuritis has been reported in three patients but in two of these gonorrhea was present and the diagnosis of Reiter's syndrome was based on a poor response to penicillin which was considered evidence for a concomitant non-specific urethritis.[35] Furthermore, in two of these cases, administration of various medications may have been related to the neurological involvement. In the third case, pain in the groin was not associated with other objective evidence of peripheral nerve involvement.

Pulmonary Involvement

Pleurisy and pneumonitis have been reported, but the rarity of such cases raises the question of whether they were instances of coincidental pulmonary infection.[20,22]

Pathology

In the early stages the histologic changes in the synovial membrane resemble a low-grade pyogenic infection.[26,52] The synovial membrane is intensely hyperemic and edematous. The inflammatory reaction is localized to the superficial, vascular zone and is characterized by a cellular infiltrate dominated by neutrophilic leukocytes and lymphocytes. Increasingly, plasma cells are frequently observed in lesions of more than two weeks' duration. Proliferation of connective tissue cells is present to a variable extent. Occasionally necrosis of the synovial cell layer is seen. Focal areas of extravasation of red blood cells are found in many cases.

Chronic arthritis of several months' duration is characterized by villous synovial hypertrophy, pannus formation and osseous erosions along the margins of the articular cartilage.[26,52] Microscopically the inflammatory lesion is non-specific, consisting of focal infiltrates of lymphocytes and plasma cells. Lymphoid nodules are observed in some cases. Foci of neutrophil infiltration also may be present. Proliferation of connective tissue cells and synovial cells is regularly present. Histologically, chronic arthritis often resembles rheumatoid arthritis.

The skin lesions are characterized by thickening of the horny layer, parakeratosis and acanthosis.[26,27,28,52] Vesicles are found in the epidermis as a result of lysis and vacuolization of the superficial prickle cells. The vesicles are filled with epithelial cells, polymorphonuclear leukocytes and lymphocytes and often resemble microabscesses. The outer layer of the corium is infiltrated with lymphocytes and plasma cells. Histologically the lesions on the mucous membranes resemble those on the skin except for the absence of keratosis.

Laboratory Findings

The white blood count is usually elevated in the range of 10,000 to 18,000 cells per cubic millimeter but occasionally leukocytosis exceeds 20,000 and, in some instances, elevations are not observed. Anemia may develop in patients who have a prolonged course but is usually not present early in the illness. The sedimentation rate is regularly elevated and usually returns to normal as the patient recovers from the acute attack. The urethral discharge contains numerous white blood cells, most of which are polymorphonuclear cells. Pyuria is regularly present and hematuria occurs in many patients.

The synovial fluid is turbid to a variable degree. In most instances the joint fluid has a grossly purulent appearance. White blood cells in the synovial fluid usually have numbered from 2,000 to 50,000 per cubic millimeter, but occasionally, larger numbers of cells are seen, even above 100,000 per cubic millimeter. The majority of the white blood cells are polymorphonuclear leukocytes in the early, acute effusions, but their proportion falls as the inflammatory reaction subsides and lymphocytes may become the predominant cells. The joint fluid sugar is usually normal but may be reduced, particularly when the leukocyte count is especially high. Joint fluid pH, pO_2 and pCO_2 have not been reported.

Joint fluid complement is higher than is usually found in other types of effusions but total synovial fluid protein is also high and the complement-protein ratio is similar to that observed with degenerative joint disease and traumatic arthritis, and contrasts with the reduction found in rheumatoid arthritis.[19,37]

Cultures of the urethral and prostatic secretions are negative for gonococci and the blood and synovial fluid are sterile. The conjunctival exudate is sterile or contains only non-pathogenic organisms. Some authors have claimed they could distinguish cases of mixed infection—namely, gonococcal urethritis and non-specific urethritis coexisting in the same patient—by the type of response to penicillin therapy. Although most patients with gonorrhea respond rapidly and are completely free of the urethral discharge within several days after initiating appropriate therapy, the variability in response makes it hazardous to conclude that a mixed infection is present unless the urethral discharge persists unabated for a prolonged period.

One observer reported finding inclusion bodies in epithelial cells obtained by urethral scrapings[49] but others have failed to confirm this observation[52] and inclusion bodies have not been seen in synovial cells.

Gonococcal and bedsonia antibodies are present in about the same frequency as in a population of venereal disease clinic patients.[25,46]

Stool cultures usually are negative for enteric pathogens in the sporadic cases, even when diarrhea has been present. In those patients in whom Reiter's syndrome has followed a dysentery epidemic, the results of stool cultures reflect the carrier rates for the interval from onset of diarrhea until cultures are obtained.[36,54]

Radiologic Changes

In the first few weeks of involvement, x-ray examination of the joints is within normal limits and milder cases may never exhibit radiologic abnormalities. Osteoporosis in areas of articular inflammation is the earliest roentgenographic change observed, and is commonly seen in patients who have been ill for two months or longer.[24] Osteoporosis has been seen as early as three weeks after onset in severe cases.[52] Erosions in the small joints of the phalanges are found when the acute attack persists for several weeks or longer.[22,24,33,52,53]

Hollander observed periosteal proliferation near involved joints in three of 25 cases of Reiter's syndrome,[24] a finding that is now recognized as a frequent feature of the condition[22,30,33,52,53] (Fig. 65-4). In a review of the x-ray changes of patients with Reiter's syndrome, periostitis was found in the os calcis, ankles, metatarsals, phalanges of the feet and hands, the knees and elbows.[53] Periostitis of the os calcis presenting as a diffuse, fluffy outline on and anterior to the plantar surface of the calcaneal tuberosity is thought to be rather characteristic though not diagnostic, of Reiter's syndrome.

Mason *et al.* compared the radiologic changes in 59 patients with either the complete or incomplete Reiter's triad to 86 patients with rheumatoid arthritis and 54 with ankylosing spondylitis.[30] Periosteal new bone formation on the malleoli occurred with equal frequency in patients with rheumatoid arthritis and Reiter's syndrome but less frequently in those with ankylosing spondylitis. However, periostitis on the plantar surface of the os calcis was observed in 20 per cent of the patients with Reiter's syndrome, but only in 4 per cent of those with rheumatoid arthritis and 5 per cent of those with ankylosing spondylitis.

Course of the Acute Illness

The clinical features of the syndrome may appear almost simultaneously or may gradually evolve over several weeks. In many patients urethritis or diarrhea precedes the second manifestation of the illness by several days to two or three weeks. In some patients the disease evolves with the development of a new manifestation at irregular intervals for weeks or months. The majority of patients recover from the initial episode within three or four months but some patients have a prolonged illness and follow a chronic course from the initial onset.

Careful follow-up has established that recurrences are especially common and probably a majority of patients have two or more attacks.[10,23,51,52] Clinical manifestations in the recurrences vary from a single feature of the illness, to the complete triad with all its complications.

Sequelae

In a few patients chronic arthritis develops during the initial illness which in these patients may persist for months or years. More often, chronic articular disease becomes apparent after several attacks. Persistent articular inflammation frequently leads to flexion contractures, limitation of motion or instability. Erosions are seen by radiologic examination in chronically involved joints and destructive changes may be seen in the small joints of the hands and feet. Bony ankylosis develops occasionally.

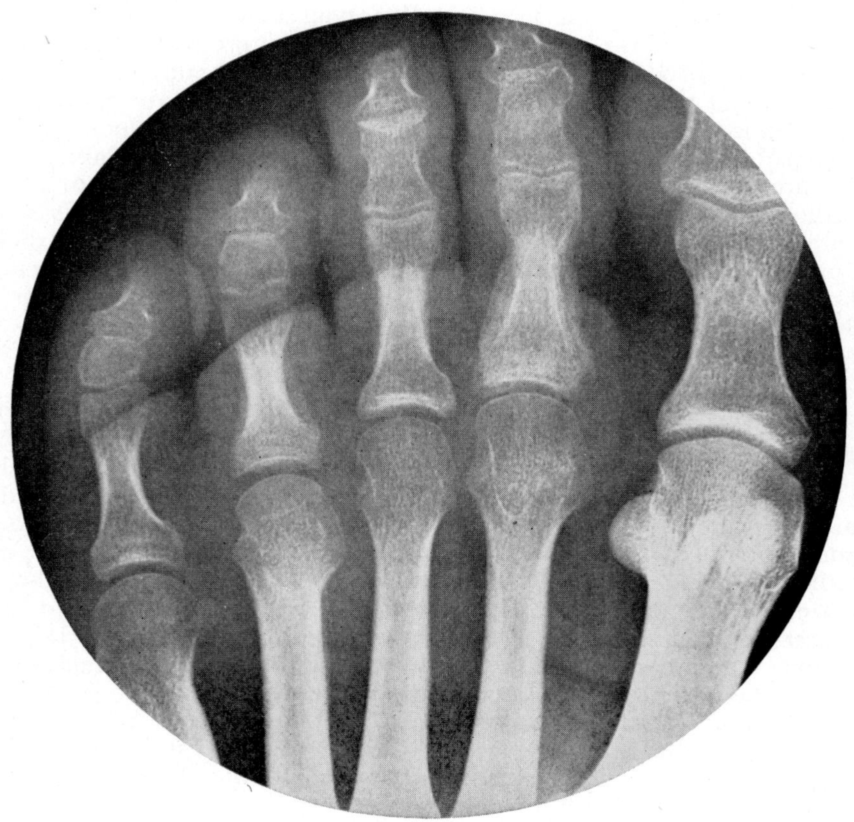

Fig. 65–4.—Radiograph of the left foot of a patient with Reiter's syndrome who had complained of pain and swelling of the foot for the preceding seven months. Periosteal new bone is visible in the shafts of the 2nd, 3rd and 4th proximal phalanges and also on the medial aspect of the distal part of the shaft of the 4th metatarsal bone.

Clinical Features Suggesting Reiter's Syndrome

Most patients are male.

Diarrhea or extramarital sexual intercourse precedes most attacks.

Patients usually febrile.

Arthritis, usually polyarticular.

Urethritis may be complicated by cystitis, prostatic abscess, or hydronephrosis.

Conjunctivitis may be complicated by keratitis, iritis, retinitis or optic neuritis.

Skin lesions include keratodermia blennorrhagica, circinate balanitis and superficial ulcerations on tongue and buccal mucosa.

EKG changes sometimes present, pericarditis infrequently seen.

Vallee in 1946 observed calcification in the lateral spinal ligament in the lower thoracic region in a patient who had had multiple recurrences of Reiter's syndrome.[51] Ford on reviewing arthritis associated with urethritis[17] and Sharp on reviewing patients with spinal disease[43] concluded that Reiter's syndrome was a cause of spondylitis. Good reported that eight of 26 cases with follow-up periods longer than two years (mean 14.5 years) had spondylitis.[21] There was progressive limitation of spinal motion in many of his patients and variable degrees of back pain were present. Radiographic abnormalities included a single syndesmophyte in one patient, extensive ankylosis of the apophyseal joints, paravertebral calcification and dense bridging. In general, patients found to have spinal disease had a longer interval from onset of Reiter's syndrome to examination, and all had bilateral radiographic changes in the sacroiliac joints. Weldon and Scalettar found lateral calcific bridging in one patient among six who had spinal films.[53]

Roentgenographic abnormalities commonly are found in the sacroiliac joints. Mason *et al.* observed bilateral changes in the sacroiliac joints in 32 per cent of 59 patients with incomplete or complete Reiter's syndrome[30] and Csonka found changes in 20 per cent of 134 patients.[8] Lovgren reported only one of 13 patients who had had either two or three attacks of Reiter's syndrome had slight changes in one sacroiliac joint.[29] However, five of 8 patients who had had more than three attacks had distinct changes in the sacroiliacs and the most pronounced changes were found in two patients who had had eight relapses. Weldon and Scalettar also observed that sacroiliac changes were usually seen in patients with multiple attacks in reporting changes in 47 per cent of 32 patients.[53] Good found bilateral changes in the sacroiliac joints in thirteen of 26 patients with the complete Reiter's syndrome whose follow-up interval was greater than two years from the initial attack.[21]

Aortic insufficiency has been attributed to Reiter's syndrome in a few instances. In 1959 Toone reported a patient with spondylitis and aortitis who had the complete Reiter's triad during one of several bouts of acute arthritis.[50] In 1960 Dixon reported another patient who had the complete triad of Reiter's syndrome preceding the development of aortic insufficiency.[15] Csonka *et al.* reported three patients with aortic insufficiency in 1961 but only one had the complete triad.[11] Rodnan attributed aortic insufficiency to Reiter's syndrome in two patients but both cases were atypical.[39] One of his patients developed keratodermia blennorrhagica, arthritis and conjunctivitis 32 years after an episode of urethritis and arthritis and three years after aortic insufficiency was first observed. Additional cases of typical Reiter's syndrome with the complete triad need to be followed closely for long intervals to define the precise relation of this condition to aortic insufficiency.

Etiology

The cause of Reiter's syndrome is unknown. At this time it is not possible to say that all cases suffering from the combination of clinical features referred to by this eponym are one disease or whether these cases incorporate two or more diseases. The unique epidemiology of this condition does require that any causative agent or pathogenetic mechanism proposed for Reiter's syndrome must take into account the apparent venereal transmission in many cases and the association with dysentery in others.

Soon after mycoplasmal species were first isolated from human beings, Dienes and others[14] reported the growth of these organisms from the urethral secretions of patients with non-gonococcal urethritis and subsequently observed mycoplasmas in the urine of patients with hemorrhagic cystitis and abacterial pyuria.[2] Subsequent studies showed mycoplasmas were common inhabitants of the genitourinary tract in asymptomatic men who lead an active sexual life and ordinary strains of mycoplasma have not been identified as the causative organism for non-gonococcal urethritis.[47] More recently Shepard[48] and Ford[18] have reported that morphologically distinct strains of mycoplasma which they refer to as "T" strains were frequently present in exudate from patients with non-specific urethritis and they have suggested that T strain mycoplasmas may be the cause of this condition. If this proves to be the case, these organisms are highly suspect as the cause of Reiter's syndrome. However, cultures of joint fluid from patients with this condition usually have failed to yield mycoplasmas.[5,45]

Schachter and his colleagues recently reported the isolation of a chlamydial* organism (psittacosis-lymphogranuloma venereum-trachoma group) from ten of 23 patients with Reiter's syndrome.[40,41,42] Five of these isolations were from synovial fluid or synovial membrane. The remaining strains were isolated from the urethra and conjunctiva. At present other laboratories have not confirmed the isolation of these organisms from the synovial fluid or synovial biopsy material of patients with Reiter's syndrome. Serologic studies have revealed antibodies to chlamydial group antigen in Reiter's syndrome and in patients with arthritis associated with urethritis in about the same frequency that they are found in a venereal disease clinic population, casting some doubt on the specific association of chlamydiae with Reiter's syndrome.[25,46] However, the usefulness of the serologic test has been questioned, since a high frequency of immunological responses has not been established in all known chlamydial infections. Regardless of the results of the serologic studies, the failure of other investigators to isolate chlamydiae from joint fluid or biopsy specimens of patients with Reiter's syndrome raises serious doubt that these organisms are the sole cause of this disease. It may be that Reiter's syndrome is due to multiple causes and Schachter may have studied a cluster of cases due to chlamydiae, thus accounting for his isolations. On the other hand, the isolated organisms may have been innocent passengers unrelated to the disease or may have been secondary invaders.

* This group was formerly known as Bedsonia.

Differential Diagnosis

If one adheres to the principle that the condition that we are discussing is a syndrome there is little difficulty in making the diagnosis. To have Reiter's syndrome, a patient must have non-gonococcal urethritis, arthritis and conjunctivitis. Further, these three manifestations of disease must be present during the same episode of illness, although not all three have to be present simultaneously. Historically, Reiter's case had diarrhea but in practice the triad has been accepted as the essential feature of the syndrome and the presence of diarrhea has not been required in the diagnosis of Reiter's syndrome.

Strict adherence to the original triad in defining Reiter's syndrome ignores the possibility that at least some patients who have only non-specific urethritis and arthritis, or who have post-dysenteric arthritis suffer from the same disease. However, until a specific etiologic agent is found, questions regarding the relationship of the incomplete cases to those with the complete triad cannot be answered.

Even lacking such information, the presence of characteristic skin lesions, namely keratodermia blennorrhagica, in combination with non-specific urethritis and arthritis, or dysentery and abacterial arthritis, provides strong evidence for a diagnosis of Reiter's syndrome. At one time keratodermia blennorrhagica was considered to be a complication of gonococcal urethritis. More recently this usually distinctive skin lesion was recognized as a component of Reiter's syndrome, and there is doubt as to whether it is ever caused by gonococci. A review of bacteriologic studies on keratodermia blennorrhagica from the early 1920's revealed that several authors found gram-negative diplococci in smears of skin lesions but cultures of these lesions were uniformly negative except for a single report.[44] Since smears of tissue granules and dead organisms commonly present on the skin are readily stained by safranin and therefore easily confused with gonococci, overwhelming evidence supports the view that keratodermia blennorrhagica is not a complication of gonococcal infection, but is specifically related to Reiter's syndrome (*see* also Chapter 64).

At present the more important diagnostic consideration is the distinction between keratodermia blennorrhagica and pustular psoriasis. Histologically the two lesions appear to be identical.[26,27,28] Clinically, patients who have the other components of Reiter's syndrome and in addition have prominent lesions on the soles of the feet and the palms of the hands, and, often in other areas of the body, are considered to have keratodermia blennorrhagica. In some cases the urethritis is transient or overlooked by the patient and conjunctivitis may be absent. In these cases, a distinction between Reiter's syndrome and psoriatic arthropathy is difficult and at times impossible (*see also* Chapter 42).

Some authors have proposed that nonspecific urethritis may occur in combination with gonococcal urethritis and have suggested that arthritis with sterile joint fluid occurring in association with gonorrhea is in fact an incomplete form of Reiter's syndrome. None of the available tests permits a clear distinction between gonococcal arthritis with sterile joint fluid cultures and Reiter's syndrome.[46] Although response to therapy in gonococcal arthritis is usually fairly prompt, some bacteriologically proven cases improve slowly, so that persistence of articular symptoms cannot be taken alone as disproving a gonococcal origin. Conversely, some patients with Reiter's syndrome have relatively brief episodes of illness, so that improvement while receiving appropriate antibotic therapy might occur as a coincidence.

Patients with Reiter's syndrome who develop chronic arthritis, must be differentiated from peripheral rheumatoid arthritis or ankylosing spondylitis depending on the site of their major involvement. If the patient is not seen during an exacerbation of the complete Reiter's triad, or if the history concerning the triad is not actively sought by the physician or clearly remembered by the patient, it may not be possible to make a straightforward diagnosis. Since rheumatoid arthritis and ankylosing spondylitis are fairly common illnesses it is also likely that these conditions occasionally will be seen coincidentally in patients who give a history of having had urethritis. The typical symmetrical small joint involvement of peripheral rheumatoid arthritis usually includes a larger number of joints than those seen in Reiter's syndrome. Subcutaneous nodules are highly specific for peripheral rheumatoid arthritis and do not occur in Reiter's syndrome. Rheumatoid factor is seen infrequently in Reiter's syndrome, probably no more often than in a control population matched for age. (*See also* Chapter 25.)

Ankylosing spondylitis usually involves a larger area of the spine than does Reiter's syndrome and involvement is more symmetrical. Localized syndesmophytes bridging one or two intervertebral spaces are seen in Reiter's syndrome after multiple attacks and long duration of illness but calcification of the anterior spinal ligament over a long course is more common in ankylosing spondylitis. Involvement of peripheral small joints may be more frequent in Reiter's syndrome than in ankylosing spondylitis. (*See also* Chapter 41.)

Behçet's disease is characterized by a variety of skin lesions, iritis, arthralgias and arthritis, thrombophlebitis, and neurologic abnormalities. Skin lesions include papules, pustules, folliculitis, cellulitis and ulcers. Oral mucous membrane ulcers and genital pustules, vesicles and ulcers are common. The absence of urethritis and the character of the eruption distinguish Behçet's disease from Reiter's syndrome. (*See also* Chapter 45.)

Treatment

There is no specific treatment for Reiter's syndrome. Salicylate is usually given for moderate discomfort and fever and usually provides some benefit. The addition of 100 to 150 mg of indomethacin, or 100 to 200 mg. of phenylbutazone, per day appears to provide further relief of pain and discomfort in many patients. In most cases these drugs, combined with either complete bed rest or very limited weight-bearing, prove to be adequate and the disease subsides in two to sixteen weeks. Recently the use of antimetabolic and cytotoxic drugs has been proposed for this condition. Since many patients suffering from Reiter's syndrome are young men who are still in the reproductive age, and since the vast majority of patients recover completely after a brief period of acute illness, these highly dangerous drugs are *not* recommended for general use. In those patients who have especially severe and prolonged episodes of Reiter's syndrome and are developing permanent residuals, the use of antimetabolic and cytotoxic drugs might be considered, provided that the patients are fully informed of the potentially serious side effects of such treatment. Even in these situations one would prefer not to use these drugs unless the patient is beyond the reproductive age. Methotrexate, 6-mercaptopurine, azathioprine and cyclophosphamide all appear to be capable of suppressing the manifestations of Reiter's syndrome in doses that are tolerable but the margin of safety in their use is limited and serious reactions including death may occur with any of these drugs. (*See also* Chapter 33.)

Some have advocated the use of antibiotics in treatment of Reiter's syndrome. I have seen no benefit from antibiotic treatment and do not use such treatment except in the early stages of illness in those cases in whom gonococcal arthritis cannot be excluded. In those instances usually penicillin therapy has been given for seven to fourteen days.

BIBLIOGRAPHY

1. Bauer, W. and Engleman, E. P.: Trans. Assoc. Amer. Phys., *57*, 307, 1942.
2. Berg, R. L., Weinberger, H. W. and Dienes, L.: Amer. J. Med., *22*, 848, 1957.
3. Brodie, B. C.: *Pathologic and Surgical Observations on Diseases of Joints*, London, Longman, 1818.
4. Burbacher, C. R. and Weiland, A. H.: J. Florida Med. Assoc., *24*, 433, 1938.
5. Claus, G., McEwen, C., Brunner, T. and Tsamparlis, G.: Brit. J. Vener. Dis., *40*, 170, 1964.
6. Colby, F. H.: J. Urol., *52*, 415, 1944.
7. Csonka, G. W.: Brit. Med. J., *1*, 1088, 1958.
8. ———: Brit. J. Vener. Dis., *35*, 77, 1959.
9. ———: Brit. J. Vener. Dis., *35*, 84, 1959.
10. ———: Arth. & Rheum., *3*, 164, 1960.
11. Csonka, G. W., Litchfield, J. W., Oates, J. K. and Wilcox, R. R.: Brit. Med. J., *1*, 243, 1961.
12. Csonka, G. W. and Oates, J. K.: Brit. Med. J., *1*, 866, 1957.
13. Culp, O. S.: J. Urol., *43*, 737, 1940.
14. Dienes, L., Ropes, M. W., Smith, W. E., Madoff, S. and Bauer, W.: New Engl. J. Med., *238*, 509; 563, 1948.
15. Dixon, A. St. J.: Ann. Rheum. Dis., *19*, 209, 1960.
16. Fiessinger, N. and LeRoy, E.: Bull. et mém. Soc. med. d. hop. de Paris, *40*, 2030, 1916.
17. Ford, D. K.: Ann. Rheum. Dis., *12*, 177, 1953.
18. Ford, D. K., Rasmussen, G. and Minken, J.: Brit. J. Vener. Dis., *38*, 22, 1962.
19. Fostiropoulos, G., Austen, K. F., and Bloch, H. J.: Arth. & Rheum., *8*, 219, 1965.
20. Gatter, R. A. and Moskowitz, R. W.: Dis. Chest, *42*, 433, 1962.
21. Good, A. E.: Ann. Intern. Med., *57*, 44, 1962.
22. Hall, W. H. and Finegold, S.: Ann. Intern. Med., *38*, 533, 1953.
23. Hancock, J. A. H.: Brit. J. Vener. Dis., *36*, 36, 1960.
24. Hollander, J. L., Fogarty, C. W., Jr., Abrams, N. R. and Kydd, D. M.: J.A.M.A., *129*, 593, 1945.
25. Kinsella, T. D., Norton, W. L. and Ziff, M.: Ann. Rheum. Dis., *27*, 241, 1968.
26. Kulka, J. P.: Arth. & Rheum., *5*, 195, 1962.

27. Lever, W. F.: *Histopathology of the Skin*, Philadelphia, J. B. Lippincott Co., 1961, p. 127.
28. Lever, W. F. and Crawford, G. M.: Arch. Dermatol. & Syphilol., *49*, 389, 1944.
29. Lovgren, O.: Acta Rheum. Scandinav., *2*, 11, 1956.
30. Mason, R. M., Murray, R. S., Oates, J. K. and Young, A. C.: J. Bone Joint Surg., *41B*, 137, 1959.
31. Mattsson, R.: Acta Ophthalmol., *33*, 403, 1955.
32. Montgomery, M. M., Poske, R. M., Barton, E. M., Foxworthy, D. T. and Baker, L. A.: Ann. Intern. Med., *51*, 99, 1959.
33. Murray, R. S., Oates, J. K. and Young, A. C.: J. Fac. Radiol., (Bristol, England), *9*, 37, 1958.
34. Noer, H. R.: J.A.M.A., *197*, 693, 1966.
35. Oates, J. K. and Hancock, J. A. H.: Amer. J. Med. Sci., *238*, 79, 1959.
36. Paronen, I.: Acta med. scandinav. (Suppl. 212), *131*, 1, 1948.
37. Pekin, T. J., Jr. and Zvaifler, N. J.: J. Clin. Invest., *43*, 1372, 1964.
38. Reiter, H.: Deutsche med. Wchnschr., *42*, 1435, 1916.
39. Rodnan, G. P., Benedek, T. G., Shaver, J. A. and Fennell, R. H., Jr.: J.A.M.A., *189*, 889, 1964.
40. Schachter, J.: Amer. J. Ophthalmol., *63*, 1082, 1967.
41. Schachter, J., Barnes, M. G., Jones, J. P., Jr., Engleman, E. P. and Meyer, K. F.: Proc. Soc. Exp. Biol. Med., *122*, 283, 1966.
42. Schachter, J., Barnes, M. G., Jones, J. P., Jr., Engleman, E. P. and Meyer, K. F.: Pan Amer. Cong. (abstract), #130, 1967.
43. Sharp, J.: Brit. Med. J., *1*, 975, 1957.
44. Sharp, J. T.: in *Vistas in Connective Tissue Diseases*, Bennett, J. C. (ed.), Springefild, Ill., Charles C Thomas, 1968, p. 155.
45. ———: Arth. & Rheum., *13*, 263, 1970.
46. Sharp, J. T., Lidsky, M. D. and Riley, W. A.: Arth. & Rheum., *11*, 569, 1968.
47. Shepard, M. C.: Amer. J. Syphil., Gonorrhea, & Vener. Dis., *38*, 113, 1954.
48. Shepard, M. C., Alexander, C. E., Lunceford, C. D. and Campbell, P. E.: J.A.M.A., *188*, 729, 1964.
49. Siboulet, A. and Galisten, P.: Brit. J. Vener. Dis., *38*, 209, 1962.
50. Toone, E. C., Jr., Pierce, E. L. and Hennigar, G. R.: Amer. J. Med., *26*, 255, 1959.
51. Vallee, B. L.: Arch. Intern. Med., *77*, 295, 1946.
52. Weinberger, H. W., Ropes, M. W., Kulka J. P. and Bauer, W.: Medicine, *41*, 35, 1962
53. Weldon, W. V. and Scalettar, R.: Amer J. Roentgen., *86*, 344, 1961.
54. Young, R. H. and McEwen, E. G.: J.A.M.A., *134*, 1456, 1947.
55. Zewi, M.: Acta Ophthalmol., *25*, 47, 1947.

Chapter 66

Tuberculous Arthritis

By Glenn M. Clark, M.D.

Tuberculous arthritis is one of the most serious diseases of the articular tissues. Because of the declining incidence of tuberculosis and of its joint manifestations, there is a growing tendency to underestimate the importance of keeping this diagnosis in mind. In contrast to many other diseases of joints, tuberculous arthritis is curable if diagnosed and treated, but may lead to complete destruction of the joint, permanent disability, and even death if not properly treated. For these reasons, the diagnosis should be considered in any case of arthritis of unknown origin, and appropriate cultures and joint biopsy should be a mandatory part of the diagnostic workup.

The incidence of tuberculous arthritis has decreased markedly in the past few years in the United States because of preventive measures and more effective early treatment of systemic tuberculosis. An analysis of bone and joint tuberculosis in a general tuberculosis hospital, prior to the advent of chemotherapy, showed that approximately 4 per cent of patients had bone and joint lesions.[48] Comparable figures from a large sanatorium in 1970 showed an incidence of less than

The Clinical Diagnosis of Tuberculous Arthritis

1. Onset: A slow insidious development of a monoarthritis (in rare cases the initial manifestation may be a transient migratory polyarthritis).[14]
2. The Order of Frequency of Joint Involvement: The spine, hip, knee, elbow, ankle, sacroiliac, shoulder and wrist.
3. Age of Onset: Most common in first three decades but may occur at any age.
4. Frequent Associated Findings: Lesions of visceral tuberculosis, positive tuberculin test, previous history of pleural effusion, a family history of tuberculosis.
5. Constitutional Symptoms: Usually absent. There may be some fever and/or weight loss.[15]
6. Localized Symptoms: Pain, stiffness and swelling of peripheral joints. When the spine is involved, there is often pain on walking, especially when stepping off a curb. With children the initial manifestations may be a limp, or severe muscular pain at night.[16,29]
7. Physical Findings: Doughy swelling of the joints with fluid accumulation, tenderness to palpation, early and *marked localized muscular atrophy*. When the spine is involved there may be deformity on physical examination or neurologic changes varying from minimal reflex changes to the full-blown Pott's paraplegia.
8. Late in the disease there may be draining sinuses in the area of the joints.

0.5 per cent.[50] In other parts of the world tuberculosis is still epidemic and tuberculous arthritis a common disease. A recent survey of 8,020 patients attending an out-patient orthopedic clinic in India showed that 580 patients (7.2 per cent) had tuberculous arthritis.[53] In a similar clinic in the United States only 8 cases of tuberculosis of the joints were identified in 32,445 patient visits.[49] Recent evidence indicates that the introduction of effective antibiotics has been followed by a marked decrease in skeletal tuberculosis in children.[15a]

DIAGNOSIS

Tuberculous arthritis may be extremely difficult to diagnose, and there are no infallible diagnostic methods, especially in early cases. Of the 25 patients with proven musculoskeletal tuberculosis seen at the Mayo Clinic in the period 1963–1967, only 5 were referred to the clinic with a presumptive diagnosis of tuberculosis. Only 3 of the patients had active infection in other organs.[35]

Laboratory Diagnosis of Tuberculous Arthritis

1. Peripheral blood count usually normal but may show a relative increase in mononuclear cells.
2. Synovial fluid leukocytosis (may be over 100,000 cells), *marked decrease in sugar content*, tubercle bacillus by smear, culture, or guinea pig inoculation.[43]
3. *The most specific diagnostic procedure is joint biopsy and should always be performed if simpler procedures leave the diagnosis in doubt.* The biopsy of adjacent lymph nodes may also be helpful.

Roentgen Findings in Tuberculous Arthritis

Although the roentgen picture is not pathognomonic, it may be very helpful. Early in the disease the x rays may be entirely normal. However, especially in weight-bearing joints, there may be marked decalcification of the bone away from the joint surfaces.

Later there is usually evidence of some subchondral invasion with marked irregularity and eventual narrowing of the joint space.

Other features are: regional atrophy of bone; decreased density of the articular cortex; and preservation of the normal cartilage space.

Especially in more advanced disease large bilateral areas of necrosis may occur at opposing points in the bones, with detachment to form "kissing sequestra."

In far-advanced cases there is widespread destruction of bone and joint surfaces with complete disorganization of the bony architecture. The identification of soft tissue shadows representing abscess formation is also helpful.

Pathology

The pathologic changes of tuberculous arthritis have been well described by various workers.[5,21,23,39,46] Allison and Ghormley believed that all cases of joint tuberculosis should be regarded as involvement of the synovial membrane, bone and cartilage.[4]

Whether the tuberculosis is primary in the synovial membrane or in the bone, there develops *a diffuse tuberculous synovitis with a pannus of granulation tissue* which tends to spread over and to destroy the articular cartilage.[47] In those joints in which the articular cartilages are in close contact over a large area of the surface, granulation is prevented from spreading over the surface of the cartilage, but erosion occurs at the margins. In other joints in which large surfaces of the cartilages are not in apposition, the granulation tissue spreads over and erodes the cartilage.

Subchondral infiltration of granulation tissue is one of the earliest changes in tuberculosis. Subchondral granulations absorb the bony articular cortex and lower portions of the cartilage and, in some cases, result in detachment. *Because of the absence of proteolytic enzymes* in tuberculous exudates, this loosened cartilage may persist for months, but is finally destroyed.

Massive bony invasion at pressure points may occur in the knee and hip, producing large bilateral areas of necrosis. True osteophyte formation does not occur at the margin of the articular cartilage in tuberculous arthritis.

Although the tuberculous process may become quiescent, it rarely heals spontaneously. If secondary sequestra are present and infection continues, bony ankylosis almost never occurs. Fibrous ankylosis may be noted when the articular cartilage is completely destroyed.

TREATMENT

Prior to the discovery of streptomycin in 1944, the treatment of tuberculosis of the bones and joints was discouraging. The articular infection usually proceeded slowly to complete destruction of the joint. Chronically draining tuberculous sinuses were common complications, and fatal hematogenous spreading of the infection was always a possibility. Orthopedists were reluctant to enter an infected joint because operation usually resulted in spreading of the infection. Reports of early conservative management showed that approximately one-fourth of the patients died, one-fourth survived with disability, and only one-half of the patients made what was considered to be a satisfactory recovery.[18]

The fact that skeletal tuberculosis is no longer a dread disease may be attributed not only to the development of effective chemotherapeutic agents but to the fact that drug therapy has made orthopedic intervention much safer and more effective.

If the infection is recognized early, before necrosis and walling off of the process with caseation and abscess formation have developed, drug therapy, combined with the usual supportive measures of rest, splinting of the lesion, and proper diet will often result in healing.[41] On the other hand, if the pathologic characteristics of the tuberculous lesion are developed to a sufficient extent that walling off, necrosis, and caseation have occurred, control of the infection may be attained with surgical intervention.[11,38] These measures include debridement of all necrotic and caseous tissue and conversion of the abscess to a freely draining sinus with gauze packing. Surgery may be undertaken as soon as the process is stabilized under the protective cover of drug therapy and without the fear of dissemination of the infection or of the production of persistently draining sinuses. In fact, operation should be undertaken as early as possible before resistance to the drugs has a chance to develop. With early operative interference combined with adequate drug therapy, normal function and motion can be obtained in a high percentage of cases.[8,11,16] If significant destruction of the joint surfaces has taken place, complete healing may not occur without surgical fusion.[9] In non-weight-bearing joints arthrodesis may be postponed to see if conservative measures alone will heal the infection. However, in weight-bearing joints, some authors[13,31] state that arrest of the disease is most rapidly and securely attained by early solid fusion of the joint, first debrided of all caseous and necrotic tissue. Drug therapy should be continued for a minimum of one year, preferably for eighteen months and in certain cases for even longer periods.[8]

In applying modern surgery and drug therapy, valuable lessons learned in the past must not be forgotten. Tuberculous arthritis is a metastatic infection, so great care must be taken to seek the primary focus and other possible metastatic lesions. Bedrest, a nutritious diet, and immobilization of the affected joint are of prime importance in increasing the resistance of the host. The recovery from tuberculosis requires adequate forces of defense to overcome tubercle bacilli, especially under circumstances in which the organisms are in a resting state. When antimicrobial agents no longer inactivate tubercle bacilli because of organism resistance or other factors, only host resistance can control the infectious agent and prevent reactivation.

Antibiotics and Chemotherapy

Understanding of the chemotherapy of tuberculosis—what it can accomplish as well as what it cannot—requires consideration of the effect of antibacterial agents on the tubercle bacillus and the circumstances under which organisms become resistant.

At present no antimycobacterial agent or combination of agents can guarantee elimination of *all* tubercle bacilli from infected tissue even when therapy is prolonged. Tubercle bacilli that are not multiplying (resting state) may not be significantly affected by present-day chemotherapy.

Most of our knowledge regarding the chemotherapy of tuberculosis has been derived from observations of effects of drugs on pulmonary tuberculosis. In this disease sputum is readily available, and it is possible to study the effect of drugs by serial examination by smear and culture of this tissue. In tuberculous arthritis, on the other hand, there is no opportunity to evaluate the effect of drugs directly except at times of surgical procedures. However, it has seemed reasonable to assume that the information obtained from chemotherapy of pulmonary tuberculosis may be applicable to the treatment of tuberculous arthritis.

The most commonly used agents in the treatment of both pulmonary tuberculosis and tuberculous arthritis are isoniazid (INH), para-aminosalicylic acid (PAS), and streptomycin.[8,9,11,34]

Isoniazid (INH).[34]—This is the most powerful established agent available. It is effective by mouth and readily diffuses into all tissues and body fluids. It penetrates into phagocytes and can thereby attack intracellular tubercle bacilli.

The recommended dose of isoniazid is 3 to 5 mg. per kilogram of body weight per day, given in two or three divided doses. The average adult receives 300 mg. a day. It is actively metabolized in the body, the acetylated form being the chief degradation product. Acetylated isoniazid does not possess antimicrobial activity and the extent to which it is produced varies widely. Thus certain patients who are rapid inactivators of INH (isoniazid) may require larger doses.

Toxic effects which include peripheral neuritis, psychosis, and convulsions are rarely observed with doses of 3 to 5 mg. per kilogram per day. Peripheral neuritis can be prevented by the concomitant administration of 50 to 100 mg. of pyridoxine (vitamin B_6) a day. Its routine use is not recommended unless daily doses greater than 300 mg. of isoniazid are to be given.

Para-aminosalicylic Acid (PAS).[34]—This preparation is now designated aminosalicylic acid, and, although relatively ineffective when used alone, is very useful as a companion drug to prevent resistance to INH. Recent evidence suggests that the efficacy of combined isoniazid and PAS therapy may in part depend on the elevation of serum levels of biologically active (non-acetylated) isoniazid. Many preparations are available, including the free acid, potassium, sodium, calcium, and calcium benzoyl salts as well as a resin absorbed form. They are prepared as a powder, compressed tablets, buffered tablets, enteric-coated tablets, granules and cachet. A lyophilized form of PAS can be given parenterally. The oral preparations are commonly dissolved in water. PAS has a very bitter taste, and at times it is helpful to administer it in milk or in citrus fruit juice. *The dose is 12 gm. of the acid daily given in three or four divided doses.* The dosage of each salt of PAS must be adjusted to correspond to 12 gm. of the acid.

Hypersensitivity reactions with fever, rash and lymphadenopathy occur. Exfoliative dermatitis, blood dyscrasias and hepatic and renal toxicity have been noted. After prolonged use there may be thyroid enlargement with or without hypothyroidism.

Streptomycin.[34] — Streptomycin, being poorly absorbed when given by mouth, is administered intramuscularly. It diffuses readily into most body tissues including the synovial fluid. *When renal insufficiency is present, high circulating blood levels and early toxicity result because the drug is excreted mainly in the urine.* Although daily use of streptomycin alone causes clinical improvement in tuberculosis, its efficacy is short-lived because of the development of bacterial resistance. In addition, alarming toxicity to the vestibular branch of the eighth nerve occurs. The vestibular effects are manifested by vertigo, nausea, vomiting, and ataxia. The ataxia, though it may be compensated for by visual mechanism, is permanent. Small doses (0.5 to 1.0 gm. daily) produce less toxicity but organism resistance develops at the same pace as with the larger doses. Toxicity is rare with 1 gm. twice weekly but efficacy is limited and significant emergence of resistant tubercle bacilli occurs.

Hypersensitivity to streptomycin and dihydrostreptomycin is evidenced by fever, urticaria, morbilliform or scarlatiniform rash, or exfoliative dermatitis.

Other Agents.[10]—Other agents, some of which pose alarming toxic potentials, include viomycin, pyrazinamide, oxitetracycline, and cycloserine. These drugs may have limited usefulness in specialized situations of resistance and/or toxicity to other drugs.

Ethionamide, introduced in 1958, seems to be an effective substitute for PAS.

Rifampin (Rimactane) shows promise of potent antituberculous activity with minimal toxicity.

Combined Drug Therapy.—It is generally agreed that a combination of agents is preferable to single drug therapy on the basis of synergistic action and the prevention of emergence of drug-resistant bacilli. When two agents are used, some of the bacteria may be resistant to one drug and some to the other. The number of mutants that are simultaneously resistant to both drugs is usually low.

Combinations of INH with either PAS or streptomycin are commonly used. Streptomycin is more effective, but certainly more toxic, than PAS as the second agent.

Although isoniazid is potent against both intracellular and extracellular organisms, streptomycin and PAS penetrate phagocytes inadequately. The acid reaction in areas of caseation necrosis inhibits streptomycin activity. Nucleic acids bind streptomycin, rendering it inert. PAS is inactivated by para-aminobenzoic acid. Metabolic acetylation of both isoniazid and PAS abolishes antimicrobial action. PAS has a sparing action on acetylation of isoniazid which may explain the synergistic activity of the two drugs.

Some orthopedists[6] prefer "triple-drug therapy" with streptomycin as a part of the therapeutic regimen during the preoperative and postoperative periods, since this drug is most effective in preventing draining sinuses.

When the major drugs are used in combination, each is given according to the dosage of the individual agent described above. When progress is unsatisfactory or resistance develops, consideration should be given to changing combinations or to adding more drugs. It is important to perform surgery before resistance has a chance to develop. Success with whatever antibiotic management is chosen is dependent on the treatment of the patient until all evidence of disease activity has disappeared. In most cases, this takes a year or more.

TUBERCULOSIS OF THE HIP JOINT

The *primary lesions* are usually in the *neck* or *head of the femur* (Fig. 66–1); these may result in complete disappearance of the head of the femur and destruction of the acetabulum. Other important points include:[22]

Early synovial invasion.

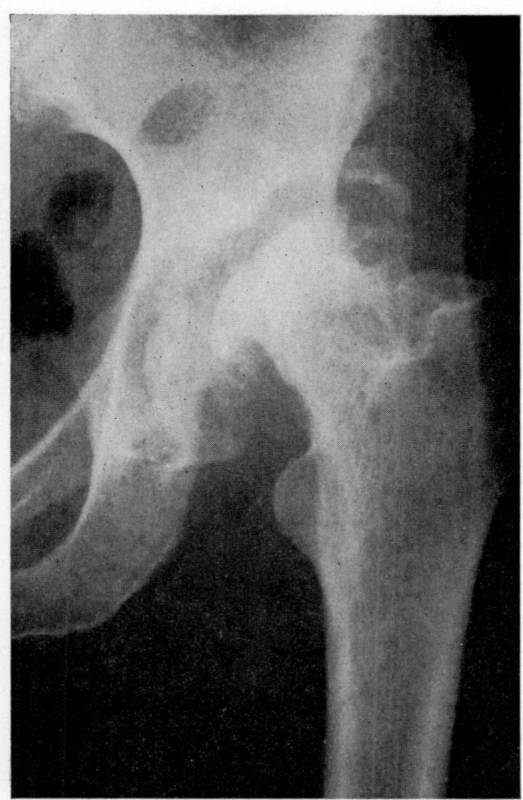

FIG. 66–1.—Far-advanced tuberculosis of the hip.

Marked rarefaction of bone with obliteration of landmarks.

Occurrence in children, in many cases, under the age of ten.

Early Symptoms

Limp, pain in the knee or thigh from pressure on the obturator and anterior crural nerves; *muscle spasm; fullness in the groin; tenderness on pressure over the hip;* slight flexion and abduction of the thigh; flattening of the buttuck and disappearance of the gluteal fold on the affected side; *limitation of all motions at the hip*, especially of rotation and abduction; at a later stage, adduction deformity of the thigh and cold abscesses or sinuses, pointing most often on the outer side of the thigh are symptoms of tuberculosis of the hip.

Treatment

If the disease is early and limited to the synovium, drug therapy combined with rest, non-weight-bearing, and leg traction may often result in arrest of the process with retention of full motion.[33] If the disease has progressed to caseation and necrosis, surgical intervention may be necessary. If the articular surfaces are intact, a radical synovectomy with removal of all necrotic and infected tissue may still preserve good joint function.[33] On the other hand, if the disease has progressed beyond the soft tissue stage and involves the bone, the joint may need fusion. Drug therapy should be continued for a minimum of one year. Cautious ambulation is started as soon as all evidence of infection has subsided. There is a tendency to encourage weight-bearing earlier than in the past.

In the past most authors have considered that the production of solid bony ankylosis gives the best results in tuberculous arthritis.[11,13,27,51,55] Recent reports have shown that with good antibiotic coverage, synovectomy and debridement produce excellent results in many cases without fusion.[58]

TUBERCULOSIS OF THE KNEE JOINT

Tuberculosis of the knee is common *in adults* (11 per cent of all tuberculous bone and joint lesions). Synovial tuberculosis progresses to bony changes in 45 per cent of cases.[45] *Tuberculous arthritis of a low grade may persist in a knee for years with very little discomfort. Local signs* include heat, swelling, deformity, stiffness, pain, limping, muscular spasm and restriction of motion. Flexion deformity of the knee and contraction of the hamstring muscles may develop. Slight jarring of the joint may produce excruciating pain.

Diagnosis of tuberculous arthritis is aided by use of synovial biopsy specimens (which may show tubercles in as high as 82 per cent of cases), and aspiration of joint fluid for cultures.

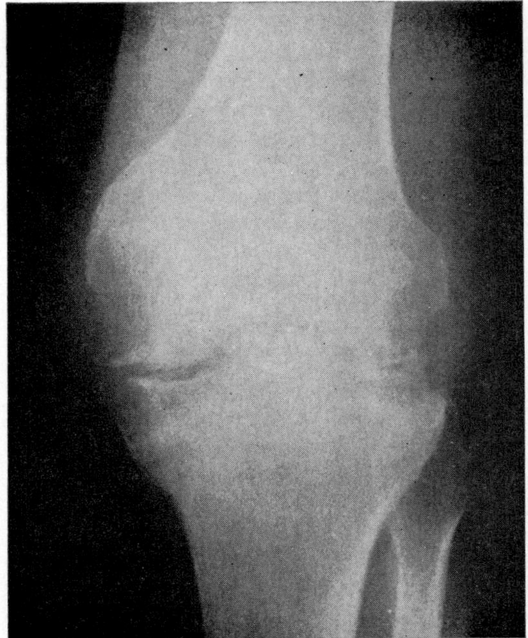

FIG. 66–2.—Early tuberculosis of the knee.

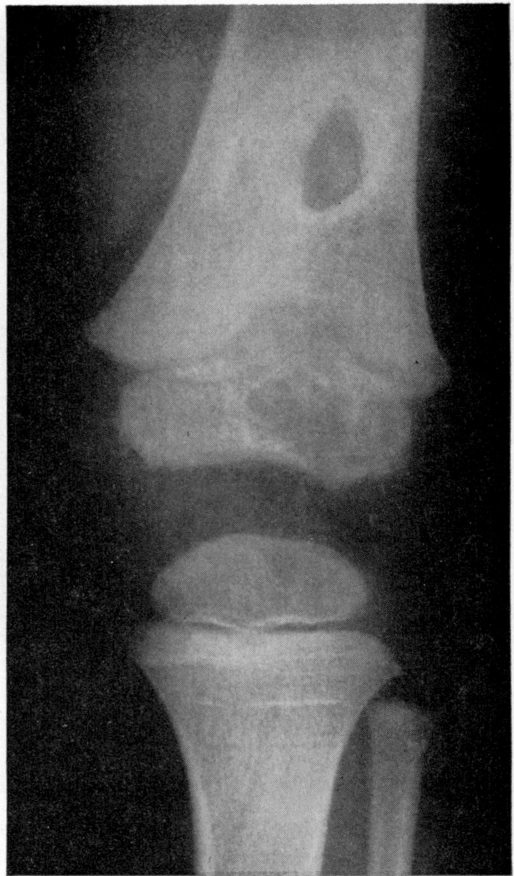

FIG. 66–3.—Tuberculosis of the knee and femur in a child.

Key summarized his findings in *adults with tuberculosis of the knee joint.*[37] *Pain* was the first symptom in 70 per cent of cases; this was usually insidious in onset. In 22 per cent of cases, *swelling* of the knee was the only initial symptom. *Stiffness* was the initial symptom in 10 per cent. Local heat was always present and there was usually *gross limitation of motion.* About 6 per cent had abscess formation.

In 87 per cent, the patient's general physical condition was good. *This disease may be confused* with rheumatoid arthritis, gonorrheal arthritis, syphilis, hemophilia, trauma and neoplasm.

Treatment

In synovial tuberculosis, especially in children and in adults without an underlying bone focus, treatment may be successful with bedrest and systemic chemotherapy.[32,33,51] If there is extensive infection of the synovium, total or partial synovectomy plus chemotherapy is often the treatment of choice. If bone and cartilage are involved, some orthopedists prefer debridement and fusion as soon as the disease is stabilized under the protective cover of dual drug therapy.[11,26,38,41,54] Drug therapy should be continued for a minimum of one year.

TUBERCULOSIS OF THE SPINE

(Pott's Disease; Tuberculous Spondylitis)

In 1940, 1 per cent of all deaths from tuberculosis in the United States were due to Pott's disease.[9] It is considered to be a local manifestation of systemic tuberculous infection.[36]

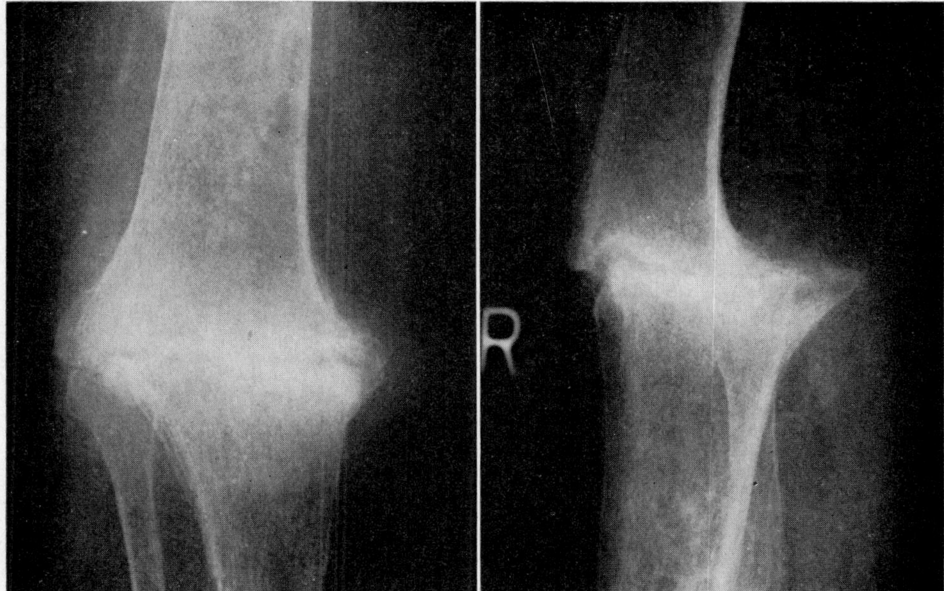

FIG. 66–4.—Far-advanced tuberculosis of the knee with nearly complete joint destruction.

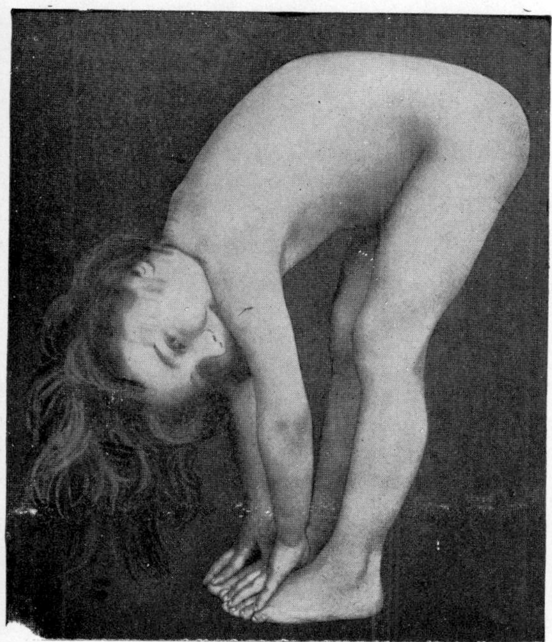

FIG. 66–5.—Incipients Pott's disease showing the break in the contour of the spine of which the normal flexibility is but slightly impaired.

The lesions occur most commonly in the bodies of the vertebrae although the intervertebral disc may be affected first.[12] The anterior border of the vertebral body is most commonly involved. A number of vertebrae (6 to 8) may be damaged. Collapse results in angulation of the spine with shortening of the trunk. Deformities are produced by caseous softening of the bodies of the vertebrae with the added pressure of weight-bearing.

Cold abscess formation and *paralysis* are the two *commonest complications.* An abscess in the cervical region may be found laterally in the neck or in the retropharyngeal space. A dorsal abscess may remain localized, or may travel along the anterior aspect of the spine forming a psoas abscess; in some cases, these point in the thigh. Psoas abscesses have been reported to be so large as to cause bulging or filling of the lower portion of the abdomen.

Symptoms and Signs

Slight *abnormalities in gait;* awkwardness in walking; listlessness.

Rigidity and upright position of the spine even when bending.

Pain and weakness in the back.

Abdominal pain (referred along the intercostal nerves); occasionally referred to the buttocks or knees.

Spinal deformity (*kyphosis*)—see Figure 66–5.

Tenderness and *muscular spasm* over the area.

Neurologic evidence of lower neuron lesions varying from muscle weakness to complete paraplegia.

Treatment

Drug therapy has greatly improved the treatment of spinal tuberculosis allowing early surgical drainage of abscesses and curettage of bony foci. Before the introduction of chemotherapy, mortality rate was 30 per cent and unstable ankylosis was common. Now practically all patients can be stabilized with drug therapy, and solid fusion obtained after surgical drainage and debridement of the diseased tissue.[3,11,20,26,27,31] Drug therapy is continued for a minimum of one year (*see* Antibiotics and Chemotherapy). Spinal fusion is still thought to be necessary by many, but may be avoided if treatment is started early.[40]

Fresh air, heliotherapy, and a high caloric diet are helpful in increasing host resistance to the tubercle bacilli and in promoting tissue healing.[42]

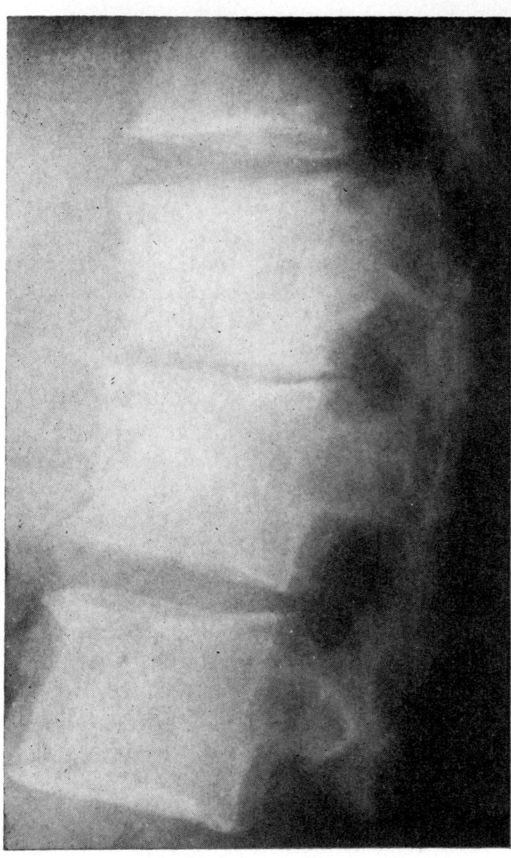

Fig. 66–6.—Early tuberculous spondylitis.

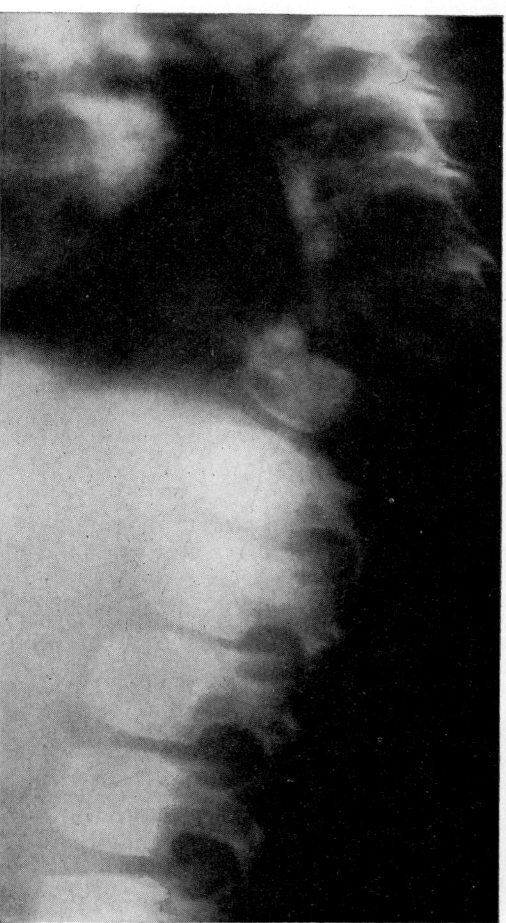

Fig. 66–7.—Tuberculous spondylitis in a child.

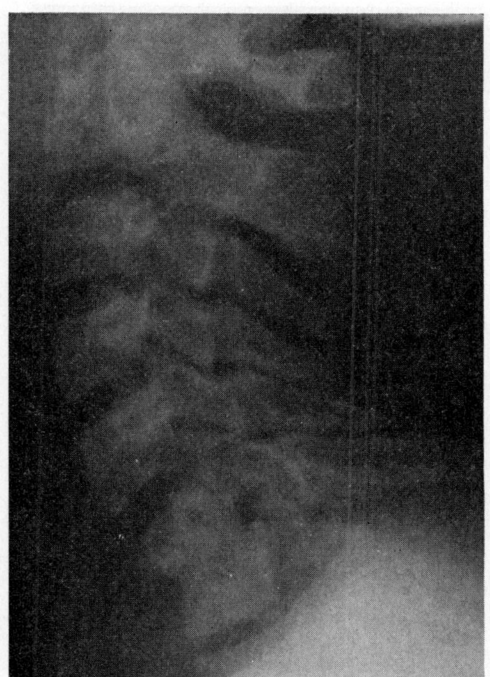

Fig. 66–8.—Tuberculosis of the cervical spine. Note collapse of C6, C7.

Ambulatory treatment may be begun only after several months of freedom from symptoms. Spinal support must always be used when the patient is up until firm fusion is obtained and all evidence of infection has subsided. A plaster jacket is best used for support when the patient is just out of bed. Later a light brace may be used for spinal support and the prevention of dangerous movements of the spine.[28]

Recent reports have indicated that many cases of tuberculosis of the spine do not require the radical surgery and prolonged immobilization still used by many orthopedists.[7,40,58] A large number of patients have been treated with oral chemotherapy, unrestricted ambulation, and surgery only to drain pointing abscesses. Although this question needs further study, the methods obtained seem comparable to those obtained with classical orthopedic treatment.

Pott's Paraplegia

Neural involvement is the most dreaded and crippling complication of spinal tuberculosis.[53] The over-all incidence in reported series ranges from 10 per cent to 30 per cent of patients with tuberculous spondylitis. Recent reports have indicated that there are a variety of reasons for paralysis, including inflammatory edema, granulation tissue, abscess formation, caseation tissue, sequestra and debris from the vertical body and discs, constriction of the cord due to narrowing of the vertebral canal, prolonged stretching of the cord or localized pressure from severe bony deformity. Tuberculosis of the cervical spine may lead to quadriparesis or quadriplegia and that of the dorsal spine to paraparesis or paraplegia.

Treatment

The introduction of chemotherapy has made surgery much safer and in some cases has made radical surgery unnecessary. When the symptoms are caused by edema or granulation tissue, chemotherapy and conservative management alone usually produce excellent results.[25,52] Abscesses and caseous tissue may require drainage and/or evacuation, but several recent reports have indicated good recovery without radical surgery. When sequestra and debris are present, operative removal is necessary, and most orthopedists recommend fusion at this time. Constriction or stretching of the cord requires operative decompression.

The principles of chemotherapy already described also apply to the medical management of tuberculous spondylitis with neurologic complications.

MISCELLANEOUS JOINTS

In non-weight-bearing joints surgical fusion, though still the surest way of arresting the disease, may be postponed while one sees if surgical debridement and a prolonged course of drug therapy plus immobilization of the joint will heal the tuberculous lesion. Partial synovectomy

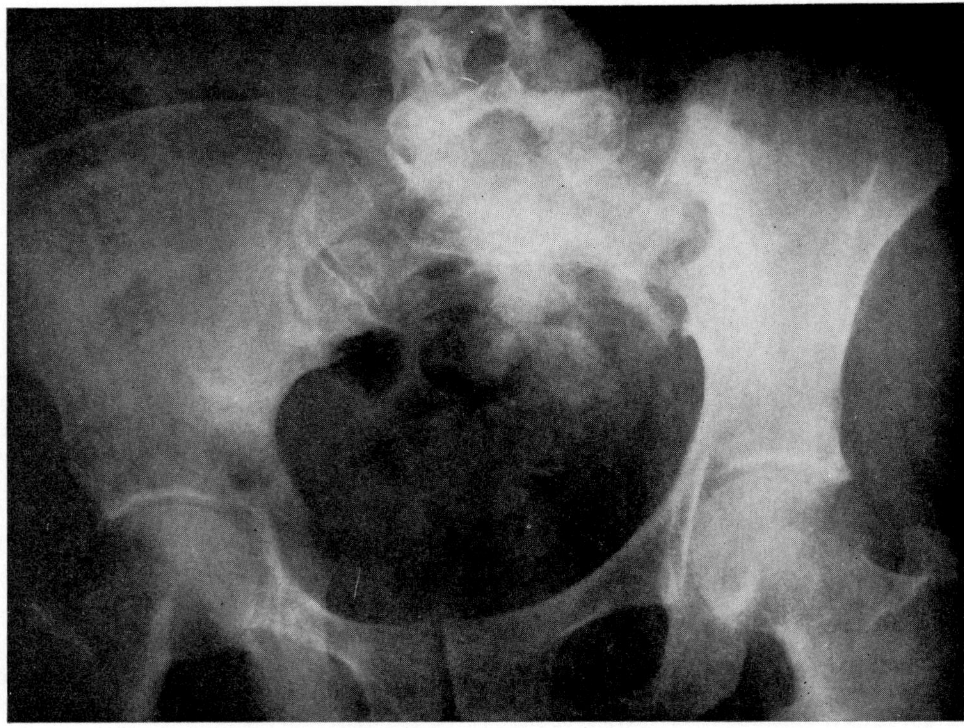

Fig. 66–9.—Unilateral tuberculous sacroiliitis.

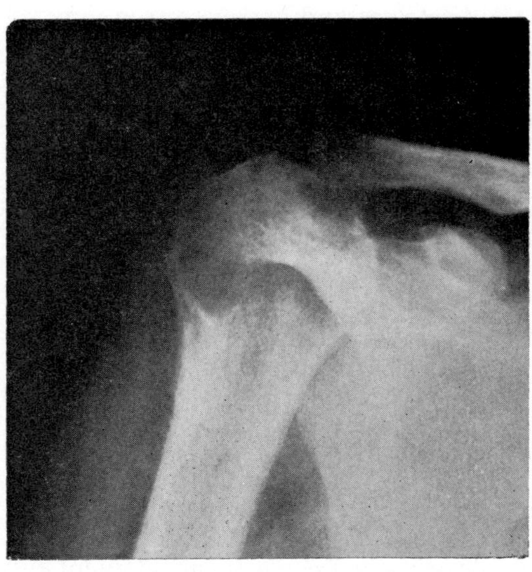

Fig. 66–10.—Tuberculosis of the shoulder. Note the atrophy of the soft tissue.

with curettage of necrotic foci have produced good results in lesions of the shoulder, elbow, wrist and ankle joint.[56] If strenuous work is not required of the individual, a pseudoarthrosis may be advisable with removal of large areas of the diseased tissue in the humerus, radius, and ulna.

Destruction of a finger joint without new bone formation in the region should be suspected as being of tuberculous origin.

Peritrochanteric bursae may be involved alone by tuberculosis.[30] Treatment is wide surgical excision under the protection of drug therapy (streptomycin and INH) which is continued for months.[26]

TUBERCULOUS TENOSYNOVITIS

This condition is rare, occurring only in 36 patients in the past forty-five years at a large general hospital.[1] The average

age incidence was thirty-six years (ranging from fifteen to seventy-five years). The right hand was involved in 22 cases (volar surface in 15, dorsal in 6, and both in 1) and the left hand in 14 cases (volar—8, dorsal—5, and both—1). None of the patients were laborers, although 30 made hard use of their hands. Thirteen of the individuals had tuberculous lesions elsewhere in the body.

The diagnosis was made by the finding of a gradually developing painless or slightly tender mass (most often on the volar aspect of the hand), with partial stiffness and inability to flex or extend the fingers completely. Grasping strength was decreased. In the later stages, finger motion occasionally produced creaking or grating due to the accumulation of rice bodies (fibrinous deposits within the tendon sheaths).

Treatment consists of rest by splinting, and if necessary, incision and drainage or resection of the involved tendon sheath. Chemotherapy should be used and continued until all evidence of activity has subsided.

BIBLIOGRAPHY

1. Adams, R., Jones, G., and Marble, H. C.: New Engl. J. Med., *223*, 706, 1940.
2. Adams, Z. B. and Decker, J. J.: J. Bone & Joint Surg., *19*, 719, 1937.
3. Allen, A. R. and Stevenson, A. W.: J. Bone & Joint Surg., *49A*, 1001, 1967.
4. Allison, N. and Ghormley, R. K.: *Diagnosis in Joint Disease*, New York, William Wood and Co., 1931.
5 Amberson, L. B., Jr.: J. Bone & Joint Surg., *22*, 807, 1940.
6. Anderson, L.: Personal communication.
7. Arct, W.: J. Bone Joint Surg., *50A*, 255, 1968.
8. Badger, T. L.: New Engl. J. Med., *261*, 30, 74, 1959.
9. Bickel, H.: Proc. Staff Meet., Mayo Clinic, *28*, 370, 1953.
10. Bowerman, E.: Personal communication.
11. Buchman, J.: Bull. Hosp. Joint Dis., *12*, 265, 1954.
12. Cave, E. F.: New Engl. J. Med., *217*, 853, 1937.
13. Chan, K. P. and Shin, J. S.: J. Bone & Joint Surg., *50A*, 1341, 1968.
14. Clark, G. M.: Tenn. State Med. J., *56*, 3, 10, 1963.
15. Cleveland, M.: Surg., Gynec. & Obst., *61*, 503, 1935.
15*a*. Davidson, P. T. and Horowitz, I.: Amer. J. Med., *48*, 77, 1970.
16. Derow, M. S. and Fisher, H.: J. Bone & Joint Surg., *24A*, 229, 1952.
17. Dickson, F. D.: J. Lab. & Clin. Med., *22*, 35, 1936.
18. Dobson, J.: J. Bone & Joint Surg., *30B*, 149, 1951.
19. Duncan, W.: Cleveland Clin. Quart., *2*, 33, 1935.
20. Fellander, M.: Acta Orthop. Scandinav. Supp. 19, 1955.
21. Fraser, J.: *Tuberculosis of the Bones and Joints in Children*, London, A. & C. Black, 1944.
22. Fripp, A. T.: J. Roy. Inst. Pub. Health & Hyg., *3*, 127, 1940.
23. Ghormley, R. K. and Deacon, A. D.: Amer. J. Roentgenol., *35*, 740, 1936.
24. Girdlestone, G. R.: *Tuberculosis of Bone and Joint*, New York, Oxford Univ. Press, 1940.
25. Guirguis, A. R.: J. Bone & Joint Surg., *49B*, 658, 1967.
26. Hald, J.: Acta Tuberc. Scandinav., *30*, 82, 1954.
27. Hallock, H. and Jones, J. B.: J. Bone & Joint Surg., *36A*, 219, 1954.
28. Harris, R. I. and Coulthard, H. S.: J. Bone & Joint Surg., *22*, 862, 1940.
29. Hency, P. S., *et al.*: Ann. Intern. Med., *11*, 1089, 1938.
30. ———: Ann. Intern. Med., *15*, 1002, 1941.
31. Hodgson, A. R. and Stock, F. E.: J. Bone & Joint Surg., *42A*, 295, 1960.
32. Houli, J. and Franca, A.: Rheumatism, *16*, 78, 1960.
33. Katayama, R., Itami, Y., and Marumo, E.: J. Bone & Joint Surg., *44A*, 897, 1962.
34. Katz, S. N.: New Engl. J. Med., *259*, 536, 732, 976, 1958.
35. Kelly, P. J. and Karlson, A. G.: Mayo Clinic Proc., *44*, 73, 1969.
36. Key, J. A.: J. Bone & Joint Surg., *22*, 799, 1940.
37. ———: Brit. Med. J., *1*, 408, 1940.
38. Kolberg, G.: Acta Orthop. Scandinav., *21*, 228, 1951.
39. Konig, F.: *Die Tuberculose der Menschlichen Gelenke, sowie der Brustwand and des Schadel* (Aug. Huschaby).
40. Konstam, P. G. and Blesosky, A.: Brit. J. Surg., *50*, 26, 1962.

41. Mackenzie, I. G.: Lancet, *1*, 652, 1954.
42. Meyerding, H. W.: J. Bone & Joint Surg., *22*, 840, 1940.
43. Mitchell, C. L. and Crawford, R. G.: J. Bone & Joint Surg., *19*, 630, 1937.
44. Murphy, J. A. and Wood, C.: J. Bone & Joint Surg., *23*, 687, 1941.
45. Murray, R. C.: Brit. Med. J., *2*, 10, 1940.
46. Nichols, E. H.: Trans. Amer. Orthop. Assn., *11*, 353, 1898.
47. Phemister, D. B.: Amer. J. Roent. & Rad. Ther., *12*, 1, 1924.
48. Rosencrantz, E., Piscitelli, A., and Bost, F. C.: J. Bone & Joint Surg., *23*, 628, 1941.
49. Statistical Report, Campbell Clinic, 1970.
50. Statistical Report, West Tenn. Chest Hospital, 1970.
51. Stevenson, F. H.: J. Bone & Joint Surg., *36A*, 5, 1954.
52. Tuli, M.: J. Bone & Joint Surg., *51A*, 680, 1969.
53. Tull, S. M., Srivastava, T. P., Varma, B. P., and Sinha, G. P.: Acta Ortho. Scandinav., *38*, 445, 1967.
54. Wilkinson, M. C.: Brit. M. Bull., *10*, 130, 1954.
55. ———: J. Bone & Joint Surg., *35B*, 209, 1953.
56. ———: J. Bone & Joint Surg., *36B*, 23, 1954.
57. ———: J. Bone & Joint Surg., *44B*, 34, 1962.
58. ———: J. Bone & Joint Surg., *51A*, 7, 1969.

Chapter 67

Syphilitic Joint Disease

By GLENN M. CLARK, M.D.

TRUE syphilitic arthritis has never been common. In large series of patients with late syphilis, it has been shown that less than 1 per cent had chronic lesions of the joints. With the decrease in the incidence of syphilis following the introduction of penicillin, luetic joint disease has become even more rare. However, there has been an alarming increase in reported cases of infectious syphilis in the past ten years.[17]

Although the reported cases of congenital syphilis in the United States has continued to decline, as shown in Table 67–1, there are still over 2,000 cases a year reported, and of even more importance, only one out of seven cases is discovered during the first year of life. It is important to remember that syphilis and luetic joint disease still exist. Syphilitic joint disease may be classified as follows:

1. In Congenital Syphilis, Early
   A. Parrot's syphilitic osteochondritis
   B. Syphilitic dactylitis
2. In Congenital Syphilis, Late
   A. Clutton's joints (symmetrical serous synovitis—hydrarthrosis)
   B. Miscellaneous forms (gummatous synovitis and suppurative joint disease)
3. In Acquired Syphilis, Early
   A. Arthralgia
   B. Polyarthritis
4. In Acquired Syphilis, Late
   A. Gummatous arthritis with involvement of soft tissues, cartilage or bone
   B. Syphilitic spondylitis
   C. Charcot's joints (tabes dorsalis)

Table 67-1.—Congenital Syphilis United States, Fiscal Years 1962-1969

	Number of Cases Reported	
Fiscal Year	*Total*	*Under One* (1) *Year of Age*
1962	4,085	330
1963	4,140	410
1964	3,737	374
1965	3,505	373
1966	3,464	370
1967	3,050	398
1968	2,596	327
1969	2,224	277

Source: U.S. Public Health Service

CONGENITAL SYPHILIS

The very fact that the incidence of congenital syphilis is rapidly declining is creating a dangerous sense of security and has decreased our vigilance in the diagnosis of luetic joint disease. It is still of crucial importance that *all bone and joint disease in children should be carefully investigated for evidence of congenital syphilis.* The hallmarks of this disease are periarticular infiltration, moderate to marked enlargement of the joints, limitation of motion, and occasionally pain on manipulation. (While it is true that many patients with syphilitic joint disease have very little or no pain on motion, the complete absence of pain is probably over-emphasized.)

Early Congenital Syphilis

Parrot's Syphilitic Osteochondritis (Parrot's pseudoparalysis).—In the first year of life the most common type of congenital syphilitic arthritis with objective findings is an osteochondritis in a juxta-epiphyseal location, which is at times accompanied by considerable periarticular swelling.[13,15] It is seen in approximately 5 per cent of children with congenital syphilis.

It is most common in the first three weeks of life and rarely begins after three months of age. The upper limbs are affected more commonly than the lower. The pathologic lesion is a gelatiniform change in the bone and cartilage, which breaks down to form a greenish yellow fluid. Complete epiphyseal separation (Parrot's pseudoparalysis) or fracture of the epiphysis may occur.

On roentgen examination[5,6,10] one sees widening of the joint space, an irregular epiphyseal line, periosteal thickening, decalcification of bone, cupping of the diaphysis and irregular density and streakiness of bone adjacent to the cartilage.

If appropriate antibiotic therapy is given in time, the joint may undergo complete recovery. Shortening or deformity occurs if the growing line has been greatly damaged.

Syphilitic Dactylitis.—This occurs chiefly in children from one to three years of age.[9] The involved fingers or toes assume a characteristic spindle shape, and the process may result in deformity and marked shortening. In some cases there is absorption of bone. This condition is extremely rare and is difficult to differentiate from Still's disease.

Late Congenital Syphilis

Clutton's Joints (chronic symmetrical synovitis with effusion).—Symmetrical synovitis of the knees as a manifestation of congenital syphilis was first reported by Clutton[4] in 1886. Subsequently several writers[1,3,7,11,18,19] have described a similar condition with chronic hydrarthrosis, usually involving one or both knees. It may be recurrent, but ordinarily runs an indolent benign course without producing damage to the joints. Since luetic synovitis may mimic either pyogenic arthritis or Still's disease, this diagnosis may be easily overlooked.[2] This is especially true if other manifestations of late congenital syphilis, such as interstitial keratitis, Hutchinson's teeth, and nerve deafness, are not present. The fact that this disease may have an acute or subacute course, may be associated with fever, and may produce heat, redness, swelling, tenderness, and limitation of motion of the involved joints presents further difficulty in establishing the diagnosis.

The symptoms usually develop insidiously and occur between the ages of six and sixteen. The involvement is almost always limited to the soft tissues. The chief sites are the knees and elbows, the knees being involved in about 85 per cent of cases. The fluid accumulates rapidly if aspirated and may persist for years without permanent damage to articular tissues. From 10,000 to 45,000 leukocytes (chiefly lymphocytes) have been found per cubic millimeter of joint fluid. Polyarticular involvement has also been reported.

Roentgen examination is usually negative except for the separation of the ends of the bones due to the synovial effusion. When doubt regarding the diagnosis exists, a joint biopsy may be helpful.

Although this condition does not respond to antibiotic therapy, and relapses are common, the condition usually responds spontaneously to conservative management resulting in complete cure. Short courses of oral steroid may be helpful in suppressing symptoms.

Miscellaneous.—In congenital syphilis one may see joint lesions which appear identical with those of the tertiary stage of acquired syphilis. Aseptic necrosis may occur, resulting in formation of "pus" within the joints. Gummata of bone, Charcot's joints, and spondylitis are rare manifestations of late congenital syphilis.

ACQUIRED SYPHILIS

Early (Infectious)

Arthritis occurring in infectious (primary and secondary) syphilis is rare.[8] Although the arthralgia seen in infectious disease is encountered in secondary syphilis, inflammation of the synovium in the presence of positive serology is much more suggestive of lupus erythematosus than of syphilitic arthritis. Older literature contains many references to arthritis resembling rheumatoid arthritis, with synovitis, hydrarthrosis, tenosynovitis,[20] and bursitis. In the cases reported by Todd,[22] the presence of keratitis in about three-fourths of the patients was impressive. However, the evidence for inflammatory disease of peripheral joints as a manifestation of primary or secondary syphilis is in general unconvincing, and, if the lesion occurs at all, it must be very rare. In support of this contention is the fact that in the past five years the incidence of acquired syphilis has trebled to a rate of over 20,000 a year, with no reported observation of inflammatory joint disease.

Late Syphilis

Chronic syphilitic arthritis with synovitis, gummatous arthritis or Charcot's joints may be found in late syphilis.

Synovial Form of Gummatous Arthritis.—This is most common in the early stages of tertiary syphilis but may also occur in children with congenital syphilis (Van Gies' joints). Larger joints are affected most frequently. Considerable amounts of painless effusion are characteristic of the process, although occasionally severe pain may occur. Other features include the presence of an irregular, lumpy, localized swelling about the joint with very little restriction of motion or muscular wasting. This gummatous process, which often resembles tuberculosis, may affect the whole joint or may remain localized. In severe cases, suppuration may be the end result.

Osseous Form of Gummatous Arthritis.—Extensive gummatous involvement of bones and joints may occur with very little impairment of motion. Although such joints may be large and tense, there is very little evidence of inflammation, muscular spasm, wasting, limitation of movement, constitutional reaction or ankylosis (unless secondary infection occurs).

Gummatous deposits may be found in perisynovial tissues, cartilage, and also in the cancellous ends of bones.[12,14] Although the bony changes are most marked, all of the joint structures are usually involved. In young individuals, the process may begin as an epiphysitis. One may see erosion and irregularity of the joint surfaces, cavitation within the bones and bony outgrowths. In adults, the condition may resemble degenerative joint disease.

Osteophytes are common. If specific therapy is not instituted, the joint may become ankylosed. Syphilis and tuberculosis should always be suspected in monoarthritis.

Juxta-articular Gummata. — These may occur in tertiary syphilis and lead to symptoms in the joint. Roentgenogram may show considerable destruction while clinically there is little heat or pain in the joint. The lesion may heal completely if there has not been complete destruction of joint surfaces.

Syphilitic spondylitis with invasion of bone and periosteum by *Treponema pallida* may occur in any portion of the spine, but has a predilection for the cervical region. As in syphilitic osteitis elsewhere, the bones most affected are those exposed to trauma or pressure. It may involve only one vertebra or several adjacent ones. The vertebrae may show evidence by x ray of bone destruction, new bone production, or a combination of both. Eburnation of the vertebral bodies occurs occasionally, and in most instances the vertebrae eventually develop secondary spur formation.

Syphilitic spondylitis may occur in congenital syphilis, or during later stages of acquired syphilis. It is characterized symptomatically by localized pain (which may be more marked at night), stiffness, and localized tenderness. Usually there are coexisting lesions in other bones such as the sternum, clavicle, tibia or radius. Gummatous lesions of the vertebral bodies have been described. Proposed diagnostic criteria have included: (1) the presence of active syphilis, (2) rapid improvement under antisyphilitic treatment, and (3) suggestive roentgenographic findings.

Charcot's joints develop in the spine, the lower lumbar region being most commonly affected. The symptoms are not characteristic. Contrary to the belief of some, the process is not necessarily painless.

The roentgenographic changes are often quite characteristic with bizarre destruction of bone occurring simultaneously with extensive (but chaotic) new bone and cartilage production. The pathologic changes reflected roentgenographically may be extreme and out of all proportion to the clinical findings.

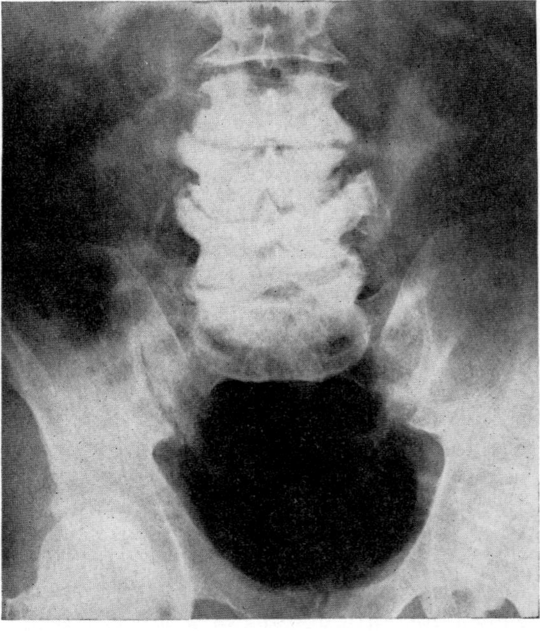

Fig. 67–1.—Charcot's joints involving the third, fourth and fifth lumbar and the first sacral vertebrae.

Charcot's joints, secondary to syphilitic lesions of the central nervous system, are discussed in Chapter 72.

DIAGNOSIS

Especially in the treatment of children, it is important to remember that despite the introduction of effective treatment of syphilis, luetic joint disease does exist and should be considered in every case of arthritis in which the etiology has not been determined. The diagnosis is made by careful evaluation of the personal and family history, a complete physical examination, including special attention to a search for other stigmata of syphilis, and laboratory examination of the blood and spinal fluid for evidence of syphilis.

Clinical points favoring the diagnosis of syphilitic joint disease include relative absence of pain, marked hydrops, free range of motion, good general health despite a long history of joint pathology, precipitation of arthritis by a blow, other evidence of syphilis, lack of response to salicylates, and favorable response to antiluetic therapy.

Too much credence should not be placed upon a single negative serologic reaction, if bone or joint syphilis is suspected. In all cases, one should x ray the long bones for additional information. No pathognomonic roentgen sign of syphilitic arthritis has been reported. However, suggestive features include erosion of bone and cartilage, with bony proliferation and periostitis in a relatively symptomless joint. When there is doubt concerning the diagnosis, a biopsy should be performed.

The demonstration of a positive serologic test result for syphilis does not necessarily incriminate this disease as the cause of joint manifestations. Biological false positive reactions occur in a number of diseases, especially in systemic lupus erythematosus.[16] Excellent tests are now available, including the *Treponema pallidum* immobilization test, the *Treponema pallidum* immune adherence test, and the *Treponema pallidum* complement-fixation test, to differentiate the presence of syphilis from a biological false positive reaction.

TREATMENT

Penicillin therapy is effective in all types of joint disease caused by syphilis, except for neurogenic arthritis and the joint manifestations of late congenital syphilis. Since most of the lesions occur in late symptomatic syphilis, the dose of penicillin should be 10 million units given over a period of three to four weeks.[21]

In patients who are sensitive to penicillin, the tetracyclines have been found to be satisfactory substitutes.

Clutton's joints respond well to conservative management with rest and physiotherapy.

Charcot's joints, secondary to syphilitic lesions of the central nervous system, are not specifically a form of syphilitic arthritis and will be discussed in Chapter 72.

BIBLIOGRAPHY

1. Blattner, R. J.: J. Pediat., *59*, 625, 1961.
2. Borella, L., Goobar, J. E., and Clark, G. M.: J.A.M.A., *180*, 190, 1962.
3. Caffey, T.: *Pediatrics X-ray Diagnosis*, Chicago, Year Book Publishers, Inc., 1961.
4. Clutton, H. H.: Lancet, *1*, 391, 1886.
5. Compere, C. L.: Urol. and Cutan. Rev., *44*, 535, 1940.
6. Dennie, C. C.: Radiology, *4*, 364, 1925.
7. Domenicone, G.: Bull Sci. Med. (Bologna), *127*, 431, 1955.
8. Hench, P. S., *et al.*: Ann. Int. Med., *28*, 66, 1948.
9. Jostes, F. A. and Roche, M. B.: J. Missouri Med. Assn., *36*, 61, 1939.
10. Klafton, E. and Priesel, R.: Roentgenstr., *47*, 59, 1933.
11. Klauder, J. V.: J.A.M.A., *103*, 236, 1934.
12. Lloyd-Williams, I. H.: Urol. & Cutan., Rev., *35*, 225, 1931.
13. McCord, J. R.: Amer. J. Obst. & Gynec., *42*, 667, 1941.
14. McEwen, C. and Thomas, E. W.: Med. Clin. North America, *22*, 1275, 1938.
15. McLean, S.: Amer. J. Dis. Child, *41*, 130, 1931.
16. Moore, J. E. and Mohr, C. F.: J.A.M.A., *150*, 46, 1952.
17. Morbidity and Mortality, Weekly Report USPH (Dec. 19, 1964), Communicable Disease Center, Atlanta, Ga.
18. Platou, R. V.: Advances Pediat., *4*, 39, 1949.
19. Rubio Garcia, J. I.: Medicina (Madr), *3*, 379, 1955.
20. Smith, C. B.: West Viginia Med. J., *34*, 111, 1938.
21. Thomas, E. W.: J. A. M. A., *162*, 1536, 1956.
22. Todd, A. H.: Brit. J. Surg., *14*, 260, 1926.

Chapter 68

Unusual Features and Special Types of Infectious Arthritis

By Frank R. Schmid, M.D.

The diagnosis and treatment of common forms of acute infectious arthritis caused by pyogenic bacteria as well as other less common but important types of joint infection as tuberculous arthritis are presented in detail in other chapters. However, a number of special problems related to infection remain for consideration. These include the unique anatomical features of sepsis in deep-seated joints such as the hip, sacroiliac and spinal joints; surgical and other considerations associated with chronic infections; and, finally, those forms of infectious arthritis caused by unusual microorganisms.

SPECIAL FEATURES OF HIP AND SPINAL MOVEMENT

Hip Involvement.—Infections of the axial joints of the body, such as the hip, shoulder and spine, present major difficulties in diagnosis and treatment. Since these joints are deep-seated, ordinary signs of inflammation are masked. Pain in these areas is all too frequently ascribed to a non-infectious cause until the process has become far advanced. In 6 patients, all with staphylococcal infections, shoulder infections were not recognized promptly because other more common causes of acute shoulder pain were considered first. As a consequence, much loss of glenohumeral joint motion resulted.[112] Diagnostic problems of this type are magnified in the hip joint. Infections occur more often here than in the shoulder, particularly in children. Of 64 patients with septic arthritis of the hip joint, 16 had the onset of the disease within the first six months of life and 11 of these were under 6 weeks old.[205] Early recognition is critical since irreversible destruction occurs within days.[63,148,194] Septic infection of the neck of the femur resulting in abscess formation with distention of the joint can rapidly deprive the femoral head of its blood supply.[205] In addition, purulent fluids cause lysis of cartilage and bone structure.

As is true for infections in other joints, hematogenous dissemination of microorganisms from a primary site of entry in the body is the usual means for inoculation of the hip joint.[63,148] In some instances, a predisposing factor such as prior disease in the joint or associated illness[28] plays a role in this process. Direct penetration also occurs. Septic arthritis of the hip developed as a complication of femoral venipuncture[10] and from intra-abdominal infection. The latter complication was seen in 5 adults[186] and 6 of 26 other individuals.[114] The infection had extended down the retroperitoneal space near the iliopsoas muscle from an abdominal abscess. Symptoms were less obvious in these cases because major interest was centered on the abdominal problem. Due to delay in diagnosis, these infections caused prolonged morbidity and poor return of function, only one third of the patients being able to return to their previous level of activity.

Symptoms of hip sepsis include a history of primary infection elsewhere in the body. Several days later patients may develop a fever of from 101° to 103° F., moderate leukocytosis and leg pain; the latter renders weight-bearing impossible. Pain in the knee is a most common complaint (due to referred pain along the obturator nerve). The thigh is usually held in flexion, adduction and internal rotation but, after a few days, in abduction, flexion and external rotation. The acute pain permits only a few degrees of motion. The joint fluid causes bulging and thickening of the capsule; the thigh appears edematous and the inguinal crease may be obliterated. Marked tenderness is experienced on local pressure.[146,114,29,141,206]

Aspiration may decompress the joint, relieve pain temporarily and aid in diagnosis. Lateral aspiration is preferred; the needle is introduced above the tip of the trochanter and is tilted down along the femoral neck. If the infection is permitted to progress, the joint cartilage undergoes autolysis and the distended capsule may rupture at its inferior mesial portion. Spontaneous dislocation of the hip may occur (posterior and upward with the head anterior).

Roentgen examination is of little aid in early diagnosis unless an adjacent site of osteomyelitis exists.[130] Roentgen-ray findings begin to develop only after the first week or two of the disease. Narrowing of the "joint space" occurs on x ray and is a measure of the damage to the articular cartilage. Hefke and Turner have called attention to the so-called obturator sign, that is, obscuring or widening and curving of the border of the obturator shadow as seen by x ray in some types of hip joint disease.[87] The obturator shadow is a soft-tissue shadow seen in the AP roentgen examination of the pelvis just medial to the acetabulum on the inner aspect of the pelvis. The upper border of the shadow begins lateral to and below the lower pole of the sacroiliac joint and follows the line of the pelvic inlet downward over the acetabulum, disappearing behind the upper ramus of the pubis. It is believed that the shadow represents the obturator internus, whose tendon is adjacent to the capsule of the hip joint. This sign may reveal the presence of septic hip joint disease at an early stage, and is of some importance in the early diagnosis of tuberculosis of the hip. It is absent in fractures, osteochondritis and other pathologic conditions of the hip.

Management of infection of the hip joint should follow the same general principles outlined in Chapter 63. These include prompt identification of the infecting microorganism, its control with appropriate antibiotics administered systemically and drainage of accumulated purulent secretions. Monitoring the course of the illness permits a rational decision to be taken for each of these components of the program. In weighing the question of open drainage rather than needle drainage of the joint, it must be borne in mind that drainage by needle from the hip presents greater technical difficulties than elsewhere. However, if sepsis is recognized within the first few days and if the organism recovered from the joint responds readily to antibiotics, for instance, the gonococcus or the pneumococcus, needle drainage is preferred since it prevents conversion of the closed-space infection into an open wound. Open wound infections are associated with greater morbidity and risk of contamination by resistant microorganisms. Should recognition of sepsis be delayed or para-articular infection, such as a pelvic abscess, be responsible for the joint disease, then open drainage is indicated. A particularly serious problem exists in children with hip disease since needle aspiration is often traumatic and symptoms of the disease difficult to interpret. In these cases, open drainage should be considered early in the treatment program, perhaps at the outset.

Surgical treatment of the late consequences of joint infection is varied.[39] Prosthetic replacement of a damaged femoral head or acetabulum can be undertaken but should be deferred a number of months until all evidence of active infection has disappeared. Acceptable results were achieved in 33 hips treated by mold arthroplasty.[103] It is conceivable that total hip replacement will be considered in the future as experience with this procedure is extended.

Spinal Involvement.—Any articulation of the spine may be affected by a septic infection. The pathogenesis is the same as for peripheral joints, the bacteria in most cases traveling via the blood stream from a distant focus of infection[161] or more rarely extending to the joint from a nearby area of osteomyelitis. Septic arthritis of the sacroiliac joint, although unusual, does occur and should be considered whenever there is unilateral sacroiliac disease. Staphylococci and other pyogenic bacteria are responsible most often[12,102,127] but brucellosis and tuberculosis may also cause sacroiliac disease.

Infectious spondylitis refers to a focal infection of one or more vertebral bodies and their adjacent disc. The adjacent apophyseal joint may also be involved, usually by direct extension of the infection. This type of localized spondylitis is a not uncommon complication in typhoid and other Salmonella infections, tuberculosis and brucellosis, though many pathogenic bacteria or fungi may be implicated.[177] In Salmonella infections these spinal lesions may appear months or years after convalescence from the original infection. Lumbar spondylitis has been reported due to a syphilitic gumma.[22]

Symptoms include primarily pain in the back, but also fever, spasm of the paraspinal or psoas muscles, tenderness over the affected area on percussion and palpation, and limitation of motion in the affected segments of the spine.

In the acute stage of the disease, roentgenograms are usually normal, but within a few months following the onset there is thinning of the involved disc or vertebra and marginal proliferation of bone. Biopsy by needle aspiration or open surgical biopsy is usually necessary for definitive diagnosis and for treatment with appropriate antibiotics.[83,145] Intervertebral disc infection often simulates hip joint disease in children and results in intercorporeal vertebral fusion.[38,162,197] Healing of an acute pyogenic lesion with bony fusion of adjacent vertebrae is illustrated in Figure 68–1.

Radiostrontium accumulates in areas

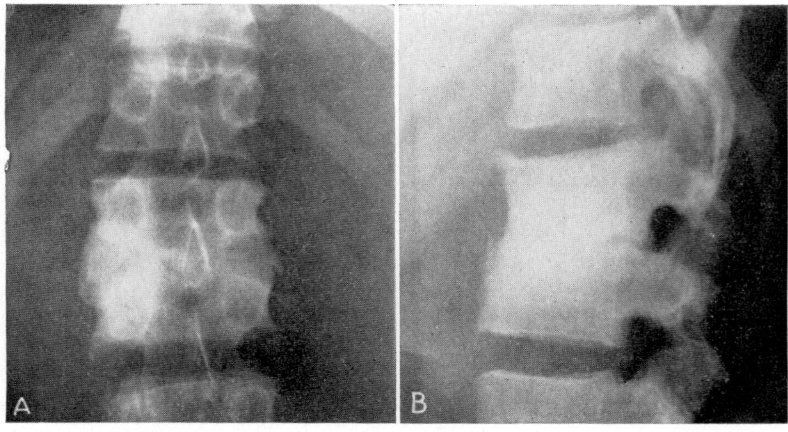

Fig. 68–1.—*A* and *B*, Specific infectious spondylitis involving lumbar vertebrae 1 and 2. The intervertebral disc has been destroyed and there is almost complete fusion of the adjacent vertebral bodies.

of osteitis or fracture because mineral metabolism in the area is increased. External counting over the spine 2 weeks after administration of this isotope may help corroborate the diagnosis in the case of dubious, early lesions or in recurrences of infection. It does not distinguish among the microorganisms responsible and the findings in tuberculosis and pyogenic infections are similar.[62]

The differential diagnosis includes osteomyelitis, post-traumatic thinning of the disc, congenital absence of the disc, osteochondrosis of the disc, tuberculosis and other specific infectious processes. Pyogenic spinal disease may be differentiated from tuberculosis by its more sudden and violent onset and by a history of a preceding acute infectious process. However, exact bacteriologic identification of the microorganism cannot be made except by smear and culture.

Prognosis in general is good for recovery, and, with suitable antibiotic therapy, little or no disability is apt to result. The spine should be immobilized in a plaster cast until evidence of healing has occurred. If abscesses develop, they should be drained. A supporting back brace should be worn for months after healing has occurred.

SPECIAL FEATURES OF CHRONIC SEPTIC ARTHRITIS

Any septic joint untreated or inadequately treated for one week or more may be considered to have developed some of the pathological changes of a chronic infection. These include damage to cartilage and bone, increase in the amount of scar tissue and ultimately destruction of the normal joint mechanism. Fortunately, the number of such cases has decreased since the modern era of antibiotic therapy has begun. In one large clinic, the number of cases of bacterial arthritis had decreased approximately 50 per cent during the period 1952 through 1957 when compared with numbers of cases from the two periods extending, respectively, from 1939 through 1945, and from 1946 through 1951. This reduction took place in the number of cases with the chronic form of the disease and not with the acute variety.[37]

Even in joint cavities that are sites of these chronic changes, diffusion of antibiotics occurs (*see* Chapter 63, Concept of a Closed-space Infection). Thus, the need to instill these drugs locally is no more indicated in chronic than in acute disease. However, some antibiotics, such as the penicillins and cephalosporins, that act by inhibition of bacterial cell wall synthesis may induce the formation of cell wall-free bacteria or protoplasts. In this form, bacteria may persist at the site of infection. Little evidence is available at present to support this potential mechanism for chronicity either by recovery of such forms from the joint or by evidence that these forms are able to exert a pathogenetic influence. In one case familiar to me, such forms as well as native bacterial forms of *S. aureus* were cultured from the necrotic remnant of a patella removed after several months of continual penicillin therapy. In the postoperative period, this patient was treated with erythromycin because this drug inhibits aspects of bacterial metabolism other than cell wall synthesis.

Whenever chronic septic arthritis occurs, a major effort should be directed toward analysis of the factor(s) responsible for this manifestation of treatment failure. Reevaluation of the bacterial status of the joint may prove helpful and, if so, cultures should be obtained after a period of withdrawal from all antibiotics. The type of antibiotic can be evaluated by utilizing a bactericidal test for its effectiveness. Finally, operation may be needed to accomplish open drainage and excision of necrotic bone and soft tissue including sinuses.[27,37,39,69,183]

Suppuration within the hip joint can run a more benign course during the first two years of life compared with the more rapid course of this disease in later childhood and adolescence; this is due in great part to the large amount of cartilage in the hip joint of young children.[81]

Recognition of this disease may be delayed until the child begins to walk, when pathologic dislocation of the hip may be observed. This condition is often misdiagnosed a superficial abscess. In the presence of a pyogenic exudate, the cartilage (which makes up the greater part of the upper femur at this age) is dissolved. Although the child apparently recovers from the infection with rapid closure of his wound (if the physician mistakes this for an abscess and drains it), the damage produced is not evident until the child becomes ambulatory at the end of the first year of life when one notices the "hip lurch" produced by the dislocation.

Harmon has described a reconstruction operation which may be done during the second and third years of life.[81]

Epiphyseal pseudoarthrosis at the hip may be seen after operative fusion of the hip, following inflammatory ankylosis of the hip or as a sequel to adolescent epiphysiolysis.[139]

In septic arthritis of the hip joint, rest of the joint should be accomplished by a double hip spica including the thigh of the opposite leg to prevent adduction and abduction of the foot on the involved side to control rotation. Windows may be provided to allow aspiration of the joint. In some cases, surgical drainage may be necessary (if the femoral head is destroyed, if thick, purulent material is present, etc.). Dependent drainage may be obtained by opening the hip joint posteriorly. Weight-bearing must not be instituted too early; follow-up orthopedic care and physical therapy are extremely important.

Heberling reviewed the results of treatment of 201 patients with acute suppurative arthritis.[86] Surgical therapy consisted of incision of the joint, under general anesthesia and suturing an appropriate-sized soft rubber drain to the capsule but not permitting this to intrude into the joint. Active motion was begun as soon as possible and was repeated every three hours. When it was necessary to replace extruded drains and reopen pockets, this could usually be done without anesthesia. In those with involvement of the knee or hip, adhesive traction with a small amount of weight was used.

Sites of incision were as follows: (1) Shoulder; anteriorly through the deltoid. (2) Elbow; posteriorly over the radiohumeral region. (3) Wrist; dorsally into the snuff-box. (4) Hip; anteriorly between the sartorius and the Tensor fasciae femoris. (5) Knee; anterior mesial and occasionally a second incision on the lateral side of the patella. (6) Ankle; posterolateral and anteromesial,

After opening the joint, it was gently flexed and extended a few times to express the contents before suturing the drain in place. Fluffed gauze was piled on loosely and secured, permitting complete joint motion. When the discharge became thin and scanty and the thickening and bogginess about the joint began to disappear, the drains were removed and the openings allowed to close gradually.

ARTHRITIS WITH SPECIFIC BACTERIAL DISEASES

Meningococcal Arthritis

Gwyn, in 1898, reported the first authentic case of meningococcal septicemia in a patient with meningitis and arthritis. Articular lesions have developed in 5 to 20 per cent of meningococcal infections in various epidemics.[106,172,196] Meningococcal infections increase in number in times of war. Conditions at large training stations are ideal for the production of a state in which these infections are endemic: men live in barracks and new recruits are constantly arriving. Bush and Bailey discussed an epidemic of meningococcal infection at a Naval Training Station.[31]

Jaeger found 37 cases of meningococcal arthritis among 1000 cases of meningococcal infection.[105] It is very likely that the true incidence of meningococcal joint involvement was much higher, inasmuch as when postmortem examination was made in 40 cases, 9 showed purulent synovitis which was not diagnosed clinically. Instances of purulent meningococcal bursitis and purulent tenosynovitis were described. This study suggests that most cases of meningococcal arthritis are instances of purulent synovitis. The wrists were involved most often; knee joints were also frequently attacked. The onset of the disease was either as a mono- or as a polyarticular involvement, the cases being about equally divided in the two groups. The prognosis was good in all cases.

During non-epidemic periods, 2 to 10 per cent of troops may be meningococcus carriers[49] while in periods of epidemics, the rate in healthy troops may reach 80 per cent. The organism probably gains entrance to the body from the nasopharynx with subsequent invasion of the blood stream, and, if not prevented by spontaneous resistance or therapy, localizes in the meninges, joints, skin, eyes or other body tissues.[94] The idea has been abandoned that meningitis is due to direct infection of the meninges through the cribriform plate except in a few cases where known trauma, with fracture, is present.

Meningococcal sepsis usually begins with prodromal symptoms of disease of the upper respiratory tract.[185] From one to many days later, acute symptoms appear such as a chill, with fever; the latter may rise suddenly or this may be gradual. Other symptoms then include weakness, malaise, muscular aches, headache, nausea, vomiting, and pains or actual inflammation in joints. The rash is the most characteristic manifestation; the most common manifestation of this is petechial or purpuric with lesions varying from 1 to 15 mm. in diameter. Many other forms of skin lesions may appear.

The articular complications of cerebrospinal fever were first reported by Welch. Osler[149] reviewed this literature and Rolleston[170] and Herrick and Parkhurst added valuable information gained during World War I.[96] Schein reported personal experience with 23 cases.[176] In World War II, Strong and Hollander[196] reported 100 cases of meningococcal infection. In their series, 11 per cent had joint symptoms and in 4 per cent suppurative arthritis developed. In 1 case the diagnosis of the infection was made by recovery of the organism from the joint fluid while blood and spinal fluid cultures were negative. Many other cases had bacteremia without meningitis. More recent reports bear out this experience.[56, 159, 213]

Pyarthrosis due to the meningococcus most commonly appears at the end of the first week of the disease, usually involving only a single joint. Meningococci may be found in the joint fluid. Intermittent migratory arthritis may occur during chronic meningococcal septicemia.[158]

Other varieties of articular involvement in meningococcal infection may be seen,[65] including arthralgias of multiple joints in the first few days of the disease during the phase of meningococcemia, that is, occurring simultaneously with the purpuric manifestations. Herrick[94] has described intra- and periarticular hemorrhages of the joints in these cases. The involvement is usually symmetrical and is often transitory in nature, producing marked pain, redness and tenderness of the joints but a minimal amount of joint swelling. Occasionally, joint manifestations may precede the meningeal signs by days or weeks (or occasionally months), rendering diagnosis difficult.[35]

Adams has discussed the arthritis which occurs with meningococcemia.[2] In the non-meningitis case, there is usually a history of respiratory symptoms and joint pains with or without redness and swelling. Large joints, such as the knees, are affected most often. These individuals will usually also have deep muscle aching in the arms and legs, and a macular or petechial eruption. In chronic meningococcemia, one or more joints may be tender.

Most observers question the existence of the so-called postmeningitic spondylitis described by Epstein and by Billington.[21, 58] Inasmuch as it is usually reported in the lower lumbar spine, Fox and Gilbert suggest that this is very likely caused by the spinal puncture needle with cellulitis or spinal osteomyelitis or herniation of the nucleus pulposus from injury of the annulus fibrosus.[65]

Treatment.—Patients should be treated by splinting of the affected joints, repeated aspirations if necessary, and, in all cases, effective antibiotics should be given. Penicillin has replaced sulfadiazine as the drug of choice in the treatment of meningococcal infections. A recent study and review of the medical literature by Leedom *et al.* indicated that fully 30 per cent of the strains studied were resistant to sulfadiazine.[126] Penicillin and ampicillin are recommended for both the treatment and prophylaxis of meningococcal infections. In meningococcal arthritis, as in other penicillin-sensitive articular infections, it is recommended that treatment be given intravenously utilizing 10 to 20 million units daily.

The prognosis is good when these drugs are used. After the acute stage of the disease has passed, adequate physical therapy (heat, massage and exercises) will be of great value and should be continued until maximum function has returned.[196]

Brucellosis

The number of cases of human brucellosis in the United States has progressively declined since World War II, largely because of an intensive educational program to eliminate the disease in cattle.[192] Brucellosis is basically a disease of animals and is very rarely transmitted from human to human. The organism gains entrance into man via the gastrointestinal tract from drinking raw milk, through minute abrasions of the skin, through mucous membranes of the eye, and probably also through the nasopharynx where there is direct contact with cattle or swine or their tissues or body fluids.[32,192] The brucella organism localizes in those tissues having an abundance of reticuloendothelial cells, especially the bone marrow, lymph nodes, liver and spleen. The bacteria invade the cells and possibly proliferate within macrophages and thus are protected from the action of antibiotics.[33,190] The incubation period in the average case varies from a few to twenty-one days but, in an occasional case, several months may elapse between the time of the exposure and the first appearance of symptoms. Among the three species of the genus *Brucella* there exist fundamental differences that have major clinical significance.[32,192] *B. melitensis* is the most invasive and produces a severe illness in man.[33,59,190] Of the human cases of brucellosis in the United States less than 10 per cent are due to *B. melitensis*, but in the world at large this species is the most common cause of brucellosis. Another 10 to 20 per cent of the cases of human brucellosis in the United States are due to *B. suis*, for which the natural reservoir is the hog. Suppurative lesions are more common with *B. suis*. The most frequent source of human brucellosis in the United States is *B. abortus* which causes about 75 per cent of all cases.[32,113,192] Eight cases of monarticular arthritis in children were ascribed to *Brucella abortus* in a study from Scotland where 23 per cent of the milk cow herds are said to be infected and pasteurization is not compulsory.[1]

Generalized aches, backache and joint pains are outstanding clinical manifestations along with weakness, sweats, chills, headache and anorexia.[90,93,192] Bone and muscle pain was present in 65 of 94 culturally proved cases of brucellosis due to *B. abortus*.[192] Definite pain over bones and joints usually indicates the presence of localized involvement. Actual joint inflammation is not common and has been reported in less than 2 per cent of one series.[80]

Bone and Joint Lesions.—Typical involvement is an osteomyelitis of the spine, long bones or pelvis. This lesion develops in the bone marrow from a localized Brucella granuloma which then infiltrates the bone and surrounding soft tissue such as the intervertebral disc. In one study, however, primary infection was thought to occur within the intervertebral disc rather than extension into it from the bony matrix.[3] Both bone and disc are destroyed by the granulation tissue with the formation of pus in some cases.[32,69,101,120] Localization in the spinal column has occurred as early as three weeks and as late as one year after the original infection. The spondylitis of brucellosis resembles tuberculous spondylitis with the exception that recovery is usually relatively rapid.[156,192] An acute or subacute serous polyarthritis or an intermittent hydrarthrosis may develop.[79,80,181] Suppurative arthritis of the sacroiliac joints or of the peripheral joints has also been reported.[93,191,193] Chronic brucellosis has not been found to be a cause of rheumatoid arthritis.[75]

Diagnosis.—The recognition of brucellosis is often first suggested by joint and muscle aches and pains, especially back pains, occurring with fever in farmers, livestock producers, veterinarians, or employees in meat-packing or rendering plants. Splenomegaly is usually present and hepatomegaly may also occur, especially in chronic or recurrent cases. The precise diagnosis is absolutely dependent upon serological and cultural evidence. Every attempt should be made to isolate the organism from the blood, bone marrow, or excised tissues or body fluids. Special culture media are necessary.[192,216] The serum agglutination test is of considerable diagnostic significance. In the vast majority of both the acute and chronic forms, the titer of agglutinins is 1:100 or more.[32,192] The complement-fixation test and the opsonophagocytic test are available but not recommended for the routine diagnostic laboratory.[192] The intradermal skin test is not diagnostic of active infection as reactions may remain positive long after the infection has been cured.

Treatment.—The ideal antibiotic or chemotherapeutic agent for the disease has not been achieved, and relapses have occurred after the use of all current antibiotics. The most successful treatment at this time consists of a daily dose of 2 gm. of tetracycline in combination with 1 or 2 gm. of streptomycin for twenty-one days.[59,68,113,216] A 20 per cent relapse rate may be expected.[216] Corticotropin or corticosteroids given for short periods have been reported to produce dramatic relief in seriously ill patients.[190] Erythromycin has been reported to be effective in 14 patients with both acute and chronic disease.[203] Bed-rest, orthopedic aids such as casts and braces, and rarely surgical procedures such as curettage were required in some patients with spine or joint involvement.[32,192]

Prophylaxis against brucellosis consists of boiling or pasteurizing all milk and destruction or treatment of infected animals.[74,192]

Bacillary Dysentery

Serous effusions containing Shiga's bacillus have been found in approximately 3 per cent of cases of bacillary dysentery.[92] This disease may involve one or multiple joints.[140,147] It appears most often within one to three weeks after the onset of the diarrhea, although it has also been noted several weeks after cessation of the diarrhea.[19] Joint involvement (usually of the knee or ankle) persists from four to six weeks and is usually followed by complete recovery of joint function.[17,73] Suppuration and resultant ankylosis have occasionally been noted.[85]

Salmonella

Bone and joint infections occur in a small number of patients with typhoid fever[137] and in perhaps a slightly larger number of patients in whom infections are caused by other Salmonella species.[164,204,207,212] The infections involve the long bones and joints, chondrosternal junction and spinal column. Arthritis (excluding spondylitis) occurred in 8.3 per cent of all Salmonella infections with *Salmonella choleraesuis* and *Salmonella typhi-*

murium being most often responsible.[45,55] The arthritis involved the knees, shoulders and hips; the hand and wrists were spared. Diagnosis required aspiration of synovial fluid with detection of the microorganism in smear and culture. At least two antibiotics, including penicillin or chloramphenicol were used in treatment.[45] *Salmonella schottmülleri* has been isolated from a sacrolumbar lesion of twenty-four years' duration.[54]

Haverhill Fever

The main characteristics of this syndrome include an abrupt onset of fever, a rubella-like or morbilliform rash, chiefly on the extremities, and polyarthritis.[161,215] Mild or marked joint redness and swelling may occur and may persist from several days to several weeks. Joint phenomena usually appear during the first several days of the illness. Marked limitation of joint function may occur but this usually clears within several months.

The organism *Haverhillia multiformis* (*Streptobacillus moniliformis*) has been demonstrated in the blood[84,151] and joint fluid[171] of some of these patients and specific agglutinins for this organism are present in the blood stream. Serum is required for its growth on artificial media.[52] The disease has been reported following a rat bite[34,66,142,178] and following drinking of (possibly) infected, raw milk. Farrell and his co-workers have reviewed the literature on this disorder.[60]

In addition to the epidemic of 86 cases, sporadic cases have been reported. Although some cases may follow a rat bite, this disease should not be called "rat-bite fever" as this term is also used to describe sodoku (*Spirillum minus* infection). Haverhill fever responds to penicillin and also to tetracycline and streptomycin.[52,66,132,142,210]

Rat-Bite Fever

There is much confusion in the literature concerning the difference between this condition and Haverhill fever.

Jeffers and his associates have discussed the etiologic and clinical relationship of *Haverhillia multiformis* septicemia to Haverhill and rat-bite fevers.[5] *Haverhillia multiformis* is the organism recovered from patients with Haverhill fever and there was no history of rat bite in the individuals in the epidemic at Haverhill in 1926. Fevers due to *Haverhillia multiformis* are characterized by septicemia with metastatic arthritis and morbilliform and petechial cutaneous eruptions. The *Spirillum minus* (*Spirochaeta morsus muris*) has been thought to be the causative agent in most patients stricken after the bite of a rat although the entirely different organism, *Haverhillia multiformis* (*Streptobacillus moniliformis*, *Streptothrix muris ratti*), was recovered from a few of these patients. Sodoku is the name given by the Japanese to infection with this motile spirillum *Spirillum minus*. Joint involvement (arthritis) has been mentioned in only a few patients with this disease.[122] Beeson reported 2 cases of rat-bite fever in which *Spirillum minus* was isolated from the blood by mouse inoculation and blood cultures for *Streptobacillus moniliformis* were negative.[18] Although neither patient showed arthritis during the period of observation, one of the patients gave a history of swelling around the wrists, elbows, knees and ankles prior to hospital admission.

Penicillin is effective in the therapy of rat-bite fever due to either organism.

Scarlet Fever

Healey reported that 3 per cent of young adults being immunized against scarlet fever developed multiple joint pains as a reaction to one or more injections of the sterile filtrate of broth cultures of scarlet fever streptococci.[85] The majority of individuals who experienced this reaction had noted joint pains previously associated with rheumatic fever or streptococcal infections of the nose and throat. The same individuals appeared to develop rheumatic affections such as heart disease, polyarthritis and erythema nodosum more often than other persons not similarly sensitized.[167]

From 1 to 5 per cent of patients with clinical scarlet fever develop joint complications, beginning from about the fourth to the tenth day of the disease. The spectrum of disease varies and may include a mild, migratory polyarthritis resembling rheumatic fever,[43,153] or recrudescence of a rheumatic fever or purulent arthritis with hemolytic streptococci cultured from the joint fluid. If a sterile joint fluid is obtained, it would be difficult to rule out the possibility of arthritis due to rheumatic fever.

Diphtheria

Acutely painful, swollen joints occur occasionally during the early stage of diphtheria from which diphtheria bacilli have been isolated. Arthritis and chorea minor have been reported accompanying diphtheria in children.[100] Penicillin is effective against diphtheria organisms, but not against the toxin they produce. In addition to penicillin, diphtheria antitoxin must be given in all virulent diphtheria infections.

Anthrax

Joint complications are rare.[50] Migratory anthralgia and serous exudates have been noted.

Leprosy

The onset of symptoms in leprosy may be accompanied by fever with generalized aching and pains in the limbs and back so severe that the patient may be unable to move. Early in the course of the disease there may be stiffness and numbness of the extremities and pain and swelling of hands and feet. It was found that 4.5 per cent of 425 patients at the Carville Leprosarium in Louisiana had had a previous diagnosis of "arthritis," "rheumatism," or acute rheumatic fever.

Contractions and distortions of fingers and toes may occur fairly early in leprosy. Later, as infiltration of nerves proceeds, trophic disorders of bones and joints as well as of muscles become apparent. Contractures of the hand are likely to assume the "main-en-griffe" appearance, with function perhaps little impaired. Sometimes only the fourth and fifth fingers show contracture. In the feet, contractures are less common. There may be excruciating pains in the toes, especially the big toe. Trophic ulcerations may combine with secondary infection. On x rays one finds partial absorption and necrosis of bones.

The pseudo-arthritis of lepers is mainly an osseous destruction; disintegration of the epiphyses and diaphyses follows destructive changes in the phalanges and metacarpal and metatarsal bones due to trophic changes. Eventually there may be spontaneous amputation of fingers or toes in whole or in part which results from secondary infection.[168] Even without ulceration, the bones of the digits may become rarefied and absorbed so that bones and joints disappear and the fingernail may be found riding back on the knuckle. With certain joints, especially the wrists and ankles, an actual neuropathic process similar to a Charcot joint may be seen, with erosion and disorganization of cartilage and bone.[152]

Epidemic Tropical Acute Polyarthritis

In September, 1942, a form of rheumatism appeared among Australian soldiers in the Darwin-Adelaide River area of northern Australia. It was characterized by acute polyarthritis, mild fever, transient rash, and lymphadenopathy. In October, 1943, Halliday and Horan of the Australian Medical Corps reported 105 cases studied in 1942.[77] The next year the disease again occurred in the northern territory as well as in Queensland and in Bougainville.

An epidemic polyarthritis in southeastern Australia occurred in 1956, similar to previous outbreaks in 1928 and in the years of World War II. The cause was unknown but the infection may have been mosquito-borne.[9]

The clinical features of all cases were similar except for minor variations. The onset was gradual, and initial symptoms were pains and sometimes swelling with redness of many peripheral joints. Involvement of midphalangeal joints of the fingers resembling rheumatoid arthritis occurred. A maculopapular rash somewhat resembling rubella usually followed and occasionally preceded the acute arthritis. Tender enlargement of lymph nodes and a mild fever (99° to 101° F.) were present. The disease was self-limited, rarely lasting more than ten to twenty days, and cleared without articular or cardiac sequelae.

The cause is unknown. Agglutination tests for Proteus OX19, XK, and OX2 and for *Brucella abortus* were negative. Cultures of blood, urine, joint fluid, stools and tonsils were also negative. The seasonal periodicity of the epidemics was of interest. It appeared each year for three successive years with the onset of the hot season and stopped abruptly with the onset of heavy rains. This suggested an insect vector but no proof was found.

In differential diagnosis, rheumatic fever, Haverhill fever and dengue were considered. Streptococcal infection did not precede the disease, and response to salicylates was poor. The rash was more extensive than that seen in dengue; pains were articular and not osseous; and post-dengue exhaustion was absent.

Treatment was symptomatic and supportive.[91]

Miscellaneous

Davidson reported a case of "infectious" polyarthritis associated with chronic bilateral bronchiectasis.[46] The association of both polyarthritis and bronchiectasis with agammaglobulinemia is well known.

Arthritis has also been caused by *Micrococcus tetragenus,*[165] *B. suipestifer,*[76,187,202] *Pseudomonas aeruginosa,*[23,64,37,160] *Pseudomonas pseudomallei,*[48] *Serratia marcescens,*[11] *Clostridium welchii,*[200] *Pasteurella multocida,*[15] an organism of the genus, *Herrellae,*[173] *Klebsiella pneumoniae,*[211] *Vibrio fetus,*[116,117,121] *Moraxella osloensis,*[61] *Micrococcus catarrhalis*[44,188] and anaerobic bacteria[217] among other unusual microorganisms. Pyarthrosis from infection with *E. coli* or *Bacterioides* organisms are becoming more common as seriously ill patients are being treated with immunosuppressive or corticosteroid drugs.[8,99,174]

Spirochetemia

Williams reported the finding of fusiform bacilli and spirochetes (of the type found in Vincent's angina) in the cultures of blood from 2 patients; in one of these patients, the organisms were recovered from the blood eleven times and successful subcultures of the organism were made.[214] These organisms were slightly pathogenic for rats. In these 2 patients with fusospirochetemia, myalgia and a migratory arthritis were observed, together with the sudden development of fever, headache and prostration. In one of these splenomegaly appeared with jaundice, pleurisy and a hemorrhagic eruption.

Causative organisms have been cultured from the blood in only a few of the spirochetal diseases.[123] Reiter cultured spirochetes from the blood of a patient with cystitis, arthritis and conjunctivitis.[166] Palmer demonstrated many times the presence of spirochetes in the blood of a patient with a prolonged illness with vague muscle and articular pains, relapsing fever, a rash resembling that of German measles, pericarditis and arthritis.[150] Juxta-articular nodules have been described in yaws.[26]

In Williams' patients, the initial symptoms resembled those of rat-bite fever, relapsing fever and Weil's disease.[214] Fever developed suddenly, associated with chilliness, prostration, headache and muscular and joint aching, followed subsequently by a migratory arthritis. The first of these patients had an intermittent type of arthritis for two years, while the second was free of arthritic symptoms after a month. In both of these patients, clinical improvement followed treatment with arsphenamine and fusiform bacilli and spirochetes apparently disappeared from the blood. Penicillin is now the treatment of choice.

ARTHRITIS IN MYCOTIC DISEASES

Coccidioidomycosis

Coccidioidomycosis is endemic in the southwestern United States, especially in the San Joaquin Valley, Mexico and South America. In the disseminated stage of the illness, bone and joint involvement is common and may be readily confused with the musculoskeletal manifestations of tuberculosis.[189]

The primary phase of the disease is usually a self-limited pulmonary infection due to inhalation of the fungus, *Coccidioides immitis*, and is characterized by malaise, anorexia, chills, fever, headache, night sweats and pleurisy. Transient joint symptoms including pain, tenderness and slight swelling without effusion occur in one-third of all pulmonary cases. Lesions of erythema nodosum may appear on the shins. No residual joint damage or deformity results from this phase which may persist approximately one month.[189]

Approximately 0.2 per cent of those with the acute illness go on to develop the second stage in which chronic granulomatous lesions are disseminated throughout the body. This is a very serious illness. In one series the mortality rate was 12.5 per cent in the Caucasian race and 77 per cent among Negroes.[136] It is in this stage of the disease that serious bone and joint lesions are fairly common. In one series of 256 cases, the joints were affected in 79 (with involvement of the ankle in 33, knee in 21, foot in 16, elbow in 11, wrist in 19, shoulder in 8, finger in 7, vertebrae in 6, hip in 5, sternoclavicular in 1, with others unspecified). The roentgen findings in these joints may mimic those of tuberculous arthritis with regions of early destruction in articular surfaces which is often accompanied by swelling of the overlying soft tissues. Articular cartilage may be destroyed with narrowing of the joint spaces. The joint spaces may completely disappear in later stages and extensive areas of destruction may be noted in articular surfaces. Ankylosis may occur in some cases.[143] The arthritis is predominantly destructive both in tuberculosis and in coccidioidal granuloma with little tendency to heal by production of bone. Pulmonary involvement is frequent in both. Coccidioidal granuloma usually attacks joints by extension from adjacent bony lesions[36] and destruction develops more rapidly than it does in tuberculosis.[198]

Coccidioidal arthritis may be suspected if progressive mono- or polyarticular arthritis occurs in individuals who have lived in or visited the San Joaquin Valley region in southern California; if serial roentgenograms show an unusually rapid progress of the destructive bony lesions, the diagnosis is more likely.[171]

Diagnosis.—There is no pathognomonic, clinical or roentgen finding. A positive skin test reaction is thought to be fairly reliable but only six weeks or more after the primary infection. It is often negative in the second or disseminated stage. A negative result early, followed by a positive result later, is conclusive.[189] A positive reaction to complement-fixation test, 1:32 or greater, usually indicates dissemination of the disease. Positive diagnosis can be established only by the demonstration of spherules in gastric washings, sputum, pleural fluid, spinal fluid, pus, or synovial fluid. Such tests should be done extremely carefully, however, since laboratory personnel have become infected very frequently.

Five cases of chronic synovitis of the knee due to *Coccidioides immitis* demonstrated the great advantage of culturing and examining synovial *tissue* in contrast to synovial *fluid* alone; the fluid showed only nonspecific changes in all 5.[175]

Treatment.—Amphotericin B has been employed successfully in the control of the systemic manifestations of the disease.[53,70,175] Its use is required over a long period of time; nephrotoxicity is a possible complication. Synovectomy and excision of the diseased soft tissue where there was no underlying bone disease apparently arrested the disease in four patients.[189,199] Amputation of a severely involved extremity was believed to have been a life-saving procedure in two patients.[136]

Histoplasmosis

It is believed that infection with *Histoplasma capsulatum* is relatively common and, with few exceptions, benign. Bone and joint involvement is rare. The majority of patients have an unrecognized primary infection which resembles "grippe" or a mild pneumonitis. Some have a non-fatal disseminated infection, and a few succumb with systemic involvement. Results of skin tests, serological tests and cultures are usually positive in chronic disease, but skin test results may be negative in acute fulminating cases.[104] Amphotericin B is effective in disseminated disease.

Key and Large reported the occurrence of involvement of a knee joint by histoplasmosis which closely resembled tuberculosis of the knee joint clinically.[115] The knee was considerably enlarged with excess fluid and thickened periarticular tissues. No redness was noted but there was a moderate increase in local heat over the joint. Roentgen examination showed thickening of the soft tissues and moderate bony atrophy with spotty atrophy of the bone structure. A thick purulent material was aspirated from the knee joint; culture of this was negative. Inoculation of the material into guinea pigs failed to show tuberculosis. The extremity was amputated as the patient did not respond to sulfonamides or other therapy. The synovial cavity of the knee was filled with thick, gray pus; the abscess extended into the calf. There was considerable erosion and necrosis of the articular surfaces of the bones. On microscopic section the synovial membrane was replaced by a mass of granulation tissue, infiltrated with giant cells and macrophages. Monocytes or mononuclear phagocytes were the predominating cells in the inflammatory exudate. Many of the phagocytic cells contained *Histoplasma capsulatum.*

Blastomycosis

Blastomyces dermatitidis has been restricted to the North American continent, especially the mid-west, the Ohio River Valley and North Carolina.[179] The disease occurs mostly in agricultural or poultry workers living under unhygienic conditions. The fungus gains access to the body through the lungs or through abraded skin. The disease usually presents as a pulmonary infection or with cutaneous manifestations but from these areas a hematogenous spread may occur to any organs including the bones and joints.[144] Blastomycotic osteomyelitis has been observed in many locations.[7] Vertebral involvement resembles that of tuberculosis, with narrowing of the disc spaces, destruction of bone with collapse of vertebral bodies and spread from segment to segment under the anterior spinal ligament.[16] Meyer and Gall have observed 12 cases of blastomycosis of the spine.[138] The clinical findings resemble those seen in actinomycosis. Moist cover-slip preparations of exudate or scrapings, stained sections, cultures, complement-fixation and skin tests are procedures used to demonstrate infection with the fungus.[57] A case of fulminating systemic blastomycosis has been reported in which the diagnosis was made by a smear of purulent joint fluid.[135] In contrast to coccidioidomycosis, joint fluid and drainage material from a bone or soft tissue abscess in *Blastomyces dermatitidis* infection are rich in organisms.[175] Successful treatment requires use of amphotericin B. Four patients, two of whom had bone lesions and all of whom were resistant to stilbamidine, have been reported cured with amphotericin B.[82,175]

Cryptococcosis (Torulosis, European Blastomycosis)

Cryptococcosis has a world-wide distribution, and has been reported throughout the southern United States from Florida to California. The usual portal of entry is the respiratory tract but the gastrointestinal tract and skin have also been suggested as possible sites of entry. While it is possible that pulmonary cryptococcosis may occur in a mild, spontaneously healing form, it is usually a progressive disease with a marked predilection for the central nervous system, lasting several years and eventually proving fatal. Bone lesions are rarer than in other systemic fungal diseases. Collins found 17 with bone lesions in his series of 200 cases.[41] One patient with initial symptoms of pain and localized swelling of the lumbar spine had an osteolytic lesion of the spinous process of the third lumbar vertebra and an extensive but asymptomatic infiltration of both lungs. The organism *Cryptococcus neoformans* was cultured from pus obtained by aspiration of the soft tissue mass overlying the third lumbar vertebra. This patient was apparently cured by aspiration of the abscess, sulfadiazine, and surgical excision of the infected spinous process. Amphotericin B has proved to be of value as it has in other deep fungal infections.[6,53]

Actinomycosis and Nocardiosis

Actinomyces israelii, the causative agent of actinomycosis, is actually a bacterium but it produces a chronic illness much like the true fungal diseases. Bone and joint involvement is common and involvement of the mandible, ribs, humerus, ilium, phalanges, and spine has been reported.[7,111,138] It is usually secondary to a focus in the respiratory or gastrointestinal tract. Cope has reported 65 cases of actinomycosis of the spine. The disease usually involved several of the vertebrae, affecting the bodies, pedicles, transverse processes and heads of neighboring ribs but sparing the discs. Dense bone sclerosis extending into the bodies and surrounding many small abscess cavities produced the "honeycomb," "lattice" or "soap bubble" appearance; long bony spurs bridging the vertebrae have been reported.[16,42] This may be mistaken for Pott's disease. Diagnosis is made by direct examination of purulent

Table 68-1.—Deep Mycotic Infections of Man that Cause Arthritis and Drugs Recommended for Treatment of Disseminated Disease

Mycoses	*Causative organism*	*Drug*
Coccidioidomycosis	*Coccidioides immitis*	Amphotericin B
Histoplasmosis	*Histoplasma capsulatum*	"
North American blastomycosis . .	*Blastomyces dermatitidis*	"
Cryptococcosis	*Cryptococcus neoformans*	"
Sporotrichosis	*Sporotrichum schenckii*	"
Actinomycosis	*Actinomyces israelii**	Penicillin G
Nocardiosis	Nocardia asteroides*	Sulfadiazine

* Bacteria, not true fungi.

material from abscesses or sinuses or by culture under anaerobic conditions.[42]

Treatment has improved with the use of several antibiotics including tetracycline, neomycin and penicillin.[98] Thorough surgical debridement of all infected tissue and bone is indicated as in other chronic infections.[42,144] Full use should be made of the bacteriologic and sensitivity tests now available to confirm diagnosis and aid in selecting the most effective antibiotic therapy.

Infection with the bacterium, *Nocardia*, has many of the features seen with the fungal diseases but responds well to sulfadiazine or other sulfa drugs.[14]

Other Fungal Diseases

Among other fungal agents, cases of bone and joint infection have been reported due to *Sporotrichum schenkii*,[133,169] *Cephalosporium* sp.[208] and *Candida albicans*.[163]

ARTHRITIS IN VIRAL DISEASES

Viral Hepatitis

During the early stages in the incubation of viral hepatitis, some patients experience polyarthritis lasting from days to occasionally months and characterized not only by pain but also by swelling that may mimic rheumatoid arthritis. When the diagnosis of hepatitis becomes overt with appearance of jaundice, the rheumatic symptoms usually disappear.

Recently, it was found that many patients with hepatitis have a virus-like particle, called Australia antigen, circulating in their blood. In some patients this material forms an immune complex with antibody. Such complexes have been shown to bind complement. By immunofluorescent techniques, Australia antigen, antibody and complement have been found in inflammatory vascular lesions in at least one patient with polyarteritis nodosa and in other patients in synovial membranes. It thus appears likely that patients who develop arthralgia in the course of hepatitis have an immune-complex disease which may account for the articular symptoms (*see also* Chapter 46).

Influenza

Monarticular or polyarticular joint involvement may complicate influenza.[25,67,134] This usually appears early in the course of the disease although it may be delayed for several weeks. Suppuration has occasionally occurred.[155] Vague joint pains have been reported in a number of such patients but the incidence of joint pathology is usually not high.[85]

Infectious Mononucleosis

Although arthralgia is unusual in this disease, joint pain and fever occasionally may be found at onset and may simulate rheumatic fever.[20]

Rubella

A self-limited form of polyarthritis that accompanies rubella (German measles) has been reported in great numbers in recent years, especially following the epidemic of the mid-1960's.[97,124,125,110,157,184] Five cases with arthritis out of 37 patients with rubella were reported by Lewis.[129] The arthritis affected primarily the small joints of the hands and cleared completely in a few weeks.[107] To date, there is no evidence that patients who develop rubella arthritis may succumb years later to rheumatoid arthritis.[110]

During testing of a rubella vaccine, a significant number of those inoculated developed a migratory polyarthralgia.[128] Again, no relationship between such reactions and a more chronic form of rheumatoid arthritis was found although one patient had joint complaints one year later.

Lymphogranuloma Venereum

Lymphogranuloma venereum is a distinct venereal disease affecting all sexes and races.[195] The primary sore which usually appears from two to five days after infective coitus is usually asymptomatic and heals spontaneously. Joint involvement may occasionally resemble rheumatic fever or purulent arthritis.[108]

The arthritis which may occur with lymphogranuloma venereum runs a variable course. In occasional cases, one may encounter tender, painful, actually swollen joints; however, the process is usually chronic and persists for weeks or months. Polyarticular involvement is common, with frequent involvement of the knees, ankles and wrists. Intermittent hydrarthrosis occurs occasionally. The Frei reaction is positive in all cases; cultures of synovial fluid are sterile.[88]

Dawson and Boots have reported a series of 24 patients (16 women and 8 men) with arthritis associated with lymphogranuloma venereum.[47] In most of these individuals there occurred a chronic indolent serous arthritis, often with intermittent hydrops. Acute flare-ups were not uncommon and there was a tendency to relapse. The disease was usually polyarticular, involving especially the knees, ankles, shoulders and wrists; occasionally, migratory joint involvement or generalized arthralgia occurred. Bilateral joint involvement was noted in 50 per cent of the cases. Patients varied from nineteen to fifty-five years of age, the majority being in the third and fourth decades.

This type of joint involvement persisted for weeks or months without destruction of bone or cartilage; swelling was usually confined to the periarticular tissues. The joint fluid was sterile on culture and was never purulent. Cell count of the synovial fluid varied from 900 to 5000 per c.mm.

Other findings in these patients included: A positive Frei reaction, other evidences of lymphogranulomatous infection (especially rectal strictures) and marked elevation of the sedimentation rate.

Grace and Rake have used a special yolk sac antigen consisting of a suspension in isotonic solutions of sodium chloride of the elementary bodies of the virus of lymphogranuloma venereum. This can be prepared with any desired concentration of virus.[71,72] Complement-fixation tests performed with this antigen were found to be more sensitive than the Frei reaction.

This disease often responds to sulfonamide therapy.[78,154,180,201] Visceral and joint manifestations usually disappeared following sulfonamide administration. Despite this, a positive Frei reaction may persist for many years after apparent healing has occurred as is the case with the tuberculin test in tuberculosis. Both tetracycline and chloramphenicol have been found to improve markedly the acute ulcerative and inguinal forms of this disease.[109]

Mumps

Slight joint swelling and effusion occur occasionally. Joint pains are not uncommon and usually disappear within a week. Acute arthritis has also followed suppurative parotitis.

Measles

Although articular complications have been reported occasionally, their association with measles has not been definitely accepted. Infectious spondylitis has occurred occasionally after an attack of measles but it is doubtful if there is any causal relationship.[13]

Smallpox

Arthritis resulting from smallpox or vaccination has been observed.[40,118,182] Suppurative arthritis and even osteomyelitis apparently are caused by secondary infection of the pustules. Lesions caused by the smallpox virus in the ends of the bones were described as necrotic areas which led to arrest of bone growth and rarely to ankylosis of a joint.

Ten days after smallpox vaccination of an adult, an acute arthritis of the knee developed with fever.[182] The joint fluid was "thick yellowish-white," showed

44,000 leukocytes/c.mm., predominantly polymorphonuclear cells, and the glucose content was 50 mg./100 ml. Bacterial cultures were sterile but vaccinia virus grew out upon inoculation into tissue culture, the first demonstration of this organism in joint tissues. The knee cleared in a week without specific therapy and follow-up x rays were negative.

Other Viral Diseases

Arthritis has been described associated with varicella and an arbovirus infection.[51,209]

ARTHRITIS IN OTHER INFECTIOUS DISEASES

Arthritis is a well-known complication in a few tropical diseases, discussed above, notably bacillary dysentery, typhoid fever, brucellosis, leprosy, the mycotic infections; it may also occur in filariasis due to *Wuchereria bancrofti*, and in the spirochetal diseases, yaws and bejel, in which gummatous lesions may involve the joints or occasionally a hydrarthrosis develops. Arthralgias, on the other hand, are very common in tropical diseases, and may occur in the rickettsial group: in typhus, Rocky Mountain spotted fever, tsutsugamushi fever, trench fever, Schara boil, Oroya fever, and verruca peruviana. Arthralgias occur in the virus group: yellow fever, dengue and sandfly fever; in the spirochetal diseases: yaws, relapsing fever and Weil's disease; in filarial infections; in onchocerciasis and dracontiasis; in malaria and African trypanosomiasis. In these groups of diseases, the spirochetal group, the rickettsial diseases, and the viral diseases, pains in the limbs and back are so severe and so regularly present as to be a helpful diagnostic aid.

ARTHRITIS RESULTING FROM THE ADMINISTRATION OF ANTIMICROBIAL AGENTS

Bone and joint pains and occasionally even joint inflammation may occur following the administration of various drugs such as serum,[95] arsenic, mepharsen, iodobismitol, gold, sulfonamides, penicillin, or other antibiotics, used to treat infections.

Long observed the occurrence of painful joints during sulfanilamide or sulfathiazole therapy.[131] A patient with chancroidal infection developed tender swollen elbows and knees during sulfathiazole therapy. The fluid was sterile and contained only a few polys per high-power field. Other manifestations of drug toxicity were also present. The joint swelling subsided with cessation of sulfonamide therapy, and recurred again a week later after administration of a test dose of 3 gm. of sulfathiazole; the joint swelling again promptly disappeared within twenty-four hours after stopping the sulfonamide.

With penicillin therapy painful polyarthritis, fever, urticaria, or sometimes erythema, and adenopathy may occur. Such reactions usually begin seven to fourteen days after therapy has been instituted and rarely as soon as forty-eight hours. The joint symptoms may subside within four or five days of stopping penicillin. The joint symptoms *per se* are not an indication for stopping penicillin therapy and usually may be controlled by pyribenzamine in doses of 50 mg. every four hours or by administration of a corticosteroid. If diffuse erythema of the skin is present it may indicate an impeding exfoliative dermatitis and penicillin administration should be terminated.

Similar reactions have occurred following other antibiotics also, and may develop one or two weeks after the agent was used. These joint reactions are believed similar to those of serum sickness (*see also* Chapter 52).

BIBLIOGRAPHY

1. Adam, A., MacDonald, A. and MacKenzie, I. G.: J. Bone & Joint Surg., *49B*, 652, 1967.
2. Adams, F. D.: Ann. Intern. Med., *20*, 33, 1944.

3. Aguilar, J. A., and Elvidge, A. R.: J. Neurosurg., *18*, 27, 1961.
4. Aidem, H. P.: J. Bone & Joint Surg., *50A*, 1663, 1968.
5. Allbritten, F. F., Sheely, R. F. and Jeffers, W. A.: J.A.M.A., *114*, 2360, 1940.
6. Allcock, E. A.: J. Bone & Joint Surg., *43B*, 71, 1961.
7. Altemeir, W. A. and Largen, T.: J.A.M.A., *159*, 1462, 1952.
8. Ament, M. E., *et al.*: Amer. J. Dis. Child., *114*, 427, 1967.
9. Anderson, S. G.: Lancet, *1*, 823, 1959.
10. Asnes, R. S. and Arendar, G. M.: Pediatrics, *38*, 837, 1966.
11. Atlas, E., and Belding, M. E.: J.A.M.A., *204*, 167, 1968.
12. Avila, L., Jr.: J. Bone & Joint Surg., *23*, 922, 1941.
13. Bade, H.: Roentgenpraxis, *11*, 461, 1939.
14. Baikie, A. G., *et al.*: Lancet, *2*, 261, 1970.
15. Barth, W. F., Healey, L. A., and Decker, J. L.: Arth. & Rheum., *11*, 394, 1968.
16. Baylin, G. J. and Wear, J. M.: Amer. J. Roentgenol., *69*, 395, 1953.
17. Bazan, F. and Maggi, R.: Archiv. Argent. de Pediat., *12*, 376, 1939.
18. Beeson, P. B.: J.A.M.A., *123*, 332, 1943.
19. Benjafield, J. D. and Halley, G. S.: Lancet, *2*, 616, 1938.
20. Bernstein, A.: Medicine, *19*, 98, 1940.
21. Billington, E. W.: J.A.M.A., *83*, 683, 1924.
22. Bingold, A. C.: Proc. Roy. Soc. Med., *55*, 354, 1962.
23. Bishop, W. A.: J. Bone & Joint Surg., *20*, 216, 1938.
24. Black, P. H., Kunz, L. J. and Swartz, M. N.: New Engl. J. Med., *262*, 811, 1960.
25. Bloise, N. L.: Arch. de Pediat. de Uruguay, *4*, 99, 1933.
26. Browne, S. G.: Ann. Trop. Med. & Parasit., *55*, 309, 1961.
27. Buchman, J.: J. Int. Coll. Surg., *24*, 300, 1955.
28. Buck, R. E.: J.A.M.A., *206*, 135, 1968.
29. Bulmer, J. H.: J. Bone & Joint Surg., *48B*, 289, 1966.
30. Burke, W. A., Kwong, O., and Halpern, R.: Calif. Med., *91*, 356, 1959.
31. Bush, F. W. and Bailey, F. R.: Ann. Intern. Med., *20*, 619, 1944.
32. Braude, A. I.: G. P., *11*, 75, 1955.
33. Braude, A. I.: J. Imm. and Infect. Dis., *89*, 76, 1951.
34. Cameron, J. M. and Izatt, M. M.: Scot. Med. J., *5*, 148, 1960.
35. Campbell, W. and Greenfield, E. C.: South African Med. J., *10*, 545, 1936.
36. Carter, R. A.: Amer. J. Roentgenol., *25*, 715, 1931.
37. Chartier, Y., Martin, W. J. and Kelly, P. J.: Ann. Intern. Med., *50*, 1462, 1959.
38. Childe, A. E. and Tucker, F. R.: J. Canad. Assoc. Radiol., *12*, 47, 1961.
39. Clayton, M. L., *et al.*: Mod. Treatm., *6*, 1093, 1969.
40. Cockshott, P. and MacGregor, M.: J. Fac. Radiol. (Lond.), *10*, 57, 1959.
41. Collins, V. P.: Amer. J. Roentgenol., *63*, 102, 1950.
42. Cope, V. Z.: J. Bone & Joint Surg., *33B*, 205, 1951.
43. Crea, M. A. and Mortimer, E. A., Jr.: Pediatrics, *23*, 879, 1959.
44. Curtis, S. H.: New York State Med. J., *32*, 672, 1932.
45. David, J. R. and Black, R. L.: Medicine, *39*, 385, 1960.
46. Davidson, M.: Post-Grad. Med. J., *18*, 166, 1942.
47. Dawson, M. H. and Boots, R. L.: J.A.M.A., *113*, 1162, 1939.
48. Diamond, H. S. and Pastore, R.: Arth. & Rheum., *10*, 459, 1967.
49. Dingle, J. H. and Finland, M.: War Medicine, *2*, 1, 1942.
50. Dobson, L., Holman, E. and Cutting, W.: J.A.M.A., *116*, 272, 1941.
51. Doherty, R. L., *et al.*: Trans. R. Soc. Trop. Med. Hyg., *64*, 740, 1970.
52. Dolman, C. E., Kerr, D. E., Chang, H., and Shearer, A. R.: Canad. J. Pub. Health, *42*, 288, 1951.
53. Dormer, B. A. and Findlay, M.: Afr. Med. J., *34*, 611, 1960.
54. Ecker, E. E., Kuehn, A. O. and Recroft, E. W.: J.A.M.A., *118*, 1296, 1942.
55. Editorial: J.A.M.A., *174*, 406, 1960.
56. Eichner, H. L., *et al.*: Arth. & Rheum., *13*, 272, 1970.
57. Elliott, G. B., Wilt, J. C. and Duggan, M.: Canad. Med. Assoc. J., *67*, 650, 1952.
58. Epstein, J.: Amer. J. Med. Sci., *163*, 401, 1922.
59. Farid, Z. and Miak, A., Jr.: Trans. Roy. Soc. Trop. Med. & Hyg., *57*, 115, 1963.
60. Farrell, E., Loroi, G. H. and Vogel, J.: Arch. Intern. Med., *64*, 1, 1939.
61. Feigin, R. D., *et al.*: J. Pediat., *75*, 116, 1969.
62. Fellander, M. and Lindberg, L.: J. Bone & Joint Surg., *48A*, 1585, 1966.
63. Fielding, J. W., and Lieber, W. A.: New York J. Med., *61*, 3916, 1961.

64. Fiset, P. E.: Canad. Med. Assoc. J., *45*, 545, 1942.
65. Fox, M. J. and Gilbert, J.: Amer. J. Med. Sci., *308*, 63, 1944.
66. Frank, W. P. and Bower, A. G.: Calif. Med., *74*, 42, 1951.
67. Freund, E.: *Gelenkerkrankungen*, Berlin, Urban, 1929.
68. Gaines, L. M. and Shulman, L. E.: Bull. Rheum. Dis., *10*, 195, 1959.
69. Ghormley, R. K.: Arch. Phys. Ther., *17*, 567, 1936.
70. Golden, H. E. and Parker, R. H.: Mod. Treatm., *6*, 1117, 1969.
71. Grace, A. W.: Arch. Dermat. & Syph., *48*, 659, 1943.
72. Grace, A. W. and Rake, G.: Arch. Dermat. & Syph., *48*, 619, 1943.
73. Graham, G.: Proc. Roy. Soc. Med., *13*, 23, 1919.
74. Green, F. B.: Texas State J. Med., *32*, 549, 1936.
75. Green, M. E. and Freyberg, R. H.: Amer. J. Med. Sci., *201*, 495, 1941.
76. Guthrie, K. J.: Arch. Dis. Child., *16*, 269, 1941.
77. Halliday, J. H. and Horan, J. P.: Med. J. Australia, *2*, 293, 1943.
78. Hamilton, G. R.: Mil. Surg., *83*, 431, 1938.
79. Hardy, A. V.: Med. Clin. North America, *21*, 1747, 1937.
80. Hardy, A. V., Jordan, C. F., Borts, I. H. and Hardy, G. C.: Pub. Health. Rep., *45*, 2433, 1930.
81. Harmon, P. H.: J. Bone & Joint Surg., *24*, 576, 1942.
82. Harrell, E. R. and Curtis, A. C.: A.M.A. Arch. Dermat., *76*, 561, 1957.
83. Hartman, J. T., *et al.*: J.A.M.A., *200*, 201, 1967.
84. Hazard, J. B. and Goodkind, R.: J.A.M.A., *99*, 534, 1932.
85. Healey, C. E.: J.A.M.A., *108*, 628, 1937.
86. Heberling, J. A.: J. Bone & Joint Surg., *23*, 917, 1941.
87. Hefke, H. W. and Turner, V. C.: J. Bone & Joint Surg., *24*, 857, 1942.
88. Hench, P. S.: Ann. Rheum. Dis., *2*, 172, 1941.
89. ————: Ann. Intern. Med., *12*, 1005, 1939.
90. Hench, P. S., *et al.*: Ann. Intern. Med., *14*, 1383, 1941.
91. ————: Ann. Intern. Med., *28*, 320, 1948.
92. ————: Ann. Intern. Med., *9*, 883, 1935.
93. Herrell, W. E. and Barber, T. S.: Postgrad. Med., *11*, 476, 1952.
94. Herrick, W. W.: J.A.M.A., *71*, 612, 1918.
95. ————: Bull. New York Acad. Med., *7*, 487, 1931.
96. Herrick, W. W. and Parkhurst, G. M.: Amer. J. Med. Sci., *158*, 473, 1919.
97. Hildebrandt, H. M., *et al.*: New Engl. J. Med., *274*, 1428, 1966.
98. Hinds, E. C. and Degnan, E. J.: Oral Surg., Oral Med. & Oral Path., *8*, 1034, 1955.
99. Hollander, J. L.: Personal communication.
100. Huber, H. G.: Monatschr. f. Kinderh., *70*, 332, 1937.
101. Huddleson, I. F.: *Brucellosis in Man and Animals*, New York, The Commonwealth Fund, 1939.
102. Hudson, O. C.: Med. Times, *63*, 342, 1935.
103. Hunt, D. D., *et al.*: J. Bone & Joint Surg., *48A*, 111, 1966.
104. Israel, H. L., DeLamater, E., Sones, M., Willis, W. D. and Mirmelstein, A.: Amer. J. Med., *12*, 252, 1952.
105. Jaeger, H. W.: Arch. de la Soc. de cir. de hosp. (Santiago, Chile), *12*, 305, 1942.
106. Jaffe, H. L.: J. Mt. Sinai Hosp., *1*, 23, 1934.
107. Johnson, R. E. and Hall, A. P.: New Engl. J. Med., *258*, 743, 1958.
108. Jones, C. A. and Rome, H. P.: Internat. Clin., 2d ser., *48*, 179, 1938.
109. Kalstone, B. M., Howell, J. A., Jr., and Cline, F. X., Jr.: J.A.M.A., *176*, 530, 1961.
110. Kantor, T. G.: Mod. Treatm., *6*, 1146, 1969.
111. Kau, L. S.: J. Clin. Med., *6*, 107, 1941.
112. Kelly, P. J., Coventry, M. B. and Martin, W. J.: Mayo Clin. Proc., *40*, 695, 1965.
113. Kelly, P. J., Martin, W. J., Schirger, A. and Weed, L. A.: J.A.M.A., *174*, 347, 1960.
114. Kelly, P. J., Martin, W. H. and Coventry, M. B.: J. Bone & Joint Surg., *47A*, 1005, 1965.
115. Key, J. A. and Large, A. M.: J. Bone & Joint Surg., *24*, 281, 1942.
116. Kilo, C., Hagemann, P. O. and Marzi, J.: Amer. J. Med., *38*, 962, 1965.
117. King, S., and Bronsky, D.: J.A.M.A., *175*, 1045, 1961.
118. Kini, M. G. and Kesavaswamy, P.: Antiseptic, *38*, 169, 1941.
119. Koshi, G., *et al.*: Indian J. Path. Bact., *7*, 264, 1964.
120. Kulowski, J. and Vinke, T. H.: J.A.M.A., *99*, 1656, 1932.
121. Kutner, L. J., *et al.*: J. Bone & Joint Surg., *52A*, 161, 1970.
122. Labendzinski, F.: Acta Rheumatol., *3*, 27, 1931.

123. Larson, W. P. and Barron, M.: J. Infect. Dis., *13*, 429, 1913.
124. Lee, P. R.: Brit. Med. J., *2*, 925, 1962.
125. Lee, P. R., Barnett, A. F., Scholer, J. F., Bryner, S. and Clark, W. H.: Calif. Med., *93*, 125, 1960.
126. Leedom, J. M., Ivler, D., Mathies, A. W., Thrupp, L. D., Portnoy, B. and Wehrle, P. F.: New Engl. J. Med., *273*, 1395, 1965.
127. L'episcopo, J. B.: Amer. J. Surg., *104*, 289, 1936.
128. Lerman, S. J., Nankevuis, G. H., Heggie, A. D. and Gold, E.: Ann. Intern. Med., *74*, 67, 1971.
129. Lewis, G. W.: Rheumatism, *10*, 70, 1954.
130. Lloyd-Roberts, G. C.: J. Bone & Joint Surg., *42B*, 706, 1960.
131. Long, P. H., *et al.*: J.A.M.A., *115*, 364, 1940.
132. Losada, M., Roeschmann, W. and Diza, E.: Arch. Inter-Amer. Rheum., *3*, 206, 1960.
133. Lynch, P. J., *et al.*: Ann. Intern. Med., *73*, 23, 1970.
134. Marsh, H.: *Diseases of Joints and Spine.* London, Cassell and Co., Ltd., 1895.
135. Marx, F. J. and Berenbaum, A. A.: New Engl. J. Med., *251*, 56, 1954.
136. Mazet, R., Jr.: Arch. Surg., *70*, 497, 1955.
137. Merwe, D. J. van der: Proc. Mine Med. Officers Assoc., *48*, 118, 1969.
138. Meyer, M. and Gall, M. B.: J. Bone & Joint Surg., *15*, 857, 1935.
139. Milch, H.: J. Bone & Joint Surg., *24*, 653, 1942.
140. Murakami, S.: Bull. Naval. Med. Assoc., Japan, *25*, 87, 1936.
141. McDonald, R.: Clin. Pediat. (Phila.), *6*, 571, 1967.
142. McGill, R. C., Martin, A. M. and Edmunds, P. N.: Brit. Med. J., *1*, 1213, 1966.
143. McMaster, P. E. and Gilfillan, C.: J.A.M.A., *112*, 1233, 1939.
144. McVay, L. V., Jr., Guthrie, R., and Sprunt, D. H.: New Engl. J. Med., *245*, 91, 1951.
145. Nagel, D. A., *et al.*: J.A.M.A., *191*, 975, 1965.
146. Nicholson, J. T.: Pennsylvania Med. J., *43*, 950, 1940.
147. Nikolskly, A. P.: Klin. Med., *13*, 1223, 1935.
148. Obletz, B. E.: Clin. Orthop., *22*, 27, 1962.
149. Osler, W.: Brit. Med. J., *1*, 1521, 1899.
150. Palmer, L.: South. Med. J., *31*, 530, 1938.
151. Parker, F., Jr. and Hudson, N. P.: Amer. J. Path., *2*, 357, 1926.
152. Paterson, D. E.: J. Fac. Radiol., London, *7*, 35, 1955.
153. Paul, J. R., Salinger, R. and Zuger, B.: J. Clin. Invest., *13*, 503, 1934.
154. Peryassu, D.: Brasil-medico, *53*, 309, 1939.
155. Peterson, J. C.: J. Pediat., *7*, 765, 1935.
156. Phalen, G. S., Prickman, L. E. and Krusen, F. H.: J.A.M.A., *118*, 859, 1942.
157. Phillips, C. A., *et al.*: J.A.M.A., *191*, 615, 1965.
158. Pinals, R. S., Ropes, M. W.: Arth. & Rheum., *7*, 241, 1964.
159. Pinelli, A.: Pediatria, *35*, 147, 1927.
160. Place, E. H. and Sutton, L. E.: Arch. Intern. Med., *54*, 659, 1934.
161. Pollack, N., Spinner, M., Richman, R.: N.Y. State Med. J., *64*, 2870, 1964.
162. Pritchard, A. E. and Robinson, M. P.: Lancet, *2*, 1165, 1961.
163. Pruitt, A. W., *et al.*: Pediatrics, *43*, 106, 1969.
164. Reeves, B. and Churchill-Davidson, D.: Postgrad. Med. J., *40*, 555, 1964.
165. Reiman, H. A.: J. Clin. Invest., *14*, 311, 1935.
166. Reiter, H.: Deutsch. Med. Wchnschr., *42*, 1535, 1916.
167. Rhoads, P. S. and Afremow, M. L.: Ann. Intern. Med., *19*, 60, 1943.
168. Riordan, D. C.: J. Bone & Joint Surg., *42A*, 683, 1960.
169. Riggs, S., *et al.*: Arch. Intern. Med., *118*, 584, 1966.
170. Rolleston, H.: Lancet, *1*, 541, 1919.
171. Rosenberg, E. F., Dockerty, M. B. and Meyerding, H. W.: Arch. Intern. Med., *69*, 238, 1942.
172. Sainton, P.: Lancet, *1*, 1080, 1919.
173. Sampson, C. C., Smith, C. D., and Robinson, H. S.: J. Nat. Med. Assoc., *51*, 360, 1959.
174. Sanders, D. Y., *et al.*: J. Pediat., *72*, 673, 1968.
175. Sanders, L. L.: Arth. & Rheum., *10*, 91, 1967.
176. Schein, A. J.: Arch. Intern. Med., *62*, 963, 1938.
177. Schirger, A., Nichols, D. R., Martin, W. H., Wellman, W. E. and Weed, L. A.: Ann. Intern. Med., *52*, 827, 1960.
178. Schottmüller, H.: Dermat. Wchnschr. (Suppl), *58*, 77, 1914.
179. Schwartz, J. and Muth, J.: Doc. Med. Geog. et Trop., *5*, 29, 1953.
180. Shaffer, L. W. and Arnold, E.: Arch. Dermat. & Syph., *38*, 705, 1938.
181. Sharpe, J. C.: Ann. Intern. Med., *9*, 1431, 1936.
182. Silby, H. M., Farber, R., O'Connell, C. J., Ascher, J. and Marine, E. J.: Ann. Intern. Med., *62*, 347, 1965.

183. Smith, A. deF.: Bull. Hosp. Joint. Dis., *12*, 459, 1951.
184. Smith, D., *et al.*: Med. J. Austral., *1*, 845, 1970.
185. Smith, H. W., Thomas, L., Dingle, J. H. and Finland, M.: Ann. Intern. Med., *20*, 12, 1944.
186. Smith, W. S. and Ward, R. M.: J.A.M.A., *195*, 1148, 1966.
187. Sokolova, Y. V., Khondu, A. A. and Kolegaeva, A. I.: Vestnik. khir., *44*, 30, 1936.
188. Solomon, W. M. and Tuchewicz, H. R.: J. Bone & Joint Surg., *20*, 1061, 1938.
189. Sotelo-Ortiz, F.: J. Bone & Joint Surg., *37A*, 49, 1955.
190. Spink, W. W.: Ann. Intern. Med., *35*, 358, 1951.
191. ———: Tr. Coll. Physicians, Philadelphia, *21*, 51, 1953.
192. ———: Seminar, *16*, 8, 1954.
193. Steinberg, C. L.: J.A.M.A., *138*, 15, 1948.
194. Stetson, J. W., De Ponte, R. J., and Southwick, W. O.: Clin. Orthop., *56*, 105, 1968.
195. Stokes, J. H., Beerman, H. and Ingraham, N. R., Jr.: Amer. J. Med. Sci., *197*, 575, 1939.
196. Strong, P. S. and Hollander, J. L.: Bull. U.S. Army Med. Dept., *78*, 68, 1944.
197. Sullivan, C. R.: Surg. Clin. North America, *41*, 1077, 1961.
198. Taylor, R. G.: Amer. J. Roentgenol., *10*, 551, 1923.
199. Thiemeyer, J. S., Jr.: J. Bone & Joint Surg., *36A*, 387, 1954.
200. Torg, J. S. and Lammot, T. R., III: J. Bone & Joint Surg., *50A*, 1233, 1968.
201. Torpin, R., Pund, E. R., Greenblatt, R. B. and Sanderson, E. S.: Amer. J. Surg., *43*, 688, 1939.
202. Tur, A. F. and Gartock, O. O.: Ztschr. f. Kinderh., *56*, 696, 1934.
203. Urteaga, O., Larrea, P. and Caldron, J.: Antibiotic Med., *1*, 513, 1955.
204. Vartiainen, J. and Hurri, L.: Acta Med. Scand., *175*, 771, 1964.
205. Wainwright, D.: Proc. Roy. Soc. Med., *52*, 864, 1959.
206. ———: Proc. Roy. Soc. Med., *61*, 1265, 1968.
207. Warren, C. P.: Ann. Rheum. Dis., *29*, 483, 1970.
208. Ward, H. P., Martin, W. H., Ivins, J. C., and Weed, L. A.: Proc. Mayo. Clin., *36*, 337, 1961.
209. Ward, J. R., *et al.*: J.A.M.A., *212*, 1954, 1970.
210. Waterson, A. P. and Wedgewood, J.: Lancet, *1*, 472, 1953.
211. Weber, R. G., and Ansell, B. A., Jr.: Ann. Intern. Med., *57*, 281, 1962.
212. Westerlund, N. C. and Bierman, A. H.: Amer. J. Clin. Path., *53*, 92, 1970.
213. Williams, D. N., *et al.*: Brit. Med. J., *2*, 93, 1970.
214. Williams, R. H.: Arch. Intern. Med., *68*, 80, 1941.
215. Willner, P., Place, E. H. and Sutton, L. E., Jr.: Med. & Surg. J., *194*, 285, 1926.
216. World Health Organization: World Health Org. Report Series, *67*, 1, 1953.
217. Ziment, I., *et al.*: Arth. & Rheum., *12*, 627, 1969.

PART XI

Miscellaneous Conditions Complicating or Producing Arthritis

Section Editor: John L. Decker, M.D.

Chapter 69

Amyloidosis

By Evan Calkins, M.D., and Alan S. Cohen, M.D.

Long regarded as an amorphous hyaline substance, amyloid is now known to represent the accumulation of increasingly well-defined connective tissue components. The most characteristic and quantitatively significant of these, the amyloid fibril, can readily be identified with the electron microscope and appears to be responsible for the distinctive histologic characteristic of amyloid. The characteristic is an amorphous-appearing eosinophilic extracellular substance which stains with special dyes, the most important of which is Congo red.[42] This imparts green birefringence when the material is viewed in the polarizing microscope.[32,56] Through use of such increasingly sensitive histologic techniques it is now realized that the occurrence of amyloid deposits is an extremely common finding.[46,53,57] Traces of amyloid have been observed in the hearts, especially auricular appendages, and the aortas of approximately one-third of people over 60 years of age. Small amounts of amyloid can also be seen in the meningeal vessels in brains of approximately half of patients in this age group and two-thirds of patients over 80 years of age.[55,57] It appears probable that the hyaline lesions in the islets of Langerhans of many patients with diabetes mellitus represent accumulations of amyloid.[24,57] Awareness of the high frequency of amyloid deposits in aged people may necessitate redefinition of the term "amyloidosis," so as to denote not merely the presence of amyloid, but also the accumulation of sufficient amounts of this substance to cause clinical manifestations, chiefly due to pressure on surrounding structures.

FREQUENCY; PREDISPOSING FACTORS

The incidence and severity of amyloidosis, both in men and animals, appear to be associated with a number of factors. Among these are (A) prolonged inflammation or repeated immunologic stimulation,[10] (B) tumors such as multiple myeloma, Hodgkin's disease and others, and (C) genetic factors.

A. Amyloid and Inflammatory Disorders ("Secondary Amyloidosis")

Since the earliest description of amyloidosis by Virchow it has been recognized that the disease is not infrequently seen in patients with tuberculosis, sepsis and rheumatoid arthritis.[37,51] In determining the incidence of amyloidosis accompanying rheumatoid arthritis one must be careful to differentiate clinically significant amyloidosis from the accumulation of traces of amyloid commonly seen in normal elderly people. In one clinical study which attempted to do this[40] only one of 50 rheumatoid patients exhibited clear-cut "secondary amyloidosis." But in a recent review it was pointed out that rectal and renal biopsy studies on rheumatoid populations suggest that amyloid is not merely an autopsy finding, but a moderately common accompaniment of clinical rheumatoid disease.[21] The true incidence and prevalence of amyloid will await further *prospective* studies of appropriate diseased and control patients in a manner similar to that reported.[40]

B. Amyloid and Multiple Myeloma

It has been known for many years that patients with multiple myeloma not infrequently exhibit amyloidosis.[38,39] Although the estimated frequency varies with different reporters, most agree that it is in the neighborhood of 15 to 20 per cent.[11] Many of these patients may exhibit enlargement of the liver and spleen and a nephrotic syndrome; others present with a variety of clinical manifestations including, for example, macroglossia and the carpal tunnel syndrome—lesions which appear to be especially characteristic of amyloidosis accompanying multiple myeloma.[7]

Application of immunochemical techniques for the detection of M-components has demonstrated their presence in the blood, urine or both in approximately one-half of patients with amyloidosis without known predisposing cause or genetic predisposition.[3,12] Most of these patients have no bone lesions and only modest increases (if any) of mature plasma cells in their bone marrow. The relationship between abnormalities in gammaglobulin metabolism and amyloidosis appears to represent a clinical and biological association of important but undefined pathogenetic significance.[38] How this will relate to the recent observation of homology in the amino acid sequence of amyloid and the variable portion of immunoglobulin light chain is not known.[27]

C. Amyloid and Genetic Factors

The third group of factors which appear to enhance the incidence of amyloidosis are genetic in nature. Numerous descriptions appear in the literature of a wide variety of syndromes in which amyloidosis involves many members of a given family.[2,35,44] The pattern of inheritance in these syndromes is usually dominant in nature (with the exception of the amyloid associated with familial Mediterranean fever which is recessive).

Amyloidosis also occurs in high frequency in several racial groups. People of Portuguese ancestry not infrequently develop a form of amyloidosis characterized by the Adie pupil, severe peripheral neuropathy, postural hypotension, diarrhea and impotence.[1] Sephardic or Iraqui Jews show, in fairly high frequency, two apparently unrelated genetic defects—one leading to so-called familial Mediterranean fever and the second to amyloidosis[30,49] (*see also* Chapter 45).

In many of the patients with amyloidosis seen in a medical center today, the condition is not accompanied or preceded by a prolonged inflammatory condition. The patients rarely give a family history consistent with amyloid. In some the involvement is widespread while in others focal lesions (in respiratory tract, urinary tract, eye, skin) may occur. These clinical aspects have recently been reviewed in detail.[19,31,34,50]

NATURE AND COMPOSITION OF AMYLOID

The most abundant single component of amyloid, representing up to 40 per cent of the dry weight of the infiltrated organ, is the amyloid fibril.[15] Characteristic fibrils have been noted in high concentration in all specimens of amyloid studied to date, whether derived from man or experimental animals.[17] Excellent techniques have been developed for the isolation and purification of these fibrils, relying, in particular, on their extraction by high speed homogenization in distilled water.[16,41]

The fibrils range from 300 to 10,000 Å in length, and in tissue section are about 100 Å in diameter.[47] They are nonbranching and in longitudinal section often appear as double-stranded structures consisting of two filaments approximately 25 Å in diameter or as cylindrical rods with 25 to 30 Å thick walls and 25 to 30 Å wide central cores. Occasionally three strands can be observed. Circular structures of diameter equal to the amyloid fibril are occasionally seen. These usually consist of 4, 5 or 6 geometrically arranged subunits, and have led to the hypothesis that the amyloid fibril is composed of 4, 5 or 6 filaments.[47] X-ray diffraction studies have shown that amyloid has a distinct cross beta pattern.

Chemical studies of the amyloid fibril protein indicate that its amino acid composition is quite distinct from collagen, elastin or fibrin.[18] Amyloid protein from different amyloid-laden organs of the same individual is identical; amyloid protein from different individuals appears to exhibit certain differences in chemical composition[28,48] and immunologic activity.[25] The carbohydrate moiety of the fibril constitutes approximately 3 to 5 per cent of the total weight.[4] It includes hexosamine, sialic acid, mannose, galactose, and glucose and a trace of fucose.

Because of the known relationship of amyloidosis with prolonged immunologic stimulation, and with multiple myeloma and myeloma-like states, numerous attempts have been undertaken to determine whether there might be some relationship between the amyloid fibrils and gammaglobulin or its fragments.[10] Although earlier immunochemical studies of crude extracts of amyloid had indicated the presence of small concentrations of gammaglobulin,[45] it was difficult to determine whether the globulin was absorbed onto the amyloid fibril or incorporated within it. Numerous efforts to demonstrate an immunologic reactivity of amyloid fibrils with antiserum directed against IgG, IgA, IgM, and light chains have been negative.[14] Recently, however, it has been shown that the amino acid sequence of the amyloid fibril protein is very similar to the amino-terminal fragment of the variable portion of an immunoglobulin light chain, a Bence Jones protein type kappa.[27]

These data, if corroborated, would be consistent with the extensive body of clinical and experimental literature documenting a relationship between the genesis of amyloidosis and disorders in the immune mechanism. The nature of the association of amyloid with the aging process,[53] with hereditary amyloid and so forth would require further study. In addition to the direct role that an abnormality in immunoglobulin synthesis or destruction may play in amyloidosis, the role of delayed hypersensitivity has begun to attract interest. It has recently been demonstrated that in casein-induced amyloid in rabbits, they retain their sensitivity to a variety of antigens while becoming tolerant to the amyloidogenic stimulus. An hypothesis concerning amyloid as a disease involving tolerance has been entertained.[13]

Recently, two groups of investigators[3a,32a] have presented evidence indicating that amyloid fiber protein isolated from patients with secondary and familial Mediterranean fever-related amyloidosis contains, as its major ingredient, a component which is similar in all cases but whose partial amino acid sequence is clearly distinct from that of any known immunoglobulin. A similar protein has also been isolated from the amyloid-laden liver of a monkey with amyloidosis secondary to chronic infection. This component does not appear to be present, at least not in large quantity, in amyloid fiber protein from patients with primary or myeloma-related amyloidosis. The nature and source of this newly described component are still unknown. This finding raises, once again, the hypothesis that there may be a difference between secondary amyloidosis and the primary or myeloma-related forms of the disease.

In addition to the amyloid fibril, electron microscopic studies have also shown the presence, in small concentrations, of an additional component, the so-called pentagonal structure or P-component.[5,26] It is a disc-like structure of distinct electron microscopic appearance, and with an apparent absence of tryptophan and a distinct x-ray diffraction picture.[4,5,22] The origin and role of this component are still not understood.

CLINICAL MANIFESTATIONS

The clinical manifestations of amyloidosis are varied, and depend entirely on the area of the body which is involved.[19,31,44] The renal involvement may consist of mild proteinuria (0.5 gm. to 3.5 gm./day) or a frank nephrosis (over 3.5 gm. of protein excretion per day) or in some cases the urinary sediment may show only a few red blood cells. The renal lesion is not reversible and in time leads to progressive azotemia and death. The prognosis does not appear to be related to the degree of the proteinuria; when azotemia finally develops, if it is due to the amyloid process and not some reversible superimposed condition, the prognosis is very grave.[7] Hypertension is rare in amyloidosis. Serial x rays of the kidneys may or may not show diminution in size. A picture of renal tubular acidosis or of renal vein thrombosis may be seen. Localized accumulation of amyloid may be noted in the ureter, bladder or other tissues of the genitourinary tract.

The liver involvement is manifested primarily by hepatomegaly, usually without jaundice.[33] Results of liver function tests may show bromsulphalein retention and definite increases in serum alkaline phosphatase. Secondary stigmata of cirrhosis are rarely present. Esophageal varices, ascites and jaundice are rare but have been described. Since painless enlargement of the liver, without jaundice, often suggests to the physician the desirability of performing a needle aspiration of the organ, it should be pointed out that this procedure has been followed by fatal intraperitoneal hemorrhage on rare occasion in patients with massive hepatomegaly due to amyloidosis.[11] Massive amyloidosis would appear to increase the hazard of needle biopsy of the liver, however, and appropriate means should be taken to exclude this diagnosis before aspiration is performed. Although the hepatomegaly may be severe, death from hepatic insufficiency is rare.

Splenic involvement results in splenomegaly, which may be massive. It usually does not cause symptoms unless traumatic rupture occurs. Amyloidosis of the spleen is not characteristically associated with leukopenia and anemia.

Cardiac manifestations consist primarily of congestive failure and cardiomegaly, either with or without murmurs and a variety of arrhythmias.[9] Although the cardiac manifestations reflect predominantly diffuse myocardial involvement, amyloid frequently also accumulates in the pericardium and in the endocardium, sometimes involving the valve leaflets. Hearts which are heavily infiltrated with amyloid may or may not exhibit an enlarged silhouette. Fluoroscopy usually shows decreased mobility of the ventricular wall; angiologic studies usually show thickened ventricular wall, decreased ventricular mobility, and, in a few cases so studied, physiologic data consistent with constrictive pericarditis. Occasionally the clinical picture resembles constrictive pericarditis. More often, cardiac amyloid presents as intractable heart failure. Electrocardiographic abnormalities include a low voltage in the QRS complex and abnormalities in atrioventricular and intraventricular conduction, often resulting in varying degrees of heart block. Due to the propensity of patients with cardiac amyloidosis to develop conduction defects and arrhythmias, they appear to be especially sensitive to digitalis and this drug should be used in small doses and with caution.

Involvement of the skin is one of the most characteristic manifestations of the so-called "primary" amyloidoses.[8] The lesions may consist of slightly raised, waxy, often translucent papules or plaques, usually clustered in the folds about the axillae, anal or inguinal regions, the face and neck, or mucosal areas such as ear or tongue (Fig. 69–1*A* and *B*). In addition, or alternatively, there may be purpuric areas, nodules or tumefactions, alopecia, a yellowish waxy discoloration, glossitis and xerostomia. The lesions are seldom pruritic. It

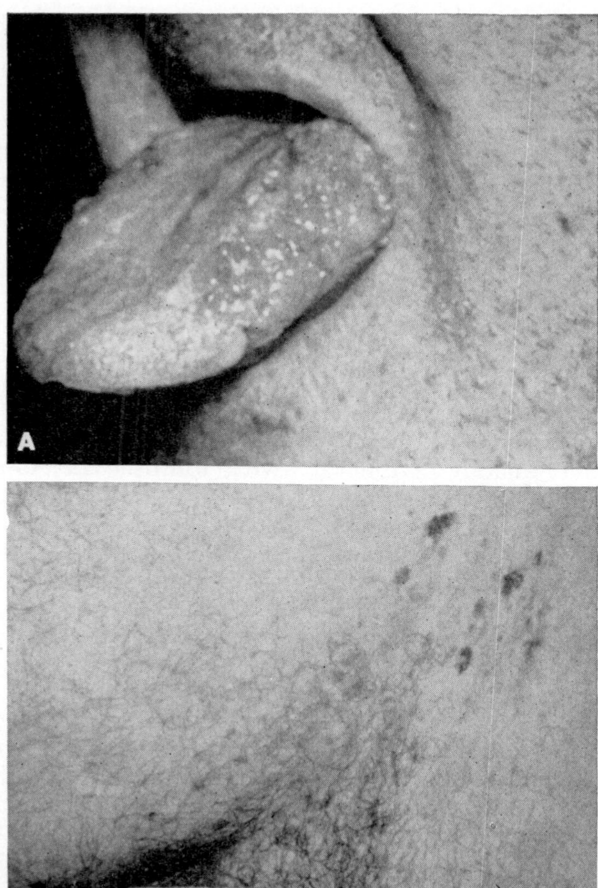

FIG. 69–1.—*A*. Fifty-five-year-old man with primary systemic amyloidosis. Note enlarged tongue with shiny papules along its lateral aspects. *B*. Left groin of the same patient showing the papules and purpuric spots in inguinal area.

should be noted that involvement of the skin or mucosa may be inapparent, even on close inspection, yet may be disclosed at biopsy. Gentle rubbing of the skin with one's finger may induce bleeding into the skin, leading to the appearance of purpura. Although uncommon, skin involvement can occur in secondary amyloidosis.

Amyloid infiltration of the gastrointestinal tract may occur at any level, resulting in a wide spectrum of manifestations. Infiltration of the tongue occasionally leads to macroglossia, which may become severely incapacitating; alternatively, the tongue, while not enlarged, may become stiffened and firm to palpation. While infiltration of the tongue is especially characteristic of primary amyloidosis or amyloidosis accompanying multiple myeloma, it is occasionally seen in the secondary form of the disease.

Amyloidosis is frequently accompanied by gastrointestinal bleeding, which may occur from any of a number of sites, notably the esophagus, stomach or large intestine and may be extremely severe and even fatal. Amyloid infiltration of the esophagus or small bowel may lead to clinical and x-ray changes of obstruction. A malabsorption syndrome is sometimes seen. Amyloidosis may develop in association with other entities involving the gastrointestinal tract, especially tuberculosis, lymphoma and Whipple's disease. Differentiation of these conditions from diffuse amyloidosis of the small bowel may be difficult. Similarly, amyloidosis of the stomach may closely mimic gastric carcinoma, with obstruction, achlorhydria and the radiologic appearance of tumor masses. The patient may exhibit cycles of constipation and diarrhea.

Neurologic manifestations are not uncommon. These may include peripheral neuropathy, postural hypotension, inability to sweat, the Adie pupil, hoarseness, and sphincter involvement.[1] Cranial nerves are generally spared except for those involving the pupillary reflexes. The protein concentration of the cerebral spinal fluid may be increased. Infiltrates of the cornea or vitreous body infrequently ensue. Amyloid may infiltrate the thyroid or other endocrine glands but rarely causes endocrine dysfunction. Local amyloid deposits almost invariably accompany medullary carcinoma of the thyroid.

The nasal sinuses, larynx, and trachea may be involved by accumulations of amyloid which block the ducts (in the case of the sinuses) or the air passage. Amyloidosis of the lung may include diffuse involvement of the bronchi or alveolar septa often accompanied by surprisingly minimal alteration of pulmonary function tests. Alternatively, amyloid may be localized in the bronchi or alveolar tissue so as to resemble a neoplasm. In these cases local excision of involved areas should be attempted, if possible, and may be followed by prolonged remissions.

Amyloid may occur in and around joints, resembling synovial tumor. It also may present as diffuse idiopathic osteoporosis. Amyloid infiltration of the muscle may lead to a pseudomyopathy.

Hematologic changes may include fibrinogenopenia, increased fibrinolysis and selective deficiency of factor X.[43]

COURSE

The course of amyloidosis is difficult to document since it is rarely possible to date the time of origin of the disease. When amyloidosis develops in patients with rheumatoid arthritis, it seldom becomes evident when the arthritis is less than two years in duration. The mean duration of arthritis before amyloidosis was detected was, in one series, 16 years.[21]

When amyloidosis develops in patients with multiple myeloma, manifestations leading to initial hospitalization are more apt to be related to the amyloid than to the myeloma.[7] In these cases prognosis is very poor and life expectancy is less than one year.

Instances have been reported of amyloidosis accompanying treatable sepsis, such as osteomyelitis, in which at least partial remission has occurred following treatment. Long-term studies of experimental amyloidosis induced in rabbits by injections of sodium caseinate have indicated that splenic amyloid accumulation, which reaches a peak after approximately 6 months of injections, is followed by resorption of amyloid from the spleen over the course of the ensuing 3 to 6 months, despite continuation of the caseinate injections. Histologic data suggest that this resorption is accomplished by phagocytosis by giant cells.[58] Amyloid deposited in the renal glomerulus and tubules does not show this tendency to spontaneous reabsorption, and giant cells are not seen. The degree to which spontaneous resorption of splenic amyloid is accomplished in man has not been well documented.

Once established, generalized amyloidosis in man while usually progressive and leading to death in several years, may have a better prognosis than once was suspected.[7]

The chief cause of death in amyloid patients is renal failure. The second most common cause is sudden death, presumably due to arrhythmias. Occasionally amyloid patients die of gastrointestinal hemorrhage or generalized sepsis.

PATHOLOGY OF AMYLOIDOSIS

When sufficiently massive to be visible, amyloid deposits have a smooth, waxy, gray or pink appearance. They endow the involved organ with a firm, rubbery texture. The gross material often will turn blue to black after the application of iodine and dilute sulfuric acid. This observation, made by Virchow, and the similarity of the reaction to that of a vegetable starch led him to name the material amyloid.

Under the microscope, amyloid has a glassy, hyaline, eosinophilic appearance, with hematoxylin and eosin. While amyloid may be suspected, based on routine hematoxylin and eosin staining, minimal deposits may be overlooked, and other eosinophilic extracellular accumulations may be confused with amyloid if special stains are not carried out.

The use of Congo red as a stain for amyloid is well known. Unless extreme care is observed in its use, the dye may adhere to dense collagenous material and give the false impression of the presence of amyloid.[42]

Considerable advances have been made in recent years in the development of new methods for localization of amyloid deposits in histologic specimens. These involve fluorescence microscopy and polarization techniques. When unstained preparations are viewed at 365 millimicrons, amyloid shows a faint auto-fluorescence. When the preparation is stained with Congo red and the slides are well decolorized, a clear-cut pink fluorescence may be observed. An even brighter fluorescence will be noted following staining tissue with thioflavin T or S.[52] This reaction should serve as a stimulus to further examination of the area in question. Positive staining with thioflavin T or S is not specific for amyloid.[36]

An apparently specific reaction involves examination of the tissue with polarized light after staining with Congo red.[32,56] Amyloid characteristically exhibits a positive birefringence in the direction of the long axis of the deposit and a color change, on rotation of the filter, between red and blue-green. Positive staining with either crystal or methyl violet provides added support to the conclusion that a given hyaline deposit is, indeed, amyloid. These histologic techniques, used together, are highly sensitive and in combination appear to be specific for the presence of amyloid. Deposits which are positive by these techniques show the typical amyloid fibrils when studied by electron microscopy.

Histologic studies of the spleen of patients with amyloidosis demonstrate diffuse or focal nodular involvement. Often accumulations of amyloid are seen in a perifollicular distribution. The splenic sinuses of the red pulp are surrounded by the material. Small and large blood vessels in the trabeculae may also be involved. In severe cases, the architecture of the organ may be completely destroyed and almost entirely replaced with amyloid.

Hepatic amyloid accumulates between the parenchymal cells and Kupffer cells lining the sinusoids (Fig. 69–2*A* and *B*). The deposition may be sufficiently marked to compress parenchymal cells and cause architectural distortion.

In the kidney the common site of deposition of amyloid is in the glomerulus (Fig. 69–3*A* and *B*). Electron microscopic studies have demonstrated that amyloid in small deposits is located in the mesangial area then between the basement membrane and endothelial cell, though in advanced disease it may also be seen on the epithelial side of the basement membrane. Involvement of renal blood vessels, as well as peritubular deposits, may be observed. Tubular casts, when found, are of interest in that they usually do not bind Congo red and are orthochromatic with crystal violet. In

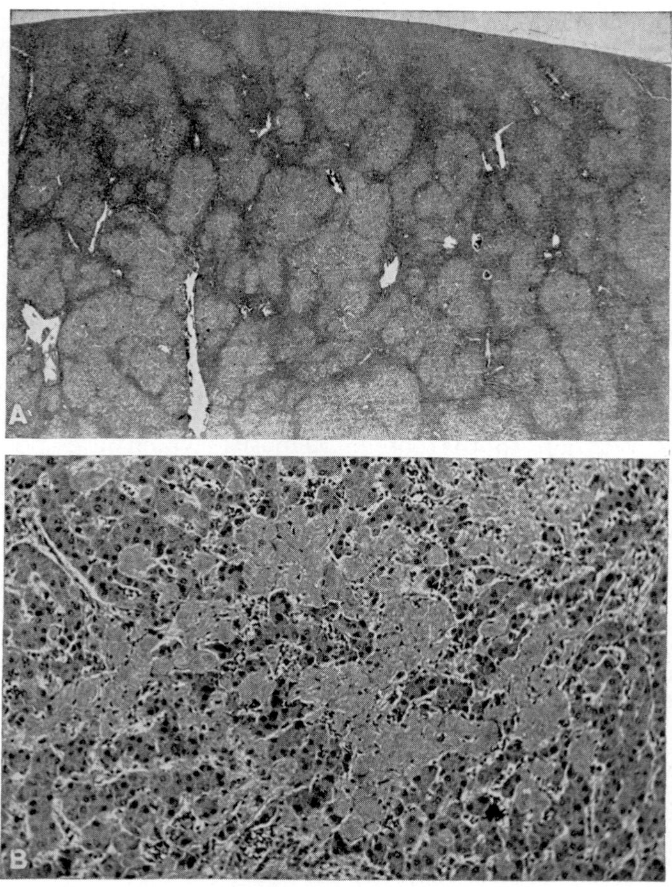

FIG. 69–2.—*A*. Forty-four-year-old man with ankylosing spondylitis of twenty-two years' duration. Postmortem examination demonstrated diffuse amyloidosis. Note pale areas of hepatic amyloidosis replacing over 50 per cent of the organ. Hematoxylin and eosin stain. Magnification $10\frac{1}{2}$ ×. *B*. Seventy-year-old man with far-advanced pulmonary tuberculosis of seven years' duration, and rheumatoid arthritis of twelve years' duration. Postmortem examination demonstrated diffuse amyloidosis. Note pale amyloid between parenchymal and Kupffer cells. Hematoxylin and eosin stain. Magnification 125 ×. (Tissue observed through the courtesy of Dr. Francis Dawson, Middlesex County Sanatorium.)

patients with amyloidosis accompanying multiple myeloma the tubular casts may show positive staining for amyloid and, on electron microscopy are seen to contain typical amyloid fibrils.

Amyloidosis of the adrenal gland may involve the zona glomerulosa, reticularis, or fasciculata. In cardiac amyloidosis, the material may be seen encircling the myocardial fibers, about the coronary vessels, or in focal deposits. Diffuse involvement of blood vessels is not uncommon (Fig. 69–4). Amyloid may also be seen in dermis, muscle, nerve, tongue, gastrointestinal tract, thyroid, pancreas, lymph nodes, lung, bone marrow, joints, and other locations.

DIAGNOSIS

As pointed out above, amyloidosis should be suspected in patients with the

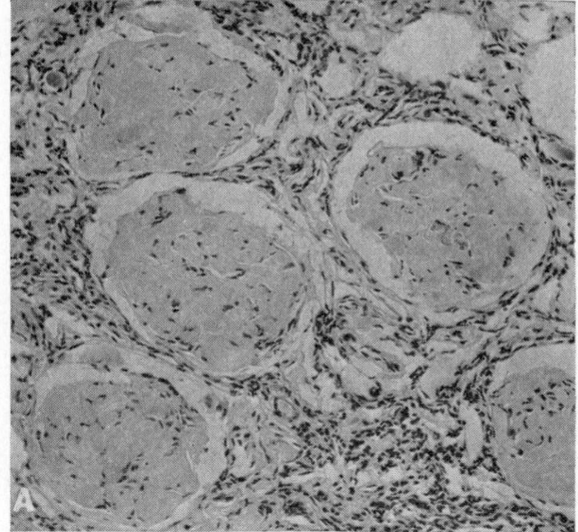

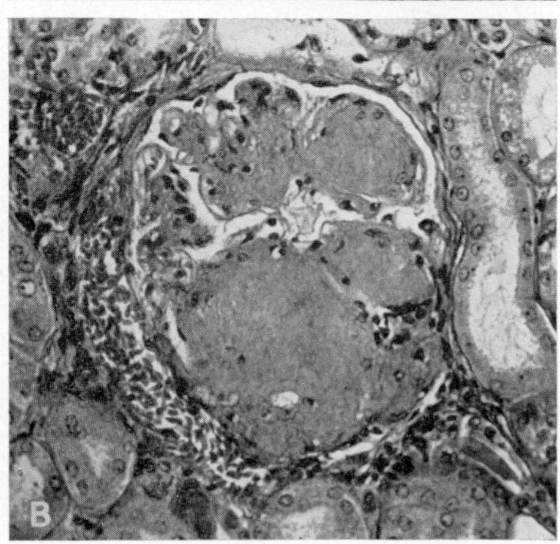

Fig. 69–3.—*A*. Amyloid involvement of kidney in primary systemic amyloidosis. Fifty-five-year-old man with nephrosis and primary systemic amyloidosis. Note almost complete replacement of glomeruli with amyloid. Hematoxylin and eosin stain. Magnification 125 ×. (Tissue obtained through the courtesy of Dr. James H. Baxter, National Heart Institute.) *B*. Amyloid involvement of kidney in ankylosing spondylitis. Same case as Figure 69–2*A*. Note marked deposition of amyloid apparently on endothelial surface occluding glomerular capillary lumen. Hematoxylin and eosin stain. Magnification 270 ×.

following clinical syndromes: (a) patients with rheumatoid arthritis, leprosy, severe prolonged osteomyelitis, or other chronic infections, who develop splenomegaly, hepatomegaly or proteinuria; (b) patients with multiple myeloma, especially those with Bence Jones proteinuria; (c) patients with polyneuropathy, cardiac failure due to diffuse myocardial involvement, or purpura accompanied by a papular, waxy skin eruption; and (d) patients with multisystem disease. The diagnosis can be confirmed only by histological demonstration of the presence of amyloid at biopsy or autopsy.

Biopsy

One of the significant advances in the clinical aspects of amyloidosis, in recent years, has been the increasing awareness of the value of biopsy technique as a means of confirming the diagnosis.[6,20] While renal biopsy probably provides the highest incidence of positive results in patients with this disease, this technique has some hazards. These may be increased in patients with massive amyloidosis due to the possibility of an accompanying defect in hemostasis. The rectal biopsy has been shown to be a convenient, safe, and quite effective procedure. In one series, rectal biopsy specimens confirmed the presence of amyloidosis in 75 per cent of cases of amyloidosis, subsequently proven at autopsy.[6]

Congo Red Test

This procedure has been regarded for many years as the prime laboratory method for confirming the diagnosis of amyloidosis. Because of its relative lack of specificity and the ease of biopsy techniques it has been to an increasing degree replaced by the latter.

THERAPY

Amyloidosis is a discouraging disease to treat. There is no specific therapy and the course may be progressively downhill. However, supportive measures, such as appropriate treatment of secondary infections and adequate diet, may contribute greatly to prolonging life. In patients with amyloidosis secondary to an underlying infection, reasonable efforts should be made to treat or

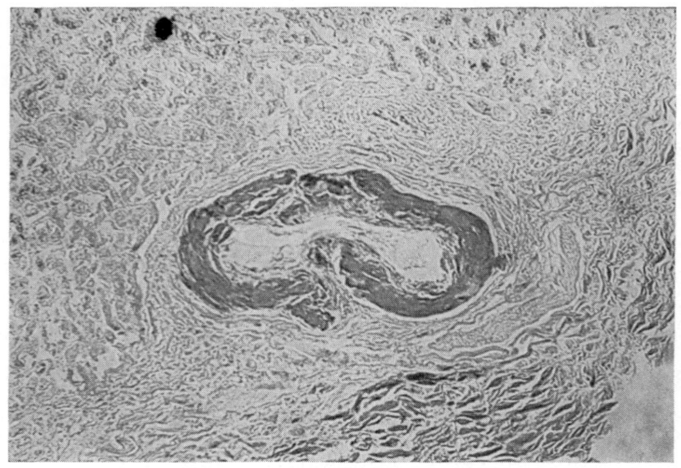

FIG. 69–4.—Amyloid involvement of blood vessel. Same case as Figure 69–2*A*. Note marked deposition of amyloid about lumen of blood vessel. Congo red stain. Magnification 125 ×.

remove the infection. The best example of this is the surgical and medical treatment of decubitus ulcers and osteomyelitis.

Crude liver therapy has been credited with inducing remissions in a number of individual cases. It is so unpalatable, however, that many patients refuse to take it and, since its beneficial effects are controversial, few physicians have persisted in its use. The usual dose is ¼ lb. of raw or light-seared liver, as a meat course, or ground in tomato juice, daily.

Although penicillamine therapy has been reportedly effective in one patient, other cases have not shown a beneficial response and the results in one controlled study in rabbits with experimental amyloidosis were not encouraging.

Increased evidence to suggest a relationship between amyloidosis and abnormalities in the immunoglobulins has provided stimulus to the use of immunosuppressive therapy. Phenylalanine nitrogen mustard has been tried in a number of cases, but clear-cut evidence of beneficial effect is not yet at hand. Some investigators recommend simultaneous treatment with phenylalanine nitrogen mustard and hydroxychloroquine. Experimental studies, on the other hand, have shown that the use of immunosuppressive agents in animals with casein-induced amyloid leads to acceleration rather than amelioration of the disease.[29]

With Dr. John Mannick one of us (ASC) has recently evaluated renal transplantation in 2 carefully selected patients dying of azotemia secondary to renal amyloid. One patient is alive and well almost 2 years post transplant while the second died 7 months postoperatively of a retroperitoneal abscess. The transplanted kidney showed no amyloid at autopsy, nor did the other transplanted kidney by biopsy 1 year after transplantation. Further evaluation of this approach is in progress.[23]

BIBLIOGRAPHY

1. ANDRADE, C.: Brain, *75*, 408, 1952.
2. ANDRADE, A., ARAKI, S., BLOCK, W. D., COHEN, A. S., JACKSON, C. E., KUROIWA, Y., MCKUSICK, V. A., NIRSIM, J., SOHAR, E. and VAN ALLEN, M. W.: Arth. & Rheum., *13*, 902, 1970.
3. BARTH, W. F., WILLERSON, J. T., WALDMANN, T. A. and DECKER, J. L.: Amer. J. Med., *47*, 259, 1969.
3*a*. BENDITT, E. P., ERIKSEN, N., HERMODSON, M. A. and ERICSSON, L. H.. FEBS Letters. *19*, 169, 1971.

4. BINETTE, P., MATSUZAKI, M., CALKINS, E., ALPER, R. and WINZLER, R. J.: Proc. Soc. Exp. Biol. Med., *137*, 165, 1971.
5. BLADEN, H. A., NYLEN, M. U. and GLENNER, G. G.: J. Ultrastruct. Res., *14*, 449, 1966.
6. BLUM, A. and SOHAR, E.: Lancet, *1*, 721, 1962.
7. BRANDT, K., CATHCART, E. S. and COHEN, A. S.: Amer. J. Med., *44*, 955, 1968.
8. BROWNSTEIN, M. H. and HELWIG, E. B.: Arch. Derm., *102*, 1, 1970.
9. BUJA, J. M., KHOI, N. B., and ROBERTS, W. C.: Amer. J. Cardiol., *26*, 394, 1970.
10. CALKINS, E.: in *Proceedings of Symposium on Amyloidosis*. E. Mandema, L. Ruinen, J. H. Scholten and A. S. Cohen, eds., Amsterdam, Excerpta Medica, 1968.
11. CALKINS, E. and COHEN, A. S.: Bull. Rheum. Dis., *10*, 215, 1958.
12. CATHCART, E. S., RITCHIE, R. F., BRANDT, K. and COHEN, A. S.: in *Proceedings of Symposium on Amyloidosis*. E. Mandema, L. Ruinen, J. H. Scholten and A. S. Cohen, eds., Amsterdam, Excerpta Medica, 1968.
13. CATHCART, E. S., MULLARKEY, M. and COHEN, A. S.: Lancet, *2*, 639, 1970.
14. CATHCART, E. S. and COHEN, A. S.: J. Immunol., *96*, 239, 1966.
15. COHEN, A. S. and CALKINS, E.: Nature, *183*, 1202, 1959.
16. ———: J. Cell Biol., *21*, 481, 1964.
17. COHEN, A. S.: in *International Review of Experimental Biology*. G. W. Richter and M. A. Epstein, eds. New York, Academic Press, 1965, volume 4.
18. ———: Lab. Invest., *15*, 66, 1966.
19. ———: New Engl. J. Med., *277*, 522, 574, 628, 1967.
20. ———: *Laboratory Diagnostic Methods in The Rheumatic Diseases*. Boston, Little, Brown and Co., 1967.
21. ———: Med. Clin. North America, *52*, 643, 1968.
22. ———: in *Chemistry and Molecular Biology of the Intracellular Matrix*. E. A. Balacz, ed., New York, Academic Press, 1970, volume 3.
23. COHEN, A. S., BRICCETTI, A., HARRINGTON, J. and MANNICK, J.: Lancet, (in Press).
24. EHRLICH, J. C. and RATNER, I. M.: Amer. J. Path., *38*, 49, 1961.
25. FRANKLIN, E. C. and PRAS, M.: J. Exp. Med., *130*, 797, 1969.
26. GLENNER, G. G. and BLADEN, H. A.: Science, *154*, 271, 1966.
27. GLENNER, G. G., TERRY, W., HARADA, M., ISERSKY, C. and PAIGE, D.: Science, *172*, 1150, 1971.
28. HARADA, M., ISERSKY, C., CUATRECASAS, P., PAIGE, D., BLADEN, H. A., EANES, E. D., KEISER, H. R. and GLENNER, G. G.: J. Histochem. Cytochem., *19*, 1, 1971.
29. HARDT, F.: Acta Path. Microbiol. Scand., Section A, *79*, 61, 1971.
30. HELLER, H., SOHAR, E., GAFNI, J. and HELLER, J.: Arch. Intern. Med., *107*, 539, 1961.
31. KENNEY, J. D. and CALKINS, E.: in *Progress in Clinical Rheumatology*. A. St. J. Dixon, ed., London, J. & A. Churchill, Ltd., 1965.
32. LADEWIG, P.: Nature, *206*, 738, 1965.

32*a*. LEVIN, M., FRANKLIN, E. C., FRANGIONE, B. and PRAS, M.: J. Clin. Invest. *51*, 1972 (in press) (abstr.).

33. LEVINE, R. A.: Amer. J. Med., *33*, 349, 1962.
34. LEVINE, R. A., PAYNE, M. D. and BURKHOLDER, P. M.: Ann. Intern. Med., *56*, 397, 1962.
35. MAHLOUDJI, M., TEASDALL, R. D., ADAMKIEWICZ, J. J., HARTMAN, W. H., LAMBIRD, P. A. and MCKUSICK, V. A.: Medicine, *48*, 1, 1969.
36. MCKINNEY, B. and GRUBB, C.: Nature, *205*, 1023, 1965.
37. MISSEN, G. A. K. and TAYLOR, J. D.: J. Path. Bact., *71*, 179, 1956.
38. OSSERMAN, E. F., TAHATSUKI, N. and TALAL, N.: in *Seminars in Hematology*. P. A. Miescher, ed., New York, Grune and Stratton, 1964.
39. OSSERMAN, E. F. and FAHEY, J. L.: Amer. J. Med., *44*, 256, 1968.
40. OZDEMIR, A. I., WRIGHT, J. R. and CALKINS, E.: New Engl. J. Med., *285*, 534, 1971.

40*a*. PEETERS, H.: Colloquium: Protides of the Biological Fluids, Brugge, Belgium, May 1972.

41. PRAS, M., SCHUBERT, M., ZUCKER-FRANKLIN, D., RIMAN, A. and FRANKLIN, E. C.: J. Clin. Invest., *47*, 924, 1968.
42. PUCHTLER, H., SWEAT, F. and LEVINE, M.: J. Histochem. Cytochem., *10*, 355, 1962.
43. REDLEAF, P. D., DAVIS, R. B., KUCINSKI, C., HOILUND, L. and GANS, H.: Ann. Intern. Med., *58*, 347, 1963.
44. RUKAVINA, J. G., BLOCK, W. D., JACKSON, C. E., FALLS, H. F., CAREY, J. H. and CURTIS, A. C.: Medicine, *35*, 239, 1956.
45. SCHULTZ, R. T., CALKINS, E., MILGROM, F. and WITEBSKY, E.: Amer. J. Path., *48*, 1, 1966.
46. SCHWARTZ, P.: Trans. New York Acad. Sci., *27*, 393, 1965.
47. SHIRAHAMA, T. and COHEN, A. S.: J. Cell Biol., *33*, 679, 1967.
48. SKINNER, M. and COHEN, A. S.: Biochim. Biophys. Acta, *236*, 183, 1971.

49. Sohar, E., Gafni, J., Pras, M. and Heller, H.: Amer. J. Med., *43*, 227, 1967.
50. Symmers, W. St. C.: J. Clin. Path., *9*, 187, 1956.
51. Teilum, G. and Lindahl, A.: Acta Med. Scand., *149*, 449, 1954.
52. Vassar, P. S. and Culling, C. F. A.: Arch. Path., *68*, 847, 1959.
53. Walford, R. L.: J. Geront., *104*, 727, 1956.
54. Walford, R. L. and Sjaarda, J. R.: J. Geront., *19*, 57, 1964.
55. Wisniewski, H., Johnson, A. B., Raine, C. S. Kay, W. T. and Terry, R. D.: Lab. Invest., *23*, 287, 1970.
56. Wolman, M. and Bubis, J. J.: Histochemie, *4*, 351, 1965.
57. Wright, J. R., Calkins, E., Breen, W. J., Stolte, G. and Schultz, R. T.: Medicine, *48*, 39, 1969.
58. Ozdemir, A. I., Matsuzaki, M., Binette, J. P. and Calkins, E.: Johns Hopkins Med. J., *130*, 278, 1972.

Chapter 70

Sarcoidosis

By H. Ralph Schumacher, M.D.

Sarcoidosis is a systemic disease characterized by a noncaseating granulomatous reaction of unknown origin. Our present concept of this syndrome has evolved from the early descriptions by Hutchinson,[10] Besnier,[2] Boeck,[3] and Schaumann.[27] Symptoms and signs depend on the organs affected. Most frequently involved tissues are lymph nodes, lungs, liver, skin and eyes. Muscle, spleen, bones, parotids, central nervous system, endocrine glands and almost any other tissue including the joints may also be involved. Although generally a chronic disease, onset can be acute with hilar adenopathy, erythema nodosum, fever and articular manifestations. This is often termed Lofgren's syndrome.[20] For unknown reasons this acute syndrome is seen more often in Europe than in the United States. In other instances sarcoidosis may present as asymptomatic hilar and right paratracheal adenopathy. Frequent laboratory alterations are impaired delayed hypersensitivity, hyperglobulinemia, hypercalcemia and elevated serum alkaline phosphatase.

Pathology

The characteristic histopathology of epithelioid tubercles with minimal necrosis and no true caseation (in contrast to tuberculosis) is the hallmark of sarcoidosis (Figs. 70–1 and 70–2). Sarcoid granulomas often contain Langhans-type

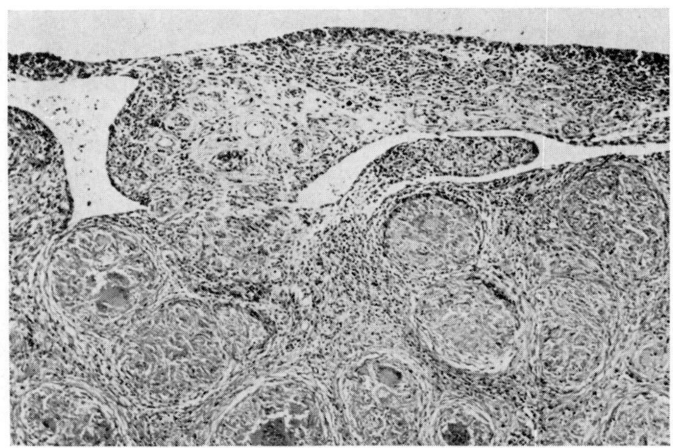

Fig. 70–1.—Granulomatous synovitis of elbow in case of chronic sarcoid arthritis. (Hematoxylin and eosin stain × 60.) The synovial tissue is crowded with discrete, noncaseating miliary tubercles. At the surface, the villi are hypertrophied and infiltrated with leukocytes and fibroblasts. The articular cartilage of this joint was intact and the subchondral bone (olecranon and lateral condyle of humerus) was free of tubercles. (Sokoloff and Bunim, courtesy of New Engl. J. Med.)

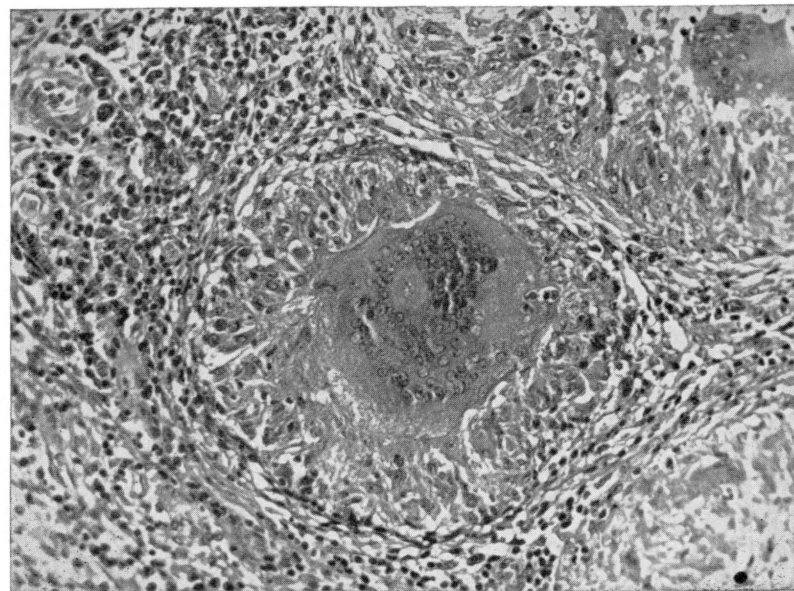

Fig. 70-2.—Multinucleated giant cell in the center of a tubercle of epithelioid cells. Surrounding the latter is a layer of fibroblasts and a cuff of lymphocytes, plasma cells and mononuclear cells. This is an area from Figure 70-1 under higher magnification (× 175). (Sokoloff and Bunim, courtesy of New Engl. J. Med.)

giant cells with three frequent types of cytoplasmic inclusions: (1) Asteroid bodies which appear to consist of criss-crossing bundles of collagen. (2) Schaumann bodies which are round or oval, laminated calcifications containing hydroxyapatite (Fig. 70–3). (3) Irregular, poorly stained, anisotropic glass-like fragments.[21] It should be emphasized that such granulomas even with the typical inclusions are not pathognomonic for sarcoidosis. Similar granulomatous tissue reactions can be seen in histoplasmosis, coccidioidomycosis, tuberculosis, lymphoma, Hodgkin's disease, bronchogenic carcinoma, foreign body granuloma, drug reactions, beryllium poisoning, syphilis and leprosy. The factor (or factors) initiating the sarcoid granuloma has not been identified although there have been isolated reports of acid-fast material in sarcoid granulomas.[33] Functional impairment in sarcoidosis appears to result from both the active granulomatous disease and secondary fibrosis.

Etiology and Prevalence

There have been a number of speculations about possible causes for this unexplained disease. There is a 4 per cent incidence of tuberculosis in sarcoidosis and an unusual reaction to mycobacterium tuberculosis or atypical mycobacteria has been one suggested mechanism. The high incidence of sarcoid in rural areas and especially regions heavily wooded with pines has suggested an unconfirmed relation to pine pollen. High titers of antibody to herpes-like virus have been reported in sarcoidosis. A similar antibody has however also been found in Burkitt lymphoma, infectious mononucleosis, and carcinoma of the posterior nasal space.[9] Despite isolated reports of sarcoidosis in several members of a family and familial coincidence of tuberculosis and sarcoidosis, there is no strong evidence for hereditary or contagious factors in causation. Several series in this country have found a higher inci-

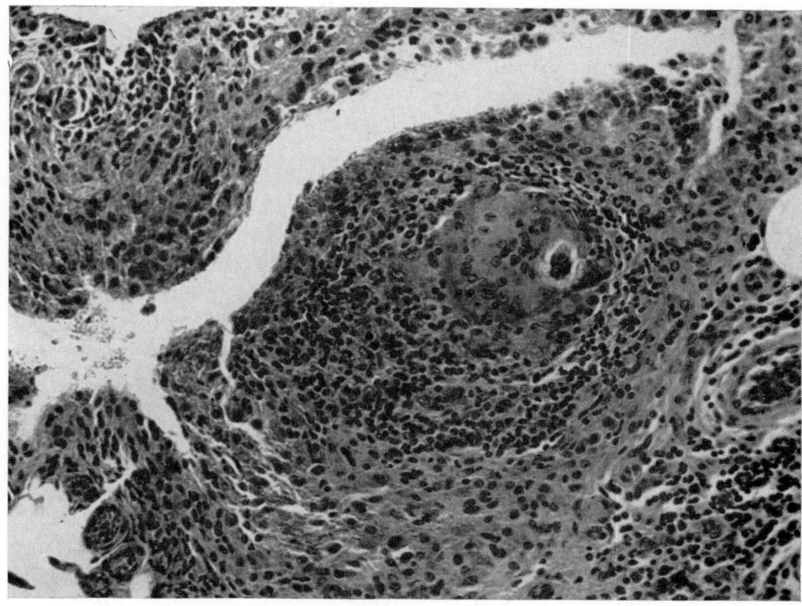

FIG. 70–3.—Granulomatous synovitis exhibiting a Schaumann-like body. This appears in the cytoplasm of a giant cell as a circular clear space and consists of a colorless crystalloid material that is doubly refractive. Section of synovial tissue from knee of a thirty-three-year-old Negro woman with sarcoid polyarthritis of about six weeks' duration. Preadmission diagnosis was rheumatic fever, later changed to rheumatoid arthritis. X ray of joint was normal and sheep cell agglutination test result negative. Antistreptolysin-O titer was normal. Random biopsy specimen of gastrocnemius disclosed numerous granulomas. No bacteria or fungi were found with Brown-Brenn, Ziehl-Neelsen or periodic acid-Schiff stains. Kveim test result was positive. Chest x rays revealed prominent bilateral hilar adenopathy. During ensuing months patient developed erythema nodosum, uveitis and parotitis. (Sokoloff and Bunim, courtesy of New Engl. J. Med.)

dence in Negro females.[22] The disease may begin at any age including infancy but is most commonly diagnosed in the third and fourth decades. Females predominate slightly over males. Sarcoidosis has a worldwide distribution with the estimated incidence of the disease reaching as high as 64/100,000 in Sweden. American veterans after World War II had an incidence of 11/100,000.

Manifestations and Prognosis

Sarcoidosis can vary from an asymptomatic chest x-ray finding to the cause of death in approximately 4 per cent. As reviewed by Mayock *et al.*[22] the most common symptoms and signs are fatigue (27%), malaise (15%), cough (30%), shortness of breath (28%) or chest pain (15%). Ninety-two per cent of patients have abnormal chest x rays. Pulmonary parenchymal involvement is more ominous than the more frequent hilar adenopathy. Restrictive lung disease and cor pulmonale can develop. A granulomatous uveitis is the most frequent visual problem. Skin lesions occur in 30 per cent of cases. They may be very nondescript but commonly are papular or nodular, erythematous or violaceous lesions and on histological examination consist of typical granulomas. Erythema nodosum is common in disease of acute onset. Liver involvement is almost always asymptomatic and is evidenced mainly by hepatomegaly. An elevated alkaline phosphatase may suggest the presence of liver granulomas. It has generally been considered that the acute sarcoidosis with erythema nodosum, hilar adenopathy and arthralgia has the best prognosis. Truelove[32] despite the similar sarcoid tissue reaction has urged separation of this syndrome from sarcoidosis. Certainly most patients with this acute syndrome go into full remission within 2 years but Israel[13] has recently emphasized that long-term follow-up has not been reported in such cases and some caution is still needed. Sarcoidosis with cutaneous granulomas and clinical evidence of other visceral involvement is more likely to cause chronic progressive disease although even some patients with advanced and disseminated granulomas may undergo spontaneous recovery.

Diagnosis

The diagnosis of sarcoidosis is established by demonstration of typical non-caseating granulomas in the absence of other identifiable causes for such granulomas. The clinical and laboratory features including the musculoskeletal manifestations described below may suggest the diagnosis. Impaired delayed hypersensitivity is characteristic but not invariably present. Impaired tuberculin sensitivity after BCG vaccination has been seen to persist even after apparent recovery from sarcoidosis. Antibody production is normal. The elevated immunoglobulins are similar to those in tuberculosis and are of little help in differential diagnosis. Leukopenia, anemia, eosinophilia and elevated sedimentation rates may be seen. Tissue diagnosis is most expeditiously established by biopsy specimen of a skin lesion or accessible superficial lymph node. With such superficial material some evidence of generalized disease is also needed, since foreign body reactions can be difficult to distinguish from sarcoidosis. Liver samples also can show granulomas, especially if the liver is palpably enlarged, but a granulomatous liver reaction is common in other liver disease and not as helpful in diagnosis as demonstration of lymph node lesions. Mediastinoscopy in experienced hands is a safe and highly reliable method of obtaining lymph node tissue for diagnosis if there is hilar adenopathy. Israel found muscle tissue positive in 89 per cent of patients with erythema nodosum or arthralgia.[11]

An intradermal injection of 0.2 cc. of a 10 per cent saline suspension of sarcoid tissue (the Kveim test) has been used for diagnosis. A positive reaction is the production of a local sarcoid granuloma at the injection site. Positive results of Kveim tests can be obtained in 80 per cent of sarcoid cases and seem positive most often in early disease with prominent adenopathy.[12] Standardization of preparations has been difficult and this material is not generally available. Kveim test results have also been reported to be positive in more than 50 per cent of patients with regional enteritis so the specificity of the test remains in doubt.[23]

MUSCULOSKELETAL MANIFESTATIONS IN SARCOIDOSIS

Muscle Sarcoid

Sarcoid granulomas in muscle are often asymptomatic but occasionally may be accompanied by local pain and tenderness or even palpable nodules. A symmetrical proximal myopathy has also been described and has been reported to occur without evident sarcoidosis in other tissues.[8,29] The involved muscles show non-caseating granulomas and also lymphocytic infiltration, muscle necrosis and regeneration.

Bone Sarcoid

Phalangeal cysts (Fig. 70–4) have often been considered a helpful diagnostic clue in sarcoidosis and were described in 14 per cent of the series collected by Mayock *et al.*[22] Although some such cysts have been shown to be due to sarcoid granulomas others may be

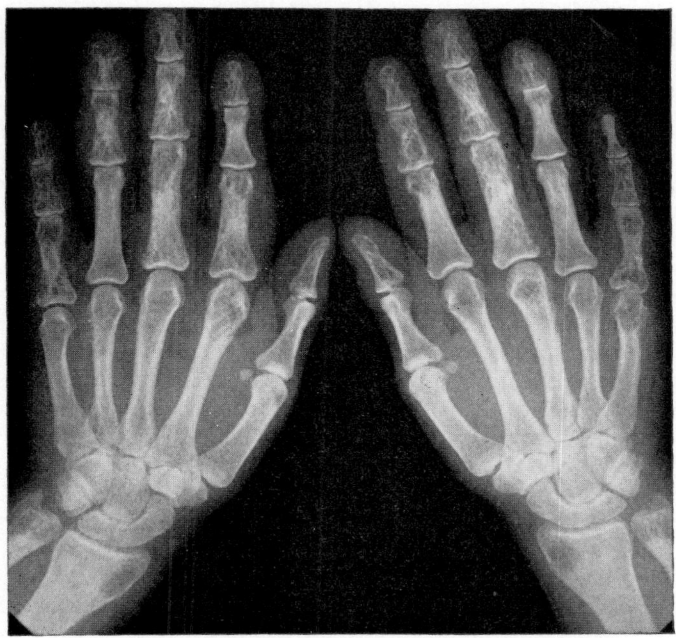

FIG. 70–4.—Roentgenograms of hands showing unusually severe bone lesions of sarcoidosis. The bone cysts have not broken through the articular cortex. The hands shown in Figure 70–5 had similar bone changes but with extension into the distal interphalangeal joints

unrelated to the sarcoidosis. Baltzer *et al.*[1] in an x-ray survey of the hands of 338 patients with sarcoidosis and 342 controls found cystic changes in 5 per cent of sarcoidosis but also in 8 per cent of controls including normals and patients with a variety of other diseases. Other bones including the skull and vertebrae[35] may also have cysts due to sarcoid granulomas. Bone sarcoidosis, especially the phalangeal cysts, is usually asymptomatic. The overlying cortex is almost always intact. Cystic bone lesions only occasionally extend into the joint but when they do they can be the cause of an arthritis.[30] Rarely, very destructive bone lesions are associated with overlying purplish red nodular cutaneous masses termed *lupus pernio.*[21]

Sarcoid Arthropathy

An arthritis was first described with sarcoidosis in 1936[4] and since then arthritis, periarthritis or arthralgia has been reported in 2 to 38 per cent of various series of patients with sarcoidosis.[22,7,28,31] The lower incidence seems to apply to chronic sarcoidosis. In acute sarcoidosis with hilar adenopathy, fever and erythema nodosum, up to 89 per cent have articular symptoms with 69 and 63 per cent having articular or periarticular swelling in the series of Lofgren,[20] and James *et al.*[14] Ankles and knees are by far most commonly involved in this acute sarcoidosis. Most other joints have occasionally been involved. Heel pad pain is not uncommon. Monoarthritis is unusual.[7] There is generally a dramatic, tender, warm, erythematous swelling that often is clearly periarticular rather than synovial. Such changes are occasionally difficult to separate from adjacent cutaneous erythema nodosum. Joint motion is often painless. The frequency of a strikingly severe, very localized tenderness has been emphasized.[16] X rays show only soft tissue swelling. Such articular findings may antedate erythema nodosum by as much as 2 weeks and suggest careful watch for the skin lesions. Ankle and knee involvement is often symmetrical and can be progressive but is not usually migratory. The acute inflammation often raises the special consideration of rheumatic fever, gonococcal or other infectious arthritis, and gout. Acute sarcoidosis is much less likely to be migratory than is rheumatic fever and the response to salicylates is not dramatic. Joint aspiration often yields no synovial fluid. When an effusion can be aspirated it is generally very mildly inflammatory with leukocyte counts of less than 1000. Cells are predominantly lymphocytes and large mononuclear cells. Viscosity is good.[18] Cultures are negative and crystals cannot be identified by compensated polarized light. Several patients with this syndrome including the first case described by Hutchinson[10] had been felt to have gout before synovial fluid crystal identification was available to confirm the presence of acute gouty arthritis.[15] Elevated uric acids have been noted in a small percentage of patients with sarcoidosis[31] with or without arthropathy but serum and urine uric acid levels have not been systematically studied nor have most series been able to exclude contributions of salicylates or diuretics to the hyperuricemia. Needle synovial biopsy specimens in acute sarcoidosis have most often shown only mild non-specific synovitis and some lining cell proliferation.[18] Although this has suggested that much of the inflammation in this acute sarcoidosis may be periarticular, synovial granulomas have occasionally been found by open surgical biopsy.[30] Caplan *et al.*[5] have described an identical periarthritis in 19 patients with hilar adenopathy none of whom had the otherwise common erythema nodosum. They found sarcoid granulomas in the subcutaneous tissue over 3 of 7 inflamed ankles but found no granulomas in an open joint biopsy.

Virtually all joint manifestations of acute sarcoidosis subside in 2 weeks to 4 months although rare cases may progress to chronic sarcoid arthritis. It should be noted that erythema nodosum and often a similar arthropathy can also be seen in lepromatous leprosy, ulcerative colitis, regional enteritis, tuberculosis, coccidioidomycosis, histoplasmosis, oral contraceptive and possibly other drug use, pregnancy, psittacosis and other infections. Other cases are idiopathic.

In sarcoidosis of more insidious onset joint manifestations are less common. In such cases even with widespread systemic granulomatous disease the arthritis may still be mild and evanescent as in acute sarcoidosis. However, arthritis can also be recurring or protracted with polysynovitis. Even with chronic synovitis joint destruction is infrequent and most x rays show only soft tissue swelling. The occasional destructive joint disease in sarcoidosis is illustrated in Figure 70–5. Such severe arthritis is most common in patients with multisystem granulomatous disease. Arthritis may occur as an initial manifestation or after years of systemic disease. Thus, such a variety of patterns can be seen that a high index of suspicion is needed to lead to biopsy and other diagnostic studies to differentiate this from rheumatoid or other types of arthritis. Synovial fluid in these cases has also shown relatively low leukocyte counts but effusions have been infrequently examined. Sokoloff and Bunim[30] found non-caseating granulomas in 3 of 5 surgical synovial biopsy specimens from patients with chronic arthritis. In addition the synovium showed diffuse chronic inflammation including plasma cells. None of their cases had any elevation of rheumatoid factor but others have found rheumatoid factor in up to 38 per cent of patients with sarcoidosis.[26] The presence of rheumatoid factor does not correlate with the presence or severity of joint disease. Sedimentation rates are commonly elevated. Tenosynovitis at the wrists and elsewhere can also be seen.

Arthritis in early childhood sarcoidosis has been described with especially large, painless, boggy synovial and tendon sheath effusions.[25] The course is indo-

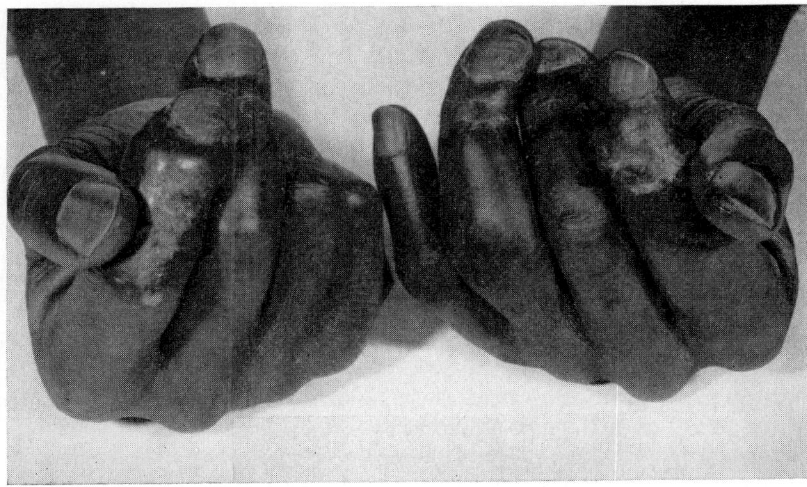

FIG. 70–5.—Hands of thirty-three-year-old Negro male with sarcoidosis of five years' duration. Depigmented skin lesions on dorsum of fingers. Distal phalanx of left fourth finger displaced. Note fusiform swelling of proximal interphalangeal joint of fourth and fifth fingers of left hand (asymmetrical). This patient did not have psoriasis. (Sokoloff and Bunim, courtesy of New Engl. J. Med.)

lent with few constitutional symptoms. Despite prolonged synovitis there were no erosive x-ray changes. Synovial effusion examinations were not described. Synovial biopsy samples showed either granulomas or non-specific inflammation. Interestingly, sarcoidosis in the young children described occurred with uveitis but not hilar adenopathy.

Diagnostic Features of Sarcoidosis

1. Non-caseating granulomas on biopsy. Must exclude other causes of granulomas.
2. Hilar and right paratracheal adenopathy in 90%.
3. Skin lesions, uveitis or involvement of almost any tissue.
4. Onset most often in third and fourth decades but cases reported at all ages.
5. Impaired delayed hypersensitivity in 85%.
6. Frequent hyperglobulinemia.

Sarcoid Arthropathy

Acute Sarcoidosis (Lofgren's Syndrome)

1. Often periarticular and very tender, warm swelling.
2. Ankles and knees almost invariably involved.
3. May be initial manifestation.
4. Joint motion may be normal.
5. Synovial effusions infrequent and mildly inflammatory when present.
6. Usually non-specific mild synovitis on synovial biopsy.
7. Self-limited in weeks to 4 months.

Chronic Sarcoidosis

1. May be acute and evanescent, recurrent or chronic.
2. Non-caseating granulomas more commonly demonstrable in synovium.
3. Usually non-destructive despite chronic or recurrent disease.
4. Rheumatoid factor titers and uric acid may be elevated.

Treatment

Many patients with minimal symptoms require no treatment. There is no curative agent. Adrenal corticosteroids are commonly used to try to suppress potentially serious active inflammatory reactions such as ocular disease, pulmonary parenchymal disease and CNS involvement and often seem to be effective. Steroids can also lower persistently elevated serum calcium levels. Initial steroid therapy when needed can be started with 20 to 40 mg. prednisone and tapered to the lowest effective maintenance dose. Objective long-term benefits from steroids have often been difficult to demonstrate[34] but improved vital capacity even in severe disease has been shown in one series.[6] Active articular disease almost always shows at least temporary improvement with steroid therapy. When steroids are used isoniazid coverage is needed in tuberculin-positive patients. However, as joint disease is often self limited, rest, salicylates and other analgesics are often all that is required. Salicylates are not as dramatically effective as in rheumatic fever. Colchicine has been observed to shorten attacks in some patients[16] but is by no means invariably effective. Chloroquine has been reported to help cutaneous sarcoidosis.[24] Uncontrolled reports of methotrexate[19] and azathioprine[17] have suggested benefit.

BIBLIOGRAPHY

1. Baltzer, G. *et al.*: Deutsch. Med. Wschr., *95*, 1926, 1970.
2. Besnier, E.: Ann. Derm. Syph., *10*, 333, 1889.
3. Boeck, C.: J. Cutan. Genitourin. Dis., *17*, 543, 1889.
4. Burman, M. S. and Mayer, L.: Arch. Surg., *32*, 846, 1936.
5. Caplan, H. I., Katz, W. A. and Rubenstein, M.: Arth. & Rheum., *13*, 101, 1970.
6. Emirgil, C., Sobol, B. J. and Williams, M. H.: J. Chron. Dis., *22*, 69, 1969.
7. Gumpel, J. M., Johns, C. J. and Shulman, L. E.: Ann. Rheum. Dis., *26*, 194, 1967.
8. Hinterbuchner, C. N. and Hinterbuchner, L. P.: Brain, *87*, 355, 1964.
9. Hirshaut, Y., *et al.*: New Engl. J. Med., *283*, 502, 1970.
10. Hutchinson, J. A.: Arch. Surg. (Lond.), *9*, 307, 1898.
11. Israel, H. L. and Sones, M.: Arch. Intern. Med., *113*, 255, 1964.
12. Israel, H. L.: Ann. Intern. Med., *68*, 1323, 1968.
13. ————: Ann. Intern. Med., *73*, 1038, 1970.
14. James, D. G., Thomson, A. D., and Wilcox, A.: Lancet, *2*, 218, 1956.
15. Kaplan, H. and Klatskin, G.: Yale J. Biol. Med., *32*, 335, 1960.
16. Kaplan, H.: New Engl. J. Med., *268*, 761, 1963.
17. Krebs, P., Abel, H., and Schonberger, W.: Munch. Med. Wsch., *111*, 2307, 1969.
18. Kitridou, R. C. and Schumacher, H. R.: Arth. & Rheum., *13*, 328, 1970.
19. Lacher, M. J.: Ann. Intern. Med., *69*, 1247, 1968.
20. Lofgren, S.: Acta Med. Scand., *145*, 424, 1953.
21. Longcope, W. T. and Freiman, D. G.: Medicine, *31*, 1, 1952.
22. Mayock, R. L., *et al.*: Amer. J. Med., *35*, 67, 1963.
23. Mitchell, D. N., *et al.*: Lancet, *2*, 571, 1969.
24. Morse, S. I., Cohn, Z. A., Hirsch, J. G. and Schaedler, R. W.: Amer. J. Med., *30*, 779, 1961.
25. North, A. F.: Amer. J. Med., *48*, 449, 1970.
26. Oreskes, I. and Siltzbach, L. E.: Amer. J. Med., *44*, 60, 1968.
27. Schaumann, J. N.: Ann. Derm. Syph., *6*, 357, 1916–1917.
28. Siltzbach, L. E. and Silverstein, J. L.: Clin. Orthop., *57*, 31, 1968.
29. Silverstein, A. and Siltzbach, L. E.: Arch. Neurol., *21*, 235, 1969.
30. Sokoloff, L. and Bunim, J. J.: New Engl. J. Med., *260*, 841, 1959.
31. Spilberg, I., Siltzbach, L. E. and McEwen, C.: Arth. & Rheum., *12*, 126, 1969.
32. Truelove, L. H.: Ann. Rheum. Dis., *19*, 174, 1960.
33. Vanek, J. and Schwarz, J.: Amer. Rev. Resp. Dis., *101*, 395, 1970.
34. Young, R. L., Harkleroad, L. E., Lordon, R. E. and Weg, J. G.: Ann. Intern. Med., *73*, 207, 1970.
35. Zener, J. C., Alpert, M., and Klainer, L. M.: Arch. Intern. Med., *111*, 62, 1963.

Chapter 71

Arthritis Associated with Hematologic Disorders, Storage Diseases and Dysproteinemias

By Gerald P. Rodnan, M.D.

There are a number of hematologic disorders, storage diseases, and dysproteinemias in which osteoarticular complaints play an important or even dominant role. In some cases these complaints are the result of direct involvement of the bones and joints in the primary disease process; in others they are a consequence of secondary metabolic or immunologic disturbances. In either event, joint symptoms may on occasion constitute the initial manifestation of disease, and require proper identification lest there may be serious delay in the recognition of the underlying disorder.

LEUKEMIA

The early manifestations of acute leukemia are extremely variable and often include symptoms indicative of rheumatic disease.[12,23,61,228,244,245] This is especially true in children, who may be thought at first to have rheumatic fever or juvenile rheumatoid arthritis.[6,23,103] There may be pain and tenderness of the bones, migratory or symmetrical polyarthralgia, and occasionally frank polyarthritis and joint effusion.[205,228] These findings occur most often in the larger peripheral articulations, but the small joints, including fingers, may also be affected. The joint symptoms are related, at least in some instances, to leukemic infiltrations or masses in the synovium, subperiosteum, and juxta-articular portions of the bones, or to hemorrhage.[46,61,108,115,140,228] Articular involvement is much less common in the chronic forms of leukemia and is seldom as dramatic. Localized proliferation of leukemic cells in the synovium may rarely give rise to arthritis.[19] Careful examination may reveal areas of bony tenderness, particularly in the sternum.[47] In both acute and chronic leukemia there is an abnormally high frequency of positive tests for antinuclear antibodies[198] and rheumatoid factor, the latter in titers up to 1:5120.[16,62,68,133,202] Rare cases of acute polymyositis occurring with leukemia have been recorded.[64] A report of a heightened frequency of chronic lymphatic leukemia in association with rheumatoid arthritis remains to be confirmed.[63]

Roentgenograms reveal a variety of skeletal changes in acute leukemia.[18,156,228,242] In children juxtaepiphyseal radiolucent bands are commonly found in long bones, close to the site of rapid bone growth. This abnormality also occurs in a number of other conditions associated with a disturbance in osteogenesis.[23,156,242] Other features of acute leukemia include osteoporosis, osteolytic lesions, cortical or periosteal defects, distortion of trabecular pattern, fractures, osteosclerosis, and subperiosteal new bone formation.[48,204,228,242] Similar although less frequent abnormalities occur in chronic leukemia[48,120,156]; the proximal portions of the femora and humeri, the bones of the pelvis, and the vertebrae are the parts most often affected. Destruction of bone may be extensive and the head of the femur may be damaged to the degree noted in Legg-Perthes disease.[245]

The joint symptoms in acute leukemia may be improved temporarily by salicylates and other anti-inflammatory agents, a reaction which has been responsible for confusion in diagnosis. The disappearance of bone and joint pain is often one of the first indications of improvement after antileukemic therapy.[228] The occurrence of secondary hyperuricemia and gout in leukemia is discussed below.

MALIGNANT LYMPHOMAS

Skeletal involvement is common in the malignant lymphomas.[77,120,156,189] In the past bony defects have been found at postmortem examination in approximately one-half of the cases of Hodgkin's disease.[66,115,140,232] Symptoms referable to these lesions are seldom prominent, however, although localized pain and tenderness (particularly in the lumbar vertebrae in Hodgkin's disease) and pathological fracture may occasionally be important or presenting complaints.[167,232] We have observed a man with a swollen, inflamed knee who had reticulum cell sarcoma which had invaded the synovium, but such direct involvement of the joints is unusual.

There have been occasional reports of positive L.E. cell tests in patients with Hodgkin's disease,[10,111] and numerous instances of individuals with systemic lupus erythematosus or rheumatoid arthritis developing lymphoma and leuemia.[10,38,54,63,87,111,135,152,159,178] In some cases the clinical and serologic evidence of lupus has disappeared during development of Hodgkin's disease.[10,159] In general, however, antinuclear antibodies and rheumatoid factor are not found in Hodgkin's disease and the other lymphomas[198,202] and it is reasonable to state that the hypothesis of an increased susceptibility of patients with connective tissue disease to the development of these conditions remains to be validated.[152,162] (*See also* below, under Myeloma.) There would seem to be little question, however, concerning the increased frequency of reticulum cell sarcoma in patients with Sjögren's syndrome.[220] The recent description of the occurrence of systemic lupus erythematosus with leukemia and lymphoma in two patients with severe hypogammaglobulinemia[152,208] adds to the increasing volume of evidence indicating an interrelationship between the connective tissue disorders, lymphomas, and immunologic competency.[78,152,165] It may be noted in this regard that Hodgkin's disease and other lymphomas are included among the malignant neoplasms which have been associated with the development of dermatomyositis in adults.[41,152,178,226] Articular symptoms may also occur in malignant lymphoma as the result of hypertrophic osteoarthropathy associated with mediastinal involvement[79,136] or because of secondary gout.[179,221]

MYELOMA

In most instances the pain that occurs in the back or the extremities and which is so frequently the earliest symptom of multiple myeloma is attributable to disease of the bone, and roentgenograms often reveal osteolytic defects.[97,104,115,140,156] There is, however, a group of patients with myeloma, usually middle-aged, who develop pain and swelling of the joints, and are found to have extensive deposits of amyloid in the synovium and para-articular tissues, including muscle.[21,53,104,144,224] The parts most often affected are the hands, antecubital fossae, shoulders and clavicles. Polyarticular involvement, particularly that associated with nodular periosteal deposits of amyloid, may closely simulate rheumatoid arthritis.[53,83,86,104,168,224] Synovial fluid in two such cases was fairly viscous and contained less than 200 and 500 cells per c.mm.[21,86] This finding together with the short duration of morning stiffness, atypical erosions of bone, and a plasmacytosis greater than 6 per cent in the bone marrow should lead to the correct diagnosis. It must be kept in mind, however, that multiple myeloma may exist without the typical serum protein electrophoretic pattern (monoclonal peak) or Bence Jones proteinuria.[21,109] In a number of cases amyloid is deposited in the carpal tunnel and compresses the median nerve (carpal tunnel syndrome).[86,96,104,164] The amyloid found in association with multiple myeloma tends to be atypical in its staining reaction with metachromatic dyes, and in most cases has an extra-articular distribution similar to that of so-called primary amyloidosis.[140] This latter condition is also marked by the occasional deposition of amyloid in and about the joints.[192] Extensive amyloid infiltration of the synovium and peri-articular tissues has also been observed in a patient with Waldenström's macroglobulinemia.[86a]

There are several reports of the association of multiple myeloma and gout.[34,104,142,221] In many of these cases joint symptoms preceded recognition of the myeloma by a lengthy period. Patients with multiple myeloma have low levels of normal serum immunoglobulins and an impairment in humoral immunity; they are peculiarly vulnerable to infection,[65] which may include septic arthritis. We have observed two patients with myeloma and pneumococcal arthritis, in both of whom there was severe hypogammaglobulinemia. There is an isolated report of a woman with multiple myeloma who developed fatal necrotizing polyarteritis of the coronary and renal vessels shortly after treatment with dexamethasone.[207]

Of great interest are recent observations on the appearance of paraproteinemia, with or without frank clinical evidence of myelomatosis (and less often, macrog obulinemia or heavy chain disease), in patients with long-standing rheumatoid arthritis.[87,104,240,254] In several of these cases it was noted that joint symptoms abated and the serum titer of rheumatoid factor fell as the myeloma progressed.[240,254] Among the hypotheses advanced in an effort to link these disorders is the suggestion that the neoplastic transformation may be closely related to, if not the direct consequence of prolonged and intense immunologic activity associated with rheumatoid arthritis.[152,254] This notion has been supported by the observation of the development of lymphoid neoplasms in New Zealand black mice with genetically dependent autoimmune disease akin to human lupus erythematosus[151] and F_1 hybrid mice recovering from a graft vs. host reaction,[195] and from the occurrence of a multiple myeloma-like condition in approximately 10 per cent of animals with Aleutian mink disease.[171] However, in view of the fact that myeloma may exist in a lanthanic form for a period of twenty or more years[109] the relationship between this disease and rheumatoid arthritis and the order of their development may be difficult to assess.

SICKLE CELL DISEASE AND OTHER HEMOGLOBINOPATHIES

The crises of sickle cell anemia are often associated with severe polyarthralgia, a finding which has been responsible for the mistaken diagnosis of rheumatic fever.[39] On occasion, the pain is accompanied by hydrarthrosis and other evidence of inflammation,[59,209] but neither the joint fluid nor synovium has been adequately examined and the nature of the arthritis remains to be clarified. The authors of a report on the occurrence of multiple hemarthroses in a patient with sickle cell trait and (coincidental) probable rheumatoid arthritis suggested that the bleeding was the result of local sickling and thrombosis induced by a decrease in oxygen tension and an increase in intra-articular temperature and hydrogen ion concentration.[40]

The skeletal lesions which are so characteristic a feature of this hemoglobinopathy may be separated into those which are related to hyperplasia of the marrow and those which are the result of local sickle cell thrombosis and infarction.[39,59,89,90,143,155,156] Included among the former are widening of medullary cavities, thinning of cortices, coarsening and irregularity of trabecular markings, and cupping of vertebral bodies. Most notable among the bone lesions believed to result from sickle cell thrombosis is avascular necrosis of the head of the femur, which may prove to be bilateral and which takes place in both the immature and mature hip. Less commonly there may be infarctions in the distal portion of the femur, the head of the humerus, radius, patella, and vertebra[39,42,59,155,156,199,222] (Fig. 71–1). Pathologic study has indicated that subchondral and intra-osseous hemorrhage contributes to the destruction of articular cartilage in the hip.[201] Necrosis of the femoral head has been noted in both the variant forms of the hemoglobinopathy (S-C, S-thalassemia, S-F) as well as in S-S disease and sickle cell trait.[17,28,42,113,114,177,182,209,210]

It has been suggested that the hip disease in these patients can be divided into three groups: (1) a Perthes-like involvement of the femoral capital epiphysis or head that runs a cyclic course of varying length with replacement of the necrotic portion of the head, a satisfactory joint being obtained if the hip is protected from weight-bearing during the period of necrosis and repair; (2) localized involvement of the femoral head, similar to osteochondritis dissecans; (3) some deformity of the femoral head in which no spontaneous improvement can be expected.[42] Although it has generally been assumed that the infarction of the femoral head is caused by sickle cell thrombosis of the fine epiphyseal vessels, it is tempting to speculate on the possibility that occlusion may be the result of fat emboli. Systemic fat embolization—apparently originating in the necrotic marrow—has been reported in hemoglobin S-C disease as well as sickle cell (S-S) anemia.[93,160,200]

In young children with sickle cell disease there may be transient swelling and tenderness of the hands and feet as a re-

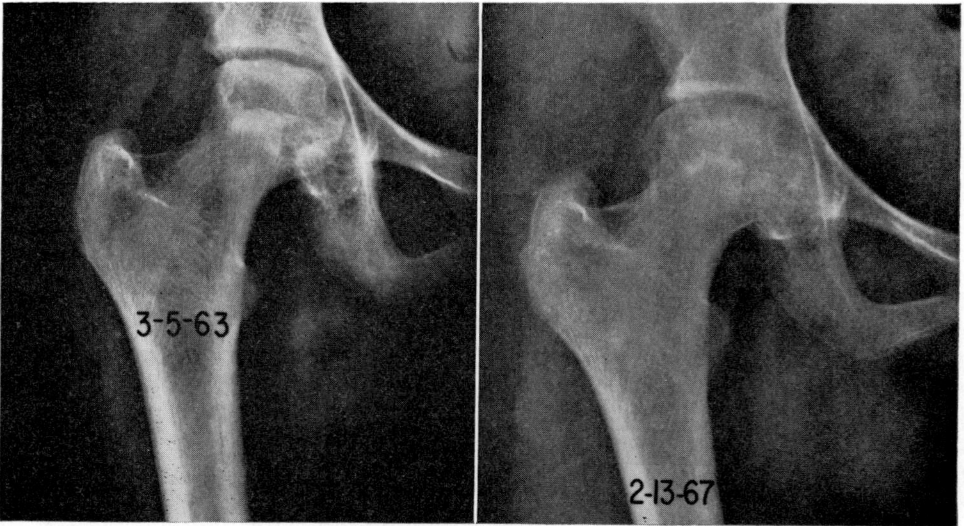

Fig. 71–1.—(*Left*) Roentgenogram of right hip of a girl, age sixteen, with sickle cell anemia (S-S hemoglobin) who complained of pain and restricted movement in the joint. Note changes indicative of avascular necrosis of the head of the right femur; (*right*) same hip, four years later. Note improvement with evidence of regeneration of articular cartilage and subchondral bone. At this time the patient was free of pain and had full motion of the joint.

sult of periostitis of the metacarpal, metatarsal, and proximal phalangeal bones (sickle cell dactylitis).[17,39,43,59,156,238] In addition to periosteal elevation and subperiosteal new bone formation, roentgenograms reveal radiolucent areas intermingled with areas of increased density, giving a moth-eaten appearance. These changes have been interpreted as evidence of infarction.[59] In most cases the integrity of the affected bones is restored to normal in several months without residual deformity or alteration in growth. The rarity of this "hand-and-foot syndrome" after the fourth year of life has been explained by the recession of red marrow from the relatively cool distal bones and its replacement by fibrous tissue.[59]

Another striking skeletal complication of sickle cell disease is salmonella osteomyelitis, which may be multi-focal.[58,59,106,112,185,199] The first sign of this infection, which usually starts in the medullary cavity of the long and tubular bones, is periosteal proliferation. This is followed by bone destruction extending throughout the shaft.[39] Septic arthritis due to salmonellae (and other organisms) has been noted.[59] The explanation for the propensity toward infection with salmonella is not clear[59] but it has been suggested that injury to the intestinal tract as a result of sickle cell thrombosis permits entry of organisms which localize in areas of ischemic necrotic bone. Staphylococci and serratia organisms have also been responsible for osteomyelitis in these patients.[59,72] Following successful treatment with antibiotics the bones tend to heal with minimal deformity.[59]

Although a third or more of patients with sickle cell anemia and hemoglobin S-C disease have been found to have hyperuricemia (usually of mild degree)[85,184,234] there are only a few reports of gouty arthritis in this group.[13,85,176,221] There is evidence that the hyperuricemia results from impaired renal function (sickle cell kidney)[235] and/or overproduction of uric acid.[13,234]

STORAGE DISEASES

Gaucher's Disease

Gaucher's disease (P. C. E. Gaucher, 1882) is a heritable disorder resulting from the deficiency of a specific glucocerebroside-cleavage enzyme and is characterized by the accumulation of large amounts of the glucocerebroside kerasin in cells of the reticuloendothelial system.[75,225] The clinical manifestations, which are fairly variable, result from the infiltration and proliferation of Gaucher cells in the spleen, liver, lymph nodes, bone marrow, and many other internal organs.[181,211,225] Symptoms may appear in early childhood or adolescence, in which case the disease tends to assume a malignant form, or may first be noted in adult life, in which case the course may prove remarkably benign.[95]

Osteoarticular complaints, resulting from infiltration of the marrow, are a prominent feature and often the earliest manifestation of Gaucher's disease.[9,206] The most common rheumatic complaint is pain in the extremities (particularly in the hip, knee and shoulder) which when accompanied by fever has been mistaken for osteomyelitis.[9,193] There may be pathologic fracture of a long bone[127] or compression deformity of vertebrae giving rise to low back pain. In rare cases there is migratory polyarthritis,[150,180,193] the nature of which is poorly understood, but for the most part joint disease is mono- or pauci-articular and appears to be related to changes in adjacent bone.[156,193,206] There are a number of reports of severe degenerative hip disease as a result of avascular necrosis and collapse of the head of the femur.[60,95,156,193,206,211,229] Recurrent avascular necrosis of the capital femoral epiphysis has been observed.[9,119] Changes in the femoral neck may lead to pathologic fracture or coxa vara deformity. On occasion, invasion of the head of the humerus has given rise to degenerative arthropathy of the shoulder.[3,128,206] Many patients with longstanding disease have elevated serum immunoglobulin levels whose increase is often monoclonal in nature.[172] One patient with Gaucher's disease is reported in whom there appears to have been a progression from monoclonal dysproteinemia to overt multiple myeloma.[169]

One of the most consistent roentgenographic features in Gaucher's disease is widening of the distal portion of the femur. This usually occurs just above the medial condyles and creates the well-known "Erlenmeyer flask" appearance.[206] Similar flaring is present less frequently in the tibia and humerus, together with changes in the other long bones, pelvis, skull, vertebrae and mandible.[153,156,180,206,225] Characteristically, areas of rarefaction are mingled with patchy sclerosis and cortical thickening resulting from new bone formation. In the case of spondylar involvement the intervertebral disc and the surfaces of adjacent vertebrae remain intact and, although there may be collapse with the formation of gibbus, the spinal cord escapes compression.[225]

The diagnosis of Gaucher's disease is established by demonstration of large kerasin-filled Gaucher cells in the bone marrow. Although most authors believe that removal of the spleen has no effect upon the occurrence or progression of skeletal lesions[60,95,229] there is a recent report which suggests that splenectomy may contribute to the progression of osseous changes by eliminating a large reservoir for Gaucher's cells.[206] There are some patients in whom bone pain has been relieved following x-irradiation or treatment with corticosteroids.[225]

Multicentric Reticulohistiocytosis

Multicentric reticulohistiocytosis, or lipoid dermatoarthritis, is an uncommon disorder which occurs in adult life and is characterized by a profusion of histiocytic nodules in the skin and mucous membranes and severe, often mutilating, polyarthritis.[7,15,30,91,141,154,163,236] The disease affects women three times as often as men and is usually insidious in onset. In approximately two-thirds of cases the first manifestation is a polyarthritis which is followed in months to years (average, 3 years) by a nodular eruption. In the remainder of patients nodules appear as the initial symptom or occur contemporaneously with joint symptoms. The polyarthritis, which tends to be symmetrical and often simulates rheumatoid arthritis, may involve virtually all the peripheral articulations (frequently including the distal interphalangeal joints of the fingers) as well as the vertebral and temporomandibular joints. Stiffness of the joints may be a prominent early complaint. The parts involved are swollen and tender and may be markedly inflamed. The course and severity of the arthritis are variable. Although there may be spontaneous remission, chronic active disease is more usual. An appreciable number of the patients suffer severe destructive changes, particularly affecting the fingers (*main en lorgnette*) and less often the hip and toe joints. In a number of cases there has been involvement of the tendon sheaths on the flexor and extensor surfaces of the wrists.

The skin lesions consist of firm, reddish-brown or yellow papulonodules which occur most commonly on the face and hands, ears, forearms and elbows, scalp, neck and chest.[15] Small tumefactions, compared to coral beads in appearance, occur around the nail fold[15] (Fig. 71–2). These lesions may remain discrete or coalesce into diffuse plaques. The nodules tend to wax and wane and to disappear without trace. Xanthelasma has been noted in a third of the patients. About half the patients have mucosal papules, which occur on the lips, tongue, buccal membrane, nasal septum, tongue, and gingiva, as well as pharynx and larynx. There may be fever and considerable weakness and weight loss during the course of this illness.

Roentgenograms of the joints have revealed extensive destructive changes with loss of cartilage and absorption of subchondral bone.[196] Examination of the cervical vertebrae in one patient showed erosion of the atlas and odontoid process, resembling the changes noted in rheumatoid arthritis.[146]

Microscopic examination shows dense infiltration of the dermis by a granulomatous proliferation of histiocytes and multinucleated giant cells which contain large amounts of periodic acid-Schiff (PAS)-positive material which appears to be a mixture of lipids, including triglycerides, cholesterol esters, and several phospholipids[14,141,163] (Fig. 71–3*A*). Similar cells have been observed in the synovium[7,91,154] (Fig. 71–3*B*) as well as bone marrow, lymph nodes, bone and

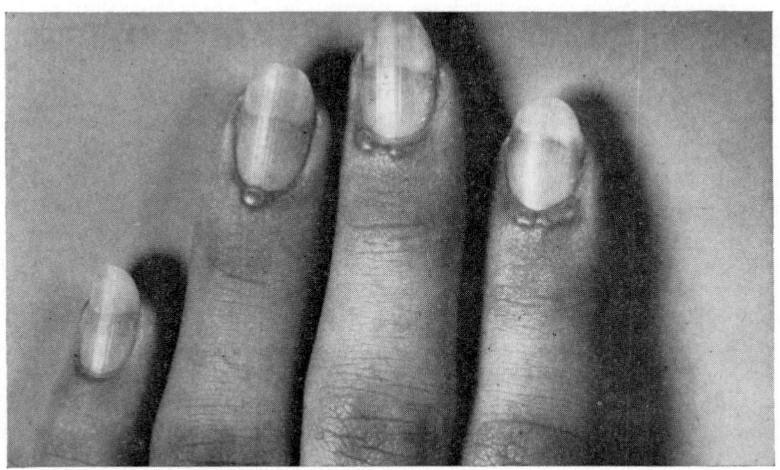

FIG. 71–2.—The fingers of a 16-year-old girl who had had polyarthritis for 8 months and these red-brown "coral beads" for 5 months. Typical infiltrates of multicentric reticulohistiocytosis were found in biopsy specimens of both skin and synovium. (J. W. Melton and R. Irby, courtesy of Arthritis and Rheumatism.)

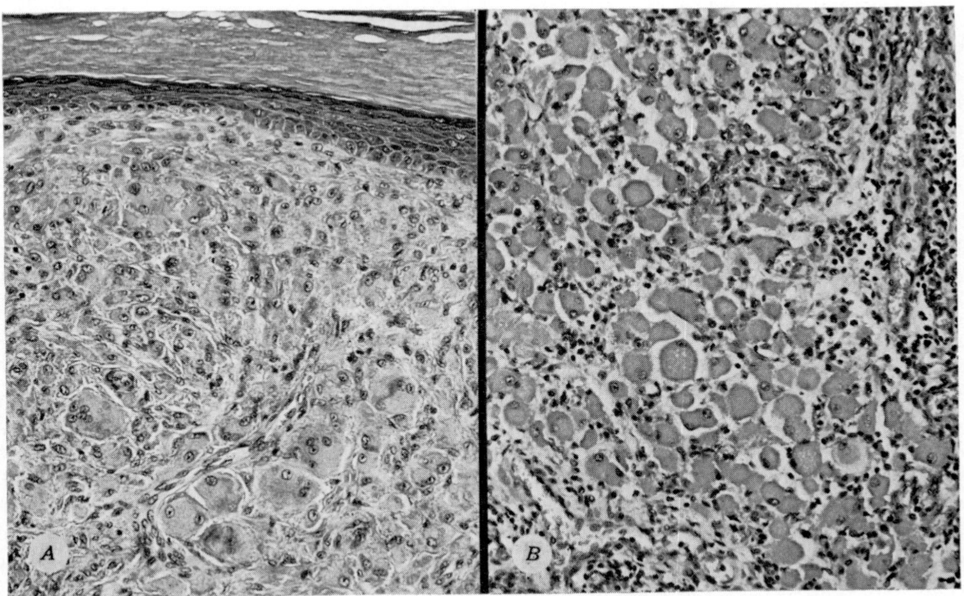

FIG. 71–3.—Photomicrograph of (*A*) skin nodule and (*B*) synovium (knee) from woman, age fifty-four, with multicentric reticulohistiocytosis. There are numerous histiocytes and multinucleated giant cells which contain large amounts of periodic acid-Schiff (PAS)-positive material. (Magnification ×185)

periosteum, muscle, larynx and endocardium.[7,236] Serum lipid abnormalities—including slight to moderate elevations in total lipid, cholesterol, phospholipid, and fatty acids, as well as changes in lipoproteins—have been found in a number of the patients.[7] The exact nature of this condition remains unknown although the evidence is strongly suggestive of a lipid storage disease. However, to date there is no indication of a familial predisposition[15] or other findings pointing toward a heritable basis for multicentric reticulohistiocytosis. The latex agglutination reaction for rheumatoid factor has been found to be negative.[7,30,163]

Several patients with multicentric reticulohistiocytosis have succumbed from cancer and we have recently observed a patient who died with complete heart block resulting from infiltration of the conducting system. In most instances, however, the disease is non-fatal and displays a tendency toward spontaneous quiescence. Although the mucocutaneous nodules may diminish in size or disappear completely, the patients are often left with serious joint disability and at times a disfigured leonine facies.[15] There is no treatment which has proven to be satisfactory. The anti-inflammatory corticosteroids may cause temporary regression of the cutaneous lesions, but have little effect on the arthritis.[7,163] In evaluating the claims for various therapies the highly variable course of the disease must be kept in mind.

Fabry's Disease

Fabry's disease, or glycolipid lipidosis (first described by J. Fabry in 1898), is an hereditary, sex-linked disorder of glycosphingolipid metabolism which is characterized by the progressive accumulation of birefringent deposits of galactosylgalactosylglucosylceramide (Gal-Gal-Gly-Cer) in endothelial, perithelial, and smooth muscle cells of blood vessels, in ganglion and perineural cells of the autonomic nervous system, in epithelial cells of the cornea, and in kidney, bone marrow and many other tissues.[219,246] This pathologic storage is due to the absence of an enzyme (ceramidetrihexosidase) required for the normal catabolism of trihexosyl ceramide (derived from kidney and the membranes of senescent erythrocytes). Death usually occurs in the fifth or sixth decade, as a result of renal failure or from the cardiac and cerebral complications of arterial hypertension or vascular disease. Heterozygous females may exhibit the disease in an attenuated form.

In addition to the characteristic rash (angiokeratoma corporis diffusum universale) males with this disease are subject to recurrent bouts of fever and of severe pain in the extremities, the latter often induced by changes in environmental temperature. There may be painful swelling of the fingers, elbows, and knees.[219] A characteristic deformity and a limitation in extension of the distal interphalangeal joints of the fingers have been described.[80,116,246] In addition there may be avascular necrosis of the head of the femur[170] or talus[71] and multiple small infarct-like opacities in the femoral head.[130] Involvement of the temporomandibular joint has been reported,[213] as well as osteoporosis of the dorsal vertebrae.[22] The diagnosis of Fabry's disease is established by observation of the characteristic rash and corneal epithelial dystrophy, demonstration of birefringent lipid material in skin and renal biopsy specimens, measurement of Gal-Gal-Gly-Cer levels, and enzymatic assay.

Farber's Disease

Farber's disease, or disseminated lipogranulomatosis (S. Farber, 1952), is a rare disorder of early life characterized by periarticular swelling, joint contractures or ankylosis, dysphonia, respiratory distress, and mental and motor retardation.[2,24,67,194] There is an accumulation of acid mucopolysaccharide, chiefly dermatan sulfate (chondroitin sulfate B) in the tissues taking the form of nodules in the skin overlying the joints, subcutaneous tissues, and viscera, and there is an increased urinary excretion of this substance. Fibroblasts, histiocytes, and macrophages with foamy cytoplasm containing material with the staining properties of lipids and glycoproteins are found in granulomatous deposits in the larynx, pleura, pericardium, synovium, bones, liver, spleen, lymph nodes, and lung; the abnormal lipid is also present in the cytoplasm of neurones of the central nervous system. Roentgenographic changes consist of generalized bony demineralization, juxta-articular erosions of long bones, and irregular disruption of trabeculae in the metacarpals and phalanges.[24,194] A brother and sister with the disease are included amongst the handful of patients described to date and it has been concluded that Farber's disease is related to other (heritable) disorders of mucopolysaccharide metabolism although the nature of the basic biochemical abnormality and explanation for the preferential involvement of joints, larynx, and subcutaneous tissues are not yet clear.

Lipochrome Histiocytosis

This rare familial disorder is marked by pulmonary infiltrates, splenomegaly, hypergammaglobulinemia, increased susceptibility to infection, and lipochrome pigment granulation of the histiocytes. In the first report of this syndrome, one of three affected sisters had juvenile rheumatoid arthritis with typical nodules, and a second had transient episodes of joint inflammation; the serum of all three contained rheumatoid factor in high titer.[73] The peripheral blood leukocytes of these patients have been found to have impaired respiration and hexose monophosphate shunt activity following phagocytosis and to be deficient in staphylocidal capacity.[186]

SECONDARY GOUT

The term "secondary gout" has been applied to those cases of gouty arthritis which occur as a complication of a variety of primary disorders in which there is a disturbance of purine or uric acid metabolism marked by prolonged hyperuricemia.[81,99,100,248] The underlying disease is usually a myeloproliferative disorder in which there is an overproduction of uric acid as a consequence of an increased turnover of nucleic acids.[13,125,142,221,252] Secondary gout is particularly frequent in polycythemia (both primary and secondary) and myeloid metaplasia,[37,51,56,100,107,137,142,212,221,237,249] and has been noted less commonly in patients with acute leukemia,[142,221] chronic granulocytic leukemia,[27,125,142,221] malignant lymphoma,[179,221] multiple myeloma,[34,104,142,221] sickle cell anemia,[13,85,176,221] thalassemia,[166,230] pernicious anemia under treatment with liver extract,[221] and megaloblastic anemia of tropical sprue.[138,221] The frequency of gout in polycythemia vera has varied in different series from 2 to 14 per cent.[56,231] The initial attack may take place during the period of active polycythemia or during or after the transition of the disease into its myeloproliferative phase.[252] The occurrence of hyperuricemia and of gout appears to be particularly frequent in those patients with polycythemia vera in whom the renal clearance of uric acid is reduced to less than 5 ml. per minute.[56] Secondary hyperuricemia and gout have also been reported in patients with disseminated carcinoma and sarcoma.[55,126,157,231]

Secondary gout is similar to primary gout in its clinical characteristics although the average age of onset and the relative frequency with which women are affected are both greater in the secondary than in the primary form of the disease.[142,221,252] In further contrast a history of familial involvement is unusual in secondary gout and there is a tendency toward higher serum urate levels and greater urinary uric acid excretion.[142,221] This excretion is often markedly excessive in those patients with good renal function. The incidence of uric acid nephrolithiasis is accordingly higher in secondary than in primary gout,[253] and a number of patients develop urinary tract infection and uremia. Large tophaceous deposits may occur in those patients whose primary disease permits prolonged survival.

Despite the similarities in the clinical and pathologic features of primary (familial) and secondary gout, there is a basic difference in the origin of the hyperuricemia in the two conditions.[13,81,125,134,197,248,249,250] When patients with secondary gout due to polycythemia or myeloid metaplasia are given labeled purine precursors, the amount of isotope which accumulates in urinary uric acid is usually much greater than that observed in normal subjects. The rate at which this incorporation occurs is slower than the rapid enrichment of urinary uric acid often found in primary gout. This observation is consistent with the belief that the hyperuricemia in these patients is the result of abnormally rapid catabolism of nucleoprotein incident to hyperactive erythropoiesis. In the case of chronic granulocytic leukemia and myeloid metaplasia the isotope enrichment of urinary uric acid following administration of sodium formate-C^{14} has been found to display a diphasic pattern, the first peak occurring 2 days after isotope administration, and the second maximum after about 12 days.[125] The initial peak has been attributed to *de novo* synthesis of uric acid, without prior incorporation of isotope into nucleic acids, and the second peak to the release of purine from degenerating leukemic cells.

Striking increases in serum urate levels may occur in patients with leukemia and malignant lymphoma as a result of rapid breakdown of cellular nucleic acids following aggressive treatment with alkylating agents, x-radiation, and adrenal corticosteroids.[94,126,142,183] The precipitation of uric acid in the renal tubules of such patients may lead to severe, sometimes fatal urinary obstruction. This hazard can be prevented or reversed by treatment with allopurinol (4-hydroxypyrazolo, [3,4-*d*] pyrimidine), an agent which has proven to be highly effective in reducing hyperuricemia in patients with leukemia, lymphoma, and cancer.[55,102,126,157,233,251] The value of dialysis as an adjunct in the management of acute obstructive uric acid nephropathy has been recorded.[145]

HYPERLIPOPROTEINEMIA

Articular and tendinous manifestations are an important feature of certain of the heritable disorders of lipid transport or lipoprotein metabolism.[76] In the case of type II hyperlipoproteinemia (essential familial hypercholesterolemia) the disease is manifested clinically by tendinous, tuberous and periosteal xanthomatosis, as well as by xanthelasma, corneal arcus, and a tendency toward early atherosclerosis. The tendinous xanthomas are located in the Achilles tendons, patellar tendons, and the extensor tendons of the hands and feet (Fig. 71–4).[105] Tendon xanthomas have also been noted in the plantar aponeurosis, the fascia and periosteum overlying the lower tibia, and the peroneal tendons[98]—all these being sites of repeated stretching, direct pressure, and trauma. These deposits are situated within the tendon fibers and not on the tendon sheath and cannot be separated from the tendon on movement (Fig. 71–5). Tuberous xanthomas are soft subcutaneous masses which occur over extensor surfaces, including the elbows, knees, and hands, as well as the buttocks.[69] Type II hyperlipoproteinemia is transmitted as a simple autosomal dominant trait with high penetrance.[76] In those individuals who are homozygous with respect to the abnormal gene, xanthomatosis usually appears in childhood and tends to be extensive; in the heterozygous condition, the serum lipid and lipoprotein abnormalities are less striking, tendinous xanthomas usually do not appear until the age of 30, and tuberous xanthomas do not develop.[105]

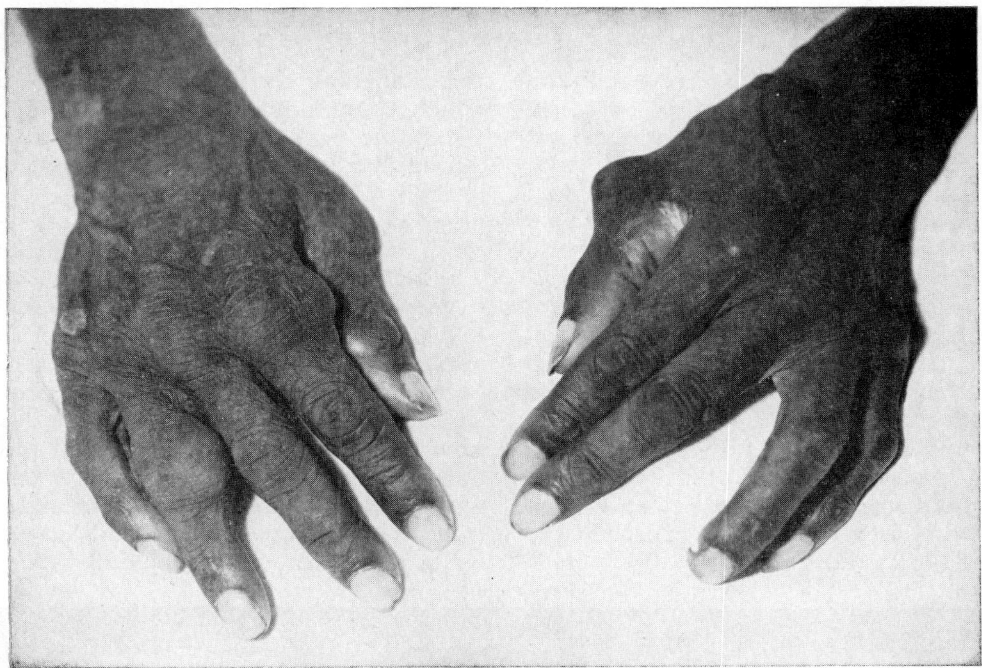

FIG. 71–4.—*Xanthoma tendinosum.* The hands of a seventy-five-year-old man with probable type II hyperlipoproteinemia, who had had nodular swellings involving extensor tendons of several fingers and both Achilles and infrapatellar tendons for more than fifty years. The patient's serum cholesterol concentration was 415 mg. per cent.

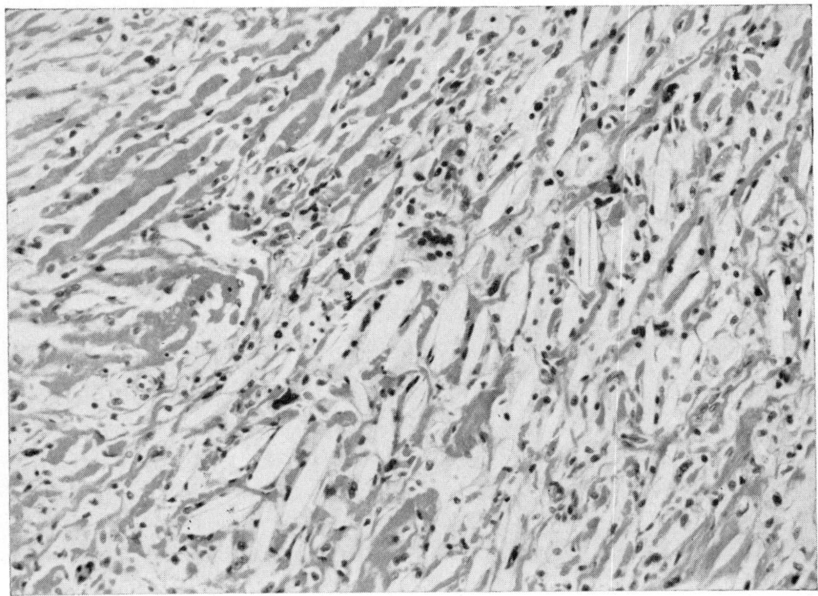

FIG. 71–5.—*Xanthoma tendinosum.* Photomicrograph of tendon nodule removed from the hand of patient illustrated in previous figure. There are numerous large lipid-filled histiocytes with pale foamy cytoplasm, strewn about in a collagenous stroma. The clefts indicate the site of deposition of crystals of cholesterol. (Magnification ×175).

Chemical analysis has revealed that tendon xanthomas are composed chiefly of cholesterol (over 90 per cent esterified) and phospholipid.[70,105] This and other evidence support the view that xanthomas are a complication resulting from elevation of plasma lipids, and their development depends upon the degree and duration of the elevation. Tendon xanthomas, which are specifically associated with hypercholesterolemia, have not been observed in individuals whose serum cholesterol levels were consistently below 300 mg. per cent.

It has been reported that patients who are homozygous with respect to type II hyperlipoproteinemia may experience repeated episodes of a migratory polyarthritis affecting the large peripheral joints which is apparently clinically similar to rheumatic fever.[123] These attacks have varied in intensity from mild joint pains without objective changes lasting a few days, to severe incapacitating pain, redness, and swelling of a month's duration. The nature of this joint inflammation is unclear; joint fluid and synovium remain to be examined. These individuals are also subject to bouts of Achilles tendinitis, occasionally accompanied by arthritis.[84] These attacks, which last two to three days, may be unilateral or bilateral and have recurred over periods of up to forty years without joint deformity or loss of motion (Fig. 71–6). Recognition of this feature, the symptoms of which frequently appear

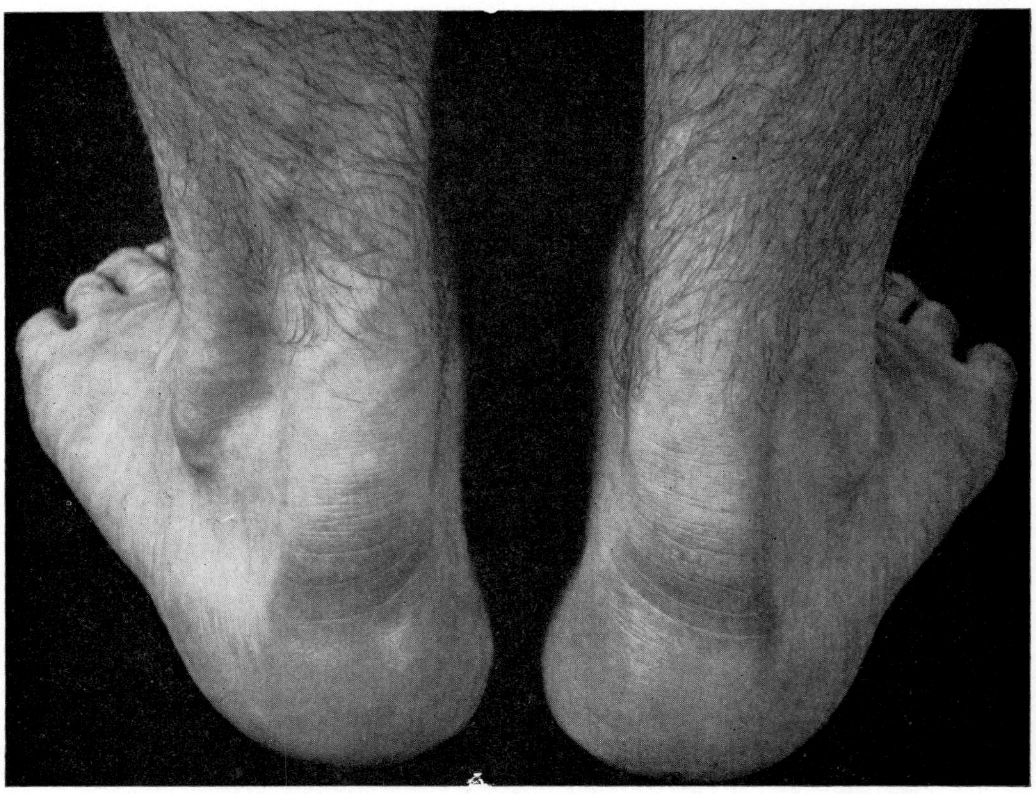

Fig. 71–6.—*Xanthoma tendinosum.* The patient, a thirty-four-year-old man with type II hyperlipoproteinemia, had had repeated episodes of acute inflammation involving the Achilles tendons, which lasted from one to three days and had led to the mistaken diagnosis of gout. The tendons were markedly enlarged, but there were no other xanthomas. This patient's serum cholesterol level varied from 330 to 485 mg. per cent.

in the second decade of life, is important in that it permits early diagnosis, family screening, and effective prophylactic treatment of the hyperlipoproteinemia.

The diagnosis of type II hyperlipoproteinemia is determined by the finding of hypercholesterolemia together with the demonstration by lipoprotein electrophoresis of a marked (familial) elevation in beta-lipoproteins which on ultracentrifugal analysis are found to be primarily S_f 0–12 and 12–20.[76]

Tendinous and tuberous xanthomas also occur in type III and type IV hyperlipoproteinemia.[69,76] Type III, in which there is an excess of lipoproteins with beta mobility but abnormally low density, is manifested by hypercholesterolemia and an elevation in plasma triglyceride levels. A peculiarly distinctive clinical feature is that of lipid deposition (plane xanthomas) in the palms of the hands.[76] In type IV hyperlipoproteinemia there is carbohydrate inducible hyperlipemia as well as a pure pre-beta lipoproteinemia. There is a recent report of the frequent occurrence of various musculoskeletal complaints, including morning stiffness, arthralgia, joint tenderness and causalgia-like hyperesthesia in association with type IV hyperlipoproteinemia.[88]

Various types of xanthomas (tendinous, tuberous, eruptive) have also been observed in patients in whom type II or type IV hyperlipoproteinemia has been associated with the development of multiple myeloma, as well as in some cases of myelomatosis without definite hyperlipoproteinemia.[76,158]

Joint changes as a result of infiltration of foam cells in subchondral bone have also been recorded in secondary hyperlipoproteinemia, such as that which develops in patients with biliary cirrhosis and hypercholesterolemia.[11]

HEMOPHILIC ARTHRITIS

Hemophilia is the collective designation for a group of heredito-familial disorders in which the deficiency of a plasma coagulation protein results in faulty fibrin clot formation[25,26,32] (Table 71–1). Patients are subject to abnormal bleeding which varies in frequency and intensity with the severity of the clotting defect. In addition to easy bruising, which is present in nearly all cases, there may be prolonged and excessive bleeding following minor injuries, recurrent bleeding from the genitourinary and gastrointestinal tracts, and hemorrhage into peripheral joints. Hemarthrosis, the most frequent and the most painful manifestation of hemophilia, has been described in all the heritable coagulation disorders (with the exception of factor V deficiency) and may also occur as an unusual complication of hypoprothrombinemia induced by anticoagulant drugs.[149] Repeated hemarthrosis is often followed by permanent disability of one or more joints.[57,64a,117,121,122,131,146,174,187,222,239]

The occurrence of joint disease in hemophilia (*bleeder's joints*) has been recognized for well over a century and was considered originally to represent a form of atypical rheumatism. Volkmann (1868) was one of the first to attribute the disturbance to the effects of hemorrhage.[122,239]

Pathogenesis and Anatomic Findings

Hemophilic hemarthrosis usually follows trauma. The injury may be trivial, however, and is often inapparent to the young patient or his parents. The changes which take place as a result of joint hemorrhage have been particularly well studied in naturally hemophilic dogs, which develop an arthropathy quite comparable to that encountered in man.[218]

The initial lesion consists of synovial or sub-synovial hemorrhage. Rupture of blood into the joint cavity provokes an inflammatory reaction which is characterized by effusion, villous hypertrophy, hyperplasia of the lining cells, and infiltration of lymphocytes and plasma cells. This reaction gradually subsides several days to weeks after the cessation of hemorrhage. Hemoglobin is released after

Table 71-1.
The heritable disorders of blood coagulation (the hemophilias) may be classified as follows:

A. Sex-linked recessive traits
  1. Factor VIII (antihemophilic factor, AHF) deficiency (classical hemophilia).
  2. Factor IX (plasma thromboplastic component, PTC) deficiency (Christmas disease).

B. Autosomal recessive traits
  1. Factor XI (plasma thromboplastic antecedent, PTA) deficiency.
  2. Factor II (prothrombin) deficiency
  3. Factor V (proaccelerin) deficiency (parahemophilia)
  4. Factor VII (proconvertin) deficiency
  5. Factor X (Stuart) deficiency
  6. Factor I (fibrinogen) deficiency
  7. Factor XII (Hageman) deficiency
  8. Factor XIII deficiency

C. Autosomal dominant traits
  1. Von Willebrand's disease (pseudohemophilia, vascular hemophilia).
  2. Congenital dysfibrinogenemia.

Factor VIII deficiency (classical hemophilia) comprises approximately 80 per cent of most large series of cases of hemophilia, while factor IX deficiency (*Christmas disease*) and factor XI (PTA) deficiency account for all but 1 to 2 per cent of the remainder. The clinical manifestations in general, and the joint involvement in particular, of patients with factor IX deficiency are quite similar to those encountered in factor VIII deficiency.

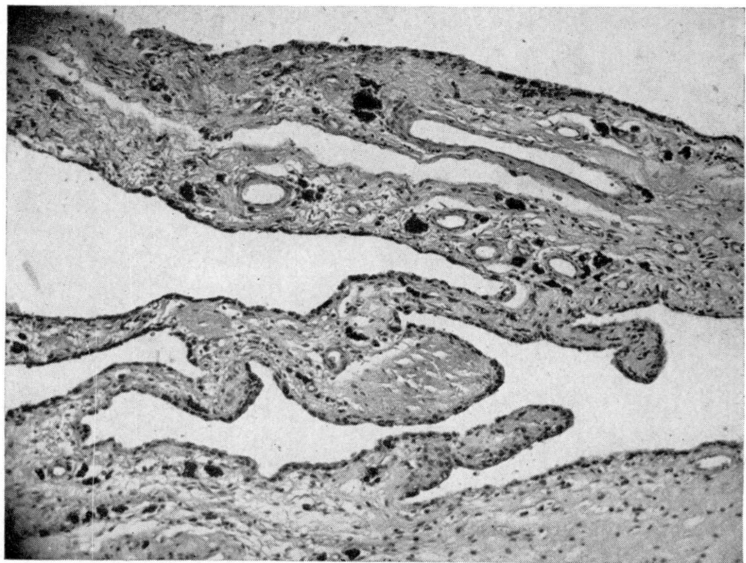

FIG. 71–7.—Photomicrograph of synovium from knee joint of hemophilic man, age seventy-six. Note heavy deposits of iron-containing pigment (hemosiderin) which is present both in lining cells and in deeper portions of the synovium. Hematoxylin and eosin stain. (Rodnan *et al.*,[188] courtesy of Arthritis and Rheumatism.)

there has been lysis of erythrocytes in the joint cavity and synovial tissues and hemosiderin remains in the synovium for an indefinitely long period, appearing as finely particulate matter within the phagocytic lining cells (Fig. 71–7). Additional coarser aggregates of this iron-containing pigment, lying free or in macrophages, are found in deeper portions of the synovium; the presence of large amounts of hemosiderin in this location is a point which distinguishes this variety of synovial siderosis from that found in hemochromatosis.[45]

Repeated hemorrhage is marked by hyperplasia of the synovial lining cells (type B) and by gradually increasing fibrosis and hemosiderosis of the synovium, which lead to rigidity of the subsynovial tissue and joint capsule.[191] Although these changes may account for some degree of limitation in motion, it is the damage to cartilage and bone which eventually proves most damaging to the joint.[57] There is both marginal erosion of the cartilage previously ascribed to encroachment of hyperplastic synovium, and more central irregular "map-like" degeneration, which has been attributed to subchondral hemorrhage.[44,122] The demonstration of plasmin (fibrinolysin) in joint fluid during the course of acute hemarthrosis[129] and the finding of numerous siderosomes suggest that the loss of cartilage may result from enzymatic degradation. (*Siderosomes* are membrane-bound bodies with aggregates of iron-containing particles, believed to be lysosomal organelles in which hemoglobin and/or its derivative are digested.) In studies of experimental hemarthrosis in the rabbit, the synthesis of both ribonucleic acid and protein by articular cartilage has been found to remain unimpaired despite the repeated daily intra-articular injection of blood.[247] The destruction of articular cartilage which occurs after repeated joint hemorrhage is accompanied by the development of cavities or "cysts" in the subchondral bone (Fig. 71–8). These lesions have been thought to be the result of intra-

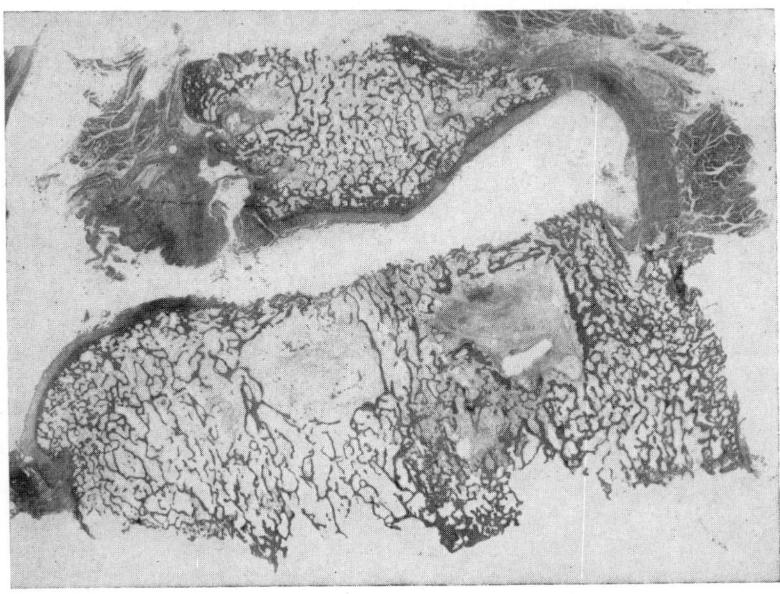

Fig. 71–8.—Sagittal section of elbow joint of the same patient described in previous figure. Note erosion of articular cartilage and the presence of several subchrondral cavities which appear to be in direct communication with the joint space (Rodnan, *et al.*,[188] courtesy of Arthritis and Rheumatism).

osseous bleeding.[44] In the study of hemophilic dogs, it was found that these "cysts" communicated with the synovial cavity at a point of cartilage and subchondral bone erosion, at the margin of the articular cartilage, or at the site of ligamentous attachments.[218] These and similar observations in human hemophilic joint disease suggest that the development of these "cysts" is related more to degenerative changes in articular cartilage and subchondral bone than to intra-osseous bleeding.[29,132,188] A striking finding in young patients is that of the accelerated maturation and hypertrophy of the epiphyses adjacent to affected joints. It has been suggested that chronic hyperemia of the epiphyseal cartilage, induced by repeated hemarthrosis, is responsible for this change.[36]

In addition to hemarthrosis, there may be bleeding into muscle and bone. The terms "hemophilic pseudotumor" or "hemophilic cyst" have been applied to the destructive hematomas resulting from massive muscle, subperiosteal, and/or intraosseous hemorrhages which occur most often in the thigh or leg.[1,74,82,147,214,223,229a] This bleeding may prove extremely dangerous because of neurovascular compression, severe destruction and contracture of muscle (including Volkmann's contracture),[64a,214,227] cyst rupture, sinus formation or chronic infection.[214] One of the most dramatic examples of hemophilic bleeding involves the iliacus.[35,92] Hemorrhage into the closed fascial compartment which contains the iliacus muscle and the femoral nerve is marked by the development of sudden severe pain in the groin and thigh which is followed by the appearance of a tender mass (hematoma) in the iliac fossa and groin, flexion contracture of the hip, and signs of femoral nerve palsy. Bleeding into the gastrocnemius or soleus muscle or both may lead to talipes equinus deformity.

Repeated bleeding in and about the joints and associated muscle atrophy thus leads to instability of the weight-bearing joints.

Clinical Features

Hemarthrosis occurs in approximately 80 to 90 per cent of patients with hemophilia[57,174,187,217,227] and constitutes the most common major hemorrhagic event in the disease. Bleeding into the joints is particularly common in those individuals in whom the level of antihemophilic globulin is less than 1 to 2 per cent of normal.[131,174,175,239] The majority of patients first experience articular symptoms between the ages of one and five and tend to have repeated hemarthroses during the remainder of the first decade of life, after which time this ordinarily becomes less and less frequent.[64a,217] Those patients with milder degrees of hemophilia experience fewer episodes of hemarthrosis and these are more often associated with severe trauma. Hemorrhage occurs most commonly in a knee, ankle, or elbow, and less frequently in the shoulders, hips, wrists, fingers, and toes.[4,217] Generally only one joint is involved in each episode, but on occasion two joints are affected simultaneously. Oftimes there is a tendency toward repeated hemorrhage in the same site.[217] The joint is swollen and warm and often becomes exquisitely painful and tender. Associated muscle spasm leads to flexion of the extremity. When hemarthrosis is severe, there may be fever and leukocytosis. In instances of milder bleeding, the normal configuration and full motion of the joint may be restored within a matter of days, the patient experiencing little more than transient stiffness on reambulation. In the case of protracted bleeding and particularly those in which re-injury of the joint leads to renewed hemorrhage, symptoms may persist for many weeks to months.

Following repeated and/or severe hemarthrosis, there is gradual failure of the joint to return to fully normal form and function. Examination now discloses thickening of the periarticular soft tissues, crepitation, atrophy of muscle which accentuates the bony enlargement of the joint, and various deformities, the most common of which are flexion contracture of the elbow and knee. The latter is frequently accompanied by posterior subluxation of the tibia. Occasionally there is fibrous and rarely bony ankylosis.[57,64a] Bleeding into the hip joint during childhood may lead to dislocation[64a] or to flattening and destruction of the capital epiphysis and deformity of the femoral neck with resultant shortening of the extremity.[243] Approximately one-half of the patients have some permanent changes in the peripheral articulations and it is the rare individual with severe hemophilia (less than 2 per cent of normal level of antihemophilic globulin) who escapes some residual deformity.[239] In most cases only a few joints are involved in this chronic arthropathy (usually knees and elbows) and many joints remain normal despite repeated bleeding.

Although the presence of hemophilia is suspected readily in the individual with a recognized bleeding tendency, the diagnosis may be much less obvious in the occasional child or adult in whom hemarthrosis is the initial symptom of the disease, or in whom minor hemorrhagic episodes have been overlooked. It is especially important that this condition be recognized before unsuspecting surgical invervention results in disastrous consequences.[122,166a]

Roentgenographic Findings

In acute intra-articular hemorrhage there is distention of the joint capsule and increased density of the soft tissues.[29] There may be evidence of an accompanying subperiosteal hemorrhage, which is followed by thickening or, in some cases, by atrophy of the underlying cortex. Subchondral hemorrhage may lead to defects in epiphyseal ossification centers.

Chronic hemophilic joint disease is characterized by irregular narrowing or obliteration of the joint space and later

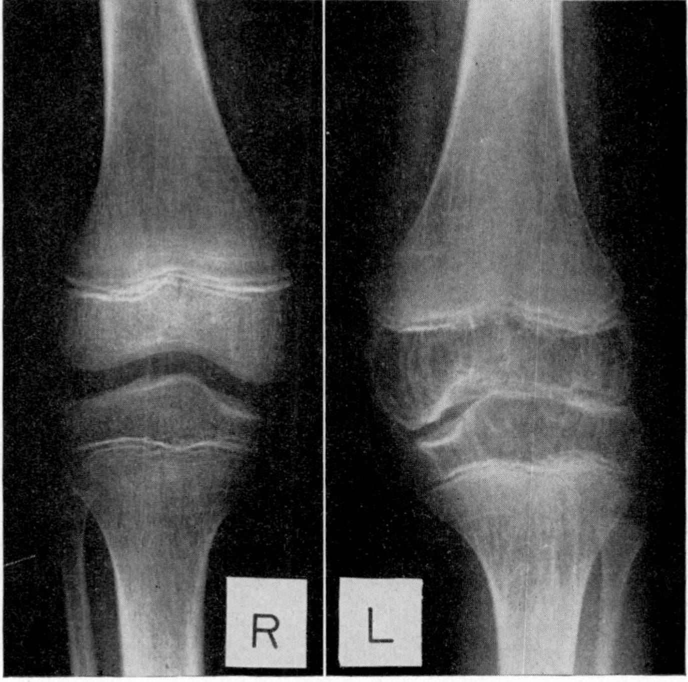

FIG. 71–9.—Roentgenograms of the knees of hemophilic boy, age nine, who had had repeated hemarthroses involving the left knee. Note loss of articular cartilage, irregularity of bony surfaces, and hypertrophy of the epiphyses of femur and tibia. The right knee appears normal.

by marginal spurring and sclerosis of bone, which often contains one or more areas of cystic translucency[29,36,57,117,156,173] (Figs. 71–9, 71–10, and 71–11). The peri-articular soft tissues may be thickened and increased in density, and occasionally contain fine opacities which have traditionally been attributed to the deposition of hemosiderin in the synovium,[36] a view which has recently been questioned.[29] Enlargement of the head of the radius is a frequent finding in patients with elbow involvement.[57,239] Flattening of the inferior portion of the patella (squared-off patella) is often noted in advanced disease of the knee and has been considered highly suggestive of hemophilic arthropathy.[117,156] Occlusion of the epiphyseal vessels as a result of intra-osseous bleeding or episodic increases in intracapsular pressure may lead to destruction and deformity of the femoral head (avascular necrosis)[29,156,243]; similar changes have been seen in the talus.[29,57]

Management

The development in recent years of highly potent cryoprecipitates and other concentrated preparations of the plasma coagulation factors has made it much easier to attain effective hemostasis and has greatly improved, indeed revolutionized, the treatment of joint and muscle bleeding.[26,90,203,215] Concentrates have been prepared from both human and animal plasma, particularly from cattle and pigs, whose blood contains factor VIII in much higher concentration than in man.[26] There are indications that maintenance of low levels (3 to 5 per cent) of factor VIII activity by the regular administration of relatively small amounts of concentrate sharply reduces the frequency of hemarthrosis and other serious

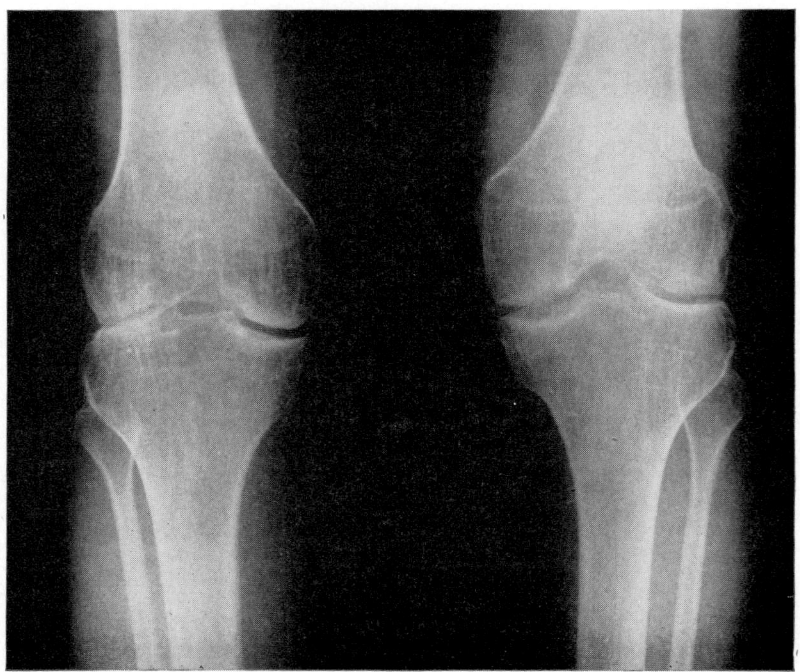

Fig. 71–10.—Roentgenograms of knees of the same patient as described in previous figure, at age seventeen. During the interval of eight years since the roentgenograms in Figure 71–9 were obtained, there were many more episodes of joint hemorrhage, involving *both* knees. Note irregular narrowing of joint space and early osteophyte formation.

hemorrhage.[5,20,118] It has been noted, furthermore, that chronic joint changes are rare in hemophilic patients with a coagulation factor content above 2 to 3 per cent of normal.[5] Hopefully we may look forward to the day when hemophilic arthropathy will be a preventable disorder.

Prophylaxis.—Every reasonable attempt should be made to avoid the trauma which may initiate joint hemorrhage. Although it is wise to interdict football and other sports which involve violent contact, it is important to keep in mind the psychological needs of the boy and value of participation in group athletics. Patients with milder degrees of hemophilia (5 per cent or more of factor VIII and 10 per cent or more of factor IX) are able to engage in rather strenuous activities with little or no difficulty. When formulating a program this should be individualized for each boy and his family, who must strive to maintain a balance between overprotecion and unwarranted liberty.[26]

Acute Hemarthrosis.—It is essential that the patient and his parents be instructed in the early recognition and immediate care of hemarthrosis so that damage to the joint is minimized and as little time as possible lost from educational and other normal pursuits.[33] Prompt treatment of hemarthrosis is the key to the prevention of the chronic disability which results from repeated joint bleeding. There is general agreement on the need for rest, which is best accomplished by putting the patient to bed and elevating the affected extremity, which should be maintained initially in the position of comfort. Ice packs are of value in lessening pain and inflammation. Aspirin should be avoided when prescribing analgesics since this drug may produce a prolongation of bleeding time and provoke or aggravate hemorrhage by interfering with platelet aggregation by connective tissue.[52,161,241]

Mild hemarthrosis is often well treated by immobilization alone. When the hemarthrosis is more severe efforts should

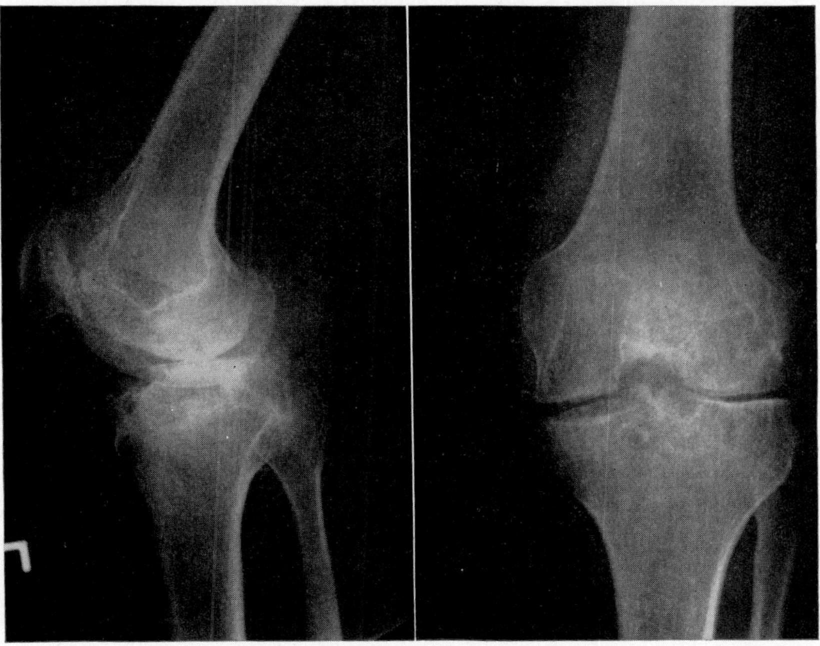

Fig. 71–11.—Roentgenograms of the left knee of a hemophilic man, age twenty-two. Note irregular narrowing of the joint space, marginal spurring of the bone, and the presence of numerous subchondral cavities in the tibia.

be made to correct the underlying defect in coagulation and thus prevent further bleeding.[8,25,26,31,50,57,175,215] In one study the prompt infusion of active plasma preparations was found to reduce the duration of incapacity from hemarthroses by over half and the incidence of new deformities by four-fifths.[8] The patient with classical hemophilia should be given cyroprecipitate or another factor VIII concentrate (or, if these are not available, quickly frozen plasma or freshly drawn blood). Concentrate of factor IX, or plasma, is used in the case of *Christmas disease.*[5,8,25,26,31,57,175] Sufficient amounts of the appropriate clotting factor should be infused so as to achieve levels of plasma activity equal initially to 10 to 20 per cent of normal, and to maintain a level of 5 to 10 per cent for a period of at least 48 to 72 hours. Relief of pain, restoration of joint mobility, and cessation of further bleeding can be expected within a few hours, provided there has been prompt administration of cryoprecipitate or other concentrates. Prolonged treatment is required in the case of severe hemorrhage.

When replacement therapy was restricted to whole blood or plasma, it was necessary to administer repeated infusions (every six to twelve hours in classical hemophilia, and daily in Christmas disease) because of the relatively short half-survival time of the coagulation factors (10 to 18 hours in the case of factor VIII[26,203] and 18 to 36 hours in the case of factor IX).[26] The volume of fluids employed was limited because of the risk of hypervolemia and only rarely could levels of factor VIII greater than 20 per cent of normal be attained with plasma.[110] In a recent study, however, satisfactory resolution of hemarthrosis in factor VIII deficiency was obtained by the use of a single dose of concentrate which yielded post-infusion levels of 40 to 50 per cent of normal.[110] This was adequate to maintain effective hemostasis throughout a 48-hour period.

Most[26,57,64a,215,229a] but not all[110] authorities favor aspiration in the case of large hemarthroses. Although some choose to intervene after the initial infusion of plasma or concentrate has been completed[57] it would seem preferable to aspirate immediately prior to or during replacement therapy, before there is clotting of the blood within the joint cavity and in order that bleeding will cease soon after the optimum amount of the effusion has been withdrawn.[26,215,229a] In any event, provided there is adequate correction of the coagulation defect, it is clear that aspiration can be carried out without danger to the patient. Careful removal of the sanguineous fluid from the tense, distended joint serves to relieve pain and stiffness, reduce the period of incapacity, and limit the damage to the synovium and cartilage.[57]

The intra-articular injection of corticosteroids is sometimes helpful in facilitating the resolution of hemarthrosis. It has been reported that a five-day course of prednisone (in doses up to 80 mg. per day) was effective in reducing the amount of specific replacement factors necessary for the treatment of acute hemarthrosis and increased the number of favorable responses to single infusions of factor VIII.[124]

As soon as pain and bleeding have been controlled (usually three to five days), normal functional position should be restored, by serial cast changes, if necessary, and muscle setting exercises are begun. When the swelling and other signs of inflammation have subsided, active exercise is encouraged in an effort to restore the normal range of motion, since this is probably the single most important factor in the prevention of permanent contracture.[57] Excessively prolonged immobilization should be avoided, since this leads to profound atrophy of the muscle. If a lower extremity is involved, the patient can be ambulated on crutches, but weight-bearing should be limited until the peri-articular soft tissues have returned to near normal and there is sufficient muscle power to stabilize the joint adequately.

Chronic Hemophilic Joint Disease.—The

joint most often chronically affected is the knee, which commonly develops a flexion contracture. This may be corrected and stable weight-bearing achieved by means of traction, wedging casts, quadriceps setting exercises, and, later, active resistive exercises.[4,5,49,57,117] The use of a long leg extension brace and crutches may be required for many months or years to prevent recurrence of the contracture.[57,117,223]

In former days the use of surgical procedures for the correction of chronic joint deformities was severely limited because of the dread of uncontrollable postoperative hemorrhage. The availability of potent concentrates of antihemophilic factors has lessened this restriction and has greatly improved the prospects for orthopedic rehabilitation.[223] The wide range of procedures which have been carried out successfully in recent years includes arthroplasty of the hip,[20] supracondylar wedge osteotomy for correction of valgus deformity of the knee,[4,5] wedge osteotomy of the tibia,[5] lengthening of the Achilles tendon and other tendons of the foot for correction of equinus contraction,[5,64a,148,217,229a] and compression arthrodesis of the knee, hip, and ankle,[26,148,229a] in addition to such heroic operations as drainage or radical excision of hematoma and the amputation of an extremity in cases of uncontrollable, life-threatening hemophilic cysts.[101,139,214,223,229a]

There is a recent report on synovectomy of the knee in a small group of patients who had had repeated hemarthrosis of this joint. Many of these were said to have enjoyed a restoration of normal joint motion and freedom from recurrent hemarthrosis. In addition there was a marked reduction postoperatively in the number and gravity of hemorrhagic episodes in both other joints and extra-articular sites.[216] The follow-up period was short, however, and much more work will have to be done before the efficacy of synovectomy can be determined.

Before any major surgery is undertaken in the patient with classical hemophilia, his plasma should be examined for the presence of an inhibitor (antibody) to factor VIII, which inactivates this protein.[26,203] Preferably both human and animal factor VIII should be used in this testing. When an inhibitor is found elective operations should be avoided. If surgery is deemed necessary, the patient should be infused with massive doses of factor VIII as rapidly as possible, choosing that variety of concentrate which is least affected by the inhibitor (an inhibitor has also been found on rare occasions in Christmas disease[26]). Sufficient factor VIII is given to establish a level of approximately 30 per cent of normal during surgery and 15 to 20 per cent in the postoperative period.[26,203] Since the potency of cryoprecipitate may vary significantly[50,203] the patient's plasma must be assayed at regular intervals by means of the thromboplastin generation test and partial thromboplastin time. Replacement therapy is given uninterruptedly until healing is well advanced, usually a period of 10 to 14 days. In more extensive procedures, however, infusions may have to be continued for 3 to 4 weeks or longer.[148]

BIBLIOGRAPHY

1. Abell, J. M., Jr., and Bailey, R. W.: Arch. Surg., *81*, 569, 1960.
2. Abul-Haj, S. K., Martz, D. G., Douglas, W. F. and Geppert, L. J.: J. Pediat., *61*, 221, 1962.
3. Adler, E. and Maybaum, S.: Ann. Rheum. Dis., *13*, 229, 1954.
4. Ahlberg, A., Nilsson, I. M. and Bauer, G. C. H.: J. Bone & Joint Surg., *47A*, 323, 1965.
5. Ahlberg, A.: Clin. Orthop., *53*, 135, 1967.
6. Aisner, M. and Hoxie, T. B.: New Engl. J. Med., *238*, 733, 1948.
7. Albert, J., Bruce, W., Allen, A. C., and Blank, H.: Amer. J. Med., *28*, 661, 1960.
8. Ali, A. M., Gandy, R. H., Britten, M. I., and Dormandy, K. M.: Brit. Med. J., *3*, 828, 1967.
9. Amstutz, H. C. and Carey, E. J.: J. Bone & Joint Surg., *48A*, 670, 1966.

10. Andreev, V. C. and Zlatkov, N. B.: Brit. J. Derm., *80*, 503, 1968.
11. Ansell, B. M. and Bywaters, E. G. L.: Ann. Rheum. Dis., *16*, 503, 1957.
12. Baldridge, C. W. and Awe, C. D.: Arch. Intern. Med., *45*, 161, 1930.
13. Ball, G. V. and Sorensen, L. B.: Arth. & Rheum., *13*, 846, 1970.
14. Barrow, M. V., Sunderman, F. W., Jr., Hackett, R. L., and Colvin, W. S.: Amer. J. Clin. Path., *47*, 312, 1967.
15. Barrow, M. V. and Holubar, K.: Medicine, *48*, 287, 1969.
16. Bartfeld, H.: Ann. Intern. Med., *52*, 1059, 1960.
17. Barton, C. J. and Cockshott, W. P.: Amer. J. Roentgenol., *88*, 523, 1962.
18. Baty, J. M. and Vogt, E. C.: Amer. J. Roentgenol., *34*, 310, 1935.
19. Bedwell, G. A. and Dawson, A. M.: Arch. Dis. Child., *29*, 78, 1954.
20. Bellingham, A., Fletcher, D., Kirwan, E. O'G., Prankerd, T. A., Jr., and Cleghorn, T.: Brit. Med. J., *4*, 531, 1967.
21. Bernhard, G. C. and Hensley, G. T.: Arth. & Rheum., *12*, 444, 1969.
22. Bethune, J. E., Landrigan, P. L. and Chipman, C. D.: New Engl. J. Med., *264*, 1280, 1961.
23. Bichel, J.: Acta Haematol., *1*, 153, 1948.
24. Bierman, S. M., Edgington, T., Newcomer, V. D. and Pearson, C. M.: Arth. & Rheum., *9*, 620, 1966.
25. Biggs, R. and Macfarlane, R. G.: *Human Blood Coagulation and Its Disorders*, 3rd ed., Philadelphia, F. A. Davis Co., 1962.
26. Biggs, R. and Macfarlane, R. G. (eds.): *Treatment of Haemophilia and Other Coagulation Disorders.* Oxford, Blackwell Scientific, 1966.
27. Blanton, F. M.: Ann. Intern. Med., *48*, 1118, 1958.
28. Blau, S. and Hamerman, D.: Arth. & Rheum., *10*, 397, 1967.
29. Boldero, J. L., and Kemp, H. S.: Brit. J. Radiol., *39*, 172, 1966.
30. Bortz, A. I. and Vincent, M.: Amer. J. Med., *30*, 951, 1961.
31. Breen, F. A., Jr. and Tullis, J. L.: J.A.M.A., *208*, 1848, 1969.
32. Brinkhous, K. M., ed.: *Hemophilia and Hemophiloid Disease.* Chapel Hill, University of North Carolina Press, 1957.
33. Britten, M. I., Spooner, R. J. D., Dormandy, K. M. and Biggs, R.: Brit. Med. J., *2*, 224, 1966.
34. Bronsky, D. and Bernstein, A.: Ann. Intern. Med., *41*, 820, 1954.
35. Brower, T. D. and Wilde, A. H.: J. Bone & Joint Surg., *48A*, 487, 1966.
36. Caffey, J. and Schlesinger, E. R.: J. Pediat., *16*, 549, 1940.
37. Cameron, E. A.: Brit. Med. J., *1*, 34, 1961.
38. Cammarata, R. J., Rodnan, G. P., and Jensen, W. N.: Arch. Intern. Med., *111*, 330, 1963.
39. Carroll, D. S.: South Med. J., *50*, 1486, 1957.
40. Casey, D. F. and Cathcart, E. S.: Arth. & Rheum., *13*, 882, 1970.
41. Christianson, H. B., Brunsting, L. A. and Perry, H. O.: Arch. Derm., *74*, 581, 1956.
42. Chung, S. M. K. and Ralston, E. L.: J. Bone & Joint Surg., *51A*, 33, 1969.
43. Cockshott, W. P.: Brit. J. Radiol., *36*, 19, 1963.
44. Collins, D. H.: *The Pathology of Articular and Spinal Diseases.* London, Edward Arnold & Co., 1949.
45. Collins, D. H.: J. Bone & Joint Surg., *33B*, 436, 1951.
46. Conybeare, E. T.: Guy's Hosp. Rep., London, *86*, 343, 1936.
47. Craver, L. F.: Amer. J. Med. Sci., *174*, 799, 1927.
48. Craver, L. F. and Copeland, M. M.: Arch. Surg., *30*, 639, 1935.
49. Crock, H. V. and Boni, V.: Brit. J. Surg., *48*, 8, 1960.
50. Dallman, P. R. and Pool, J. G.: New Engl. J. Med., *278*, 199, 1968.
51. Damon, A., Holub, D. A., Melicow, M. M. and Uson, A. C.: Amer. J. Med., *25*, 182, 1958.
52. Davies, D. T. P., Hughes, A. and Tonks, R. S.: Brit. J. Pharmacol., *36*, 437, 1969.
53. Davis, J. S., Jr., Weber, F. C., and Bartfeld, H.: Ann. Intern. Med., *47*, 10, 1957.
54. Deaton, J. G. and Levin, W. C.: Arch. Intern. Med., *120*, 345, 1967.
55. DeConti, R. C. and Calabresi, P.: New Engl. J. Med., *274*, 481, 1966.
56. Denman, A. M., Szur, L. and Ansell, B. M.: Ann. Rheum. Dis., *23*, 139, 1964.
57. DePalma, A. F.: Clin. Orthop., *52*, 145, 1967.
58. DeTorregrosa, M. V., Dapena, R. B., Hernandez, H., and Ortiz, A.: J.A.M.A., *174*, 354, 1960.
59. Diggs, J. W.: Clin. Orthop., *52*, 119, 1967.
60. Draznin, S. Z. and Singer, K.: Amer. J. Roentgenol., *60*, 490, 1948.
61. Dresner, E.: Quart. J. Med., *19*, 339, 1950.
62. Dresner, E. and Trombly, P.: New Engl. J. Med., *261*, 981, 1959.

63. DRUET, PH., DRYLL, A., RYCKEWAERT, A., DESÈZE, S. and KAHN, M.-F.: Sem. Hôp. Paris, *45*, 489, 1969.
64. EVANS, F. J. and HILTON, J. H. B.: Canad. Med. Assoc. J., *91*, 1272, 1964.
64*a*. EYRING, E. J., BJORNSON, D. R. and CLOSE, J. R.: Clin. Orthop., *40*, 95, 1965.
65. FAHEY, J. L., SCOGGINS, R., UTZ, J. P., and SZWED, C. F.: Amer. J. Med., *35*, 698, 1963.
66. FALCONER, E. H. and LEONARD, M. E.: Ann. Intern. Med., *29*, 1115, 1948.
67. FARBER, S., COHEN, J., and UZMAN, L. L.: J. Mount Sinai Hosp., *24*, 816, 1957.
68. FINKEL, H. E., BRAUER, M. J., TAUB, R. N., and DAMESHEK, W.: Blood, *28*, 634, 1966.
69. FLEISCHMAJER, R.: Dermatologica, *128*, 113, 1964.
70. FLETCHER, R. F. and GLOSTER, J.: J. Clin. Invest., *43*, 2104, 1964.
71. FONE, D. J. and KING, W. E.: Austral. Ann Med., *13*, 339, 1964.
72. FONK, J. and COONROD, J. D.: J.A.M.A., *217*, 80, 1971.
73. FORD, D. K., PRICE, G. E., CULLING, C. F. A., and VASSAR, P. S.: Amer. J. Med., *33*, 478, 1962.
74. FRAENKEL, G. J., TAYLOR, K. B., and RICHARDS, W. C. D.: Brit. J. Surg., *46*, 383, 1959.
75. FREDRICKSON, D. S.: Cerebroside lipidosis: Gaucher's disease. In *The Metabolic Basis of Inherited Disease*, 2nd edition. Stanbury, J. B., Wyngaarden, J. B. and Fredrickson, D. S., Eds., New York, Blakiston-McGraw-Hill Book Company, 1966, pp. 565–585.
76. FREDRICKSON, D. S., LEVY, R. I. and LEES, R. S.: New Engl. J. Med., *276*, 32, 94, 148, 215, and 273, 1967.
77. FUCILLA, I. S. and HAMANN, A.: Radiology, *77*, 53, 1961.
78. FUDENBERG, H. H.: Arth. & Rheum., *9*, 464, 1969.
79. GALY, P., BRUNE, J., DORSIT, G., and DUPONT, J.-C.: Lyon Méd., *217*, 715, 1967.
80. GARCIN, R., HEWITT, J., GODLEWSKI, S., LAUDAT, P., DEMONTERA, H., and EMILE, J.: Presse Méd., *75*, 435, 1967.
81. GARDNER, F. H. and NATHAN, D. G.: Med. Clin. North America, *45*, 1273, 1961.
82. GHORMLEY, R. K. and CLEGG, R. S.: J. Bone & Joint Surg., *30A*, 589, 1948.
83. GLENCHUR, H., ZINNEMAN, H. H., and HALL, W. H.: Arch. Intern. Med., *103*, 173, 1959.
84. GLUECK, C. J., LEVY, R. I., and FREDRICKSON, D. S.: J.A.M.A., *206*, 2895, 1968.
85. GOLD, M. S., WILLIAMS, J. C., SPIVACK, M. and GRANN, V.: J.A.M.A., *206*, 1572, 1968.
86. GOLDBERG, A., BRODSKY, I. and MCCARTY, D.: Amer. J. Med., *37*, 653, 1964.
86*a*. GOLDBERG, L. S., FISHER, R., CASTRONOVA, E. A. and CALABRO, J. J.: New Engl. J. Med., *281*, 256, 1969.
87. GOLDENBERG, G. J., PARASKEVAS, F. and ISRAELS, L. G.: Arth. & Rheum., *12*, 569, 1969.
88. GOLDMAN, J. A., STEINER, P., ABRAMS, N. R., GLUECK, C. J. and HERMAN, J. H.: Arth. & Rheum., *14*, 384, 1971 (abstract).
89. GOLDRING, J. S. R.: Ann. Roy. Coll. Surg. Engl., *19*, 296, 1956.
90. GOLDRING, J. S. R., MACIVER, J. E. and WENT, L. N.: J. Bone & Joint Surg., *41B*, 711, 1959.
91. GOLTZ, R. W. and LAYMON, C. W.: Arch. Derm. & Syph., *69*, 717, 1954.
92. GOODFELLOW, J., FEARN, C. B. D'A, and MATTHEWS, J. M.: J. Bone & Joint Surg., *49B*, 748, 1967.
93. GRABER, S.: South Med. J., *54*, 1395, 1961.
94. GREENBAUM, D. and STONE, H. F. H.: Lancet, *1*, 73, 1959.
95. GROEN, J. and GARRER, A. H.: Blood, *3*, 1221, 1948.
96. GROSSMAN, L. A., KAPLAN, H. J., OWNBY, F. D. and GROSSMAN, M.: J.A.M.A., *176*, 259, 1961.
97. GROSSMAN, R. E. and HENSLEY, G. T.: Amer. J. Roentgenol., *101*, 872, 1967.
98. GURAVICH, J. L.: Amer. J. Med., *26*, 8, 1959.
99. GUTMAN, A. B.: Ann. Intern. Med., *39*, 1062, 1953.
100. GUTMAN, A. B. and YÜ, T. F.: Ann. Intern. Med., *56*, 675, 1962.
101. HALL, M. R. P., HANDLEY, D. A., and WEBSTER, C. U.: J. Bone & Joint Surg., *44B*, 781, 1962.
102. HALL, T. C.: J. Clin. Pharmacol., *7*, 156, 1967.
103. HALLIDIE-SMITH, K. A. and BYWATERS, E. G. L.: Arch. Dis. Child., *33*, 350, 1958.
104. HAMILTON, E. B. D. and BYWATERS, E. G. L.: Ann. Rheum. Dis., *20*, 353, 1961.
105. HARLAN, W. R., JR., GRAHAM, J. B. and ESTES, E. H.: Medicine, *45*, 77, 1966.
106. HENDRICKSE, R. G. and COLLARD, P.: Lancet, *1*, 80, 1960.
107. HICKLING, R. A.: Lancet, *1*, 175, 1958.
108. HINDMARSH, J. R. and EMSLIE-SMITH, D.: Brit. Med. J., *1*, 593, 1953.
109. HOBBS, J. R.: Brit. Med. J., *3*, 699, 1967.
110. HONIG, G. R., FORMAN, E. N., JOHNSTON, C. A., SEELER, R. A., ABILDGAARD, C. F. and SHULMAN, I.: Pediatrics, *43*, 26, 1969.

111. Howqua, J. and Mackay, I. R.: Blood, *22*, 191, 1963.
112. Hughes, J. G. and Carroll, D. S.: Pediatrics, *19*, 184, 1957.
113. Hurwitz, D. and Roth, H.: Arth. & Rheum., *13*, 422, 1970.
114. Jacob, G. F. and Raper, A. B.: Brit. J. Haematol., *4*, 138, 1958.
115. Jaffe, H. L.: *Tumors and Tumorous Conditions of the Bones and Joints*. Philadelphia, Lea & Febiger, 1958.
116. Johnston, A. W., Weller, S. D. and Warland, B. J.: Arch. Dis. Child., *43*, 73, 1968.
117. Jordan, H. H.: *Hemophilic Arthropathies*. Springfield, Charles C Thomas, 1958.
118. Kasper, C. K., Dietrich, S. L. and Rapaport, S. I.: Arch. Intern. Med., *125*, 1004, 1970.
119. Katz, J. F.: J. Bone & Joint Surg., *49A*, 514, 1967.
120. Kellerhouse, L. E. and Limarzi, L. R.: Med. Clin. North America, *49*, 203, 1965.
121. Kerr, C. B.: Med. Hist., *7*, 359, 1963.
122. Key, J. A.: Ann. Surg., *95*, 198, 1932.
123. Khachadurian, A. K.: Arth. & Rheum., *11*, 385, 1968.
124. Kisker, C. T. and Burke, C.: New Engl. J. Med., *282*, 639, 1970.
125. Krakoff, I. H.: Arth. & Rheum., *8*, 772, 1965.
126. Krakoff, I. H.: Cancer, *19*, 1489, 1966.
127. Kroboth, F. J., Jr., and Johnson, E. W., Jr.: Surg. Clin. North America, *32*, 1141, 1952.
128. Kulowski, J.: Amer. J. Roentgenol., *63*, 840, 1950.
129. Lack, C. H.: J. Bone & Joint Surg., *41B*, 384, 1959.
130. Lacroux, R.: Bull. Soc. franç. Dermat. Syph., *67*, 474, 1960.
131. Landbeck, G. and Kurme, A.: Mschr. Kinderheilk., *118*, 29, 1970.
132. Landells, J. W.: J. Bone & Joint Surg., *35B*, 643, 1953.
133. Lane, J. J., Jr. and Decker, J. L.: J.A.M.A., *173*, 982, 1960.
134. Laster, L. and Muller, A. F.: Amer. J. Med., *15*, 857, 1953.
135. Lea, A. J.: Ann. Rheum. Dis., *23*, 480, 1964.
136. Lewis, B. S.: Brit. Med. J., *2*, 27, 1955.
137. Lewis, J. G.: Brit. Med. J., *1*, 24, 1961.
138. ———: Ann. Rheum. Dis., *21*, 284, 1962.
139. Lewis, J. H., Cottington, G. M. and Brower, T. D.: J. Bone & Joint Surg., *47A*, 333, 1965.
140. Lichtenstein, L.: *Bone Tumors*. 3rd ed. St. Louis, C. V. Mosby Company, 1965.
141. Lyell, A. and Carr, A. J.: Brit. J. Derm., *71*, 12, 1959.
142. Lynch, E. C.: Arch. Intern. Med., *109*, 639, 1962.
143. Macht, S. H. and Roman, P. W.: Radiology, *51*, 697, 1948.
144. Magnus-Levy, A.: Acta Med. Scand., *95*, 217, 1938.
145. Maher, J. F., Rath, C. E. and Schreiner, G. E.: Arch. Intern. Med., *123*, 198, 1969.
146. Martel, W., Abell, M. R. and Duff, I. F.: Radiology, *77*, 613, 1961.
147. Fernandez de Valderrama, J. A. and Matthews, J. M.: J. Bone & Joint Surg., *47B*, 256, 1965.
148. Mazza, J. J., Bowie, E. J. W., Hagedorn, A. B., Didisheim, P., Taswell, H. F., Peterson, L. F. A. and Owen, C. A., Jr.: J.A.M.A., *211*, 1818, 1970.
149. McLaughlin, G. E., McCarty, D. J., Jr. and Segal, B. L.: J.A.M.A., *196*, 1020, 1966.
150. Melamed, S. and Chester, W.: Arch. Intern. Med., *61*, 798, 1938.
151. Mellors, R. C.: Blood, *27*, 435, 1966.
152. Miller, D. G.: Ann. Intern. Med., *66*, 507, 1967.
153. Moch, W. S.: Oral Surg., Oral Med., and Oral Path., *6*, 1250, 1953.
154. Montgomery, H., Polley, H. F. and Pugh, D. G.: Arch. Derm., *77*, 61, 1958.
155. Moseley, J. E. and Manly, J. B.: Radiology, *60*, 656, 1953.
156. Moseley, J. E.: *Bone Changes in Hematologic Disorders*. New York, Grune & Stratton, 1963.
157. Muggia, F. M., Ball, T. J., Jr. and Ultmann, J. E.: Arch. Intern. Med., *120*, 12, 1967.
158. Neufeld, A. H., Morton, H. S. and Halpenny, G. W.: Canad. Med. Assoc. J., *91*, 374, 1964.
159. Nilsen, L. B., Missal, M. E. and Condemi, J. J.: Cancer, *20*, 1930, 1967.
160. Ober, W. B., Bruno, M. S., Simon, R. M. and Weiner, L.: Amer. J. Med., *27*, 647, 1959.
161. O'Brien, J. R.: Lancet, *1*, 779, 1968.
162. Oleinick, A.: Blood, *29*, 144, 1967.
163. Orkin, M., Goltz, R. W., Good, R. A., Michael, A. and Fisher, I.: Arch. Derm., *89*, 640, 1964.
164. Osserman, E. F.: New Engl. J. Med., *261*, 952, 1006, 1959.
165. Page, A. R., Hansen, A. E. and Good, R. A.: Blood, *21*, 197, 1963.
166. Paik, C. H., Alavi, I., Dunea, G. and Weiner, L.: J.A.M.A., *213*, 296, 1970.

166a. Pappas, A. M., Barr, J. S., Salzman, E. W., Britten, A. and Riseborough, E. J.: J.A.M.A., *187*, 772, 1964.
167. Paquet, E. and Delage, J.-M.: Canad. Med. Assoc. J., *76*, 927, 1957.
168. Perl, A. F.: Canad. Med. Assoc. J., *79*, 122, 1958.
169. Pinkhas, J., Djaldetti, M. and Yaron, M.: Israel J. Med. Sci., *1*, 537, 1965.
170. Pittelkow, R. B., Kierland, R. R. and Montgomery, H.: Arch. Derm., *72*, 556, 1955.
171. Porter, D. D., Dixon, F. J. and Larsen, A. E.: Blood, *25*, 736, 1965.
172. Pratt, P. W., Estren, S. and Kochwa, S.: Blood, *31*, 633, 1968.
173. Prip Buus, C. E.: Acta Radiol., *16*, 503, 1935.
174. Ramgren, O.: Acta Med. Scand., *171*, 237, 1962.
175. ———: Acta Med. Scand., suppl. 379, 1962.
176. Ransone, J. W. and Lange, R. D.: Ann. Intern. Med., *46*, 420, 1957.
177. Ratcliff, R. G. and Wolf, M. D.: Ann. Intern. Med., *57*, 299, 1962.
178. Razis, D. V., Diamond, H. D. and Craver, L. F.: Amer. J. Med. Sci., *238*, 327, 1959.
179. Recant, L. and Lacy, P.: Amer. J. Med., *36*, 936, 1964.
180. Reed, J. and Sosman, M. C.: Radiology, *38*, 579, 1942.
181. Reich, C., Seife, M. and Kessler, B. J.: Medicine, *30*, 1, 1951.
182. Reich, R. S. and Rosenberg, N. J.: J. Bone & Joint Surg., *35A*, 894, 1953.
183. Rieselbach, R. E., Bentzel, C. J., Cotlove, E., Frei, E., III and Freireich, E. J.: Amer. J. Med., *37*, 872, 1964.
184. River, G. L., Robbins, A. B. and Schwartz, S. O.: Blood, *18*, 385, 1961.
185. Roberts, A. R. and Hilburg, L. E.: J. Pediat., *52*, 170, 1958.
186. Rodey, G. E., Park, B. H., Ford, D. K., Gray, B. H. and Good, R. A.: Amer. J. Med., *49*, 322, 1970.
187. Rodnan, G. P., Lewis, J. H., Brower, T. D. and Warren, J. E.: Bull. Rheum. Dis., *8*, 137, 1957.
188. Rodnan, G. P., Brower, T. D., Hellstrom, H. R., Didisheim, P. and Lewis, J. H.: Arth. & Rheum. *2*, 152, 1959.
189. Rosenberg, S. A., Diamond, H. D., Jaslowitz, B. and Craver, L.: Medicine, *40*, 31, 1961.
190. Rothermel, J. E. and Raney, R. B.: South. Med. J., *62*, 1340, 1969.
191. Roy, S. and Ghadially, F. N.: Ann. Rheum. Dis., *28*, 402, 1969.
192. Rukavina, J. G., Block, W. D., Jackson, C. E., Falls, H. F., Carey, J. H. and Curtis, A. C.: Medicine, *35*, 239, 1956.
193. Schein, A. J. and Arkin, A. M.: J. Bone & Joint Surg., *24*, 396, 1942.
194. Schultze, G. and Lang, E. K.: Radiology, *74*, 428, 1960.
195. Schwartz, R. S. and Beldotti, L.: Science, *149*, 1511, 1965.
196. Schwarz, E. and Fish, A.: Amer. J. Roentgenol., *83*, 692, 1960.
197. Seegmiller, J. E., Laster, L. and Howell, R. R.: New Engl. J. Med., *268*, 712, 764, 821, 1963.
198. Seligmann, M., Cannat, A. and Hamard, M.: Ann. N.Y. Acad. Sci., *124*, 816, 1965.
199. Serjeant, G. R.: West Indian Med. J., *19*, 1, 1970.
200. Shelley, W. M. and Curtis, E. M.: Bull. Johns Hopkins Hosp., *103*, 8, 1958.
201. Sherman, M.: South. Med. J., *52*, 632, 1959.
202. Sherry, M. G.: Amer. J. Clin. Path., *50*, 398, 1968.
203. Shulman, N. R., Cowan, D. H., Libre, E. P., Watkins, S. P., Marder, V. J., Jr.: Ann. Intern. Med., *67*, 856, 1967.
204. Silverman, F. N.: Amer. J. Roentgenol., *59*, 819, 1948.
205. Silverstein, M. N. and Kelly, P. J.: Ann. Intern. Med., *59*, 637, 1963.
206. ———: Amer. J. Med. Sci., *253*, 569, 1967.
207. Skoog, W. A. and Adams, W. S.: Amer. J. Med., *34*, 417, 1963.
208. Smith, C. K., Cassidy, J. T. and Bole, G. G.: Amer. J. Med., *48*, 113, 1970.
209. Smith, E. W. and Conley, C. L.: Bull. Johns Hopkins Hosp., *94*, 289, 1954.
210. Smith, E. W. and Krevans, J. R.: Bull. Johns Hopkins Hosp., *104*, 17, 1959.
211. Snapper, I.: *Bone Diseases in Medical Practice*. New York, Grune & Stratton, 1957.
212. Somerville, J.: Brit. Heart J., *23*, 31, 1961.
213. Spaeth, G. L. and Frost, P.: Arch. Ophthal., *74*, 760, 1965.
214. Steel, W. M., Duthie, R. B., and O'Connor, B. T.: J. Bone & Joint Surg., *51B*, 614, 1969.
215. Sterndale, H.: Proc. Roy. Soc. Med., *60*, 37, 1967.
216. Storti, E., Traldi, A., Tosatti, E. and Davoli, P. G.: Acta Haematol., *41*, 193, 1969.
217. Stuart, J., Davies, S. H., Cummings, R. A., Girdwood, R. H. and Darg, A.: Brit. Med. J., *2*, 1624, 1966.

218. Swanton, M. C.: In *Hemophilia and Hemophiloid Disease*, Brinkhous, K. M., Ed., Chapel Hill, University of North Carolina Press, 1957, pp. 219–224.
219. Sweeley, C. C., Klionsky, B., Desnick, R. J. and Krivit, W.: In *The Metabolic Basis of Inherited Disease*, 3rd edition. Stanbury, J. B., Wyngaarden, J. B. and Fredrickson, D. S., Eds. New York, Blakiston-McGraw-Hill Book Company, in press.
220. Talal, N., Sokoloff, L. and Barth, W. F.: Amer. J. Med., *43*, 50, 1967.
221. Talbott, J. H.: Medicine, *38*, 173, 1959.
222. Tanaka, K. R., Clifford, G. O. and Axelrod, A. R.: Blood, *11*, 998, 1956.
223. Tarnay, T. J.: *Surgerv in the Hemophiliac*. Springfield, Charles C Thomas, 1968.
224. Tarr, L. and Ferris, H. W.: Arch. Intern. Med., *64*, 820, 1939.
225. Thannhauser, S. J.: *Lipidoses. Disease of the Intracellular Lipid Metabolism*. 3rd edition. New York, Grune & Stratton, 1958.
226. Thiers, H., Moulin, G., Fayolle, J. and Tuaillon, J.: Lyon Méd., *221*, 954, 1969.
227. Thomas, H. B.: J. Bone & Joint Surg., *18*, 140, 1936.
228. Thomas, L. B., Forkner, C. E., Jr., Frei, E. III, Besse, B. E., Jr. and Stabenau, J. R.: Cancer, *14*, 608, 1961.
229. Todd, R. M. and Keidan, S. E.: J. Bone & Joint Surg., *34B*, 447, 1952.
229*a*. Trueta, J.: In *Treatment of Haemophilia and Other Coagulation Disorders*. Biggs, R. and Macfarlane, R. G., Eds.: Oxford, Blackwell Scientific, 1966, pp. 229–323.
230. Tsachalos, P.: Rev. Rhum., *27*, 414, 1960.
231. Ultmann, J. E.: Cancer, *15*, 122, 1962.
232. Vieta, J. O., Friedell, H. L. and Craver, L. F.: Radiology, *39*, 1, 1942.
233. Vogler, W. R., Bain, J. A., Huguley, C. M., Jr., Palmer, H. G., Jr. and Lowrey, M. E.: Amer. J. Med., *40*, 548, 1966.
234. Walker, B. R. and Alexander, F.: J.A.M.A., *215*, 255, 1971.
235. Walker, B. R., Alexander, F., Birdsall, T. R. and Warren, R. L.: J.A.M.A., *215*, 437, 1971.
236. Warin, R. P., Evans, C. D., Hewitt, M., Taylor, A. L., Price, C. H. G. and Middlemiss, J. H.: Brit. Med. J., *1*, 1387, 1957.
237. Wasserman, L. R. and Bassen, F.: J. Mt. Sinai Hosp., *26*, 1, 1959.
238. Watson, R. J., Burko, H., Magas, H. and Robinson, M.: Pediatrics, *31*, 975, 1963.
239. Webb, J. B. and Dixon, A. St. J.: Ann. Rheum. Dis., *19*, 143, 1960.
240. Weglius, O., Skrifvars, B. and Anderson, L.: Acta Med. Scand., *187*, 133, 1970.
241. Weiss, H. J., Aledort, L. M. and Kochwa, S.: J. Clin. Invest., *47*, 2169, 1968.
242. Willson, J. K. V.: Radiology, *72*, 672, 1959.
243. Winston, M. E.: J. Bone & Joint Surg., *34B*, 412, 1952.
244. Wintrobe, M. M. and Mitchell, D. M.: Quart. J. Med., *9*, 67, 1940.
245. Wintrobe, M. M.: *Clinical Hematology*, 6th ed. Philadelphia, Lea & Febiger, 1967.
246. Wise, D., Wallace, H. J. and Jellinek, E. H.: Quart. J. Med., *31*, 177, 1961.
247. Wolf, C. R. and Mankin, H. J.: J. Bone & Joint Surg., *47A*, 1203, 1965.
248. Wyngaarden, J. B.: In *The Metabolic Basis of Inherited Disease*, 2nd edition. New York, Blakiston-McGraw-Hill Book Company, 1966, pp. 667–728.
249. Yü, T. F., Wasserman, L. R., Benedict, J. D., Bien, E. J., Gutman, A. B. and Stetten, DeW., Jr.: Amer. J. Med., *15*, 845, 1953.
250. Yü, T. F., Weissmann, B., Sharney, L., Kupfer, S. and Gutman, A. B.: Amer. J. Med., *21*, 901, 1956.
251. Yü, T. F. and Gutman, A. B.: Amer. J. Med., *37*, 885, 1964.
252. Yü, T. F.: Arth. & Rheum., *8*, 765, 1965.
253. Yü, T. F. and Gutman, A. B.: Ann. Intern Med., *67*, 1133, 1967.
254. Zawadzki, Z. A. and Benedek, T. G.: Arth. & Rheum., *12*, 555, 1969.

Chapter 72

Neuropathic Joint Disease (Charcot Joints)

By Gerald P. Rodnan, M.D.

Neuropathic joint disease (Charcot joints) is a form of chronic progressive degenerative arthropathy affecting one or more peripheral and/or vertebral articulations which develops as a result of a disturbance in normal sensory innervation of the joints. The arthropathy represents a complication of a variety of neurologic disorders, the most common of which are syphilitic tabes dorsalis, diabetic neuropathy, and syringomyelia.

HISTORICAL NOTE

Credit for the recognition of neuropathic arthropathy rests with J-M. Charcot, who in 1868 provided an incisive account of the indolent swelling and instability of the knees occurring in patients with *l'ataxie locomotrice progressive* (tabes dorsalis).[14] The relationship between syringomyelia and neuropathic joint disease was established by Sokoloff in 1892.[58] Clinical appreciation of diabetic neuropathy as a cause of this arthropathy dates from the report of Jordan in 1936.[30]

PATHOPHYSIOLOGY

It was apparent to Charcot that this condition was not a *primary* affection of the joints, but was rather a consequence of disease of the nervous system. He noted what he believed to be a similar disorder following other types of cord injury, and postulated that the articular disease was due to the damage or interruption of nerves which exerted a trophic influence on the tissues of the joint. This concept was soon challenged and the hypothesis advanced that the arthropathy resulted from traumatization of a joint deprived of its sensory innervation.[17,70] The latter view was supported by the studies of Eloesser (1917),[19] who observed the development of lesions corresponding to those of human neuropathic joint disease in cats which remained active, although ataxic, after section of posterior nerve roots. Destructive changes appeared with particular rapidity in a number of animals in which radicotomy was followed by cauterization of an area of femoral condyle. Of considerable interest with reference to the question of pathogenesis is the frequent occurrence of fractures and of destructive arthropathy in children and young adults with congenital insensitivity to pain[41,55] (including that associated with familial dysautonomia[10]). The parts most often affected in this condition are the ankles and tarsal joints. In some cases there has been involvement of the knee[1,39,69] and there is a report of a pain-insensitive woman who showed severe degeneration of a knee and upper lumbar vertebrae at age seventeen, and later, similar destructive changes in a hip and lower dorsal vertebrae.[46]

It appears that neuropathic arthropathy follows upon a loss of proprioceptive and/or pain sensation which leads to relaxation of supporting structures and chronic instability of the joint. Under these circumstances, the joint (or, in the case of insensitivity to pain, the entire patient) is deprived of normal protective reactions when exposed to the stress of everyday motion and to the additional trauma to which the joint is liable because of underlying neurologic disease. Severe and/or cumulative injury results in damage to articular cartilage and fracture of subchondral bone which eventuate in degeneration and disorganization of the joint. The existence of an "acute neuroarthropathy" without antecedent trauma in which symptoms appear suddenly and severe disintegration of the joint takes place within a period of a few weeks to months[42,65] has suggested the possibility that vascular insufficiency may play a role in the pathogenesis of certain cases.[65]

PATHOLOGIC FINDINGS

In instances of advanced disease, the Charcot joint presents a combination of destructive and hypertrophic changes which are similar in many respects to those found in ordinary non-neuropathic degenerative joint disease. These changes include fibrillation and erosion of articular cartilage, destruction of menisci, formation of loose bodies, and the growth of marginal osteophytes.[35,47] These latter are more exuberant and grotesque in neuropathic arthropathy than in ordinary degenerative joint disease, perhaps, as has been suggested,[16] because of the hypermobility of the joint. New bone growth may extend up the shaft of the bone well beyond the confines of the joint, and into ligaments and muscles.[47] Areas of dense bone formation also occur in the zone of provisional calcification beneath the articular surface, where there is proliferation and calcification of cartilage. Subluxation is common as are various intra- and juxta-articular fractures which may involve articular facets, osteophytes, epicondyles or condyles, and lead to the formation of additional callus.[29]

Neuropathic joint disease which affects large peripheral articulations is often accompanied by bulky, frequently sanguineous, effusions. The composition of

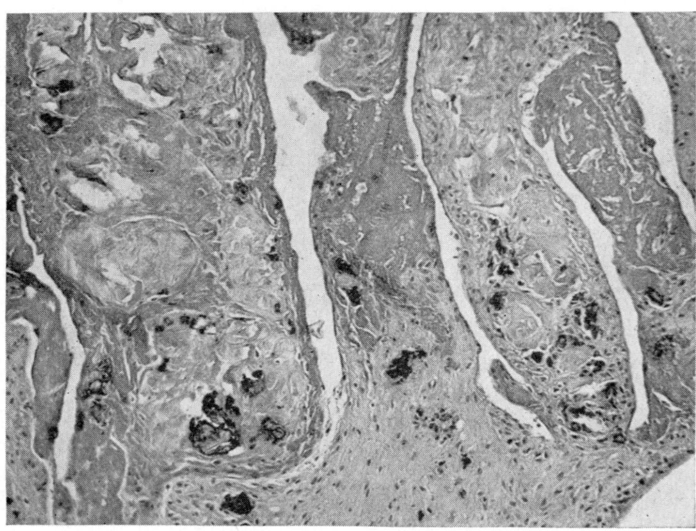

Fig. 72–1.—Photomicrograph of synovium from right hip of man, age thirty-one, with neuropathic disease secondary to syphilitic tabes dorsalis (congenital syphilis). (*See* roentgenogram, Fig. 72–3.) Note surface hyalinization, dense fibrosis, and scattered areas of calcification. Hematoxylin and eosin stain.

the fluid is similar to that of other types of traumatic synovitis. When studied by means of the intra-articular injection of a tracer quantity of iodine 131-labeled protein, the absorption of serum albumin from a Charcot knee joint was found to be the same as that from the normal knee.[51] The synovium usually shows a mild inflammatory reaction and frequently contains bits of calcified cartilage and metaplastic bone, as well as deposits of hemosiderin[16,28,50] (Fig. 72–1). These abnormalities, while not restricted to the Charcot joint, should serve to suggest this diagnosis when found in synovium from patients with degenerative joint disease.

CLINICAL FEATURES

General Observations[18,21,34,59,63,65,71]

Charcot joints occur more often in men than women, and usually develop past the age of forty. The distribution of affected joints is determined by the underlying neurologic lesion (see below). Changes characteristically commence in a single large joint or group of neighboring small joints, *e.g.* the tarsus, and frequently follow trauma to the part. The onset of symptoms is usually insidious, the patient noting progressive enlargement of an effusion and/or increasing instability of the joint. Although the swelling is often painful, presumably because of stretching of overlying soft tissues, the discomfort tends to be disproportionately mild compared to the degree of distention and destructive changes which may be present. Thus the patient may continue to use the joint freely and not seek medical attention. In some cases the occurrence of an intra- or juxta-articular fracture evokes presenting symptoms with dramatic suddenness. Careful questioning usually reveals evidence of antecedent neurologic abnormalities, although it is surprising how often the presence of the underlying disease of the nervous system, particularly tabes dorsalis, remains long unsuspected.

Examination of the joint early in the course of the disease usually reveals *hypermobility*, a finding which should always alert one to the possibility of neuropathic arthropathy. In the presence of effusion, there is increased warmth, and, not uncommonly, tenderness and pain on motion, although these findings are much less intense than would be expected from the marked distention of the joint. Synovial effusions may persist for many weeks or months and yield large amounts of fluid. Later, there is increasing enlargement, deformity, and instability of the joint, and coarse crepitation as a result of the overgrowth of bone, loss of articular cartilage, and the formation of loose bodies. Palpation of the latter has been described as like feeling a "bag of bones." When the feet, hips, or vertebrae are involved, abnormalities in articular form and function may be much less apparent. The presence of Charcot spine is to be suspected chiefly on circumstantial evidence (*e.g.* the presence of tabes dorsalis), for although vertebral changes often result in root pain and the formation of a kyphos, some patients complain of only mild back pain and show little that is unusual on physical examination.[11,25,67]

The diagnosis of neuropathic arthropathy requires identification of an underlying neurologic disorder. Patients who have monoarticular disease with marked joint effusion, hypermobility of the joint and disproportionately little pain should be particularly suspect.

Tabes Dorsalis

Neuropathic joint disease was first associated with locomotor ataxia,[14] and for many years recognition of this arthropathy was limited almost solely to its occurrence in patients with syphilitic tabes dorsalis. In view of the ease with which involvement of the vertebral column may be overlooked, previous estimates of an incidence of Charcot joints in 5 per cent of tabetic patients may well have been erroneously low.[63] Tabes dorsalis remains one of the most common causes of Charcot joints, despite the declining incidence of late syphilis and the wider recognition of neuropathic arthropathy of other origin.[11,21,34,63,65,71] The development of neuropathic joint disease may be one of the earliest manifestations of tabes, and some patients may remain free of obvious ataxis or other complaints referable to neurologic dysfunction for long periods.[34,71] It should be stressed that the presence of neither the classically complete form of Argyll Robertson pupils nor positive serologic test results is essential to the diagnosis of syphilitic tabes dorsalis. The irregularity in pupillary size and reaction (described by D. Argyll Robertson in 1868) may be slight and it is more important that careful sensory examination be stressed. Conventional procedures measuring reagin often revert to negative, with treatment and time,[59,63,71] although reactions to more sensitive tests for specific antibody, utilizing spirochetal antigen or treponema immobilization, may remain positive indefinitely.

In the case of tabes dorsalis, the neuropathic joint disease is characteristically monoarticular at the onset. The parts most frequently affected are the knee, hip, ankle, and the joints between bodies of lumbar and lower dorsal vertebrae (Figs. 72–2 and 72–3). Cervical vertebral arthropathy has been noted.[7] On

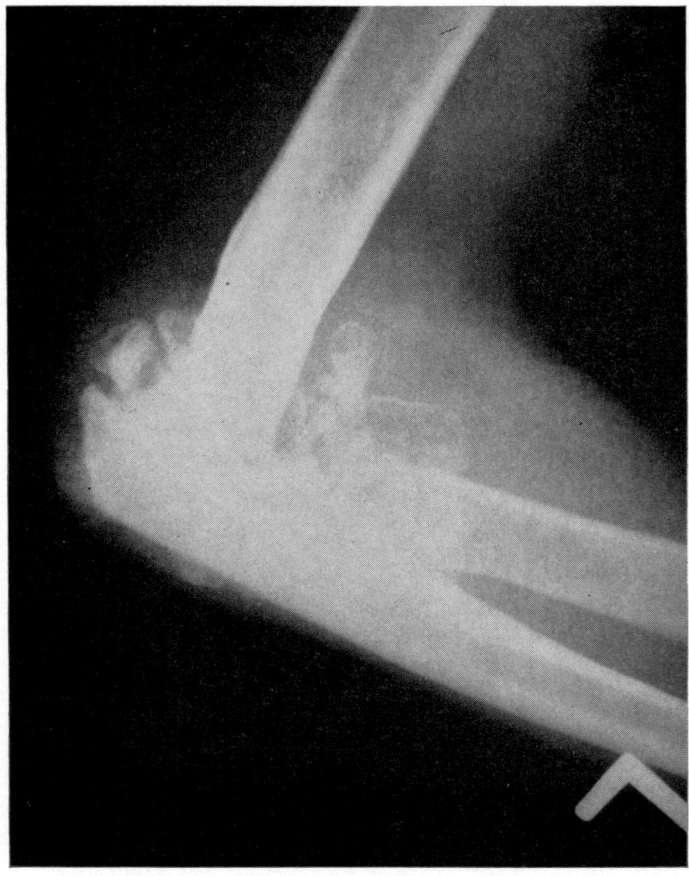

Fig. 72–2.—Neuropathic disease of the elbow in man, age forty-two, with syphilitic tabes dorsalis. Note marked fragmentation and erosion of articular margins of humerus and ulna, and new bone formation.

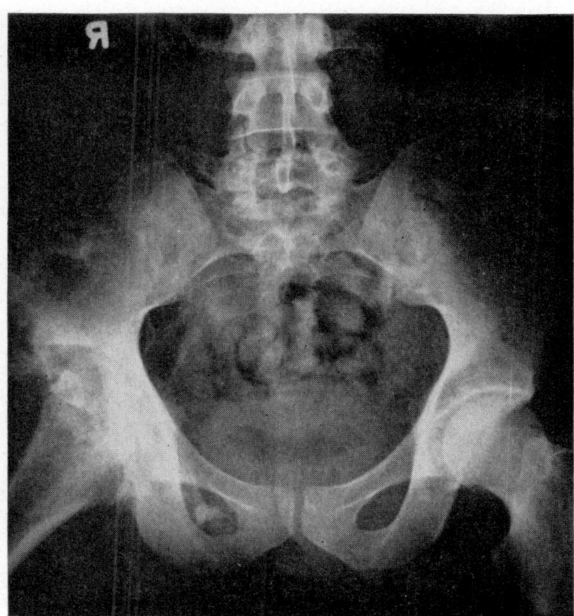

FIG. 72–3.—Neuropathic disease of the right hip in a man, age thirty-one, with tabes dorsalis as a result of congenital syphilis. Note loss of articular cartilage, marked sclerosis of subchondral bone, and deformity of the femur and acetabulum.

occasion, there may be polyarticular involvement including joints of the upper as well as lower extremity.[5] In such cases one must take care to exclude the possibility of other rheumatic disorders. The eventual involvement of more than a single joint is commonplace, but seldom are more than three affected in one individual. Damage to the knee leads to an increase in lateral motion and varus or valgus or genu recurvatum deformity. There may be partial or complete dislocation. Pyemic staphylococcal infection of a Charcot knee has been reported.[36] Disease of the hip is often complicated by fracture[59] and the absorption of bone may be striking. Vertebral osteoarthropathy leads to kyphosis or kyphoscoliosis; local tenderness may be lacking and movement, although restricted, may be painless despite the deformity.

Diabetic Neuropathy

Diabetic neuropathy constitutes an increasingly frequent basis for Charcot joint disease and now ranks a close second if not equal to tabes dorsalis in this respect.[4,6,38,49,54] The patients who develop this arthropathy have usually been known to have diabetes mellitus of long standing, and commonly show evidence of severe sensory impairment in the feet. Low-grade infection of the joints may play a pathogenetic role. Destructive changes, which are ordinarily unilateral, occur chiefly in the tarsal bones and the tarsometatarsal and metatarsophalangeal joints, and much less often in the ankles or knees. Polyarticular disease is unusual but has been reported, including involvement of the fingers, wrists, and elbows.[5,20] The presence of Charcot disease of the lumbar vertebrae has been reported in a patient with diabetic taboneuropathy.[73] Extensive and severe cervical and lumbar vertebral arthropathy may occur with little or no evidence of sensory loss, however, and it has been suggested that metabolic factors associated with diabetes mellitus render the intervertebral disks particularly prone to degeneration.[7]

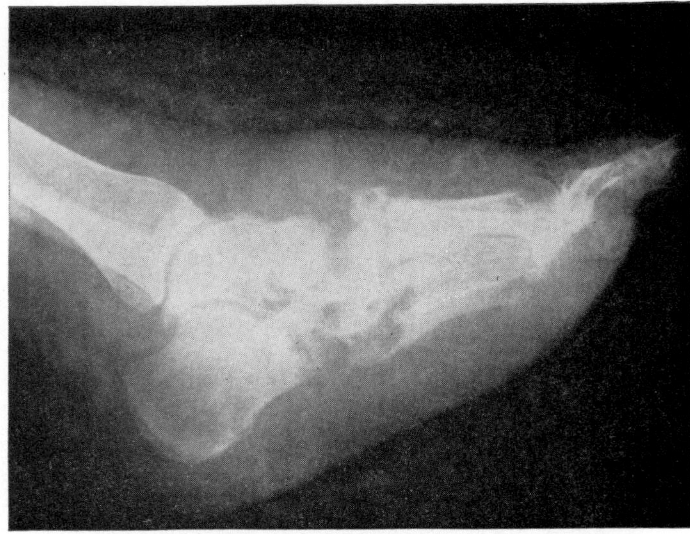

FIG. 72–4.—Neuropathic joint disease of the foot in a woman, age fifty-eight, with diabetic neuropathy. Note the almost complete destruction of the mid tarsus and proximal portions of the metatarsal bones.

Typically, there is painless swelling of the foot, accompanied by little if any redness or warmth. Some cases are complicated by local infection, and in such circumstances destructive changes may be in part the result of osteomyelitis.[24] Progressive disintegration of the joints leads to shortening and deformity of the foot which tends to become everted (Fig. 72–4).

Syringomyelia

Neuropathic joint disease develops in approximately one-fourth of patients with syringomyelia, usually involving a shoulder or elbow and less commonly the more distal joints of the upper extremity.[48,56,62] Brain and Wilkinson found roentgenographic evidence of cervical vertebral osteoarthropathy in nearly half their patients.[7] There was osteoporosis and flattening of the vertebral bodies, narrowing of intervertebral disks, and a tendency towards the formation of florid osteophytes—findings representative of the final stages of a process which earlier in its course appeared indistinguishable from ordinary cervical spondylosis. They concluded that these changes were due to the same causes as cervical spondylosis, but that the process of degeneration was intensified by the neurologic disease. When the shoulder and elbow are affected, there tend to be large effusions and, later, striking disintegration of bone which often occurs with striking rapidity (Fig. 72–5).[37,42,56]

Myelomeningocele

Sensory impairment resulting from myelomeningocele is the most frequent basis of neuropathic arthropathy in childhood, affecting the ankle and tarsal joints.[12,21,49] It is those individuals who retain the power of locomotion who are particularly liable to this complication, which has been observed in children as young as five years (Fig. 72–6).

Miscellaneous

Charcot joints have been described in patients with a variety of other spontaneous and traumatic disorders of the central and peripheral nervous system which cause sensory impairment in the

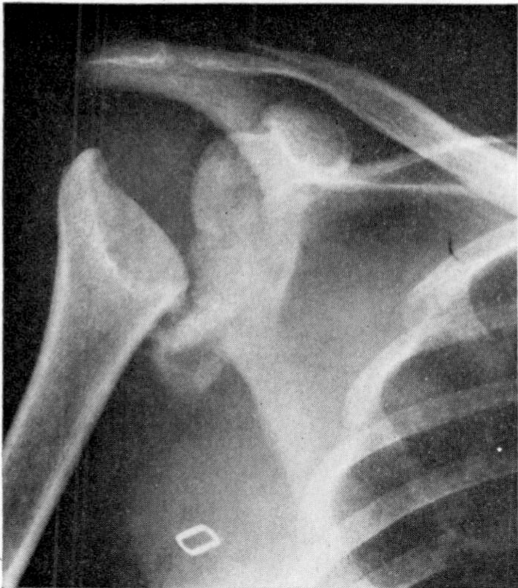

Fig. 72–5.—Neuropathic disease of the shoulder in a woman age 54, with syringomyelia. Note loss of bony substance of humeral head and cloud-like calcification in the periarticular soft tissues. The patient had first noted painless swelling of the shoulder only two weeks before this roentgenogram was obtained.

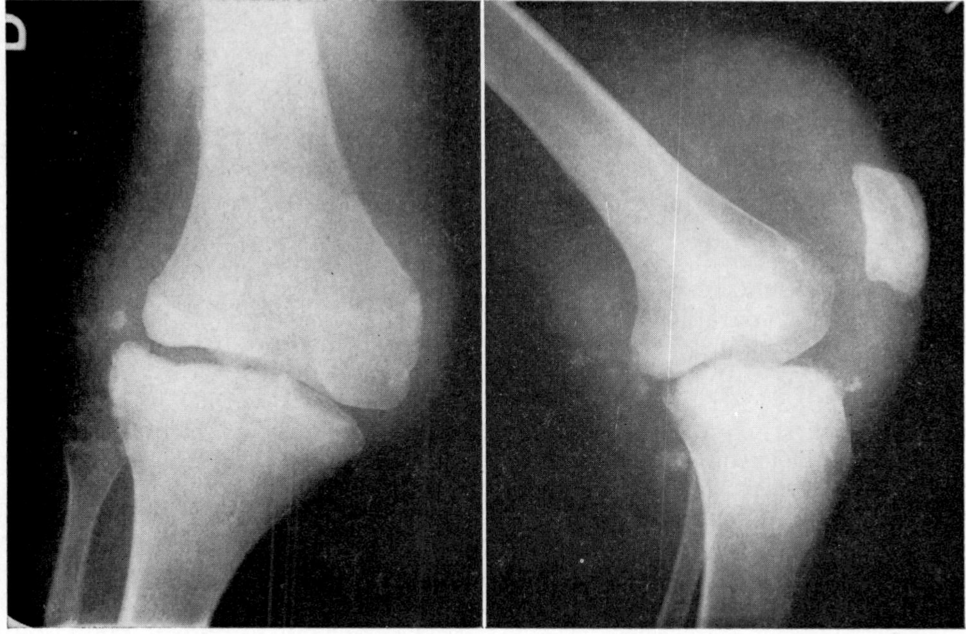

Fig. 72–6.—Neuropathic disease of the right knee in a man, age eighteen, with myelomeningocele. Note erosion of the lateral condyle of the femur and the lateral portion of the tibial plateau, the numerous calcified bodies, and evidence of a large effusion. Pathologic examination of the synovium revealed changes similar to those illustrated in Figure 72–1. Compression arthrodesis was performed and the joint has now remained fused for a period of more than six years.

Table 72-1—Primary Diseases Responsible for the Development of Neuropathic Arthropathy

Neurologic Disorder	*Joints Most Frequently Affected by Neuropathic Arthropathy*
Syphilitic tabes dorsalis	Knee, hip, ankle, lumbar and lower dorsal vertebrae
Diabetic neuropathy	Tarsus, tarsometatarsal, metatarsophalangeal
Syringomyelia	Shoulder, elbow, cervical vertebrae
Myelomeningocele	Ankle, tarsus
Congenital insensitivity to pain (including familial dysautonomia)	Ankle, tarsus
Miscellaneous	
Myelopathy of pernicious anemia	
Spinal cord trauma	
Paraplegia	
Hereditary sensory neuropathy	
Charcot-Marie-Tooth disease	
Familial interstitial polyneuropathy of Déjerine and Sottas	
Injury of peripheral nerve	
Leprous neuropathy	
Late yaws	
Progressive arthropathy following intra-articular injection of corticosteroids	Hip, knee

limbs. These conditions include congenital insensitivity to pain and familial dysautonomia (*see* above),[1,10,39,41,46,55,69] myelopathy of pernicious anemia,[22] spinal cord injury,[33] paraplegia,[64] hereditary sensory neuropathy,[23,43] Charcot-Marie-Tooth disease (J. M. Charcot and P. Marie, 1886; H. H. Tooth, 1886),[9] familial interstitial hypertrophic polyneuropathy of Déjerine and Sottas (described by J. J. Déjerine and J. Sottas in 1890),[52] peripheral nerve injury,[21,32,65] the neuropathy of leprosy,[45] and late yaws.[57]

Progressive Arthropathy Following Intra-Articular Injection of Corticosteroids

There have been a number of reports of the rapid deterioration of a hip or knee following the repeated intra-articular injection of hydrocortisone, with clinical and roentgenographic findings similar to those of neuropathic arthropathy.[2,13,61,66] It has been suggested that the relief of pain provided by such treatment permits excessive weight-bearing and mobility and interferes with normal protective processes, thereby accelerating the progress of the underlying joint disease (usually rheumatoid arthritis or osteoarthritis). Although this hypothesis may appear attractive, the question of a neuropathic basis for these joint changes remains a controversial matter, since steroid-treated patients retain normal sensibility to pain. There is evidence, too, that corticosteroids may directly inhibit the formation of protein polysaccharide (matrix) by articular cartilage.[35a] Hollander, Jessar, and Brown found that the extent of deterioration in injected knees of patients with rheumatoid arthritis or osteoarthritis was no greater over a seven-year period than that observed in untreated joints.[26] Instability of a weight-bearing joint developed in less than 1 per cent of their patients and in only four joints (of approximately 4000 patients) did they observe extensive absorption of bone. In at least one instance of so-called "cortisone arthropathy of the hip" in a patient receiving cortisone orally, the joint destruction appears to have been the result of staphylococcal infection.[40]

ROENTGENOGRAPHIC FINDINGS

Roentgenographic examination is important in the evaluation of the degree of joint damage, and essential to the detection of involvement in such inaccessible articulations as those of the vertebral column. It is important to realize, however, that the x-ray findings in the early stages of the Charcot joint may be normal, except perhaps for changes due to synovial effusion and/or evidence of bony detritus in the para-articular soft tissue.[31,42]

In more advanced cases the roentgenograms show varying degrees and combinations of destructive and hypertrophic changes. There is loss of articular cartilage, fragmentation and absorption of subchondral bone, and proliferation of new bone at the joint margins. The bony overgrowth, which is often bizarre in configuration, may be so great as to surround the joint like a spongy mass. The periarticular tissues are increasingly dense and may contain scattered calcifications.

Pathological fractures are common and usually involve the articular surface. They vary from "chips" or minute fragments of the articular margins which give rise to irregular free bodies within the joint, to extensive fractures in the condyle of the tibia or the neck of the femur. There may be considerable destruction of epiphyseal substance (tapering) accompanied by fragmentation of bone, while the bone which remains is markedly condensed. Ultimately there may be complete disintegration of the osseous structures. Findings such as these are present to greater or lesser degree in Charcot joints regardless of location or of the different primary neurologic disorders responsible for their development. Although the changes just described tend to evolve slowly, there are a number of patients with neuropathic arthropathy of diverse origin in whom severe joint destruction has been observed to occur within a period of a few weeks to months.[42]

Similar changes are encountered in the Charcot spine—destruction and collapse of the vertebral bodies and formation of large, beaked osteophytes (*les becs des perroquets*), or massive paravertebral bone growths which may lead to ankylosis.[11,67] The most common deformity is that of kyphoscoliosis; spondylolisthesis may occur.

In the pedal arthropathy complicating diabetic neuropathy, there is degeneration of the articular cartilage and subchondral bone of the tarsal and metatarsal articulations. The metatarsal shafts often become sharply tapered ("sucked candy-stick" osteolysis[49]) and may fracture. There tends to be little or no new bone formation in this variety of neuropathic arthropathy.

It will be appreciated that in their general character these abnormalities are quite similar to those encountered in non-neuropathic degenerative joint disease. It is the exaggerated degree of the changes which lends distinctiveness to the radiographic appearance of the Charcot joint. In any event, suspicion aroused by roentgenographic findings must be carefully corroborated by clinical evidence before diagnosis can be considered established.

MANAGEMENT

The nature of most of the neurologic diseases responsible for neuropathic arthropathy is such that treatment of these conditions can be expected to have little if any influence upon the progression of the joint disease. Immobilization of the affected joint and restriction of weight-bearing are basic principles in management. Mechanical devices should be fitted with great care and readjusted frequently since the patient may be unable to judge the efficiency of the appliance. Immobilization of the vertebral column is attempted by corset or brace. The patient with a Charcot joint of the lower extremity can be placed in a caliper walking splint. Crutches are helpful when the hips are involved. Surprising improvement may occur at times in the early stages of neuropathic arthropathy if complete immobilization can be provided by casts.

Operative procedures may include amputation or arthrodesis of weight-bearing joints. Amputation may become advisable in disease of the foot or knee, especially when complicated by septic arthritis which fails to respond to appropriate treatment with antibiotics. Amputation in the case of genicular involvement is to be considered only when there is advanced disintegration of the joint and when the process has remained unilateral.

Arthrodesis of Charcot joints often proves difficult. There have been many failures in the past because of infection or non-union, or both.[8,18,28,60,72] There have been occasional reports of successful fusions of the hip, knee, ankle (extra-articular) and vertebrae although the period of follow-up observation has often been relatively brief.[15,27,53,68,72] The apparent improvement in efforts at arthrodesis of the knee has been attributed to the introduction of better methods of internal fixation and use of a compression technique.[27,53] Despite the difficulties, the improvement which results from arthrodesis makes the attempt worthwhile, especially in a relatively young patient (Fig. 72–6).

Although gradual progressive breakdown and lysis of bone are the general rule in the arthropathy of the foot secondary to diabetic neuropathy, an occasional patient shows improvement when placed in a walking cast or short leg brace.[3] Arrest of bone destruction has been reported in two cases following lumbar sympathectomy,[44] but this has not been found by others.

BIBLIOGRAPHY

1. ABELL, J. M., JR., and HAYES, J. T.: J. Bone & Joint Surg., *46A*, 1287, 1964.
2. ALARCON-SEGOVIA, D. and WARD, L. E.: J.A.M.A., *193*, 1052, 1965.
3. ANTES, E. H.: J.A.M.A., *156*, 602, 1954.
4. BAILEY, C. C. and ROOT, H. F.: New Engl. J. Med., *236*, 397, 1947.
5. BEETHAM, W. P., JR., KAYE, R. L., and POLLEY, H. F.: Ann. Intern. Med., *58*, 1002, 1963.
6. BOEHM, H. J., JR.: New Engl. J. Med., *267*, 185, 1962.
7. BRAIN, R. and WILKINSON, M.: Brain, *81*, 275, 1958.
8. BRASHEAR, H. R.: Amer. J. Surg., *87*, 63, 1954.
9. BRUCKNER, F. E. and KENDALL, B. E.: Ann. Rheum. Dis., *28*, 577, 1969.
10. Brunt, P. W.: Brit. Med. J., *4*, 277, 1967.
11. CAMPBELL, D. J. and DOYLE, J. O.: Brit. Med. J., *1*, 1018, 1954.
12. CARR, T. L.: Postgrad Med. J., *32*, 201, 1956.
13. CHANDLER, G. N., JONES, D. T., WRIGHT, V., and HARTFALL, S. J.: Brit. Med. J., *1*, 952, 1959.
14. CHARCOT, J-M.: Arch. de Physiol. Norm. et Path., *1*, 161 and 379, 1868.
15. CLEVELAND, M. and WILSON, H. J., JR.: J. Bone & Joint Surg., *41A*, 336, 1959.
16. COLLINS, D. H.: *The Pathology of Articular and Spinal Diseases*, Baltimore, The Williams & Wilkins Co., 1950.
17. DELANO, P. J.: Amer. J. Roent. & Rad. Ther., *56*, 189, 1946.
18. EICHENHOLTZ, S. N.: *Charcot Joints*, Springfield, Charles C Thomas, 1966.
19. ELOESSER, L.: Ann. Surg., *66*, 201, 1917.
20. FELDMAN, M. J., BECKER, K. L., REEFE, W. E. and LONGO, A.: J.A.M.A., *209*, 1690, 1969.
21. FLOYD, W., LOVELL, W., and KING, R. E.: South Med. J., *52*, 563, 1959.
22. HALONEN, P. I. and JARVINEN, K. A. J.: Ann. Rheum. Dis., *7*, 152, 1948.
23. HELLER, I. H. and ROBB, P.: Neurology, *5*, 15, 1955.
24. HODGSON, J. R., PUGH, D. G., and YOUNG, H. H.: Radiology, *50*, 65, 1948.
25. HOLLAND, H. W.: Proc. Roy. Soc. Med., *46*, 747, 1953.

26. Hollander, J. L., Jessar, R. A., and Brown, E. M., Jr.: Bull. Rheum. Dis., *11*, 239, 1961.
27. Holt, E. P.: South Med. J., *50*, 1215, 1957.
28. Horwitz, T.: J. Bone & Joint Surg., *30A*, 579, 1948.
29. Johnson, J. T. H.: J. Bone & Joint Surg., *49A*, 1, 1967.
30. Jordan, W. R.: Arch. Intern. Med., *57*, 307, 1936.
31. Katz, I., Rabinowitz, J. G., and Dziadiw, R.: Amer. J. Roent., *86*, 965, 1961.
32. Kernwein, G. and Lyon, W. F.: Ann. Surg., *115*, 267, 1942.
33. Kettunen, K. O.: Ann. Chir. Gynaec. Fenn., *46*, 95, 1957.
34. Key, J. A.: Amer. J. Syph., *16*, 429, 1932.
35. King, E. J. S.: Brit. J. Surg., *18*, 113, 1930.
35*a*. Mankin, H. J. and Conger, K. A.: J. Bone & Joint Surg., *48A*, 1383, 1966.
36. Martin, J. R., Root, H. S., Kim, S. O., and Johnson, L. G.: Arth. & Rheum., *8*, 389, 1965.
37. Meyer, G. A., Stein, J., and Poppel, M. H.: Radiology, *69*, 415, 1957.
38. Miller, D. S. and Lichtman, W. F.: Arch. Surg., *70*, 513, 1955.
39. Mooney, V. and Mankin, H. J.: Arth. & Rheum., *9*, 820, 1966.
40. Moynihan, F. J.: Guy's Hosp. Rep., *111*, 388, 1962.
41. Murray, R. O.: Brit. J. Radiol., *30*, 2, 1957.
42. Norman, A., Robbins, H. and Milgram, J. E.: Radiology, *90*, 1159, 1968.
43. Pallis, C. and Schneeweiss, J.: Amer. J. Med., *32*, 110, 1962.
44. Parsons, H. and Norton, W. S., II: New Engl. J. Med., *244*, 935, 1951.
45. Paterson, D. E.: J. Fac. Radiol., London, *7*, 35, 1955.
46. Petrie, J. G.: J. Bone & Joint Surg., *35B*, 399, 1953.
47. Potts, W. J.: Ann. Surg., *86*, 596, 1927.
48. Rataj, R.: Neurol. Neurochir. Psychiat. pol., *14*, 439, 1964.
49. Robillard, R., Gagnon, P. A., and Alarie, R.: Canad. Med. Assoc. J., *91*, 795, 1964.
50. Rodnan, G. P., Yunis, E. J., and Totten, R. S.: Ann. Intern. Med., *53*, 319, 1960.
51. Rodnan, G. P., and MacLachlan, M. J.: Arth. & Rheum., *3*, 152, 1960.
52. Russell, W. R. and Garland, H. G.: Brain, *53*, 376, 1930.
53. Samilson, R. L., Sankaran, B., Bersani, F. A., and Smith, A. D.: Arch. Surg., *78*, 115, 1959.
54. Semb, H. and Turner, N.: Nord. Med., *71*, 613, 1964.
55. Silverman, F. N. and Gilden, J. J.: Radiology, *72*, 176, 1959.
56. Skall-Jensen, J.: Acta Radiol., *38*, 382, 1952.
57. Smith, F. H.: U.S. Naval Med. Bull., *46*, 1832, 1946.
58. Sokoloff, N. A.: Deut. Ztschr. f. Chirurgie, *34*, 505, 1892.
59. Soto-Hall, R. and Haldeman, K. O.: J.A.M.A., *114*, 2076, 1940.
60. Stack, J. K.: Amer. J. Surg., *83*, 291, 1952.
61. Steinberg, C. L., Duthie, R. B., and Piva, A. E.: J.A.M.A., *181*, 851, 1962.
62. Steinberg, V. L.: Ann. Phys. Med., *3*, 103, 1956.
63. Steindler, A.: J.A.M.A., *96*, 250, 1931.
64. Stepanek, V. and Stepanek, P.: Radiol. Clin. (Basel), *29*, 28, 1960.
65. Storey, G.: Brit. J. Vener. Dis., *40*, 109, 1964.
66. Sweetham, D. R., Mason, R. M., and Murray, R. O.: Brit. Med. J., *1*, 1392, 1960.
67. Thomas, D. F.: J. Bone & Joint Surg., *34B*, 248, 1952.
68. Vallis, J.: J. Bone & Joint Surg., *40B*, 148, 1958.
69. Van der Houwen, H.: J. Bone & Joint Surg., *43B*, 314, 1961.
70. Westphal, C.: Berl. Klin. Wchschr., *18*, 413, 1881.
71. Wile, U. J. and Butler, M. G.: J.A.M.A., *94*, 1053, 1930.
72. Wiseman, L. W.: Clin. Orthop., *8*, 218, 1956.
73. Zucker, G. and Marder, M. J.: Amer. J. Med., *12*, 118, 1952.

Chapter 73

Heritable and Developmental Disorders of Connective Tissues and Bone

By VICTOR A. MCKUSICK, M.D.

WHENEVER one undertakes to survey the role of genetic factors in the disorders of a given system, one finds three categories:

1. Some are "caused" primarily by a single mutant gene as indicated by the fact that they display simple Mendelian pedigree patterns, *e.g.*, autosomal dominant, autosomal recessive, or X-linked recessive.[86] These disorders are individually rare but there are many of them[87] so that in the aggregate they represent a significant category of disease. The heritable disorders of connective tissue are examples of this category.
2. Other disorders have a multifactorial basis. Multiple environmental and genetic (polygenic) factors collaborate in etiopathogenesis. The genetic factors represent a predisposition to the particular disorder. Disorders in this category tend to be relatively common. A priori, for example, one would anticipate a multifactorial basis of osteoarthritis.
3. In a third category, the disorder results from an abnormality of chromosome number or structure identifiable by the relatively gross techniques of karyotyping now available. These disorders are for the most part complex malformations involving multiple organ systems. The connective tissue system shows abnormality in the case of the XO Turner syndrome, trisomy 21 Down's syndrome (mongolism) and others but these are mostly of minor functional significance.

The discussion here concerns mainly disorders in the first category. Readers are referred elsewhere for a discussion of genetic principles.[86]

Heritable disorders of connective tissue are generalized defects involving primarily one element of connective tissue—collagen, elastin or mucopolysaccharide—and transmissible in a simple Mendelian manner.

The following heritable disorders of connective tissue have significant changes relevant to clinical rheumatology:

1. Marfan syndrome — loosejointedness, scoliosis, joint contractures.
2. Homocystinuria—reduced joint mobility, osteoporosis.
3. The Weill-Marchesani syndrome—stiff joints.
4. Ehlers-Danlos syndrome — loosejointedness, habitual dislocation of joints, hemarthroses, spondylolisthesis.
5. Osteogenesis imperfecta — osteoporosis, scoliosis.
6. The mucopolysaccharidoses — reduced joint mobility.

Each disorder is discussed in more detail below. Even alkaptonuria would be considered a heritable disorder of connective tissue if the colored substance noted in the urine had not called attention first to the existence of the inborn error of metabolism—this having been the first disorder to which Garrod applied this designation. If it were not for the alkaptonuria and black pigmentation of cartilage and collagen, the progressive arthropathy, cardiovascular involvement and Mendelian inheritance would have qualified the condition as a heritable disorder of connective tissue.

Vitamin D-resistant (hypophosphatemic) rickets is a simply inherited disorder which in the adult sometimes leads to ankylosing arthropathy. Multiple epiphyseal dysplasia and the X-linked late spondylo-epiphyseal dysplasia[70] are disorders which characteristically are accompanied by precocious osteoarthrosis especially of the hips. Legg-Perthes disease is almost certainly not a single entity and does not have a simple genetic basis. Sometimes it is merely the predominant feature of a generalized disorder such as multiple epiphyseal dysplasia.

Among their features fibrodysplasia (formerly "myositis") ossificans progressiva has progressive ankylosis and arthrogryposis multiplex congenita has congenital underdevelopment of joints. The "chondrodystrophies," more legitimately called osteochondrodysplasias, of which achondroplasia and the Morquio syndrome are prototypes, have arthritic manifestations or features simulating arthritis.

HERITABLE DISORDERS OF CONNECTIVE TISSUE

The Marfan Syndrome[87]

Patients with the Marfan syndrome may have major abnormalities in three

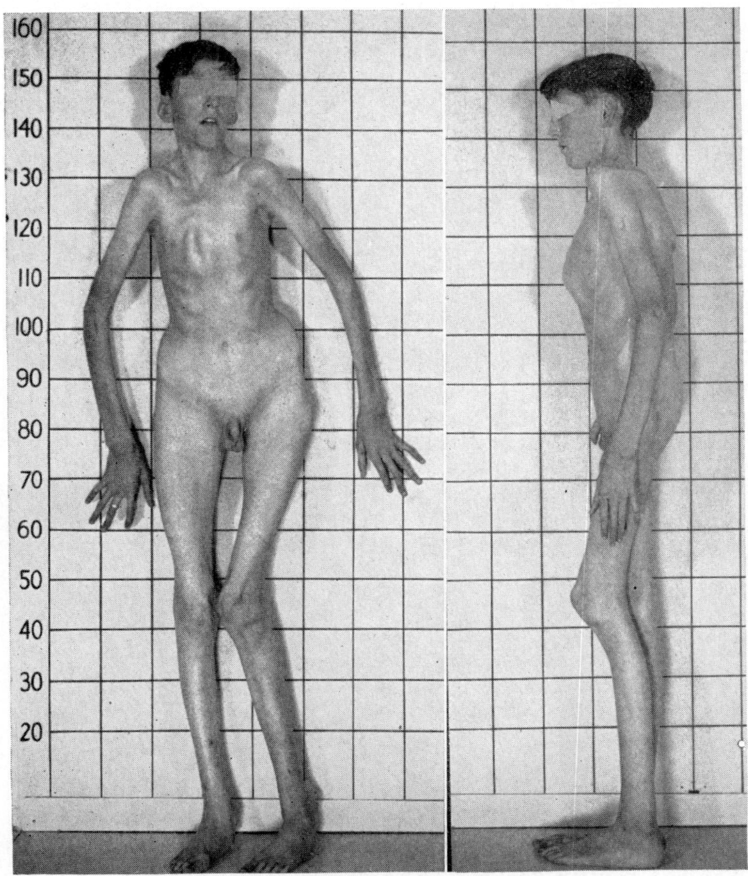

FIG. 73–1.—Marfan syndrome in 14-year-old boy. Note excessive height, pectus carinatum, sparse subcutaneous fat, arachnodactyly, left genu valgum and flat feet. The patient died of aortic rupture at the age of 15 years. Ectopia lentis was present.

areas: the eye, especially dislocation of the lenses; the skeletal system, namely excessive length of the extremities, loosejointedness, kyphoscoliosis, and anterior chest deformity; and the cardiovascular system, notably aortic aneurysm (diffuse and/or dissecting) and mitral valve redundancy with regurgitation. The disorder is inherited as an autosomal dominant.

Skeletal Features.—Patients with the Marfan syndrome (Fig. 73–1) are excessively tall, or at least taller than unaffected relatives. Body proportions are irregular with an abnormally low ratio of the upper segment to the lower segment. The segments are measured below and above the top of the pubic symphysis. In practice two measurements are made with the patient standing: height and lower segment (top of pubic symphysis to floor). In adult white persons the mean ratio is about 0.92; in adult American Negro persons it is about 0.87. The excessive length of the lower extremities is primarily responsible for the abnormally low upper segment to lower segment ratio (US/LS) in the Marfan syndrome. Shortening of the trunk by kyphoscoliosis further depresses the US/LS and makes its interpretation difficult. Indeed, kyphoscoliosis of any cause usually results in an abnormally low US/LS. In the presence of more than minimal kyphoscoliosis, the US/LS should not be used in support of the diagnosis of Marfan's syndrome. The upper extremities also show excessive length; the arm span of patients with Marfan's syndrome is usually greater than the height. The metacarpal index, based on the ratio of length to width of metacarpals, is said to be useful but requires a radiograph of the hands.

The ribs seem to undergo the same excessive longitudinal growth as do the bones of the extremities. Depression of the sternum (pectus excavatum) or projection (pectus carinatum) or an asymmetrical deformity of the anterior chest results.

Loosejointedness is often striking in patients with the Marfan syndrome. Flatfootedness, hyperextensibility at the knees (genu recurvatum) and elbows, and dislocation of joints, including congenital dislocation of the hip in the newborn, are manifestations of the loosejointedness. Because of both the loosejointedness and the long extremities the patient is often able to touch his umbilicus with his right hand passed around his back, and approaching his umbilicus from the left. A relatively narrow palm of the hand with long thumb and loosejointedness is the basis for Steinberg's thumb sign (Fig. 73–2): the thumb apposed across the palm extends well beyond the ulnar

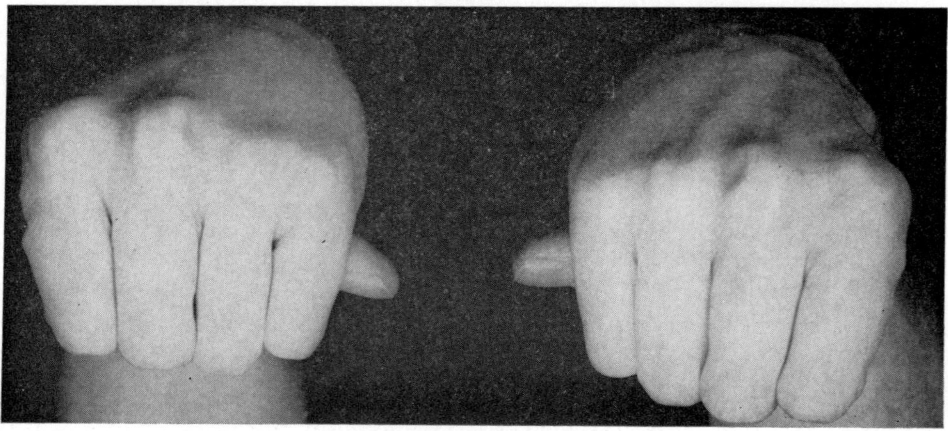

Fig. 73–2.—The Steinberg thumb sign in a patient with the Marfan syndrome. (Thumb grasped in clenched fist protrudes on ulnar side.)

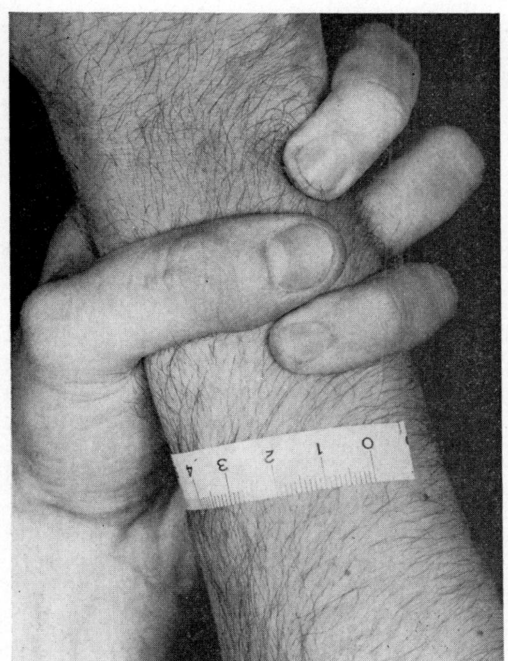

Fig. 73–3.—The wrist sign in a patient with the Marfan syndrome.

margin of the hand. Another simple test is that for the wrist sign[132]: when the Marfan patient puts his thumb and index finger around his wrist they overlap appreciably (*see* Fig. 73–3).

Other Features.—Most patients with the Marfan syndrome have myopia and about 75 per cent have subluxation of the lenses. In the aorta the ascending portion bears the main brunt in the Marfan syndrome. Progressive dilatation begins in the region of the sinuses of Valsalva with development of significant aortic regurgitation despite lack of aortic enlargement by ordinary radiography. Dissecting aneurysm with aortic rupture is also a complication and mitral regurgitation is sometimes the functionally dominant cardiovascular lesion. Hernias are frequent, cystic changes in the lungs lead to pneumothorax, and striae distensae over the pectoral and deltoid areas and thighs are often seen in teen-age patients.

Other Observations on the Joints in the Marfan Syndrome.—Scoliosis can reach very severe proportions in the Marfan syndrome. The feet are often markedly flat. Despite genu recurvatum and habitual dislocation of joints, the patients are remarkably little inconvenienced by the joint abnormalities.

Camptodactyly (volar contracture) of the fifth fingers occurs frequently in patients with the Marfan syndrome and sometimes the contracture extends in progressively diminishing severity to the 4th, 3rd and 2nd fingers. In rare patients other joints such as the elbows show limitation in extension rather than hyperextensibility as is usually the case.

In the *differential diagnosis* of the Marfan syndrome one must consider "contractural arachnodactyly" as described by Beals and Hecht[9a] and by others—Marfan's patient may have had this rather than the Marfan syndrome! Also the Marfanoid hypermobility syndrome[131] seems to be distinct. The Marfan syndrome remains a clinical diagnosis since no specific laboratory test is available. The diagnosis is most secure if ectopia lentis and/or a positive family history accompany the other features. These are not present, however, in all bona fide cases, namely about 25 per cent who lack the ectopia lentis (*see* above) and about 15 per cent of cases which originate through new mutation.

The nature of the basic defect of connective tissue in the Marfan syndrome is not known.

Standard operative procedures such as Harrington rodding have been used with success for the scoliosis. Early induction of puberty with a physiologic estrogen-progesterone program is useful in preventing grotesquely excessive growth in girls with the Marfan syndrome. In both sexes, hormonal induction of puberty with early termination of growth may have usefulness in preventing development of severe scoliosis.

Homocystinuria[88]

Homocystinuria (Fig. 73–4) is an inborn error in the metabolism of methio-

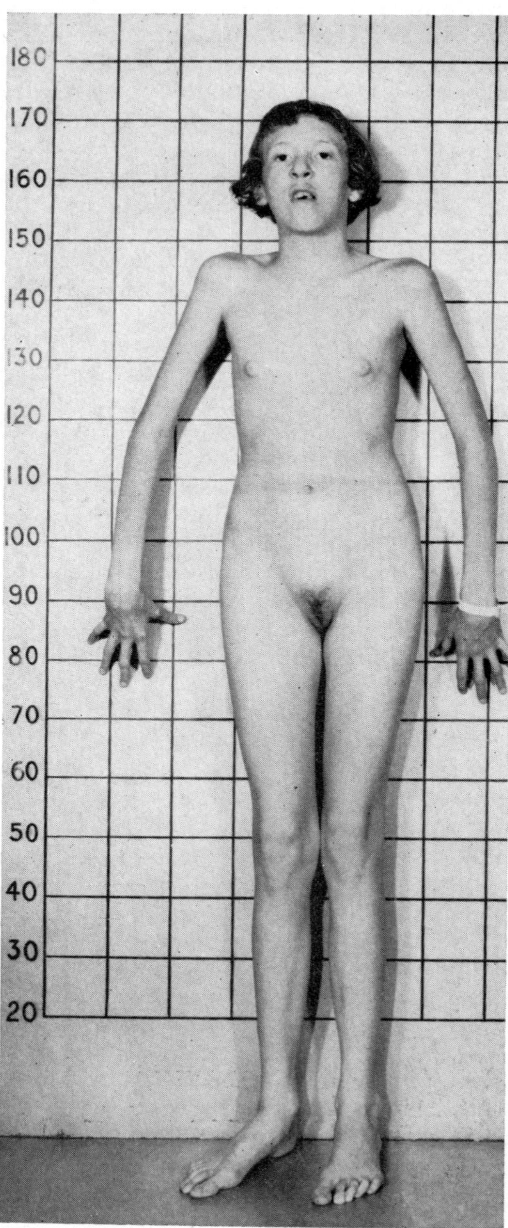

Fig. 73–4.—Homocystinuria in a 12-year-old girl. Note excessive height, long, narrow feet and mild anterior chest deformity. Joints generally showed moderate restriction of motion. The teeth were crowded. Ectopia lentis was present and the patient has had several episodes of probable pulmonary embolism.

nine. Activity of the enzyme cystathionine synthase is deficient. Clinical features include ectopia lentis, dolichostenomelia (long, thin limbs), and chest and spinal deformity, as in the Marfan syndrome. Generalized osteoporosis, "tight" joints, arterial and venous thrombosis, malar flush, and mental retardation are features of homocystinuria usually not found in the Marfan syndrome. Aortic aneurysm and mitral regurgitation are not features of homocystinuria. Back pain due to osteoporosis occurs in some patients. The hand in homocystinuria has a "tight feel" and joints generally tend to have reduced mobility.

The mechanisms of the three cardinal groups of manifestations —mental retardation, connective tissue disorder (ectopia lentis, osteoporosis, "tight" joints), thrombosis—are not understood. It is suspected that sulfhydryl groups of homocysteine or other substances which accumulate proximal to the block interfere with cross-linking in collagen, thus accounting for the connective tissue manifestations. If true, this is a form of thiolism such as occurs from prolonged administration of penicillamine, which bears a structural similarity to homocysteine.

Homocystinuria is an autosomal recessive disorder, like all other Garrodian inborn errors of metabolism, and unlike the Marfan syndrome which is a dominant.

Treatment consists of supplemental vitamin B_6 (pyridoxine), 300 to 500 mg. a day, to which about half the patients respond with clearing of homocystine from the urine and apparent clinical improvement in terms of mental capacity and behavior and avoidance of thrombotic episodes. Low methionine diet (with supplementary cystine) is another therapeutic approach.

Weill-Marchesani Syndrome[88]

The Weill-Marchesani syndrome (Fig. 73–5) is another systemic disorder with ectopia lentis as a conspicuous feature.

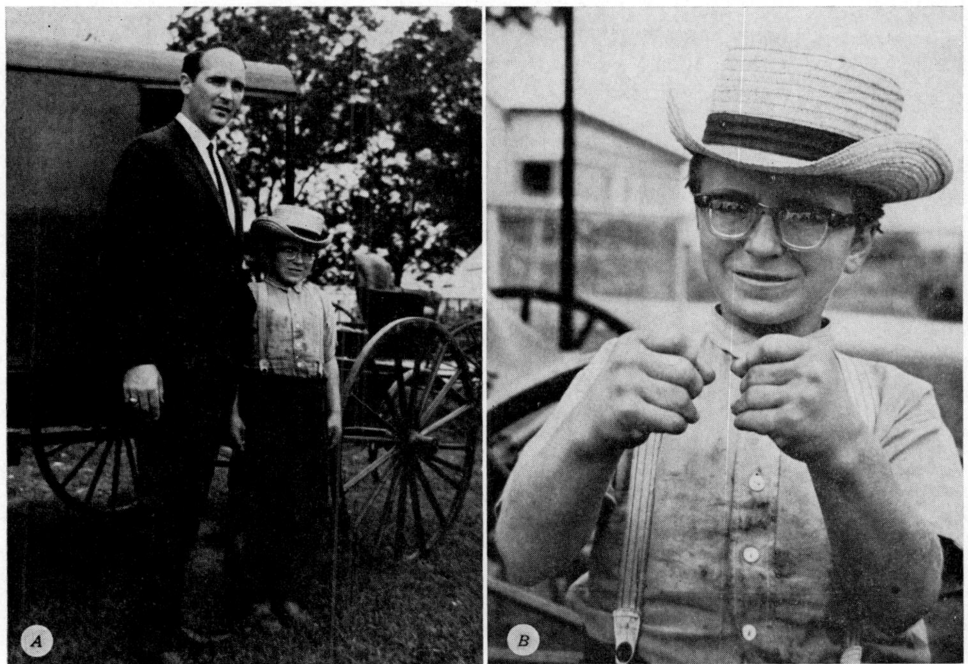

FIG. 73–5.—Weill-Marchesani syndrome in a 15½-year-old Amish boy. *A*. Shown with normal adult male. Ectopia lentis was present and attacks of acute glaucoma had occurred. *B*. The fingers are short with knobby joints and restricted finger flexion. Flattening of the thenar eminence was consistent with carpal tunnel compression.

The skeletal features are the antithesis of those in Marfan's syndrome: The patients are short of stature, with particularly short hands and feet, and many have stiff joints, especially in the hands. The hands sometimes show atrophy of the abductor pollicis brevis muscle consistent with carpal tunnel compression. The Weill-Marchesani syndrome is autosomal recessive, but heterozygotes are short of stature.[65]

Ehlers-Danlos Syndrome[11,88]

Cardinal features relate to the joints and skin: loosejointedness (Fig. 73–6) and bruisability, stretchability, and fragility of skin. Internal features include rupture of great vessels, hiatal hernia, diverticulum of the gastrointestinal tract, spontaneous rupture of the bowel and "spontaneous" pneumothorax.

Clinical Features.—Generalized hyperextensibility of joints, together with stretchability of skin, leads to characterization of the affected persons as "India rubber men." Other features are bruisability of the skin and fragility with many gaping wounds from minor trauma and poor holding of sutures. Congenital dislocation of the hips in the newborn, habitual dislocation of selected joints in later life, joint effusions, deformity of the feet of clubfoot type, and spondylolisthesis are all consequences of the loosejointedness. Hemarthroses and "hemarthrotic disability" have been described and are comparable to the bruisability of the skin and bleeding at other sites which occur in this syndrome. Scoliosis is sometimes severe. Severe leg cramps occurring while watching television or in bed have been troublesome to some patients.

A defect in collagen, quantitative

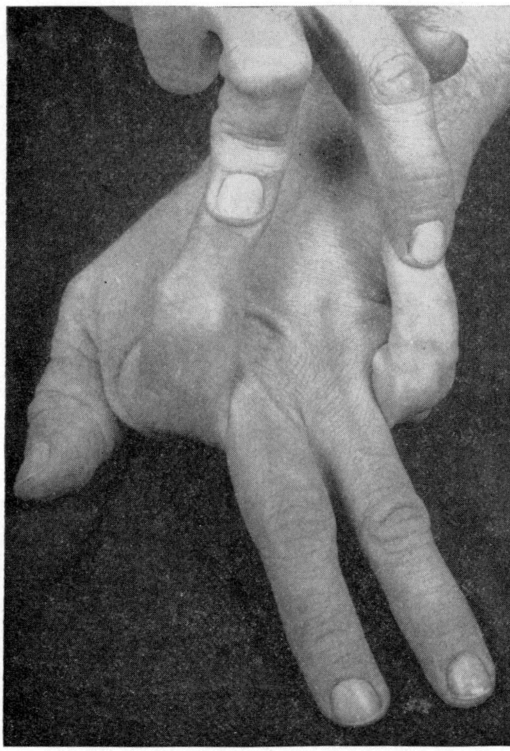

Fig. 73–6.—Joint hypermobility in the Ehlers-Danlos syndrome. Recurrent dislocation of the right hip, relaxation of right radiocarpal joint and disability of the knee were major problems.

and/or qualitative in nature, appears to be responsible for the several forms of the Ehlers-Danlos syndrome.

It is now clear that the Ehlers-Danlos syndrome is in fact a category which encompasses several distinct entities. A classic form with typical loosejointedness and with fragility, stretchability and bruisability of skin is inherited as an autosomal dominant. Mild and severe forms are distinguishable and "breed true" within families. A dangerous form with thin, fragile, bruisable skin and friable tissues and with spontaneous rupture of the bowels and fatal rupture of large arteries is probably also an autosomal dominant. Some families with clear X-linked recessive transmission have been noted.[10]

Arthrochalasis multiplex congenita, "simple joint hypermobility," and the *Larsen syndrome* are examples of familial and congenital joint hypermobility. Families with simple joint hypermobility have been reported.[23–25] Arthrochalasis multiplex congenita, as described by Hass and Hass[54] who suggested this term, is difficult to distinguish from the severe form of the disorder which others termed "simple joint hypermobility." Some reported cases of simple hypermobility of joints may be instances of the Ehlers-Danlos syndrome, *e.g.*, those in photographs in the report who show "cigarette-paper" scars over the knees typical of the Ehlers-Danlos syndrome.[62] (*See* Fig. 73–7 for a method of evaluating joint laxity.)

The Larsen syndrome is characterized by multiple congenital dislocations and characteristic facies — prominent forehead, depressed nasal bridge and widely spaced eyes. Dislocation occurs at the knees (characteristically anterior displacement of the tibia on the femur), hips and elbows. The metacarpals are short with cylindrical fingers lacking the usual tapering. Cleft palate, hydrocephalus and abnormalities of spinal segmentation have occurred in some. Several instances of multiple affected sibs with normal parents are known to me, suggesting autosomal recessive inheritance, but parent-child involvement has also been seen[75] suggesting dominant inheritance.

Osteogenesis Imperfecta[88]

The clinical features are mainly osseous, ocular and aural.

Skeletal Features.—"Brittle bones" are a familiar and dramatic feature of osteogenesis imperfecta. Sometimes fractures occur in utero, and the antenatal diagnosis is possible by x ray of the unborn child. In such cases the extremities are likely to be short and bent at birth. Other patients escape fractures although they have blue sclerae and deafness and may suffer rupture of the Achilles or patellar

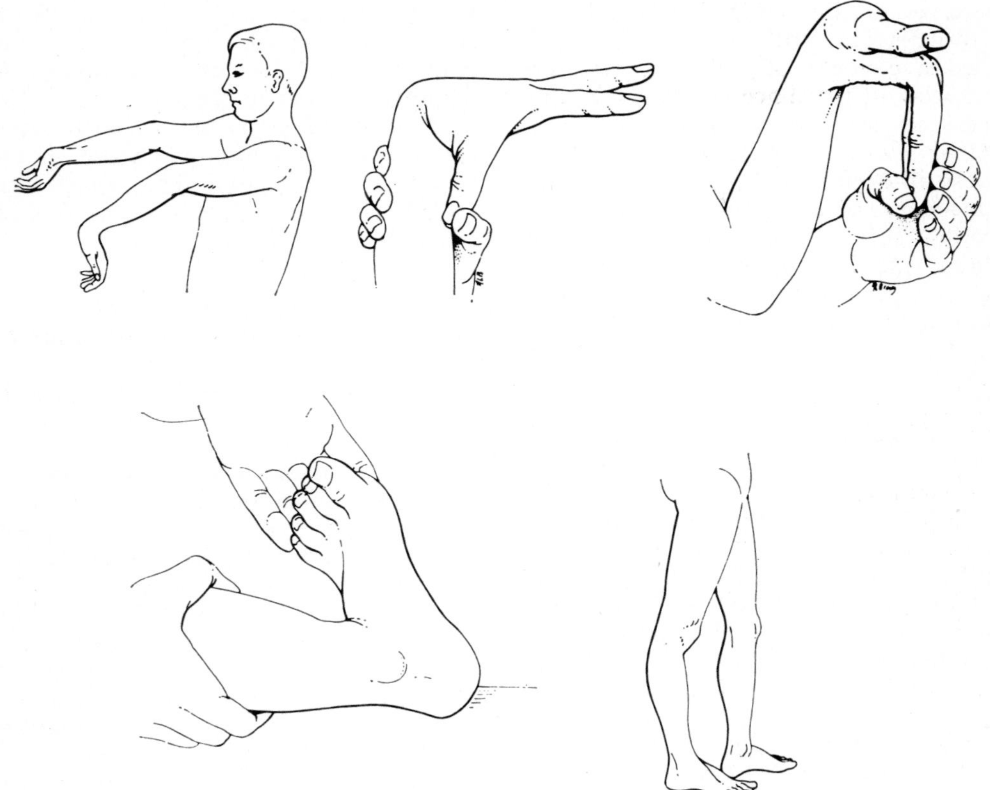

FIG. 73–7.—A method for evaluating joint mobility.[25,139] Excessive joint laxity is judged to be present when at least three of the following five conditions obtain: elbows and knees extended beyond 180 degrees, thumb touching the forearm on flexing the wrist, the fingers parallel to the forearm on extending the wrist and metacarpophalangeal joints, the foot dorsiflexed to 45 degrees or more. Courtesy of Ruth Wynne-Davies and *J. Bone & Joint Surg.*

tendon. Brittle bones result from a defect in the collagenous matrix of bone. The skeletal aspect of osteogenesis imperfecta is, therefore, a hereditary form of osteoporosis. "Codfish vertebrae" (hollowing out of vertebral bodies by pressure from the expansile intervertebral disc) or flat vertebrae are observed particularly in older patients in whom senile or postmenopausal changes exaggerate the change, or young patients who are immobilized after fractures or osteotomies. Usually the frequency of fractures decreases at puberty. Because of failure of union of fractures, pseudoarthrosis, *e.g.*, of humerus or femur, occurs in some. Hypertrophic callus occurs frequently in patients with osteogenesis imperfecta and is often difficult to distinguish from osteosarcoma. Loosejointedness is sometimes striking in osteogenesis imperfecta patients. Dislocation of joints can be a problem.

Ocular Features.—Blue sclerae are almost always present and represent a valuable clue to the diagnosis. The cornea is, like the sclera, abnormally thin. The ocular features are usually not of great functional importance.

Aural Features.—Deafness develops in many of the patients by the second decade of life. Audiologically the deafness is usually indistinguishable from that of otosclerosis, although some patients have an element of cochlear, or nerve, deafness and there are histological differences between the two processes.

Other Features.—Patients with osteogenesis imperfecta may have thin, rather translucent skin. It may resemble the atrophic skin of the aged. By study of surgical incisions in these patients, healing of skin wounds has been found to result in wider scars than usual. Macular atrophy of the skin has been described in patients with osteogenesis imperfecta. This may be comparable to the spotty blueness of the sclera seen in some patients.

Unusual bruisability occurs in some of the patients. This is probably due to a defect in the connective tissue in the walls of small blood vessels or in the supporting connective tissues. No consistent defect of the coagulation mechanism has been demonstrated.

The dental involvement in osteogenesis imperfecta is termed dentinogenesis imperfecta. (A clinically distinguishable form of dentinogenesis imperfecta also occurs as an isolated genetic defect.) The teeth may be stunted and discolored. Both primary and secondary dentition may be affected. Minimal involvement may consist merely of a bluish, semitranslucent appearance of the incisor teeth near the occlusive margin. Often the inferior incisor teeth are most severely affected and they tend to wear away with unusual ease.

Abnormality of the aortic and/or mitral valves with regurgitation has been observed.

Genetics.—Many families demonstrate autosomal dominant inheritance with the variability characteristic of dominants. Attempts to separate two or more types of osteogenesis imperfecta on the basis of severity and age of onset—congenita, tarda gravis, and tarda levis—are unconvincing. A majority of osteogenesis imperfecta cases are sporadic. Many of these may represent new dominant mutations. Others may represent a recessive form of the disease. Multiple affected sibs and parental consanguinity have been observed in only a relatively few instances, however. Skipped generations or multiple affected sibs with both parents ostensibly unaffected can have at least two different explanations: reduced penetrance in one parent and recessive inheritance.

THE GENETIC MUCOPOLYSACCHARIDOSES

This class of disorder is characterized particularly by mucopolysacchariduria and by deposits of mucopolysaccharides in various tissues. Six distinct types of mucopolysaccharidoses[88] can be distinguished on the basis of combined phenotypic (*i.e.*, clinical), genetic, and biochemical analysis. Table 73–1 summarizes the distinctive features of each. These six almost certainly do not exhaust the heterogeneity in mucopolysacchariduria. Furthermore, genetic disturbances of mucopolysaccharide metabolism without mucopolysacchariduria have been clearly identified. All six of the best delineated disorders are recessives, five being autosomal and one X-linked.

Leading constituents of the ground substance, acid mucopolysaccharides (glycosaminoglycans),* are macromolecular substances, most of which consist of repeating units of hexosamine and a hexuronic acid, bound to protein. Excessive urinary excretion of three mucopolysaccharides—dermatan sulfate, heparan sulfate and keratan sulfate—has been found in various types of genetic mucopolysaccharidosis.

Mucopolysacchariduria is identified by screening tests. One is based on the for-

* The term recommended by Jeanloz[57] was "glycosaminoglycuronoglycan." Further recommendations were chondroitin-4-sulfate for chondroitin sulfate A, chondroitin-6-sulfate for chondroitin sulfate C, dermatan sulfate for chondroitin sulfate B, heparan sulfate for heparitin sulfate, and keratan sulfate for keratosulfate. These terms for the individual mucopolysaccharides have been adopted here.

Table 73-1.
The Genetic Mucopolysaccharidoses with Mucopolysacchariduria

	MPS	*Clinical Features*	*Genetics*	*Urinary MPS's*
I	(The Hurler Syndrome)	Early clouding of cornea, grave manifestations	Autosomal recessive	Dermatan sulfate Heparan sulfate
II	(The Hunter Syndrome)	No clouding of cornea, milder	X-linked recessive	Dermatan sulfate Heparan sulfate
III	(The Sanfilippo Syndrome)	Mild somatic, severe central nervous system effects	Autosomal recessive	Heparan sulfate
IV	(The Morquio Syndrome)	Severe bone changes of distinctive types cloudy cornea, intellect +/−, aortic regurgitation	Autosomal recessive	Keratan sulfate
V	(The Scheie Syndrome)	Stiff joints, coarse facies, cloudy cornea, intellect +/−, aortic regurgitation	Autosomal recessive	Dermatan sulfate Heparan sulfate
VI	(The Maroteaux-Lamy Syndrome)	Severe osseous and corneal change, normal intellect	Autosomal recessive	Dermatan sulfate

mation of a precipitate when cetyltrimethylammonium bromide (CAB) or cetylpyridinium chloride (CPC) is added to urine. Another turbidity test involves addition of acidified bovine albumin to the urine. The Berry reaction is positive if metachromasia results when a urine spot on filter paper is stained with toluidine blue.

Fractionation and characterization of the urinary mucopolysaccharides are useful in separating the several types of mucopolysaccharidoses: for example, the Sanfilippo syndrome (the heparan sulfate excretors) and the Morquio syndrome (the keratan sulfate excretors) in young subjects may be distinguished from the other types, especially the Hurler syndrome, only by the chemical analysis.

Demonstration of metachromatically staining material in the cytoplasm of lymphocytes is also a useful diagnostic method.

Fibroblasts grown from biopsy specimens of skin of patients with the mucopolysaccharidoses display cytoplasmic metachromasia secondary to accumulations of mucopolysaccharides.[28,29] Studies with radioactive sulfate indicate accumulation of label in fibroblasts and delayed washout, compatible with the conclusion that these disorders are due to a degradative defect.[39] More specifically, they are lysosomal disorders. What specific lysosomal enzyme is deficient in each is unknown. Like other lysosomal disorders—over a dozen conditions, *e.g.*, Tay-Sachs disease, have been related to deficiency of specific lysosomal enzyme—the mucopolysaccharidoses have six distinctive characteristics:

1. Storage of material occurs.

2. The storage material is heterogeneous since the degradative enzymes are not strictly specific. Predominantly ganglioside is deposited in brain and predominantly mucopolysaccharide in the liver, and two mucopolysaccharides are excreted in the urine.

3. Deposition is vacuolar, *i.e.*, is membrane bound, when viewed with the electron microscope.

4. Many tissues are affected.

5. The disorder is clinically progressive.

6. Replacement therapy is at least theoretically possible, through getting the missing enzyme into cells by the process of endocytosis. The possibility of replacement therapy in the mucopolysaccharidoses is more than theoretic. Normal cells or the medium in which they have grown, when mixed with MPS fibroblasts, correct the metabolic defect.[40] This indicates the production of a diffusible correction factor by normal cells. It is found also in normal urine.

By a combination of clinical, genetic and biochemical study, it is possible to distinguish at least six mucopolysaccharidoses with mucopolysacchariduria. The differential features of these are summarized in Table 73–1 and clinical features of MPS I, MPS II and MPS V are illustrated in Figures 73–8, 73–9, and 73–10, respectively. The nosologic validity of this classification is supported by the findings of co-cultivation of fibroblasts: mutual correction of their metabolic defects occurs when fibroblasts from I and II, I and III, II and III, I and VI, II and VI, III and VI, and II and V are mixed. Surprisingly, cross correction does not occur when fibroblasts from MPS's I and V are mixed.[135] Clinically these are clearly distinct; the lack of cross correction is interpreted as meaning that these conditions are due to the homozygous state of different, although allelic (at the same locus), mutant genes. To draw an analogy from the hemoglobinopathies, the Hurler syndrome might be compared to SS disease and the Scheie syndrome to CC disease.

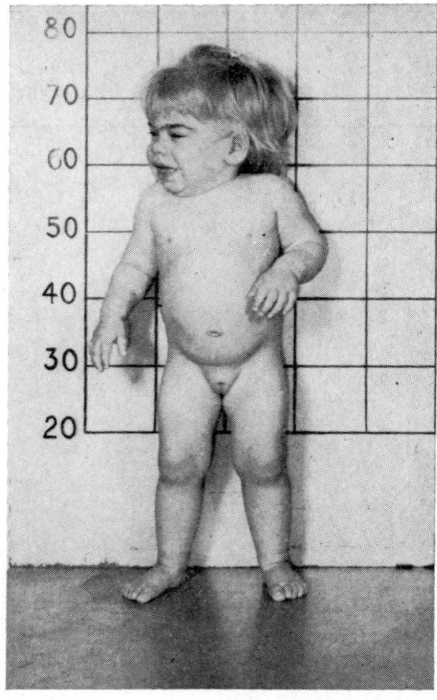

Fig. 73–8.—The Hurler syndrome (MPS I) in a 2-year-old child. Note coarse facial features, prominent abdomen from hepatosplenomegaly, claw hands. The joints generally had moderate restriction of motion.

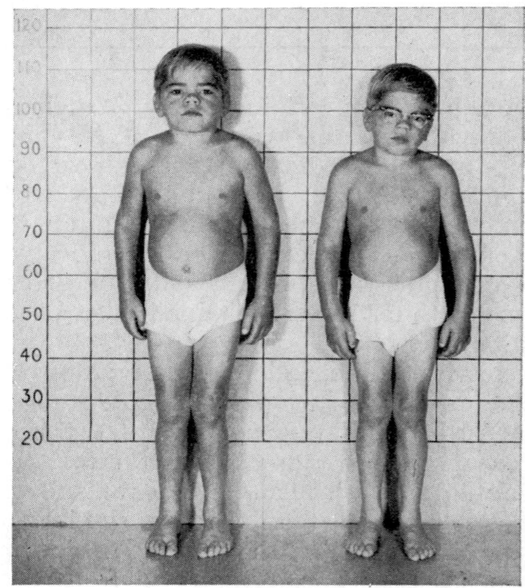

Fig. 73–9.—The Hunter syndrome (MPS II) in brothers, aged 7 and 6 years. Note short stature, coarse facies, prominent abdomen and genu valgum.

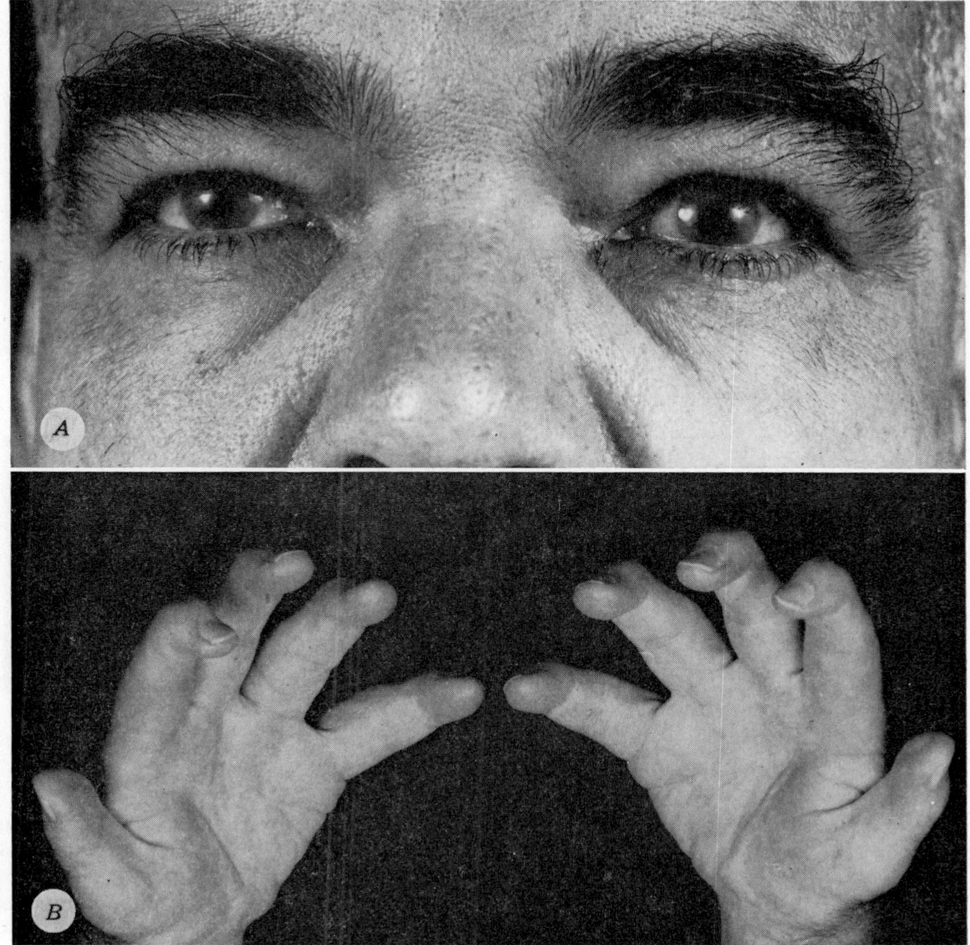

FIG. 73–10.—The Scheie syndrome (MPS V) in a 54-year-old attorney. *A*, Clouding is densest in the peripheral part of the cornea. *B*, The hands are clawed. Atrophy of the lateral aspect of the thenar eminences indicates carpal tunnel compression.

Stiff joints are a more or less striking feature of all except MPS IV. Like the other somatic features it is less striking in MPS III than in the others. In the Scheie syndrome stiff hands lead, together with clouding of the cornea, to the main disability. In that condition, as in the others, carpal tunnel syndrome contributes to the disability. Early decompression can be beneficial. Presumably collagenous overgrowth secondary to the excessive mucopolysaccharides is the basis of the median nerve compression in the carpal tunnel. (Amyloid neuropathy of the Rukavina or Indiana type[82] is another genetic disorder of which carpal tunnel compression is a leading feature and it occurs also in the Weill-Marchesani syndrome, p. 1344.)

Therapy with fresh plasma is under trial in the treatment of the severe forms of mucopolysaccharidosis and purified correction factors are likely to become available within the next few years.

Pseudo-Hurler polydystrophy (Fig. 73–11) is a mucopolysaccharidosis without muco-

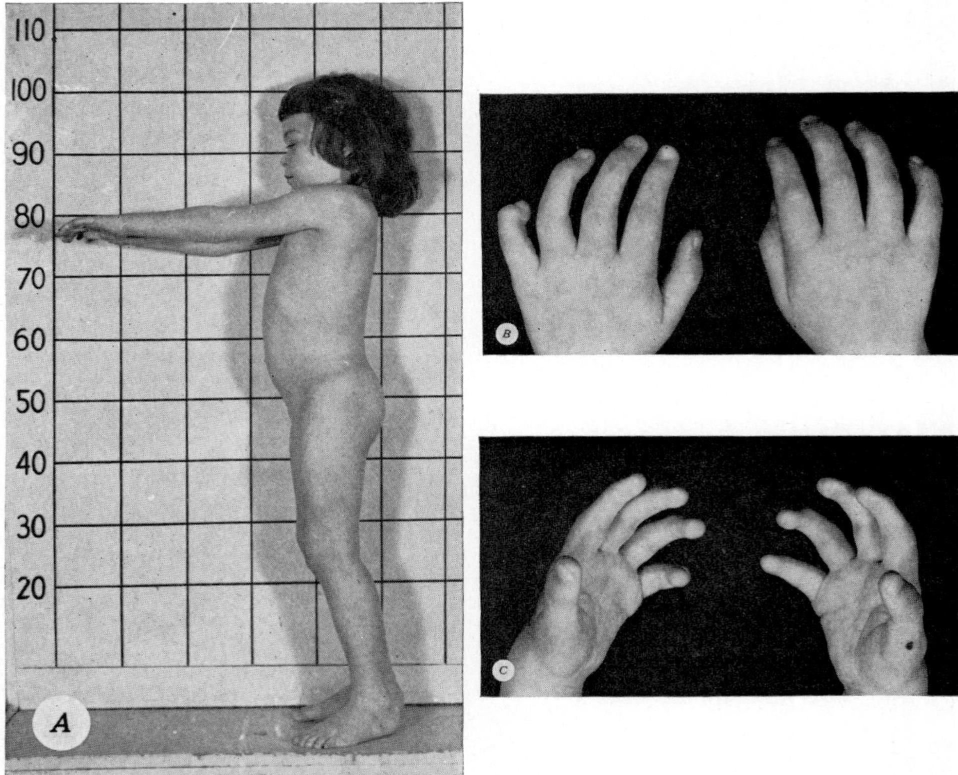

FIG. 73–11.—Pseudo-Hurler polydystrophy in a 6-year-old child. *A*. Note short stature and limitation in elevation of the arms. The facies were coarse. Mild clouding of the cornea, the murmur of aortic regurgitation, restriction in motion of all joints and mild intellectual deficiency were other findings. *B*, *C*. The hands are clawed and atrophy of the thenar eminences indicates carpal tunnel compression, for which operation was performed at age 13 years, with some benefit.

polysacchariduria. (Others[120] have classed it as a mucolipidosis.) Stiffness of all joints is the first and leading feature. The carpal tunnel sydnrome occurs with this disorder also. Later mild clouding of the cornea and involvement of the aortic valve with aortic regurgitation appear. The affected persons are short of statute, have somewhat coarse facies with wide spacing of the teeth, and are mildly retarded intellectually. This disorder is an autosomal recessive. Its nature as a disturbance of mucopolysaccharide metabolism is supported by the finding of cytoplasmic metachromasia.

Selected Genetic Disorders Simulating Arthritides

Ankylosing Arthropathy in Vitamin D-Resistant Hypophosphatemic Rickets. Adults (Fig. 73–12) with this X-linked dominant disorder, especially males and especially if untreated, develop ankylosing spondylosis as well as ankylosis of some peripheral joints. Some such patients have been given x-ray therapy to the spine on the basis of a mistaken diagnosis.[97] As in Reiter's disease the patient with hypophosphatemia shows calcaneal spurs, roughening of the ischium and capsular calcification at the hip.

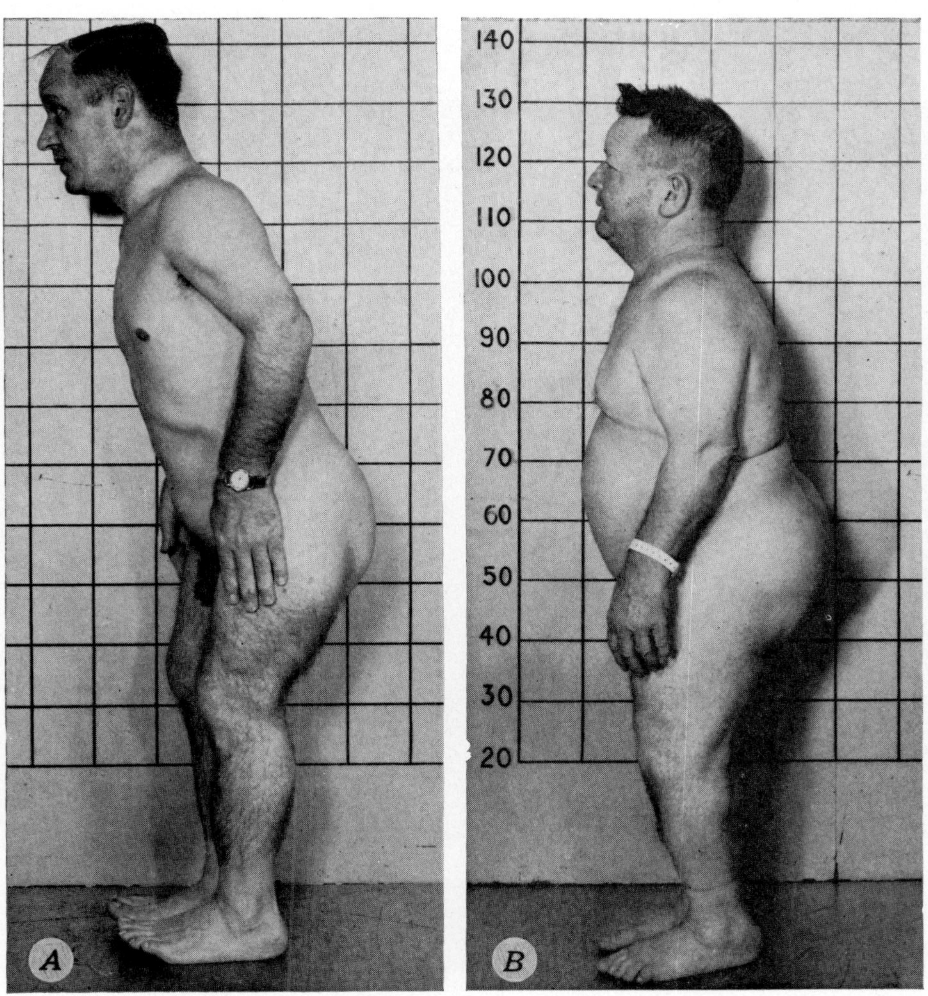

FIG. 73–12.—See legend on page 1355.

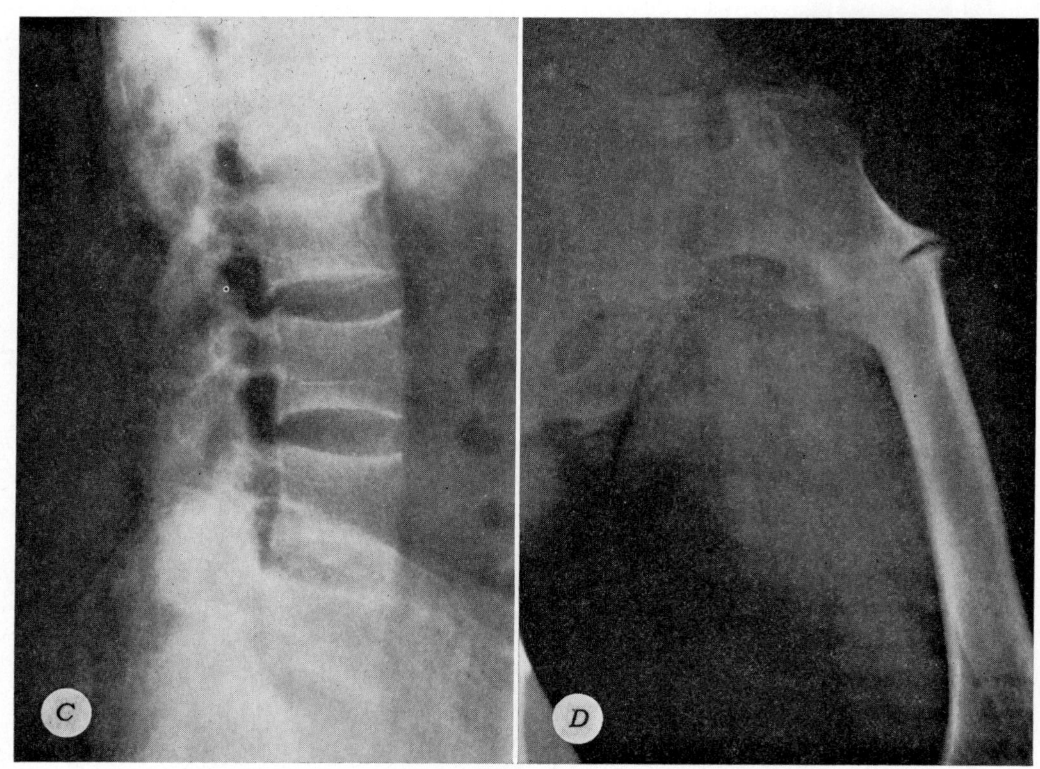

Fɪɢ. 73–12.—See legend on facing page.

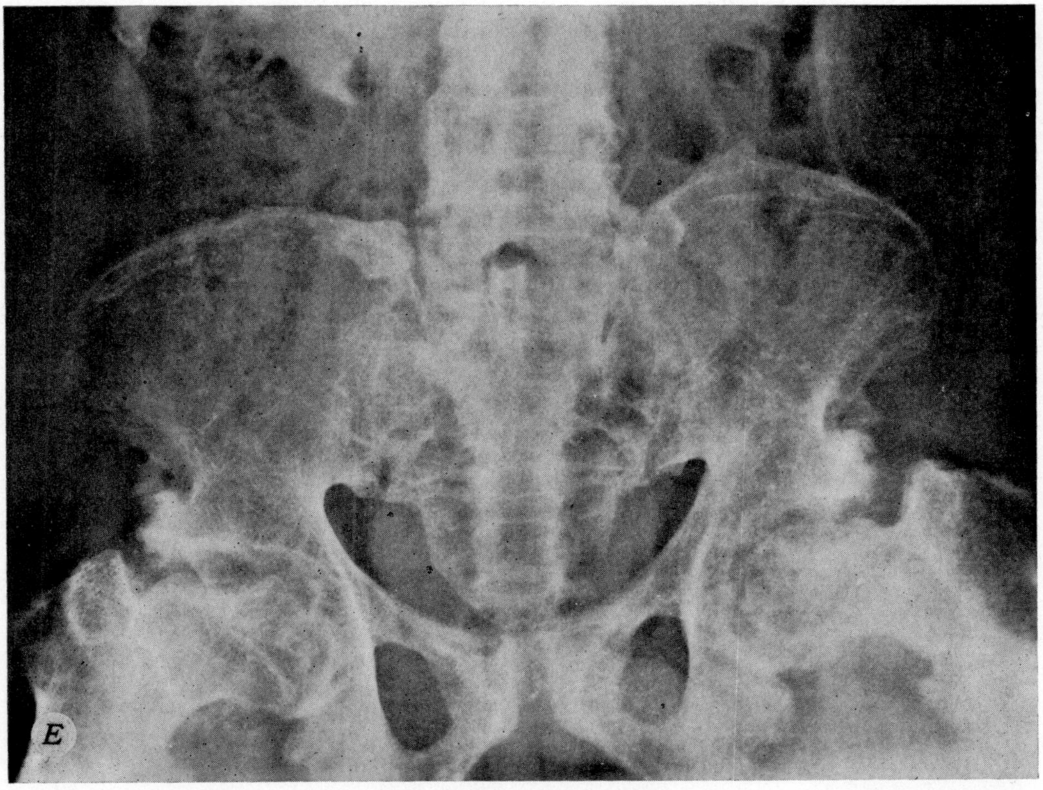

FIG. 73–12.—Ankylosing arthropathy in two men with vitamin D-resistant rickets *A*. 41-year-old man. *B*. 61-year-old man. The younger man is the more severely affected but both have almost complete ankylosis of the spine and similar changes in some peripheral joints. Note short stature. *C*. Lower spine, lateral, in older man. *D*. Left femur in the 41-year-old man. Pseudofractures were situated symmetrically in the subtrochanteric area of both femurs. *E*. Pelvis of the 41-year-old man.

Farber's lipogranulomatosis,[26] an autosomal recessive disorder, first manifests itself in the first few weeks of life with irritability, hoarse cry and nodular, erythematous swelling of the wrists and other sites, particularly those subject to trauma. Masses around the joints suggest rheumatoid nodules (Fig. 73–13).

Fibrodysplasia (formerly myositis) ossificans progressiva[88] is characterized by progressive ossification of ligaments, tendons and aponeuroses. It begins in the first year or so of life usually with a seemingly inflammatory process and nodule formation on the back of the thorax, neck or scalp. Local heat, as well as leukocytosis and elevated sedimentation rate is observed at this stage and acute rheumatic fever is sometimes diagnosed. A valuable clue to the correct diagnosis is short thumb and hallux, often with hallux valgus. In the first two decades of life the ossification usually progresses to produce almost total immobilization. This disorder is an autosomal dominant. Most cases are the consequence of new mutation. The average age of fathers of such cases is over 6 years higher than that of fathers generally.

Symphalangism is the term given by Harvey Cushing to a condition of hereditary ankylosis of the proximal interphalangeal joints.[122a] Fusion of carpal and tarsal bones is an accompanying feature. Inheritance is autosomal dominant.

Camptodactyly was mentioned earlier as a rather frequent feature of the Marfan syndrome. It is found as part of several other syndromes,[44] but occasionally is an isolated abnormality inherited as an autosomal dominant.[136] It consists of limitation of extension at the proximal interphalangeal joints without limitation of flexion, typically accompanied by hyperextension at the metacarpophalangeal joints and sometimes at the distal

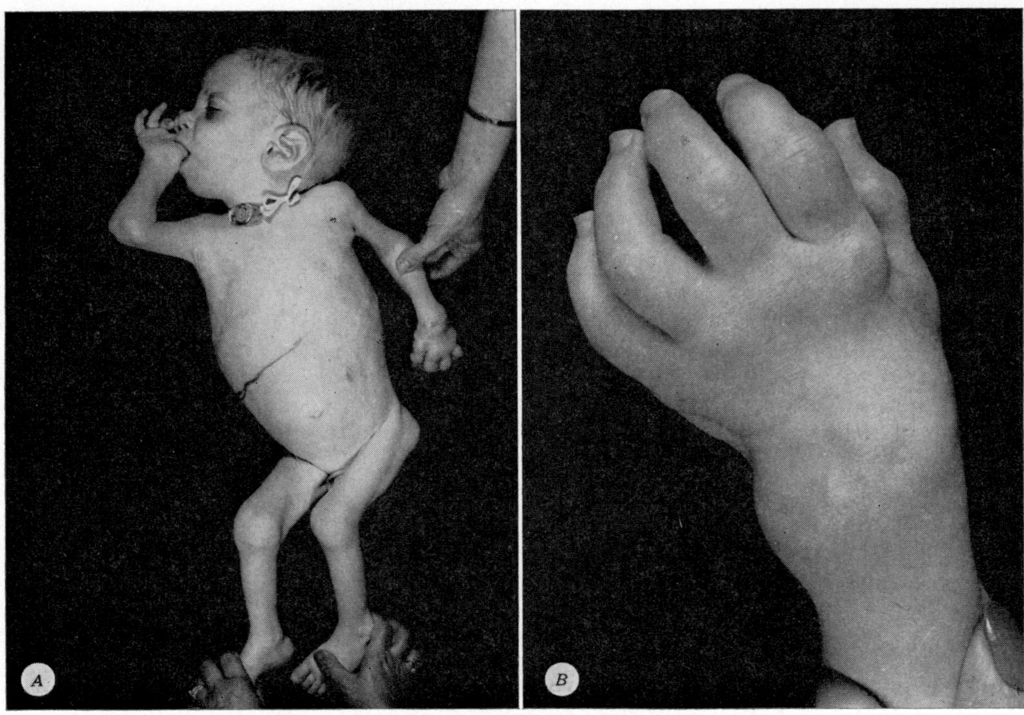

FIG. 73–13.—Farber's lipogranulomatosis in an 18-month-old boy. Note the swelling and nodes of the wrists, hands, fingers, and elbows as well as the signs of grave illness. Tracheostomy was necessitated by the laryngeal involvement. (Autospy findings were reported by Abul-Haj *et al.*[1])

interphalangeal joint. It may be limited to the fifth finger or the other fingers may be involved as well, in descending order of severity, fingers IV, III and II, but the thumb is probably always spared. A contracture band can often be felt on the volar surface of the affected proximal interphalangeal joint and the transverse skin creases are invariably absent there. Camptodactyly is present from birth or early childhood and shows little tendency to progression. Because of compensatory hyperextension at the metacarpophalangeal joints, the contracture causes little disability. As was pointed out by Archibald Garrod, camptodactyly, when it involves multiple fingers, is often accompanied by "knuckle pads," thickened skin on the dorsal aspect of the proximal interphalangeal joints.[136] Camptodactyly is sometimes confused with Dupuytren's contracture which is late in onset and has the primary site of contracture in the palm.

Genetic disorders which are the substrate for precocious osteoarthritis of the hips. Lloyd-Roberts[78] found that 26 of 124 cases of early osteoarthritis of the hips could be related to subluxation. Of the 51 cases (out of 124) in which an etiologic factor was evident, this was, then, a predominant one. Familial joint laxity, discussed above, is one factor in subluxation of the hip and acetabular dysplasia is another, apparently unrelated,[139] factor. Subluxation of the hip which comes to light soon after birth is usually that related to familial joint laxity; that which is recognized later is related to acetabular dysplasia.

Multiple epiphyseal dysplasia (MED) comes to medical attention in the child because of short stature, somewhat stiff joints, or changes in the heads of the femurs like Legg-Perthes disease leading to abnormality of gait. In the 20's or 30's, the patient develops osteoarthritis of the hips (Fig. 73–14) and to a lesser extent of other joints. Suspicion that multiple epiphyseal dysplasia underlies precocious osteoarthritis of the hips may come from short stature and be corroborated by the finding of sloping at the distal end of the tibia. This condition is a Mendelian dominant.

Some families with multiple epiphyseal dysplasia show especially striking changes in the hands with short fingers and painless deformity at the proximal interphalangeal joints. This may be the disorder which has been described as "familial osteoarthropathy of the fingers,"[2] or the Thiemann epiphyseal type of acrodysplasia (*see* Table 73–2).

Hereditary progressive arthro-ophthalmopathy is the designation used[122] for an autosomal dominant disorder characterized by (1) premature degenerative changes in various joints with abnormal epiphyseal development and hyperextensibility of some joints and (2) progressive myopia leading to retinal detachment.

Genetic factors in Heberden's nodes are discussed elsewhere (see p. 1025).

Arthrogryposis multiplex congenita (AMC) is a syndrome which probably has more than one origin and is characterized by congenital rigidity of multiple joints. The hands and feet are usually clubbed. The disorder is essentially a malformation of joints resulting from immobilization of the developing fetus so that the proper stimulus for joint development is lacking.[32] The cause of the immobilization may be a prenatal disorder of brain, spinal cord, peripheral nerves or muscle. The affected baby is born with the arms and legs fixed in postures dictated by the position of the embryo and fetus in development. In addition to joint rigidity, dislocation of the hips and micrognathia are frequent findings. The Drachman theory of fetal immobilization as the "cause" of AMC was developed from studies of the effects on chick embryos of neuromuscular blocking agents. His theory is supported by observation of AMC in an infant born of a mother who received tubocurarine in early pregnancy for treatment of tetanus.[56a]

Disorders of the Bony Skeleton.—The osseous skeleton, the largest specialized connective tissue, participates in many of

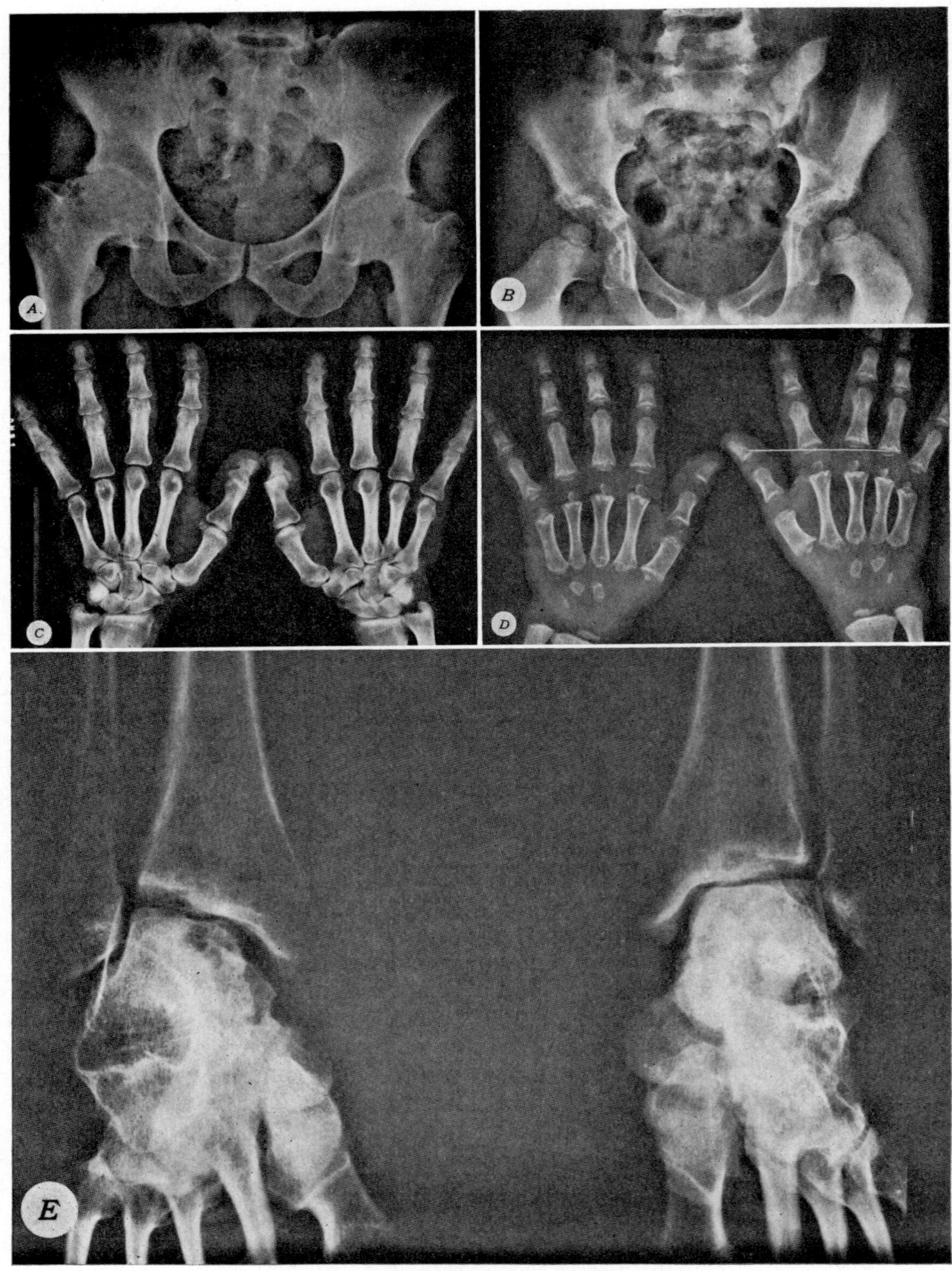

FIG. 73–14.—See legend on facing page.

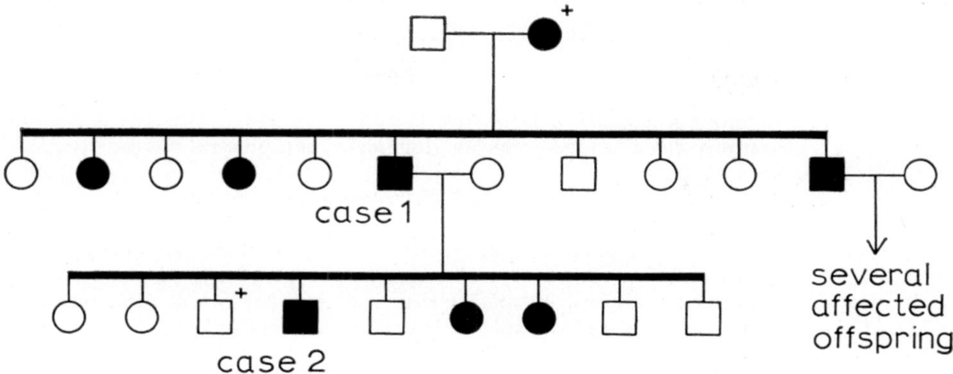

■ ● Male, female with MED

+ Deceased

(F)

Fig. 73–14.—Multiple epiphyseal dysplasia in father and son. Both were short of stature, the father being 61½ inches tall. *A.* Hips in the father at age 44 years showing advanced degenerative changes. *B.* Hips in the son at age 10 years showing small femoral capital epiphyses and irregularities of the acetabulum. *C.* Hands of the father showing brachydactyly and degenerative joint disease. The carpus is short. *D.* Hands of the son (aged 10 years) showing dysplastic epiphyses and delayed development of the carpal bones. *E.* Sloping of the distal tibia is a clue to the diagnosis of MED in the adult. *F.* Pedigree. Cases 1 and 2 are the father and son illustrated here. Typical autosomal dominant pedigree pattern is demonstrated.

Table 73-2.
A Nomenclature for Constitutional (Intrinsic) Disorders of Bone

I. Constitutional Diseases of Bones with Unknown Pathogenesis: OSTEOCHONDRODYSPLASIAS (abnormalities of cartilage and/or bone growth and development)

A. **Defects of growth of tubular bones and/or spine**

1. *Manifest at birth*
   - *a.* Achondroplasia[72]
   - *b.* Achondrogenesis[99]
   - *c.* Thanatophoric dwarfism[73]
   - *d.* Chondrodysplasia punctata (formerly stippled epiphyses chondrodystrophia calcificans congenita), several forms[119]
   - *e.* Metatrophic dwarfism[74]
   - *f.* Diastrophic dwarfism[69]
   - *g.* Chondroectodermal dysplasia (Ellis-van Creveld)[89]
   - *h.* Asphyxiating thoracic dysplasia (Jeune)[71]
   - *i.* Spondyloepiphyseal dysplasia, congenital[118a]
   - *j.* Mesomelic dwarfism
     - (1) Nievergelt type[118]
     - (2) Langer type[68]
   - *k.* Cleidocranial dysplasia (formerly cleidocranial dysostosis)[38]

Table 73-2.—(Continued)

2. *Manifest in later life*
   - *a.* Hypochondroplasia[9]
   - *b.* Dyschondrosteosis[37]
   - *c.* Metaphyseal chondrodysplasia (formerly metaphyseal dysostosis), Jansen type[76]
   - *d.* Metaphyseal chondrodysplasia (formerly metaphyseal dysostosis), Schmidt type[104]
   - *e.* Metaphyseal chondrodysplasia, McKusick type (formerly cartilage-hair hypoplasia)[90]
   - *f.* Metaphyseal chondrodysplasia with malabsorption and neutropenia[114]
   - *g.* Metaphyseal chondrodysplasia with thymolymphopenia[41]
   - *h.* Spondylometaphyseal dysplasia (Kozlowski)[66]
   - *i.* Multiple epiphyseal dysplasia (several forms)[35,126]
   - *j.* Hereditary arthro-ophthalmopathy[122]
   - *k.* Pseudoachondroplastic dysplasia (formerly pseudoachondroplastic type of spondyloepiphyseal dysplasia)[51]
   - *l.* Spondyloepiphyseal dysplasia tarda[70]
   - *m.* Acrodysplasia
     - (1) Trichorhinophalangeal syndrome (Giedion)[42]
     - (2) Epiphyseal type (Thiemann)[2,16]
     - (3) Epiphysometaphyseal type (Brailsford)[18]

B. **Disorganized development of cartilage and fibrous components of the skeleton**

1. Dysplasia epiphysealis hemimelica[106]
2. Multiple cartilaginous exostoses[117]
3. Enchondromatosis (Ollier)[106]
4. Enchondromatosis with hemangioma (Maffucci)[4]
5. Fibrous dysplasia (Jaffe-Lichtenstein)[20]
6. Fibrous dysplasia with skin pigmentation and precocious puberty (McCune-Albright)[1]
7. Cherubism[59]
8. Multiple fibromatosis[109]

C. **Abnormalities of density, of cortical diaphyseal structure and/or of metaphyseal modeling**

1. Osteogenesis imperfecta congenita (Vrolik, Porak-Durante)[88]
2. Osteogenesis imperfecta tarda (Lobstein)[88]
3. Juvenile idiopathic osteoporosis[30]
4. Osteopetrosis with precocious manifestations[34]
5. Osteopetrosis with delayed manifestations[58]
6. Pyknodysostosis[5]
7. Osteopoikilosis[12]
8. Melorheostosis[22]
9. Diaphyseal dysplasia (Camurati-Engelmann)[43]
10. Craniodiaphyseal dysplasia[53]
11. Endosteal hyperostosis (Van Buchem and other forms)[129]
12. Tubular stenosis (Kenny-Caffey)[21]
13. Osteodysplasia (Melnick-Needles)[92]
14. Pachydermoperiostosis[101]
15. Osteoectasia with hyperphosphatasia[7]
16. Metaphyseal dysplasia (Pyle)[94]
17. Craniometaphyseal dysplasia (several forms)[56,93]
18. Frontometaphyseal dysplasia[45]
19. Oculo-dento-osseous dysplasia (formerly oculo-dento-digital syndrome)[46]

Table 73-2.—(Continued)

II. CONSTITUTIONAL DISEASES OF BONE WITH UNKNOWN PATHOGENESIS: DYSOSTOSES (malformation of individual bones, singly or in combination)

A. **Dysostoses with cranial and facial involvement**

1. Craniosynostosis, several forms[27,113]
2. Craniofacial dysostosis (Crouzon)[130]
3. Acrocephalosyndactyly (Apert)[108]
4. Acrocephalopolysyndactyly (Carpenter)[124]
5. Mandibulofacial dysostosis (Treacher-Collins, Franceschetti and others)[105]
6. Mandibular hypoplasia (includes Pierre Robin syndrome)[116]
7. Oculomandibulofacial syndrome (Hallermann-Streiff-François)[36]
8. Nevoid basal cell carcinoma syndrome[100]

B. **Dysostoses with predominant axial involvement**

1. Vertebral segmentation defects (including Klippel-Feil)[50]
2. Cervico-oculo-acoustic syndrome (Wildervanck)[63]
3. Sprengel deformity[110]
4. Spondylocostal dysostosis (several forms)[94,103]
5. Oculovertebral syndrome (Weyers)[137]
6. Osteo-onychodysostosis (formerly nail-patella syndrome)[79]

C. **Dysostoses with predominant involvement of extremities**[124a]

1. Amelia
2. Hemimelia (several types)
3. Acheiria
4. Apodia
5. Adactyly and oligodactyly
6. Phocomelia
7. Aglossia-adactylia syndrome[93a]
8. Congenital bowing of long bones (several types)[5a]
9. Familial radioulnar synostosis[53a]
10. Brachydactyly (several types)[124a]
11. Symphalangism[122a]
12. Polydactyly (several types)[124a]
13. Syndactyly (several types)[124a]
14. Polysyndactyly (several types)[124a]
15. Campodactyly[136]
16. Clinodactyly[124a]
17. Biedl-Bardet syndrome[3,64]
18. Popliteal pterygium syndrome[48]
19. Pectoral aplasia-dysdactyly syndrome (Poland)[133]
20. Rubinstein-Taybi syndrome[107]
21. Pancytopenia-dysmelia syndrome (Fanconi)[60]
22. Thrombocytopenia-radial-aplasia syndrome[52]
23. Orofaciodigital (OFD) syndrome (Papillon-Léage)[47,102]
24. Cardiomelic syndrome (Holt-Oram and others)[98]

III. CONSTITUTIONAL DISEASES OF BONE WITH UNKNOWN PATHOGENESIS: IDIOPATHIC OSTEOLYSES

A. **Acro-osteolysis**

1. Phalangeal type[67]
2. Tarsocarpal form, with or without nephropathy[128]

Table 73-2.—(Continued)

B. **Multicentric osteolysis**[127]

IV. PRIMARY DISTURBANCES OF GROWTH
- A. Primordial dwarfism (without associated malformations)[14,134]
- B. Cornelia de Langes syndrome[96]
- C. Bird-headed dwarfism (Virchow, Seckel)[91]
- D. Leprechaunism[123]
- E. Russell-Silver syndrome[55]
- F. Progeria[81]
- G. Cockayne syndrome[80]
- H. Bloom syndrome[15]
- I. Geroderma osteodysplastica[19]
- J. Spherophakia-brachymorphia syndrome (Weill-Marchesani)[111]
- K. Marfan syndrome[88]

V. CONSTITUTIONAL DISEASES OF BONES WITH KNOWN PATHOGENESIS: Chromosomal Aberrations

VI. CONSTITUTIONAL DISEASES OF BONES WITH KNOWN PATHOGENESIS: Primary Metabolic Abnormalities

A. **Disorders of calcium/phosphorus metabolism**
1. Hypophosphatemic familial rickets[13,130]
2. Pseudo-deficiency rickets (Royer, Prader)[31]
3. Late rickets (McCance)[85]
4. Idiopathic hypercalciuria
5. Hypophosphatasia (several forms)[8]
6. Idiopathic hypercalcemia[61]
7. Pseudohypoparathyroidism (normo- and hypocalcemic forms)[83]

B. **Mucopolysaccharidoses**[88]
1. Mucopolysaccharidosis I (Hurler)
2. Mucopolysaccharidosis II (Hunter)
3. Mucopolysaccharidosis III (Sanfilippo)
4. Mucopolysaccharidosis IV (Morquio)
5. Mucopolysaccharidosis V (Scheie)
6. Mucopolysaccharidosis VI (Maroteaux-Lamy)

C. **Mucolipidoses**[120] **and lipidoses**
1. Mucolipidosis I (Spranger-Wiedemann)[121]
2. Mucolipidosis II (Leroy)[77]
3. Mucolipidosis III (Pseudo-Hurler polydystrophy)[112]
4. Fucosidosis[33]
5. Mannosidosis[95]
6. Generalized Gml gangliosidosis (several forms)[94a]
7. Sulfatidosis with mucopolysacchariduria (Austin; Thieffry)[6,125]
8. Cerebrosidosis including Gaucher's disease[17]

D. Other metabolic extra-osseous disorders

VII. BONE ABNORMALITIES SECONDARY TO DISTURBANCES OF EXTRA-SKELETAL SYSTEMS
- A. Endocrine, e.g., hypothyroidism
- B. Hematologic, e.g., thalassemia
- C. Neurologic, e.g., sensory neuropathy
- D. Renal, e.g., cystinosis
- E. Gastrointestinal, e.g., celiac disease
- F. Cardiopulmonary, e.g., hypertrophy osteoarthropathy

the generalized heritable disorders of connective tissue discussed earlier. In addition it is subject to a large number of gene-determined derangements with primary effects apparently limited to bone and cartilage.

The bone dysplasias represent a difficult category of hereditary disease because the types are legion; each is rare or fairly rare so that most physicians, even specialists such as orthopedists, radiologists and rheumatologists, encounter them rarely; nothing is known of etiopathogenesis and little even of the standard histopathology; no definitive therapy is available for most; and nomenclature is chaotic.

Most of the skeletal dysplasias fall into the category of disproportionate dwarfism (called dwarfs by the layman), contrasted with proportionate dwarfs (called midgets by the layman), who often have deficiency of growth hormone. Disproportionate dwarfs tend further to fall into short-limb or short-trunk groups, of which achondroplasia and the Morquio syndrome are, respectively, prototypes. In individual patients many different conditions have often been labeled either achondroplasia or Morquio syndrome. In recent years recognition of the heterogeneity in the skeletal dysplasia[106] delineation of many simulating but distinct disorders and better definition of the prototype disorders, achondroplasia and Morquio syndrome, have led to much better understanding of this category although much remains to be learned.

In these disorders the application of biochemical, including enzymatic, and ultrastructural methods to biopsy material or fibroblasts or chondrocytes in culture promises to lead to important advances in the near future.

To bring some order out of the terminologic and nosologic chaos of the skeletal dysplasias a working group met in Paris in 1969[91a] and prepared a suggested nomenclature, which unavoidably was to some extent also a classification (Table 73–2).

The classification made a distinction between osteochondrodysplasias (abnormalities of cartilage and/or bone growth and development) and dysostoses (malformations of individual bones, singly or in combination). For some disorders the distinction was difficult or to some extent arbitrary. Pyknodysostosis, for example, has mandibular malformation, a dysplasia, and increased bone density, a dysostosis.

A special effort was made to avoid eponyms. Only those were retained which are in wide use for conditions which lack another satisfactory eponym. Some new terms were suggested, e.g., *metaphyseal chondrodysplasia* for *metaphyseal dysostosis* and *cleidocranial dysplasia* for *cleidocranial dysostosis*.

Key references for most of the disorders are provided. A description of each and further references are available in McKusick's *Mendelian Inheritance in Man*.[87]

BIBLIOGRAPHY

1. Abul-Haj, S. K., Martz, D. G., Douglas, W. F. and Geppert, L. J.: J. Pediat., *61*, 221, 1962.

1a. Albright, F., Butler, A. M., Hampton, A. O., and Smith, P.: New Engl. J. Med., *216*, 727, 1937.

2. Allison, A. C. and Blumberg, B. S.: J. Bone & Joint Surg., *401B*, 538, 1958.

3. Amman, F.: J. Génét. hum., *18* (Suppl.), 1, 1970.

4. Anderson, I. F.: S. Afr. Med. J., *39*, 1066, 1965.

5. Andren, L., Dymling, J. F., Hogeman, K. E. and Wendeberg, B.: Acta Chir. Scand., *124*, 496, 1962.

5a. Angle, C. R.: Pediatrics, *13*, 193, 1954.

6. Austin, J. H.: In, *Medical Aspects of Mental Retardation*. Ed., C. C. Carter, Springfield, Ill., Charles C Thomas, 1965.

7. Bakwin, H., Golden, A , and Fox, S.: Amer. J. Roentgenol., *91*, 609, 1964.

7a. Bannerman, R. M.: In, *Clinical Delineation of Birth Defects*. IV. *Skeletal Dysplasias*, Bergsma, D. (ed.), New York: National Foundation-March of Dimes, 1969.

8. Bartter, F. C.: In, *The Metabolic Basis of Inherited Disease*. Stanbury, J. B., Wyngaarden, J. B. and Fredrickson, D. S., eds. New York, McGraw-Hill, (2nd Ed.) pp. 1015–1023, 1966.

9. Beals, R. K.: J. Bone & Joint Surg., *51A*, 728, 1969.
9a. Beals, R. K. and Hecht, F.: J. Bone & Joint Surg., *53A*, 1071, 1971.
10. Beighton, P.: Brit. Med. J., *3*, 409, 1968.
11. Beighton, P.: *The Ehlers-Danlos Syndrome.* London, William Heinemann Medical Books Ltd., 1970.
12. Berlin, R., Hedensio, B., Lilja, B., and Linder, L.: Acta Med. Scand., *181*, 305, 1967.
13. Bianchine, J. W., Stambler, A. A. and Harrison, H. E.: In, *Clinical Delineation of Birth Defects. X. Endocrine System*, Bergsma, D., Ed., Baltimore, Williams and Wilkins, 1971.
14. Black, J.: Arch. Dis. Child., *35*, 633, 1961.
15. Bloom, D.: J. Pediat., *68*, 103, 1966.
16. Bohme, A.: Z. gesam. inn. Med., *18*, 491, 1963.
17. Brady, R. O.: New Engl. J. Med., *275*, 312, 1966.
18. Brailsford, J. F.: Amer. J. Surg., *7*, 404, 1929.
19. Brocher, J. E. W., Klein, D., Bamatter, F., Franceschetti, A., and Boreux, G.: Fortsch. Roentgenstr., *109*, 185, 1968.
20. Caffey, J.: *Pediatric X-Ray Diagnosis*, 5th Ed., Chicago, Year Book Medical Publishers, 1967.
21. ———: Amer. J. Roentgenol., *100*, 1, 1967.
22. Campbell, C. J., Papademetriou, T., and Bonfiglio, M.: J. Bone & Joint Surg., *50A*, 1281, 1968.
23. Carter, C. O. and Sweetnam, R.: J. Bone & Joint Surg., *40B*, 664, 1958.
24. ———: J. Bone & Joint Surg., *42B*, 721, 1960.
25. Carter, C. O. and Wilkinson, J.: J. Bone & Joint Surg., *46B*, 40, 1964.
26. Clausen, J. and Rampini, S.: Acta neurol. Scand., *46*, 313, 1970.
27. Cross, H. E. and Opitz, J.: J. Pediat., *75*, 1037, 1969.
28. Danes, B. S., and Bearn, A. G.: Science, *149*, 987, 1965.
29. ———: Lancet, *1*, 241, 1967.
30. Dent, C. E. and Friedman, M.: Quart. J. Med., *34*, 177, 1965.
31. Dent, C. E., Friedman, M. and Watson, L.: J. Bone & Joint Surg., *50B*, 708, 1968.
32. Drachman, D. B.: In, *Clinical Delineation of Birth Defects.* VIII. *Muscle.* Bergsma, D. (ed.), Baltimore: Williams and Wilkins, 1971.
33. Durand, P., Barrone, C. and Della Cella, G.: J. Pediat., *75*, 665, 1969.
34. Elsbach, L.: J. Bone & Joint Surg., *41B*, 514, 1959.
35. Fairbank, T.: Brit. J. Surg., *34*, 225, 1947.
36. Falls, H. F. and Schull, W. J.: Arch. Ophthal., *63*, 409, 1960.
37. Felman, A. H. and Kirkpatrick, J. A., Jr.: Radiology, *93*, 1037, 1969.
38. Forland, M.: Amer. J. Med., *33*, 792, 1962.
39. Fratantoni, J. C., Hall, C. W., and Neufeld, E. F.: Proc. Nat. Acad. Sci., *60*, 699, 1968.
40. Fratantoni, J. C., Hall, C. W., and Neufeld, E. F.: Science, *162*, 570, 1968.
41. Gatti, R. A., Platt, N., Pomerance, H. H., Hong, R., Langer, L. O., Kay, H. E. M. and Good, R. A.: J. Pediat., *75*, 675, 1969.
42. Giedion, A.: Helv. Paediat. Acta, *21*, 475, 1966.
43. Girdany, B. R.: Clin. Orthop., *14*, 102, 1959.
44. Gordon, H., Davies, D. and Berman, M.: J. Med. Genet., *6*, 266, 1969.
45. Gorlin, R. J. and Cohen, M. M., Jr.: Amer. J. Dis. Child., *118*, 487, 1969.
46. Gorlin, R. J., Meskin, L. H. and St. Geme, J. W.: J. Pediat., *63*, 69, 1963.
47. Gorlin, R. J. and Pindborg, J. J.: In, *Syndromes of the Head and Neck.* New York: McGraw-Hill Book Co., 1964. pp. 438–446.
48. Gorlin, R. J., Sedano, H. O. and Cervenka, J.: Pediatrics, *41*, 503, 1968.
49. Gorlin, R. J., Spranger, J. and Koszalka, M. F.: In, *Clinical Delineation of Birth Defects.* Vol. 5, Part IV. *Skeletal Dysplasias.* Birth Defects: Original Article Series. New York, National Foundation-March of Dimes, 1969. pp. 79–95.
50. Gunderson, C. H., Greensplan, R. H., Glaser, G. H. and Lubs, H. A., Jr: Medicine, *46*, 491, 1967.
51. Hall, J. G. and Dorst, J. P.: In, *The Clinical Delineation of Birth Defects.* Part IV. *Dysplasias.* New York, National Foundation-March of Dimes, 1969, pp. 242–259.
52. Hall, J. G., Levin, J., Kuhn, J. P., Offenheimer, E. J., Van Berkum, K. A. P., and McKusick, V. A.: Medicine, *48*, 411, 1969.
53. Halliday, J. A.: Brit. J. Surg., *37*, 52, 1949.
53a. Hansen, O. H. and Andersen, N. O.: Acta orthop. Scand., *41*, 225, 1970.
54. Hass, J., and Hass, R.: J. Bone & Joint Surg., *40A*, 663, 1958.
55. Holden, J. D.: Develop. Med. Child. Neurol., *9*, 457, 1967.
56. Holt, J. F.: Ann. Radiol., *9*, 209, 1966.
56a. Jago, R. H.: Arch. Dis. Child., *45*, 277, 1970.

57. JEANLOZ, R. W.: Arth. & Rheum., *3*, 233, 1960.
58. JOHNSTON, C. C., JR., LAVY, N., LORD, T., VELLIOS, F., MERRITT, A. D. and DEISS, W. P., JR.: Medicine, *47*, 149, 1968.
59. JONES, W. A.: Oral Surg. Oral Med. & Oral Pathol., *20*, 648, 1965.
60. JUHL, J. H., WESENBERG, R. L. and GWINN, J. L.: Radiology, *89*, 646, 1967.
61. KENNY, F. M., ACETO, T., JR., PURISCH, M., HARRISON, H. E., HARRISON, H. C. and BLIZZARD, R. M.: J. Pediat., *62*, 531, 1963.
62. KEY, J. A.: J.A.M.A., *88*, 1710, 1927.
63. KIRKHAM, T. H.: Arch. Dis. Child, *44*, 504, 1969.
64. KLEIN, D. and AMMANN, F.: J. Neurol. Sci., *9*, 479, 1969.
65. KLOEPFER, H. W., and ROSENTHAL, J. W.: Amer. J. Hum. Genet., *7*, 398, 1955.
66. KOZLOWSKI, K., MAROTEAUX, P. and SPRANGER, J.: Presse med., *75*, 2769, 1967.
67. LAMY, M. and MAROTEAUX, P.: Arch. Franç. Pediat., *18*, 693, 1961.
68. LANGER, L. O.: Radiology, *89*, 654, 1967.
69. LANGER, L. O., JR.: Amer. J. Roentgen., *93*, 399, 1965.
70. ————: Radiology, *82*, 833, 1964.
71. ————: Radiology, *91*, 447, 1968.
72. LANGER, L. O., JR., BAUMANN, P. A., and GORLIN, R. J.: Amer. J. Roentgen., *100*, 12, 1967.
73. LANGER, L. O., JR., SPRANGER, J. W., GREINACHER, I. and HERDMAN, R. C.: Radiology, *92*, 285, 1969.
74. LAROSE, J. H. and GAY, B. B., JR.: Amer. J. Roentgen., *106*, 156, 1969.
75. LATTA, R. J., GRAHAM, C. B., AASE, J., SCHAM, S. M. and SMITH, D. W.: J. Pediat., *78*, 291, 1971.
76. LENZ, W. D. and HOLT, J. F.: In, *Clinical Delineation of Birth Defects*. Part IV. *Skeletal Dysplasias*. New York, National Foundation-March of Dimes, 1969. pp. 71–75.
77. LEROY, J. G., DEMARS, R. I. and OPITZ, J. M.: In, *Clinical Delineation of Birth Defects*. Part V. *Birth Defects*: *Skeletal Dysplasias*, New York, National Foundation-March of Dimes, 1969, pp. 174–185.
78. LLOYD-ROBERTS, G. C.: J. Bone & Joint Surg., *37B*, 8, 1955.
79. LUCAS, G. L. and OPITZ, J. M.: J. Pediat., *68*, 273, 1966.
80. MACDONALD, W. B., FITCH, K. D. and LEWIS, I. C.: Pediatrics, *25*, 997, 1960.
81. MACLEOD, W.: Brit. J. Radiol., *39*, 224, 1966.
82. MAHLOUDJI, M., TEASDALL, R. D., ADAMKIEWICZ, J. J., HARTMANN, W. H., LAMBIRD, P. A. and MCKUSICK, V. A.: Medicine, *48*, 1, 1969.
83. MANN, J. B., ALTERMAN, S. and HILLS, A. G.: Ann. Intern. Med., *56*, 315, 1962.
84. MAROTEAUX, P.: Ann. Radiol., *13*, 455, 1970.
85. MCCANCE, R. A.: Quart. J. Med., *16*, 33, 1947.
86. MCKUSICK, V. A.: *Human Genetics*, (2nd. ed.) Englewood Cliffs, N.J., Prentice-Hall, 1969.
87. MCKUSICK, V. A.: *Mendelian Inheritance in Man. Catalogs of Autosomal Dominant, Autosomal Recessive and X-linked Phenotypes*, (3rd. ed.), Baltimore, Johns Hopkins Press, 1971.
88. MCKUSICK, V. A.: *Heritable Disorders of Connective Tissue* (4th ed.). St. Louis, Mosby, 1972.
89. MCKUSICK, V. A., EGELAND, J. A., ELDRIDGE, R. and KRUSEN, D. E.: Bull. J. Hopkins Hosp., *115*, 306, 1964.
90. MCKUSICK, V. A., ELDRIDGE, R., HOSTETLER, J. A., RUANGWIT, U. and EGELAND, J. A.: Bull. J. Hopkins Hosp., *116*, 285, 1965.
91. MCKUSICK, V. A., MAHLOUDJI, M., ABBOTT, M. H., LINDENBERG, R. and KEPAS, D.: New Engl. J. Med., *277*, 279, 1967.
91*a*. MCKUSICK, V. A. and SCOTT, C. I.: J. Bone & Joint Surg., *53A*, 978, 1971.
92. MELNICK, J. C. and NEEDLES, C. F.: Amer. J. Roentgenol., *97*, 39, 1966.
93. MILLARD, D. R., JR., MAISELS, D. O., BATSTONE, J. H. F. and YATES, B. W.: Amer. J. Surg., *113*, 615, 1967.
93*a*. NEVIN, N. C., DODGE, J. A. and KERNOHAN, D. C.: Oral Surg., *29*, 443, 1970.
94. HORUM, R. A.: In, *Clinical Delineation of Birth Defects*. Part IV. *Skeletal Dysplasias*. Birth Defects: Original Article Series, New York, National Foundation-March of Dimes. pp. 326–329, 1969.
94*a*. O'BRIEN, J.: J. Pediat., *75*, 167, 1969.
95. OCKERMAN, P. A.: Lancet, *2*, 239, 1967.
96. PASHAYAN, H., WHELAN, D., GUTTMAN, S. and FRASER, F. C.: J. Pediat., *75*, 853, 1969.
97. PATTON, J. T.: In, *Symposium Ossium*, Jelliffe, A. M. and Strickland, B. (eds.) Edinburgh and London, E. & S. Livingstone, 1970, p. 299.
98. POZNANSKI, A. K., GALL, J. C., JR., and STERN, A. M.: Radiology, *94*, 45, 1970.
99. QUELCE-SALGADO, A.: Acta Genet. Statist. Med., *14*, 63, 1964.
100. RATER, C. J., SELKE, A. C. and VAN EPPS, E. F.: Amer. J. Roentgen., *103*, 589, 1968.
101. RIMOIN, D. L.: New Engl. J. Med., *272*, 923, 1965.

102. Rimoin, D. L. and Edgerton, M. T.: J. Pediat., *72*, 94, 1967.
103. Rimoin, D. L., Fletcher, B. D. and McKusick, V. A.: Amer. J. Med., *45*, 948, 1968.
104. Rosenbloom, A. L. and Smith, D. W.: J. Pediat., *66*, 857, 1965.
105. Rovin, S., Dachi, S. F., Borenstein, D. B. and Cotter, W. B.: J. Pediat., *65*, 215, 1964.
106. Rubin, P.: *Dynamic Classification of Bone Dysplasias*. Chicago, Year Book Publishers, Inc., 1964.
107. Rubinstein, J. H.: In *Clinical Delineation of Birth Defects*. Part II. *Birth Defects*: Original Article Series, New York National Foundation-March of Dimes, 1968, pp. 25–41.
108. Schauerte, E. W. and St. Aubin, P. M.: Amer. J. Roentgen, *97*, 67, 1966.
109. Schnitka, T. K., Asp, D. M. and Horner, R. H.: Cancer, *11*, 627, 1958.
110. Schwarzweller, F.: Z. Menschl. Vererb. Konstitutionsl., *20*, 341, 1937.
111. Scott, C. I.: In, *Clinical Delineation of Birth Defects*. Part II. *Malformation Syndromes*, New York: National Foundation-March of Dimes. 1969, pp. 238–240.
112. Scott, C. I., Jr. and Grossman, M. S.: In, *Clinical Delineation of Birth Defects*. Part V. *Birth Defects: Skeletal Dysplasias*, New York, National Foundation-March of Dimes. 1969, pp. 349–355.
113. Shillito, J., Jr. and Matson, D. D.: Pediatrics, *41*, 829, 1968.
114. Shmerling, D. H., Prader, A., Hitzig, W. H., Giedion, A., Hadorn, B. and Kuhni, M.: Helv. Paediat. Acta, *24*, 547, 1969.
115. Silverman, J. L.: Ann. Intern. Med., *110*, 191, 1962.
116. Smith, J. L. and Stowe, F. R.: Pediatrics, *27*, 128, 1961.
117. Solomon, L.: J. Bone & Joint Surg., *45B*, 292, 1963.
118. Solonen, K. A. and Sulamaa, M.: Annales Chir. Gynaec Fenniae, *47*, 142, 1958.
118*a*. Spranger, J. and Langer, L. O., Jr.: Radiology, *94*, 313, 1970.
119. Spranger, J. W., Opitz, J. M. and Bidder, U.: In, *Clinical Delineation of Birth Defects*. Part XII. *Birth Defects: Skin, Hair and Nails*, Baltimore, Williams and Wilkins, 1971.
120. Spranger, J. W. and Wiedemann, H. R.: Humangenetik, *9*, 113, 1970.
121. Spranger, J., Wiedemann, H. R., Tolksdorf, M., Graucob, E. and Caesar, R.: Ztsch. Kinderheilk., *103*, 285, 1968.
122. Stickler, G. B. and Pugh, D. G.: Mayo Clin. Proc., *42*, 495, 1967.
122*a*. Strasburger, A. K., Hawkins, M. R., Eldridge, R., Hargrave, R. L. and McKusick, V. A.: Bull. Johns Hopkins Hosp., *117*, 108, 1965.
123. Summitt, R. L. and Favara, B. E.: J. Pediat., *74*, 601, 1969.
124. Temtamy, S. A.: J. Pediat., *69*, 111, 1966.
124*a*. Temtamy, S. A. and McKusick, V. A.: In, *Clinical Delineation of Birth Defects*. Bergsma, D. (ed.): Part III. *Limb Malformations*, New York, National Foundation-March of Dimes, 1969.
125. Thieffry, S., Lyon, G., and Maroteaux, P.: Arch. Franç. Pediat., *24*, 425, 1967.
126. Tips, R. L. and Lynch, H. T.: Acta Paediat., *51*, 585, 1962.
127. Torg, J. S., DiGeorge, A. M., Kirkpatrick, J. A., Jr. and Trujillo, M. M.: J. Pediat., *75*, 243, 1969.
128. Torg, J. S. and Steel, H. H.: J. Bone & Joint Surg., *50A*, 1629, 1968.
129. Van Buchem, F. S. P., Hadders, H. N., Hansen, J. F. and Woldring, M. G.: Amer. J. Med., *33*, 387, 1962.
130. Vulliamy, D. G. and Normandale, P. A.: Arch. Dis. Child., *41*, 375, 1966.
131. Walker, B. A., Beighton, P. H. and Murdoch, J. L.: Ann. Intern. Med., *71*, 349, 1969.
132. Walker, B. A. and Murdoch, J. L.: Arch Intern. Med., *126*, 276, 1970.
133. Walker, J. C., Jr., Meijer, R. and Aranda, D.: J. Ped. Surg., *4*, 569, 1969.
134. Warkany, J., Monroe, B. B. and Sutherland, B. S.: Amer. J. Dis. Child., *102*, 249, 1961.
135. Weismann, U. and Neufeld, E. F.: Science, *169*, 72, 1970.
136. Welch, J. P. and Temtamy, S. A.: J. Med. Genet., *3*, 104, 1966.
137. Weyers, H. and Thier, C. J.: J. Génét. hum., *7*, 143, 1958.
138. Williams, T. F., Winters, R. W. and Burnett, C. H.: In, *The Metabolic Basis of Inherited Disease*. Stanbury, J. B., Wyngaarden, J. B. and Fredrickson, D. S., Eds. (2nd ed.). New York, McGraw-Hill, 1966, pp. 1179–1199.
139. Wynne-Davies, R.: J. Bone & Joint Surg., *52B*, 704, 1970.

Chapter 74

Hypertrophic Osteoarthropathy

By David S. Howell, M.D.

HYPERTROPHIC OSTEOARTHROPATHY

Familial Idiopathic Hypertrophic Osteoarthropathy, Marie-Bamberger's Syndrome, Osteoarthropathie Hypertrophiante and Pneumique, Secondary Hypertrophic Osteoarthropathy

Few clinical abnormalities manifest so ancient a vintage as clubbing—yet little more is known of its pathogenesis today than when recorded circa 400 B.C. by Hippocrates.[12] In addition to clubbing, bone and joint changes were noted by Bamberger and Marie (1889, 1890, respectively).[1,19] The term *hypertrophic osteoarthropathy* refers to a syndrome including clubbing of fingers and toes, periostitis with new osseous formation at the ends of long bones, arthritis, and signs of autonomic disorders, such as flushing, blanching, and profuse sweating —most severe in hands and feet. The syndrome is classified: (1) *secondary* to other diseases, (2) *hereditary* or (3) *idiopathic* (pachydermoperiostosis).[30] The syndrome is to be distinguished from the isolated firm thickening of distal phalanges with clubbing of congenital origin. Clubbing associated with various extrathoracic diseases, discussed below, wherein periosteal ossification and arthritis rarely develop,[13] may be, in some instances, a forme fruste of hypertrophic osteoarthropathy or may bear no direct relationship to it.

Pathology

Pathologic changes develop at the distal end of metacarpal, metatarsal and long bones of the forearms and legs.[8] In severe disease, ribs, clavicles, scapulae, pelvis and malar bones sometimes are afflicted. The earliest histologic alterations are round cell infiltration and edema of the periosteum, synovial membrane, articular capsule and neighboring subcutaneous tissues. These changes are associated with lifting of the periosteum, deposition of osteoid matrix beneath it, and subsequent mineralization. Such foci enlarge so that eventually distal parts of the long bones become ensheathed with a cuff of new bone (Fig. 74–1). Concurrent with thickening, there is accelerated resorption of endosteal and

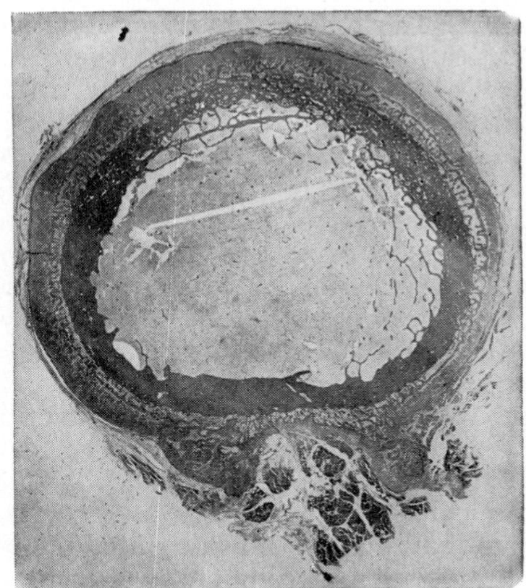

Fig. 74–1.—Cross section through a metatarsal of a patient with hypertrophic osteoarthropathy. The periosteum shows thickening with an irregular cuff of new bone deposited over the cortex. (F. C. Bartter and W. Bauer in Cecil and Loeb, *Textbook of Medicine*, courtesy of W. B. Saunders Company.)

Haversian bone so that the resultant structure is weakened and pathologic fractures may occur. With advancing disease, the pathologic alterations spread proximally along the shafts. Synovial membranes adjoining the involved bones often are edematous and infiltrated with lymphocytes, plasma cells and a few polymorphonuclear leukocytes. Advancing proliferative fibrous tissue at joint margins sometimes is associated with cartilage degeneration. In clubbed phalanges, there is edema of the soft parts, thickening of the blood vessel walls, cellular infiltration, fibroblastic proliferation and growth of new collagenous tissue. These changes result in the uniform enlargement of terminal segments. Similar histopathologic changes have been found both in the hereditary and secondary forms.

Etiology

This syndrome usually appears secondary to other systemic diseases—particularly neoplasms or suppurative conditions of the lungs, mediastinum and pleura. In a small proportion of patients the disorder is hereditary, whereas in others it is idiopathic. Hypertrophic osteoarthropathy has been observed in 5 to 10 per cent of patients with intrathoracic neoplasms.[17,5,31] The most frequent tumor is bronchogenic carcinoma: tumors of the pleura rank high but metastatic lesions are an uncommon cause of osteoarthropathy.[32] The syndrome often accompanies lung abscess, bronchiectasis and empyema, but with improved therapy of chronic infections incidence of osteoarthropathy due to suppurative states has declined. Hypertrophic osteoarthropathy is associated occasionally with chronic pneumonitis, pneumoconiosis, pulmonary tuberculosis, and mediastinal Hodgkin's disease.

For lack of convincing evidence of its separate nature, thyroid achropachy may be considered as a secondary form of hypertrophic osteoarthropathy. The full syndrome of hypertrophic osteoarthropathy has been rarely documented in the presence of cyanotic heart disease[23] and various other extrathoracic diseases. Unless there is also periosteal and synovial involvement in such cases, the term "clubbing" rather than hypertrophic osteoarthropathy is preferable.[13]

Among diseases of the heart accompanied by this syndrome, congenital malformations predominate, yet it seldom is seen in congenital heart disease without cyanosis, unless there is a complicating chronic pulmonary infection or bacterial endocarditis. Clubbing is a sign of the latter disease only with left-sided heart lesions and probably indicates embolization. Hypertrophic osteoarthropathy sometimes appears with a rare disease, primary cholangiolitic cirrhosis, but is found in lower incidence with toxic, biliary or portal cirrhosis.[2] Clubbing has been described in the presence of secondary hepatic amyloidosis but a suppurative process may have been instrumental.[20] Among gastrointestinal diseases leading to osteoarthropathy diarrheal states predominate. These include ulcerative colitis, regional enteritis, intestinal tuberculosis, amoebic or bacillary dysentery, idiopathic steatorrhea, sprue, neoplasms of the small intestine, multiple colonic polyposis, as well as carcinoma of the colon. Clubbing has developed following thyroidectomy for Graves' disease, in hyperparathyroidism and, rarely, in a miscellaneous group of disorders in which the diagnosis of arthropathy is often questionable.[20,5,27] *Unilateral* clubbing results from aneurysms of the aorta, subclavian or innominate artery, as well as axillary tumors, subluxations of the shoulder, apical lung cancer, and brachial arteriovenous aneurysm. *Unidigital* clubbing is reported following injury to the median nerve, in sarcoidosis and tophaceous gout. "Paddle fingers" occasionally develop in bass violin players.

Pathogenesis

The nature of the genetic factors operative in the idiopathic form of hypertrophic osteoarthropathy is unknown. In the secondary type it has been postulated that the vascular proliferation and osteogenesis may be produced by: (1) obscure autonomic reflexes stimulated at the site of underlying disease, (2) a high local arteriolar pulse pressure [possibly also involving (1) or (3)], (3) toxins liberated by primary malignant lesions, and (4) osteoblastic-stimulating agents released at the site of malignant pulmonary lesions or by pluripotential cells of pleural membranes.

Factors which might condition susceptibility of an individual with intrathoracic disease to develop the hypertrophic osteoarthropathy are unknown. But there is evidence for the participation of a local circulatory disorder.[20,22] Increased vascularity of clubbed fingers (secondary type) has been shown by measurement of skin temperature, infrared photography, nailbed capillaroscopy and postmortem arteriography.[11,25] Mendlowitz clearly demonstrated elevated digital pulse pressure and blood flow in patients with the condition and a return to normal pressures following removal of pulmonary lesions.[20,21] Evidence for growth hormone production by bronchogenic carcinomas provides a possible explanation for joint marginal bony overgrowth observed in some afflicted patients.[3,7] Ginsburg noted that abnormal vascular responses to intravenous infusion of epinephrine disappeared after excision of lung tumor.[9] Striking resolution of symptoms and signs in such cases attends simple denervation of the hilum or vagotomy on the same side as the lesion;[13,26,5] thoracotomy alone is ineffective.

Dogs with pulmonary metastases from extrathoracic tumors frequently develop hypertrophic osteoarthropathy. Such dogs have been the subject of cross-circulation studies, but in one type of experiment the data failed to demonstrate any factor in the blood of the donor (osteoarthropathic) dog that would produce peripheral vascular effects, at least as measured by plethysmography, in the normal recipient animal.[28] Further study of such animal preparations seems warranted with the hope of unraveling pathophysiologic mechanism of hypertrophic osteoarthropathy.

Clinical Description

Clubbing, alone, produces no symptoms except for occasional burning or warmth of the fingertips. For this reason, the physician generally precedes the patient in observing the deformity. At the beginning of the disease one observes increased convexity of the nailbeds in sagittal and cross-sectional planes. Loss of the normal 15-degree angle between the nail's proximal portion and dorsal surface of the phalanx also is an early sign. Excessive sweating or warmth of the fingertips, eponychia, paronychia, breaking or loosening of the nail, hangnails and accelerated nail or cuticle growth are frequent. The nail base will rock on pressure due to softening from the underlying proliferative tissue. In advanced stages, fingers may assume a drumstick appearance and the distal interphalangeal joints show hyperextensibility (Fig. 74–2). Similar changes occur in the toes. There may be spade-like enlargement of the hands and feet. Also, coarsening of the facial features and thickened furrowed skin of the face (leonine facies) and scalp may develop.

In regard to bones and joints, symptoms range widely from mild arthralgias (often there are asymptomatic periosteal reactions) to severe, deep-seated aching or burning pain and tenderness over the long bones, progressive clumsiness of hands and awkwardness of gait. Concomitant with these symptoms is variable heat, erythema, swelling with effusion of the wrists, elbows, metacarpophalangeal joints, knees, ankles, and other regions discussed under Pathology, restricted joint motion and ankylosis. Aggravation of bone pain on dependency of the limbs is a unique feature suggesting that local vascular stasis may play a role in production of pain. Gynecomastia, as well as

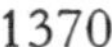

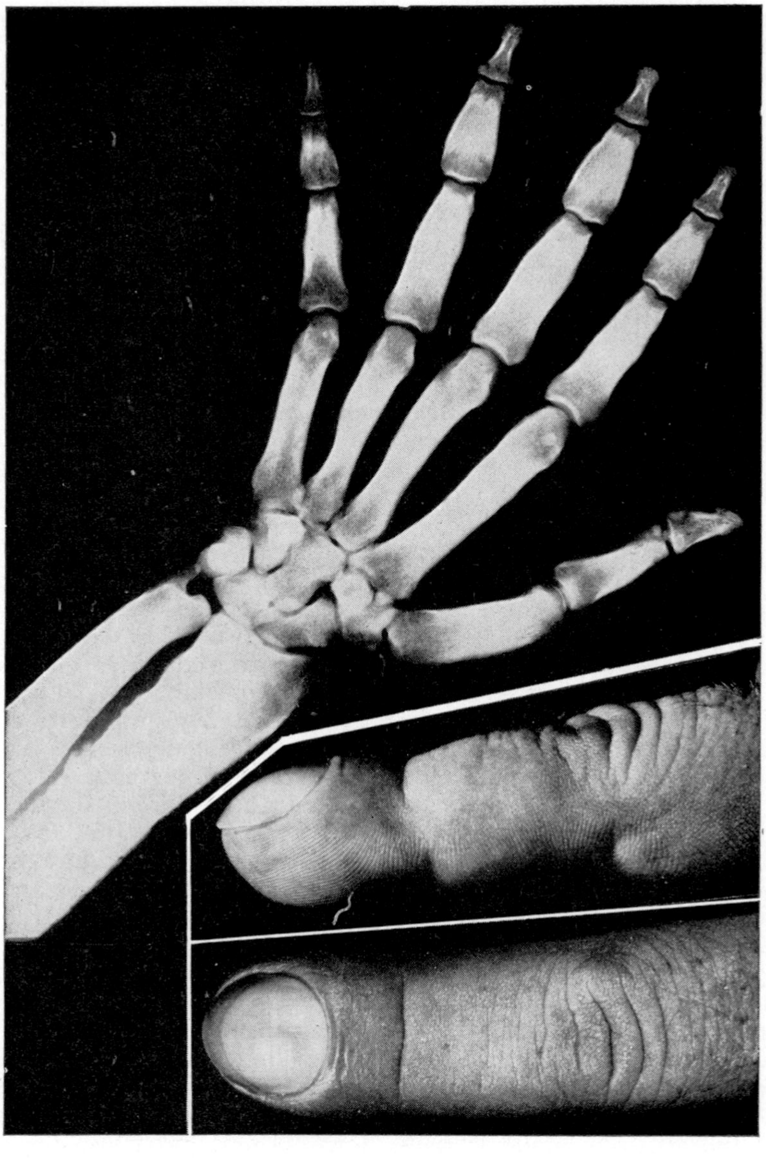

FIG. 74-2.—Hippocratic finger and roentgenogram of hand showing the characteristic features of hypertrophic osteoarthropathy. (Campbell *et al.*, Proc. Staff Meet. Mayo Clin.)

elevation of urinary estrogen excretion, is noted sometimes in patients with hypertrophic osteoarthropathy, but the significance is obscure.[9,16] Insidious development of symptoms and signs over a period of months or years generally characterizes osteoarthropathy associated with suppurative disease of the lungs, and rheumatic complaints are mild. In contrast, a rapidly progressing syndrome with prominent joint pain and stiffness is common with malignant diseases.

Efforts should be exerted to exclude primary disease before relegating patients to the ill-defined hereditary or idiopathic groups. This is emphasized because of the danger of overlooking a resectable tumor or other treatable lesions. In either hereditary or idiopathic osteoarthropathy there is often onset of the syndrome after puberty, a self-limited clinical course after one to two decades, and detection in other members of the family.[3] Findings in these cases range from clubbing, alone, to widespread periosteal thickening of the long bones, metacarpals, metatarsals, and distal phalanges, with limitation of joint motion and ankle edema; usually bone and joint pain is absent. Some of these patients have shown gynecomastia, thickening of the skin over the face and limbs (cutis verticis gyrata), feminine distribution of hair, striae, acne vulgaris, and hypertrophy or atrophy of the ungual tufts of the fingers, all of which become manifest at adolescence.[28,29,30] The hereditary form is transmitted as a Mendelian dominant trait. Thyroid achropachy is manifested by (present or past) hyperthyroidism, pretibial myxedema, exophthalmos, clubbing and periosteal elevation of phalanges, metacarpals and metatarsals.[6]

Differential Diagnosis

The presence of clubbing simplifies diagnosis and a primary disease is sought. Yet, if acute polyarthritis precedes clubbing by months or years, search for an asymptomatic pulmonary neoplasm may be neglected and the case mislabeled rheumatoid arthritis.[15,24] In most instances, x rays reveal elevation of the periosteum and evidence of new bone growth (Fig. 74–3). To be differentiated are periosteal elevations resulting from tumors, lymphangitis, syphilis and hemorrhages of trauma or scurvy (Fig. 74–4). Swelling and tenderness of the lower legs may falsely suggest thrombophlebitis,

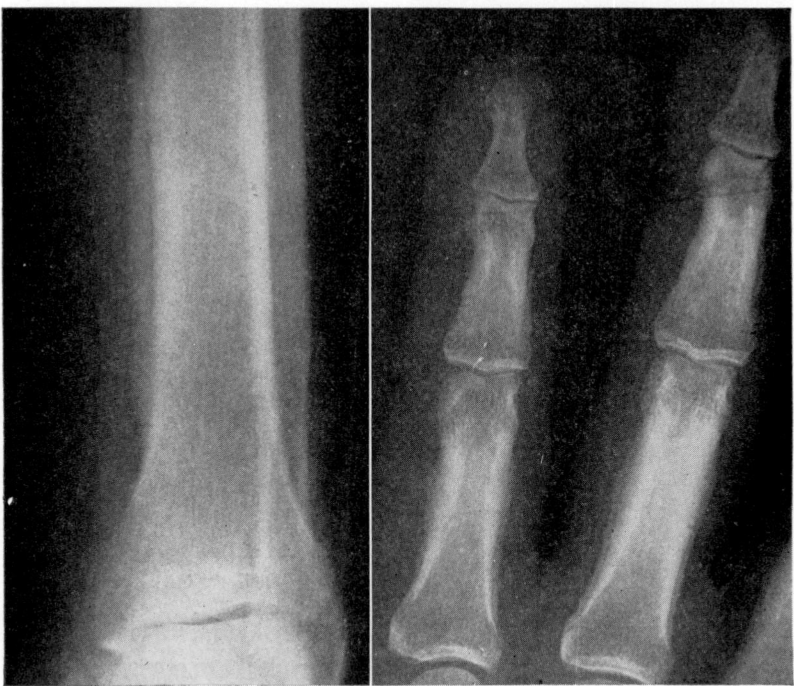

Fig. 74–3.—Hypertrophic osteoarthropathy. Radiodense bands along a margin of the shaft indicate new osseous formation beneath the elevated periosteum. Appearance of these typical lesions is similar in phalanges (*right*) to that of long bones (*left*). (Courtesy of the late Dr. J. J. Bunim.)

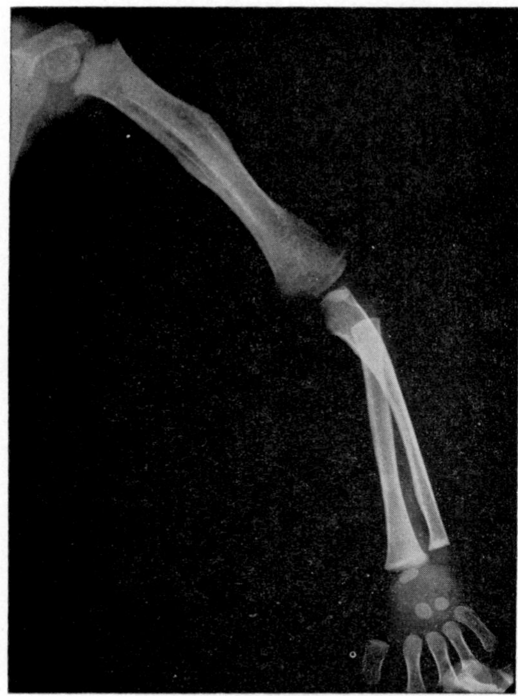

Fig. 74–4.—Periosteal reaction in a patient with scurvy (following recent antiscorbutic treatment). Trauma, syphilis or scurvy, although a cause of proliferative periostitis, should rarely be confused with hypertrophic osteoarthropathy. (From Stein, Stein and Beller, *Living Bone in Health and Disease*, courtesy of J. B. Lippincott Company.)

and bony pains be misinterpreted as peripheral neuritis. Spoon-shaped nails of hypochromic anemia should be readily distinguishable.

Treatment

Clubbing (for lack of symptoms) usually requires no treatment. Disabling symptoms related to joints and bones generally respond with dramatic promptness to removal of the primary pulmonary lesion or to intrathoracic vagotomy.[13,5,18] Supportive analgesic measures, or, in some instances, treatment with adrenocortical steroid derivatives may be useful.[13] Complete disappearance of hypertrophic osteoarthropathy is described after appropriate therapy for empyema, lung abscess, bronchiectasis and pneumonia. Treatment of the idiopathic form is symptomatic.

BIBLIOGRAPHY

1. Bamberger, E. von: Wein. Klin. Wschr., *2*, 226, 1891.
2. Buchan, D. J., and Mitchell, D. M.: Ann. Intern. Med., *66*, 130, 1967.
3. Cameron, D. P., Burger, H. G., Dekretzer, D. M., Catt, K. J., and Best, J. B.: Austral. Ann. Med., *18*, 143, 1969.
4. Camp, J. D. and Scanlan, R. L.: Radiology, *50*, 581, 1948.
5. Christian, C. S.: Arthritis and Rheumatism (Nineteenth Rheumatism Review) Arth. & Rheum. *13*, No. 5, 1970.
6. Diamond, M. T.: Ann. Intern. Med., *50*, 206, 1959.
7. DuPont, B.: Acta Med. Scand., *188*, 25, 1970.
8. Gall, E. A., Bennett, G. A., and Bauer, W.: Amer. J. Path., *27*, 349, 1951.
9. Ginsburg, J.: Quart, J. Med., *27*, 335, 1958.
10. Ginsburg, J. and Brown, J. B.: Lancet, *2*, 1274, 1961.
11. Harter, J. S.: Discussion to van Hagel. J. Thoracic Surg., *9*, 505, 1939–40.
12. Hippocrates (c. 400 B.C.): The Genuine Works of Hippocrates, Translated by F. Adams, Vol. 1, p. 249, New Syndenham Society.
13. Holling, H. E. and Brodey, R. S.: J.A.M.A., *178*, 977, 1961.
14. Holling, H. E., Brodey, R. S., and Boland, H. C. Lancet, *2*, 7215, 1961.
15. Holmes, H. H., Bauman, E., and Ragan, C.: Ann. Rheum. Dis., *9*, 169, 1950.
16. Jao, J. Y., Barlow, J. J., and Krant, M. J.: Ann. Intern. Med., *70*, 581, 1969.
17. Lansbury, J.: Geriatrics, *9*, 319, 1954.
18. LeRoux, B. T.: South African Med. J., *42*, 1074, 1968.
19. Marie, P.: Rev. Medicine, *10*, 1, 1890.
20. Mendlowitz, M.: Medicine, *21*, 269, 1942.
21. ———: J. Clin. Invest., *20*, 113, 1941.
22. Mendlowitz, M. and Leslie, A.: Amer. Heart J., *24*, 141, 1942.
23. McLaughlin, G. E., McCarty, D. J., Jr., and Downing, D. F.: Ann. Intern. Med., *67*, 579, 1967.
24. Polley, H. F., Clagett, O. T., McDonald, J. R., and Schmidt, H. W.: Ann. Rheum. Dis., *11*, 314, 1952.

25. Rominger, E.: Deutsche Med. Wchnschr., *46*, 148, 1920.
26. Semple, T. and McCluskie, R. A.: Brit. Med. J., *1*, 754, 1955.
27. Souders, C. R. and Manuell, J. L.: New Engl. J. Med., *250*, 594, 1954.
28. Touraine, A., Solente, A., and Gole, L.: Presse Med., *43*, 1820, 1935.
29. Vogl, A., Blumenfeld, S., and Gutner, L. B.: Amer. J. Med., *18*, 51, 1955.
30. Vogl, A. and Goldfischer, S.: Amer. J. Med., *33*, 166, 1962.
31. Wierman, W. H., Clagett, O. T., and McDonald, J. R.: J.A.M.A., *155*, 1459, 1954.
32. Yacoub, M. H., Simon, G., and Ohnsorge, J.: Thorax, *22*, 226, 1967.

Chapter 75

Tumors of Synovial Joints, Bursae, and Tendon Sheaths

Revised by Alan S. Cohen, M.D.

Neoplasms and other tumorous conditions of the articular structures are relatively uncommon in rheumatologic practice. It is important, nevertheless, that these disorders be given prominent consideration, particularly in cases of monarticular disease, lest there be undue delay in proper diagnosis and treatment. The suspicion of neoplasm usually calls for surgical exploration of the joint.

We shall make no attempt to cover the broad subject of bone tumors in this chapter, although osseous lesions which are located close to articular structures often give rise to symptoms which may be mistaken as evidence of primary joint disease. The reader who is particularly interested in bone tumors is referred to the comprehensive works of Jaffe and of Lichtenstein.[35,48]

PIGMENTED VILLONODULAR SYNOVITIS, BURSITIS, AND TENOSYNOVITIS

Pigmented villonodular synovitis, a term suggested by Jaffe, Lichtenstein, and Sutro (upon whose work much of the following description is based), represents a group of interrelated benign tumorous disorders which involve the linings of joints, bursae, and tendon sheaths and/or the fascial and ligamentous tissues adjacent to tendons.[3,35,36,43,47,62] These lesions consist of villous or nodular growths which are marked by the presence of variable amounts of hemosiderin and cholesterol crystals and variable numbers of multinucleated giant cells embedded in a stroma of loosely or densely packed connective tissue. Although the exact nature of pigmented villonodular synovitis is presently unknown, the condition appears to be basically an inflammatory granuloma rather than a true neoplasm. Repeated hemorrhage into the joints and tendon sheaths has been postulated as an etiologic factor, but the studies have not been conclusive.[33]

There may be either localized or diffuse involvement of the affected tissues. This feature of the disease together with the complex pattern of the histologic findings has led to a bewildering variety of nosologic devices, including benign (giant cell) synovioma, giant cell tumor of tendon sheath or synovium, xanthoma, xanthogranuloma, hemorrhagic villous synovitis, etc.

Pigmented Villonodular Synovitis

This condition occurs chiefly in young adults, and is more frequent in men than women. The joint usually affected is the knee, followed by much less common involvement of the hip, ankle, tarsus, carpus, and elbow.[12,13,35,74] The principal symptoms are pain and swelling, which may be mild and intermittent for a long period of time, and recurrent locking of the joint, which gradually becomes increasingly swollen by effusion. Focal masses are occasionally palpable in or about the joint. The joint fluid is usually sanguineous or dark brown, not viscous and usually does not clot.[14,70] The average white cell count in one series was about 3,000 per cu. mm. with an average of 26 per cent polymorphonuclears. The red cell count varied from 43,000 to 1,780,000. The mucin test varied from fair to good. Roentgenographic examination, in addition to showing evidence of increased amounts of joint fluid, may reveal lobulation and thickening of the synovial tissues, and erosion of neighboring bone.[8,27,56,74] In the case of involvement of the hip and elbow (and on occasion wrist and finger), there may be considerable narrowing of the joint space, bone erosions and uni- and multiloculated cysts in the subchondral bone.[8,13] Arthrograms of the knee have demonstrated enlargement and distortion of the suprapatellar bursa with numerous recesses and filling defects.[69]

The synovial membrane shows a diffuse brownish discoloration and is covered by thick beard-like growth of long tangled villi, fusion and compaction of which lead to the formation of clumps of pedunculated or sessile nodules of varying size.[35] Whether the lesion be localized or diffuse, and predominantly villous or villonodular in its gross appearance, the histological pattern is essentially similar. Both villi and nodules are covered by a thin layer of synovial lining cells and supported by a stroma of connective tissue containing a variably dense collection of round or polyhedral cells (Fig. 75–1). Granules of hemosiderin and crystals of cholesterol are present both as free aggregates and as inclusions in the cytoplasm of superficially and deeply situated cells. There are varying numbers of pigment-bearing multinucleated giant cells in the nodular lesions. The nuclei of these large histiocytes are usually concentrated in the middle of the cell, but may be dispersed about the periphery. In most lesions there also is evidence of fibrosis giving the lesion a complex appearance with spongy

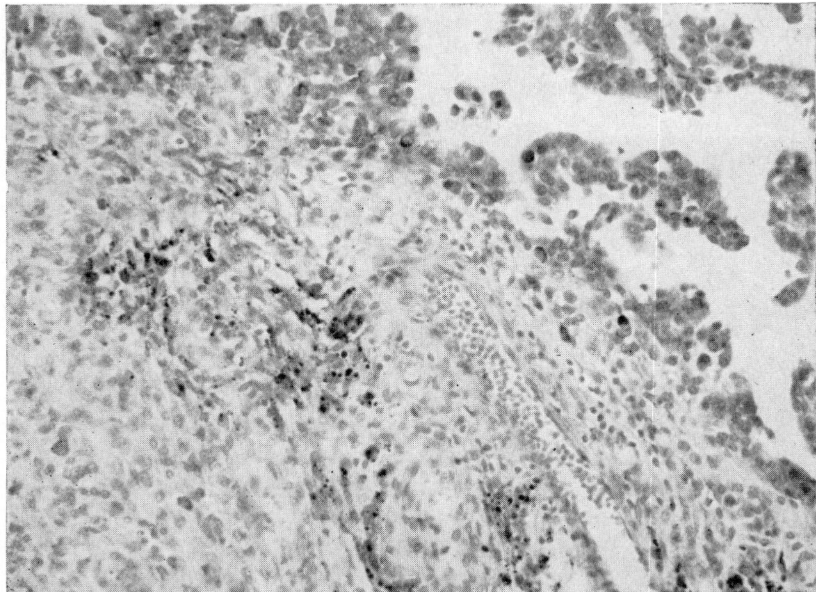

FIG. 75–1.—*Pigmented villonodular synovitis.* Photomicrograph of synovium from knee of a twenty-two-year-old man who had had recurrent pain, swelling, and sanguineous effusion for four years. There are papillary projections covered by synovial lining cells and an abundance of hemosiderin pigment. (Magnification ×175.)

and densely matted areas. An electron microscopic study of the stroma of one case demonstrated that two predominant cell types existed. One resembled the fibroblast of connective tissue and had the organelles usually associated with protein (collagen) synthesis, although some lipid and dense inclusions were also present. The second cell contained electron dense inclusions, hemosiderin and occasionally lipid and was comparable to the macrophage.[83] The fine structure of two additional cases of "giant cell tumor" of tendon sheath also suggested that there were two cell types present and that these macrophage-like and fibroblast-like cells were consistent with a derivation from normal synovial cells.[18]

Localized Nodular Synovitis

Localized involvement of the synovium is more common than the diffuse form of the disease. Here again the joint most commonly affected is the knee, and the patient is usually an adult, who has had symptoms for many months or years before the diagnosis is established. The symptoms may be similar to those of the diffuse disease, but, as would be expected, are less severe. The clinical findings are often considered to be indicative of an internal derangement of the knee, and the true nature of the disturbance not suspected before the joint is examined at surgery and found to contain one or more sessile or stalked yellow-brown nodular growths (Fig. 75–2). The symptoms are often acute and episodic and consist of pain, locking and giving way of the joint. The physical findings are small to moderate effusions and occasional limited range of motion. The synovial fluid is less likely to be sanguineous. X ray of the joint usually shows no abnormality.[26] In the knee, the tumor frequently originates from synovial membrane near a menisco-capsular junction, but it may be located almost anywhere within the joint. Compression of the nodule may lead to fibrosis or necrosis, but the pattern of histologic changes is otherwise quite similar to that encountered in the larger nodules in cases of diffuse villonodular synovitis (Fig. 75–3).

Pigmented Villonodular Bursitis

This is an uncommon lesion, which may be found in the popliteal and certain

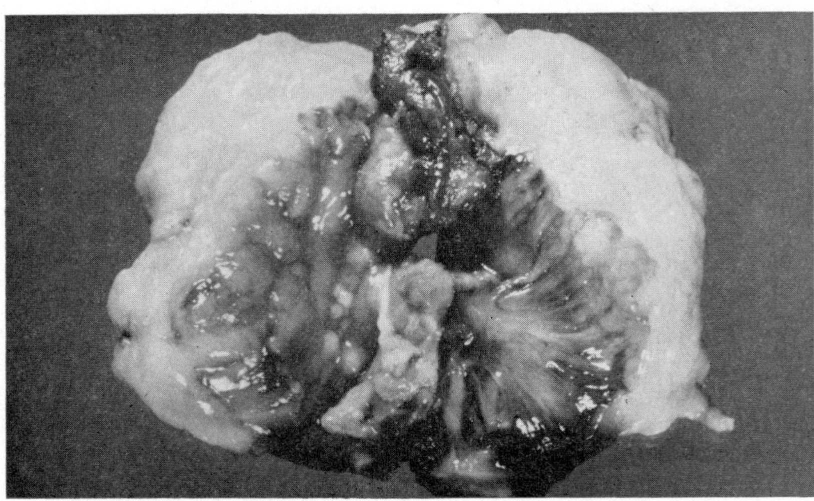

FIG. 75–2.—*Localized nodular synovitis.* Portion of lining tissue from knee joint of a thirteen-year-old boy showing a 1 × 2 cm. pigmented tumor. The patient had had recurrent effusion in the knee for eight months.

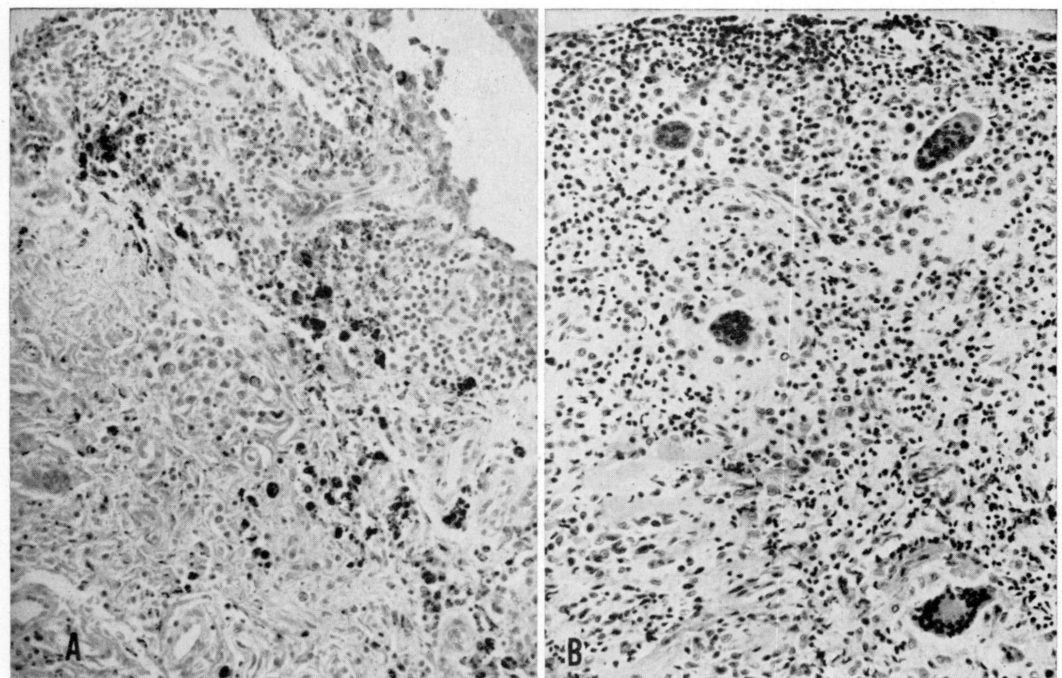

FIG. 75–3.—*Localized nodular synovitis.* Photomicrographs of nodular lesion illustrated in Figure 75–2. (*A*) Large deposits of hemosiderin pigment in richly cellular connective tissue stroma. (*B*) Multinucleated giant cells amid dense infiltrate of small round cells and large cells with pale, spindle-shaped nuclei. (Magnification ×175.)

other bursae, including those about the ankle, and is marked clinically by a slowly enlarging mass. The pathologic findings are similar to those described in pigmented villonodular synovitis.

Localized Nodular Tenosynovitis

This constitutes by far the most common form of the disorder under consideration.[22,24,53,66,73,81] The majority of patients are young or middle-aged adults, and women are affected more often than men. The part most frequently involved is a finger, more often the index or middle, on the volar or dorsal or lateral aspect of which there develops a firm, nodular mass. Less often this lesion is found near a metacarpophalangeal joint, wrist, ankle or toe. In the case of larger lesions, there may be extensive erosion of adjacent bone.[22,49] It is uncommon to find more than a single site affected. Patients with multiple nodules, particularly involving the Achilles tendon and extensor tendons, are more likely to have *xanthoma tuberosum multiplex*, a complication of familial hypercholesterolemia or of hyperlipemia (Figs. 75–4 and 75–5).[21] Nodular tenosynovitis is always benign, and there appears to have been no case in which this lesion has been proven to have undergone malignant change.[66]

The exact site of origin of these growths is a matter of dispute. Clearly, many arise from the linings of the fibrous sheaths of tendons and/or the fascial and ligamentous tissue adjacent to tendons. In some cases, however, the source of the lesion may lie in the dorsal prolongation of the synovial membrane of the distal interphalangeal joint.[81] The growth may consist of a single globular nodule, but is often lobulated and sepa-

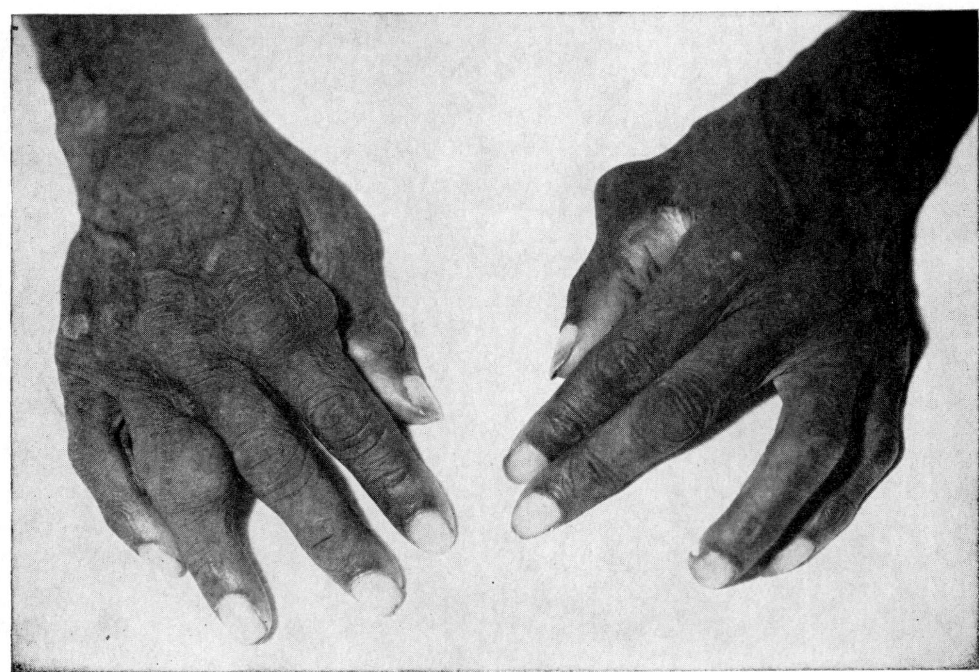

FIG. 75–4.—*Xanthoma tendinosum.* The hands of a seventy-five-year-old man with probable type II hyperlipoproteinemia, who had had nodular swellings involving extensor tendons of several fingers and both Achilles and infrapatellar tendons for more than fifty years. The patient's serum cholesterol concentration was 415 mg. per cent.

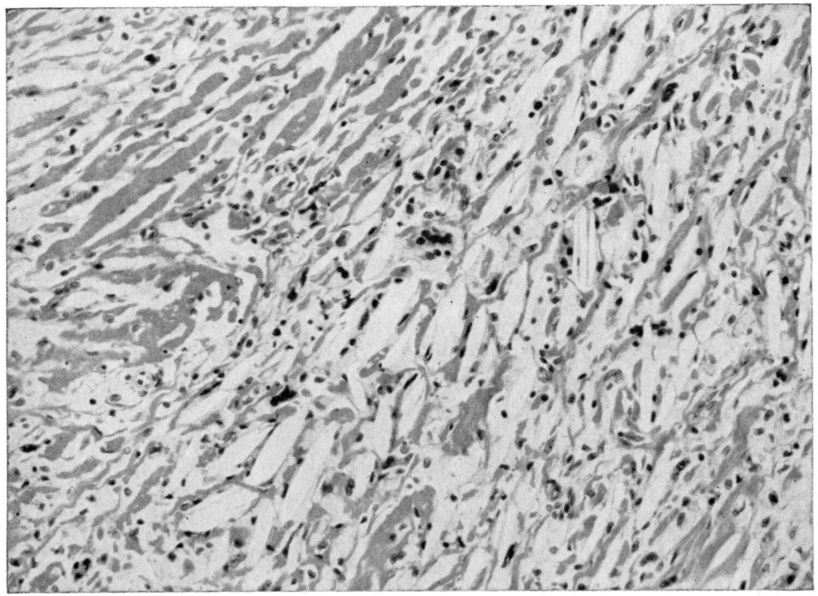

FIG. 75–5.—*Xanthoma tendinosum.* Photomicrograph of tendon nodule removed from the hand of patient illustrated in previous figure. There are numerous large lipid-filled histiocytes with pale foamy cytoplasm, strewn about in a collagenous stroma. The clefts indicate the site of deposition of crystals of cholesterol. (Magnification ×175).

rable into a number of smaller masses, which are gray, yellow or reddish-brown in color, depending upon the relative abundance of fibrous tissue, cholesterol, and hemosiderin. In some cases, histologic examination reveals the pigmented villous proliferation which represents the early stage of this lesion.[35] Most often, however, the pattern is that of the fused cellular nodule, or of the hypocellular fibrous nodule which constitutes the end stage of the inflammatory process.

Pigmented Villonodular Tenosynovitis

Occasionally there is diffuse involvement of the tendon sheaths of the hand and foot, in which the lesions may grow to a large size and cause erosion of neighboring bone.[54]

Pathogenesis

Controversy has centered about the question of whether this condition represents a true neoplasia of synovial tissue (benign giant cell synovioma)[81] or some form(s) of obscure chronic inflammation.[35,49,76] The occasional erosion of adjacent bone by these lesions, their recurrence following incomplete extirpation, and the presence of clefts and of spaces surrounded by synovial lining cells have been held to support the theory of neoplasm. However, Jaffe, who is a strong proponent of the theory of inflammatory hyperplasia, believes that the spaces and clefts in these lesions are due to entrapment of hyperplastic villi following their infolding and fusion, and suggests that exuberant growth represents merely an aggravation of the original proliferative process, which may result from intralesional bleeding.[35] Whatever its nature, the origin of pigmented villonodular synovitis remains unclear. Although in a number of cases there is a history of local injury, neither trauma nor infection appears to play a fundamental role in the origin of this lesion.[66] Changes resembling those of the human disease have been produced experimentally in the knee joints of dogs by repeated intra-articular injection of blood.[84] Although this would appear to support the theory that this condition is the result of intra-articular hemorrhage, it should be noted that the patients show no (other) evidence of a hemorrhagic disorder and that the synovial changes in hemophilic joint disease do not have the histological features observed in villonodular synovitis (*see* Chapter 71).

Treatment

Surgical resection of the lesion, be it localized or diffuse, is the prime treatment.[66] If the extirpation is incomplete, there is likely to be a recurrence of the lesion,[81] which tends to become more florid and is sometimes evident within a few weeks, and requires there be additional surgical intervention. If synovectomy fails in the case of pigmented villonodular synovitis, the patient should receive x-ray therapy. Tissue radiation of between 1500 and 3000 r, given in divided doses, has been followed by prompt improvement and apparent cure.[23,35] Irradiation has also been used (in larger doses) in the treatment of nodular tenosynovitis.

SYNOVIAL CHONDROMATOSIS

In synovial chondromatosis, there are focal metaplastic growths of normal-appearing cartilage in the synovium of a joint (or rarely in a bursa, tendon sheath, joint capsule, or para-articular connective tissue).[35,59,85] Bits of these growths may become detached from the synovium and persist and grow as viable loose bodies within the joint cavity.[20,35,39] When this cartilage becomes calcified and ossified, the condition has been called *synovial osteochondromatosis.* The origin of the disorder is unknown.

Synovial chondromatosis occurs most often as a monarticular disturbance in young or middle-aged adults and is more common in men than women.[60] The joint most frequently involved is the knee, followed by the hip and elbow and shoulder.[55,60,86] Osteochondromatosis of the temporomandibular joint has been reported.[19] In those unusual cases of oligoarticular disease, it is usually both knees which are affected.

The patient may have pain, swelling, and limitation in motion of the joint or may be asymptomatic, and the lesion be discovered quite by accident. Examination of the joint often reveals the presence of loose bodies and increased amounts of synovial fluid. The diagnosis is usually established by the roentgenographic examination, which discloses several small rounded opacities within the confines of the cavity of the joint which may otherwise appear normal[86] (Fig. 75–6). The roentgenogram may be of little aid, however, in those cases of chondromatosis in which the cartilage has not yet become calcified. When the number of loose bodies is very large (joint mice) and/or there is evidence of severe degenerative changes in the joint, synovial chondromatosis is less likely to be the correct diagnosis than some other condition associated with loose joint bodies, such as osteochondritis dissecans and neuropathic arthropathy.

Gross examination of the affected joint reveals variably large and compact clusters of flat or pedunculated cartilaginous nodules protruding from the thickened synovial membrane and variable numbers of loose bodies within the cavity. Microscopic study has indicated that the cartilage found in synovial chondromatosis develops as a result of metaplastic transformation of the synovial connective tissue[26,35,38,39] (Fig. 75–7). The nodules of cartilage are often richly

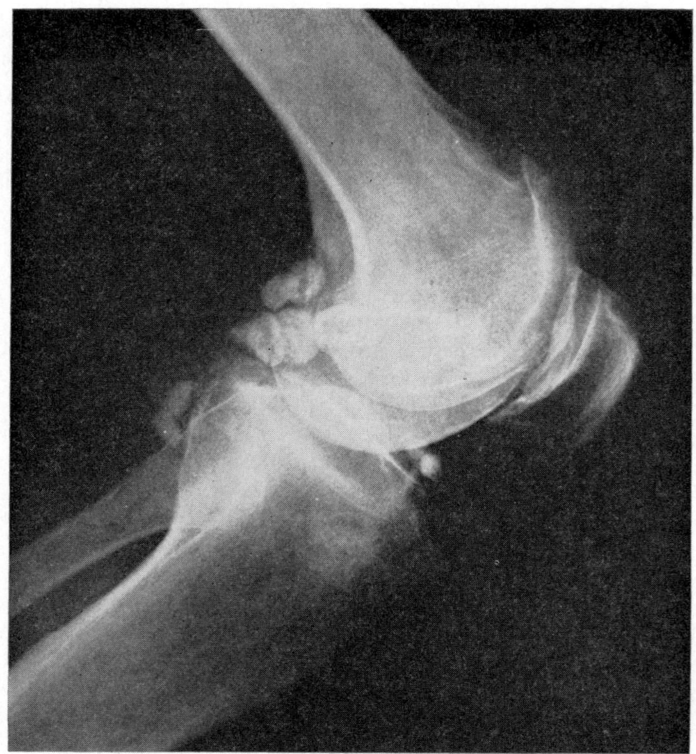

Fig. 75–6.—*Synovial osteochondromatosis.* Lateral roentgenogram of right knee of seventy-two-year-old man who had had intermittent pain and locking of the joint for twenty years. The left knee was not involved

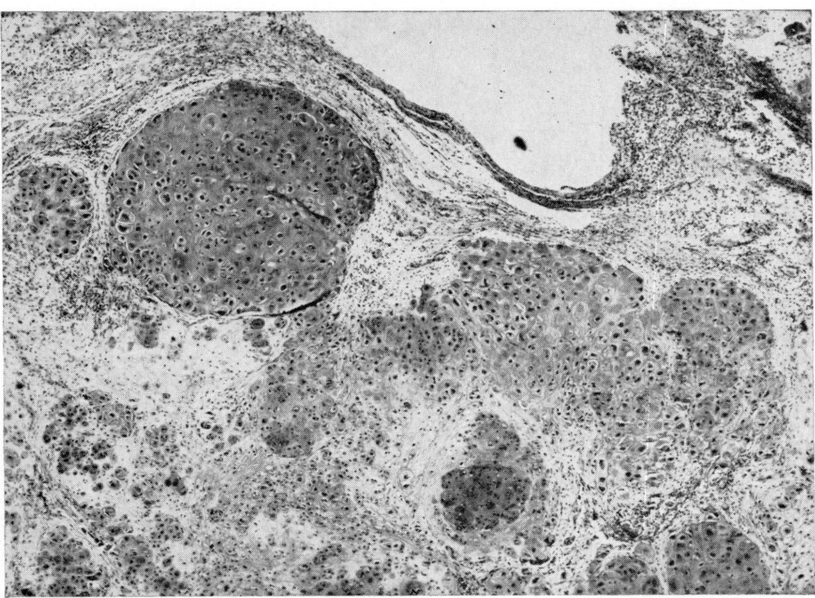

FIG. 75-7.—*Synovial chondromatosis.* Photomicrograph of synovium showing several small islands of relatively highly cellular cartilage lying just beneath the surface of the membrane. (Magnification ×25.)

cellular prior to calcification. In later stages of the development of this lesion, there is invasion by blood vessels followed by the deposition of layers of lamellar bone, which may eventually contain a bit of fatty marrow. Synovial chondromatosis is a benign lesion and rarely, if ever, undergoes malignant change.[25,63]

Treatment

Synovectomy is indicated for relief of pain and disability and should be radical in extent in order to reduce the likelihood of recurrence of the chondromatosis.

BENIGN NEOPLASMS OF THE JOINTS

Hemangioma

The tissue usually affected is the synovial membrane of the knee.[9,29,34,35,40,45,71] In cases in which the joint capsule is diseased, the adjacent soft tissues and bone may become involved. This tumor occurs most often in adolescents or young adults, many of whom have symptoms from the time of childhood, suggesting that the lesion may represent a congenital vascular malformation.[35] The affected joint tends to be periodically painful and swollen, and may contain bloody fluid. There may be repeated locking or buckling. These symptoms often follow mild trauma. If an A–V shunt is present in connection with the hemangioma, there may be increased leg length. In some cases there is a tender doughy joint mass which decreases in size upon elevation of the limb. The roentgenographic examination may show a tumor which contains phlebolithic densities, but is ordinarily of little specific value. When hemangioma is suspected arteriography or phlebography may help to localize the lesion and rule out arteriovenous shunt.[29]

The hemangioma within the joint often takes the form of a dark grape-like mass which is either circumscribed or diffuse in its extent. The circumscribed lesion may be sessile or stalked and commonly originates from the infrapatellar fat pad. In some cases it is difficult to differentiate diffuse hemangiomatous involvement of the synovium from hemorrhagic villonodular synovitis.[35] In circumscribed lesions the histologic pattern is usually that of a capillary and/or cavernous hemangioma, while in the diffuse variety the vascular channels appear venous in nature. Surgical excision, which is usually simple and effective in the case of a circumscribed hemangioma, often proves less satisfactory when there is diffuse involvement of the synovial membrane and regional soft tissues, and the likelihood of recurrence is high. The capsular hemangioma remains benign, however, in its cytologic features.

Hemangiomas may also occur in tendon sheaths and grow to involve both the tendon itself and surrounding structures.[4,30] There is usually a soft compressible swelling which changes when the limb is elevated or a tourniquet is placed above the mass. The roentgenographic examination frequently reveals many calcified phleboliths. The hand, forearm, and ankle are the sites favored by this lesion, which is treated by surgical excision and irradiation.

Lipoma

This is a rare neoplasm, almost all examples of which have been found in the knee joint, usually originating in the subsynovial fat on either side of the patellar ligament or on the anterior surface of the femur.[2,35] Lipomas are also found in tendon sheaths of the hands, wrists, feet, and ankles.[78] Extensor tendons appear to be affected more often than flexor tendons and there may be bilateral involvement. "Lipoma aborescens" represents a villous or polypoid synovial proliferation in response to chronic irritation of the synovium. It is often associated with degenerative joint disease and should not be classified as a neoplasm.

Fibroma

Jaffe has suggested that most of the cases reported as fibromas of joint and tendon sheaths in the older literature were probably examples of the late fibrous stage of pigmented villonodular synovitis.[35] True fibromatous neoplasm appears to be a great rarity.

MALIGNANT NEOPLASMS OF THE JOINTS

These may be either primary or secondary. The former are uncommon and are represented almost solely by the neoplasm known as *synovial sarcoma* or *malignant synovioma*. Secondary involvement of the articular structures, which is less unusual in general experience, occurs as a complication of the contiguous spread of malignant bone tumors (among which the most common are reticulum cell sarcoma, osteogenic sarcoma and chondrosarcoma) or from metastasis of carcinoma.

Synovial Sarcoma

This is a highly malignant and histologically complex neoplasm of connective tissue which is generally found near one or another of the larger joints.[6,10,11,16,28,31,52,64,65,79,80,82] The tumor seldom originates within the joint itself. This lesion has been described under many different names, including malignant synovioma, synovial fibrosarcoma, sarcoendothelioma, and mesothelioma[10] and has been observed in certain domestic animals, including the dog and cow.[17] The reader is referred to the excellent recent monograph by Cade, who has had an extensive personal experience with synovial sarcoma, based upon the care of 100 patients.[10]

Synovial sarcoma occurs most often in an adolescent or young adult, but has been observed at all ages from birth to eighty years. There is a preponderance in men. The lower limb (thigh, leg, foot, knee) is more commonly the site of primary involvement than the upper limb (arm, forearm, hand). Other primary sites have included the buttock, trunk (back), neck, chest or abdominal wall, and orbit.[10,15,31,37,50,52,57,64,75] The characteristic history is that of a slowly growing mass which, in the case of a more deeply situated lesion, may reach considerable size before its detection. When located on the hand or foot, the tumor may resemble a ganglion or distended bursa. Pain is not marked unless the lesion is so placed that it interferes with normal movement of the joint. It is important to note, however, that synovial sarcoma is usually located in the soft tissues at some distance from a joint.

The typical roentgenographic appearance of malignant synovioma is that of (1) a para-articular soft tissue mass of homogeneous density, which has a sharp, discrete border and may be lobulated.[15,72] Less often the mass is irregular in outline and not clearly separable from the surrounding tissues. (2) In some cases the tumor may contain clusters or small foci of calcification.[15,46] (3) Secondary invasion of contiguous bone which produces osteolytic defects[15,72,77] may occur, as well as periosteal reaction nearby. Arteriographic examination has shown greatly increased vascularity, particularly in rapidly growing tumors.[10]

Although there is some variability in the rate of growth and rapidity of metastatic spread, the disease characteristically follows a highly malignant, occasionally fulminating, course.[1,10] The progress of the neoplasm often appears to become more rapid following biopsy or incomplete surgical resection. The sarcoma spreads by direct extension, by invasion of regional lymph nodes, and by visceral and skeletal metastases. The most common site of visceral metastasis is the lung, in which the lesions take the form of multiple large densities ("cannon balls") or a diffuse infiltrate. Osteolytic lesions are more common than sclerotic changes in skeletal metastases.

Synovial sarcomas most commonly originate in peri- and para-articular tissues, including the joint capsule, tendon sheaths, bursae, intermuscular septa and the fascia separating muscles and ligaments. It appears that they may also develop within the substance of bone.[32,44,67] Only rarely does this neoplasm lie within a joint cavity. In those locations which are normally devoid of synovial elements, the tumor presumably arises from metaplastic transformation of primitive tissue or from embryonally segregated synovioblastic cells. The gross appearance of a synovial sarcoma depends upon its place of origin, the duration and rapidity of its growth, and its cellular composition. The color of the tumor, which may be from 1 to 20 or more cm. in diameter, varies from a pale gray-yellow to deep red which is usually the result of hemorrhage. The tumor may be homogeneously firm in consistency when there is a predominance of spindle cell elements (*see* below), or it may be soft and contain cystic spaces filled with mucoid secretions in those cases in which the epithelioid cell type predominates. Compression of surrounding tissues may give rise to the mistaken belief that the tumor is enclosed by a capsule.

Synovial sarcomas are characteristically highly pleomorphic tumors in which fusiform spindle and cuboidal or columnar epithelioid cells are combined in such a way as to form what has been described as a "caricature" of normal synovium[28,35,41,48,61,82] (Fig. 75–8). The relative proportion of these two cell types—which are believed to be derived from a single progenitor, the spindle cell—varies in different parts of the tumor. In places where there is a preponderance of spindle cells, the appearance is that of a fibrosarcoma. In other areas there may be large numbers of epithelial-like synovioblasts, cuboidal or columnar in shape, one or more layers thick and gathered in compact masses or arranged in the form of small villi or in a papillary structure. There is no basement membrane subjacent to these structures. The most distinctive histologic feature of synovial sarcoma is the presence of clefts and cystic spaces which are lined by cuboidal or columnar-shaped cells and contain a mucin-rich secretion, which has been identified as hyaluronic acid.[51]

Treatment.—The possibility of syno-

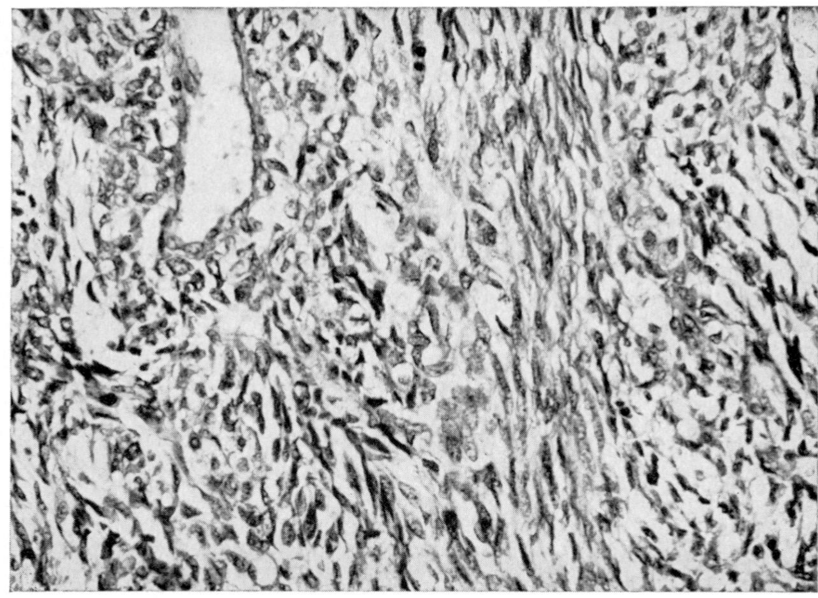

FIG. 75-8.—*Synovioma* (*synovial sarcoma*). Photomicrograph of lung tumor from a thirty-one-year-old woman who had had a synovial sarcoma removed from her left mid-foot six years before. Closely packed oval and spindle-shaped cells are arranged in interlacing fascicles. The nuclei of these cells are highly pleomorphic and there are numerous mitotic figures. There are other cells, more polygonal in form, which are arranged in solid cords or in gland-like aggregates surrounding cystic spaces. (Magnification ×250.) This histologic pattern was similar to that observed in the primary tumor of the foot.

vial sarcoma should be suspected in the case of any tumor in the soft parts of the hand or foot, or in the vicinity of the knee, elbow, and shoulder joints, especially. Once considered, the diagnosis should be confirmed by histological examination. However, it is imperative that biopsy of the tumor not be undertaken unless there are adequate facilities for immediate histological study and prompt radical treatment if warranted by the findings. The all too frequent practice of partial exploration and incomplete resection of the tumor has been strongly condemned.[10,65]

There is general agreement on the need for wide excision of the primary growth in the case without visceral metastases.[1,10,65,68] The magnitude of resection depends upon the location, extent, and aggressiveness of the neoplasm, which is usually found to be intimately adherent to surrounding structures. In practice, this requires amputation of the limb at an appropriate level according to the site of the tumor (*a*) in the case of deep-seated lesions of the hands or feet or joints, (*b*) in the event of local recurrence of the neoplasm, and (*c*) for bulky growths, adequate removal of which would result in a functionless part.[1,10,65] When the neoplasm originates in the upper thigh, disarticulation at the hip joint or hemipelvectomy may prove necessary. Radical dissection of the regional lymph nodes is included as a regular practice in the initial surgical treatment of synovial sarcoma in many centers, but has often failed to control the disease if there has been malignant invasion of these glands. Although there have been a number of patients who may have been cured by irradiation, synovial sarcomas as a group have not proven sufficiently radiosensitive to warrant reliance on irradiation alone.[28,65] It appears well established, however, that prognosis is improved when postoperative irradiation of the tumor area and regional lymph nodes, in a total dose of 2500 to 5000 r, is included as part of primary definitive treatment.[1,7,10,65,68]

Irradiation may also be useful in the palliation of patients with inoperable recurrences or metastatic visceral disease.[1,7,10,68] Chemotherapy has often proven disappointingly ineffective in this situation,[1] but Cade believes that chlorambucil, actinomycin D (given intravenously), and vinblastine sulfate may be of some value.[10]

Prognosis.—Berman reviewed the outcome of 314 cases of synovial sarcoma reported in the older literature, and found that there were only 39 patients who were known to have lived five years or longer from the time of initial treatment. Twenty-three of these survivors were apparently free of disease after (radical) excision and/or irradiation, but in 16 there had been a recurrence of the tumor.[7] According to Wright, the prognosis is worse in those individuals whose tumors show a poorly differentiated histologic structure,[82] but this is a matter which requires additional study.[16] The prognosis appears to be somewhat better in children than in adults.[10,16] Ariel and Pack have noted a five-year "cure" rate of 29 per cent in a group of 25 recently treated patients,[1] while in Cade's series of 46 patients who were free of distant metastases when treated by combined wide local excision and irradiation, the five-year disease-free survival rate was 50 per cent.[10] These figures must be accepted with some reservation, however, since the metastases of synovial sarcoma have been known to appear after a latent period of ten years or more following removal of the primary neoplasm.[47]

Synovial Chondrosarcoma

On rare occasions, chondrosarcoma may arise in the synovial lining of a joint (knee), tendon sheath, and, possibly, even a bursa.[25] Although the lesion may simulate chondromatosis in its gross appearance, synovial chondrosarcoma does not ordinarily appear to develop through malignant transformation of the benign condition.[42,58] Cytologic study of the malignant tumor indicates atypical growth of cartilage. There are greatly enlarged cells with bizarre hyperchromatic nuclei as well as binucleated and occasional multinucleated forms. Radical excision or amputation is the treatment of choice. Some believe that irradiation should be avoided.[42]

Metastatic Neoplasm of the Joints

This is a rare problem which is most likely to occur as a result of metastases to small peripheral bones, such as the patella and phalanges, in which the lesion is necessarily close to a joint.[5] Most often the primary neoplasm has been carcinoma of the lung. In a recent case in which there was total destruction of the patella, invasion of the knee joint was marked by the development of pain, swelling, and a bloody effusion which was found to contain malignant cells.[5]

BIBLIOGRAPHY

1. Ariel, I. M. and Pack, G. T.: New Engl. J. Med., *268*, 1272, 1963.
2. Arzimanoglu, A.: J. Bone & Joint Surg., *39A*, 976, 1957.
3. Atmore, W. G., Dahlin, D. C. and Ghormley, R. K.: Minn. Med., *39*, 196, 1956.
4. Bate, T. H.: J. Bone & Joint Surg., *36A*, 104, 1954.
5. Benedek, T. G.: Arth. & Rheum., *8*, 560, 1965.
6. Bennett, G. A.: J. Bone & Joint Surg., *29*, 259, 1947.
7. Berman, H. L.: Radiology, *81*, 997, 1963.
8. Breimer, C. W. and Freiberger, R. H.: Amer. J. Roentgenol., *79*, 618, 1958.
9. Brodsky, A. E.: Bull. Hosp. Joint Dis., *17*, 58, 1956.
10. Cade, S.: J. Roy. Coll. Surg. Edinburgh, *8*, 1, 1962.
11. Cadman, N. L., Soule, E. H. and Kelly, P. S.: Cancer, *18*, 613, 1965.
12. Carr, C. R., Berley, F. V., and Davis, W. C.: J. Bone & Joint Surg., *36A*, 1007, 1954.

13. Chung, S. M. K. and Janes, J. M.: J. Bone & Joint Surg., *47A*, 293, 1965.
14. Clark, W. S.: Bull. Rheum. Dis., *8*, 161, 1958.
15. Craig, R. M., Pugh, D. G., and Soule, E. H.: Radiology, *65*, 837, 1955.
16. Crocker, D. W. and Stout, A. P.: Cancer, *12*, 1123, 1959.
17. Dungworth, D. L., Wilson, M. R., Gruchy, C. L., and McCallum, G.: J. Path. & Bact., *88*, 83, 1964.
18. Eisenstein, R.: J. Bone & Joint Surg., *50A*, 476, 1968.
19. Feist, J. H. and Gibbons, T. G.: Radiology, *74*, 291, 1960.
20. Fisher, A. G. T.: Brit. J. Surg., *8*, 35, 1920–21.
21. Fleischmajer, R.: Dermatologica, *128*, 113, 1964.
22. Fletcher, A. G., Jr., and Horn, R. C., Jr.: Ann. Surg., *133*, 374, 1951.
23. Friedman, M. and Schwartz, E. E.: Bull. Hosp. Joint Dis., *18*, 19, 1957.
24. Galloway, J. D. B., Broders, A. C., and Ghormley, R. K.: Arch. Surg., *40*, 485, 1940.
25. Goldman, R. L. and Lichtenstein, L.: Cancer, *17*, 1233, 1964.
26. Granowitz, S. P. and Mankin, H. J.: J. Bone & Joint Surg., *49A*, 122, 1967.
27. Greenfield, M. M. and Wallace, K. M.: Radiology, *54*, 350, 1950.
28. Haagensen, C. D. and Stout, A. P.: Ann. Surg., *120*, 826, 1944.
29. Halborg, A., Hansen, H. and Sneppen, H. D.: Acta orthop. scand., *39*, 209, 1968.
30. Harkins, H. N.: Arch. Surg., *34*, 12, 1937.
31. Harrison, E. G., Black, B. M. and Devine, K. D.: Arch. Path., *71*, 137, 1961.
32. Hicks, J. D.: J. Path. & Bact., *67*, 151, 1954.
33. Hoaglund, F. T.: J. Bone & Joint Surg., *49A*, 285, 1967.
34. Jacobs, J. E. and Lee, F. W.: J. Bone & Joint Surg., *31A*, 831, 1949.
35. Jaffe, H. L.: *Tumors and Tumorous Conditions of the Bones and Joints*, Philadelphia, Lea & Febiger, 1958.
36. Jaffe, H. L., Lichtenstein, L., and Sutro, C. J.: Arch. Path., *31*, 731, 1941.
37. Joffe, N.: Brit. J. Radiol., *32*, 619, 1959.
38. Jones, H. T.: J. Bone & Joint Surg., *6*, 407, 1924.
39. ————: J. Bone & Joint Surg., *9*, 310, 1927.
40. Karlholm, S. and Stjernsward, J.: Acta orthop. scand., *33*, 306, 1963.
41. King, E. S. J.: J. Bone & Joint Surg., *34B*, 97, 1952.
42. King, J. W., Spjut, H. J., Fechner, R. E. and Vanderpool, D. W.: J. Bone & Joint Surg., *49A*, 1389, 1967.
43. Larmon, W. A.: Med. Clin. North America, *49*, 141, 1965.
44. Lederer, H. and Sinclair, A. J.: J. Path. & Bact., *67*, 163, 1954.
45. Lewis, R. C., Coventry, M. B., and Soule, E. H.: J. Bone & Joint Surg., *41A*, 264, 1959.
46. Lewis, R. W.: Radiology, *49*, 26, 1947.
47. Lichtenstein, L.: Cancer, *8*, 816, 1955.
48. ————: *Bone Tumors*, 3rd. ed., St. Louis, C. V. Mosby Co., 1965.
49. Litwer, H.: Radiology, *69*, 247, 1957.
50. Lord, G. A. and Goodale, F.: Arch. Surg., *81*, 1020, 1960.
51. Luse, S. A.: Cancer, *13*, 312, 1960.
52. Marsh, H. O., Shellito, J. G. and Callahan, W. P.: J. Bone & Joint Surg., *45A*, 151, 1963.
53. Martens, V. E.: J.A.M.A., *157*, 888, 1955.
54. Mason, M. L.: Surg., Gynec. & Obst., *64*, 129, 1937.
55. McIvor, R. R. and King, D.: J. Bone & Joint Surg., *44A*, 87, 1962.
56. McMaster, P. E.: J. Bone & Joint Surg., *42A*, 1170, 1960.
57. Moses, R., Chomet, B., and Gibbel, M.: Amer. J. Surg., *97*, 120, 1959.
58. Mullins, F., Berard, C. W. and Eisenberg, S. H.: Cancer, *8*, 1180, 1965.
59. Murphy, A. F. and Wilson, J. N.: J. Bone & Joint Surg., *40A*, 1236, 1958.
60. Murphy, F. P., Dahlin, D. C. and Sullivan, C. R.: J. Bone & Joint Surg., *44A*, 77, 1962.
61. Murray, M. R., Stout, A. P., and Pogogeff, I. A.: Ann. Surg., *120*, 843, 1944.
62. Nilsonne, U. and Moberger, G.: Acta orthop. scand., *40*, 448, 1969.
63. Nixon, J. E., Frank, G. R., and Chambers, G.: U.S. Armed Forces Med. J., *11*, 1434, 1960.
64. Pack, G. T. and Ariel, I. M.: Surgery, *28*, 1047, 1950.
65. ————: *Tumors of the Soft Somatic Tissues*, New York, Hoeber-Harper, 1958.
66. Phalen, G. S., McCormack, L. J., and Gazale, W. J.: Clin. Orthop., *15*, 140, 1959.
67. Price, C. H. G. and Valentine, J. C.: J. Clin. Path., *7*, 231, 1954.
68. Raben, M., Calabrese, A., Higinbothan, N. L., and Phillips, R.: Amer. J. Roentgenol., *93*, 145, 1965.
69. Rein, B. I., Bilodeau, L. P., and Johanson, P.: Amer. J. Roentgenol., *92*, 1322, 1964.
70. Ropes, M. W. and Bauer, W.: *Synovial Fluid Changes in Joint Disease*, Cambridge, Harvard University Press, 1953.

71. Sabanas, A. O. and Ghormley, R. K.: Proc. Staff Meet. Mayo Clinic, *30*, 171, 1955.
72. Sherman, R. S. and Chu, F. C. H.: Amer. J. Roentgenol., *67*, 80, 1952.
73. Sherry, J. B. and Anderson, W.: J. Bone & Joint Surg., *37A*, 1005, 1955.
74. Smith, J. H. and Pugh, D. G.: Amer. J. Roentgenol., *87*, 1146, 1962.
75. Somerville-Large, L. B. and O'Meara, R. A. Q.: Amer. J. Ophth., *45*, 631, 1958.
76. Spencer, H. and Whimster, I. W.: J. Path. & Bact., *62*, 411, 1950.
77. Strickland, B. and MacKenzie, D. H.: J. Fac. Radiol. (Lond), *10*, 64, 1959.
78. Sullivan, C. R., Dahlin, D. C., and Bryan, R. S.: J. Bone & Joint Surg., *38A*, 1275, 1956.
79. Tillotson, J. F., McDonald, J. R., and Janes, J. M.: J. Bone & Joint Surg., *33A*, 459, 1951.
80. Vincent, R. G.: Ann. Surg., *152*, 777, 1960.
81. Wright, C. J. E.: Brit. J. Surg., *38*, 257, 1951.
82. ————: J. Path. & Bact., *64*, 585, 1952.
83. Wyllie, J. C.: Arth. & Rheum., *12*, 205, 1969.
84. Young, J. M. and Hudacek, A. G.: Amer. J. Path., *30*, 799, 1954.
85. Zadek, I.: Bull. Hosp. Joint Dis., *5*, 12, 1944.
86. Zimmerman, C. and Sayegh, V.: Amer. J. Roentgenol., *83*, 680, 1960.

PART XII

Regional Disorders of Joints and Related Structures

Section Editor: THEODORE A. POTTER, M.D.

Chapter 76

Traumatic Arthritis and Allied Conditions

By Robert S. Pinals, M.D.

In its broadest sense the term "traumatic arthritis" circumscribes a diverse collection of pathologic and clinical states which develop after single or repetitive episodes of trauma (Table 76–1). Although these conditions may be encountered frequently by the rheumatologist, interest in the area has been casual, and studies of basic mechanisms of disease few as compared with those in the other rheumatic diseases. Since surgeons are more likely to deal with the sequelae of trauma it is not surprising that the most significant contributions are to be found in the orthopedic literature. The credulous assignment of etiologic roles to trauma in early writings stands in sharp contrast to modern attitudes on the subject. Rheumatoid arthritis, tuberculous arthritis, gout and other rheumatic diseases were formerly attributed to trauma, which might alter the structural integrity of

TABLE 76-1
A Classification of Traumatic Arthritis and Allied Conditions

I. Articular Trauma, single episode.
   A. Traumatic synovitis, without disturbance of articular cartilage or disruption of major supporting structures. This includes acute synovitis, with or without hemarthrosis, and most sprains. Healing would be expected within several weeks, without permanent tissue damage.
   B. Disruptive trauma, with infraction of the articular cartilage or complete rupture of major supporting structures. This includes intra-articular fractures, meniscal tears, and severe sprains.
   C. Post-traumatic osteoarthritis. This includes cases of disruptive trauma in which major residual damage is present. Patients may have deformity, limited motion or instability of joints.

II. Repetitive Articular Trauma. This includes a variety of conditions related to occupation, sports etc. and results in localized chronic arthritis.

III. Induction or aggravation of another specific rheumatic disease by acute or repetitive trauma.

IV. Conditions in which trauma may be one of several etiologic factors, or in which a relationship has been suggested but not established: osteochondritis dissecans, osteitis pubis, Tietze's syndrome and others.

V. Disorders of extra-articular structures such as tendons, bursae and muscles, in which trauma commonly plays an etiologic role.

VI. Non-mechanical types of trauma: arthropathy following frostbite, radiation and decompression.

joints, predisposing them to inflammation.[89] As other pathogenetic mechanisms have been revealed, it has become less necessary to invoke "unrecognized trauma," which was previously such a convenient explanation for poorly understood disorders. Even in osteoarthritis, once the bellwether of traumatic disorders, considered by some to be synonymous with traumatic arthritis, increasing emphasis is being placed on altered cartilage metabolism, leaving an even smaller role for "multiple microtraumata."

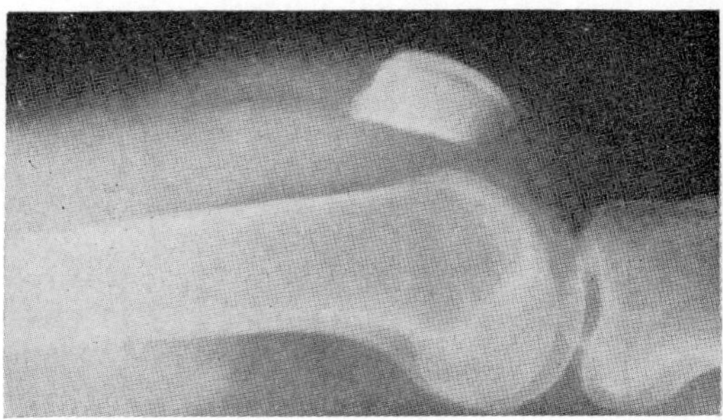

Fig. 76–1.—Traumatic hemarthrosis. Liquid fat and a fat-blood level are visible in the joint. (From Berk, R. N., New Engl. J. Med., *277*, 1411, 1967.)

ACUTE TRAUMATIC SYNOVITIS

Following a direct blow or forced inappropriate motion to a joint, swelling and pain may develop. Since the knee is most commonly affected, the following discussion will be directed at that joint, but a similar approach might also be taken toward a traumatic synovitis in the elbow, shoulder, ankle or elsewhere. On examination there is usually evidence of an effusion, which should be aspirated to determine whether hemarthrosis is present and to aid in further examination of the joint. Hemarthrosis is usually present if fluid appears within two hours after the injury;[94] in about half the cases swelling occurs within 15 minutes.[18] On the other hand, non-bloody effusions usually appear 12 to 24 hours after injury.[18] With hemarthrosis there is usually more pain, and at times a low-grade fever. Fractures, internal derangements or major ligamentous tears must be ruled out by examination and radiographs, which should include stress, skyline and intercondylar views. In one series of patients with traumatic hemarthrosis, 66 had fractures or ligamentous rupture, and 20 did not.[94] There may be detachment or laceration of cartilage and capsular tears which may not be discovered in this manner. It has been suggested, on the basis of calcification which developed later in the median parapatellar area, that lateral subluxation of the patella, tearing the medial retinaculum, may be the source of joint hemorrhage in some cases.[94] The presence of fat globules floating on the surface of bloody fluid usually indicates a fracture. At times, sufficient fat may be present to be detectable on a lateral knee radiograph as a radiolucent layer in the suprapatellar pouch[5] (Fig. 76–1). Hemorrhagic fluid usually does not clot; Smillie believes that coagulation indicates more profound tissue damage and a poorer prognosis.[79]

In the absence of gross bleeding, examination of the fluid reveals a variable number of red blood cells and from 50 to 1000 white blood cells, of which only a few are neutrophils. The protein content is two or three times that of normal fluid, mostly albumin. Viscosity is slightly reduced but the mucin clot is good.[72] Synovial biopsy reveals some vasodilatation, edema and an occasional small focus of synovial cell proliferation with mild lymphocytic infiltration. An electronmicroscopic study has shown evidence of increased protein synthesis by synovial cells, perhaps accounting for a portion of the excessive protein content in post-traumatic effusions.[73]

Treatment may include such measures as cold packs initially and heat later; compression dressings[30,79] or posterior splints; graded quadriceps exercises; repeated aspiration if significant volumes of fluid reaccumulate; and a period of bedrest or partial weight-bearing, depending upon the severity of the injury. Prognosis is excellent in the absence of improper treatment, such as cylinder cast immobilization, which may result in muscle atrophy and loss of motion,[79] or premature weight-bearing which may lead to an extended duration of synovitis. A study of experimental hemarthrosis in rabbits has shown that there is no deleterious effect on articular cartilage, even from repeated hemarthroses, although the synovium may show a mild inflammatory process and iron accumulation.[101]

SPRAINS

A sprain may be defined as a stretching or tearing of a supporting ligament of a joint by forced movement beyond its normal range. In its simplest form there is minimal disruption of fibers, swelling, pain and dysfunction. Severe sprains may cause total rupture of ligaments, marked swelling and hemorrhage, and joint instability, which may be permanent if untreated. Sprains occur most frequently in the ankle but are also common in the knee, low back and neck.

Ankle Sprains.—Most ankle sprains result from unintentional weight-bearing on the inverted, plantar-flexed foot, with partial or total disruption of one or more of the three main lateral supporting structures, which unite the fibula above with the calcaneus and talus below (Fig. 76–2). Rupture of the anterior talofibular ligament is most common; this structure prevents anterior displacement of the talus out of the ankle joint mortise. With additional force the calcaneofibular ligament, which prevents excessive inversion, may also rupture. The third ligament, the posterior talofibular ligament, is seldom torn with the usual type of injury; a completely unstable ankle would result. Stretching of the medial supporting structures usually results in fracture and avulsion of the medial malleolus rather than a sprain.

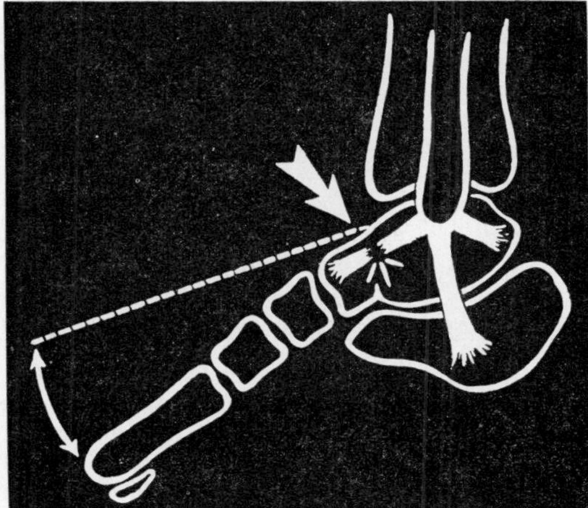

Fig. 76–2.—A severe ankle sprain, occurring in equinus and inversion, may result in rupture of the anterior talofibular ligament. (From Pipkin, G.: Clin. Orthop., *3*, 8, 1954.)

The patient presents with severe pain and swelling on the outer aspect of the foot and ankle. Much of the early swelling is due to hemorrhage, resulting in ecchymosis several hours later. A history of something snapping, giving away or slipping out of place may suggest a complete ligament rupture. The nature of the treatment is largely dependent upon assessment of the integrity of these ligaments. This is most easily accomplished soon after the injury, before swelling and pain make forced motion difficult. Local anesthesia may be required for proper examination. Some orthopedists insist upon stress roentgenograms in all severe sprains.[97]

Early treatment of simple sprains may include elevation, ice packs and compression dressing to prevent swelling; injection of local anesthetics to permit early motion; and adhesive strapping. Full weight-bearing is permitted on the following day. A lift on the outer border of the heel will maintain eversion and prevent strain on the injured ligament. Strapping, or later an elastic support, is continued until healing is complete, usually for three to six weeks.[1,97]

Severe sprains may demand additional treatment, such as a walking plaster for four to six weeks when the anterior talofibular ligament is ruptured, and early surgical repair when, in addition, the calcaneofibular ligament is torn.[1]

Other Sprains.[68]—Knee sprains are considered in Chapter 77 and low back sprains in Chapter 82. Shoulder "sprain" is actually a subluxation of the acromioclavicular joint, commonly seen in body contact sports. Wrist "sprain" is usually a fractured navicular, often missed on initial roentgenograms. Traumatic torticollis may be called a neck sprain. Following a sudden twist or wrenching of the neck, pain and muscle spasm may result in involuntary assumption of a "wry neck" position. Spontaneous remission occurs after one or two weeks. Such measures as a cervical collar, traction and heat may be helpful. The actual structures involved in neck sprain have not been well defined.

PELLEGRINI-STIEDA SYNDROME

Following acute knee trauma a linear calcific density may develop in the area of the medial collateral ligament (Fig. 7–51). Its exact anatomic location is uncertain but it lies between the deep fascia and the femoral periosteum. A hematoma may be the initial event. Calcification is noted on roentgenograms obtained as early as three or four weeks after the injury.[60] Few biopsies have been obtained in the early stages; those done later show bone rather than a calcific deposit. The initial injury may be minor or may produce a fracture, torn meniscus or ligamentous rupture. Initial signs and symptoms, as well as subsequent disability, are related more to this associated trauma than to the Pellegrini-Stieda lesion itself.[41] However, persistent tenderness and some swelling are often found on the medial aspect of the knee. Local corticosteroid injections have been advocated in these cases. This is said to accelerate disappearance of the metaplastic bone,[41] but spontaneous resolution occurs eventually in many cases. Surgical excision has been attempted in occasional instances in which limited motion has been attributed to the lesion, but recurrences have been noted in some.

DISRUPTIVE ARTICULAR TRAUMA; POST-TRAUMATIC OSTEOARTHRITIS

Permanent joint damage may be the end result of various types of trauma, including fractures through the articular surface; dislocations; internal derangements; major ligamentous ruptures; and wounds, often with sepsis and foreign body implantation (Fig. 76–3). There may be structural alterations of a permanent or progressive nature: deterioration of articular cartilage, limitation of joint motion, instability, or angular deviation. Detailed consideration of these injuries and their treatment is beyond the scope of this book. Pathologically and radiographically the condition has most of the characteristics of osteoarthritis.

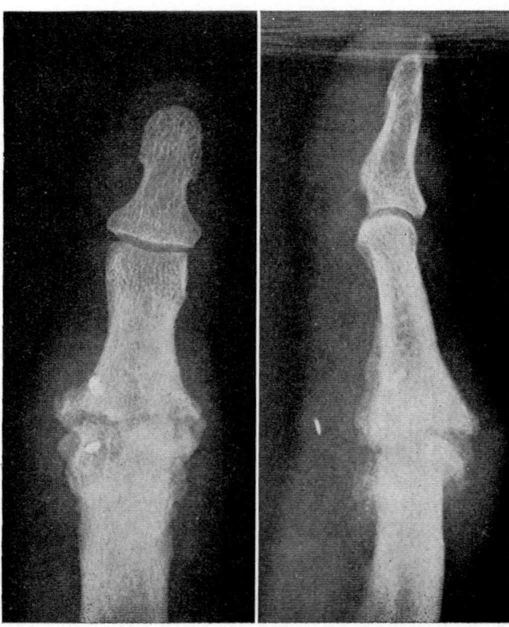

Fig. 76–3.—Arthritis due to foreign body. A piece of steel lodged in this index finger of the patient four years before. Swelling of the finger began about two years later and has continued to date. Roentgenograph shows marked deformity of the proximal interphalangeal joint of the right index finger. This consists of marked hypertrophic changes with possible ankylosis of the joint. There are two small opaque foreign bodies in relation to the palmar and radial aspects of the joint.

However, a specific traumatic episode should not be definitely accepted as etiologically related to osteoarthritis unless there is evidence establishing the following points: (1) the joint was normal prior to injury; (2) records document either an effusion or structural damage shortly after the injury; (3) similar disease has not occurred in non-traumatized joints. Other points favoring a traumatic origin are the occurrence of significant isolated osteoarthritis in a joint usually not involved by the idiopathic variety (such as ankle, wrist, elbow or metacarpophalangeal joint) and radiologic demonstration of foreign bodies and healed fractures near the joint in question.

REPETITIVE ARTICULAR TRAUMA

Osteoarthritis may develop in joints repeatedly traumatized as a result of certain occupations and sports. Radiographic abnormalities, such as joint space narrowing, subcortical cysts and marginal osteophytes, are common in some groups studied, but many of the affected individuals are asymptomatic. These changes occur in the hands and wrists of boxers[11] and of stone workers using pneumatic hammers,[47] in the ankles of soccer players[81] and in the first metatarsophalangeal joints of ballet dancers.[61]

ROLE OF TRAUMA IN OTHER TYPES OF ARTHRITIS

Trauma plays an important role in the development of neuropathic joint disease (Chapter 72). Attacks of gouty arthritis often develop in recently injured joints. Rheumatoid arthritis occasionally starts in a joint which has been injured or subjected to a surgical procedure. A history of recent or old trauma to the affected joint is sometimes obtained from patients with septic or tuberculous arthritis. However, the evidence in these situations is anecdotal and difficult to evaluate. Data have not been gathered in an organized fashion and there is little understanding of the mechanisms involved. In many instances the trauma has been minimal, perhaps representing an unrelated antecedent to the joint disease.[32]

Williams and Scott[95] have reported three patients in whom trauma to a finger joint was followed by chronic polyarthritis with most prominent involvement of the injured joint. On reviewing the literature they concluded that trauma is a precipitating factor in about 5 per cent of patients with rheumatoid arthritis. It was suggested that the mechanism might be similar to that in experimental arthritis in rabbits, induced by intra-articular fibrin injections.[24]

Preexisting arthritis may certainly be aggravated by trauma, but the dimensions of this statement are an unknown quantity and each case must be considered on its own merits.[26] Only minor force would be required to cause rupture of a frayed wrist extensor tendon or collateral ligament in a patient with rheumatoid arthritis. Other acute episodes, such as abrupt increase in joint swelling or rupture of the posterior knee joint capsule, are commonly associated with unusual resistive exercise. Sanguineous joint fluid is sometimes aspirated from a knee or shoulder in patients with rheumatoid arthritis who report sudden increase in pain and swelling following relatively minor trauma. It is presumed that pinching or compression of the hypertrophied synovium may result in bleeding. In such cases the synovial fluid hematocrit is fairly low, usually less than 10 per cent.

TEMPOROMANDIBULAR JOINT SYNDROME

Pain in the ear, face and temple may be caused by dysfunction or structural change in the temporomandibular joint. Symptoms are usually intermittent and unilateral. Tense young women are particularly susceptible, but the syndrome may also follow trauma to the mandible, repeated dislocation, dental manipulation with forceful opening of the mouth, prolonged cervical traction, compulsive gum chewing and bruxism, malocclusion, loss of teeth and use of ill-fitting dentures.[21,29,36,93]

In most cases a click or snap is palpable on motion of the jaw, excursion is somewhat limited, and there may be mild tenderness over the joint. The muscles of mastication may also be tender on the affected side, particularly the pterygoids, which function in opening the mouth and may be palpated only from within the buccal cavity. Biting with the incisors on a firm morsel, such as a cotton-wool roll, increases pain by compressing the joint. However, when the roll is placed between the molars of the affected side, biting does not increase the pain, and may indeed relieve it, since the articulating surfaces are distracted by this maneuver.[14]

Asymmetry and incoordination of temporomandibular joint motion results in deviation of the chin toward the painful side.[29] With cineradiography it can be demonstrated that one condyle remains in the fossa for a longer interval than the other, snapping out suddenly at a time corresponding to the click which the examiner may note.[93] Standard radiographs may reveal an irregular contour of the mandibular condyle and narrowing of the joint space. Corresponding structural changes have been found in joints subjected to surgery; attrition and partial detachment of the meniscus are common. However, since the syndrome often occurs in the absence of any structural change, a myofascial trigger mechanism with referred pain and reflex muscle spasm has been proposed.[31] Chronic muscle spasm may thus result in a variety of self-inflicted traumatic arthritis.

Costen reported a number of other symptoms which he felt were commonly associated with temporomandibular joint dysfunction ("Costen's syndrome"). These include occipital headache; impaired hearing; nystagmus; burning or dryness in the throat, mouth or tongue; and herpes of the external auditory canal. In most recent reports these symptoms have not been emphasized and their pathogenesis is uncertain. Ward *et al.*[93] found diminished hearing in 15 of 40 patients but the audiograms were typical of presbycusis; no definite relationship to the temporomandibular joint syndrome could be established.

Conservative treatment is generally successful.[93] It consists of reassurance, exercise to stretch spastic muscles and restore coordinated motion, and occasional use of tranquilizers and intra-articular corticosteroid injections.[21] (*See also* Chapter 32.) Correction of malocclusion and replacement of dentures are appropriate in some cases. A few patients, who have pronounced structural changes or frequent dislocation and locking, may require a surgical procedure, such as menisectomy, arthroplasty, condylectomy or grafts of bone and fascia.[21]

ACUTE BONE ATROPHY (SUDECK'S ATROPHY; REFLEX DYSTROPHY)

After trauma to an extremity a few patients develop severe pain, edema, vasomotor abnormalities and atrophy of bone, muscle and skin. Many labels have been applied to this syndrome, depending upon the feature of particular interest to the describer: *Sudeck's atrophy*, *Leriche's post-traumatic osteoporosis*, *Weir Mitchell's causalgia*, *peripheral trophoneurosis*, *reflex dystrophy* and *chronic traumatic edema*. The term "causalgia" should probably be reserved for cases in which there has been injury to a major nerve trunk, but the resulting intense burning pain is not confined to the distribution of the nerve and may not differ from that which occurs in reflex dystrophy without nerve injury.[23] Another variant, the "shoulder-hand syndrome," is usually not related to trauma and is described in detail in Chapter 80.

The antecedent injury may be a fracture but is often fairly trivial, such as a sprain or laceration, and may occur with about equal frequency in an upper or lower extremity.[23] Pain, of a quality and degree quite inappropriate for the injury, may start immediately or not until several weeks after the trauma.[77] Disinclination to move the extremity is also an early feature and is inextricably linked to the pain; the limb is painful on motion and may have striking cutaneous hyperalgesia and cold sensitivity. A hyperemic stage may be noted in some cases, but a cold, moist, cyanotic, edematous hand or foot is more typical after two or three months. Roentgenograms may be normal during the first month but later show patchy osteopenia, often periarticular in distribution initially, but diffuse later. With continued immobility, muscle and skin atrophy occur and joint motion is lost.

Pathogenesis and management are discussed in Chapter 80. It should be emphasized that early identification of patients and restoration of active motion are the key to successful treatment. Early cases may respond well to a simple conservative approach, including graded active exercises, heat and elevation.[69] Long-standing disease, with advanced atrophy of skin, muscle and bone, may be largely irreversible. In one study of patients with fractures it was suggested that active exercise to joints which do not require immobilization may prevent Sudeck's atrophy. Osteopenia developed in only 0.6 per cent of the exercised group and in 17.4 per cent of those who were not so instructed.[10]

Another syndrome characterized by pain and osteopenia has been described in several reports since 1967[25,43,52,87] under the following titles: *migratory osteolysis*, *regional migratory osteoporosis*, and *transient osteoporosis of the hip*. The patients are usually middle-aged men, who develop painful swelling in one region of a lower extremity, rarely with preceding trauma.[87] Either the hip, knee or foot may be involved. Pain is often severe, especially on motion and weight-bearing. Although radiographs may be normal during the first two or three weeks of symptoms, severe osteoporosis in the painful region is readily apparent thereafter. This is unlikely to be related to disuse since uptake of a bone-seeking radioisotope is increased in the affected area during the first week, prior to immobilization of the extremity.[62] The disorder is self-limited, with resolution of signs and symptoms in several months and eventual return of bone density to normal. Subsequent attacks may occur in other areas but not in previously involved joints. Nothing is known of the pathogenesis of this syndrome, but its resemblance to Sudeck's atrophy has been noted.[52,87]

OSTEOCHONDRITIS DISSECANS

This local disorder of subchondral bone is most commonly found in the knees of adolescents and young adults. A devitalized fragment of bone, with its articular cartilage still present, demarcates from its original site, usually on the lateral portion of the medial femoral condyle. Partial or complete detachment may occur eventually, with resulting signs and symptoms of a "loose body" in the joint; less frequently, the fragment may lodge in the intercondylar notch and remain clinically silent.

Antecedent trauma is common but seems to be only one of several etiologic factors. Smillie,[80] who has reviewed this controversial topic in great detail, believes that anomalous ossification centers, locally deficient blood supply and genetic factors[38] are particularly important in the younger age group, whereas trauma plays a greater role in adults. The trauma involved may be "endogenous," such as repeated contact between an unusually prominent tibial spine or aberrantly situated cruciate ligament and the femoral condyle.

The clinical picture in cases with knee involvement consists of mild discomfort rather than pain. This is aggravated by exercise but there may also be some aching at rest. With separation of the fragment the patient may complain of instability or "giving-way." Often an unusual stance, due to external rotation of the tibia, may be noted.[98] This diminishes contact between the tibial spine and the usual site of osteochondritis on the medial condyle, near the intercondylar notch. A physical sign which correlates with this may be demonstrated by forcing the tibia into internal rotation while slowly extending the knee from 90° of flexion. At about 30° the patient complains of pain which is relieved immediately by external rotation of the tibia.

Roentgenograms may be normal for as long as six months after the injury; the typical picture is that of a bony sequestrum lodged in a sharply defined cavity (Fig. 76–4). The lesion has a similar appearance when it occurs in other locations such as the elbow (capitellum), ankle (talus), hip and metatarsal head. Occasionally multiple sites are involved, particularly in individuals from predisposed families.[38]

Treatment is conservative if the fragment remains in place. Loose fragments may be treated surgically, with either removal or fixation.[80] The immediate prognosis is good but some patients may develop osteoarthritis later in life.

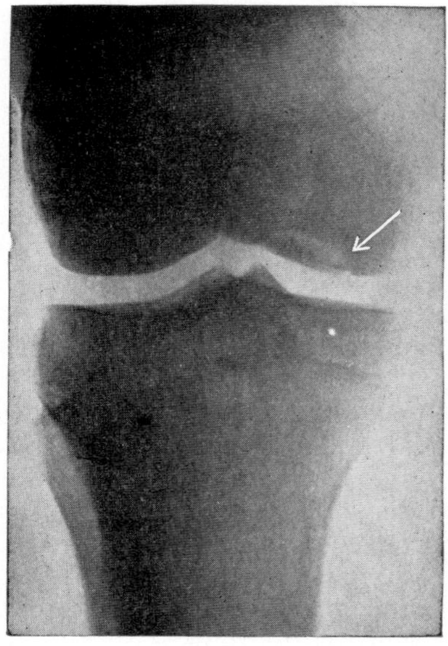

Fig. 76–4.—Osteochondritis dissecans. (Holmes and Robbins.)

Epiphyseal Osteochondritis.—Necrosis of an entire epiphysis is a common localized disorder in childhood. Vascular insufficiency is thought to be the most significant etiologic factor; trauma is often mentioned but seldom established as a contributing cause. In the hip (*Legg-Calve-Perthes disease*) osteochondritis occurs in younger children (age two to ten years), usually presenting with a limp rather than with pain. In the knee (*Osgood-Schlatter disease*) older children (age nine to 15) develop pain and swelling in the tibial tubercle. Osteochondritis of the vertebrae (*Scheuermann's disease*) presents with kyphosis and is described in Chapter 82.

TIETZE'S SYNDROME

In 1921 Tietze described a benign condition in which painful enlargement develops in the upper costal cartilages.[91] In the most recent review of the literature Levey and Calabro[53] found that 290 cases had been reported. The syndrome occurs with the same frequency in both sexes and on both sides of the chest. Involvement of only a single costal cartilage is found in 80 per cent of patients, the second and third being most often affected. Onset of pain is either acute or insidious, usually without prior injury, with the exception of trauma which may have occurred during vigorous coughing in a minority of cases. Pain is sometimes severe, is aggravated by motion of the rib cage and may radiate to the shoulder and arm. Palpation of a firm tender fusiform swelling of the costal cartilage confirms the diagnosis. Biopsy usually shows normal cartilage, occasionally some edema of the perichondrium and rarely non-specific chronic inflammation in the surrounding tissues. The duration is variable, from a week to several years. Some patients have multiple episodes but spontaneous remission is the rule. The swelling has been attributed to cartilaginous hypertrophy by some and to abnormal angulation by others, but nothing is known of the pathogenesis. Treatment may include analgesics, heat, local infiltration with corticosteroids, intercostal nerve block and reassurance that symptoms are not due to heart disease.

Other disorders may produce pain, tenderness or evidences of inflammation in the costochondral junctions, but not a hard swelling as in Tietze's syndrome. They include rheumatoid arthritis, fibrositis, gout, pyogenic infection and the anterior chest wall syndrome which may follow myocardial infarction.

OSTEITIS PUBIS

Surgical trauma in the retropubic area may occasionally provoke an inflammatory process in the pubic symphysis and adjacent bone.[3,15,74,100] Osteitis pubis may occur after prostate or bladder surgery and, more rarely, following herniorrhaphy or childbirth. Several weeks postoperatively the patient develops pain over the symphysis radiating down the inner aspects of the thighs, often aggravated by coughing and straining. Physical findings include an antalgic gait, point tenderness over the symphysis, spasm in the abdominal and hip adductor muscle groups and a low-grade fever. Radiographs may be normal initially but rarefaction and osteolysis develop around the symphysis within two to four weeks. A sterile chronic inflammatory process is usually noted on biopsy,[15] but a true osteomyelitis may be discovered in a minority of patients, generally those with more marked bone destruction and fever.[74] Tuberculosis and metastatic disease must also be considered in the differential diagnosis. Similar radiographic findings may be observed in ankylosing spondylitis and occasionally in chondrocalcinosis or in other types of polyarthritis, but pain is minimal or absent. Although spontaneous remission may be expected in osteitis pubis, disabling symptoms may persist for many months. The gamut of anti-inflammatory drugs has been used with varying success, and other measures such as immobilization, wearing a tight pelvic belt, surgical debridement[74] and radiotherapy have been advocated. The pathogenesis is uncertain, but there is general agreement that one or more factors, in addition to trauma, must contribute. Neurogenic, hormonal, vascular and infectious factors have been proposed but none has been substantiated.

SYNOVIAL CYSTS OF THE POPLITEAL SPACE; "BAKER'S CYSTS"

There are six primary bursae associated with muscles and tendons on the posteromedial aspect of the knee. Communications between two bursae and between a bursa and the knee joint are common. Popliteal cysts may arise in three ways: (1) accumulation of fluid in a noncommunicating bursa; (2) distention of a bursa by fluid originating as a result of a lesion in the knee joint; (3) posterior herniation of the joint capsule in response to increased intra-articular pressure. The communication between joint and cyst is generally narrow and the anatomy such that a flap-valve mechanism may be operative, allowing free passage of fluid from knee to cyst but not in the opposite direction.[79]

Popliteal cysts may be seen at all ages. Those in children are usually unassociated with joint disease and are often bilateral. In about half of all cases there is evidence of some abnormality in the knee joint. In one study of 198 patients, 40 had osteoarthritis, 27 had rheumatoid arthritis, 11 had cartilage tears or osteochondromatosis and 11 had a variety of other conditions.[7] Only ten patients had a history of trauma. In most patients with knee joint disease a connection between the cyst and joint could be demonstrated. The cyst itself usually causes only mild discomfort; other symptoms may be related to associated joint lesions. A fluctuant swelling is present in the popliteal area, occasionally extending well into the calf and presenting superficially at the medial border of the gastrocnemius. The differential diagnosis includes aneurysms, benign neoplasms, varicosities and thrombophlebitis. Arthrograms may be helpful if the cyst communicates with the knee joint.[39] The histopathologic characteristics of the cysts are varied, and do not particularly correspond to the presumed origin, bursal or hernial.[7] Most have a thin fibrous wall, lined by a single layer of flat cells. Others have structural characteristics of a synovial membrane, particularly those occurring in patients with rheumatoid arthritis. A few have a thickened, inflamed wall coated with fibrin but no villus formation.

Treatment is essentially surgical.[79] In some cases correction of knee joint pathology (such as synovectomy in a patient with rheumatoid arthritis) may result in spontaneous disappearance. Aspiration of the cyst and corticosteroid injections are often palliative (*see* Chapter 32).

Synovial cysts in rheumatoid arthritis are seen in many other joints.[63] Occasionally a communicating cyst of traumatic or non-specific origin may be seen elsewhere. For instance, a cyst connecting with the hip joint may present anteriorly as a mass in the groin or posteriorly with sciatic pain.[44]

GANGLION

A ganglion is a cystic swelling which may be found near and often attached to a tendon sheath or joint capsule, and is believed to be derived from these structures.[55] The thick mucoid material within the ganglion contains hyaluronic acid, although there is no direct communication between the ganglion and tendon sheath.[4] The most common location is on the dorsum of the wrist (Fig. 76–5), but ganglia are also frequently noted on the fingers and dorsum of the foot. They have been reported near many other joints and also attached to the tibial periosteum.[8] In most instances there has been no definite relationship to trauma. There are few symptoms other than unsightly swelling and slight discomfort on motion.

Ganglia may disappear spontaneously[12] and treatment is not necessarily required but is often demanded by the patient for cosmetic reasons. Successful treatment in about 80 per cent of cases has been reported after multiple punctures of the cyst wall with a large bore needle, aspiration of the contents and injection of a corticosteroid preparation.[19,48] If there is recurrence after this procedure surgical excision may be performed.

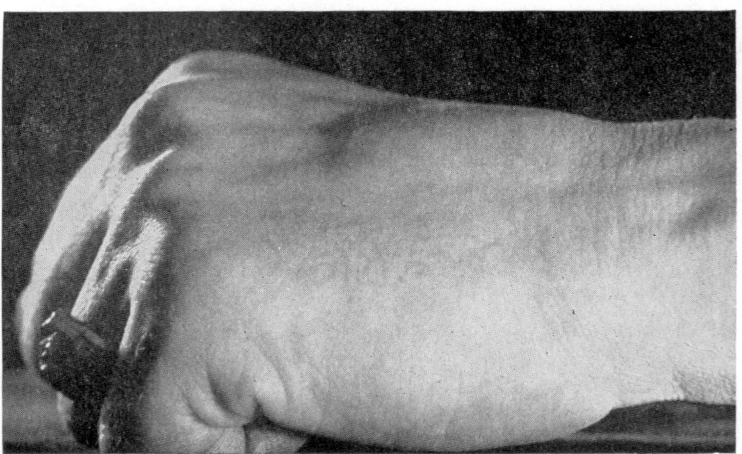

Fig. 76–5.—Ganglion arising from extensor tendon sheaths—oval and flattened cystic mass on dorsum of hand. (Brunschwig's *Surgery,* courtesy of C. V. Mosby Company.)

TENOSYNOVITIS; STENOSING TENOVAGINITIS

Tenosynovitis is an inflammation of the cellular lining membrane of the fibrous tube (vagina) through which a tendon moves. It may be produced by various diseases (rheumatoid arthritis, gout, gonococcal arthritis) but even more commonly by trauma. This may be from a direct blow, from abnormal pressure upon a tendon (such as from the stiff counter of a new shoe on the Achilles tendon) or, most often, from a short period of unusual activity involving a certain muscle-tendon unit. In one industrial study of 88 cases, the wrist and thumb extensors were involved in 71 per cent and the dorsiflexors at the ankle in 18 per cent. Most were related to a new type of repetitive work or to resumption of work after vacation.[99] The condition is identified by tenderness, swelling and palpable crepitus over the tendon as it is moved (*peritendinitis crepitans*). Remission usually occurs if the affected part is rested for a few days.

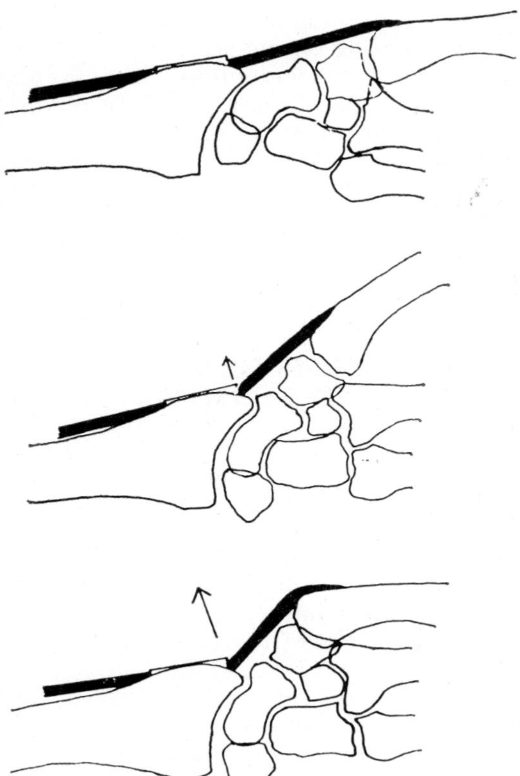

FIG. 76–6.—(*Top*) Wrist and thumb in neutral position, tendons relaxed. (*Center*) Radial deviation of wrist with thumb relaxed, minor tearing stress applied to retinaculum. (*Bottom*) Radial deviation of wrist while gripping, strong tearing stress applied to retinaculum. (From Muckart, R. D., Clin. Orthop., *33*, 204, 1964.)

Stenosing tenovaginitis is primarily a disorder of the fibrous wall of the tendon sheath, particularly at locations where the tendon passes through a fibrous ring or pulley. Generally an osseous groove comprises part of the ring, which is completed by a thickening of the tendon sheath. Such arrangements are found over bony prominences such as the radial styloid (Fig. 76–6), and the flexor surfaces of the metacarpal and metatarsal heads. With prolonged mechanical stress from either tendon motion under an excessive load or external pressure, such as from the handles of pruning shears, there is abnormal proliferation of fibrous tissue in the ring, constricting the lumen of the tendon sheath. Secondary changes may then occur in the tendon usually with enlargement distal to the constriction. There may be a snapping sensation with movement of the enlarged segment of tendon through the narrowed ring ("*trigger finger*"; "*snapping thumb*"). Further progression may produce locking in flexion; the tendon may be pulled through the constriction by its own flexor muscle but not by its weaker extensor antagonist. When extension is forced the bulbous portion suddenly pops back through the constriction and the digit "unlocks." Tenosynovitis due to mechanical stress may also contribute to pain and loss of motion.

Stenosing tenovaginitis of the abductor pollicis longus and extensor pollicis brevis at the radial styloid is known as "*De Quervain's disease*."[59,102] It is a fairly common disorder among women who perform repetitive manual tasks involving grasping with the thumb accompanied by movement of the hand in a radial direction (Fig. 76–6). Symptoms include pain in the area of the radial styloid and weakness of grip. On examination there is tenderness and thickening over the involved tendons and limited excursion of the thumb; locking and snapping seldom occur. The classical test is the demonstration of *Finkelstein's sign.* The thumb is placed in the palm of the hand and grasped by the fingers; ulnar deviation of the wrist elicits a sharp pain if inflammation of the tendon sheath is present.

The most common locations for stenosing tenovaginitis are the thumb flexor and extensor tendons and the finger flexors, but occasionally other sites are involved. These include the flexor carpi radialis tendon, resulting in pain at the base of the thenar eminence,[28] the common peroneal sheath, causing pain on the lateral aspect of the ankle[65] and the tibialis posterior tendon,[96] presenting with pain below and behind the medial malleolus after prolonged standing and walking.

Treatment of Stenosing Tenovaginitis.—Conservative measures such as (1) cessation of the repetitive activity thought to have provoked the condition, (2) immobilization with splints and (3) local corticosteroid injections often result in improvement, but recurrences are common. Tenosynovitis may subside, but the area of fibrous constriction is unlikely to be greatly altered by this approach, and it is sometimes necessary to resort to surgical excision of this portion of the sheath. In all of the locations the operation is fairly simple and results in permanent remission, even allowing resumption of full activity in most cases.

Carpal Tunnel Syndrome.—Tenosynovitis in the flexor compartment of the wrist, where the tendons are enclosed in a bony canal, roofed by a rigid transverse carpal ligament, may result in compression and degeneration of the median nerve which shares this space.[71] Trauma is only one of many causes of this syndrome; others include rheumatoid arthritis, amyloidosis, myxedema, benign tumors, pregnancy, Raynaud's disease and diabetes.[16,66,88] In one report, about half of the patients had been engaged in prolonged activity involving forceful flexion of the fingers with the wrist held in flexion or moving through an arc of flexor motion.[88] In another larger series, only 16 per cent of patients had a history of possibly related trauma, including fractures and sprains as well as excessive use.[66]

The patient complains of paresthesias and pain in the first three fingers of the hand, often worse at night. Physical findings may include sensory loss in the median nerve distribution, weakness in abduction and opposition of the thumb, atrophy of the thenar musculature and a tender swelling on the volar aspect of the wrist. Nerve conduction time across the wrist is almost always prolonged; this measurement may be of value in confirming the diagnosis in atypical cases. Immobilization and local corticosteroid injections into the tendon sheaths often bring about a remission, but surgical division of the transverse carpal ligament is the definitive treatment.[16]

OTHER FORMS OF TENDINITIS AND BURSITIS

Painful conditions attributed to strain or injury of tendons and their attachments to bone are often loosely described by the term tendinitis. The supraspinatus and bicipital tendons of the shoulder are commonly affected, and are discussed in Chapter 80. Frequently tendinitis is related to a particular occupation or sport. For instance, a baseball pitcher, at the end of his delivery, stretches the attachment of the long head of the triceps to the inferior glenoid rim. This results in pain in the posterior axillary fold. It is presumed that inflammatory changes occur in the tendon attachment; treatment includes rest, local corticosteroid injections and ultrasound.[57] Baseball pitchers and golfers may also develop a similar condition at the *medial* epicondyle of the elbow.

TENNIS ELBOW (EPICONDYLITIS)

This is a common condition, most often found in middle-aged men, in which pain derives from the origin of the wrist and finger extensors at the lateral epicondyle. Although first described in tennis players, most cases are not related to that sport, but may be provoked by any exercise or occupation which involves repeated and forcible wrist extension or pronation-supination. The right elbow is involved more often than the left; the condition is seldom bilateral.[49] Pain is usually gradual in onset, but is sometimes related to a specific traumatic incident; it often radiates to the forearm and dorsum of the hand. Physical examination reveals point tenderness at or near the lateral epicondyle, with little or no swelling. Elbow joint motion is unrestricted and painless, but resisted wrist extension results in accentuation of pain. Many thoughts have been expressed about the pathogenesis,[34] including tendon rupture, radiohumeral synovitis, periostitis, neuritis, aseptic necrosis and displacement of the orbicular ligament. A detailed pathologic study, including a control group of autopsied individuals with apparently normal elbows, revealed no evidence of a bursa in the area of the common extensor insertion, but rather a subtendinous space containing loose areolar connective tissue. In patients with tennis elbow this space showed granulation tissue, increased vascularity and edema. Periostitis and tendon tears were not noted.[34]

Many treatments have been proposed; these include massage, ultrasound, anti-inflammatory drugs, braces and several surgical procedures. However, the most common approach, local corticosteroid injection, is usually successful.[17,78,49]

BURSITIS

Bursae are closed sacs, lined with a cellular membrane resembling synovium. They serve to facilitate motion of tendons and muscles over bony prominences. There are approximately 78 bursae on each side of the body.[9] Many are nameless and additional ones may form at almost any point subjected to frequent irritation. Excessive frictional forces or, at times, direct trauma may result in an inflammatory process in the bursal wall, with excessive vascularity, exudation of increased amounts of viscous bursal fluid and fibrin-coating of the lining membrane. Only small numbers of inflammatory cells are found in bursal fluid in traumatic bursitis, but there may be a greater leukocyte response in bursitis secondary to other rheumatic diseases, such as rheumatoid arthritis or gout. Septic bursitis is usually caused by organisms introduced through punctures, wounds or cellulitis in the overlying skin. Traumatic bursitis may be complicated by infection or hemorrhage; "*beat knee*"[76] and "*beat shoulder*"[92] in miners are examples of this. Continuous abrasion of the skin with stone dust results in cellulitis, and repeated scraping of the bursa against rough stone surfaces leads to hemorrhage. With modification of occupations and habits, many of the classical forms of bursitis are encountered less frequently, *e.g.*, "*housemaid's knee*," "*weaver's bottom*" and "*policeman's heel*."

Subdeltoid bursitis, which is described in detail in Chapter 80, is the most common bursitis; other types which are frequently seen are:

Trochanteric Bursitis, an inflammation of one or more of the bursae about the gluteal insertion on the femoral trochanter.[35] This is usually insidious in onset, preceded by apparent trauma in only about a fourth of the cases. Aching pain on the lateral aspect of the hip and thigh is aggravated by lying on the affected side. There is tenderness posterior to the trochanter and pain with external rotation of the hip and with active abduction against resistance, but not with flexion and extension.

Olecranon Bursitis, an inflammation with effusion at the point of the elbow, occurring frequently with rheumatoid arthritis and gout as well as after trauma. Pain is usually minimal except when pressure is exerted on the swollen bursa. Elbow motion is unimpaired and usually painless. The swelling will often subside if further trauma is prevented with a sponge ring.

Achilles Bursitis, an inflammation of the bursa just above the attachment of the Achilles tendon to the os calcis, often related to trauma from tight shoes ("pump bumps") and perhaps to an unusual configuration of the posterior calcaneus[20] (*see* Chapter 78).

Calcaneal Bursitis, an inflammation of a bursa at the point of attachment of the plantar fascia to the os calcis (*see* Chapter 78).

Bunion, a painful bursitis over the medial surface of the first metatarsophalangeal joint, usually with a hallus valgus (*see* Chapter 78).

Ischial Bursitis, an inflammation of the bursa separating the gluteus maximus from the underlying ischial tuberosity, usually produced by prolonged sitting on hard surfaces ("*weaver's bottom*").

Prepatellar Bursitis, a swelling between the skin and lower patella or patellar tendon, resulting from frequent kneeling (Figure 76–7). Pain is usually slight unless there is direct pressure on the swollen area.

Anserine Bursitis, an inflammation of the sartorius bursa on the medial aspect of the tibia.[58] This is said to occur in women whose legs are disproportionately large. The characteristic complaint is pain with stair climbing. Inflammation in another, nameless bursa located at the anterior edge of the medial collateral ligament[83] also gives pain on the inner aspect of the knee, but with point tenderness in a different area.

Iliopectineal Bursitis, an inflammation of a bursa between the iliopsoas and inguinal ligament.[42] The patient complains of groin pain, radiating to the knee, and often adopts a shortened stride to prevent hyperextension of the hip while walking. Examination reveals tenderness just below the inguinal ligament, lateral to the femoral pulse, and pain on hyperextension of the hip.

Treatment.—In general, therapy includes protection from irritation and trauma, either by modifying the patient's activities or by the use of appropriate padding. Anti-inflammatory drugs, heat and ultrasound are also commonly employed. Local corticosteroid injections are usually successful. Surgical excision is reserved for refractory cases.

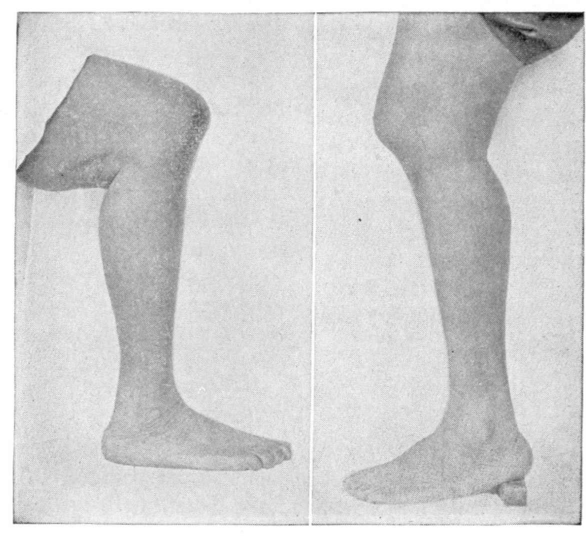

Fig. 76–7.—Bilateral prepatellar bursitis (housemaid's knee) in a scrubwoman. (Lewin, *Orthopedic Surgery for Nurses*, courtesy of W. B. Saunders Company.)

Calcific Tendinitis and Periarthritis.—Some cases of tendinitis and bursitis are associated with calcific deposits, most commonly with subdeltoid bursitis and trochanteric bursitis, but occasionally with tendinitis, bursitis, or periarthritis around the wrist, knee, elbow and elsewhere.[67,75] In these instances the attacks are less likely to be preceded by recognized trauma and tend to be abrupt in onset with intense local inflammatory signs, resembling an attack of gout.[54,67,84,90] The calcific deposit may be present before the acute attack and may disappear within several weeks thereafter.[67] It would appear that calcium hydroxyapatite is deposited initially in a tendon, for reasons which are not presently known. The deposit, which has a pasty consistency, enlarges but often causes no symptoms or, depending upon its size and location, chronic symptoms with pain on certain motions, as in the supraspinatus tendon. The resolution of the calcification following an acute inflammatory attack may suggest that release of hydroxyapatite crystals from a ruptured deposit into the bursa or peritendinous tissues is responsible for provoking the inflammation.[54,67] There is no direct evidence to support this possibility, although crystals have been identified in the exudate, some within leukocytes.[54] Most patients have acute attacks of calcific tendinitis in only one area but a few have involvement in multiple sites.[67] There is no evidence of a generalized disorder of calcium metabolism; serum calcium, phosphorus and alkaline phosphatase are normal.

INJURIES TO MUSCLES AND TENDONS

Haldeman and Soto-Hall[37] discussed certain features of injuries to muscles and tendons. Features which they found very suggestive of rupture of muscles included:

1. A history of a sudden sharp pain or snapping sensation occurring during violent muscular effort.
2. Inability to perform certain definite movements following this.
3. The diagnosis is more certain if one sees the appearance of a defect in the belly of the muscle or in the tendon, with subsequent ecchymosis.
4. Roentgenogram of soft tissues often reveals a defect in the shadow cast by the muscle; in some cases, a small chip of bone is seen attached to a tendon which has been torn from its insertion.
5. Electrical stimulation of the muscle will cause it to contract and produce pain at the site of a tear in either the muscle or tendon.
6. Local injection of procaine will eliminate pain and will permit testing of muscular function in those cases in which the diagnosis is difficult.

The supraspinatus muscle or tendon is the most likely to be torn in the upper extremity and the quadriceps is the most vulnerable in the lower extremity. The average age of patients with tears of muscles or tendons was forty-two years, corresponding to the period in which the greatest physical activity overlaps with degenerative changes.

Attrition of the musculotendinous cuff, secondary to local trauma by pulley systems and bony prominences, may lead to necrobiotic changes which predispose to rupture.[6] Trauma is the immediate and direct cause of rupture; sudden application of a stretching force on a strongly contracting muscle results in tearing of muscle fibers, followed by hemorrhage, edema and localized spasm ("*charley horse*"). In some cases extreme passive stretching of a tendon attachment is the primary mechanism, such as the avulsion of the adductor insertion in the groin in a water skier falling with widely abducted hips. Muscle fatigue results in incomplete relaxation and predisposes to stretch injuries. Therefore, these are more likely to occur in poorly conditioned athletes.[6]

Tendon rupture is common in rheumatoid arthritis, caused by the lytic effect of tenosynovial inflammation and, in addition, mechanical abrasion of tendons due to disruption of the contiguous bone. Injection of corticosteroids for tendinitis has also been said to predispose to tendon rupture, especially in the Achilles tendon.[85]

McMaster's experiments on the breaking weight and site of rupture of a preparation of muscle and tendon showed that normal tendon does not rupture but that the rupture occurs at the attachment of tendon to bone, the musculotendinous junction or through the muscle substance.[56]

Codman has emphasized the importance and frequency of *tears of the supraspinatus tendon.*[13] They occur in older individuals and it is presumed that attrition and trauma both contribute to the rupture (Chapter 80).

Rupture of the long head of the biceps may be the final result of chronic frictional attrition of the tendon within the bicipital groove (Chapter 80). The rupture may be accompanied by transient pain over the anterior aspect of the shoulder. The belly of the muscle assumes a spherical shape and lies closer to the elbow than normal. Surgical repair is often possible but not mandatory, since disability is generally mild.

The rhomboideus major or minor muscles may be strained by a sudden incoordinated movement of the shoulder; this occurs frequently in industrial practice. These muscles arise from the ligamentum nuchae and the spinous process of the seventh cervical to the fifth dorsal vertebrae and insert into the vertebral border of the scapula. Contraction of these muscles draws this border of the scapula upward.

Following injury to the rhomboid muscles there is a localized tenderness between the mid-dorsal spine and the scapula; pain occurs at this point if the shoulder is passively flexed forward or if it is extended against resistance. Treatment consists of partial immobilization of the scapula by drawing it backward and upward with adhesive. Physical therapy (heat and light massage) should be started when the signs of injury have disappeared.

Other muscles arising from the spinous processes and inserting on the scapula or humerus include the *levator scapulae, latissimus dorsi and trapezius muscles*; strains of these muscles give a clinical picture which is somewhat similar to injury to the rhomboids.

Rupture of the pectoralis major muscle is usually due to an abrupt traction injury, with sudden sharp pain in the shoulder and a snapping sensation.[64] A tender mass is felt in the muscle and there is ecchymosis of the overlying skin. Evacuation of the hematoma and surgical repair are the treatment of choice.

Rupture of the rectus abdominis muscle may at times be mistaken for intraperitoneal disease (such as appendicitis). Rupture of this muscle may occur following a severe bout of coughing or sneezing, during pregnancy or labor or following influenza or typhoid fever (with degeneration of the muscle fibers). A large hematoma may form due to tears of branches of the epigastric vessels. The hematoma may require evacuation surgically.

Rupture of the quadriceps muscle or tendon is relatively common. This occurs at the point of attachment of the tendon to the patella or at the musculotendinous junction; occasionally, a tear may occur through the purely tendinous or muscular portions. The usual cause of this condition is a violent contraction of the muscle, such as falling on a flexed knee. The injury occurs in both young and aged. There is inability to actively extend the knee and a hiatus is seen in the tendon or muscle. Partial tears of the muscle may leave only a depression in the muscle substance without permanent disability. These usually heal readily following splinting of the leg in full extension for three or four weeks, with gradual mobilization following this. Complete tears of the quadriceps muscle or tendon should be repaired surgically.

When the *patellar tendon* is ruptured, the patella lies higher than usual, a gap is noted, active knee extension is lost and joint effusion is usually present. A roentgenogram will confirm the diagnosis.

Partial rupture of one of the calf muscles has been termed "*tennis leg*"; this usually involves the plantaris muscle, but may affect a belly of the gastrocnemius. Symptoms include a snap with sudden burning pain in the calf during a strong muscular contraction. The pain may extend to the popliteal space; it is aggravated by passive dorsiflexion of the ankle. Treatment includes adhesive strapping to immobilize the ankle in plantar flexion for several weeks, following which heat, massage and exercises are used.

Spontaneous rupture of the posterior tibial tendon results in pain, tenderness and swelling behind and below the medial malleolus, with loss of stability of the foot. It is usually preceded by chronic symptoms suggestive of tenosynovitis and is often associated with planovalgus feet. Treatment is either surgical repair, in cases diagnosed early, or an arch support.[45]

Injury to the Achilles tendon may occur after violent exercise (as in boxers or sprinters) or in middle-aged men, unaccustomed to exertion, who indulge in weekend athletics involving jumping (such as basketball and volleyball). There may be rupture at the musculotendinous junction or avulsion at the attachment to the calcaneus. Examination reveals a depression over the tendon and inability to plantar flex the ankle against resistance. In partial rupture the pain may be fairly mild; swelling and ecchymosis may conceal the depression usually noted with complete tears. Partial ruptures may be treated conservatively with immobilization of the foot in plantar flexion; complete tears usually require surgical intervention.[33,86]

The anterior tibial compartment syndrome is an ischemic necrosis of muscle due to swelling after unaccustomed exercise. The muscles in this compartment are confined by a tight fascial sheath, resulting in a compromised blood supply when swelling occurs. On examination there is marked weakness of the involved muscle and local swelling and erythema. Sensation in the first two toes is often lost due to compression of the deep peroneal nerve. Immediate fasciotomy must be performed to prevent irreversible destruction of muscle.[51,82]

ARTHROPATHY FOLLOWING NON-MECHANICAL TRAUMA

Caisson Disease

Men who work in pressurized chambers, such as the caissons used in tunnel construction, may be exposed to repeated episodes of excessively rapid decompression. Release of bubbles of nitrogen gas into the tissues and vascular space may cause acute throbbing pain in the extremities, known as "*the bends*." Since nitrogen is very soluble in lipid, the fatty marrow of long bones is particularly liable to injury. Bubbles released into this rigid closed space raise intramedullary pressure, interfere with blood supply and may result in infarction. Bubbles obstructing terminal arteries may cause avascular necrosis, particularly in both femoral epiphyses, the humeral head and the proximal tibia. In one recent study 47 of 241 tunnel workers had radiographic evidence of avascular necrosis; its occurrence was a function of the number of exposures to decompression and the height of pressure.[2] There is usually little or no pain in affected joints until collapse of necrotic bony trabeculae results in deformity of the articular surface. Radiographically, caisson disease resembles avascular necrosis and bone infarction caused by other conditions.[70] Aviators subjected to sudden decompression may rarely experience "the bends" and, in one case, avascular necrosis has been reported.[40]

Radiation Arthropathy

Joints exposed to irradiation may sustain injury which is usually not symptomatic until several years later.[46] The changes resemble degenerative arthritis and are found only in joints which had been included in the field of radiation. Radiographic findings include narrowing of the joint space, marginal new bone formation and periarticular osteoporosis. Occasionally chondrocalcinosis and ankylosis may occur. A few examples of "rheumatoid-like" arthritis with soft tissue swelling were also noted. The spine may be involved, showing narrowing and calcification of intervertebral discs.

Irradiation of the rib cage may result in osteochondritis, with pain and swelling in the costal cartilages. This may suggest metastatic malignancy or Tietze's syndrome but, in contrast to these conditions, there is erythema in the tender area.[50]

Frostbite Arthropathy

Severe frostbite may cause destruction of the phalangeal epiphyses, resulting in short fingers,[22] or asymptomatic bony enlargement, resembling Heberden's nodes.[27]

BIIBLOGRAPHY

1. Anderson, K. J., LeCocq, J. F. and Clayton, M. L.: Clin. Orthop., *23*, 146, 1962.
2. Barnes, R.: Manitoba Med. Rev., *47*, 547, 1967.
3. Barnes, W. C. and Malament, M.: Surg., Gyn. & Obstet., *117*, 277, 1963.
4. Begg, M. W. and Scott, J. E.: Ann. Rheum. Dis., *25*, 145, 1966.
5. Berk, R. N.: New Engl. J. Med., *277*, 1411, 1967.
6. Brewer, B. J.: Clin. Orthop., *23*, 30, 1962.
7. Burleson, R. J., Bickel, W. H. and Dahlin, D. C.: J. Bone & Joint Surg., *38A*, 1265, 1956.
8. Byers, P. D. and Wadsworth, T. G.: J. Bone & Joint Surg., *52B*, 290, 1970.
9. Bywaters, E. G. L.: Ann. Rheum. Dis., *24*, 215, 1965.
10. Carstensen, E. and Giebel, M. G.: Deutsche med. Wchnschr., *86*, 2114, 1961.
11. Cermak, J. and Bilek, F.: Cas. Lek. ces., *104*, 151, 1965.
12. Cherry, J. H. and Ghormley, R. K.: Amer. J. Surg., *52*, 319, 1941.
13. Codman, E. A.: *The Shoulder*, Boston, Thomas Todd Company, 1934.
14. Coffin, F.: J. Laryngol., *74*, 155, 1960.
15. Coventry, M. B. and Mitchell, W. C.: J.A.M.A., *178*, 898, 1961.
16. Cseuz, K. A., Thomas, J. E., Lambert, E. H., Love, J. G. and Lipscomb, P. R.: Mayo Clin. Proc., *41*, 232, 1966.
17. Cyriax, J.: *Textbook of Orthopaedic Medicine*, 5th ed., Baltimore, Williams & Wilkins, 1969.
18. Davie, B.: Med. J. Australia, *1*, 1355, 1969.
19. Derbyshire, R. C.: Amer. J. Surg., *112*, 635, 1966.
20. Dickinson, P. H., Coutts, M. B., Woodward, E. P. and Handler, D.: J. Bone & Joint Surg., *48A*, 77, 1966.
21. Dingman, R. O. and Constant, E.: Plastic & Reconstructive Surg., *44*, 119, 1969.
22. Dreyfuss, J. R. and Glimcher, M. J.: New Engl. J. Med., *253*, 1065, 1955.
23. Drucker, W. R., Hubay, C. A., Holden, W. D. and Bokovnic, J. A.: Amer. J. Surg., *97*, 454, 1959.
24. Dumonde, D. C. and Glynn, L. E.: Brit. J. Exp. Path., *43*, 373, 1962.
25. Duncan, H., Frame, B., Frost, H. M. and Arnstein, A. R.: Ann. Intern. Med., *66*, 1165, 1967.
26. Durman, D. C.: J. Mich. Med. Soc., *51*, 301, 1955.
27. Ellis, R., Short, J. G. and Simonds, B. D.: Radiol., *93*, 857, 1969.
28. Fitton, J. M., Shea, F. W. and Goldie, W.: J. Bone & Joint Surg., *50B*, 359, 1968.
29. Foged, J.: Lancet, *2*, 1209, 1949.
30. Forrester, C. R. G.: Amer. J. Surg., *28*, 145, 1935.
31. Freese, A. S.: Arch. Otolaryngol., *70*, 309, 1959.
32. Gelfand, L. and Merliss, R.: Ann. Intern. Med., *50*, 999, 1959.
33. Gillies, H. and Chalmers, J.: J. Bone & Joint Surg., *52A*, 337, 1970.
34. Goldie, I.: Acta Chir. Scand., supp. 339, 1964.
35. Gordon, E. J.: Clin. Orthop., *20*, 193, 1961.
36. Gozum, E.: Ann. Otol., *69*, 348, 1960.
37. Haldeman, K. O. and Soto-Hall, R.: J.A.M.A., *104*, 2319, 1935.
38. Hanley, W. B., McKusick, V. A. and Barranco, F. T.: J. Bone & Joint Surg., *49A*, 925, 1967.
39. Harvey, J. P., Jr. and Corcos, J.: Arth. & Rheum., *3*, 218, 1960.
40. Hodgson, C. J., Davis, J. C., Randolph, C. L., Jr. and Chambers, G. H.: Aerospace Med., *39*, 417, 1968.

41. Houston, A. N., Roy, W. A., Faust, R. A., Ewin, D. M. and Espenan, P. A.: South. M. J., *61*, 113, 1968.
42. Hucherson, D. C. and Freeman, G. E.: Amer. J. Orthop., *4*, 220, 1962.
43. Hunder, G. G. and Kelly, P. J.: Ann. Intern. Med., *68*, 539, 1968.
44. Johnson, E. W. and Granberry, W. M.: Amer. J. Orthop., *4*, 216, 1962.
45. Kettelkamp, D. B. and Alexander, H. H.: J. Bone & Joint Surg., *51A*, 759, 1969.
46. Kolar, J., Vrabec, R. and Chyba, J.: J. Bone & Joint Surg., *49A*, 1157, 1967.
47. Kouba, R.: Zbl. Arbeitsmed., *17*, 67, 1967.
48. Lapidus, P. W. and Guidotti, F. P.: Bull. Hosp. Joint Dis., *28*, 50, 1967.
49. Lapidus, P. W. and Guidotti, F. P.: Industr. Med., *39*, 171, 1970.
50. Lau, B. P.: Radiol., *89*, 1090, 1967.
51. Leach, R. E., Hammond, G. and Stryker, W. S.: J. Bone & Joint Surg., *49A*, 451, 1967.
52. Lequesne, M.: Ann. Rheum. Dis., *27*, 463, 1968.
53. Levey, G. S. and Calabro, J. J.: Arth. & Rheum., *5*, 261, 1962.
54. McCarty, D. J. and Gatter, R. A.: Arth. & Rheum., *9*, 804, 1966.
55. McEvedy, B. V.: Brit. J. Surg., *49*, 585, 1962.
56. McMaster, P. E.: J. Bone & Joint Surg., *15*, 705, 1933.
57. Middleman, I. C.: Amer. J. Surg., *102*, 627, 1961.
58. Moschcowitz, E.: J.A.M.A., *109*, 1362, 1937.
59. Muckart, R. D.: Clin. Orthop., *33*, 201, 1964.
60. Nachlas, I. W.: Clin. Orthop., *3*, 121, 1954.
61. Nikolaev, I. A. and Najdenov, S.: Arch. Mal. Prof., *31*, 39, 1970.
62. O'Mara, R. E. and Pinals, R. S.: Radiol., *97*, 579, 1970.
63. Palmer, D. G.: Ann. Intern. Med., *70*, 61, 1969.
64. Park, J. Y. and Espiniella, J. L.: J. Bone & Joint Surg., *52A*, 577, 1970.
65. Parvin, R. W. and Ford, L. T.: J. Bone & Joint Surg., *38A*, 1352, 1956.
66. Phalen, G. S.: J. Bone & Joint Surg., *48A*, 211, 1966.
67. Pinals, R. S. and Short, C. L.: Arth. & Rheum., *9*, 566, 1966.
68. Pipkin, G.: Clin. Orthop., *3*, 8, 1954.
69. Plewes, L. W.: J. Bone & Joint Surg., *38B*, 195, 1956.
70. Poppel, M. H. and Robinson, W. T.: Amer. J. Roentgenol., *76*, 74, 1956.
71. Robbins, H.: J. Bone & Joint Surg., *45A*, 953, 1963.
72. Ropes, M. W. and Bauer, W.: *Synovial Fluid Changes in Joint Disease*, Cambridge, Harvard University Press, 1953.
73. Roy, S., Ghadially, F. N. and Crane, W. A. J.: Ann. Rheum. Dis., *25*, 259, 1966.
74. Samellas, W. and Finkelstein, P.: J. Urol., *87*, 553, 1962.
75. Sandstrom, C.: Amer. J. Roentgenol., *40*, 1, 1938.
76. Sharrard, W. J. W.: Brit. J. Industr. Med., *20*, 24, 1963.
77. Shumaker, H. B. and Abramson, D. I.: Surg. Gynec. & Obstet., *88*, 417, 1949.
78. Sinclair, A.: Brit. J. Industr. Med., *22*, 144, 1965.
79. Smillie, I. S.: *Injuries of the Knee Joint*, 3rd ed., Baltimore, Williams & Wilkins, 1962.
80. Smillie, I. S.: *Osteochondritis Dissecans*, E. & S. Livingstone Ltd., Edinburgh, 1960.
81. Solonen, K. A.: Ann. Chir. Gynaec. Fenn., *55*, 176, 1966.
82. Stark, W. A.: Clin. Orthop., *62*, 180, 1969.
83. Stuttle, F. L.: Clin. Orthop., *15*, 197, 1959.
84. Swannell, A. J., Underwood, F. A. and Dixon, A. St. J.: Ann. Rheum. Dis., *29*, 380, 1970.
85. Sweetnam, R.: J. Bone & Joint Surg., *51B*, 397, 1969.
86. Swenson, S. A. and Smith, W.: J. Trauma, *10*, 334, 1970.
87. Swezey, R. L.: Arth. & Rheum., *13*, 858, 1970.
88. Tanzer, R. C.: J. Bone & Joint Surg., *41A*, 626, 1959.
89. Thomas, H. O.: *Diseases of the Hip, Knee and Ankle Joints, with their Deformities, treated by a New and Efficient Method*, 3rd ed., London, H. K. Lewis, 1878.
90. Thompson, G. R., Ming Ting, Y., Riggs, G. A., Fenn, M. E. and Denning, R. M.: J.A.M.A., *203*, 464, 1968.
91. Tietze, A.: Berlin. Klin. Wchnschr., *58*, 829, 1921.
92. Turnbull, V. H.: Brit. J. Industr. Med., *19*, 222, 1962.
93. Ward, J. R., Dolowitz, D. A., Baukol, J. L., Smith, C. and Fingerle, C. O.: Ann. Intern. Med., *112*, 693, 1963.
94. Wilkinson, A.: Lancet, *2*, 13, 1965.
95. Williams, K. A. and Scott, J. T.: Ann. Rheum. Dis., *26*, 532, 1967.
96. Williams, R.: J. Bone & Joint Surg., *45B*, 542, 1963.

97. Wilson, J. D.: Clin. Orthop., *3*, 109, 1954.
98. Wilson, J. N.: J. Bone & Joint Surg., *49A*, 477, 1967.
99. Wilson, R. N. and Wilson, S.: Practitioner, *178*, 612, 1957.
100. Wiltse, L. L. and Frantz, C. H.: J. Bone & Joint Surg., *38A*, 500, 1956.
101. Wolf, C. R. and Mankin, H. J.: J. Bone & Joint Surg., *47A*, 1203, 1965.
102. Younghusband, O. Z. and Black, J. D.: Canad. Med. Ass. J., *89*, 508, 1963.

Chapter 77

Internal Derangement of the Knee Joint

By PHILIP D. WILSON, JR., M.D., and DAVID B. LEVINE, M.D.

Definition

Internal derangement of the knee (IDK) is an ambiguous term, which covers a multitude of lesions having in common only the fact that they interfere with the normal mechanics (*i.e.*, function) of the knee joint. Many of the potential causes have been discussed in other chapters (*i.e.*, Osteochondritis Dissecans, Osgood-Schlatter's Disease, Prepatellar Bursitis, Baker's Cyst, Pellegrini-Stieda's calcification, Osteoarthritis, "Traumatic Arthritis," Rheumatoid Arthritis and Pigmented Villonodular Synovitis).

ANATOMICAL CONSIDERATIONS

The knee is a hinge joint, which relies on ligaments and muscles for its stability. The major muscle in this respect is the *quadriceps*, which extends by a tendinous expansion across the joint, to be inserted into the tibia.[15] The major *ligaments* are the *tibial* and *fibular collaterals* and the *anterior* and *posterior cruciates*, which act together to limit abduction and adduction movements, anterior or posterior displacement and twisting strains of the tibia on the femur.[3]

Although the movements of this articulation appear to be simple flexion and extension, for these movements to be accomplished smoothly, a certain amount of rotation of one condylar surface on another must occur. To extend the knee fully, the tibia must twist outward in relation to the femur, and the reverse is necessary to begin the action of flexion. The joint is well lubricated by fluid secreted from the largest synovial surface in the body. Much of this membrane is contained in the suprapatellar pouch, which extends 3 finger-breadths above the patella. Diffusion of the synovial fluid is facilitated by two fibrocartilaginous menisci which are anchored to the tibia by the coronary ligaments, and in the case of the medial meniscus, to the collateral ligament as well. These structures occupy the chinks created by the incongruity of the tibial and femoral condylar surfaces. In the rotation movements that accompany flexion and extension of the knee they follow the action of the femoral condyles and it is this flexibility that accounts for their ready displacement and rupture during strain or injury.

The *prime movers of the joint* are the *hamstrings* behind, and the *quadriceps* in front. The quadriceps forms a tendinous expansion which partially envelops the anterior surface of the knee. In its center lies a large sesamoid bone, the *patella*, which glides over the intercondylar (or patellar) groove of the femur. Multiple bursae are scattered about to facilitate movement. The semimembranosus bursa which often communicates with the knee joint cavity,[6,30] the prepatellar bursa and the anserine bursa are the three of chief clinical interest.

In the examination of no other joint is a knowledge of the surface anatomy so important, since much of it is readily accessible to palpation.

GENERAL CONSIDERATIONS OF DIAGNOSIS

Lesions of the knee usually manifest themselves by *pain, interference with mechanics of motion* (*i.e.*, snapping, locking, giving way, or buckling), *loss of movement, local tenderness, thigh atrophy* and *joint swelling.* It should be remembered, however, that *hip disease* often manifests itself by pain in the knee and the hip should always be checked during the course of examination.

Points of pain and tenderness should be localized as accurately as possible and also the angle of flexion at which mechanical derangement seems to occur. Range of motion can be accurately recorded by goniometric measurement and compared to the opposite side. Muscle atrophy is readily apparent and can be checked by circumferential thigh measurements. The presence of fluid is detected by an anteromedial fullness when slight, or by gross distention, fluctuation and ballottement of the patella against the femoral condyles, when pronounced. If questionable, it can be confirmed by careful examination of the shadow of the synovial pouch in x-ray examination.[17] Even the most experienced examiner, however, cannot determine the character of the fluid unless aspiration is carried out (*see* Chapter 6, p. 67 and Chapter 32, p. 526).

Locking, buckling (*i.e.*, giving way) and snapping are symptoms frequently experienced by the patient with internal derangement. True locking is experienced at the immediate moment of injury, whether slight or severe, and commonly involves some twisting strain. The knee is suddenly prevented from extending, not so much by pain as by an actual internal physical obstruction. Flexion is not usually so noticeably affected. The locked position interferes with, but does not necessarily prevent, walking and may persist indefinitely or correct itself by some sudden twist, blow, or manipulative movement. It is typical of a torn *displaced* meniscus, but may be due to a loose body or incomplete dislocation of the patella. It should be distinguished from the *gradually* developed attitude of fixed flexion, which arises from synovial distention whether it be exudative or from hemorrhage. Buckling is a delayed and not an immediate manifestation of injury. It is a symptom of the "trick knee" and can be caused by quadriceps weakness, tears, or abnormal mobility of the menisci or ligamentous weakness. Snapping is a symptom usually not associated with appreciable disability. It is often both audible and palpable, and in the adolescent is most frequently caused by a discoid lateral meniscus, while in the adult it most usually represents softening, fissuring and roughening of the patellar articular surface (chondromalacia). When possible, these symptoms should be reproduced at the time of examination. Even a minor degree of locking can easily be detected by failure of the patient to extend the joint fully when walking or standing, and a rubbery resistance to full extension when the heel is supported and the knee rocked gently while the patient is supine. Buckling is difficult to reproduce, but ligamentous instability can be demonstrated. To test the collateral ligaments properly, the knee must be fully extended (in flexion, a small amount of adduction is possible since the fibular collateral ligament is taut only in full extension) and the knee forcibly abducted or adducted. There should be no difference between the two sides. This can be checked by an AP x ray made while abduction or adduction strain is applied to both knees. The cruciate ligaments are best tested with the knee flexed to 90 degrees. The tibia is firmly grasped and suddenly pulled forward (anterior cruciate) or pushed backward (posterior cruciate) on the femur. Again, the patient should be relaxed, the force suddenly and strongly applied, and the affected knee checked against its opposite. Small degrees of excursion are not necessarily significant, particularly in the presence of quadriceps atrophy.

Various special maneuvers have been

devised to reproduce snapping, momentary locking and catching. They are not usually applicable, however, to the acutely traumatized patient, and are only helpful, not absolute, signs in the chronic one. Deep knee bending will often reproduce the snap of the discoid meniscus. Flexion and extension of the knee, or passive movements of the patella while it is compressed against the femur will often reproduce the crepitus due to roughening of its articular surface. Forced rotation while the knee is carried from full flexion to extension (McMurray's sign)[21] will often produce a palpable and sometimes audible snapping in the presence of a torn meniscus. It is often accompanied by a painful twinge. Rotation movements of the tibia, while the knee is held in 90 degrees flexion, will sometimes help to distinguish meniscal tears if the pain produced is localized to one side of the joint line.

Passive limitation of side-to-side and up-and-down excursion of the patella is often a sign of arthritic change; also palpable lipping of the articular margins. The bulbous nodular and thickened synovium of chronic synovitis can usually be distinguished from the soft fluctuant membrane characteristic of recent or early effusion. Here, x-ray examination will often be of great diagnostic aid. To be complete, it should include four views: AP or PA in full extension, PA in flexion (*i.e.*, tunnel or Holmbladt view), lateral, and vertical (axial) view with the knee flexed to show the patella and its joint space. Lewis[17] has stressed the importance of adequate investigation of the soft tissue shadows for early x-ray diagnosis of many knee joint lesions.

Aspiration of the Knee

When fluid is present after injury, aspiration is usually indicated. This should always be done under the strictest sterile precautions. If bloody fluid is obtained, a capsular or ligamentous tear or osteochondral fracture is most likely; if the fluid is clear, one should think more of a meniscal tear or simple sprain. If the fluid is cloudy, beware of infection; do *not* inject a steroid compound until the fluid has been analyzed and cultured (*see also* Chapters 6 and 32).

GENERAL CONSIDERATIONS OF TREATMENT

Rest

Protection of the knee after acute injury is of paramount importance in healing. Bedrest and traction are required if the knee cannot be fully straightened, but if this is not feasible, certainly non-weight-bearing on crutches. A padded elastic bandage placed circumferentially for a distance four inches above and below the joint line and reinforced by strips of felt or basswood is usually most useful. If full extension is possible, immobilization in a plaster cylinder may also be considered, but is only practical when the period of protection is to be for two weeks or more.

Quadriceps Setting

Atrophy of the quadriceps occurs surprisingly rapidly following injury. It is mandatory to instruct every patient in ways and means of preventing this. Weight-resistance exercise (*see* Chapter 34) cannot be instituted until a diagnosis is made, and suitable treatment well under way. Setting of the quadriceps, however, can be started almost immediately. The patient will usually be helped by being shown the method of exercise on the unaffected side first, and the examiner should not leave until he is satisfied that it is being correctly performed. This is not a job for the physiotherapist alone, though in difficult cases, his help may be most useful.

As the knee improves, the exercise can be graduated first to straight leg raising, then to knee extension without resistance, and finally to extension against resistance. Early institution of and proper observation of a good knee exercise program will do more than almost anything else to shorten disability.

Operation

Arthrotomy should be carefully considered in all healthy active patients whose injuries are due to acute violence. It is definitely indicated when one or more of the following factors are present: sustained locking with its inception at the time of injury or immediately afterward; gross anteroposterior and/or lateral instability (demonstrated under anesthesia if necessary); and inability to extend the knee actively against gravity, when passively it can be straightened. In the first instance, a displaced torn meniscus, loose body or tangential osteochondral fracture is to be expected. In the second, a major ligamentous tear is probably present; and in the third, the extensor mechanism most likely has been disrupted.

Prior to operation, of course, diagnosis should be established as accurately as possible by the various measures already discussed. Aspiration and x-ray exam-

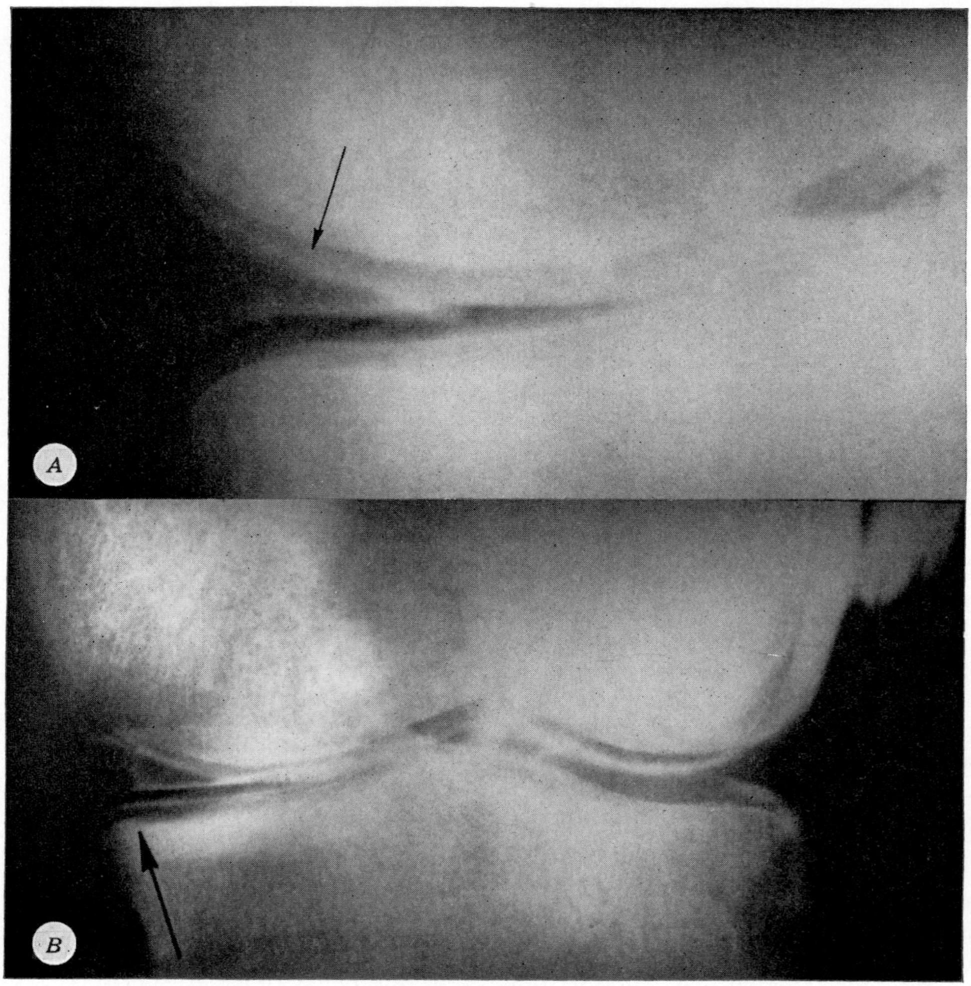

Fig. 77–1.—Double contrast arthrogram of the knee illustrates (*A*) normal medial meniscus and (*B*) vertical tear in the medial meniscus. (Courtesy of Dr. Robert H. Freiberger.)

ination are particularly important in this respect. Arthrography of the knee has proven to be a most valuable diagnostic procedure.[21a] The technique of double contrast arthrography consists of injection of air into the knee followed by injection of Renografin 60. No complications of this procedure have been reported and preoperative diagnostic accuracy has been approximately 90 per cent (Fig. 77–1). Early operation, under the above conditions, is the best and often the only way of restoring unrestricted activity. It will not only save the patient much time, but may prevent permanent disability, which in many instances cannot be overcome by later reconstruction.[22]

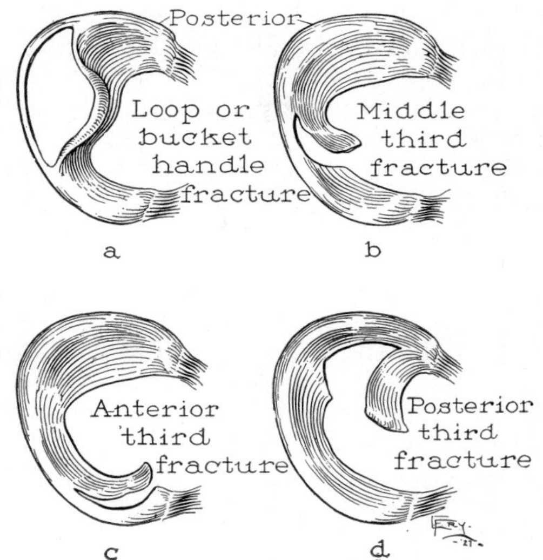

FIG. 77–2.—Types of injury to the semilunar cartilage. (Henderson, courtesy of Surg. Gynec. & Obst.)

COMMON CAUSES OF INTERNAL DERANGEMENT

Tears of the Menisci[25]

The medial meniscus is much more prone to laceration than the lateral. The typical cause of injury is a blow against the lateral aspect of the knee while it is flexed and the foot fixed on the ground in an outwardly twisted position. This is obviously very likely to occur in contact sports and the injured person, therefore, likely to be young and athletically active. Not uncommonly, however, and especially in later adult life, tears may be produced by much less severe trauma. Individuals who work in a crouched position much of the time are particularly susceptible, and tearing may occur as they stand up from a deep-knee-bend position.

At the moment of injury, the individual is aware of a painful tearing at the medial side of his knee and cannot extend his leg fully thereafter. He may continue this way until finally relieved by operation, or he may suddenly find the locked position corrected by a twist, a blow against the inner side of the joint, or by some other such manipulation. Locking is caused by a displacement of the torn portion of the meniscus so that it jams the knee and prevents movement. The symptoms vary with the location of the tear and the extent of displacement. The so-called bucket handle tear (*see* Fig. 77–2) usually is accompanied by a permanent locking which can be relieved only by operation. Manipulation of these cases only causes completion of the tear, not reduction of the torn portion and, therefore, is not recommended. Tears of the anterior or posterior horns, transverse tears of the middle portion and horizontal fissures are more compatible with continuing function and are the types that lead to recurring symptoms ("trick knee"). When the individual pivots, the knee is likely to lock momentarily and to give way. There may be little attendant reaction unless the catching leads to further tearing and especially to a displacement of the torn segment in the joint, in which case the initial sypmtoms may be repeated even to the point of sustained locking. Most meniscal tears have little power to heal since they are situated in relatively avascular fibrocartilage. Relief, therefore, must usually come about by surgical removal, erosion of the torn tab by constantly repeated minor traumata or curtailment of activities. Tears near the periphery, on the other hand, may heal if protected sufficiently after the initial episode.[16]

The history of the injury and subsequent events is obviously all-important in making a diagnosis. X rays are of little value except to exclude other lesions such as osteochondritis dissecans. More recently, we have come to rely on the arthrograms as a valuable aid in arriving at a diagnosis. Physical examination will usually show a mild degree of effusion, joint line tenderness, and, if soon after injury, the locked position or a resistance to full extension, with pain when forced. Twisting of the knee will usually aggravate or reproduce pain. This can sometimes be accentuated by compressing the articular surfaces as the tibia is rotated on the femur. Occasionally, exact diagnosis is not possible.[19] It has been reported that *arthroscopy* has been most valuable for difficult diagnostic problems.[6a] The technique is not without its limitations since considerable experience is necessary before the procedure is satisfactory and general anesthesia has been required.

The major indication for arthrotomy is locking, and operation should not be delayed when this is definitely present. If the knee is not locked, conservative management is in order until the true nature of the lesion is established by failure to improve or by later recurrences. The patient should be kept off his leg during the acute phase of symptoms. After weight-bearing has commenced, the joint should be protected by suitable bandaging until swelling and pain have completely subsided. Exercise is started immediately after injury by quadriceps setting and then graduated to resisted extension according to the rate of recovery. The interval between injury and recovery will vary on an individual basis; therefore, no set time for return to full activity, especially sports, should be established. The best practice is to delay resumption of athletics until the quadriceps has recovered strong power. In this way over-all morbidity is reduced and more serious injury prevented.

Cysts of the Menisci[2,4]

Unlike tears, cysts are much more commonly seen arising from the lateral meniscus than from the medial. They are usually manifested by a swelling noted most readily with the knee in right angle flexion. Their causation is not perfectly understood, but from a pathologic point of view, they closely resemble multilocular ganglions. Although trauma sometimes antecedes the development of a cyst, less than half of the cases have associated tears of the menisci, and in these, it is seldom if ever possible to determine whether the tear is cause or effect of the condition.

Onset is characterized by well-localized aching pain with gradual appearance of a tender swelling most frequently at the midlateral joint line. Variation from this set pattern is not unusual; the cysts often fluctuate in size, may occasionally enlarge rapidly, and sometimes extend below or above the joint for a considerable distance. Locking, snapping and buckling are not necessarily associated and synovial effusion is uncommon. Symptoms are usually aggravated by activity and may be severe enough to interfere with sleep.

X rays will often show the soft tissue bulging in an anteroposterior view and particularly in the "tunnel view," since it is taken with the knee in a flexed position. Diagnosis can sometimes be confirmed by local aspiration, and especially so in the case of the larger cysts. If so, considerable improvement may ensue from instillation of a steroid compound into the lesion. Recurrence cannot be prevented until all pathologically involved tissue (*i.e.* capsule containing the cysts and underlying meniscus) is removed. After adequate excision, full recovery can be expected.

Discoid Meniscus

This is a condition of late adolescence or early adult life in which the meniscus (usually the lateral) is found to be discoid rather than semilunar in shape. Whether it is congenital or traumatic in origin is a matter of debate.[14] It is not infrequently bilateral and is associated with a snapping sound during movement. It may be otherwise asymptomatic and often does not interfere with joint mechanics. The most characteristic finding is a widened lateral joint space shown on x ray. Symptoms are usually initiated by trauma, even though of minor severity, and result from tearing. When a tear is present, differentiation from the usual type of meniscal injury is difficult unless there is a past history of snapping or the opposite knee is also involved. Operative excision is the treatment of choice.[9,26]

Calcified Meniscus

This is a rare lesion and not necessarily of symptomatic significance. When the calcification is localized, differentiation from a loose osteochondritic body is difficult to make.[8] If associated with significant symptoms removal is indicated. Chondrocalcinosis of the meniscus is a finding suggesting pseudogout (*see* Chapter 60).

Ligamentous Tears[1,22,23]

Severe tears or ruptures of the major ligaments of the knee are almost always brought on by injuries of considerable violence. They occur usually during athletics and are particularly common in football players and skiers. Athletes who have been classified as having a generalized ligamentous hyperelasticity incur a special risk of ligament ruptures from injuries.[21b] A major tear should always be suspected in the presence of hemarthrosis unless x rays indicate a fracture involving the joint surface. Early diagnosis is essential to proper management. These types of injury obviously do not often come to the attention of the rheumatologist, since they are referred directly from the scene of accident to a surgeon, who is known locally for his interest in these problems. Prompt surgical repair is the treatment of choice, but good results have also been reported from simple immobilization.[24a]

Milder Sprains (Incomplete Tears)

These present a more universal problem and one which is more difficult to differentiate from tears of the menisci. The mechanisms of injury are very much the same, and by the time the patient reaches a physician, there is often associated swelling which prevents full extension, thus simulating a locked position. A careful history as to the sequence of events is necessary and it will usually be found that only after swelling had appeared did the knee fail to extend. Tenderness is usually less well localized than is the case in a meniscal tear and swelling greater. Because of pain and because the knee cannot be extended, tests for stability are difficult to evaluate.[24] Aspiration of the knee is sometimes helpful, since the presence of blood indicates a capsular injury, and hemarthrosis is less likely to occur in an uncomplicated meniscal tear.

Facility in diagnosis of these cases is attained only after considerable experience. It is better, therefore, to perform examination under heavy sedation or even anesthesia, whenever there is doubt. If stability is not significantly impaired, conservative treatment is in order, including splint-bandaging of the knee, application of cold during the acute phase and heat in the convalescent period, graduated quadriceps exercise and guarded resumption of activity.

A relaxed knee following ligamentous injury is a common cause of chronic disability. A careful examination will usually reveal an associated quadriceps atrophy, and it is often surprising how much improvement can come from strengthening of this muscle alone. By and large, late surgical reconstructions of the ligaments give disappointing results, and are only indicated in the presence of marked instability. The use of a knee cage type brace (Fig. 77–3) made of plastics, leather or corseting and elastic

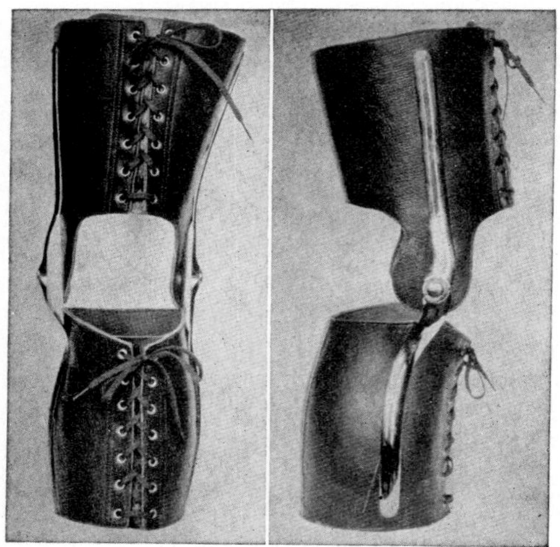

Fig. 77–3.—Jones knee cage for after-care in knee injuries. (Bennett, courtesy of Amer. J. Surg.)

may be helpful in protecting such a joint. However, these are difficult to fit properly and, for the grossly unstable knee, a long leg brace with shoe caliper is required.

Fractures of the tibial plateaus, like ligamentous tears, usually result from abduction or adduction strains and sometimes the two conditions may be associated in a single case. The recognition of the depressed plateau fractures is not difficult, but the undisplaced linear ones may be missed unless a careful x-ray examination, including obliques, is made. The suspicion of the examiner should be aroused by the presence of marked swelling (hemarthrosis) and tenderness over the involved bony condyle rather than over the joint line. The management of a joint fracture of this kind demands the best of orthopedic care since operative intervention is definitely indicated in some cases, whereas others may be better treated by immobilization or early exercise in a suspension apparatus.[12]

Injuries to the Extensor Mechanism (Tears of the Patellar or Quadriceps Tendons. Fracture of the Patella)

These injuries are usually sustained as the result of a blow against the anterior aspect of the knee while the extensor mechanism is under tension with the knee flexed 90 degrees or more. They are recognized by tenderness and ecchymosis anteriorly and by marked joint swelling. Inability to extend the knee actively or the palpation of a defect indicates significant separation and operative repair is indicated. X rays should obviously be obtained. Bipartite ossification of the patella should not be mistaken for a fracture. The irregularity of contours of the tendinous structures will sometimes make it possible to confirm the diagnosis of a tendon rupture in the absence of a patellar fracture.[17] If the patellar fracture fragments are not separated and complete *active* extension is possible, treatment by immobilization in extension alone will be sufficient.

Loose Bodies.—"Joint mice" may develop in four ways: osteochondritis dissecans (Chapter 76), osteoarthritis (Chapters 55 and 56), synovial chondromatosis and tangential osteocartilaginous fractures. The bodies may be cartilaginous or osteocartilaginous, thus invisible or visible on x rays (Fig. 77–4). When completely loose, they are free to wander about the joint, and to jam it during movement, leading to intermittent catching, locking or giving way. The larger they are, the more likely they are to be tucked in some cranny of the joint (posteriorly or in the suprapatellar pouch) and the less likely to produce symptoms. Even partially attached bodies may cause derangement; in the case of osteochondritis dissecans, by raising or softening or fissuring the overlying cartilage or if the attached synovial stalk is long, by wandering far enough to interfere with movement. Unless the patient or examiner is fortunate enough to palpate the body, or if the loose body is not visible roentgenographically, exact diagnosis is next to impossible. When causing derangement, early removal is advisable, with the one exception that an osteochondritic body-in-situ in childhood may heal with immobilization alone.[31]

When surgery is undertaken for the

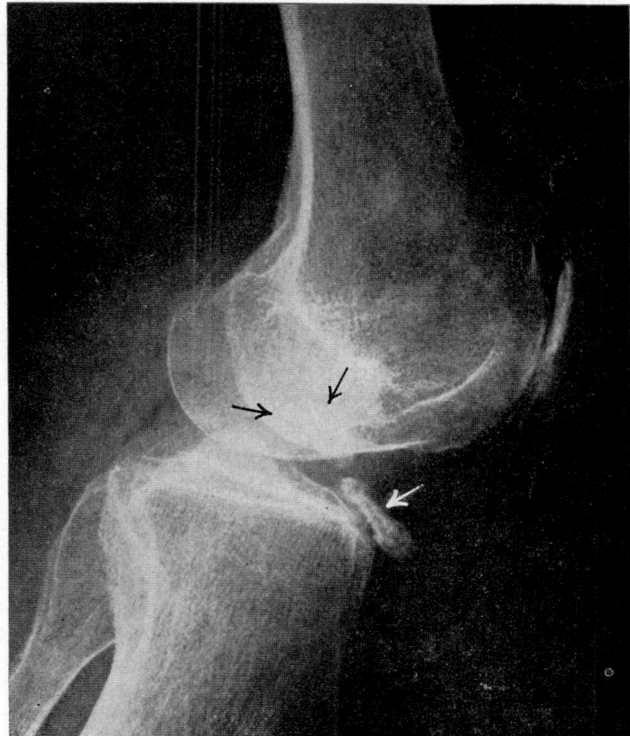

Fig. 77–4.—Loose bodies in a knee joint.

removal of one loose body, more should always be suspected, and looked for. The causative lesion should be corrected lest more fragments loosen. In osteochondritis dissecans, or osteoarthritis, this means removal or debridement of loose cartilaginous tabs, projecting marginal spurs and sometimes patellectomy.

In synovial chondromatosis, loose bodies may form in great numbers (Fig. 77–5), and total synovectomy is necessary for relief. Diagnosis of this condition in its early phases is difficult, but it should be suspected in the presence of a chronic persisting synovitis especially if faint calcifications are seen roentgenographically. Differentiation from synovial sarcoma (Chapter 75) may be difficult if the calcific shadow is small and isolated.

Chondromalacia Patellae[5,7,28]

Because it is subjected to so much friction, the patellofemoral joint compartment is particularly prone to cartilaginous attrition. This produces the crepitus so familiar to all when the knee is being extended. When roughening is marked, pain, snapping and catching develop leading to synovial reaction. At first, this is confined to a circumferential zone around the patella only, but eventually the whole joint may be involved and effusion becomes marked. Symptoms are initiated or aggravated by forceful extension of the knees as when climbing steps or arising from the sitting or, worse still, the crouched position. The condition is especially prone to give rise to symptoms in women in adult life. Early onset, however, is favored by a relaxed quadriceps mechanism, which permits *recurrent subluxation or dislocation.* The tendency to dislocation or subluxation should, therefore, be corrected surgically as soon as it is recognized.[11,13,18] Any young adolescent girl who complains of

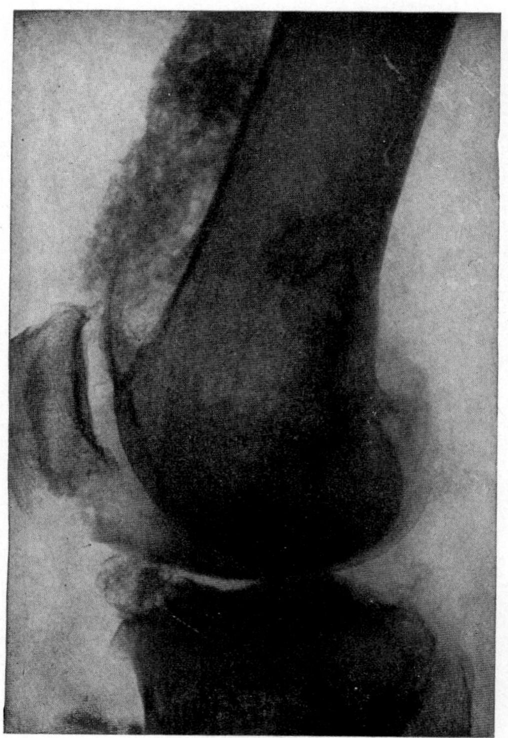

Fig. 77–5.—Multiple calcified bodies in knee joint (osteochondromatosis). (Holmes and Robbins.)

recurring painful sensations in her knees should be suspected of having the condition, which is more often than not bilateral. Lateral migration of the patella during active extension, peripatellar tenderness, and a marked apprehension of the patient when the patella is forced laterally are characteristic findings, which should lead to diagnosis. Since the patella tends to displace laterally, medial transfer of the patellar tendon insertion, plication of the medial capsule and correction of valgus alignment, used either singly or in combination, are the usual means of correction.

Once chondromalacia has developed, treatment must be directed toward relieving strain by restricting, insofar as possible, stair climbing, crouching and prolonged standing or sitting. Bandaging and resistive exercises will often aggravate the condition rather than help it; therefore, simple quadriceps setting and straight leg raising only are indicated. When symptoms are pronounced, the condition can best be relieved by patellectomy, after which useful and painless function is usually restored.

Traumatic Synovial Effusions

Despite one's best efforts to arrive at a diagnosis, the cause of synovial effusion following trauma may sometimes remain obscure (Chapter 76). Direct contusion or pinching of the synovial membrane or of the infrapatellar fat pad may be responsible for some of these cases. Although hemorrhagic and cystic lesions of the fat pad have occasionally been found to be responsible for such effusions, by and large, hypertrophy and tenderness of the infrapatellar fat pad should lead one to suspect some more subtle pathologic change in the knee.

A persistent increase of synovial fluid in the knee joint will frequently lead to recurrent clicking of the patella on movement. This is due to loosening of the quadriceps expansion secondary to chronic distention of the joint capsule and quadriceps wasting. If, in addition, there is a slight limitation of joint motion and especially of extension, differentiation from other types of "trick knee" may be difficult. A careful history is usually most helpful in this respect.

In conclusion, the reader should remember that IDK is not a single entity, but a symptom complex, some components of which are found in almost all lesions of the knee joint. Only the more common of these have been discussed here. More comprehensive discussions are available in textbooks of orthopedic surgery or monographs on this subject.[25]

BIBLIOGRAPHY

1. Abbott, L. C., Saunders, J. B. deC., Bost, F. C. and Anderson, C. E.: J. Bone & Joint Surg., *26*, 503, 1944.
2. Bonnin, J. G.: Brit. J. Surg., *40*, 558, 1953.
3. Brantigen, O. C. and Voshell, A. F.: J. Bone & Joint Surg., *23*, 44, 1941.

4. Breck, L. W.: Clin. Orth., *3*, 27, 1954.
5. Bronitsky, J.: J. Bone & Joint Surg., *29*, 931, 1947.
6. Burleson, R. I., Bickel, W. H. and Dahlin, D. C.: J. Bone & Joint Surg., *38A*, 1265, 1956.
6*a*. Casscells, S. W.: J. Bone & Joint Surg., *53A*, 287, 1971.
7. Cave, E. F. and Rowe, C. R.: J. Bone & Joint Surg., *32A*, 542, 1950.
8. Cave, E. F.: J. Bone & Joint Surg., *25*, 53, 1943.
9. Cave, E. F. and Staphles, O. S.: Amer. J. Surg., *54*, 371, 1941.
10. Childress, H. B.: J. Bone & Joint Surg., *36A*, 1233, 1954.
11. Harrison, M. H. M.: J. Bone & Joint Surg., *37B*, 559, 1955.
12. Hohl, M. and Luck, J. V.: J. Bone & Joint Surg., *38A*, 1001, 1956.
13. Houkom, S. S.: Arch. Surg., *44*, 1026, 1942.
14. Kaplan, E. B.: J. Bone & Joint Surg., *39A*, 77, 1957.
15. ———: J. Bone & Joint Surg., *39A*, 1223, 1957.
16. King, D.: J. Bone & Joint Surg., *18*, 333, 1936.
17. Lewis, R. W.: Amer. J. Roentg. & Rad. Ther., *65*, 200, 1951.
18. MacNab, I.: J. Bone & Joint Surg., *34A*, 957, 1952.
19. Murdock, G.: J. Bone & Joint Surg., *39B*, 503, 1957.
20. Mussey, R. D. and Henderson, M. S.: J. Bone & Joint Surg., *31A*, 619, 1949.
21. McMurray, T. P.: Brit. J. Surg., *29*, 407, 1942.
21*a*. Nicholas, J. A. and Freiberger, R. H.: J. Bone & Joint Surg., *52A*, 203, 1970.
21*b*. Nicholas, J. A.: J.A.M.A., *212*, 2236, 1970.
22. O'Donoghue, D. H.: J. Bone & Joint Surg., *32A*, 721, 1950.
23. ———: J. Bone & Joint Surg., *37A*, 1, 1955.
24. ———: Am. Acad. Orth. Surg. Instruct Course Lect., *15*, 105, 1958.
24*a*. Richman, R. M. and Barnes, K. O.: J. Bone & Joint Surg., *28*, 473, 1946.
25. Smillie, J. S.: *Injuries of the Knee Joint*, Baltimore, The Williams & Wilkins Co., 1962.
26. Smillie, J. S.: J. Bone & Joint Surg., *30B*, 671, 1948.
28. Wiles, P.: J. Bone & Joint Surg., *38B*, 95, 1956.
29. Wilmoth, C. L.: J. Bone & Joint Surg., *23*, 367, 1941.
30. Wilson, P. D., Eyre-Brooke, A. S. and Francis, J. D.: J. Bone & Joint Surg., *20*, 963, 1938.
31. Wiberg, G.: Acta. Orthop. Scand., *14*, 270, 1943.

Chapter 78

Painful Feet

By Theodore A. Potter, M.D.

The feet will show swelling, stiffness, and pain in most patients suffering from rheumatoid arthritis. Evidence of osteoarthritis, often symptomless, will be found in x rays of the feet in most of the patients over sixty years of age. In gout and in many of the "collagen diseases" the feet are involved frequently and disabilities occur. The majority of painful feet not associated with arthritis are caused by weak muscles, relaxed ligaments, and deformity. These are called static disabilities. Most of the static disabilities of the feet respond readily to treatment. Arthritis in the foot responds more slowly but in most instances a painless, useful foot can be obtained. Painful feet will be considered under these categories: static disabilities, traumatic disabilities, inflammatory conditions, congenital deformities, disturbances of growth, and circulatory disturbances.

Over 90 per cent of painful feet are caused by static disabilities. These usually begin as a mild weakness and slowly progress, if untreated, to serious disability with deformities in the bones, muscles and ligaments.[1] Traumatic disabilities give little difficulty in diagnosis. They usually require immediate treatment and in most instances recovery is prompt.[20] Congenital disabilities usually come under the care of orthopedic surgeons early if they are at all serious. The milder ones can usually be treated like static disabilities. Infections in the foot usually require avoidance of weight-bearing, except in the milder cases. Antibiotics are often required. Most developmental disabilities are self-limited and require treatment only if there are symptoms. Circulatory disturbances are most commonly found in the aged. While most of these can be helped, few of them can be cured and treatment at best is palliative.[8] Neoplasms are rare in the feet.

Systemic diseases which must be considered in the etiology of pain in the foot include diabetes mellitus, arteriosclerosis, intermittent claudication, deficiency of

Predisposing Causes of Foot Strain
Congenital relaxation of ligaments
Disturbances in weight carriage—genu valgum, coxa vara, dislocation of the hip
Poor posture
Badly fitting shoes and stockings (especially short shoes and stockings)
Prolonged illness (prolonged bed rest)
Obesity
Occupations requiring prolonged standing and walking
Circulatory impairment
Systemic diseases which produce weakness or malnutrition

vitamin B_1, arthritis, (tuberculous, gonorrheal, rheumatoid, etc.), syphilis, rheumatic fever, gout, Raynaud's disease, Buerger's disease, poliomyelitis, spastic paralysis, erythromelalgia, cardiac and nephritic disease. Pain in the sole of the foot may be caused also by: deformities; injuries; neoplasms; contractions; scar tissue; absorption of fat from pressure or after prolonged illness; and plantar neuralgia.

Circulatory disorders of the foot which may present cutaneous manifestations include: obliterating arteriosclerosis, thromboangiitis obliterans, acrocyanosis, Raynaud's syndrome, erythromelalgia, immersion foot and vascular anomalies (such as port wine or capillary angioma, spider nevus, small cavernous angiomas, lymphangiomas and diffuse lymphangiomatosis of the leg and foot).

NORMAL PHYSIOLOGY OF THE FEET

The center of gravity of the body is normally balanced over the triangular weight-bearing area of the foot, with its apex posteriorly. This weight is divided equally between the heads of the metatarsal bones and the tuberosity of the os calcis. The anterior shift of the center of gravity which accompanies poor posture disturbs the muscle balance in the foot, and causes a strain on one group of these, leading to what is known as the weak foot.[33] Physicians desiring detailed anatomic or physiologic data on this subject are referred to the works of Dickson and Dively,[10] Morton, Lake, Lewin,[22] Hauser,[15] Kelikian,[18] and Giannestras.[12]

The foot is in part like a spring, com-

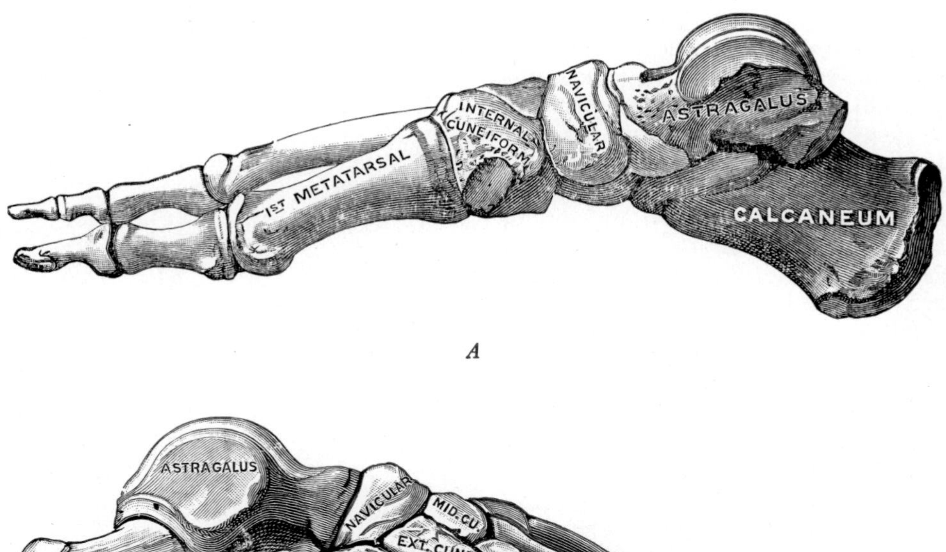

Fig. 78–1.—*A*, The bones of the right foot, viewed from the inner side. *B*, The bones of the right foot, viewed from the outer side.

posed of a bony framework with arches that are maintained by the physiologic tone of muscles, ligaments and fascia. The whole weight of the body in walking and standing comes down on an elastic arch composed of small bones joined by ligaments and connected by muscles. Unfortunately this complicated structure is not left free to perform its function, but is encased from childhood in a distorting leather covering which may compress and deform the forefoot and weaken its muscles. Inasmuch as the shape of the shoe very seldom corresponds to the shape of the adult foot, the shoe is one of the most important factors contributing to foot strain.

Physicians commonly speak of a *longitudinal* and a *transverse arch* of each foot. The longitudinal arch runs anteroposteriorly along the inner border of the foot from the tuberosity of the os calcis to the heads of the metatarsals, centering about the inner three metatarsals, cuneiforms, scaphoid, astragalus and the calcaneus. The medial portion of the longitudinal arch rests upon the os calcis and the head of the first metatarsal.[5] The anterior transverse metatarsal arch passes through the necks of the second, third and fourth, and the heads of the first and fifth metatarsals. It becomes flattened on weight-bearing, but returns to its arched position when the weight is removed. All of the heads of the metatarsals rest upon the ground in weight-bearing so that no transverse arch is present at that time.

The longitudinal and transverse arch form a composite system. The longitudinal arch blends into the transverse arch behind the metatarsal heads and the transverse arch passes imperceptibly into the longitudinal arch as one approaches the base of the metatarsal bones. When the feet are brought together the arches of both feet resemble a shallow, inverted bowl.

The ligaments which aid in maintaining the integrity of the longitudinal arch include the "spring" ligament (or inferior calcaneoscaphoid) which is the main ligamentous support on the inner side,

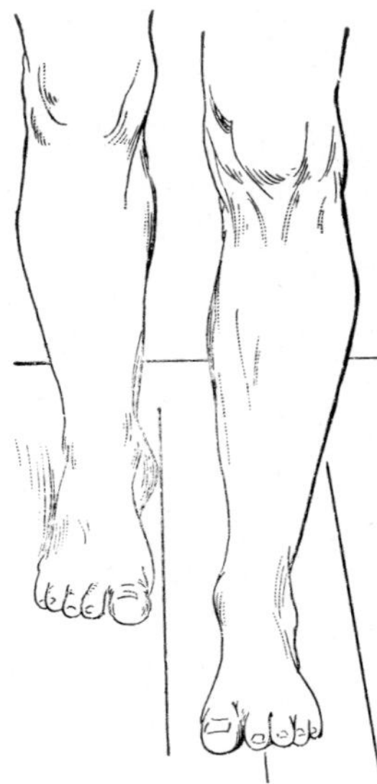

Fig. 78–2.—Illustrating the automatic adduction of the forefoot on the right side, due to the obliquity of the bearing surface of the metatarsus, in the proper attitude for walking.

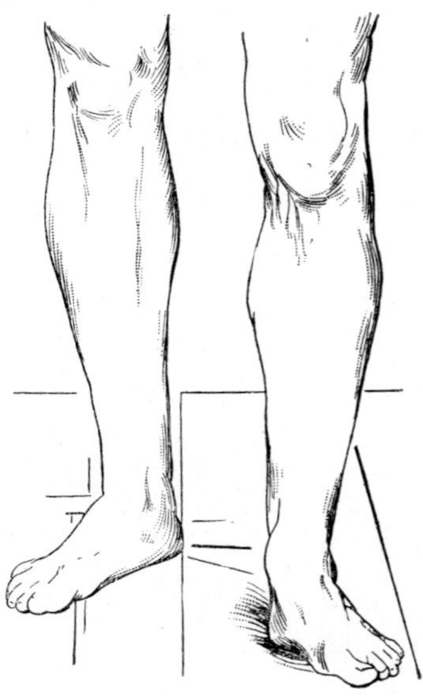

Fig. 78–3.—The improper attitude of outward rotation of the limbs usually accompanied by eversion of the feet, in which there is disuse of the leverage function.

Definitions of Positions of Foot

Adduction: Forefoot displaced inward in relation to midline of limb.
Abduction: Forefoot displaced outward in relation to midline of limb.
Inversion: Sole of foot turned inward.
Eversion: Sole of foot turned outward.
Adduction and inversion and abduction and eversion are often combined.
Valgus: Deformity of the foot in abduction and eversion.
Varus: Deformity of the foot in adduction and inversion.
Calcaneus: Deformity of the foot in dorsiflexion.
Equinus: Deformity of the foot in plantar flexion.
Supination: Same as inversion.
Pronation: Same as eversion.

Examination of the Foot

History of pain or preexisting arthritis. Relation of pain to standing and walking. Pain while resting. Stiffness on arising. Relation to work.

History should include duration and course of the disability and the type and result of treatment.

The gait should be observed.

See that the patient's shoe is not too short, long, narrow or wide. Note the points of greatest wear on the shoe. With short tendo Achilles the tips of the soles are scuffed and worn. In simple eversion the inner side of the heel is worn. With abduction the outer side of the heel is worn lower. With depression of the metatarsal bones a hole may be worn in the anterior part of the sole. If any part of the foot is displaced a distortion will show in that part of the shoe.

See that the stockings are not too tight for the foot.

Examine the posture of the body particularly excessive lordosis and flexion and rotation at the hip and flexion or genu valgum at the knee. Are the legs of equal length?

Examine the foot at rest and on weight-bearing. Look for prominences on the inner side of foot, spread of the forefoot, shape and position of toes.

See if the heel is held in varus or valgus.

Look for corns and calluses, prominence of metatarsal heads on sole of foot, bony prominences at side or dorsum of the foot, swelling about the malleoli, thickening over any tendon, plantar warts, varicose veins, ulceration, blueness or coldness of the feet.

Palpate the joints for swelling or tenderness.

Look for tenderness under the calcaneal fat pad, in the plantar fascia, the inner and outer side of the ankle.

See to what extent the longitudinal and transverse arches are depressed with weight-bearing.

Examine the range of motion at the ankle, tarsal and toe joints. If the ankle joint dorsiflexes to a right angle when the knee is straight there is no contracture of the tendo Achilles.

Examine the skin for color, warmth and excessive perspiration. Look for epidermophytosis between the toes.

Palpate the dorsalis pedis and posterior tibial arteries.

Look for deformities of the nails and irritation at sides of nails.

X-ray examination is indicated if any gross variation from the normal is found.

and the long and short calcaneocuboid or plantar ligaments (supporting the middle and outer part).

The strength and importance of the plantar fascia are demonstrated in paralysis of the extensor muscles of the foot. A pes cavus develops with extreme contracture of the plantar fascia.

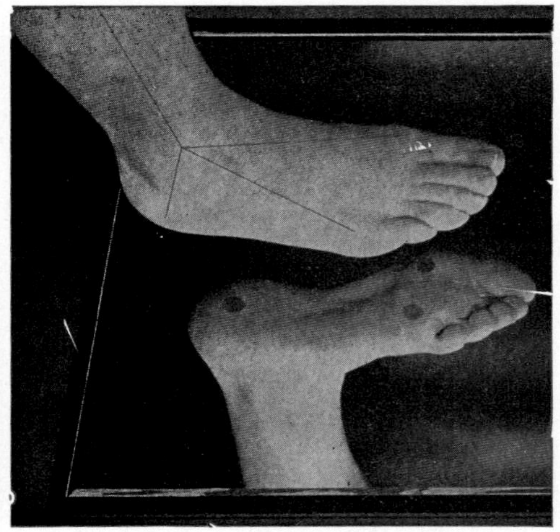

FIG. 78–4.—Distribution of weight to the foot. (Geo. E. Keith Company.)

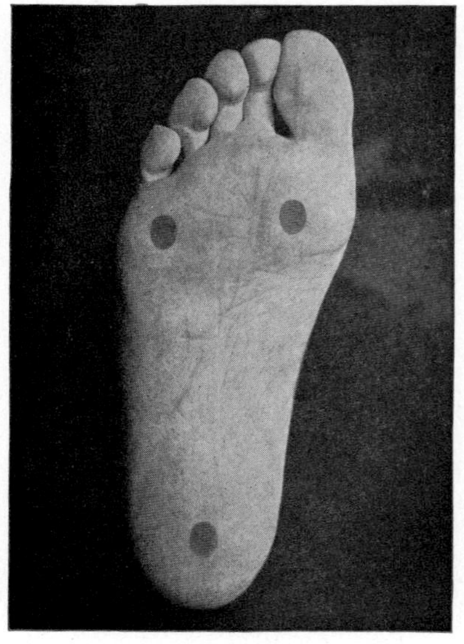

FIG. 78–5.—Weight-bearing points of the foot. (Geo. E. Keith Company.)

The muscles are important structures in the foot. The plantar flexors are approximately 5 times as strong as the dorsal flexors and the gastrocnemius and soleus are 3 times as powerful as the remainder of the foot muscles combined.[29] The chief movements of the foot are carried out by the tibial and peroneal muscles. The tibialis anterior elevates and the peroneus longus depresses the first metatarsal. The tibialis posterior produces inversion and adduction. The peroneal muscles aid eversion and abduction.[26] The chief evertors of the foot are the peroneus longus and peroneus brevis. The invertors are chiefly the tibialis anterior and tibialis posterior. The normal ratio of strength of the invertors to the evertors should be 6:5.

STATIC DISABILITIES

Flat (Weak) Feet

Flat feet may be congenital or acquired. The latter may be classified as flaccid (or static), spastic and rigid. In the flaccid type of flat foot, the main or longitudinal arch is depressed only with weight-bearing and assumes a normal contour when the weight is removed. It has been suggested that a better name for this type of flat foot might be abducted or weak foot because some of these patients may have high arches yet may suffer greatly. During activity these individuals turn their feet outward so that the weight-bearing line prolonged downward through the center of the patella along the crest of the tibia no longer falls in the normal position between the first and second toes, but may be to the inner side of the first metatarsal.[17]

If the flaccid flat foot is untreated, peroneal muscular spasm may occur, producing the spastic flat foot resulting in tenderness over the peroneal tendons and limitation of inversion (which is very painful).

The rigid flat foot is an end stage, with the foot firmly fixed in abduction by contractures and adhesions in which simple measures will not restore the

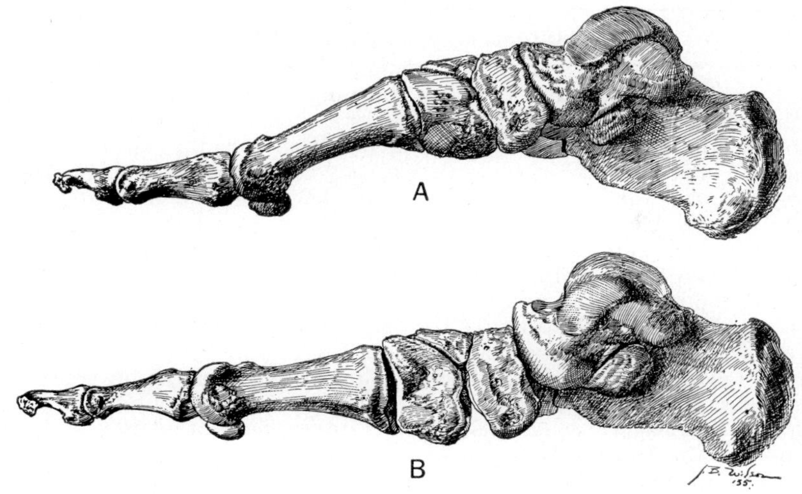

Fig. 78–6.—Medial aspect of the foot: *A*, Normal longitudinal arch. *B*, Arch in flat foot. (Shands, *Orthopedic Surgery*, courtesy of the C. V. Mosby Company.)

normal balance of the foot. Many of these patients have severe pain.

The causes of weak feet are legion but they can be grouped into congenital, developmental, occupational, systemic, traumatic and neurological categories. In those seen in early childhood there is usually a congenital relaxation or weakness of muscles and ligaments. In the developmental group in addition to faulty posture, abnormal development in tarsal or metatarsal bones is sometimes seen. This disturbs the normal balance of the foot. Obesity leads to a slow tiring and overstretching of muscles and ligaments. Systemic diseases involving the bones and joints of the feet lead to weakening, distortion and limitation of motion in these structures.

Trauma may include a fracture of the os calcis, sprained ankle, Potts' fracture, short leg, favoring one foot after injury or because of a wart on the sole, Morton's toe, corns, and the like.

Vocational flat feet may develop from standing on hard surfaces for long periods, as in policemen, mailmen, physicians, dentists, waiters, teachers, barbers and bakers.

Failure of the tibialis anterior and posterior (which maintains the longitudinal arch of the foot) throws strain upon and stretches the ligaments with weight-bearing; this leads to the pain in early flat foot. Foot strain is common in

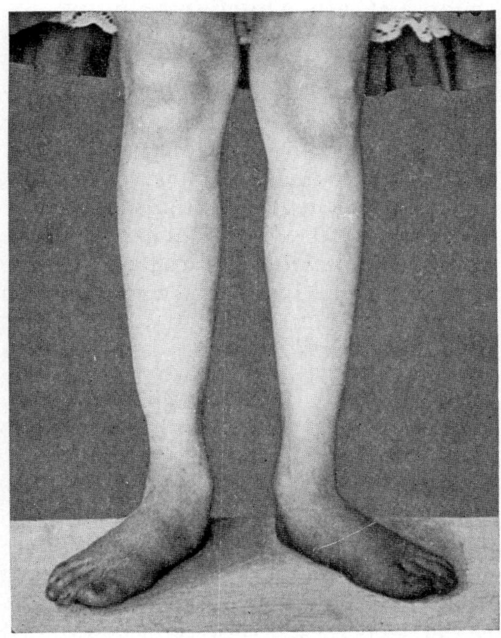

Fig. 78–7.—The ordinary type of weak foot in a child. The degree of abduction indicated by the relation of the patellae to the feet.

Symptoms of Weak, Painful Feet

Weakness in the feet; pain, dull or sharp, burning or stabbing, especially on the medial side of the feet; *ready tiring of the feet* or ankles varying widely in character; coldness, numbness or severe cramps, generalized over the ball of the foot or localized in one joint; *aching or cramps in the calf at night or occasionally during the day,* or pain in the ankle, knee (especially on the inner side from strain of the medial collateral ligament), thigh, hip and lumbar region following weight-bearing or activity; pain along the longitudinal arch and inner border of the foot (due to ligamentous strain); pain in the calf; pain on the inferior and medial aspect of the head of the first metatarsal bone, occasionally with numbness of the toe and pain near the origin of the plantar fascia in the heel and at or under the external malleolus, in weak feet.

One may have pain in the feet, legs and low back for hours on retiring; this usually disappears by morning.

Burning or callus formation on the soles of the feet under the heads (distal ends) of the second and third metatarsals.

Tendency to sit more, and to walk and stand less than previously.

adolescence and early adult life, particularly in those who stand for long periods.[5] If these individuals are treated as soon as pain or tiredness of the feet is noted, one may prevent the development of a deformity.

Flat feet are caused mainly by improper shoes, overstrain and debilitating illness. Foot strain may be alleviated by proper shoes and snugly fitting supports for weak feet or strained arches but foot exercises and training in correct walking are required to develop the foot muscles and relieve symptoms entirely.[6]

Before flat feet can occur, a severe strain must have been placed on the ligaments. The ligaments, together with the muscles, act as safeguards to keep the arches from flattening. Ligamentous strain is preceded by muscular fatigue and weakness. It is only after both the muscles and ligaments give way that flat feet occur.

Strain of the anterior arches is due mainly to cramping of the forefoot; this will usually not occur if one wears shoes which are wide enough, and properly fitting stockings; treatment includes raising the arch by pads, or by a metatarsal bar, and by exercises.

Most of the patients with symptoms of foot disorder have developed a moderate degree of pronation.[11] Normal feet may be strained by excessive loads or long hours of standing, because one naturally assumes a neutral position in standing (with the toes turned outward about 15 degrees), so that strain falls upon the ligaments. Increased strain falls upon the inner side of the foot when the feet are turned out in walking.

In the strained foot there is overstretching of the inferior calcaneoscaphoid ligament, plantar fascia and plantar ligaments and straining of the muscles controlling the inner side of the foot.[9]

Treatment of the Weak (Flat) Foot

Pain and impaired function are indications for treatment. If pain is present at rest or if there is an associated arthritis, prohibit weight-bearing until pain subsides if this is economically possible; use a light removable plaster cast to maintain the foot in inversion, the forefoot in adduction and to support the longitudinal arch. It may be removed each day to permit exercise of the invertor muscles of the foot; exercises must not cause muscular fatigue or pain.

Many individuals with weak, pronated, painful feet may be markedly benefited by a longitudinal arch pad of felt, cork

Signs of Painful, Flat (Strained) Feet

Abduction, dorsiflexion and supination of the forefoot. The weight-bearing line (dropped from the middle of the patella) should come between the first and second toes in the normal foot; in flat feet this line often falls mesial to the great toe.

Prominence of the internal malleoli with a prominent convex curve along the inner and inferior aspects of the arch.

Pain and tenderness beneath the scaphoid, head of the astragalus, sustentaculum tali and internal malleolus and along the plantar surface of the inner border of the foot and over the central portion of the plantar fascia.

Lengthening of the inner borders of the feet (because of separation of the os calcis and scaphoid, stretching of the spring ligament, and dropping of the head of the astragalus between the two bones).

A downward and outward position of the tendo Achilles (instead of the normal directly downward position).

Swelling of the feet, especially anterior to the internal and external malleoli. List of the foot to the inner side; leg seems displaced medially.

Marked wear of the soles of the shoes along the inner side. Weight is borne on the inner side of the foot.

Knock knee may be an early sign of development of flat foot.

In weak feet with peroneal spasm, there is slight or marked limitation to adduction or turning in of the foot when the leg is extended. The flat foot is actually a valgus foot, *i.e.*, abducted and everted.

Secondary signs include: *tenderness and callus formation under the first metatarsophalangeal joint* and the inner side of the heel; callus formation beneath the prominent scaphoid bone (if marked relaxation of the longitudinal arch occurs); and an awkward gait.

If not relieved, eversion and abduction lead to osseous, irreducible flat foot. When rigid flat foot has occurred, there is no spring in the gait and patients use their lower extremities like pedestals.

Deformities secondary to flat feet include hallux valgus, hallux rigidus and hammer toe.

Roentgen examinations of the feet may aid in establishing an accurate diagnosis. Findings of importance in such films include:

- *Shortness of the first metatarsal*, noting the position of its head in comparison to the head of the second metatarsal.
- Partial union of astragalus and os calcis, or other bony union.
- Navicular-cuneiform sag.
- Supernumerary bones may be present, especially an accessory scaphoid.
- Loss of cartilage and development of bony ridges and deformities in the intertarsal and metatarsophalangeal joints in most cases.

Outline of Treatment in Early, Flaccid Flat (Weak) Foot

No weight-bearing if pain is present at rest.

Proper shoes, with heel and sole wedges, if indicated.

Temporary use of arch supports in some cases (especially if markedly overweight or if required to stand or walk for long periods).

Correct posture in standing and walking.

Physical therapy and *exercises* for the muscles of the foot and leg.

Foot baths, particularly contrast baths.

Reduction of weight if indicated.

Night plaster boot with ankle at right angle and foot in slight inversion if there is persistent muscular spasm.

or rubber, averaging $\frac{3}{16}$ inch (beveled to $\frac{1}{32}$ inch on the lateral side) and a heel wedge at the rand (just beneath the sole). The proper placing of the rand wedge is extremely important, lest one turn the heel of the shoe and not the foot. The physician must insist that the entire heel be taken off, the wedge placed next to the sole (heel rand) and that the heel then be replaced. This wedge averages $\frac{1}{4}$ inch in thickness with its highest point at the breast of the heel (anteriorly on the mesial aspect), running to $\frac{1}{32}$ inch posteriorly and laterally.[15]

In mild cases or those associated with knock knee, throw the weight toward the outer side of the foot, by using a crooked and elongated heel, or by raising the inner border of the sole and heel of a flexible shoe approximately $\frac{1}{4}$ inch. Shaping of the heels and soles to produce inversion of the foot in weight-bearing may prove useful.

In very flexible weak feet the patient often obtains greater comfort with the use of a pronatory inner wedge under the heel and a supinatory outer wedge under the little toe. These are not used in rigid or in juvenile flat foot. The wedge raises the inner border of the heel so that the os calcis is placed squarely on the ground. In addition, in order to equalize any tendency to excessive supination in the forefoot, a short cleat is applied to the outer side of the forepart of the shoe. If the varus position of the heel can be maintained until the weight of the body has been transmitted to the head of the fifth metatarsal through the mid-foot, this provides security from strain-provoking pronation.[14]

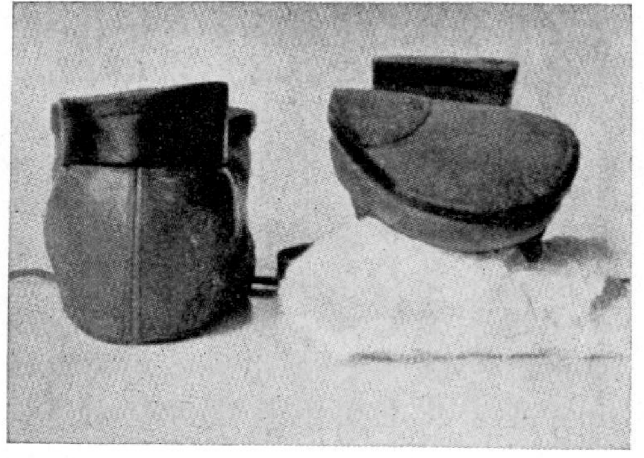

Fig. 78–8.—Shoes corrected with cleats; inner wedge heel and outer patch over toes. (Steindler, J. Bone & Joint Surg.)

In patients with short Achilles tendons, the whole heel must be raised temporarily to relieve this strain.

If necessary, an arch support is used temporarily when the patient becomes ambulatory; *properly made supports are comfortable, support the arch, favor walking on the outer rather than the inner border of the foot,* and toeing straight ahead or slightly inward. The altered heel or arch supports are used for several months after the patient can perform a day's work or exercise without fatigue or pain in the feet. In severely deformed feet and in elderly individuals the supports must often be used permanently.

Arch Supports

These are very useful appliances in the relief of the symptoms from weak feet. In general two types are used; tempered steel plates and leather inlays with raises under the arch of felt or sponge rubber. These stainless steel plates are molded to support the longitudinal and transverse arches. They are most satisfactory when made from plaster impressions of the non-weight-bearing foot. About one-half of those which are used are manufactured in a small number of standard sizes. While these can be obtained readily from surgical supply houses, they rarely fit accurately and do not give as much relief as those which are made from plaster impressions of the patient's foot.

Leather inlays fit in the shoe like insoles. In these the arches are supported by molded areas of felt, sponge rubber or cork which are incorporated in the inlays under the arches of the foot. Both of these types of arch supports have the advantage that they can be adjusted to fit the changing need of support as the foot becomes less strained and fatigued. In this they are superior to any rigid support.[20]

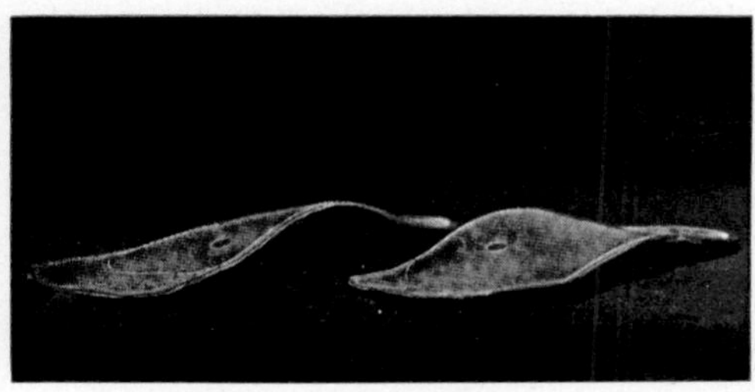

FIG. 78–9.—Type of metal foot plate sometimes used to support the arches. (Kuhns, courtesy of Rheumatism.)

Foot supports are used to relieve the strain on the foot by raising the arches a little, to aid in foot balance and thus lessen muscular fatigue and gradually to bring the foot into a more efficient position for function. Usually steel plates are better for most adults and for feet that do not come into varus readily. In children and in those with circulatory disturbances, relatively soft leather inlays are more comfortable and satisfactory in most cases. Generally, the foot supports give only slight pressure under the arches of the feet at first. As symptoms subside and the foot becomes more flexible, more pressure is exerted. In plates this is done by pounding or bending up the raised portion of the steel plate further. At the same time an attempt is made to hold the foot in slight varus and slight adduction. In leather insoles or "foot pads" more felt or rubber can be put under the arches until symptoms are completely relieved and the foot is held in a good position for weight-bearing. While arch supports are being worn, exercises and foot baths are also prescribed.[21] In the uncomplicated case of weak feet, supports are usually worn for a number of months and are gradually given up as normal strength and alignment return to the foot. In older patients and in those whose feet cannot be made normal, arch supports may be required all of the patient's life.

In the milder forms of foot strain, pads cut from felt or firm sponge rubber can be fitted into the shoe under the arches of the foot and held in place with glue or rubber cement.

If the patient can rest for days or weeks with practically no weight-bearing, to relieve strain, and then is given exercises and proper footwear, often no arch support may be required. But few individuals can rest for a sufficiently long period to achieve this end.

Muscular and ligamentous strain and not merely lowering of the arches of the foot are the cause of pain and disability. A foot with a high arch is more likely to give trouble since it is more readily strained than a foot with a low arch. The rationale of arch supports is the relief of this strain with support of the fatigued and weakened muscles and ligaments. When this is relieved one attempts to secure a normal position of the foot in walking. The elevation in the arch support should extend from the anterior portion of the heel (sustentaculum tali) to the head of the first metatarsal bone. They should extend laterally about $\frac{3}{4}$ of the width of the foot. They should extend only to the fifth metatarsal bone. The height should conform in both longitudinal and transverse arches to the height of these regions when no weight is borne.

Deficiency of the First Metatarsal Segment

Morton reported that the main disturbance in disorders of the longitudinal arch and of the anterior portion of the foot is a "functional deficiency of the first metatarsal segment," so that excessive load and strain are placed upon the second metatarsal segment and its tarsal joints (part of which are normally borne by the first metatarsal segment).

For treatment of this condition, one places a support of sufficient height under the head of the first metatarsal so that contact is made by this metatarsal at the same time as this occurs with the other metatarsals; thus the first metatarsal segment again carries its portion of the burden, and allows the second metatarsal

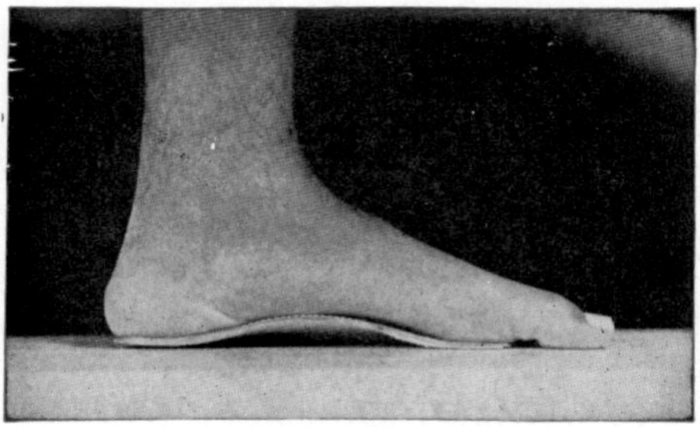

Fig. 78–10.—Metal plate beneath the foot. (Kuhns, courtesy of Rheumatism.)

segment to support only its normal share of the body weight. For this purpose, there has been devised a compensating insole which fits into the shoe with a "platform-like projection" just under the head of the first metatarsal bone. This may also be useful in cases of foot strain due to a congenitally short first metatarsal bone. The height of the small platform thus placed can be determined only by trial, as the "compensating insole" can be removed easily for adjustment of the height of this portion. In some cases however, any support under the first metatarsal head causes midtarsal pain and tends to throw weight to the outer aspect of the foot causing irritation of the fifth metatarsal.

Proper Shoes

Well-fitting shoes of proper construction are necessary for walking under present-day conditions.[3] Soft moccasins or boots were adequate for warmth and protection when man walked on soft yielding earth, but feet will not withstand prolonged use upon hard pavements and floors without adequate protection. Many shoes now being worn do not protect the feet in the present unnatural environment in which most of us must live.

The proper shoe should fit. If shoes are persistently uncomfortable they should not be worn regardless of their quality or beauty. New shoes can be secured readily but foot disabilities cannot be discarded readily and their correction often requires long time and effort. Shoes are now made over a relatively large number of standard lasts. There are few feet which cannot be fitted properly in ready-made shoes if a few general instructions are followed.[3]

Standard lasts with their insole patterns are available for determining the length of heel to great toe as well as the width and other pecularities of foot shape. Fitting shoes requires careful measurement from heel to ball and from heel to toe. This is essential for support and for function of the muscles on the inner side of the foot. Cramping of the toes leads to weakness and is soon followed by depression of the transverse arch. Insufficient space in the mid-foot may weaken and depress the longitudinal arch. Insufficient cuboid space does not give proper seating of this bone, leading to fatigue and faults in walking.[12]

Sometimes one foot is a little longer or broader than the other foot. An insole or a slight correction where the one shoe is too large will often lead to a comfortable fit. For those with a large variation in the size of the feet, many large shoe stores will fit with individual sizes for each foot. Those with very severe deformity can often only be fitted adequately by a maker of orthopedic shoes. These men can also make adjustments in the shoe for fixed deformities of the heel, forefoot or toes.

In order to fit the shoe properly and to order modifications intelligently one must know something about its manufacture and the various parts of a shoe. The *last* of a shoe is a wooden model, similar to the shape of the foot, over which the shoe is built. A *combination last* means that the shoe is made with several different *combinations of widths, i.e.*, at the heel, waist, tread measurements and ball measurement. The heel is always narrower than the ball of the foot. The toe cap is the part covering the toes and may be either soft or firm. The vamp is the upper part of the shoe anterior to the laces. The quarter is the remainder of

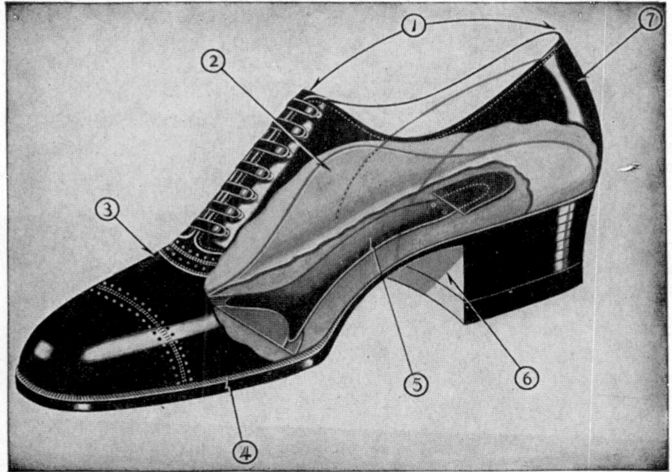

Fig. 78–11.—Shoe showing *shank* (*5*) of a shoe extending from the heel to the forepart of the foot. (Geo. E. Keith Company.)

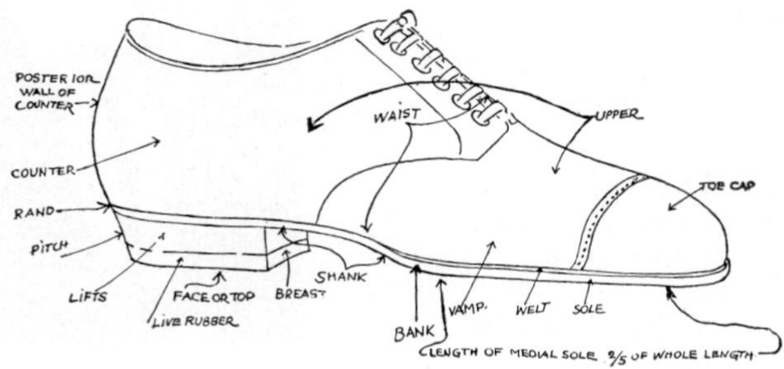

Fig. 78–12.—External parts of a shoe. (Ashley, courtesy of Medical Record.)

the upper behind the vamp. The waist is the portion of the upper immediately in front of the heel. This part is often too tight in high-arched feet. The shank is a thin supportive bar, usually steel, placed above the sole running from the anterior third of the heel forward almost to the metatarsal heads.

Shoe Corrections

The shoe correction most frequently prescribed is a raise in the front inner corner of the heel $\frac{1}{8}$ to $\frac{3}{8}$ of an inch. This is indicated in mild valgus of the os calcis. It is often combined, especially in children with relaxed feet, with arch supports. Usually in children the raise varies between $\frac{1}{8}$ and $\frac{1}{4}$ inch. In adults usually $\frac{1}{4}$ inch is prescribed. Such raises are usually placed just beneath a rubber heel but may be put inside the shoe beneath the insole. A *Thomas heel*, often combined with a raise of the front inner corner of the heel, is a forward extension of the heel on the medial side $\frac{1}{2}$ to $\frac{3}{4}$ of an inch. This gives added support to the shank of the shoe and lessens fatigue in the region of the longitudinal arch.[4]

A *metatarsal bar* (*Jones bar*) is a strip of leather fixed to the sole of the shoe transversely just behind the metatarsal heads. It is usually $\frac{1}{8}$ to $\frac{1}{4}$ of an inch in thickness and about $\frac{3}{8}$ of an inch wide.

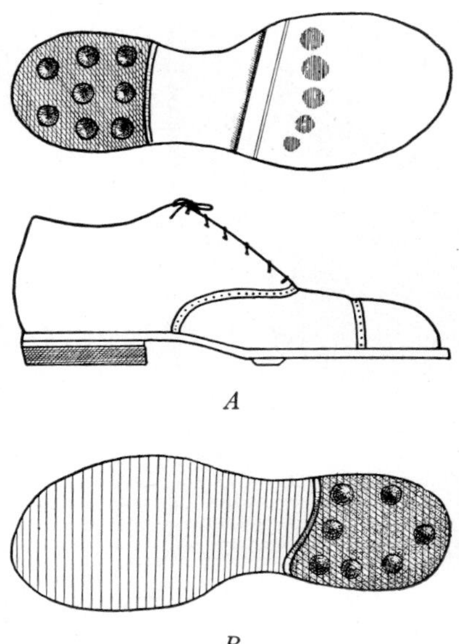

Fig. 78–13.—*A*, Metatarsal bar. *B*, Thomas heel; note the forward extension of the heel along the inner margin. (Shands, *Orthopedic Surgery*, courtesy of the C. V. Mosby Company.)

It is used chiefly in rigid depressions of the transverse arch associated with contracture of the extensor tendons and hammer toe deformity. It shifts the weight back to the bar from the metatarsal heads and usually affords comfort from severe anterior arch strain.[15]

A *cuboid wedge* is a raise ⅛ to ⅜ of an inch placed under the cuboid region on the lateral side of the sole. It is used to aid the correction of an adduction of the forefoot. It is of much value only in feet that are flexible.

Corrections can be added to high shoes (boots) or low shoes (oxfords). The shoe should be a well-fitting laced shoe.

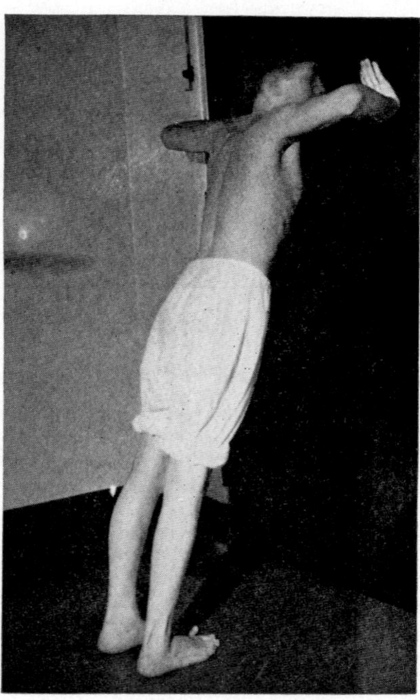

Fig. 78–14.—Usual exercise for stretching a contracted or tight tendo Achilles. The heels should remain on the floor and the knees should not bend during the exercise.

Proper Standing and Walking Positions

Feet 4 inches apart.

Toes pointing straight ahead.

Weight on the midlongitudinal axis of the feet.

Arches cupped as the palm of the hand.

Head up, abdomen in.

To demonstrate good posture: Stand with the back against a wall, with the head, shoulders, buttocks touching the wall and the heels slightly forward. Place the hand between the small of the back and the wall. Abnormal lumbar lordosis produces a large space here. Flatten the lumbar spine by pushing the small of the back against the hand.

Do not keep one position for a long period of time.

Exercises and Postural Aids for Weak, Painful Feet[15]

Exercise is more important than mechanical supports in the treatment of weak feet. Exercises strengthen the lifting muscles on the medial border and transverse portion of the arch (*i.e.*, the tibialis anterior and posterior, flexor longus hallucis, flexor longus digitorum, interossei and peroneus longus). Proper function of the foot muscles prevents painful lowering of the arch and renders mechanical support unnecessary. Exercises must not be instituted in the acute stages of foot strain as they may aggravate the condition.

Foot exercises aim to strengthen plantar flexors and adductors and to stretch the dorsiflexors and pronators. Plantar flexors are strengthened by rising on the toes, while rolling onto the outer sides of the feet strengthens the supinators.

Foot exercises should be performed barefooted. The following exercises may be used in patients with weak, pronated feet. Exercises are instituted gradually, are done slowly and regularly, and must never cause fatigue or pain. At the onset, one or two exercises may be performed 5 times once or twice a day. Exercises should be given first without weight-bearing. As the symptoms become less severe, sitting and standing exercises should be given. Later the exercises are performed less frequently as normal strength returns.

1. Spread and flex the toes sharply downward; this may be done with the shoes off or on.
2. Stand on the toes with these turned inward, roll out on the sides and return to a flat position.
3. Place about 12 small marbles on the floor. While sitting with the bare feet pick up 1 marble at a time with the foot and place it in the opposite hand (*i.e.*, right foot to the left hand and vice versa). Repeat this several times a day using a dozen marbles each time with each foot. This is particularly useful in children.
4. Walk on the outer borders of the bare feet along a straight line.
5. Stand with the toes pointing inward and attempt to externally rotate the knees without lifting the big toe from the floor.
6. While seated on the floor, bring one sole into contact with the other as much as possible.
7. Sit with feet pointing forward, curl all toes slowly, relax.
8. Sit squarely, roll feet outward until soles are almost parallel, relax.
9. Sitting cross kneed, push foot downward, roll foot inward and then pull foot upward describing a circle with the foot.
10. For stretching tight tendo Achilles stand facing the wall, 2 feet from the wall, sway toward the wall keeping heels on floor. Do not bend at the knees.

If it is necessary to stand for long periods, rise on the toes and put weight on the outer border of feet, about every ten minutes.

Children should be encouraged to walk in bare feet on sand or grass.

Corrections should not be applied in pumps or high-heeled shoes. Corrections on shoes or firm corrective shoes are worn until symptoms subside and examination shows disappearance of the weakness or deformity.

Adhesive Strapping for the Weak Foot

Pain may be relieved temporarily by the proper application of strips of adhesive to the weak foot. Such strapping should not be continued for long periods because of the danger of irritation to the skin.

As a temporary measure for relief of pain in the transverse arch, place a small felt or sponge rubber pad on the sole just proximal to the heads of the second and third metatarsal bones; hold this in place by adhesive. This pad must be skived at all margins. In most adults, it should average 2 inches in length, $1\frac{1}{2}$ to $1\frac{3}{4}$ inches in width and $\frac{3}{16}$ inch in height (at its highest point). Circular strapping of the bare feet behind the metatarsal heads may also relax the overstretched transverse ligaments.

Adhesive strapping may be used temporarily in patients with weak feet. In addition, the inner border of the heel may be raised about $\frac{1}{4}$ inch to relieve strain on the dressing and to get the patient used to carrying weight on the outside of the foot.

A simple form of adhesive dressing may be applied as follows: (1) Paint the skin with compound tincture of benzoin. (2) Have the patient hold the foot in slight inversion and at right angles to the leg. (3) Apply a strip of adhesive about 18

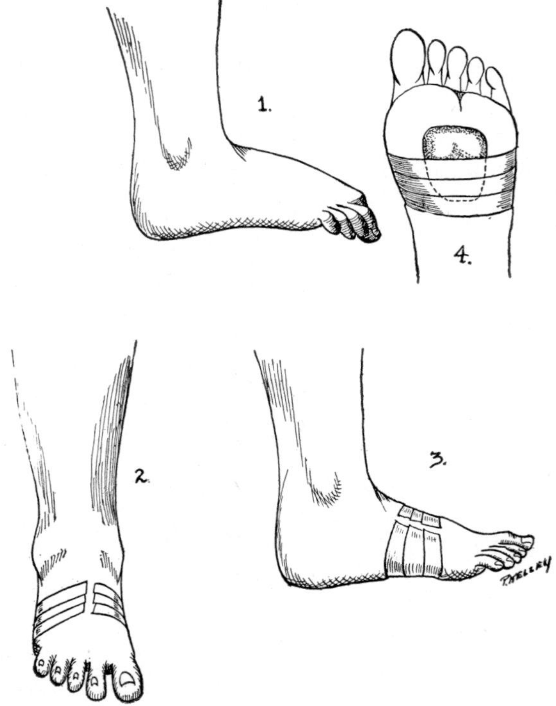

Fig. 78–15.—Anterior (metatarsal arch) strapping. Soft foot pad (as in 4) may be incorporated into strapping. Distal border of the pad must be proximal to the metatarsophalangeal joints. The pad lies over the second, third and fourth (but not the first or fifth) metatarsals. (Dickson and Diveley, *Functional Disorders of the Foot,* courtesy of J. B. Lippincott Company.)

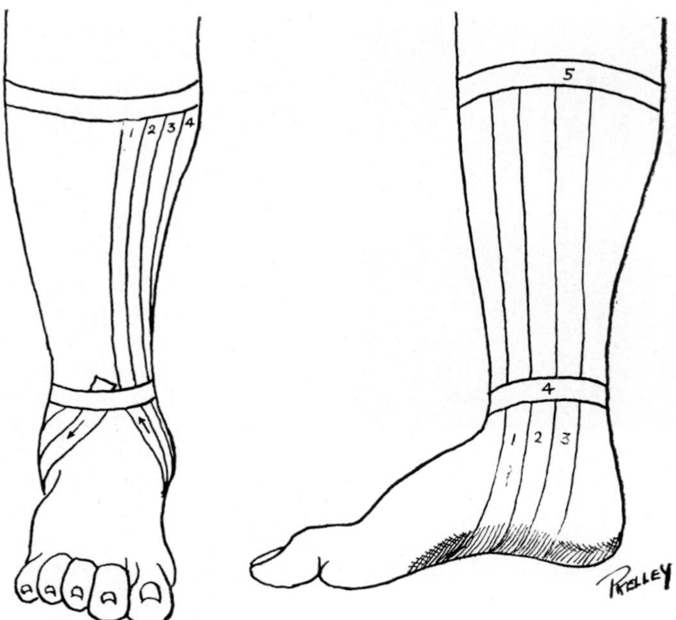

FIG. 78–16.—Strapping of the longitudinal arch useful in acute foot strain. Straps *1*, *2* and *3* are applied firmly. Transverse straps (*4* and *5*) are applied lightly so that no circulatory constriction results. The transverse strips need not encircle the leg but may be of only sufficient length to cover the free ends of *1*, *2* and *3*, and prevent these from slipping. (Dickson and Diveley, *Functional Disorders of the Foot*, courtesy of J. B. Lippincott Company.)

inches long and 2 inches wide, beginning on the outer aspect of the foot, passing under the foot and running up the inner side of the leg to mid-calf. (4) A second longitudinal strip may be applied slightly anterior to the first strip. (5) Continue the strips forward until the metatarsal heads are reached. Leave 1 inch free from adhesive on the dorsum of the foot to prevent edema. (6) Gauze is applied around the adhesive to hold this firmly to the skin and to prevent damage to the stocking. The gauze may be removed in twenty-four hours. Do not apply adhesive if there is marked eczema, many thin varicose veins or skin sensitivity.[31]

Additional Aids in the Treatment of Painful (Weak) Feet Include: (1) elastic or leather metatarsal strips with a metatarsal pad for patients with metatarsalgia; (2) the elastic web band where there is effusion in the mid-tarsal joints causing pain along the branches of the median plantar nerve; and (3) sponge rubber heel inserts for patients with tenderness of the tuberosity of the os calcis. (4) A figure-of-8 leather strap about the ankle is helpful for a weak ankle. (5) Physical therapy in the form of heat, massage and exercises aids in breaking up adhesions and reestablishing a normal circulation.

Surgery of Painful Feet

When the aforementioned procedures do not relieve the symptoms surgical treatment should be considered. Manipulation under anesthesia is of value particularly if adhesions or contractures are present.[22] The deformities usually helped by manipulation are spastic flat foot and deformities of the toes. After manipulation the foot is held in the

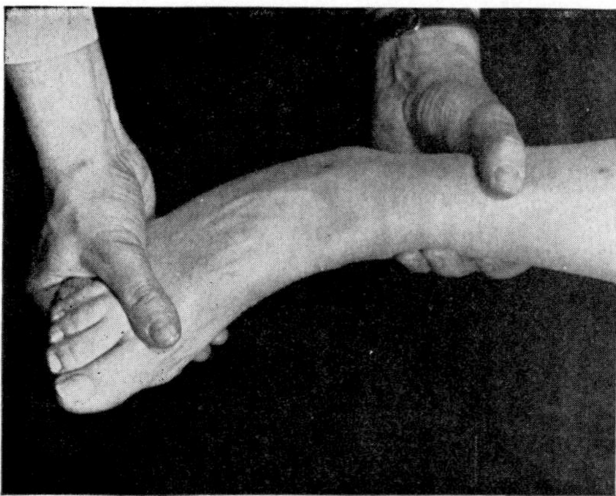

FIG. 78–17.—Manipulation of the foot. Short leverage is used. The forefoot is inverted, and posterior tarsal joints are manipulated.

corrected position by a plaster cast for one week, then physiotherapy and supports are resumed.[23] The surgical procedures employed in painful feet are fusion of the medial tarsal joints to hold a very weak longitudinal arch. A wedge osteotomy through the tarsal bones with its widest part on the dorsum of the foot may be necessary if there is much cavus of the foot.[27] There are numerous operations for hallux valgus and hammer toe deformities. For hallux valgus the removal of the exostosis and osteotomy of the neck of the first metatarsal bone with medial displacement of the distal fragment are the procedure of choice. Resection of the distal half of the proximal phalanx is preferred for correction of hammer toes.[19]

Sprains of the Anterior Arch of the Foot

The anterior arch of the foot, the space behind the distal ends of the metatarsal bones, is often depressed and sprained. This condition often accompanies flat foot. The anterior arch acts as a shock absorber for the anterior part of the foot. Its integrity depends chiefly upon the normal strength of the flexor muscles of the toes. This condition is found most often in adults, especially women who wear high-heeled, poorly fitted shoes.

The usual symptoms are pain in the forepart of the foot and toes, often with swelling about the metatarsophalangeal joints. There are tenderness and callus formation under the metatarsal heads. Hallux valgus and hammer toe deformity usually accompany sprain of the anterior arch of the foot.

Treatment includes: (1) removal of the painful callus under the metatarsal heads; (2) heat, particularly foot soaks if the tissues are very tender; (3) felt or sponge rubber metatarsal pads from $\frac{1}{4}$ to $\frac{1}{2}$ inch thick as a temporary measure; (4) strapping of the anterior arch or an elastic or leather cuff around the foot behind the metatarsal heads; (5) a metatarsal bar and (6) properly fitting shoes; (7) exercises to strengthen the flexor and extensor muscles of the toes and thus aid the metatarsal arch.[13]

Many individuals with tender second, third and fourth metatarsal heads are greatly relieved by a metatarsal bar, particularly if there is any contracture of the extensor muscles of the toes. A strip of leather approximately $\frac{3}{4}$ inch wide and $\frac{3}{16}$ inch thick running across the outer sole from just proximal to the first metatarsal head to a point proximal to the fifth metatarsal head is attached to the sole or inserted between the layers of the sole. Operative removal of the depressed metatarsal heads is sometimes necessary.

COMMON ABNORMALITIES OF THE FEET

Hammer Toe

This may begin in childhood and is most common in the second toe (although sometimes it is a congenital defect). It consists of extension at the metatarsophalangeal joint with flexion at the proximal interphalangeal joint; this is usually caused by pressure of a short narrow shoe or tight, short sock. Pain results from the development of a callus or corn on the top of the proximal joint. Therapy consists of manipulation,[26] splinting and the use of felt pads about or behind the affected joints in the early

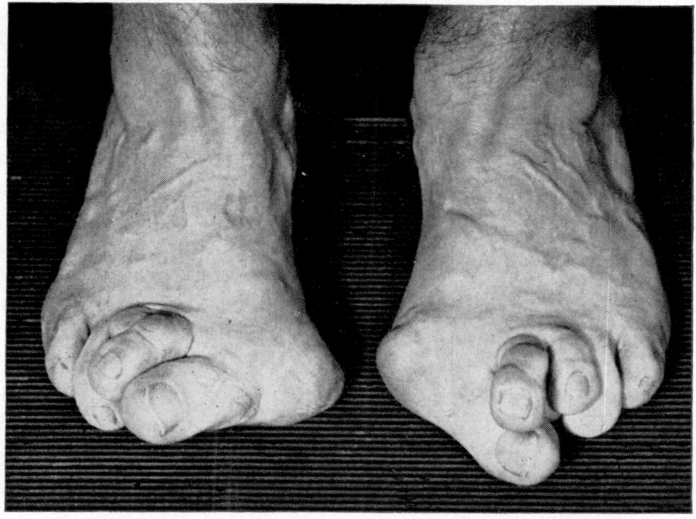

FIG. 78–18.—Hallux valgus, with marked spread of forefoot, exostosis and bursa at first metatarsophalangeal joint.

mild cases, and surgical resection in the more advanced cases.[24]

Hallux Valgus

The great toe is abducted so that it lies on top of, or under the other toes. Associated with this is marked prominence of the first metatarsophalangeal joint, with bony enlargment of the inner side of the first metatarsal head, over which a bursa may form (due to pressure from the shoe). This bursa is commonly called a bunion. Inflammation may occur in the bursa, occasionally with suppuration.[30]

Hallux valgus may be present without the formation of a bunion and without marked discomfort even in the presence of marked deformity.[28] Short, narrow, pointed shoes or snugly fitting socks are a common cause of hallux valgus. A congenital metatarsus varus may precede hallux valgus. It is often associated with a depressed metatarsal arch.

In mild cases with slight discomfort relief may be obtained by the use of proper shoes, insertion of a pad between the first and second toes, stretching of the great toe, and proper arch supports and exercises. A metatarsal cuff will often correct the alignment of the toe in mild cases.

Severe deformity of hallux valgus and hallux rigidus can be corrected usually by removal of the exostoses from the metatarsal head and excision of a small portion of the proximal phalanx.[2] There are many surgical procedures for the correction of this deformity.[10]

Hallux Rigidus

This is a limitation of plantar or dorsiflexion of the great toe usually resulting from bony proliferation at the margins of the metatarsophalangeal joints.

In hallux rigidus, permanent subjective relief may be obtained in early cases by a properly made shoe with pads, supports and a metatarsal bar.[29] A stiff sole or a long arch support will at times relieve symptoms. A shoe with a soft toe cap should be worn. Surgical procedures include removal of the osteophytic ridges with remodeling of the metatarsal head, or fusion of the first metatarsophalangeal joint.

Anterior Metatarsalgia

This condition may occur in the foot with a high longitudinal arch, the foot with a short Achilles tendon, the abducted foot, or without evident pathologic change; this latter has been called *Morton's metatarsalgia.*[20] It is often seen with a depressed metatarsal arch. It is characterized by the sudden onset (while walking) of a severe crampy pain in the anterior portion of the foot forcing the patient to remove the shoe at once, and to move and rub the toes until the pain is eased.

This disorder is often unilateral, affecting women more frequently than men.[7] It is due mainly to lateral compression of the forefoot forcing the head of the fifth metatarsal inward and behind the head of the fourth, thus causing pressure on the large superficial branch of the external plantar nerve which lies between the heads of these two bones.[17] This results in a neuralgic pain. With prolonged irritation of the nerve a neuroma may develop.[11]

Symptoms of this disorder include:

1. Burning, numbness, tingling or cramplike pain in the forepart of the foot, often under the fourth metatarsal head occurring when wearing shoes (in most instances).[16]
2. Pain may be so intense as to require sudden removal of the shoe and rubbing of the foot to obtain relief; it is often relieved by squeezing the metatarsals together. A sense of soreness persists at night in some cases, keeping the patient awake. In long-standing cases, a traumatic neuritis is set up causing pain whether the shoe is worn or not.
3. Tenderness and numbness may persist for several days in the forepart of the foot or toes especially about the head of the second, third, or fourth metatarsals.
4. Pain may radiate up the foot or leg, or to the end of the toe.
5. In some cases, the only discomfort may be an aching across the metatarsal arch.
6. Painful callus is frequently seen under the metatarsal head.
7. Sensory disturbance in the web between the fourth and fifth or third and fourth toes may be found.

Treatment consists of the use of felt pads placed just proximal to the head of the fourth metatarsal bone and a metatarsal elastic strap to decrease splaying of the foot; if the pain persists, a metatarsal bar may be tried.

In the treatment of some of these patients it may be necessary to inject from 2 to 3 cc. of 1 per cent procaine hydrochloride into the dorsum of the

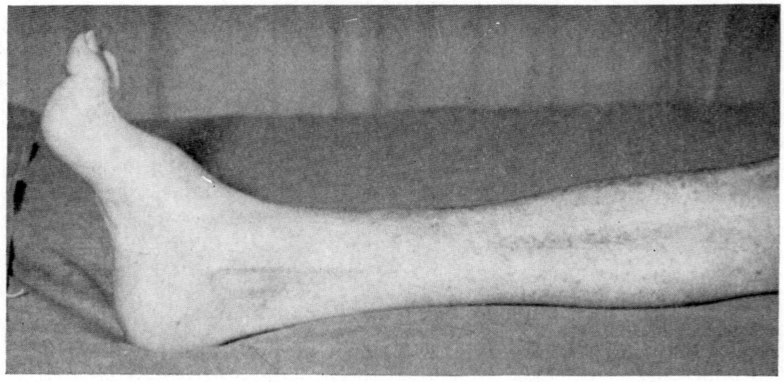

Fig. 78–19.—Cavus of the foot. There is contracture of the plantar fascia. The dorsal portion of the mid-foot is prominent. The toes are held in extension.

foot or to the painful area near the sole of the foot.

Morton's metatarsalgia possibly is caused by a tumor involving the most lateral branch of the medial plantar nerve; these tumors are neurofibromas or angioneurofibromas. If symptoms are severe, the tumor is excised.

Achillodynia

This is an inflammation of the bursa which lies between the os calcis and the tendo Achilles at the point of attachment of the tendon. Symptoms include pain over the bursa with swelling, especially during walking. Treatment consists mainly of rest, removal of pressure from shoes and heat to the bursa; in some cases it may be necessary to inject this with procaine for relief. A felt or sponge rubber pad under the heel affords some relief. Surgical removal of the bursa or rheumatoid nodules within it may be necessary.

Painful Heel

This may be caused by traumatic rupture of the Achilles tendon, inflammation of the retrocalcaneal bursa, exostoses, degenerative joint disease, strain on the attachment of the plantar fascia or inflammation of a bursa (occasionally present between the tendo Achilles and the skin) or degeneration of the calcaneal fat pad.

Pain on the sole at the center of the heel on walking may be due to the presence of an exostosis, an inflamed bursa or undue trauma to the tissues in this area.[10] *If no exostosis is present* (as seen by x ray), *relief is usually obtained by 1 per cent procaine injections* (*1 to 3 cc.*) *into the painful region and insertion into the heel of the shoe of a soft rubber doughnut*, *i.e.*, a piece of rubber approximately ¼ inch thick with an area about 1½ inches in diameter cut out in its center portion. An arch plate may be made with a hole in the central portion of the heel and padding around the edge of the heel.

Bony Spurs

Bony spurs occur on the anterior plantar surface of the os calcis or on the dorsal surface of the foot. Many result from chronic strain at points of ligamentous attachments. Relief of strain and procaine infiltration usually cause symptoms to disappear. Surgery is rarely necessary.

Pes Cavus

In this condition, there is an abnormally high arch and a tendency for the foot to roll outward. This may be due to unbalanced muscular action or to a congenital abnormality (with a short, contracted plantar fascia). Many neurological disturbances and especially poliomyelitis may cause muscular disturbances which permit the development of this deformity. Most of the weight is borne on the heel and ball of the foot.

Symptoms of pes cavus include pain in the ball of the foot, a sense of tiredness in the longitudinal arch, cramping in the calf, sprain of the forefoot, calluses under the metatarsal heads, and hammer toe deformities.

Therapy of this disorder includes arch supports high in longitudinal arch, with a support for the anterior arch of the foot. Exercises are of value in lessening deformity. When the cavus is severe a wedge osteotomy through the tarsal bones with its base on the dorsum of the foot will usually correct the deformity. Resection of the heads of the metatarsal bones is of value in relieving symptoms in the forefoot.

OTHER CAUSES OF PAINFUL FEET

There are a large number of painful feet not due to static disturbances. The largest group are the traumatic lesions: contusions, sprains, and fractures. Here there is almost always a definite history of injury to the foot. Other articulations will not be involved. These lesions usually respond promptly to treatment. Inflammatory lesions of the foot include infections of the bones or soft tissues, the various forms of articular inflammation and inflammations of the skin. Congenital deformities, the most common of which are club foot, deformities of the toes, metatarsus primus varus and cavus deformity can usually be diagnosed by their characteristic deformity and a history of their presence since infancy. All of these become progressively worse if untreated. The great majority of them are corrected in early childhood. Circulatory disturbances of the feet may be either venous or arterial.[32] Disturbances in the venous return of the blood are observed in a large number of patients with arthritic deformities of the legs. One observes stasis, later eczema, and finally ulceration of the skin usually over the lower leg and dorsum of the foot. A pressure bandage or an elastic stocking may be necessary. Correction of flexion deformities improves the circulation greatly. When ulceration has occurred, elevation, an Unna paste boot,

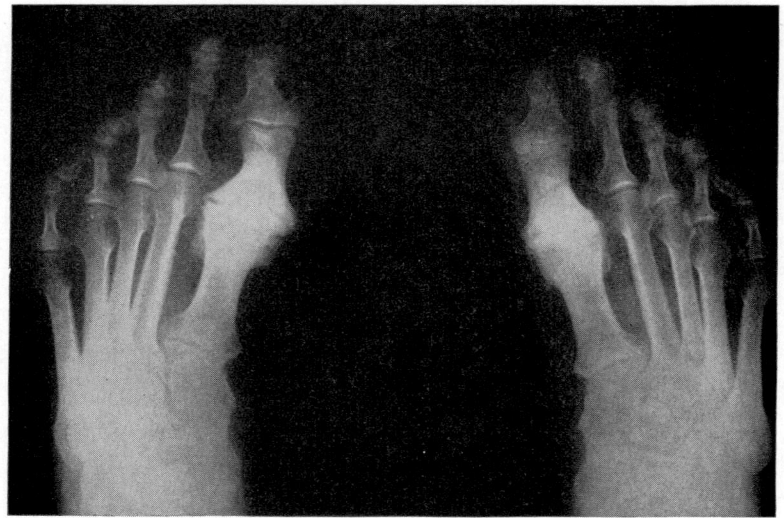

Fig. 78–20.—A severe hallux rigidus, osteoarthritis in the first metatarsophalangeal joint.

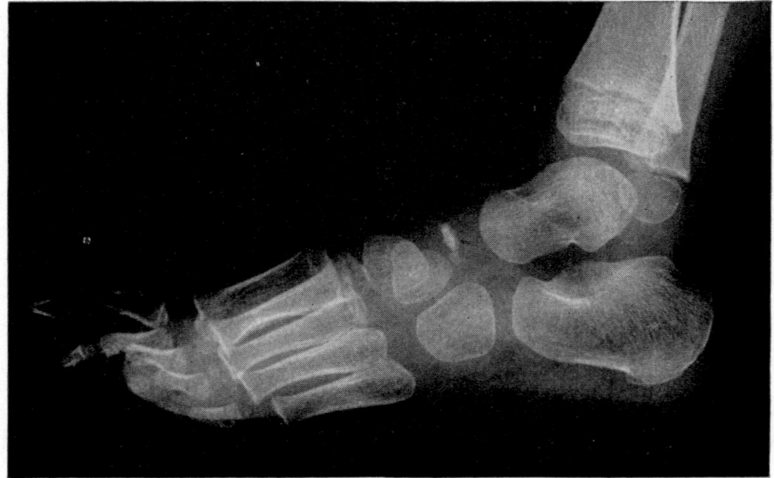

Fig. 78–21.—Köhler's disease. Note thin, dense tarsal scaphoid.

sterile wet dressings or skin grafting may be required. Arterial disturbances may be caused either by vasospasm or by the narrowing of the lumen of the artery. Vasculitis has been reported with increasing frequency since the use of steroids in the treatment of rheumatoid arthritis. There are a number of surgical procedures available in the treatment of arterial disturbances.

Brief mention should be made of disturbances of growth, particularly epiphyseal disturbances, which later may be precursors of arthritic disabilities in the feet. The common ones are the involvement of the tarsal scaphoid, called Köhler's disease, osteochondritis of the second metatarsal bone, called Freiberg's disease, and involvement of the epiphysis of the os calcis. Temporary protection of these areas is usually all the treatment that is necessary but, despite this, deformity sometimes occurs.

BIBLIOGRAPHY

1. Aitken, J. T.: Brit. J. Phys. Med., *12*, 92, 1949.
2. Bailey, E. T. and Harrens, B. S.: Lancet, *2*, 490, 1946.
3. Baker, D. M.: Brit. J. Phys. Med., *11*, 87, 1948.
4. Bingold, A. C. and Collins, D. H.: J. Bone & Joint Surg., *32*, 214, 1950.
5. Bivings, L.: Amer. J. Dis. Child., *76*, 440, 1948.
6. Blomfield, L. B.: Ann. Phys. Med., *6*, 274, 1962.
7. Brattström, H. and Brattström, M.: Acta Orthop. Scand., *41*, 213, 1970.
8. Calabro, J. J.: Arth. & Rheum., *5*, 19, 1962.
9. Compere, E. L.: Med. Clin. North Amer., *30*, 635, 1946.
10. Dickson, F. D. and Diveley, R. L.: *Functional Disorders of the Foot*, Philadelphia, J. B. Lippincott Co., 1949.
11. Duthie, J. J.: Practitioner, *186*, 729, 1961.
12. Giannestras, N. J.: *Foot Disorders, Medical and Surgical Management*. Philadelphia, Lea & Febiger, 1967.
13. Gum, R. E.: Brit. J. Phys. Med., *18*, 273, 1955.
14. Harris, R. I. and Beath, T.: J. Bone & Joint Surg., *31*, 553, 1949.
15. Hauser, E. W. D.: Indust. Med., *18*, 326, 1949.
16. Joplin, R. J.: J. Bone & Joint Surg., *32*, 779, 1950.
17. Joplin, A. H.: Surg. Clin. N. Amer., *49*, 847, 1969.
18. Kelikian, H.: *Hallux valgus, Allied Disorders of the Forefoot and Metatarsalgia*. Philadelphia, W. B. Saunders Co., 1965.
19. Key, J. A.: Amer. J. Surg., *79*, 667, 1950.
20. Kuhns, J. G.: J.A.M.A., *120*, 329, 1942.
21. Lapidus, P. W.: J. Bone & Joint Surg., *28*, 126, 1946.
22. Lewin, P.: *The Foot and Ankle*, 4th ed., Philadelphia, Lea & Febiger, 1959.
23. Marmor, L.: *Surgery of the Rheumatoid Foot*. Philadelphia, Lea & Febiger, 1967.
24. McKeever, D. C.: J. Bone & Joint Surg., *34*, 129, 1952.
25. Mennell, J.: *Science and Art of Joint Manipulation*. London, J. & A. Churchill Ltd., 1949.
26. Osgood, R. B.: New Engl. J. Med., *226*, 552, 1942.
27. Potter, T. A.: Surg. Clin. N. Amer., *49*, 883, 1969.
28. Rose, G. K.: J. Bone & Joint Surg., *44*, 647, 1962.
29. Schwartz, R. P. and Heath, A. L.: J. Bone & Joint Surg., *19*, 431, 1937.
30. Steindler, A.: Military Surgeon, *86*, 379, 1940.
31. Swaim, L. T. and Kuhns, J. G.: J.A.M.A., *94*, 1743, 1930.
32. Thompson, C.: J. Bone & Joint Surg., *46*, 1117, 1964.
33. Woolworth, J.: Med. J. Australia, *2*, 851, 1954.

Chapter 79

The Syndrome of Cervical Nerve Root Compression

By Ruth Jackson, M.D.

The term *cervical syndrome* has been used by the author for more than twenty years to designate a group of symptoms and clinical findings which results from irritation or compression of the cervical nerve roots, within the intervertebral foramina or canals before the nerve trunks divide into anterior and posterior primary rami.

ANATOMICAL CHARACTERISTICS

A knowledge of the anatomical characteristics of the cervical portion of the spine is imperative for adequate interpretation and treatment of the symptoms and the clinical findings resulting from irritation or compression of the cervical nerve roots.

The cervical spine is placed vulnerably between the relatively immobile thoracic spine and the skull, which is an 8 pound weight that must be balanced upon the cervical spine, and which is held in place by the supporting ligamentous, capsular, muscular and fibrocartilaginous structures. The special design of the bones and joints of the cervical spine permits a marked degree of mobility. Its great range of motion is dependent upon the composite movement between all the vertebrae. The slight flexibility of the intervertebral discs, the shape and inclination of the primary articulations and their incomplete apposition, as well as the laxity of the ligamentous and capsular structures, determine the range of normal motion.

The architectural design of the atlas and the axis permits nodding, rotation and lateral bending of the head. The head and the atlas move very much as one unit on the axis, in rotation and lateral bending. The shape of the atlanto-occipital articulations and the laxness of their capsules permit fairly free nodding movements, backward nodding being greater than forward nodding.

As rotation of the head and atlas takes place upon the axis, the inferior facets of the atlas slip forward and backward over the superior facets of the axis. However, in radiographs made with the head rotated, the lateral masses of the atlas maintain a constant relationship to the odontoid process of the axis.

Motion in the other cervical joints consists of forward flexion, hyperextension, lateral bending and rotation. However, the plane of the articular surfaces prevents lateral bending from occurring without some degree of rotation, or rotation from occurring without some degree of lateral bending.

The normal laxity of the ligamentous and capsular structures permits a free range of motion. Undue laxity allows subluxations of the joints, or an abnormal range of motion or slipping between the articular surfaces (Fig. 79–1).

The two apophyseal or posterior joints and the fibrocartilaginous disc joints are characteristic of all areas of the spine below the atlanto-axial articulations. In addition, the cervical spine has two lateral interbody joints. These small articulations are formed by the upward posterolateral projections on the superior surfaces of the vertebral bodies and the adjacent beveled surfaces on the inferior portion of the vertebral bodies (Fig. 79–2).

Von Luschka[10] described these joints between the bodies of the cervical vertebrae in 1858, hence they have been called the *joints of Luschka*. However, in 1892, Trolard called them *articulations uncoverte-*

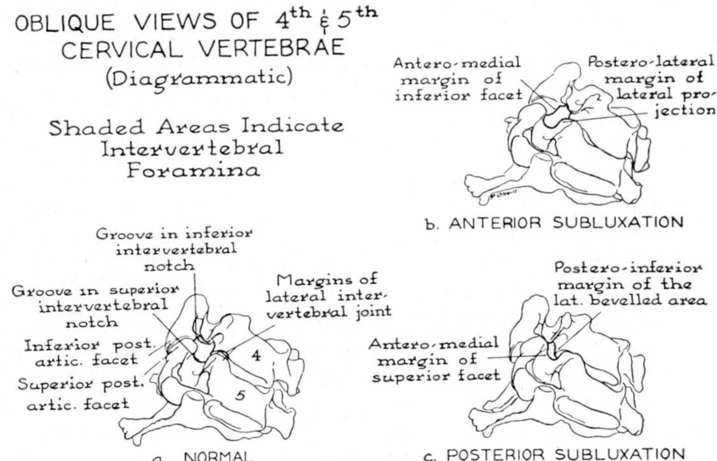

Fig. 79–1.—A normal intervertebral canal and its boundaries (*a*). Foraminal changes from subluxations of the cervical vertebrae (*b* and *c*). (Jackson, *The Cervical Syndrome*, courtesy of Charles C Thomas.)

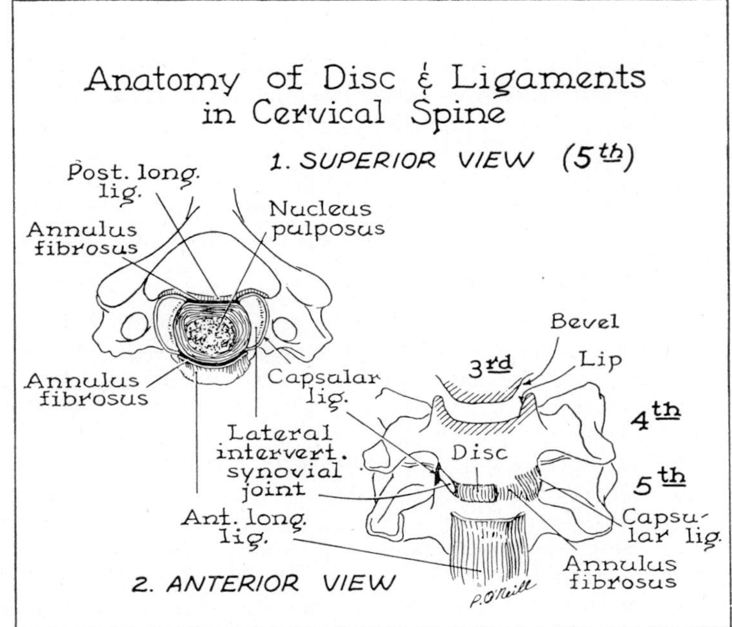

Fig. 79–2.—The lateral interbody joints and their relationship to the cervical discs. (Jackson, *The Cervical Syndrome*, courtesy of Charles C Thomas.)

brales. These terms are used interchangeably. I prefer to call these small articulations the *lateral interbody joints*, which is a correct anatomical description and avoids any confusion concerning them.

The lateral interbody joints are of great significance. Their presence prevents the exposure of the intervertebral discs at the posterolateral margins of the vertebral bodies. These joints and the adjacent surfaces of the bodies of the vertebrae form the anterior walls of the intervertebral canals through which the cervical nerve roots pass. Motion occurs here and contributes somewhat to the great range of motion in the cervical spine. Their capsular ligaments are short and taut and they are, therefore, extremely vulnerable to sprain. It is at the margins of these joints that the greatest amount of arthrosis (osteoarthritic change) occurs. The close proximity of the cervical nerve roots to these joints makes them unusually vulnerable to irritation or compression from any derangement in or about the joints. These joints prevent the extrusion of disc material posterolaterally, which is the favorite site of extrusion in other areas of the spine. However, the seventh and the sixth vertebrae may not have well-developed upward lips, in which event disc material may be extruded posterolaterally.

The bodies of the cervical vertebrae are flat posteriorly, and the anterior surfaces are curved, with the inferior margins jutting downward. The posterior vertical diameter is greater than the anterior vertical diameter. To assure the normal forward curve in the cervical spine, the vertical diameter of the posterior portion of the intervertebral discs is much less than the anterior diameter.

The intervertebral foramina from the second to the seventh vertebrae are actual bony canals which are somewhat ovoid in shape, and which have greater vertical diameters than anteroposterior diameters. The grooves in the vertebral arches form the roofs and floors of the canals. The posterior articulations and the lateral interbody joints form the posterior and the anterior walls of the canals (Figs. 79–1 and 79–2).

The nerve roots rest upon the floors of the canals and fill the anteroposterior diameter of the canals, but they do not fill the vertical diameter. The upper one-eight to one-fourth of the canals is filled with areolar and fatty tissues, small veins, the spinal branches of the vertebral arteries, the recurrent meningeal nerves and their sympathetic connections.

The ventral and dorsal nerve roots arise from the corresponding surfaces of the spinal cord on a level with the vertebral bodies. Small intervals, which are on a level with the intervertebral discs, exist between the origins of the nerve root fibers, so that the nerve root fibers do not cross the intervertebral discs as they do in other areas of the spine (Fig. 79–6). As the nerve root fibers leave the spinal canal, they carry with them a dural covering from the dura spinalis, and they enter the intervertebral canals immediately, where they join to form the nerve trunks. They are, therefore, well protected from posterior extrusion of disc material, but they are extremely vulnerable to any derangement within the intervertebral canals.

Textbooks of anatomy have indicated that the cervical spinal nerves are composed of sensory and motor fibers only, and they do not contain the white rami communicantes of the sympathetic system, as do the dorsal and upper two lumbar nerves; they communicate with the sympathetic nervous system through the white rami communicantes of the first and second thoracic nerves, which join the sympathetic trunk by way of their anterior primary rami and proceed upward to the cervical sympathetic ganglia; from these ganglia postganglionic fibers, or gray rami communicantes, pass to the anterior rami of the cervical nerves to be distributed with their branches. However, Laruelle has demonstrated the presence of sympathetic cell bodies in the cervical portion of the spinal cord in the mediolateral gray matter of the base of the anterior horn from the fourth through the eighth nerve root levels. The preganglionic sympathetic fibers leave the spinal cord with the somatic motor nerve fibers in the ventral roots of C5 through T1. One part of the preganglionic neurons forms a synaptic connection with the postganglionic neurons in the small ganglia of a deep sympathetic chain which has been described by Delmas and his associates. The other preganglionic neurons traverse

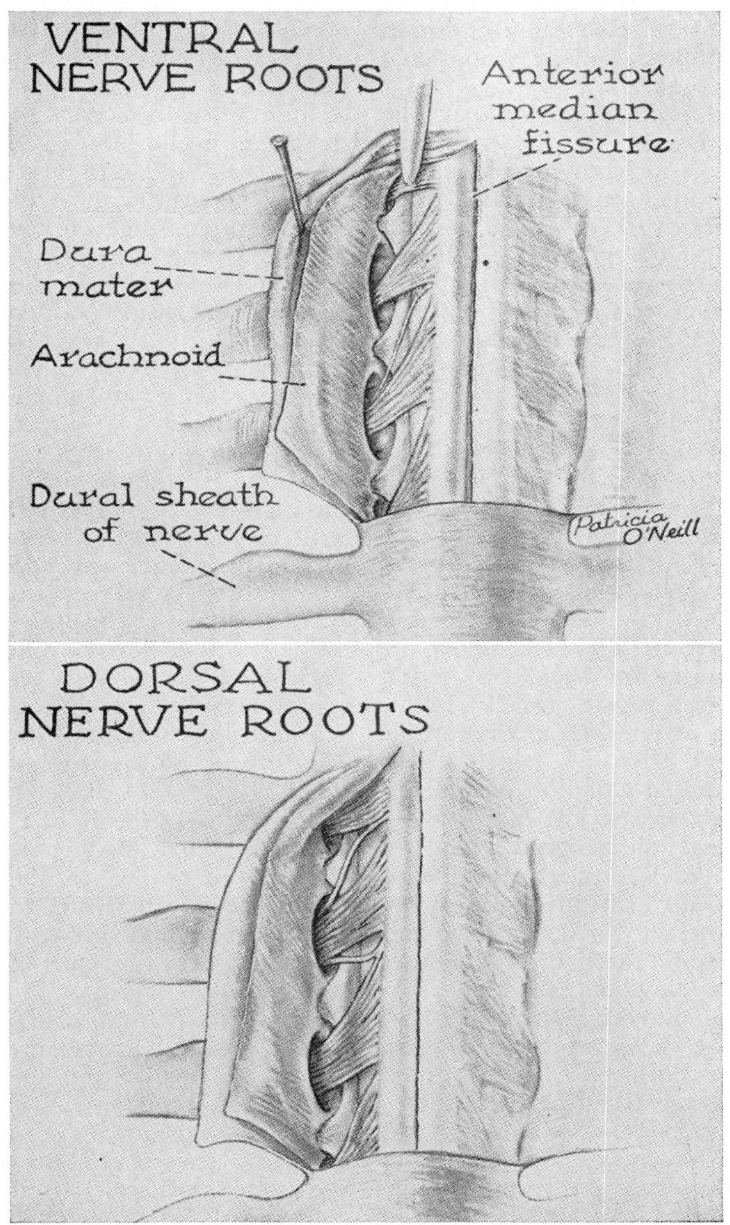

FIG. 79–3.—The origin of the ventral and dorsal nerve roots from the spinal cord and their exit through the dura spinalis. (Jackson, *The Cervical Syndrome*, courtesy of Charles C Thomas.)

the deep chain of small sympathetic ganglia situated in the transverse foramina and join the vertebral nerve. The deep chain consists of a tangled web of sympathetic fibers and of macroscopically visible ganglia. It ascends along the posterior aspect of the vertebral artery from C7 to C4. It is the continuation in the neck of the thoracolumbar sympathetic ganglionated trunk.

In the cervical area, the sympathetic trunk is composed of the superior, middle and inferior ganglia which are connected by intervening cords. The efferent branches proceed to the viscera of the neck and chest and the afferent branches form the vertebral nerve. Communicating rami connect the superior ganglion with the ninth, tenth and twelfth cranial nerves. Gray rami communicantes join the anterior rami of the upper four cervical nerves. The internal carotid nerve passes upwards with the internal carotid artery and forms a plexus about the artery. Pharyngeal branches communicate with the superior laryngeal nerve and join the pharyngeal plexus. The external carotid nerve forms a plexus around the external carotid artery, and cardiac branches follow the carotid artery into the thorax on the left side and on the right side branches follow the trachea to end in the deep cardiac plexus.

From the middle ganglion postganglionic fibers are given to the inferior thyroid artery and the thyroid gland; a cardiac branch ends in the cardiac plexus and another branch, the ansa subclavius, descends to the subclavian artery and then ascends to join the inferior ganglion.

The inferior ganglion sends fine filaments to the subclavius plexus and larger filaments to the vertebral artery to form the vertebral plexus. A cardiac branch reaches the deep cardiac plexus.

According to Tinel the fifth cervical nerve root carries sympathetic fibers which join the carotid plexus to give sympathetic innervation to the arteries of the head and neck. The sixth root carries sympathetic fibers which go to the subclavian artery and the brachial plexus. From the seventh nerve root, fibers reach the cardio-aortic plexus and the subclavian and axillary arteries, as well as the phrenic nerve.

Other postganglionic fibers communicate with the recurrent spinal meningeal nerves. The fibers which invest the internal carotid arteries give branches to the back of the orbit, the dilator muscle of the pupil and to the smooth muscle of the upper eyelid. Some of the branches which surround the vertebral arteries supply the vestibular portion of the ears.

Pain-conducting, afferent spinal nerve fibers from the blood vessels of the head, neck and upper extremities traverse the sympathetic trunk and communicating rami.

These facts are of importance in the consideration of cervical nerve root irritation, inasmuch as stimulation of the sympathetic fibers gives rise to symptoms and clinical findings which may confuse the picture. Stimulation of the cervical sympathetic fibers may cause vasoconstriction and aggravation of pain caused by irritation of the cervical nerve roots. Interruption or paralysis of the sympathetic fibers may relieve pain by paralyzing the afferent pain-conducting spinal nerve fibers which traverse the sympathetic trunk and the communicating rami, or by the relief of vasoconstriction.

The dural covering of the spinal cord is firmly fixed to the margins of the foramen magnum, to the second and third cervical vertebrae, and to the periosteum on the back of the coccyx. It is separated from the walls of the vertebral canal by the cavum epidurale, which is filled with soft fat and a plexus of thin-walled veins. The spinal dura is, therefore, fairly free within the spinal canal and its attachments do not interfere with the free movement of the vertebral column. As the spinal nerve roots pierce the dura, they carry with them a tubular covering of the dura spinalis (Fig. 79–3). Injuries or inflammatory reactions of the dural sleeves of the nerve roots may result in the formation of adhesions between the sleeves and the adjacent capsular ligaments. In the dissection of anatomical specimens the author has found this to be true and has found, in addition, the spinal dura bound completely to the posterior longitudinal ligament at definite areas of localized pathological changes.

The relationship of the vertebral arteries and their branches to the spinal nerves and the bony structures is of importance. These arteries and their surrounding plexuses of sympathetic fibers may be injured by subluxations of the vertebrae or by the changes which occur at the anterior portions of the lateral interbody joints. Angiographic studies have shown obliteration of these arteries caused by changes in position of the head and neck. Actual constrictions of these arteries, especially at the level of the upper cervical vertebrae, may occur.

The posterior longitudinal ligament in the cervical area is composed of two distinct layers, in contradistinction to its structure below this area. The superficial layer, which is absent below the cervical area, is a strong ligamentous structure which extends vertically downward from the skull, dorsal to the deep layer. It extends laterally to the intervertebral foramina (Fig. 79–4) and it is firmly adherent to the structures anterior to it. The deep layer has the denticulated appearance of the posterior ligament distal to the cervical area. Some of the fibers of the capsular ligaments of the lateral interbody joints take origin from the deep layer, as well as from the adjacent bone of the vertebral bodies. This strong ligament acts as a barrier to extrusion of disc material in the midline posteriorly, although disc extrusion can occur here, depending upon the severity of an injury and the integrity of the ligament.

The greatest amount of stress and strain in the cervical spine occurs at the level of the fourth and fifth cervical vertebrae when the neck is in hyperextension, and at the level of the fifth and sixth cervical vertebrae when the neck is in hyperflexion. Limitation of motion from muscle spasm or fixation will alter the points of greatest stress and strain, depending upon the degree and level of fixation. This accounts for the fact that the greatest amount of degenerative change in the intervertebral discs and in the lateral interbody joints occurs at these levels. However, such changes may take place at any level.

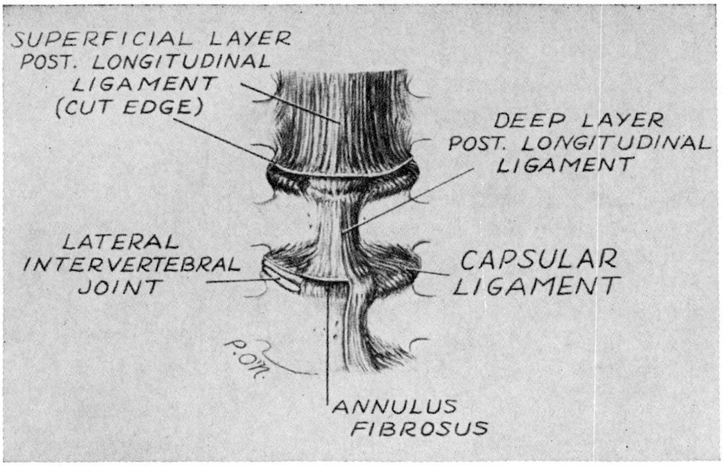

FIG. 79–4.—The two-layered posterior longitudinal ligament and the capsular ligaments of the lateral interbody joints. (Jackson, *The Cervical Syndrome*, courtesy of Charles C Thomas.)

CAUSATIVE FACTORS

The cervical spine, because of its position, structure and great mobility, is much more vulnerable to injury than is any other portion of the spine, and, hence, to the changes initiated by trauma.

Approximately 90 per cent of all cervical nerve root irritation is the result, either directly or indirectly, of sprain injuries of the ligamentous and capsular structures of the cervical spine. Sprain injuries of these structures permit subluxations. Anteroposterior narrowing of the intervertebral canals results in immediate or delayed irritation or compression of the cervical nerve roots. Sixty per cent of these injuries give rise to some immediate symptoms, whereas the other 40 per cent give rise to symptoms days, weeks or months later.

Symptoms which occur immediately or within a few hours following injury may be due to actual compression of the nerve roots within their bony canals as the joints are subluxated, or they may be due to swelling and hemorrhage of the adjacent capsular ligaments.

Delayed symptoms are the result of foraminal narrowing initiated by the original trauma and by repeated stress and strain of continued movement in the joints. As time goes on, osteophytic formations, or spurs, occur at the margins of the lateral interbody joints and/or the posterior joints. The ligamentous and capsular structures become thickened and lose their normal elasticity. Such foraminal encroachment may cause gradual compression of the nerve roots and perineural fibrosis. Inasmuch as these changes take place relatively slowly, the nerve roots may become adjusted to, or tolerant of, their narrowed canals, until some apparently trivial incident sets off a response which is manifested by pain and disability.

The extent and degree of nerve root irritation vary. Some fibers within a nerve root may escape involvement, while others may sustain variable degrees of irritation or compression. There may be individual differences of susceptibility of nerve fibers to trauma, and some may be better protected than others. The symptoms and clinical findings will, therefore, vary with the location and extent of the irritation or compression.

Vehicular crash accidents are responsible for the greatest percentage of neck sprains. The "whip-lash" mechanism (Fig. 79–5), which may be described as any sudden forceful movement of the neck in any direction with a recoil in the opposite direction, accounts for eighty to ninety per cent of these sprain injuries. The lashing effect is greatest when the muscles are caught off guard, which occurs frequently in rear-end collisions. However, sprain injuries may occur in strenuous sports; in falls; from sudden, forceful pulls on the arms; from sudden,

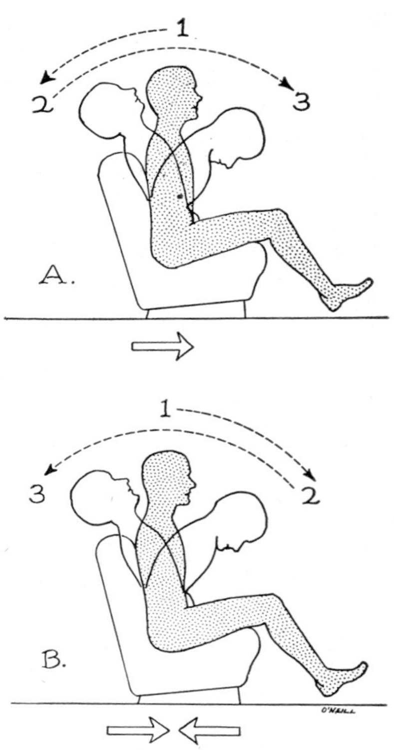

FIG. 79–5.—The "whip-lash" mechanism. Rear-end collison (*A*) and head-on collision (*B*). (Jackson, *The Cervical Syndrome,* courtesy of Charles C Thomas.)

thrusting forces against the arms; and from blows on the head or chin.

A diagnosis of *cervical disc* is made frequently following sprain injuries with nerve root involvement. This term implies pressure upon a nerve root from posterolateral disc extrusion. However, the nerve roots are protected by the lateral interbody joints, and the nerve root fibers are protected by *safety zones*, or the vertebral bodies (Fig. 79–6). When disc extrusion occurs posteriorly in the cervical spine, it causes pressure upon the spinal cord itself. Some of the upper or lower fibers of the ventral portion of the nerve roots may suffer compression, if the disc material is large, or if it is forced upward or downward in the spinal canal. The cervical discs do not extend to the posterolateral margins of the vertebral bodies (Fig. 79–2) because of the presence of the lateral interbody joints. Thickening of the capsular ligaments and osteophytic formations at the margins of the lateral interbody joints give the appearance of a bulging disc ventral to the nerve root as it lies within the intervertebral canal. This represents the so-called *hard disc*, which is removed frequently by surgical measures. The projecting spurs are lined on their adjacent surfaces by cartilage, but this cartilage does not have the characteristics of disc cartilage, either microscopically or macroscopically.

Sprain injuries may and do cause damage to one or more cervical discs, resulting in disc degeneration and narrowing, which imposes greater strain upon the lateral interbody joints. Osteoarthritic and chondromalacic changes occur as motion is continued. Osteophytic formations develop at the anterior margins of the vertebral bodies at the attachments of the anterior longitudinal ligament. It is not unusual to find these formations bridging the vertebral bodies. This bridging, however, is unlike the ossification of the joints and the ligaments, which is seen in ankylosing spondylitis (Fig. 79–7). In the latter instance, foraminal narrowing does not occur usually, except by swelling of the adjacent capsular and ligamentous structures from inflammation.

Inflammatory joint changes, fractures of the articular processes, the vertebral arches, the posterior arches, the vertebral bodies, and the lateral masses or articulations of the first two vertebrae produce symptoms of cervical nerve root irritation in approximately ten per cent of the cases.

Certain other conditions may aggravate the symptoms and clinical findings associated with irritation of the cervical nerve roots. These conditions include emotional tension, fatigue, poor postural attitudes and activities, as well as changes in the weather.

In general, it can be stated that foraminal narrowing from mechanical derangements or from inflammatory changes may cause irritation of the cervical nerve roots. The extent of the

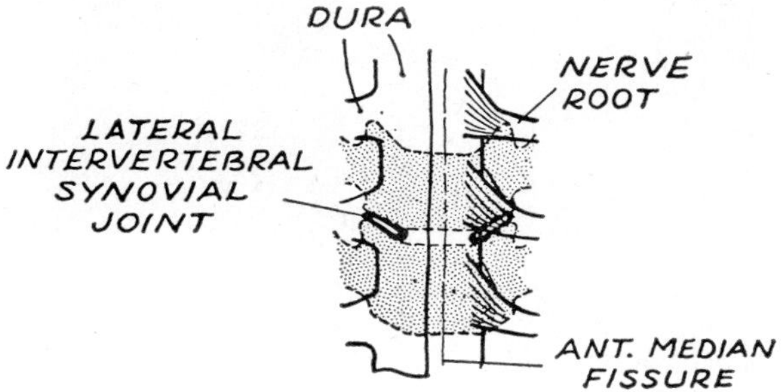

Fig. 79–6.—The "safety zone" for the cervical nerve roots, which is the corresponding vertebral body. The nerve roots do not pass over the intervertebral discs. (Jackson, *The Cervical Syndrome*, courtesy of Charles C Thomas.)

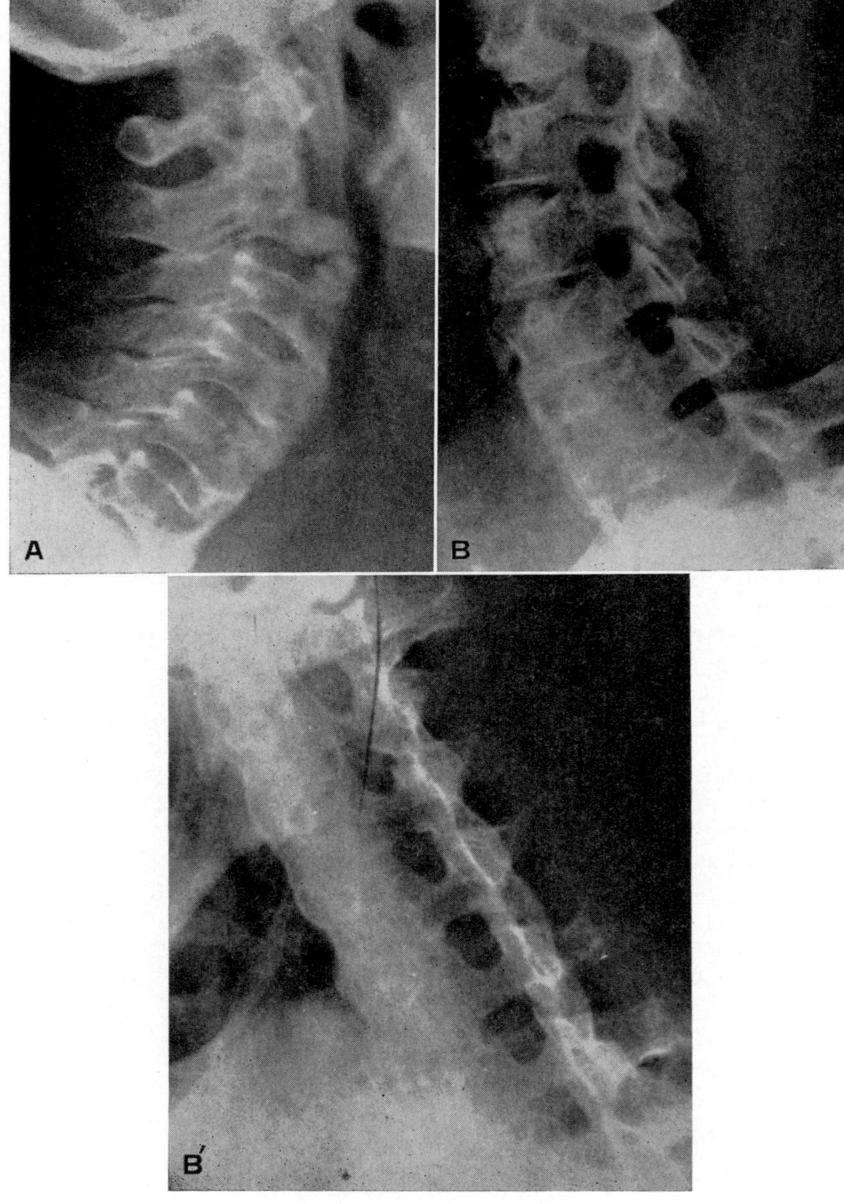

FIG. 79–7.—Ankylosing spondylitis involving the anterior portion of the vertebral bodies (*A*), the anterior longitudinal ligament (*B*), and the joints (*B′*). Note the lack of foraminal narrowing in *B* and *B′*. (Jackson, *The Cervical Syndrome*, courtesy of Charles C Thomas.)

mechanical derangement as evidenced by radiographic studies is no indication of the severity of the symptoms, nor the extent of the clinical findings. The problem is made more complex by virtue of the involvement of the sympathetic nerve supply, as well as the associated injury or involvement of the vertebral arteries and their branches.

SYMPTOMS AND SIGNS OF NERVE ROOT IRRITATION

Irritation or compression of the cervical nerve roots is manifested by pain and/or sensory, motor and trophic changes anywhere along the segmental distribution of the nerve or nerves. Areas of localized deep tenderness and muscle spasm are found at the painful sites. The reflexes in the upper extremities may be absent, diminished or normal. The overlapping of the segmental nerve supply makes the exact localization of the nerve roots which are involved somewhat difficult.

Irritation of the cervical sympathetic nerve supply may give rise to dilatation of a pupil, loss of balance, palpitations, nausea, vomiting, tinnitus, circulatory changes, and reflex dystrophy.

Irritation or compression of the cervical nerve roots may cause variable degrees of limitation of neck motion. Figure 79–8 shows the normal range of motion. In rare instances glenohumeral motion may be limited due to voluntary immobilization because of pain, or it may be limited due to reflex sympathetic dystrophy, which gives rise to degenerative changes, tendinitis and adhesive capsulitis. Calcareous deposits in the musculotendinous cuff are found in approximately 8 per cent of cases who have cervical nerve root irritation. Whether or not these deposits are coincidental has not been determined. Humeral epicondylitis and fibrotic changes in the palmar fascia may be the result of reflex sympathetic dystrophy. Variations in the blood pressure readings in the arms may be present. This, too, is probably due to stimulation of the sympathetic nerve supply, or to spasm of the proximate muscles.

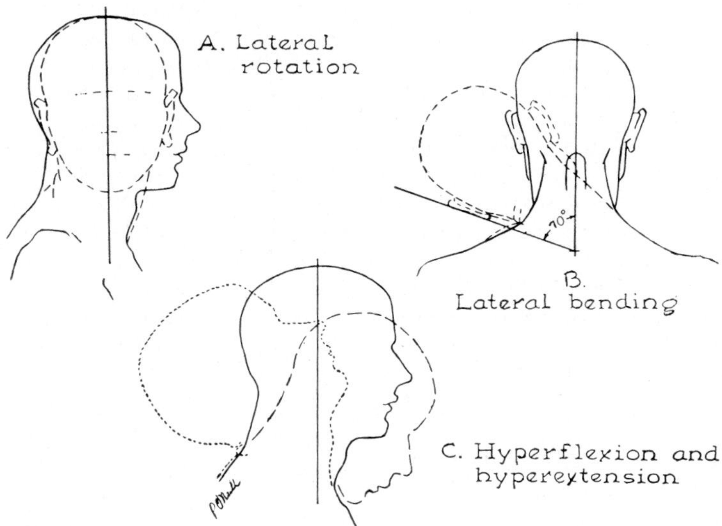

Fig. 79–8.—The range of normal neck motion. The head can be rotated so that the chin is parallel with the shoulder (*A*); it can be bent laterally seventy to eighty degrees (*B*); it can be flexed so that the chin rests upon the upper portion of the sternum, and it can be extended so that the occiput touches the spinous process of the first thoracic vertebra (*C*). (Jackson, *The Cervical Syndrome*, courtesy of Charles C Thomas.)

RADIOGRAPHIC FINDINGS

Adequate radiographic studies should be made in all cases of suspected cervical pathologic changes. Correct interpretation of such studies is impossible unless the symptoms and clinical findings are correlated with the x-ray findings. Minimal changes noted in the radiographs may give rise to severe symptoms, whereas marked changes may give rise to minimal symptoms and clinical findings. Multiple views are necessary.

The three upright lateral views suggested by Davis[3] should be made routinely. Seventy-eight per cent of these cases show a loss of the normal forward curve in the straight lateral view, and a reversal of the curve will be found in 20 per cent of these (Fig. 79–9). Spasm or contraction of the muscles which straighten the neck causes the loss of the forward curve. Steindler[8] has called this the *antalgic position*, because the patient experiences some relief of pain due to the enlargement of the intervertebral canals. This is an involuntary reaction. If sharp posterior angulation at a specific level is noted, tearing of the interspinous ligament and/or the posterior longitudinal ligament has occured or there has been a rupture of the intervertebral disc anteriorly. Forward subluxation of the posterior articulations with widening of the joint spaces and separation of the contiguous spinous processes may account for the sharp posterior angulation (Fig. 79–9).

The forward flexion view and the hyperextension view show the amount and location of motion and the presence of subluxations. All lateral views show the presence or absence of fractures of the vertebral bodies, of the spinous processes and of the laminae. If a persistent forward subluxation is noted in all the views, oblique flexion and extension views should be made to show the site of the disruption of the posterior elements.

The forward flexion view may show separation of the anterior arch of the atlas from the odontoid process, if there is relaxation of the transverse ligament.

Degenerated or narrowed intervertebral discs, and hypertrophic spurring or osteophytic formations can be seen in the lateral views.

Oblique views may show foraminal narrowing, if ligamentous instability is present or if osteophytic formations are present at the margins of the lateral interbody joints or the posterior joints. The exact amount of foraminal narrowing cannot always be determined. Anatomical specimens show that the greatest amount of osteophytic formation occurs at the margins of the lateral interbody joints. In lateral views these formations may appear to be projections on the posterior margins of the vertebral bodies, but in most instances they are on the margins of the joints (Fig. 79–10).

The lateral oblique views and the 30-degree caudad-angled anteroposterior view, as recommended by Abel,[1] show the posterior joints, the interarticular isthmi and the laminae. These views are of great diagnostic value in locating fractures of the posterior elements of the cervical spine, and for showing spurring about the posterior joints.

Anteroposterior views made with the tube tilted at an angle of 25 degrees toward the head demonstrate the upward lateral projections of the vertebral bodies. Narrowing or widening of the joint spaces and spur formations about the lateral interbody joints can be demonstrated in this projection (Fig. 79–10). A compression fracture of an upward lateral projection may be seen in the anteroposterior view.

An anteroposterior view of the upper two cervical vertebrae may reveal fractures, subluxations and rotational deformities of these vertebrae.

Myelographic studies may be indicated if the clinical findings are suggestive of a space-occupying lesion or if conservative treatment fails to give relief of the symptoms. Such studies must be correctly done and interpreted. Kaplan and Kennedy[5] have shown the effect of head posture on the obstruction and flow of radiopaque material in the spinal fluid. An apparent blockage may be caused by

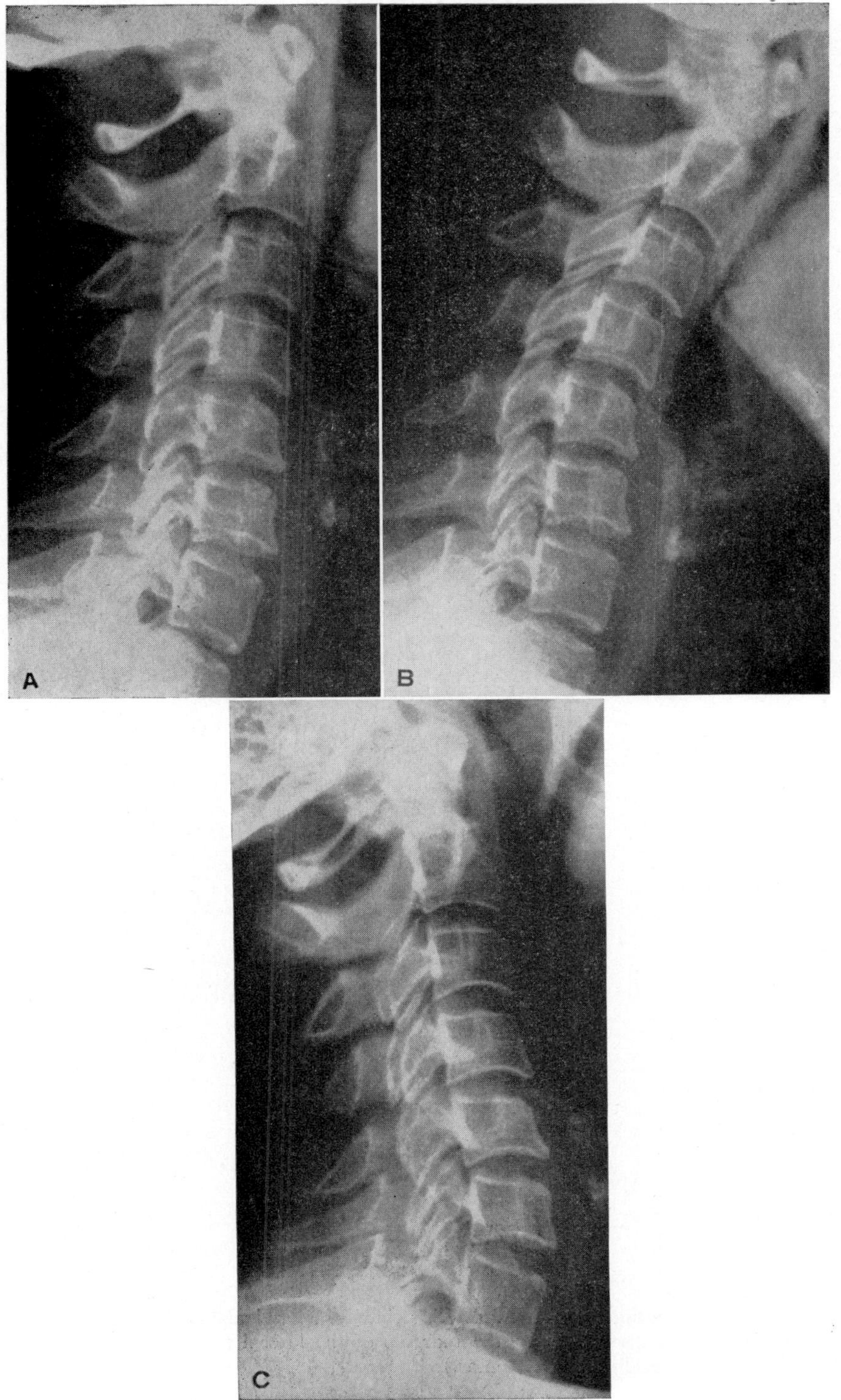

Fig. 79–9.—The Davis series of lateral radiographs. (Jackson, *The Cervical Syndrome*, courtesy of Charles C Thomas.)

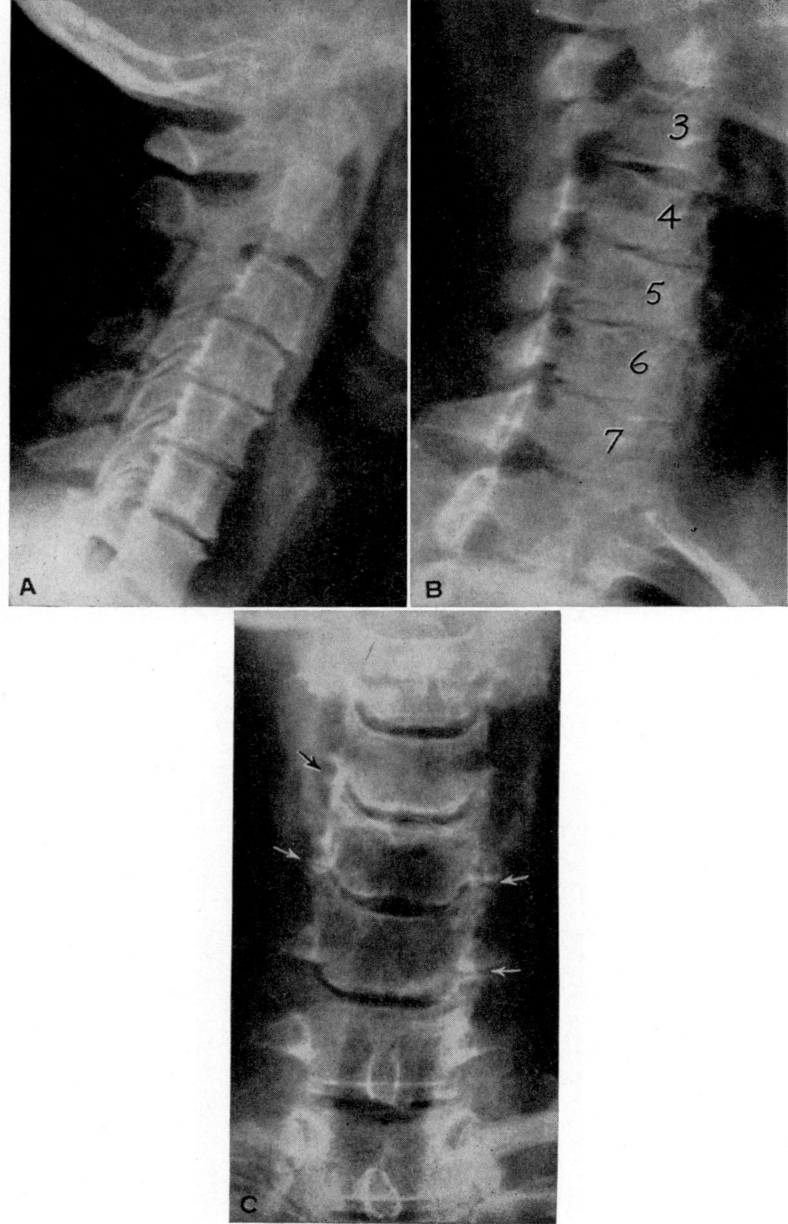

Fig. 79–10.—Lateral, oblique and anteroposterior views of a cervical spine, which show hypertrophic changes with marked spur formations at the margins of the lateral interbody joints. (Jackson, *The Cervical Syndrome*, courtesy of Charles C Thomas.)

spur formations at the margins of the lateral interbody joints or on the posterior surface of a vertebral body.

Discographic studies have gained in popularity, and they are of much greater diagnostic value in cervical disc disorders than are myelographs. Scanigrams may be necessary in some instances to demonstrate occult or questionable fractures and lesions of the bony structures.

Radiographs of a recently injured cervical spine, which show degenerative changes of long standing, should be regarded with respect. The ligamentous and capsular structures of a degenerated joint, or of a joint showing hypertrophic changes, are more subject to sprain injuries than are those of a normal joint. Motion is limited in such joints, and any sudden movement beyond the tolerance of these joints may, in the words of Vernon Luck, "take a heavy toll."[7]

DIFFERENTIAL DIAGNOSIS

Pain caused by irritation of the cervical nerve roots must be differentiated from the following: pain reflexly referred from somatic and visceral structures which have the same segmental nerve supply; pain resulting from involvement of a nerve or its branches; pain caused by lesions of the spinal cord and of the brain; and pain of psychogenic origin.

Differentiation is based on certain neurological considerations. Pain which is caused by irritation of a nerve root or a nerve trunk is referred to various points along the segmental distribution of that nerve root or nerve trunk. At the sites of pain, deep tenderness and muscle spasm are found. Irritation of a nerve or its branches may cause pain which is referred to the periphery, either proximal or distal to the site of involvement, but the painful areas are not tender to deep palpation. Pain which originates in a somatic or visceral structure may be referred along the segmental distribution of the nerve supply of such structures, but these areas of pain are not tender on deep palpation. Hyperalgesia or superficial tenderness may be present. Sensory, motor and trophic changes do not involve the region of reflexly referred pain. Pain which results from lesions of the cervical spinal cord and of the brain follows no definite nerve root pattern and is ill defined and indistinctly demarcated. Coughing, sneezing and straining usually aggravate the pain. Spasticity or hypertonia and hyperreflexia are the rule, whereas lesions affecting the nerve roots cause hypotonia and decreased reflexes.

TREATMENT

Treatment must be individualized, and the patient must be taught to live with the altered mechanics of his neck.

Some form of heat is gratifying to most patients. Hot moist packs and diathermy give the best results (*see* Chapter 34).

Traction is indicated in most instances of nerve root irritation. Skeletal traction is indicated in certain fractures and fracture dislocations for a period of six to eight weeks. Brace or collar immobilization can be used at the end of this time, in most instances (*see also* Chapter 37).

Some of the acute neck sprains are best treated in a hospital, by use of constant head-halter traction for a period of a few days. Six to 10 pounds of weight can be tolerated usually. The patient should be placed in a jack-knife position for comfort and for effectiveness of the traction (Fig. 79–11*B*). When the patient becomes ambulatory, some type of brace or collar immobilization which keeps the patient's neck straight, and which does not produce hyperextension of the neck, is indicated for a period of a few weeks.

Motorized intermittent traction, which can be given in the doctor's office or in a physical therapy department, gives the best results (Fig. 79–11*A*). This method of traction application can be controlled in amount and in duration. It provides

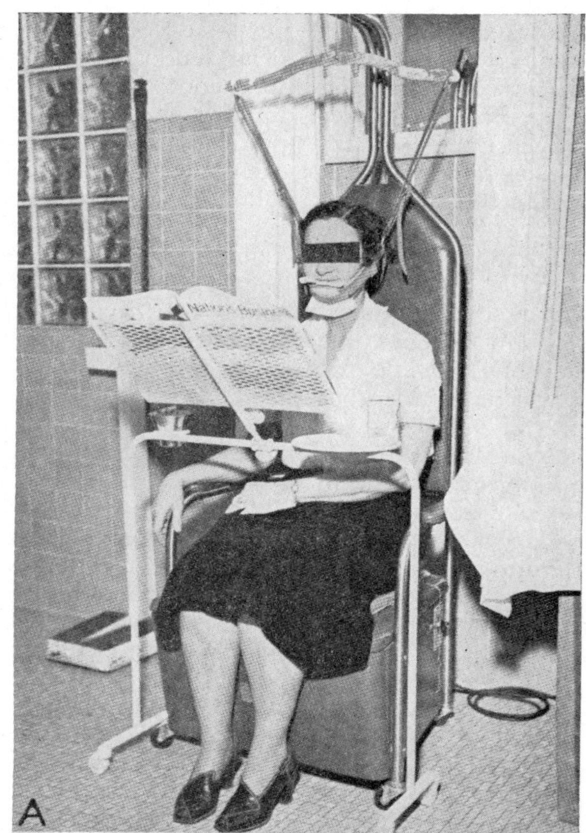

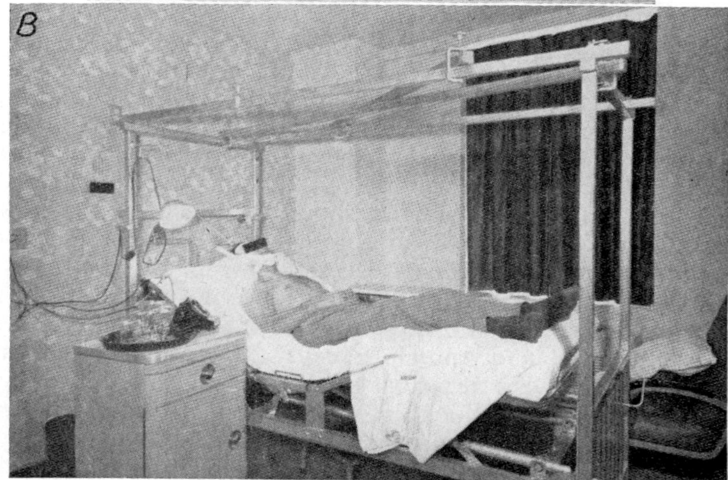

Fig. 79–11.—Traction: motorized intermittent traction (*A*), and constant bed traction (*B*). (Jackson, *The Cervical Syndrome*, courtesy of Charles C Thomas.)

the maximum pull, with a minimum amount of discomfort to the patient's jaw and chin.

I have shown by cineradiography that 10 pounds of traction lifts the weight of the head from the neck, but produces no visible distraction of the vertebrae. Twenty-five to 35 pounds of traction produces definite distraction of the vertebrae and causes straightening of the forward curve.

This method of traction prevents the formation of adhesions between the dural sleeves of the nerve roots and the adjacent structures. It may free adhesions in some instances. It relieves muscle spasm and pain, and many patients fall asleep during the treatment. Traction should be continued at regular intervals as long as indicated.

In some instances it may be necessary to permit the patient to use traction at home. Medication to relieve muscle spasm and pain may be necessary. Measures to improve the patient's general health are essential.

In acute sprain injuries, correct collar or brace immobilization should be used for a period of six to eight weeks. Chronic cases may need immobilization for short intervals only.

If localized pain and muscle spasm persist, dramatic relief can be obtained by the injection of a ½ per cent local anesthetic (*e.g.* procaine) into the painful areas. Paralysis of the pain receptors and conductors breaks the pain reflex and gives relief for days, weeks or months.

Poor postural habits should be corrected. The patient should be taught to avoid hyperextension and hyperflexion of the neck in his everyday activities, inasmuch as the intervertebral canals are of maximum size when the neck is straight. Shoulder braces may be indicated to correct drooping shoulders and to help straighten the cervical spine.

The cervical contour pillow, as designed by me, is an important adjunct in the treatment of cervical spine conditions (Fig. 79–12). It assures correct positioning of the neck during sleep, whether the patient sleeps on his back or on his side. Sleeping in the prone position is forbidden, because this position keeps the neck turned to one side for prolonged periods of time, which aggravates the symptoms.

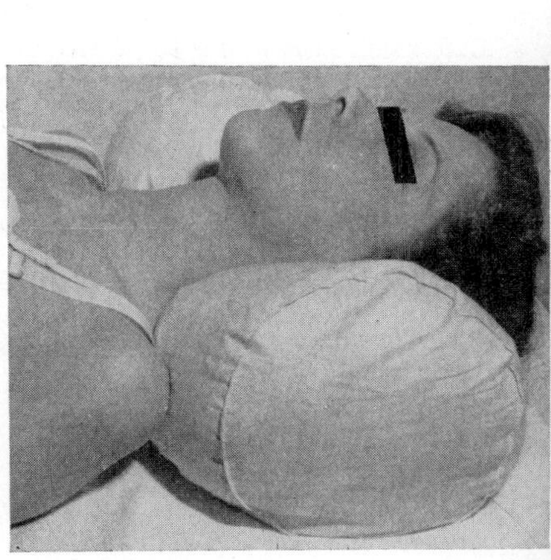

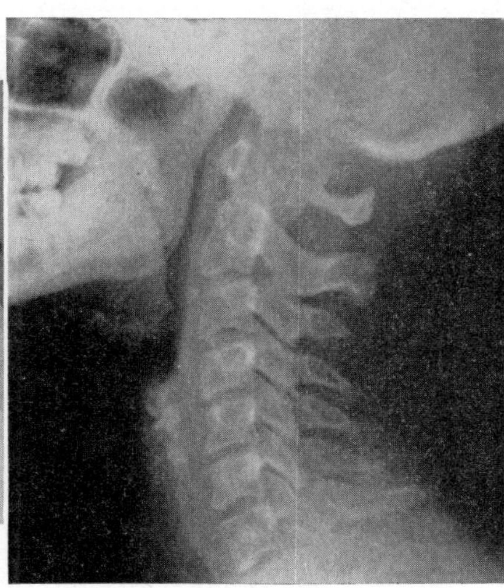

Fig. 79–12.—The cervical contour pillow for correct sleeping posture. The radiograph shows the position of the vertebrae with the neck on the pillow. (Jackson, *The Cervical Syndrome*, courtesy of Charles C Thomas.)

Inasmuch as emotional stress and strain may aggravate the symptoms, these factors should be eliminated as much as possible.

Surgical procedures on the cervical spine should be reserved for those patients who do not respond to conservative measures, or for those who have definite evidence of cord compression from epidural space-occupying lesions or from subarachnoid space-occupying lesions.

In some patients in whom there are overriding spinous processes, removal of these processes may be necessary.

Persistent and resistant nerve root irritation may be relieved by a simple facet fenestration, the purpose of which is to remove the posterior wall of the intervertebral canal to decompress the nerve root.

Removal of degenerated disc material and spur formations by the anterior route, followed by an intervertebral body graft for fusion, is gaining in popularity. Most surgeons who fuse the cervical spine by the anterior route utilize discography for localization of the offending disc, and to determine the site for fusion. However, much controversy has arisen concerning the advisability and the fallacy of discography. A degenerated or creviced disc may not be the true cause of the symptoms, which explains the reason for the second and third operations which are often done in an effort to relieve the symptoms.

Removal of foraminal osteophytes by facetectomy, followed by fusion, via the posterior route is much preferred by some surgeons, in spite of the acclaimed advantages of the anterior method.

CONCLUSIONS

The importance of cervical investigation for any patient who has head, neck, chest, shoulder or arm pain is emphasized. Diagnoses of arthritis, bursitis, neuritis, muscular rheumatism, fibrositis, fascitis, tendinitis, pseudoangina or migraine should be avoided until cervical nerve root involvement has been eliminated as the causative factor.

Conservative measures give gratifying results in the majority of cases. Treatment should be individualized and definitive. Surgical measures are rarely necessary. Such treatment should be reserved for those patients who do not respond to adequate conservative treatment and who have definite indications for operative procedure.

BIBLIOGRAPHY

1. ABEL, M. S.: Clinical Orthopaedics, *72*, 189, 1958.
2. DELMAS, J. *et al.*: Comment atteinare les fibres preganglionares du membre supérieur. Gaz. méd. de France, *54*, 703, 1947.
3. DAVIS, A. G.: J.A.M.A., *127*, 149, 1944.
4. JACKSON, R.: *The Cervical Syndrome*, Springfield, Charles C Thomas, 1971.
5. KAPLAN and KENNEDY: Brain, *73*, 337, 1956.
6. LARUELLE, L. L.: Les Bases anatomiques du système autonome cortical et bulbo-spinal. Rev. neurol., *72*, 349, 1940.
7. LUCK, J. V.: *Bone and Joint Diseases*, Springfield, Charles C Thomas, 1950.
8. STEINDLER, A.: *Instructional Course Lectures*, Ann Arbor, Edwards Brothers, 1957.
9. TINEL, J.: *Le Système Nerveux Végétatif*. Paris, Masson & Cie, 1937.
10. VON LUSCHKA, H.: *Die Halbergelenke des Menschlechen Korpers*, G. Reimer, 1858.

Chapter 80

The Painful Shoulder

By Otto Steinbrocker, M.D.

Introduction

The title of this chapter arises from the symptom which usually leads patients with disorders of the shoulder to seek medical care. In most of them pain is associated with some degree of disturbed or limited motion. The shoulder area, of course, may be the site of any lesion or symptoms occurring in the musculoskeletal system, whether generalized or local. Disturbances of the shoulder may arise from the shoulder joint itself—the scapulohumeral articulation, from its overlying periarticular structures, from adjacent or distant musculoskeletal, neural, vascular or visceral lesions, or even as a somatization (Table 80–1). The conditions derived locally, directly from the structures of the shoulder joint or its intimately related musculotendinous, capsular, bursal and other periarticular soft tissues, may conveniently be classified as "intrinsic." Those arising outside this area, transmitting symptoms from distant disorders to the shoulder region, may be termed "extrinsic."[148] Pain in the shoulder does not necessarily mean disease arising there, as can be readily seen from the host of extraneous sources listed in Table 80–1.

The intrinsic, nonarticular syndromes of the shoulder are the most frequent and are characteristic of that location.[13,18,49] Apart from acute traumatic lesions, such as fractures, dislocations, contusions, sprains and ruptured tendons, 85 to 90 per cent of painful disabilities of the shoulder are due to acute or chronic calcific tendinitis and bursitis, adhesive capsulitis, bicipital tendinitis and lesions of the musculotendinous cuff.[49,148] They, therefore, will be the chief subjects of this chapter.

Except for patients suffering from generalized arthropathies, arthritis of the shoulder joint, in spite of the frequent impression to the contrary, causes less than 5 per cent of painful shoulders.[49,97]

Although the painful shoulder due to intrinsic lesions is encountered generally in the later decades, it often occurs earlier among baseball pitchers, paper hangers, violinists, orchestra conductors and those who use their arms vigorously and repetitively.[49,93]

Anatomic and Physiologic Factors

The shoulder joint is a part of the rather intricate musculoarticular mechanism constituting the shoulder girdle.[13,56,97] The "shoulder joint" generally brings to mind the scapulohumeral joint. Actually, however, the shoulder normally functions by the action of its muscles through a "joint complex" consisting of four independent articulations—the glenohumeral, acromioclavicular and sternoclavicular, as well as the scapulothoracic surface relationship and the motion of the bicipital tendon. Each of these is capable of separate, independent motion, but all participate simultaneously in the movements of the upper extremity. These functions revolve about the action of the scapulohumeral articulation as a nearly universal joint, synchronized with motion at its associated mobile units. Ankylosis of any of the joints causes a permanent

Table 80-1.—Intrinsic and Extrinsic Pain Syndromes of the Shoulder

- Musculoskeletal
  - Nonarticular (soft tissue lesions)
    - Definitive intrinsic syndromes
      - Calcareous tendinitis and bursitis
      - Adhesive capsulitis
      - Bicipital tenosynovitis
      - Musculotendinous cuff lesions
    - Fibromyopathies and myalgias
      - Traumatic fibromyopathy or myalgia
      - "Fibrositis syndrome"
      - Miscellaneous fibromyalgias and myalgias
        - Focal myalgias, "trigger point" and "tender point" disorders
  - Articular (shoulder or cervical spine)
      - (Systemic or localized)
      - Inflammatory
      - Infectious
      - Degenerative
      - Metabolic
      - Neuropathic
      - Traumatic
  - Neurovascular
    - Compression syndromes
      - ("Thoracic outlet syndromes")
      - Cervical rib, scalenus anticus, or first rib
      - Costoclavicular
      - Hyperabduction
    - Reflex neurovascular syndromes
      - Shoulder-hand syndrome
      - Circumscribed reflex dystrophy
  - Vascular, predominantly
    - Arterial
      - Acute arterial occlusion
      - Chronic occlusive arterial disease
      - Aneurysm
      - Arteriovenous fistula
      - Erythromelalgia
      - Raynaud's disease
    - Venous
      - Acute thrombosis or thrombophlebitis
      - Chronic venous insufficiency
    - Lymphatic
      - Acute lymphangitis
      - Chronic lymphedema
  - Osseous
    - Traumatic
      - Fracture, dislocation, subluxation of humerus, scapula, clavicle, vertebra, disc (herniation)
      - Congenital anomalies
      - Infectious, inflammatory or metabolic
      - Neoplastic, primary or metastatic
  - Neurological, predominantly
    - Central
      - Cervical osteophyte or disc
      - Herpes zoster neuropathy
      - Neoplasm of brain or cord
      - Primary disease—multiple sclerosis, etc.
      - Radiculitis
      - Syringomyelia
      - Vascular occlusion or hemorrhage
      - Trauma to brain or cord
    - Peripheral
      - Cervicobrachial and peripheral neuralgia and neuropathy
      - Dysesthesias
        - Brachialgia paresthetica
        - Acroparesthesias
        - Carpal tunnel syndrome
  - Systemic (non-rheumatic) diseases with local features
    - Connective tissue diseases
      - Dermatomyositis
      - Diffuse vasculitis
      - Scleroderma
  - (Post) infectional and (post) viral states
  - Relapsing nodular panniculitis
  - Serum sickness
  - Hormonal imbalance
  - Nutritional deficiencies
- Viscerogenic (referred)
- Psychogenic
- Idiopathic
  - Myalgia, arthralgia, neuralgia
  - Polymyalgia rheumatica

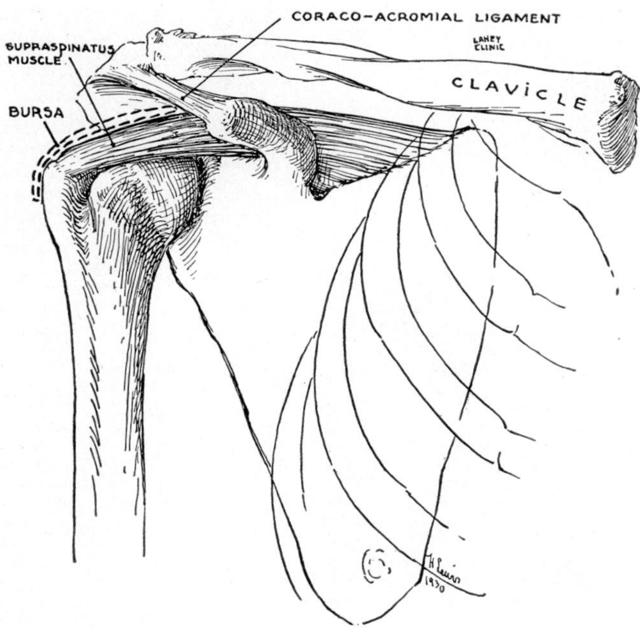

FIG. 80–1.—Drawing showing relation of subacromial bursa to supraspinatus tendon, coracoacromial ligament and greater tuberosity of the humerus. (Haggart and Allen, courtesy of Surg. Clin. North America.)

loss in degree of movement in direct proportion to the amount of motion that joint should have contributed to complete mobility.

The functions of the scapulohumeral joint and its related articulations and moving parts also are dependent upon the state and performance of the periarticular structures. Smooth, rhythmic motion of the upper extremity is produced by the coordinated action of the muscles surrounding, and attached to, the osseous components of the shoulder joints—the clavicle, scapula and humerus. Their normal function, or "scapulohumeral rhythm"—usually disturbed in the common shoulder disorders—is derived from sound musculoarticular action.

In addition, good shoulder function requires unhampered movement at certain gliding surfaces of the periarticular structures—the musculotendinous cuff, the subdeltoid bursa and the long head of the biceps. Pathologic changes in these periarticular components or "soft tissues" chiefly are responsible for the conditions to be discussed here.

Overlying the scapulohumeral joint and its surrounding articular capsule are three strata of periarticular structures apt to become the seat of lesions. The innermost is the musculotendinous cuff, or conjoined tendon, consisting of the rotator tendons joined together by a webbing of fibrous tissue. It is partially attached to the articular capsule. The supraspinatus tendon lies under the floor of the middle stratum, the subacromial bursa, which rests between the musculotendinous cuff and the outer stratum or "sleeve," the deltoid muscle (Fig. 80–1). Spreading over it, as a delicate, membranous flattened sac, with an inner synovial layer and a slight amount of fluid, lies the bursa, sometimes as large as the palm of the hand (Fig. 80–2). The tendon of the supraspinatus, and its adjacent tissues, notably the overlying bursa, rest and function in a space between the acromion, humerus and

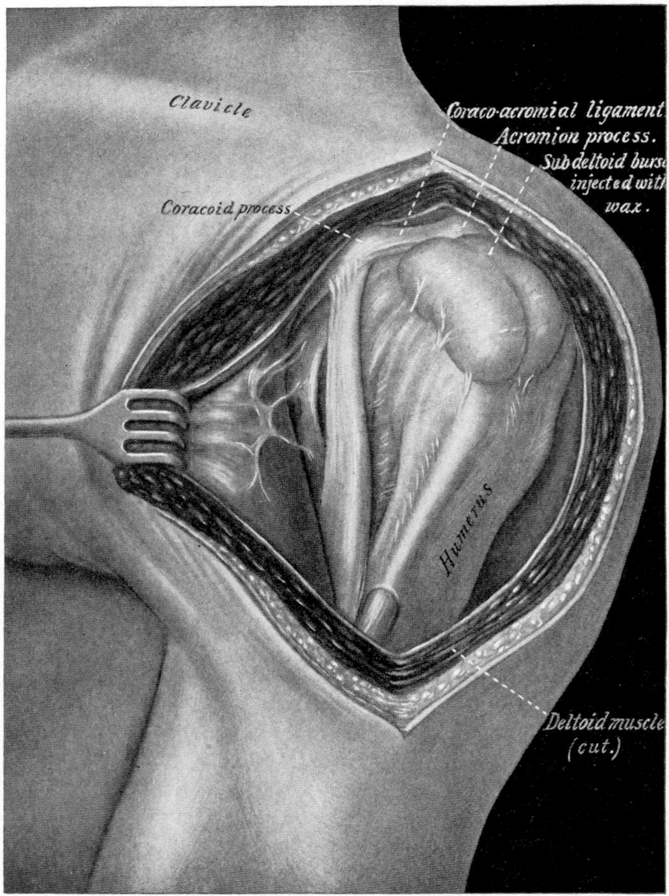

FIG. 80–2.—The subdeltoid bursa. (Baer.)

coracoacromial ligament, which barely is free during elevation of the extremity. There the tendon is subjected to pressure and friction during strenuous activities. It is important, too, that the floor of the bursa forms part of the tendon sheath and is included in the contiguous peritendinous tissues of the supraspinatus tendon.[13]

Just below the bursa and the musculotendinous cuff, from within the joint capsule, emerges the long head of the biceps to run through the bicipital groove. It is a long, movable tendon with a synovial sheath, an extension of the scapulohumeral synovium. Each of these structures must function adequately as a gliding surface for normal movement at the scapulohumeral joint and its related articulations. The capsule of the scapulohumeral joint is loose, particularly its inferior part where redundant folds provide freedom of mobility and also constitute its most vulnerable portion.[105]

Pathophysiology

The shoulder area is the crossroad for vascular stimuli to the extremity from the brain, spinal cord and many segmentally related viscera. The pendulous upper extremity continually is subjected to the pull of gravity. The versatile mobility of the shoulder, often congenitally or functionally imperfect, exposes its abundant connective tissue, bursa(e), capsule and musculotendinous cuff to more direct and cumulative stress and strain than any other articulation.[13,56]

Predisposing and active pathologic lesions of various degees are found in the diseased shoulder. These consist of the evidence of "aging" degeneration, "wear and tear," minute and gross tears and attrition of tendons and cuff tissue, low-grade inflammation, localized or extensive, in the form of latent or florid tendinitis, tenosynovitis, bursitis and capsulitis. Such predisposing alterations often are due to past gross or minute injuries, minimum habitual or occupational trauma, repetitive injury from congenital anomalies or hypertrophic osseous changes or, possibly, from "irritative" local metabolic or circulatory disturbance.

The precipitating factor often is trauma—direct injury, a sudden effort, unaccustomed or prolonged exertion, or exercise; even a usual motion may seem to be "the last straw." Not infrequently the incitement is blamed on exposure to environmental factors, such as chilling (air conditioning), wind (electric fan), or dampness. The physical condition of the patient may appear to bear a provocative relationship to shoulder symptoms—in depletion, exhaustion, systemic illness, nutritional and hormonal deficiency, and in acute emotional crises or prolonged tension states. In some patients confined to bed for long periods, painful, or even painless, disability may occur for no other ascribable reason.

When pain arises at the shoulder, a vicious circle of gross physiologic disturbances long has been known to lead to disability and to the "frozen shoulder." Ordinarily, this reaction seems, during clinical observation, to be initiated by the pain with its protective muscle spasm and limitation of mobility, further aggravated by the pathologic process and its adhesions. Muscle atrophy may develop and, often, osteoporosis. Limited function or prolonged disuse, "inactivity," may constitute a final, local depleting factor.

Pain referred to the shoulder is encountered frequently in disturbed persons, sometimes with obvious characteristics and relationship to an emotional conflict or crisis which create no etiologic or diagnostic difficulty. In neurotic and psychotic patients presenting localized subjective or objective symptoms, and more often in those whose symptoms are well masked, the clinical talents of the examiner may be severely taxed to arrive at correct conclusions. How great a part conscious or subconscious emotional conflicts may take in the definitely organic, disabling syndromes of the shoulder is not clear at this time. It is noted commonly that in some subjects, with demonstrable intrinsic disease from persistent shoulder symptoms, emotional trends tend to be stirred up and to color the symptom picture. In others, with little apparent pathologic basis, the severity of the complaints appears to be closely bound up with the patient's psychodynamics.

That somatizations, partly or completely immobilizing a shoulder, may in that way promote specific, intrinsic disease in some individuals already predisposed by latent pathologic alterations, has not been proved. It is suggested by clinical as well as psychiatric observations.[38,83,128,134]

Examination of the Patient

To examine the shoulders, the patient is seated on a stool, in a good light and stripped to the waist. A comparison is made of both shoulders, anteriorly and posteriorly, for swelling, muscular atrophy or tenderness over the trapezius, deltoid, scapular, pectoral and paravertebral muscles. Palpation for tender points and trigger points is carefully carried out at symmetrical areas on both sides, starting at the normal side to give the patient a comparative idea of the response of sound tissues. Palpation of the neck muscles also is helpful to determine the extent of irritation or hypersensitivity to the stimulus. The scalenus muscles also should be tested, by pressure behind the sternomastoid muscle, over the first rib. The recognition and delineation of cutaneous hyperesthesia by pinch, scratch and prick may be informative, particularly in radicular syndromes and in the hyperreactive psychoneuroses. In acute conditions palpation should be especially cautious and gentle, and in hyperacute disorders it should be kept to a minimum.

Full elevation of the arm includes rotation of the humerus upward on the scapula and of the scapula on the chest wall. When the arm is fully elevated the glenoid faces outward. The greater tuberosity of the humerus slides under the acromion during elevation of the arm, requiring a normal subacromial bursal sac, rotator cuff and capsule for smooth, painless and unlimited performance. If adhesions at these structures are not present, the arm can be elevated horizontally as a result of the rotation of the scapula on the chest. If the physician stands on the unaffected side he can control the motion of the opposite, involved scapula by clasping the hands below the axilla, thereby determining how much of the limitation of motion is due to lost movement of the humerus. This scapulohumeral rhythm also may be observed by inspection.

The patient carries out standard motions of the head at the cervical spine, in rotation to each side, in flexion (chin to chest) and extension. Limited mobility in any of these ranges may be the first evidence of cervical spinal changes or muscular dysfunction responsible for, or contributing to, the complaints described at the shoulder (*see* Chapter 79).

The hands are examined for palmar (Dupuytren's) changes, tenderness, vasomotor disturbances, swelling, digital atrophy and functional disability which may be related to the source of shoulder symptoms or other pathology.

Special tests for pain, tenderness, compression or circulatory response may be helpful, such as Yergason's for bicipital tendinitis (*see* p. 1478), Adson's for the scalenus syndrome (p. 1487), bilateral blood pressures, hyperabduction or exaggerated military position of the shoulders.

The Definitive Intrinsic Syndromes of the Shoulder

The major intrinsic syndromes of the shoulder are generally accepted now to consist of:

Calcareous tendinitis (and
  subacromial bursitis)
Adhesive capsulitis
Bicipital tenosynovitis
Lesions of the musculotendinous cuff

These conditions present many similarities and frequently overlap in symptomatology, course, predisposing and precipitating factors, as well as responsiveness or refractoriness to similar therapeutic agents. Multiple intrinsic lesions, and sometimes all of them, may be encountered in the same shoulder. In longstanding, chronic disease, identifying the predominant or instigating lesion frequently becomes a matter of interpretation. Progress in the demarcation of these syndromes therefore has been hampered by the similarities and overlapping. A multiplicity of terminology also has added to the confusion which still prevails regarding these processes as clinical entities, in spite of the constructive, pioneering contributions of Codman and others.[140,148]

"*Subacromial*" *or* "*subdeltoid bursitis*" *and* "*bursitis of the shoulder*," terms widely used to designate any or all of these disorders, have created great confusion. Actually, bursitis rarely is encountered as an isolated, local disturbance due to direct or violent injury, traumatic rupture and hemorrhage, fractures, infection, granuloma or inflammation initiated within the confines of the bursa. In fact, bursal "irritation" or inflammation has been found, in many observations at open operations and explorations of involved shoulders, arising generally as a secondary reaction to underlying or adjacent supraspinatus tendinitis, usually calcareous.[13,86,90,97] Calcific material sometimes can be seen to have perforated the bursal sac and discharged into it. Codman long ago pointed out that often, owing to the peculiar mechanics of the shoulder, "the inert and avascular supraspinatus tendon is the most vulnerable part of this joint complex, and inflammation within it may be painless until the adjacent bursa is involved. There, owing to the abundant bursal vessels and nerves, symptoms are produced."

Bursal inflammation, with acute, subacute and chronic infiltration, thickening of the bursal sac, adhesive changes within and about it, may occur, with little or great effusion. Early bursal lesions generally are associated with, and related to, acute calcific tendinitis, while late changes are a part of widespread involvement of other periarticular structures also extending to the bursa. "Bursitis," therefore, when present, often is a secondary, incidental part of the effect of disease starting in other, adjacent structures.[13,41,86]

In generalized arthritis, such as rheumatoid, acute or chronic, secondary inflammation of the subacromial bursa sometimes occurs, occasionally with large effusion, and even communication with the concomitantly involved scapulohumeral joint.

Whether bursal involvement at the shoulder is "primary" or "secondary," it constitutes the most frequent cause of the painful shoulder as well as the most common bursitis of the 140 or more bursae in the body (33 in each upper and 37 in each lower extremity). Subdeltoid bursitis accompanying calcific tendinitis obviously is the most frequent form.[49,90,97]

In the discussion to follow, in accordance with the weight of all available evidence, *subdeltoid bursitis is to be assumed as a probable, secondary pathologic and clinical concomitant of calcareous tendinitis and, at times, of the other intrinsic syndromes.*

CALCAREOUS TENDINITIS (WITH SUBACROMIAL BURSITIS)

Calcareous tendinitis is a symptomatic, inflammatory involvement of one or more of the rotator tendons due to inflammation associated with deposition of calcium in and about the tendon, most often the supraspinatus. It first was described in the same year (1907) by Painter and by Baer in this country as "subdeltoid bursitis."[44,97]

Frequency

Calcific deposits, in and about the rotator tendons, are the most frequent abnormal radiologic and clinicopathologic findings in the painful shoulder.[10,41] Many calcifications, however, do not provoke complaints.[10]

When calcium deposits become provocative, they produce the most painful shoulder involvement. Calcific tendinitis also is the most frequent source of acute or hyperacute symptoms at the shoulder. The right shoulder is the active site with $1\frac{1}{2}$ to 2 times the frequency of the left; occasionally both sides may be symptomatic. Men are affected somewhat more often than women, between the ages of thirty-six to sixty years, with the peak during the fifth decade. The subjects usually do relatively sedentary work, requiring partial, repeated abduction, such as tailors, typists, clerks and "white collar" workers more than laborers or factory workers.[10,41,86]

Etiology and Pathogenesis[86,114]

Apart from trauma, actual or assumed, the calcium and the inflammatory reaction it provokes are the two chief factors known in symptomatic calcareous tendinitis. In spite of many explanations as a working basis, the exact method by which calcium is deposited remains obscure. An initial, severe enough injury to any of the rotator tendons may start pathologic changes. From gross and microscopic studies of tissues removed from shoulders at necropsy and during surgical exploration an understandable picture of the pathogenesis emerges.[10,13,17,86,90,97,114]

"Use destruction" produces a circumscribed area of "avascular necrosis" in the tendon where collagen fibrils degenerate and disappear. Continued "wear and tear" increase the extent of necrosis and fraying of tendon fibers and loss of vascularity. The degenerating, necrotic tissue is replaced by a fibrinoid mass surrounded by leukocytes and histiocytes. Calcium is deposited by a mechanism not clear at this time. The enlarging calcareous deposit may encroach on the more responsive tendon sheath or subacromial bursa, the floor of which forms part of the tendon sheath of the supraspinatus.

Repeated motion of the extremity or sudden stress of the tendon may arouse an inflammatory reaction at the calcified site. Fluid collects within the tendon sheath about the deposit to produce pressure, pain and muscle spasm. The clinical picture is patterned by the severity and rapidity of these reactions.

Symptomatology

The symptoms may be *acute*, *subacute* or *chronic*.[41,86,97,127,140,148]

The *cardinal symptoms* of calcareous tendinitis at any of the rotator tendons are *pain, tenderness and limited mobility* at the shoulder in acute cases, less pronounced in subacute disorders, and usually milder in chronic cases, where motion often is not impaired.[41,86,97,148]

Calcareous tendinitis of the supraspinatus generally produces the symptoms, so it will serve as the typical picture to be described. Involvement of this tendon particularly is apt to be associated with some degree of secondary subacromial bursitis which contributes to the severity of the acute picture.[13]

Acute supraspinatus tendinitis is characterized by sudden onset of pain, or the acute flare-up of previous discomfort, located at the shoulder tip. As a rule, the patient presents a first attack without previous knowledge of any local disease. The pain is severe, sometimes agonizing, interfering with rest and sleep, and is provoked and increased by motion. The individual with hyperacute symptoms fears any handling of the extremity by the examiner and pleads to avoid it. The extremity is voluntarily fixed, adducted to the side with the forearm flexed. The slightest abduction and external rotation are distressing. The pain is felt at the upper humerus in the subacromial area, radiates often to the insertion of the deltoid, in severe cases even up to the occiput and downward along the extremity to the fingertips. Tenderness is exquisite at the lateral area of the humeral head, below the acromion, and often at and above the insertion of the deltoid. Sometimes fluctuation may be felt, or swelling seen, below the acromial border. Fever, leukocytosis and an elevated sedimentation rate occasionally accompany an acute attack.

X-ray films show a calcific deposit in or at the line of the supraspinatus tendon, below the acromion over the head of the humerus, or at the site of any other rotator tendon that may be the source of symptoms (Fig. 80–3). Two views, one in slight, internal rotation, the other in slight, external rotation, are most informative. The calcific material usually is dense, may be amorphous, irregular in shape, of large or medium size, as a rule. It may be in several fragments. Acute reactions with edema or effusion tend to create lighter portions. Such material, when aspirated, comes out with the consistency of toothpaste. In chronic deposits it is a dry powdery substance. Rupture of the calcium into the bursa produces a diffuse opacity in the bursal cavity.

The acute symptoms may remain at their peak for days, at times. Spontaneous diminution of their severity may occur abruptly or gradually. Sometimes they assume a subacute form.

Chronic calcific tendinitis is characterized by pain during certain motions, or an

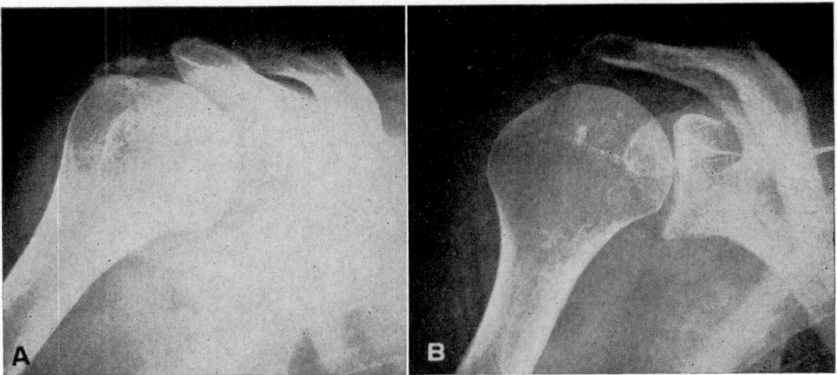

FIG. 80–3.—Roentgenograms showing: *A*, Acute calcareous supraspinatus tendinitis of right shoulder. *B*, Same shoulder, one day after two-needle irrigation, with disappearance of calcium.

"awareness" of the shoulder in abduction and internal rotation while getting into jackets and overcoats, and similar motions of daily living. The pain may be steady, nagging, or only a stab of soreness or aching during motion, or a throbbing discomfort at night. Usually, there is no limitation of motion. Some tenderness to palpation is likely to be found at the subacromial area of the humerus, with supraspinatus involvement. A dense calcification is seen on x-ray films. This pattern may go on for many months or years with periods of spontaneous relief. The pathology represents a potential source of an acute or subacute flare-up, when exposed to adequate provocation, or gradual periarticular extension of inflammation spreading to and from the musculotendinous cuff and the bursa.

Treatment of Acute Calcific Tendinitis and Bursitis and Other Intrinsic Syndromes

The Specificity of Therapeutic Measures.— The choice of therapy in this extremely common condition has seemed to depend in large part upon the field of specialization of the writers. The roentgenologist claimed excellent results with roentgen-ray therapy; the physical therapist stated that diathermy, galvanism or iontophoresis was the treatment of choice; the anesthesiologist advocated nerve blocks; the surgeon preferred a surgical procedure; the orthopedist suggested a regimen including splints and traction or surgical correction, while internists (and some orthopedists and surgeons) found that good results followed procaine injection and "washing out" the bursa by needle irrigation, or multiple punctures in the wall of the bursa. The variety of treatments recommended strongly suggests that none is specific.[49] Many are outmoded now by new and simpler procedures.

Calcium deposition in tendons provokes an inflammation which is reversible. Unless they are large, deposits often are absorbed by any process producing acute hyperemia. Many deposits disappear rather rapidly after almost any or no treatment. An adequate trial of simple, conservative measures, therefore, is recommended.

Acute, or hyperacute, tendinitis with bursitis is likely to proceed to a tolerable, natural recovery, if the discomfort of the patient is alleviated long enough by a selective program of *basic measures* (Table 80–2). In addition, when the patient clamors for relief, or when spontaneous resolution is unbearably delayed, it becomes necessary to introduce one of the supplementary *"specific" procedures to accelerate response.*

Table 80-2.—Basic Conservative Measures Used in Shoulder Syndromes

Objectives: Relief of pain and muscle spasm, restoration of motion and prevention of secondary, inflammatory ankylosing changes.

1. *Limited use of extremity* during painful period.
   - Complete rest for hyperacute symptoms
   - Arm in sling (adducted) in acute and subacute stages; forearm and hand elevated.
2. *Analgesics* (and sedatives)
   - Salicylates
   - Acetophenetidin
   - Phenylbutazone (Butazolidin)
   - Narcotics for severe symptoms
   - Barbiturates, relaxants
3. *Physical therapy:*
   - *Heat or cold:*
     - *Home:* Infrared, electric pad, hot packs, liniment rub (*cold applications* superior in *many acute cases*)
     - *Office:* Diathermy, ultrasonic
     - *Hospital:* Underwater therapy, wheel, pulley and other devices.
     - *Spa:* In refractory, selected cases.
   - *Special Exercises* (Fig. 80–4)
4. *Treatment of associated or underlying condition*
5. *Psychological aid* (in chronic cases)
   - Reassurance, encouragement
   - Psychotherapy, selective
6. *Elimination of provocative activities or positions.*

Conservative Basic Measures in the Management of Calcareous Tendinitis and Other Painful Shoulder Disabilities

The chief consideration in the choice of the treatment program is whether the condition is acute (or hyperacute), subacute or chronic. All measures are planned to relieve pain, restore function as rapidly as possible, and prevent residual subacute or chronic progression, according to the requirements of the situation.

Rest in some form is the first basic measure. It requires complete or partial immobilization in the acute or hyperacute conditions. In the milder forms, limitation of the use of the extremity, with the arm carried in a sling until the acute or subacute symptoms have abated, will suffice. Chronic disorders do not require immobilization of the extremity.

Analgesics in ample dosage are indicated, notably in acute onsets of painful disability. Hyperacute and acute symptoms justify the use of narcotics, orally or hypodermically for the first few days. Codeine sulfate, 0.015 to 0.03 gm. ($\frac{1}{4}$ to $\frac{1}{2}$ gr.) 3 or 4 times daily, may be required to supplement conventional analgesics during acute episodes of any of these disorders. Salicylates, 4 to 6 gm. daily, in divided doses, usually help. If not, phenylbutazone (Butazolidin), starting with two 100-mg. tablets 3 times daily then reduced, with response, to low maintenance doses, may give superior results in painful shoulder disturbances. A five- to seven-day trial serves as a reliable index as to whether it deserves to be continued, with the precautions it imposes.

Physical therapy and exercises may give additional palliation and accelerated recovery of function. The most generally useful of these procedures is the introduction of the standard exercises[51] (Fig.

80–4). These must be demonstrated to the patient and started at an opportune time. Certainly, they should not be initiated during acute symptoms under any circumstances, particularly when motion increases pain. They are carried out gently, and increased in number and duration every few days until they can be done for a period of five to ten minutes once a day, and later twice daily. Exercises which are followed by more than one hour of increased soreness or pain on motion are excessive. Pulley exercises are especially helpful when pain has subsided.

To control the pain of active symptoms and to promote mobility at all stages, physical modalities include[11,25,51,69,130,148] hot applications or infrared radiation to the shoulder. Cold applications often prove to be more effective in the acute attack. Diathermy is favored by some, but may exacerbate acute symptoms. Ultrasonic therapy has been reported helpful, but this has not been established.[39,98]

Patients who, for personal or environmental reasons, have difficulty in carrying out a treatment program, particularly physical measures, should be hospitalized, if practical, for supervised, intensive physical therapy. In subacute or chronic conditions, refractory to therapy on an ambulatory basis, one to three weeks of an intramural treatment program may initiate improvement.

Treatment of underlying conditions must be continued, particularly diabetes, cardiovascular and other disease. Their relationship in the choice of agents like corticosteroids, phenylbutazone or injection procedures must be considered.

Psychological aids in the simple form of reassurance and encouragement and psychiatric assistance in severe emotional states must be part of a thorough program.

SPECIAL MEASURES IN ACUTE DISEASE OF THE SHOULDER

The *acute* phase has been found particularly responsive to one or more of several

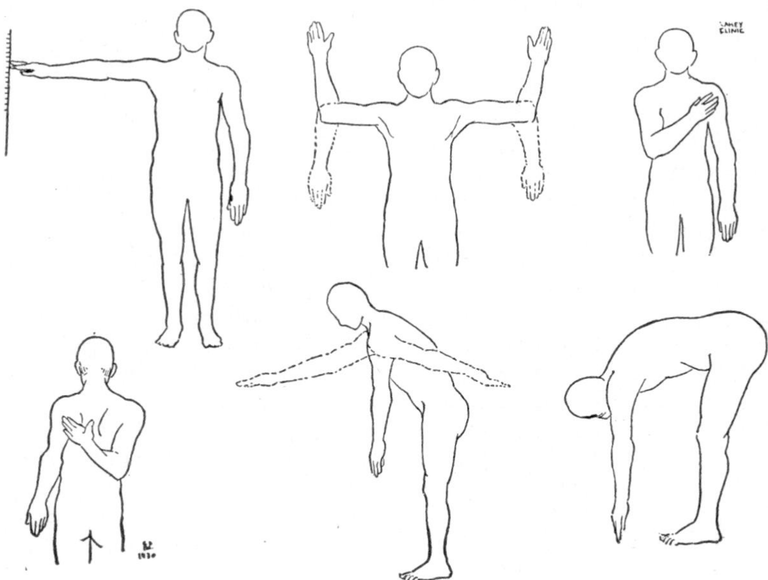

Fig. 80–4.—Exercises useful in redeveloping shoulder muscle power; of special value are climbing the wall with the fingers of the outstretched abducted arm, and swinging the arms anteroposteriorly and also mediolaterally (not shown) with the trunk flexed. (Haggart and Allen, courtesy of Surg. Clin. North America.)

forms of treatment, not necessarily in the following order of preference, but according to circumstances: (1) *x-ray therapy*, (2) *local* (subacromial) *injection of hydrocortisone or other corticosteroid suspension*, (3) *two-needle irrigation of a calcific deposit* with ½ per cent procaine solution, (4) *corticosteroids* (*or ACTH*) *administered systemically*, (5) *multiple needling of the calcareous deposit* (*and bursa*).

The choice of each of the special methods of treatment must depend on the attitude of the patient and the skill of the physician in the use of these techniques.

X-ray therapy has been noted by many observers to be helpful in over 60 per cent of cases although recent controlled studies have been presented to show that the effectiveness is a form of "suggestion."[11, 62, 116, 127, 140] A course of 3 to 6 treatments usually is given. Pain may be aggravated for twenty-four hours after a treatment. This form of therapy has been abandoned by most rheumatologists.

Corticosteroids (*and ACTH*), given systemically, although not constituting the simplest approach to a local condition, have been found of distinct value in the treatment of acute, or subacute tendinitis and bursitis, with or without calcium deposits, in 50 to 60 per cent of the cases.[7, 29, 137, 143, 148] In subacute and chronic conditions, prolonged corticotherapy becomes necessary for months, often with recurrence of symptoms when the hormone is discontinued. *Many rheumatologists now regard direct infiltration as a simpler approach to a local inflammation, particularly in the acute and subacute phases.*

Local Injection of Corticosteroid.—This probably is the most widely used special method at this time. Since first reported by Hollander,[54] its place as a simple, effective procedure has been rapidly established.[9, 11, 14, 21, 71, 73, 97, 111, 120, 126, 130, 143, 144, 167] Hydrocortisone acetate, or the more satisfactory tertiary-butyl-acetate (t.b.a.), prednisolone t.b.a., or newer equivalents, may be used. The suspension is given in doses of (25 to 50 mg. of hydrocortisone) 1 to 2 ml. at standard concentrations marketed for intra-articular injection, every three to ten days, if needed. The approach for injection of the shoulder bursa for calcific tendinitis is shown in Figure 80–5. General technique is described in Chapter 32. A 22-gauge needle is inserted at the point of maximum tenderness.

Aspiration first is done, before injecting, to release any calcific material or fluid present. For the usual case of acute or subacute calcific tendinitis this procedure is adequate and is tolerated well by the average patient, even when repeated infiltrations are required. As a rule one injection of corticosteroid suspension suffices for acute attacks, in combination with basic measures. Corticosteroid infiltrations are so effective, that unpleasant and repeated probing or needling for decompression, or to reach and withdraw calcareous material or fluid, ordinarily is not required.

In hyperacute cases the same procedure is followed, but the injection of corticosteroid suspension is preceded by the instillation of 5 to 10 ml. of 1 per cent procaine solution for better anesthesia and quicker analgesia. (A history of satisfactory tolerance of procaine always should be obtained before its use.) After this step, the syringe containing the corticosteroid suspension is attached to the inserted needle and the compound is injected.

Two-needle irrigation of the calcareous deposit with 0.25 per cent procaine solution in an effort to "wash out" the soft, calcific material, as described by Darrach and Patterson, may the most promptly effective therapeutic method, and the most thorough.[16] Calcium may disappear shortly after any manner of treatment, or spontaneously, but it actually is removed, in great part, at once by this technique. Its disadvantage is that it must be carried out in the hospital under intravenous (or inhalation) anesthesia, owing to the excruciating tenderness of the acutely affected shoulder. It also requires some degree of skill to locate the deposit.

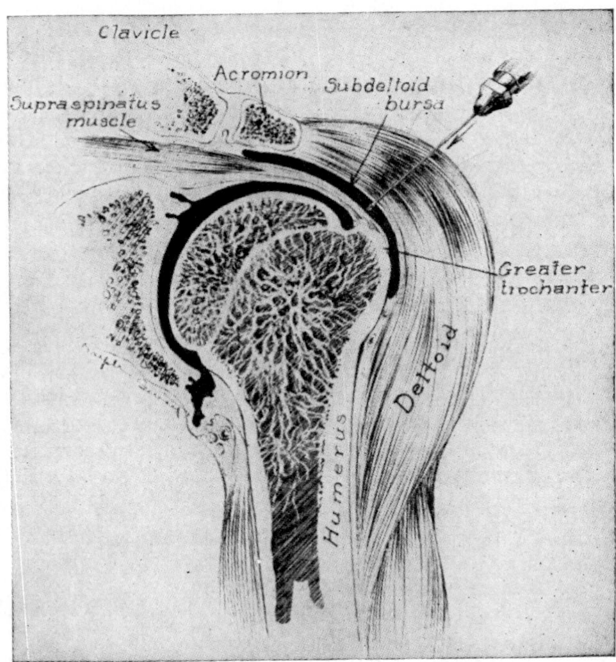

Fig. 80–5.—Injection of subdeltoid bursa. (Haldemann and Soto-Hall, courtesy of J.A.M.A.)

Multiple Punctures of the Bursa.—Flint first suggested needling the subdeltoid bursa in 1913 for acute, traumatic subdeltoid bursitis.[35a] More than thirty years ago Weeks and his co-workers found that the mere passage of the needle through the bursa relieved the symptoms whether fluid could be withdrawn or not.[161a] Simple multiple punctures of the bursal sac resulted in relief of symptoms in a large percentage of their patients, regardless of the presence or absence of calcareous material.[49] This procedure was the most popular for some time and led to the use of procaine injections and finally the injection of corticosteroid suspensions.

Surgery.—Excision or drainage of calcific material is reserved, in acute conditions, for large deposits responsible for repeated, acute attacks in spite of other treatment. The operation is simple, being performed under anesthesia (local infiltration, brachial plexus block, or general if desired).

The postoperative care of the patients includes either rest in bed for a period of one or two days, or carrying the affected arm in a sling. In either case, one of the most important points in follow-up treatment is the opportune and discreet use of active exercises, usually begun within forty-eight hours after the operation.[51a]

Other therapeutic procedures and agents have been reported to be useful in acute tendinitis and bursitis. A number of observers have effectively applied nerve blocks—suprascapular, brachial plexus and stellate ganglion, with procaine solution, usually in series.[45,46] Good results have been reported from such varied remedies as intravenous administration of 2-benzylimidazoline-HCl (Priscoline), intravenous iron cacodylate, intravenous procaine, ultraviolet irradiation of the blood, adenosine-5-monophosphate, trypsin, vitamin A and vitamin B_{12}, and undoubtedly a number of others which have escaped the writer.[3,58] The difficulty of evaluating therapy in acute conditions and the lack of confirmatory observations do not permit recommendation of any of these preparations for a treatment program.

A disability lag, after relief of acute pain, for one to five weeks following any method of treatment, often is encountered. It probably represents the period required for resolution of inflammation sufficient to overcome the reflex spasm and inhibition of motor function in the muscles of the shoulder area. Progressively increasing restoration of mobility tends to come naturally and is accelerated by the judicious use of basic measures, physical therapy and, especially, gently graduated *exercises*. When necessary, manipulative or assistive motion in skilled hands proves helpful.

Subacute calcareous tendinitis with bursitis does not respond as frequently to two-needle irrigation or any of the needling or injection procedures used in the acute attacks. If the patient is needle-shy or suffers from complicating disease requiring a careful approach, the same considerations and order of choice prevail in the subacute as in the acute disorders. The simplest special measures, added to the basic management program, are *local infiltration of corticosteroid suspension*, or the *systemic use of corticosteroids. Surgery is a last resort* in refractory cases, usually when the condition threatens to become chronic, in the presence of the calcific abnormalities mentioned for the acute stage.

Chronic calcific tendinitis with bursitis consists of pain, with or without localized tenderness, little or no disability and a calcific deposit visible on x-ray films. There may be only occasional, minor discomfort or prolonged soreness, throbbing or aching, especially at night, or brought on by certain ranges of motion. *Chronic calcific tendinitis exhibits less consistent response to all forms of treatment used in the acute phase.*

Any of the *special methods* of choice may be employed to complement the basic conservative measures, particularly *local injections* of *corticosteroid suspension*. About 50 per cent of the patients respond to one or another of the "specific" procedures. If the patient does not derive enough benefit to live tolerably with the chronic symptoms, *surgery* is indicated. Surgical removal of troublesome calcific deposits follows the same considerations as in the other phases.

In patients with refractory chronic shoulder symptoms, the presence of bicipital tenosynovitis, capsulitis, or musculotendinous inflammation makes the calcific deposit a minor and innocent manifestation of multiple pathologic lesions or extensive involvement of the periarticular structures. A better diagnostic evaluation of such chronically troublesome shoulders, apart from the calcification, therefore becomes desirable, and treatment is directed accordingly.

ADHESIVE CAPSULITIS

(Frozen Shoulder, Scapulohumeral Periarthritis, Adhesive Bursitis, Periarticular Fibrositis)

Adhesive capsulitis is an inflammatory disorder of the capsule of the scapulohumeral joint, often with involvement of other periarticular soft tissues, associated with pain and disability of the shoulder. Duplay described this condition first in 1872 as scapulohumeral periarthritis,[24] but over the many years it has acquired a bewildering number of synonyms. Although each of the intrinsic lesions, especially bicipital tenosynovitis, may produce a frozen shoulder, capsulitis is most prone to proceed to a relentless, disabling, chronic course.[10,13,14,18,86,105]

Frequency

Women, especially housewives, are affected by this disorder twice as often as men. It is seen in people over forty years, most commonly in the sixth decade, rarely before the menopause. In men, it occurs most frequently in the sixth and seventh decades, in elderly sedentary workers, rather than those in strenuous occupations.[42,86,105,148]

Etiology

As in all intrinsic shoulder disorders, some correlation with an injury, too trivial or vague to seem significant, is likely to be offered. A history of definite trauma, including contusions, sprains, possible injury to the shoulder-cuff and fractures requiring immobilization or casts, is given in 12 to 15 per cent of the cases. In a great proportion of the patients no specific cause is demonstrable. Calcific tendinitis, bicipital tenosynovitis in acute or chronic form, as well as lesions and disorders of the musculotendinous cuff, may precede the evolution of a full-blown frozen shoulder. Longstanding focal pain at the shoulder, visceral referred pain and reflex phenomena in myocardial infarction and chronic pulmonary disease, thyrotoxicosis, and cervical radicular pain radiating to the shoulder area, immobilization for fractures, even prolonged "inactivity" in some bedridden individuals, may be followed by, or associated with, shoulder disability resembling adhesive capsulitis.[36,44,74,122,125,140a,156]

The occurrence of the disorder during such illnesses emphasizes the probable importance of "inactivity" or "disuse" brought about by immobilization or by the muscle spasm of painful disability which, when prolonged, asserts some deleterious influence, as yet not clear, in shoulders already the site of pathologic alterations. The suggestive contribution of the disturbed physiology of reflex neurovascular imbalance arising in visceral disease, and of muscle spasm in anxiety and depression, has been noted recently.[31,95,134,149]

Pathogenesis

Adhesive capsulitis, from tissue studies and exploratory examination, has been reported by different observers (McLaughlin, Neviaser, Simmonds) to arise from the joint lining itself in a primary form, or spreading to it secondarily from any of the constituents of the extra-articular joint structures.[10,86,105,121,138] The predisposing role of "aging" and subclinical alterations, as in other intrinsic disorders (p. 1465), is noted in these observations. Similar demonstrations by radiopaque visualization, confirmed by open surgery, have been described.[66,90]

Symptomatology and Course[2,13,18,95,135,167]

The onset of capsulitis may be *acute* or *subacute*, usually following some real or fancied trauma or strain. *A period of gradually increasing soreness* of the shoulder, during abduction and internal rotation especially, building up to a peak of *constant pain*, *disability* and *disturbed sleep*, is characteristic of the history. The pain may be at the upper humerus, radiating along the arm to the forearm, sometimes posteriorly to the scapular area, at times with neuralgic distribution to the hands and fingers. Stiffness accompanies the pain and increases with it. Slight to complete disability may be presented in some or all ranges of motion. *Scapulohumeral fixation* soon is noticeable. The arm is kept adducted, supported or favored by the patient. *Point tenderness to palpation*, single or multiple, during early phases may be found in the subacromial, bicipital and other areas about the shoulder.

The duration of pain varies among the patients seeking medical care. It may last weeks or months, when a natural termination often occurs. It is not unusual for a patient to present herself for persistent disability, after the pain has receded or terminated spontaneously. The disability continues for some time afterwards, even in the most favorable situations. Pain may continue to be provoked only during certain movements, especially abduction and internal rotation, and sleep is disturbed when the patient turns on the shoulder or rests on it. A chronic, moderately uncomfortable or, in due time, entirely painless disability may persist during a long chronic stage.

No diagnostic x-ray changes occur at any time, except demineralization after the first two to three months, at the head and upper portion of the humerus, increasing with continued limitation of motion. Atrophy of the biceps and the muscles of the shoulder girdle gradually occurs in prolonged disability, if some function is not maintained. The duration of the chronic disability is unpredictable in individual cases, persisting in the majority for months to two years. Careful follow-up observations have shown that in over 30 per cent of cases the disability lasts longer than two years, and in about 8 to 10 per cent over four years, probably with irreversible changes in most of the latter group.[95] The occurrence of more prolonged disability has been reported by De Palma, observed in some individuals for four to eight years.[18]

Treatment of Adhesive Capsulitis

Acute symptoms are managed expectantly with a *selective conservative program* (Table 80–2), particularly in early cases presenting a short history of active symptoms, and only limited impairment of motion. Early capsulitis may respond satisfactorily to conservative measures, including well-regulated exercises. This phase, generally the first two to three months of symptoms, also provides the best results obtained with nearly all therapeutic measures said to be useful. As in tendinitis and bursitis, when conservative methods already have been used without sufficient benefit, *special additional procedures* are indicated. Unlike acute calcareous tendinitis and bursitis, however, once the diagnosis is made *in adhesive capsulitis, a chronic course with prolonged disability is more likely*, unless effective therapeutic approaches are introduced at once.

Psychological aids may be especially important in the treatment program in capsulitis. The nature and chronicity, but ultimately favorable outlook, in the average case must be explained. In the chronic stage, especially after a number of ineffective forms of treatment, a sympathetic, encouraging atmosphere is important to bolster the patient's morale. A receptive attitude and conscientious adherence to the program, chiefly the exercise routine, must be stressed. Emotional disturbances should receive attention.

Special Measures

There is so much difference of opinion about special forms of treatment, unfortunately even on the same methods, that adhesive capsulitis is one of the most *controversial* therapeutic outposts of rheumatology. It therefore has been stated that "most patients recover within twelve to eighteen months, with or without treatment."[42] There are available, nevertheless, some informative, controlled as well as conventional, observations demonstrating the value of special measures in relieving pain and accelerating recovery of function. There is a possibility of spontaneous resolution at some time or other, unpredictable in individual cases, as in all of the intrinsic lesions of the shoulder. The significance of the symptoms to the patient in terms of uncomfortable living and activity and the extent of handicap at work or other functions, must be weighed and discussed before initiating special procedures, particularly surgery.

Special Measures in Capsulitis

When response to a conservative program is unsatisfactory, the following special measures are employed.

X-ray therapy is less frequently effective than in acute calcareous tendinitis, but worth a trial if other measures are contraindicated.

Systemic corticosteroids are prescribed as in acute calcareous bursitis. In 40 to 60 per cent of patients oral corticotherapy alone has been observed to give satisfactory results.[29,137] No definite information is available for the acute phase alone. The systemic administration of corticosteroids and their injection locally[7] have been found to reduce the need for manipulation, one of the surgical procedures used in this condition, to be discussed later.

Needling and local injections of procaine solution are useless, if discrete tender points are not palpable, as often happens.

Local injection of hydrocortisone, or equivalent corticosteroid suspension, has been applied in conventional and controlled studies.[124,133] Direct infiltration of this material at the strategic points of involvement, as employed by Crisp and Kendall,[15] has given the author the best and quickest results in a confirmatory series of 42 "idiopathic," "frozen" shoulders, in a 1 to 5 year follow-up.[149a] At each session we alternately injected two of the three sites utilized by them—"anteriorly into the subacromial area, anterolaterally at the tendon of the long head of the biceps and posteriorly into the joint capsule."[15] At each we introduced depot triamcinolone, 20 mg. (with 1 to 3 ml. of lidocaine), repeated 1 to 3 times every 3 to 4 days to control pain, then weekly or longer. Six to 10 sessions restored 75 per cent or more mobility in over 85 per cent of the series.[149a] Shoulder exercises were started when pain was controlled.

Surgery

Closed manipulation of the affected extremity under general (sodium pentobarbital or gas) anesthesia formerly was the method of choice for surgical treatment. It has been the subject of vigorous condemnation by some of the most eminent orthopedists, for the damage observed by them in studies during open manipulation, and the tendency of the disability to recur afterwards.[17,18,38,86,97] Its proponents insist that modifications have made it a more dependable method of treatment. When the manipulation was done in 2 or 3 stages, during ten days of hospitalization, with intensive physical therapy, and a return later for one to three days for the final maneuver, few failures were seen, even after long follow-up.[51] Manipulation, it is agreed by all, if it is to be done, should be carried out only in the "cold," chronic stage, in patients otherwise fit for the procedure.

Manipulation with simultaneous injection of hydrocortisone suspension, 100 mg. into the scapulohumeral joint and at the lower portion of its capsule immediately after the manipulation, has been reported to yield superior results.[121] In controlled studies, similar injections to the scapulohumeral joint simultaneously with manipulations gave results superior to those with concomitant lignocaine injection, manipulation alone, or only conservative measures including physical therapy.[80,100]

Open surgery is done for adhesive capsulitis when bicipital tenosynovitis is suspected to be the predominant lesion.[18,78]

Acromionectomy has been successfully employed.[89]

BICIPITAL TENOSYNOVITIS

This condition is an inflammatory disorder of the synovial sheath of the tendon of the long head of the biceps muscle, and of the peritendinous connective tissue, often with erosion and inflammation of the tendon as well as extensive adhesions. This process frequently leads to, or is associated with, similar involvement of other periarticular structures. The role of predisposing pathologic changes of the bicipital tendon (p. 1465) was suggested by the observations of Meyer[88] at necropsies, later by Olsson and De Palma, but it first was recognized and described as a clinically significant disorder by Pasteur.[112]

Frequency

Bicipital tendinitis is a common source of shoulder disability, more often affecting women. Its importance as a special entity has been one of the late developments in our understanding of the intrinsic disorders of the shoulder. It is regarded by De Palma as the most frequent cause of pain and disability at the shoulder.[17,18,19] Its importance as a distinctive condition has been confirmed by Lippmann.[78]

Etiology and Pathogenesis[19,44,78,97]

As in the other intrinsic disorders of the shoulder, clinical observations and studies of local tissue pathology indicate that the provocation may arise from, or is attributed to, minor strain, exposure to temperature changes and dampness, direct or violent trauma with partial rupture, or dislocation of the tendon. Whether the local inflammation of the tendon sheath is from systemic disease, or "idiopathic" inflammation starting in the tendovaginal tissues, the inflammatory or "irritative" process produces a serofibrinous exudate. When progressive, it involves the tendon, synovium and surrounding tissues, ultimately with fibrinous deposition, fibrous and adhesive changes binding the tendon and sheath to each other and to the floor of the sulcus.[18] The process may be localized at the start, but usually is part of extensive periarticular involvement of neighboring structures as well.

A traumatizing anatomic abnormality sometimes accounts for the start of the lesion in the bicipital tendon, such as a roughening or excrescence on the floor of the bicipital groove.[53,88] The latter may become irregular following a fracture. The sulcus may be abnormally shallow, or its walls may slope too widely, predisposing the tendon to traumatizing recurrent dislocation or excessive functional stress.

Symptomatology[18,19,97,152]

Disturbances of the bicipital tendon and their symptoms vary in severity.

Acute pain and disability at the shoulder may appear suddenly after a trivial exposure, strain or injury, or without any apparent provocation. Often the symptoms build up insidiously. The *pain* radiates along the biceps and to the forearm. It may be especially disturbing at night when the patient rests on the shoulder during sleep. *Disability*, chiefly in abduction and internal rotation, varies with the pain, but may be felt from the start. *Tenderness* and pain are provoked by palpation at the anterior area of the humeral head *over the bicipital groove, increased by rolling the bicipital tendon under the fingertips*. In mild cases, the tendon on the normal side first is palpated as a basis of comparison. *Yergason's sign* is positive in acute cases, but in only about 50 per cent of those with mild or chronic symptoms. This test is performed with the patient seated. With the elbow held against the side by one hand of the examiner, the forearm and hand to be tested are supinated against the resistance of the examiner's other hand clasping the patient's.

Subacute symptoms then develop or frequently arise gradually as a milder version of the acute phase.

The *chronic stage* usually consists of moderate to great disability with little or no pain. Discomfort wanes or disappears over a period of weeks or months, leaving many of these patients with relatively painless disability as the chief complaint. Atrophy of the biceps and of the muscles of the shoulder girdle develops with prolonged limitation of function. The clinical picture then becomes indistinguishable from adhesive capsulitis, except for the persistent, palpable *tenderness at the bicipital tendon*, possibly with a positive Yergason's sign. Natural resolution may take place in many individuals over a period of six to twenty-four months, or longer,[18] as in adhesive capsulitis (p. 1475).

Treatment of Bicipital Tenosynovitis

At all stages *the basic program* should be given an adequate trial. *Special measures*, when needed, are introduced along the lines discussed in adhesive capsulitis and calcareous tendinitis, with the considerations peculiar to this condition.

Systemic corticosteroids are indicated especially during the acute stage. In severe or stubborn cases they may be combined with local injections at the bicipital tendon. The local approach is so simple that, for the practitioner willing to do so, it probably is sounder to apply it before using systemic corticotherapy.

Local injections of hydrocortisone suspension or equivalents, 50 mg. in 5 to 10 ml. of 1 per cent procaine solution (mixed in the same syringe), are given through a procaine wheal in the skin over the maximum tender point, at the bicipital tendon, and distributed along it, fanwise, at intervals of three to seven days or longer.[63a,148] Procaine solution, 5 to 15 ml. of 1 per cent solution, may produce nearly the same results.[148,152] Physical therapy, particularly graded exercises, is introduced at once.

Surgery

Manipulation is employed by some orthopedists in the chronic stage. Others have observed that frozen shoulders usually are released in manipulation only by internal tears, chiefly rupture of the bicipital tendon, with later recurrence of disability; therefore they oppose the procedure.[18,86,97]

Exploratory surgery of the shoulder has been found to yield good results, by transplantation of the tendon to the coracoid process or to the floor of the bicipital groove.[18,53,78]

MUSCULOTENDINOUS CUFF LESIONS

The great mobility of the shoulder and the versatility of the upper extremity expose its periarticular soft tissues to a variety of violent and minor traumata, as well as the alterations of attrition, and of "aging" tissues in the cumulative "wear and tear" of normal activities at a vulnerable location.[13,88] The tendons of the shoulder, the rotators in their conjoining connective tissue webbing as the musculotendinous cuff, get the brunt of these reactions.[13] It is doubtful, from observations that have accumulated, that the usual injuries can damage a normal rotator cuff.[97] The weight of evidence indicates that tears as well as calcific deposits occur only in a tendon already diseased.[13,86] Postmortem and exploratory studies have revealed that function is compatible with massive avulsion of the cuff, provided the balance between the deltoid muscle and the remaining intact portion of the rotator cuff is not seriously impaired.[17,19]

Changes produced by gross violence, lesser trauma or "use destruction" may provide the nidus of further tendinous degeneration, necrosis, and inflammation which spread to produce intrinsic, active disease.[13,88,139] Before and while such extension occurs, symptoms of injury or involvement of constituents of the shoulder cuff produce the clinical picture of musculotendinous lesions. Minor injuries, "strains" or jarring may cause little or no demonstrable new damage, yet may serve in some cases to stir up long resident subclinical lesions in the musculotendinous cuff.[97]

Rupture of the Supraspinatus and Other Tendons.[13,44,88,97]—Injuries of the constituents of the musculotendinous cuff are its most common lesions. The supraspinatus tendon is most frequently ruptured. Rupture of this tendon is brought about by a sudden strain in abduction, by a blow on the shoulder or a fall on it, usually in middle-aged or elderly males doing strenuous work. Codman regarded complete rupture of the supraspinatus tendon as the most common form of industrial accident to the shoulder, and incomplete ruptures as the basis of the majority of minor shoulder disabilities. Partial tears are more frequent.

A complete rupture of the supraspinatus, the most severe effect of trauma, consists of a tear across all of the fibers of its tendon, and includes the floor of the bursa lying over it, as well as the roof of the joint capsule on its under surface. It may arise spontaneously after a long history of shoulder symptoms, or suddenly after heavy lifting.

The chief clinical features of a ruptured supraspinatus tendon include a history of injury (usually a fall), often a "snap" is felt, local discoloration, sudden pain, apt to be followed by a pain-free interval of hours, then a recurrence of severe pain and disability, inability to raise the arm, tenderness over the greater tuberosity (shoulder tip), a sulcus at the point of tear, soft crepitation to palpation as the tuberosity slides under the acromion when the extremity is elevated, faulty scapulohumeral rhythm and negative x-ray findings. Pain is typically severe. Occasionally, however, patients with already pathological tendons feel little or no pain after the episode and the impaired abduction brings to their attention the extent of the injury that has occurred.[13,44,97] In any case the patient is *unable to initiate abduction* in elevating the extremity. With help, it comes up with faulty scapulohumeral rhythm and a painful arc of motion between about 70 to 110 degrees as the lesion impinges on the acromion. The arm can be lowered smoothly and without pain to a right angle or a little more, but then it falls to the side. During this sudden motion pain again is felt at the point of rupture. As a probable diagnostic aid in doubtful cases of supraspinatus rupture, injection of 1 per cent procaine solution at the site of suspected rupture permits abduction of the arm, but it cannot be maintained against resistance, when the extremity is dropped in the presence of a rupture.[97]

Minor or partial tears produce pain, stiffness and disability in which the severity and duration are proportionate to the damage.

Acute and *subacute* symptoms usually follow trauma. These vary from minor, transient pain or uncomfortable mobility, to the moderate or severe pain indicative of real, new damage.

Chronic symptoms of intermittent or steady "awareness" of soreness at the shoulder, discomfort or pain with or without stiffness or impaired mobility during certain movements or in turning over at night, of varying severity, may continue at the same bearable level for years or become troublesome following a more active acute or subacute incident. The appearance, and certainly the progression, of stiffness and disability are indicative of extending pathology and may be forerunners of a frozen shoulder.

Treatment of Musculotendinous Lesions

Severe tear or complete rupture of the supraspinatus tendon requires surgical evaluation and treatment. *Rupture of the biceps tendon*, sometimes encountered in elderly individuals, is treated conservatively.[13,97] *Other disorders* of the musculotendinous cuff, with or without a history of trauma during the acute phase, usually are controlled by a program of *conservative measures*, sufficient to relieve pain and to overcome disability, or to prevent it. *When symptoms persist* and include localized tenderness, the *special measures* employed for adhesive capsulitis may be applied.

FIBROMYOPATHIES AND MYALGIAS OF THE SHOULDER

A number of less well-defined shoulder disorders have come to be regarded as forms of non-articular soft tissue lesions, or disturbances — "fibromyopathies," "myopathies," "myalgias" or localized "fibrositis."[37,89,163] Some of these will be briefly considered.

Localized muscular pain and stiffness at the shoulder, *with or without disability*, may be transient phenomena, or may persist as part of a disseminated disorder, such as the fibrositis syndrome (*see* Chapter 49). They also may accompany or follow a variety of seasonal or systemic conditions, infectional (including viral), hematogenous, rheumatic, allergic and any of the generalized diseases with musculoskeletal features. Painful disorders of the shoulder may predominate in some extensive disturbances not clearly understood, such as vasomotor imbalance ("hypersympatheticotonia"), metabolic, toxic and psychomotor states. Neurologic disorders, such as the muscular dystrophies, may produce localized pain and disability of the shoulder before more widespread features are recognizable.

External Environmental Factors.—Cold, damp, temperature changes, air currents, especially when the shoulder is unduly exposed, may be the source of temporary or prolonged pain, stiffness, and even disability. *The internal environment*, e.g. emotional tension states, may cause shoulder pain.

Traumatic myalgia, myopathy or fibromyalgia, due to trauma with known or unnoticed injury, such as contusions, sprains, ruptures of muscle tissue, fascia or sheath, or organized hemorrhage involving these tissues, may produce pain, stiffness and disability at the shoulder.

Tender points and "*trigger points*" frequently are described at the shoulder region as well as elsewhere. By definition, a trigger point is a spot in a muscle which, when palpated, (1) reproduces the patient's pain and its radiation, (2) reproduces these characteristics when penetrated with a needle, (3) loses this reactivity when infiltrated with 1 to 5 ml. of procaine solution, (4) leaving the patient free of the previous tenderness to palpation, pain and sometimes the disability during motion of the part.[149b]

The delineation of various muscular and myofascial syndromes exhibiting a typical reaction-pattern, pain distribution and other features, with a trigger point as the cardinal sign, resulting from a variety of predisposing and precipitating factors, has been the subject of a number of interesting reports, especially by Travell and co-workers. The effective use of local freezing sprays and procaine injections to trigger points for the relief of these conditions has been described by her and others.[37,47,69,157,158]

Local infiltration of circumscribed tenderness in supportive tissues with procaine and other analgesic substances has a background of application for several decades.[4,20,145] Experimental observations, as well as clinical application, have appeared to provide a rational basis.[65] Controlled studies are not available to provide more exact pharmacologic and clinical appraisal of the contribution of these widely used procedures.[117] More recently, the infiltration of corticosteroid suspension is replacing procaine or is combined with it.[89]

Conservative treatment consists of *analgesics*, weight control, *correction of deficiencies*, possibly a *sedative* or relaxant. *Exposure* to provocative environmental factors, physical and emotional, must be *minimized or eliminated*. *Mechanical, postural*, habitual or occupational *strain is removed or corrected*, as far as is practical. *Heat* is a helpful adjunct. *Psychologic aids* are important in tension states.

When circumscribed tenderness to palpation is present in acutely painful trauma or at a stubborn or chronic site of pain, relief often is hastened or initiated by local injection of the tender spot with procaine solution, 1 to 5 ml., or a corticosteroid in suspension, 15 to 25 mg., or both in combination, depending on the point to be infiltrated or the extent of diffusion desired. If improvement occurs for one to two days, the procedure may be repeated once or twice a week, provided increasing intervals of response follow. When a *somatization of hysteria*, severe anxiety state or other emotional conflict, is suspected in the myalgias, especially in younger individuals, a *psychiatric evaluation* should precede any repeated or intensive course of treatment.

The scapulocostal syndrome is a term originated by Michele and his co-workers to designate the "postural drag paradox" which he believes characterizes "the pain-pattern distributions in about 50 per cent of all middle-aged individuals presenting shoulder symptoms on a traumatic or non-traumatic basis," frequently due to postural, habitual and occupational strain.

The condition presents a gradual, insidious onset, with deep shoulder pain as the first symptom. The pain may be associated with a number of patterns of radiation. Accompanying the pain, the

Table 80-3.—Summary of the Intrinsic, Painful Shoulder Syndromes

The Intrinsic Syndromes.—Calcareous tendinitis and bursitis, adhesive capsulitis, bicipital tenosynovitis and musculotendinous cuff lesions, (with calcareous tendinitis, the occurrence of bursitis is common, sometimes in the other disorders).

Synonyms.—Subacromial and subdeltoid bursitis, periarthritis, frozen shoulder, adhesive bursitis.

Pathogenesis.—Predisposing pathologic changes usually are combined with precipitating factors.

Predisposing Pathology.—"Wear and tear" of deteriorating aging tissue, minute or severe past trauma to tendons or musculotendinous cuff, circumscribed tendon necrosis, surrounding latent inflammation, extensive low-grade, silent or intermittently active inflammation of tendons, sheaths, bursa, capsule.

Precipitating Factors.—Definite trauma or strain, cumulative minor occupational or habitual stress, overexertion, fatigue, depletion states, severe illness, disuse after fractures or violent trauma, organic conditions with referred pain or reflex neurovascular disturbances, such as cervical discogenic disease, thoracic visceral disease, or even emotional crises, sometimes no demonstrable precipitating factor.

Stages and Course.—Acute (or hyperacute), subacute and chronic.

Acute symptoms are apt to resolve spontaneously in 70 to 85 per cent of patients with calcareous tendinitis, if symptoms are tolerable and their quicker relief not requested, less frequently in bicipital tendinitis and capsulitis. With conservative treatment, pain is relieved in days or weeks, disability taking somewhat longer, unless a subacute or chronic course develops.

Subacute symptoms are less severe than the acute, but prolonged for two to three months, not usually encountered in calcific tendinitis, but in adhesive capsulitis, bicipital tenosynovitis and lesions of the musculotendinous cuff.

Chronic symptoms are most characteristic of adhesive capsulitis and bicipital tenosynovitis often build up insidiously, may follow acute or subacute phases of all, pain varies, but disability leads to muscle atrophy. Capsulitis may be primary, or secondary to chronic calcific tendinitis, bicipital tenosynovitis and inflammation of the shoulder cuff; spontaneous recovery may occur in months to two years, but in 10 per cent the course is more prolonged.

most important diagnostic sign is the trigger point to palpation located at or under the upper medial angle of the scapula at the posterior thoracic wall, resembling the features of local disorders reported also by others.

The pain is described by Michele as presenting a number of characteristic patterns delineated by him: (1) along the neck upward to the occiput and the side of the head, (2) along the posterior area of the arm downward, often to the forearm, wrist and hand, (3) about the chest, chiefly along the distribution of the 4th and 5th intercostal nerves, and (4) combinations of these patterns.

The scapulocostal syndrome has been the subject of confirmatory and dissenting observations by others.[72,89,131]

Treatment recommended by Michele consists chiefly of an organized program of the measures stated in the management of myalgias, with emphasis on physical therapy, especially massage, postural and special exercises for the shoulders, and the use of ethyl chloride spray or injection of procaine or hydrocortisone suspension at the characteristic "trigger point."[89] He has noted that firm, sustained digital pressure over the "trigger-point or tension tenderness" often is followed by "immediate mitigation of acute symptomatology."

EXTRINSIC CAUSES OF PAINFUL SHOULDER

Many diseases and disorders in nearby or distant structures (Table 80–1) may refer symptoms to the shoulder, or serve as a source of secondary disorder there. The diagnostic possibilities thereby presented must guide efforts to arrive at the causes of atypical or persistent shoulder complaints. Nearly all of these extraneous causes are uncommon or rare, but may pose problems of interpretation and recognition.

The cervical spine by neural irritation, foraminal encroachment or discogenic compression, is the most frequent extraneous source of shoulder pain and disability.[50,57] Vascular abnormalities, brain tumors and peripheral nerve lesions occasionally may be responsible.[155] Psychogenic disturbances frequently provoke pain and muscle spasm at the neck and shoulder.[31,83]

Viscerogenic pain at the shoulder is particularly important in diagnosis. The associated or reflexly painful, stiff shoulder, resembling or regarded as adhesive capsulitis, and reflex neurovascular phenomena, notably the shoulder-hand syndrome, are generally known complications of visceral disease of the chest, central nervous system and the upper abdominal viscera and diaphragm.[5,95,135,149] *Pain in the deltoid area usually reflects intrinsic disease of the shoulder, rarely is viscerogenic.* Pains at the shoulder region without such specific local manifestations frequently have a viscerogenic origin.[12] The role of pulmonary, cardiovascular, intraabdominal, and even genitourinary disease in producing referred shoulder pain has been repeatedly observed.[12,75,96,139]

Visceral pain is referred to the shoulder at fairly typical locations through the cervicothoracic outflow of sympathetic innervation, or the brachial plexus at the superior thoracic outlet or the phrenic nerves. The long route of the phrenic nerve through the thoracic outlet along the pericardium and entire length of the mediastinum provides many locations for disease to produce afferent pain stimuli. The inferior and superior surfaces of the diaphragm, innervated by the phrenic, give ample sources of morbidity appearing as shoulder pain.[75,96]

Location of referred pain has been found rather characteristically *at the trapezius ridge* for *intrathoracic*, *intraabdominal*, or *pericardial disease*, but most frequently is reported there after *pulmonary infarction* (Fig. 80–6).

The pain of *myocardial ischemia* usually is referred to the *left pectoral region* and the *ulnar surface of the left arm. When shoulder pain is a prominent symptom in myocardial infarction, simultaneous anterior chest pain* is apt to be acknowledged or described.

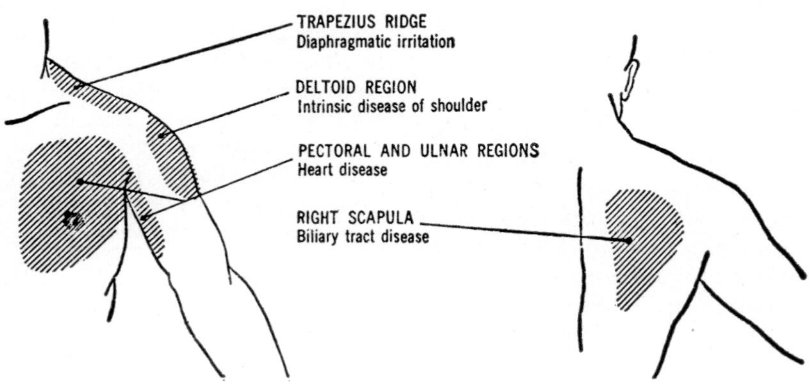

Fig. 80–6.—Sites of reference about the shoulder in viscerogenic pain. (Morgan, courtesy of Modern Medicine.)

Pain from disease of the *ascending arch of the aorta* generally is felt at the *right side of the neck and shoulder.* Pain arising at the *transverse or descending portions of the aortic arch* is transmitted to the *left side of the back and shoulder.*

Pain emanating from *diffuse esophageal spasm* may be experienced *in the arms. Hiatal hernia* may simulate cardiac pain by extension to the *infraclavicular area* and the *inner arm*, or it may be described at the *ridge of the trapezius.*

A *perforated viscus* often produces *pain felt at one or both shoulders.* Pain of the *same character* may be encountered *when air is left in the peritoneum after laparotomy.*

Shoulder pain of biliary origin is reflected, as a rule, *at the right side. Irritation of right phrenic afferent components* distributed *in the coronary and falciform ligaments, the gallbladder, the hepatic capsule and the liver itself* may cause *pain at the right trapezius ridge. Pain at the shoulder* may indicate *irritation of the diaphragm by a liver abscess. Stimulation of visceral afferent fibers* in the major splanchnic nerves with central communications in the sixth through ninth thoracic segments produces *right scapular pain, associated usually with deep epigastric* discomfort.[96]

In pancreatic disease pain in the shoulder generally represents a secondary extension of abdominal pain.

Other occasional viscerogenic sources of shoulder pain are ectopic pregnancy with intraperitoneal hemorrhage and metastatic disease of the head of the humerus from carcinoma of the renal cortex.[96]

Management of viscerogenic pain obviously must be directed *first* to the *treatment of the underlying visceral disease.* Sometimes, when such pathology presents no urgent problem, and the referred symptoms are annoying, basic and local measures discussed for myalgia may be utilized for added palliation, while the visceral condition is under treatment. Freezing sprays and procaine infiltration, in troublesome complaints with consistent local tenderness, have been found useful, particularly in myocardial ischemic and post-infarctional pain at the shoulder and anterior chest wall.[157,158]

Acute and chronic arthritis of the scapulohumeral joint occurs more often as part of generalized inflammatory or degenerative arthritis. Rarely, a monarthropathy, due to suppurative infection, tuberculosis or syphilis may produce such localized pathology. The same diagnostic and therapeutic considerations prevail as in the discussions elsewhere of these joint diseases.

Acromioclavicular separation may produce local symptoms. The lesion is detected by x-ray films taken with the arm in a position of abduction and another in adduction, while the patient is standing.[70]

Acromioclavicular arthritis is reflected in the x-ray features of rheumatoid involvement or, more likely, degenerative articular disease with narrowing of the joint space responsible for the symptoms. Swelling and tenderness of the joint are detectable clinically.

Conservative measures are employed, supplemented by local periarticular and intraarticular *injections* of procaine or corticosteroids, occasionally *surgery.*[97]

NEUROVASCULAR COMPRESSION SYNDROMES OF THE SHOULDER AREA AND UPPER EXTREMITY ("THORACIC OUTLET SYNDROME")

The neurovascular syndromes are among the most perplexing and difficult musculoskeletal disorders affecting the shoulder and upper extremity. *Pain, paresthesias, hyperesthesia* or *vasomotor disturbances* may occur in any of them, but these symptoms in combination are characteristic of few, chiefly the neurovascular syndromes.[40]

Anatomy

The anatomy is complex, so only its main features will be mentioned here. The normal components of this area include the first rib, the scalene muscles (anterior, medial, occasionally inferior),

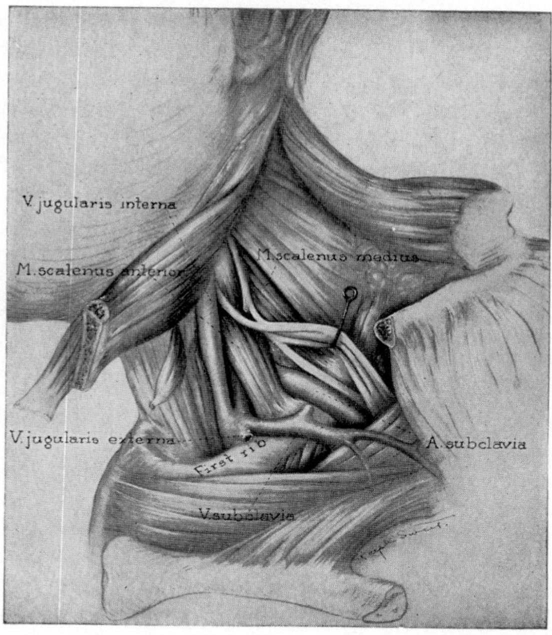

FIG. 80–7.—Dissection of the neck to show the arrangement of the brachial plexus, subclavian artery and the scalenus anticus muscle. (Naffziger and Grant, courtesy of Surg., Gynec. & Obst.)

the clavicle and subclavius muscle, the coracoid process and pectoralis minor muscle. Added to these, at times, may be encountered bony deformities of the first rib and the clavicle, superimposed cervical ribs, gross deformities due to kyphoscoliosis, thoracoplasty or injury, bizarre insertions of the scalene muscles and assorted congenital fibrous bands, vascular anomalies, lymph node enlargements, tumors, etc. The key to the whole problem consists of the size and adaptability of the thoroughfare, the "thoracic outlet" and the contiguous space, through which the neurovascular bundle must pass in close relationship to the anatomic constituents already mentioned. In the vast majority of people this short distance is traversed without difficulty, even in the presence of anomalous structures. In some, however, the bundle is impinged upon, in one way or another, to produce the symptoms characterizing the syndromes under discussion.[81]

Normally, the subclavian artery hooks up and over the first rib, lying between the insertions of the scalenus anterior and medius muscles, passes down under the coracoid process and then into the axilla. The subclavian vein runs a parallel route, except that it proceeds between the scalenus anterior and the clavicle. The brachial plexus in this region tends to course along the artery and is represented primarily by fibers from C8–T1. *The prominent points of compression* have given their names to the syndromes they provoke.

Contributory or Provocative Factors[103,108,154]

Contributory, predisposing factors in all of these syndromes include the great mobility of the shoulder which, even in normal structures, permits compression of the neurovascular bundle in certain positions. Anatomic anomalies are important in predisposing some individuals to compressive symptoms. As people age there is a tendency toward a reduction in muscle mass and a loss of tone with a drooping of the shoulders. Strain from postural defects, disturbed body mechanics or associated, degenerative cervical spinal changes frequently must be reckoned with. Generally, these are responsible for symptoms only when there is superimposed some precipitating trauma or the strain from prolonged maintenance of bizarre positions, as in work, sleep, etc. Arteriosclerosis with loss of pliability often is a factor predisposing to vascular complications from compression in the older age groups.[27,28]

THE CERVICAL RIB, SCALENUS ANTICUS AND FIRST RIB SYNDROME

Historically, the first of these to be described was the cervical rib syndrome.[101,164] Cervical ribs occur as anomalous appendages in approximately .05 per cent of individuals, with more than half being bilateral. They are two to three times more common in women. Usually they are incidental findings, with only some 10 per cent of them causing any difficulty. The size, shape and insertion of the rib will frequently be the determining factors in the production of symptoms. Most patients do not present symptoms until they reach the twenty to forty year age group. Often there is arterial compression, with poststenotic dilatation and incipient thrombosis.[27,102,136]

Cervical Rib

The approach to this problem, in the more severe cases, has been surgical removal of the rib, initiated by Coste in 1861. This procedure, although surgically sound, too often was attended by various complications which resulted in equally severe symptoms, sometimes worse. The scalenus muscles may or may not be important in the activation of symptoms.[35] Their participation, however, frequently cannot be determined with certainty preoperatively. Law in 1920,[159] and Adson and Coffey in 1947, nevertheless, suggested resection of the scalenus anticus muscle as an easier method of decompression. They found in an impressive series that simple tenotomy was quite effective.[1] Today, *scalenotomy* is performed, *with partial resection* of the rib, if necessary.

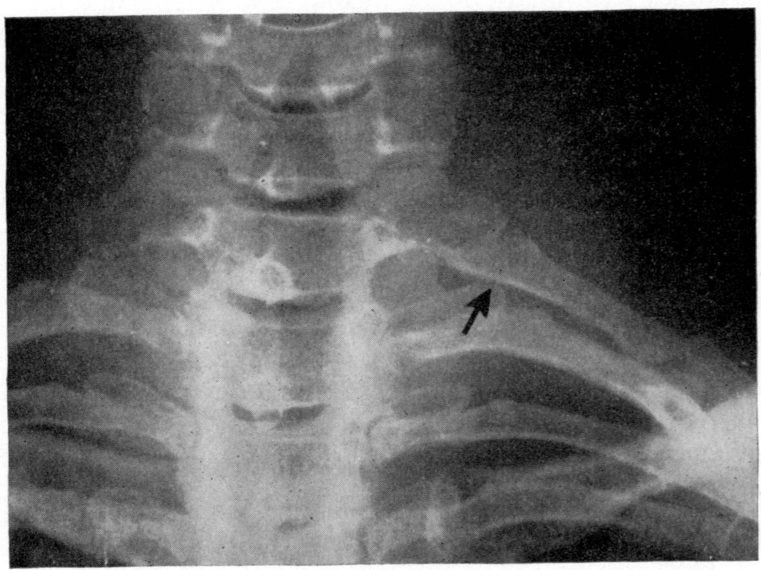

FIG. 80–8.—Cervical rib on left, associated with postural imbalance, which was asymptomatic.

Scalenus Anticus (and First Rib) Syndrome

This syndrome was suggested or implied by numerous workers during the past fifty years, who were impressed by the presence of the "cervical rib syndrome in the absence of cervical rib." Observers during the 1903–1917 period attributed these cases to stretching of the brachial plexus over the first rib due to drooping of the shoulder girdle from an increased lateral diameter of the chest with age. In 1933 Adson emphasized the possible responsibility of the scalenus anticus muscle. The "scalenus anticus syndrome" was given its present formulation in 1935 by Naffziger and Grant,[103] as well as Ochsner, Gage and De Bakey.[108] The basic concept is the deduction that, in the presence of a normal shoulder girdle, the scalenus anticus muscle compresses the neurovascular bundle against the first rib and a normal scalenus medius muscle through a process of spastic irritability and hypertrophy. This concept holds that the scalenus anticus is irritated in some fashion, so bringing about spasticity, whereby it compresses the brachial plexus. The compression reflexly increases the spasm of the scalenus anticus. These reactions are believed to produce a vicious circle. The corollary, in the thesis of the originators, is breaking the circle by sectioning the scalenus anticus muscle.

Symptoms of a scalenus anticus syndrome regarded as diagnostic consisted of pain extending from the neck to the hand, usually along the ulnar side, neuralgic in character, or pain over the deltoid down the arm and often greatest at the elbow; tiredness or weakness of the extremity; paresthesias or anesthesia, at times hyperesthesia, at the distribution of tenderness or pain; cramps of the fingers, vasomotor disturbances, coldness, numbness, or tingling of the hand and digits, discoloration of the hand and digits; symptoms worsened by work and exercise. Specific signs were considered to be evidence *of a tender scalenus anticus* at its lower third, the *dampening of the pulse* of the affected extremity by certain maneuvers (*Adson maneuver*: With the examiner's fingers on the pulse of the seated patient's hand held at the side, the subject takes a deep breath and holds it, then fully extends the neck, then turns the head toward the involved side; sometimes more effectively on the opposite side), and the *partial relief of symptoms by procaine injection of the anticus muscle.*[59,72a,103,108] Sometimes a bruit may be heard in the supraclavicular area.[28]

The general view today is that the scalenus anticus syndrome, as postulated in the 1930's, does not occur and that relief of symptoms by surgical tenotomy is secondary to simple decompression of the neurovascular bundle and elimination of secondary effects. This relief, according to present opinions, arises from the removal of one arm of a passive vise, or to the simpler fact that the patient receives, together with the surgery, a period of bed rest and change in usual habits.[24a,104,115] The more severe symptomatic failures, when restudied, often were found to have other mechanisms or sources of compression.

Costoclavicular Syndrome

In 1943, Falconer and Weddell described the costoclavicular syndrome.[33] In restudying 3 cases of scalenotomy failure, they found the principal site of compression located between the clavicle and the first rib. They were able to demonstrate that *backward and downward bracing of the shoulders, as in the exaggerated military posture*, would approximate the two bony structures and *compress the neurovascular elements*. That this mechanism could occur in a normal shoulder had been appreciated by earlier workers. It has been reaffirmed by others.[81,160,165] *The pulse can be dampened in some 60 per cent of people by an exaggerated military posture.*

This syndrome was common during the war, when heavy packs could not be worn by many young men owing to the severe pain, paresthesias, venous congestion and edema which would develop, due to direct costoclavicular compression. Interestingly, many of these young soldiers were able to sustain the packs following six to eight weeks of army life and training. In the absence of deformities or exogenous factors this is not a common syndrome. Walshe, however, cites repetitive costoclavicular compression as a frequent contributor to symptoms.[161]

Hyperabduction Syndrome

Wright described the mechanism of the hyperabduction syndrome in 1945.[165] In this group of patients with clearcut neurovascular symptoms, predominantly vascular, the principal points of compression were found to be under the coracoid process and between the clavicle and first rib. *The symptoms* were demon-

Table 80-4.—Neurovascular Syndromes of the Shoulder Girdle*
(Steinbrocker and Argyros, courtesy of Med. Clinics North America.[149])

	History	*Pulse*	*Neurologic Signs*	*Diagnostic Test*	*Therapeutic Response*
Costoclavicular Syndrome	Symptoms associated with shoulders forced downward for long periods	Reduced in abnormal shoulder position	None	Forced abnormal position of shoulder—reproduces signs and symptoms	Elimination of postural defects giving relief
Hyperabduction Syndrome (Costoclavicular Syndrome)	Hyperabduction in sleep or at work for long periods	Reduced in hyperabd. (also B. P. and oscillometry)	None	Hyperabduction—reproduction of signs and symptoms	Correction of sleeping or working position giving relief
Scalenus Anticus Syndrome and Cervical Rib	No special postural features	Reduced in resting position or brought on by Adson maneuver	Reflexes reduced or absent on affected side; noted weakness in same	Supraclav. bruit (?) Adson maneuver reproduces musculoskeletal, neuritic and vascular signs Tender point at scalenus anticus	Injection of procaine into ant. scalenus gives relief; scalenotomy effective
Shoulder-Hand Syndrome (Reflex Dystrophy)	Trauma, intrathoracic disease or idiopathic, no special postural features	Sometimes reduced	Increased or decreased reflexes of part; hyperesthesia	Stellate ganglion block produces transient or prolonged relief	Repeated blocks; effective in earlier stages Steroids(orally) also

* *Symptoms common* to some or all in each disorder; pain of shoulder, arm and/or hand; numbness, paresthesias of fingers; swelling of hand(s), fingers; discoloration of hand(s); Raynaud's phenomenon; weakness of hand(s).

strated to occur *by laterally circumducting the arms and clasping the hands over the head.* The neurovascular bundle becomes taut as it crosses the coracoid process and the head of the humerus. It is further compressed by the clavicle and the muscular action of the pectoralis minor. Some reduction of the pulse by this maneuver has been observed in 60 to 80 per cent of normal individuals. The original paper reported 8 patients in whom the principal factor was this persistent posture in sleep. Symptoms were relieved by a change in the habit. Most individuals affected have been found to maintain a hyperabducted position of the extremity in sleep or in certain occupations—ballet dancers, painters, grease-pit mechanics, and others. Subsequent observations also have shown the presence of Raynaud's phenomenon in about 50 per cent of the patients.[6] In some cases symptoms included superficial gangrene of the fingertips which healed readily.

Diagnosis in Compression Syndromes

Diagnostic evaluation requires a careful history and physical examination to investigate the characteristic points mentioned in each compression disorder. Inspection, palpation, auscultation at the neck for a bruit (in first rib-scalenus syndrome), for cervical ribs, long transverse processes, thoracic deformities, bulges or distortions in the supraclavicular area, evidence of vascular disturbance or disease, and the specific postural tests for compression; x-ray films of the cervical spine (with oblique views), and of the shoulder and hand, may be necessary, as well as special tests for bizarre compression arising from tumor, enlarged lymph nodes, etc.

Management of Compression Syndrome

For many years surgical intervention has been emphasized more than medical measures. The many incomplete results or failures have created a trend toward the *full and extensive utilization of conservative measures, with surgical procedures as the last resort.*[24a,104,115]

Conservative management begins with the elimination of *provocative, exogenous factors,* such as strain from pushing, pulling, lifting, carrying heavy objects, etc. Postural correction may help. When shoulder drooping is due to poor posture, age and related factors, muscle development may be indicated. *Exercises,* to develop weak muscles, are important when practical, with *physical therapy* in some form of heat. *Analgesics* may help resolve residual soreness of muscles. *Sedation* and *psychological aids* may prove useful, in some cases even *psychotherapy.* When *surgery* is performed, the current tendency is to do a thorough exploration in order to decompress the neurovascular canal adequately by combined procedures, where necessary—scalenotomy with clavicular removal; possibly resection of the first rib or of a cervical rib; or section of the pectoralis minor muscle in some severe cases of hyperabduction disorder.[10a,81,82]

THE SHOULDER-HAND SYNDROME AND REFLEX NEUROVASCULAR DYSTROPHY OF THE UPPER EXTREMITY

Reflex neurovascular dystrophy is a disorder of a limb due to some form of injury producing pain, reflex vasomotor reactions, disability, with peripheral swelling, tenderness and osteoporosis, usually at the hands or feet.[3,52,56,76,104,150] Other parts, the face, spine and different localities at the extremities occasionally may be involved. These conditions are of particular concern to internists and practitioners, because they so closely simulate arthritis or related conditions for which they usually are treated ineffectively.

At the upper extremity the most frequent and extensive manifestation in medical patients is the shoulder-hand syndrome.[5,129,149] Accumulating clinical evidence strongly suggests that this disorder belongs among the reflex dystrophies.[8,127,140] It is characterized by painful disability of the shoulder preceding, accompanying or following the involvement of the hand by stiffness, painful disability, vasomotor changes with swelling, or dystrophic (peculiar atrophic) alterations in the later phases.[146] Only the shoulder or hand or fingers may be affected in some circumscribed cases of a reflex dystrophy.

The shoulder-hand syndrome, in the great majority of cases seen in general practice or internal medicine,[18] is associated chiefly with medical lesions. These patients present more or less the same features which for generations surgeons especially have called Sudeck's atrophy, post-traumatic osteoporosis, reflex dystrophy or reflex sympathetic dystrophy, to mention only the more common terminology. Within the last few decades internists have reported disturbances of the upper extremity with similar clinical characteristics associated with internal lesions variously described as "a syndrome of painful disability of the shoulder and hand following coronary occlusion,"[3,26] "post-infarctional sclerodactylia,"[59] "the swollen, atrophic hand associated with osteoarthritis,"[110] vasomotor disturbances and edema in hemiplegia,[30] and others. It has become clear from these reports and recent studies that the shoulder-hand syndrome and other manifestations resembling reflex dystrophy may follow internal lesions with symptom patterns more or less similar to, and probably pathogenetically and clinically identical with, those produced by external trauma. These are clinical presumptions not yet entirely established.

The term "dystrophy," applied by de Takats, characterizes the peculiar nutritional and atrophic changes of the skin, underlying tissues and adjacent articulations, apparently induced by the prolonged neural and circulatory disturbances.[22]

The reflex neurovascular disorders are properly designated as "reflex"[32] because they usually are provoked by, or appear to be the aftermath of,[146] definite surgical, orthopedic, neurologic or medical conditions. However, in 15 to 30 per cent of the cases reported, no etiology is demonstrable.[129,149]

Frequency

The shoulder-hand syndrome affects both sexes almost equally, with women slightly predominant, except post-infarctional syndromes which are more frequent in men.[72,129,131] Few are engaged in strenuous occupations. Over 90 per cent of the patients are past fifty years of age.[129,149] The condition therefore is encountered following, or in association with, the etiologic factors frequent in the older age groups, particularly myocardial

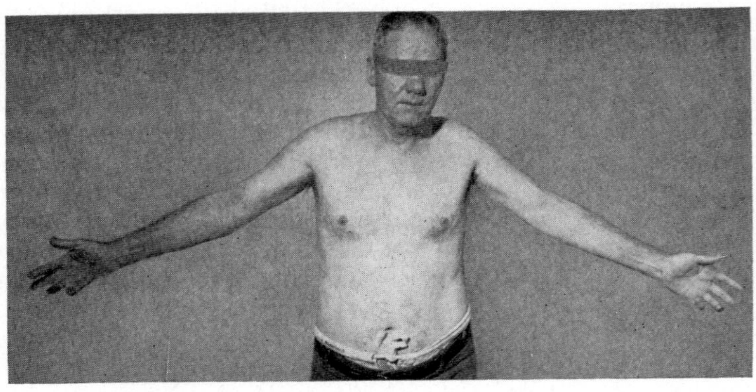

Fig. 80–9.—Shoulder-hand syndrome: Inability to abduct at shoulder joints, contracture of fingers.

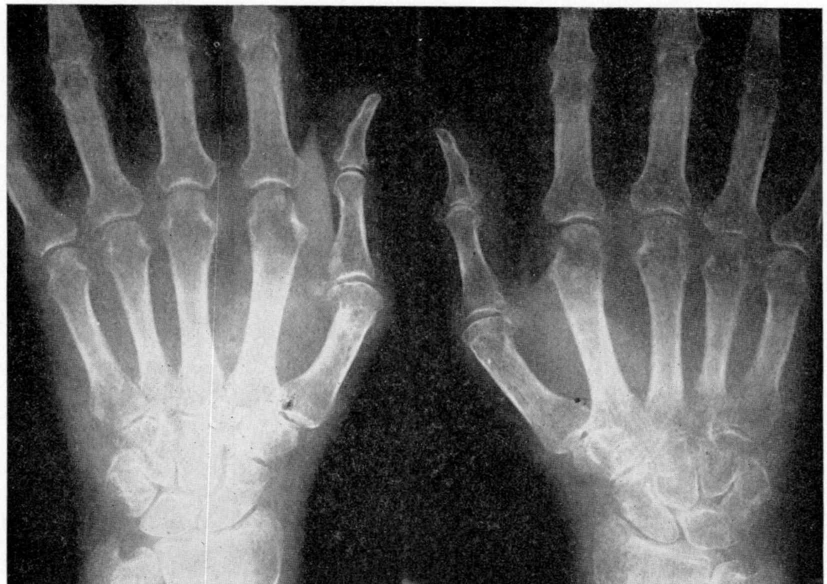

Fig. 80–10.—Shoulder-hand syndrome: x ray showing the marked osteoporosis in bones of right wrist and fingers.

infarction in medical cases.[3,26,59,63,64,30,151]

Symptomatology[5,23,129,147,149]

The *onset* of symptoms may consist of stiffness and discomfort, possibly weakness, for days or weeks, at the shoulder or hand, or it may arise as sudden pain and stiffness, followed shortly at the hand by swelling, vasomotor changes, hyperesthesia and disability. These symptoms may follow quickly after an external injury or in weeks or months after a myocardial infarction.

The clinical picture for convenience has been *divided* rather *roughly into three stages* (Table 80–5). Phases overlap in many patients. In the first stage, there is the full-blown shoulder and hand involvement, lasting three to six months. The second stage is characterized by partial or complete resolution of the swelling and vasomotor disorder (instability, vasospasm or vasodilatation), possibly with the appearance of early trophic changes and beginning contractures. This phase may continue from three to six months. In the third stage, the tenderness, vasomotor disturbance and swelling usually have resolved, but to a lesser or greater degree there are apt to be atrophic, or "dystrophic," alterations of the soft tissues of the fingers and hand, obliteration of the dorsal skin creases, with contractures of the fingers of varying extent, usually "frozen" in partial flexion, occasionally a "frozen" shoulder with some atrophy of the overlying muscle, and demineralization of the upper humerus. The final stage varies in duration, continuing in exceptional cases for years to produce irreversible changes and contractures. Rapid telescoping of all stages within a short time in severe progression occasionally may be encountered.

Characteristic radiographic changes generally occur throughout the clinical course, although sometimes they may not be discernible in the early stages—spotty demineralization early, a diffuse demineralization later, at the head of the humerus, at the carpus and often at the phalanges.

Table 80-5.—Clinical Evolution of the Shoulder-Hand Syndrome

Stage 1	*Stage 2*	*Stage 3*
Shoulder		
Pain	Pain and disability resolving or persisting	Residual pain infrequently
Disability in all ranges		
Tenderness, diffuse (localized early)	Possible atrophy of muscles	Disability sometimes
Osteoporosis, patchy at humeral head sometimes	Osteoporosis, patchy then ground-glass	Ground-glass, diffuse osteoporosis
Hand and Fingers		
Pain	Symptoms resolving or continuing with early dystrophic changes	Persistent pain, rarely
Tenderness, diffuse		Residual dystrophy and contractures
Cutaneous hyperesthesia		
Disability		
Massive dorsal swelling	Often induration of cutis and subcutis	
Digital Changes		
Dermal swelling, diffuse	Firm induration with obliteration of dorsal skin creases	Rarely increased
Sometimes early, shiny cutis and trophic changes as in next stage	Shiny, trophic skin surface	Dull, diffuse atrophy of skin and subcutis
	Trophic nail changes initiated sometimes	Marked occasionally
	Dorsal hypertrichosis sometimes	Increased sometimes
Incomplete, painful digital flexion	Resolving or impending digital atrophy and contractures	Residual contractures and distortions
Vasomotor Changes		
Vasodilatation or vasospasm	Vasospasm often with hyperhidrosis	Vasomotor imbalance occasionally
Color changes		Usually absent with dystrophic changes
Hyperhidrosis at palms		
Roentgenographic Changes		
Spotty osteoporosis of humeral head, wrist	More marked	Ground-glass diffuse osteoporosis of humeral head, wrist and fingers

The opposite shoulder or hand, or both, also may be affected in some 25 per cent of the patients. The whole clinical picture may undergo spontaneous resolution at any time, with or without residual changes or disability, such as contractures of the fingers. For so far unexplained reasons, the elbow generally escapes involvement.

Systemic signs do not occur, unless some complication is present. The blood count is not elevated. The sedimentation rate may be increased in over 20 per cent of the patients, usually by other assumed or demonstrable disturbances.[135,149]

Etiology

Reflex neurovascular disturbances of the upper extremity may be due to, or coincidental with, any of a variety of provocative or "benign" associated disorders or diseases, sometimes multiple, as listed in Table 80–6. Whether the simultaneous presence of some "pathologic" condition necessarily implies an activating relationship often cannot be definitely determined by present clinical methods.

Any neurally related visceral, musculoskeletal, neurologic or vascular pathology is a potential source of reflex neurovascular symptoms. Reflex disorders, particularly in their early phase, frequently are overlooked in the presence of more serious problems. Incipient reflex neurovascular reactions may resolve unnoticed. In some cases, however, even with serious causative disease, such as myocardial infarction, the reflex phenomena may so rapidly progress in severity and disability as to overshadow the underlying condition in diagnostic and therapeutic importance, at least from the patient's viewpoint.

Pathophysiology

The nature and mechanism of the shoulder-hand symptom complex, like all reflex neurovascular syndromes, are still obscure. In fact there is no clinching evidence that the shoulder-hand syndrome is necessarily a reflex neurovascular or sympathetic disorder, or dystrophy.

A number of theories have been originated in the past few decades, chiefly to account for the striking and painful, reflex neurovascular phenomena appear-

Table 80-6.—Shoulder-Hand Syndrome: Provocative or Associated Conditions (146 Cases*) (Steinbrocker and Argyros Courtesy of Med. Clinics North America[149])

		No.	*Per Cent*
Idiopathic		33	23
Postinfarctional		30	20
Cervical—discogenetic or intraforaminal spurring		29	20
Post-traumatic		15	10
Multiple, inconclusive		16	11
Posthemiplegic		9	6
Miscellaneous		14	10
Post-herpes zoster	3		
Calcific tendinitis of shoulder	2		
Pancoast-type tumor	3		
Diffuse vasculitis	2		
Brain tumor	2		
Febrile panniculitis	1		
Gonococcal arthritis	1		

* Includes 35 with circumscribed involvement.

ing in a small percentage of individuals suffering battle wounds (causalgia) and injuries of extremities (Sudeck's atrophy, post-traumatic osteoporosis).[8,23,52,76,92,100,107]

The most widely accepted explanation is the theory of the "internuncial pool," derived from experimental observations by Lorente de No,[84] elaborated and applied clinically to causalgia and related syndromes by Livingston.[79] It assumes that an injury or lesion of tissue provokes a flow of painful impulses through afferent pathways to the spinal cord where the bombardment initiates a cycle of reflexes spreading through the interconnecting pool of neurons, upward, downward and across the cord, in short and long circuits of various extent. These, by their transmission of impulses, provide a continuous flow of stimulation to the lateral and anterior tracts. From them efferent autonomic and motor stimulation goes out to the peripheral tissues to produce the reflex symptoms. These are abnormal, disturbing local reactions of circulation and muscle spasm and thereby add noxious stimuli to reinforce those already arising from the original, peripheral or visceral lesion. *A "vicious circle"* may be established in that way, Livingston has pointed out, and what today may be called "feedback" circuits, which prolong the stimulation and reaction, and their clinical features, unless they cease spontaneously or are interrupted by therapy, nerve block or surgery.

In 1944 Doupe, Cullen and Chance suggested the possibility that causalgic pain is due to activation of sensory fibers by sympathetic impulses, postulating a conjunction of sympathetic and sensory nerve fibers with cross stimulation, either at the site of injury or peripheral to it, through defective insulation or actual union of nerve fibers.[23a] About this time Granit, Leksell and Skoglund showed that fiber interaction is a normal process at an injured portion of a mammalian nerve, and that any further injury to the nerve considerably facilitates the transmission of the impulse across this point of interaction or "artificial synapse."[49a]

From the clinical standpoint, the shoulder involvement of the shoulder-hand syndrome behaves like a "frozen shoulder" or adhesive capsulitis. In the complete syndrome the clinical picture and physiologic disturbance suggest the simultaneous presence of periarthritis of the shoulder with reflex dystrophy (Sudeck's atrophy) of the hand.[8,95,135,166] These features have led to the suggestion that the symptoms at the shoulder and hand merely represent a coincidental occurrence of two separate disorders, or that the provocative disturbance occurs at the shoulder, with or without symptoms there.

This theory seems to be fortified by the occurrence of shoulder disability and even the shoulder-hand syndrome in individuals long bedridden by illness, particularly cardiac and pulmonary disease. It must be assumed by this idea that "inactivity," or predisposing lesions of the shoulder, or both, determine the occurrence of this disturbance. In the literature of causalgia, the most painful reflex syndrome, the author has not found any mention of shoulder involvement in causalgic upper extremities.

Another explanation postulates that the involvement of the shoulder, which lends itself readily to being favored by the apprehensive individual, often reflects symptoms due to psychosomatic factors, the "periarthritic personality."[14] Many of the patients in the older age groups subject to the shoulder-hand syndrome are anxious, tense people whose symptoms are greatly influenced or exaggerated by their emotional state and hypersensitivity to pain.

Chemotherapeutic agents, notably antituberculous, especially *isoniazid*, recently have been reported to provoke the shoulder-hand syndrome as well as other rheumatic complaints.[75a,85a,135a] Reduced dosage or discontinuance has been observed to bring about quick spontaneous resolution of symptoms.[75a,85a] Contractures of the digital tendons have persisted in some cases. The role of *phenobarbital* in predisposing to the shoulder-hand syndrome has been impressively suggested by a carefully controlled statistical series.[159a] Ethionamid, related to isoniazid, and *radioactive iodine* also have been said to be responsible.[75a,135a] These are provocative observations deserving further controlled study. The mechanism remains to be clarified.

Pathology

Limited histologic examination of digital skin and muscle and palmar fascia has been uninformative in the late stages of the shoulder-hand syndrome.[149] Biopsies of tissue from the shoulder in the disorder have been found to show inflammatory and proliferative changes similar to those in nonspecfic periarthritis and capsulitis.[87,106] In lesions removed from the fingers in post-traumatic reflex dystrophy and the shoulder-hand syndrome there was edema of the subcutis with shrinkage of fat, areas of minute hemorrhage, cellular infiltration with perivascular localization as the outstanding feature.[74a] In early publications Sudeck described the osseous changes as due to an increased vascularization of the affected bone.[150]

Diagnosis

The outlook and management of the patient, as well as accurate diagnosis, require the earliest possible differentiation of the shoulder-hand syndrome. In bedridden patients especially, the insidious development of reflex symptoms may evade recognition for some time. When the usual acute onset occurs, the question of diagnosing such manifestations arises early.

In the early stages and throughout the progression of the syndrome to its terminal changes, rheumatoid arthritis is most closely simulated. The involvement of only the shoulder and hand in one extremity, except when bilateral, the characteristic diffuse edema rather than

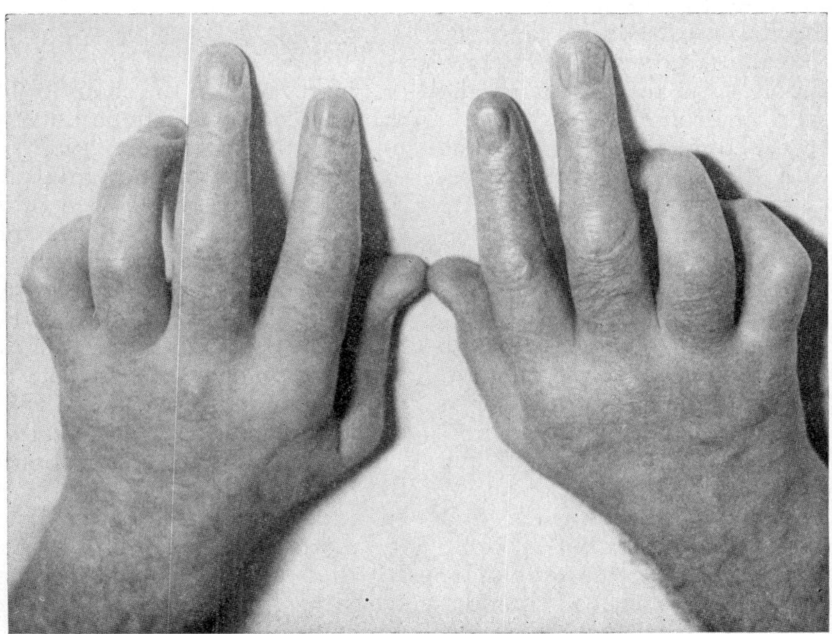

Fig. 80–11.—Shoulder-hand syndrome: Dorsal view of hands showing trophic changes in skin, flexion contractures of fingers.

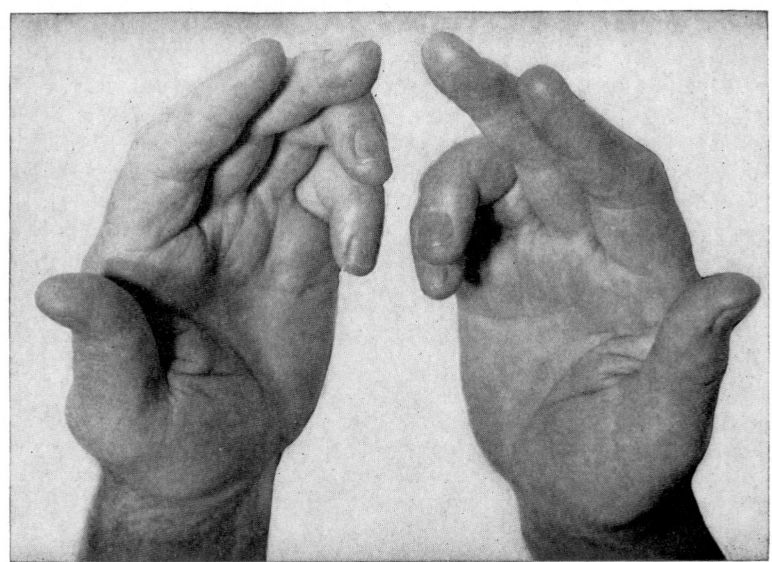

Fig. 80–12.—Shoulder-hand syndrome: Bilateral palmar fascial contractures resembling Dupuytren's contracture.

articular swelling, the usually normal sedimentation rate, negative tests for rheumatoid factor, the absence of involvement at the lower extremities, and the frequently obvious, provocative, underlying condition serve to distinguish the shoulder-hand syndrome.

The early shoulder-hand syndrome starting with *shoulder* involvement resembles "bursitis" or periarthritis. The presence of active visceral or other disease (Table 80–6) favors a reflex disorder. The onset of *hand* signs clinches the diagnosis.

Acute or early involvement of the hand suggests acute arthritis or gout. The lack of systemic symptoms, or a normal blood uric acid and the ineffectiveness of a therapeutic trial of colchicine, should clarify the situation.

Indurated swelling of the hand and fingers and, later, the peculiar atrophy and digital contractures may simulate sclerodactylia. A history of shoulder involvement or its appearance, as well as the clinical evolution associated with an underlying factor, establishes the differentiation of the reflex syndrome from the local variant of scleroderma.

Prognosis

The severity of the shoulder-hand syndrome is not proportionate to the extent of the provocative condition. For example, mild and uneventful infarction sometimes may be followed by the most troublesome and prolonged reflex syndrome, or minor trauma may induce severe reflex features and terminal dystrophy. The onset usually is evidenced by pain of troublesome degree, often acute. The course is variable, therefore unpredictable, as to extent, severity and duration in any individual case.

It is believed by many observers that the earlier the syndrome is recognized and treated the better the outlook for more rapid resolution of symptoms. In the post-infarctional shoulder-hand syndrome, Edeiken reported that his patients uniformly recovered without any specific therapy in two years or less on a conservative program including physical therapy and wall-climbing exercises.[26] Nevertheless, residual contractures of the fingers have been observed in a small number of patients three to six years after myocardial infarction and in others with various causes of their shoulder-hand syndromes.[149] Nearly half of the patients are seen first in the later stages, without previous treatment.[129,149] Whether the prognosis, particularly regarding therapeutic or spontaneous recovery and residua, varies with etiology has not been established.

Management of the Shoulder-Hand Syndrome

Present Status.—Treatment cannot be based on any entirely satisfactory specific therapeutic agent. Numerous methods of therapy have been advocated, as for other reflex neurovascular disorders. Our own observations agree with those of others that the earlier stages are the most favorable for therapy.[129]

Treatment of Any Underlying Condition

Myocardial infarction, trauma, degenerative spondylosis, or any other condition susceptible to therapy or correction should, of course, receive the attention it requires. Strenuous therapeutic or surgical measures in the management of the reflex symptoms are not helpful. The presence of cervical degenerative disc changes or spondylosis with encroachment on foramina, or both, may prove difficult to evaluate in these older groups. When symptoms and limited cervical mobility point to active cervical osteoarthritis, measures as outlined in Chapter 79 are indicated.

Analgesics

Pain may require supplementary analgesics. Salicylates in large amounts in divided doses, 4 to 6 grams daily, may give some palliation. Codeine or other narcotics may become necessary for temporary relief of acute symptoms. *Sedation* often helps. Meprobamate and other "relaxants" may be useful.

Reassurance always is desirable. More definite *psychotherapy sometimes is in order.*

Therapeutic Procedures of Possible Value

Physical therapy may give temporary palliation. *X-ray therapy* has been advocated and deprecated.[52,97]

Local analgesic iniections of "trigger points" or "tender points" at the shoulder or other parts of the extremity may prove effective at sites of trauma, when performed *early* after injury.[146]

Procedures Not Advisable

Worsening of the symptoms may follow manipulation of the shoulder under anesthesia or the application of casts for reflex syndromes.[146]

Measures of Definite Value

Exercises of the shoulder and hand, passive and active, particularly when adjusted to the comfort and tolerance of the patient have been most useful. They recently were combined with physical modalities "overloading the sensory circuits," reported to give "successful results" within 6 weeks in the first 8 patients.[59b] Heat or cold is used twice daily, continously for 6 to 7 hours, interrupted for exercises, then on alternate days, shorter periods and continued at home.[59b]

The most effective measures have been the systemic administration of corticosteroids and stellate ganglion blocks.

Corticosteroids,[129,139,147,149] such as prednisolone, or newer equivalents, are more easily utilized, but practitioners must be familiar with their use. The same schedule of administration is followed as for a patient with rheumatoid arthritis of similar severity. Generally, as a start, 15 mg. daily of prednisolone may be prescribed, in divided doses, increasing or decreasing this amount according to the response of the patient, reducing the daily total by modest weekly decrements with the onset of improvement. The usual precautions and contraindications to corticosteroids prevail here (*see* Chapter 31). If there is any doubt or contra-indication, stellate ganglion blocks should be used instead.

Stellate ganglion (sympathetic) blocks have the advantage of presenting no contra-indications, except hypersensitivity to procaine or related substances, even in the older age groups generally subject to the shoulder-hand syndrome.[5b,9,22,32,58,147,151] If three or four successive blocks do not show increasing responsiveness between infiltrations, there is no advantage in continuing them. An average of 7 may be required, although as many as 14 sympathetic blocks have been given. The anterior (paratracheal) route is used,[34] starting with a test injection of 10 ml. of 0.5 per cent procaine solution; thereafter, 20 to 30 ml. of 1 per cent solution. The procedure may be utilized on an ambulatory basis. Continuous block is carried out in the hospital.[5b] Sympathetic blocks require special technique.

In patients seen *in the later stages*, only persistent and troublesome pain justifies the use of corticosteroids or stellate blocks. A *rehabilitation program and exercises* provide the most useful measures to overcome disability due to advanced changes. For long-standing irreversible contractures, *special orthopedic surgical reconstruction occasionally* may be required. In severe, refractory syndromes, in the earlier stages, *sympathectomy rarely* may be indicated.

Even with serial blocks or corticosteroids, which have given approximately similar results in comparable series of patients, complete recovery or major improvement (abolition or great diminution of pain, swelling and other signs, complete or marked recovery of function at the shoulder and hand) has been reported in 32 to 50 per cent of those treated in the early stages.[129,149] In another 25 to 45 per cent there was appreciable benefit (partial relief or abolition of pain), and at least half of these patients derived some increased function.

Follow-up studies have disclosed few recurrences and well-sustained benefits, with only minor complaints, in those recovering.[129,149] The similarity of results with both corticosteroids (or ACTH) and sympathetic blocks raises the question whether the improvement is not spontaneous. In comparison with the trend of recovery in a small control group, not receiving any of these therapeutic measures, the actively treated patients appeared to have been made more comfortable and derived benefits more quickly,[149] possibly with less frequent contractures.

Prevention of the Shoulder-Hand Syndrome and Reflex Neurovascular Disorders

Although the mechanism by which reflex dystrophies are produced may not be clear, clinical observations suggest preventive measures worthy of application in certain conditions:

1. *The prompt evaluation of intercurrent, atypical or different pain, with or without disability,* at a shoulder or hand following trauma, internal disease, previous disorder or involvement of the extremity. Physicians treating wounds, injuries or intrathoracic diseases, particularly myocardial infarction, should be alert for swelling, vasomotor phenomena and reflex symptoms concurrent with or following these conditions.
2. *Avoidance of casts, splints or manipulations* in the management of painful symptoms associated with neurovascular features.
3. *Injection of definite local "trigger point(s)"* with procaine solution in traumatic or post-traumatic disorders, especially in the presence of suggestive reflex neurovascular symptoms.
4. *Gently graduated exercises, whenever feasible* and tolerable, for the

shoulders and hands of patients suffering from lesions known to provoke reflex syndromes, particularly when prolonged bed rest is required in middle-aged or elderly individuals.

BIBLIOGRAPHY

1. Adson, A. W. and Coffey, J. R.: Surg., Gynec. & Obst., *85*, 675, 1947.
2. Arlet, J. and Mole, J.: Rheumatism, *21*, 580, 1954.
3. Askey, J. M.: Amer. Heart J., *22*, 1, 1941.
4. Barany, R.: Nord. Med. Tidskr., *7*, 295, 1934.
5. Bayles, T. B., Judson, W. E. and Potter, T. A.: J.A.M.A., *144*, 537, 1950.

5*b*. Betcher, A. M. and Casten, D. F.: Anesthesiology, *16*, 994, 1955.

6. Beyer, J. A. and Wright, I. S.: Circulation, *4*, 2, 1951.
7. Blockey, N. J., Wright, J. K. and Kellgren, J. H.: Brit. Med. J., *1*, 1455, 1954.
8. Blumensaat, Carl: *The Present Status of the Sudeck Syndrome*, Berlin, Springer, 1956.
9. Bonica, J. J.: *The Management of Pain*, Philadelphia, Lea & Febiger, 1953.
10. Bosworth, D. M.: New York Acad. Med., *20*, 460, 1944; J.A.M.A., 116, 2477, 1941.

10*a*. Brannon, E. W.: J. Bone & Joint Surg., *45*, 977, 1963.

11. Caldwell, G. A. and Unkauf, B. M.: Ann. Surg., *132*, 432, 1950.
12. Capps, J. A. and Coleman, C. H.: *Clinical Study of Pain in Pleura, Pericardium and Peritoneum*, New York, The Macmillan Co., 1932.
13. Codman, E. A.: *The Shoulder*: Rupture of the Supraspinatus Tendon and Other Lesions in or about the Subacromial Bursa. Boston, Thomas Todd Co., 1934.
14. Coventry, M. B.: Proc. Staff. Meet. Mayo Clin., *29*, 58, 1954; J.A.M.A., *151*, 177, 1943.
15. Crisp, E. J. and Kendall, P. H.: Lancet, *1*, 476, 1955; *ibid*, 975; Brit. Med. J., *1*, 500, 1955.
16. Darrach, W. and Patterson, R. L., Jr.: J. Bone & Joint Surg., *19*, 993, 1937.
17. DePalma, A. F., Collery, G. and Bennett, G. A.: The Amer. Orthop., Instructional Course Lectures. Ann. Arbor Mich., J. W. Edwards, *6*, 255, 149; *7*, 168, 1956.
18. DePalma, A. F.: Ann. Surg., *35*, 193, 1952; *Surgery of the Shoulder*, Philadelphia, J. B. Lippincott Co., 1950.
19. DePalma, A. F. and Callery, G. E.: Clinical Orthop., *3*, 69, 1954.
20. DeSeze, S.: Presse Med., *143*, 96, 1936.
21. DeSeze, S., Robin, J. and DeBeyrne, N.: Rev. Rheumatisme, *19*, 35, 1952; *ibid*, 119, 329.
22. DeTakats, G. and Miller, D. S.: Arch. Surg., *16*, 469, 1943.
23. DeTakats, G.: J.A.M.A., *128*, 699, 1945.

23*a*. Doupe, J., Cullen, C. H. and Chance, G. Q.: Neurol., Neurosurg. & Psych., *7*, 33, 1934.

24. Duplay, S.: Arch. gen. de. med., *2*, 513, 1872.

24*a*. Eaton, L. M.: Surg. Clin. North America, *26*, 810, 1946; also discussion of 115.

25. Echtman, J.: New York State J. Med., *36*, 503, 1936.
26. Edeiken, J.: Circulation, *16*, 14, 1957.
27. Eden, K. C.: Brit. J. Surg., *27*, 111, 1939.
28. Edwards, E. A. and Levine, H. D.: New Engl. J. Med., *247*, 79, 1942.
29. Ehrlich, M., Carp, C., Berkowitz, S., Spitzer, N., Silver, M., and Steinbrocker, O.: Ann. Rheumat. Dis., *10*, 482, 1951.
30. Ellis, L. B. and Weiss, S.: Arch. Neurol. & Psychiat., *36*, 362, 1936.
31. Engel, G. L.: Amer. J. Med., *17*, 899, 1959.
32. Evans, J. A.: J.A.M.A., *130*, 620, 1946.
33. Falconer, Murray, A. and Weddell, G.: Lancet, *1*, 245, 539, 1943.
34. Findley, T. and Patzer, R.: J.A.M.A., *128*, 1271, 1945.
35. Fiske, L. G.: J.A.M.A., *149*, 758, 1952.

35*a*. Flint, J. M.: J.A.M.A., *61*, 1224, 1913.

36. Franklin, C. J. and Nemcik, F. J.: Amer. J. Med. Sci., *227*, 601, 1954.
37. Freese, A. S.: New York State J. Med., *49*, 278, 1959.
38. Freiberg, J. A.: Postgraduate Medicine, *16*, 104, 1954.
39. Friedland, F.: Amer. J. Phys. M., *34*, 379, 1955.
40. Friedman, H. A., Argyros, T. G. and Steinbrocker, O.: Postgraduate Medicine, *35*, 397, 1959.
41. Friedman, M. S.: Amer. J. Surg., *94*, 56, 1957.
42. Furlong, R.: Practitioner, *173*, 90, 1954.
43. Gamble, S. G.: Arch. Phys. Med., *32*, 516, 1951.
44. Ghormley, R. K.: Rocky Mount. Med. J., *54*, 706, 1957.
45. Goldner, J. L.: South. Med. J., *45*, 1125, 1952.
46. Gordon, E. J.: South. Med. J., *45*, 1131, 1952.

47. Gorrell, R. L.: J.A.M.A., *142*, 537, 1950; Journ.-Lancet, *75*, 32, 1955.
48. Graham, W.: Personal communication.
49. ———: In *Arthritis and Allied Conditions*, ed. by Hollander, J. L., Philadelphia, Lea & Febiger, 6th Ed., 1960.
49*a*. Granit, R., Leksell, L. and Skoglund, C. R.: Brain, *64*, 197, 1941.
50. Gross, S. W.: Amer. J. Med., *91*, 869, 1956.
51. Haggert, G. E., Dignam, R. J. and Sullivan, T. S.: J.A.M.A., *161*, 1217, 1958; J.A.M.A., *137*, 508, 1948.
51*a*. Haggert, G. E. and Allen, H. A.: Surg. Clin. North America, *15*, 1537, 1935.
52. Hermann, L. G., Reineke, H. G., and Caldwell, J. A.: Amer. J. Roentgenol., *47*, 353, 1942.
53. Hitchcock, H. H. and Bechtol, C. O.: J. Bone & Joint Surg., *30A*, 263, 1948.
54. Hollander, J. L., Brown, E. M., Jr., Jessar, R. A. and Brown, C. Y.: J.A.M.A., *147*, 1629, 1951; J. Bone & Joint Surg., *35A*, 983, 1953.
55. Homans, J.: New Engl. J. Med., *222*, 870, 1940.
56. Inman, V. T., Saunders, J. B. de C. M. and Abbott, L. C.: J. Bone & Joint Surg., *26A*, 261, 1944.
57. Jackson, R.: *The Cervical Syndrome*, Springfield, Charles C Thomas, 1956.
58. Jesperson, K.: Ann. Rheum. Dis., *8*, 220, 1949.
59. Johnson, A. C.: Ann. Int. Med., *19*, 433, 1943.
59*a*. Johnson, D. A.: J.A.M.A., *159*, 1567, 1955.
59*b*. Johnson, E. W. and Pannozzo, A. N.: J.A.M.A., *195*, 152, 1966.
60. Judovich, B., Bates, W., and Drayton, W., Jr.: *Pain Syndromes*, Philadelphia, F. A. Davis Co., 1953.
61. Judovich, B.: Pensonal communication.
62. Kahlmeter, G.: Brit. J. Phys. Med., *7*, 242, 1933.
63. Kammerling, E., Lewis, G. N. and Ehrlich, L.: New Engl. J. Med., *242*, 701, 1950.
63*a*. Kaplan, I. W. and Tyler, J.: Louisiana Med. Soc., *106*, 351, 1954.
64. Kauther, R.: Med. Klin., *48*, 1750, 1953.
65. Kellgren, J. H.: Clin. Sci., *3*, 175, 1938.
66. Kernwin, G. A., Berth, R. and Sneed, W. B., Jr.: J. Bone & Joint Surg., *39A*, 1267, 1957.
67. Kelly, M.: Med. J. Australia, *1*, 48, 1942; *1*, 330, 1953.
68. Kovacs, R.: Arch. Phys. Ther., *23*, 341, 1942.
69. Krauss, H.: J.A.M.A., *116*, 2582, 1941.
70. Kuhns, J. G.: New Engl. J. Med., *219*, 516, 1938.
71. Kyle, J. and Allen, F. C. O.: Ulster Med. J., 26 (2), 1957.
72. Laine, V. A.: Ann. Rheumat. Dis., *12*, 315, 1953.
72*a*. Lambert, C.: J. Bone & Joint Surg., *45*, 997, 1963.
73. Lapidus, B. W. and Guidotti, F. F.: Indust. Med. & Surg., *26*, 234, 1957.
74. Legrand, R. and Desruellas, J.: Echo. Med. Du. Nord., *24*, 313, 1953.
74*a*. Lehman, E. D.: Arch. Surg., *39*, 92, 1934.
75. Leland, J. L.: Bull. Hosp. Joint Dis., *14*, 71, 1953.
75*a*. Lequesne, M.: Sem. Hop. Paris, *42*, 2581, 1967.
76. Leriche, R.: *The Surgery of Pain*, Baltimore, The Williams & Wilkins Co., 1939.
76*a*. Lewis, Thos.: *Pain*, New York, The Macmillan Co., 1942.
77. Lipkin, E.: Proc. North. End. Clinic., Detroit, 1940.
78. Lippmann, R. X.: New York State J. Med., *44*, 2235, 1944.
79. Livingston, W. K.: *Pain Mechanisms*, New York, The Macmillan Co., 1943.
80. Lloyd-Roberts, G. C. and French, P. R.: Brit. Med. J., *1*, 1569, 1959.
81. Lord, J. W., Jr., and Rosati, L. M.: Clinical Symposia, *10*, 2, March-April, 1958.
82. Lord, J. W. and Stone, P. W.: Circulation, *13*, 537, 1956.
83. Lorenz, T. H. and Messer, M. J.: Ann. Int. Med., *37*, 1232, 1952.
84. Lorente de No, R.: J. Neurophys., *1*, 207, 1938.
85. Mauvoisin, F. and Bernard, J.: Toulouse med., *55*, (6), 597, 1954.
85*a*. McKusick, A. B. and Hsu, J. M.: Arth. & Rheum., *4*, 426, 1961.
86. McLaughlin, H. L.: Ann. Surg., *124*, 354, 1946; J. Bone & Joint Surg., *33A*, 76, 1951.
87. ———: Personal communication.
88. Meyer, W.: Arch. Surg., *35*, 1, 1937.
89. Michele, A. A.: New York State J. Med., *33*, 2485, 1955, and discussors.
90. Michotte, L. J.: Brit. J. Phys. Med., *1*, 77, 1957.
91. Miller, D. S. and de Takats, G.: Surg., Gyn. & Obst., *75*, 558, 1941.
92. Mitchell, S., W., Morehouse, G. R. and Keen, W. W.: *Wounds and Other Injuries of Nerves*, Philadelphia, J. B. Lippincott Company, 1864.
93. Mizumachi, S. and Toreyame, N.: Yokahoma Med. Bull., *6*, 93, 1955.

94. Moberg, E.: Acta Chir. Scandinav., *109*, 284, 1955.
95. Mogensen, E. F.: Act. Med. Scand., *145*, 1, 1953; *155*, 195, 1956; *156*, 15, 1956.
96. Morgan, E. H.: J.A.M.A., *169*, 804, 1959.
97. Moseley, H. F.: *Shoulder Lesions*, Springfield, Charles C Thomas, 1945; Clin. Symposia, *11*, 75, 1959.
98. Mueller, E. E., Mead, S., Schulz, B. F. and Vaden, M. R.: Amer. J. Phys. Med., *40*, 1145, 1954.
99. Mumford, E. D.: J. Bone & Joint Surg., *20*, 949, 1938.
100. Murnaghan, G. H. and McIntosh, D.: Lancet, *2*, 789, 1955.
101. Murphy, T.: Australian Med. J., *15*, 582, 1910.
102. Murphy, J. B.: Ann. Surg., *41*, 399, 1955.
103. Naffziger, H. C. and Grant, W. T.: Surg. Gyn., & Obst., *67*, 722, 1938.
104. Nelson, P. A.: J.A.M.A., *163*, 1570, 1957.
105. Neviaser, J. S.: J. Bone & Joint Surg., *27*, 211, 1943; Amer. Acad. Orthop. Surg., Instructional Course *6*, 281, 1949.
106. ————: Personal communication.
107. Noble T. P. and Hauser, R.: Arch. Surg., *17*, 75, 1926.
108. Ochsner, A., Gage, M. and de Bakey, M.: Amer. J. Surg., *28*, 689, 1938.
109. Olsson, Olof: Acta chir. Scand. Suppl., *181*, 1, 1955.
110. Oppenheimer, A.: Surg. Gyn. & Obst., *76*, 454, 1938; J. Bone & Joint Surg., *25*, 867, 1943.
111. Overton, L. M.: Clin. Orthop., *4*, 115, 1954.
112. Pasteur, F.: J. Radiologie et Electrol., *16*, 419, 1932.
113. Paull, R.: Amer. Heart J., *32*, 32, 1946.
114. Pederson, H. E. and Key, J. A.: Arch. Surg., *62*, 50, 1951.
115. Peet, R., Henriksen, J. D., Anderson, T. P., and Martin, G. M.: Proc. Staff Meet. Mayo Clinic, *31*, 281, 1956.
116. Plenk, H. P.: Radiology, *59*, 384, 1952.
117. Pratt, J. H., Golden, L. A. and Rosenthal, J.: Tr. Assoc. Amer. Phys., *46*, 313, 1941.
118. Prewitt, G.: Portland Clin. Bull., *8*, 111, 1955.
119. Pruce, A. M., Miller, J., Jr. and Berger, T. R.: Clin. Symposia, *10*, 1, 1958.
120. Quigley, T. B. and Renold, A. R.: New Engl. J. Med., *246*, 1012, 1952.
121. Quigley, T. B.: Clinical Orthoped., *10*, 182, 1957; J.A.M.A., *161*, 850, 1956.
122. Ravault, P., Vignon, G. and Ponsonnet, G.: Rev. Rheumat., *22*, 421, 1955; Rev. Lyon Med., *4*, 403, 1956.
123. Reg, L.: J. do Medico, *22*, 570, 1953.
124. Reynolds, F. C. and Ramsey, R. H.: South. Med. J., *47*, 209, 1954.
125. Robecchi, A.: *Periarthritis of the Shoulder*, Valecchi, Florence, 1952; Rheumatismo, *7*, 153, 1955.
126. Robecchi, A. and Daneo, V.: Minerva Med., *98*, 1802, 1953.
127. Robinson, W. D., *et al.*: Eleventh Review of Rheumatism and Arthritis, Ann. Int. Med. *45*, 831, 1956.
128. Rome, H. P.: Med. Clin. North America, *29*, 106, 1949.
129. Rosen, P. S. and Graham, W.: Can. Med. Assoc. J., *77*, 86, 1957.
130. Russek, H. J.: Med. Clin. North America, *42*, 1555, 1959.
131. Russek, A. S.: J.A.M.A., *156*, 1575, 1954.
132. Russell, J. J., Russek, H. I., Doerner, A. A. and Zohman, B. L.: Arch. Int. Med., *91*, 457, 1953.
133. Sacks, S.: South African Med. J., *27*, 335, 1956.
134. Scheifley, O. H.: Proc. Staff Meet. Mayo Clin., *29*, 363, 1954.
135. Schwartz, M. and Meulengracht, E.: Nord. Med., *40*, 1629, 1951.
135*a*. Serre, H., Simon, L. and Caillens, J. P.: Rev. Rhum., *29*, 165, 1962.
136. Shenkin, H. A.: J.A.M.A., *165*, 335, 1957.
137. Sigler, J. W. and Ensign, D. C.: J. Mich. M. Soc., *50*, 1038, 1954; Ann. Rheum. Dis., *10*, 484, 1951.
138. Simmonds, F. A.: J. Bone & Joint Surg., *31B*, 426, 1949.
139. Smith, L. A.: Postgrad. Med., *26*, 272, 1959.
140. Smyth, C. J., *et al.*: Twelfth Rheumatism Review, Ann. Int. Med., *50*, 366, 1959.
140*a*. Snorassen, E.: Nord. Med., *20*, 1798, 1943.
141. Soulie, P., Tricot, R. and DeGeorges: Semaine hop. Paris, *26*, 4141, 1950.
142. Stammers, F. A. R.: Lancet, *1*, 603, 1950.
143. Stein, I., Stein, R. O. and Bellar, M. L.: Amer. J. Surg., *85*, 215, 1953.
144. Steinberg, C. L. and Roodenburg, C. I.: J.A.M.A., *149*, 1458, 1952.
145. Steinbrocker, O.: Ann. Int. Med., *12*, 1917, 1939; *Arthritis in Modern Practice*, Philadelphia, W. B. Saunders Company, 1941, pp. 344–414.
146. Steinbrocker, O., Spitzer, N. and Friedman, H. H.: Ann. Int. Med., *29*, 22, 1948.
147. Steinbrocker, O., Neustadt, D., and Lapin, L.: J.A.M.A., *153*, 788, 1953.
148. Steinbrocker, O., Neustadt, D. and Bosch, S. J.: Med. Clin. North America, *33*, 1, 1955.

149. Steinbrocker, O. and Argyros, T. G.: Med. Clin. North America, *42*, 1533, 1958.
149*a*. Steinbrocker, O.: In preparation.
149*b*. Steindler, A. and Luck, J. V.: J.A.M.A., *110*, 106, 1938.
150. Sudeck, P.: Arch. f. klin. chir., *62*, 147, 1900; Roentgenstr., *5*, 277, 1901.
151. Swan, D. M. and McGowan, J. M.: J.A.M.A., *146*, 774, 1951; Neurology, *4*, 480, 1954.
152. Tarsy, J. M.: New York State J. Med., *46*, 996, 1946.
153. Telford, R. D. and Mottershead, S.: Brit. Med. J., *1*, 325, 1947; J. Bone & Joint Surg., *30B*, 249, 1948.
154. Theis, F. V.: Surg., *6*, 112, 1939.
155. Thompson, W. A. L. and Kopell, H. P.: J.A.M.A., *260*, 1261, 1959.
156. Thompson, R. G. and Compere, E. L.: J.A.M.A., *109*, 945, 1959.
157. Travell, J., Rinzler, S. and Herman, M.: J.A.M.A., *120*, 417, 1942.
158. Travell, J.: New York State J. Med., *48*, 2050, 1948.
159. Upmalis, I. H.: Internat. Abst. Surg., *107*, 521, 1958.
159*a*. Van der Korst, J. K., Colenbrander, H. and Cats, A.: Ann. Rheum. Dis., *25*, 553, 1968.
160. Vishnevsky, A. V.: Novy Khir. Arch., *38*, 392, 1937.
161. Walshe, F. N. R.: *Modern Trends in Neurology*, Edited by Feling, A., London, Butterworth, 1951, p. 542.
161*a*. Weeks, A. and Delprati, G. D.: Internat. Cl., *3*, 40, 1936.
162. Whitcomb, W. P.: Radiology, *66*, 237, 1956.
163. Williamson, Paul: Am. Pract. & Dig. of Treat., *9*, 1225, 1958.
164. Willshire: Lancet, *2*, 633, 1860.
165. Wright, I. S.: Amer. Heart J., *29*, 1, 1945.
166. Young, J. H. and Pearson, A. T.: Med. J. Australia, *1*, 776, 1952.
167. Young, H. H., Ward, L. E. and Henderson, E. O.: J. Bone & Joint Surg., *36A*, 602, 1954.
168. Editorial: G. P., *12*, 198, 1955.

Chapter 81

Dupuytren's Contracture

By John W. Sigler, M.D.

Contraction of the palmar fascia was described by Plater in 1610, and Sir Astley Cooper described correction by fasciotomy in 1818. Dupuytren's classic description of fascial contracture, flexion deformities of the fingers, and loss of function appeared in the Lancet for 1834.[12] Reviews of the literature have periodically come forth.[10,11,24,28,29,34,41,42,45,46,48,49]

Etiology

The etiology of this condition is unknown. Numerous factors have been incriminated among which the most important are: heredity,[32,33,39,48] trauma,[43] focal hypertrophy of connective tissue originating in vessel walls,[5,34] fibroblastic proliferation,[24,32,34,43] disturbances of sympathetic tone,[44] nervous system lesions, rupture of fibers in the palmar aponeurosis with subsequent deposition of iron pigment[33,48] and various disease states. Histological similarity to other fibroplasias such as fascial desmoids, and induratio penis plastica (Peyronie's disease) has been noted.[7,18,27]

In recent years trauma is considered to have no etiologic relationship to Dupuytren's contracture, but it may represent an aggravating factor in those individuals with a predisposition to the disease. The importance of trauma has probably been exaggerated in the past due to Dupuytren's original observations, and by patients still insisting on associating the onset of their disease with explicit injury or occupational wear and tear on the hand.

Dupuytren's contracture has been observed in several generations of the same family usually on the male side and a high familial incidence has been noted in several large series.[32,34,44,47,48] The role of heredity in Dupuytren's contracture is being acknowledged with increasing frequency. Evidence of heredity varies proportionally with the effort of the examiner to pursue the stigmata through the various members of the patient's family. Ling, after examining 832 relatives of 50 patients, found a familial incidence in 68 per cent and strong hearsay evidence indicating the percentage to be even higher. In Skoog's own group of 50 cases of Dupuytren's contracture, involvement in other members of the family was shown to be present in 44 per cent. In this series, men were affected 9 times as frequently as women. More recent work indicates the male and female ratio to be approximately 6:1.[13] It may be assumed that hard manual labor is related in view of this sex disproportion; but the majority of authors discount occupational trauma, and also the male and female disproportion becomes less in the older age groups.[35] The normal aging process and chronic invalidism are worthy of mention in connection with Dupuytren's contracture. Hueston has shown a gradual increase in the incidence of this disease with age. In patients over 40 years of age, Dupuytren's contracture was found with increasing frequency in each decade. He noted that after sixty years of age, 25 per cent of all persons examined had palmar thickening to suggest Dupuytren's contracture.[19,20,21]

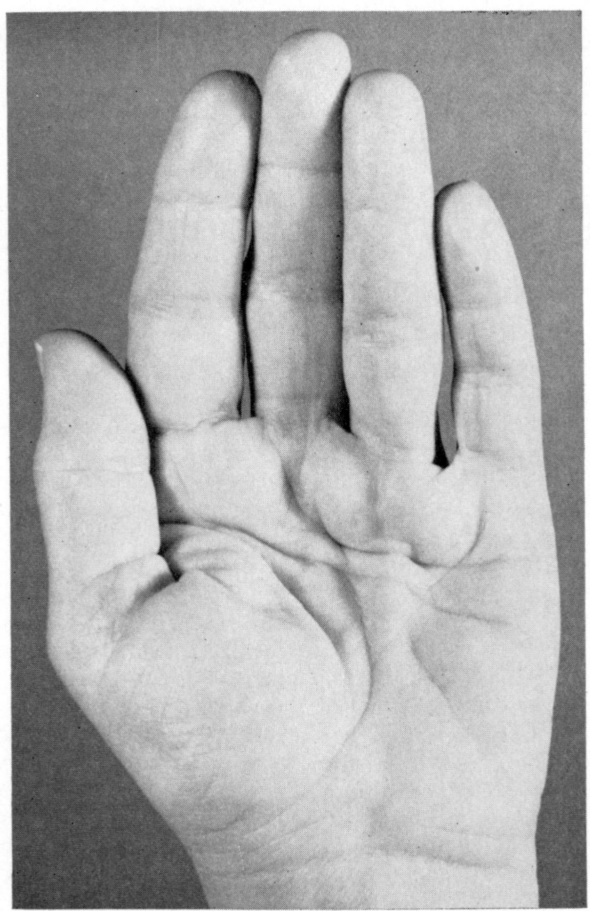

Fig. 81–1.—Dupuytren's contracture. Puckering of the palmar skin and contraction of the palmar fascial bands extending to the base of the fourth metacarpophalangeal joint causing early flexion contracture of the fourth finger.

Chronic invalids have been found to have a higher incidence of Dupuytren's contracture regardless of their general health status. Specific disease groups who more frequently have Dupuytren's contracture include epileptics, patients with pulmonary tuberculosis, chronic alcoholics, and diabetics. A great incidence of Dupuytren's contracture in these groups is thought to be due to an aging population group under physician observation. However, the high incidence of diabetic glucose tolerance curves in association with palmar contractures is worthy of further investigation.[50a] Barbiturate usage has been suspected as a common factor in many of these chronic disease states.[23,30] Recent studies noted an association of Dupuytren's contracture with abnormal liver function (excretory enzymes) in patients with alcoholism and epilepsy.[44a]

A curious, and perhaps significant, association between Dupuytren's contracture and epilepsy has been described by Lund.[1,37] He reported contractures of the hand in 50 per cent of 190 male epileptics, and in 25 per cent of 171 females with the convulsive state. Skoog subsequently studied 207 afflicted males and found palmar contractures in 42 per cent. Concurrent hereditary predisposition toward both of these conditions may be the common denominator for this unusual association. Barbiturates are again mentioned as a possible contributing factor in these studies.

Increased sympathetic tone has been suggested as a cause,[44] and Hale Powers has placed Dupuytren's contracture in the same category as scleroderma, hypertrophic pulmonary osteoarthropathy, and other trophic disturbances.[45] A few cases have been seen associated with Raynaud's phenomenon. A reflex dystrophy involving the shoulder and the hand has been observed with increasing frequency in recent years.[2,29,41,51] This has been aptly termed the *shoulder-hand syndrome* by Steinbrocker, who regards Dupuytren's contracture as part of a reflex neurovascular dystrophy. It is most frequently seen after myocardial infarctions, hemiplegias, splinting, minor injuries to the shoulder, manipulation, cervical arthritis, and occasionally completely alone. Pain in the shoulder with associated swelling of the finger pads and palm may appear within a few weeks to a year after coronary occlusion. Gradually the shoulder disability improves, but the hand changes may become more pronounced with considerable pain, stiffness, numbness, tingling, coldness, livid discoloration, and inability to either extend or flex the fingers fully.[23,25,27,29] In one series, changes in the hands were not noted prior to the infarction. As the condition progresses, the skin becomes shiny, taut, and pale; but congestion may, at times, be striking. Demineralization of varying degrees can be seen in films of both the shoulder and hand in well-established cases. No obliteration of the joint spaces or bony proliferation occurs. It is presumed that, in the presence of a myocardial infarction, pain impulses originating in the heart pass up sensory fibers to the "internuncial pool" of the lower cervical-upper dorsal cord and are relayed down the inside of the arm and side of the chest via the first, second, and third thoracic sympathetic rami. For a more complete discussion of the shoulder-hand syndrome see the chapter on the Painful Shoulder, page 1489.

It has also been suggested that palmar contractures may originate as a *tendinous or aponeurotic degeneration* in vestigial remnants of the superficial flexores brevis muscle; this set of muscles is present in many of the lower mammals in which it serves as a third set of flexors. Krogius has described islets of this muscle in the palmar aponeurosis of the newborn,[33] but the persistence of the atavistic muscle in man has been denied by others.

Symptoms

One or both hands may be affected.[17] It was unilateral in half of one series,[27] but more commonly bilateral in the experiences of other observers.[34] The right hand is apt to be affected more often than the left in unilateral disease. Males are predominantly affected, and the incidence rises sharply in the fourth decade with little leveling off through the seventh. The ring finger is most frequently involved; the little, middle and index fingers follow in that order. When several fingers are affected, the involvement may not occur at the same time and may not progress at the same rate.[50] Occasionally the nodules may be dorsal in the proximal interphalangeal area, or, more rarely still, have characteristic puckering associated with these changes.

Diagnosis

The diagnosis is made by visual inspection and palpation. Congenital or spastic contractures or those following injury or infection can be differentiated by having the patient flex his wrist; this maneuver relieves shortening of the flexor tendons and permits full extension of the fingers. In Dupuytren's contracture, extension of the fingers is not possible after bending the wrist. When associated with the shoulder-hand syndrome, the hands may at times resemble those seen in scleroderma and Raynaud's disease.

Hypertrophic scarring of the palms secondary to burns or other injury may rarely be confused with Dupuytren's contracture. Knuckle pads, plantar fibromatosis (Fig. 81–2) and Peyronie's disease are associated disease processes that should be sought in the patient with Dupuytren's contracture.

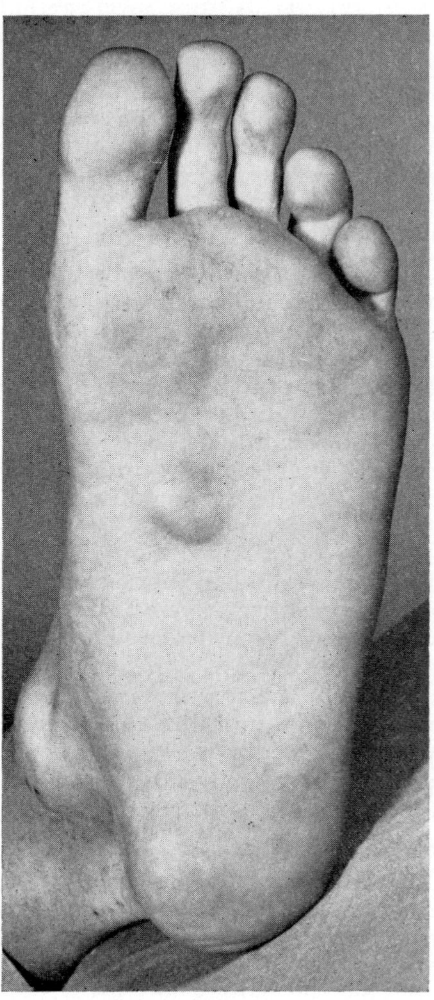

FIG. 81–2.—Plantar fibromatosis associated with Dupuytren's contracture histologically may be mistaken for fibrosarcoma, prompting unnecessary radical surgical procedures and even amputation in isolated instances.

Pathology

Normally, the palmar fascia or aponeurosis is a triangular membrane consisting of four layers with its apex at the transverse carpal ligament. The superficial layer separates into four bundles one of which goes to each of the fingers; the thumb may receive a tiny band.[33] They attach to the deeper layers of the skin proximal to the webs and extend into the bases of the fingers. Some fibers run vertically and obliquely binding the skin to the aponeurosis, and giving rise to creases at the level of the metacarpal heads. Transverse fasciculi communicate beneath with the three deeper fascial layers, the metacarpal bones, phalanges, and interphalangeal joints.[26,27,28] The palmar aponeurosis serves as a protection for the important compartments of the hand and helps to stabilize the skin so that it does not slide loosely on its base when the hand is used.

Early changes consist of small palmar nodules or plaque-like thickening arising in the palmar connective tissues overlying the tendons of the fourth and fifth fingers. The process may extend to the third, first, and second digits sequentially. This nodular phase is the first or cellular phase advanced by Luck.[36] The overlying skin becomes puckered and adherent to the fascia. In many instances the fibrosis may remain stationary for months or years and may never affect the palmar fascia beyond the distal palmar crease. McCallum and Hueston have adopted the viewpoint expressed by Goyrand that the nodule arises primarily in the fibro-fatty tissues overlying the palmar fascia rather than in the fascia proper.[15,38] The arguments put forth for this thesis are strong, but the palmar fascia becomes involved so rapidly in the process that from a clinical point of view the origin of the nodule appears relatively unimportant.

The second or involutional phase is a lessening of the cellularity of the nodule and the appearance of fibrous bands extending centrifugally from the nodule.

Signs of Dupuytren's Contracture

Small nodules or plaque-like thickening of the palmar connective tissues overlying the tendons of the fourth and fifth fingers.
Puckering of the palmar skin.
Appearance of fibrous bands extending centrifugally from the palmar nodule.
Extension of fascial bands from the concavity of the palm to metacarpophalangeal and proximal interphalangeal joints.
Progressive involvement of the palmar skin and fingers.
Dupuytren's contracture may progress to involve the greater portion of the palmar fascia and all of the fingers, leading to marked flexion contracture of the fingers.
In many instances, the fibrosis may remain stationary for months or years and may never affect visibly the palmar fascia beyond the distal palmar crease.

Once the fascial bands extend to the base of the fourth and fifth fingers, contractures of the metacarpophalangeal and proximal interphalangeal joints occur (Fig. 81–1).

In the third or residual phase, the nodule involutes, leaving dense fibrous bands connecting the skin and palmar fascia along the lines of maximum tension. There is some contention as to whether the fibrous cord is an actively formed structure or whether it represents a fibrous contraction developing secondary to finger motion. It is worthwhile to reiterate that nodule formation and various stages of involution may be present simultaneously in several areas of the involved hand.

Treatment

Therapy should first be directed toward reassuring the patient of the benign nature of the disease. The patient appearing with a primary complaint of a painful nodule in the palm most often finds the discomfort negligible after an adequate explanation. In the occasional patient who has persistent pain, a single ten-day course of ultrasound may prove effective. In some instances, ultrasonic therapy may temporarily lessen the degree of a palmar contracture in early cases. Other forms of heat along with stretching exercises have been used for symptomatic relief. Corticosteroids (either systemic or local), drugs and radiation therapy are not usually beneficial in Dupuytren's contracture. Local steroid injections into the affected tendon sheaths may be worthy of trial in early cases.

However, in those cases of Dupuytren's contracture associated with the shoulder-hand syndrome, shoulder motion may be re-established by the concurrent use of corticosteroids and intensive physical therapy. For details of the program of management of the shoulder-hand syndrome see Chapter 80, p. 1497.

The surgical management of Dupuytren's contracture should be carried out after contracture begins. The intelligent patient is instructed to return when beginning limitation of extension of the fingers is noted, but the less reliable patient should be examined at regular intervals to determine the extent of the contracture. The presence of nodules, puckering and skin involvement may remain static for a number of years and does not represent a valid indication for surgical intervention.

Surgical treatment is currently accomplished by:

1. Subcutaneous Fasciotomy
2. Limited Fasciectomy
3. Radical Fasciectomy
4. Digital Amputation

The type and extent of involvement, the overall health and the needs of the patient determine which procedure is most suitable. A minimal procedure which offers the patient the most function with the least threat of complication and reasonable freedom from recurrence is chosen.

The subcutaneous fasciotomy, reported by Sir Astley Cooper in 1823, is most suitable for the single hand contracture, particularly when the active disease has subsided.[9] Luck, who has been a student of this malady for a number of years and is responsible for the re-introduction of this form of treatment, believes that the procedure of nodule excision from the palm or proximal finger represents adequate and definitive treatment for a large percentage of patients with Dupuytren's disease.[36] The recurrences have not been significantly higher than in those with more radical forms of treatment. It also has a distinct place in the treatment of less suitable contractures in those patients in whom the severity of concomitant disease makes a minimal procedure the most desirable.[31]

The limited fasciectomy is suitable for most patients seeking surgical relief for Dupuytren's contracture. The procedure, which received its main impetus from the work of Hamlin,[16] has been employed increasingly over the past decade. It is generally performed through staggered incisions, or linear incisions converted to Z-plastys over the maximal areas of involvement.[22] Visualization of important structures, especially the digital nerves, is excellent, and undermining of skin with the threat of hematoma or skin slough is minimal. The morbidity is only a few days more than for the fasciotomy patient. Light forms of work can be handled in four to five days.

Radical fasciectomy, the procedure of choice of surgeons for several decades, had as its goal the complete removal of the palmar fascia. The attainment of this ideal would cure the patient of contracture and relieve him of the prospect of recurrence. The radical procedure, however, did not prevent recurrences, and extensions into unoperated areas were common. The morbidity was long and many hands never recovered mobility. The loss of flexion was more disabling than the original complaint. Rumblings of discontent among the surgeons began.[6,14,31,52] Clarkson presented the case against the radical fasciectomy in detail.[8] The radical procedure, however, has a definite place in the treatment of Dupuytren's contracture. The current concept of the procedure is to remove all the diseased fascia in the palm and fingers in a single operative session. Closure may be a problem because of the sacrifice of damaged skin or in elasticity when it is retained. Skin grafts or rotated dorsal flaps are sometimes necessary for closure. McCash has reported two series wherein the palm was left open to heal secondarily, primary attention being directed to maintaining finger motion.[40] The open palm technique is similar to Baron Dupuytren's original operative approach.

Few surgeons still attempt to clear all the fascia, both diseased and grossly normal. Most surgeons reserve the procedure for patients in the younger age groups in whom the disease has a more rapid course and involvement tends to be more widespread. The edema following the procedure may be severe and slow to resolve, but if cases are properly selected this problem is less formidable.[3] Seldom is the patient able to return to any but the most sedentary occupation in less than two months and to manual labor in about four months.

Finger amputation is a useful procedure for the patient with severe digital deformity. In some cases the proximal interphalangeal joint has been destroyed by continued severe flexion deformities. An extensive procedure restoring excellent metacarpophalangeal joint mobility fails to clear the finger from its obstructing position. In this type of case simple amputation of one or more digits can make the hand more useful than can the more radical operations. Filleting of a finger to create a pedicle flap for coverage of a palmar defect may enable the surgeon to obtain excellent release of remaining digits.

In summary, treatment of Dupuytren's contracture is surgical; the proper selection of patient and procedure affords excellent relief of the disability associated with this malady. Surgical treatment cannot be said to be curative any more than insulin cures diabetes mellitus. If the physician thinks of surgery in this context, he can better prepare the patient for the repeated limited surgical procedures that have gained favor over the single radical operative attack.

Postoperative Therapy

When the skin incision is well healed, whirlpool (water temperature at 92–98 °F.) may be used once or twice daily for thirty minutes during which the patient's fingers may be passively extended. Assisted active exercise is then instituted, and later active flexions and extensions are carried out repeatedly throughout each day. Occasionally, for the patient who is not progressing satisfactorily, posterior extension splints may be worn at night and during inactive daytime periods until good function can be demonstrated.

BIBLIOGRAPHY

1. Arieff, A. J. and Bell, J. L.: Neurology, *6*, 115, 1956.
2. Askey, J. M.: Amer. Heart J., *22*, 1, 1941.
3. Barclay, T. R.: Plast. Reconstruct. Surg., *23*, 348, 1959.
4. Baxter, H., Johnson, L., Mader, V. and Schiller, C.: Canad. Med. Ass. J., *63*, 540, 1950.
5. Broadbent, T. R.: Rocky Mountain Med. J., *52*, 1087, 1955.
6. Brunner, J. M.: Trans. Int. Soc. Plast. Surg. Second Congress, London, E. & S. Livingstone, 1959.
7. Bunnell, S.: *Surgery of the Hand*, 2nd ed., Philadelphia, J. B. Lippincott Co., 1949.
8. Clarkson, P.: Brit. J. Plast. Surg., *16*, 273, 1963.
9. Cooper, Astley: *Treatise on Dislocations and on Fractures at the Joints*, 2nd Ed., London, Longmans, p. 521, 1823.
10. Cordrey, J. L.: Geriatrics, *11*, 440, 1956.
11. Desplas, B. and Meillere, J.: Bull. et mem. Soc. nat. de. chir., *58*, 424, 1932.
12. Dupuytren, B.: Lancet, *2*, 222, 1834.
13. Early, P. F.: J. Bone & Joint Surg., *44b*, 602, 1962.
14. Furlong, R.: Practitioner, *180*, 498, 1958.
15. Goyrand, G.: Cited by ref. 17.
16. Hamlin, E., Jr.: Ann. Surg., *155*, 454, 1962.
17. Hohmann, G.: Ztschr. f. Orthop., *73*, 45, 1941.
18. Horwitz, T.: Arch. Surg., *44*, 687, 1942.
19. Hueston, J. T.: *Dupuytren's Contracture*, Baltimore, The Williams & Wilkins Co., 1963.
20. Hueston, J. T.: Med. J. Aust., *1*, 1962.
21. ———: Med. J. Aust., *2*, 999, 1960.
22. Iselin, M. and Dieckmann, D. G.: Presse Med., *59*, 1394, 1951.
23. Jacobson, H. S.: Personal communication.
24. Janssen, P.: Arch. f. klin. Chir., *67*, 761, 1902.
25. Johnson, A. C.: Ann. Int. Med., *19*, 433, 1943.
26. Kalberg, W.: Anat. Anz., *81*, 149, 1935.
27. Kanavel, A. B., Koch, S. L. and Mason, M. L.: Surg., Gynec. & Obstet., *48*, 145, 1929.
28. Kaplan, E. B.: Surgery, *4*, 415, 1949.
29. Kehl, K. C.: Ann. Int. Med., *19*, 213, 1943.
30. Kelly, A. P.: Personal communication.
31. Kelly, A. P. and Clifford, R. H.: Plast. Reconstr. Surg., *24*, 505, 1959.
32. Kostia, J.: Ann. Chir. et Gyn. fenn., *46*, 351, 1957.
33. Krogius, A.: Zentralbl. f. Chir., *47*, 914, 1920.
34. Larsen, R. D. and Posch, J. L.: J. Bone & Joint Surg., *40A*, 773, 1958.
35. Ling, R. S. M.: J. Bone & Joint Surg., *45b*, 709, 1963.
36. Luck, J. V.: J. Bone & Joint Surg., *41a*, 635, 1959.
37. Lund, M.: Acta Psychiat. et. Neurol., *16*, 465, 1941.
38. MacCallum, P. and Hueston, J. T.: Australia & New Zealand J. Surg., *31*, 241, 1962.
39. Manson, J. S.: Brit. Med. J., *2*, 11, 1931.
40. McCash, C. R.: Brit. J. Plast. Surg., *17*, 271, 1964.
41. Meyer, J. C. and Binswanger, H. F.: Amer. Heart J., *23*, 715, 1942.
42. Meyerding, H. W.: Arch. Surg., *32*, 320, 1936.
43. Niederland, W.: Med. Welt, *7*, 126, 1933.

44. NIPPERT: Deutsche Ztschr. f. Chir., *216*, 289, 1929.

44a. POJER, J., RADIVOJEVIC, M. and WILLIAMS, T. F.: A.M.A. Arch. Int. Med., *129*, 561, 1972.

45. POWERS, H.: J. Nerv. Ment. Dis., *80*, 386, 1934.

46. ROODENBURG, A. T.: A.M.A. Arch. Int. Med., *101*, 551, 1958.

47. SCHRODER, C. H.: Arch. f. Orthop. u. Unfall-Chir., *35*, 125, 1934.

48. SKOOG, T.: Acta chir. Scand., *96* (Supp. 139), 1, 1948.

49. ————: Postgrad. Med., *21*, 91, 1957.

50. SMITH, N.: Brit. Med. J., *1*, 603, 1884.

50a. SPRING, M., FLECK, H. and COHEN, B. D.: New York State J. Med., *70*, 1037, 1970.

51. STEINBROCKER, O.: Amer. J. Med., *3*, 402, 1947.

52. WEBSTER, G. V.: Amer. J. Surg., *100*, 372, 1960.

Chapter 82

Low Back Pain and Sciatica

By Philip D. Wilson, Jr., M.D., and David B. Levine, M.D.

The symptom of pain in the low back with or without radiation into the lower extremities is an extremely common one. It can be most disabling and is a major cause of loss of time from work.[24a,55]

Despite the past four decades of massive research which has led to a better understanding of the pathologic entities involved in this syndrome, current diagnostic procedures continue to be hampered by their complexity, hazardous nature and lack of precision, so that early accurate pathologic diagnosis is often difficult to establish in the individual patient. Loose diagnostic categories, therefore, continue to be useful to the physicians. "Lumbago," "sciatica" and "lumbosacral strain" should be recognized for the ambiguous terms they are. While "degenerative disc disease," "herniated disc," and "arthritis" refer to more specific entities, there is a tendency to use them too casually and without adequate basis.

The prime duty of the physician is to maintain an orderly approach to the problems presented by a patient with a low back pain syndrome. First of all, he should determine as well as possible whether the lesion is primarily musculoskeletal, neurological or visceral. When one or the other of these has been established, then the working diagnosis should be carried only as far as the physical, roentgenological and laboratory findings warrant. If a definite diagnosis is necessary, as for a medical form or compensation report, it should be defined as fully as possible in terms of the actual findings. For instance, all patients with leg radiation of pain do not suffer from nerve root compression and, therefore, such a diagnosis is only presumed until actual neurological deficit or myelographic changes are demonstrated. Generally speaking, two broad classifications of diagnosis are applicable to intrinsic low back pain and sciatica syndromes: *lumbosacral sprain* and *nerve root compression*. These can then be further subdivided into the more specific causes which are described in this chapter. The discussion has been arranged in the following sections:

I. Anatomy and physiology
II. History, examination and x ray
III. Lumbosacral sprain syndromes
IV. Nerve root compression syndromes
V. Other conditions

ANATOMY AND PHYSIOLOGY

Anatomical Considerations

The Segmented Column.—Each vertebra is composed of an anterior portion, the body, and a posterior part, the neural arch. From the latter there are several processes of importance. These are the transverse processes, one on each side; superior and inferior articular processes (facets), one above and below on each side; and one spinous process. The portion of the neural arch connected to the body and anterior to the articular processes is called the root or pedicle; that behind is called the lamina; that part between the superior and inferior articular facets has come to be known as the pars interarticularis or isthmus.

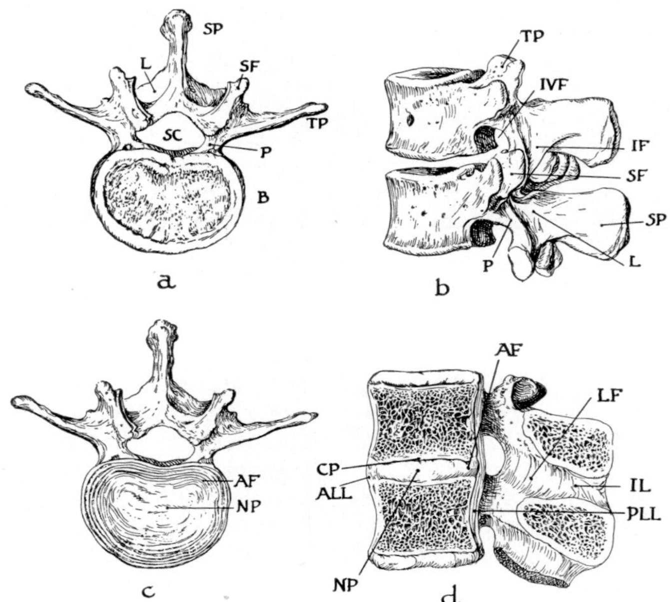

FIG. 82–1.—Anatomy of the lumbar vertebrae and their articulations. *a*, Superior view of a stripped lumbar vertebra. *b*, Lateral view of two articulated lumbar vertebrae. *c*, Superior view of a horizontal section of a lumbar disc. *d*, Lateral view of a sagittal section of two articulated lumbar vertebrae.

Key:
B—body
SC—spinal canal
IVF—intervertebral foramen
IF—inferior articular facet
SF—superior articular facet
P—pedicle
TP—transverse process
SP—spinous process
L—lamina
AF—annulus fibrosus
NP—nucleus pulposus
CP—cartilage plate
ALL—anterior longitudinal ligament
PLL—posterior longitudinal ligament
LF—ligamentum flavum
IL—interspinous ligament

The vertebrae are articulated together by a system of joints, three for each level. The disc lies between two adjacent vertebral bodies, and is composed of a tough fibrocartilaginous outer ring, the annulus fibrosus, with a central viscus core, the nucleus pulposus. It is bounded above and below by hyaline cartilaginous plates that blend with the annulus fibrosus. The transitions from cartilaginous plate to annulus and from annulus to nucleus are gradual. The fibers of the annulus are arranged concentrically and in multiple layers. In the lumbar discs the layers are thicker anteriorly and laterally than posteriorly, and the nucleus is closer to the posterior aspect of the disc. Posteriorly, one for each side, there are true diathrodial joints. These lie between the inferior facets of one vertebra above and the superior facets of the next below.

The ligamentous support of the spine is provided by the massive anterior longitudinal and the narrow posterior longitudinal ligaments. In a study of 35 autopsy specimens at the level of the L5 vertebral body the average width of the anterior longitudinal ligament was found to be 2 cm. and average thickness 1.9 mm. while the average width of the posterior longitudinal ligament was 0.7 cm. and average thickness 1.3 mm.[48a] These are situated around the margins of the vertebral bodies and lend strong support to the discs except posteriorly on either side of the midline where their fibers are much attenuated or nonexistent. In contrast to the anterior ligaments which can be easily separated from the underlying annulus fibrosus, the posterior longitudinal ligament is strongly attached to the annulus fibers. Additional support is provided by the ligamentum flavum, an elastic structure which bridges the interlaminal spaces and reinforces the facet joint capsules, and the interspinous, intertransverse and iliolumbar ligaments.

Embryology.—The anlage of the spine forms in a right and left column on each side of the primitive notochord just anterior to the neural tube.[3] At a later stage of development the two halves fuse anteriorly and posteriorly around the developing spinal cord. It is failure of this process that accounts for the relatively frequent incidence of fusion defects; various degrees of spina bifida when posteriorly, and various degrees of platyspondyly and butterfly vertebrae when anteriorly. The latter conditions have a much rarer incidence than the former.

At the same time the vertebrae are formed also from a fusion of two embryonic parts in another plane; that is the lower portion of one sclerotome with the subjacent upper part of another.[11] Disturbances of this stage of development produce incomplete and asymmetrical segmentation and hemivertebrae.

As the lateral halves of the vertebral body fuse in the midline the notochord is forced above and below where its remnants concentrate to aid in the formation of the nucleus pulposus. This process when imperfect leads to defects in the cartilaginous plates. The annulus fibrosus which encloses the nucleus pulposus takes its origin from the mesenchyme left as the cephalad and caudad portions of the sclerotome separate to form the vertebral bodies.

The Sacrum and Pelvis.—The anatomical details of the sacrum do not warrant special description. The articulation between it and the fifth lumbar vertebra follows the pattern described above. The sacrum articulates with the pelvis by means of the two sacroiliac joints which are partly fibrous and partly diarthrodial. The surfaces of the fibrous portion of these joints are irregular and fit closely and snugly together. In the female pelvis there is less bony apposition than in the male and the ligaments are stronger. The cartilaginous surface of the sacrum is thicker and hyaline, that of the ilium thinner and fibrous. In both sexes some motion can and does take place but, with the exception of the late stages of pregnancy, the range is small and physiologically insignificant. The motion is in a rotary plane and is resisted in one direction by the wedge shape of the sacrum and in the other by the sacrotuberous and sacrospinous ligaments. We do believe, however, that increased compensatory motion can occur at the sacroiliac joints in cases that have had previous surgical fusions of the lumbar spine. Since the joint is supported by some of the densest ligaments of the body, it is doubtful that sacroiliac strain or "slipping" can occur without extensive injury, pregnancy, or disease. However, that portion of the joint which is lined, although imperfectly, by synovium is subject to all the diseases of diarthrodial joints, and is a common site of involvement for arthritic disease, whether infectious, rheumatoid, or degenerative.

The coccyx is composed of four segments, the first one of which is often free from the others. Motion can and does take place between the sacrum and coccyx. There is little ligamentous support of this joint and it is vulnerable to injury, but it is so situated as to be fairly well protected.

The Neural Structures.—The neural arch of each vertebra encloses the spinal cord, together with its supporting structures. Originally, the distal end of the cord extends to the caudal end of the dural sac at about the level of the third sacral segment, but it retracts upward as the spine grows in length to reach a final adult position at the level of the first

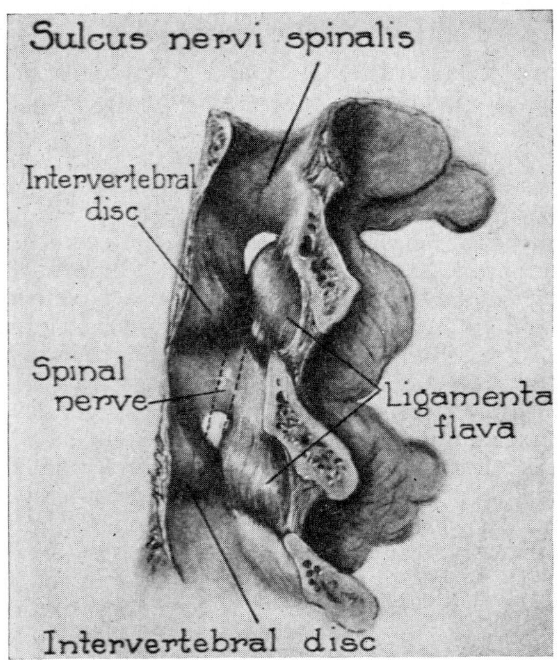

Fig. 82–2.—The relations of a typical lumbar nerve root. View of the 3rd and 4th intervertebral foramina from within the spinal canal. The vertebrae have been cut tangentially. Note the relation of the 4th lumbar nerve root (dotted lines) to the 3rd lumbar disc. At this level the root has less space than it does when opposite the 4th lumbar disc. It is thus more readily affected by protrusion of the 3rd lumbar disc than one of the 4th. Note also its relation to the facets, here hidden by the underlying portion of the capsule, the fibers of which blend with those of the ligamentum flavum. The nerve root is also in close contact with the pedicle. (Naffziger, Inman and Saunders, courtesy of Surg., Gynec. & Obst.)

lumbar vertebra. The nerve roots of the lumbosacral plexus are drawn up with the cord and lie within the dura, forming the cauda equina. A slender filament, the filum terminale, loosely anchors the distal end of the cord to the coccyx. Cephalad the cord is held by its origin from the brain. It is also fixed by the succession of spinal nerves which pass out through the intervertebral foramina. It is supported everywhere by its dural and arachnoidal membranes. Over this relatively immobile neural tube the spinal segments must move smoothly to perform their physiological functions.

Each nerve root leaves the spinal canal under its corresponding vertebral arch except in the cervical spine, where it leaves above. That is to say, the first cervical nerve root passes out *above* the first cervical vertebral arch, whereas the fifth lumbar nerve root leaves the canal *below* the fifth lumbar vertebral arch. The difference is made up by the presence of eight cervical nerves as opposed to seven cervical vertebrae, the 8th cervical nerve passing out of the intervertebral foramen between C7 and T1.

A nerve root is in intimate relation with several parts of the vertebra and discs as it passes from the dural sac to without the neural canal.[7,40,44] In the lower lumbar spine each nerve root, together with a sheath of dura, becomes separated from the remainder of the cauda equina at the level of the disc above, courses laterally as it passes distally across its corresponding vertebral body and reaches the intervertebral foramen at a point opposite its disc of the same numerical designation. For instance, the fifth lumbar nerve leaves the cauda equina just above the level of the fourth lumbar disc (the disc between L4 and L5), passes diagonally laterally, posterior to the 5th lumbar body to reach the intervertebral foramen between L5 and the sacrum. In the foramen it is held against the medial and inferior surfaces of the pedicle (in this case, of L5) lying in a groove called the sulcus nervi spinalis. Anteriorly, lies the body (of L5), inferiorly the bulging (5th) lumbar disc and posteriorly, shielded by ligamentum flavum, the inferior facet (of L5). Although the nerve root moves fairly freely in the intervertebral foramen, pathologic or traumatic disturbances of any of these structures (pedicle, body or facet) can obstruct its passage and cause pressure. More recently, transforaminal ligaments (reducing available space for passage of the nerve root through the lumbar intervertebral foramina) have been described.[19a] It is important to remember that the extradural courses of the lower lumbar roots are related to two discs: the one above and the one below their corresponding vertebrae.

Spinal Function

In utero the spine is formed in one long curve with its convexity directed posteriorly. After birth and with the gradual assumption of vertical posture, this curve is altered. Since the thoracic segment is relatively immobile, because of its attached ribs, the kyphosis (curve with convexity posteriorly) persists in this area. However, as strength develops to allow the infant to raise its head and then sit and finally stand, lordoses (curves with their convexities directed anteriorly) develop first in the cervical segment and then in the lumbar segment. By this means balance is achieved and the weight of the trunk is carried directly over its base. As long as the curves anteriorly and posteriorly balance each other, the erect position can be maintained with surprisingly little muscular effort. The lordotic curves are entirely functional, and can be reversed by bending forward, in contrast to the kyphotic thoracic curve which is relatively fixed.

There are two essential forces which are responsible for the development of these curves. One is the anterior tilt of the pelvis produced by the downward pull of the iliopsoas muscles and hip capsules, and the other the extending force of the massive erector spinae. However, once the spine is balanced in the erect position, the muscular forces in various directions become purely stabilizing in effect. Thus, if the normal erect posture is not disturbed, it is possible to stand with little or no muscular effort and the ligaments act mainly as check-reins to prevent excessive motion.

In the cervical region, the motion is remarkably free in all planes. The vertebral bodies are small, the discs relatively thick and the planes of the facets more nearly horizontal. In the thoracic region there is relatively little motion in any plane since the rib cage restricts the lateral and rotary motions, the discs are thin and the vertebral bodies relatively large in diameter, but the facets are oriented to guide motion mainly in the direction of flexion and extension. In the lumbar spine motion is largely in flexion and extension. On bending forward, the lumbar lordosis is reversed and on extension it is accentuated. Lateral inclination and rotation occur mainly at the thoracolumbar junction.

Generally speaking, those muscles which lie anterior to the small posterior articulations, including the abdominals especially, act as flexors, and those posterior as extensors. The actions of the muscle groups on one side result in lateral inclination. Rotation is produced by more complex muscle combinations. It is important to remember, however, that since many of the spinal motions are performed in the erect position, that the force of gravity can never be discounted and, once started, the muscles opposing that motion performed are the ones called into play in order to prevent loss of balance. For instance, on bending to the right the muscles on the left side of the spine must act in order to prevent falling to the right. This description of function represents a great oversimplification of spinal kinesiology, but will serve as a basis for understanding the principles discussed elsewhere in this chapter.

The Nature of Pain in Somatic Structures

There is one more basic item to be discussed in relation to low back pain in order to understand it more clearly, and that is the source and character of the pain itself.[29,36]

The foremost differentiation to be made is that between pain from deep skeletal structures and pain from direct nerve pressure.[13] Almost everyone is familiar with the nature of the latter as seen in the "funny or crazy bone" sensation after the ulnar nerve is suddenly bumped. Faradic stimulation of a peripheral mixed nerve results in the same sensation. The onset of pain is rapid, it follows the distribution of the sensory portion of the ulnar nerve and is associated with numbness and tingling when severe. If we substitute for the peripheral mixed ulnar nerve a single spinal nerve root, we will find that the sensation is the same in character, but confined to the peripheral representation or dermatome of that nerve root. The pain is sharp, lancinating and accompanied by paresthesia and numbness. It may be accompanied by muscle cramps. This is "*neuralgia*."

If the pressure is severe and prolonged, the nerve is deadened, the property of conduction is lost even though the fibers are still in continuity. The larger nerve fibers, that is, those mediating touch and motor stimuli, lose their function first, followed in order by the progressively smaller ones. Pain fibers, though large and small, are, in general, smaller than those for touch and motor conduction, and their function may be unimpaired if pressure is relieved soon enough.

The properties described above hold only for sudden forceful pressure on a nerve. In the case of gradual or intermittent pressure, the stimulus may not be sufficient at any time to excite the nerve tissue and its presence may remain undetected until paresis develops. This is not infrequently the case in gradually developing gibbus consequent to tuberculosis.

Quite different is the pain produced by stimuli within deep skeletal structures (ligaments, fascia, muscle and periosteum). Here the pain is vaguely localized, aching in character, radiating over great distances, slow in onset and long in duration. When severe it is often accompanied by sweating, nausea and vomiting. The patterns of radiation are consistent for one point of stimulation, but the extent of radiation depends on the intensity of stimulation. Experimental data have accumulated which show that the pattern of radiation is fairly consistent from one individual to another. Although these "sclerotomes" appear to have a segmental representation, they do not follow the patterns of corresponding dermatomes. The sclerotome and dermatome coincide more nearly in the midportion of the trunk than they do in the extremities.

The pain thresholds of different somatic structures are variable.[26] The periosteum is most sensitive, followed by ligaments and fibrous joint capsules, tendons, fascia and muscle in that order. Ligaments and capsules are particularly sensitive at points close to their osseous attachments. Bone for the most part is insensitive, although its endosteal surface apparently contains some pain perceptive nerves.

It is important to understand the difference between this "deep" pain and the "superficial" pain of skin. The difference can be readily demonstrated by pinching a small piece of skin (superficial pain) and squeezing a web space between the fingers (deep pain). This simple experiment is not completely accurate since the modality of touch in the skin helps to localize the deep pain elicited. From experimental evidence it would appear that the more superficially situated deep structures show fairly accurate localization of pain source. Thus, stimulation of periosteum overlying the subcutaneous surface of the tibia can be pointed out relatively accurately by the subject. However, pain from deeply situated periosteum, as in the spine, is poorly localized and diffuse with radiation to considerable distance from the source.

In this respect another point to be stressed is that a stimulus in any one portion of a segmental sclerotome may give rise to pain which, for the subject, will not vary though the stimulus be applied at different points. Thus, Kellgren[30] has shown that pain provoked from the testis, abdominal obliques, and multifidus (1st lumbar segment) was of a similar pattern and character, though usually a little more intense near the site of stimulation. Further observations by Lewis and Kellgren[37] have shown that the sclerotomal pain is accompanied by superficial tenderness and muscle rigidity. Clinicians familiar with these phenomena in visceral disease are often less cognizant of the fact that skeletal lesions often behave similarly.

HISTORY AND EXAMINATION

Medical History

A patient who consults a physician because of a sudden twist of the spine with subsequent low back pain does not present a diagnostic problem from the point of view of cause and effect. But in the majority of cases the pain is spontaneous in onset and a carefully taken history will help greatly to ascertain the cause.

A general appraisal should include sex, age, race, economic and social background, past medical history and a general system review. The type of work and daily habits are important to ascertain. Relevant points in the family history should be sought.

An analysis of the pain itself is then necessary, and should proceed along two lines: one concerned with the chronological aspect (*i.e.*, onset, development and reaction to previous treatment), the other, with the character. Chronologically, one should ascertain when and where the pain began; also was its onset associated with injury or illness? If there was an injury, was it on the job or involving liability? Has the pain remained the same, gotten worse or better? Is it intermittent or have there been periods of amelioration or exacerbation? Has there been any change in the site of pain, or has it extended to involve hitherto painless areas? Have there been aggravating incidents since its onset and if so what? Has there been any kind of treatment, self-administered or otherwise and with what effect?

The character of the pain may be analyzed in various ways:

1. *Severity.*—This is an individually variable factor and should be interpreted with caution. Useful indices include inability to work, confinement to bed and sleeplessness.
2. *Quality.*—This is also variable and depends much on previous experience. Therefore its usefulness is somewhat questionable. However, one should differentiate somatic from nerve root pain insofar as possible (*see* page 1516).
3. *Localization.*—This is most important though it is often hard for the patient to locate his pain accurately. A point of origin will usually be recognized. Distal radiation is often present. The extent of radiation in many instances may be used as a rough index of the severity of the lesion. The type of radiation should be distinguished again into either a nerve root type or into the vaguely localized deep aching pain that is so characteristic of irritation of skeletal structures.

4. *Duration.*—Here it is determined whether the pain is steady in duration or intermittent. If it is steady, is it at all times the same or does it have periods of exacerbation? If it is intermittent, at what times do the pains seem to occur? Is it a night or early morning pain suggesting a joint source? Is it a pain associated with work or with being active, suggesting strain, or does it occur only with certain movements?
5. *Reduplication.* — Has the patient found he can, during the time of the examination, reduplicate his pain or can it be produced by some technique of examination?
6. *Aggravation.*—Is the pain aggravated by coughing or sneezing, by bending or lifting, and if so is it reproduced in full or only in part?
7. *Alleviation.*—Is the pain relieved by rest, or by any particular types of medication? Is it relieved by manipulation, by gentle activity, or by vigorous exercise?

General Appraisal.—In general, it will be sufficient to note whether the individual is stocky and heavy-set with heavy musculature and strong ligaments and tight joints, or whether he is sthenic, tall and lithe, with relatively relaxed joint structure, ligaments and muscles. Are the legs well aligned? Are the feet pronated? Are the knees bowed, straight or in some valgus? Are there any abnormal or suggestive skin pigmentations? A café-au-lait mark may signify an underlying neurofibromatosis.

If, in the history, any points of suspicion have come up relative to other systems, these should be investigated before proceeding with the specific examination of the back.

Stance and Posture.—The posterior aspect of the back is first viewed. It should be noted whether the iliac crests are level, whether the spine is straight or curved and whether there is a list to one side or the other. In the human being there is a strong reflex to keep the head centered over the feet and the eyes level. Thus, in the normal individual a deviation of the spinal column from the vertical is compensated by an opposite deviation elsewhere whenever possible. From the point of view of the spine, full compensation signifies that the first thoracic vertebra is centered over the sacrum, no matter what the spine does in between. If the spine is uncompensated, that is, if the first thoracic vertebra is not centered over the sacrum, the patient is spoken of as having a list. A convenient measurement of list is that of dropping a perpendicular from the first thoracic spine and measuring how far to right or left of the gluteal cleft it falls. If a list is present, a lateral curvature of the spine (scoliosis) must be present also. The scoliosis may be classified as structural or nonstructural. In the former, intrinsic structural changes of the vertebral column and thoracic rib cage will be present and may commonly be detected by asking the patient to bend forward and viewing the trunk from behind. Asymmetry will be noted with the high side on the convex side of the curve. In nonstructural scoliosis no intrinsic anatomical changes occur and no asymmetry will be found on forward bending. It is the latter that commonly occurs secondary to pain and may be termed "sciatic scoliosis."

A scoliosis is designated right or left depending on the direction of its convexity (right scoliosis—curve convex to right). The curve pattern of the scoliosis is designated by the apex of the curve (thoracic curve—apex at thoracic level, thoracolumbar curve—apex at junction of thoracic and lumbar spine, lumbar curve—apex at lumbar level). Usually the pelvis is level in nonstructural and structural scoliosis. If not, some other causes for the pelvic obliquity should be sought, such as a gross decompensation of the curves or a short leg or a hip contracture.

The patient is then viewed from the side. The posture is noted. It is normal to stand with a slight degree of lumbar lordosis (anterior curve) and dorsal kyphosis (posterior curve). Increase or

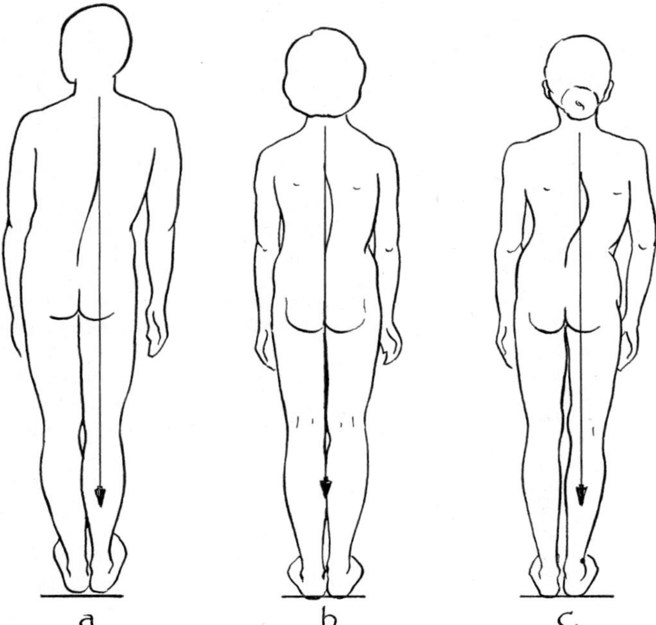

Fig. 82–3.—Compensated and uncompensated deviations of posture. A plumb line dropped from the 1st thoracic spinal process indicates a right list (*a*); a compensated right thoracolumbar scoliosis (*b*); and an uncompensated right thoracic, left lumbar scoliosis with right list (*c*). List, or decompensation, causes prominence of the hip opposite to the direction of the list.

decrease of these curves should be noted. Very often the muscle spasm in acute low back pain will cause flattening of the lumbar lordosis. In the sagittal plane, as well as in the transverse, man shows a very strong tendency to maintain balance, that is, to have the head centered over the feet. The curves in between will tend to balance one another. Thus, if the dorsal kyphosis is increased, the lumbar lordosis is usually increased. Sometimes, such a state of affairs does not exist and in order to balance an increased dorsal kyphosis, the patient will stand with a posterior over-carriage, that is, leaning backwards. Over-carriage is to the sagittal plane, what list is to the transverse.

The degree of forward inclination of the pelvis should be noted. Is the abdomen pendulous and is the chest well developed or does the patient stand with a very narrow anteroposterior thoracic diameter? There is a tendency for the sthenic body type to have a narrow chest and for the heavy body type to have just the opposite.

An analysis of the position in stance is completed by a brief survey from the front. Here again list may be noted and the anterior superior iliac spines palpated to check whether the pelvis is level or not. It should be added that slight degrees of curvature of the spine are difficult to detect especially in heavy-set individuals. Certain things may lead one to suspect the presence of a structural scoliosis; that is, a prominent hip, a flank crease on one side or the other, prominence of one side of the chest or of the opposite shoulder blade, or a high shoulder.

Spinal Motions.—The spine is now analyzed in movement. Again viewing the patient from the back, he is asked to bend forward. The lordotic curve of the lumbar spine should first flatten and

THE DORSAL AND LUMBAR SPINE (FLEXION)

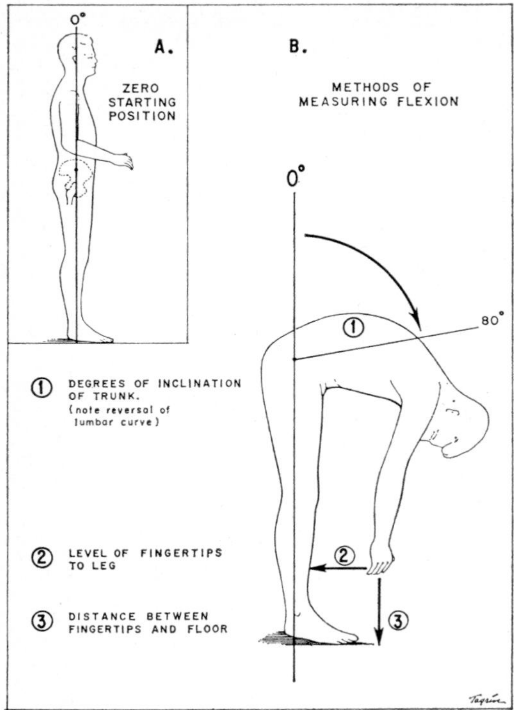

FIG. 82–4.—Measurement of spinal motion.

A.
ZERO STARTING POSITION: The correct standing position.

B.—Flexion

Four clinical methods of estimating the range of spinal flexion.

1. By measuring the degrees of forward inclination of the trunk in relation to the longitudinal axis of the body. The examiner should "fix" the pelvis with his hands. The loss (or not) of lordosis should also be noted.
2. By indicating the level the fingertips reach along the patient's leg. For instance, fingertips to the patella; or fingertips to midtibia.
3. By measuring the distance in inches or centimeters between the fingertips and the floor.
4. By the steel or plastic tape measure method.

(Contination)
METHODS OF
MEASURING
SPINAL
FLEXION

C7

S1

④ THE STEEL TAPE MEASURING METHOD

C. THE PATIENT STANDING ERECT

C.—The Steel Tape Measure Method

4. This is perhaps the most accurate clinical method of measuring true motion of the spine in flexion. The flexible steel or plastic tape adjusts very accurately to the thoracic and lumbar contours of the spine.

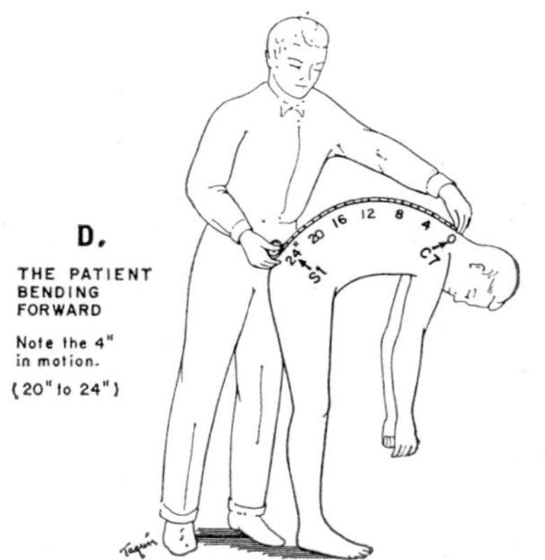

D.—

As the patient bends forward, if the lumbar curve reverses, and the spinous processes spread, this will be indicated by lengthening of the tape measure. In the normal healthy adult, there is, on the average, an increase of 4 inches in forward flexion. If the patient bends forward with his back straight (as in rheumatoid spondylitis), the tape will not record motion. One is able to record motion of the thoracic spine per se, by taping from the spinous process of C7 to T12. Likewise, motion of the lumbar spine can be measured from the spinous process of T12 to S1. Usually, if the total spine in flexion is 4 inches the examiner will find that 1 inch occurs in the dorsal spine, and 3 inches occurs in the lumbar spine.

THE DORSAL AND LUMBAR SPINE
LATERAL BENDING

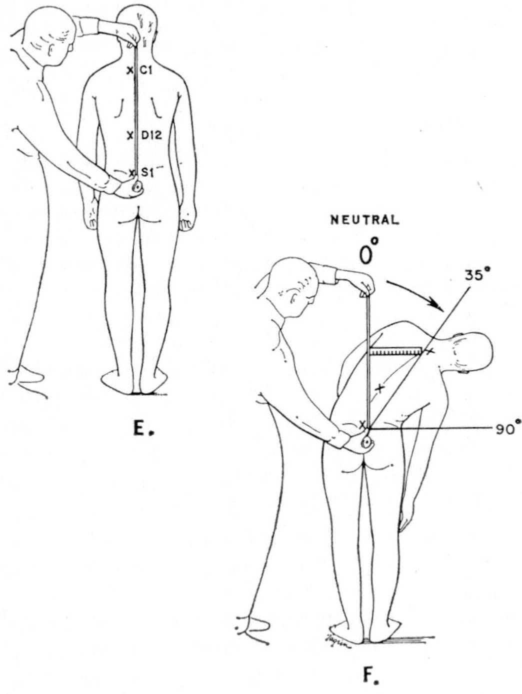

E and F.—Lateral Bending

The vertical steel tape, if held firmly and straight, may also aid in measuring the motion of lateral bending. This can be estimated in:

(1) The degrees of lateral inclination of the trunk, or,
(2) By noting position of spinous process of C7 with relation to pelvis.
(3) Note level of lumbar spine reflecting base of lateral motion. This level may be lumbosacral or higher and may vary from right to left in the same patient.
(4) The knee joint may be used as fixed point. Record distance of fingertips from the knee joint on lateral bending (see F).

THE DORSAL AND LUMBAR SPINE (EXTENSION)

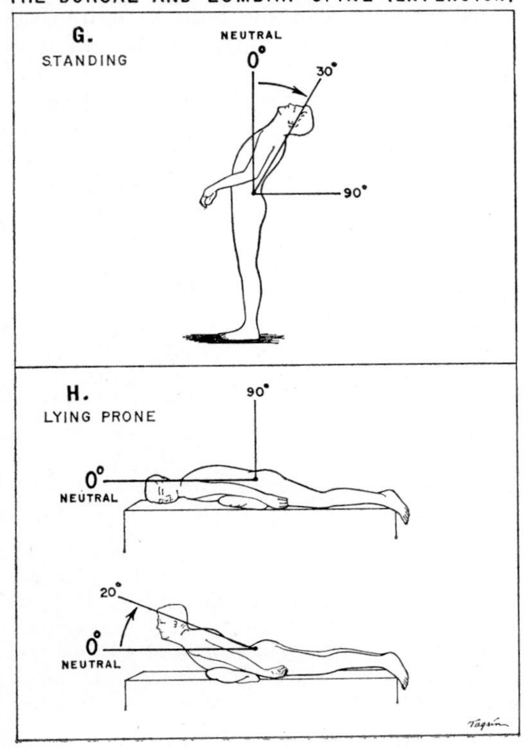

G.—Extension Standing

The range of extension is recorded by degrees.

H.—Extension Lying Prone

The range of motion in this position is measured by degrees, in relation to the position of the spinous process of C7.

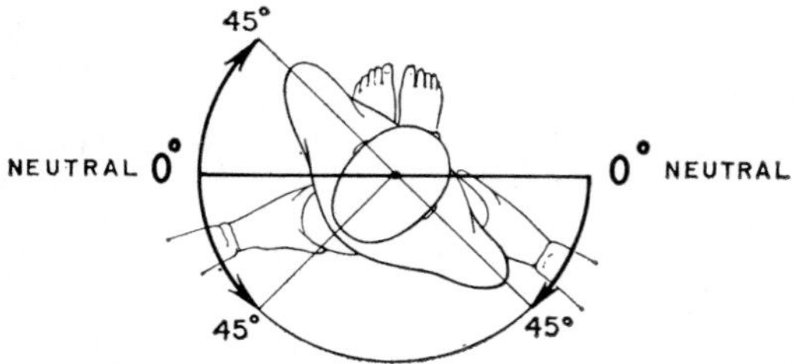

I.—Rotation

To estimate the degrees of rotation of the spine, the pelvis must be held firmly by the examiner's hands, and the patient is instructed to rotate to the right or left. This motion is recorded in degrees, or in percentages of motion, as compared to individuals of similar age and physical build.

then reverse slightly as the degree of forward bending increases. If it does not do so, the motion is limited, even though the patient is able to touch the floor. The patient should be watched to see if he bends straight forward or whether he tends to list off to one side or the other as he bends forward. If he does so, it may suggest some restriction of straight-leg raising on the opposite side. If a scoliosis has been detected in the erect position, this should again be checked in the flexed position to determine whether it is structural. The associated rotation of the vertebrae will produce a prominence of the thorax and overlying scapula on the side of convexity. In a lumbar scoliosis the rotation is not so readily evident but can be detected by prominence of the paravertebral muscles on the side of the convexity and a depression of those on the opposite side. In cases of very slight degree of scoliosis, forward flexion is the best position for detection since the deformity is accentuated. When the patient is bent forward it is also wise to view his back from the side. There is usually a smooth curve with its convexity posteriorly extending from the base of the skull to the sacrum. If the curve is broken and becomes more sharply angular at any point, it should be recorded. This is very often the case in structural round back (*i.e.*, "epiphysitis" of the spine).

The degree of backward bending is

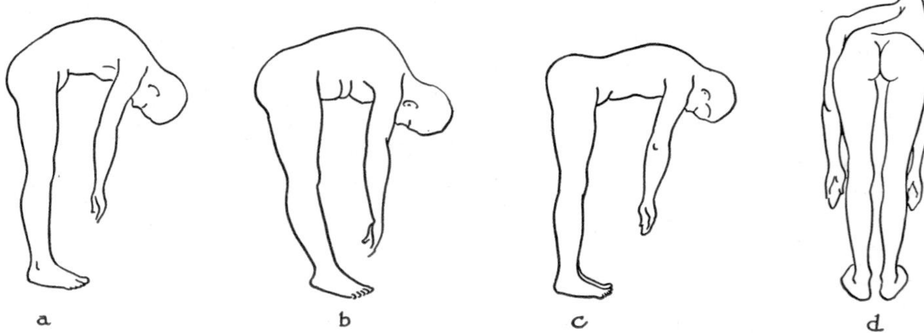

FIG. 82–5.—Forward bending. *a*, Normally on forward bending there is an even contour of the spine when viewed laterally. *b*, An accentuation of the dorsal kyphosis indicates a dorsal round back, especially when the apex of the curve is sharp and angular. *c*, A persistence of the lumbar lordotic curve in the position of forward bending indicates that the lumbar spine has lost its flexibility. The flexion is all taking place at the hip joints. *d*, When viewed posteriorly minor degrees of structural scoliosis can readily be detected in the position of forward bending. The convex rotation of the thoracic vertebrae is easily recognized since it is accentuated by the rib deformity or hump. Similar rotation of the lumbar segment is more difficult to detect.

then determined. This will be accompanied by an increase in the lordotic curve. If the degree of lordosis does not increase, then the motion is limited. After returning to the upright position, the patient is asked to bend to one side and then to the other. The normal one will show an equivalent degree of bending to both sides with a smooth curve starting at the sacrum. Limitation of motion can be detected in one of two ways. The maximum degree of motion may not be as much to one side as to the other, or the curve on bending to one side may be broken and begin at a higher level than it does to the other side.

In examination of the lower back, the motions of flexion, extension and lateral bending are those most important to analyze. However, it is often wise to check the whole spine and the patient should be asked to demonstrate the degree of rotation lacing his fingers behind his neck. This motion will occur chiefly in the thoracic region. The degree of cervical lordosis and cervical motions should also be noted. The findings are rechecked in the sitting position, where normally the lordosis will flatten and a scoliosis, if functional, will tend to disappear.

Measurements.—The patient is next asked to lie supine on the examining table. A patient with acute pain can be made more comfortable by placing a pillow under the knees. Measurements of the thigh and calf at equivalent points above and below the patellae should be made and recorded. If there is atrophy, it may be due to disuse or to neuromuscular disease. The patient is next carefully positioned so that the pelvis is level and the hips are placed in a neutral degree of abduction and adduction. The leg lengths are then recorded using the bony landmarks of the anterior superior iliac spine and medial malleolus. In the presence of a fixed deformity of one hip or the other the measurement loses some of its significance and, to be accurate, the lower extremities must have equivalent relationships to the pelvis.

Hip Motions.—The hip movements are now analyzed. Flexion contracture is noted by maximally flexing the opposite hip to flatten the lumbar lordosis and measuring the degree of the angle between the horizontal surface of the table and the maximally extended extremity. The movements of each hip in abduction, adduction, internal and external rotation should be measured. The arcs of rotation are usually most easily obtained rotating the foot and leg inward (external rotation), and outward (internal rotation) with the hips flexed to 90°.

Passive Spinal Movements.—Movements of the lumbar spine are now performed passively by grasping both legs with the knees bent, and flexing the spine maximally. Keeping the hips flexed to 90° the pelvis is then inclined laterally and then rotated on the spine. Note is made if these motions produce pain.

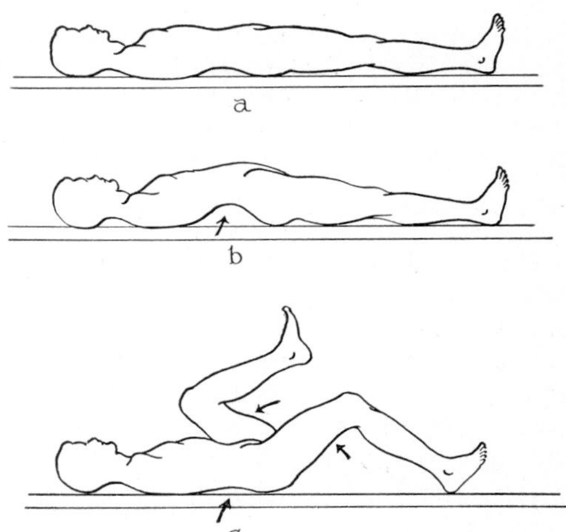

FIG. 82–6.—Lumbar lordosis and hip flexion contracture. An inability to fully extend one or both hips may produce an increase in the lumbar lordosis in the standing or lying positions. The angle of the deformity can be determined by flattening the lordosis. This is brought about by maximum flexion of the opposite hip. *a*, Normal. *b*, Flexion deformity of the hip is masked by increase in the lumbar lordosis. *c*, Flexion of the opposite hip flattens the lumbar spine to the table and indicates the true situation.

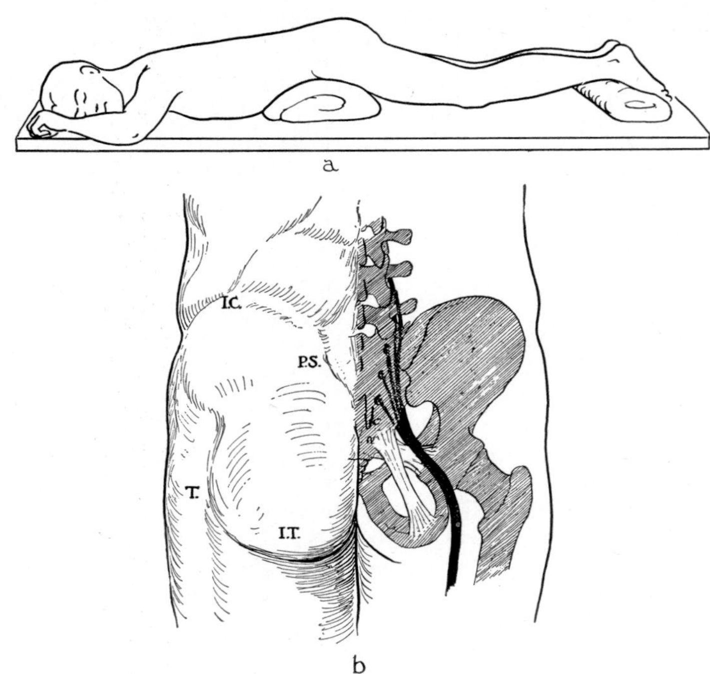

FIG. 82–7.—Palpation of the back. *a*, Good positioning is necessary for adequate examination. When the lumbar spine is flat, the bony elements are more easily distinguished from one another. The interspinous and interlaminal spaces are opened. *b*, Useful landmarks include the iliac crest (I.C.), the posterior superior iliac spine (P.S.), the greater trochanters (T) and the ischial tuberosities (I.T.). The position of the sacrosciatic notch and course of the sciatic nerve should always be kept in mind. The lumbar roots are shielded from palpation in their extraspinal course.

Palpation and Tenderness.—The patient is next asked to lie prone with a pillow under his abdomen. The thickness of the pillow should be sufficient to flatten the lumbar lordosis. The lower spine and structures of the back are carefully palpated. Tightness or spasm of paravertebral muscles is noted. At all times the patient must be fully relaxed. Points of tenderness are recorded. Just as in examination of the abdomen, the anatomical structures under the examining finger must constantly be kept in mind. The spine of each lumbar vertebra is pressed and the interspaces between are palpated. It is sometimes advantageous to examine the patient acutely flexed lying on his side in order to more easily palpate the bony spinous processes and the interspinous ligaments. Adjacent spinous processes can be grasped from the side by the examiner and rotated in opposite directions in order to better differentiate the source of pain. Useful landmarks are the iliac crests; a horizontal from these usually runs across the fourth lumbar process; and the posterior superior iliac spines which lie opposite the second sacral spine. The sacrosciatic notch is palpated where tenderness may indicate irritation of one or more roots of the sciatic nerve. The thighs and calves must also be palpated in any case where there is extension of pain into the legs. The region of the trochanters should also be examined.

Percussion Tenderness.—Pressure or percussion over the interlaminal spaces, may, in the cases of disc herniation, produce sharp lancinating pain radiating into the lower extremities. Since in the position of extension the lumbar lordosis is increased, the vertebral spinous processes are brought closer together and it is difficult to distinguish the separate processes. For this reason, it is most important to have the back flattened or the lumbar lordosis reversed. If this cannot be achieved in the prone position with a pillow under the abdomen, the patient may be asked to bend over the examining table. He can usually do this despite the presence of pain, if the knees are flexed and the weight is borne upon the abdomen.

Rectal Examination.—A rectal examination is usually advisable and especially in those cases with coccygeal pain. The coccyx may be grasped between the finger in the rectum, and the thumb outside and moved about. Its angle of inclination should be noted; the freedom of movement should be noted; also the presence of pain on movement. The levator ani and coccygeus muscles, sacrotuberous and sacrospinalis ligaments are palpated on either side of the sacrum and tenderness noted. In thin individuals the region of the sacrosciatic notch can often be reached and bimanual palpation of this region is possible. The rectal examination is completed with palpation of the pelvic viscera. Tenderness in the sacroiliac joint may be elicited by pressure exerted over it. This joint lies between the posterior inferior spine and superior border of the sciatic notch.

Vaginal Examination. — Bimanual vaginal examination with cytological smear should be performed in indicated cases. For the physician who does not feel qualified in such an examination the patient may be referred to a gynecologist.

Neurological Examination.—It is important to analyze the knee and ankle jerks. The best position for eliciting the knee jerks is one of sitting with the legs hanging free: that for the ankle jerks is one of kneeling on a chair with a pillow under the legs, the feet projecting out from the edge of the seat. The reflexes can be reinforced if necessary by the patient contracting the muscles of the upper extremities with the fingers locked together. If the reflexes are tested carefully in this fashion, small discrepancies will be of much greater significance than if the testing is done casually. Gluteus maximus, medial hamstring and posterior tibial reflex responses should also be determined. However, they are more difficult to elicit and, therefore, most significant when absent on one side, and present on the other. Babinski's sign is also tested.

Sensory examination is performed with the point of a pin and light stroke of the finger or cotton.[28] Significant zones of sensory disturbance will be found in this manner and if so the examination can be repeated in more detail including heat and cold sensation.

Atrophy of the buttocks must be determined from inspection and palpation. Although atrophy of the thigh (especially the quadriceps) and that of the calf (especially the triceps surae) may be visible, circumferential measurements may be helpful in detecting them. The ability to walk on tiptoe and on the heel, the ability to do a deep knee bend, and the ability to stand on one leg alone should be tested. The manner of walking should be observed and the cause of limp, if one is present, determined. More accurate analysis of motor function is done by testing the strength of muscle action in various planes, but may be omitted for practical purposes unless some previous point of history or physical examination leads one to suspect nerve root compression. The power of dorsiflexion of the great toe, of the lateral four toes, and of the entire foot should be analyzed and compared on the two sides. Similarly, the forces of inversion, eversion, and plantar flexion of the foot and of the toes can be tested. Power of hip flexion when sitting, and of knee extension when supine are easily determined. When the patient is in a good deal of pain, or when movement is accompanied by pain, weakness of function should be given less significance. Also the inability of some patients, and especially that of older ones, to coordinate may interfere with muscle examination of this kind.

Special Tests.—Many special tests have been championed for their usefulness in pinpointing the source of back pain. They are usually titled by the name of their originator, or by that of their latest avid supporter. The signs of Lasegue, Goldthwaite, and Faber are some well-known examples. Although these tests have varying degrees of useful-

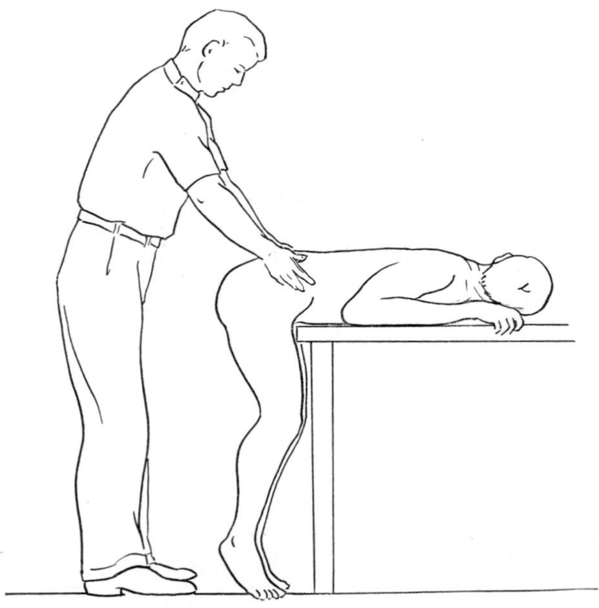

Fig. 82–8.—Percussion test. With the patient positioned as shown the interlaminal spaces are opened as much as possible. In the case of irritation of a nerve root, sharp percussion or deep pressure may reproduce the sciatic distribution of pain. This is especially true in the presence of disc herniation since the nerve root is forced posteriorly in the spinal canal. This position is also a good one for palpation of the back.

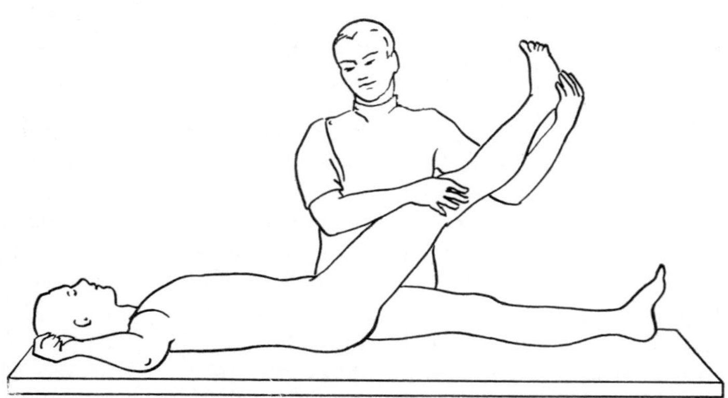

Fig. 82–9.—Straight leg raising. The leg being tested should be utterly relaxed and resting in the examiner's hand. The knee is fully extended and kept from flexing by gentle pressure against the patella.

ness, we have found that in practice the methods of performing them vary tremendously. To avoid confusion, it is best to describe the maneuvers one uses as accurately as possible and to include one's interpretation of them. For example, the phrase "straight leg raising of 45 degrees causes pain radiating to the calf" means much more than "Lasegue sign, positive." The preciseness of such reporting is well worth the time and space given to it.

Straight Leg Raising Test of Lasegue.[16]—This is without doubt one of the most useful maneuvers in analysis of low back disorders. It does two things. First, it stretches the roots of the lumbosacral plexus by putting tension on the sciatic nerve, a tension that increases as the leg is raised higher. Secondly, it flattens the lumbar spine by putting tension on the extensor muscles of the hip and hamstrings as they pass from the pelvis to the femur and tibia. Thus, a nerve root lesion is not prerequisite for painful or restricted straight leg raising. On the other hand, it is quite true that the restriction of straight leg raising is usually much more marked in lesions affecting the nerve roots than it is in purely skeletal ones. The angle of straight leg raising, which is limited by tightness of the hamstring muscles, is normally less in sthenic than it is in asthenic individuals.

The test is performed passively by the examiner and the patient must be made to relax. The knee is held extended and the leg is raised gradually from the table until the point of pain is reached. Not only is this point important to record but the patient should also be asked to describe the extent and radiation of the pain. In nerve root lesions, the typical pattern of radiation may be reproduced.

Sitting Knee Extension Test.—While the patient is sitting, one knee is extended. The patient should be observed to see if and at what angle of extension he leans backward. He should be asked whether the test is painful and if so, whether the pain is localized to his back, or whether it radiates. The maneuver is repeated on the other side and the two sides then compared. Occasionally extension of one knee will cause aggravation of "sciatica" in the opposite leg. This test is very similar to the straight leg raising one, but with one major difference, and that is that in the sitting position the lumbar lordosis is usually largely obliterated.

Popliteal Compression.—When radiating pain is produced, either by sitting knee-extension or by straight leg raising, it can often be aggravated by pressure over the

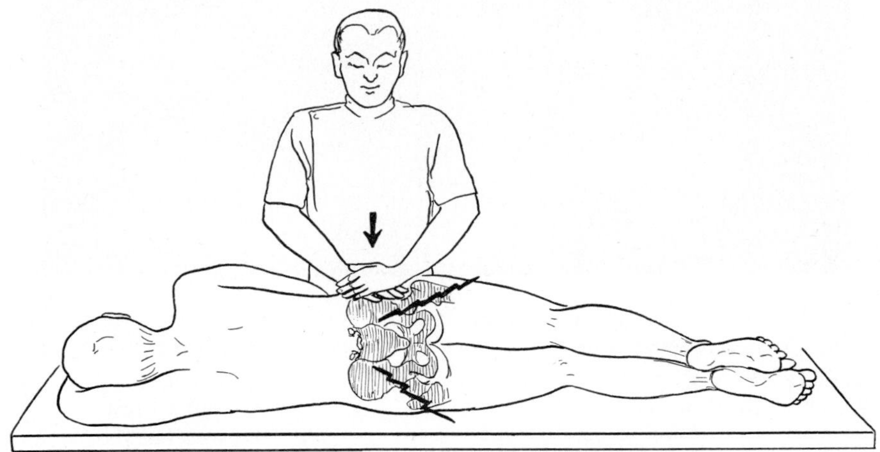

Fig. 82–10.—The iliac compression test. The position of lateral recumbency is the most satisfactory in which to elicit the pain of sacroiliac disease. Compression of the joint is produced by downward pressure of the examiner's hands.

course of the tibial nerve through the popliteal space. When this is so, it is an additional finding in favor of root compression.

Jugular Compression (*Naffziger*[40]).—This test should be performed wherever there is suspected involvement of the spinal cord or nerve roots. It is performed by placing a blood pressure cuff about the neck and inflating it to 40 mm. Hg and holding it there for the length of one minute. By this method cerebrospinal fluid pressure is increased. The patient is asked to indicate when and if his pain is reproduced and if it is reproduced accurately. When the exact pattern of the patient's leg pain is reproduced, the test is practically pathognomonic of an intraspinal lesion. A negative test, however, is not as significant.

Iliac Compression Test.—Of all the tests that have been described as pathognomonic of sacroiliac disease, the test of iliac compression is the most sensitive. It is performed most easily with the patient lying on his side. The examiner applies firm pressure against the uppermost iliac crest. When positive, pain will be produced in the region of the involved sacroiliac joint. Other signs which suggest sacroiliac disease are: pain in the region of that joint on passive abduction of one or both hips while they are flexed; tenderness along the superior bony margin of the sacroiliac notch; lower quadrant abdominal tenderness; and tenderness in the region of the joint on rectal examination.

Passive Extension Test.—This test is performed with the patient lying on his

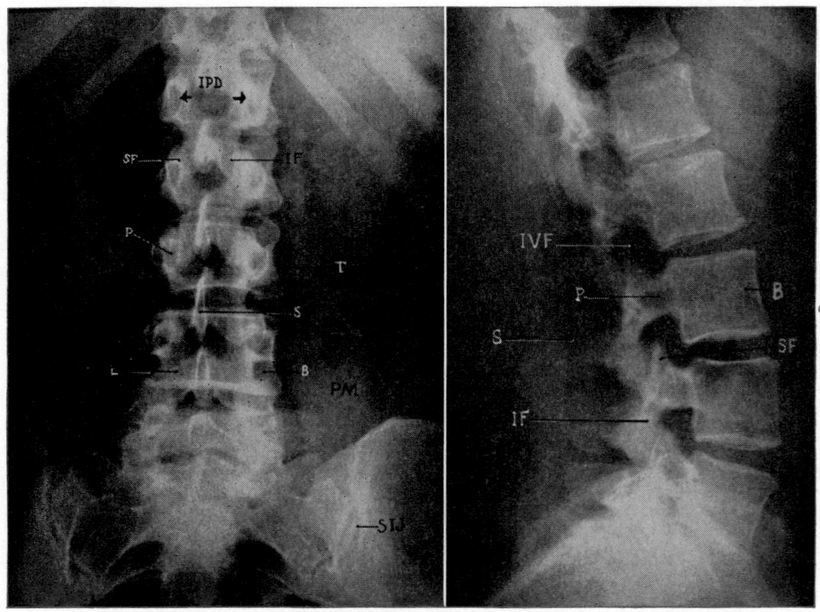

Fig. 82–11.—X rays of normal spine. A.P. and lateral x rays of lumbar spine—see page 1529 of text for technique. Note good detail of most of lumbar spine but obscurity of lumbosacral region.

Legend:
B—body
D—disc space
I—isthmus or pars interarticularis
IF—inferior facet
IVF—intervertebral foramen
L—lamina
P—pedicle
PM—psoas margin
S—spinous process
SF—superior facet
SIJ—sacroiliac joint
T—transverse process
IPD—interpedicular diameter

back at the foot of the examining table. The extremities are supported by the examiner with the hips and knees flexed. First, the uninvolved lower extremity is lowered. There is no pain. The involved leg is then gradually lowered extending the spine and pain develops. The unaffected extremity is then flexed maximally, thus flattening the lumbar spine, and the pain is relieved. If this test produces pain with radiation similar to that which the patient experiences spontaneously it is highly suggestive of root compression. Other lesions of the back, however, may be associated with pain on hyperextension.

The back examination is now finished. As can be seen, it requires considerable exertion by the patient. In acute cases it will not always be possible to do it completely. However, it will often be found that after a day or two of rest and sedation, a more satisfactory analysis can be carried out.

X-ray Examination

A routine examination of the back is not complete unless x rays have been made. To the trained observer, an A.P. and a lateral view of the entire lumbar spine and sacrum often suffice. First A.P. and lateral views are made of the lumbar spine with the x-ray tube centered at the upper lumbar region and inclined slightly distally (10°). A true or 45° A.P. of the lumbosacral region is then obtained. For this view the direction of the tube is adjusted to the inclination of the sacrum. The actual angle of the tube is usually nearer 30° than 45°. The tube itself is centered opposite the third or fourth lumbar vertebra. If the technique is good, detail of the vertebral bodies, sacrum, sacroiliac and intervertebral joints should be good enough for the detection of significant abnormalities including defects of the neural arch and facets.

Special roentgenographic views are used only to obtain better detail of spinal parts or to detect the presence of specific pathologic processes. Oblique views show the intervertebral foramina and lesions of the neural arch and facets exceptionally well. The x-ray technique is difficult, however. A P.A. film made with the patient standing and bending

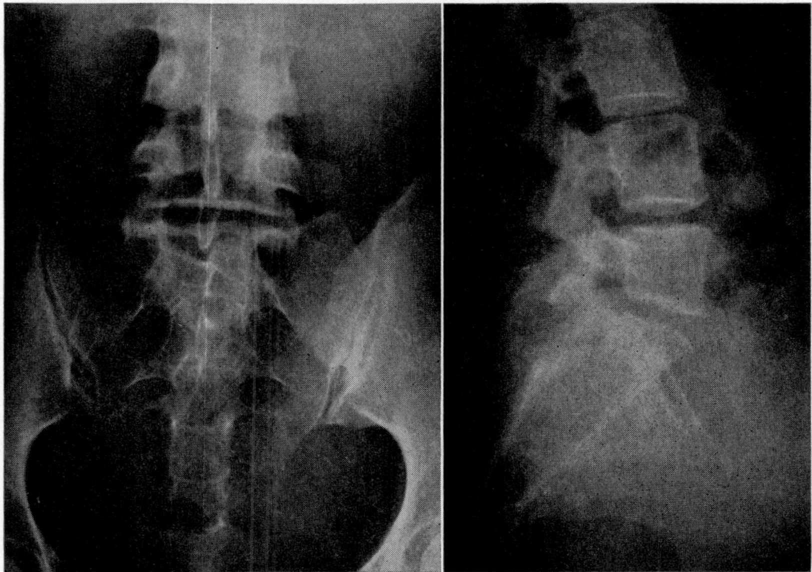

Fig. 82–12.—45° A.P. and lateral x rays of lumbosacral level and sacrum. Note good detail of 5th lumbar vertebra, sacrum, lumbosacral disc space and sacroiliac joints.

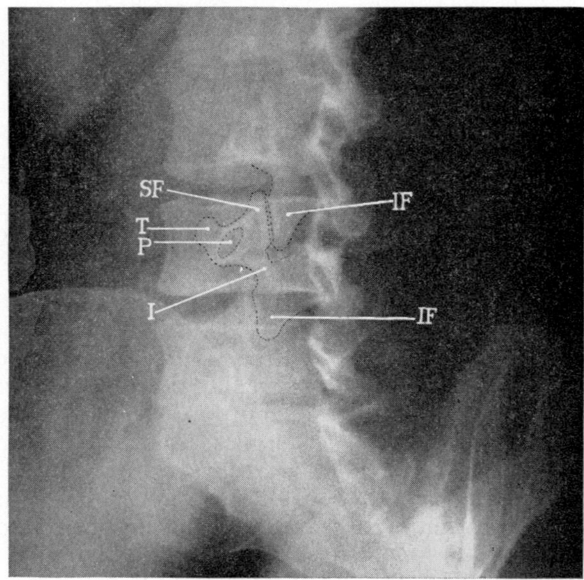

FIG. 82–13.—Oblique x ray of lumbar spine. Note good detail of facets and pars interarticularis. (See Fig. 82–11 for legend.)

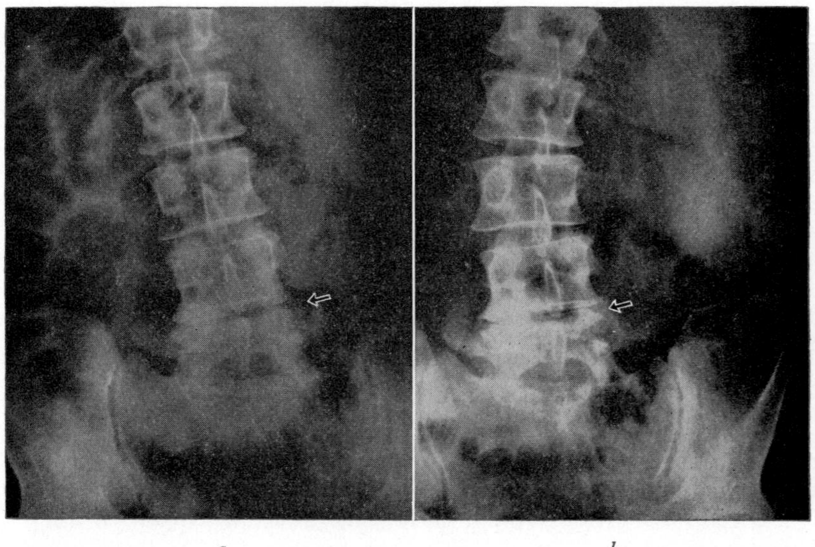

FIG. 82–14.—Lateral bending films. P.A. x rays of lumbar spine in left (*a*) and right (*b*) bending. In *a* the entire spine bends to the left and all the interspaces are wider on the right than on the left. In *b* the 4th lumbar space (*arrow*) does not close on the right indicating disc protrusion. The fifth lumbar disc space is not well visualized, but there is usually little lateral motion at this level.

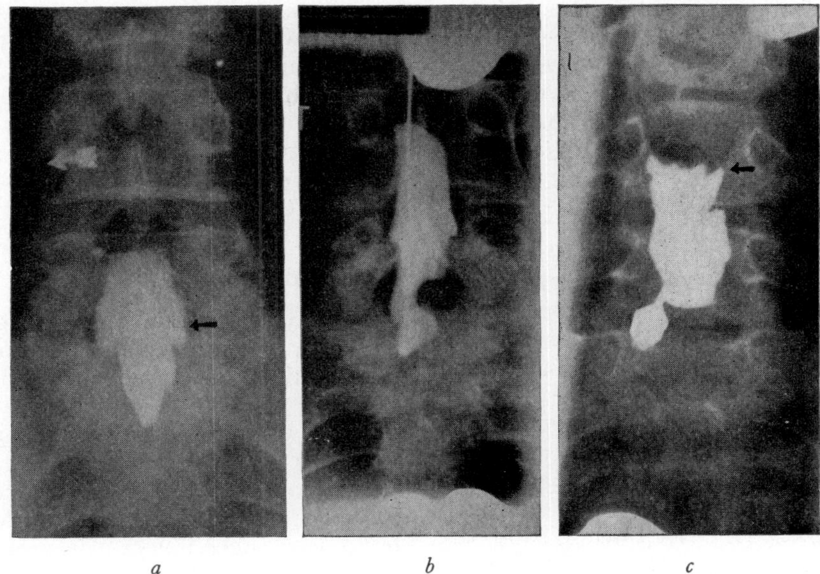

FIG. 82–15.—Pantopaque myelogram. *a*, There is normal filling of the lower end of the dural sac. The axillary pouches (nerve root sheaths) are well visualized at the lumbosacral level (*arrow*). In order to complete the examination each intervertebral level must be similarly visualized until the lower end of the cord is reached. *b*, There is a filling defect on the left side at the level of the fifth lumbar disc. A disc herniation is likely, though cyst or tumor are not ruled out. *c*, There is complete block of the spinal canal by which the pantopaque cannot pass. Such a block indicates a tumor of the cauda equina. It is rarely seen in disc herniation.

first to the right and then to the left is often helpful in diagnosing the level of a disc lesion. If the restriction of lateral movement is diffuse throughout the lumbar spine, the x rays are of no help, but if the restriction of lateral bending seems to be confined to one disc space and to one side only, it suggests a pathologic condition at this level.[9] Lateral films of the lumbosacral spine in full flexion and extension are occasionally useful to demonstrate an anterior-posterior instability in the early stages of disc degeneration, but are mainly indicated for postoperative study of spinal lesions.

Pantopaque Myelography

This type of x-ray examination is the most sensitive test yet devised for the determination of the presence and level of disc herniations.[35] It is also useful to differentiate such lesions from tumors and to detect partial or complete blocks secondary to degeneration of the intervertebral joint complexes, when such degeneration is complicated by spondylolisthesis and osteophyte formation. Where nerve root, conus or cauda equina compression is suspected, a myelogram is indicated.

To be sure there are certain disadvantages to the use of pantopaque, and other substances have been tried. In the article in which Harvey and Freiberger have presented their results with myelography using a water-soluble contrast agent, there is an excellent comparison of the advantages and disadvantages of these various myelographic agents.[21]

Myelography has the undeserved reputation of being an arduous and painful examination, but in skilled hands this is rarely so, and it certainly is not a reason to forego its use. False-positive and false-negative examinations do occur in a small percentage of cases. Instances of arachnoiditis have been reported; therefore, myelograms should be confined to patients who have not responded to conservative measures of treatment, or to those whose pains or neurologic deficits are severe enough to justify this risk.

Discography

The visualization of the internal structure of the disc by the injection of radiopaque absorbable compounds may be helpful in the diagnosis of disc degeneration when routine x-ray studies show no abnormality.[2] However, degeneration can occur at one or more levels with little or no symptomatic consequences and this detracts from their value especially in older patients. In our opinion this technique should be reserved for difficult and atypical syndromes.

Electromyography

Muscular paresis can be shown by alteration of electromyographic pattern when gross muscle weakness cannot be detected. The technique has been proposed, therefore, as a means of diagnosis and of localizing the level or root compression due to herniated discs.[32] In our experience its use has not been helpful enough to recommend it routinely, although it certainly is indicated in the differential diagnosis of certain atypical pain syndromes such as early amyotrophic lateral sclerosis. But, the clinical picture is often suggestive enough in such instances to make the use of electromyography confirmatory rather than diagnostic.

LUMBOSACRAL SPRAIN SYNDROMES

For the sake of convenience all conditions creating a structural weakness of the back will be described under this heading. Although the therapeutic approach may have to be altered to fit certain peculiarities of each condition, the overall principles of treatment are the same and will be described in general under the subheadings of "Acute Sprain" and "Subacute or Chronic Sprain." When there is complicating nerve root or cauda equina involvement, further treatment measures, as described under "Degenerative Disc Disease and Disc Herniation" will apply.

Physicodynamics

In order to understand the principles of strain in relation to causation of low back pain, one must reconsider for a moment the physiology of the spine in relation to stance, movement and work.

It has already been pointed out that under normal conditions the spine is well balanced in the erect position. The head is centered over the feet and the successive spinal curves neutralize one another. The ligaments, assisted by the superincumbent weight of the body, exert a contractile force which is counterbalanced by the inherent expansile turgor of the discs. In addition, the intervertebral joints are held midway between their extremes of motion. A cushioning zone is thus provided in which the muscles may first provide a buffering action and the ligaments finally a checking action. The normal spine, therefore, is a resilient structure, prepared amazingly well for the shocks and excessive pressures to which it is continually subjected.

The normal physiological state can be upset, however, by faulty posture or disease. If posture is poor, the intervertebral joints lie near one extreme of motion. The muscles and ligaments are shortened on one side and lengthened on the other. The buffering mechanism is markedly impaired. If, by specific disease processes, or by the degenerative effects of wear and tear, the resiliency of the discs is lost, the spine can no longer respond efficiently to sudden disturbances of its equilibrium. Thus, any and every pathological change that may occur will leave its mark upon the spine and it becomes more prone to injury.

Very few people are aware of the tremendous mechanical forces that are at play in the spine during normal daily life. Any movement is associated with changes of pressure that defy calculation, but these are as nothing when compared to the leverage forces produced by such acts as sneezing, bending or lifting. It requires very little knowledge of physical laws to understand that these pressures are greatest in the lower lumbar region and it is here that one finds the most marked signs of wear and tear.

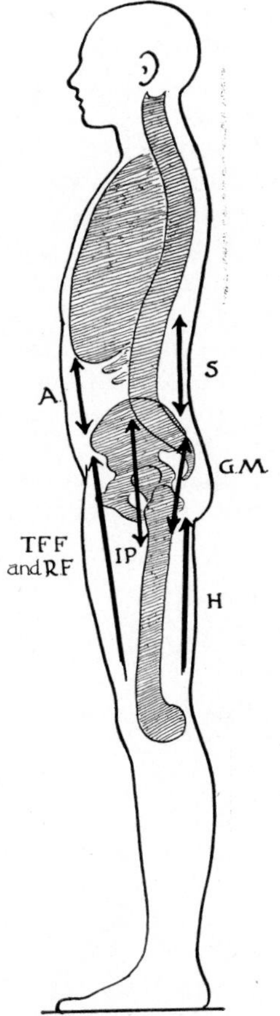

Fig. 82–16.—The important muscles in relation to posture of the lumbar spine. Contraction of the abdominals (A) and gluteus maximus (GM) reduces the lumbar lordosis by flexion of the lumbar spine and by reducing the forward tilt of the pelvis. Contraction of the other muscles increases the lordosis. The rectus femoris (RF), the tensor fascia femoris (TFF), and the iliopsoas (IP) flex the hip and increase the forward tilt of the pelvis. The sacrospinalis (S) extends the spine and thereby increases the lumbar lordosis. The hamstrings (H) are also illustrated since they frequently become shortened in cases of low back pain and sciatica.

Putting all these facts together, one can understand how overstrain of the back occurs so easily, and in the presence of such trivial initiating injuries. In many instances the pain of overstrain may seemingly appear spontaneous, but it is the summation of inherent degenerative processes with repeated subclinical traumata that brings the pathological lesion to clinical significance.

Pathogenesis.—What is the pathology of sprain? Unfortunately this is a hard question to answer since it is seldom that fresh material is available for examination. Much of it occurs in the disc and will be subsequently described. There are acute tears of ligaments, muscles and fascia. Occasionally there are avulsion fractures as of the transverse or spinous processes. However, of greater significance are the less violent reactions, such as the wearing of cartilaginous joint surfaces; the minor microscopic tears of ligaments and muscles; and the gradual fibrosis of the various specialized connective tissues. These are the changes of aging, which themselves are rarely symptomatic, but may predispose to symptoms by causing mechanical weakness.

One more thing must be explained for adequate understanding of the subject of sprain. Many of the underlying changes of wear and tear begin and progress to advanced stages, with little or no objective evidence. Furthermore, x rays are often entirely negative, or the changes present of equivocal significance.

CONDITIONS PREDISPOSING TO SPRAIN SYNDROMES

Faulty Posture.—As is widely known bad posture is relatively prevalent.[34] It can be classified into two groups. The first of these is a *functional* one in which the position of faulty posture is correctable. It is extremely common in children and progressively less so in older age groups. The second is a *structural* group in which the deformity is fixed. The cervical lordosis is increased. The thoracic spine is rounded and its motion limited. The exaggerated lordotic lumbar curve may become fixed due to shortening of the sacrospinalis muscles. If so, the interspinous ligaments become contracted so that the tips of the spinous processes and facets "kiss." Conversely the abdominal muscles overstretch and relax, a process which may be accelerated by pregnancies and overweight. The pelvis tilts more anteriorly than normal and the hip flexors shorten. The lumbosacral angle increases. When the patient is asked to bend forward he will not obliterate his lumbar curve as he normally should. Often there are secondary degenerative changes on x ray.

In the purely functional state, faulty posture is rarely painful; at most it may cause some fatigue and backache. But when the position becomes fixed, then the symptoms are more likely to be significant and bothersome.

Spondylolisthesis. — Generically this term means a slipped vertebra but clinically it is associated only with anterior displacement of one vertebra upon the next below (*see* Figs. 82–17 and 18).

Congenital or Spondylolytic Type.—Defects of ossification are present in the isthmic portions of the vertebral arch, that is in the parts lying between the superior and inferior articular processes. The defect may be unilateral and without consequence, but when bilateral the anterior and posterior halves of the vertebra are held together by fibrous tissue instead of bone. The anterior half may slip forward with the superincumbent spine while the posterior half remains behind, and a true spondylolisthesis results. If the defect is present only unilaterally, or is

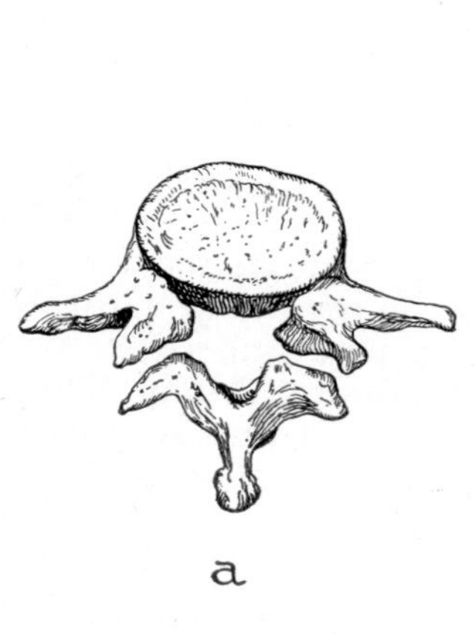

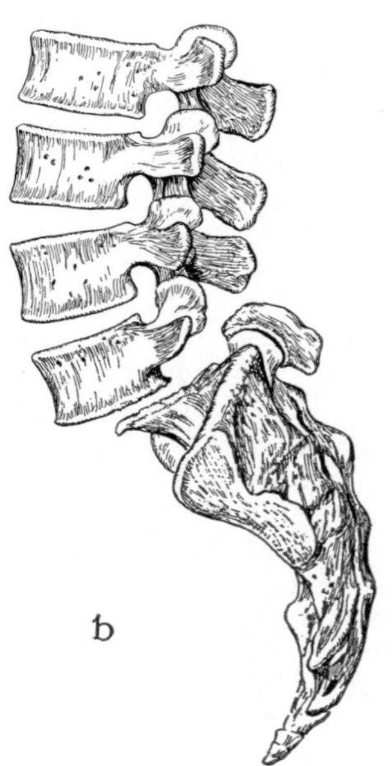

Fig. 82–17.—Spondylolisthesis. *a*, Vertebra showing failure of ossification of the interarticular portions of the neural arch. Without forward slip of the involved vertebra, this is called spondylolysis. (Willis, courtesy of J. Bone Joint Surg.) *b*, The deformity (spondylolisthesis) which may occur as the result of the above. The defect is in the arch of L5. The posterior portion of the arch including the inferior facets remains with the sacrum while the rest of the 5th lumbar vertebra slips forward, carrying with it the entire spine. All degrees of slipping are seen.

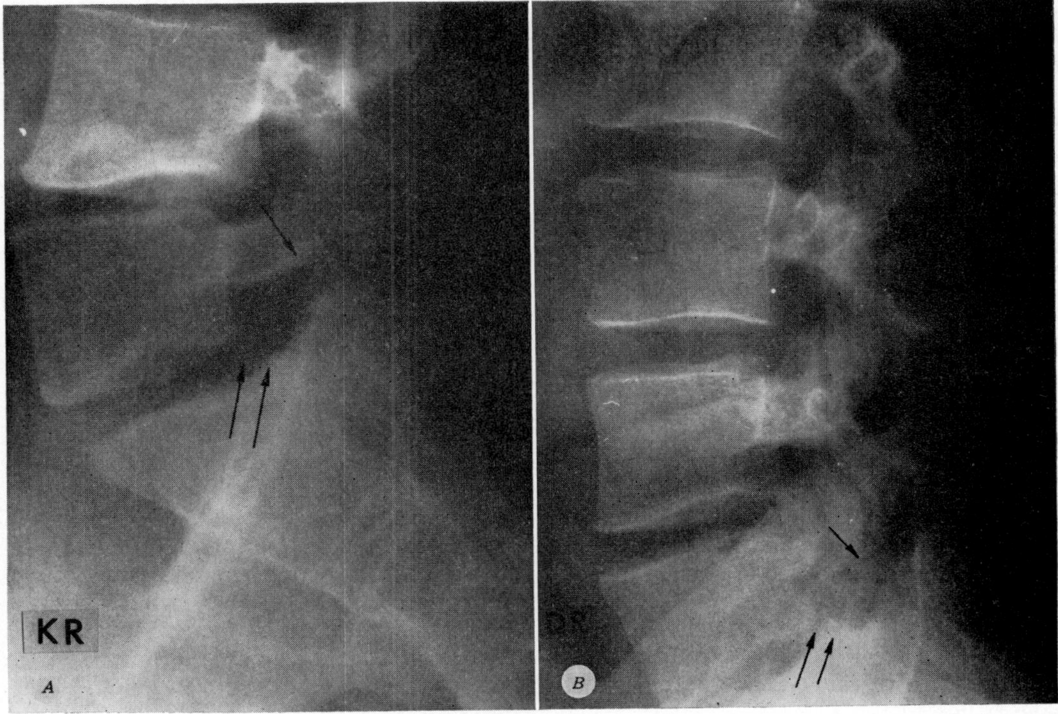

Fig. 82–18.—Identical twins with spondylolisthesis of L5-S1. *A*, Lateral x ray of lumbosacral area of K.R., who had progressive back pain requiring spinal fusion. *B*, Lateral x ray of twin, D.R., who never had any back symptoms.

present bilaterally but without forward slip, the condition is termed *spondylolysis.*

The cause of the basic lesion, the neural arch defects, is still the subject of some controversy. Willis found spondylolysis in 4 per cent of adult skeletal specimens, yet not in fetal skeletons.[51] Friberg[18] has traced it through a family tree, and we have encountered it in identical twins and in several members of the same family. Hitchcock[24] has shown that hyperextension of the back of the newborn can produce fractures of the pars interarticularis. Harris[20] has shown that such defects can arise in a previously normal vertebra above an intact fusion mass. Logically, these facts can be put together to mean that a predisposing factor, such as vulnerability of the pars interarticularis, is congenital in origin and may be genetically determined and, therefore, inheritable; while the final fully manifest condition is produced by wear and tear or trauma.[56]

Spondylolisthesis is usually qualified by the amount of forward displacement; first degree for one-quarter anteroposterior-vertebral-diameter displacement and fourth degree for full diameter displacement. Although it is uncommon to see the condition progress in adults, it is not unusual to see it do so in children. The fibrous tissue bridging the defects, the structure of the disc, and the intervertebral ligaments must give and stretch so that the vertebral body, pedicles and superior facets can slip away from the detached portion of the neural arch which includes the laminae, spinous process and inferior facets. Pseudoarthroses may develop in the sites of defective ossification if the degree of slipping is minimal, since movements of the spine cause false motion between the two vertebral segments.

From a clinical standpoint several types of syndromes are caused by spondylolisthesis. First of all, the condition may be silent or the symptoms associated with it inconsequential. Second, back pain may arise from the pseudoarthrosis or from wear and tear of the disc joint which has slipped. In this connection, herniation of such a disc has been described, but we have not encountered it. Third, unilateral or bilateral sciatica may be caused by root impingement due to hypertrophy of the fibrous tissue in one or both defects, or by traction on the roots secondary to forward displacement, especially when the defects are situated low in the superior articular processes. Fourth, the displacement may be so severe that a lesion of the whole cauda equina is produced, in part due to traction and in part due to compression. This severest of the syndromes is usually seen in adolescents.

Although the astute clinician can often make the diagnosis from a visible or palpable prominence of the spine of the affected vertebra, noticed most readily when the patient is bent forward, final diagnosis depends on x-ray demonstration of the neural arch defects. When slipping is sufficient these may be visible in a routine lateral film if the tube is well centered (Fig. 82–18). However, in the presence of minimal slipping, oblique views are necessary (Fig. 82–13). Occasionally, although a defect is present, slippage may not be evident on the routine lateral recumbent x ray of the lumbosacral junction but if the x ray is taken with the patient standing slippage becomes apparent.

Treatment varies with the syndrome encountered. Postural measures sometime suffice for the more minimal symptoms and especially if there is no nerve involvement. However, spinal fusion is indicated when the symptoms of sprain are more severe, persist or begin before maturity. When the nerve roots or cauda equina is involved, decompression is the most important part of the operation and is indicated at the time of or before spinal fusion. Occasionally, simple removal of the loose neural arch and hypertrophic tissue in the defects (*i.e.* foraminatomy) will afford relief,[19] but the outcome in our experience is too uncertain to recommend this routinely.

Degenerative or Articular Type.—Spondylolisthesis can also occur in the presence of congenital or acquired *abnormalites of the facets.*[41] The congenital lesion is a rare one in which the facet joints are oriented in a horizontal plane so that they do not prevent forward slip. The

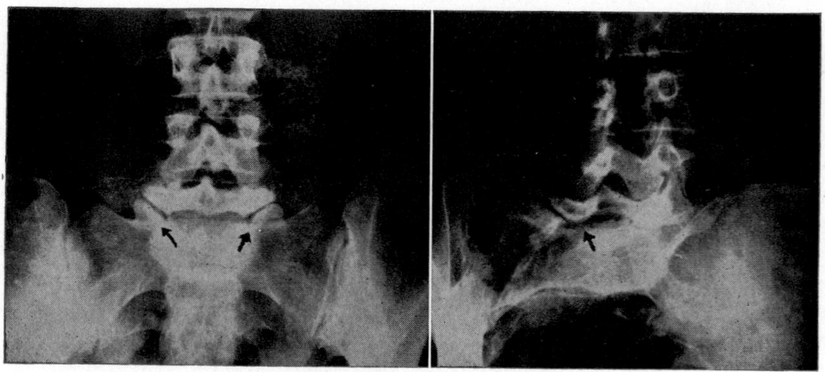

FIG. 82–19.—Abnormal facets. A.P. and oblique x rays in a case of low back pain. Note the abnormal plane of the facets between the fifth lumbar vertebra and the sacrum. There is less bony stability and actual spondylolisthesis may occur. Sometimes the instability may be detected roentgenographically only with flexion or extension of the spine.

much more common acquired form is one in which osteoarthritic changes of the facets combined with disc degeneration result in forward displacement. These conditions are diagnosed by x ray, especially by oblique views. Treatment is planned in very much the same way as for congenital spondylolisthesis. Complicating compression of nerve roots or cauda equina should be looked for and given precedence in the therapeutic plan.

Trauma.—Each spinal injury that occurs tends to weaken the spine and predispose to further injury, regardless of type and extent of damage. This is especially the case where protection of the injured part is not adequate. Ligaments and muscles heal only by scar formation and the annulus fibrosus is almost powerless to heal tears of its substance. These circumstances, unfortunately, are beyond the control of the physician, but the patient should be warned to protect his back following injury.

Disc Degeneration.—The pathologic aspects of this condition are also discussed later (p. 1543). Besides predisposing to herniation (*see* p. 1544), disc degeneration also weakens the structure of the intervertebral joint predisposing it to sprain syndromes.[3,22] When the degeneration is localized little loss of stability results and the normal width of the disc space may be preserved. A patient with such a back may have few or no symptoms, and it is for this reason that some patients do very well after simple removal of herniated disc material.

When the degeneration is more massive, however, narrowing of disc space follows (Figs. 82–29 and 32). If this occurs slowly over the course of years there may be little pain or other evidence of it. Stability and vertebral alignment are preserved by marginal spur formation and by adaptive changes in the facets and intervertebral ligaments (Fig. 82–31). Occasionally, such patients give a history of several acute episodes of back pain many years before, but frequently they are unaware of any previous back trouble.

If massive disc degeneration occurs more rapidly, however, it is likely to be continuously painful, whether or not

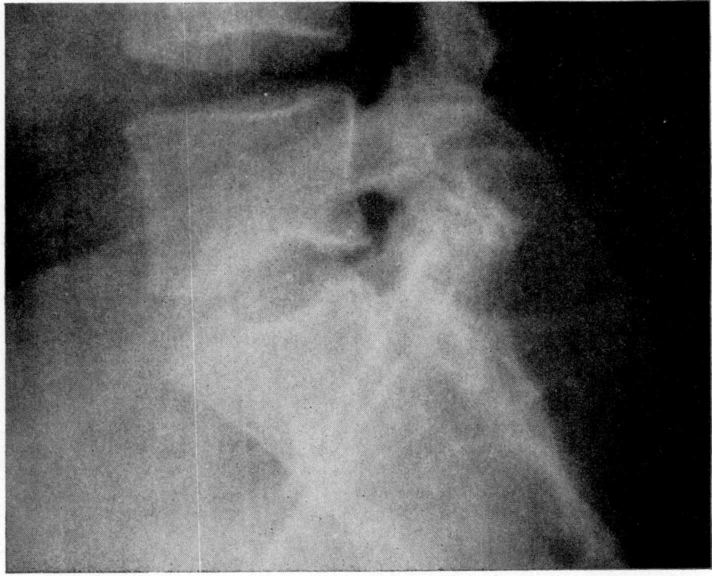

Fig. 82–20.—Retrodisplacement. Lateral x ray of a case with slight narrowing of the 5th lumbar disc and retrodisplacement of the 5th lumbar vertebra on the sacrum. This condition is often called reverse spondylolisthesis. It is often associated with pain.

herniation and root compression are associated. Instability of such joints either leads to backward shift of the superior vertebra on the inferior as the facets telescope on each other (Fig. 82–20), or to forward displacement as the structure of the articular facets gives way, *i.e.* articular spondylolisthesis (*see* above).

During the course of collapse of the disc space, not only the disc itself but also the intervertebral joint is *unstable* and therefore prone to give symptoms of sprain; but when the intervertebral space becomes narrowed and arthritic it is again relatively stable and back pain may subside. However, later symptoms may develop from projection of marginal osteophytes against the nerve roots either posteriorly in the neural canal, or laterally in the narrowed intervertebral foramina (*see* root compression syndromes).

Stages in the Phylogenetic Shortening of the Spine.—The structure of the lowest lumbar vertebra and the first sacral segment is quite variable. Either may take on some or all of the characteristics of the other. When this happens the vertebrae are spoken of as *transitional*.

Willis found that the fifth lumbar vertebra was partially sacralized in 4.7 per cent and completely sacralized in 1.5 per cent of nearly 1500 skeletons.[52] In the same study he found that the first segment of the sacrum was partially lumbarized in 1.2 per cent and completely lumbarized in 4.1 per cent of the spines. Certainly complete fusion or sacralization of the fifth lumbar vertebra does not predispose to strain. It is also hard to see how complete lumbarization of the first sacral segment could do so.

However, in cases in which the changeover is incomplete, the situation is somewhat different. One finds a unilaterally enlarged transverse process articulating with the sacrum and asymmetrical facets; that is, the facets are in different planes on the two sides.[53] These changes reduce intervertebral mobility and, therefore, may predispose to sprain. They are not incompatible, on the other hand, with normal existence, and the fact is that if trouble occurs, the joint above is

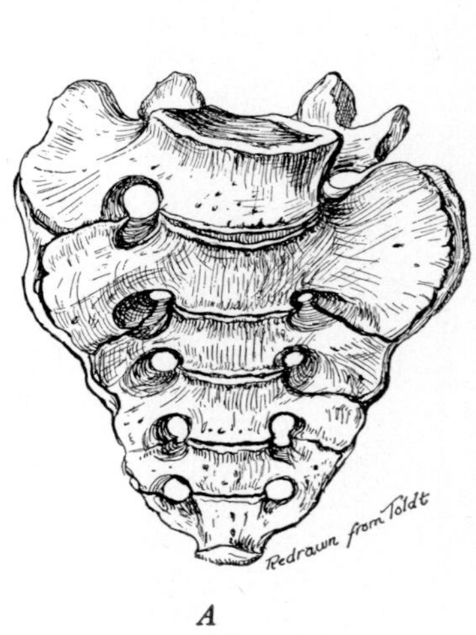

A

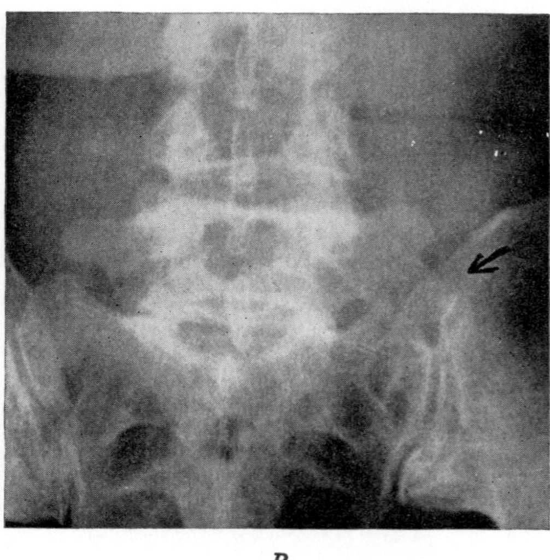

B

FIG. 82–21.—Articulating transverse process. *A*, An incompletely sacralized fifth lumbar vertebra is shown with an articulating transverse process on the right. The intervertebral disc is usually congenitally narrow in these cases. *B*, An articulating transverse process on the left side of the 5th lumbar vertebra. The articulation is usually a fibrous one. This congenital anomaly is not uncommon and is not necessarily associated with pain.

very often the one involved. If the transitional vertebra itself is ever responsible for pain, the symptom probably arises from a sclerosing osteitis of the pseudoarthrosis between the enlarged transverse process and the sacrum.

Spina Bifida Occulta.—This condition is a failure of fusion between the right and left halves of the neural arch and is extremely common in the fifth lumbar and first sacral segments. It is in no way a predisposing factor to sprain. Occasionally the remnants of the spinous processes may appear roentgenographically as loose ossicles, but they are embedded in fibrous tissue and it is very unlikely that they produce symptoms in any way.

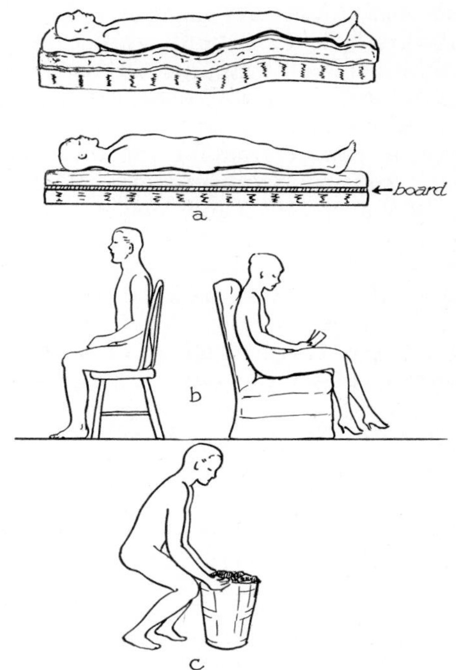

FIG. 82–22.—Postural principles. Patients should be instructed in some simple principles to avoid unnecessary back strain. *a*, The bed should be hard in order to avoid sagging of the buttocks with increase in the lumbar lordosis. *b*, A hard straight-back chair is desirable. Arm rests are not contraindicated. *c*, Lifting should be avoided whenever possible. When unavoidable the legs should do most of the work. The elbows can be buttressed by the thighs.

Clinical Picture of Sprain Syndromes

Low back sprain may be acute, subacute, or chronic. The acute syndrome usually follows an injury or trivial strain, is of relatively short duration, and self limited enough to respond gratifyingly to treatment (the type does not seem to be very important). The chronic form, on the other hand, is usually of relatively long duration, often is devoid of history of initiating trauma, and tends to be refractory to treatment. Recurrences of the acute form are not uncommon.

Acute Sprain.—The pain is usually severe, and diffuse over the lower back and associated with paravertebral muscle spasm. The patient adopts a protective attitude of moderate flexion and perhaps some list. Any motion is painful and associated with aggravation of the spasm.

Complete examination is out of the question but is carried as far as possible. X rays should be made if the patient can cooperate well enough. If not, they can be safely deferred until he can.

The patient should be put to bed, preferably a bed with a thin sponge rubber or hair mattress reinforced by an underlying board (Fig. 82–22). If such a board is not available, shifting the mattress to the floor will often substitute. A pillow behind the knees often assists in relaxation. "Muscle relaxants" and salicylates are usually helpful; but narcotics are sometimes necessary. No particular drug combination will fit all patients. Heat in the form of hot moist packs should be applied to the back, since it is effective in relieving muscle spasm. Light massage is often helpful in this respect, but deep massage should be avoided. Sometimes procaine infiltration of the tight muscles is helpful, but injection of a locally acting steroid into the disc has a very questionable value.[12] Traction has been used for acute low back symptoms for many years and has been thought only to keep a restless patient still. If applied directly to the pelvis, there is no doubt that such forces may be transmitted to the spine and cause a stretching effect. Countertraction may be provided by positioning the patient with the foot of the bed elevated or by applying countertraction on the head. In the routine management of scoliosis the effects of head and pelvic traction have been documented by x rays of the spine showing the stretching effect. Constant pelvic traction may be used with weights up to 35 or 40 pounds while intermittent pelvic traction of 65 to 70 pounds has been of value in treating patients with acute back symptoms.[24b] If traction is necessary then we believe that this should be carried out at first while the patient is hospitalized. It is difficult to instruct a patient initially in the correct use of traction unless he is in the hospital.

As the pain subsides more complete examination can be carried out. As soon as straight leg raising is free through an arc of 45° or more, the patient may be allowed up. His back must be protected until his symptoms have subsided completely. If the sprain has been severe,

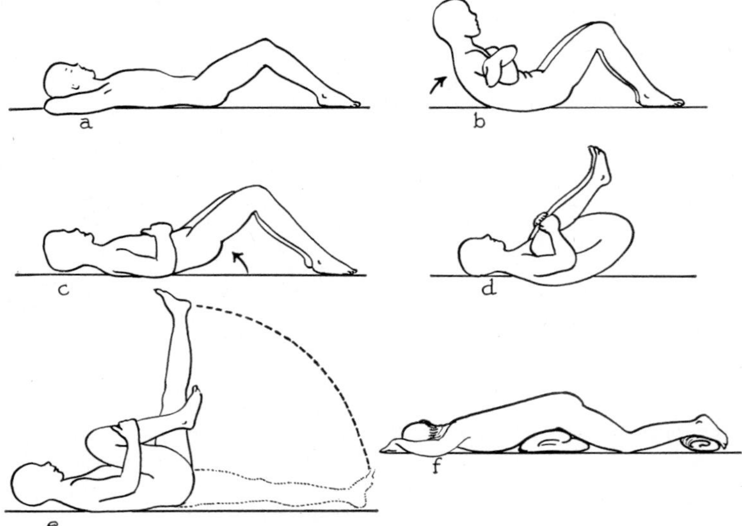

Fig. 82–23.—Postural exercises. Carefully supervised exercises will do more for the patient with a weak back than almost any other conservative measure. They should be graduated carefully and the routine varied as indicated by the patient's response. The exercises are exaggerated in the illustrations. The method of doing the exercise is described with each.

a, Lying, hands at back of neck, breathe deeply, raising chest; hold chest up and exhale by drawing upper abdomen in. Take next breath against the uplifted chest. 10 breaths. This is a good rest position.

b, Lying in the same position, knees bent, contract the lower abdominal muscles; relax. Repeat 10 times. It is better to do the exercise without actually raising the shoulders.

c, Lying in the same position, knees bent, flatten back against the floor by contracting the lower abdominal muscles and tightening the buttocks. Relax. Repeat 10 times. This may be painful at first and should be approached cautiously.

d, Lying on back, hug both knees to the chest and repeat 10 times. This is only indicated where there is a fixed lordosis. Since it is a spinal stretching exercise, it should be done lightly at first.

e, Lying in the same position, hug one knee to chest. Raise other leg straight and lower slowly, keeping abdomen in. 5 times on each leg. Also a stretching exercise, the patient should not be fórced to do it early.

f, Lying in the prone position, pillow under abdomen, tighten buttock. Relax. Repeat 10 times. (Figures *b*, *c*, *d* are redrawn from Posture and Its Relationship to Orthopaedic Disabilities. Posture Committee of American Academy of Orthopaedic Surgery, Chicago, Ill.)

a brace or lumbosacral corset may be advisable. Before normal activities are resumed, the patient should be checked to see if he has regained full motion. Exercises should be instituted not only to restore motion and strength, but also to stretch out contracted muscles and ligaments. Exercises must be started gradually, and gauged to pain tolerance (Fig. 82–23).

Many acute attacks are not so severe as the one painted above. In these cases ambulatory treatment may be sufficient. Adhesive strapping (Fig. 82–24), procaine injection and physiotherapy including heat and massage are all useful measures of treatment. Again the patient should be watched for developing contractures. These should be corrected with exercises whenever present.

Chronic Sprain. — This syndrome which is probably the most common of low back conditions is extremely variable. In its milder form it is characterized by a very mild low backache aggravated by bending and lifting and improved by rest. On the other hand, the pain may be more severe and cause the patient to be most uncomfortable. Rarely is it severe for more than short periods at a time, subsiding in between to a nagging, diffuse low backache with radiation into one or both thighs. It is almost always aggravated by activity and improved by rest.

The physical signs are also quite variable. In the mild cases there may be no limitation of motion, but usually the extremes of motion are painful. There is almost always tenderness at some point over the lower spine. As the severity of the syndrome increases one notes additional signs such as partial restriction of straight leg raising, loss of motion, abnormal postural attitudes and muscle spasm particularly in response to movement.

In severe cases a period of bedrest may be indicated, in which case the measures are the same as described for acute low back sprain. In milder cases the patient should be instructed in proper postural principles.[25] The proper sleeping and sitting positions are shown. He is taught to avoid bending and lifting, or proper methods for doing these in order to minimize the pressure on his back. He is instructed in postural exercises, which have as their principle the reduction of lumbar lordosis and the strengthening of the trunk. Stretching of shortened hamstring and sacrospinalis muscles may be advisable but should be done cautiously.[34,50]

Frequently external support will be helpful, and many different types of braces have been designed to achieve the

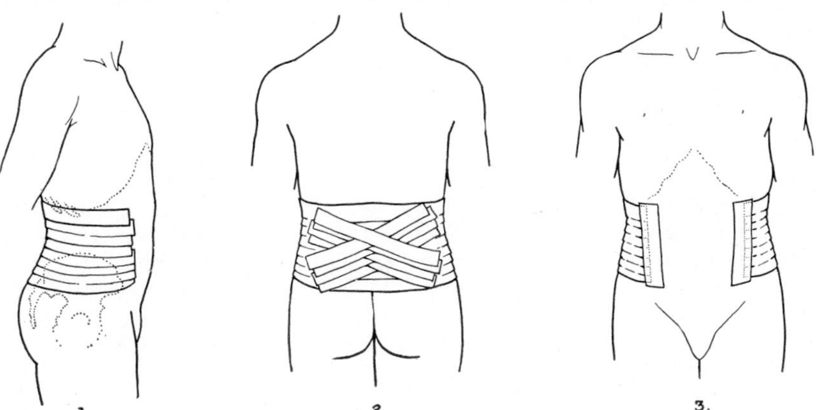

Fig. 82–24.—Strapping of the low back. 1. Overlapping horizontal adhesive strips. 2. Diagonal layer of overlapping strips. 3. Final layer of horizontal strips with anchoring anterior vertical strips.

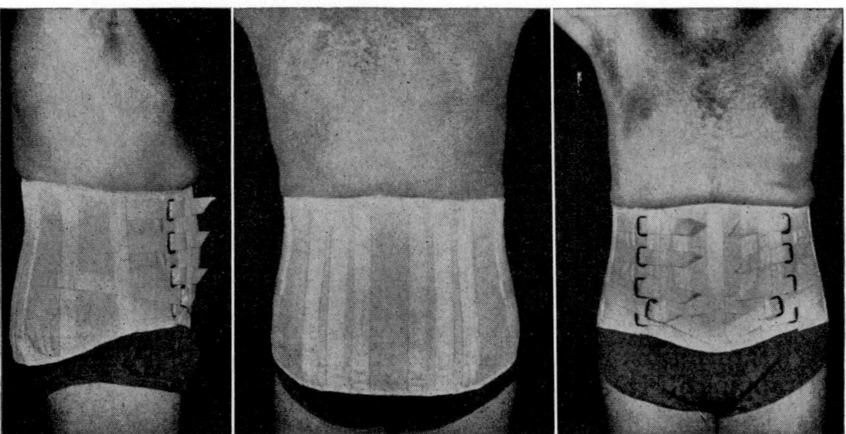

Fig. 82–25.—Lumbosacral corset. Steel stays are incorporated into the back of the support. It must extend from the iliac crests to just over the costal margins.

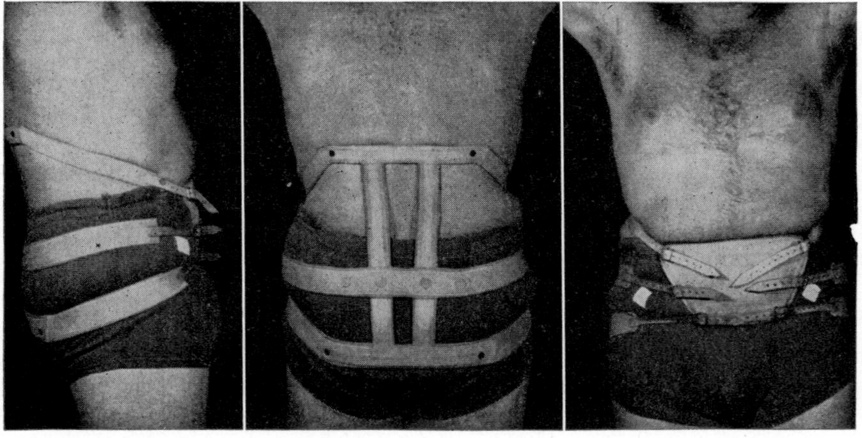

Fig. 82–26.—Goldthwaite brace. A light support that incorporates the principles of good posture. The lowest strap should come just over the trochanters and under the anterior superior iliac spines (marked). The vertical steels in back are bent to a position of slight lordosis.

desired goals of abdominal compression and restricted spinal movement (Figs. 82–25 and 26). In principle, they should reach from pubic level to the lower costal margins and support the abdomen, particularly the lower abdomen. The central back uprights, if present, should be contoured to fit comfortably when the patient is seated erect. Pressure into the lumbosacral hollow is not necessary and in fact should be avoided.

When conservative therapy fails, a lumbosacral fusion operation should be considered. This operation is one in which two or more vertebrae are induced to grow together so as to put the intervening joint at rest, and many techniques have been devised (Fig. 82–27). Although newer methods have shortened morbidity, the incidence of pseudoarthroses is still bothersome; and rarely, following a successful fusion, the intervertebral joint above may become troublesomely painful due to the additional wear and tear

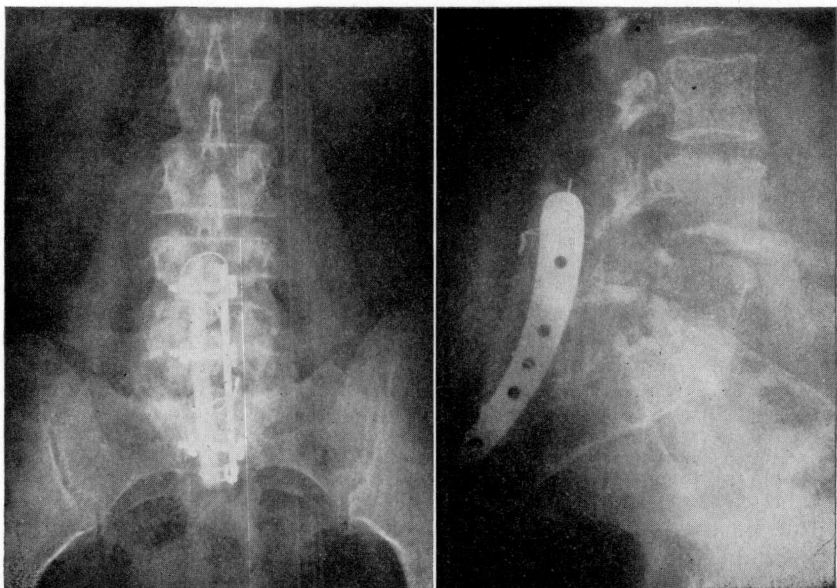

FIG. 82–27.—Spinal fusion. Spinal fusion is sometimes necessary to relieve low back pain. The 4th and 5th lumbar vertebrae have been united to the sacrum by bone grafts. The Wilson metallic plate serves as fixation to prevent motion while the bone is healing. Once the fusion is consolidated the plate and bolts may remain without causing harm. This is only one of many useful techniques.

placed on it. Since the operation is elective, the decision to proceed should be left up to the patient after the advantages and disadvantages have been explained to him.

NERVE ROOT COMPRESSION SYNDROMES

Degenerative Disc Disease and Herniated Disc

Since Mixter and Barr first clearly described the syndrome of nerve root compression due to herniated disc in 1934,[39] it has become clear that lesions of the disc are responsible for much of idiopathic low back pain.[31]

Pathogenesis.—While a single trauma, if severe enough, can cause rupture of a hitherto normal annulus and prolapse of disc substance with disastrous effect on the cauda equina, this is a rare occurrence. More commonly the trauma (or strain) acts only as a triggering mechanism. Underlying asymptomatic biomechanical and biochemical changes usually first weaken the disc structure. The course of these changes has been traced anatomically, and alteration and weakening of the discs are part of the aging process.[23,38] Since the discs have no innervation and no blood supply, such degeneration can take place silently and with little appreciable repair. When the annulus has weakened enough, the interior disc substance (nucleus pulposus and degenerating annular fibers) will tend to prolapse in the direction of greatest weakness. Because of the forces involved and certain anatomic factors already described (*see* p. 1512), the directions of greatest weakness for the lumbar discs are to right and left of the posterior midline (Fig. 82–30). Lumbar disc herniations, therefore, follow these two directions. They are favored by radially oriented annular tears or fissures, which develop either as the result of normal wear and tear, or perhaps as the result of one or more excessive strains.

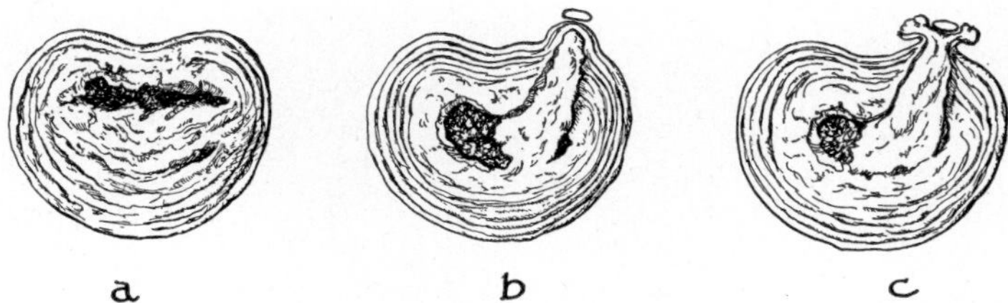

FIG. 82–28.—Types of disc degeneration. *a*, Degeneration of the disc. There is fissuring of the annulus, and the nucleus is loosened and desiccated. There is no herniation. This is the preliminary phase of degenerative disc disease. *b*, There is degeneration but there is partial posterolateral rupture of the annulus and nerve root pressure is produced by *protrusion*. At surgery the posterior longitudinal ligament and intact annular fibers must be incised before the degenerated disc fragments can be removed. *c*, Again there is degeneration, but here there is a complete rupture and disc material has been *extruded*. Loose tabs will still be present in the disc space and should be curetted to prevent subsequent recurrence.

When these herniations approach the surface they distend the superficial fibers and longitudinal ligaments where pain perceptive nerve endings are situated.[48] This deep pain is poorly localized and can radiate into the buttocks and perhaps even into the lower extremities (*see* p. 1516). The source of the pain is further obscured by the fact that spasm of the lumbar and hamstring muscles frequently develops and this spasm in itself is painful. If herniation proceeds, the lumbar nerve roots or cauda equina may next become involved; the smaller the diameter of the neural canal and the larger the herniation, the more likely is this to occur and when it occurs, to be consequential to nerve root functions. If the herniation does not rupture through the longitudinal ligament it is called a *protrusion*, and if it does, an *extrusion*. In either case the root or roots are displaced and compressed (Fig. 82–28). Disc fragments may herniate from the disc space and come to lie above or below it and still not extrude.

Because of all these variables, the manifestations of disc herniation are quite different from one patient to the next. Most commonly, the root compression is localized and the neurological deficit relatively minor. In rare instances, however, the prolapse may be massive and involve several roots or the entire cauda equina. As the site of herniation comes closer to the midline, the more likely it is that more than one root is involved; as the site shifts laterally the more likely is involvement to be confined to one nerve root.

Clinical Picture.—Although any of the lumbar discs can herniate, one or the other or sometimes both of the lowest (L4–5 and L5–S1) are responsible for symptoms in the majority of instances.[54] L3–4 is occasionally involved and other lumbar levels rarely.

If nerve root compression is *minimal* there may be no localizing physical or x-ray findings and conclusive diagnosis depends on doing a myelogram. In many instances, however, symptoms and signs may subside with bedrest (*see* p. 1546), and a myelogram therefore can be deferred. We have followed the practice of recommending myelograms only when the syndrome is atypical or operative intervention is being contemplated. Because of the lack of definitive diagnosis such patients should be carried under the diagnosis of "Acute Lumbosacral Sprain" (*see* p. 1539). The additional diagnosis of "Degenerative Disc Disease" is justified if routine x-ray studies of the low back show such changes, but the diagnoses of "Root Compression" and "Herniated Disc" should not be used. They should be reserved for those patients showing con-

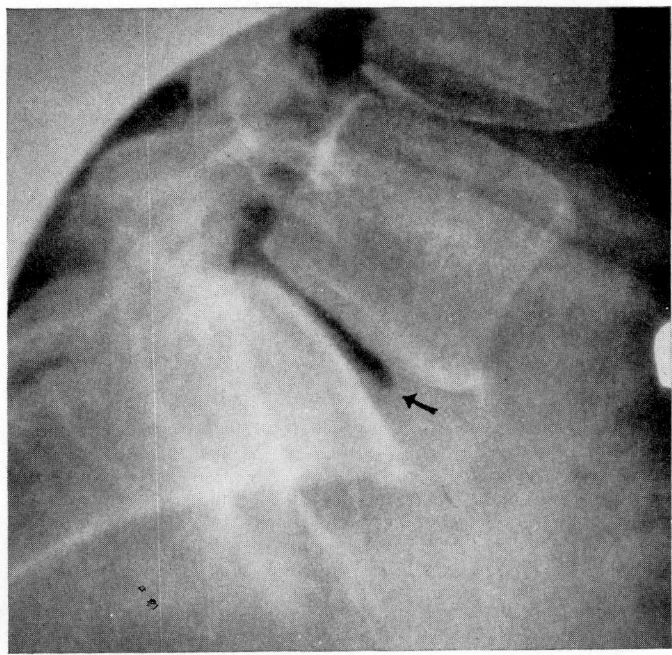

Fig. 82–29.—Phantom nucleus. This phenomenon is seen occasionally and is said to be due to a negative pressure produced in the nucleus by sudden distraction of the vertebral bodies. However, it may be a sign of fatty degeneration or of ochronosis. In this case there is some narrowing of the disc as well.

clusive findings or for those in whom myelograms are positive.

Classical cases of root compression due to herniated disc are difficult to overlook. The patients are otherwise healthy and often vigorous men or women of mid-adult age. There is often a previous history of backache or of one or more acute lumbosacral sprains from which there have been complete recoveries. Usually the present attack of pain begins after a back injury, but not necessarily a severe one; in fact, it is sometimes so minor that it is difficult for the patient to recall it. Frequently a snap is felt before the back pain begins. Once started, the pain increases in intensity and after an interval radiates distally into one or other lower extremity. As radiation begins, the back pain may subside. The sciatica, on the other hand, increases and is associated with numbness and paresthesias. The patient cannot stand straight and the involved leg is too sensitive to bear weight. Examination shows a patient in a great deal of pain with paravertebral muscle spasm, who stands with a flattened lumbar lordosis and list to the side opposite the pain, and who walks only with difficulty. All spinal movements are limited, particularly bending to the side of the pain. Straight leg raising is markedly restricted on the involved side and often this leg cannot be straightened out. The patient prefers the sitting or flexed position to any other. There is marked paravertebral tenderness with reproduction of sciatica on percussion or deep palpation.

Neurological signs are variable for the reasons already described, but certain combinations of them suggest specific root involvements. Loss or suppression of ankle jerk, sensory deficit in the lateral

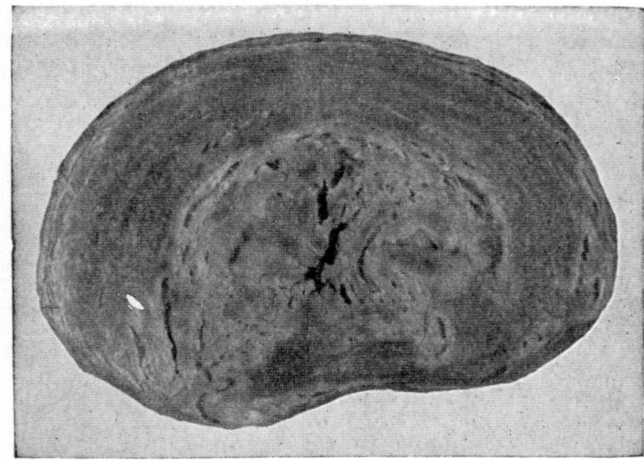

Fig. 82–30.—Disc herniation. Transverse section of a disc with central degeneration and with rupture through the posterolateral fibers of the annulus. Extrusion has occurred.

border and sole of the foot and toes, and weakness and atrophy of the calf suggest S1 root compression. No reflex change, sensory deficit in the lateral leg and mediodorsal aspect of the foot, and weakness of the toe extensors suggest L5 root compression. Loss or suppression of the knee jerk, sensory deficit along the shin, and weakness of knee extension suggest L4 root compression.[1,47] Most commonly S1 root compression is the result of herniation of the L5–S1 disc, L5 root compression of the L4–5 disc, and L4 root compression of the L3–4 disc. When neurological findings are profound, however, it is wise to suspect that more than one root is involved and a myelogram should be done to confirm the level of involvement in all instances where operation is being contemplated.

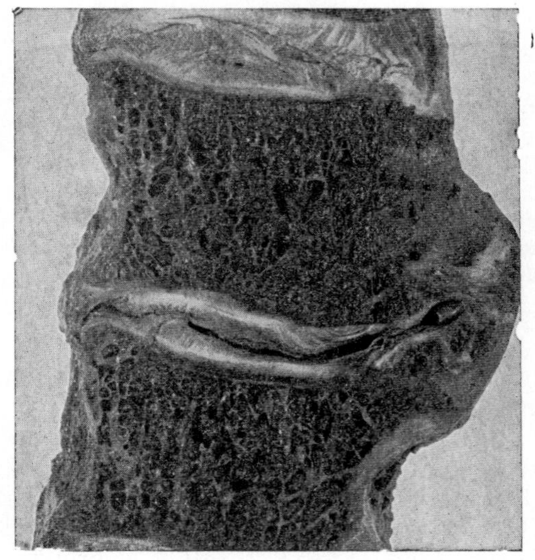

Fig. 82–31.—A longitudinal section of the spine showing an advanced stage of degeneration with narrowing of the disc and spurring anteriorly. Note less advanced degeneration of the upper disc.

Treatment.—Thanks to improvement of myelographic technique, diagnosis can be definitely established in the overwhelming majority of patients. Operative intervention is elective unless there is important nerve deficit or intractable pain. Even in the presence of definite signs of root compression the majority of patients will respond to conservative treatment. A trial of two or three weeks of bedrest in the hospital is indicated for most patients with acute symptoms before advising operation.[10] When the syndrome is subacute, there may be less value to bedrest, but a sustained course of outpatient treatment is indicated before considering operation.

When pain is relieved by conservative treatment, it is probable that the relief is due largely to subsidence of root edema and to limited repair of the superficial layers of the annulus and posterior longitudinal ligament. It is doubtful that the herniated disc material is ever fully absorbed, but it must shrink and/or become pocketed somewhere in the neural canal so that it no longer compresses nerve tissue. This is more likely to happen where the lumbar neural canal is proportionately large in comparison to the cauda equina. Along with subsidence of pain there is often improvement in the neurological picture. However, some neurological changes of little functional significance may persist.

When operative treatment is advised, the question is whether to be content with root decompression only, or whether to proceed with spinal fusion. That is to say, should the degenerative disc process be controlled by fusing the involved joint at the same time that loosened disc tissue is removed? On this point there is still considerable difference of opinion, and there are good arguments on both sides. Our own thinking has undergone some change over the past several years, and may continue to do so. In cases of rupture of the intervertebral discs in adolescence, in acute ruptures for the first time, and in intervertebral disc ruptures with previous history of symptoms but little x-ray changes, when surgery becomes necessary we prefer to decompress the involved disc space without fusion. If, however, repeat operation is necessary or if there are advanced changes of degenerative arthritis spinal fusion may be considered. When there exists questionable situations we prefer not to fuse. This is because the decompression operation is less extensive, convalescence is usually easier, and, if a fusion fails to heal properly and a pseudoarthrosis develops, the situation can be worse than if no fusion had been done. We try to review these various aspects of the problem with the patient and, if we are uncertain, request that we be allowed to make the final decision at the time of operation.

Complications.—If the indications for operative intervention are conservative, and the type of operation precisely fitted to the circumstances, the results will be satisfying.[43,45,54] Complications are rare.[39a] However, one particularly deserves mention. This is a spondylitis or osteitis which sometimes develops in the operated disc space. It is manifested by recurrence of back pain which begins three to four weeks after operation, and elevation of the ESR. Other manifestations of inflammation such as fever and leukocytosis are absent and infection, the primary concern, cannot be demonstrated. In time, x rays show sclerosis of the adjacent vertebral margins and localized areas of bone absorption. The cause of this complication has not been

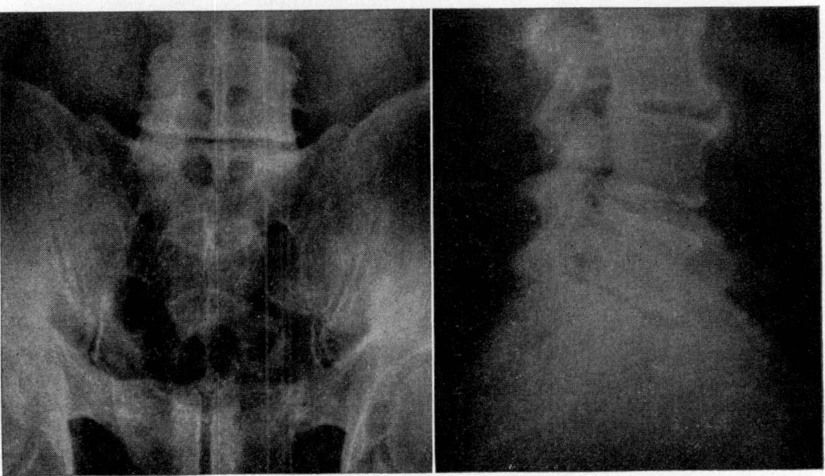

Fig. 82–32.—X rays showing an advanced stage of degenerative disc disease.

definitely established, but the condition is almost always self-limited and subsides with bedrest.

Recurrences of root compression from fresh herniation of degenerated disc tissue can occur, but are infrequent. Because the mobility of the root and dura has been reduced by postoperative scarring, such herniations do not have to be large to irritate the nerve tissue. In such cases, treatment by bedrest is well worth a trial, but if it fails, reoperation for decompression is indicated and the question of also doing a fusion should be carefully reconsidered. It is probably wise to advise it, and especially so if the degenerative disease is still localized to one disc level.

Degenerative Disc Disease and Osteoarthritis

Another type of root compression syndrome can occur in the late phases of degenerative disc disease, especially when it is associated with osteoarthritis of the facets and articular spondylolisthesis. If the pain or root signs become disabling a trial of conservative treatment is indicated, but root compression of this type does not respond so easily to bedrest and bedrest must be used judiciously since these patients are in the older age groups. When conservative treatment fails, operative decompression is indicated. In these cases the decompression has to be carried well into the involved intervertebral foramina, requiring the sacrifice of much of the facets, but because of the preexistent narrowing of the disc spaces and marginal spurring of the vertebral bodies, stability of the spine is usually not appreciably impaired.

Spina Bifida with Enlargement of the Superseding Spinous Process.—Root compression may rarely be caused by impingement of an enlarged fifth lumbar spinous process against the neural tube, through an open upper sacral spina bifida. Such compression is difficult to diagnose because it is intermittent, occurring only during the act of hyperextension of the back.

OTHER CONDITIONS PRODUCING LOW BACK PAIN

Infections

1. It is not uncommon for backache to occur as part of the toxemia of a generalized infection. In these cases diagnosis

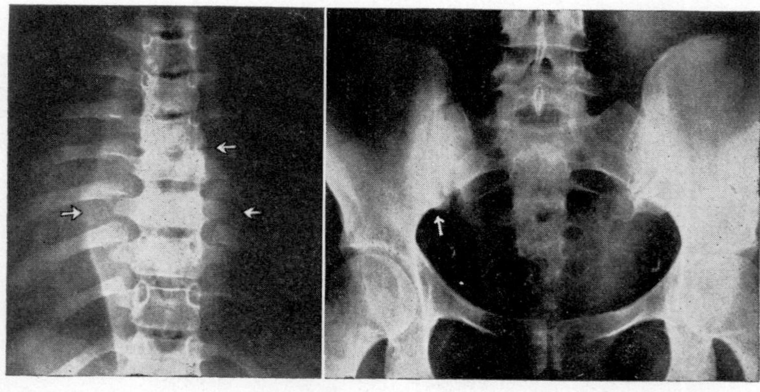

a *b*

FIG. 82–33.—Tuberculosis. *a*, Tuberculous spondylitis. Note abscess (*arrow*). There is destruction of the 6th dorsal intervertebral disc space. This case is too high to cause pain in the lower back. When involvement is in the lumbar spine, the abscesses frequently follow the plane of the psoas muscle and x rays will show distention of the muscle border. *b*, Sacroiliac tuberculosis. Note sclerosis and irregularity of right sacroiliac joint.

will usually not be a problem. Except for muscle soreness, there are few if any localizing signs. More important is the back pain that accompanies meningeal irritation. There is usually in these cases a generalized spasm of the erector spinae which may be detected by Kernig's maneuver or by limitation of straight leg raising. When severe, as in infectious meningitis, it will produce opisthotonus.

2. Infections may cause backache by direct involvement of spinal structures. Non-tubercular infections are now more prevalent, and are seen most commonly in the aged. The infection usually begins in the disc space and spreads to involve the bone secondarily. X-ray changes may be slow to develop. At first an abscess shadow may appear, followed by gradual destruction of the contiguous vertebral margins, with final obliteration of the disc space.

The organism may be obtained from culture of blood, or from aspiration biopsy of the disc space itself. Sometimes the spine may become involved from an infection elsewhere, such as the urinary tract, and culture from the suspected source may reveal the organism. Treatment by bedrest, spinal bracing, and suitable chemotherapy is best. Operation is rarely necessary, since the involved vertebrae often undergo spontaneous fusion.

3. Perhaps of a greater interest in the differential diagnosis are the granulomatous infections. By far the most important of these is tuberculosis, though brucellosis and fungal (particularly coccidioidomycosis) infections also occur.

Pott's disease (*tuberculosis*) is extremely variable in its symptomatology because of the marked individual variation of resistance. Back pain may be present for several months before other characteristic changes of the disease occur. Systemic signs, particularly otherwise *unexplained weight loss*, should make one suspicious. Night pain, night cries, fever, previous pulmonary tuberculosis all help to make the diagnosis. Paraplegia is not an uncommon complication. *Elevation of the erythrocyte sedimentation rate* is the most helpful laboratory clue. A tuberculin test should always be done. Even though a positive test is not conclusive evidence to support the diagnosis, a negative one will certainly start the search elsewhere.

X-ray changes are usually present, though early in the disease they may be hard to find. Tomograms may be helpful. Narrowing of the disc space with destruction of neighboring vertebrae and *soft tissue abscess* are the most typical changes. Diagnosis can be made from culture of aspirated pus.

It is important to remember that this disease often involves the sacroiliac joints. Here again x-ray evidence of bone destruction is the most important diagnostic finding.

4. *Herpes Zoster*.—Infection of the dorsal lumbar root ganglions by the herpes zoster virus may cause severe sciatica. Early diagnosis is difficult, but the absence of trauma and presence of fever should make one suspicious. As soon as the vesicular eruption appears the diagnosis becomes evident.

Fractures and Dislocations

1. Characteristic wedge fractures of the vertebral bodies caused by injuries in flexion are not difficult to recognize or treat. However, fractures of the posterior elements (pedicles, laminae and articular processes) may be complicated by severe cord or root damage and especially when accompanied by subluxation or dislocation. Immediate exploration and fixation of the region of injury are indicated and these patients require around-the-clock special care to avoid pressure sores, urinary tract infection, and increased neurological damage, all of which can take place very quickly, with improper management. Later, rehabilitation also is a special problem.

2. Fractures of the spinous processes are rare in the lumbar spine. Separations of the posterior elements with or without fractures of the vertebral body or neural arch have been sustained by persons in-

volved in automobile accidents when wearing the automobile lap-type seat belt.[46a] However, fractures of one or more transverse processes are common. They are usually caused by simultaneous local contusion and strain, and usually respond well to supportive treatment (*i.e.* rest, sedation and strapping). Sometimes injection of the injured area with procaine provides remarkable relief.

3. Fractures of the sacrum usually result from direct trauma. Localized tenderness and superficial hematomata help to make the diagnosis. These fractures are difficult to demonstrate by x ray. Fractures of the pelvic ring are sometimes associated with dislocation of the sacroiliac joints. Proper x-ray evaluation is not difficult.

4. *Pathologic Fracture.*—Because of the great forces brought to bear upon the spine, it is not surprising that destruction or weakening of the vertebral trabecular structure is followed by vertebral fracture. However, it is surprising that much bone substance may be lost without roentgenographic evidence of it. Not infrequently the pain of the fracture will be the first indication of the pathologic process. Lack of adequate trauma should cause one to suspect this diagnosis. The following lesions are those most likely to lead to collapse of a vertebra:

a. Metastatic malignancy, such as breast, kidney, thyroid or lung in the adult, or neuroblastoma in children. Occasionally the primary source cannot be found.

b. Primary neoplasms, such as multiple myeloma.

c. Metabolic dyscrasias, particularly senile, postmenopausal, or "steroid-induced" osteoporosis. Rarely from osteomalacia or hyperparathyroidism.

d. Tuberculosis

e. Other conditions, such as Gaucher's disease and eosinophilic granuloma.

Differential diagnosis of these conditions depends on a complete history and physical examination and full use of laboratory and radiographic techniques.[42] Radioactive bone scanning has proved to be quite effective in distinguishing various lesions of the spine. Sr^{85} as an aid in the diagnosis of skeletal lesions was first introduced in 1959.[2a] The method has been developed so that differentiation between recent and old compression fractures can be made; detection of occult metastasis to the spine is possible; and activity of an infectious spondylitis may be evaluated.[7a] Biopsy of the lesion itself should be done whenever possible. If the lesion is accessible without hazard to adjacent viscera, blood vessels or nerves, the technique of needle biopsy is a practical method of obtaining material for section.[5,49] If not, open biopsy is necessary unless the clinical, laboratory and radiographic findings are sufficiently conclusive.

Rheumatic Diseases

Ankylosing spondylitis is a common cause of low back pain in young men with involvement of the sacroiliac joints early in the disease. It can be diagnosed by diminished chest expansion and reduced spinal mobility. A useful sign to look for is the contraction of the ipsilateral spinal musculature when bending to the side (Forestier's bowstring sign).[15] Normally the contralateral musculature tightens. The ESR is usually elevated and x rays show narrowing and sclerosing osteitis of the sacroiliac joints. Later the joints may become ankylosed, but in this advanced stage there is usually bony bridging of other intervertebral joints as well. It is important to prevent flexion deformity of the spine. The use of pillows should be avoided. Instead the patient should recline flat on a hard mattress on top of bedboards. Postural exercises and sometimes an extension spinal brace may be helpful. Not infrequently this condition may result in a severe spinal deformity of acute flexion (kyphosis) of both the thoracic and lumbar spine so that restoration of balance by a spinal osteotomy may be the only hope. This type of operation, by its nature, can be hazardous and we have been able to restore balance by the use of a compensatory osteotomy at the level of the pelvis.[55a] The medical management is described in Chapter 41.

Osteitis condensans ilii is a term applied to the roentgenographic demonstration of sclerotic changes on the iliac sides of the sacroiliac joints. It is particularly common in postpartum women and may be related to the strain that delivery places on these joints. Where such changes occur, however, a more exact diagnosis should be sought, since they are also seen in osteoarthritis, in early ankylosing spondylitis, and in the presence of a nearby osteoid osteoma. The clinical picture is not characteristic and the condition is said to respond to conservative therapy identical to that for low back sprain.[46]

Occasionally, late in pregnancy, women may develop low back pain as the result of relaxation of the sacroiliac joints. The pubic symphysis is also involved and tender. The syndrome can be very troublesome and the pain severe enough to force the patient to bed. Although it may be aggravated during delivery, the pain usually subsides afterward and the joints resume their former stability. Rarely the pain and instability may persist, requiring sacroiliac fusion for relief.

Metabolic Bone Disease

1. **Osteoporosis — Post-menopausal (or Senile Osteoporosis).**—Osteoporosis is a troublesome demineralizing syndrome that is commonly associated with back pain. Diagnosis can be made only after complete x ray and laboratory work-up (*see* Chapter 62 for details).

2. **Osteomalacia.**—In the adult skeleton where growth has ceased, vitamin D deficiency causes a picture very similar to that of senile osteoporosis. This condition is fortunately rare in civilized areas, except as the result of the malabsorption syndrome. The changes are more widespread than the average case of senile osteoporosis and careful laboratory analysis will lead to diagnosis (*see* Chapter 62 for details).

3. **Hyperparathyroidism.** — Osteitis fibrosa cystica, as hyperparathyroid changes in the skeleton are termed, leads to a clinical picture similar to the two previously mentioned syndromes. Again the changes are much more widespread and drastic than in the average case of senile osteoporosis and again laboratory analysis leads to proper diagnosis (*see* Chapter 62 for details).

4. **Paget's Disease.**—This peculiar affliction of bone not infrequently involves the pelvis and spine. Confusion with senile osteoporosis, osteomalacia and hyperparathyroidism is not likely, since the x-ray changes are quite characteristic. The trabecular pattern is coarsened, the bone hypertrophies, and there is loss of the denser lines of stress. The condition is often asymptomatic and when causing pain the possibility of a superimposed osteogenic sarcoma should not be forgotten. Laboratory work-up and full x-ray studies are indicated (*see* Chapter 62).

Neoplastic Disease

Certain tumors show a predilection for the spine.

1. **Intraspinal Lesions.**—There are very few men experienced in spinal surgery who have not at one time or another encountered an intraspinal tumor causing backache and sciatica. A report from the Mayo Clinic[6] has shown the incidence of various lesions. Neurofibroma and ependymoma each occurred 3 times in over 1000 cases. Carcinoma metastatic to the spinal cord and its supporting structures occurs as well as other primary tumors. These conditions develop quite frequently in the *absence* of neurologic signs. Pantopaque examination is necessary for diagnosis.

2. **Lesions of Vertebral Column.**—*a.* Of the malignant tumors by far the most common are *multiple myeloma* and *metastatic carcinoma.* Both often have a very similar appearance on x ray and can lead to surprisingly extensive bone destruction. Both are often widespread. Differentiation depends on the demon-

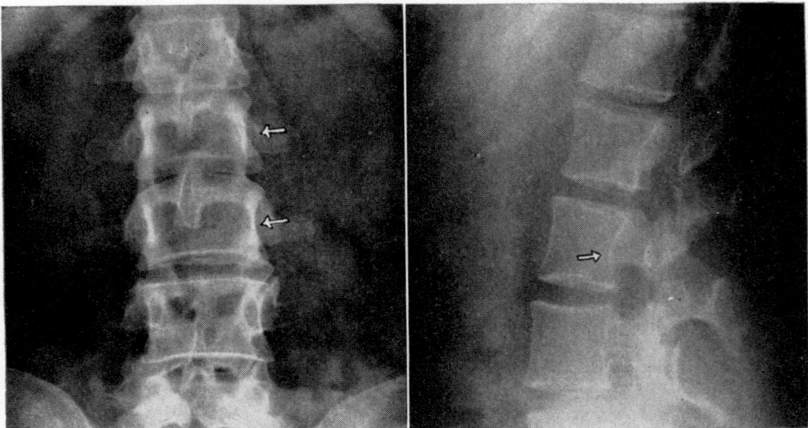

Fig. 82–34.—Spinal cord tumor. Note widening of interpedicular diameter and flattening of pedicles (*arrow*). There is pressure erosion of the posterior portions of the vertebra in the lateral view.

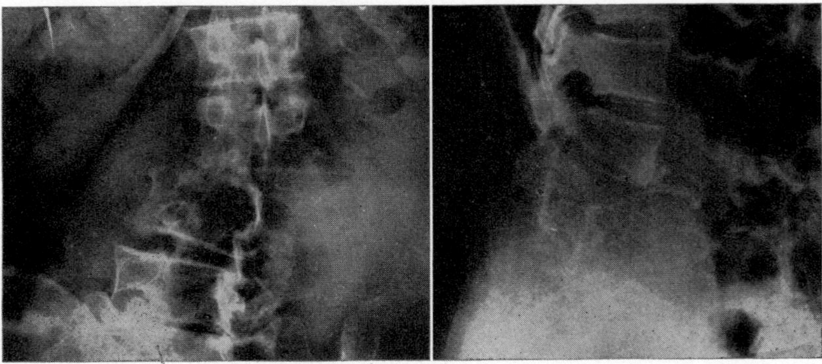

Fig. 82–35.—Multiple myeloma. The 3rd lumbar vertebra is completely destroyed. This is rarefaction and partial destruction of L2 and L4. The associated neurological changes were surprisingly few.

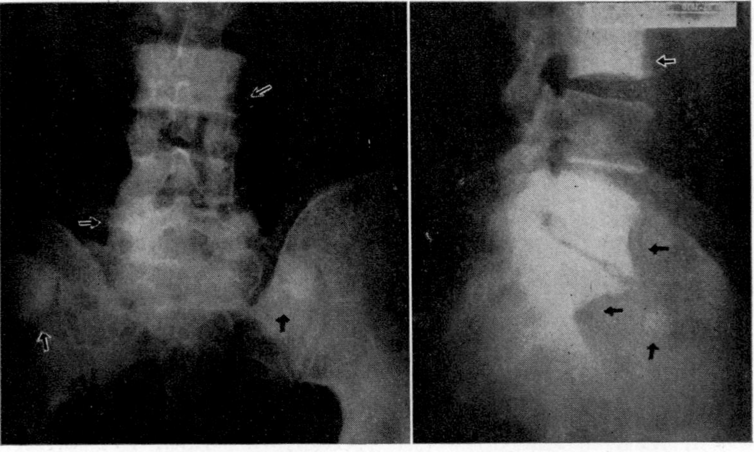

Fig. 82–36.—Prostatic carcinoma with scattered osteoblastic metastases (*arrows*).

stration of a primary source (prostate, breast, kidney, thyroid and lung most frequently) in the case of metastatic disease and of abnormal gamma globulins in the case of multiple myeloma. Plasma electrophoresis is immensely valuable in the early diagnosis of the latter condition.[33] Not infrequently there is an associated anemia. Rarely both metastatic carcinoma and multiple myeloma can cause cord and root compression. Chordoma is a rare malignant tumor largely confined to the sacrococcygeal and cranial portions of the axial skeleton. It arises from remnants of the primitive notochord, and is locally invasive. It is quite resistant to both surgical and roentgen therapy.

b. Benign tumors of the spine are rather uncommon. Giant cell tumor, bone cysts, osteochondromas and chondromas may occur, but hemangiomas, aneurysmal bone cysts, and osteoid osteomas are the most common. It is probably wrong to classify all hemangiomas as benign since some lead to quite extensive bone destruction. However, many of these tumors respond very favorably to irradiation. The x-ray picture when typical is easily recognized. There are vertical striations in the vertebral body which is often partially crushed so as to be broadened in all dimensions but the vertical.[4] Aneurysmal bone cysts involve the posterior elements and form large paraspinal masses with scattered calcific deposits. Although biopsy is required for definitive diagnosis, they are quite radiosensitive and are therefore best treated by irradiation.[8]

Osteoid osteoma[17] is a painful tumor in which a small focus of osteogenetic activity develops and leads to extensive surrounding sclerosis of bone. It usually arises in the posterior vertebral elements and is therefore difficult to demonstrate roentgenographically. Tomograms are helpful to demonstrate the typical lesion, a zone of dense bone surrounding a small radiolucent nidus. The pain may be severe and often occurs at night. It is so dramatically relieved by aspirin that this is used as a helpful diagnostic test.

Epiphysitis, or Scheuermann's disease, is a painful back condition of adolescence, the cause of which is obscure. It is more common in boys than in girls and involves the thoracic spine much more frequently than the lumbar. Although structural round back, increased anteroposterior diameter of the chest and tight hamstrings form part of the syndrome, this symptom triad is frequently seen without pain. In fact,

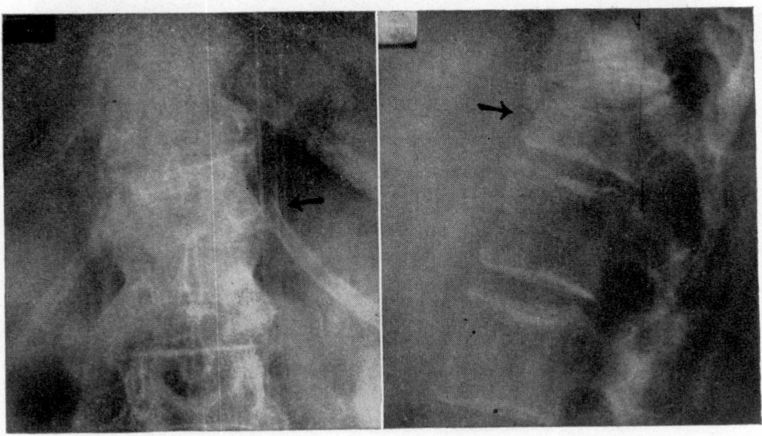

Fig. 82–37.—An osteolytic metastasis with pathologic compression fracture of D12 (*arrow*). These may be difficult to recognize before collapse occurs. The source of the metastasis was a carcinoma of the breast, operated twenty years previously.

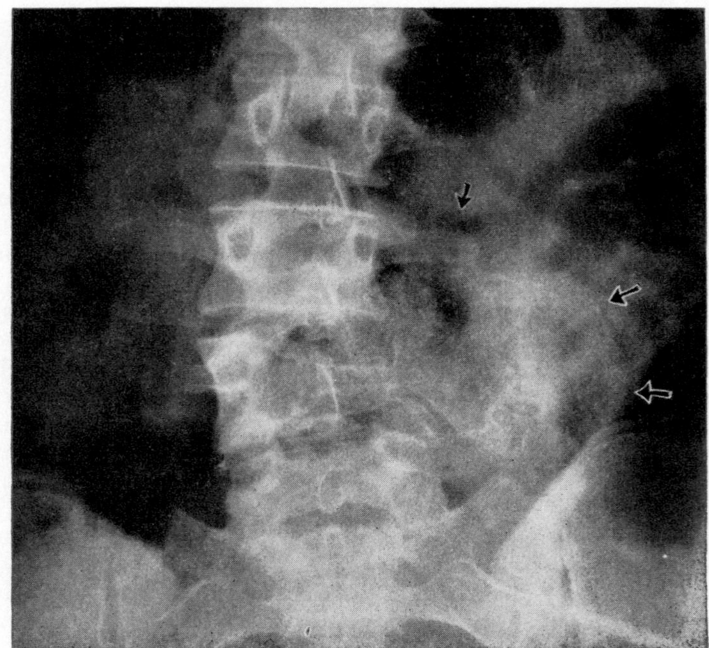

Fig. 82–38.—Aneurysmal bone cyst. The lesion is not always so extensive, but the blown-out appearance is typical.

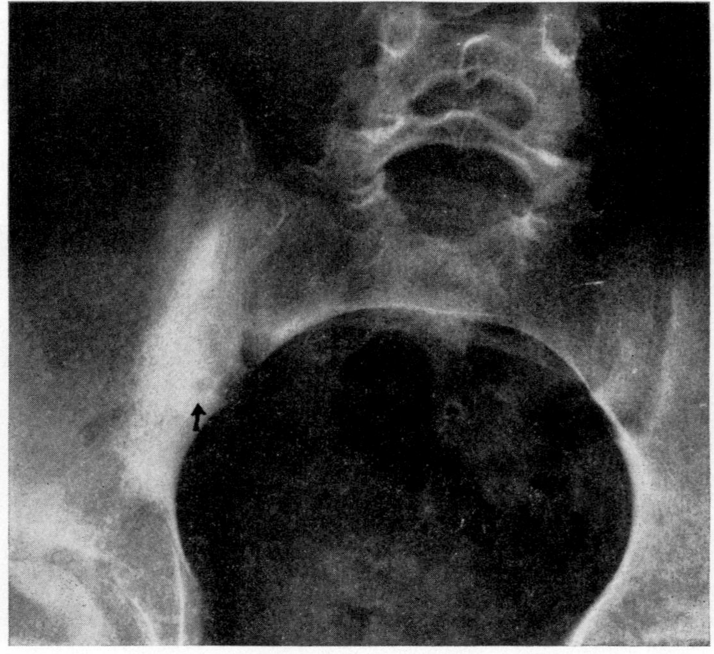

Fig. 82–39.—Osteoid osteoma. An osteoid osteoma involving the ilium near the sacroiliac joint. The central nidus (*arrow*) is well visualized. The lesion was associated with low back pain. Only the nidus must be removed for operation to be successful.

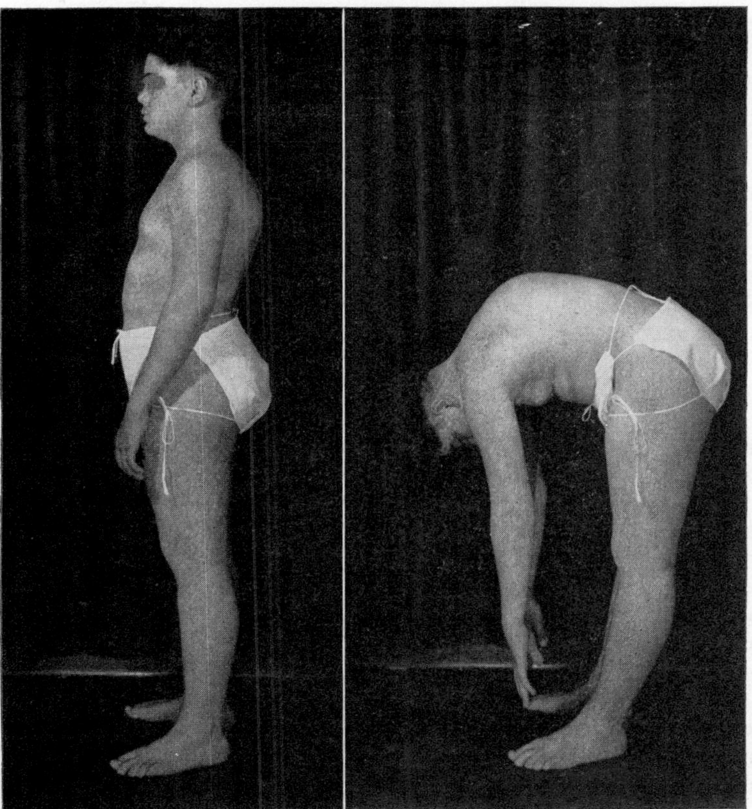

FIG. 82–40.—Dorsal round back. The photographs show the abnormal dorsal curve and the deformity is accentuated by forward bending.

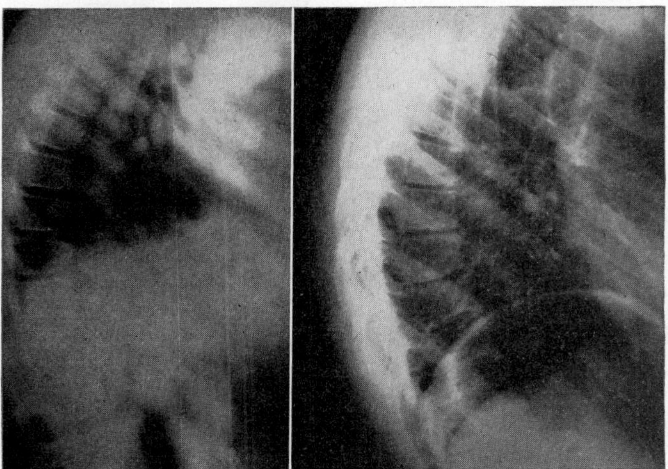

FIG. 82–41.—X rays of dorsal round back. There is anterior wedging of several of the dorsal vertebrae in the x rays which were made four years apart.

we have seen it much more frequently without pain than with, the usual presenting complaint of the patients being that of poor posture. The so-called typical x-ray findings of several mildly wedged vertebrae, narrowed disc spaces and irregular vertebral margins are also not exclusively limited to patients with pain (Figs. 82–40 and 41). Schmorl has pointed out that these are caused by faults in the cartilaginous end plates which permit herniation of the disc material into the spongiosa.

Treatment, therefore, must be different for patients whose primary problem is deformity, from that for those who present themselves because of pain. In the first case the use of a firm mattress reinforced by a bed board and postural exercises are indicated when the deformity is mild. When there is a significant thoracic kyphosis and the patient has not completed growth, the use of a Milwaukee brace is most gratifying (Fig. 82–42). Frequently after wearing this brace for only a period of six months full time and an equal duration part time, a noticeable improvement of the round back is apparent. In those patients in whom pain is present with little deformity more simplified bracing or the use of plaster jacket for a few months may be all that is necessary for successful treatment.

The intent of postural treatment is not to correct deformity, but to prevent its progression, and whether this goal can actually be achieved or not is open to some question since the condition in many instances is self-limiting. The problem of such treatment is actually to accomplish reduction of the thoracic or thoracolumbar kyphosis instead of just increasing the lumbosacral lordosis (*see* section on Spinal Function, p. 1515). When an exercise program is considered, therefore, the usual lumbar flattening exercises (Fig. 82–23) are not only recommended, but in addition, a special one is added to extend the thoracic spine. The patient is asked to flatten his lumbar spine by flexing his hips over the end of a hard table, and to hold this position while he raises his head and shoulders.

If a plaster jacket or brace is used, the same principles again apply: the lumbar

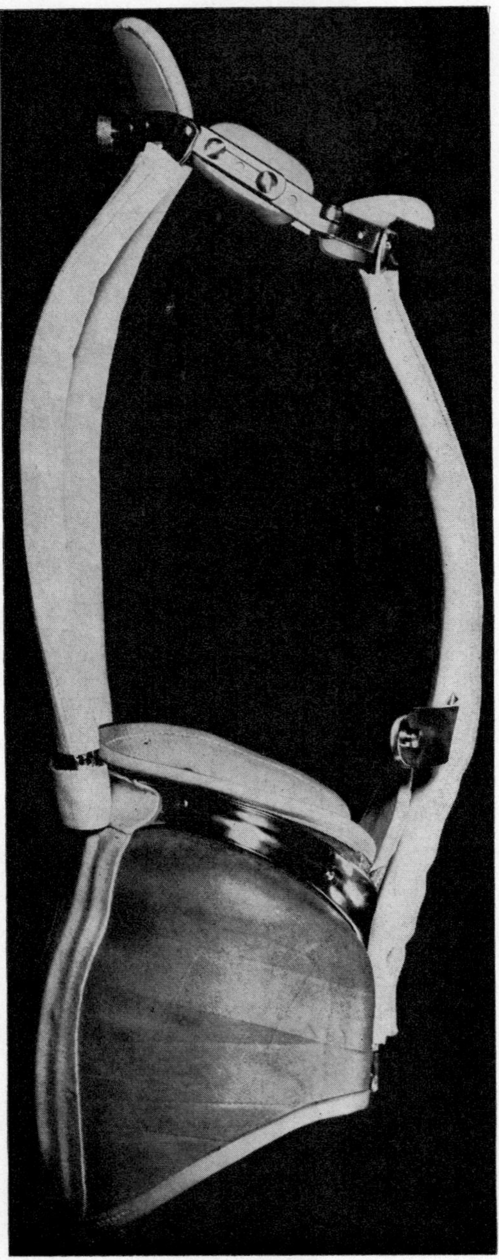

Fig. 82–42.—A Milwaukee brace may be used to correct mild spinal deformities during the growing years.

lordosis must first be flattened and then the thoracic kyphosis extended. Immobilization of this kind is more likely to be helpful to patients whose pain is subacute. For those whose pain is severe, however, spinal fusion should not be delayed since it is not only the best way of relieving the pain, but also is the most effective means of controlling progression of deformity. Operative reduction of kyphosis is difficult to accomplish, but may take place with further spinal growth, once a strong fusion has been obtained.

Scoliosis

In the past it has been taught that lateral curvature of the spine was rarely ever painful. On the contrary, we have found that 40 per cent of patients with adolescent idiopathic scoliosis have pain.[40a] The problem of pain in the older patient with scoliosis can sometimes be most challenging. Pain may exist at the level of the apex of the curve secondary to osteoarthritis which occurs in the growing child. In lumbar curves low back pain with leg radiation simulates disc type of symptoms. The usual operative management of excision of the disc is doomed to fail. Such patients should be treated by external support with the use of lumbosacral corsets. If no relief is obtained a course of traction supplemented by a more rigid brace (Fig. 82–43) is often helpful. In those patients responding to conservative treatment, reduction of the curve and spinal fusion will relieve the pain.

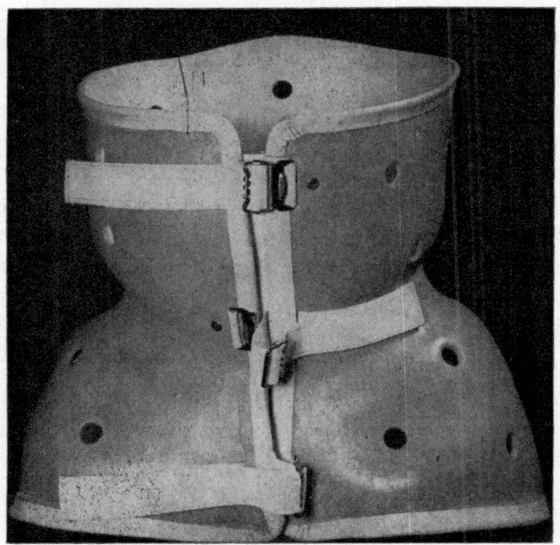

Fig. 82–43.—This thermal setting isoprene brace was fabricated from a plaster model taken with the patient in traction. It is particularly helpful in treating older patients with painful scoliosis.

While idiopathic scoliosis does not usually progress after full maturation of the spine, we have seen several patients in whom lumbar curves have worsen during middle age. Such symptomatic curves may best be treated initially by correction and fusion as these will continue to progress throughout life. Those patients with untreated progressive painful scoliosis over the age of 65 are most difficult to manage.

Coccygodynia

Pain in the coccygeal area is often troublesome from point of view of diagnosis and treatment. It may be of three separate types.

1. **Primary Coccygeal Abnormality.**—As the result of direct trauma or childbirth, the coccyx may be fractured or the sacrococcygeal joint severely strained.

2. **Primary Low Back Pathology.**—It is not uncommon for coccygodynia to develop as a secondary phenomenon in a patient with low back pain. The mechanism is not understood, but the pain is most likely of referred type.

3. **Visceral Lesion.**—It is not uncommon for patients with rectal or genitourinary disease to develop coccygeal pain. This is of a referred type and sometimes associated with "spasm" of the muscles of the pelvic floor.

It is only by careful evaluation that these three entities may be separated. The back must always be examined since trauma to the coccyx cannot usually occur without simultaneously involving the low back. Rectal examination should include palpation of pelvic structures as well as of the coccyx and its adjacent structures (*i.e.*, the coccygeus and levator ani muscles, sacrospinous and sacrotuberous ligaments).

Proctological, gynecological and urological evaluation may be indicated. In those cases where examination points to primary pathology in the sacrococcygeal articulation, coccygectomy may be effective if conservative therapy fails. Every effort should be made to avoid irritation of the painful area. Soft chairs are usually worse than hard and the patient should sit with good posture. A rubber ring may be necessary. Sometimes a strapping or "sacroiliac belt" will be helpful by pulling fatty tissues over the nonpadded coccygeal region. Massage and diathermy may provide symptomatic relief.

Camptocormia

Hysterical back pain characterized by extreme flexion of the spine and pain in the lumbar area has been termed "camptocormia."[43a] The diagnosis is made by normal findings on orthopaedic and neurological examinations, a deformity that disappears in recumbency and the disappearance of the deformity by suggestion.

Although this condition is not that common, psychological overlay in the patient with back pain is almost always present. Such anxiety frequently confuses the clinical picture and often is transferred to the treating physician which then makes diagnosis and successful treatment difficult.

When evaluating the patient with low back pain the physician must be aware of the possibility of secondary gain such as associated with liability cases, compensation cases, avoidance of military draft, and malingering.

Pain from Stenosis of the Aortic Bifurcation and Iliac Arteries.—When pain is centered in the buttocks, groins and thighs and brought on by walking, but relieved quickly by rest, one should think of the possibility of intermittent claudication due to stenosis of the iliac arteries. Palpation of the femoral arteries should provide a quick diagnosis. The condition is common enough so that palpation of the arterial trunks should be included as part of the routine back examination.[14]

Pain from Hip Joint Disease

Occasionally it is quite difficult to distinguish the pain of hip disease from that of the spine, since both may radiate along the same pathways. Intra-articular disease often causes pain radiating down the inner aspects of the thighs to the knees, whereas the pain of a trochanteric bursitis may follow the more usual "sciatic" distribution. For this reason it is most important to analyze hip joint movements in all patients with sciatica and especially those in whom the findings in the lower back are equivocal.

Referred Pain from Visceral Structures

It is imperative to remember that a lesion in one of the pelvic organs or the retroperitoneal structures can cause pain referred to the back. In women, the most usual condition is one of a retroverted uterus, but disease of the ovaries and tubes may also be at fault. The pain in these cases tends to be worse during menses. In men, referred low back pain is usually the result of a prostatic lesion. Stones within the urinary tract are easily diagnosed in the presence of typical ureteral colic, but at other times may be a more obscure cause of back pain. In the presence of associated anorexia and weight loss a retroperitoneal neoplasm must always be considered. In most such patients the back findings are insufficient to explain the symptoms but in elderly patients, there may be associated lower back lesions to complicate the picture and to test severely the diagnostic acumen of the attending physician.

BIBLIOGRAPHY

1. Aronson, H. A. and Dunsmore, R. H.: J. Bone & Joint Surg., *45A*, 311, 1963.

2. BAUER, D. DE F.: *Lumbar Discography and Low Back Pain*, Springfield, Charles C Thomas, 1960.

2a. BAUER, G. C. H.: J. Bone & Joint Surg., *41B*, 558, 1959.

3. BUCHMAN, J.: Arch. Surg., *34*, 23, 1937.

4. COLEY, B. L.: *Neoplasms of Bone*, 2nd Ed., New York, Paul B. Hoeber, Inc., p. 143, 1960.

5. CRAIG, F. S.: J. Bone & Joint Surg., *38A*, 93, 1956.

6. CRAIG, W. MCK., SVIEN, H. J., DODGE, J. W., JR., and CAMP, J. D.: J.A.M.A., *149*, 250, 1952.

7. DANFORTH, M. S. and WILSON, P. D.: J. Bone & Joint Surg., 7, 109, 1925.

7a. DEFIORE, J. C., LINDBERG, L., and RANAWAT, N. S.: J. Bone & Joint Surg., *52A*, 21, 1970.

8. DONALDSON, W. F.: J. Bone & Joint Surg., *44A*, 25, 1963.

9. DUNCAN, W. and HOEN, T. I.: Surg. Gynec. & Obstet., *75*, 257, 1942.

10. DUNNING, H. S.: Arch. Neurol. & Psych., *55*, 573, 1946.

11. EHRENHAFT, J. L.: Surg., Gynec. & Obstet., *75*, 257, 1942.

12. FEFFER, H. L.: J. Bone & Joint Surg., *38A*, 585, 1956.

13. FEINSTEIN, B., LUCE, J. C., and LANGTON, J. N. K.: In Klopstey, P. E. and Wilson, P. D. *et al.*, *Human Limbs and their Substitutes*, New York, McGraw-Hill Book Co. Inc., 1954, pp. 101–120.

14. FILTZER, D. L. and BAHNSON, H. T.: J. Bone & Joint Surg., *41B*, 244, 1959.

15. FORESTIER, J., JACQUELINE, F. and ROLES-QUEROL, J.: *Ankylosing Spondylitis*, Springfield, Charles C Thomas, 1956.

16. FORST, J. J.: *Contribution a l'etude clinique de la Sciatique*. Paris, These *33*, 1881.

17. FREIBERGER R. H.: Radiology, *75*, 232, 1960.

18. FRIBERG, S.: Acta Chir. Scand., *82*, Suppl. 55, 1939.

19. GILL, G. G., MANNING, J. G., and WHITE, H. L.: J. Bone & Joint Surg., *37A*, 493, 1955.

19a. GOLUB, B. S. and SILVERMAN, B.: J. Bone & Joint Surg., *51A*, 947, 1969.

20. HARRIS, R. I. and WILEY, J. J.: J. Bone & Joint Surg., *45A*, 1159, 1963.

21. HARVEY, J. P., JR. and FREIBERGER, R. H.: J. Bone & Joint Surg., *47A*, 397, 1965.

22. HENDRY, N. G. C.: J. Bone & Joint Surg., *40B*, 132, 1958.

23. HIRSCH, C.: J. Bone & Joint Surg., *41B*, 237, 1959.

24. HITCHCOCK, H. H.: J. Bone & Joint Surg., *22*, 1, 1940.

24a. HAKELIUS, A.: Acta Orthop. Scand. Suppl., *129*, 59, 1970.

24b. HOOP, L. B. and CHRISMAN, D.: Physical Therapy, *48*, 21, 1968.

25. HOWORTH, M. B.: J. Bone & Joint Surg., *45A*, 1487, 1963.

26. INMAN, V. T. and SAUNDERS, J. B. DEC.: J. Nerv. & Ment. Dis., *99*, 660, 1944.

27. JOUCK, L. M.: J. Bone & Joint Surg., *43B*, 362, 1961.

28. KEEGAN, J. J.: J.A.M.A., *126*, 868, 1944.

29. KELLGREEN, J. H.: Clin. Science, *3*, 182, 1937–38.

30. ————: Clin. Science, *4*, 33, 1939.

31. KEY, J. A.: Bull. Johns Hopkins Hosp., *80*, 217, 1947.

32. KNUTSSON, B.: Acta Orthop. Scand. Suppl., *49*, 1961.

33. KORNGOLD, L., VANLeenwen, G. and ENGLE, R. L., JR.: Ann. New York Acad Med., *101*, 203, 1962.

34. KUHNS, J. G., *et al.*: *Posture and Its Relationship to Orthopaedic Disabilities*, Ann Arbor, Edwards Bros., 1942.

35. LANSCHE, W. E. and FORD, L. T.: J. Bone & Joint Surg., *42A*, 193, 1960.

36. LEWIS, T.: *Pain*, New York, The Macmillan Co., 1942.

37. LEWIS, T. and KELLGREN, J. H.: Clin. Science, *4*, 48, 1939.

38. MITCHELL, P. E. G., HENDRY, N. G. C., and BILLEWICZ, W. Z.: J. Bone & Joint Surg., *43B*, 141, 1961.

39. MIXTER, W. J. and BARR, J. S.: New Engl. J. Med., *211*, 210, 1934.

39a. MORGAN, H. C.: J. Bone & Joint Surg., *50A*, 411, 1968.

40. NAFFZIGER, J., INMAN, V. T. and SAUNDERS, J. B.: Surg. Gynec. & Obstet., *66*, 288, 1938.

40a. NASTASI, A., LEVINE, D. B., and VELISKAKIS, K.: Presented at Sixth Annual Meeting Scoliosis Research Society, Hartford, 1970.

41. NEWMAN, P. H.: J. Bone & Joint Surg., *45B*, 39, 1963.

42. NICHOLAS, J. A., WILSON, P. D., and FREIBERGER, R.: J. Bone & Joint Surg., *42A*, 127, 1959.

43. REYNOLDS, F. C., MCGINNIS, A. E., and MORGAN, H. C.: J. Bone & Joint Surg., *41A*, 223, 1959.

43a. ROCKWOOD, C. A. and EILERT, R. E.: J. Bone & Joint Surg., *51A*, 553, 1969.

44. SAUNDERS, J. C. DEC. and INMAN, V. I.: Arch. Surg., *40*, 389, 1940.

45. SCHLESINGER, E. B.: J. Trauma, *2*, 162, 1962.

46. SHIPP, F. L. and HAGGART, G. E.: J. Bone & Joint Surg., *32A*, 841, 1950.

46a. SMITH, W. S. and KAUFER, H.: J. Bone & Joint Surg., *51A*, 239, 1969.
47. SPURLING, R. G. and THOMPSON, T. C.: Surgery, *15*, 387, 1944.
48. STEINDLER, A.: J.A.M.A., *110*, 106, 1938.
48a. TKACZUK, H.: Acta Orthop. Scand. Suppl., *115*, 16, 1968.
49. VALS, J., OTTOLENGHI, C. E., and SCHAJOWICZ, F.: J.A.M.A., *136*, 376, 1948.
50. WILLIAMS, P. C.: Amer. Acad. Orthop. Surg. Instruct. Course Lect., *10*, 90, 1953.
51. WILLIS, T. A.: J. Bone & Joint Surg., *13*, 709, 1931.
52. ———: J. Bone & Joint Surg., *23*, 410, 1941.
53. ———: J. Bone & Joint Surg., *41A*, 935, 1959.
54. WILSON, P. D.: Rhode Island Med. J., *43*, 167, 1960.
55. WILSON, P. D., JR.: Arch. Environmental Health, *5*, 505, 1962.
55a. WILSON, P. D., JR. and LEVINE, D. B.: J. Bone & Joint Surg., *51A*, 142, 1969.
56. WILTSE, L. L.: *A.A.O.S. Symposium on Spine*, St. Louis, C. V. Mosby Co., 1969.

Index

Page numbers followed by t indicate tables.

B

D

E

I

P

Q

R

S

T

U